# 海外医疗
# 实用药物手册

## Practical Pharmacy Handbook for
## Overseas Medical Treatment

主 编 张 沂 费舒扬

河南科学技术出版社
郑 州

# 内容提要

本书是一部由中文、英文、法文和西班牙文4种文字构成的药学工具书，共收载临床常用的20类1000余种药品。内容包括：中-英文、中-法文及中-西班牙文对照的药品分类及名称表；4种文字对照的药品临床使用说明，包括药品类别、名称、适应证、用法用量和剂型规格；4种文字对照的麻醉及精神药品目录；4种文字对照的妊娠危险等级药品目录；4种文字对照的运动员禁忌药品目录；常用中成药临床使用说明（中文）；临床用药常用单位换算表及计算公式；缩略语（含处方常用）对照表；4种文字的药品名称索引。本书可以满足中外医务人员在国际医疗援助及学术交流中对药品临床应用的中、英、法、西班牙4种文字的需求，以解决国际医疗合作与交流中药学专业语言的困难。

## 图书在版编目（CIP）数据

海外医疗实用药物手册/张沂，费舒扬主编．—郑州：河南科学技术出版社，2022.9
ISBN 978-7-5725-0858-5

Ⅰ．①海…　Ⅱ．①张…②费…　Ⅲ．①药物—手册　Ⅳ．① R97-62

中国版本图书馆 CIP 数据核字（2022）第 124358 号

---

**出版发行**：河南科学技术出版社

北京名医世纪文化传媒有限公司

地址：北京市丰台区万丰路 316 号万开基地 B 座 115 室　　邮编：100161

电话：010-63863186　010-63863168

**策划编辑**：梁紫岩　杨磊石

**文字编辑**：杨永岐

**责任审读**：周晓洲

**责任校对**：张　娟

**封面设计**：吴朝洪

**版式设计**：吴朝洪

**责任印制**：程晋荣

**印　　刷**：河南瑞之光印刷股份有限公司

**经　　销**：全国新华书店、医学书店、网店

**开　　本**：889mm×1194mm　1/16　**印张**：84.5　**字数**：2720 千字

**版　　次**：2022 年 9 月第 1 版　　2022 年 9 月第 1 次印刷

**定　　价**：598.00 元

---

# 主编简介

张沂　主任药师，硕士研究生导师，毕业于海军军医大学药学院（原第二军医大学药学系）。历任中国人民解放军第八届、九届、十届医学科学技术委员会药学专业委员会常务委员，北京药学会药物经济学专业委员会、北京药理学会精准药学专业委员会副主任委员，国家教育部学位中心、北京市自然科学基金评审专家。从事医院药学和临床药理学研究、教学及工作近40年。承担国家自然科学基金、首都医学发展基金及军队科研项目10余项，获得北京市和军队科技进步二等奖3项，发表研究论文100余篇。

费舒扬　医师，硕士研究生，内科学心血管专业，毕业于首都医科大学临床医学院。现任首都医科大学附属北京同仁医院重症医学科医师。从事心血管疾病及危重症患者临床诊疗、科研工作。作为项目组成员完成北京市自然科学基金2020年项目1项："钙库操纵性钙通道Orai 1/$Ca^{2+}$径路在动脉粥样硬化斑块延展和易损性中的作用"。在《心肺血管病杂志》等期刊发表"重组腺病毒载体敲减$ApoE^{-/-}$小鼠血管平滑肌细胞Orai1基因模型的构建""钙库操纵性钙通道蛋白在心血管疾病中的研究进展"等研究论文8篇。

# 编 委 名 单

# 前　言

《海外医疗实用药物手册》（Practical Pharmacy Handbook For Overseas Medical Treatment）是一部由中文、英文、法文和西班牙文4种语言文字构成，以中-英文、中-法文、中-西班牙文对照形式编纂的药物临床应用说明的药学工具书。迄今，国内外在该专业领域未见同类书出版。

书中收录了临床常用的20类1000余种药品。内容包括：①中文-英文、中文-法文及中文-西班牙文4种语言文字对照的药品分类及名称表；②药品临床使用说明，包括药品类别、名称、适应证、用法用量和剂型规格；③4种文字对照的麻醉及精神药品目录；④4种文字对照的妊娠危险等级药品目录；⑤4种文字对照的运动员禁忌药物（临床常用）目录；⑥常用中成药临床使用说明（中文）；⑦临床用药常用单位换算表及计算公式；⑧缩略语（含处方常用）对照表；⑨4种文字的药品名称索引。

本书可满足中外医务人员在国际医疗援助、救援及学术交流中对药品临床应用的中、英、法、西4种语言文字的需求。

早在20世纪50年代，中国政府开始了国际人道主义医疗援助，始于1956年的中国援助非洲医疗队一直延续至今。2014年西非3个国家暴发埃博拉出血热疫情，中国先后派出近1000名医务人员的医疗队进入疫区开展国际医疗救助。2010年以来，中国海军"和平方舟"医院船的海外医疗、国际人道主义医疗救助，以及医学学术交流的航迹遍及五大洲三大洋40多个国家。至今，数以万计中国医务工作者先后参加国际医疗援助和救助，彰显了国际人道主义精神和勇于奉献的医者风范，向世界展示了中国负责任大国的担当，做出了举世瞩目和卓有成效的贡献。

本书主编从事医院药学工作和临床药理学研究30余年，并曾多次参加和完成中国海军"和平方舟"医院船的海外医疗和国际人道主义医疗救助中的药学保障任务。深感中方医务人员在与外方患者及外方医务人员进行药物治疗和药品使用的交流沟通时，存在专业语言文字的困难，影响诊疗和交流的顺利进行。为此，于2011年编写了《海外医疗实用药物手册》。本书在"和平方舟"医院船执行的多次"和谐使命"海外医疗、国际人道主义医疗救助及联合演习中，在与外方医务人员及患者沟通交流中发挥了重要作用，已列为"和平方舟"医院船的常备工具书之一，2016年已由人民军医出版社出版，全书约273万字。

《海外医疗实用药物手册》经过进一步修订完善，由河南科学技术出版社再次出版发行。

随着中国对外交流的不断增加，相信本书一定能够为中外医学、药学同行及与患者的沟通交流中，提供有效的中、英、法、西班牙4种文字医药学专业语言文字支持，为中外国际医疗合作与交流做出贡献。

张　沂

解放军总医院第六医学中心（原海军总医院）

解放军第十届医学科学委员会药学专业委员会常务委员

2021年10月29日

# 目　录

# 第1章
# 中、英、法、西班牙文药品分类及名称

| 药品名称 | Drug Names | Dénomination du Médicament | Denominación del Medicamento |
|---|---|---|---|
| 1. 抗生素 Antibiotics | | | |
| 1.1 青霉素类 Benzylpenicillins | | | |
| 青霉素 | Penicillin | Pénicilline | Penicilina |
| 青霉素 V | Phenoxymethylpenicillin | Phenoxymethylpenicilline | Fenoximetilpenicilina |
| 苯唑西林钠 | Oxacillin Sodium | Oxacilline sodique | Oxacilina sódica |
| 氯唑西林钠 | Cloxacillin Sodium | Cloxacilline sodique | Cloxacilina sódica |
| 氟氯西林 | Flucloxacillin | Flucloxacilline | Flucloxacilina |
| 氨苄西林 | Ampicillin | Ampicilline | Ampicilina |
| 阿莫西林 | Amoxicillin | Amoxicilline | Amoxicilina |
| 哌拉西林钠 | Piperacillin Sodium | Pipéracilline sodique | Piperacilina sódica |
| 替卡西林 | Ticarcillin | Ticarcilline | Ticarcilina |
| 美洛西林钠 | Mezlocillin Sodium | Mézlocilline sodique | Mezlocilina sódica |
| 阿洛西林钠 | Azlocillin Sodium | Azlocilline sodique | Azlocilina sódica |
| 磺苄西林钠 | Sulbenicillin Sodium | Sulbénicilline sodique | Sulbenicilina sódica |
| 阿帕西林钠 | Apalcillin Sodium | Apalcilline sodique | Apalcilina sódica |
| 1.2 头孢菌素类 Cephalosporins | | | |
| 头孢氨苄 | Cefalexin | Céfalexine | Cefalexina |
| 头孢唑林钠 | Cefazolin Sodium | Céfazoline sodique | Cefazolina sódica |
| 头孢羟氨苄 | Cefadroxil | Céfadroxil | Cefadroxilo |
| 头孢拉定 | Cefradine | Céfradine | Cefradina |
| 头孢呋辛钠 | Cefuroxime Sodium | Céfuroxime sodique | Cefuroxima sódica |
| 头孢呋辛酯 | Cefuroxime Axetil | Céfuroxime axétil | Cefuroxima axetilo |
| 头孢克洛 | Cefaclor | Céfaclor | Cefaclor |
| 头孢噻肟钠 | Cefotaxime Sodium | Céfotaxime sodique | Cefotaxima sódica |
| 头孢匹胺钠 | Cefpiramide Sodium | Céfpiramide sodique | Cefpiramida sódica |
| 头孢曲松钠 | Ceftriaxone Sodium | Céftriaxone sodique | Ceftriaxona sódica |
| 头孢哌酮钠 | Cefoperazone Sodium | Céfoperazone sodique | Cefoperazona sódica |
| 头孢他啶 | Ceftazidime | Céftazidime | Ceftazidima |
| 头孢美唑 | Cefmetazole | Céfmétazole | Cefmetazol |
| 头孢克肟 | Cefixime | Céfixime | Cefixima |
| 头孢西丁钠 | Cefoxitin Sodium | Céfoxitine sodique | Cefoxitina sódica |

**续 表**

| 药品名称 | Drug Names | Dénomination du Médicament | Denominación del Medicamento |
|---|---|---|---|
| 头孢米诺钠 | Cefminox Sodium | Céfminox sodique | Cefminox sódico |
| 头孢吡肟 | Cefepime | Céfepime | Cefepima |
| 头孢布烯 | Ceftibuten | Céftibutene | Ceftibuteno |
| 头孢丙烯 | Cefprozil | Céfprozil | Cefprozilo |
| 头孢泊肟酯 | Cefpodoxime Proxetil | Céfpodoxime Proxetil | Cefpodoxima Proxetilo |
| 头孢托仑匹酯 | Cefditoren Pivoxil | Céfditorène pivoxil | Cefditoren pivoxilo |
| 头孢地嗪钠 | Cefodizime Sodium | Céfodizime sodique | Cefodizima sodica |
| 头孢硫脒 | Cefathiamidine | Céfathiamidine | Cefatiamidina |
| 头孢替安 | Cefotiam | Céfotiam | Cefotiam |
| 头孢替坦 | Cefotetan | Céfotetan | Cefotetán |
| 头孢唑肟 | Ceftizoxime | Céftizoxime | Ceftizoxima |
| 头孢孟多 | Cefamandole | Céfamandol | Cefamandol |
| 头孢尼西钠 | Cefonicid Sodium | Céfonicide sodique | Cefonicida sodica |
| 拉氧头孢钠 | Latamoxef Sodium | Latamoxef sodique | Latamoxef de sodio |
| 氟氧头孢钠 | Flomoxef Sodium | Flomoxef sodique | Flomoxef de sodio |

### 1.3 β- 内酰胺酶抑制剂及其与 β- 内酰胺类抗生素配伍的复方制剂 β-lactamase inhibitors and its Co. preparation with β-lactamase antibiotics

| | | | |
|---|---|---|---|
| 克拉维酸钾 | Clavulanate Potassium | Clavulanate de potassium | Clavulanato de potasio |
| 舒巴坦钠 | Sulbactam sodium | Sulbactam sodique | Sulbactam sodica |
| 他唑巴坦 | Tazobactam | Tazobactam | Tazobactam |
| 阿莫西林 - 克拉维酸钾 | Amoxillin and Clavulanate Potassium | Amoxicilline et Clavulanate de potassium | Amoxicilina y Clavulanato de potásico |
| 替卡西林钠 - 克拉维酸钾 | Ticarcillin Sodium and Clavulanate Potassium | Ticarcilline de sodium et clavulanate de potassium | Ticarcilina de sodio y clavulanato de potasio |
| 氨苄西林钠 - 舒巴坦钠 | Ampicillin Sodium and Sulbactam Sodium | Ampicilline de sodium et Sulbactam de sodium | Ampicilina sódica y sulbactam sódico |
| 舒他西林 | Sultamicillin | Sultamicilline | Sultamicilina |
| 哌拉西林钠 - 他唑巴坦钠 | Piperacillin Sodium and Tazobactam Sodium | Pipéracilline de sodium et tazobactam de sodium | Piperacilina sódico y tazobactam sódico |

### 1.4 碳青霉烯类和其他 β- 内酰胺类 Carbapenems and other β-lactamase antibiotics

| | | | |
|---|---|---|---|
| 亚胺培南 - 西司他汀钠 | Imipenem and Cilastatin Sodium | Imipénèm et cilastatine sodique | Imipenem y cilastatina sódica |
| 美罗培南 | Meropenem | Méropénèm | Meropenem |
| 帕尼培南 - 倍他米隆 | Panipenem and Betamipron | Panipénèm et bétamipron | Panipenem y betamiprón |
| 厄他培南 | Ertapenem | Ertapénèm | Ertapenem |
| 比阿培南 | Biapenem | Biapénèm | Biapenem |
| 法罗培南钠 | Faropenem Sodium | Faropénèm sodique | Faropenem de sódio |
| 氨曲南 | Aztreonam | Aztréonam | Aztreonam |

**续　表**

| 药品名称 | Drug Names | Dénomination du Médicament | Denominación del Medicamento |
| --- | --- | --- | --- |
| 1.5 氨基糖苷类 Aminoglycosides | | | |
| 卡那霉素 | Kanamycin | Kanamycine | Kanamicina |
| 阿米卡星 | Amikacin | Amikacine | Amikacina |
| 妥布霉素 | Tobramycin | Tobramycine | Tobramicina |
| 庆大霉素 | Gentamicin | Gentamicine | Gentamicina |
| 西索米星 | Sisomicin | Sisomicine | Sisomicina |
| 奈替米星 | Netilmicin | Nétilmicine | Netilmicina |
| 小诺米星 | Micronomicin | Micronomicine | Micronomicina |
| 异帕米星 | Isepamicin | Isépamicine | Isepamicina |
| 依替米星 | Etimicin | Etimicine | Etimicina |
| 大观霉素 | Spectinomycin | Spectinomycine | Espectinomicina |
| 1.6 四环素类 Teracyclines | | | |
| 四环素 | Tetracycline | Tétracycline | Tetraciclina |
| 土霉素 | Oxytetracycline | Oxytétracycline | Oxitetraciclina |
| 多西环素 | Doxycycline | Doxycycline | Doxiciclina |
| 米诺环素 | Minocycline | Minocycline | Minociclina |
| 替加环素 | Tigecycline | Tigécycline | Tigeciclina |
| 1.7 林可霉素类 Lincomycins | | | |
| 林可霉素 | Lincomycin | Lincomycine | Lincomicina |
| 克林霉素 | Clindamycin | Clindamycine | Clindamicina |
| 氯霉素 | Chloramphenicol | Chloramphénicol | Cloramfenicol |
| 甲砜霉素 | Thiamphenicol | Thiamphénicol | Tiamfenicol |
| 1.8 大环内酯类 Macrolides | | | |
| 红霉素 | Erythromycin | Erythromycine | Eritromicina |
| 琥乙红霉素 | Erythromycin Ethylsuccinate | Ethylsuccinate de Erythromycine | Eritromicina Etilsuccinato |
| 罗红霉素 | Roxithromycin | Roxithromycine | Roxitromicina |
| 克拉霉素 | Clarithromycin | Clarithromycine | Claritromicina |
| 阿奇霉素 | Azithromycin | Azithromycine | Azitromicina |
| 泰利霉素 | Telithromycin | Télithromycine | Telitromicina |
| 地红霉素 | Dirithromycin | Dirithromycine | Diritromicina |
| 吉他霉素 | Kitasamycin | Kitasamycine | Kitasamicina |
| 麦迪霉素 | Midecamycin | Midécamycine | Midecamicina |
| 乙酰麦迪霉素 | Acetylmidecamycin | Acétylmidécamycine | Acetilmidecamicina |
| 交沙霉素 | Josamycin | Josamycine | Josamicina |
| 麦白霉素 | Meleumycin | Méleumycine | Meleumicina |
| 罗他霉素 | Rokitamycin | Rokitamycine | Rokitamicina |
| 乙酰螺旋霉素 | Acetylspiramycin | Acetylspiramycine | Acetilspiramicina |

**续 表**

| 药品名称 | Drug Names | Dénomination du Médicament | Denominación del Medicamento |
|---|---|---|---|
| **1.9 糖肽类 Glycopeptides** | | | |
| 去甲万古霉素 | Norvancomycin | Norvancomycine | Norvancomicina |
| 万古霉素 | Vancomycin | Vancomycine | Vancomicina |
| 替考拉宁 | Teicoplanin | Teicoplanine | Teicoplanina |
| **1.10 其他抗菌抗生素 Others antibiotics** | | | |
| 磷霉素 | Fosfomycin | Fosfomycine | Fosfomicina |
| 达托霉素 | Daptomycin | Daptomycine | Daptomicina |
| 利福昔明 | Rifaximin | Rifaximine | Rifaximina |
| 多黏菌素 B | Polymyxin B | Polymyxine B | Polimixina B |
| 黏菌素 | Colistin | Colistine | Colistina |
| 夫西地酸钠 | Fusidate Sodium | Fusidate sodique | Fusidato de sódio |
| **2. 化学合成的抗菌药 Chemical Synthetic Antibacterial Drugs** | | | |
| **2.1 磺胺类 Sulfonamides** | | | |
| 磺胺嘧啶 | Sulfadiazine | Sulfadiazine | Sulfadiazina |
| 磺胺甲噁唑 | Sulfamethoxazole | Sulfaméthoxazole | Sulfametoxazol |
| 柳氮磺吡啶 | Sulfasalazine | Sulfasalazine | Sulfasalazina |
| **2.2 甲氧苄啶类 Trimethoprim** | | | |
| 甲氧苄啶 | Trimethoprim | Triméthoprime | Trimetoprima |
| **2.3 硝基呋喃类 Nitrofurans** | | | |
| 呋喃妥因 | Nitrofurantoin | Nitrofurantoïne | Nitrofurantoin |
| 呋喃唑酮 | Furazolidone | Furazolidone | Furazolidona |
| **2.4 喹诺酮类 4-Quinolones** | | | |
| 吡哌酸 | Pipemidic Acid | Acide pipémidique | Ácido pipemídico |
| 诺氟沙星 | Norfloxacin | Norfloxacine | Norfloxacina |
| 氧氟沙星 | Ofloxacin | Ofloxacine | Ofloxacina |
| 左氧氟沙星 | Levofloxacin | Lévofloxacine | Levofloxacina |
| 依诺沙星 | Enoxacin | Enoxacine | Enoxacina |
| 环丙沙星 | Ciprofloxacin | Ciprofloxacine | Ciprofloxacina |
| 洛美沙星 | Lomefloxacin | Lomefloxacine | Lomefloxacina |
| 培氟沙星 | Pefloxacin | Péfloxacine | Pefloxacina |
| 芦氟沙星 | Rufloxacin | Rufloxacine | Rufloxacina |
| 司帕沙星 | Sparfloxacin | Sparfloxacine | Sparfloxacina |
| 氟罗沙星 | Fleroxacin | Fleroxacine | Fleroxacina |
| 莫西沙星 | Moxifloxacin | Moxifloxacine | Moxifloxacina |
| 加替沙星 | Gatifloxacin | Gatifloxacine | Gatifloxacina |
| 帕珠沙星 | Pazufloxacin | Pazufloxacine | Pazufloxacina |
| 托氟沙星 | Tosufloxacin | Tosufloxacine | Tosufloxacina |

**续　表**

| 药品名称 | Drug Names | Dénomination du Médicament | Denominación del Medicamento |
|---|---|---|---|
| **2.5 硝基咪唑类 Nitroimidazoles** | | | |
| 甲硝唑 | Metronidazole | Métronidazole | Metronidazol |
| 替硝唑 | Tinidazole | Tinidazole | Tinidazol |
| 奥硝唑 | Ornidazole | Ornidazole | Ornidazol |
| 塞克硝唑 | Secnidazole | Secnidazole | Secnidazol |
| **2.6 噁唑烷酮类 Oxazolidinones** | | | |
| 利奈唑胺 | Linezolid | Linézolide | Linezolida |
| **3. 抗结核药 Antituberculosis Drugs** | | | |
| 异烟肼 | Isoniazid | Isoniazide | Isoniacida |
| 对氨基水杨酸钠 | Sodium Aminosalicylate | Aminosalicylate de Sodium | Aminosalicilato de Sodio |
| 利福平 | Rifampicin | Rifampicine | Rifampicina |
| 利福定 | Rifandin | Rifandine | Rifandina |
| 利福喷丁 | Rifapentine | Rifapentine | Rifapentina |
| 利福霉素钠 | Rifamycin Sodium | Rifamycine de Sodium | Rifamicina de Sodio |
| 链霉素 | Streptomycin | Streptomycine | Estreptomicina |
| 乙胺丁醇 | Ethambutol | Ethambutol | Etambutol |
| 乙硫异烟胺 | Ethionamide | Ethionamide | Etionamida |
| 丙硫异烟胺 | Protionamide | Protionamide | Protionamida |
| 吡嗪酰胺 | Pyrazinamide | Pyrazinamide | Pirazinamida |
| **4. 抗麻风病药及抗麻风病反应药 Anti-Leprosy Drugs and Anti-Leprosy Reaction Drugs** | | | |
| 氨苯砜 | Dapsone | Dapsone | Dapsona |
| 醋氨苯砜 | Acedapsone | Acédapsone | Acedapsona |
| 苯丙砜 | Solasulfone | Solasulfone | Solasulfona |
| 氯法齐明 | Clofazimine | Clofazimine | Clofazimina |
| 沙利度胺 | Thalidomide | Thalidomide | Talidomida |
| **5. 抗真菌药 Antifungal Drugs** | | | |
| 两性霉素 B | Amphotericin B | Amphotericine B | Anfotericina B |
| 伊曲康唑 | Itraconazole | Itraconazole | Itraconazol |
| 氟康唑 | Fluconazole | Fluconazole | Fluconazol |
| 伏立康唑 | Voriconazole | Voriconazole | Voriconazol |
| 泊沙康唑 | Posaconazole | Posaconazole | Posaconazol |
| 氟胞嘧啶 | Flucytosine | Flucytosine | Flucitosina |
| 特比奈芬 | Terbinafine | Terbinafine | Terbinafina |
| 美帕曲星 | Mepartricin | Mépartricine | Mepartricina |
| 阿莫罗芬 | Amorolfine | Amorolfine | Amorolfina |
| 醋酸卡泊芬净 | Caspofungin Acetate | Acétate de Caspofungine | Acetato de Caspofungina |
| 米卡芬净 | Micafungin | Micafungine | Micafungina |

**续 表**

| 药品名称 | Drug Names | Dénomination du Médicament | Denominación del Medicamento |
| --- | --- | --- | --- |
| 阿尼芬净 | Anidulafungin | Anidulafungine | Anidulafungina |
| 制霉菌素 | Nystatin | Nystatine | Nistatina |
| 咪康唑 | Miconazole | Miconazole | Miconazol |
| 6. 抗病毒药 Antiviral Drugs | | | |
| 阿昔洛韦 | Aciclovir | Aciclovir | Aciclovir |
| 更昔洛韦 | Ganciclovir | Ganciclovir | Ganciclovir |
| 伐昔洛韦 | Valaciclovir | Valaciclovir | Valaciclovir |
| 泛昔洛韦 | Famciclovir | Famciclovir | Famciclovir |
| 奥司他韦 | Oseltamivir | Oseltamivir | Oseltamivir |
| 达拉他韦 | Daclatasvir | Daclatasvir | Daclatasvir |
| 阿舒瑞韦 | Asunaprevir | Asunaprevir | Asunaprevir |
| 扎那米韦 | Zanamivir | Zanamivir | Zanamivir |
| 阿巴卡韦 | Abacavir | Abacavir | Abacavir |
| 阿糖腺苷 | Vidarabine | Vidarabine | Vidarabina |
| 利巴韦林 | Ribavirin | Ribavirine | Ribavirina |
| 齐多夫定 | Zidovudine | Zidovudine | Zidovudina |
| 拉米夫定 | Lamivudine | Lamivudine | Lamivudina |
| 阿德福韦酯 | Adefovir dipivoxil | Adéfovir dipivoxil | Adefovir dipivoxil |
| 恩替卡韦 | Entecavir | Entécavir | Entecavir |
| 替比夫定 | Telbivudine | Télbivudine | Telbivudina |
| 聚乙二醇干扰素 α-2a | Peginterferon alfa-2a | Intérféron pégylé alfa-2a | Peginterferón alfa-2a |
| 奈韦拉平 | Nevirapine | Névirapine | Nevirapina |
| 司他夫定 | Stavudine | Stavudine | Stavudina |
| 利托那韦 | Ritonavir | Ritonavir | Ritonavir |
| 膦甲酸钠 | Foscarnet Sodium | Foscarnét de sodium | Foscarnet de sodio |
| 去羟肌苷 | Didanosine | Didanosine | Didanosina |
| 茚地那韦 | Indinavir | Indinavir | Indinavir |
| 替诺福韦 | Tenofovir | Ténofovir | Tenofovir |
| 恩曲他滨 替诺福韦 | Emtricitabine and Tenofovir | Emtricitabine et Ténofovir | Emtricitabina y Tenofovir |
| 奈韦拉平 | Nevirapine | Névirapine | Nevirapina |
| 依非韦伦 | Efavirenz | Efavirénz | Efavirenz |
| 洛匹那韦 利托那韦 | Lopinavir and Ritonavir | Lopinavir et Ritonavir | Lopinavir y Ritonavir |
| 达芦那韦 | Darunavir | Darunavir | Darunavir |
| 拉替拉韦 | Raltegravir | Raltégravir | Raltegravir |
| 多替拉韦 | Dolutegravir | Dolutégravir | Dolutegravir |

**续　表**

| 药品名称 | Drug Names | Dénomination du Médicament | Denominación del Medicamento |
|---|---|---|---|
| 金刚烷胺 | Amantadine | Amantadine | Amantadina |
| 7. 抗寄生虫病药 Antiparasitic Drugs | | | |
| 7.1　抗疟药 Antimalarial drugs | | | |
| 氯喹 | Chloroquine | Chloroquine | Cloroquina |
| 羟氯喹 | Hydroxychloroquine | Hydroxychloroquine | Hidroxicloroquina |
| 青蒿素 | Artemisinin | Artémisinine | Artemisinina |
| 青蒿素哌喹 | Artemisinin and Piperaquine | Artémisinine et Pipéraquine | Artemisinina y Piperaquina |
| 双氢青蒿素 | Dihydroartemisinin | Dihydroartémisinine | Dihidroartemisinina |
| 双氢青蒿素磷酸哌喹 | Dihydroartemisinin and Piperaquine Phosphate | Dihydroartémisinine et Phosphate de Pipéraque | Dihidroartemisinina y Piperaquina fosfato |
| 蒿甲醚 | Artemether | Arteméther | Arteméter |
| 奎宁 | Quinine | Quinine | Quinina |
| 伯氨喹 | Primaquine | Primaquine | Primaquina |
| 乙胺嘧啶 | Pyrimethamine | Pyriméthamine | Pirimetamina |
| 7.2　抗阿米巴药 Anti-Amebicide drugs | | | |
| 双碘喹啉 | Diiodohydroxyquinoline | Diiodohydroxyquinoline | Diiodohidroxiquinolina |
| 依米丁 | Emetine | Emétine | Emetina |
| 7.3　抗滴虫药 Anti-Trichomonal drug | | | |
| 甲硝唑 | Metronidazole | Métronidazole | Metronidazol |
| 7.4　抗血吸虫药 Anti-Schistosmomicide drugs | | | |
| 吡喹酮 | Praziquantel | Praziquantel | Praziquantel |
| 7.5　抗其他吸虫药 Anti other fluke drug | | | |
| 硫氯酚 | Bithionol | Bithionol | Bitionol |
| 7.6　抗丝虫药 Antifilarial | | | |
| 乙胺嗪 | Diethylcarbamazine | Diethylcarbamazine | Dietilcarbamacina |
| 7.7　抗利什曼原虫药 Antileishmania drug | | | |
| 葡萄糖酸锑钠 | Sodium Stibogluconate | Stibogluconate sodique | Estibogluconato sodio |
| 7.8　驱肠虫药 Intestinal anthelmintics | | | |
| 哌嗪 | Piperazine | Pipérazine | Piperazina |
| 左旋咪唑 | Levamisole | Lévamisole | Levamisol |
| 阿苯达唑 | Albendazole | Albendazole | Albendazol |
| 尼可刹米 | Nikethamide | Nicéthamide | Niketamida |
| 8. 主要作用于中枢神经系统的药物 Drugs Mainly Acting on the Central Nervous System | | | |
| 8.1　中枢神经系统兴奋药 Drugs exciting central nervous system | | | |
| 洛贝林 | Lobeline | Lobéline | Lobelina |
| 戊四氮 | Pentetrazole | Pentétrazole | Pentetrazol |
| 贝美格 | Bemegride | Bémégride | Bemegrida |

续　表

| 药品名称 | Drug Names | Dénomination du Médicament | Denominación del Medicamento |
|---|---|---|---|
| 咖啡因 | Caffeine | Caféine | Cafeína |
| 甲氯芬酯 | Meclofenoxate | Méclofénoxate | Meclofenoxato |
| 乙哌立松 | Eperisone | Epérisone | Eperisona |
| 细胞色素 C | Cytochrome C | Cytochrome C | Citocromo C |
| 8.2　镇痛药 Analgesics | | | |
| 吗啡 | Morphine | Morphine | Morfina |
| 哌替啶 | Pethidine | Péthidine | Petidina |
| 美沙酮 | Methadone | Méthadone | Metadona |
| 芬太尼 | Fentanyl | Fentanyl | Fentanilo |
| 阿芬太尼 | Alfentanil | Alfentanil | Alfentanilo |
| 舒芬太尼 | Sufentanil | Sufentanil | Sufentanilo |
| 瑞芬太尼 | Remifentanil | Rémifentanil | Remifentanilo |
| 布桂嗪 | Bucinnazine | Bucinnazine | Bucinazina |
| 喷他佐辛 | Pentazocine | Pentazocine | Pentazocina |
| 羟考酮 | Oxycodone | Oxycodone | Oxicodona |
| 地佐辛 | Dezocine | Dézocine | Dezocina |
| 普瑞巴林 | Pregabalin | Prégabaline | Pregabalina |
| 曲马多 | Tramadol | Tramadol | Tramadol |
| 四氢帕马丁 | Tetrahydropalmatine | Tétrahydropalmatine | Tetrahidropalmatina |
| 罗通定 | Rotundine | Rotundine | Rotundina |
| 麦角胺 | Ergotamine | Ergotamine | Ergotamina |
| 乙酰乌头碱 | Acetylaconitine | Acetylaconitine | Acetilaconitina |
| 洛美利嗪 | Lomerizine | Lomérizine | Lomerizina |
| 齐考诺肽 | Ziconotide | Ziconotide | Ziconotida |
| 他喷他多 | Tapentadol | Tapentadol | Tapentadol |
| 阿片全碱 | Papaveretum | Papaveretum | Papaveretum |
| 荷包牡丹碱 | Dicentrine | Dicentrine | Dicentrina |
| 山豆碱 | Total Alkaloids of Sophora Tonkinesis | Total Alcali de Sophora Tonkinesis | Total Alcali de Sophora Tonkinesis |
| 匹米诺定 | Piminodine | Piminodine | Piminodina |
| 西马嗪 | Simazine | Simazine | Simazina |
| 千金藤啶碱 | Stepholidine | Stépholidine | Estefolidina |
| 高乌甲素 | Lappaconitine | Lappaconitine | Lappaconitina |
| 美西麦角 | Methysergide | Méthysergide | Metisergida |
| 氨酚氢可酮 | Paracetamol and Hydrocodone Bitartrate | Paracétamol et Hydrocodone Bitartrate | Paracetamol y Hidrocodona Bitartrato |
| 8.3　解热镇痛抗炎药 Non-steroidal anti-inflammatory drugs | | | |
| 阿司匹林 | Aspirin | Aspirine | Aspirina |

**续　表**

| 药品名称 | Drug Names | Dénomination du Médicament | Denominación del Medicamento |
| --- | --- | --- | --- |
| 阿司匹林精氨酸盐 | Aspirin-arginine | Aspirine arginine | Aspirina-arginina |
| 阿司匹林赖氨酸盐 | Aspirin-DL-lysine | Aspirine-DL-lysine | Aspirina-DL-lisina |
| 美沙拉秦 | Mesalazine | Mésalazine | Mesalazina |
| 对乙酰氨基酚 | Paracetamol | Paracetamol | Paracetamol |
| 吲哚美辛 | Indometacin | Indométacine | Indometacina |
| 双氯芬酸 | Diclofenac | Diclofénac | Diclofenaco |
| 萘普生 | Naproxen | Naproxène | Naproxeno |
| 布洛芬 | Ibuprofen | Ibuprofène | Ibuprofeno |
| 酮洛芬 | Ketoprofen | Kétoprofène | Ketoprofeno |
| 芬布芬 | Fenbufen | Fenbufène | Fenbufeno |
| 吡洛芬 | Pirprofen | Pirprofène | Pirprofeno |
| 阿明洛芬 | Alminoprofen | Alminoprofène | Alminoprofeno |
| 洛索洛芬 | Loxoprofen | Loxoprofène | Loxoprofeno |
| 吡罗昔康 | Piroxicam | Piroxicam | Piroxicam |
| 美洛昔康 | Meloxicam | Méloxicam | Meloxicam |
| 氯诺昔康 | Lornoxicam | Lornoxicam | Lornoxicam |
| 塞来昔布 | Celecoxib | Célécoxib | Celecoxib |
| 帕瑞昔布 | Parecoxib | Parécoxib | Parecoxib |
| 尼美舒利 | Nimesulide | Nimésulide | Nimesulida |
| 安乃近 | Metamizole Sodium | Metamizole sodique | Metamizol sódico |
| 保泰松 | Phenylbutazone | Phénylbutazone | Fenilbutazona |
| 萘丁美酮 | Nabumetone | Nabumétone | Nabumetona |
| 来氟米特 | Leflunomide | Léflunomide | Leflunomida |
| 复方骨肽 | Compound Ossotide | Composée d'ossotide | Ossotida Compuesto |
| 硫辛酸 | Lipoic Acid（Thioctic Acid） | Acide Lipoique | Ácido Lipoico |
| 氟比洛芬 | Flurbiprofen | Flurbiprofène | Flurbiprofeno |
| 醋氯芬酸 | Aceclofenac | Acéclofénac | Aceclofenaco |
| 8.4　抗痛风药 Gout suppressant | | | |
| 秋水仙碱 | Colchicine | Colchicine | Colchicina |
| 丙磺舒 | Probenecid | Probénécide | Probenecida |
| 苯溴马隆 | Benzbromarone | Benzbromarone | Benzbromarona |
| 别嘌醇 | Allopurinol | Allopurinol | Alopurinol |
| 非布司他 | Febuxostat | Febuxostat | Febuxostat |
| 8.5　抗癫痫药 Antiepileptics | | | |
| 苯妥英钠 | Phenytoin Sodium | Phénytoïne sodium | Fenitoína Sódica |
| 卡马西平 | Carbamazepine | Carbamazépine | Carbamazepina |

| 药品名称 | Drug Names | Dénomination du Médicament | Denominación del Medicamento |
|---|---|---|---|
| 奥卡西平 | Oxcarbazepine | Oxcarbazépine | Oxcarbazepina |
| 托吡酯 | Topiramate | Topiramate | Topiramato |
| 乙琥胺 | Ethosuximide | Ethosuximide | Etosuximida |
| 丙戊酸钠 | Sodium Valproate | Valproate sodique | Valproato de sódio |
| 拉莫三嗪 | Lamotrigine | Lamotrigine | Lamotrigina |
| 加巴喷丁 | Gabapentin | Gabapentine | Gabapentina |
| 左乙拉西坦 | Levetiracetam | Lévétiracétam | Levetiracetam |
| 扑米酮 | Primidone | Primidone | Primidona |
| **8.6 镇静药、催眠药和抗惊厥药 Sedative, Hypnotics and Anticonvulsants** | | | |
| 咪达唑仑 | Midazolam | Midazolam | Midazolam |
| 苯巴比妥 | Phenobarbital | Phénobarbital | Fenobarbital |
| 异戊巴比妥 | Amobarbital | Amobarbital | Amobarbital |
| 司可巴比妥 | Secobarbital | Sécobarbital | Secobarbital |
| 佐匹克隆 | Zopiclone | Zopiclone | Zopiclona |
| 唑吡坦 | Zolpidem | Zolpidem | Zolpidem |
| 水合氯醛 | Chloral Hydrate | Hydrate de chloral | Hidrato de cloral |
| 扎来普隆 | Zaleplon | Zaleplon | Zaleplón |
| 艾司佐匹克隆 | Eszopiclone | Eszopiclone | Eszopiclona |
| 溴化钾 | Potassium Bromide | Bromure de potassium | Bromuro de potasio |
| 戊巴比妥钠 | Pentobarbital Sodium | Pentobarbital sodique | Pentobarbital sódico |
| **8.7 抗帕金森病药 Antiparkinsonian Drugs** | | | |
| 左旋多巴 | Levodopa | Lévodopa | Levodopa |
| 卡比多巴 | Carbidopa | Carbidopa | Carbidopa |
| 苄丝肼 | Benserazide | Bénsérazide | Benserazida |
| 多巴丝肼 | Levodopa and Benserazide | Lévodopa et Bénsérazide | Levodopa y Benserazida |
| 溴隐亭 | Bromocriptine | Bromocriptine | Bromocriptina |
| 普拉克索 | Pramipexole | Pramipexole | Pramipexol |
| 司来吉兰 | Selegiline | Sélégiline | Selegilina |
| 雷沙吉兰 | Rasagiline | Rasagiline | Rasagilina |
| 苯海索 | Trihexyphenidyl | Trihéxyphénidyl | Trihexifenidilo |
| 金刚烷胺 | Amantadine | Amantadine | Amantadina |
| 美金刚 | Memantine | Mémantine | Memantina |
| **8.8 抗精神病药 Antipsychotic Drugs** | | | |
| 氯丙嗪 | Chlorpromazine | Chlorpromazine | Clorpromazina |
| 奋乃静 | Perphenazine | Pérphénazine | Perfenazina |
| 氟奋乃静 | Fluphenazine | Fluphénazine | Flufenazina |
| 三氟拉嗪 | Trifluoperazine | Trifluopérazine | Trifluoperazina |

**续　表**

| 药品名称 | Drug Names | Dénomination du Médicament | Denominación del Medicamento |
| --- | --- | --- | --- |
| 硫利达嗪 | Thioridazine | Thioridazine | Tioridazina |
| 氟哌啶醇 | Haloperidol | Halopéridol | Haloperidol |
| 氟哌利多 | Droperidol | Dropéridol | Droperidol |
| 氯哌噻吨 | Clopenthixol | Clopénthixol | Clopentixol |
| 氟哌噻吨 | Flupentixol | Flupéntixol | Flupentixol |
| 氟哌噻吨美利曲辛 | Flupentixol and Melitiacen | Flupéntixol et Mélitiacén | Flupentixol y Melitraceno |
| 舒必利 | Sulpiride | Sulpiride | Sulpirida |
| 氯氮平 | Clozapine | Clozapine | Clozapina |
| 奥氮平 | Olanzapine | Olanzapine | Olanzapina |
| 喹硫平 | Quetiapine | Quétiapine | Quetiapina |
| 利培酮 | Risperidone | Rrispéridone | Risperidona |
| 帕潘立酮 | Paliperidone | Palipéridone | Paliperidona |
| 齐拉西酮 | Ziprasidone | Ziprasidone | Ziprasidona |
| 五氟利多 | Penfluridol | Pénfluridol | Penfluridol |
| 阿立哌唑 | Aripiprazole | Aripiprazole | Aripiprazol |
| 曲美托嗪 | Trimetozine | Trimétozine | Trimetozina |
| 癸氟奋乃静 | Fluphenazine Decanoate | Fluphénazine décanoate | Decanoato de Flufenazina |
| **8.9 抗焦虑药 Antianxietic Drugs** | | | |
| 地西泮 | Diazepam | Diazépam | Diazepam |
| 奥沙西泮 | Oxazepam | Oxazépam | Oxazepam |
| 硝西泮 | Nitrazepam | Nitrazépam | Nitrazepam |
| 氟西泮 | Flurazepam | Flurazépam | Flurazepam |
| 氯硝西泮 | Clonazepam | Clonazépam | Clonazepam |
| 劳拉西泮 | Lorazepam | Lorazépam | Lorazepam |
| 氟硝西泮 | Flunitrazepam | Flunitrazépam | Flunitrazepam |
| 艾司唑仑 | Estazolam | Estazolam | Estazolam |
| 阿普唑仑 | Alprazolam | Alprazolam | Alprazolam |
| 奥沙唑仑 | Oxazolam | Oxazolam | Oxazolam |
| 美沙唑仑 | Mexazolam | Méxazolam | Mexazolam |
| 谷维素 | Oryzanol | Oryzanol | Orizanol |
| **8.10 抗躁狂药 Antimanic Drugs** | | | |
| 碳酸锂 | Lithium Carbonate | Carbonate de lithium | Carbonato de litio |
| 卡马西平 | Carbamazepine | Carbamazépine | Carbamazepina |
| 丙戊酸钠 | Sodium Valproate | Valproate sodique | Valproato de sodio |
| **8.11 抗抑郁药 Antidepressants** | | | |
| 丙米嗪 | Imipramine | Imipramine | Imipramina |

**续 表**

| 药品名称 | Drug Names | Dénomination du Médicament | Denominación del Medicamento |
|---|---|---|---|
| 氯米帕明 | Clomipramine | Clomipramine | Clomipramina |
| 阿米替林 | Amitriptyline | Amitriptyline | Amitriptilina |
| 多塞平 | Doxepin | Doxépine | Doxepina |
| 吗氯贝胺 | Moclobemide | Moclobémide | Moclobemida |
| 氟西汀 | Fluoxetine | Fluoxétine | Fluoxetina |
| 氟伏沙明 | Fluvoxamine | Fluvoxamine | Fluvoxamina |
| 帕罗西汀 | Paroxetine | Paroxétine | Paroxetina |
| 舍曲林 | Sertraline | Sértraline | Sertralina |
| 西酞普兰 | Citalopram | Citalopram | Citalopram |
| 艾司西酞普兰 | Escitalopram | Escitalopram | Escitalopram |
| 8.12 抗脑血管病药 Anti-Cerebrovascular Disease Drugs | | | |
| 尼莫地平 | Nimodipine | Nimodipine | Nimodipina |
| 桂利嗪 | Cinnarizine | Cinnarizine | Cinarizina |
| 氟桂利嗪 | Flunarizine | Flunarizine | Flunarizina |
| 降纤酶 | Defibrase | Défibrase | Defibrasa |
| 巴曲酶 | Defibrin | Defibrine | Defibrina |
| 倍他司汀 | Betahistine | Bétahistine | Betahistina |
| 罂粟碱 | Papaverine | Papavérine | Papaverina |
| 己酮可可碱 | Pentoxifylline | Péntoxifylline | Pentoxifilina |
| 丁咯地尔 | Buflomedil | Buflomédil | Buflomedil |
| 尼麦角林 | Nicergoline | Nicérgoline | Nicergolina |
| 川芎嗪 | Ligustrazine | Ligustrazine | Ligustrazina |
| 丁苯酞 | Butylphthalide | Butylphtalide | Butilftalida |
| 奥扎格雷 | Ozagrel | Ozagrél | Ozagrel |
| 曲克芦丁 | Troxerutin | Troxérutine | Troxerutina |
| 维生素 E 烟酸酯 | Vitamin E Nicotinate | Niacine de Vitamine E | Niacina de Vitamina E |
| 灯盏花素 | Breviscapine | Bréviscapine | Breviscapina |
| 地芬尼多 | Difenidol | Difénidol | Difenidol |
| 长春西汀 | Vinpocetine | Vinpocétine | Vinpocetina |
| 依达拉奉 | Edaravone | Edaravone | Edaravona |
| 血塞通 | Xuesaitong | Xuesaitong | Xuesaitong |
| 七叶皂苷钠 | Sodium Aescinate | Aéscinate sodique | Aescinato sódico |
| 葛根素 | Puerarin | Puérarin | Puerarina |
| 8.13 抗老年痴呆药和改善脑代谢药 Anti-Senile Dementia Drugs and Improving Brain Metabolic Drugs | | | |
| 加兰他敏 | Galanthamine | Galantamine | Galantamina |
| 美金刚 | Memantine | Mémantine | Memantina |
| 吡拉西坦 | Piracetam | Piracétam | Piracetam |

**续 表**

| 药品名称 | Drug Names | Dénomination du Médicament | Denominación del Medicamento |
|---|---|---|---|
| 茴拉西坦 | Aniracetam | Aniracétam | Aniracetam |
| 奥拉西坦 | Oxiracetam | Oxiracétam | Oxiracetam |
| 银杏叶提取物 | Ginkgo Biloba Leaf Extract | Sextrait de Ginkgo biloba Feuille | Extracto de Ginkgo Biloba Hoja |
| 阿米三嗪/萝巴新 | Almitrine/Raubasine | Almitrine/Raubasine | Almitrina/Raubasina |
| 吡硫醇 | Pyritinol | Pyritinol | Piritinol |
| 小牛血去蛋白提取物 | Deprotenized Hemoderivative of Calf Blood | Extrait déprotéinisé du sang de veau | Derivados de desproteinización de la sangre de ternero |
| 胞磷胆碱 | Citicoline | Citicoline | Citicolina |
| 单唾液酸四己糖神经节苷脂 | Monosialoteterahexosyl Ganglioside | Monosialaté de térahéxose Ganglioside | Gangliosidos monosialicos de tetrahexosina |
| 脑蛋白水解物 | Cerebroprotein Hydrolysate | Hydrolysats de protéines du cerveau | Hidrolizados de proteínas del cerebro |
| 赖氨酸 | Lysine | Lysine | Lisina |
| **8.14 麻醉药及其辅助用药 Anesthetics and Their Supplementary Drugs** | | | |
| 恩氟烷 | Enflurane | Enflurane | Enflurano |
| 异氟烷 | Isoflurane | Isoflurane | Isoflurano |
| 七氟烷 | Sevoflurane | Sévoflurane | Sevoflurano |
| 硫喷妥钠 | Thiopental Sodium | Thiopental sodique | Tiopental Sódico |
| 氯胺酮 | Ketamine | Kétamine | ketamina |
| 依托咪酯 | Etomidate | Etomidate | Etomidato |
| 羟丁酸钠 | Sodium Hydroxybutyrate | Hydroxybutyrate sodique | Hidroxibutirato sódico |
| 丙泊酚 | Propofol | Propofol | Propofol |
| 普鲁卡因 | Procaine | Procaïne | Procaína |
| 丁卡因 | Tetracaine | Tétracaïne | Tetracaína |
| 利多卡因 | Lidocaine | Lidocaïne | Lidocaína |
| 布比卡因 | Bupivacaine | Bupivacaïne | Bupivacaína |
| 罗哌卡因 | Ropivacaine | Ropivacaïne | Ropivacaína |
| 达克罗宁 | Dyclonine | Dyclonine | Diclonina |
| 泮库溴铵 | Pancuronium Bromide | Bromure de pancuronium | Bromuro de pancuronio |
| 罗库溴铵 | Rocuronium Bromide | Bromure de rocuronium | Bromuro de rocuronio |
| 维库溴铵 | Vecuronium bromide | Bromure de vecuronium | Bromuro de vecuronio |
| 阿库氯铵 | Alcuronium Chloride | Chlorure d'alcuronium | Cloruro de alcuronio |
| 哌库溴铵 | Pipecuronium Biomide | Bromure de pipecuronium | Bromuro de pipecuronio |
| 阿曲库铵 | Atracurium | Atracurium | Atracurio |
| 顺阿曲库铵 | Cisatracurium | Cisatracurium | Cisatracurio |
| 琥珀胆碱 | Succinylcholine | Succinylcholine | Succinilcolina |

| 药品名称 | Drug Names | Dénomination du Médicament | Denominación del Medicamento |
| --- | --- | --- | --- |
| 9. 作用于自主神经系统的药物 Drugs Mainly Acting on the Autonomic Nervous System | | | |
| 9.1　拟胆碱药和抗胆碱药 Cholinergic Drugs and Anticholinergic Drugs | | | |
| 卡巴胆碱 | Carbachol | Carbachol | Carbachol |
| 毛果芸香碱 | Pilocarpine | Pilocarpine | Pilocarpina |
| 毒扁豆碱 | Physostigmine | Physostigmine | Fisostigmina |
| 新斯的明 | Neostigmine | Néostigmine | Neostigmina |
| 溴吡斯的明 | Pyridostigmine Bromide | Bromure de Pyridostigmine | Bromuro de Piridostigmina |
| 石杉碱甲 | Huperzine A | Hupérzine A | Huperzina A |
| 多奈哌齐 | Donepezil | Donépézil | Donepezil |
| 加兰他敏 | Galanthamine | Galantamine | Galantamina |
| 阿托品 | Atropine | Atropine | Atropina |
| 东莨菪碱 | Scopolamine | Scopolamine | Escopolamina |
| 山莨菪碱 | Anisodamine | Anisodamine | Anisodamina |
| 托吡卡胺 | Tropicamide | Tropicamide | Tropicamida |
| 颠茄 | Belladonna | Belladone | Belladona |
| 后马托品 | Homatropine | Homatropine | Homatropina |
| 9.2　拟肾上腺素药和抗肾上腺素药 Adrenergic Drugs and Adrenoceptor Antagonists | | | |
| 萘甲唑啉 | Naphazoline | Naphazoline | Nafazolina |
| 米多君 | Midodrine | Midodrine | Midodrina |
| 拉贝洛尔 | Labetalol | Labétalol | Labetalol |
| 卡维地洛 | Carvedilol | Carvédilol | Carvedilol |
| 酚妥拉明 | Phentolamine | Phéntolamine | Fentolamina |
| 妥拉唑林 | Tolazoline | Tolazoline | Tolazolina |
| 酚苄明 | Phenoxybenzamine | Phénoxybenzamine | Fenoxibenzamina |
| 普萘洛尔 | Propranolol | Propranolol | Propranolol |
| 噻吗洛尔 | Timolol | Timolol | Timolol |
| 索他洛尔 | Sotalol | Sotalol | Sotalol |
| 阿替洛尔 | Atenolol | Aténolol | Atenolol |
| 美托洛尔 | Metoprolol | Métoprolol | Metoprolol |
| 比索洛尔 | Bisoprolol | Bisoprolol | Bisoprolol |
| 倍他洛尔 | Betaxolol | Bétaxolol | Betaxolol |
| 艾司洛尔 | Esmolol | Esmolol | Esmolol |
| 10. 主要作用于心血管系统的药物 Drugs Mainly Acting on the Cardiovascular System | | | |
| 10.1　钙通道阻滞药 Calcim Channel Blockers | | | |
| 维拉帕米 | Verapamil | Vérapamil | Verapamilo |
| 硝苯地平 | Nifedipine | Nifédipine | Nifedipina |
| 尼卡地平 | Nicardipine | Nicardipine | Nicardipina |

**续　表**

| 药品名称 | Drug Names | Dénomination du Médicament | Denominación del Medicamento |
|---|---|---|---|
| 尼群地平 | Nitrendipine | Nitrendipine | Nitrendipina |
| 尼莫地平 | Nimodipine | Nimodipine | Nimodipina |
| 非洛地平 | Felodipine | Félodipine | Felodipina |
| 氨氯地平 | Amlodipine | Amlodipine | Amlodipina |
| 左氨氯地平 | Levamlodipine | Lévoamlodipine | Levamlodipina |
| 西尼地平 | Cilnidipine | Cilnidipine | Cilnidipina |
| 拉西地平 | Lacidipine | Lacidipine | Lacidipina |
| 地尔硫䓬 | Diltiazem | Diltiazem | Diltiazem |
| 桂利嗪 | Cinnarizine | Cinnarizine | Cinarizina |
| 氟桂利嗪 | Flunarizine | Flunarizine | Flunarizina |
| 利多氟嗪 | Lidoflazine | Lidoflazine | Lidoflazina |
| 10.2　治疗慢性心功能不全的药物 Drugs Treating Chronic Cardiac Insufficiency | | | |
| 洋地黄毒苷 | Digitoxin | Digitoxine | Digitoxina |
| 地高辛 | Digoxin | Digoxine | Digoxina |
| 毛花苷 C | Lanatoside C | Lanatoside C | Lanatosida C |
| 去乙酰毛花苷 | Deslanoside | Déslanoside | Deslanósida |
| 毒毛花苷 K | Strophanthin K | Strophantin K | Strofantin K |
| 氨力农 | Amrinone | Amrinone | Amrinona |
| 米力农 | Milrinone | Milrinone | Milrinona |
| 奈西利肽 | Nesiritide | Nésiritide | Nesiritida |
| 左西孟旦 | Levosimendan | Lévosiméndan | Levosimendan |
| 伊伐布雷定 | Ivabradine | Ivabradine | Ivabradina |
| 托伐普坦 | Tolvaptan | Tolvaptane | Tolvaptan |
| 沙库巴曲缬沙坦钠 | Sacubitril and Valsartan Sodium | Sacubitril et Valsartan sodique | Sacubitril y Valsartan sodico |
| 10.3　抗心律失常药 Antiarrhythmics | | | |
| 奎尼丁 | Quinidine | Quinidine | Quinidina |
| 普鲁卡因胺 | Procainamide | Procaïnamide | Procainamida |
| 丙吡胺 | Disopyramide | Disopyramide | Disopiramida |
| 利多卡因 | Lidocaine | Lidocaïne | Lidocaína |
| 苯妥英钠 | Phenytoin Sodium | Phénytoïne sodium | Fenitoína Sódica |
| 美西律 | Mexiletine | Méxilétine | Mexiletina |
| 普罗帕酮 | Propafenone | Propafénone | Propafenona |
| 恩卡尼 | Encainide | Encaïnide | Encainida |
| 氟卡尼 | Flecainide | Flécaïnide | Flecainida |
| 胺碘酮 | Amiodarone | Amiodarone | Amiodarona |
| 索他洛尔 | Sotalol | Sotalol | Sotalol |

**续 表**

| 药品名称 | Drug Names | Dénomination du Médicament | Denominación del Medicamento |
|---|---|---|---|
| 伊布利特 | Ibutilide | Ibutilide | Ibutilida |
| 依地酸二钠 | Disodium Edetate | Edétate disodique | Edetato disódico |
| 门冬氨酸钾镁 | Potassium Aspartate and Magnesium Aspartate | Aspartate de magnésium et Aspartate de potassium | Aspartato de magnesio y Aspartato potasio |
| **10.4 防治心绞痛药 Antianginal Drugs** | | | |
| 硝酸甘油 | Nitroglycerin | Nitroglycérine | Nitroglicerina |
| 戊四硝酯 | Pentaerythritol Tetranitrate | Tétranitrate de Pentaérythritol | Tetranitrato de Pentaeritritolo |
| 硝酸异山梨酯 | Isosorbide Dinitrate | Dinitrate d'Isosorbide | Dinitrato de Isosorbida |
| 单硝酸异山梨酯 | Isosorbide Mononitrate | Mononitrate d'Isosorbide | Mononitrato de Isosorbida |
| 曲美他嗪 | Trimetazidine | Trimétazidine | Trimetazidina |
| 双嘧达莫 | Dipyridamole | Dipyridamole | Dipiridamol |
| 丹参酮ⅡA磺酸钠 | Sodium Tanshinon ⅡA Sulfonate | Sulfonate de sodium de tanshinone IIA | Tanshinon ⅡA Sulfonato sódico |
| 川芎嗪 | Ligustrazine | Ligustrazine | Ligustrazina |
| 葛根素 | Puerarin | Puérarin | Puerarina |
| 银杏叶提取物 | Ginkgo Biloba Leaf Extract | Extrait de féuilles de Ginkgo biloba | Extracto de Ginkgo Biloba |
| 辅酶Ⅰ | Coenzyme Ⅰ | Coénzyme Ⅰ | Coenzima Ⅰ |
| **10.5 周围血管舒张药 Peripheral Vasodilators** | | | |
| 二氢麦角碱 | Dihydroergotoxine | Dihydroérgotoxine | Dihidroergotoxina |
| 烟酸 | Nicotinic Acid | Acide nicotinique | Ácido Nicotínico |
| 尼莫地平 | Nimodipine | Nimodipine | Nimodipina |
| 烟酸肌醇酯 | Inositol Nicotinate | Nicotinate d'Inositol | Nicotinato de Inositol |
| 桂利嗪 | Cinnarizine | Cinnarizine | Cinarizina |
| 氟桂利嗪 | Flunarizine | Flunarizine | Flunarizina |
| 维生素E烟酸酯 | Vitamin E Nicotinate | Niacine de Vitamine E | Niacina de Vitamina E |
| 罂粟碱 | Papaverine | Papavérine | Papaverina |
| 西地那非 | Sildenafil | Sildénafil | Sildenafil |
| 环扁桃酯 | Cyclandelate | Cyclandélate | Ciclandelato |
| 长春西汀 | Vinpocetine | Vinpocétine | Vinpocetina |
| 倍他司汀 | Betahistine | Bétahistine | Betahistina |
| 地芬尼多 | Difenidol | Difénidol | Difenidol |
| 血管舒缓素 | Kallidinogenase | Kallidinogénase | Kalidinogenasa |
| 二氢麦角胺 | Dihydroergotamine | Dihydroérgotamine | Dihidroergotamina |
| 依前列醇 | Epoprostenol | Epoprosténol | Epoprostenol |
| 尼麦角林 | Nicergoline | Nicérgoline | Nicergolina |
| 长春胺 | Vincamine | Vincamine | Vincamina |

续 表

| 药品名称 | Drug Names | Dénomination du Médicament | Denominación del Medicamento |
|---|---|---|---|
| **10.6 抗高血压药 Antihypertensive Drugs** | | | |
| 可乐定 | Clonidine | Clonidine | Clonidina |
| 莫索尼定 | Moxonidine | Moxonidine | Moxonidina |
| 利美尼定 | Relmenidine | Relménidine | Relmenidina |
| 噻美尼定 | Tiamenidine | Tiaménidine | Tiamenidina |
| 托洛尼定 | Tolonidine | Tolonidine | Tolonidina |
| 哌唑嗪 | Prazosin | Prazosine | Prazosina |
| 特拉唑嗪 | Terazosin | Térazosine | Terazosina |
| 多沙唑嗪 | Doxazosin | Doxazosine | Doxazosina |
| 布那唑嗪 | Bunazosin | Bunazosine | Bunazosina |
| 阿呋唑嗪 | Alfuzosin | Alfuzosine | Alfuzosina |
| 乌拉地尔 | Urapidil | Urapidil | Urapidilo |
| 米诺地尔 | Minoxidil | Minoxidil | Minoxidilo |
| 吡那地尔 | Pinacidil | Pinacidil | Pinacidilo |
| 利血平 | Reserpine | Réserpine | Reserpina |
| 肼屈嗪 | Hydralazine | Hydralazine | Hidralazina |
| 双肼屈嗪 | Dihydralazine | Dihydralazine | Dihidralazina |
| 硝普钠 | Sodium Nitroprusside | Nitroprusside de sodium | Nitroprusito Sódico |
| 阿利吉仑 | Aliskiren | Aliskiréne | Aliskirena |
| 卡托普利 | Captopril | Captopril | Captopril |
| 依那普利 | Enalapril | Enalapril | Enalapril |
| 贝那普利 | Benazepril | Bénazépril | Benazepril |
| 培哚普利 | Perindopril | Périndopril | Perindopril |
| 氯沙坦 | Losartan | Losartan | Losartán |
| 缬沙坦 | Valsartan | Valsartan | Valsartán |
| 厄贝沙坦 | Irbesartan | Irbésartan | Irbesartán |
| 坎地沙坦 | Candesartan | Candésartan | Candesartán |
| 替米沙坦 | Telmisartan | Télmisartan | Telmisartán |
| 奥美沙坦酯 | Olmesartan Medoxomil | Olmésartan Médoxomil | Olmesartan Medoxomil |
| 阿利沙坦酯 | Allisartan Isoproxil | Allisartan Isoproxil | Allisartan Isoproxil |
| 依普沙坦 | Eprosartan | Eprosartan | Eprosartan |
| 吲达帕胺 | Indapamide | Indapamide | Indapamida |
| 甲基多巴 | Methyldopa | Méthyldopa | Metildopa |
| 胍乙啶 | Guanethidine | Guanéthidine | Guanetidina |
| 倍他尼定 | Betanidine | Bétanidine | Betanidina |
| 异喹胍 | Debrisoquine | Débrisoquine | Debrisoquina |
| 阿拉普利 | Alacepril | Alacepril | Alacepril |

**续 表**

| 药品名称 | Drug Names | Dénomination du Médicament | Denominación del Medicamento |
| --- | --- | --- | --- |
| 莫维普利 | Moveltipril | Movéltipril | Moveltipril |
| 佐芬普利 | Zofenopril | Zofénopril | Zofenopril |
| 群多普利 | Trandolapril | Trandolapril | Trandolapril |
| 赖诺普利<br>氢氯噻嗪 | Lisinopril and Hydrochlorothi-azide | Lisinopril et Hydrochlorothi-azide | Lisinopril y Hidroclorotiazida |
| 西拉普利 | Cilazapril | Cilazapril | Cilazapril |
| 喹那普利 | Quinapril | Quinapril | Quinapril |
| 雷米普利 | Ramipril | Ramipril | Ramipril |
| 咪达普利 | Imidapril | Imidapril | Imidapril |
| 赖诺普利 | Lisinopril | Lisinopril | Lisinopril |
| 福辛普利 | Fosinopril | Fosinopril | Fosinopril |
| 10.7 抗休克的血管活性药 Anti-Shock Vasoactive Drugs | | | |
| 去甲肾上腺素 | Norepinephrine(Noradrenaline) | Norépinéphrine(Noradrénaline) | Norepinefrina(Noradrenalina) |
| 去氧肾上腺素 | Phenylephrine | Phényléphrine | Fenilefrina |
| 甲氧胺 | Methoxamine | Méthoxamine | Metoxamina |
| 间羟胺 | Metaraminol | Métaraminol | Metaraminol |
| 肾上腺素 | Epinephrine(Adrenaline) | Epinéphrine(Adrénaline) | Epinefrina(Adrenalina) |
| 多巴胺 | Dopamine | Dopamine | Dopamina |
| 多巴酚丁胺 | Dobutamine | Dobutamine | Dobutamina |
| 美芬丁胺 | Mephentermine | Méphéntérmine | Mefentermina |
| 血管紧张素胺 | Angiotensinamide | Angioténsinamide | Angiotensinamida |
| 10.8 调节血脂药及抗动脉粥样硬化药 Blood Lipid Regulating Drugs and Antiatherosclerosis Drugs | | | |
| 氯贝丁酯 | Clofibrate | Clofibrate | Clofibrato |
| 阿昔莫司 | Acipimox | Acipimox | Acipimox |
| 非诺贝特 | Fenofibrate | Fénofibrate | Fenofibrato |
| 环丙贝特 | Ciprofibrate | Ciprofibrate | Ciprofibrato |
| 洛伐他汀 | Lovastatin | Lovastatine | Lovastatina |
| 辛伐他汀 | Simvastatin | Simvastatine | Simvastatina |
| 普伐他汀 | Pravastatin | Pravastatine | Pravastatina |
| 氟伐他汀 | Fluvastatin | Fluvastatine | Fluvastatina |
| 阿托伐他汀 | Atorvastatin | Atorvastatine | Atorvastatina |
| 瑞舒伐他汀 | Rosuvastatin | Rosuvastatine | Rosuvastatina |
| 匹伐他汀 | Pitavastatin | Pitavastatine | Pitavastatina |
| 普罗布考 | Probucol | Probucol | Probucol |
| 考来烯胺 | Colestyramine | Coléstyramine | Colestiramina |
| 依折麦布 | Ezetimibe | Ezétimibe | Ezetimiba |
| 地维烯胺 | Divistyramine | Divistyramine | Divistiramina |
| 考来维仑 | Colesevelam | Colésevelam | Colesevelam |

| 药品名称 | Drug Names | Dénomination du Médicament | Denominación del Medicamento |
|---|---|---|---|
| 阿利西尤单抗 | Alirocumab | Alirocumab | Alirocumab |
| 依洛尤单抗 | Evolocumab | Evolocumab | Evolocumab |
| 洛美他派 | Lomitapide | Lomitapide | Lomitapida |
| 米泊美生 | Mipomersen | Mipomérsén | Mipomersen |
| 11. 主要作用于呼吸系统的药物 Drugs Mainly Acting on the Respiratory System ||||
| 11.1 祛痰药 Expectorants ||||
| 氯化铵 | Ammonium Chloride | Chlorure d'ammonium | Cloruro de Amonio |
| 溴己新 | Bromhexine | Bromhexine | Bromhexina |
| 氨溴索 | Ambroxol | Ambroxol | Ambroxol |
| 乙酰半胱氨酸 | Acetylcysteine | Acétylcystéine | Acetilcisteína |
| 羧甲司坦 | Carbocysteine | Carbocystéine | Carbocisteína |
| 厄多司坦 | Erdosteine | Erdostéine | Erdosteina |
| 福多司坦 | Fudosteine | Fudostéine | Fudosteina |
| 标准桃金娘油 | Gelomyrtol | Gélomyrtol | Gelomirtol |
| 碘化钾 | Potassium Iodide | Iodure de potassium | Yoduro de Potasio |
| 美司钠 | Mesna | Mésna | Mesna |
| 11.2 镇咳药 Antitussives ||||
| 可待因 | Codeine | Codéine | Codeína |
| 福尔可定 | Pholcodine | Pholcodine | Folcodina |
| 喷托维林 | Pentoxyverine | Péntoxyvérine | Pentoxiverina |
| 氯哌斯汀 | Cloperasteine | Clopérasteine | Cloperasteina |
| 苯丙哌林 | Benproperine | Bénpropérine | Benproperina |
| 二氧丙嗪 | Dioxopromethazine | Dioxoprométhazine | Dioxoprometazina |
| 苯佐那酯 | Benzonatate | Bénzonatate | Benzonatato |
| 左丙氧芬 | Levopropoxyphene | Lévopropoxyphéne | Levopropoxifeno |
| 地美索酯 | Dimethoxanate | Diméthoxanate | Dimetoxanato |
| 替培啶 | Tipepidine | Tipépidine | Tipepidina |
| 依普拉酮 | Eprazinone | Eprazinone | Eprazinona |
| 普罗吗酯 | Promolate | Promolate | Promolato |
| 左羟丙哌嗪 | Levodropropizine | Lévodropropizine | Levodropropizina |
| 右美沙芬 | Dextromethorphan | Déxtrométhorphane | Dextrometorfano |
| 11.3 平喘药 Antiasthmatics ||||
| 麻黄碱 | Ephedrine | Ephédrine | Efedrina |
| 异丙肾上腺素 | Isoproterenol (Isoprenaline) | Isoprotérénol (Isoprenaline) | Isoproterenol (Isoprenalina) |
| 沙丁胺醇 | Salbutamol | Salbutamol | Salbutamol |
| 特布他林 | Terbutaline | Térbutaline | Terbutalina |
| 氯丙那林 | Clorprenaline | Clorprénaline | Clorprenalina |

| 药品名称 | Drug Names | Dénomination du Médicament | Denominación del Medicamento |
|---|---|---|---|
| 海索那林 | Hexoprenaline | Héxoprénaline | Hexoprenalina |
| 克伦特罗 | Clenbuterol | Clénbutérol | Clenbuterol |
| 妥洛特罗 | Tulobuterol | Tulobutérol | Tulobuterol |
| 茚达特罗 | Indacaterol | Indacatérol | Indacaterol |
| 福莫特罗 | Formoterol | Formotérol | Formoterol |
| 丙卡特罗 | Procaterol | Procatérol | Procaterol |
| 沙美特罗 | Salmeterol | Salmétérol | Salmeterol |
| 班布特罗 | Bambuterol | Bambutérol | Bambuterol |
| 甲氧那明 | Methoxyphenamine | Méthoxyphénamine | Metoxifenamina |
| 异丙托溴铵 | Ipratropium Bromide | Bromure d'Ipratropium | Bromuro de Ipratropio |
| 噻托溴铵 | Tiotropium Bromide | Bromure de Tiotropium | Bromuro de Tiotropio |
| 异丙东莨菪碱 | Isopropylscopolamine | Isopropylscopolamine | Isopropilscopolamina |
| 氨茶碱 | Aminophylline | Aminophylline | Aminofilina |
| 多索茶碱 | Doxofylline | Doxofylline | Doxofilina |
| 二羟丙茶碱 | Diprophylline | Diprophylline | Diprofilina |
| 色甘酸钠 | Sodium Cromoglicate | Cromoglicate de sodium | Cromoglicato Sódico |
| 酮替芬 | Ketotifen | Kétotifène | Ketotifeno |
| 曲尼司特 | Tranilast | Tranilast | Tranilast |
| 氮䓬斯汀 | Azelastine | Azélastine | Azelastina |
| 倍氯米松 | Beclomethasone | Béclométhasone | Beclometasona |
| 布地奈德 | Budesonide | Budésonide | Budesonida |
| 氟替卡松 | Fluticasone | Fluticasone | Fluticasona |
| 曲安奈德 | Triamcinolone Acetonide | Triamcinolone Acétonide | Acetónido de Triamcinolona |
| 糠酸莫米松 | Mometasone Furoate | Furoate de mométasone | Furoato de Mometasona |
| 扎鲁司特 | Zafirlukast | Zafirlukast | Zafirlukast |
| 孟鲁司特钠 | Montelukast Sodium | Montélukast de sodium | Montelukast Sódico |
| 普仑司特 | Pranlukast | Pranlukast | Pranlukast |
| 吡嘧司特 | Pemirolast | Pémirolast | Pemirolast |
| 阿吉片 | Compound Opioid and Platycodon Grandiflorum Tablet | Comprimés Opiacées et platycodon Grandiflorum Composés | Combinaciones Opiata y Platycodon Grandiflorum Comprimidos |
| 异丁司特 | Ibudilast | Ibudilast | Ibudilast |
| 齐留通 | Zileuton | Ziléuton | Zileuton |
| 12. 主要作用于消化系统的药物 Drugs Mainly Acting on the Digestive System | | | |
| 12.1 抗酸药 Antacids | | | |
| 氢氧化铝 | Aluminium Hydroxide | Aluminium Hydroxide | Hidróxido de Aluminio |
| 铝碳酸镁 | Hydrotalcite | Hydrotalcite | Hidrotalcito |
| 氧化镁 | Magnesium Oxide | Oxyde de magnésium | Óxido de magnesio |
| 碳酸钙 | Calcium Carbonate | Carbonate de calcium | Carbonato de Calcio |
| 12.2 胃酸分泌抑制剂 Inhibitors of Gastric Acid Secretion | | | |
| 西咪替丁 | Cimetidine | Cimétidine | Cimetidina |

**续　表**

| 药品名称 | Drug Names | Dénomination du Médicament | Denominación del Medicamento |
| --- | --- | --- | --- |
| 雷尼替丁 | Ranitidine | Ranitidine | Ranitidina |
| 枸橼酸铋雷尼替丁 | Bismuth Citrate and Ranitidine | Citrate de Bismuth et Ranitidine | Citrato de Bismuto y Ranitidina |
| 法莫替丁 | Famotidine | Famotidine | Famotidina |
| 尼扎替丁 | Nizatidine | Nizatidine | Nizatidina |
| 罗沙替丁醋酸酯 | Roxatidine Acetate | Acétate de Roxatidine | Acetato de Roxatidina |
| 拉呋替丁 | Lafutidine | Lafutidine | Lafutidina |
| 奥美拉唑 | Omeprazole | Oméprazole | Omeprazol |
| 兰索拉唑 | Lansoprazole | Lansoprazole | Lansoprazol |
| 泮托拉唑 | Pantoprazole | Pantoprazole | Pantoprazol |
| 雷贝拉唑 | Rabeprazole | Rabéprazole | Rabeprazol |
| 艾司奥美拉唑 | Esomeprazole | Esoméprazole | Esomeprazol |
| 哌仑西平 | Pirenzepine | Pirénzépine | Pirenzepina |
| 丙谷胺 | Proglumide | Proglumide | Proglumida |

## 12.3 胃黏膜保护药 Gastric Mucosa Protectives

| | | | |
| --- | --- | --- | --- |
| 枸橼酸铋钾 | Bismuth Potassium Citrate | Citrate de Bismuth Potassium | Citrato de Potasio Bismuto |
| 胶体果胶铋 | Colloidal Bismuth Pectin | Colloïdale Bismuth Pectine | Pectina de Bismuto Coloidal |
| 胶体酒石酸铋 | Colloidal Bismuth Tartrate | Colloïdal Bismuth Tartrate | Tartrato de Bismuto Coloidal |
| 米索前列醇 | Misoprostol | Misoprostol | Misoprostol |
| 硫糖铝 | Sucralfate | Sucralfate | Sucralfato |
| 甘珀酸钠 | Carbenoxolone Sodium | Carbenoxolone de Sodium | Carbenoxolona Sódico |
| 麦滋林 -S | Marzulene-S | Marzulene-S | Marzulena-S |
| 替普瑞酮 | Teprenone | Téprenone | Teprenona |
| 吉法酯 | Gefarnate | Géfarnate | Gefarnato |
| 甘草锌 | Licorzinc | Licorzinc | Licorzinc |
| 瑞巴派特 | Rebamipide | Rébamipide | Rebamipida |
| 伊索拉丁 | Irsogladine | Irsogladine | Irsogladina |
| 复方铝酸铋 | Compound Brismuth Aluminate | Aluminate de Bismuth Composé | Compuestas de Aluminate Bismuto |

## 12.4 胃肠解痉药 Drugs Relieving Gastrointestinal Spasm

| | | | |
| --- | --- | --- | --- |
| 丁溴东莨菪碱 | Scopolamine Butylbromide | Butylbromure de Scopolamine | Butilbromuro de Escopolamino |
| 曲美布汀 | Trimebutine | Trimébutine | Trimebutina |
| 匹维溴铵 | Pinaverium Bromide | Bromure de Pinaverium | Bromuro de Pinaverio |
| 奥替溴铵 | Otilonium Bromide | Bromure de Otilonium | Bromuro de Otilonio |
| 屈他维林 | Drotaverine | Drotavérine | Drotaverina |
| 阿尔维林 | Alverine | Alvérine | Alverina |
| 溴甲阿托品 | Atropine Methylbromide | Méthylbromure d'Atropine | Metilbromuro de Atropina |
| 苯羟甲胺 | Diphemin | Diphémine | Difemina |
| 曲匹布通 | Trepibutone | Trépibutone | Trepibutona |

**续 表**

| 药品名称 | Drug Names | Dénomination du Médicament | Denominación del Medicamento |
|---|---|---|---|
| 间苯三酚 | Phloroglucinol | Phloroglucinol | Floroglucinol |
| 罂粟碱 | Papaverine | Papavérine | Papaverina |
| 溴丙胺太林 | Propantheline Bromide | Bromure de Propanthéline | Bromuro de Propantelina |
| **12.5 助消化药 Digestants** | | | |
| 多酶 | Multienzyme | Multienzyme | Multienzimá |
| 复方慷彼申 | Compound Combizym | Composés de Combizym | Combinación de Combizim |
| 复方阿嗪米特 | Compound Azintamine | Composé Azintamine | Compuesto Azintamina |
| 干酵母 | Dried Yeast | Levures séchées | Levadura seca |
| **12.6 促胃肠动力药 Gastrointestinal Excitomotors** | | | |
| 甲氧氯普胺 | Metoclopramide | Métoclopramide | Metoclopramida |
| 多潘立酮 | Domperidone | Dompéridone | Domperidona |
| 西沙必利 | Cisapride | Cisapride | Cisaprida |
| 伊托必利 | Itopride | Itopride | Itoprida |
| 莫沙必利 | Mosapride | Mosapride | Mosaprida |
| **12.7 止吐药和催吐药 Antiemetics and Emetics** | | | |
| 昂丹司琼 | Ondansetron | Ondansétron | Ondansetrón |
| 托烷司琼 | Tropisetron | Tropisétron | Tropisetrón |
| 格拉司琼 | Granisetron | Granisétron | Granisetrón |
| 雷莫司琼 | Ramosetron | Ramosetron | Ramosetron |
| 阿扎司琼 | Azasetron | Azasétron | Azasetrón |
| 阿扑吗啡 | Apomorphine | Apomorphine | Apomorfina |
| 氯波必利 | Clebopride | Clebopride | Cleboprida |
| 普芦卡比利 | Prucalopride | Prucalopride | Prucaloprida |
| 地芬尼多 | Difenidol | Difénidol | Difenidol |
| **12.8 泻药 Laxatives** | | | |
| 硫酸镁 | Magnesium Sulfate | Sulfate de magnésium | Sulfato de Magnesio |
| 甘油 | Glycerol | Glycérol | Glicerina |
| 开塞露 | Enema Glycerini | Enéma Glycérini | Enema Glicerini |
| 硫酸钠 | Sodium Sulfate | Sulfate de sodium | Sulfato de sodio |
| 比沙可啶 | Bisacodyl | Bisacodyl | Bisacodil |
| 聚乙二醇 | Polyethylene Glycol | Polyéthylene Glycol | Polietileno Glicol |
| 多库酯钠 | Docusate Sodium | Docusate de Sodium | Docusato de Sódico |
| 乳果糖 | Lactulose | Lactulose | Lactulosa |
| 聚卡波非钙 | Calcium Polycarbophil | Polycarbophil de Calcium | Policarbofil de Calcio |
| 液状石蜡 | Liquid Paraffin | Paraffine Liquide | Líquido de Parafina |
| **12.9 止泻药 Antidiarrheal Drugs** | | | |
| 双八面体蒙脱石 | Dioctahedral Smectite | Sméctite Dioctahédrique | Esmectita Dioctahedrica |
| 鞣酸蛋白 | Tannalbin | Tannalbin | Tannalbin |

**续　表**

| 药品名称 | Drug Names | Dénomination du Médicament | Denominación del Medicamento |
|---|---|---|---|
| 地芬诺酯 | Diphenoxylate | Diphénoxylate | Difenoxilato |
| 洛哌丁胺 | Loperamide | Lopéramide | Loperamida |
| 药用炭 | Medicinal Charcoal | Charbon Médicinal | Carbón Medicinal |
| 消旋卡多曲 | Racecadotril | Racécadotril | Racecadotril |
| 碱式碳酸铋 | Bismuth Subcarbonate | Subcarbonate de Bismuth | Subcarbonato de Bismuto |
| **12.10　微生态药物 Microecological Drugs** | | | |
| 地衣芽孢杆菌活菌 | Live Bacillus Licheniformis | Bacillus Lichéniformis, Viable | Licheniformis, Bacillus Viable |
| 双歧杆菌活菌 | Live Bifidobacteria | Bifidobactérium, Viable | Bifidobacteria, Viable |
| 枯草杆菌活菌 | Live Bacillus Subtilis | Bacillus Subtilis, Viable | Bacillus Subtilis, Viable |
| 蜡样芽孢杆菌活菌 | Live Bacillus Cereus | Bacillus Céréus, Viable | Bacillus Cereus, Viable |
| 凝结芽孢杆菌 | Bacillus coagulans | Bacillus Coagulans | Bacillus Coagulans |
| 酪酸梭菌活菌 | Live Clostridium Butyricum | Clostridium Butyricum Viable | Clostridium Butyricum, Viable |
| 布拉氏酵母菌 | Saccharomyces Boulardii | Saccharomycés Boulardii | Saccharomices Boulardii |
| 嗜酸乳杆菌 | Lactobacillus LB | Lactobacillus LB | Lactobacillus |
| 复合乳酸菌 | Lactobacillus Complex | Lactobacillus Complex | Lactobacillus Compuestos |
| 双歧杆菌嗜酸乳杆菌肠球菌三联活菌 | Live Combined Bifidobacterium, Lactobacillus and Enterococcus | Combined Bifidobactérium, Lactobacillus et Entérococcus, Viable | Bifidobacterium, Lactobacillus y Enterococcos Combinados, Viable |
| 双歧杆菌四联活菌 | Combined Bifidobacterium, Lactobacillus, Enterococcus and Bacilluscereus, Live | Combined Bifidobactérium, Lactobacillus, Entérococcus and Bacilluscéréus, Viable | Combined Bifidobacterium, Lactobacillus, Enterococcus y Bacilluscereus, Viable |
| 乳酶生 | Lactasin | Lactasine | Lactasina |
| **12.11　治疗肝性脑病药 Drugs Treating Hepatic Encephalopathy** | | | |
| 乳果糖 | Lactulose | Lactulose | Lactulosa |
| 谷氨酸钠 | Sodium Glutamate | Glutamate de Sodium | Glutamato de Sodio |
| 支链氨基酸 | Branched Amino Acid | Acides Aminés Ramifiés | Aminoácidos de Cadena Ramificada |
| 谷氨酸钾 | Potassium Glutamate | Glutamate de Potassium | Glutamato de Potasio |
| 精氨酸 | Arginine | Arginine | Arginina |
| 谷氨酸 | Glutamic Acid | Acide Glutamique | Glutámico Acido |
| **12.12　治疗肝炎辅助用药 Adjuvant Drugs Treating the Hepatitis** | | | |
| 联苯双酯 | Bifendate | Bifendate | Bifendato |
| 门冬氨酸钾镁 | Potassium Magnesium Aspartate | Aspartate de Potassium Magnésium | Aspartato de Potasio y Magnesio |
| 水飞蓟宾 | Silibinin | Silibinine | Silibinina |
| 牛磺酸 | Taurine | Taurine | Taurina |
| 促肝细胞生长因子 | Hepatocyte Growth-Promoting Factor | Facteur de Croissance des Hépatocytes | Factores de Promoción de Crecimiento de Hepatocitos |
| 多烯磷脂酰胆碱 | Polyene Phosphatidylcholine | Polyene Phosphatidylcholine | Polieno Fosfatidilcolina |

**续 表**

| 药品名称 | Drug Names | Dénomination du Médicament | Denominación del Medicamento |
|---|---|---|---|
| 甘草酸二铵 | Diammonium Glycyrrhizinate | Glycyrrhiate de diammonium | Glicirrato de diamonio |
| 异甘草酸镁 | Magnesium Isoglycyrrhizinate | Isoglycyrrhizate de Magnésium | Isoglicirato de Magnesio |
| 硫普罗宁 | Tiopronin | Tiopronine | Tiopronina |
| 葡醛内酯 | Glucurolactone | Glucurolactone | Glucurolactona |
| 谷胱甘肽 | Glutathione | Glutathion | Glutation |
| 辅酶 A | Coenzyme A | Coenzyme A | Coenzima A |
| 12.13 利胆药 Choleretic Drugs | | | |
| 熊去氧胆酸 | Ursodeoxycholic Acid | Acide Ursodésoxycholique | Acido Ursodesoxicólico |
| 鹅去氧胆酸 | Chenodeoxycholic Acid | Acide Chenodeoxycholique | Acido Cenodeoxicolico |
| 12.14 治疗炎症性肠病药 Drugs Treating Inflammatory Bowel Disease | | | |
| 美沙拉秦 | Mesalazine | Mésalazine | Mesalazina |
| 柳氮磺吡啶 | Sulfasalazine | Sulfasalazine | Sulfasalazina |
| 巴柳氮钠 | Balsalazide Sodium | Balsalazine sodique | Balsalazida sódica |
| 奥沙拉秦 | Olsalazine | Olsalazine | Olsalazina |
| 12.15 其他消化系统用药 Other Drugs of Digestive System | | | |
| 奥曲肽 | Octreotide | Octréotide | Octreotida |
| 生长抑素 | Somatostatin | Somatostatine | Somatostatina |
| 抑肽酶 | Aprotinin | Aprotinine | Aprotinina |
| 加贝酯 | Gabexate | Gabexate | Gabexato |
| 乌司他丁 | Ulinastatin | Ulinastatine | Ulinastatina |
| 盐酸小檗碱 | Berberine Hydrochloride | Chlorhydrate de Bérbérine | Clorhidrato de Berberina |
| 二甲硅油 | Dimethicone | Diméthicone | Dimeticona |
| 13. 影响血液及造血系统的药物 Drugs Mainly Acting to Blood and Hematopoietic System | | | |
| 13.1 促凝血药 Coagulants | | | |
| 亚硫酸氢钠甲萘醌 | Menadione Sodium Bisulfite | Bisulfite de Ménadione Sodium | Bisulfito de Menadiona Sodio |
| 维生素 $K_1$ | Phytomenadione (Vitamin $K_1$) | Phytoménadione (Vitamine $K_1$) | Fitomenadiona (Vitamina $K_1$) |
| 矛头腹蛇血凝酶 | Hemocoagulase Bothrops Atrox | Hémaglutinase de Bothrops Atrox | Hemaglutinasa de Bothrops Atrox |
| 蛇毒血凝酶 | Hemocoagulase Venin | Hémaglutinase de Vénine | Hemaglutinasa de Venina |
| 尖吻腹蛇血凝酶 | Hemocoagulase Agkistrodon | Hémaglutinase de Agkistrodon | Hemaglutinasa de Agkistrodon |
| 重组人凝血因子Ⅷ | Recombinant Human Coagulation Factor Ⅷ | Facteur Ⅷ de coagulation humaine recombinante | Factor Ⅷ de Coagulación Humana Recombinante |
| 重组人凝血因子IX | Recombinant Human Coagulation Factor IX | Facteur de coagulation humaine recombinant IX | Factor de Coagulación Humana Recombinante IX |
| 重组人凝血因子VII a | Recombinant Human Coagulation Factor VII a | Facteur de coagulation humaine recombinant VII a | Factor de Coagulación Humana Recombinante VII a |
| 人纤维蛋白原 | Human Fibrinogen | Fibrinogène Humain | Fibrinógeno Humano |

**续　表**

| 药品名称 | Drug Names | Dénomination du Médicament | Denominación del Medicamento |
| --- | --- | --- | --- |
| 抑肽酶 | Aprotinin | Aprotinine | Aprotinina |
| 氨基己酸 | Aminocaproic Acid | Acide Aminocaproïque | Acido Aminocaproico |
| 氨甲苯酸 | Aminomethylbenzoic Acid | Acide Aminométhylbenzoïque | Acido Aminometilbenzoico |
| 血凝酶 | Hemocoagulase | Hémocoagulase | Hemocoagulasa |
| 聚桂醇 | Lauromacrogol | Lauromacrogol | Lauromacrogol |
| 酚磺乙胺 | Etamsylate | Etamsylate | Etamsilato |
| 卡巴克洛 | Carbazochrome | Carbazochrome | Carbazocromo |
| 重组人凝血因子Ⅷ | Recombinant Human Coagulation Factor Ⅷ | Facteur Ⅷ de Coagulation Humain Recombinante | Factor Ⅷ de Coagulación Humana Recombinante |
| 重组人血小板生成素 | Recombinant Human Thrombopoietin | Thrombopoïétine Humaine Recombinante | Trombopoietina Humana Recombinante |
| 重组人白细胞介素 -11 | Recombinant Human Interleukin-11 | Interleukine-11 Humaine Recombinante | Interleucina -11 Humana Recombinante |
| 云南白药 | Yunnan Baiyao | YunNan BaiYao | YunNan BaiYao |
| 氨甲环酸 | Tranexamic Acid | Acide Tranexamique | Ácido Tranexamico |
| 鱼精蛋白 | Protamine | Protamine | Protamina |
| 凝血酶 | Thrombin | Thrombine | Trombina |
| 凝血酶原复合物 | Prothrombin Complex | Complexe de Prothrombine | Complejo Protrombina |

## 13.2　抗凝血药 Anticoagulants

| 药品名称 | Drug Names | Dénomination du Médicament | Denominación del Medicamento |
| --- | --- | --- | --- |
| 枸橼酸钠 | Sodium Citrate | Citrate Sodique | Citrato de Sodio |
| 肝素钠 | Heparin Sodium | Héparine Sodique | Sódico de Heparina |
| 肝素钙 | Heparin Calcium | Héparine Calcique | Cálcica de Heparina |
| 低分子量肝素 | Low Molecular Weight Heparin | Héparine de Faible Poids Moléculaire | Heparina de bajo peso Molecular |
| 华法林 | Warfarin | Warfarine | Warfarina |
| 利伐沙班 | Rivaroxaban | Rivaroxaban | Rivaroxaban |
| 磺达肝癸钠 | Fondaparinux Sodium | Fondaparinux Sodique | Fondaparinux Sódica |
| 舒洛地特 | Sulodexide | Sulodéxide | Sulodexida |
| 阿加曲班 | Argatroban | Argatroban | Argatroban |
| 达比加群酯 | Dabigatran Etexilate | Dabigatran Etexilate | Dabigatran Etexilato |
| 阿哌沙班 | Apixaban | Apixaban | Apixaban |
| 奥扎格雷 | Ozagrel | Ozagrel | Ozagrel |
| 重组链激酶 | Recombinant Streptokinase | Streptokinase Recombinante | Estreptokinasa Recombinante |
| 尿激酶 | Urokinase | Urokinase | Uroquinasa |
| 阿替普酶 | Alteplase | Alteplase | Alteplasa |
| 瑞替普酶 | Reteplase | Retéplase | Reteplasa |
| 降纤酶 | Defibrase | Defibrase | Defibrasa |
| 蚓激酶 | Lumbrukinase | Lumbrokinase | Lumbroquinasa |

**续　表**

| 药品名称 | Drug Names | Dénomination du Médicament | Denominación del Medicamento |
| --- | --- | --- | --- |
| 13.3　血浆代用品 Blood Substitutes | | | |
| 右旋糖酐 40 | Dextran 40 | Dextrane 40 | Dextrano 40 |
| 右旋糖酐 70 | Dextran 70 | Dextrane 70 | Dextrano 70 |
| 右旋糖酐 10 | Dextran 10 | Dextrane 10 | Dextrano 10 |
| 琥珀酰明胶 | Succinylated Gelatin | Gélatine Succinylee | Gelatina Succinilato |
| 羟乙基淀粉 200/0.5 | Hydroxyethyl Starch 200/0.5 | Hydroxyéthyl Amidon 200/0.5 | Almidón Hidroxietil 200/0.5 |
| 羟乙基淀粉 130/0.4 | Hydroxyethyl Starch 130/0.4 | Hydroxyéthyl Amidon 130/0.4 | Almidón Hidroxietil 130/0.4 |
| 包醛氧淀粉 | Coated Aldehyde Oxystarch | Aldéhyde oxygène amidon | Almidón de Oxígeno Aldehído |
| 聚维酮 | Polyvidon | Polyvidone | Polividona |
| 羟乙基淀粉 40 | Hydroxyethyl Starch 40 | Hydroxyéthyl Amidon 40 | Almidón Hidroxietil 40 |
| 人血白蛋白 | Human Albumin | Albumine Humaine | Albúmina Humana |
| 13.4　抗贫血药 Drugs Treating Anemia | | | |
| 硫酸亚铁 | Ferrous Sulfate | Sulfate Ferreux | Sulfato Ferroso |
| 葡萄糖酸亚铁 | Ferrous Gluconate | Gluconate Ferreux | Gluconato Ferroso |
| 蔗糖铁 | Iron Sucrese | Saccharose Fer | Hierro Sacarosa |
| 叶酸 | Folic Acid | Acide Folique | Ácido Fólico |
| 氰钴胺（维生素 $B_{12}$） | Cyanocobalamin (Vitamin $B_{12}$) | Cyanocobalamine (Vitamine $B_{12}$) | Cianocobalamina (Vitamina $B_{12}$) |
| 腺苷钴胺 | Cobamamide | Cobamamide | Cobamamida |
| 甲钴胺 | Mecobalamin | Mécobalamine | Mecobalamina |
| 重组人红细胞生成素 | Recombinant Human Erythropoietin | Erythropoïétin Humain Recombinant | Eritropoyetina Humana Recombinante |
| 琥珀酸亚铁 | Ferrous Succinate | Succinate ferreux | Succinato Ferroso |
| 富马酸亚铁 | Ferrous Fumarate | Fumarate ferreux | Fumarato Ferroso |
| 枸橼酸铁铵 | Ferric Ammonium Citrate | Citrate d' Ammonium Ferrique | Citrato de Amonio Férrico |
| 右旋糖酐铁 | Iron Dextran | Fer-dextran | Hierro Dextrano |
| 山梨醇铁 | Iron Sorbitex | Fer sorbitol | Hierro Sorbitol |
| 去铁胺 | Desferrioxamine | Desferrioxamine | Desferrioxamina |
| 亚叶酸钙 | Calcium Folinate | Folinate de calcium | Folinato Calcio |
| 13.5　促白细胞增生药 Drugs Promoting Leukocytosis | | | |
| 腺嘌呤（维生素 $B_4$） | Adenine(Vitamin $B_4$) | Adenine (Vitamine $B_4$) | Adenina(Vitamina $B_4$) |
| 重组人粒细胞集落刺激因子 | Recombinant Human Granulocyte Colony- Stimulating Factor | Facteur stimulant de colonie de granulocytes humains recombinant | Factor Estimulante de Colonias de Granulocitos Humanos Recombinante |
| 重组人粒细胞-巨噬细胞集落刺激因子 | Recombinant Human Granulocyte-Macrophage Colony- Stimulating Factor | Facteur de stimulation des colonies de macrophages dans les granulocytes humains recombinant | Factor Estimulante de Colonias de Granulocitos-Macrófago Humanos Recombinante |

**续　表**

| 药品名称 | Drug Names | Dénomination du Médicament | Denominación del Medicamento |
| --- | --- | --- | --- |
| 地菲林葡萄糖苷 | Diphyllin Glycoside | Diphylline Glucoside | Difilina Glucósidos |
| 苦参总碱 | Alkaloids Sophora | Alcaloïdes du Sophora | Sophora de Alcaloides |
| 鲨肝醇 | Batilol | Batilol | Batilol |
| 利可君 | Leucogen | Léucogen | Leucogen |
| 肌苷 | Inosine | Inosine | Inosina |
| 氨肽素 | Aminopolypeptide | Aminopolypéptide | Aminopolipeptida |
| **13.6 抗血小板药物 Antiplatelet Drugs** | | | |
| 阿司匹林 | Aspirin | Aspirine | Aspirina |
| 双嘧达莫 | Dipyridamole | Dipyridamole | Dipiridamol |
| 氯吡格雷 | Clopidogrel | Clopidogrél | Clopidogrel |
| 西洛他唑 | Cilostazol | Cilostazol | Cilostazol |
| 噻氯匹啶 | Ticlopidine | Ticlopidine | Ticlopidina |
| 普拉格雷 | Prasugrel | Prasugrél | Prasugrel |
| 沙格雷酯 | Sarpogrelate | Sarpogrélate | Sarpogrelato |
| 依前列醇 | Epoprostenol | Epoprosténol | Epoprostenol |
| 贝前列素 | Beraprost | Béraprost | Beraprost |
| 伊洛前列素 | Iloprost | Iloprost | Iloprost |
| 依替巴肽 | Eptifibatide | Eptifibatide | Eptifibatida |
| 替罗非班 | Tirofiban | Tirofiban | Tirofibán |
| 奥扎格雷 | Ozagrel | Ozagrél | Ozagrel |
| 曲克芦丁 | Troxerutin | Troxérutine | Troxerutina |
| 氯贝丁酯 | Clofibrate | Clofibrate | Clofibrato |
| **14. 主要作用于泌尿系统的药物 Drugs Mainly Acting on Urinary System** | | | |
| **14.1 利尿药 Diuretics** | | | |
| 呋塞米 | Furosemide | Furosémide | Furosemida |
| 依他尼酸 | Ethacrynic Acid | Acide Ethanique | Ácido etanínico |
| 吡咯他尼 | Piretanide | Pirétanide | Piretanida |
| 阿佐塞米 | Azosemide | Azosémide | Azosemida |
| 依普利酮 | Eplerenone | Eplérénone | Eplerenona |
| 双氯非那胺 | Diclofenamide | Diclofénamide | Diclofenamida |
| 醋甲唑胺 | Methazolamide | Méthazolamide | Metazolamida |
| 布美他尼 | Bumetanide | Bumétanide | Bumetanida |
| 托拉塞米 | Torasemide | Torasémide | Torasemida |
| 氢氯噻嗪 | Hydrochlorothiazide | Hydrochlorothiazide | Hidroclorotiazida |
| 环戊噻嗪 | Cyclopenthiazide | Cyclopénthiazide | Ciclopentiazida |
| 吲达帕胺 | Indapamide | Indapamide | Indapamida |
| 螺内酯 | Spironolactone | Spironolactone | Espironolactona |

| 药品名称 | Drug Names | Dénomination du Médicament | Denominación del Medicamento |
|---|---|---|---|
| 氨苯蝶啶 | Triamterene | Triamtérène | Triamtereno |
| 阿米洛利 | Amiloride | Amiloride | Amilorida |
| 乙酰唑胺 | Acetazolamide | Acétazolamide | Acetazolamida |
| 14.2　脱水药 Dehydrants | | | |
| 甘露醇 | Mannitol | Mannitol | Manitol |
| 葡萄糖 | Glucose | Déxtrose | Glucosa |
| 甘油果糖氯化钠 | Glycerin Fructose and Sodium Cloride | Glycérine-fructose et Chlorure de Sodium | Glicerina Fructosa y Cloruro sódico |
| 14.3　治疗尿崩症用药 Drugs Treating Diabetes Insipidus | | | |
| 鞣酸加压素 | Vasopressin Tanate | Vasopréssine Tannique | Tanina Vasopresina |
| 氯磺丙脲 | Chlorpropamide | Chlorpropamide | Clorpropamida |
| 氯贝丁酯 | Clofibrate | Clofibrate | Clofibrato |
| 垂体后叶粉 | Powdered Posterior Pituitary | Poudre Hypophyse Postérieure | Polvo de Pituitaria Posterior |
| 去氨加压素 | Desmopressin | Désmopréssine | Desmopresina |
| 14.4　治疗良性前列腺增生症药 Drugs Treating Benign Prostatic Hyperplasia | | | |
| 酚苄明 | Phenoxybenzamine | Phénoxybénzamine | Fenoxibenzamina |
| 特拉唑嗪 | Terazosin | Térazosine | Terazosina |
| 阿夫唑嗪 | Alfuzosin | Alfuzosine | Alfuzosina |
| 多沙唑嗪 | Doxazosin | Doxazosine | Doxazosina |
| 坦洛新 | Tamsulosin | Tamsulosine | Tamsulosina |
| 赛洛多辛 | Silodosin | Silodosine | Silodosina |
| 非那雄胺 | Finasteride | Finastéride | Finasterida |
| 依立雄胺 | Epristeride | Epristéride | Epristerida |
| 度他雄胺 | Dutasteride | Dutastéride | Dutasterida |
| 普适泰 | Prostat | Prostate | Prostato |
| 谷丙甘氨酸 | Glutamate Acid, Alanine and Glycine | Acide Glutamique, Alanine et Glycine | Ácido Glutámico, Alanina y Glicina |
| 15. 主要作用于生殖系统的药物 Drugs Mainly Acting on the Reproductive System | | | |
| 15.1　子宫收缩药及引产药 Uterine Tonics and Drugs Induced Labor | | | |
| 垂体后叶素 | Pituitrin | Pituitrine | Pituitrina |
| 缩宫素 | Oxytocin | Ocytocine | Oxitocina |
| 卡贝缩宫素 | Carbetocin | Carbétocine | Carbetocina |
| 麦角新碱 | Ergometrine | Ergométrine | Ergometrina |
| 甲麦角新碱 | Methylergometrine | Méthylérgométrine | Metilergometrina |
| 硫前列酮 | Sulprostone | Sulprostone | Sulprostona |
| 地诺前列素 | Dinoprost | Dinoprost | Dinoprost |
| 卡前列素氨丁三醇 | Carboprost Tromethamine | Carboprost Trométhamine | Carboprost Trometamina |

**续　表**

| 药品名称 | Drug Names | Dénomination du Médicament | Denominación del Medicamento |
|---|---|---|---|
| 卡前列素 | Carboprost | Carboprost | Carboprost |
| 吉美前列素 | Gemeprost | Géméprost | Gemeprost |
| 卡前列甲酯 | Carboprost Methylate | Carboprost Méthylate | Carboprost Metilato |
| 米非司酮 | Mifepristone | Mifépristone | Mifepristona |
| 地诺前列酮 | Dinoprostone | Dinoprostone | Dinoprostona |
| 米索前列醇 | Misoprostol | Misoprostol | Misoprostol |
| 依沙吖啶 | Ethacridine | Ethacridine | Etacridina |
| **15.2 促进子宫颈成熟药 Drugs Promoting Cervix Uterus Maturity** | | | |
| 普拉睾酮 | Prasterone | Prastérone | Prasterona |
| 地诺前列酮 | Dinoprostone | Dinoprostone | Dinoprostona |
| **15.3 抗早产药 Drugs of Anti- Premature Delivery** | | | |
| 利托君 | Ritodrine | Ritodrine | Ritodrina |
| 沙丁胺醇 | Salbutaline | Salbutaline | Salbutalina |
| 特布他林 | Terbutaline | Térbutaline | Terbutalina |
| 硫酸镁 | Magnesium Sulfate | Sulfate de magnésium | Sulfato de magnesio |
| 烯丙雌醇 | Allylestrenol | Allyléstrenol | Alilestrenol |
| 阿托西班 | Atosiban | Atosiban | Atosiban |
| **15.4 退乳药物 Lactation Suppression Medication** | | | |
| 溴隐亭 | Bromocriptine | Bromocriptine | Bromocriptina |
| 甲麦角林 | Metergoline | Métérgoline | Metergolina |
| **16. 主要作用于内分泌系统药物 Drugs Mainly Acting on Endocrine System** | | | |
| **16.1 肾上腺皮质激素和促肾上腺皮质激素 Adrenocortical Hormones and Adrenocorticotropic Hormone** | | | |
| 氢化可的松 | Hydrocortisone | Hydrocortisone | Hidrocortisona |
| 泼尼松 | Prednisone | Prednisone | Prednisona |
| 泼尼松龙 | Prednisolone | Prednisolone | Prednisolona |
| 甲泼尼龙 | Methylprednisolone | Méthylprédnisolone | Metilprednisolona |
| 曲安西龙 | Triamcinolone | Triamcinolone | Triamcinolona |
| 曲安奈德 | Triamcinolone Acetonide | Acétonide de triamcinolone | Acetónida de Triamcinolona |
| 布地奈德 | Budesonide | Budésonide | Budesónida |
| 氟替卡松 | Fluticasone | Fluticasone | Fluticasona |
| 莫米松 | Mometasone | Mométasone | Mometasona |
| 地塞米松 | Dexamethasone | Dexaméthasone | Dexametasona |
| 倍他米松 | Betamethasone | Bétaméthasone | Betametasona |
| 氟氢可的松 | Fludrocortisone | Fludrocortisone | Fludrocortisona |
| 氯倍他索 | Clobetasol | Clobétasol | Clobetasol |
| 氟轻松 | Fluocinolone | Fluocinolone | Fluocinolona |
| 倍氯米松 | Beclomethasone | Béclométhasone | Beclometasona |

**续 表**

| 药品名称 | Drug Names | Dénomination du Médicament | Denominación del Medicamento |
|---|---|---|---|
| 哈西奈德 | Halcinonide | Halcinonide | Halcinonida |
| 氟米龙 | Fluorometholone | Fluorométholone | Fluorometolona |
| 卤米松 | Halometasone | Halométasone | Halometasona |
| 可的松 | Cortisone | Cortisone | Cortisona |
| 促肾上腺皮质激素 | Corticotrophin | Corticotrophine | Corticotrofina |

**16.2 雄激素及同化激素 Androgen and Protein Anabolic Hormone**

| | | | |
|---|---|---|---|
| 丙酸睾酮 | Testosterone Propionate | Propionate de Téstostérone | Propionato de Testosterona |
| 甲睾酮 | Methyltestosterone | Méthyltestostérone | Metiltestosterona |
| 苯丙酸诺龙 | Nandrolone Phenylpropionate | Phénylpropionate de Nandrolone | Nandrolona Fenilpropionato |
| 十一酸睾酮 | Testosterone Undecanoate | Undécanoate de Téstostérone | Undecanoato de Testosterona |
| 司坦唑醇 | Stanozolol | Stanozolol | Estanozolol |
| 达那唑 | Danazol | Danazol | Danazol |

**16.3 雌激素及其类似合成药物 Estrogen and its Similar Synthetic Drugs**

| | | | |
|---|---|---|---|
| 雌二醇 | Estradiol | Estradiol | Estradiol |
| 苯甲酸雌二醇 | Estradiol Benzoate | Bénzoate de Estradiol | Estradiol de Benzoato |
| 戊酸雌二醇 | Estradiol Valerate | Valérate de Estradiol | Valerato de Estradiol |
| 炔雌醇 | Ethinylestradiol | Ethinyléstradiol | Etinilestradiol |
| 雌三醇 | Estriol | Estriol | Estriol |
| 尼尔雌醇 | Nilestriol | Niléstriol | Nilestriol |
| 结合雌激素 | Conjugated Estrogens | Combinaison de Oestrogène | Combinación de Estrógeno |
| 氯烯雌醚 | Chlorotrianisene | Chlorotrianisene | Clorotrianisena |
| 普罗雌烯 | Promestriene | Proméstriene | Promestrieno |
| 己烯雌酚 | Diethylstilbestrol | Diéthylstilbéstrol | Dietilstilbestrol |

**16.4 孕激素类 Progestogens**

| | | | |
|---|---|---|---|
| 黄体酮 | Progesterone | Progestérone | Progesterona |
| 甲羟孕酮 | Medroxyprogesterone | Médroxyprogestérone | Medroxiprogesterona |
| 炔孕酮 | Ethisterone | Ethistérone | Etisterona |
| 环丙孕酮 | Cyproterone | Ciprotérone | Ciproterona |
| 地屈孕酮 | Dydrogesterone | Dydrogésterone | Didrogesterona |
| 替勃龙 | Tibolone | Tibolone | Tibolona |
| 烯丙雌醇 | Allylestrenol | Allyléstrenol | Alilestrenol |
| 屈螺酮 | Drospirenone | Drospirénone | Drospirenona |

**16.5 雌激素受体调节剂 Estrogen Receptor Modulators**

| | | | |
|---|---|---|---|
| 雷洛昔芬 | Raloxifene | Raloxiféne | Raloxifeno |

**16.6 促性腺激素 Gonadotrophin**

| | | | |
|---|---|---|---|
| 绒毛膜促性腺激素 | Chorionic Gonadotrophin | Gonadotropine Corionique | Gonadotropina Coriónica |

续　表

| 药品名称 | Drug Names | Dénomination du Médicament | Denominación del Medicamento |
|---|---|---|---|
| 尿促性素 | Menotrophin | Ménotrophine | Menotropina |
| 氯米芬 | Clomiphene | Clomifène | Clomifeno |
| 戈那瑞林 | Gonadorelin | Gonadoréline | Gonadorelina |
| 普罗瑞林 | Protirelin | Protiréline | Protirelina |
| 亮丙瑞林 | Leuprorelin | Léuproreline | Leuprorelina |
| 戈舍瑞林 | Goserelin | Goséréline | Goserelina |
| 丙氨瑞林 | Alarelin | Alaréline | Alarelina |
| 曲普瑞林 | Triptorelin | Triptoréline | Triptorelina |
| 16.7　短效口服避孕药 Short-Acting Oral Contraceptives | | | |
| 炔诺酮 | Norethindrone | Noréthindrone | Noretindrona |
| 甲地孕酮 | Megestrol | Mégéstrol | Megestrol |
| 左炔诺孕酮 | Levonorgestrel | Lévonorgéstrel | Levonorgestrel |
| 去氧孕烯 | Desogestrel | Désogéstrél | Desogestrel |
| 孕二烯酮 | Gestodene | Géstodéne | Gestodena |
| 孕三烯酮 | Gestrinone | Géstrinone | Gestrinona |
| 炔诺孕酮 | Norgestrel | Norgéstrél | Norgestrel |
| 16.8　长效避孕药 Short-Acting Contraceptives | | | |
| 氯地孕酮 | Chlormadinone | Chlormadinone | Clormadinona |
| 羟孕酮 | Hydroxyprogesterone | Hydroxyprogéstérone | Hidroxiprogesterona |
| 庚酸炔诺酮 | Norethisterone Enanthate | Enanthate Norethisterone | Enantato Noretisterona |
| 16.9　外用避孕药 External Use Contraceptives | | | |
| 壬苯醇醚 | Nonoxinol | Nonoxinol | Nonoxinol |
| 16.10　男用避孕药 Male Contraceptive | | | |
| 棉子酚 | Gossypol | Gossypol | Gossipol |
| 16.11　高血糖素 Glucagon | | | |
| 高血糖素 | Glucagon | Glucagon | Glucagón |
| 16.12　胰岛素 Insulin | | | |
| 胰岛素 | Insulin | Insuline | Insulina |
| 门冬胰岛素 | Insulin Aspartate | Insuline Aspartate | Insulina Aspartico |
| 赖脯胰岛素 | Insulin Lispro | Insuline lispro | Insulina Lispro |
| 谷赖胰岛素 | Insulin Glulisine | Insulin Glulisine | Insulina Glulisina |
| 低精蛋白锌胰岛素 | Isophane Insulin | Isophane Insuline | Isophana Insulina |
| 精蛋白锌胰岛素 | Protamine Zinc Insulin | Insuline Protamine Zinc | Insulina Protamina Zinc |
| 甘精胰岛素 | Insulin Glargine | Insuline glargine | Insulina Glargina |
| 地特胰岛素 | Insulin Detemir | Insuline Détémir | Insulina Detemir |
| 德古胰岛素 | Insulin Degludec | Insuline Dégludéc | Insulina Degludec |
| 胰岛素预混制剂 | Insulin Premix | Insuline Prémix | Insulina Premix |

**续 表**

| 药品名称 | Drug Names | Dénomination du Médicament | Denominación del Medicamento |
|---|---|---|---|
| 胰岛素类似物预混制剂 | Insulin Analogue Premix | Insuline Analogue Prémix | Insulina Analogos Premix |

### 16.13 口服及其他降糖药 Oral and other Antidiabetics

| 药品名称 | Drug Names | Dénomination du Médicament | Denominación del Medicamento |
|---|---|---|---|
| 甲苯磺丁脲 | Tolbutamide | Tolbutamide | Tolbutamida |
| 格列本脲 | Glibenclamide | Glibénclamide | Glibenclamida |
| 格列吡嗪 | Glipizide | Glipizide | Glipizida |
| 格列齐特 | Gliclazide | Gliclazide | Gliclazida |
| 格列喹酮 | Gliquidone | Gliquidone | Gliquidona |
| 格列美脲 | Glimepiride | Glimépiride | Glimepirida |
| 二甲双胍 | Metformin | Métformine | Metformina |
| 苯乙双胍 | Phenformin | Phenformine | Fenformina |
| 瑞格列奈 | Repaglinide | Répaglinide | Repaglinida |
| 那格列奈 | Nateglinide | Natéglinide | Nateglinida |
| 罗格列酮 | Rosiglitazone | Rosiglitazone | Rosiglitazona |
| 吡格列酮 | Pioglitazone | Pioglitazone | Pioglitazona |
| 阿卡波糖 | Acarbose | Acarbose | Acarbosa |
| 伏格列波糖 | Voglibose | Voglibose | Voglibosa |
| 艾塞那肽 | Exenatide | Exénatide | Exenatida |
| 利拉鲁肽 | Liraglutide | Liraglutide | Liraglutida |
| 西格列汀 | Sitagliptin | Sitagliptine | Sitagliptina |
| 沙格列汀 | Saxagliptin | Saxagliptine | Saxagliptina |
| 维格列汀 | Vidagliptin | Vidagliptine | Vidagliptina |
| 利格列汀 | Linagliptin | Linagliptine | Linagliptina |
| 阿格列汀 | Alogliptin | Alogliptine | Alogliptina |
| 达格列净 | Dapagliflozin | Dapagliflozine | Dapagliflozina |
| 卡格列净 | Canagliflozin | Canagliflozine | Canagliflozina |
| 恩格列净 | Empagliflozin | Empagliflozine | Empagliflozina |

### 16.14 抗肥胖症药 Anti-Obesity Drug

| 药品名称 | Drug Names | Dénomination du Médicament | Denominación del Medicamento |
|---|---|---|---|
| 奥利司他 | Orlistat | Orlistat | Orlistat |

### 16.15 影响骨代谢药物 Drugs Affecting Bone Metabolism

| 药品名称 | Drug Names | Dénomination du Médicament | Denominación del Medicamento |
|---|---|---|---|
| 依替膦酸二钠 | Etidronate Disodium | Étidronate Disodique | Etidronato Disódico |
| 氯膦酸二钠 | Clodronate Disodium | Clodronate Disodique | Clodronato Disódico |
| 帕米膦酸二钠 | Pamidronate Disodium | Pamidronate Disodique | Pamidronato Disódico |
| 阿仑膦酸钠 | Alendronate Sodium | Aléndronate Sodique | Alendronato Sódico |
| 伊班膦酸钠 | Ibandronate Sodium | Ibandronate Sodique | Ibandronato Sódico |
| 利塞膦酸钠 | Risedronate Sodium | Risédronate Sodique | Risedronato Sódico |
| 唑来膦酸 | Zoledronic Acid | Acide Zolédronique | Ácido Zoledrónico |
| 英卡磷酸二钠 | Incadronate Disodium | Incadronate Disodique | Incadronato Disódico |
| 依普黄酮 | Ipriflavone | Ipriflavone | Ipriflavona |

**续　表**

| 药品名称 | Drug Names | Dénomination du Médicament | Denominación del Medicamento |
|---|---|---|---|
| 雷洛昔芬 | Raloxifene | Raloxifene | Raloxifeno |
| 降钙素 | Calcitonin | Calcitonine | Calcitonina |
| 骨化三醇 | Calcitriol | Calcitriol | Calcitriol |
| 阿法骨化醇 | Alfacalcidol | Alfacalcidol | Alfacalcidol |
| 碳酸钙 | Calcium Carbonate | Carbonate de calcium | Carbonato de calcio |
| 特立帕肽 | Teriparatide | Tériparatide | Teriparatida |
| 维生素 D | Vitamin D | Vitamine D | Vitamina D |
| 雷奈酸锶 | Strontium Ranelate | Ranélate de Srontium | Ranelato de estroncio |
| 四烯甲萘醌 | Menatetrenone | Ménatetrenone | Menatetrenona |
| 氨基葡萄糖 | Glucosamine | Glucosamine | Glucosamina |
| 16.16 甲状腺激素类药物 Thyroid Hormones Drugs | | | |
| 左甲状腺素 | Levothyroxine | Lévothyroxine | Levotiroxina |
| 甲状腺片 | Thyroid Tablets | Thyroide en Comprimés | Tabletas de Tiroideo |
| 碘赛罗宁 | Liothyronine | Liothyronine | Liotironina |
| 促甲状腺素 | Thyrotrophin | Thyrotropine Stimulante | Tirotropina |
| 16.17 抗甲状腺药 Anti-Thyroid Drugs | | | |
| 丙硫氧嘧啶 | Propylthiouracil | Propylthiouracil | Propiltiouracilo |
| 甲巯咪唑 | Thimazole | Thimazole | Tiamazol |
| 17. 主要影响变态反应和免疫功能的药物 Drugs Mainly Affecting Allergy and Immune Function | | | |
| 17.1 抗变态反应药物 Antiallergic Drugs | | | |
| 苯海拉明 | Diphenhydramine | Diphénhydramine | Difenhidramina |
| 异丙嗪 | Promethazine | Prométhazine | Prometazina |
| 去氯羟嗪 | Decloxizine | Décloxizine | Decloxizina |
| 阿伐斯汀 | Acrivastine | Acrivastine | Acrivastina |
| 左卡巴斯汀 | Levocabastine | Lévocabastine | Levocabastina |
| 咪唑斯汀 | Mizolastine | Mizolastine | Mizolastina |
| 曲吡那敏 | Tripelennamine | Tripélénnamine | Tripelenamina |
| 美喹他嗪 | Mequitazine | Méquitazine | Mequitazina |
| 司他斯汀 | Setastine | Sétastine | Setastina |
| 非尼拉敏 | Pheniramine | Phéniramine | Feniramina |
| 多西拉敏 | Doxylamine | Doxylamine | Doxilamina |
| 安他唑啉 | Antazoline | Antazoline | Antazolina |
| 氯环利嗪 | Chlorcyclizine | Chlorcyclizine | Clorciclizina |
| 羟嗪 | Hydroxyzine | Hydroxyzine | Hidroxizina |
| 奥沙特米 | Oxatomide | Oxatomide | Oxatomida |
| 阿扎他定 | Azatadine | Azatadine | Azatadina |
| 左西替利嗪 | Levocetirizine | Lévocétirizine | Levocetirizina |
| 奥洛他定 | Olopatadine | Olopatadine | Olopatadina |

**续 表**

| 药品名称 | Drug Names | Dénomination du Médicament | Denominación del Medicamento |
|---|---|---|---|
| 卢帕他定 | Rupatadine | Rupatadine | Rupatadina |
| 氯马斯汀 | Clemastine | Clémastine | Clemastina |
| 特非那定 | Terfenadine | Térfénadine | Terfenadina |
| 非索非那定 | Fexofenadine | Féxofénadine | Fexofenadina |
| 依美斯汀 | Emedastine | Emédastine | Emedastina |
| 依匹斯汀 | Epinastine | Epinastine | Epinastina |
| 贝他斯汀 | Bepotastine | Bépotastine | Bepotastina |
| 曲普利啶 | Triprolidine | Triprolidine | Triprolidina |
| 多赛平 | Doxepin | Doxépine | Doxepina |
| 吡嘧司特钾 | Pemirolast Potassium | Pémirolast de Potassium | Pemirolast de Potasio |
| 赛庚啶 | Cyproheptadine | Cyprohéptadine | Ciproheptadina |
| 氯雷他定 | Loratadine | Loratadine | Loratadina |
| 西替利嗪 | Cetirizine | Cétirizine | Cetirizina |
| 依巴斯汀 | Ebastine | Ebastine | Ebastina |
| 地氯雷他定 | Desloratadine | Désloratadine | Desloratadina |
| 氮䓬斯汀 | Azelastine | Azélastine | Azelastina |
| 溴苯那敏 | Brompheniramine | Bromphéniramine | Bromfeniramina |
| 氯苯那敏 | Chlorpheniramine | Chlorpheniramine | Clorfeniramina |
| 茶苯海明 | Dimenhydrinate | Diménhydrinate | Dimenhidrinato |
| 色甘酸钠 | Sodium Cromoglicate | Cromoglycate de sodium | Cromoglicato sódico |
| 酮替芬 | Ketotifen | Kétotifène | Ketotifeno |
| 曲尼司特 | Tranilast | Tranilast | Tranilast |
| 塞曲司特 | Seratrodast | Sératrodast | Seratrodast |
| 倍他司汀 | Betahistine | Bétahistine | Betahistina |
| **17.2 免疫抑制药 Immunosuppressants** | | | |
| 环孢素 | Cyclosporin | Cyclosporine | Ciclosporina |
| 他克莫司 | Tacrolimus | Tacrolimus | Tacrolimus |
| 西罗莫司 | Sirolimus | Sirolimus | Sirolimus |
| 依维莫司 | Everolimus | Evérolimus | Everolimus |
| 吗替麦考酚酯 | Mycophenolate Mofetil | Mycophénolate mofétil | Micofenolato mofetil |
| 咪唑立宾 | Mizoribine | Mizoribine | Mizoribina |
| 来氟米特 | Leflunomide | Léflunomide | Leflunomida |
| 泼尼松 | Prednisone | Prédnisone | Prednisona |
| 硫唑嘌呤 | Azathioprine | Azathioprine | Azatioprina |
| 羟基脲 | Hydroxycarbamide (Hydroxyurea) | Hydroxycarbamide (Hydroxyurée) | Hidroxicarbamida (Hidroxiurea) |
| 羟氯喹 | Hydroxychloroquine | Hydroxychloroquine | Hidroxicloroquina |

**续　表**

| 药品名称 | Drug Names | Dénomination du Médicament | Denominación del Medicamento |
|---|---|---|---|
| 艾拉莫德 | Iguratimod | Iguratimod | Iguratimod |
| 甲氨蝶呤 | Methotrexate | Méthotréxate | Metotrexato |
| 环磷酰胺 | Cyclophosphamide | Cyclophosphamide | Ciclofosfamida |
| 苯丁酸氮芥 | Chlorambucil | Chlorambucil | Clorambucil |
| 抗人 T 细胞免疫球蛋白 | Antihuman T Lymphocyte Immunoglobulin | Immunoglobuline Anti-Céllules T Humaines | Inmunoglobulina Anti-Celulas T Humanas |
| 兔抗人胸腺细胞免疫球蛋白 | Rabbit Anti-Human Thymocyte Immunoglobulin | Immunoglobuline Rabbit Anti-Thymocyte Humaines | Immunoglobulina Rabbit Anti Thymocyte Humanas |
| 抗人 T 细胞 CD3 鼠单抗 | Mouse Monoclonal Antibody Against Human CD3 Antigen of T Lymphocyte | Anticorp Monoclonaux de Rat Résistant à l' Antigène CD3 Humain Lymphocytes T | Anticuerpo Monoclonal de Rata Contra el Antígeno CD3 Humano Linfocitos T |
| 巴利昔单抗 | Basiliximab | Basiliximab | Basiliximab |
| 曲妥珠单抗 | Trastuzumab | Trastuzumab | Trastuzumab |
| 西妥昔单抗 | Cetuximab | Cetuximab | Cetuximab |
| 利妥昔单抗 | Rituximab | Rituximab | Rituximab |
| 英夫利昔单抗 | Infliximab | Infliximab | Infliximab |
| 雷公藤多苷 | Tripterygium Glycosides | Tripterygium Glycosides | Tripterigio Glicosida |
| 托法替布 | Tofacitinib | Tofacitinib | Tofacitinib |
| 阿普斯特 | Apremilast | Apremilast | Apremilast |
| 吡非尼酮 | Pirfenidone | Pirfénidone | Pirfenidona |
| 沙利度胺 | Thalidomide | Thalidomide | Talidomida |
| 麦考酚钠 | Mycophenolate Sodium | Mycophenolate de Sodium | Micofenolato Sódico |
| 重组人 II 型肿瘤坏死因子受体 - 抗体融合蛋白 | Recombinant Human Type II Tumor Necrosis Factor Receptor-Antibody Fusion Protein | Recombinant Human Type II Récepteur du Facteur de Nécrose Tumorale- Protéine de Fusion des Anticorps | Recombinant Human Tipo II Receptor del Factor de Necrosis Tumoral-Proteína de Fusión de Anticuerpos |
| 青霉胺 | Penicillamine | Penicilamine | Penicilamina |
| **17.3 免疫增强药 Immunostimulants** | | | |
| 香菇多糖 | Lentinan | Lentinan | Lentinan |
| 咪喹莫特 | Imiquimod | Imiquimod | Imiquimod |
| 胸腺法新 | Thymalfasin | Thymalfasine | Timalfasina |
| 胸腺素 | Thymosin | Thymosine | Timosina |
| 重组人白细胞介素 -2 | Recombinant Human Interleukin-2 | Interleucine-2 Humaine Recombinante | Interleucina-2 Recombinante Humana |
| 重组人白细胞介素 -11 | Recombinant Human Interleukin-11 | Interleucine-11 Humaine Recombinante | Interleucina-11 Recombinante Humana |
| 重组人干扰素 | Recombinant Human Interferon (rh IFN) | Interféron Humain Recombinant (rh IFN) | Interferón Recombinante Humana (rh IFN) |

**续 表**

| 药品名称 | Drug Names | Dénomination du Médicament | Denominación del Medicamento |
|---|---|---|---|
| 重组人干扰素 α-2a | Recombinant Human Interferon α-2a (rh IFNα-2a) | Interféron α -2a Humain Re-combinant | Interferón α-2a Recombinante Huma-na |
| 重组人干扰素 α-1b | Recombinant Human Interferon α-1b (rh IFNα-1b) | Interféron α -1b Humain Re-combinant | Interferón α--1b Recombinante Hu-mana |
| 重组人干扰素 α-2b | Recombinant Human Interferon α-2b (rh IFNα-2b) | Interféron α -2b Humain Re-combinant | Interferon α-2b Recombinante Huma-na |
| 重组人干扰素 β | Recombinant Human Interferon-β (rh IFN-β) | Interféron-β Humain Recombi-nant | Interferon-β Recombinante Humana |
| 重组人干扰素 γ | Recombinant Human Interfer-on-γ (rh IFN-γ) | Interféron-γ Humain Recombi-nant | Interferon-γ Recombinante Humana |
| 人免疫球蛋白 | Human Immunoglobulin | Immunoglobuline Humaine | Inmunoglobulina Humana |
| 聚乙二醇干扰素 α-2a | Peginterferon alfa-2a | Péginterféron alfa -2a | Peginterferón alfa-2a |
| 聚乙二醇干扰素 α-2b | Peginterferon alfa-2b | Péginterféron alfa -2b | Peginterferón alfa-2b |
| 乌苯美司 | Ubenimex | Ubénimex | Ubenimex |
| 白芍总苷 | Total Glucosides of Paeony | Glucoside Total de Paeonia Alba | Glucosido Total de Peoniaceae |
| 匹多莫德 | Pidotimod | Pidotimod | Pidotimod |
| 奥马珠单抗 | Omalizumab | Omalizumab | Omalizumab |

18. 维生素类，酶类及生化制剂，调节水、电解质和酸碱平衡药物，肠内营养药物，肠外营养药物 Vitamins, Enzymes and Biochemical Preparation, Drugs Regulating Balance of Water Electrolyte and Acid-Base, Enternal Nutrition Drugs, Total Parenteral Nutrition(TPN)

### 18.1 维生素类 Vitamins

| | | | |
|---|---|---|---|
| 维生素 A | Vitamin A (Retinol) | Vitamine A (Retinol) | Vitamina A (Retinol) |
| 维生素 D | Vitamin D | Vitamine D | Vitamina D |
| 维生素 AD | Vitamin AD | Vitamine AD | Vitamina AD |
| 复合维生素 B | Vitamin B Complex | Composés Vitamine B | Compuestos Vitamina B |
| 骨化三醇 | Calcitriol | Calcitriol | Calcitriol |
| 阿法骨化醇 | Alfacalcidol | Alfacalcidol | Alfacalcidol |
| 维生素 $B_1$ | Vitamin $B_1$ (Thiamine) | Vitamine $B_1$ (Thiamine) | Vitamina $B_1$ (Tiamina) |
| 维生素 $B_2$ | Vitamin $B_2$ (Riboflavin) | Vitamine $B_2$ (Riboflavine) | Vitamina $B_2$ (Riboflavina) |
| 烟酸 | Nicotinic Acid | Acide Nicotinique | Ácido Nicotínico |
| 烟酰胺 | Nicotinamide | Nicotinamide | Nicotinamida |
| 维生素 $B_6$ | Vitamin $B_6$ (Pyridoxine) | Vitamine $B_6$ (Pyridoxine) | Vitamina $B_6$ (Piridoxina) |
| 干酵母 | Dried Yeast | Levures Séchées | Levaduras Secas |
| 维生素 C | Vitamin C (Ascorbic acid) | Vitamine C (Acide Ascorbique) | Vitamina C (Acido Ascorbico ) |
| 维生素 E | Vitamin E (Tocopherol) | Vitamine E (Tocopherol) | Vitamina E (Tocoferol) |

### 18.2 酶类和其他生化制剂 Enzymes and Biochemical Preparation

| | | | |
|---|---|---|---|
| 胰蛋白酶 | Trypsin | Trypsine | Tripsina |
| 糜蛋白酶 | Chymotrypsin | Chymotrypsine | Quimotripsina |

**续　表**

| 药品名称 | Drug Names | Dénomination du Médicament | Denominación del Medicamento |
|---|---|---|---|
| 抑肽酶 | Aprotinin | Aprotinine | Aprotinina |
| 玻璃酸酶 | Hyaluronidase | Hyaluronidase | Hialuronidasa |
| 三磷酸腺苷 | Adenoside Triphosphate | Adénosine Triphosphate | Adenosína Trifosfato |
| 18.3　调节水、电解质和酸碱平衡用药 Drugs Regulating Balance of Water Electrolyte and Acid-Base ||||
| 氯化钠 | Sodium Chloride | Chlorure de Sodium | Cloruro Sódico |
| 氯化钾 | Potassium Chloride | Chlorure de Potassium | Cloruro Potásico |
| 门冬氨酸钾镁 | Potassium Magnesium Aspartate | Aspartate de Potassium Magnésium | Aspartato de Potasio y Magnesio |
| 枸橼酸钾 | Potassium Citrate | Citrate de Potassium | Citrato de potasio |
| 氯化钙 | Calcium Chloride | Chlorure de Calcium | Cloruro de calcio |
| 碳酸钙 | Calcium Carbonate | Carbonate de Calcium | Carbonato de calico |
| 葡萄糖酸钙 | Calcium Gluconate | Gluconate de Calcium | Gluconato de Calcio |
| 乳酸钙 | Calcium Lactate | Lactate de Calcium | Lactato de Calcio |
| 甘油磷酸钠 | Sodium Glycerophosphate | Glycérophosphate de Sodium | Glicerofosfato Sódico |
| 硫酸镁 | Magnesium Sulfate | Sulfate de Magnésium | Sulfato de Magnesio |
| 乳酸钠 | Sodium Lactate | Lactate de Sodium | Lactato sódico |
| 葡萄糖 | Glucose | Glucose | Glucosa |
| 果糖 | Fructose | Fructose | Fructosa |
| 乳酸钠林格液 | Sodium Lactate Ringer's Solution | Lactate de Sodium Ringer's Solution | Lactato de Sodio Ringer's solucion |
| 腹膜透析液 | Peritoneal Dialysis Solution | Solution de Dialyse Péritoneale | Solución de Diálisis Peritoneal |
| 18.4　肠内营养药物 Enternal Nutrition(EN) ||||
| 安素 | Ensure | Ensure | Ensure |
| 肠内营养粉剂(TP) | Enteral Nutritional Powder(TP) | Poudrés Entéral Nutritional(TP) | Polvos Enteral Nutritional(TP) |
| 肠内营养乳剂(TP) | Enteral Nutritional Emulsion(TP) | Emulsion Nutritive Entérale(TP) | Emulsion Nutricional Enteral (TP) |
| 肠内营养乳剂(TPF) | Enteral Nutritional Emulsion(TPF) | Emulsion Nutritive Entérale(TPF) | Emulsion Nutricional Enteral (TPF) |
| 18.5　肠外营养药物 Total Parenteral Nutrition(TPN) ||||
| 水解蛋白 | Protein Hydrolysate | Protéines Hydrolysées | Hidrolizado de Proteínas |
| 复方氨基酸注射液 (18AA) | Compound Amino Acid Injection(18AA) | Injéction Composés d'acides Aminés (18AA) | Inyeccion de Aminoácidos Compuestos (18AA) |
| 复方氨基酸注射液 (9AA) | Compound Amino Acid Injection (9AA) | Injéction Composée d'acide Aminé (9AA) | Inyeccion de Aminoácidos Compuestos (9AA) |
| 复方 α- 酮酸 | Compound α Ketoacid | Composés α-Acide Cétone | Compuesto α-Cetoácido |
| 复方氨基酸注射液 (3AA) | Compound Amino Acid Injection (3AA) | Injéction Composée d' Acide Aminé (3AA) | Inyeccion de Aminoácidos Compuestos (3AA) |
| 复方氨基酸注射液 (15AA) | Compound Amino Acid Injection (15AA) | Injéction Composée d'acide Aminé (15AA) | Inyeccion de Aminoácidos Compuestos (15AA) |

续　表

| 药品名称 | Drug Names | Dénomination du Médicament | Denominación del Medicamento |
|---|---|---|---|
| 脂肪乳注射液 | Fat Emulsion Injection | Injection d' émulsion de Graisse | Inyección de Emulsión de Grasas |
| ω-3鱼油脂肪乳注射剂 | ω-3 Fish Oil Emulsion Injection | Injéction d' émulsion d' Huile de Poisson ω-3 | Inyección de Emulsión Grasa de Aceite de Pescado ω-3 |
| 多种微量元素注射液（Ⅰ） | Multi Trace Element Injection（Ⅰ） | Multi-Oligo-éléments Injéction（Ⅰ） | Inyección de Múltiples Elementos Traza(Ⅰ) |
| 多种微量元素注射液（Ⅱ） | Multi Trace Element Injection（Ⅱ） | Multi-Oligo-éléments Injéction（Ⅱ） | Inyección de Múltiples Elementos Traza(Ⅱ) |
| 脂溶性维生素注射液（Ⅰ） | Fat-Soluble Vitamin Injection（Ⅰ） | Injéction de Vitamine Liposoluble (I) | Inyección de Vitaminas Liposoluble (I) |
| 脂溶性维生素注射液（Ⅱ） | Fat-soluble Vitamin Injection（Ⅱ） | Injéction de Vitamine Liposoluble (II) | Inyección de Vitaminas Liposoluble (II) |
| 注射用水溶性维生素 | Water-Soluble Vitamin for Injection | Vitamines Soluble dans l'eau Pour Injéction | Vitaminas solubles en agua |
| 19. 专科用药 Specialist Drugs | | | |
| 19.1 治疗骨质疏松、骨质增生，前列腺增生症及老年性白内障药物 Drugs for Osteoporosis, Bone Hyperlasia, Prostatic Hyperplasia and Senile Cataract | | | |
| 帕米膦酸二钠 | Pamidronate Disodium | Pamidronate Disodique | Pamidronato Disódico |
| 阿仑膦酸钠 | Alendronate Sodium | Aléndronate Sodique | Alendronato sódico |
| 伊班膦酸钠 | Ibandronate Sodium | Ibandronate Sodique | Ibandronato Sódico |
| 利塞膦酸钠 | Risedronate Sodium | Risédronate Sodique | Risedronato Sódico |
| 降钙素 | Calcitonin | Calcitonine | Calcitonina |
| 骨化三醇 | Calcitriol | Calcitriol | Calcitriol |
| 阿法骨化醇 | Alfacalcidol | Alfacalcidol | Alfacalcidol |
| 碳酸钙 | Calcium Carbonate | Carbonate de Calcium | Carbonato de Calcio |
| 替勃龙 | Tibolone | Tibolone | Tibolona |
| 雌二醇 | Estradiol | Estradiol | Estradiol |
| 雷洛昔芬 | Raloxifene | Raloxifène | Raloxifeno |
| 氨基葡萄糖 | Glucosamine | Glucosamine | Glucosamina |
| 酚苄明 | Phenoxybenzamine | Phénoxybénzamine | Fenoxibenzamina |
| 特拉唑嗪 | Terazosin | Térazosine | Terazosina |
| 坦洛新 | Tamsulosin | Tamsulosine | Tamsulosina |
| 非那雄胺 | Finasteride | Finastéride | Finasterida |
| 舍尼通 | Cernilton | Cérnilton | Cernilton |
| 依立雄胺 | Epristeride | Epristéride | Epristerida |
| 谷丙甘氨酸 | Glutamate Acid, Alanine and Glycine | Acide Glutamique Alanine et Glycine | Ácido glutámico,Alanina y Glicina |
| 吡诺克辛 | Pirenoxine | Pirénoxine | Pirenoxina |

**续　表**

| 药品名称 | Drug Names | Dénomination du Médicament | Denominación del Medicamento |
|---|---|---|---|
| **19.2 消毒防腐收敛药 Drugs for Sterilizing, Antisepsis and Convergence** | | | |
| 过氧乙酸 | Peracetic Acid | Acide Peracétique | Ácido Peracético |
| 聚维酮碘 | Povidone Iodine | Povidone iodée | Povidona yodada |
| 氯己定 | Chlorhexidine | Chlorhéxidine | Clorhexidina |
| 戊二醛 | Glutaraldehyde | Glutaraldéhyde | Glutaraldehído |
| 鞣酸 | Tannic Acid | Acide Tannique | Acido Tanico |
| 苯酚 | Phenol | Phénol | Fenol |
| 鱼石脂 | Ichthammol | Ichthammol | Ictamol |
| 乙醇 | Ethanol | Ethanol | Etanol |
| 甲紫 | Methylrosanilinium | Méthylrosanilinium | Metilrosanilinium |
| 依沙吖啶 | Ethacridine | Ethacridine | Etacridina |
| 高锰酸钾 | Potassium permanganate | Permanganate de Potassium | Permanganato de potasio |
| 过氧化氢溶液 | Hydrogen Peroxide Solution | Solution de Péroxyde d'Hydrogène | Solución de Peróxido de Hidrógeno |
| 苯甲酸 | Benzoic Acid | Acide Bénzoique | Acido Benzoico |
| 苯扎溴铵 | Benzalkonium Bromide | Bromure de Bénzalkonium | Bromuro de Benzalconio |
| 呋喃西林 | Furacilin | Furacilline | Furacilina |
| **19.3 皮肤科用药 Drugs for Dermatology** | | | |
| 莫匹罗星 | Mupirocin | Mupirocine | Mupirocina |
| 夫西地酸 | Fusidic Acid | Acide Fusidique | Ácido Fusídico |
| 环吡酮胺 | Ciclopirox Olamine | Ciclopirox Olamine | Ciclopirox Olamina |
| 联苯苄唑 | Bifonazole | Bifonazole | Bifonazolo |
| 奥昔康唑 | Oxiconazole | Oxiconazole | Oxiconazol |
| 芬替康唑 | Fenticonazole | Fénticonazole | Fenticonazol |
| 克霉唑 | Clotrimazole | Clotrimazole | Clotrimazol |
| 酞丁安 | Ftibamzone | Ftibamzone | Ftibamzona |
| 克罗米通 | Crotamiton | Crotamiton | Crotamitón |
| 维 A 酸 | Tretinoin | Trétinoine | Tretinoina |
| 异维 A 酸 | Isotretinoin | Isotrétinoine | Isotretinoína |
| 他扎罗汀 | Tazarotene | Tazaroténe | Tazarotena |
| 阿达帕林 | Adapalene | Adapaléne | Adapalena |
| 糠酸莫米松 | Mometasone Furoate | Furoate de Mométasone | Furoato de Mometasona |
| **19.4 眼科用药 Drugs for Ophthalmology** | | | |
| 吡诺克辛 | Pirenoxine | Pirénoxine | Pirenoxina |
| 布林佐胺 | Brinzolamide | Brinzolamide | Brinzolamida |
| 拉坦前列腺素 | Latanoprost | Latanoprost | Latanoprost |
| 他氟前列素 | Tafluprost | Tafluprost | Tafluprost |
| 托吡卡胺 | Tropicamide | Tropicamide | Tropicamida |

**续　表**

| 药品名称 | Drug Names | Dénomination du Médicament | Denominación del Medicamento |
|---|---|---|---|
| 吡嘧司特 | Pemirolast | Pémirolast | Pemirolast |
| 卡巴胆碱 | Carbachol | Carbachol | Carbacol |
| 依美斯汀 | Emedastine | Emédastine | Emedastina |
| 普拉洛芬 | Pranoprofen | pranoprofène | Pranoprofeno |
| 雷珠单抗 | Ranibizumab | Ranibizumab | Ranibizumab |
| 康柏西普 | Conbercept | Conbércépt | Conbercept |
| 阿柏西普 | Aflibercept | Aflibércépt | Aflibercept |
| 玻璃酸钠 | Sodium Hyaluronate | Hyaluronate de Sodium | Hialuronato de sodio |
| **19.5　耳鼻喉科和口腔科用药 Drugs for Otolaryngology and Dental** | | | |
| 羟甲唑啉 | Oxymetazoline | Oxymétazoline | Oximetazolina |
| 西地碘 | Cydiodine | Cydiodine | Cidiodina |
| 左卡巴斯汀 | Levocabastine | Levocabastine | Levocabastina |
| 氯霉素滴耳液 | Chloramphenicol Auristillae | Chloramphénicol gouttes pour oreilles | Gotas para los oidos de Cloranfenicol |
| 氧氟沙星滴耳液 | Ofloxacin Auristillae | Ofloxacine gouttes pour oreilles | Gotas para los oidos de Ofloxacina |
| 酚甘油滴耳液 | Phenol Glycerol Auristillae | Phénoglycérol gouttes pour oreilles | Gotas para los oidos de Fenolglicerol |
| 硼酸滴耳液 | Boric Acid Auristillae | Acide Borique gouttes pour oreilles | Gotas para los oidos de Ácido Bórico |
| 碳酸氢钠滴耳液 | Sodium Bicarbonate Auristillae | Bicarbonate de Sodium gouttes pour oreilles | Gotas para los oidos de Bicarbonato Sódico |
| 碘甘油 | Iodine Glycerin | Iode Glycérine | Iodoglicerina |
| 呋喃西林/麻黄碱滴鼻液 | Furacilin/ Ephedrine Naristillae | Furacilline/Ephédrine gouttes nasales | Gotas nasales de Furacilina/ Efedrina |
| 复方薄荷滴鼻液 | Compound Mint Naristillae | Composés Menthe gouttes nasales | Gotas nasals de Compuesto de Mentol |
| 盐酸麻黄碱滴鼻液 | Ephedrine Hydrochloride Naristillae | Chlorhydrate d' Ephédrine gouttes nasales | Gotas nasales de Clorhidrato de Efedrina |
| 呋喃西林片（漱口） | Furacilin Tablet(for Gargle ) | Furacilline Comprimé (pour Bouche) | Tabletas de gargara be Furacilina |
| 复方硼砂片 | Compound borax tablet(for Gargle) | Comprimes de borax composé (Pour Bouche) | Tabletas de borax compuesto(Gargarizar) |
| **19.6　妇科外用药 Drug for Gynaecology** | | | |
| 硝呋太尔/制霉素 | Nifuratel/Nystatin(Vaginal use) | Nifuratel/Nystatine(Pour vagin) | Nifuratel/Nistatina(Para uso vaginal) |
| 地瑞舒林 | Dicresulene | Dicrésuléne | Dicresulena |
| 普罗雌烯 | Promestriene | Proméstriene | Promestrieno |
| **20. 其他类药物 Other Drugs** | | | |
| **20.1　解毒药 Alexipharmac** | | | |
| 谷胱甘肽 | Glutathione | Glutathion | Glutatión |
| 二巯丙醇 | Dimercaprol | Dimércaprol | Dimercaprol |

**续　表**

| 药品名称 | Drug Names | Dénomination du Médicament | Denominación del Medicamento |
| --- | --- | --- | --- |
| 二巯丁二钠 | Sodium Dimercaptosuccinate | Dimércaptosuccinate de Sodium | Dimercaptosuccinato Sodio |
| 二巯丙磺钠 | Sodium Dimercaptopropane Sulfonate | Dimercaptopropane sulfonate de Sodium | Dimercaptopropane sulfonato Sodio |
| 依地酸钙钠 | Calcium Disodium Edetate | Edetate de Disodique et Calcium | Edetato de Calcio y disodico |
| 青霉胺 | Penicillamine | Pénicilamine | Penicilamina |
| 去铁胺 | Deferoxamine | Déféroxamine | Deferoxamina |
| 碘解磷定 | Pralidoxime Iodide | Iodure de Pralidoxime | Pralidoxima Yoduro |
| 氯解磷定 | Pralidoxime Chloride | Chlorure de Pralidoxime | Pralidoxima Cloruro |
| 阿托品 | Atropine | Atropine | Atropina |
| 东莨菪碱 | Scopolamine | Scopolamine | Escopolamina |
| 戊乙奎醚 | Penehyclidine | Pénéhyclidine | Penehiclidina |
| 亚甲蓝 | Methylthioninium Chloride | Chlorure de Méthylthionine | Cloruro de metiltioninio |
| 硫代硫酸钠 | Sodium Thiosulfate | Thiosulfate de sodium | Tiosulfato de Sodio |
| 亚硝酸钠 | Sodium Nitrite | Nitrite de Sodium | Nitrito de Sodio |
| 亚硝酸异戊酯 | Isoamyl Nitrite | Nitrite d'Isopéntyle | Nitrito de Isopentilo |
| 乙酰胺 | Acetamide | Acétamide | Acetamida |
| 氟马西尼 | Flumazenil | Flumazénil | Flumazenil |
| 纳洛酮 | Naloxone | Naloxone | Naloxona |
| 纳美芬 | Nalmefene | Nalméféne | Nalmefeno |
| 乙酰半胱氨酸 | Acetylcysteine | Acétylcystéine | Acetilcisteína |
| 亚叶酸钙 | Calcium Folinate | Folinate de Calcium | Folinato de calcio |

**20.2　防治放射病药物 Drugs for Prophylaxis and Treatment of Radiation Sickness**

| | | | |
| --- | --- | --- | --- |
| 巯乙胺 | Mercaptamine | Mércaptamine | Mercaptamina |
| 半胱氨酸 | Cysteine | Cystéine | Cisteína |

**20.3　诊断用药 Drugs for Diagnosis**

| | | | |
| --- | --- | --- | --- |
| 碘海醇 | Iohexol | Iohexol | Iohexol |
| 碘佛醇 | Ioversol | Ioversol | Yoversol |
| 碘帕醇 | Iopamidol | Iopamidol | Iopamidol |
| 碘克沙醇 | Iodixanol | Iodixanol | Iodixanol |
| 碘比醇 | Iobitridol | Iobitridol | Iobitridol |
| 碘普罗胺 | Iopromide | Iopromide | Iopromida |
| 碘美普尔 | Iomeprol | Iomeprol | Iomeprol |
| 硫酸钡 | Barium Sulfate | Sulfate de Baryum | Sulfato de Bario |
| 碘化油 | Iodinated Oil | Huile iodée | Aceite Yodado |
| 复方泛影葡胺 | Compoud Meglumine Diatrizoate | Composé Diatrizoate de Méglumine | Compuesto Meglumina Diatrizoato |
| 钆喷酸葡胺 | Gadopentetate Dimethyl Meglumine | Gadopentétate Diméthylglumine | Gadopentetato Dimetiglumina |
| 钆双胺 | Gadodiamide | Gadodiamide | Gadodiamida |
| 钆贝葡胺 | Gadolinium Meglumine | Gadolinium Meglumine | Gadolinium Meglumina |

| 药品名称 | Drug Names | Dénomination du Médicament | Denominación del Medicamento |
|---|---|---|---|
| 钆布醇 | Gadobutrol | Gadobutrol | Gadobutrol |
| 钆特酸葡胺 | Gadoteric Acid Meglumine | Acide Gadolétrique Meglumine | Ácido Gadoterico Meglumina |
| 钆塞酸二钠 | Gadoxetic Acid Disodium | Acide Gadolésique Disodique | Ácido Gadolesato Disódico |
| 六氟化硫 | Sulfur Hexafluoride | Hexafluorure de Soufre | Hexafluoruro de Azufre |
| 组胺 | Histamine | Histamine | Histamina |
| 吲哚菁绿 | Indocyanine Green | Indocyanine Vert | Verde de Indocianina |
| 荧光素钠 | Fluorescein Sodium | Fluorescéine de sodium | Fluoresceína sódica |
| **20.4 生物制品 Biological Products** | | | |
| 人用狂犬病疫苗 (vero 细胞 ) | Rabies Vaccine for Human Use (vero Cell) | Vaccins Antirabiquesà Usage Humain (Cellules vero) | Vacunas Antirrábicas para Uso Humano (vero Células) |
| 破伤风抗毒素 | Tetanus Antitoxin | Antitoxine Tétanique | Tétanos Antitoxina |
| 抗蛇毒血清 | Antivenin | Antivenin | Antiveneno |
| 抗狂犬病血清 | Rabies Antiserum | Sérum Antirabique | Suero Antirrábico |
| 人血白蛋白 | Human Albumin | Albumine Humaine | Albúmina Humana |
| 人免疫球蛋白 | Human Immunoglobulin | Immunoglobuline Humaine | Inmunoglobulina Humana |
| 乙型肝炎人免疫球蛋白 | Human Hepatitis B Immunoglobulin | Immunoglobuline Humaine Hépatite B | Inmunoglobulina Humana Hepatitis B |
| 破伤风人免疫球蛋白 | Human Tetanus Immunoglobulin | Humaine Tétanos Immunoglobuline | Inmunoglobulina Humana de Tétanos |
| 狂犬病人免疫球蛋白 | Human Rabies Immunoglobulin | Humaine Rabique Immunoglobuline | Inmunoglobulina Rabia humana |
| 人纤维蛋白原 | Human Fibrinogen | Fibrinogène Humain | Fibrinógeno humano |
| 凝血酶原复合物 | Prothrombin Complex | Complexe Prothrombin | Complejo Protrombina |
| 重组人干扰素 α- 1b | Recombinant Human Interferon α -1b | Interféron Humain Recombinant α- 1b | Interferón α-1b recombinante Humana |
| 重组人白细胞介素 -2 | Recombinant Human Interleukin-2 | Interleukine-2 Humain recombinant | Interleucina -2 Recombinante Humana |
| 结核菌素纯蛋白衍生物 | Purified Protein Derivative of Tuberculin (TB-PPD) | Dérivés Protéiques purs de la Tuberculine(TB-PPD) | Derivado Proteico purificado de la Tuberculina (TB-PPD) |
| 卡介苗纯蛋白衍生物 | Purified Protein Derivative of BCG (BCG-PPD) | Dérivés Protéiques purs de la BCG (BCG-PPD) | Derivado Proteico purificado de BCG (BCG-PPD) |
| 布氏菌纯蛋白衍生物 | Purified Protein Derivative of Brucellin (BR-PPD) | Dérivés Protéiques purs de la Brucella (BR-PPD) | Derivado Proteico purificado de Brucella (BR-PPD) |

# 第2章

# 中文—英文对照药品临床使用说明

## Instructions for Clinical Application of Drugs In Chinese - English

| 1. 抗生素 Antibiotics | |
|---|---|
| 1.1　青霉素类 Penicillins | |
| 药品名称 Drug Names | 青霉素 Penicillin |
| 适应证<br>Indications | 青霉素用于敏感菌所致的急性感染，如：菌血症、败血症、猩红热、丹毒、肺炎、脓胸、扁桃体炎、中耳炎、蜂窝织炎、疖、痈、急性乳腺炎、心内膜炎、骨髓炎、流行性脑膜炎（流脑）、钩端螺旋体病（对本病早期疗效较好）、奋森咽峡炎、创伤感染、回归热、气性坏疽、炭疽、淋病、放线菌病等。治疗破伤风、白喉宜与相应的抗毒素联用。<br><br>普鲁卡因青霉素吸收缓慢，肌内注射30万U，血药浓度峰值约2U/ml，24小时仍可测得。适用于梅毒和一些敏感菌所致的慢性感染。<br><br>苄星青霉素吸收极缓慢，血药浓度低，适用于需长期使用青霉素预防的患者，如慢性风湿性心脏病患者。<br><br>Benzylpenicillin is used to treat acute infection caused by susceptible strains, such as: bacteremia, Septicemia, scarlet fever, erysipelas, pneumonia, empyema, tonsillitis, otitis media, cellulitis, boils, carbuncles, acute mastitis, endocarditis, osteomyelitis, meningococcal meningitis (ECM), leptospirosis (the response for early stage of the disease is better), vincents angina, wound infection, relapsing fever, gas gangrene, anthrax, gonorrhea, actinomycetes, etc. Using for treatment of tetanus and diphtheria should be combined with appropriate antitoxin.<br><br>The absorption for Procaine penicillin is slow, when the intramuscular injection is 30 million units and the peak plasma concentration is about 2 units/ml, it still can be measured after 24 hours. It can be used for syphilis, and some chronic infection caused by susceptible strains.<br><br>Since the very slow absorption and low plasma concentration of Benzathine, the patients who need long-term use of penicillin prophylaxis, for example, patients with chronic rheumatic heart disease. |
| 用法、用量<br>Dosages | 青霉素钠常用于肌内注射或静脉滴注．肌内注射成人一日量为80万～320万U，儿童一日量为3万～5万U/kg，分为2～4次给予。静脉滴注适用于重病，如感染性心内膜炎、化脓性脑膜炎患者。成人一日量为240万～2000万U，儿童一日量为20万～40万U/kg，分4～6次加至少量输液中做间歇快速滴注。输液的青霉素（钠盐）浓度一般为1万～4万U/ml。青霉素钾通常用于肌内注射，由于注射局部较痛，可以用0.25%利多卡因注射液作为溶剂（2%苯甲醇注射液已不用）。钾盐也可静脉滴注，但必须注意患者体内血钾浓度和输液的钾含量（每100万U青霉素G中含钾量为65mg，与氯化钾125mg中的含钾量相近），并注意滴注速度不可太快。<br><br>普鲁卡因青霉素仅供肌内注射，1次量40万～80万U，一日1次。苄星青霉素仅供肌内注射，1次60万U，10～14日1次；1次120万U，14～21日1次。<br><br>Sodium penicillin is commonly used in intramuscular injection or intravenous infusion. The amount of intramuscular injection for an adult is 800, 000 to 3.2 million units per day, but for a child, it's 30, 000 to 50, 000 U / kg per day by two to four times. While, intravenous infusion is used to treat serious illness, such as infective endocarditis and purulent meningitis. The amount of intravenous infusion for an adult is 240 million to 20 million units per day, but for a child, it's 200, 000 to 40 million U / kg per day by adding at least 4 to 6 times into the infusion as intermittent rapid drips. The concentration of penicillin (sodium salt) for infusion generally ranges from 10, 000 to 40, 000 U / ml. Penicillin potassium is usually used for intramuscular injection. As the injection site will be in great pain, 0.25% lidocaine injection can be used as a solvent (parenteral solution of 2% benzyl alcohol has been in disuse). Potassium can also be used for intravenous infusion, but care must be taken in patient's |

potassium concentration, the potassium content in parenteral solution (the potassium content is 65mg per 1 million units of penicillin G potassium, which is similar to the potassium content in 125mg potassium chloride), and the infusion speed which can not be too fast.

Procaine penicillin can be used only for intramuscular injection; the amount for every injection is 400,000 to 800,000, one time a day. Benzathine is also used for intramuscular injection only, the 600,000 units per time, amount for every injection is 600,000 units, one time every 10 to 14 days or one time of 1.2 million units, but every 14 to 21days.

| 剂型、规格<br>Preparations | 注射用青霉素钠：每支（瓶）0.24g（40 万 U）、0.48g（80 万 U）或 0.6g（100 万 U）。<br>注射用青霉素钾：每支 0.25g（40 万 U）。<br>注射用普鲁卡因青霉素：每瓶 40 万 U 者，含普鲁卡因青霉素 30 万 U 及青霉素钾盐或钠盐 10 万 U；每瓶 80 万 U 者其含量加倍。既有长效，又有速效作用。每次肌内注射 40 万～80 万 U，一日 1 次。<br>注射用苄星青霉素（长效青霉素，长效西林）：每瓶 120 万 U，肌内注射。<br><br>Sodium penicillin for injection: 0.24g (40 million units), 0.48g (80 million units) or 0.6g (100 million units) per vial.<br>Potassium penicillin for injection: 0.25g (40 million units) per vial.<br>Procaine penicillin for injection: with 400,000 units per vial contains 300,000 units of procaine penicillin and 100,000 units of penicillin potassium or sodium; with 800,000 units per vial doubles the former contents. It is not only long-acting, but quick acting. The amount for Intramuscular injection every time is 400,000 to 800,000 units, once a day.<br>Benzathine penicillin (long-acting penicillin, long-acting amoxicillin) for injection: 1.2 million units per vial, intramuscular injection. |
|---|---|
| 药品名称 Drug Names | 青霉素 V Phenoxymethylpenicillin |
| 适应证<br>Indications | 青霉素用于敏感菌所致的急性感染，如：菌血症、败血症、猩红热、丹毒、肺炎、脓胸、扁桃体炎、中耳炎、蜂窝织炎、疖、痈、急性乳腺炎、心内膜炎、骨髓炎、流行性脑膜炎（流脑）、钩端螺旋体病（对本病早期疗效较好）、奋森咽峡炎、创伤感染、回归热、气性坏疽、炭疽、淋病、放线菌病等。治疗破伤风、白喉宜与相应的抗毒素联用。<br>普鲁卡因青霉素吸收缓慢，肌内注射 30 万 U，血药浓度峰值约 2U/ml，24 小时仍可测得。适用于梅毒和一些敏感菌所致的慢性感染。<br>苄星青霉素吸收极缓慢，血药浓度低，适用于需长期使用青霉素预防的患者，如慢性风湿性心脏病患者。<br><br>Benzylpenicillin is used to treat acute infection caused by susceptible strains, such as: bacteremia, Septicemia, scarlet fever, erysipelas, pneumonia, empyema, tonsillitis, otitis media, cellulitis, boils, carbuncles, acute mastitis, endocarditis, osteomyelitis, meningococcal meningitis (ECM), leptospirosis (the response for early stage of the disease is better), Fen Sen angina, wound infection, relapsing fever, gas gangrene, anthrax, gonorrhea, actinomycetes, etc. Using for treatment of tetanus and diphtheria should be combined with appropriate antitoxin.<br>The absorption for Procaine penicillin is slow, when the intramuscular injection is 30 million units and the peak plasma concentration is about 2 U / ml, it still can be measured after 24 hours. It can be used for syphilis, and some chronic infection caused by susceptible strains.<br>Since the slow absorption and low plasma concentration of Benzathine, the patients who need long-term use of penicillin prophylaxis, for example, patients with chronic rheumatic heart disease. |
| 用法、用量<br>Dosages | 口服。成人：125～500mg（20 万～80 万 U）/ 次，每 6～8 小时 1 次。儿童：每日 15～50mg/kg，分 3～6 次服用。<br><br>Oral medication: for adults, give 125～500mg (20 million to 80 million units) a time, every 6 to 8 hours; for children: give daily 15～50mg/kg in divided 3 to 6 doses. |
| 剂型、规格<br>Preparations | 片剂、胶囊剂：每片或粒 125mg（20 万 U）；250mg（40 万 U）；500mg（80 万 U）。还有颗粒剂或口服干糖浆。<br><br>Tablets, capsules: each is125mg (20 million units), 250mg (40 million units) or 500mg (80 million units). There are also granules and oral dry syrups. |

**续　表**

| 药品名称 Drug Names | 苯唑西林钠 Oxacillin Sodium |
|---|---|
| 适应证<br>Indications | 本品主要用于产酶的金黄色葡萄球菌和表皮葡萄球菌的周围感染，包括内脏、皮肤和软组织等部位的感染，但对耐甲氧西林金黄色葡萄球菌（MSRA）感染无效。对中枢感染不适用。<br><br>This product is mainly used for the peripheral infection caused by enzyme producing staphylococcus aureus and staphylococcus epidermidis, including infection of internal organs, skins,, soft tissue, and etc. But for methicillin-resistant staphylococcus aureus (MSRA) infection, it is ineffective. And so does the central nervous system infection. |
| 用法、用量<br>Dosages | 静脉滴注：1 次 1 ~ 2g，必要时可用到 3g，溶于 100ml 输液内滴注 0.5 ~ 1 小时，一日 3 ~ 4 次。小儿每日用量 50 ~ 100mg/kg，分次给予。肌内注射：1 次 1g，一日 3 ~ 4 次。口服、肌内注射均较少用。肾功能轻中度不足者可按正常用量，重度不足者应适当减量。<br><br>Intravenous infusion: 1 ~ 2g per time, or 3g, if necessary, and make it dissolve in 100ml infusion. Give 3 to 4 times a day and each time should be within 0.5 ~ 1hour. For children, give daily 50 ~ 100mg/kg in divided doses. Intramuscular injection: 1g per time, 3 to 4 times a day. Oral medication and intramuscular injections are less common. Patients with mild or moderate renal insufficiency could be administered by normal dosage, while the severe ones need appropriate reductions. |
| 剂型、规格<br>Preparations | 注射用苯唑西林钠：每瓶 0.5g；1g（效价）。<br>Oxacillin sodium for injection: 0.5g or 1g (titer) per bottle. |
| 药品名称 Drug Names | 氯唑西林钠 Cloxacillin Sodium |
| 适应证<br>Indications | 主要用于产酶金黄色葡萄球菌或不产酶葡萄球菌所致的败血症、肺炎、心内膜炎、骨髓炎或皮肤软组织感染等。但对耐甲氧西林金黄色葡萄球菌（MSRA）感染无效。<br><br>It is mainly used for pneumonia, endocarditis, osteomyelitis, or skin soft tissue infection and etc. caused by enzyme producing staphylococcus aureus or enzyme non-producing staphylococcus. But for methicillin-resistant Staphylococcus aureus (MSRA) infection, it is ineffective. |
| 用法、用量<br>Dosages | 肌内注射：1 次 0.5 ~ 1g，一日 3 ~ 4 次。静脉滴注：一次 1 ~ 2g，溶于 100ml 输液中，滴注 0.5 ~ 1 小时，一日 3 ~ 4 次。小儿每日用量 30 ~ 50mg/kg，分次给予。口服剂量：每次 0.25 ~ 0.5g，一日 4 次，空腹服用。<br><br>Intramuscular injection: 0.5 ~ 1g per time, 3 to 4 times a day. Intravenous infusion: 1 ~ 2g per time, make it dissolve in 100ml infusion, give 3 to 4 times a day and each time should be within 0.5 to 1 hour, . For children, give daily 30 ~ 50mg/kg in divided doses. Oral dosage: 0.25 ~ 0.5g per time, 4 times a day, on an empty stomach. |
| 剂型、规格<br>Preparations | 注射用氯唑西林钠：每瓶 0.5g（效价）。<br>胶囊剂：每胶囊 0.125g；0.25g；0.5g。<br>颗粒剂：50mg。<br><br>Cloxacillin sodium for injection: 0.5g per bottle (titer).<br>Capsules: 0.125g, 0.25g, 0.5g per capsule.<br>Granules: 50mg. |
| 药品名称 Drug Names | 氟氯西林 Flucloxacillin |
| 适应证<br>Indications | 主要应用于葡萄球菌所致的各种周围感染，但对耐甲氧西林金黄色葡萄球菌（MSRA）感染无效。<br><br>It is mainly used in treatment of various infections caused by Staphylococcus, but for methicillin-resistant Staphylococcus aureus (MSRA) infection, it is ineffective. |
| 用法、用量<br>Dosages | 口服（用游离酸）：常用量为每次 250mg，一日 3 次；重症用量为每次 500mg，一日 4 次，于食前 0.5 ~ 1 小时空腹服用。<br>肌内注射：常用量为每次 250mg，一日 3 次；重症用量为每次 500mg，一日 4 次。静脉注射：每次 500mg，一日 4 次，将药物溶于 10 ~ 20ml 注射用水或葡萄糖输液中使用，每 4 ~ 6 小时 1 次。一日量不超过 8g。<br>儿童：2 岁以下按成人量的 1/4；2 ~ 10 岁按成人量的 1/2，根据体重适当调整。也可按照每日 25 ~ 50mg/kg，分次给予。 |

|  |  |
| --- | --- |
|  | Oral medication (with free acid): the usual dose is 250mg singly, 3 times a day; while the individual dose for severe case is 500mg, 4 times a day and take it on an empty stomach, 0.5 to 1 hour before meals.<br>Intramuscular injection: the usual dose is 250mg singly, 3 times a day; while the dose for severe case is 500mg singly, 4 times a day. Intravenous: the single dose is 500mg, 4 times a day. Make it dissolve in 10 ~ 20ml injection water or glucose infusion for the dose given every 4 to 6 hours. 8g is the maximum dosage for one single day.<br>For children under the age of 2, give a quarter of the adult dosage, while for children of 2 to 10 years old, give half of the adult dosage and make appropriate adjustments according to the weight. Or give daily 25 ~ 50mg/kg in divided doses. |
| 剂型、规格<br>Preparations | 片剂（游离酸）：每片125mg。<br>注射用氟氯西林钠：每瓶500mg；1000mg。<br><br>Tablets (free acid): 125mg per tablet.<br>Flucloxacillin sodium for injection: 500mg, 1000mg per vial. |
| 药品名称 Drug Names | 氨苄西林 Ampicillin |
| 适应证<br>Indications | 本品主要用于敏感菌所致的泌尿系统、呼吸系统、胆道、肠道感染以及脑膜炎、心内膜炎等。<br>This product is mainly used to treat infection of urinary system, respiratory system, biliary tract and intestinal tract, as well as meningitis, endocarditis and etc., which are all caused by susceptible strains. |
| 用法、用量<br>Dosages | 口服：一日50 ~ 100mg/kg，分成4次空腹服用；儿童一日50 ~ 100mg/kg，分成4次。<br>肌内注射：1次0.5 ~ 1g，一日4次；儿童一日50 ~ 100mg/kg，分成4次。<br>静脉滴注：1次1 ~ 2g，必要时可用到3g，溶于100ml输液中，滴注0.5 ~ 1小时，一日2 ~ 4次，必要时每4小时1次；儿童一日100 ~ 150mg/kg，分4次给予。<br>Oral medication: give daily 50 ~ 100mg/kg in divided four doses on an empty stomach; for children, give daily 50 ~ 100mg/kg in divided four doses. Intramuscular injection: the single 0.5 ~ 1g, 4 times a day; for children, give daily 50 ~ 100mg/kg in divided four doses.<br>Intravenous infusion: the single dose is 1 ~ 2g, or 3g if necessary. Dissolve it in 100ml infusion, give 2 to 4 times or once every 4 hours a day if necessary, and each infusion time should be within 0.5 to 1 hour; for children, give daily 100 ~ 150mg / kg in divided 4 doses. |
| 剂型、规格<br>Preparations | 胶囊剂：每胶囊0.25g。<br>注射用氨苄西林钠：每瓶0.5g；1.0g。<br><br>Capsules: 0.25g per capsule.<br>Ampicillin sodium for injection: 0.5g, 1.0g per vial. |
| 药品名称 Drug Names | 阿莫西林 Amoxicillin |
| 适应证<br>Indications | 常用于敏感菌所致的呼吸道、尿路和胆道感染以及伤寒等。<br>It is commonly used to treat infection of respiratory tract, urinary tract and biliary tract, as well as typhoid, which are all caused by susceptible strains. |
| 用法、用量<br>Dosage | 口服：成人每日1 ~ 4g，分3 ~ 4次服。儿童每日50 ~ 100mg/kg，分3 ~ 4次服。肾功能严重不足者，应延长用药间隔时间；肾小球滤过率（GFR）为10 ~ 30ml/min者，每12小时给药1次；<10ml/min者，每24小时给药1次。<br>Oral medication: for adults, give daily 1 ~ 4g, in divided 3 to 4 doses; for children, give daily 50~100mg/kg, in divided 3 to 4 doses. While for severe renal insufficiency patients, the interval should be extended; for patients whose glomerular filtration rate (GFR) was 10 ~ 30ml/min, give once every 12 hours, and the ones with less than 10ml/min GFR, every 24 hours. |
| 剂型、规格<br>Preparations | 片剂（胶囊）：每片（粒）0.125g；0.25g（效价）。<br>Tablets (capsules): 0.125g, 0.25g (titer) per tablet (capsule). |
| 药品名称 Drug Names | 哌拉西林钠 Piperacillin Sodium |
| 适应证<br>Indications | 临床上用于上述敏感菌中所引起的感染（对中枢感染疗效不确切）。<br>It is clinically used to treat the above mentioned infection caused by susceptible strains (efficacy for the central nervous system infection remains uncertainty). |

**续　表**

| 用法、用量<br>Dosage | 尿路感染，1 次 1g，一日 4 次，肌内注射或静脉注射。<br>　其他部位（呼吸道、腹腔、胆道等）感染：一日 4 ～ 12g，分 3 ～ 4 次静脉注射或静脉滴注。严重感染一日可用 10 ～ 24g。<br>　Urinary tract infection: give 1g per time, 4 times a day, by intramuscular injection or intravenous injection.<br>　Infection of other parts (respiratory tract, abdominal cavity, biliary tract, etc.): give daily 4 ～ 12g, in divided 3 to 4 doses, by intravenous injection or intravenous infusion. Dosage of 10 ～ 24g a day can be administered in serious infection case. . |
|---|---|
| 剂型、规格<br>Preparations | 注射用哌拉西林钠：每瓶 0.5g；1.0g（效价）。<br>Piperacillin Sodium for Injection: 0.5g, 1.0g (titer) per vial. |
| **药品名称 Drug Names** | 替卡西林 Ticarcillin |
| 适应证<br>Indications | 主要用于革兰阴性菌感染，包括变形杆菌、大肠埃希菌、肠杆菌属、淋球菌、流感杆菌等所致全身感染，对尿路感染的效果好。对于铜绿假单胞菌感染，常需与氨基糖苷类抗生素联合应用。本品不耐酶，对 MRSA 也无效。<br>　It is mainly used to treat Gram-negative bacterial infection, as well as systemic infection caused by Proteus, E. coli, Enterobacter, Neisseria gonorrhoeae, Haemophilus influenzae, etc. Besides, it is of good efficacy for urinary tract infection treatment. In the treatment of Pseudomonas aeruginosa infection, it is often used in combination with aminoglycosides. This product is resistant to the enzyme, so it is ineffective against MRSA. |
| 用法、用量<br>Dosage | 成人一日 200 ～ 300mg/kg，分次给予或 1 次 3g，根据病情，每 3、4 或 6 小时 1 次。按每 1g 药物用 4ml 溶剂溶解后缓缓静脉注射或加入适量溶剂中静脉滴注 0.5 ～ 1 小时。泌尿系统感染可肌内注射给药，1 次 1g，每日 4 次，用 0.25% ～ 0.5% 利多卡因注射液 2 ～ 3ml 溶解后深部肌内注射。<br>　儿童一日为 200 ～ 300mg/kg。婴儿一日为 225mg/kg，7 日龄以下婴儿则一日 150mg/kg，均分 3 次给予。<br>　For adults, give 200 ～ 300mg/kg per day in divided doses or 3g per time, every 4 or 6 hours according to patients' conditions. Dissolve every 1g of the drug in 4ml solvent for slowly intravenous injection, or add appropriate amount of solvent for intravenous infusion, lasting 0.5 to 1 hour. Urinary tract infection can be administered intramuscularly, 1g per time, 4 times a day, by using 2 ～ 3ml of the 0.25% to 0.5% lidocaine solution to dissolve the drug for deep intramuscular injection.<br>　For children, give daily 200 ～ 300mg/kg. For infants, give daily 225mg/kg, while for infants born less than 7days, give daily 150mg/kg in equally 3 divided doses. |
| 剂型、规格<br>Preparations | 注射用替卡西林钠：每瓶 1g；3g；6g（效价）。<br>Ticarcillin sodium for injection: 1g, 3g, 6g (titer) per vial. |
| **药品名称 Drug Names** | 美洛西林钠 Mezlocillin Sodium |
| 适应证<br>Indications | 本品主要用于一些革兰阴性病原菌，如假单胞菌、克雷伯菌、肠杆菌属、沙雷菌、变形杆菌、大肠埃希菌、嗜血杆菌，以及拟杆菌和其他一些厌氧菌（包括革兰阳性的粪链球菌）所致的下呼吸道、腹腔、胆道、尿路、妇科、皮肤及软组织部位感染以及败血症。<br>　This product is mainly used for infection of lower respiratory tract, abdominal cavity, biliary tract, urinary tract, gynecology, skin and soft tissue and septicaemia caused by some Gram-negative pathogens such as Pseudomonas, Klebsiella, Enterobacter, Serratia, Proteus, E. coli, Haemophilus, and as well as Bacteroides and other anaerobes (including gram-positive Streptococcus faecalis). |
| 用法、用量<br>Dosage | 用氯化钠液、葡萄糖液或乳酸钠林格液溶解后静脉注射或静脉滴注，也可肌内注射给药。<br>　成人一般感染每日 150 ～ 200mg/kg，或每次 2 ～ 3g，每 6 小时 1 次；重症感染每日 200 ～ 300mg/kg，或每次 3g，每 4 小时 1 次；极重感染可用到每日 24g 分 6 次用；淋球菌尿道炎，1 ～ 2g，只用 1 次，用前 0.5 小时服用丙磺舒 1g。<br>　新生儿用量：≤ 7 日龄者，每日 150mg/kg 或 75mg/kg，每 12 小时 1 次。> 7 日龄者，根据体重不同可按每日 225 ～ 300mg/kg，或每次 75mg/kg，每日 3 ～ 4 次。肾功能受损者：肌酐清除率 >30ml/min 者，可按正常用量；10 ～ 30ml/min 者，按疾病轻重每次 1.5 ～ 3g，每 8 小时 1 次；<10ml/min 者，用 1.5g，每 8 小时 1 次，重症可用到 2g，每 8 小时 1 次。 |

**续　表**

| | 手术预防感染给药：每次 4g，与术前 1 小时及术后 6 ~ 12 小时各给药 1 次。 |
|---|---|
| | Dissolve the drug by solutions of Sodium chloride, glucose or Ringer lactate for intravenous injection or intravenous infusion. |
| | Administering intramuscularly is also allowed. For adults with moderate infection, give daily 150 ~ 200mg/kg, or 2 ~ 3g singly, every 6 hours; for ones with severe infection, give daily 200 ~ 300mg/kg, or 3g singly, every 4 hours; while if the patients are infected extremely severe, give daily 24g in 6 doses. For patients infected gonococcal urethritis, give 1 ~ 2g singly for only once, with 1g probenecid half an hour before taking. |
| | For newborns less than 7 days, give daily 150mg/kg or 75mg/kg, every 12 hours; for ones more than 7 days, give daily 225 ~ 300mg/kg, or every 75mg/kg singly, 3 to 4 times a day according to body weight. For patients of impaired renal function: if the creatinine clearance rate is more than 30ml/min, give them normal dosage; if the rate is 10 ~ 30ml/min, give them 1.5 ~ 3g singly, every 8 hours according to patients' conditions; if the rate is less than10ml/min, give them 1.5 g singly, every 8 hours, or 2g, every 8 hours for severe ones. |
| | Surgery to prevent infection administration: 4g singly, both an hour before surgery and 6 to 12 hours after it. |
| 剂型、规格<br>Preparations | 粉针剂：每瓶 1g。<br>Powder injection: 1g of each. |
| **药品名称 Drug Names** | 阿洛西林钠 Azlocillin Sodium |
| 适应证<br>Indications | 主要用于铜绿假单胞菌与其他革兰阴性菌所致的系统感染，如败血症、脑膜炎、肺炎及尿路和软组织感染。必要时可与氨基糖苷类联合以加强抗铜绿假单胞菌的作用。<br><br>It is mainly used to treat system infection caused by Pseudomonas aeruginosa and other Gram-negative bacteria, such as Septicemia, meningitis, pneumonia, urinary tract infection and soft tissue infection. It is used in combination with the aminoglycoside if necessary, to strengthen the function of anti-Pseudomonas aeruginosa. |
| 用法、用量<br>Dosage | 尿路感染：每日 50 ~ 100mg/kg；重症感染，成人每日 200 ~ 250mg/kg，儿童每日 50 ~ 150mg/kg。<br><br>以上量分 4 次，静脉注射或静脉滴注，也可肌内注射给予。可用氯化钠注射液、葡萄糖液或乳酸钠林格液溶解后给予，也可加入墨菲管中，随输液进入（但要掌握速度，不宜过快）。<br><br>Urinary tract infection: give daily 50 ~ 100mg/kg; Severe infection: for adults, give daily 200 ~ 250mg/kg; for children, give daily 50 ~ 150mg/kg.<br><br>Both adults and children are administered in 4 divided doses by intravenous injection, intravenous infusion or intramuscular injection. The drug can be either dissolved by Sodium Chloride Injection, Ringer lactate solution or glucose for usage or added into Murphy tube for the infusion (but the speed should not be too fast). |
| 剂型、规格<br>Preparations | 粉针剂：每支 2g；3g；4g。<br>Powder injection: 2g, 3g, 4g of each. |
| **药品名称 Drug Names** | 磺苄西林钠 Sulbenicillin Sodium |
| 适应证<br>Indications | 临床上用于敏感的铜绿假单胞菌、某些变形杆菌属，以及其他敏感革兰阴性菌所致肺炎、尿路感染、复杂性皮肤软组织感染和败血症等。对本品敏感菌所致腹腔感染、盆腔感染宜与抗厌氧菌药物联合应用。<br><br>It is clinically used for pneumonia, urinary infection, complicated skin and soft tissue infection, Septicemia and etc. caused by sensitive Pseudomonas aeruginosa, some Proteus and other sensitive gram-negative bacteria. In the treatment of abdominal infection and pelvic infection caused by bacteria which are susceptible this drug, it should be used in combination with anti-anaerobic drugs. |
| 用法、用量<br>Dosage | 中度感染，成人一日 8g，重症感染或铜绿假单胞菌感染时剂量需增至一日 20g，分 4 次静脉滴注或静脉注射；儿童根据病情每日剂量按 80 ~ 300mg/kg，分 4 次给药。<br><br>For adults with moderate infection, give daily 8g; infection, for adults with severe infection or Pseudomonas aeruginosa infection, the dosage should be increased to 20g by 4 divided intravenous infusion or intravenous injection. For children, give daily 80 ~ 300mg/kg, in 4 divided doses. |
| 剂型、规格<br>Preparations | 注射用磺苄西林钠：每瓶 1.0g；2g；4g。<br>Sulbenicillin sodium for injection: 1.0g, 2g, 4g per vial. |

**续　表**

| 药品名称 Drug Names | 阿帕西林钠 Apalcillin Sodium |
|---|---|
| 适应证<br>Indications | 临床可用于敏感革兰阳性或阴性菌感染，如呼吸道、尿路、胆道、妇科感染，也可用于术后感染和五官科感染的治疗。<br><br>It is clinically used to treat sensitive gram-positive or-negative bacterial infection, such as respiratory infection, urinary tract infection, biliary tractinfection and gynecological infection, as well as postoperative infection and ENT infection. |
| 用法、用量<br>Dosage | 成人 1 次 2 ～ 3g，一日 3 次，肌内或静脉给药。10 岁以下儿童，一日 60 ～ 220mg/kg，分 3 ～ 4 次静脉滴注。10 岁以上儿童剂量同成人。<br><br>For adults, give 2 ～ 3g singly, 3 to 4 times a day, by intramuscular or intravenous administration. For children under the age of 10, give daily 60 ～ 220mg/kg in 3 to 4 divided doses by intravenous infusion. For children over the age of 10, give the same dosage as adults. |
| 剂型、规格<br>Preparations | 注射用阿帕西林钠：每瓶 1g；3g。<br>Apalcillin sodium for injection: 1g, 3g per vial. |

## 1.2　头孢菌素类 Cephalosporins

| 药品名称 Drug Names | 头孢氨苄 Cefalexin |
|---|---|
| 适应证<br>Indications | 用于敏感菌所致的呼吸道、泌尿道、皮肤和软组织、生殖器官（包括前列腺）等部位的感染，也常用于中耳炎。<br><br>It is used to treat infection of respiratory tract, urinary tract, skin and soft tissue, reproductive organs (including prostate) and other parts caused by susceptible strains. It is also commonly used for treatment of otitis media. |
| 用法、用量<br>Dosage | 成人：一日 1 ～ 2g，分 3 ～ 4 次服用，空腹服用。小儿：一日 25 ～ 50mg/kg，分 3 ～ 4 次服用。<br><br>For adults, give daily 1 ～ 2g in 3 to 4 divided doses, on an empty stomach. For children, give daily 25 ～ 50mg/kg in 3 to 4 divided doses a. |
| 剂型、规格<br>Preparations | 片（胶囊）剂：每片（粒）0.125g；0.25g。<br>颗粒剂：1g 含药 50mg。<br>Tablets (capsules): 0.125g, 0.25g per tablet (capsule).<br>Granules: 50mg of Cefalexin contained in1g of the drug. |

| 药品名称 Drug Names | 头孢唑林钠 Cefazolin Sodium |
|---|---|
| 适应证<br>Indications | 用于敏感菌所致的呼吸道、泌尿生殖系、皮肤软组织、骨和关节、胆道等感染，也可用于心内膜炎、败血症、咽和耳部感染。<br><br>It is intended to treat infection of respiratory tract, urogenital system, skin and soft tissue, bone and joint, biliary tract and other infection caused by susceptible strains, as well as endocarditis, septicemia, throat infection and ear infection. |
| 用法、用量<br>Dosage | 肌内注射或静脉注射，1 次 0.5 ～ 1g，一日 3 ～ 4 次。革兰阳性菌所致轻度感染一日 0.5g，一日 2 ～ 3 次；中度或重症感染：1 次 0.5 ～ 1g，一日 3 ～ 4 次；极重感染：1 次 1 ～ 1.5g，一日 4 次。泌尿系统感染：1 次 1g，一日 2 次。儿童一日量为：20 ～ 40mg/kg，分 3 ～ 4 次给予；重症可用到一日 100mg/kg。新生儿 1 次不超过 20mg/kg，一日 2 次。<br><br>Intramuscular or intravenous injection: give 0.5 ～ 1g singly, 3 to 4 times a day. For mild Gram-positive bacteria infected adults, give 0.5g singly, 2 to 3 times a day; for moderate or severe infected ones, give 0.5 ～ 1g singly, 3 to 4 times a day; for extremely severe infected ones, give 1 ～ 1.5g singly, 4 times a day. Urinary tract infection: 1g per time, 2 times a day. For children, give 20 ～ 40mg/kg a day, in 3 to 4 divided doses; and the severe ones can be administered 100mg/kg a day. For newborns, single does can not exceed 20mg/kg, 2 times a day. |
| 剂型、规格<br>Preparations | 注射用头孢唑林钠：每瓶 0.5g；1g；2g。<br>Cefazolin Sodium for Injection: 0.5g, 1g, 2g per vial. |

| 药品名称 Drug Names | 头孢羟氨苄 Cefadroxil |
|---|---|
| 适应证<br>Indications | 用于呼吸道、泌尿道、咽部、皮肤等部位敏感菌感染。<br><br>It is intended to treat infection of respiratory tract, urinary tract, throat, skin and etc. caused by susceptible strains. |

| 用法、用量<br>Dosage | 成人平均用量：一日 1 ~ 2g，分 2 ~ 3 次口服，泌尿道感染时，也可 1 次服下。小儿一日量 50mg/kg，分 2 次服用。<br><br>肾功能不全者，首次服 1g，以后按肌酐清除率制订给药方案：肌酐清除率为 25 ~ 50ml/min 者，每 12 小时服 0.5g；10 ~ 25ml/min 者，每 24 小时服 0.5g；<10ml/min 者，每 36 小时服 0.5g。<br><br>The average dosage for adults is 1 ~ 2g a day in 2 to 3 divided doses orally, while the urinary tract infected adults can take all for once. For children, give 50mg/kg a day, in 2 divided doses.<br><br>For Renal insufficiency patients, give 1g for the first time, and the afterward administration should depend on the creatinine clearance rate. If the rate is 25 ~ 50ml/min, give 0.5g every 12 hours; if the rate is 10 ~ 25ml/min, give 0.5g every 24 hours ; if the rate is less than10ml/min, give 0.5g every 36 hours. |
|---|---|
| 剂型、规格<br>Preparations | 片剂（胶囊剂）：每片（粒）0.125g；0.25g。<br>Tablets (capsules): 0.125g, 0.25g per tablet (capsule). |
| 药品名称 Drug Names | 头孢拉定 Cefradine |
| 适应证<br>Indications | 用于呼吸道、泌尿道、咽部、皮肤等部位的敏感菌感染，注射剂也可用于败血症和骨感染。<br><br>It is intended to treat infection of respiratory tract, urinary tract, throat, skin and other parts caused by susceptible strains, and the injection can be used for Septicemia and bone infection. |
| 用法、用量<br>Dosage | 口服：成人一日 1 ~ 2g，分 3 ~ 4 次服用。小儿每日 25 ~ 50mg/kg，分 3 ~ 4 次服用。<br>肌内注射、静脉注射或滴注：成人一日 2 ~ 4g，分 4 次注射。小儿每日 50 ~ 100mg/kg，分 4 次注射。<br>肾功能不全者按患者肌酐清除率制订给药方案：肌酐清除率为 >20ml/min 者，每 6 小时服 500mg；15 ~ 20ml/min 者，每 6 小时服 250mg；<15ml/min 者，每 12 小时服 250mg。<br><br>Oral medication: for adults, give 1 ~ 2g a day, in 3 to 4 divided doses; for children, give 25 ~ 50mg/kg a day, in 3 to 4 divided doses.<br><br>Intramuscular injection or intravenous infusion: for adults, give 2 ~ 4g a day, in 4 divided doses; for children, give 50 ~ 100mg/kg a day, in 5 divided doses.<br><br>Renal dysfunction patients should be administered by creatinine clearance rate: if the c rate is more than 20ml/min, give 500mg every 6 hours; if the rate is 15 ~ 20ml/min, give 250mg every 6 hours; if the rate is less than 15ml/min, give 250mg every 12 hours. |
| 剂型、规格<br>Preparations | 胶囊剂：每粒 0.25g；0.5g。<br>干混悬剂：0.125g；0.25g。<br>注射用头孢拉定（添加碳酸钠）：每瓶 0.5g；1g。<br>注射用头孢拉定 A（添加精氨酸）：每瓶 0.5g；1g。<br><br>Capsules: 0.25g, 0.5g per capsule.<br>Suspension: 0.125g, 0.25g.<br>Cefradine for njection (sodium carbonate added): 0.5g, 1g per vial.<br>Cefradine A for injection (arginine added): 0.5g, 1g per vial. |
| 药品名称 Drug Names | 头孢呋辛钠 Cefuroxime Sodium |
| 适应证<br>Indications | 临床应用于敏感的革兰阴性菌所致的下呼吸道、泌尿系统、皮肤和软组织、骨和关节、女性生殖器等部位的感染。对败血症、脑膜炎也有效。<br><br>It is clinically intended to treat infection of the lower respiratory tract, urinary tract, skin and soft tissues, bones and joints, female genitals and etc. caused by sensitive Glenn negative bacteria. It is also effective in treatment of Septicemia meningitis. |
| 用法、用量<br>Dosage | 肌内注射或静脉注射，成人：1 次 750 ~ 1500mg，一日 3 次；对严重感染，可按 1 次 1500mg，一日 4 次。应用于脑膜炎，一日剂量在 9g 以下。儿童：平均一日量为 60mg/kg，严重感染可用到 100mg/kg，分 3 ~ 4 次给予。<br><br>肾功能不全者按患者肌酐清除率制订给药方案：肌酐清除率为 >20ml/min 者，每日 3 次，每次 0.75 ~ 1.5g；10 ~ 20ml/min 者，每次 0.75g，一日 2 次；<10ml/min 者，每次 0.75g，一日 1 次。<br><br>肌内注射：1 次用 0.75g，加注射用水 3ml，振摇使成混悬液，用粗针头做深部肌内注射。 |

**续　表**

| | |
|---|---|
| | 　　静脉给药：每 0.75g 本品，用注射用水约 10ml，使溶解成澄明溶液，缓慢静脉注射或加到墨菲管中随输液滴入。<br><br>　　Intramuscular injection or intravenous injection: for adults, give 750 ~ 1500mg singly, 3 times a day; for severely infected ones, give 1500mg singly, 4 times a day; in treatment of meningitis, the daily maximum dose is 9g; for children, give 60mg/kg on average, or 100mg/kg a day in 3 to 4 divided doses for the severely infected.<br><br>　　The administration to renal insufficiency patients should depend on the creatinine clearance: creatinine clearance > 20ml/min, 0.75 ~ 1.5g singly, 3 times a day; creatinine clearance =10 ~ 20ml/min, 0.75g singly, twice a day; creatinine clearance <10ml/min, 0.75g singly, once a day.<br><br>　　Intramuscular injection: give 0.75g singly; add 3ml water for injection into the drug, shake it into a suspension, and make the deep intramuscular injection with a thick needle.<br><br>　　Intravenous administration: dissolve every 0.75g of the drug into approximately 10ml water for injection and make it into a clear solution for slow intravenous injection or add into Murphy tube for infusion. |
| 剂型、规格<br>Preparations | 注射用头孢呋辛钠：每瓶 0.75g；1.5g。<br>Cefuroxime Sodium for Injection: 0.75g, 1.5g per vial. |
| 药品名称 Drug Names | 头孢呋辛酯 Cefuroxime Axetil |
| 适应证<br>Indications | 临床用用于敏感菌所致的上、下呼吸道及泌尿系统、皮肤和软组织等部位的感染。<br><br>　　It is clinically intended to treat infection of lower respiratory tract, urinary tract, skin and soft tissue and etc. caused by susceptible strains. |
| 用法、用量<br>Dosage | 成人每次口服 250mg，1 日 2 次，重症可用到每次 500mg。儿童每次 125mg，1 日 2 次。一般疗程为 7 日。<br><br>　　For adults, give orally 250mg each time, twice a day; for the severe infected ones, give 500mg singly. For children, give 125mg singly, twice a day. The general course of treatment is 7 days. |
| 剂型、规格<br>Preparations | 片剂（薄膜衣片）：每片 125mg；250mg。<br>Tablets (film coated): 125mg, 250mg per tablet. |
| 药品名称 Drug Names | 头孢克洛 Cefaclor |
| 适应证<br>Indications | 用于敏感菌所致的呼吸道、泌尿道和皮肤、软组织感染，以及中耳炎等。<br><br>　　It is intended to treat infection of respiratory tract, urinary tract, skin and soft tissues caused by susceptible strains mentioned above, as well as otitis media. |
| 用法、用量<br>Dosage | 成人口服常用量为 250mg，每 8 小时 1 次。重症或微生物敏感性较差时，剂量可加倍，但一日量不可超过 4g。儿童：一日口服剂量为 20mg/kg，分 3 次（每 8 小时 1 次）；重症可按一日 40mg/kg 给予，但一日量不超过 1g。<br><br>　　For adults, the usual oral dose is 250mg, once every 8 hours. And for severe patients or when the microbial sensitivity is poor, the dose could be doubled, but the daily maximum dose can not exceed 4g. For children, the daily oral dose is 20mg/kg, in 3 divided doses.(every 8 hours). And for the severe, give 40mg/kg a day, but the daily maximum dose can not exceed 1g |
| 剂型、规格<br>Preparations | 胶囊剂（片剂）：每粒（片）0.125g；0.25g。<br>干混悬剂：0.125g；1.5g。<br>Capsules (tablets): 0.125g, 0.25g per capsule (tablet).<br>Suspension: 0.125g, 1.5g. |
| 药品名称 Drug Names | 头孢噻肟钠 Cefotaxime Sodium |
| 适应证<br>Indications | 用于敏感菌所致的呼吸道、泌尿道、骨和关节、皮肤和软组织、腹腔、胆道、消化道、五官、生殖器等部位的感染，对烧伤、外伤引起的感染以及败血症、中枢感染也有效。<br><br>　　It is intended to treat infection of respiratory tract, urinary tract, bone and joints, skin and soft tissue, abdominal cavity, biliary tract, digestive tract, facial features, genitals and etc. caused by susceptible strains. It is also effective in treatment of infection in burn and trauma, Septicemia and central nervous system infection. |

| 用法、用量<br>Dosage | 临用前，加灭菌注射用水使溶解，溶解后立即使用。<br><br>成人：肌内或静脉注射，1 次 0.5 ~ 1g，一日 2 ~ 4 次。一般感染用 2g/d，分成 2 次肌内注射或静脉注射；中等或较重感染 3 ~ 6g/d，分为 3 次肌内注射或静脉注射；败血症等 6 ~ 8g/d，分为 3 ~ 4 次静脉给药，极重感染一日不超过 12g，分为 6 次静脉给药；淋病用 1g 肌内注射（单次给药已足）。静脉滴注，2 ~ 3g/d。<br><br>小儿：肌内注射或静脉注射一日量为 50 ~ 100mg/kg，分成 2 ~ 3 次给予。婴幼儿不能肌内注射。<br><br>Before being used, the drug should be dissolved by sterile water for injection. And then put it into use immediately after the dissolution.<br><br>For adults, give 0.5 ~ 1g singly, 2 to 4 times a day by intramuscular or intravenous injection. General infection: 2g a day in 2 divided doses; Moderate or severe infection: 3 ~ 6g a day in 3 divided doses. Septicemia: 6 ~ 8g a day in 3 to 4 divided doses intravenously; severe Septicemia patients: 12g maximum a day in 6 divided doses intravenously. Gonorrhea: 1g, intramuscular injection (single dose is enough).<br><br>Intravenous infusion: 2 ~ 3g a day for children, give daily 50 ~ 100mg/kg in divided 2 to 3 doses by intramuscular injection or intravenous injection. Infants can not be administered by intramuscular injection. |
| --- | --- |
| 剂型、规格<br>Preparations | 注射用头孢噻肟钠：每瓶 0.5g；1g；2g。<br>Cefotaxime sodium for injection: 0.5g, 1g, 2g per vial. |
| 药品名称 Drug Names | 头孢匹胺钠 Cefpiramide Sodium |
| 适应证<br>Indications | 用于敏感菌所致的下呼吸道、胆道、泌尿道、生殖系统、皮肤和软组织等部位的感染及败血症，腹腔炎时与甲硝唑或克林霉素合用。<br><br>It is used in combination with metronidazole or clindamycin in treating infection of lower respiratory tract, biliary tract, urinary tract, reproductive system, skin and soft tissue, etc. caused by susceptible strains, as well as, sepsis and abdominal inflammation. |
| 用法、用量<br>Dosage | 成人：轻中度感染，口服，一日 1 ~ 2g，分 2 次给予；肌内注射，用 0.5% ~ 1% 利多卡因注射液作为溶剂，进行深部肌内注射；静脉注射，溶于 5% 的葡萄糖注射液或 0.9% 氯化钠注射液中，缓慢滴注 30 ~ 60 分钟。重度感染，一日剂量 4g，用法同上。<br><br>儿童：静脉给药，轻中度感染，一日 20 ~ 80mg/kg，分成 2 ~ 3 次给予；重度感染，一日剂量增至 150mg/kg，分 2 ~ 3 次缓慢静脉注射或静脉滴注。<br><br>For mild and moderate infected adults: give 1 ~ 2g a day in 2 divided doses for oral medication; dissolve the drug in 0.5% to 1% lidocaine injection for deep intramuscular injection; dissolve the drug in 5 % dextrose injection or 0.9% sodium chloride injection for slowly intravenous injection, lasting 30 to 60 minutes. For Severe infected ones. Give 4g a day by the usage mentioned above.<br><br>For children, give intravenous administration: the mild to moderate infected, 20 ~ 80mg/kg a day in 2 or 3 divided doses; the severe infected, 150mg/kg a day for an increase, in 2 to 3 doses, by slow intravenous injection or intravenous infusion . |
| 剂型、规格<br>Preparations | 注射用头孢匹胺钠：每瓶 0.5g；1g。<br>Cefpiramide for injection: 0.5g, 1g per vial. |
| 药品名称 Drug Names | 头孢曲松钠 Ceftriaxone Sodium |
| 适应证<br>Indications | 对罗氏芬敏感的致病菌引起的感染，如脓毒血症，脑膜炎，播散性莱姆病（早、晚期），腹部感染（腹膜炎、胆道及胃肠道感染），骨、关节、软组织、皮肤及伤口感染，免疫力低下病人之感染，肾脏及泌尿道感染，呼吸道感染，尤其是肺炎、耳鼻咽喉感染，生殖系统感染，包括淋病，术前预防感染。<br><br>It is intended to treat infection caused by Pathogens which are susceptible to Ceftriaxone, such as septicemia, meningitis, disseminated Lyme disease (early and terminal), abdominal infection (peritonitis, biliary tract infection and gastrointestinal infection), infection of bones, joints, soft tissue, skin and wound, infection of patients with low immune mechanism, infection of kidneys and urinary tract, respiratory tract infection especially pneumonia and ENT infections, reproductive tract infection, as well as gonorrhea and infection of preoperative prevention. |

**续　表**

| 用法、用量<br>Dosage | 　　一般感染，每日 1g，1 次肌内注射或静脉注射。严重感染，每日 2g，分 2 次给予。<br>　　脑膜炎，可按一日 100mg/kg（但总量不超过 4g），分 2 次给予。淋病，单次用药 250mg 即足。儿童用量一般按成人量的 1/2 给予。<br>　　肌内注射：将 1 次药量溶于适量 0.5% 盐酸利多卡因注射液中做深部肌内注射。<br>　　静脉注射：按 1g 药物用 10ml 灭菌注射用水溶解，缓缓注入，历时 2 ~ 4 分钟。<br>　　静脉滴注：成人 1 次量 1g 或一日量 2g，溶于等渗氯化钠注射液或 5% ~ 10% 葡萄糖液 50 ~ 100ml 中，于 0.5 ~ 1 小时滴入。<br>　　General infection: give1g a day, once only, by intramuscular injection or intravenous injection. Severe infection: give 2g a day, in 2 divided doses.<br>　　Meningitis: give 100mg/kg a day (but the maximum total does can not exceed 4g), in 2 divided doses. Gonorrhea: a single dose of 250mg is enough. For children, give half of the adult dose.<br>　　Intramuscular injection: dissolve1 single dose in 0.5% lidocaine hydrochloride injection for deep intramuscular injection.<br>　　Intravenous injection: dissolve every 1g of the drug in 10ml sterile water for slowly injection, lasting 2 to 4 minutes.<br>　　Intravenous infusion: give adults 1g singly or 2g a day; dissolve the drug in isotonic sodium chloride injection or 50 ~ 100ml of 5% ~ 10% glucose solution for infusion lasting 0.5 to 1 hour. |
| 剂型、规格<br>Preparations | 　　注射用头孢曲松钠：每瓶 0.5g；1g；2g。<br>　　Ceftriaxone for injection: 0.5g, 1g, 2g per vial. |
| **药品名称 Drug Names** | **头孢哌酮钠 Cefoperazone Sodium** |
| 适应证<br>Indications | 　　用于各种敏感菌所致的呼吸道、泌尿道、腹膜、胸膜、皮肤和软组织、骨和关节、五官等部位的感染，还可用于败血症和脑膜炎等。<br>　　It is intended to treat infection of respiratory tract, urinary tract, peritoneum, pleura, skin and soft tissues, bones and joints, facial features and etc., caused by a variety of susceptible strains, as well as septicemia and meningitis. |
| 用法、用量<br>Dosage | 　　肌内或静脉注射，成人 1 次 1 ~ 2g，一日 2 ~ 4g。严重感染，1 次 2 ~ 4g，一日 6 ~ 8g。小儿每日 50 ~ 100mg/kg，分 2 ~ 4 次注射。<br>　　Intramuscular or intravenous injection: for adults, give 1g ~ 2g singly, 2g ~ 4g a day; for the severe infected, give 2g ~ 4g singly, 6g ~ 8g a day; for children, give 50 ~ 100mg/kg a day, in 2 to 4 divided doses of injections. |
| 剂型、规格<br>Preparations | 　　注射用头孢哌酮钠：每瓶 0.5g；1g；2g。<br>　　注射用头孢哌酮钠 / 舒巴坦（1 ：1；2 ：1；4 ：1；8 ：1）。<br>　　Cefoperazone Sodium for injection: 0.5g, 1g, 2g per vial.<br>　　Cefoperazone Sodium / sulbactam for injection :(1 ：1; 2 ：1; 4 ：1; 8 ：1). |
| **药品名称 Drug Names** | **头孢他啶 Ceftazidime** |
| 适应证<br>Indications | 　　用于革兰阴性菌的敏感菌所致的下呼吸道、皮肤和软组织、骨和关节、胸腔、腹腔、泌尿生殖系及中枢等部位感染，也用于败血症。<br>　　It is intended to treat infection of lower respiratory tract, skin and soft tissues, bones and joints, thoracic cavity, abdominal cavity, urogenital system, central nervous system and etc. caused by sensitive strains of Gram-negative bacteria, as well as septicemia. |
| 用法、用量<br>Dosage | 　　轻症一日剂量为 1g，分 2 次肌内注射。<br>　　中度感染一次 1g，一日 2 ~ 3 次肌内注射或静脉注射。<br>　　重症一次 2g，一日 2 ~ 3 次，肌内注射或静脉注射。<br>　　本品可加入氯化钠注射液、5% ~ 10% 葡萄糖注射液、含乳酸钠的输液、右旋糖酐输液中。<br>　　Mild infection: 1g a day, in 2 divided doses, by intramuscular injection<br>　　Moderate infection: 1g singly, 2 or 3 times a day, by intramuscular injection or intravenous injection<br>　　Severe infection: 2g singly, two or three times a day, by intramuscular injection or intravenous injection<br>　　Sodium chloride injection, 5% to 10% glucose injection, infusion with sodium lactate, dextran infusion can be added into the drug. |

**续 表**

| 剂型、规格<br>Preparations | 注射用头孢他啶：每瓶 1g；2g。<br>Ceftazidime for injection: 1g, 2g per vial. |
|---|---|
| **药品名称 Drug Names** | **头孢美唑钠 Cefmetazole Sodium** |
| 适应证<br>Indications | 用于葡萄球菌、大肠埃希菌、克雷伯杆菌、吲哚阴性和阳性杆菌、拟杆菌等微生物的敏感菌株所致的肺炎、支气管炎、胆道感染、腹膜炎、泌尿系统感染、子宫及附件感染等。<br><br>It is intended to treat pneumonia, bronchitis, biliary tract infection, peritonitis, urinary tract infection, uterine and accessories infection, etc. caused by susceptible strains of microorganisms, such as staphylococcus aureus, Escherichia coli, Klebsiella, indole negative and positive bacteria, Bacteroides and etc. |
| 用法、用量<br>Dosage | 成人，一日 1～2g，分 2 次静脉注射或静脉滴注。小儿，一日 25～100mg/kg，分 2～4 次静脉注射或者静脉滴注。重症或顽症时，成人可用到一日 4g，儿童可用到一日 150mg/kg。溶剂可选用等渗氯化钠注射液或 5% 葡萄糖液，静脉注射时还可用灭菌注射用水（但不可用于滴注，因渗透压过低）。<br><br>For adults, give 1～2g a day, in 2 divided doses, by intravenous injection or intravenous infusion. For children, give 25～100mg/kg a day, in 2 to 4 divided doses, by intravenous injection or intravenous infusion. Severe infection or stubborn and chronic disease: give adults 4g a day and children 150mg/kg a day. The solvent could be isotonic sodium chloride injection or 5% glucose solution, and sterile water for injection is available for intravenous infusion (but not for infusion because of low osmotic pressure). |
| 剂型、规格<br>Preparations | 注射用头孢美唑钠：每瓶 0.25g；0.5g；1g；2g（效价）。<br>Cefmetazole Sodium for injection: 0.25, 0.5g, 1g, 2g (titer) per vial. |
| **药品名称 Drug Names** | **头孢克肟 Cefixime** |
| 适应证<br>Indications | 用于上述敏感菌所引起的肺炎、支气管炎、泌尿道炎、淋病、胆囊炎、胆管炎、猩红热、中耳炎、副鼻窦炎。<br><br>It is intended to treat pneumonia, bronchitis, urethritis, gonorrhea, cholecystitis, cholangitis, scarlet fever, otitis media and sinusitis caused by susceptible strains mentioned above. |
| 用法、用量<br>Dosage | 成人及体重为 30kg 以上的儿童：1 次 50～100mg，一日 2 次；重症 1 次口服量可增至 200mg。体重为 30kg 以下的儿童：1 次 1.5～3mg/kg，一日 2 次；重症 1 次量可增至 6mg/kg。<br><br>For adults and children over 30kg: give 50～100mg singly, two times a day; the severe infected can be given an increased dose of 200mg orally.<br><br>For children under 30kg: give 1.5～3mg/kg singly, twice a day; the severe infected can be given an increased dose of 6mg/kg. |
| 剂型、规格<br>Preparations | 胶囊剂：每粒 50mg 或 100mg；<br>颗粒：每 1g 中含本品 50mg（效价）。<br>Capsules: 50mg, 100mg per capsule.<br>Particles: 50mg of the drug contained in 1g (titer). |
| **药品名称 Drug Names** | **头孢西丁钠 Cefoxitin Sodium** |
| 适应证<br>Indications | 临床应用于敏感的革兰阴性菌或厌氧菌所致的下呼吸道、泌尿生殖系、腹腔、骨和关节、皮肤和软组织等部位感染，也可用于败血症。<br><br>It is clinically used to treat infection of lower respiratory tract, urogenital system, abdominal cavity, bones and joints, skin and soft tissues, etc. caused by sensitive gram-negative bacteria or anaerobic bacteria, as well as septicemia. |
| 用法、用量<br>Dosage | 成人：1 次 1～2g，一日 3～4 次。肾功能不全者按患者肌酐清除率制订给药方案：肌酐清除率为 30～50mg/min 者，每 8～12 小时用 1～2g；10～29ml/min 者，每 12～24 小时用 1～2g；5～9ml/min 者，每 12～24 小时用 0.5～1g；<5ml/min 者，每 24～48 小时用 0.5～1g。<br><br>For adults: give1～2g singly, 3 to 4 times a day. Administration for Renal insufficiency patients should depend on the creatinine clearance rate: if the rate is 30～50mg/min, give 1～2g singly, every 8 to 12 hours; if the rate is 10～29ml/min, give 1～2g singly, every 12 to 24 hours; if the rate is 5～9ml/min, give0.5～1g singly, every 12 to 24 hours; if the rate is less than 5ml/min, give 0.5～1g singly, every 24 to 48 hours. |

**续　表**

| | |
|---|---|
| 剂型、规格<br>Preparations | 注射用头孢西丁钠：每瓶 1g。<br>Cefoxitin sodium for injection: 1g per vial. |
| **药品名称 Drug Names** | 头孢米诺钠 Cefminox Sodium |
| 适应证<br>Indications | 用于上述敏感菌所致的扁桃体、呼吸道、泌尿道、胆道、腹腔、子宫等部位的感染，也可用于败血症。<br><br>　　It is intended to treat infection of tonsils, respiratory tract, urinary tract, biliary tract, abdominal cavity, uterine and etc. caused by susceptible strains mentioned above, as well as septicemia. |
| 用法、用量<br>Dosage | 　　静脉注射或静脉滴注。成人每次 1g，一日 2 次；儿童每次 20mg/kg，一日 3 ～ 4 次。败血症时，成人一日可用到 6g，分 3 ～ 4 次给予。本品静脉注射，每 1g 药物用 20ml 注射用水、5% ～ 10% 葡萄糖液或 0.9% 氯化钠液溶解。滴注时，每 1g 药物溶于输液 100 ～ 200ml 中，滴注 1 ～ 2 小时。<br><br>　　Intravenous injection or intravenous infusion: for adults, give 1g singly, twice a day; for children, give 20mg/kg singly, 3 to 4 times a day. For septicemia adult patients, give 6g a day, in3 to 4 divided doses. Intravenous injection: dissolve every 1g of the drug injection in 20ml of water for injection, 5% to 10% glucose solution or 0.9% sodium chloride. Infusion: 1g of drug was dissolved by 100 ～ 200ml of the infusion; and the time for infusion is 1 to 2 hours. |
| 剂型、规格<br>Preparations | 注射用头孢米诺钠：每瓶 0.5g；1g（效价）。<br>Sodium cefminox for injection: 0.5g, 1g per vial (titer). |
| **药品名称 Drug Names** | 头孢吡肟 Cefepime |
| 适应证<br>Indications | 用于敏感菌所致的下呼吸道、皮肤和骨组织、泌尿系、妇科和腹腔感染以及菌血症等。<br><br>　　It is intended to treat infection of lower respiratory tract, skin and bone tissue, urinary tract, gynecology and abdominal cavity caused by susceptible strains, as well as bacteremia. |
| 用法、用量<br>Dosage | 　　常用剂量每日 2 ～ 4g，分 2 次给予。治疗泌尿系感染每日 1g。极严重感染每日 6g，分 3 次给予。可用 0.9% 氯化钠、5% ～ 10% 葡萄糖、0.16mol/L 乳酸钠、林格液等溶解。溶解液在室温 24 小时内应用。<br><br>　　The usual dose is 2 ～ 4g a day, in two divided doses. Urinary tract infection: 1g a day; the severe infected: 6g a day, in 3 divided doses It is available to dissolve the drug by 0.9% sodium chloride, 5% to 10% glucose, 0.16mol / L sodium lactate, Ringer's solution and etc... The solution should be used at room temperature within 24 hours. |
| 剂型、规格<br>Preparations | 粉针剂：每瓶 0.5g；1g；2g。<br>Powder: 0.5g, 1g, 2g per vial. |
| **药品名称 Drug Names** | 头孢布烯 Ceftibuten |
| 适应证<br>Indications | 主要用于上述敏感菌所致的呼吸道感染，如慢性气管炎急性发作、咽炎、扁桃体炎、泌尿道感染等。<br><br>　　It is mainly used to treat respiratory tract infection, such as acute exacerbation of chronic bronchitis, pharyngitis and tonsillitis, as well asurinary tract infection caused by susceptible strains mentioned above. |
| 用法、用量<br>Dosage | 　　成人和体重 45kg 以上儿童：一日 1 次 400mg。儿童：体重 10kg 服 90mg，20kg 服 180mg，40kg 服 360mg。服用混悬剂必须避开进食（食前 1 小时或食后 2 小时服用）；胶囊剂则无碍。肾功能不全者，肌酐清除率 >50ml/min 者，可按正常剂量服用（9mg/kg 或 400mg，一日 1 次）；肌酐清除率 30 ～ 49ml/min 者，照上量减半；肌酐清除率为 5 ～ 29ml/min 者，给上量 1/4。<br><br>　　For adults and children over 45kg: give 400mg singly, once a day. For children with 10kg, the dose is 90mg; with 20kg, the dose is 180mg; with 40kg, the dose is 360mg. Taking suspensions must avoid eating (an hour before eating or two hours after eating), while capsules do not have to. For patients with renal dysfunction: if the creatinine clearance rate is more then 50ml/min, give normal dose (9mg/kg or 400mg/QD); if the rate is 30 ～ 49ml/min, give half of the normal dose; if the rate is 5 ～ 29ml/min, give 1/4 of the normal dose. |

**续　表**

| 剂型、规格<br>Preparations | 胶囊剂：每粒 200mg，400mg。<br>混悬剂：90mg/5ml、180mg/5ml，每瓶 30ml、60ml、120ml。<br>Capsules: 200mg, 400mg per capsule.<br>Suspension: 90mg/5ml, 180mg/5ml; 30ml, 60ml, 120ml per vial. |
| --- | --- |
| **药品名称 Drug Names** | **头孢丙烯 Cefprozil** |
| 适应证<br>Indications | 用于敏感菌所致上呼吸道、下呼吸道、中耳、皮肤和皮肤组织、尿路等部位感染。<br>It is intended to treat infection of upper respiratory tract, lower respiratory tract, middle ear, skin and skin tissue, urinary tract and etc. caused by susceptible strains. |
| 用法、用量<br>Dosage | 成人（含 13 岁以上）：上呼吸道感染，每次 500mg，一日 1 次；下呼吸道感染，每次 500mg，一日 2 次；皮肤感染，250mg，一日 1 次（重症每日 2 次）。儿童（2 ~ 12 岁）：上呼吸道感染，每次 7.5mg/kg，一日 2 次；皮肤感染，每次 20mg/kg，一日 2 次；中耳炎，每次 15mg/kg，一日 2 次。肾功能不全：肌酐清除率小于 30mg/min 者，用量减半。<br>Adults (including children over the age of 13) with upper respiratory tract infection: 500mg singly, once a day; with lower respiratory tract infection: 500mg singly, twice a day; with skin infection: 250mg singly, once a day (or twice for the severe infected). Children (age of 2 to 12) with upper respiratory tract infection: 7.5mg/kg singly, two times a day; with skin infection: 20mg/kg singly, two times a day; with otitis media: 15mg/kg singly, two times a day. For renal insufficiency patients whose. creatinine clearance rate is less than 30mg/min, give half of the dosage |
| 剂型、规格<br>Preparations | 片剂：每片 250mg；500mg。<br>干混悬剂：每瓶 2.5g、5g，加水后成为 125mg/5ml 和 250mg/5ml。<br>Tablets: 250mg, 500mg per tablet<br>Suspension: 2.5g, 5g; 125mg/5ml 250mg/5ml (after water added) per bottle |
| **药品名称 Drug Names** | **头孢泊肟酯 Cefpodoxime Proxetil** |
| 适应证<br>Indications | 用于敏感菌所致支气管炎、肺炎、泌尿系统、皮肤组织、中耳、扁桃体等部位的感染。<br>It is used to treat bronchitis, pneumonia and infection of urinary tract, skin, middle ear, tonsils, etc. caused by susceptible strains. |
| 用法、用量<br>Dosage | 成人（或大于 12 岁儿童）用量：一般感染，每日 200mg；重度感染，每日 400mg；皮肤及皮肤组织感染，每日 800mg，以上均分为 2 次服用。妇女淋球菌感染，服用单剂量 200mg。儿童：每日 10mg/kg，一般分为 2 次给予（单次剂量不超过 400mg）。<br>肾功能严重不全（肌酐清除率 <30ml/min）者给药间隔延长至 24 小时（按以上每日剂量的一半），透析患者于透析后每日给药 3 次。<br>Adult (or children over the age of 12) with moderate infection: 200mg a day; with severe infection: 400mg a day; with skin and skin structure infection: 800mg a day, all in 2 divided doses. Female with gonococcal infection: 200mg singly. Children: 10mg/kg a day, in generally 2 divided doses (single dose can not exceed 400mg).<br>For patients with severe renal insufficiency (creatinine clearance rate <30ml/min), the interval between doses should be extended to 24 hours (half of daily dose above); for dialysis patients, give 3 times a day after dialysis. |
| 剂型、规格<br>Preparations | 片剂：每片 100mg；200mg。<br>干混悬剂：每瓶 1000mg，加水至 100ml，得 50mg/5ml 混悬剂。<br>Tablets: 100mg, 200mg per tablet.<br>Suspension: 1000mg per bottle; 50mg/5ml (after 100ml water added). |
| **药品名称 Drug Names** | **头孢托仑匹酯 Cefditoren Pivoxil** |
| 适应证<br>Indications | 临床用于敏感菌引起的皮肤感染、乳腺炎、肛周脓肿、泌尿生殖系统感染、胆囊炎、胆管炎、中耳炎、鼻窦炎、牙周炎、睑腺炎、泪囊炎、咽喉炎、扁桃体炎、急慢性支气管炎。<br>It is clinically used to treat skin infection, mastitis, abscess, urogenital infections, cholecystitis, cholangitis, otitis media, sinusitis, periodontitis, hordeolum, dacryocystitis, pharyngitis, tonsillitis, acute and chronic bronchitis caused by susceptible strains. |

**续 表**

| 用法、用量<br>Dosage | 口服：成人每次 200 ～ 400mg，一日 2 次，连续用药 10 ～ 14 天。肾功能不全者，肌酐清除率 <30ml/min 者，每次用量不应超过 200mg，一日 1 次，肌酐清除率为 30 ～ 49ml/min 者，每次用量不应超过 200mg，一日 2 次。<br><br>Oral medication: give adults 200mg ～ 400mg singly, twice a day, for continuous 10 to 14 days. For patients with renal insufficiency: if the creatinine clearance rate is less than 30ml/min, the singlw dose should not exceed 200mg, once a day; if the rate is 30 ～ 49ml/min, the single dose should not exceed 200mg, twice a day. |
|---|---|
| 剂型、规格<br>Preparations | 片剂：每片 100mg；200mg。<br>Tablets: 100mg, 200mg per tablet. |

| 药品名称 Drug Names | 头孢地嗪钠 Cefodizime Sodium |
|---|---|
| 适应证<br>Indications | 临床用于敏感菌所致的下呼吸道、泌尿系感染。<br>It is clinically used to treat infection of lower respiratory tract and urinary tract caused by susceptible strains. |
| 用法、用量<br>Dosage | 成人：每次 1g（重症可用到 2g），溶于注射用水 10ml，再加入其他输液中，使成 50 ～ 100ml，静脉滴注，一日 2 次。肌内注射：用注射用水 4ml 溶解，也可用 0.5% ～ 1% 利多卡因注射液溶解，以减轻疼痛。淋病的治疗只注射 1 次，用量 0.5g。<br><br>For adults, give 1g ( 2g for the severe) singly; dissolve the drug in 10ml water for injection, then add other fluids to 50 ～ 100ml for intravenous infusion, twices a day. If for intramuscular injection, dissolve the drug by 4ml water for injection, or 0.5% ～ 1% lidocaine injection to ease pain. Treatment of gonorrhea needs injection only once, with 0.5g of the drug. |
| 剂型、规格<br>Preparations | 粉针剂：每瓶 1g；2g。<br>Powder: 1g, 2g of each. |

| 药品名称 Drug Names | 头孢硫脒 Cefathiamidine |
|---|---|
| 适应证<br>Indications | 用于敏感菌所引起的呼吸道、泌尿道、胆道、皮肤及软组织感染，对心内膜炎、败血症也有较好疗效。<br>It is intended to treat infection of respiratory tract, urinary tract, biliary tract, skin and soft tissues caused by susceptible strains mentioned above. And it is also effective in treatment of endocarditis and septicemia. |
| 用法、用量<br>Dosage | 成人：一日 2 ～ 4g，分 2 ～ 4 次给药，肌内注射或静脉滴注，严重者可增至一日 8g。<br>儿童：一日 50 ～ 100mg/kg，分 2 ～ 4 次给药，肌内注射或静脉滴注。先用生理盐水或注射用水溶解后，再用生理盐水或 5% 葡萄糖注射液 250ml 稀释。<br><br>For adults, give 2 ～ 4g a day, in 2 to 4doses, by intramuscular injection or intravenous infusion. The daily dose for the severe case can be increased to 8g.<br>For children, give 50 ～ 100mg/kg a day, in 2 to 4 doses, by intramuscular injection or intravenous infusion. Dissolve the drug by normal saline or water injection first and then dilute it with.saline or 250ml 5% glucose injection |
| 剂型、规格<br>Preparations | 注射用头孢硫脒：每瓶 0.5g；1g。<br>Cefathiamidine for injection: 0.5g, 1g per vial. |

| 药品名称 Drug Names | 头孢替安 Cefotiam |
|---|---|
| 适应证<br>Indications | 用于敏感菌所引起的术后感染、烧伤感染、皮肤软组织感染、骨及关节感染、呼吸系统扁桃体炎、肺炎、支气管炎、泌尿道炎、前列腺炎、胆囊炎、胆管炎，以及子宫内膜炎、盆腔炎。<br>It is intended to treat postoperative infection, burn infection, skin and soft tissue infection, bone sand joints infection, respiratory system infection, tonsillitis, pneumonia, bronchitis, urethritis, prostatitis, cholecystitis and cholangitis caused by susceptible strains, as well as endometrial inflammation and pelvic inflammatory disease. |

**续 表**

| 用法、用量<br>Dosage | 成人：静脉给药，一日 1 ～ 2g，2 ～ 4 次缓慢静脉注射或静脉滴注；严重感染增至一日 4g。<br>儿童：一日 40 ～ 80mg/kg，分 3 ～ 4 次静脉给药；重症时剂量可增至一日 160mg/kg。<br>For adults, by intravenous administration, give 1 ～ 2g a day, in 2 ～ 4 divided doses, by intravenous injection or intravenous infusion; in severe infected cases, the dose can be increased to 4g.<br>For children, give 40 ～ 80mg/kg a day, in 3 to 4 divided doses intravenously; daily dose in severe infection cases can be increased on 160mg/kg. |
|---|---|
| 剂型、规格<br>Preparations | 注射用盐酸头孢替安：每瓶 0.25g；0.5g；1g。<br>Cefotiam Hydrochloride for injection: 0.25g, 0.5g, 1g per vial. |
| **药品名称 Drug Names** | 头孢替坦 Cefotetan |
| 适应证<br>Indications | 用于敏感菌所引起的呼吸道、肺部感染、腹部感染、尿路感染、妇科感染及皮肤软组织感染。<br>It is used to treat respiratory tract infection lung infection, abdominal infection, urinary tract infection, gynecological infection and skin and soft tissue infection caused by susceptible strains. |
| 用法、用量<br>Dosage | 深部肌内注射、静脉注射或静脉滴注。成人：常用量每次 1 ～ 2g，每 12 小时 1 次，每日最大剂量不超过 6g。儿童：每日 40 ～ 60mg/kg，病情严重者可增至 100mg/kg，分 2 ～ 3 次。<br>The drug is administered by deep intramuscular injection, intravenous injection or intravenous infusion. For adults, give 1 ～ 2g singly as the usual dose, every 12 hours, and the maximum daily dose can not exceed 6g. For children, give 40 ～ 60mg/kg a day and dose for the severe case can be increased to 100mg/kg, in 2 to 3 divided doses. |
| 剂型、规格<br>Preparations | 注射用头孢替坦二钠：每瓶 1g；2g；10g。<br>Cefotetan disodium for injection: 1g, 2g, 10g per vial. |
| **药品名称 Drug Names** | 头孢唑肟 Ceftizoxime |
| 适应证<br>Indications | 敏感菌所致的下呼吸道感染、尿路感染、腹腔感染、盆腔感染、败血症、皮肤软组织感染、骨和关节感染、肺炎链球菌或流感嗜血杆菌所致脑膜炎和单纯性淋病。<br>It is intended to treat lower respiratory tract infection, urinary tract infection, abdominal infection, pelvic infection, septicemia, skin and soft tissue infection, bone and joint infection caused by susceptible strains, as well as meningitis and simple gonorrhea caused by treptococcus pneumoniae or haemophilus influenzae . |
| 用法、用量<br>Dosage | 静脉滴注静脉注射。成人：1 次 1 ～ 2g，每 8 ～ 12 小时 1 次；严重感染者的剂量可增至 1 次 3 ～ 4g，每 8 小时一次；治疗非复杂性尿路感染时，1 次 0.5g，每 12 小时 1 次。6 个月及 6 个月以上的婴儿及儿童常用量：按体重 1 次 50mg/kg，每 6 ～ 8 小时 1 次。<br>The drug is administered by intravenous infusion or intravenous infection. For adults, give 1 ～ 2g singly, every 8 to 12 hours; and the dose in severe case can be increased to 3 ～ 4g singly, every 8 hours; in treatment of uncomplicated urinary tract infection, give 0.5g singly, every 12 hours. The usual dose for children and infants of 6 months and above is 50mg/kg, every 6 to 8 hours. |
| 剂型、规格<br>Preparations | 注射用头孢唑肟钠：每瓶 0.5g；1g。<br>Ceftizoxime for injection: 0.5g, 1g per vial. |
| **药品名称 Drug Names** | 头孢孟多 Cefamandole |
| 适应证<br>Indications | 临床应用于敏感的革兰阴性菌所致的呼吸道、泌尿生殖系、皮肤和软组织、骨和关节、耳鼻咽喉等部位感染，以及腹膜炎、败血症等。对胆道和肠道感染有较好疗效。<br>It is clinically used to treat infection of respiratory, genitourinary system, skin and soft tissues, bones and joint, ENT, as well as peritonitis and septicemia caused by sensitive Gulen negative bacteria. It is also effective in treatment of biliary react infeciotn and intestinal infection. |
| 用法、用量<br>Dosage | 静脉注射或静脉滴注。成人，一般感染 1 次 0.5 ～ 1g，一日 4 次；较重感染 1 次 1g，一日 6 次；极严重感染一日可用到 12g。儿童，一日剂量为 50 ～ 100mg/kg；极重感染可用到 150mg/kg，分 3 ～ 4 次给予。<br>The drug is administered by intravenous injection or intravenous infusion. General infected adults: 0.5 ～ 1g singly, 4 times a day; Severe infected adults: 1g singly, 6 times a day; Extremely severe infected adults: 12g a day; Children: 50 ～ 100mg/kg a day; Extremely severe infected children: 150mg/kg a day, in 3to 4 divided doses. |

**续 表**

| | |
|---|---|
| 剂型、规格<br>Preparations | 注射用头孢孟多甲酸酯钠：每瓶 0.5g、1g。每 1g 药物添加碳酸钠 63mg。<br>Cefamandole sodium formate for injection: 0.5g, 1g per vial; Add 63mg sodium carbonate in every 1g of the drug. |
| **药品名称 Drug Names** | **头孢尼西钠 Cefonicid Sodium** |
| 适应证<br>Indications | 用于敏感菌所致的下呼吸道感染、尿路感染、败血症、皮肤软组织感染、骨和关节感染。也可用于手术预防感染。<br>It is intended to treat lower respiratory tract infection, urinary tract infection, septicemia, skin and soft tissue infection, bone and joint infection caused by susceptible strains mentioned above. It is also be used in preventing surgical infection. |
| 用法、用量<br>Dosage | 一般轻度至中度感染成人每日剂量为 1g，一日 1 次；在严重感染或危及生命的感染中，可每日 2g，每 24 小时给药 1 次；无并发症的尿路感染：每日 0.5g，每 24 小时 1 次；手术预防感染：手术前 1 小时单剂量给药 1g，术中和术后没有必要再用。必要时如关节成形手术或开胸手术可重复给药 2 天；剖宫产手术中，应在脐带结扎后再给予本品。<br>Adults with mild or moderate infection: 1g singly, once a day; with severe of life-threatening infection: 2g a day, every 24 hours; with uncomplicated urinary tract infection: 0.5g a day, every 24 hours. Preventing surgical infection: 1g singly, an hour before surgery, no administration intraoperatively and postoperatively. If necessary, in arthroplasty surgery or thoracic surgery, the drug could be administered for two days. and in cesarean surgery, the drug should be administered after the umbilical cord ligation. |
| 剂型、规格<br>Preparations | 注射用头孢尼西钠：每瓶 0.5g；1g；2g。<br>Cefonicid Sodium for injection: 0.5g, 1g, 2g per vial. |
| **药品名称 Drug Names** | **拉氧头孢钠 Latamoxef Sodium** |
| 适应证<br>Indications | 用于敏感菌所致肺炎、气管炎、胸膜炎、腹膜炎，以及皮肤和软组织、骨和关节、五官、创面等部位的感染，还可用于败血症和脑膜炎。<br>It is used to treat pneumonia, bronchitis, pleurisy, peritonitis, skin and soft tissue infection, bone and joint infection, facial features infection, wound infections, etc. caused by susceptible strains, as well as sepsis and meningitis. |
| 用法、用量<br>Dosage | 肌内注射：1 次 0.5 ~ 1g，一日 2 次，用 0.5% 利多卡因注射液溶解，做深部肌内注射。静脉注射：1 次 1g，一日 2 次，溶解于 10 ~ 20ml 液体中，缓缓注入。静脉滴注：1 次 1g，一日 2 次，溶于液体 100ml 中滴入，重症可加倍量给予。儿童用量：一日 40 ~ 80mg/kg，分 2 ~ 4 次。静脉注射和静脉滴注可用等渗氯化钠溶液或 5% ~ 10% 葡萄糖注射液、灭菌注射用水、低分子右旋糖酐注射液等作溶剂，但不得与甘露醇注射液配伍。<br>Intramuscular injection: 0.5 ~ 1g singly, 2 times a day, 0.5% lidocaine injection as solvent for deep intramuscular injection. Intravenous injeciton: 1g singly, twice a day, 10 ~ 20ml liquid as solvent for slow injection. Intravenous infusion: 1g singly, twice a day, 100ml liquid as solvent. And the dose could be doubled for severe cases. For children, give 40 ~ 80mg/kg a day, in 2 to 4 divided doses. In intravenous injection and intravenous infusion, the drug can use isotonic sodium chloride solution, 5% to 10% glucose injection, sterile water for injection, low molecular weight dextran injection as solvent, but it can not be used in combination with mannitol injection. |
| 剂型、规格<br>Preparations | 注射用拉氧头孢钠：每瓶 0.25g；0.5g；1g。<br>Latamoxef Sodium for injection: 0.25g, 0.5g, 1g per vial. |
| **药品名称 Drug Names** | **氟氧头孢钠 Flomoxef Sodium** |
| 适应证<br>Indications | 用于敏感菌所致的咽炎、扁桃体炎、支气管炎、肺炎、肾盂肾炎、膀胱炎、前列腺炎、胆道感染、腹膜炎、盆腔炎、子宫及附属组织炎症、中耳炎、创口感染、心内膜炎及败血症等。<br>It is intended to treat pharyngitis, tonsillitis, bronchitis, pneumonia, pyelonephritis, cystitis, prostatitis, biliary tract infection, peritonitis, pelvic inflammatory disease, uterine and affiliated organizations inflammation, otitis media, wound infections, endocarditis and septicemia caused by susceptible strains mentioned above. |

**续 表**

| | |
|---|---|
| 用法、用量<br>Dosage | 　　轻症：成人一日量 1 ~ 2g，分成 2 次静脉注射；儿童一日 60 ~ 80mg/kg，分 2 次静脉注射或静脉滴注。重症：成人一日 4g，分 2 ~ 4 次用；儿童一日 150mg/kg，分 3 ~ 4 次用。<br>　　Mild infection case: for adults, give 1 ~ 2g a day in 2 divided doses by intravenous injection; for children, give 60 ~ 80mg/kg a dya in 2 divided doses by intravenous injection or intravenous drip. Severe infection case: for adults, give 4g a day in 2 to 4 doses; for children, givw 150mg/kg a day in 3to4 doses. |
| 剂型、规格<br>Preparations | 　　注射用氟氧头孢钠：每瓶 0.5g；1g；2g。<br>　　Flomoxef Sodium for injection: 0.5g, 1g, 2g per vial. |

1.3 β- 内酰胺酶抑制剂及其与 β- 内酰胺类抗生素配伍的复方制剂 β-lactamase inhibitors and their compound preparation with antibiotics of β- lactamase

| 药品名称 Drug Names | 克拉维酸钾 Clavulanate Potassium |
|---|---|
| 适应证<br>Indications | 　　与 β- 内酰胺类抗生素联用用于敏感菌所致的下呼吸道感染、耳鼻咽喉感染、尿路感染、腹腔感染、盆腔感染、骨和关节感染、皮肤软组织感染、血流感染及败血症等<br>　　And β- lactam antibiotics combined with, for the treatment of lower respiratory tract infections caused by susceptible strains, ENT infections, urinary tract infections, abdominal infections, pelvic infections, bone and joint infections, skin and soft tissue infections, bloodstream infections and septicemia. |
| 用法、用量<br>Dosage | 　　本药单用无效，常与 β- 内酰胺类抗生素组成复方制剂应用。各复方制剂的具体用法与用量参见"阿莫西林克拉维酸钾""替卡西林钠克拉维酸钾"。<br>　　The drug alone ineffective, often with β- lactam antibiotics composition compound preparation applications. Specific usage and the amount of each compound preparation See "amoxicillin and clavulanate potassium, " "Ticarcillin sodium clavulanate potassium." |
| 剂型、规格<br>Preparations | 　　参见"阿莫西林克拉维酸钾""替卡西林钠克拉维酸钾"的相关项。<br>　　See "amoxicillin and clavulanate potassium, " "Ticarcillin sodium potassium clavulanate" related items. |
| 药品名称 Drug Names | 舒巴坦钠 Sulbactam Sodium |
| 适应证<br>Indications | 　　与青霉素类或头孢菌素类药联用用于治疗敏感菌所致的败血症、尿路感染、肺部感染、支气管感染、胆道感染、腹腔感染、盆腔感染、皮肤软组织感染及耳鼻咽喉部感染等<br>　　The drugs and the penicillins or cephalosporins combined with, for the treatment of sepsis caused by susceptible strains, urinary tract infections, lung infections, bronchial infections, biliary tract infections, abdominal infections, pelvic infections, skin and soft tissue infections and ear, nose, throat infections |
| 用法、用量<br>Dosage | 　　静脉滴注与氨苄西林联用，本药一日 1 ~ 2g，氨苄西林一日 2 ~ 4g，分 2 ~ 3 次给药。<br>　　Intravenous infusion, and ampicillin in conjunction with, the drug day 1-2g, ampicillin day 2 ~ 4g, 2 ~ 3 doses. |
| 剂型、规格<br>Preparations | 　　注射用舒巴坦钠：0.5g；1g。<br>　　Sulbactam for injection: 0.5g, 1g. |
| 药品名称 Drug Names | 他唑巴坦 Tazobactam |
| 适应证<br>Indications | 　　参见"哌拉西林钠 - 他唑巴坦钠"的相关项<br>　　See "sodium piperacillin - tazobactam sodium" related items |
| 用法、用量<br>Dosage | 　　参见"哌拉西林钠 - 他唑巴坦钠"的相关项<br>　　See "sodium piperacillin - tazobactam sodium" related items |
| 剂型、规格<br>Preparations | 　　参见"哌拉西林钠 - 他唑巴坦钠"的相关项。<br>　　See "sodium piperacillin - tazobactam sodium" related items |
| 药品名称 Drug Names | 阿莫西林 - 克拉维酸钾 Amoxillin and Clavulanate Potassium |
| 适应证<br>Indications | 　　用于敏感菌所致的下呼吸道、中耳、鼻窦、皮肤组织、尿路等部位感染。对肠杆菌属尿路感染也有效。<br>　　It is intended to treat infection of lower respiratory tract, middle ear, sinus, skin, urinary tract and etc. caused by susceptible strains mentioned above. It is also effective in treatment of urinary tract infection for Enterobacter. |

**续　表**

| | |
|---|---|
| 用法、用量<br>Dosage | 　　一般感染：用 2：1 比例片，每次 1 片，每 8 小时 1 次。重症或呼吸道感染，用 4：1 比例片，每次 1 片，每 6～8 小时 1 次。注射应用见阿莫西林。<br>　　General infection case: 1 tablet of 2：1 singly, every 8 hours. Severe infection or respiratory infection case: 1 tablet of 4:1 ratio, every 6 to 8 hours. See item of amoxicillin for dosage of injection. |
| 剂型、规格<br>Preparations | 　　片剂：0.375g（2：1）；0.625g（4：1）；0.3125g（4：1）；0.475g（7：1）；1.0g（7：1）。<br>　　注射用阿莫西林钠 - 克拉维酸钾：1.2g/ 瓶（5：1）。<br>　　Tablets: 0.375g（2：1）, 0.625g（4：1）, 0.3125g（4：1）, 0.475g（7：1）, 1.0g（7：1）.<br>Amoxicillin and Clavulanate Potassium for injection: 1.2g per vial（5：1）. |
| 药品名称 Drug Names | 替卡西林钠 - 克拉维酸钾 Ticarcillin Sodium and Clavulanate Potassium |
| 适应证<br>Indications | 　　本品适用于敏感菌引起的呼吸道、骨和关节、皮肤组织、尿路等部位的感染以及败血症、骨髓炎和各种手术后感染。<br>　　This product is intended to treat infection of respiratory tract, bones and joints, skin, urinary tract and etc., as well as septicemia, osteomyelitis and a variety of post-surgical infections caused by susceptible strains mentioned above. |
| 用法、用量<br>Dosage | 　　每次注射 3g，每 4～6 小时 1 次，溶于 13ml 等渗盐水或灭菌注射用水中，缓缓静脉推注，或溶于适量溶剂中静脉滴注，30 分钟内滴完。<br>　　Give 3g for each injection, every 4 to 6 hours. Dissolve the drug in 13ml of isotonic saline or sterile water for injection for slow injection or dissolve it in an appropriate amount of solvent for intravenous drip within 30 minutes. |
| 剂型、规格<br>Preparations | 　　注射用替卡西林钠 - 克拉维酸钾：3g（3：0.1）；3g（3：0.2）。<br>　　Ticarcillin Sodium and Clavulanate Potassium for injection: 3g（3：0.1）, 3g（3：0.2）. |
| 药品名称 Drug Names | 氨苄西林钠 - 舒巴坦钠 Ampicillin Sodium and Sulbactam Sodium |
| 适应证<br>Indications | 　　可用于治疗敏感菌所致的下呼吸道、泌尿道、胆道、皮肤和软组织、中耳、鼻窦等部位感染。<br>　　It is infection of used to treat infection of the lower respiratory tract, urinary tract, biliary tract, intestinal tract, skin and soft tissue, middle ear, sinus and etc. caused by susceptible strains mentioned above. |
| 用法、用量<br>Dosage | 　　氨苄西林和舒巴坦钠以 2：1（效价）的比率联合应用。肌内注射：一次 0.75g（氨苄西林 0.5g 和舒巴坦钠 0.25g），一日 2～4 次。静脉注射或静脉滴注：1 次 1.5g，一日 2～4 次。静脉滴注时以 100ml 等渗氯化钠液或注射用水溶解，滴注 0.5～1 小时。<br>　　Ampicillin and sulbactam should be used by the ratio 2：1 (titer) in combination. Intramuscular injection: 0.75g singly (0.5g ampicillin and 0.25g sulbactam), 2 to 4 times a day. Intravenous injection or intravenous infusion: 1.5g singly, 2 to 4 times a day. In intravenous infusion, dissolve the drug in 100ml of isotonic sodium chloride solution or water for injection, and the infusion lasts for 0.5 to 1 hour. |
| 剂型、规格<br>Preparations | 　　注射用氨苄西林钠 - 舒巴坦钠：0.75g；1.5g [ 含氨苄西林钠和舒巴坦钠（重量效价比）2：1]。<br>　　Ampicillin Sodium and Sulbactam Sodium for injection: 0.75g, 1.5g [containing ampicillin sodium and sulbactam sodium (weight titer) 2：1]. |
| 药品名称 Drug Names | 舒他西林 Sultamicillin |
| 适应证<br>Indications | 　　用于治疗敏感细菌引起的下列感染：<br>　　(1) 上呼吸道感染：鼻窦炎、中耳炎、扁桃体炎等。<br>　　(2) 下呼吸道感染：支气管炎、肺炎等。<br>　　(3) 泌尿道感染及肾盂肾炎。<br>　　(4) 皮肤、软组织感染。<br>　　(5) 淋病。<br>　　For the treatment of the following infections caused by sensitive bacteria:<br>(1) Upper respiratory tract infections: sinusitis, otitis media, tonsillitis.<br>(2) Lower respiratory tract infections: bronchitis, pneumonia .<br>(3) Urinary tract infections and pyelonephritis.<br>(4) Skin and soft tissue infections.<br>(5) gonorrhea. |

**续 表**

| | |
|---|---|
| 用法、用量<br>Dosage | 1 次 375mg，一日 2～4 次，在餐前 1 小时或餐后 2 小时服用。<br>375mg singly, 2 to 4 times a day, 1 hour before or 2 hours after meals. |
| 剂型、规格<br>Preparations | 片剂：375mg（效价）。<br>Tablets: 375mg (titer). |
| **药品名称 Drug Names** | 哌拉西林钠 - 他唑巴坦钠 Piperacillin Sodium and Tazobactam Sodium |
| 适应证<br>Indications | 临床主要用于敏感菌所致下呼吸道、腹腔、妇科、泌尿、骨及关节、皮肤组织等部位感染和败血症。也可用于多种细菌的混合感染和患中性粒细胞缺乏者的感染。<br><br>It is clinically used to treat lower respiratory tract infection, abdominal infection, gynecological infection, urological infection, bone and joint infection, skin infection, septicemia and etc. caused by susceptible strains. It can also be used to treat mixed infection by several bateria and infection of those who have neutrophil deficiency. |
| 用法、用量<br>Dosage | 成人和 12 岁以上儿童的常用量为：每次 4.5g，每日 3 次静脉滴注（滴注 30 分钟），也可静脉注射。<br><br>The usual dose for adults and children over the age of 12 is 4.5g singly, three times a day, by intravenous infusion (for 30 minutes), or intravenous injection. |
| 剂型、规格<br>Preparations | 注射用哌拉西林钠 - 他唑巴坦：2.25g（8：1）；4.5g（8：1）。<br>Piperacillin Sodium and Tazobactam Sodium for Injection: 2.25g (8：1), 4.5g (8：1). |

1.4　碳青酶烯类和其他 β- 内酰胺类 Carbapenems and other antibiotics of β- lactamase

| | |
|---|---|
| **药品名称 Drug Names** | 亚胺培南 - 西司他汀钠 Imipenem and Cilastatin Sodium |
| 适应证<br>Indications | 用于敏感菌所致的腹膜炎、肝胆感染、腹腔内脓肿、阑尾炎、妇科感染、下呼吸道感染、皮肤和软组织感染、尿路感染、骨和关节感染以及败血症等。<br><br>It is intended to treat peritonitis, liver and gallbladder infection, intra-abdominal abscesses, appendicitis, gynecological infection, lower respiratory tract infection, skin and soft tissue infection, urinary tract infection, bone and joint infection and septicemia caused by susceptible strains. |
| 用法、用量<br>Dosage | 静脉滴注或肌内注射。用量以亚胺培南计，根据病情，一次 0.25～1g，一日 2～4 次，对中度感染一般可按 1 次 1g，一日 2 次给予。静脉滴注可选用等渗氯化钠注射液、5%～10% 葡萄糖液作溶剂。每 0.5g 药物用 100ml 溶剂，制成 5mg/ml 液体，缓缓滴入。肌内注射用 1% 利多卡因注射液为溶剂，以减轻疼痛。<br><br>对肾功能不全者应按肌酐清除率调整剂量：肌酐清除率为 31～70ml/min 的患者，每 6～8 小时用 0.5g，每日最高剂量为 1.5～2g；肌酐清除率为 21～30ml/min 的患者，每 8～12 小时用 0.5g，每日最高剂量为 1～1.5g；肌酐清除率为 <20ml/min 的患者，每 12 小时用 0.25～0.5g，每日最高剂量为 0.5～1g。<br><br>The drug is administered by intravenous infusion or intramuscular injection. The administration dose is measured by imipenem. Give 0.25～1g singly, 2 to 4times a day according to patients' condition. For moderate infected patients, give1g singly, two times a day. In intravenous infusion, isotonic sodium chloride injection and 5% to 10% glucose solution could be used as solvent. Dissolve every 0.5g of the drug in 100ml solvent; make it into the liquid 5mg/ml for slow infusion. In intramuscular injection, 1% lidocaine is used as solvent to relieve the pain.<br><br>The dose for renal dysfunction patients should depend on the creatinine clearance rate: if the rate is 31～70ml/min, give 0.5g every 6 to 8 hours with the maximum daily dose of 1.5～2g; if the rate is 21～30ml / min, give 0.5g every 8 to 12 hours with the maximum daily dose of 1～1.5g; if the rate is less than 20ml/min, give 0.25～0.5g every 12 hours with, the maximum daily dose of 0.5～1g. |
| 剂型、规格<br>Preparations | 注射用亚胺培南 - 西司他汀：每支 0.25g；0.5g；1g（以亚胺培南计量）。其中含有等量的西司他汀钠。<br><br>Imipenem/Cilastatin Sodium for injection: 0.25g, 0.5g, 1g (measured by imipenem) per vial, with the same amount of Cilastatin sodium. |

**续　表**

| 药品名称 Drug Names | 美罗培南 Meropenem |
| --- | --- |
| 适应证<br>Indications | 用于敏感菌所致的呼吸道、尿路、肝胆、外科、骨科、妇科、五官科感染以及腹膜炎、皮肤化脓性疾病等。本品可适用于敏感菌所致脑膜炎。<br><br>It is intended to treat respiratory tract infection, urinary tract infeciton, hepatobiliary infeciton, surgical infeciton, orthopedics infeciton, gynecological infeciton, ENT infection, peritonitis, purulent skin disease, meningitis and etc.caused by susceptible strains. |
| 用法、用量<br>Dosage | 成人每日 0.5 ~ 1g，分为 2 ~ 3 次，稀释后静脉滴注每次 30 分钟。重症每日剂量可增至 2g。连续应用不超过 2 周。本品每 0.5g 用生理盐水约 100ml 溶解，不可用注射用水。<br>儿童（3 月龄以上）推荐用量：周围感染 20mg/kg，每 8 小时 1 次；脑膜炎 40mg/kg，每 8 小时一次。肾功能减退者应按肌酐清除率调整剂量：肌酐清除率为 26 ~ 50ml/min 的患者，每 12 小时用 1g；肌酐清除率为 10 ~ 25ml/min 的患者，每 12 小时用 0.5g；肌酐清除率为 <10ml/min 的患者，每 24 小时用 0.5g。<br><br>For adults, give 0.5 ~ 1g a day, in 2 or 3 divided doses, by intravenous infusion. Each infusion lasts 30 minutes and the drug should be diluted before administration. The daily dose could be increased to 2g in severe cases. Continuous administration should be within 2 weeks.Every 0.5g of the drug is dissolved in 100ml saline, but not in water for injection.<br>Recommended dosage for Children (aging 3 months and above): in treatment of peripheral infection, give 20mg/kg, every 8 hours; in treatment of meningitis, give 40mg/kg, every 8 hours. The dose for renal dysfunction patients should depend on creatinine clearance rate: if the rate is 26 ~ 50ml/min, give1g every 12 hours; if the rate is 10 ~ 25ml/min, give 0.5g every 12 hours; if the rate is less than10/min patients, give 0.5g every 24 hours. |
| 剂型、规格<br>Preparations | 粉针剂：每瓶 0.5g；1g。<br>Powder: 0.5g, 1g of each. |
| 药品名称 Drug Names | 帕尼培南 - 倍他米隆 Panipenem and Betamipron |
| 适应证<br>Indications | 用于治疗敏感菌引起的呼吸系统、泌尿生殖系统、腹内、眼科、皮肤及软组织、骨及关节的感染。如急慢性支气管炎、肺炎、肺脓肿、胆囊炎、腹膜炎、肝脓肿、肾盂肾炎、前列腺炎、子宫内感染、角膜溃疡、眼球炎、丹毒、蜂窝织炎、骨髓炎、关节炎等。还可用于败血症、感染性心内膜炎等严重感染。<br><br>It is intended to treat infection of respiratory system, genitourinary system, abdominal cavity, eyes, skin and soft tissue, bone and joint caused by susceptible strains. For example, acute or chronic bronchitis, pneumonia, lung abscess, cholecystitis, peritonitis, liver abscesses, pyelonephritis, prostatitis, intrauterine infection, corneal ulcers, eye inflammation, erysipelas, cellulitis, osteomyelitis, arthritis and etc. It also can be used to treat severe infection like septicemia and endocarditis. |
| 用法、用量<br>Dosage | 静脉滴注：成人，一般感染，每次 0.5g，每日 2 次，用不少于 100ml 的生理盐水或 5% 葡萄糖注射液溶解后，于 30 ~ 60 分钟滴注；重症或顽固性感染，剂量为每次 1g，每日 2 次，静脉滴注时间不少于 1 小时。儿童，每日 30 ~ 60mg/kg，分 2 ~ 3 次，每次 30 分钟静脉滴注；严重感染可增加至每日 100mg/kg，分 3 ~ 4 次。<br><br>Intravenous infusion: for adults' general infection, give 0.5g singly, two times a day, dissolve the drug in at least100ml saline or 5% dextrose injection, and the infusion time should be within 30 to 60 minutes; for adults' severe or persistent infection, give 1g singly, two times a day, and the infusion time should be at least one hour; for children, give 30 ~ 60mg/kg a day in two to three divided doses and each infusion lasts 30minutes; for severe infected children, give100mg/kg a day in three to four divided doses. |
| 剂型、规格<br>Preparations | 注射用帕尼培南 - 倍他米隆：250mg/ 瓶；500mg/ 瓶。帕尼培南与等量倍他米隆配伍，以帕尼培南含量计。<br><br>Panipenem and Betamipron for injection: 250mg, 500mg per vial. Panipenem is used in combination with the same amount of betamipron with panipenem as the content measure. |

**续 表**

| 药品名称 Drug Names | 厄他培南 Ertapenem |
|---|---|
| 适应证<br>Indications | 用于治疗敏感菌引起的呼吸系统、泌尿生殖系统、腹腔、皮肤及软组织、盆腔等部位的感染。<br>It is intended to treat infection of respiratory system, genitourinary system, abdominal cavity, skin and soft tissue, pelvic cavity and etc. caused by susceptible strains. |
| 用法、用量<br>Dosage | 静脉滴注：成人，每日 1g，用不少于 100ml 的生理盐水稀释。肾功能不全者，肌酐清除率＜30ml/min，每日剂量 0.5g。3 个月及以上的儿童每日 2 次按 15mg/kg 给予肌注或静脉滴注，日剂量不超过 1g。<br>For adults, give 1g a day, by intravenous infusion; dilute the drug with at least 100ml of saline. Renal dysfunction patients: if the creatinine clearance rate is less than 30ml/min, give 0.5g a day. For children aging 3 months and above, give 15mg/kg singly, twice a day by intramuscular injection or intravenous infusion, and the daily dose can not exceed 1g. |
| 剂型、规格<br>Preparations | 注射用厄他培南：每支 1g。<br>Ertapenem for injection: 1g per vial. |
| 药品名称 Drug Names | 比阿培南 Biapenem |
| 适应证<br>Indications | 用于肠杆菌属、假单胞属、不动杆菌、枸橼酸杆菌、脆弱拟杆菌所致慢性呼吸道感染急性发作、肺炎、肺脓肿、腹膜炎、复杂性膀胱炎、女性生殖器感染。对某些革兰阳性菌也有效。<br>It is intended to treat acute exacerbation of chronic respiratory infection, pneumonia, lung abscess, peritonitis, complicated cystitis and female genital infection caused by Enterobacter, Pseudomonas species, Acinetobacter, Citrobacter and Bacteroides fragilis. It is also effective to treat infection by some Gram-positive bacteria. |
| 用法、用量<br>Dosage | 静脉滴注：成人一般感染，每次 0.3g，每日 2 次。可根据病情增加剂量，但每日不可超过 1.2g。用 0.9% 的生理盐水或 5% 葡萄糖注射液稀释。<br>Adults' general infection: 0.3g singly, two times a day. The dose can be increased according to patients' condition, but the daily dose can not exceed 1.2g. The drug should be diluted with 0.9% saline or 5% dextrose injection. |
| 剂型、规格<br>Preparations | 注射用比阿培南：每支 300mg。<br>Biapenem for injection: 300mg per vial. |
| 药品名称 Drug Names | 法罗培南钠 Faropenem Sodium |
| 适应证<br>Indications | 用于皮肤及软组织、呼吸系统、泌尿生殖系统及眼、耳、鼻、喉、口腔等部位的敏感菌感染。<br>It is intended to treat infection of skin and soft tissue, respiratory system, urogenital system, as well as eye, ear, nose, throat, mouth and etc.caused by susceptible strains. |
| 用法、用量<br>Dosage | 口服：成人常用量每次 150～200mg，一日 3 次。重症每次 200～300mg，一日 3 次。<br>Oral medication: adults' usual dose is 150～200mg singly, three times a day; dose for the severe infected is 200～300mg singly, three times a day. |
| 剂型、规格<br>Preparations | 片剂：每片 150mg；300mg。<br>Tablets: 150mg; 300mg per tablet. |
| 药品名称 Drug Names | 氨曲南 Aztreonam |
| 适应证<br>Indications | 用于敏感的革兰阴性菌所致的感染，包括肺炎、胸膜炎、腹腔感染、胆道感染、骨和关节感染、皮肤和软组织炎症，尤适用于尿路感染，也用于败血症。由于本品有较好的耐酶性，因此，当细菌对青霉素类、头孢菌素类、氨基糖苷类等药物不敏感时，可试用本品。<br>It is intended to treat infection caused by sensitive gram-negative bacteria, including pneumonia, pleurisy, abdominal infection, biliary tract infection, bone and joint infection, skin and soft tissue inflammation, septicemia, especially urinary tract infection. Since this product has good resistance to enzymes, it can be used when the bacteria are not sensitive to penicillins, cephalosporins, aminoglycosides and etc. |

**续　表**

| | |
|---|---|
| 用法、用量<br>Dosage | 　　肌内注射、静脉注射、静脉滴注。成人，一般感染，3～4g/d，分2～3次给予；严重感染，1次2g，一日3～4次，一日最大剂量为8g；无其他并发症的尿路感染，只需用1g，分1～2次给予。儿童，每次30mg/kg，一日3次，重症感染可增加至一日4次给药，一日最大剂量为120mg/kg。肌内注射：每1g药物，加液体3～4ml溶解。静脉注射：每1g药物，加液体10ml溶解，缓慢注射。静脉滴注：每1g药物，加液体50ml以上溶解（浓度不超过2%），滴注时间20～60分钟。<br><br>　　注射时，下列药液可用于本品的溶解 - 稀释液：灭菌注射用水、等渗氯化钠注射液、林格液、乳酸钠林格液、5%～10%葡萄糖液、葡萄糖氯化钠注射液等。用于肌内注射时，还可用含苯甲醇的氯化钠注射液作溶剂。<br><br>　　The drug is administered by intramuscular injection, intravenous injection and intravenous infusion. Adults' general infection: 3 ~ 4g a day, in 2 to 3 divided doses; severe infection: 2g singly, 3 to 4 times a day, with maximum daily dose of 8g; urinary tract infection with no complications: 1g only, in1 or 2 divided doses. Children: 30mg/kg singly, three times a day or 4 times a day in severe infection case, with maximum daily dose of 120mg/kg. Intramuscular injection: dissolve every 1g of the drug in 3 ~ 4ml of the liquid. Intravenous injection: dissolve every 1g of the drug in 10ml of the liquid for slow injection. Intravenous infusion: dissolve every 1g of the drug in over 50ml of the liquid (concentration can not exceed 2%), and the infusion time lasts 20 to 60 minutes.<br><br>　　In injection, the following can be used to dissolve or dilute the drug: sterile water for injection, isotonic sodium chloride injection, Ringer's solution, lactated Ringer's solution, 5% to 10% glucose solution, glucose and sodium chloride injection. While in intramuscular injection, the solvent could be sodium chloride injection with benzyl alcohol. |
| 剂型、规格<br>Preparations | 　　注射用氨曲南：每天1g（效价）。内含精氨酸0.78g（稳定、助溶用）。<br><br>　　Aztreonam for injection: 1g per vial (titer), containing 0.78g of arginine (for stabilization and solubilization). |

### 1.5　氨基糖苷类 Aminoglycosides

| 药品名称 Drug Names | 卡那霉素 Kanamycin |
|---|---|
| 适应证<br>Indications | 　　口服用于治疗敏感菌所致的肠道感染及用作肠道手术前准备，并有减少肠道细菌产生氨的作用，对肝硬化消化道出血患者的肝性脑病有一定防治作用。肌内注射用于敏感菌所致的系统感染，如肺炎、败血症、尿路感染等，常与其他抗菌药物联合应用。<br><br>　　By oral medication, it is intended to treat intestinal infection caused by susceptible strains, or used in preoperative preparation of intestinal surgery. It can weaken the function of intestinal bacteria to produce ammonia, and prevent hepatic encephalopathy of gastrointestinal bleeding in cirrhotic patients. By intramuscular, it is often in combination with other antimicrobial drugs to treat system injection caused by susceptible strains, such as pneumonia, septicimia, urinary tract infection and etc. |
| 用法、用量<br>Dosage | 　　肌内注射或静脉滴注：1次0.5g，一日1～1.2g；小儿每日15～25mg/kg，分2次给予。静脉滴注时应将一次用量以输液约100ml稀释，滴入时间为30～60分钟，切勿过速。口服：用于防治肝性脑病，一日4g，分次给予。腹部手术前准备：每小时1g，连续4次（常与甲硝唑联合应用）后，改为每6小时1次，连服36～72小时。<br><br>　　Intramuscular injection or intravenous infusion: 0.5g singly, 1 ~ 1.2g a day; children with 15 ~ 25mg/kg a day, in 2 divided doses. Intravenous infusion: the single dose of drug should be diluted with 100ml of infusion; the infusion time is 30 to 60 minutes, and the speed can not be too fast. Oral medication: for preventing hepatic encephalopathy, 4g a day, in several divided dose. Preoperative preparation of abdominal surgery: give 1g every an hour, 4 times in a row (often in combination with metronidazole), afterwards give once every 6 hours for 36 to 72 hours. |

**续 表**

| | |
|---|---|
| 剂型、规格<br>Preparations | 注射用硫酸卡那霉素：每瓶 0.5g；1g。<br>注射液（含单硫酸卡那霉素）：每支 500mg（2ml）。<br>滴眼液：8ml（40mg）。<br>Kanamycin sulfate for injection: 0.5g, 1g per vial.<br>Injection (containing kanamycin sulfate): 500mg (2ml) per vial.<br>Drops: 8ml (40mg). |
| **药品名称 Drug Names** | 阿米卡星 Amikacin |
| 适应证<br>Indications | 临床主要用于对卡那霉素或庆大霉素耐药的革兰阴性杆菌所致的尿路、下呼吸道、腹腔、软组织、骨和关节、生殖系统等部位的感染，以及败血症等。<br>It is clinically used to treat infection of urinary tract, lower respiratory tract, abdominal cavity, soft tissue, bonesand joint, reproductive system and etc, as well as septicemia caused by kanamycin or gentamicin-resistant Gram-negative bacteria. |
| 用法、用量<br>Dosage | 肌内注射或静脉滴注：成人 7.5mg/kg，每 12 小时一次，每日总量不超过 1.5g，可用 7～10 日；无并发症的尿路感染，每次 0.2g，每 12 小时一次；小儿，开始用 10mg/kg，以后 7.5mg/kg，每 12 小时一次；较大儿童可按成人用量。<br>给药途径以肌内注射为主，也可用 100～200ml 输液稀释后静脉滴注，30～60 分钟进入体内，儿童则为 1～2 小时。疗程一般不超过 10 日。<br>肾功能不全者首次剂量 7.5mg/kg，以后则调整使血药峰浓度为 25μg/ml，谷浓度 5～8μg/ml。<br>The drug can be administered by intramuscular injection or intravenous infusion. Adults: 7.5mg/kg every 12 hours, with maximum daily dose of 1.5g, for 7 to 10 days; Uncomplicated urinary tract infection: 0.2g singly, every 12 hours Children: start with 10mg/kg, then give 7.5mg/kg, every 12 hours; older children can be given the adult dose.<br>The drug is administered mainly by intramuscular injection. It can also be given by intravenous infusion after diluting the drug with 100～200ml of the infusion. Time of infusion for adults is 30 to 60 minutes, while for children is 1 to 2 hours. The course of treatment is generally within 10 days.<br>Renal insufficiency patients: first dose is 7.5mg/kg, afterwards make adjustment to insure the peak plasma concentration is 25μg/ml and trough concentrations is 5～8μg/ml. |
| 剂型、规格<br>Preparations | 注射液：每支 0.1g（1ml）；0.2g（2ml）。<br>注射用硫酸阿米卡星：每瓶：0.2g。<br>Injection: 0.1g (1ml), 0.2g (2ml) per vial.<br>Amikacin sulfate for injection: 0.2g per vial. |
| **药品名称 Drug Names** | 妥布霉素 Tobramycin |
| 适应证<br>Indications | 临床主要用于铜绿假单胞菌感染。如烧伤、败血症等。对其他敏感革兰阴性杆菌所致的感染也可应用。与庆大霉素间存在较密切的交叉耐药性。<br>It is clinically used to treat Pseudomonas aeruginosa infection, such as burns and septicemia, as well as infection caused by other sensitive gram-negative bacilli. And it has cross-resistance with gentamicin. |
| 用法、用量<br>Dosage | 肌内注射或静脉滴注，一日 4.5mg/kg，分为 2 次给予，一日剂量不可超过 5mg/kg。静脉滴注时 1 次量用输液 100ml 稀释，于 30 分钟左右滴入。新生儿一日量 4mg/kg，分为 2 次给予。一般用药不超过 7～10 日。<br>Intramuscular injection or intravenous infusion: 4.5mg/kg a day, in 2 divided doses, with maximum daily dose of 5mg/kg. In intravenous infusion, dilute the single dose of the drug with 100ml of the infusion, and the time for infusion lasts 30 minutes. Newborns: 4mg/kg a day, in 2divided doses. Generally, the administraiton continues 7 to 10 days. |
| 剂型、规格<br>Preparations | 注射液：每支 80mg（2ml）。<br>Injection: 80mg (2ml) per vial. |

**续　表**

| 药品名称 Drug Names | 庆大霉素 Gentamicin |
|---|---|
| 适应证<br>Indications | 　临床主要用于大肠埃希菌、痢疾杆菌、克雷伯肺炎杆菌、变形杆菌、铜绿假单胞菌等革兰阴性菌引起的系统或局部感染（对中枢感染无效）。<br><br>　It is clinically used to treat system infection or local infection (excluding central nervous infection) caused by gram-negative bacteria,　such as E. coli, Shigella, Klebsiella pneumoniae, Proteus mirabilis, Pseudomonas aeruginosa and etc. |
| 用法、用量<br>Dosage | 　肌内注射或静脉滴注，一次 80mg，一日 2～3 次（间隔 8 小时）。对于革兰阴性杆菌所致重症感染或铜绿假单胞菌全身感染，一日量可用到 5mg/kg。静脉滴注给药可将 1 次量（80mg），用输液 100ml 稀释，于 30 分钟左右滴入。小儿一日 3～5mg/kg，分 2～3 次给予。<br>　口服：一次 80～160mg，一日 3～4 次。小儿每日 10～15mg/kg，分 3～4 次服，用于肠道感染或术前准备。<br><br>　Intramuscular injection or intravenous infusion: 80mg singly, 2 or 3 times a day (with interval of 8 hours). Severe infection caused by Gram-negative bacteria or systemic infection caused by Pseudomonas aeruginosa: the daily dose can be 5mg/kg. In intravenous infusion, dilute the single dose (80mg) with 100ml of the infusion, and the time for infusion is about 30 minutes. For children, give 3～5mg/kg a day, in 2 to 3 divided doses. Oral medication: 80～160mg singly, 3 to 4 times a day. Children: 10～15mg/kg a day, in 3 to 4 divided doses, for treating intestinal infection and preoperative preparation. |
| 剂型、规格<br>Preparations | 　注射液：每支 20mg（1ml）；40mg（1ml）；80mg（2ml）。<br>　片剂：每片 40mg。<br>　滴眼液：8ml（40mg）。<br><br>　Injection: 20mg (1ml), 40mg (1ml), 80mg (2ml) per vial.<br>　Tablets: 40mg per tablet.<br>　Drops: 8ml (40mg). |
| 药品名称 Drug Names | 西索米星 Sisomicin |
| 适应证<br>Indications | 　临床主要用于大肠埃希菌、痢疾杆菌、克雷伯杆菌、变形杆菌等革兰阴性菌引起的局部或系统感染（对中枢感染无效），对尿路感染作用尤佳。<br><br>　It is clinically used to treat system infection or local infection (excluding central nervous infection) caused by gram-negative bacteria, such as E. coli, Shigella, Klebsiella, Proteus and etc..It is. especially effective in treating urinary tract infection. |
| 用法、用量<br>Dosage | 　成人一日量 3mg/kg，分为 3 次，肌内注射。疗程不超过 7～10 日。<br><br>　For adults, give 3mg/kg a day, in 3 divided doses, by intramuscular injection. The course of treatment continues 7 to 10 days. |
| 剂型、规格<br>Preparations | 　注射液：每支 75mg（1.5ml）；100mg（2ml）。<br>　Injection: 75mg (1.5ml), 100mg (2ml) per vial. |
| 药品名称 Drug Names | 奈替米星 Netilmicin |
| 适应证<br>Indications | 　临床主要用于大肠埃希菌、克雷伯杆菌、变形杆菌、肠杆菌属、枸橼酸杆菌、沙雷杆菌、流感嗜血杆菌、沙门杆菌、志贺杆菌、奈瑟球菌等革兰阴性菌所致呼吸道、消化道、泌尿生殖系、皮肤和软组织、骨和关节、腹腔、创伤等部位的感染，也适用于败血症。<br><br>　It is clinically used to treat infection of respiratory tract, alimentary canal, urogenital system, skin and soft tissue, bone and joint, abdominal cavity, trauma and etc. caused by Gram-negative bacteria, such as E. coli, Klebsiella, Proteus, Enterobacter, Citrobacter, Serratia bacteria, Haemophilus influenzae, Salmonella, Shigella, Neisseria and etc. It is also effective in treating septicemia. |
| 用法、用量<br>Dosage | 　单纯泌尿系感染：成人一日量为 3～4mg/kg，分为 2 次。较严重的系统感染：成人一日量为 4～6.5mg/kg，分为 2～3 次给予；新生儿（6 周龄以内）：一日 4～6.5mg/kg；婴儿和儿童：一日 5～8mg/kg，分为 2～3 次给予，肌内注射给药。如必须静脉滴注，则将 1 次药量加入 50～200ml 输液中，缓慢滴入。有报道，本品一日按 4.5～6mg/kg 量，1 次肌内注射，效果好，且不良反应少。 |

**续 表**

| | Simple urinary tract infection: for adults, give 3 ~ 4mg/kg a day, in 2 divided doses. Severe infection: for adults, give 4 ~ 6.5mg/kg a day, in 2 or 3 divided doses; for newborns, (within 6 weeks), give 4 ~ 6.5mg/kg a day; for infants and children: give 5 ~ 8mg/kg a day, in 2 to 3 divided doses, by intramuscular injection. If intravenous infusion is needed, add the single dose in 50 ~ 200ml of the infusion for slow infusion. It has been reported that the dosage of 4.5 ~ 6mg/kg a day by one time intramuscular injection has better effect and less side effect. |
|---|---|
| 剂型、规格<br>Preparations | 注射液：每支 150mg（1.5ml）。<br>Injection: 150mg (1.5ml) per vial. |

| 药品名称 Drug Names | 小诺米星 Micronomicin |
|---|---|
| 适应证<br>Indications | 临床主要用于大肠埃希菌、克雷伯杆菌、变形杆菌、肠杆菌属、沙雷杆菌、铜绿假单胞菌等革兰阴性杆菌引起的呼吸道、泌尿道、腹腔以及外伤感染，也适用于败血症。<br>It is clinically used to treat urinary tract infection, abdominal infection and trauma infection caused by gram-negative bacteria, such as E. coli, Klebsiella, Proteus, Enterobacter, Serratia respiratory tract bacteria, Pseudomonas aeruginosa and etc.. And it is also effective in teating septicemia. |
| 用法、用量<br>Dosage | 泌尿道感染：1 次 120mg，肌内注射，一日 2 次。其他感染：1 次 60mg，一日 2 ~ 3 次，肌内注射。用药疗程一般不超过 2 周。<br>Urinary tract infection: 120mg singly, by intramuscular injection, 2 times a day. Other infection: 60mg singly, 2 or 3 times a day, by intramuscular injection. The course of treatment is generally within two weeks. |
| 剂型、规格<br>Preparations | 注射液：每支 60mg（2ml）。<br>Injection: 60mg (2ml) per vial. |

| 药品名称 Drug Names | 异帕米星 Isepamicin |
|---|---|
| 适应证<br>Indications | 临床适用于不敏感菌所致外伤或烧伤创口感染、肺炎、支气管炎、肾盂肾炎、膀胱炎、腹膜炎及败血症。<br>It is clinically used to treat trauma infection or burns of wound infection, pneumonia, bronchitis, pyelonephritis, cystitis, peritonitis and septicemia caused by susceptible strains mentioned above. |
| 用法、用量<br>Dosage | 成人一日量 400mg，通常分为 2 次（或每日 1 次）肌内注射或静脉滴注。静脉滴注速度控制为 0.5 ~ 1 小时滴毕，按年龄、体质和症状适当调整。<br>Adults: 400mg a day, usually in 2 divided doses (or once a day), by intramuscular injection or intravenous drip. Infusion time should be controlled as 0.5 to 1 hour, and make appropriate adjustments according to age, physical condition and symptoms. |
| 剂型、规格<br>Preparations | 注射液：每支 200mg（2ml）。<br>Injection: per 200mg (2ml). |

| 药品名称 Drug Names | 依替米星 Etimicin |
|---|---|
| 适应证<br>Indications | 临床主要用于革兰阴性杆菌、大肠埃希菌、肺炎克雷伯菌、沙雷菌属、奇异变形杆菌、沙门菌属、流感嗜血杆菌等敏感菌所引起的呼吸道、泌尿生殖系统、腹腔、皮肤和软组织等部位的感染及败血症。<br>It is clinically used to treat infection of respiratory tract, urogenital system, abdomimal cavity, skin and soft tissue, septicemia and etc. caused by susceptible strains, such as Gram-negative bacteria, Escherichia coli, Klebsiella pneumoniae, Serratia, Proteus mirabilis, Salmonella, Haemophilus influenzae, etc. |
| 用法、用量<br>Dosage | 成人量每日 200mg，一次加入输液（0.9% 氯化钠液或 5% 葡萄糖液）100ml 中，静脉滴注 1 小时，每日只用 1 次，连用 3 ~ 7 日。<br>For adults, give 200mg a day, by intravenous infusion. Add 100ml of the infusion (0.9% sodium chloride or 5% glucose solution) in the drug for intravenous infusion of 1 hour. It is administeder only once a day for 3 to 7 days. |

**续　表**

| | |
|---|---|
| 剂型、规格<br>Preparations | 注射用粉针：每支 50mg；100mg。<br>注射液：50mg（1ml）；100mg（2ml）。<br>Powder for injection: 50mg, 100mg of each.<br>Injection: 50mg (1ml), 100mg (2ml). |
| 药品名称 Drug Names | 大观霉素 Spectinomycin |
| 适应证<br>Indications | 临床主要应用于淋球菌所引起的泌尿系感染，适用于对青霉素、四环素等耐药的病例。<br>It is clinically intended to treat urinary tract infection caused by Neisseria gonorrhoeae, as well as cases which are resistant to penicillin and tetracycline. |
| 用法、用量<br>Dosage | 1 次肌内注射 2g。将特殊稀释液（0.9% 苯甲醇溶液）3.2ml 注入药瓶中，猛力振摇，使成混悬液（约 5ml），用粗针头注入臀上部外侧深部肌肉内。一般只用 1 次即可。对于使用其他抗生素治疗而迁延未愈的患者，可按 4g 剂量给药，即 1 次用药 4g，分注于两侧臀上外侧肌内，或 1 次肌内注射 2g，一日内用药 2 次。<br>The single dose for intramuscular injection is 2g. Add 3.2ml of the special diluent (0.9% benzyl alcohol solution) into the bottle, shake vigorously to make a suspension (about 5ml), then use a thick needle to injected into the deep muscle outside of the upper buttock. Usually, give only one times. For unhealed patients who has been given other antibiotics: give 4g dose, ie, a second medication 4g, on the outside of both sides of the superior gluteal intramuscular injection or an intramuscular injection 2g, medication twice a day. |
| 剂型、规格<br>Preparations | 注射用盐酸大观霉素：每支 2g；4g（附 0.9% 苯甲醇注射液 1 支）。<br>Spectinomycin Hydrochloride for injection: 2g, 4g (with 1 bottle of 0.9% benzyl alcohol injection) per vial. |

1.6　四环素类 Teracyclines

| | |
|---|---|
| 药品名称 Drug Names | 四环素 Tetracycline |
| 适应证<br>Indications | 现主要用于立克次体病、布氏杆菌病、淋巴肉芽肿、支原体肺炎、螺旋体病、衣原体病，也可用于敏感的革兰阳性球菌或革兰阴性杆菌所引起的轻症感染。<br>It is now mainly used to treat for rickettsial diseases, brucellosis, lymphogranuloma venereum, mycoplasma pneumonia, leptospirosis, chlamydia, as well as mild infection caused by susceptible Gram-positive cocci or gram-negative bacilli. |
| 用法、用量<br>Dosage | 口服：成人一日 3 ~ 4 次，1 次 0.5g；8 岁以上小儿一日 30 ~ 40mg/kg，分 3 ~ 4 次用。<br>Oral medication: for adults, give 0.5g singly, 3 to 4 times a day; for children over the age of 8, give 30 ~ 40mg/kg singly, in 3 to 4 divided doses. |
| 剂型、规格<br>Preparations | 片剂：每片 0.125g；0.25g。<br>胶囊剂：每粒 0.25g。<br>Tablets: 0.125g, 0.25g per tablet.<br>Capsules: 0.25g per capsule. |
| 药品名称 Drug Names | 土霉素 Oxytetracycline |
| 适应证<br>Indications | 现主要用于立克次体病、布氏杆菌病、淋巴肉芽肿、支原体肺炎、螺旋体病、衣原体病，也可用于敏感的革兰阳性球菌或革兰阴性杆菌所引起的轻症感染。<br>It is now mainly used to treat for rickettsial diseases, brucellosis, lymphogranuloma venereum, mycoplasma pneumonia, leptospirosis, chlamydia, as well as mild infection caused by susceptible Gram-positive cocci or gram-negative bacilli. |
| 用法、用量<br>Dosage | 口服：1 次 0.5g，一日 3 ~ 4 次。8 岁以上小儿每日 30 ~ 40mg/kg，分 3 ~ 4 次服。<br>Oral medication: 0.5g singly, 3 to 4 times a day; children over the age of 8: 30 ~ 40mg/kg a day, in 3 to 4 divided doses. |
| 剂型、规格<br>Preparations | 片剂：每片 0.125g；0.25g（1mg= 盐酸土霉素 1000U）。<br>Tablets: 0.125g, 0.25g per tablet (1mg = 1000 units of oxytetracycline hydrochloride). |

**续　表**

| 药品名称 Drug Names | 多西环素 Doxycycline |
|---|---|
| 适应证<br>Indications | 临床主要用于敏感的革兰阳性球菌和革兰阴性杆菌所致的上呼吸道感染、扁桃体炎、胆道感染、淋巴结炎、蜂窝织炎、老年慢性支气管炎等，也用于斑疹伤寒、恙虫病、支原体肺炎等。尚可用于治疗霍乱，也可用于预防恶性疟疾和钩端螺旋体感染。<br><br>It is clinically used to treat upper respiratory infection, tonsillitis, biliary tract infection, lymphadenitis, cellulitis, chronic bronchitis and etc. caused by susceptible gram-positive cocci and gram-negative bacteria, as well as typhus, scrub typhus and mycoplasma pneumonia, etc.. It is also can be used in treating cholera and preventing Falciparum malaria and leptospira infection. |
| 用法、用量<br>Dosage | 口服，首次 0.2g，以后每次 0.1g，一日 1～2 次。8 岁以上儿童，首次 4mg/kg，以后每次 2～4mg/kg，一日 1～2 次。一般疗程为 3～7 日。预防恶性疟：每周 0.1g；预防钩端螺旋体病：每周 2 次，每次 0.1g。<br><br>Oral medication: give first dose of 0.2g, afterwards 0.1g singly, 1 to 2 times a day; children over the age of 8: give the first dose of 4mg/kg, afterwards 2～4mg/kg singly, 1 or 2 times a day. The general course of treatment is 3 to 7 days. Falciparum malaria prevention: 0.1g a week; leptospira infection prevention: 0.1g singly, 2 times a week. |
| 剂型、规格<br>Preparations | 片剂：每片 0.05g；0.1g。<br>胶囊剂：每粒 0.1g（1mg= 盐酸多西环素 1000U）。<br>Tablets: 0.05g, 0.1g per tablet.<br>Capsules: 0.1g per capsule (1mg = doxycycline hydrochloride 1000 units). |
| 药品名称 Drug Names | 米诺环素 Minocycline |
| 适应证<br>Indications | 临床主要用于立克次体病、支原体肺炎、淋巴肉芽肿、下疳、鼠疫、霍乱、布氏杆菌病（与链霉素联合应用）等引起的泌尿系、呼吸道、胆道、乳腺及皮肤软组织感染。<br><br>Clinically, it is mainly used to treat rickettsial diseases, mycoplasma pneumonia, lymphogranuloma venereum, urinary chancre, plague, cholera, as well as infection of urinary tract, respiratory tract, biliary tract, breast, skin and soft tissue caused by brucellosis (in combination with streptomycin). |
| 用法、用量<br>Dosage | 成人一般首次量 200mg，以后每 12 小时服 100mg。或在首次量后，每 6 小时服用 50mg。<br><br>Adults: general first dose is 200mg, afterwards give100mg every 12 hours; or give 50mg every 6 hours after the first dose. |
| 剂型、规格<br>Preparations | 片剂：每片 0.1g（效价）。<br>Tablets: 0.1g (titer) per tablet. |

1.7　林可霉素类 Lincomycins

| 药品名称 Drug Names | 氯霉素 Chloramphenicol |
|---|---|
| 适应证<br>Indications | 临床主要用于伤寒、副伤寒和其他沙门菌、脆弱拟杆菌感染。与氨苄西林合用于流感嗜血杆菌性脑膜炎。由脑膜炎球菌或肺炎链球菌引起的脑膜炎，在患者不宜用青霉素时，也可用本品。外用治疗沙眼或化脓菌感染。<br><br>Clinically, it is mainly used to treat typhoid and paratyphoid, as well as other Salmonella infection and Bacteroides fragilis infection. It can treat meningitis caused by haemophilus influenzae when used in combination with ampicillin. In treatment of meningitis caused by meningococcus or streptococcus pneumoniae, if the patients are not suggested to use penicillin, this drug can be used. External use can treat trachoma or pyogenic bacteria infection. |
| 用法、用量<br>Dosage | 口服：成人 1 次 0.25～0.5g，一日 1～2g；小儿每日 25～50mg/kg，分 3～4 次服；新生儿每日不超过 25mg/kg。<br>　静脉滴注：一日量为 1～2g，分 2 次注射。以输液稀释，1 支氯霉素（250mg）至少用稀释液 100ml。氯霉素注射液（含乙醇、甘油或丙二醇等溶媒），宜用干燥注射器抽取，边稀释边振荡，防止析出结晶。症状消退后应酌情减量或停药。<br><br>Oral medication: for adults, give 0.25～0.5g singly, 1～2g a day; for children, give 25～50mg/kg a day, in 3 to 4 divided doses; for newborns, daily dose can not exceed 25mg/kg.<br>　Intravenous infusion: 1～2g a day, in 2divided doses. Dilute every 1 bottle of chloramphenicol (250mg) with at least 100ml of the infusion. Chloramphenicol injection (containing ethanol, glycerol |

**续　表**

| | or propylene glycol solvent): use dried syringe to get drawn out, shake while diluting to prevent crystallization. When symptoms subside, reduce the drug dose or suspend medication appropriately. |
|---|---|
| 剂型、规格<br>Preparations | 片（胶囊剂）：每片（粒）0.25g。<br>注射液：每支 0.25g（2ml）。<br>滴眼液：8ml（20mg）。<br>滴耳液：10ml（0.25g）。<br>眼膏：1%；3%。<br>Tablets (capsules): (tablets) 0.25g per tablet.<br>Injection: 0.25g (2ml) per vial.<br>Drops: 8ml (20mg).<br>Eardrops: 10ml (0.25g).<br>Ointment: 1%; 3%. |
| **药品名称 Drug Names** | 林可霉素 Lincomycin |
| 适应证<br>Indications | 用于葡萄球菌、链球菌、肺炎链球菌引起的呼吸道感染、骨髓炎、关节和软组织感染及胆道感染。对一些厌氧菌感染也可应用。外用治疗革兰阳性菌化脓性感染。<br><br>It is intended to treat respiratory tract infection, osteomyelitis, joint and soft tissue infection and biliary tract infection caused by Staphylococcus, Streptococcus, and Streptococcus pneumoniae. It is also effective in treating infection by some of anaerobes. External use of the drug can treat purulent infection by Gram-positive bacteria. |
| 用法、用量<br>Dosage | 口服（空腹）：成人，1 次 0.25 ~ 0.5g（活性），一日 3 ~ 4 次；小儿一日 30 ~ 50mg（活性）/kg，分 3 ~ 4 次服用。肌内注射：成人 1 次 0.6g（活性），一日 2 ~ 3 次；小儿一日 10 ~ 20mg（活性）/kg，分 2 ~ 3 次给药。静脉滴注：成人 1 次 0.6g（活性），溶于 100 ~ 200ml 输液内，滴注 1 ~ 2 小时，每 8 ~ 12 小时 1 次。<br><br>Oral medication (on an empty stomach): for adults, give 1 0.25 ~ 0.5g (activity) singly, 3 to 4 times a day; for children, give 30 ~ 50mg (activity) / kg, 3 to 4 times a day. Intramuscular injection: for adults, give 0.6g (activity) singly, 2 to 3 times a day; for children, give 10 ~ 20mg (activity) / kg a day, in 2 to 3 divided doses. Intravenous infusion: give adults 0.6g (activity) singly, every 8 to 12 hours. Dissolve the drug in 100 ~ 200ml of the infusion. And the time for infusion is 1 to 2 hours. |
| 剂型、规格<br>Preparations | 片（胶囊）剂：每片（粒）0.25g（活性）；0.5g（活性）。<br>注射液：每支 0.2g（活性）（1ml）；0.6g（活性）（2ml）。<br>滴眼液：每支 3%（8ml）。<br>Tablets (capsules): 0.25g (activity), 0.5g (activity) per tablet (capsule).<br>Injection: 0.2g (activity) (1ml), 0.6g (activity) (2ml) per bottle.<br>Drops: 3% (8ml) per bottle. |
| **药品名称 Drug Names** | 克林霉素 Clindamycin |
| 适应证<br>Indications | 主要用于厌氧菌（包括脆弱拟杆菌、产气荚膜杆菌、放线菌等）引起的腹腔和妇科感染（常需与氨基糖苷类联合以消除需氧病原菌）。还用于敏感的革兰阳性菌引起的呼吸道、关节和软组织、骨组织、胆道等感染及败血症、心内膜炎等。本品是金黄色葡萄球菌骨髓炎的首选治疗药物。<br><br>It is mainly used to treat abdominal infection and gynecological infection (often used in combination with aminoglycoside to eliminate aerobic pathogens) caused by anaerobic bacteria (including Bacteroides fragilis, Clostridium perfringens, actinomycetes and etc.). It is also intended to treat infection of respiratory tract, joint and soft tissue, bone tissue, biliary tract and etc., as well as septicemia, endocarditis and etc. caused by susceptible Gram-positive bacteria. This product is the preferred choice for treating Staphylococcus aureus osteomyelitis. |

**续　表**

| | |
|---|---|
| 用法、用量<br>Dosage | 　　盐酸盐口服：成人，一次 0.15 ~ 0.3g（活性），一日 3 ~ 4 次；小儿，一日 10 ~ 20mg（活性）/kg，分 3 ~ 4 次给予。棕榈酸酯盐酸盐（供儿童应用）：一日 8 ~ 12mg/kg，极严重时可增至 20 ~ 25mg/kg，分为 3 ~ 4 次给予；10kg 以下体重的婴儿可按一日 8 ~ 12mg/kg 用药，分为 3 次给予；磷酸酯（注射剂）：成人革兰阳性需氧菌感染，一日 600 ~ 1200mg，分为 2 ~ 4 次肌内注射或静脉滴注；厌氧菌感染，一般用一日 1200 ~ 2700mg，极严重感染可用到 4800mg/d。儿童（1 月龄以上），重症感染一日量 15 ~ 25mg/kg，极严重可按 25 ~ 40mg/kg，均分为 3 ~ 4 次应用。<br>　　肌内注射量一次不超过 600mg，超过此量应静脉给予。静脉滴注前应先将药物用输液稀释，600mg 药物应加入不少于 100ml 输液中，至少输注 20 分钟。1 小时输注的药量不应超过 1200mg。<br>　　Hydrochloride Oral medication: for adults, give 0.15 ~ 0.3g (activity) singly, 3 to 4 times a day; for children, give 10 ~ 20mg (activity) / kg a day, in 3 to 4divided doses. Palmitate hydrochloride (for children): give 8 ~ 12mg/kg a day; or 20 ~ 25mg/kg a day, in divided 3 to 4 divided doses in very severe case; for children weighting under10kg, give 8 ~ 12mg/kg a day, in 3 divided doses. Phosphate (injection): Adults' aerobic Gram-positive infection, give 600 ~ 1200mg a day, in 2 to 4divided doses, by intramuscular injection or intravenous infusion; anaerobes infection: usually give 1200 ~ 2700mg a day or 4800mg a day in very severe infection case. Children (over the age of 1 month): in severe infection cases, give 15 ~ 25mg/kg a day, in 3 to 4 divided doses; in extremely severe case, increase the daily dose to 25 ~ 40mg/kg, in 3 to 4 divided doses.<br>　　Single dose for intramuscular injection should not exceed 600mg; if the single dose is more than this amount should be administered intravenously. Before intravenous infusion, dilute the drug with the infusion, and every 600mg of the drug needs at least 100ml of the infusion. The time for infusion is at least 20 minutes. Single dose for a one-hour infusion should not exceed 1200mg. |
| 剂型、规格<br>Preparations | 　　盐酸克林霉素胶囊剂：每胶囊 75mg（活性）；150mg（活性）。<br>　　盐酸克林霉素注射液：每支 150mg（2ml）；300mg（2ml）；600mg（4ml）。<br>Clindamycin Hydrochloride Capsules: 75mg (activity), 150mg (activity) per capsule.<br>Clindamycin Hydrochloride injection: 150mg (2ml), 300mg (2ml), 600mg (4ml) per vial. |
| 药品名称 Drug Names | 甲砜霉素 Thiamphenicol |
| 适应证<br>Indications | 　　临床主要用于伤寒、副伤寒和其他沙门菌感染，也用于敏感菌所致的呼吸道、胆道、尿路感染。<br>　　Clinically, it is mainly used to treat typhoid, paratyphoid and other salmonella infection, as well as infection of respiratory tract, biliary tract and urinary tract caused by susceptible strains. |
| 用法、用量<br>Dosage | 　　1 次 0.25 ~ 0.5g，一日 3 ~ 4 次。<br>0.25 ~ 0.5g singly, 3 to 4 times a day. |
| 剂型、规格<br>Preparations | 　　片剂 / 胶囊剂：0.125g；0.25g。<br>Tablets/ Capsules: 0.25, 0.5g per tablet/capsule. |

### 1.8　大环内酯类 Macrolides

| 药品名称 Drug Names | 红霉素 Erythromycin |
|---|---|
| 适应证<br>Indications | 　　临床主要应用于链球菌引起的扁桃体炎、猩红热、白喉及带菌者、淋病、李斯特菌病、肺炎链球菌下呼吸道感染（以上适用于不耐青霉素的患者）。对于军团菌肺炎和支原体肺炎，本品可作为首选药应用。尚可应用于流感杆菌引起的上呼吸道感染、金黄色葡萄球菌皮肤及软组织感染、梅毒、肠道阿米巴病等。<br>　　Clinically, it is mainly used to treat Tonsillitis, scarlet fever, diphtheria and carriers, gonorrhea, are Streptococcus listeriosis and streptococcus pneumoniae lower respiratory tract infection caused by streptococcus (suitable for patients who are intolerant of penicillin). In treatment of Legionella pneumonia and mycoplasma pneumonia, it can be the preferred drug. It can also be applied in treating respiratory tract infection caused by Haemophilus influenzae, Staphylococcus aureus skin and soft tissue infection, syphilis, and other intestinal amebiasis, etc. |

**续 表**

| | |
|---|---|
| 用法、用量<br>Dosage | 　　口服：成人一日 1 ～ 2g，分 3 ～ 4 次服用，整片吞服；小儿，每日 30 ～ 50mg/kg，分 3 ～ 4 次服用。静脉滴注：成人一日 1 ～ 2g，分 3 ～ 4 次滴注；小儿每日 30 ～ 50mg/kg，分 3 ～ 4 次滴注。用时，将乳糖酸红霉素溶于 10ml 灭菌注射用水中，再添加到输液 500ml 中，缓慢滴入（最后稀释浓度一般小于 0.1%）。不能直接用含盐输液溶解。<br><br>　　Oral medication: for adults, give 1 ～ 2g a day, in 3 to 4 divided doses, by swallowing the whole tablet; for children, give 30 ～ 50mg/kg a day, in 3 to 4 divided doses. Intravenous infusion: for adults, give 1 ～ 2g a day, in 3 to 4 divided doses; for children, give 30 ～ 50mg/kg a day, in 3 to 4 divided doses. When using the erythromycin lactobionate, dissolve it in 10ml of sterile water for injection, then add into 500ml of the infusion for slow infusion (final concentration after dilution is generally less than 0.1%). It can not be directly dissolved in saline infusion. |
| 剂型、规格<br>Preparations | 　　片剂（肠溶）：每片 0.1g（10 万 U）；0.125g（12.5 万 U）；0.25g（25 万 U）。<br>　　注射用乳糖酸红霉素：每瓶 0.25g（25 万 U）；0.3g（30 万 U）。<br>　　红霉素软膏：1%。<br>　　红霉素眼膏：0.5%。<br><br>　　Tablets (enteric-coated): 0.1g (10 million units), 0.125g (12.5 million units), 0.25g (25 million units) per tablet.<br>　　Erythromycin lactobionate for injection: 0.25g (25 million units), 0.3g (30 million units) per vial.<br>　　Erythromycin ointment: 1%.<br>　　Erythromycin eye ointment: 0.5%. |
| 药品名称 Drug Names | 琥乙红霉素 Erythromycin Ethylsuccinate |
| 适应证<br>Indications | 　　临床主要应用于链球菌引起的扁桃体炎、猩红热、白喉及带菌者、淋病、李斯特菌病、肺炎链球菌下呼吸道感染（以上适用于不耐青霉素的患者）。对于军团菌肺炎和支原体肺炎，本品可作为首选药应用。尚可应用于流感杆菌引起的上呼吸道感染、金黄色葡萄球菌皮肤及软组织感染、梅毒、肠道阿米巴病等。<br><br>　　Clinically, it is mainly used to treat Tonsillitis, scarlet fever, diphtheria and carriers, gonorrhea, are Streptococcus listeriosis and streptococcus pneumoniae lower respiratory tract infection caused by streptococcus (suitable for patients who are intolerant of penicillin). In treatment of Legionella pneumonia and mycoplasma pneumonia, it can be the preferred drug. It can also be applied in treating respiratory tract infection caused by Haemophilus influenzae, Staphylococcus aureus skin and soft tissue infection, syphilis, and other intestinal amebiasis, etc. |
| 用法、用量<br>Dosage | 　　口服：成人一次 0.25 ～ 0.5g，一日 3 ～ 4 次；小儿一日量 30 ～ 50mg/kg，分 3 ～ 4 次用。或按下列方案应用：体重 <5kg 者，1 次 40mg/kg，一日 4 次；5 ～ 7kg 者，1 次 50mg，一日 4 次；7 ～ 11kg 者，1 次 100mg，一日 4 次；11 ～ 23kg 者，1 次 200mg，一日 4 次；23 ～ 45kg 者，1 次 300mg，一日 4 次；>45kg 者，按成人量给予。<br><br>　　Oral medication: for adults, give 0.25 ～ 0.5g singly, 3 to 4 times a day; for children, give 30 ～ 50mg/kg a day, in 3 to 4 divided doses. Or use the following dosage regimen for children: under 5kg: 40mg/kg singly, 4 times a day; 5 ～ 7kg: 50mg singly, 4 times a day; 7 ～ 11kg: 100mg singly, 4 times a day; 11 ～ 23kg: 200mg singly, 4 times a day; 23 ～ 45kg: 300mg singly, 4 times a day; over 45kg: as adult dosage. |
| 剂型、规格<br>Preparations | 　　片剂：每片 0.1g；0.125g（按红霉素计）。<br>　　颗粒剂：每袋 0.05g；0.1g；0.125g；0.25g（按红霉素计）。<br><br>　　Tablets: 0.1g, 0.125g per tablet (measured by erythromycin).<br>　　Granules: 0.05g, 0.1g, 0.125g, 0.25g per bag (measured by erythromycin). |
| 药品名称 Drug Names | 罗红霉素 Roxithromycin |
| 适应证<br>Indications | 　　临床应用于敏感菌所致的呼吸道、泌尿道、皮肤和软组织、五官科感染。<br>　　It is clinically used to treat infection of respiratory tract, urinary tract, skin and soft tissue, and ENT caused by susceptible strains. |

| | |
|---|---|
| 用法、用量<br>Dosage | 成人一次 150mg，一日 2 次，餐前服。幼儿：每次 2.5 ~ 5mg/kg，一日 2 次。老年人与肾功能一般减退者不需要调整剂量。严重肝硬化者，每日 150mg。<br><br>Adults: 150mg singly, 2 times a day, before meals. Children: 2.5 ~ 5mg/kg singly, 2 times a day. Elderly patients and patients with general renal insuffiency do not need to make adjustment on the dose. Severe cirrhosis: 150mg a day. |
| 剂型、规格<br>Preparations | 片剂：每片 150mg；250mg；300mg。<br>Tablets: 150mg, 250mg, 300mg per tablet. |
| 药品名称 Drug Names | 克拉霉素 Clarithromycin |
| 适应证<br>Indications | 临床用于化脓性链球菌所致的咽炎和扁桃体炎，肺炎链球菌所致的急性中耳炎、肺炎和支气管炎，流感嗜血杆菌、卡他球菌所致支气管炎，支原体肺炎以及葡萄球菌、链球菌所致皮肤及软组织感染。<br><br>It is clinically uesd to treat pharyngitis and tonsillitis caused by Streptococcus pyogenes, acute otitis media, pneumonia and bronchitis caused by Streptococcus pneumoniae,, bronchitis and mycoplasma pneumonia caused by Haemophilus influenzae and catarrhal cocci and skin and soft tissue infection bronchitis caused by Staphylococcus aureus and Streptococcus. |
| 用法、用量<br>Dosage | 轻症：每次 250mg，重症每次 500mg，均为 12 小时 1 次口服，疗程 7 ~ 14 日。12 岁以上儿童按成人量。6 个月以上小儿至 12 岁以下儿童用量每日 15mg/kg，分为 2 次；或按以下方法口服给药：8 ~ 11kg 体重每次 62.5mg，12 ~ 19kg 体重每次 125mg，20 ~ 29kg 体重每次 187.5mg，30 ~ 40kg 体重每次 250mg，按上量每日用药 2 次。<br><br>Mild case: give 250mg singly, every 12 hours, orally; severe case: give 500mg singly, every 12 hours, orally. The course of treatment is 7 to 14 days. Children over the age of 12: give adult dosage. Children over 6 months or under the age of 12: give15mg/kg a day, in 2 divided doses. or use the following dosage regimen for oral medication: weight of 8 ~ 11kg: 62.5mg singly, twice a day; 12 ~ 19kg: 125mg singly, twice a day; 20 ~ 29kg: 187.5mg singly, twice a day; 30 ~ 40kg: 250mg singly, twice a day. |
| 剂型、规格<br>Preparations | 片剂：每片 250mg 或 500mg。<br>Tablets: 250mg or 500mg per tablet. |
| 药品名称 Drug Names | 阿奇霉素 Azithromycin |
| 适应证<br>Indications | 临床应用于敏感微生物所致的呼吸道、皮肤和软组织感染。<br><br>It is clinically used to treat infection of respiratory tract, skin and soft tissue caused by susceptible microorganisms. |
| 用法、用量<br>Dosage | 每日只需服 1 次，成人 500mg；儿童 10mg/kg，连用 3 日。<br>重症可注射给药，每日 1 次，每次 500mg，以注射用水 5ml 溶解后，加入 0.9% 氯化钠液或 5% 葡萄糖液中使成 1 ~ 2mg/ml 浓度，静脉滴注 1 ~ 2 小时，约 2 日症状控制后改成口服巩固疗效。<br><br>Adults: 500mg singly, only once a day Children: 10mg/kg singly, only once a day, for 3 days<br>Severe infected patients can be given injection: 500mg singly, once a day. Dissolve the drug in 5ml of water for injection, then add in 0.9% sodium chloride or 5% glucose solution until its concentration become 1 ~ 2mg/ml, afterwards five intravenous infusion for 1 to 2 hours. After about 2 days, if the symptom get well controlled, the patients can be given oral medication for consolidation. |
| 剂型、规格<br>Preparations | 片剂（胶囊）：每粒 250mg 或 500mg。<br>乳糖酸阿奇霉素（冻干粉针）：每支 500mg。<br>Tablets (capsules): 250mg or 500mg per tablet (capsule).<br>Lactose azithromycin (lyophilized powder for injection): 500mg of each. |

| 药品名称 Drug Names | 泰利霉素 Telithromycin |
| --- | --- |
| 适应证<br>Indications | 临床主要用于敏感菌所致的呼吸道感染，包括社区获得性肺炎、慢性支气管炎、急性上颌窦咽炎及扁桃体炎。<br>Clinically, it is mainly used to treat respiratory tract infection caused by susceptible strains, including community-acquired pneumonia, chronic bronchitis, acute maxillary sinus pharyngitis and tonsillitis. |
| 用法、用量<br>Dosage | 口服，一日 1 次 800mg，疗程为 5 ～ 10 日。<br>Oral medication: 800mg a day, with treatment course of 5 to 10 days |
| 剂型、规格<br>Preparations | 片剂：400mg；800mg。<br>Tablets: 400mg, 800mg. |
| 药品名称 Drug Names | 地红霉素 Dirithromycin |
| 适应证<br>Indications | 本品适用于敏感菌所致的轻、中度感染，慢性支气管炎（包括急性发作）、社区获得性肺炎、咽炎、扁桃体炎等。<br>It is intended to treat mild infection, moderate infection, chronic bronchitis (including acute attack), community-acquired pneumonia, pharyngitis, tonsillitis and etc. caused by susceptible strains. |
| 用法、用量<br>Dosage | 每次 500mg，每日 1 次，餐时服用，疗程根据病情为 7 ～ 14 日。<br>Take it when eating meals; and the course of treatment is 7 to 14 days according to patients' condition. |
| 剂型、规格<br>Preparations | 片剂（肠溶衣片）：每片 250mg。<br>Tablets (enteric-coated): 250mg per tablet. |
| 药品名称 Drug Names | 吉他霉素 Kitasamycin |
| 适应证<br>Indications | 可作为红霉素的替代品，用于敏感菌所致的口咽部、呼吸道、皮肤和软组织、胆道等感染。<br>It can be a substitute for Erythromycin. It is intended to treat infection of oropharynx, respiratory tract, skin and soft tissue, biliary tract and etc. caused by susceptible strains mentioned above. |
| 用法、用量<br>Dosage | 口服：每次 0.3 ～ 0.4g，每日 3 ～ 4 次。静脉注射：1 次 0.2 ～ 0.4g，一日 2 ～ 3 次，将 1 次用量溶于 20ml 氯化钠注射液或葡萄糖液中，缓慢注射。<br>Oral medication: 0.3 ～ 0.4g singly, 3 to 4 times a day. Intravenous: 0.2 ～ 0.4g singly, 2 to 3 times a day; dissolve to the single dose in 20ml of sodium chloride injection or glucose solution for slow injection. |
| 剂型、规格<br>Preparations | 片剂：每片 0.1g。<br>注射用酒石酸吉他霉素：每瓶 0.2g。<br>Tablets: 0.1g per tablet.<br>Tartrate Kitasamycin for injection: 0.2g per vial. |
| 药品名称 Drug Names | 麦迪霉素 Midecamycin |
| 适应证<br>Indications | 可作为红霉素的替代品，用于上述敏感菌所致的口咽部、呼吸道、皮肤和软组织、胆道等感染。<br>It can be a substitute for Erythromycin. It is intended to treat infection of oropharynx, respiratory tract, skin and soft tissue, biliary tract and etc. caused by susceptible strains mentioned above. |
| 用法、用量<br>Dosage | 口服，成人一日量 0.8 ～ 1.2g，分 3 ～ 4 次用。儿童一日量 30mg/kg，分 3 ～ 4 次给予。<br>Oral medication: for adults, give 0.8 ～ 1.2g a day, in 3 to 4 divided doses; for children, give 30mg/kg a day, in 3 to 4 divided doses. |
| 剂型、规格<br>Preparations | 麦迪霉素片：每片 0.1g。<br>Tablets: 0.1g per tablet. |
| 药品名称 Drug Names | 乙酰麦迪霉素 Acetylmidecamycin |
| 适应证<br>Indications | 主要适用于金黄色葡萄球菌、溶血性链球菌、肺炎球菌等所致的呼吸道感染及皮肤、软组织感染，也可用于支原体肺炎。<br>Mainly applicable to respiratory tract infections and skin and soft tissue infections by Staphylococcus aureus, hemolytic streptococcus pneumoniae bacteria caused, can also be used for Mycoplasma pneumonia. |

| 用法、用量<br>Dosage | 成人：一日 300 ～ 900mg，分 3 ～ 4 次服。<br>儿童：一日 15 ～ 30mg/kg，分 3 ～ 4 次给予。<br>Adults: 300 ~ 900mg a day, in 3 to 4 divided doses.<br>Children: 15 ~ 30mg/kg a day, in 3 to 4 divided doses. |
|---|---|
| 剂型、规格<br>Preparations | 醋酸乙酰麦迪霉素颗粒剂：1.0g：0.2g；干混悬剂：0.1g。<br>Acetyl acetate Midecamycin granules: 1.0g: 0.2g; dry suspension: 0.1g. |
| **药品名称 Drug Names** | **交沙霉素 Josamycin** |
| 适应证<br>Indications | 临床应用于敏感菌所致的口咽部、呼吸道、肺、鼻窦、中耳、皮肤及软组织、胆道等部位的感染。<br>It is clinically used to treat infection of oropharynx, respiratory tract, lungs, sinus, middle ear, skin and soft tissue, biliary tract and etc. caused by susceptible strains. |
| 用法、用量<br>Dosage | 成人：一日量 0.8 ～ 1.2g，分 3 ～ 4 次应用。儿童：一日量为 30mg/kg，分 3 ～ 4 次给予。空腹服用吸收好。<br>Adults: 0.8 ~ 1.2g a day, in 3 to 4divided doses. Children: 30mg/kg a day, in 3 to 4 divided doses. Well absorbed on an empty stomach. |
| 剂型、规格<br>Preparations | 交沙霉素片剂：每片 0.1g。<br>丙酸交沙霉素散剂：每包含药 0.1g（效价）。<br>Josamycin tablets: 0.1g per tablet.<br>Propionate Josamycin powder: 0.1g per bag (titer). |
| **药品名称 Drug Names** | **麦白霉素 Meleumycin** |
| 适应证<br>Indications | 用于敏感菌所致的呼吸道感染、皮肤感染、软组织感染、胆道感染、支原体性肺炎等。<br>Respiratory tract infections, skin infections, soft tissue infections, biliary tract infection, mycoplasma pneumonia, caused by the susceptible strains. |
| 用法、用量<br>Dosage | 成人一日量 0.8 ～ 1.2g，分 3 ～ 4 次服。儿童一日量 30mg/kg，分 3 ～ 4 次服。<br>Adults: 0.8 ~ 1.2g a day, in 3 to 4 divided doses. Children: 30mg/kg a day, in 3 to 4divided doses. |
| 剂型、规格<br>Preparations | 片剂：每片 0.1g。<br>Tablets: 0.1g per tablet. |
| **药品名称 Drug Names** | **罗他霉素 Rokitamycin** |
| 适应证<br>Indications | 临床应用于敏感菌所致的咽、扁桃体、支气管、肺、中耳、鼻旁窦、牙周、皮肤及软组织等部位的感染。<br>It is clinically used to treat infection of pharynx, tonsils, bronchi, lungs, middle ear, paranasal sinuses, periodontium, skin and soft tissue and etc. caused by susceptible strains mentioned above. |
| 用法、用量<br>Dosage | 口服，成人每次 200mg，一日 3 次。儿童：一日量 20 ～ 30mg/kg，分 3 次服。<br>Oral medication: for adults, give 200mg singly, 3 times a day; for children, give 20 ~ 30mg/kg a day, in 3 divided doses. |
| 剂型、规格<br>Preparations | 片剂：每片 100mg。<br>Tablets: 100mg per tablet. |
| **药品名称 Drug Names** | **乙酰螺旋霉素 Acetylspiramycin** |
| 适应证<br>Indications | 适用于敏感菌所致的扁桃体炎、支气管炎、肺炎、咽炎、中耳炎、皮肤和软组织感染、乳腺炎、胆囊炎、猩红热、牙科和眼科感染等。<br>It is intended to treat tonsillitis, bronchitis, pneumonia, pharyngitis, otitis media, skin and soft tissue infection, mastitis, cholecystitis, scarlet fever, dental infection and eye infection caused by susceptible strains mentioned above. |
| 用法、用量<br>Dosage | 成人一次 0.2g，一日 4 ～ 6 次。重症一日可用至 1.6 ～ 2g。儿童一日量 30mg/kg，分 4 次给予。<br>Adults: 0.2g singly, 4 to 6 times a day; or 1.6 ~ 2g a day in severe cases. Children: 30mg/kg a day, in 4 divided doses. |

**续　表**

| 剂型、规格<br>Preparations | 乙酰螺旋霉素片（肠溶）剂：每片 0.1g（效价）。<br>Tablets (enteric-coated): 0.1g per tablet (titer). |
| --- | --- |

## 1.9　糖肽类 Glycopeptides

| 药品名称 Drug Names | 去甲万古霉素 Norvancomycin |
| --- | --- |
| 适应证<br>Indications | 主要用于葡萄球菌（包括产酶株和耐甲氧西林株）、肠球菌（耐氨苄西林株）、难辨梭状芽孢杆菌等所致的系统感染和肠道感染，如心内膜炎、败血症，以及假膜性肠炎等。<br><br>It is mainly used to treat systemic infection and intestinal infection, such as endocarditis, septicemia and pseudomembranous colitis, caused by staphylococci (including enzyme-produced strains and methicillin-resistant strains), enterococci (ampicillin-resistant strains), Clostridium difficile and etc. |
| 用法、用量<br>Dosage | 口服（治疗假膜性肠炎）：成人一次 0.4g，每 6 小时 1 次，每日量不可超过 4g；儿童酌减。静脉滴注：成人一日量 0.8 ~ 1.6g，1 次或分次给予；小儿一日量 16 ~ 24mg/kg，1 次或分次给予。一般将 1 次量的药物先用 10ml 灭菌注射用水溶解，再加入到适量等渗氯化钠注射液或葡萄糖输液中，缓慢滴注。如采取连续滴注给药，则可将一日量药物加到 24 小时内所用的输液中给予。<br><br>Oral medication (treatment for pseudomembranous colitis): for adults, give 0.4g singly, every 6 hours, with the maximum daily dose of 4g; children dosage shoud be reduced accordingly. Intravenous infusion: for adults, give 0.8 ~ 1.6g a day, in 1 dose or several divided doses; for children, give 16 ~ 24mg/kg a day, in 1 dose or several divided doses. Dissolve single dose of the drug in 10ml of the sterile water for injection, then add it into an appropriate amount of isotonic sodium chloride or glucose infusion for slow infusion. If the drug is administered by continuous infusion, daily dose of the drug can be added into the infusion which will be used within 24 hours. |
| 剂型、规格<br>Preparations | 注射用盐酸去甲万古霉素：每瓶 0.4g（40 万 U）[相当万古霉素约 0.5g（50 万 U）]。<br>Norvancomycin Hydrochloride for injection: 0.4g per vial (40 million units) [equals about 0.5g (50 million units) of norvancomycin ]. |
| 药品名称 Drug Names | 万古霉素 Vancomycin |
| 适应证<br>Indications | 临床用于革兰阳性菌严重感染，尤其是对其他抗菌药耐药的耐甲氧西林菌株。血液透析患者发生葡萄球菌属所致的动静脉分流感染。口服用于对甲硝唑无效的假膜性结肠炎或多重耐药葡萄球菌小肠结肠炎。<br><br>It is clinically used to treat severe Gram-positive bacteria infection, especially methicillin-resistant strains which are resistant to other antibacterial. It is also effective in treatment of Hemodialysis patients' arteriovenous shunt infection caused by Staphylococcus.. Oral medication can treat pseudomembranous colitis which is ineffective for metronidazole or multidrug-resistant staphylococcus enterocolitis. |
| 用法、用量<br>Dosage | 口服：每次 125 ~ 500mg，每 6 小时 1 次，每日剂量不宜超过 4g，疗程 5 ~ 10 天；小儿 1 次 10mg/kg，每 6 小时 1 次，疗程 5 ~ 10 天。<br>静脉滴注：全身感染，成人每 6 小时 7.5mg/kg，或每 12 小时 15mg/kg。严重感染，可一日 3 ~ 4g 短期应用；新生儿（0 ~ 7 日）首次 15mg/kg，以后 10mg/kg，每 12 小时给药 1 次；婴儿（7 日 ~ 1 个月）首次 15mg/kg，以后 10mg/kg，每 8 小时给药 1 次；儿童每次 10mg/kg，每 6 小时给药 1 次，或每次 20mg/kg，每 12 小时 1 次。<br><br>Oral medication: for adults, 125 ~ 500mg singly, every 6 hours, with maximum daily dose of 4g and treatment course of 5 to 10 days; for children, 10mg/kg singly, every 6 hours, with treatment course of 5 to 10 days.<br>Intravenous infusion: in treatment of systemic infection, give adults 7.5mg/kg every 6 hours, or 15mg/kg every 12 hours; give 3 ~ 4g a day for short-term use in severe infection case; for newborns (0 to 7 days), give first dose of 15mg/kg, afterwards 10mg/kg every 12 hours; for infants (7 to 30 days), give first dose 15mg / kg, afterwards 10mg/kg every 8 hours; for children, give 10mg/kg every 6 hours, or 20mg/kg every 12 hours. |
| 剂型、规格<br>Preparations | 胶囊：每粒 20mg；250mg。<br>注射用盐酸万古霉素：每支 0.5g；1.0g。<br><br>Capsules: 20mg; 250mg per capsule.<br>Vancomycin Hydrochloride for Injection: 0.5g, 1.0g per vial. |

**续 表**

| 药品名称 Drug Names | 替考拉宁 Teicoplanin |
|---|---|
| 适应证<br>Indications | 临床用于耐甲氧西林金黄色葡萄球菌和耐氨苄西林肠球菌所致的系统感染（对中枢感染无效）。<br><br>本类药物（万古霉素与本品）现用于上述适应证，其目的是防止过度应用（即用于其他抗生素能控制的一些病原菌感染而造成耐药菌滋生）。<br><br>It is clinically used to treat systemic infection (ineffective in treating central nervous system infection) caused by methicillin-resistant Staphylococcus aureus and ampicillin-resistant Enterococcus.<br><br>This kind of drug (referring to vancomycin and Teicoplanin ) is now used for these indications, in order to prevent excessive use (its use for Pathogen infection which can be controlled by other antibiotics leads to the growing of drug-resistant bacteria). |
| 用法、用量<br>Dosage | 首剂（第一日）400mg，次日开始每日 200mg，静脉注射或肌内注射；严重感染，每次 400mg，每日 2 次，3 日后减为一日 200 ～ 400mg。<br><br>用前以注射用水溶解，静脉注射应不少于 1 分钟。若采取静脉滴注，则将药物加入 0.9% 氯化钠溶液中，静脉滴注不少于 30 分钟。也可采用肌内注射。<br><br>Give first dose (on the first day) of 400mg, afterwards 200mg a day, by intravenous injection or intramuscular injection; in severe infection case, give 400mg singly, 2 times a day, reduce to 200 ～ 400mg after 3 days.<br><br>Before use, dissolve the drug in water for injection. The time for intravenous injection should be no less than one minute. If it is administered by intravenous infusion, add the drug in 0.9% sodium chloride solution. And the time for infusion is at least 30 minutes. Intramuscular injection can also be used. |
| 剂型、规格<br>Preparations | 粉针：每支 200mg；400mg。<br>Powder for injection: 200mg, 400mg of each. |

### 1.10　其他抗菌抗生素 Other antibiotics

| 药品名称 Drug Names | 磷霉素 Fosfomycin |
|---|---|
| 适应证<br>Indications | 临床主要用于敏感菌引起的尿路、皮肤及软组织、肠道等部位感染。对肺部、脑膜感染和败血症也可考虑应用。可与其他抗生素联合治疗由敏感菌所致重症感染。也可与万古霉素合用治疗 MRSA 感染。<br><br>Clinically, it is mainly used to treat infection of urinary tract, skin and soft tissue and intestineal tract and etc. caused by susceptible strains. Treating lungs infection, meningeal infection and septicemia may also consider using this drug. It can be used in combination with other antibiotics to treat severe infection caused by susceptible strains, or with vancomycin to treat MRSA infection. |
| 用法、用量<br>Dosage | 口服磷霉素钙，适用于尿路感染及轻症感染，成人 2 ～ 4g/d，儿童一日量为 50 ～ 100mg/kg，分 3 ～ 4 次服用。静脉注射或静脉滴注磷霉素钠，用于中度或重度系统感染，成人 4 ～ 12g/d，重症可用到 16g/d；儿童一日量为 100 ～ 300mg/kg，均分为 2 ～ 4 次给予。1g 药物至少应用 10ml 溶剂，如一次用数克，则应按每 1g 药物用 25ml 溶剂的比率进行溶解，予以静脉滴注或缓慢静脉注射。适用的溶剂有：灭菌注射用水、5% ～ 10% 葡萄糖液、0.9% 氯化钠注射液、含乳酸钠的输液等。<br><br>Oral medication of fosfomycin calcium I intended to treat urinary tract infection and mild infection. For adults, give 2 ~ 4g a day; for children, give 50 ~ 100mg/kg a day, in 3 to 4 divided doses. Intravenous injection or intravenous infusion of fosfomycin is intended to treat moderate infection and severe systemic infection. For adults, give 4 ~ 12g a day, and increase to 16g a day in severe case; for children, give 100 ~ 300mg/kg a day, in 2 ~ 4 divided doses. Dissolve 1g of the drug in at least 10ml of the solvent. If the single dose is more than 1g, dissolve every 1g of drug in 25ml of the solvent for intravenous infusion or slow intravenous injection. The solvent could be sterile water for injection, 5% to 10% glucose solution, 0.9% sodium chloride injection, infusion with sodium lactate and etc. |
| 剂型、规格<br>Preparations | 磷霉素钙胶囊：每粒 0.1g；0.2g；0.5g。<br>注射用磷霉素钠：每瓶 1g；4g。<br><br>Fosfomycin Calcium Capsules: 0.1g, 0.2g, 0.5g per capsule.<br>Fosfomycin sodium for injection: 1g, 4g per vial. |

**续 表**

| 药品名称 Drug Names | 达托霉素 Daptomycin |
| --- | --- |
| 适应证<br>Indications | 临床用于复杂性皮肤及皮肤软组织感染。<br>It is clinically used to treat complicated skin and soft tissue of skin infection. |
| 用法、用量<br>Dosage | 静脉注射：每次 4mg/kg，每日 1 次，连续用药 7 ～ 14 天。肌酐清除率低于 30ml/min 者，每次 4mg/kg，每 2 天 1 次。<br>Intravenous injection: 4mg/kg singly, once a day, for 7 to 14 days of continuous treatment. Patients with creatinine clearance less than 30ml/min: 4mg/kg singly, once every 2 days. |
| 剂型、规格<br>Preparations | 注射用达托霉素：每支 250mg；500mg。<br>Daptomycin for injection: 250mg, 500mg per vial. |
| 药品名称 Drug Names | 利福昔明 Rifaximin |
| 适应证<br>Indications | 临床用于敏感菌所致的肠道感染，预防胃肠道围术期感染性并发症，也可用于高氨血症的辅助治疗。<br>It is clinically used to treat intestinal infections caused by susceptible strains, prevent infectious complications gastrointestinal perioperative period, and assist in the treatment of hyperammonemia. |
| 用法、用量<br>Dosage | 口服，肠道感染：成人每次 200mg，一日 4 次，连续使用 5 ～ 7 天。6 ～ 12 岁儿童，每次 100 ～ 200mg，一日 4 次。手术前后预防感染：成人每次 400mg，6 ～ 12 岁儿童每次 200 ～ 400mg，一日 2 次，在手术前 3 天给药。高氨血症的辅助治疗：成人每次 400mg，疗程 7 ～ 21 天。6 ～ 12 岁儿童每次 200 ～ 300mg，一日 3 次。<br>The drug is administered orally. Intestinal infection: for adults, give 200mg a day, 4 times a day, for 5 to 7 days of continuous treatment; for. children aging 6 to 12, give 100 ~ 200mg singly, 4 times a day. Pre-and postoperative infection prevention: for adults, give 400mg singly, 2 times a day, before surgery; for children aging 6 to 12, give 200 ~ 400mg singly, 2 times a day, before surgery. Adjuvant treatment for hyperammonemia: for adults, give 400mg singly, for 7 to 21 days of treatment course; for children from 6 to 12 years old, give 200 ~ 300mg singly, 3 times a day. |
| 剂型、规格<br>Preparations | 片剂（胶囊剂）：每片（粒）200mg。<br>Tablets (capsules): 200mg per tablet (capsule). |
| 药品名称 Drug Names | 多黏菌素 B　Polymyxin B |
| 适应证<br>Indications | 临床主要应用于铜绿假单胞菌及其他假单胞菌引起的创面、尿路以及眼、耳、气管等部位感染，也可用于败血症。鞘内注射用于铜绿假单胞菌脑膜炎。<br>Clinically, it is mainly used to treat infection of wound, urinary tract, eyes, ears, trachea and etc. caused by Pseudomonas aeruginosa and Pseudomonas, as well as septicemia. Intrathecal injection of the drug is intended to treat Pseudomonas aeruginosa meningitis. |
| 用法、用量<br>Dosage | 静脉滴注：成人及儿童肾功能正常者一日 1.5 ～ 2.5mg/kg（一般不超过 2.5mg/kg），分 2 次给予，每 12 小时滴注 1 次。每 50mg 本品，以 5% 葡萄糖液 500ml 稀释后滴入。婴儿肾功能正常者可耐受一日 4mg/kg 的用量。肌内注射：成人及儿童一日 2.5 ～ 3mg/kg，分次给予，每 4 ～ 6 小时用药 1 次。婴儿一日量可用到 4mg/kg，新生儿可用到 4.5mg/kg，滴眼液浓度 1 ～ 2.5mg/ml。<br>Intravenous infusion: for adults and children with normal renal function, give1.5 ~ 2.5mg/kg a day (usually not exceed 2.5mg/kg), in 2 divided doses, every 12 hours. Dilute every 50mg of the drug with 500ml of 5% glucose solution for infusion. Infants with normal renal function can be given 4mg/kg a day. Intramuscular injection: for both adults and children, give 2.5 ~ 3mg/kg, in several divided doses, every 4 to 6 hours. The daily dose for infants is 4mg/kg, while for newborns could be 4.5mg/kg. The concentration of drops is 1 ~ 2.5mg/ml. |
| 剂型、规格<br>Preparations | 注射用硫酸多黏菌素 B：每瓶 50mg（1mg=10 000U）。<br>Polymyxin B for injection: 50mg (1mg = 10 000units) per vial. |

| 药品名称 Drug Names | 黏菌素 Colistin |
|---|---|
| 适应证<br>Indications | 用于治疗大肠埃希菌性肠炎和对其他药物耐药的菌痢。外用于烧伤和外伤引起的铜绿假单胞菌局部感染和耳、咽等部位敏感菌感染。<br><br>It is intended to treat enteritis by E. coli and dysentery by bcteria which are resistant to other drugs. External use can treat Pseudomonas aeruginosa local infection caused by burns and trauma, as well as susceptible infection of ear, throat and etc. |
| 用法、用量<br>Dosage | 口服：成人一日 150 万～ 300 万 U，分 3 次服。儿童 1 次量 25 万～ 50 万 U，一日 3 ～ 4 次。重症时上述剂量可加倍。外用：溶液剂 1 万～ 5 万 U/ml，氯化钠注射液溶解。<br><br>Oral medication: for adults, give 1.5 million to 300 million units a day, in 3 divided doses; for children, give 250, 000 to 500, 000 units singly, 3 to 4 times a day. The above dosage could be doubled in severe infection case. External use: the solution is 10, 000 to 50, 000 units / ml, dissolved by sodium chloride injection. |
| 剂型、规格<br>Preparations | 片剂：每片 50 万 U；100 万 U；300 万 U。<br>灭菌粉剂：每瓶 100 万 U，供制备溶液用（1mg=6500U）。<br>Tablets: 500, 000 units, 1, 000, 000 units, 3, 000, 000 units per tablet.<br>Sterile powders: 1, 000, 000 units per bottle, for the preparation of solution (1mg = 6500 units). |

| 药品名称 Drug Names | 夫西地酸钠 Fusidate Sodium |
|---|---|
| 适应证<br>Indications | 主治由各种敏感细菌，尤其是葡萄球菌引起的各种感染，如骨髓炎、败血症、心内膜炎、反复感染的囊性纤维化、肺炎、皮肤及软组织感染，外科及创伤性感染等。<br><br>It is mainly intended to treat different kinds of infection caused by a variety of sensitive bacteria, especially the infection caused by Staphylococcus aureus, such as osteomyelitis, septicemia, endocarditis, recurrent cystic fibrosis, pneumonia, skin and soft tissue infection, surgical infection and traumatic infection. |
| 用法、用量<br>Dosage | 口服：每 8 小时 500mg，重症感染可加倍服用；儿童 1 岁以下，每日 50mg/kg，分次给予；1 ～ 5 岁，每次 250mg，一日 3 次；5 ～ 12 岁，可按成人量给予。静脉滴注：成人每次 500mg，一日 3 次；儿童及婴儿每日 20mg/kg，分 3 次给药。将本品 500mg 溶于 10ml 所附的无菌缓冲溶液中，然后用氯化钠注射液或 5% 葡萄糖注射液稀释至 250 ～ 500ml 静脉输注。若葡萄糖注射液过酸，溶液会呈乳状，如出现此情况即不能使用。输注时间不应少于 2 ～ 4 小时。<br><br>Oral medication: give 500mg every 8 hours, and the dose can be doubled in severe infection case; for children under the age of 1, give 50mg/kg a day, in several divided doses; at the age of 1 to 5, give 250mg singly, three times a day; at the age of 5 to 12, give adult dosage. Intravenous infusion: for adults, give 500mg singly, 3 times a day; for children and infants, give 20mg/kg a day, in 3 divided doses. Dissolve 500mg of the drug in the attached 10ml of sterile buffer solution, then dilute it with sodium chloride injection or 5% dextrose injection to 250 ~ 500ml for intravenous infusion. If glucose injection is too acid, the solution will be milky which can not be used. The time for Infusion should not be less than 2 to 4 hours. |
| 剂型、规格<br>Preparations | 片剂：每片 250mg。<br>注射用夫西地酸：每瓶 500mg（钠盐）；580mg（二乙醇胺盐）。<br>Tablets: 250mg per tablet.<br>Fusidic acid for injection: 500mg (sodium salt), 580mg (diethanolamine salt) per vial. |

## 2. 化学合成的抗菌药 Chemical synthetic antibacterial drugs

### 2.1 磺胺类 Sulfonamides

| 药品名称 Drug Names | 磺胺嘧啶 Sulfadiazine |
|---|---|
| 适应证<br>Indications | 防治敏感脑膜炎球菌所致的流行性脑膜炎。<br>It is used to prevent meningococcal meningitis caused by susceptible meningococcal. |
| 用法、用量<br>Dosage | 口服：成人：预防脑膜炎，1 次 1g，一日 2g；治疗脑膜炎：1 次 1g，一日 4g。儿童：一般感染，可按一日 50 ～ 75mg/kg，分为 2 次用；流脑：则按一日 100 ～ 150mg/kg 应用。<br><br>缓慢静脉注射或静脉滴注：治疗严重感染，成人 1 次 1 ～ 1.5g，一日 3 ～ 4.5g。本品注射液为钠盐，需用灭菌注射用水或等渗氯化钠注射液稀释，静脉注射时浓度应低于 5%；静脉滴注时浓度约为 1%（稀释 20 倍），混匀后应用。 |

**续　表**

| | Oral medication: in adults' meningitis prevention, give1g singly, 2g a day; in adults' meningitis treatment, give 1g singly, 4g a day; in children's general infection, give 50 ~ 75mg/kg a day, in 2 divided doses; in meningococcal meningitis, give 100 ~ 150mg/kg a day. |
|---|---|
| | Slow intravenous injection or intravenous infusion: in severe infection, give adults 1 ~ 1.5g singly, 3 ~ 4.5g a day. This drug's injection is sodium salt, so it needs to be diluted with sterile water for injection or isotonic sodium chloride injection. The injection's concentration should be less than 5%; while the infusion's is about 1% (diluted 20 times), used after mixing evenly. |
| 剂型、规格<br>Preparations | 片剂：每片 0.5g。<br>磺胺嘧啶混悬液：10%。<br>磺胺嘧啶钠注射液：每支 0.4g（2ml）；1g（5ml）。<br>注射用磺胺嘧啶钠：每瓶 0.4g；1g。<br>复方磺胺嘧啶（双嘧啶，SD-TMP）片：每片含磺胺嘧啶（SD）400mg 和甲氧苄啶（TMP）50mg。<br>本品的治疗效果约与复方磺胺甲噁唑（SMZ-TMP）片相近。<br>Tablets: 0.5 g per tablet.<br>Sulfadiazine suspension: 10% (g / ml).<br>Sulfadiazine Sodium injection: 0.4g (2ml), 1g (5ml) per vial.<br>Sulfadiazine sodium for injection: 0.4g, 1g per vial.<br>Compound sulfadiazine (bispyrimidine, SD-TMP) tablets: containing 400mg of sulfadiazine (SD) and 50mg of trimethoprim (TMP) per tablet.<br>And it has the similar therapeutic effect with sulfamethoxazole (SMZ-TMP) tablets. |
| 药品名称 Drug Names | 磺胺甲噁唑 Sulfamethoxazole |
| 适应证<br>Indications | 用于急性支气管炎、肺部感染、尿路感染、伤寒、布氏杆菌病、菌痢等，疗效与氨苄西林、氯霉素、四环素等相近。<br>It is intended to treat acute bronchitis, lungs infection, urinary tract infection, typhoid fever, brucellosis, dysentery and etc..It has the similiar efficacy with ampicillin, chloramphenicol, tetracycline and etc. |
| 用法、用量<br>Dosage | 一日 2 次，每次服 1g。<br>1g singly, 2 times a day. |
| 剂型、规格<br>Preparations | 片剂：每片 0.5g。<br>复方磺胺甲噁唑（复方新诺明，SMZ-TMP）片：每片含 SMZ0.4g、TMP0.08g。<br>联磺甲氧苄啶片（增效联磺片）：每片含 SMZ0.2g、SD0.2g、TMP0.08g<br>复方磺胺甲噁唑（复方新诺明；SMZ-TMP）注射液：每支 2ml，含 SMZ0.4g、TMP0.08g。<br>Tablets: 0.5g per tablet.<br>Sulfamethoxazole tablets (Bactrim, SMZ-TMP): containing 0.4g of SMZ and 0.08g of TMP per tablet.<br>Sulfamethoxazole trimethoprim tablets (SMZ-SD-TMP tablets): containing 0.2g of SMZ, 0.2g of SD and 0.08g of TMP per tablet.<br>Sulfamethoxazole (Bactrim; SMZ-TMP) Injection: 2ml per vial, containing 0.4g of SMZ and 0.08g of TMP. |
| 药品名称 Drug Names | 柳氮磺吡啶 Sulfasalazine |
| 适应证<br>Indications | 用于治疗轻中度溃疡性结肠炎，活动期的克罗恩病，类风湿关节炎。<br>It is intended to treat mild and moderate ulcerative colitis, active Crohn's disease and rheumatoid arthritis. |
| 用法、用量<br>Dosage | 口服：治疗溃疡性结肠炎，1 次 0.5 ~ 1g，一日 2 ~ 4g。如需要可逐渐增量至一日 4 ~ 6g，好转后减量为一日 1.5g，直至症状消失。也可用于灌肠，每日 2g，混悬于生理盐水 20 ~ 50ml 中，做保留灌肠，也可添加白及粉以增大药液黏滞度。治疗类风湿关节炎：用肠溶片，每次 1g（4 片），每日 2 次。<br>直肠给药：重症患者，1 次 0.5g，早、中、晚各 1 次。轻、中度患者，早、晚各 0.5g。症状明显改善后，每晚或隔日睡前 0.5g。用药后需侧卧半小时。 |

续　表

| | |
|---|---|
| | Oral medication: in ulcerative colitis treatment, give 0.5 ~ 1g singly, 2 ~ 4g a day. If necessary, the dose can be gradually increased to 4 ~ 6g a day, then reduced to 1.5g a day after improvement until the symptoms disappear. It is also can be used for enema: give 2g a day, suspend the drug in 20 ~ 50ml of the saline as retention enema or add Bletilla striata powder to increase the viscosity of the liquid. In rheumatoid arthritis treatment, give 1g (4 enteric-coated tablets) singly, twice a day.<br><br>Rectal administration: for patients with severe disease, give 0.5g singly, 3 times(in the morning, noon and evening)a day; for patients with mild and moderate disease, give 0.5g singly, twice(in the morning and evening ) a day. When symptoms get improved, give0.5g singly, in the evening or before sleeps every other day. Patients need to lie on the side for half an hour after medication. |
| 剂型、规格<br>Preparations | 片剂：每片 0.25g。<br>栓剂：每个 0.5g。<br>肠溶片：每片 0.25g。<br><br>Tablets: 0.25g per tablet.<br>Suppositories: 0.5g of each.<br>Enteric-coated tablets: 0.25g per tablet. |

## 2.2　甲氧苄啶类 Trimethoprim

| 药品名称 Drug Names | 甲氧苄啶 Trimethoprim |
|---|---|
| 适应证<br>Indications | 常与磺胺药合用（多应用复方制剂）于治疗肺部感染、急慢性支气管炎、菌痢、尿路感染、肾盂肾炎、肠炎、伤寒、疟疾等，也与多种抗生素合用。本品单独可应用于大肠埃希菌、奇异变形杆菌、肺炎克雷伯杆菌、肠杆菌属、凝固酶阴性的金黄色葡萄球菌所致单纯性尿路感染。本品单用易引起细菌耐药，故不宜单独用。<br><br>It is often associated with sulfa drugs (multi-application compound preparation) to treat pulmonary infection, acute and chronic bronchitis, dysentery, urinary tract infection, pyelonephritis, enteritis, typhoid, malaria and so on. It is also used in combination with a variety of antibiotics. This product can be used alone to treat uncomplicated urinary tract infection caused by Escherichia coli, Proteus mirabilis, Klebsiella pneumoniae, Enterobacter, and coagulase-negative Staphylococcus aureus. But it is not suggested because it would lead to bacteria's resistance. |
| 用法、用量<br>Dosage | 口服，每次 0.1 ~ 0.2g，一日 0.2 ~ 0.4g。<br>Oral administration: 0.1 ~ 0.2g singly, 0.2 ~ 0.4g a day. |
| 剂型、规格<br>Preparations | 片剂：每片 0.1g。<br>Tablets: 0.1g per tablet. |

## 2.3　硝基呋喃类 Nitrofurans

| 药品名称 Drug Names | 呋喃妥因 Nitrofurantoin |
|---|---|
| 适应证<br>Indications | 本品主要应用于敏感菌所致的泌尿系统感染。一般地说，微生物对本品不易耐药，如停药后重新用药，仍可有效。但近年来耐药菌株有一定程度发展。必要时可与其他药物（如TMP）联合应用以提高疗效。<br><br>It is mainly used to treat urinary tract infection caused by susceptible strains. Generally, since microorganisms are not liable to be resistant to this drug, it still remains effective when reused after withdrawal. But resistant strain has been developed in recent years, so if necessary, it can be used in combination with other drugs (such as TMP) to improve efficacy. |
| 用法、用量<br>Dosage | 每次 0.1g，一日 0.2 ~ 0.4g，至尿内检菌阴性再继续用 3 日。但连续应用不宜超过 14 日。<br>Give 0.1g singly, 0.2 ~ 0.4g a day, until urine examination of bacteria is negative; afterwards continue administration for 3 days. However, the consecutive medication should not exceed 14 days. |
| 剂型、规格<br>Preparations | 肠溶片：每片 0.05g；0.1g。<br>Enteric-coated tablets: 0.05g, 0.1g per tablet. |
| 药品名称 Drug Names | 呋喃唑酮 Furazolidone |
| 适应证<br>Indications | 主要用于菌痢、肠炎，也可用于伤寒、副伤寒、梨形鞭毛虫病和阴道滴虫病。<br>It is mainly used to treat dysentery, enteritis, as well as typhoid, paratyphoid, pear-shaped giardiasis and vaginal trichomoniasis. |

**续　表**

| | |
|---|---|
| 用法、用量<br>Dosage | 常用量 1 次 0.1g，一日 3 ～ 4 次，症状消失后再服 2 日。梨形鞭毛虫病疗程为 7 ～ 10 日。<br>The usual dose is 0.1g singly, 3 to 4 times a day; continue administration for 2 days after symptoms disappear.<br>Treatment course of pear-shaped giardiasis is 7 to 10 days. |
| 剂型、规格<br>Preparations | 片剂：每片 0.1g。<br>Tablets: 0.1g per tablet. |

## 2.4　喹诺酮类 4-Quinolones

| 药品名称 Drug Names | 吡哌酸 Pipemidic Acid |
|---|---|
| 适应证<br>Indications | 临床主要应用于敏感革兰阴性杆菌和葡萄球菌所致尿路、肠道和耳道感染，如尿道炎、膀胱炎、菌痢、肠炎、中耳炎等。<br>Clinically, it is mainly used to treat infection of urinary tract, intestinal tract and ear canal, such as urethritis, cystitis, dysentery, enteritis, otitis media and etc., caused by susceptible Gram-negative bacilli and staphylococci. |
| 用法、用量<br>Dosage | 成人口服：1 次 0.5g，一日 1.5 ～ 2g，分次给予，一般不超过 10 日。<br>Oral medication for adults: 0.5g singly, 1.5 ～ 2g a day, in several doses, generally for no more than 10 days. |
| 剂型、规格<br>Preparations | 片剂：每片 0.25g；0.5g。<br>胶囊剂：每胶囊 0.25g。<br>Tablets: 0.25g, 0.5g per tablet.<br>Capsules: 0.25g per capsule. |
| 药品名称 Drug Names | 诺氟沙星 Norfloxacin |
| 适应证<br>Indications | 本品应用于敏感菌所致泌尿道、肠道、耳鼻喉科、妇科、外科和皮肤科等感染性疾病。<br>It is intended to treat infectious diseases, such as urinary tract infection, intestinal infection, ENT infection, gynecological infection, surgical infection and skin infection, etc., caused by susceptible strains. |
| 用法、用量<br>Dosage | 口服，成人 1 次 0.1 ～ 0.2g，一日 3 ～ 4 次。空腹服药吸收较好。一般疗程为 3 ～ 8 日，少数病例可达 3 周。对于慢性泌尿道感染病例，可先用一般量 2 周，再减量为 200mg/d，睡前服用，持续数月。<br>　严重病例及不能口服者静脉滴注。用量：每次 200 ～ 400mg，每 12 小时 1 次。将一次量加于输液中，滴注 1 小时。<br>Oral medication for adults: 0.1 ～ 0.2g singly, 3 to 4 times a day. Taking the drug on empty stomach can absorb well. The general course of treatment is 3 to 8 days, while a few cases may last three weeks. For chronic urinary tract infection, give usual dose for two weeks, and then reduce to 200mg a day, before sleep, for several months.<br>In severe disease cases, patients who are unable to take oral medication could be administered by intravenous drip. The dose is 200 ～ 400mg singly, every 12 hours. Add single dose of the drug into the infusion before use, and the time for infusion is 1 hour. |
| 剂型、规格<br>Preparations | 胶囊：每粒 100mg。<br>输液：每瓶 200mg/100ml（尚有其他规格）。<br>滴眼液：8ml（24mg）。<br>软膏：1%。<br>Capsules: 100mg per capsule.<br>Infusion: 200mg/100ml per bottle (there are other specifications).<br>Drops: 8ml (24mg).<br>Ointment: 1%. |
| 药品名称 Drug Names | 氧氟沙星 Ofloxacin |
| 适应证<br>Indications | 主要用于革兰阴性菌所致的呼吸道、咽喉、扁桃体、泌尿道（包括前列腺）、皮肤及软组织、胆囊及胆管、中耳、鼻窦、泪囊、肠道等部位的急、慢性感染。<br>It is mainly used to treat acute and chronic infection of respiratory tract, throat, tonsils, urinary tract (including prostate), skin and soft tissue, gallbladder and bile ducts, middle ear, sinus, lacrimal sac, intestinal tract and etc. caused by Gram-negative bacteria mentioned above. |

续 表

| 用法、用量<br>Dosage | 口服：每日 200 ～ 600mg，分 2 次服。根据病情适当调整剂量。抗结核用量为每日 0.3g，顿服。控制伤寒反复感染：每日 50mg，连用 3 ～ 6 个月。滴注给药：每次 200 ～ 400mg，每 12 小时 1 次，以适量输液稀释，滴注 1 小时。<br><br>Oral medication: give 200 ～ 600mg a day, in 2 divided doses; make appropriate adjustment according to patients' condition. Daily dosage for anti-TB is 0.3g; take at a draught. Control typhoid repeated infections: Daily 50mg, once every 3 to 6 months. Infusion administration: per 200 ～ 400mg, every 12 hours, in order to dilute the amount of the infusion, infusion of 1 hour. |
| --- | --- |
| 剂型、规格<br>Preparations | 片剂：每片 100mg。<br>注射液：每支 400mg/10ml（用前需稀释）。<br>输液：每瓶 400mg/100ml（可直接输注）。<br><br>Tablets: 100mg per tablet.<br>Injection: 400mg/10ml per vial (diluted before use).<br>Infusion: 400mg/100ml per bottle (directly use is permissible). |
| 药品名称 Drug Names | 左氧氟沙星 Levofloxacin |
| 适应证<br>Indications | 主要用于革兰阴性菌所致的呼吸道、咽喉、扁桃体、泌尿道（包括前列腺）、皮肤及软组织、胆囊及胆管、中耳、鼻窦、泪囊、肠道等部位的急、慢性感染。<br><br>It is mainly used to treat acute and chronic infection of respiratory tract, throat, tonsils, urinary tract (including prostate), skin and soft tissue, gallbladder and bile ducts, middle ear, sinus, lacrimal sac, intestinal tract and etc. caused by Gram-negative bacteria mentioned above. |
| 用法、用量<br>Dosage | 口服：每次 100mg，每日 2 次，根据感染严重程度可增量，最多每次 200mg，每日 3 次。静脉滴注，一日 200 ～ 600mg，分 1 ～ 2 次静脉滴注。<br><br>Oral medication: give 100mg singly, 2 times a day; the dose can be increased according to the severity of the infection, but maximum dosage is 200mg singly, 3 times a day. Intravenous infusion: 200 ～ 600mg a day, in 1 to 2 divided doses. |
| 剂型、规格<br>Preparations | 片剂：每片 100mg；200mg；500mg。<br>注射液：200mg（100ml）；300mg（100ml）；500mg（100ml）。<br>Tablets: 100mg, 200mg, 500mg per tablet.<br>Injection: 200mg (100ml), 300mg (100ml), 500mg (100ml). |
| 药品名称 Drug Names | 依诺沙星 Enoxacin |
| 适应证<br>Indications | 用于敏感菌所致的咽喉、支气管、肺、尿路、前列腺、胆囊、肠道、中耳、鼻旁窦等部位感染，也可用于脓皮病及软组织感染。<br><br>It intended to treat infection of throat, bronchus, lung, urinary tract, prostate, gallbladder, intestinal tract, middle ear and paranasal sinus and other parts caused by susceptible strains, as well as pyoderma and soft tissue infection. |
| 用法、用量<br>Dosage | 成人常用量一日 400 ～ 600mg（按无水物计量）。分 2 次给予。<br>Adults' usual dose is 400 ～ 600mg a day (measured by anhydride), in 2 divided doses. |
| 剂型、规格<br>Preparations | 片剂：每片 100mg（标示量以无水物计，相当于含水物 108.5mg）；200mg（相当于含水物 217mg）。<br><br>Tablets: 100mg (measured by anhydride, equivalent to 108.5mg of the hydride), 200mg (equivalent to 217mg of hydride) per tablet. |
| 药品名称 Drug Names | 环丙沙星 Ciprofloxacin |
| 适应证<br>Indications | 适用于敏感菌所致的呼吸道、尿道、消化道、胆道、皮肤和软组织、盆腔、眼、耳、鼻、咽喉等部位的感染。<br><br>It is intended to treat infection of respiratory tract, urinary tract, digestive tract, biliary tract, skin and soft tissue, pelvic, eye, ear, nose, throat and other parts caused by susceptible strains. |

**续　表**

| 用法、用量<br>Dosage | 口服：成人 1 次 250mg，一日 2 次，重症者可加倍量。但一日最高量不可超过 1500mg。肾功能不全者（肌酐清除率低于 30ml/min）应减少服量。<br>静脉滴注：1 次 100 ～ 200mg，一日 2 次，预先用等渗氯化钠或葡萄糖注射液稀释，滴注时间不少于 30 分钟。<br>Oral medication: for adults, give 250mg singly, 2 times a day; the dose can be doubled in severe case, but daily dose can not exceed the1500mg; for patients with renal insufficiency (creatinine elimination rate less than 30ml/min), the dose should be reduced.<br>Intravenous infusion: give 100 ~ 200mg singly, 2 times a day; before use, dilute the drug with isotonic sodium chloride or dextrose injection and the time for infusion time is at least 30 minutes. |
|---|---|
| 剂型、规格<br>Preparations | 片剂：每片（标示量按环丙沙星计算）为 250mg；500mg；750mg（含盐酸盐一水合物量分别为 291mg、582mg 和 873mg）。<br>注射液：每支 100mg（50ml）；200mg（100ml）（含乳酸盐分别为 127.2mg 和 254.4mg）。<br>Tablets: 250mg, 500mg, 750mg per tablet (calculated by ciprofloxacin) (with hydrochloride monohydrate is 291mg, 582mg, 873mg).<br>Injection: 100mg (50ml), 200mg (100ml) per vial (with lactate is 127.2mg, 254.4mg). |
| 药品名称 Drug Names | 洛美沙星 Lomefloxacin |
| 适应证<br>Indications | 应用于敏感菌所致的下呼吸道、尿道感染。本品对链球菌、肺炎链球菌、洋葱假单胞菌、支原体和厌氧菌均无效。<br>It is intended to treat lower respiratory tract infection and urinary tract infection caused by susceptible strains mentioned above. It is ineffective at Streptococcus pneumoniae, Pseudomonas cepacia, mycoplasma and anaerobes. |
| 用法、用量<br>Dosage | 口服：每日 1 次 400mg，疗程为 10 ～ 14 日。手术感染的预防，手术前 2 ～ 6 小时，1 次服 400mg。静脉滴注：每次 200mg，一日 2 次，或每次 400mg，一日 1 次。每 100mg 药物需用 5% 葡萄糖液或 0.9% 氯化钠液 60 ～ 100ml 稀释后缓慢滴注。<br>肾功能不全者的用量，按血清肌酐值，依下式计算：男性： ［体重（kg） × （140- 年龄）］ / ［72× 血清肌酐值（mg/dl）］ 女性：按男性结果 ×0.85<br>Oral medicaton: give 400mg singly, once a day; with treatment course of 10 to 14 days; for surgical infection prevention, give 400mg, 2 to 6 hours before surgery. Intravenous infusion: give 200mg singly, 2 times a day or 400mg singly, once a day. Dilute every 100mg of the drug with 60 ~ 100ml of 5% glucose solution or 0.9% sodium chloride solution for slow infusion.<br>Patient with renal insufficiency should be administered according to serum creatinine values. The formula is Male: [weight (kg) × (140 - Age)] / [72 × serum creatinine (mg / dl)]; women: male result × 0.85. |
| 剂型、规格<br>Preparations | 薄膜衣片：每片 400mg。<br>注射液（盐酸盐或天冬氨酸盐）：每支 100mg/2ml；每瓶 200mg/100ml、400mg/250ml。<br>Film-coated tablets: 400mg per tablet.<br>Injection (hydrochloride or aspartate): 100mg/2ml; bottle 200mg/100ml, 400mg/250ml per vial. |
| 药品名称 Drug Names | 培氟沙星 Pefloxacin |
| 适应证<br>Indications | 用于治疗革兰阴性菌和金黄色葡萄球菌引起的中度或重度感染。如：泌尿系统、呼吸道、耳鼻喉、生殖系统、腹部和肝、胆系统感染，脑膜炎、骨和关节感染，败血症和心内膜炎。<br>It is intended to treat moderate or severe infection, caused by gram-negative bacteria and Staphylococcus aureus, such as infection of urinary tract, respiratory tract, ENT, reproductive system, abdomen, hepatobiliary system infection, meningitis, bone and joint infeciton, septicemia and endocarditis. |
| 用法、用量<br>Dosage | 口服：成人每日 400 ～ 800mg，分 2 次给予。静脉滴注：一次 0.4g，加入 5% 葡萄糖注射液 250ml 中，缓慢滴入，滴注时间不少于 60 分钟，每 12 小时 1 次。<br>Oral medicaiotn: give adults 400 ~ 800mg a day, in 2 divided doses. Intravenous infusion: give 0.4g singly, every 12 hours; add the drug into 250ml of 5% glucose injection for slow infusion, and the time for infusion is at least 60 minutes. |

| | |
|---|---|
| 剂型、规格<br>Preparations | 片剂：每片 200mg。<br>注射液（甲磺酸盐）：每支 400mg（5ml）。<br>Tablets: 200mg per tablet.<br>Injection (mesylate): 400mg (5ml) per vial. |
| 药品名称 Drug Names | 芦氟沙星 Rufloxacin |
| 适应证<br>Indications | 临床用于敏感菌引起的下呼吸道及尿道感染。如肺炎、急慢性支气管炎、急慢性肾盂肾炎、急性膀胱炎、尿道炎以及皮肤软组织化脓性感染。<br>It is clinically used to treat lower respiratory tract and urinary tract infection caused by susceptible strains, such as pneumonia, acute and chronic bronchitis, acute and chronic pyelonephritis, acute cystitis, urethritis and purulent infection of skin's soft tissue. |
| 用法、用量<br>Dosage | 成人每日 1 次，每次 200mg，早餐后服。5 ～ 10 日为 1 个疗程。前列腺炎的疗程可达 4 周。<br>Adults: give 200mg singly, once a day, after breakfast. One course of treatment is 5 to 10 days, while the course for Prostatitis could be 4 weeks. |
| 剂型、规格<br>Preparations | 片剂：每片 200mg。<br>胶囊剂：每粒 100mg。<br>Tablets: 200mg per tablet.<br>Capsules: 100mg per capsule. |
| 药品名称 Drug Names | 司帕沙星 Sparfloxacin |
| 适应证<br>Indications | 临床用于敏感菌所致的咽喉、扁桃体、支气管、肺、胆囊、尿道、前列腺、肠道、子宫、中耳、鼻旁窦等部位感染，还可用于皮肤、软组织感染及牙周组织炎。<br>It is clinically used to treat infection of throat, tonsils, bronchus, lung, gallbladder, urethra, prostate, intestine, uterus, middle ear, paranasal sinus infections and other parts caused by susceptible strains, as well as skin infection, soft tissue infection and periodontal tissue inflammation. |
| 用法、用量<br>Dosage | 口服：成人每次 100 ～ 300mg，最多不超过 400mg，一日 1 次。疗程一般为 5 ～ 10 日。<br>Oral medication: for adults, give 100 ～ 300mg singly, once a day, with maximum daily dose of 400mg. The course of treatment is usually 5 to 10 days. |
| 剂型、规格<br>Preparations | 胶囊剂：每粒 100mg。<br>Capsules: 100mg per capsule. |
| 药品名称 Drug Names | 氟罗沙星 Fleroxacin |
| 适应证<br>Indications | 用于敏感菌所致的呼吸系统、泌尿生殖系统、消化系统的感染，以及皮肤软组织、骨、关节、耳鼻喉、腹腔、盆腔感染。<br>It is intended to treat infection of respiratory system, urinary system, reproductive system and digestive system, as well as infection of, skin soft tissue, bone, joint, ENT, abdominal cavity, pelvic cavity caused by susceptible strains. |
| 用法、用量<br>Dosage | 口服：每日 0.4g，一次顿服。疗程视感染不同而定：复杂性尿路感染 1 ～ 2 周；呼吸道感染 1 ～ 3 周；皮肤、软组织感染 4 至 3 周；骨髓炎、化脓性关节炎 2 ～ 12 周；伤寒 1 ～ 2 周；沙眼衣原体尿道炎 5 日；单纯性尿路感染、细菌性痢疾、淋球菌尿道炎（宫颈炎）只用 1 次。静脉滴注：一次 200 ～ 400mg，一日 1 次，加入 5% 葡萄糖注射液 250ml 中，避光缓慢滴注（每 100ml 滴注至少 45 ～ 60 分钟）。<br>Oral medication: 0.4g a day, at draught. The course of treatment varies for different infection: complicated urinary tract infection is 1 to 2 weeks; respiratory infection is 1 to 3 weeks; skin and soft tissue infections is 4 ～ 12 days; osteomyelitis, and septic arthritis is 2 to 12 weeks; typhoid is 1 ～ 2 weeks; Chlamydia trachomatis urethritis is 5 days. In treatment of uncomplicated urinary tract infection, dysentery and gonorrhea urethritis (cervicitis), give only once. Intravenous infusion: give 200 ～ 400mg singly, once a day; add the drug into 250ml of 5% glucose injection for slow infusion, away from light (every 100ml of the infusion needs at least 45 to 60 minutes) |
| 剂型、规格<br>Preparations | 胶囊剂：每粒 200mg；400mg。<br>Capsules: 200mg, 400mg per capsule. |

**续　表**

| 药品名称 Drug Names | 莫西沙星 Moxifloxacin |
| --- | --- |
| 适应证<br>Indications | 适用于敏感菌所致的呼吸道感染，包括慢性支气管炎急性发作，轻度或中度的社区获得性肺炎，急性鼻窦炎等。<br><br>It is intended to treat respiratory tract infections caused by susceptible strains, including acute exacerbation of chronic bronchitis, mild or moderate community-acquired pneumonia, acute sinusitis and etc. |
| 用法、用量<br>Dosage | 成人每日 1 次 400mg，连用 5～10 日，口服或静脉滴注。滴注时间为 90 分钟。<br><br>Adult: give 400mg a day, for 5 to 10 days, by oral medicaiton or intravenous infusion. The time of each infusion is 90 minutes. |
| 剂型、规格<br>Preparations | 片剂 400mg。<br>注射液 250ml（莫西沙星 0.4g）。<br>Tablets: 400mg per tablet.<br>Injection: 250ml (0.4g of moxifloxacin). |
| 药品名称 Drug Names | 加替沙星 Gatifloxacin |
| 适应证<br>Indications | 用于敏感菌所致的慢性支气管炎急性发作、急性鼻窦炎、社区获得性肺炎、尿路感染、急性肾盂肾炎、女性淋球菌性宫颈感染。<br><br>It is intended to treat acute chronic bronchitis attack, acute sinusitis, community-acquired pneumonia, urinary tract infection, acute pyelonephritis and female cervical gonococcal infection caused by susceptible strains. |
| 用法、用量<br>Dosage | 静脉给药：成人每次 200～400mg，一日 1 次，疗程一般 5～10 日。治疗中由静脉给药改为口服给药时，无须调整剂量。治疗非复杂性淋球菌尿路或直肠感染和女性淋球菌性宫颈感染，400mg 单次给药。中度肝功能不全者，无须调整剂量；中、重度肾功能不全者，应减量使用。<br><br>Intravenous administration: for adults, give 200～400mg singly, once a day, with general treatment course of 5 to 10 days. Oral administration uses the same dose of intravenous administration. In treatment of uncomplicated urinary tract infection, rectal infeciotn and female cervical gonococcal infection, give 400mg singly, only once. Patients with moderate hepatic insufficiency do need dose adjustment; whiel patients with moderate or severe renal insufficiency need dose reduction. |
| 剂型、规格<br>Preparations | 片剂：每片 100mg；200mg；400mg。<br>注射液：100mg（100ml）；200mg（100ml）；400mg（40ml）。<br>Tablets: 100mg, 200mg, 400mg per tablet.<br>Injection: 100mg (100ml), 200mg (100ml), 400mg (40ml). |
| 药品名称 Drug Names | 帕珠沙星 Pazufloxacin |
| 适应证<br>Indications | 用于敏感菌所致的呼吸道感染、泌尿道感染，妇科、外科、耳鼻喉科和皮肤科等感染性疾病。<br><br>It is intended to treat respiratory tract infection, urinary tract infection and infectious disease in gynecology, surgery, ENT and dermatology, etc. caused by susceptible strains. |
| 用法、用量<br>Dosage | 静脉滴注，每次 300mg，滴注时间为 30～60 分钟，一日 2 次，疗程为 7～14 日。肾功能不全者应调整剂量：肾清除率 >44.7ml/min，每次 300mg，一日 2 次；肾清除率为 13.6～44.7ml/min，每次 300mg，一日 1 次；透析患者用量为每次 300mg，每 3 日 1 次。<br><br>Intravenous infusion: give 300mg singly, 2 times a day, with treatment course of 7 to 14 days; the infusion time needs 30 to 60 minutes. Administration for renal insufficiency patients should make adjustment on the dose: renal clearance rate> 44.7ml/min, give 300mg singly, 2 times a day; renal clearance rate=13.6～44.7ml/min, give 300mg singly, once a day; dialysis patients, give 300mg singly, every 3 days. |
| 剂型、规格<br>Preparations | 甲磺酸帕珠沙星注射液：100mg（10ml）；150mg（10ml）；200mg（100ml）；300mg（100ml）。<br>Mesylate Pazufloxacin injection: 100mg (10ml), 150mg (10ml), 200mg (100ml), 300mg (100ml). |

续　表

| 药品名称 Drug Names | 托氟沙星 Tosufloxacin |
| --- | --- |
| 适应证<br>Indications | 临床用于敏感菌引起的呼吸系统、泌尿系统、胃肠道、皮肤软组织感染，以及中耳炎、牙周炎、眼睑炎等。<br><br>It is clinicaly used to treat infection of respiratory system, urinary system, gastrointestinal tract, and skin soft tissue caused by susceptible strains, as well as otitis media, periodontitis and blepharitis. |
| 用法、用量<br>Dosage | 口服每次 75 ~ 150mg，一日 2 ~ 3 次，一般疗程为 3 ~ 7 日；最多每日剂量 600mg，分 2 ~ 3 次服用，疗程为 14 日。<br><br>Oral medication: give 75 ~ 150mg singly, 2 to 3 times a day, with general treatment course of 3 to 7 days. The maximum daily dose is 600mg, in 2 to 3 divided doses. The course of treatment is 14 days. |
| 剂型、规格<br>Preparations | 托西酸托氟沙星片：每片 75mg；150mg；300mg。<br>甲苯磺酸托氟沙星片：每片 150mg。<br><br>Tosi acid tosufloxacin tablets: 75mg; 150mg; 300mg per tablet.<br>Toluenesulfonic tosufloxacin tablets: 150mg per tablet. |

2.5　硝基咪唑类 Nitroimidazoles

| 药品名称 Drug Names | 甲硝唑 Metronidazole |
| --- | --- |
| 适应证<br>Indications | 主要用于治疗或预防厌氧菌引起的系统或局部感染，如腹腔、消化道、女性生殖系、下呼吸道、皮肤及软组织、骨和关节等部位的厌氧菌感染，对败血症、心内膜炎、脑膜感染，以及使用抗生素引起的结肠炎也有效。治疗破伤风常与破伤风抗毒素（TAT）联用。还可用于口腔厌氧菌感染。<br><br>It is mainly used to treat or prevent systemic infection and local infection caused by anaerobic bacteria mentioned above, such as anaerobic infection of abdominal cavity, gastrointestinal tract, female reproductive system, lower respiratory tract, skin and soft tissue, bone and joint and other parts. It is also effective in treatment of septicemia, endocarditis, meningeal infection and colitis by use of antibiotics. It is often associated with tetanus antitoxin (TAT) to treat Tetanu. It can be also used to treat oral anaerobic infection. |
| 用法、用量<br>Dosage | 厌氧菌感染：口服，1 次 0.2 ~ 0.4g，一日 0.6 ~ 1.2g；静脉滴注，1 次 500mg，8 小时 1 次，每次滴注 1 小时。7 日为 1 个疗程。预防用药：用于腹部或妇科手术前一天开始服药，1 次 0.25 ~ 0.5g，一日 3 次。治疗破伤风：一日量 2.5g，分次口服或滴注。<br><br>Anaerobic infection: give 0.2 ~ 0.4g singly, 0.6 ~ 1.2g a day, by oral medication; or give, 500mg singly, every8 hours, by intravenous infusion, one hour for each infusion; one course of treatment is seven days. Prophylaxis: give 0.25 ~ 0.5g singly, 3 times a day, one day before abdominal surgery or gynecological surgery.. Tetanus: give 2.5g a day, in divided doses or by infusion. |
| 剂型、规格<br>Preparations | 片剂：每片 0.2g。<br>注射液：50mg（10ml）；100mg（20ml）；500mg（100ml）；1.25g（250ml）；500mg（250ml）。<br>甲硝唑葡萄糖注射液：250ml，含甲硝唑 0.5g 及葡萄糖 12.5g。栓剂：每个 0.5g；1g。<br>甲硝唑阴道泡腾片：每片 0.2g。<br><br>Tablets: 0.2g per tablet.<br>Injection: 50mg (10ml), 100mg (20ml), 500mg (100ml), 1.25g (250ml), 500mg (250ml) Metronidazole glucose injection: 250ml (with 0.5g of metronidazole and 12.5g of glucose) Suppositories: 0.5g, 1g of each.<br>Metronidazole vaginal effervescent tablets: 0.2g per tablet. |
| 药品名称 Drug Names | 替硝唑 Tinidazole |
| 适应证<br>Indications | 用于厌氧菌的系统与局部感染，如腹腔、妇科、手术创口、皮肤软组织、肺、胸腔等部位感染及败血症、肠道或泌尿生殖道毛滴虫病、梨形鞭毛虫病，以及肠道和肝阿米巴病。<br><br>It is intended to treat systemic infection and local infection caused by anaerobic bacteria, such as infeciotn of abdominal cavity, gynecology, surgical wounds, skin soft tissue, lung, chest and other parts, as well as septicemia, intestinal or genitourinary trichomoniasis, giardiasis and intestinal and hepatic amebiasis. |

**续　表**

| 用法、用量<br>Dosage | 厌氧菌系统感染：口服每日 2g；重症可静脉滴注，每日 1.6g，1 次或分为 2 次给予。手术感染的预防：术前 12 小时服 2g，手术间或结束后输注 1.6g（或口服 2g）。非特异性阴道炎：每日 2g，连服 2 日。急性牙龈炎：1 次口服 2g。泌尿生殖道毛滴虫病：1 次口服 2g，必要时重复 1 次；或每次 0.15g，一日 3 次，连用 5 日。需男女同治以防再次感染。儿童 1 次 50 ～ 75mg/kg，必要时重复 1 次。合并白念珠菌感染者须同时进行抗真菌治疗。梨形鞭毛虫病：1 次 2g。肠阿米巴病：每日 2g，服 2 ～ 3 日。儿童每日 50 ～ 60mg，连用 5 日。肝阿米巴病：每日 1.5 ～ 2g，连用 3 日，必要时可延长至 5 ～ 10 日。应同时排出脓液。口服片剂应于餐间或餐后服用。<br><br>静脉滴注每 400mg(200ml) 应不少于 20 分钟。<br><br>Anaerobic infection: give 2g a day, by oral medication; for severe infection casse, give 1.6g a day, in 1 or 2 divided doses, by intravenous infusion. Surgical infection prevention: give 2g 12 hours before surgery, and 1.6g intravenously (or 2g orally), in or after the surgery. Nonspecific vaginitis: give 2g a day, for 2 days. Acute gingivitis: give single dose of 2g orally. Urogenital trichomoniasis: give single dose of 2g orally, repeat the dose if necessary ; or 0.15g singly, 3 times a day, for 5 days. Both men and women need to be treated at the same time to prevent re-infection. For children, give 50 ～ 75mg/kg singly, repeat the dose if necessary. Candida albicans infected patients, antifungal therapy are required at the same time. Giardiasis: give 2g each time. Intestinal amebiasis: give 2g a day, for 2 to 3 days; for children, give 50 ～ 60mg a day, for 5 days. Hepatic amebiasis: give 1.5 ～ 2g a day, for 3 days; extend to 5 to 10 days if necessary. Pus should be discharged at the same time. Oral tablets should be taken after or with the meal.<br><br>Every 400mg (200ml)of the drug needs at least 20 minutes' intravenous infusion. |
|---|---|
| 剂型、规格<br>Preparations | 片剂：每片 0.25g；0.5g。<br>注射液：每瓶 400mg/200ml 或 800mg/400ml （含葡萄糖 5.5%）。<br>栓剂：每个 0.2g。<br>Tablets: 0.25g, 0.5g per tablet.<br>Injection: 400mg/200ml, 800mg/400ml(containing 5.5% of glucose) per vial.<br>Suppositories: 0.2g of each. |
| **药品名称 Drug Names** | **奥硝唑 Ornidazole** |
| 适应证<br>Indications | 用于由厌氧菌感染引起的多种疾病。男女泌尿生殖道毛滴虫、贾第鞭毛虫感染引起的疾病。还用于肠、肝阿米巴病。<br><br>It is intended to treat a variety of disease caused by anaerobic infections, as well as disease caused by urogenital Trichomonas vaginalis infeciotn and Giardia infection. It is also used to treat intestinal and hepatic amebiasis. |
| 用法、用量<br>Dosage | 口服：预防术后厌氧菌感染，术前 12 小时服用 1500mg，以后每次 500mg，每日 2 次，至术后 3 ～ 5 日；治疗厌氧菌感染，每次 500mg，一日 2 次；急性毛滴虫病，于夜间单次服用 1500mg；慢性毛滴虫病，1 次 500mg，一日 2 次，共用 5 日；贾第鞭毛虫病，于夜间顿服 1500mg，用药 1 ～ 2 日；阿米巴痢疾，于夜间顿服 1500mg，用药 3 日；其他阿米巴病，1 次 500mg，一日 2 次。静脉滴注：预防术后厌氧菌感染，术前 1 ～ 2 小时给药 1000mg，术后 12 小时给药 500mg，24 小时再给药 500mg；治疗厌氧菌感染，初始剂量为 500 ～ 1000mg，以后每 12 小时 500mg，疗程为 3 ～ 6 日。<br><br>The drug is administered by oral medication. Postoperative anaerobic infection prevention: give 1500mg 12 hours before surgery, afterwards 500mg singly, 2 times a day, until 3 to 5 days after surgery. Anaerobic infection: give 500mg singly, 2 times a day. Acute trichomoniasis: give single dose of 1500mg at night. Chronic trichomoniasis: give 500mg singly, 2 times a day, for five days. Giardiasis: give 1500mg singly, at a draught, at night, for 1 to 2 days Amoebic dysentery: give 1500mg singly, at a draught, at night, for3 days. Other amebiasis: give 500mg singly, 2 times a day. The drug is administered by intravenous infusion. Postoperative anaerobic infection prevention: give 1000mg 1 to 2 hours before surgery, 500mg 12 hours after surgery, and another 500mg after 24 hours. Anaerobic infection: give a first dose of 500 ～ 1000mg, afterwards 500mg every 12 hours, with treatment course of 3 to 6 days. |

| 剂型、规格<br>Preparations | 片剂（胶囊剂）：每片（粒）0.25g。<br>注射液：0.25g（5ml）。<br>奥硝唑氯化钠（葡萄糖）注射液：0.25g（100ml）；0.5g（100ml）。<br>Tablets (capsules): 0.25g per tablet (capsule).<br>Injection: 0.25g (5ml).<br>Ornidazole sodium chloride (dextrose) injection: 0.25g (100ml), 0.5g (100ml). |
|---|---|
| **药品名称 Drug Names** | 塞克硝唑 Secnidazole |
| 适应证<br>Indications | 主要用于由阴道毛滴虫引起的尿道炎和阴道炎，肠阿米巴病，肝阿米巴病及贾第鞭毛虫病。<br>It is mainly used to treat urethritis and vaginitis by Trichomonas vaginalis, intestinal amebiasis, hepatic amebiasis and giardiasis. |
| 用法、用量<br>Dosage | 口服，成人 2g，单次服用。治疗阴道滴虫病和尿道滴虫病，配偶应同时服用。肠阿米巴病：有症状的急性阿米巴病，成人 2g，单次服用；儿童 30mg/kg，单次服用；无症状的急性阿米巴病，成人一次 2g，一日 1 次，连服 3 日；儿童一次 30mg/kg，一日 1 次，连服 3 日。肝脏阿米巴病：成人一日 1.5g，一次或分次口服，连服 5 日；儿童一次 30mg/kg，一次或分次口服，连服 5 日。贾第鞭毛虫病：儿童 30mg/kg，单次服用。<br>Oral medication: give adults 2g, single dose only. In treatment of vaginal and urethral trichomoniasis, spouses should also receive the therapy. Symptomatic acute intestinal amebiasis with symptoms: give adults 2g, single dose only; give children 30mg/kg, single dose only. Asymptomatic acute amebiasis: give adults 2g singly, once a day, for 3 days; give children 30mg/kg singly, once a day, for 3 days. Hepatic amebiasis: give adults 1.5g a day orally, in 1 or several divided doses, for 5 days; give children 30mg/kg singly, in 1or several divided doses, for 5 days. Giardiasis: give children 30mg/kg, single dose only. |
| 剂型、规格<br>Preparations | 片剂（胶囊）：每片 / 粒 0.25g；0.5g。<br>Tablets (capsules): 0.25g, 0.5g per tablet (capsule). |

2.6　噁唑烷酮类 Oxazolidinones

| **药品名称 Drug Names** | 利奈唑胺 Linezolid |
|---|---|
| 适应证<br>Indications | 主要用于控制耐万古霉素粪肠球菌所致的系统感染，包括败血症、肺炎及复杂性皮肤和皮肤组织感染等。<br>It is mainly used to control systemic infection caused by vancomycin-resistant Enterococcus Faecium, including septicemia, pneumonia and complicated skin and skin structure infection. |
| 用法、用量<br>Dosage | 口服与静脉滴注剂量相同。成人和超过 12 岁儿童，每次 600mg，每 12 小时 1 次。治疗耐万古霉素肠球菌感染疗程为 14 ～ 28 日。肺炎、菌血症及皮肤软组织感染疗程为 10 ～ 14 日。儿童（出生至 11 岁者），每次 10mg/kg，每 12 小时 1 次，疗效欠佳可增至每 8 小时 1 次，口服或静脉给药。<br>Oral dose and intravenous dose is same. Adults and children over the age of 12: give 600mg singly, every 12 hours. Treatment course of vancomycin-resistant enterococci infection is 14 to 28 days, while Pneumonia, bacteremia, and skin and soft tissue infection is 10 to 14 days. Children ( under the age of 11, including newborns): give 10mg/kg singly, every 12 hours; if with poor efficacy, increase to once every 8 hours, by oral or intravenous administration. |
| 剂型、规格<br>Preparations | 片剂：每片 600mg。<br>注射液：600mg（300ml）。<br>Tablets: 600mg per tablet.<br>Injection: 600mg (300ml). |

**续　表**

| 3. 抗结核药 Antituberculous Drugs | |
|---|---|
| 药品名称 Drug Names | 异烟肼 Isoniazid |
| 适应证<br>Indications | 　　主要用于各型肺结核的进展期、溶解播散期、吸收好转期，尚可用于结核性脑膜炎和其他肺外结核等。本品常需和其他抗结核病药联合应用，以增强疗效和克服耐药菌。此外，对痢疾、百日咳、麦粒肿等也有一定疗效。<br>　　It is mainly used in advanced stage, dissolution and spread stage, absorption and remission stage of various kinds of tuberculosis, as well as in treatment of tuberculous meningitis and other extrapulmonary tuberculosis. It is often used in combination with other anti-TB drugs to enhance efficacy and overcome resistant bacteria. In addition, it also has effect in treatment of dysentery, pertussis, stye and etc. |
| 用法、用量<br>Dosage | 　　口服：成人 1 次 0.3g，1 次顿服；对急性粟粒性肺结核或结核性脑膜炎，1 次 0.2 ～ 0.3g，一日 3 次。静脉注射或静脉滴注：对较重度浸润结核，肺外活动结核等，1 次 0.3 ～ 0.6g，加 5% 葡萄糖注射液或等渗氯化钠注射液 20 ～ 40ml，缓慢推注；或加入输液 250 ～ 500ml 中静脉滴注。<br>　　百日咳：一日按 10 ～ 15mg/kg，分为 3 次服。<br>　　麦粒肿：一日按 4 ～ 10mg/kg，分为 3 次服。<br>　　局部（胸腔内注射治疗局灶性结核等）：1 次 50 ～ 200mg。<br>　　Oral medication: give adults 0.3g singly, once only, at a draught; for acute miliary tuberculosis or tuberculous meningitis, give 0.2 ～ 0.3g singly, 3 times a day. Intravenous injection or intravenous infusion: for severe infiltration tuberculosis, extrapulmonary active tuberculosis and etc., give 0.3 ～ 0.6g singly, add 20 ～ 40ml of 5% dextrose injection or isotonic sodium chloride injection for slow injection or 250 ～ 500ml of the infusion for intravenous infusion.<br>Pertussis: give 10 ～ 15mg/kg a day, in 3 divided doses.<br>Stye: give 4 ～ 10mg/kg a day, in 3 divided doses.<br>Locally (intrathoracic injection therapy for focal tuberculous, etc.): give 50 ～ 200mg singly. |
| 剂型、规格<br>Preparations | 　　片剂：每片 0.05g；0.1g；0.3g。<br>　　注射液：每支 0.1g（2ml）。<br>Tablets: 0.05g, 0.1g, 0.3g per tablet.<br>Injection: 0.1g (2ml) per vial. |
| 药品名称 Drug Names | 对氨基水杨酸钠 Sodium Aminosalicylate |
| 适应证<br>Indications | 　　本品很少单独应用，常配合异烟肼、链霉素等应用，以增强疗效并避免细菌产生耐药性。也可用于甲状腺功能亢进症。对于甲亢合并结核患者较适用，在用碘剂无效而影响手术时，可短期服用本品为手术创造条件。本品尚有较强的降血脂作用。<br>　　This product is rarely used alone, often associated with isoniazid, streptomycin and so on to enhance the efficacy and avoid bacterial resistance. It can also be used to treat hyperthyroidism. For hyperthyroidism -TB patients, it can be short term used to create the conditions for operation when iodine has no effect . Besides, it has strong lipid-lowering effect. |
| 用法、用量<br>Dosage | 　　口服：每次 2 ～ 3g，一日 8 ～ 12g，饭后服。小儿每日 200 ～ 300mg/kg，分 4 次服。<br>　　静脉滴注：每日 4 ～ 12g（先从小剂量开始），以等渗氯化钠注射液或 5% 葡萄糖液溶解后，配成 3% ～ 4% 浓度滴注。小儿每日 200 ～ 300mg/kg。<br>　　胸腔内注射：每次 10% ～ 20% 溶液 10 ～ 20ml（用等渗氯化钠注射液溶解）。<br>　　甲状腺功能亢进症手术前：一日 8 ～ 12g，分 4 次服，同时服用维生素 B、维生素 C。服药时间不可过长，以防毒性反应出现。<br>　　Oral medication: give 2 ～ 3g singly, 8 ～ 12g a day, after meals; give children 200 ～ 300mg/kg a day, in 4 divided doses. Intravenous infusion: give 4 ～ 12g (start with small dose) a day, dissolve the drug in the same amount of isotonic sodium chloride injection or 5% glucose solution and make its concentration of 3% to 4% for infusion; give children 200 ～ 300mg/kg a day. Intrathoracic injection: give 10 ～ 20ml of 10% to 20% solution (dissolved by isotonic sodium chloride injection solution). Hyperthyroidism before surgery: give 8 ～ 12g a day, in 4 divided doses, with vitamin B and C taken. The drug can not be administered for a long time, in case of toxic reaction. |

| | |
|---|---|
| 剂型、规格<br>Preparations | 片剂：每片 0.5g。<br>注射用对氨基水杨酸钠：每瓶 2g；4g；6g。<br><br>Tablets: 0.5g per tablet.<br>Sodium aminosalicylate for injection: 2g, 4g, 6g per vial. |
| **药品名称 Drug Names** | 利福平 Rifampicin |
| 适应证<br>Indications | 主要应用于肺结核和其他结核病，也可用于麻风病的治疗。此外也可考虑用于耐甲氧西林金黄色葡萄球菌（MRSA）所致的感染。抗结核治疗时应与其他抗结核药联合应用。<br><br>It is mainly used to treat Tuberculosis and other tuberculosis, as well asleprosy. It can also be considered to treat infection caused by methicillin-resistant Staphylococcus aureus (MRSA). In treatment of anti-TB, it should be combined with other anti-TB drugs. |
| 用法、用量<br>Dosage | 肺结核及其他结核病：成人，口服，1 次 0.45 ~ 0.6g，一日 1 次，于早饭前服，疗程约 6 个月；1 ~ 12 岁儿童 1 次量为 10mg/kg，一日 2 次；新生儿 1 次 5mg/kg，一日 2 次。<br>其他感染：一日量 0.6 ~ 1g，分 2 ~ 3 次给予，饭前 1 小时服用。<br>沙眼及结膜炎：用 0.1% 滴眼剂，一日 4 ~ 6 次。治疗沙眼的疗程为 6 周。<br><br>Tuberculosis and other tuberculosis: for adults, give 0.45 ~ 0.6g singly, once a day, before breakfast, with treatment course of about six mònths ; for children aging 1 to 12, give 10mg/kg singly, 2 times a day; for newborns, give 5mg/kg singly, 2 times a day.<br>Other infection: give 0.6 ~ 1g a day, in 2 to 3 divided doses, 1 hour before meals.<br>Trachoma and conjunctivitis: give 0.1% eye drops, 4 ~ 6 times a day; the reatment course of trachoma is 6 weeks. |
| 剂型、规格<br>Preparations | 片（胶囊）剂：每片（粒）0.15g；0.3g；0.45g；0.6g。<br>口服混悬液：20mg/ml。<br>复方制剂：RIMACTAZIDE（含利福平及异烟肼）；RIMATAZIDE+Z（含利福平、异烟肼及吡嗪酰胺）。<br><br>Tablets (capsules): 0.15g, 0.3g, 0.45g, 0.6g pertablet (capsule).<br>Oral suspension: 20mg/ml.<br>Compound preparation: RIMACTAZIDE (containing rifampicin and isoniazid), RIMATAZIDE + Z (containing rifampin, isoniazid and pyrazinamide). |
| **药品名称 Drug Names** | 利福定 Rifandin |
| 适应证<br>Indications | 用于各型肺结核和其他结核病，包括对多种抗结核药物已产生耐药性患者。亦用于麻风病及敏感菌感染性皮肤病等。<br><br>It is intended to treat various kinds of tuberculosis and other tuberculosis, as well as patients who are resistant to many other anti-TB drugs. It is also used to treat leprosy and infectious skin diseases caused by susceptible stains. |
| 用法、用量<br>Dosage | 成人每日 150 ~ 200mg，早晨空腹一次服用。儿童按 3 ~ 4mg/kg，一次服用。治疗肺结核病的疗程为 6 个月至 1 年。眼部感染采取局部用药（滴眼剂浓度 0.05%）。<br><br>Adults: 150 ~ 200mg a day, one dose only, on empty stomach in the morning. Children: 3 ~ 4mg/kg, in one dose. Treatment course of TB is 6 to 12 months. Eye infection: topical administration (0.05% of eye drops concentration). |
| 剂型、规格<br>Preparations | 胶囊：每粒 75mg；150mg。<br>Capsules: 75mg, 150mg per capsule. |
| **药品名称 Drug Names** | 利福喷丁 Rifapentine |
| 适应证<br>Indications | 主要用于治疗结核病（常与其他抗结核药联合应用）。<br>It is mainly used to treat tuberculosis (often in combination with other anti-TB drugs). |
| 用法、用量<br>Dosage | 1 次 600mg，每周只用 1 次（其作用约相当于利福平 600mg，一日 1 次）。必要时可按上量，每周 2 次。<br><br>Give 600mg singly, only once a week (as the same effect with approximately 600mg of rifampicin). If necessary, give 600mg singly, 2 times a week. |

**续 表**

| 剂型、规格<br>Preparations | 片（胶囊）剂：每片（粒）150mg；300mg。<br>Tablets (capsules): 150mg, 300mg per tablet (capsule). |
|---|---|
| 药品名称 Drug Names | 利福霉素钠 Rifamycin Sodium |
| 适应证<br>Indications | 用于不能口服用药的结核患者和耐甲氧西林金葡菌（MRSA）感染，以及难治性军团菌病。<br>It can be used for patients who can not receive oral medication to treat Tuberculosis. And it is intended to treat methicillin-resistant Staphylococcus aureus (MRSA) infection, as well as refractory Legionnaires' disease. |
| 用法、用量<br>Dosage | 肌内注射：成人 1 次 250mg，每 8 ～ 12 小时 1 次。静脉注射（缓慢注射）：1 次 500mg，一日 2 ～ 3 次；小儿一日量 10 ～ 30mg/kg。此外亦可稀释至一定浓度局部应用或雾化吸入。重症患者宜先静脉滴注，待病情好转后改肌内注射。用于治疗肾盂肾炎时，每日剂量在 750mg 以上。对于严重感染，开始剂量可酌增到一日 1000mg。<br>Intramuscular injection: give adults 250mg singly, every 8 to 12 hours. Intravenous injection (slow injection): give 500mg singly, 2 or 3 times a day; give children 10 ～ 30mg/kg a day. It can also be diluted into a certain concentration for topical administration or inhalation. For patients with severe disease, it is recommended to give intravenous infusion and then change into intramuscular injection after an improvement. Pyelonephritis: give more than 750mg a day; for severe infection case, appropriately increase first dose to 1000mg. |
| 剂型、规格<br>Preparations | 注射用利福霉素钠：每瓶 250mg。<br>注射液：每支 0.25g（5ml）（供静脉滴注用）；0.125g（2ml）（供肌内注射用）。<br>Rifamycin sodium for injection: 250mg per bottle.<br>Injection: 0.25g (5ml) (for intravenous infusion), 0.125g (2ml) (for intramuscular injection) per vial. |
| 药品名称 Drug Names | 链霉素 Streptomycin |
| 适应证<br>Indications | 主要用于结核杆菌感染，也用于布氏杆菌病、鼠疫及其他敏感菌所致的感染。<br>It is mainly used to treat Mycobacterium tuberculosis infection, as well as infection brucellosis, plague and other infection caused by susceptible strains. |
| 用法、用量<br>Dosage | 口服不吸收，只对肠道感染有效，现已少用。系统治疗需肌内注射，一般应用 1 次 0.5g，一日 2 次，或 1 次 0.75g，一日 1 次，1 ～ 2 周为 1 个疗程。用于结核病，一日剂量为 0.75 ～ 1g，1 次或分成 2 次肌内注射。<br>儿童一般一日 15 ～ 25mg/kg，分 2 次给予；结核病治疗则一日 20mg/kg，隔日用药。新生儿一日 10 ～ 20mg/kg。<br>用于治疗结核病时，常与异烟肼或其他抗结核药联合应用，以避免耐药菌株的产生。<br>Oral medication is effective only at intestinal infection, so it has been seldom adopted. Systemic treatment requires intramuscular injection, and the general dosage is 0.5g singly, twice a day or 0.75g singly, once a day, with treatment course of.1 to 2 weeks. The dosage for tuberculosis is 0.75 ～ 1g, in 1 or 2 divided doses, by intramuscular injection.<br>Children: generally, give 15 ～ 25mg/kg a day, in 2 divided doses; in tuberculosis treatment, give 20mg/kg a day, every other day. Newborns: give 10 ～ 20mg/kg a day.<br>In treatment of tuberculosis, it is often associated with isoniazid or other anti-TB drugs to avoid drug-resistant strains. |
| 剂型、规格<br>Preparations | 注射用硫酸链霉素：每瓶 0.75g；1g；2g；5g。<br>Streptomycin Sulfate for injection: 0.75g, 1g, 2g, 5g per vial. |
| 药品名称 Drug Names | 乙胺丁醇 Ethambutol |
| 适应证<br>Indications | 为二线抗结核药，可用于经其他抗结核药治疗无效的病例，应与其他抗结核药联合应用。以增强疗效并延缓细菌耐药性的产生。<br>It is a second-line anti-TB drugs and can be used for patients who are resistant to other anti-TB drugs. It should be combined with other anti-TB drugs to enhance efficacy and delay bacteria's drug resistance. |

**续　表**

| 用法、用量<br>Dosage | 结核初治：一日 15mg/kg，顿服；或每周 3 次，每次 25 ～ 30mg/kg（不超过 2.5g）；或每周 2 次，每次 50mg/kg（不超过 2.5g）。<br>结核复治，每次 25mg/kg，一日 1 次顿服，连续 60 日，继而按每次 15mg/kg，一日 1 次顿服。<br>非典型分枝杆菌感染，按每次 15 ～ 25mg/kg，一日一次顿服。<br>In initial treatment of TB, give 15mg/kg a day, at a draught or 25 ～ 30mg/kg (less than 2.5g) singly, 3 times a week..<br>In retreatment of TB, give 25mg/kg singly, once a day, at a draught, for 60 days; afterwards give 15mg/kg singly, once a day, at a draught.<br>Atypical mycobaterial infection: give 15 ～ 25mg/kg singly, once a day, at a draught. |
|---|---|
| 剂型、规格<br>Preparations | 片剂：每片 0.25g。<br>Tablets: 0.25g per tablet. |
| **药品名称 Drug Names** | 乙硫异烟胺 Ethionamide |
| 适应证<br>Indications | 单独应用少，常与其他抗结核病药联合应用以增强疗效和避免病菌产生耐药性。<br>It is rarely used alone, often associated with other anti-TB drugs to enhance the efficacy and avoid bacteria resistance. |
| 用法、用量<br>Dosage | 一日量 0.5 ～ 0.8g，一次服用或分次服（以一次服效果为好），必要时也可从小剂量（0.3g/d）开始。<br>The daily dose is 0.5 ～ 0.8g, in one or several divided doses (one dose has good effect); if necessary, start with small dose (0.3g a day). |
| 剂型、规格<br>Preparations | 肠溶片：每片 0.1g。<br>Enteric-coated tablets: 0.1g per tablet. |
| **药品名称 Drug Names** | 丙硫异烟胺 Protionamide |
| 适应证<br>Indications | 本品仅对分枝杆菌有效，与其他抗结核药联合用于结核病经一线药物（如链霉素、异烟肼、利福平和乙胺丁醇）治疗无效者。<br>This product is only effective at mycobacteria, and it is used in combination with other anti-TB drugs for patients who are resistant to first-line anti-TB drugs (such as streptomycin, isoniazid, rifampicin and ethambutol). |
| 用法、用量<br>Dosage | 口服，成人常用量，与其他抗结核药物合用，一次 250mg，一日 2 ～ 3 次。小儿常用量，与其他抗结核药合用，一次按体重口服 4 ～ 5mg/kg，一日 3 次。<br>Oral medication (in combination with other anti-TB drugs): give adults 250mg singly, 2 to 3 times a day; give children 4 ～ 5mg/kg singly, 3 times a day. |
| 剂型、规格<br>Preparations | 肠溶片：每片 0.1g。<br>Enteric-coated tablets: 0.1g per tablet. |
| **药品名称 Drug Names** | 吡嗪酰胺 Pyrazinamide |
| 适应证<br>Indications | 与其他抗结核药联合用于经一线抗结核药（如链霉素、异烟肼、利福平和乙胺丁醇）治疗无效的结核病。本品仅对分枝杆菌有效。<br>It is used in combination with other anti-TB drugs to treat Tuberculosis which is resistant to first-line anti-TB drugs (such as streptomycin, isoniazid, rifampicin and ethambutol).This product is only effective at mycobacteria. |
| 用法、用量<br>Dosage | 口服。成人常用量，与其他抗结核药联合，每 6 小时按体重 5 ～ 8.75mg/kg，或每 8 小时按体重 6.7 ～ 11.7mg/kg 给予，最高一日 3g。治疗异烟肼耐药菌感染时可增加至一日 60mg/kg。<br>Oral medication (in combination with other anti-TB drugs), give adults 5 ～ 8.75mg/kg singly, every 6 hours or 6.7 ～ 11.7mg/kg singly, every 8 hours, with maximum daily dose of 3g. Isoniazid-resistant infection: increase daily dose to 60mg/kg. |
| 剂型、规格<br>Preparations | 肠溶片：每片 0.25g；0.5g。<br>Enteric-coated tablets: 0.25g, 0.5g per tablet. |

**续　表**

| 4. 抗麻风病药及抗麻风病反应药 Anti-Leprosy Drugs and Anti-Leprosy Reaction Drugs | |
|---|---|
| 药品名称 Drug Names | 氨苯砜 Dapsone |
| 适应证<br>Indications | 主要用于治疗各型麻风病。近年试用本品治疗系统性红斑狼疮、痤疮、银屑病、带状疱疹等。<br><br>It is mainly used to treat various types of leprosy. In recent years, it is on trial to treat systemic lupus erythematosus, acne, psoriasis, herpes zoster and etc. |
| 用法、用量<br>Dosage | 治疗麻风病，口服，1 次 50 ~ 100mg，一日 100 ~ 200mg。可于开始一日 12.5 ~ 25mg，以后逐渐加量到一日 100mg。由于本品有蓄积作用，故每服药 6 日后停药一日，每服 10 周停药 2 周。必要时，可与利福平每日 600mg 联合应用。儿童剂量一日 1.4mg/kg。治疗红斑狼疮，一日 100mg，连用 3 ~ 6 个月；痤疮，一日 50mg；银屑病或变应性血管炎一日 100 ~ 150mg；带状疱疹，一日 3 次，1 次 25mg，连服 3 ~ 14 日；糜烂性扁平苔藓，一日 50mg，连用 3 个月。以上治疗中，均遵循服药 6 日，停药一日的原则。<br><br>Leprosy: give adults 150 ~ 100mg singly, 100 ~ 200mg a day, orally; start with 12.5 ~ 25mg a dya, then gradually increase to 100mg a day. Since this drug has accumulated effect, it discontinued the medication for one day after 6 days of taking and for two weeks after 10. If necessary, it could be used in combination with 600mg of rifampicin a day. For children, give 1.4mg/kg a day. Lupus: give 100mg a day, for 3 to 6 months. Acne: give 50mg a day. Psoriasis or allergic vasculitis: give 100 ~ 150mg a day. Shingles: give 25mg singly, three times a day, for 3 to 14 days. Erosive lichen planus: give 50mg a day, for 3 months. The above treatment must follow the rule of one-day withdrawal after 6-day medication. |
| 剂型、规格<br>Preparations | 片剂：每片 50mg；100mg。<br>Tablets: 50mg, 100mg per tablet. |
| 药品名称 Drug Names | 醋氨苯砜 Acedapsone |
| 适应证<br>Indications | 用于各型麻风病。<br>It is intended to treat all types of leprosy. |
| 用法、用量<br>Dosage | 肌内注射，1 次 0.225g，隔 60 ~ 75 日注射 1 次，疗程长达数年。为了防止长期单用本品导致细菌产生耐药性，可在用药期间加服氨苯砜 0.1 ~ 0.15g，每周 2 次。<br><br>Intramuscular injection: give 0.225g singly, every 60 to 75 days, with treatment course of years. Long-term medication of this drug may lead to bacteria's drug-resistance, so FDA can be used during the medication: 0.1 ~ 0.15g singly, 2 times a week. |
| 剂型、规格<br>Preparations | 油注射液：每支 225mg（1.5ml）；450mg（3ml）；900mg（6ml）。为 40% 苯甲酸苄酯及 60% 蓖麻油的混悬剂。用前振摇均匀，用粗针头吸出，注入臀肌。<br><br>Oil Injection: 225mg (1.5ml), 450mg (3ml), 900mg (6ml) per vial. It is a suspension with 40% of benzyl benzoate and 60% of castor oil. Shake before use; draw it out by a thick needle; inject into gluteus. |
| 药品名称 Drug Names | 苯丙砜 Solasulfone |
| 适应证<br>Indications | 主要用于治疗各型麻风病。近年试用本品治疗系统性红斑狼疮、痤疮、银屑病、带状疱疹等。<br><br>It is mainly used to treat various types of leprosy. In recent years, it is on trial to treat systemic lupus erythematosus, acne, psoriasis, herpes zoster and etc. |
| 用法、用量<br>Dosage | 肌内注射：每周 2 次，第 1 ~ 2 周每次 100 ~ 200mg，以后每 2 周每次递增 100mg，至第 14 ~ 16 周，每次量为 800mg，继续维持，每用药 10 周后，停药 2 周。<br>口服：300mg/d，逐渐增量至 3g。每服药 10 周，停药 2 周。<br><br>Intramuscular injection: give 2 times a week, 100 ~ 200mg singly for the first 1 to 2 weeks; afterwards increase 100mg singly every two weeks; until 14 to 16 weeks, give 800mg singly. Every 10 weeks of medication needs two weeks' withdrawal.<br>Oral medication: give 300mg a day, gradually increase to 3g. Every 10 weeks of medication needs two weeks' withdrawal. |

**续　表**

| 剂型、规格<br>Preparations | 注射液：每支 2g（5ml）；4g（10ml）。<br>片剂：每片 0.5g。<br>Injection: 2g (5ml), 4g (10ml) per vial.<br>Tablets: 0.5g per tablet. |
|---|---|
| **药品名称 Drug Names** | **氯法齐明 Clofazimine** |
| 适应证<br>Indications | 对于瘤型麻风病和其他型麻风病均有一定疗效，对耐砜类药物麻风杆菌感染也有效。可用于因用其他药物而引起急性麻风反应的病例。<br><br>It is effective in treatment lepromatous leprosy and other types of leprosy, as well as sulfone drug-resistant M. leprae infection. It also can be associated with other drugs to treat acute leprosy reaction. |
| 用法、用量<br>Dosage | 口服。对麻风病，每日 100mg；对麻风反应，一日 200 ~ 400mg，麻风反应控制后，逐渐减量至每日 100mg。<br><br>The drug is administered orally. Leprosy: give 100mg a day. Leprosy reaction: give 200 ~ 400mg a day; after leprosy reaction is controlled, gradually reduce to 100mg a day. |
| 剂型、规格<br>Preparations | 胶囊：每粒 50mg；100mg。<br>胶丸（油蜡或聚乙二醇基质）：每丸 50mg。<br>Capsules: 50mg; 100mg per capsule.<br>Soft capsules (oil wax or polyethylene glycol matrix): 50mg per capsule. |
| **药品名称 Drug Names** | **沙利度胺 Thalidomide** |
| 适应证<br>Indications | 用于麻风结节性红斑。在 2006 年美国 FDA 批准用于治疗多发性骨髓瘤。中华医学会认可：除了可以治疗麻风结节性红斑外，在《临床诊疗指南·血液学分册》中沙利度胺可以治疗多发性骨髓瘤；在《临床诊疗指南·风湿学分册》中沙利度胺可以治疗强直性脊柱炎和白塞病。<br><br>It is intended to treat erythema nodosum leprosy. In 2006, FDA approved that it can be used to treat multiple myeloma. Chinese Medical Association confirmed that: *Clinical Practice Guidelines & Hematology Volum*, suggests thalidomide can treat multiple myeloma except for rythema nodosum leprosy; *Clinical Practice Guidelines & Rheumatology Volume* suggests thalidomide can treat treat ankylosing spondylitis and Behcet's disease. |
| 用法、用量<br>Dosage | 口服每日 100 ~ 200mg，分 4 次服。对严重反应，可增至 300 ~ 400mg（反应得到控制即逐渐减量）。对长期反应者，需要较长期服药，每日或隔日服 25 ~ 50mg。<br>移植后用药：一日 800 ~ 1600mg，分 4 次服，治疗可持续 2 ~ 700 日（平均为 240 日）。治疗完全有效的患者，再持续 3 个月以后逐渐减量（每 2 周减少 25%）；部分有效的患者，再观察到最大效应后还应再治疗 6 个月。<br><br>Give 100 ~ 200mg a day, in 4 divided doses, orally; for patients with severe reaction, increase to 300 ~ 400mg (gradually reduce dose after reaction is controlled); for patients with long-term reaction, require long-term medication: 25 ~ 50mg every day or every other day.<br>Medication after transplantation: give 800 ~ 1600mg a day, in 4 divided doses, for 2 to 700 days (240 days on average). If the treatment has complete effect, make gradual dose reduction (25% reduction every 2 weeks) after 3 months continuous medication; if has partial effect, continue treatment for 6 months after greatest effect is observed. |
| 剂型、规格<br>Preparations | 片剂：每片 25mg；50mg。<br>Tablets: 25mg, 50mg per tablet. |

5. 抗真菌药 Antifungal Drugs

| **药品名称 Drug Names** | **两性霉素 B　Amphotericin B** |
|---|---|
| 适应证<br>Indications | 用于隐球菌、球孢子菌、荚膜组织胞浆菌、芽生菌、孢子丝菌、念珠菌、毛霉、曲霉等引起的内脏或全身感染。<br><br>It is intended to treat viscera or systemic infection caused by Cryptococcus, Coccidioides, Histoplasma capsulatum, Blastomyces, sporotrichosis, Candida, Mucor, Aspergillus and etc. |

**续　表**

| 用法、用量<br>Dosage | 临用前加灭菌注射用水适量使溶解（不可用氯化钠注射液溶解与稀释），再加入 5% 葡萄糖注射液（pH>4.2）中浓度每 1ml 不超过 1mg。<br><br>　　静脉滴注：开始用小剂量 1 ~ 2mg，逐日递增到一日 1mg/kg。每日给药一次，滴注速度通常为每分钟 1 ~ 1.5ml。疗程总量：白念珠菌感染约 1g，隐球菌脑膜炎约 3g。<br><br>　　鞘内注射：对隐球菌脑膜炎，除静脉滴注外尚需鞘内给药。每次从 0.05 ~ 0.1mg 开始，逐渐递增至 0.5 ~ 1mg（浓度为 0.1 ~ 0.25mg/ml）。溶于注射用水 0.5 ~ 1ml 中，按鞘内注射法常规操作，共约 30 次，必要时可酌加地塞米松注射液以减轻反应。<br><br>　　雾化吸入：适用于肺及支气管感染病例。一日量 5 ~ 10mg，溶于注射用水 100 ~ 200ml 中，分 4 次用。<br><br>　　局部病灶注射：浓度 1 ~ 3mg/ml，3 ~ 7 日用 1 次，必要时可加普鲁卡因注射液少量；对真菌性脓胸和关节炎，可局部抽脓后，注入药 5 ~ 10mg，每周 1 ~ 3 次。<br><br>　　局部外用：浓度 2.5 ~ 5mg/ml。<br><br>　　腔道用药：栓剂 25mg。<br><br>　　眼部用药：眼药水 0.25%；眼药膏 1%。<br><br>　　口服：对肠道真菌感染一日 0.5 ~ 2g，分 2 ~ 4 次服。<br><br>Before use, dissolve the drug in appropriate amount of sterile water for injection to (sodium chloride injection is not available in dissolution or dilution), then add it ito 5% glucose injection (pH>4.2) and the concentration can not exceed 1mg in every 1ml of the liquid .<br><br>Intravenous infusion: start with a small dose of 1 ~ 2mg, then increase gradually to 1mg/kg a day, once a day; the infusion rate is generally 1 ~ 1.5ml per minute. The total dose for Candida albicans infection is approximately 1g, for cryptococcal meningitis is about 3g.<br><br>In treatment of cryptococcal meningitis, intrathecal injection is still needed except for intravenous infusion. Intrathecal injection: start with 0.05 ~ 0.1mg, then gradually increase to 0.5 ~ 1mg (with concentration of 0.1 ~ 0.25mg/ml). Dissolve the drug in 0.5 ~ 1ml of water for injection, then give intrathecal injection by common practice, about 30 times in total; if necessary, add dexamethasone injection to reduce reaction.<br><br>Pulmonary and bronchial infection can be administered by inhalation. Inhalation: give 5 ~ 10mg a day; dissolve the drug in 100 ~ 200ml of water for injection, in 4 divided doses.<br><br>Localized lesion injection: give once every 3 ~ 7 days, with concentration of 1 ~ 3mg/ml; if necessary, add a small amount of procaine injection; for Fungal pleural empyema and arthritis, inject 5 ~ 10mg after local pus pumping,, 1 ~ 3 times a week.<br><br>Topical external use: concentration of 2.5 ~ 5mg/ml.<br>Cavity medication: 25mg of suppositories.<br>Eye medication: 0.25% of eye drops; 1% of eye ointment.<br>Oral medication: for intestinal fungal infection, give 0.5 ~ 2g a day, in 2 to 4 divided doses. |
| 剂型、规格<br>Preparations | 注射用两性霉素 B（脱氧胆酸钠复合物）：每支 5mg；25mg；50mg。<br>Amphotericin B for injeciotn (sodium deoxycholate complex): 5mg, 25mg, 50mg per vial. |
| 药品名称 Drug Names | 伊曲康唑 Itraconazole |
| 适应证<br>Indications | 主要应用于深部真菌所引起的系统感染如类球孢子菌病、组织胞浆菌病、芽生菌病、着色真菌病、孢子丝菌病等。也可用于念珠菌病和曲霉病。<br><br>It is mainly used to treat systemic infection caused by deep fungus, such as coccidioidomycosis, histoplasmosis, blastomycosis, colored fungal disease, sporotrichosis, and etc.. It can also be used to treat candidiasis and aspergillosis. |
| 用法、用量<br>Dosage | 一般为一日 100 ~ 200mg，顿服，一般疗程为 3 个月，个别情况下疗程延长到 6 个月。<br>　　短程间歇疗法：1 次 200mg，一日 2 次，连服 7 日为 1 个疗程。停药 2 日，开始第 2 个疗程，指甲癣服 2 个疗程，趾甲癣服 3 个疗程，治愈率分别为 97% 和 69.4%。<br><br>Generally, give 100 ~ 200mg a day, at a draught and have, the treatment course of 3 months or extend to 6 months on rare occasion. Short-course intermittent therapy: give 200mg singly, 2 times a day, with a treatment course of 7 days, then stop drug 2 days and begin the second course afterwards. Medication for fingernail tinea is 2 courses, while toenail tinea is 3 courses. The cure rate is 97% and 69.4% respectively. |

**续 表**

| 剂型、规格<br>Preparations | 片剂：每片 100mg；200mg。<br>注射液：25ml：250mg。<br>Tablet: 100mg, 200mg per tablet.<br>Injection: 25ml:250mg. |
|---|---|
| **药品名称 Drug Names** | 氟康唑 Fluconazole |
| 适应证<br>Indications | 应用于敏感菌所致的各种真菌感染，如隐球菌性脑膜炎、复发性口咽念珠菌病等。<br><br>It is used to treat a variety of fungal infection caused by susceptible strains, such as cryptococcal meningitis, recurrent oropharyngeal candidiasis and etc. |
| 用法、用量<br>Dosage | 念珠菌性口咽炎或食管炎：第一日口服 200mg，以后每日服 100mg，疗程 2 ～ 3 周（症状消失仍需用药），以免复发。<br><br>念珠菌系统感染：第 1 天 400mg，以后每天 200mg。疗程 4 周或症状消失后再用 2 周。<br><br>隐球菌性脑膜炎：第 1 天 400mg，以后每天 200mg。如患者反应正常，也可用每日 1 次 400mg，至脑脊液细菌培养阴性后 10 ～ 12 周。<br><br>肾功能不全者，减少用量。肌酐清除率 >50ml/min 者用正常量；肌酐清除率为 21 ～ 50ml/min 者用 1/2 量；肌酐清除率为 11 ～ 20ml/min 者用 1/4 量。口服和静脉输注用量相同。静脉滴注速度约为 200mg/h。可加入到葡萄糖液、生理氯化钠液、乳酸钠林格液中滴注。<br><br>Candidal oropharyngeal infection or esophagitis: give orally 200mg in the first day, afterwards 100mg a day, with a treatment course of 2 to 3 weeks (medication is still needed after symptoms disappear to avoid recurrence).<br><br>Candida systemic infection: give 400mg in the first day, afterwards 200mg a day, with a treatment course of 4 weeks or with continuous treatment for another 2 weeks after the disappearance of symptoms..<br><br>Cryptococcal meningitis: give 400mg in the first day, afterwards 200mg a day. If patients have normal response, give 400mg a day until another 10 to 12 weeks after cerebrospinal fluid bacteria is negative.<br><br>The dosage for renal insufficiency patients should be reduced. Patients with creatinine clearance> 50ml/min, give normal dose; with creatinine clearance rate of 21 ～ 50ml/min, give 1/2 of the dose; with creatinine clearance rate of 11 ～ 20 ml / min, give 1/4 of the dose. Oral medication and intravenous infusion has the same dose. Infusion rate is about 200mg / h. it can be added into glucose solution, physiological sodium chloride solution and Ringer's lactate solution for infusion. |
| 剂型、规格<br>Preparations | 片剂（胶囊）：每片（粒）50mg；100mg；150mg 或 200mg。<br>注射剂：每瓶 200mg/100ml。<br>Tablets (capsules): 50mg, 100mg, 150mg, 200mg per tablet (capsule).<br>Injection: 200mg/100ml per bottle. |
| **药品名称 Drug Names** | 伏立康唑 Voriconazole |
| 适应证<br>Indications | 用于治疗侵入性曲霉病，以及对氟康唑耐药的严重进入性念珠菌病感染及由足放线病菌属和镰刀菌属引起的严重真菌感染。主要用于进行性、致命危险的免疫系统受损的 2 岁以上患者。<br><br>It is intended to treat invasive aspergillosis, candidiasis with severe accessibility of fluconazole-resistance and severe fungal infection caused by actinomycetes bacteria genus and fusarium. .it is mainly used in the progressive and fatal dangerous immune system damage whose patients are over the age of 2. |
| 用法、用量<br>Dosage | 负荷剂量：第 1 天静脉滴注每次 6mg/kg，12 小时 1 次；口服每次 400mg（体重 ≥ 40kg）或 200mg 每次（体重 <40kg），每 12 小时一次。维持剂量：第 2 天起静脉滴注 4mg/kg 一日 2 次，或 200mg 一日 2 次（体重 ≥ 40kg），或 100mg 一日 2 次（体重 <40kg）。均为 12 小时 1 次。治疗口咽、食管、白念珠菌病：口服，一次 200mg，一日 2 次；静脉注射，每次 3 ～ 6mg/kg，12 小时 1 次。<br><br>Loading dose: give infusion of 6mg/kg/second in thefirst day, every 12 hours or oral medication of 200mg(body weight ≥ 40kg) or 400mg (weight <40kg) singly, every 12 hours. Maintenance dose: from the second day, give infusion of 4mg/kg, every 12 hours or oral medication of 200mg (body weight ≥ 40kg) or 100mg (weight <40kg) singly, every 12 hours. Oropharyngeal infection and esophagitis by candidia: give 200mg singly, twice a day, orally or 3 ～ 6mg/kg singly, every 12 hours, intravenous injection. |

续　表

| 剂型、规格<br>Preparations | 片剂：每片 50mg；200mg。<br>注射用伏立康唑：每支 200mg。<br>Tablets: 50mg, 200mg per tablet.<br>Voriconazole for injection: 200mg per vial. |
|---|---|
| 药品名称 Drug Names | 氟胞嘧啶 Flucytosine |
| 适应证<br>Indications | 用于念珠菌和隐球菌感染，单用效果不如两性霉素 B，可与两性霉素 B 合用，以增疗效（协同作用）。<br>It is intended to treat candidia infection and cryptococcal infection; it is not as effective as amphotericin B when used alone, so it could be combined with amphotericin B to increase the efficacy (synergy). |
| 用法、用量<br>Dosage | 口服：一日 4 ～ 6g，分 4 次服，疗程为数周至数月。静脉注射，一日 50 ～ 150mg/kg，分 2 ～ 3 次。单用本品时真菌易产生耐药性，宜与两性霉素 B 合用。<br>Oral:4 ～ 6g one day, 4 times daily, courses from several weeks to several months.Intravenous injection, 50 ～ 150mg/kg one day, 2 to 3 times.When using this fungus is easy to produce single-drug resistance, should better used in combination with amphotericin B. |
| 剂型、规格<br>Preparations | 片剂：每片 250mg；500mg。<br>注射液：2.5g（250ml）。<br>Tablets: 250mg, 500mg per tablet.<br>Injection: 2.5g (250ml). |
| 药品名称 Drug Names | 特比奈芬 Terbinafine |
| 适应证<br>Indications | 用于浅表真菌引起的皮肤、指甲感染，如毛癣菌、犬、小孢子菌、絮状表皮癣菌等引起的体癣、股癣、足癣、甲癣，以及皮肤白念珠菌感染。<br>It is used to treat the skin infection and nail infection caused by superficial fungus, such as tinea corporis, tines cruris, tinea pedis, onychomycosis and skin candida albicans caused by trichophyton, dogs, small spores, Epidermophyton floccosum, and etc. |
| 用法、用量<br>Dosage | 口服，一日 1 次 250mg，足癣、体癣、股癣服用 1 周；皮肤念珠菌病 1 ～ 2 周；指甲癣 4 ～ 6 周，趾甲癣 12 周（口服对花斑癣无效）。<br>外用（1% 霜剂）用于体癣、股癣、皮肤念珠菌病、花斑癣等，一日涂抹 1 ～ 2 次，疗程不定（1 ～ 2 周）。<br>Oral medication: give 250mg a day. Patients with tinea pedis, tinea corporis and tinea cruris need medication for one week; with skin candidiasis, for1 to 2 weeks; with nail ringworm, for 4 to 6 weeks; with nail ringworm, for12 weeks (oral medication is ineffective at tinea versicolor).<br>Topical external use (1% cream): it can used in treatment of body ringworm, jock itch, skin candidiasis, tinea versicolor, and etc.; give 1 to 2 times a day, with uncertain treatment course (about 1 to 2 weeks). |
| 剂型、规格<br>Preparations | 片剂：每片 125mg 或 250mg。<br>霜剂：1%。<br>Tablets: 125mg. 250mg per tablet.<br>Cream: 1%. |
| 药品名称 Drug Names | 美帕曲星 Mepartricin |
| 适应证<br>Indications | 用于白念珠菌阴道炎和肠道念珠菌病，也可用于阴道或肠道滴虫病。本品在肠道内与甾醇类物质结合成不吸收的物质，可用于治疗良性前列腺肿大。<br>It is intended to treat Candida albicans vaginitis and intestinal candidiasis, as well as vaginal or intestinal trichomoniasis. Nonabsorb material may be compounded in the intestine when it is combined with sterols, which can be used to treat benign prostate enlargement. |
| 用法、用量<br>Dosage | 阴道或肠道念珠菌感染或滴虫病（用含十二烷基硫酸钠的复合片）：1 次 100 000U（2 片），每 12 小时 1 次，连用 3 日为 1 个疗程。对于复杂性病例，疗程可酌情延长。宜食后服用。<br>治疗前列腺肿大或肠道念珠菌病、滴虫病（用不含十二烷基硫酸钠的片剂）：一日 1 次，每次 100 000U。 |

**续 表**

| | Vaginal or intestinal candidiasis and vaginal or intestinal trichomoniasis (sodium dodecyl sulfate compound tablets used):give 100 000 units once(2 tablets) singly, every 12 hours, after meals, with a treatment course of three days .For complex cases, treatment course can be extended as required.<br><br>Prostate enlargement and intestinal candidiasis or trichomoniasis (non sodium dodecyl sulfate tablets used): give 100, 000 units singly, once a day. |
|---|---|
| 剂型、规格<br>Preparations | 肠溶片：每片 50 000U。<br>阴道片：每片 25 000U。<br>乳膏：供黏膜用。<br><br>Enteric-coated tablets: 50, 000 units per tablet.<br>Vaginal tablets: 25, 000 units per tablet.<br>Cream: for mucosal use. |
| 药品名称 Drug Names | 阿莫罗芬 Amorolfine |
| 适应证<br>Indications | 用于治疗皮肤及黏膜浅表真菌感染，如体癣、手癣、足癣、甲真菌病及阴道白念珠菌病等。<br><br>It is intended to treat superficial fungal infection of skin and mucous membranes, such as tinea corpris, tinea magnum, tinea pedis, onychomycosis, vaginal candidiasis and so on. |
| 用法、用量<br>Dosage | 甲真菌病：挫光病甲后将搽剂均匀涂抹于患处，每周 1 ~ 2 次。指甲感染一般连续用药 6 个月，趾甲感染持续用药 9 ~ 12 个月。皮肤浅表真菌感染：用 0.25% 乳膏局部涂抹，一日 1 次，至临床症状消失后继续治疗 3 ~ 5 日。阴道念珠菌病：先用温开水或 0.02% 高锰酸钾无菌溶液冲洗阴道或坐浴，再将一枚栓剂置于阴道深处。<br><br>Onychomycosis: smear the liniment evenly over the affected area after polishing the illness nail, 1 ~ 2 times a week. Nail infection generally need continuous medication for 6 months, toenail infection need for 9 to 12 months. Superficial fungal skin infection: smear 0.25% creamtopically, once a day; continue treatment for another 3 to 5 days after clinical symptoms disappear. Vaginal candidiasis: before use, use warm water or a sterile solution of 0.02% potassium permanganate for vaginal washing or sitz bath, then put one suppository into the vagina. |
| 剂型、规格<br>Preparations | 搽剂：每瓶 125mg（2.5ml）。<br>乳膏剂：每支 0.25%（5g）。<br>栓剂：每枚 25mg；50mg。<br><br>Liniment: 125mg (2.5ml) of each.<br>Cream: 0.25% (5g) of each.<br>Suppository: 25mg; 50mg of each. |
| 药品名称 Drug Names | 醋酸卡泊芬净 Caspofungin Acetate |
| 适应证<br>Indications | 用于治疗对其他治疗无效或不能耐受的侵袭性曲霉菌病；对疑似真菌感染的粒缺伴发热患者的经验治疗；口咽及食管念珠菌病。侵袭性念珠菌病，包括中性粒细胞减少症及非中性粒细胞减少症患者的念珠菌血症。<br><br>It is intended to treat invasive aspergillosis which is resistant or intolerant to other therapy, as well as oropharyngeal and esophageal candidiasis. It can be used in empirical therapy of febrile neutropenic patients who are suspected to get fungal infection, Invasive candidiasis, including neutropenic and non-neutropenic patients' candidemia. |
| 用法、用量<br>Dosage | 第一天给予单次 70mg 负荷剂量，随后每天给予 50mg 的剂量。本品约需要 1 小时的时间经静脉缓慢输注给药。疗程取决于患者疾病的严重程度、被抑制的免疫功能恢复情况以及对治疗的临床反应。对于治疗无临床反应而对本品耐受性良好的患者可以考虑将每日剂量加大到 70mg。<br><br>Give a single loading dose of 70mg in the first day, afterwards 50mg a day. Administration by slow intravenous infusion needs to take about an hour. The course of treatment varies according to the severity of the disease, suppressed immune function recovery and clinical response to treatment. For patients who have no clinical response to treatment but well tolerance to the drug, it can be considered to increase the daily dose to 70mg. |
| 剂型、规格<br>Preparations | 注射用醋酸卡泊芬净：50mg；70mg（以卡泊芬净计）。<br>Caspofungin Acetate injection: 50mg, 70mg (calculated by caspofungin net content). |

**续　表**

| 药品名称 Drug Names | 米卡芬净 Micafungin |
|---|---|
| 适应证<br>Indications | 用于治疗食管念珠菌感染，预防造血干细胞移植患者的念珠菌感染。<br>It is intended to treat esophageal candidiasis and prevent candida infections of hematopoietic stem cell transplantation patients. |
| 用法、用量<br>Dosage | 治疗食管念珠菌病的推荐剂量为 150mg/d，预防造血干细胞移植患者的念珠菌感染的推荐剂量为 50mg/d。平均疗程分别为 15 日和 19 日。<br>只能用生理盐水（可用 5% 葡萄糖注射液代替）配制和稀释。每 50mg 米卡芬净钠先加入 5ml 生理盐水溶解。为减少泡沫的产生，须轻轻转动玻璃瓶，不可用力振摇。随后将已溶解好的米卡芬净钠溶液加入到 100ml 生理盐水中滴注给药，给药时间至少 1 小时。<br>Esophageal candidiasis: give recommended dose of 150mg a day. Hematopoietic stem cell transplant patients' candida infection prevention: give recommended dose of 50mg a day. The course of treatment is 15 days and 19 days on average respectively.<br>It can only be formulated and diluted with saline (5% Dextrose Injection can be substitude). Add 5ml of saline solution in every 50mg of micafungin sodium for dissolution. In order to reduce the generation of foam, turn the bottle lightly; shaking vigorously is not aloowed. Then add the dissolved micafungin sodium into 100ml of saline for infusion, the time for which is at least an hour. |
| 剂型、规格<br>Preparations | 米卡芬净钠冻干粉针：每瓶 50mg；100mg。<br>Micafungin sodium lyophilized powder: 50mg, 100mg of each. |
| 药品名称 Drug Names | 阿尼芬净 Anidulafungin |
| 适应证<br>Indications | 用于治疗食管念珠菌感染，念珠菌性败血症，念珠菌引起的腹腔脓肿及念珠菌性腹膜炎。<br>It is intended to treat esophageal candidiasis, candida septicemia, abdominal abscess by Candida albicans and Candida peritonitis. |
| 用法、用量<br>Dosage | 静脉给药：食管念珠菌病，第 1 日 100mg，随后每天 50mg 疗程至少 14 日，且至少持续至症状消失后 7 日。念珠菌性败血症等，第一日 200mg，随后每天 100mg，疗程持续至最后一次阴性培养后至少 14 日。<br>The drug is administered intravenously. Esophageal candidiasis: give 100mg in the first day, afterwards 50mg a day; the treatment course is at least 14 days, and continues until at least 7 days after symptoms disappear. Candida septicemia: give 200mg in the first day, afterwards 100mg a day; the treatment course continues until 14 days after the bacteria is negative. |
| 剂型、规格<br>Preparations | 注射用阿尼芬净：每瓶 50mg；100mg。<br>Anidulafungin for injection: 50mg, 100mg per vial. |
| 药品名称 Drug Names | 制霉菌素 Nystatin |
| 适应证<br>Indications | 口服用于治疗消化道念珠菌病。<br>Taking orally is intended to treat gastrointestinal candidiasis. |
| 用法、用量<br>Dosage | 消化道念珠菌病：口服，成人 1 次 50 万～ 100 万 U，一日 3 次。小儿每日按体重 5 万～ 10 万 U/kg，分 3 ～ 4 次服。<br>Gastrointestinal candidiasis: give adults 50 to 100 million units singly, three times a day, orally; give children 5 to 10 million units / kg a day, in 3 to 4 divided doses. |
| 剂型、规格<br>Preparations | 片剂：50 万 U。<br>软膏：每克 10 万 U。<br>栓剂：每枚 10 万 U。<br>Tablets: 500, 000 units.<br>Ointment: 100, 000 units per gram.<br>Suppository: detachment 100, 000 units. |
| 药品名称 Drug Names | 咪康唑 Miconazole |
| 适应证<br>Indications | 局部治疗念珠菌性外阴阴道病和革兰阳性细菌引起的双重感染。<br>It is intended to treat local vulvovaginal candidiasis and dual infection caused by Gram-positive bacteria. |

| | |
|---|---|
| 用法、用量<br>Dosage | 静脉给药：治疗深部真菌病一日常用量为 600 ~ 1800mg，分 3 次给予。局部用药：常作为全身用药的补充。<br><br>Intravenous administration: in treatment of deep mycoses, give 600 ~ 1800mg a day, in 3 divided doses. Topical administration: often as a supplement to systemic administration |
| 剂型、规格<br>Preparations | 注射液：200mg；<br>栓剂：100mg；<br>霜剂：15g<br><br>Injection: 200mg.<br>Suppository: 100mg.<br>Cream: 1%. |

## 6. 抗病毒药 Antiviral Drugs

| 药品名称 Drug Names | 阿昔洛韦 Aciclovir |
|---|---|
| 适应证<br>Indications | 用于防治单纯疱疹病毒 HSV1 和 HSV2 的皮肤或黏膜感染，还可用于带状疱疹病毒感染。<br><br>It is intended to prevent and treat skin or mucous membrane infection by herpes simplex virus HSV1 and HSV2, as well as herpes zoster virus infection. |
| 用法、用量<br>Dosage | 口服：1 次 200mg，每 4 小时 1 次或一日 1g，分次给予。疗程根据病情不同，短则几天，长者可达半年。肾功能不全者酌情减量。静脉滴注：1 次用量 5mg/kg，加入输液中，滴注时间为 1 小时，每 8 小时 1 次，连续 7 日。12 岁以下儿童 1 次按 250mg/ 用量给予。急性或慢性肾功能不全者，不宜用本品静脉滴注，因为滴速过快时可引起肾衰竭。<br>国内治疗乙型肝炎的用法为 1 次滴注 7.5mg/kg，一日 2 次，溶于适量输液，维持滴注时间约 2 小时，连续应用 10 ~ 30 日。<br>治疗生殖器疱疹，1 次 0.2g，一日 4 次，连用 5 ~ 10 日。<br><br>Oral medication: give 200mg singly, every four hours or 1g a day, in divided doses; the treatment course varies for different disease, from a few days to six months; renal insufficiency patients need appropriate dose reduction.<br>Intravenous infusion: give 5mg/kg singly, every 8 hours, for 7 days; add the drug into the infusion, and the infusion time is 1 hour. For children under the age of 12, give 250mg/ m² singly. For acute or chronic renal insufficiency patients, do not use this product for intravenous infusion because too fast drip may cause kidney failure. In domestic treatment of hepatitis B, give 7.5mg/kg, 2 times a day, for 10 to 30 days; dissolve the drug in the appropriate amount of fluid, ; the infusion time lasts about 2 hours.<br>Genital herpes: 0.2g singly, 4 times a day, for 5 to 10 days. |
| 剂型、规格<br>Preparations | 胶囊剂：每粒 200mg；<br>注射用阿昔洛韦（冻干制剂）：每瓶 500mg（标示量，含钠盐 549mg，折合纯品 500mg）。<br>滴眼液：0.1%。<br>眼膏：3%。<br>霜膏剂：5%。<br><br>Capsules: 200mg per capsule.<br>Acyclovir for injection (lyophilized formulations): 500mg per bottle (labeled amount, containing 549mg of sodium which is equivalent to 500mg purely).<br>Drops: 0.1%.<br>Ointment: 3%.<br>Ointment cream: 5%. |
| 药品名称 Drug Names | 更昔洛韦 Ganciclovir |
| 适应证<br>Indications | 用于巨细胞病毒感染的治疗和预防，也可适用于单纯疱疹病毒感染。<br><br>It is used in the treatment and prevention of cytomegalovirus infection, as well as to treat herpes simplex virus infection. |

续　表

| | |
|---|---|
| 用法、用量<br>Dosage | 诱导治疗：静脉滴注 5mg/kg（历时至少 1 小时），每 12 小时 1 次，连用 14 ～ 21 日（预防用药则为 7 ～ 14 日）；<br>维持治疗：静脉滴注，5mg/kg，一日 1 次，每周用药 7 日；或 6mg/kg，一日 1 次，每周用药 5 日。<br>口服，每次 1g，一日 3 次，与食物同服，可根据病情选用其中之一。 输液配制：将 500mg 药物（钠盐），加 10ml 注射用水振摇，使其溶解，液体应澄明无色，此溶液在室温时稳定 12 小时，切勿冷藏。进一步可用 0.9% 氯化钠、5% 葡萄糖、林格或乳酸钠林格等输液稀释至含药量低于 10mg/ml，供静脉滴注 1 小时。<br>Induction therapy: by intravenous infusion, give 5mg/kg (which lasts at least an hour), every 12 hours, for 14 to 21 days (7 to 14 days for prophylactic medication).<br>Maintenance therapy: by intravenous infusion, give 5mg/kg a day, seven days a week or 6mg/kg, once a day, 5 days a week.<br>Oral medication: give 1g a day, 3 times a day, with food. Either can be chosen according to the disease. Infusion preparation:, add 10ml of water for injection in 500mg of drug (sodium salt) and shake it to dissolution, the liquid should be clear and colorless; keep the solution stable at room temperature for 12 hours and do not freeze. Further, use 0.9% sodium chloride, 5% dextrose, Ringer's or lactated Ringer's for dilution and make drug content less than 10mg/ml for intravenous infusion, which lasts 1 hour. |
| 剂型、规格<br>Preparations | 胶囊剂：每粒 250mg。<br>注射剂（冻干粉针）：每瓶 500mg。<br>Capsules: 250mg per capsule.<br>Injection (lyophilized powder): 500mg per vial. |
| 药品名称 Drug Names | 伐昔洛韦 Valaciclovir |
| 适应证<br>Indications | 本品主要用于治疗带状疱疹，也可用于治疗 HSV1 和 HSV2 感染。<br>It is mainly used in the treatment of herpes zoster, as well as HSV1 or HSV2 infection. |
| 用法、用量<br>Dosage | 口服，成人每日 0.6g，分 2 次服，疗程为 7 ～ 10 日。<br>Oral medication: give adults 0.6g a day, in 2 divided doses, for 7 to 10 days. |
| 剂型、规格<br>Preparations | 片剂：每片 200mg；300mg。<br>Tablets: 200mg, 300mg per tablet. |
| 药品名称 Drug Names | 泛昔洛韦 Famciclovir |
| 适应证<br>Indications | 用于治疗带状疱疹和原发性生殖器疱疹。<br>It is used in treatment of shingles and primary genital herpes. |
| 用法、用量<br>Dosage | 口服，成人一次 0.25g，每 8 小时 1 次，治疗带状疱疹的疗程为 7 日，治疗原发性生殖器疱疹的疗程为 5 日。<br>Oral medication: give adults 0.25g a day, every 8 hours; the treatment course for herpes zoster is 7 days, for primary genital herpes is 5 days. |
| 剂型、规格<br>Preparations | 片剂：每片 125mg；250mg；500mg。<br>Tablets: 125mg, 250mg, 500mg per tablet. |
| 药品名称 Drug Names | 奥司他韦 Oseltamivir |
| 适应证<br>Indications | 用于成人和 1 岁及 1 岁以上儿童的甲型和乙型流感的治疗（磷酸奥司他韦能够有效治疗甲型和乙型流感，但是乙型流感的临床应用数据尚不多）。用于成人和 13 岁及 13 岁以上青少年的甲型和乙型流感的预防。<br>It is intended to treat influenza A or B infection in adults and children of 1 year old and above (oseltamivir phosphate can effectively treat influenza A and B, but the clinical application data of influenza B is insufficient). It also can be used to prevent influenza A and B in adults and adolescents of 13 years old and above. |

**续 表**

| 用法、用量<br>Dosage | 成人推荐量，每次 75mg，一日 2 次，共 5 日。肾功能不全者：肌酐清除率 <30ml/min 者每日 75mg，共 5 日。肌酐清除率 <10ml/min 者尚无研究资料，应慎重使用。<br><br>Adults: give recommended dose of 75mg singly, 2 times a day, for 5 days. Renal insufficiency patients: with creatinine clearance <30ml/min, give 75mg a day, for 5 days; with creatinine clearance <10ml/min, use with caution because of no existence of research data. |
|---|---|
| 剂型、规格<br>Preparations | 胶囊剂：每粒 75mg（以游离碱计）。<br>Capsules: 75mg (calculated by free base) per capsule. |
| **药品名称 Drug Names** | **扎那米韦 Zanamivir** |
| 适应证<br>Indications | 用于治疗流感病毒感染及季节性预防社区内 A 和 B 型流感。<br><br>It is used in treatment of influenza virus infection, as well as in seasonal prevention of community influenza A and B. |
| 用法、用量<br>Dosage | 成人和 12 岁以上的青少年，一日 2 次，间隔约 12 小时。每日 10mg，分 2 次吸入，一次 5mg，经口吸入给药，连用 5 日。随后数日，两次的服药时间尽可能保持一致，剂量间隔 12 小时。季节性预防社区内 A 和 B 型流感：成人 10mg，一日 1 次，用 28 日，在流感暴发 5 日内开始治疗。<br><br>Adults and adolescents over the age of 12: by inhalation, give 5mg singly, 2 times a day, every 12 hours, for 5 days; in the next few days, keep the intervals as 12 hours. Seasonal prevention of community influenza A and B: give adults 10mg a day, once a day, for 28 days; treatment starts within 5 days from the influenza outbreak. |
| 剂型、规格<br>Preparations | 吸入粉雾剂：每个泡囊含扎那米韦（5mg）和乳糖（20mg）的混合粉末。<br>Powders for inhalation: containing vesicles zanamivir (5mg) and lactose (20mg). |
| **药品名称 Drug Names** | **阿巴卡韦 Abacavir** |
| 适应证<br>Indications | 本品常与其他药物联合用于艾滋病的治疗。<br>It is often combined with other drugs to treat AIDS. |
| 用法、用量<br>Dosage | 与其他抗反转录酶药物合用。成人：一次 300mg，一日 2 次。3 月龄至 16 岁儿童：一次 8mg/kg，一日 2 次。<br><br>It is used in combination with other antiretroviral drugs.<br>Adults:300mg singly, 2 times a day.<br>Children aging 3 months to 16 years old: 8mg/kg singly, 2 times a day. |
| 剂型、规格<br>Preparations | 片剂：300mg（以盐基计）。<br>口服液：20mg/ml。<br>Tablets: 300mg (calculated by salt).<br>Oral liquid: 20mg/ml. |
| **药品名称 Drug Names** | **阿糖腺苷 Vidarabine** |
| 适应证<br>Indications | 有抗单纯疱疹病毒 HSV1 和 HSV2 作用，用以治疗单纯疱疹病毒性脑炎，也用以治疗免疫抑制患者的带状疱疹和水痘感染。但对巨细胞病毒则无效。本品的单磷酸酯有抑制乙肝病毒复制的作用。<br><br>It has effect in anti-herpes simplex virus HSV1 and HSV2, so it can treat of herpes simplex virus encephalitis, as well as immune suppressed patients' herpes zoster and varicella infection. But it is ineffective at cytomegalovirus. Monophosphate contained in this drug can inhibit HBV replication. |
| 用法、用量<br>Dosage | 单纯疱疹病毒性脑炎：一日量为 15mg/kg，按 200g 药物、500ml 输液（预热至 35 ～ 40℃）的比率配液，做连续静脉滴注，疗程为 10 日。<br>带状疱疹：10mg/kg 连用 5 日，用法同上。<br><br>Herpes simplex virus encephalitis: give15mg/kg a day, by continuous intravenous infusion, for 10 days as a treatment course; every 200g of the drug needs 500ml of the infusion (preheated to 35 ～ 40℃ ).<br>Shingles: give10mg/kg, for 5 days; drug usage is the same with the above. |

**续　表**

| | |
|---|---|
| 剂型、规格<br>Preparations | 注射液（混悬液）：200mg（1ml）；1000mg（5ml）。加入输液中滴注用。<br>注射用单磷酸阿糖腺苷：每瓶 200mg。<br><br>Injection (suspension): 200mg (1ml), 1000mg (5ml); added into the infusion for drip.<br>Vidarabine monophosphate for injection: 200mg per vial. |
| **药品名称 Drug Names** | 利巴韦林 Ribavirin |
| 适应证<br>Indications | 用于呼吸道合胞病毒引起的病毒性肺炎与支气管炎，皮肤疱疹病毒感染。<br><br>It is intended to treat viral pneumonia and bronchitis caused by respiratory syncytial virus, as well as skin's herpesvirus infection. |
| 用法、用量<br>Dosage | 口服：一日 0.8 ~ 1g，分 3 ~ 4 次服用。肌内注射或静脉滴注：一日 10 ~ 15mg/kg，分 2 次，静脉滴注宜缓慢。<br>用于早期出血热，每日 1g，加入输液 500 ~ 1000ml 中静脉滴注，连续应用 3 ~ 5 日。<br>滴鼻：用于防治流感，用 0.5% 溶液（以等渗氯化钠溶液配制），每小时 1 次。<br>滴眼：治疗疱疹感染，浓度 0.1%，一日数次。<br><br>Oral medication: give 0.8 ~ 1g a day, in 3 to 4 divided doses. Intramuscular injection or intravenous infusion: give 10 ~ 15mg/kg a day, in 2 divided doses, for slow intravenous infusion.<br>Early hemorrhagic fever: give 1g a day, for 3 to 5 days; add into 500 ~ 1000ml of the infusion for intravenous infusion.<br>Intranasal medication: in influenza prevention and treatment, give 0.5% solution (isotonic sodium chloride solution preparation), once every hour.<br>Eye drops: for treating herpes infection, with the concentration of 0.1%, several times a day. |
| 剂型、规格<br>Preparations | 片剂：每片 50mg；100mg。<br>颗粒剂：每袋 50mg；100mg。<br>注射液：100mg（1ml）；250mg（2ml）。<br><br>Tablets: 50mg, 100mg per tablet.<br>Granules: 50mg, 100mg per bag.<br>Injection: 100mg (1ml), 250mg (2ml). |
| **药品名称 Drug Names** | 齐多夫定 Zidovudine |
| 适应证<br>Indications | 用于治疗获得性免疫缺陷综合征（AIDS）。患者有并发症（卡氏肺囊虫病或其他感染）时尚需应用对症的其他药物联合治疗。<br><br>It is used in the treatment of acquired immunodeficiency syndrome (AIDS). If the patients have complications (carinii disease or other infections), it is required to be used in combination with other symptomatic drugs. |
| 用法、用量<br>Dosage | 成人常用量：1 次 200mg，每 4 小时 1 次，按时间给药。有贫血的患者：可按 1 次 100mg 给药。<br><br>Adults: 200mg singly, every four hours, with ontime administeration. Patients with anemia: 100mg singly. |
| 剂型、规格<br>Preparations | 胶囊剂：每粒 100mg。<br>Capsules: 100mg per capsule. |
| **药品名称 Drug Names** | 拉米夫定 Lamivudine |
| 适应证<br>Indications | 用于乙型肝炎病毒所致的慢性乙型肝炎，与其他抗反转录病毒药联用用于治疗人类免疫缺陷病毒感染。<br><br>It is intended to treat chronic hepatitis B caused by hepatitis B virus. Combining with other anti-retroviral drugs can treat human immunodeficiency virus infection. |
| 用法、用量<br>Dosage | 成人：慢性乙型肝炎，一日 1 次，100mg 口服；HIV 感染，推荐剂量一次 150mg，一日 2 次，或一次 300mg；一日 1 次。<br><br>Adults: for chronic hepatitis B, give 100mg orally, once a day; for HIV infection, give recommended dose of 150mg singly, 2 times a day or 300mg singly, once a day. |

| 剂型、规格<br>Preparations | 片剂：每片 100mg；150mg。<br>Tablets: 100mg; 150mg per tablet. |
|---|---|
| **药品名称 Drug Names** | 阿德福韦酯 Adefovir dipivoxil |
| 适应证<br>Indications | 用于乙型肝炎病毒感染，人类免疫缺陷病毒感染。<br>It is intended to treat hepatitis B virus infection and human immunodeficiency virus infection. |
| 用法、用量<br>Dosage | 成人口服：慢性乙型肝炎，一日 1 次，每次 10mg；HIV 感染，一日 1 次，每次 125mg，疗程 12 周。静脉滴注：HIV 感染，每次 1 ~ 3mg/kg，一日 1 次或每周 3 次，每次给药时间不少于 30 分钟。皮下注射剂量同静脉滴注。<br><br>Adults' oral medication: for chronic hepatitis B, give10mg singly, once a day; for HIV infection, give 125mg singly, once a day, for 12 weeks. Intravenous infusion: for HIV infection, give 1 ~ 3mg/kg singly, once a day or 3 times a week, and each infusion time is not less than 30 minutes. Subcutaneous injection is with the same dose of intravenous infusion. |
| 剂型、规格<br>Preparations | 阿德福韦酯片（胶囊）：每片（粒）10mg。<br>Adefovir dipivoxil tablets (capsules): 10mg per tablet (capsule). |
| **药品名称 Drug Names** | 恩替卡韦 Entecavir |
| 适应证<br>Indications | 用于病毒复制活跃，血清转氨酶 ALT 持续升高或肝脏组织学显示有活动性病变的慢性成人乙型肝炎的治疗。<br>It is intended to treat adults' chronic hepatitis B, which has active viral replication, persistently elevated serum transaminases ALT or displayed pathological changes in liver histology. |
| 用法、用量<br>Dosage | 口服，每天 1 次，每次 0.5mg。拉米夫定治疗时发生病毒血症或出现拉米夫定耐药突变的患者推荐剂量为一日 1 次，每次 1.0mg，空腹服用。<br><br>Oral medication: give 0.5mgsingly, once a day. In lamivudine treatment, if the patients have Viremia or lamivudine-resistant mutation, the recommended dose is 1.0mg singly, once a day, on an empty stomach. |
| 剂型、规格<br>Preparations | 片剂：每片 0.5mg。<br>Tablets: 0.5mg per tablet. |
| **药品名称 Drug Names** | 替比夫定 Telbivudine |
| 适应证<br>Indications | 用于有病毒复制证据，血清转氨酶（ALT 或 AST）持续升高或肝组织学显示有活动性病变的慢性成人乙型肝炎的患者。<br>It is intended to treat adults' chronic hepatitis B, which has evidence for viral replication, persistently elevated serum transaminase (ALT or AST) or displayed pathological changes in liver histology. |
| 用法、用量<br>Dosage | 成人和青少年（≥16 岁）推荐剂量为 600mg，一日 1 次口服，餐前或餐后均可，不受进食影响。<br>Adults and adolescents ( ≥ 16 years): give the recommended dose of 600mg, once a day, orally, before or after meals; administration is not affected by meals. |
| 剂型、规格<br>Preparations | 片剂：每片 600mg。<br>Tablets: 600mg per tablet. |
| **药品名称 Drug Names** | 聚乙二醇干扰素 α -2a Peginterferon α -2a |
| 适应证<br>Indications | 用于肝硬化代偿期或无肝硬化的慢性乙型或丙型肝炎的治疗。<br>It is used in treatment of liver cirrhosis in decompensate stage and chronic hepatitis B or C without liver cirrhosis. |
| 用法、用量<br>Dosage | 皮下注射，推荐剂量为一次 180μg，每周 1 次，共用 48 周。发生中度和重度不良反应的患者，应调整剂量，初始剂量一般减至 135μg，有些病例需减至 90μg 或 45μg。随不良反应的减轻，逐渐增加或恢复至常规剂量。<br><br>Subcutaneous injection: give the recommended dose of 180μg singly, once a week, for 48 weeks. If patients have moderate and severe adverse reaction, make an adjustment on dosage. Usually, the staring dose is reduced to 135μg; in some cases, it may need to be reduced to 90μg or 45μg. With the reduction of adverse reactions, gradually increase the dose or return to regular dose. |

| 剂型、规格<br>Preparations | 注射液：每支 180μg（1ml）；135μg（1ml）。<br>Injection: 180μg (1ml), 135μg (1ml) per vial. |
|---|---|
| **药品名称 Drug Names** | 奈韦拉平 Nevirapine |
| 适应证<br>Indications | 常与其他药物联合应用于治疗Ⅰ型 HIV 感染。单独用本品则病毒可迅速产生耐药性。<br>It is often combined with other drugs to treat HIV infection Ⅰ. Using it alone may lead to rapid emergence of virus's drug resistance. |
| 用法、用量<br>Dosage | 成人：先导期剂量，每日 1 次 200mg，用药 14 日（以减少皮疹发生）；以后每日 2 次，2 次 200mg。儿童：2 个月至 8 岁，一日一次 4mg/kg，用药 14 日，以后一日 2 次，每次 7mg/kg；儿童：8 岁以上，一日一次 4mg/kg，用药 14 日，以后一日 2 次，每次 4mg/kg。所有患者的用量每日不超过 400mg。<br>Adults: in pilot stage, give 200mg singly, once a day, for 14 days (to reduce skin rash); afterwards 200mg singly, two times a day. Children: from two months to 8 years old, give 4mg/kg, once a day, for14 days and afterwards 7mg/kg, 2 times a day; over the age of 8, give 4mg/kg, once a day, for 14 days snd afterwards 2 4mg/kg times a day, once a day.Daily dosage of all patients can not exceed 400mg. |
| 剂型、规格<br>Preparations | 片剂（胶囊剂）：每片（粒）200mg。<br>Tablets (capsules): 200mg per tablet (capsule). |
| **药品名称 Drug Names** | 司他夫定 Stavudine |
| 适应证<br>Indications | 用于治疗Ⅰ型 HIV 感染。<br>It is intended to treat HIV infection Ⅰ. |
| 用法、用量<br>Dosage | 成人：体重 ≥ 60kg 者，口服一次 40mg，一日 2 次（相隔 12 小时）；体重 <60kg 者，口服一次 30mg，一日 2 次。儿童：体重 ≥ 30kg 者，按成人剂量；体重 <30kg 者，一次 1mg/kg，一日 2 次。肾功能低下者，需根据其肌酐清除率调整剂量。<br>Adults: ≥ 60kg, give orally 40mg singly, 2 times a day (every 12 hours); <60kg, give orally 30mg singly, 2 times a day. Children: ≥ 30kg, give adult dose; <under 30kg, give1mg/kg, 2 times a day. Renal insufficiency patients need dose adjustment according to creatinine clearance. |
| 剂型、规格<br>Preparations | 胶囊剂：每粒 20mg；30mg；40mg。<br>Capsules: 20mg, 30mg, 40mg per capsule. |
| **药品名称 Drug Names** | 利托那韦 Ritonavir |
| 适应证<br>Indications | 单独使用或与其他反转录酶抑制药联合用于治疗 HIV 感染。<br>It is used alone or with other reverse transcriptase inhibitors to treat HIV infection. |
| 用法、用量<br>Dosage | 口服：成人初始剂量一次 300mg，一日 2 次，之后每 2～3 日每次用量增加 100mg，直至达推荐剂量每次 600mg，一日 2 次。2 岁以上儿童初始剂量一次 250mg/m²，一日 2 次，之后每 2～3 日每次用量增加 50mg/m²，直至达推荐剂量每次 400mg/m²，一日 2 次。最大剂量不超过每次 600mg，一日 2 次。<br>Oral medication: give adults initial dose of 300mg singly, 2 times a day, afterwards increase 100mg singly every 2 to 3 days until it comes to recommended dose of 600mg singly, 2 times a day. Children over the age of 2: give the starting dose of 250mg/ m² singly, 2 times a day, afterwards increase by 50mg/ m² every 2 to 3 days, until it comes to the recommended dose of 400mg/ m²，2 times a day. Maximum dose can not exceed 600mg singly, 2 times a day. |
| 剂型、规格<br>Preparations | 软胶囊：每粒 100mg。<br>Soft Capsule: 100mg per capsule. |

| 药品名称 Drug Names | 膦甲酸钠 Foscarnet Sodium |
|---|---|
| 适应证<br>Indications | 　　主要用于免疫缺陷者（如艾滋病患者）发生的巨细胞病毒性视网膜炎的治疗。也可用于对阿昔洛韦耐药的免疫缺陷者（如 HIV 感染患者）的皮肤黏膜单纯疱疹病毒感染或带状疱疹病毒感染。<br>　　It is mainly used in treatment of cytomegalovirus retinitis by immunodeficiency (such as AIDS) patients. .It can also be used to treat acyclovir-resistant immunodeficiency patients (such as HIV-infected patients) mucocutaneous herpes simplex virus infection or herpes zoster virus infection. |
| 用法、用量<br>Dosage | 　　静脉滴注：初始剂量 60mg/kg，每 8 小时 1 次，至少需 1 小时恒速滴入，用 2 ～ 3 周；剂量、给药间隔、连续应用时间须根据患者的肾功能与用药耐受程度予以调整。维持量为每日 90 ～ 120mg/kg，静脉滴注 2 小时。<br>　　Intravenous infusion: give starting dose 60mg/kg, every 8 hours, by at least 1 hour of constant rate infusion, for 2 to 3 weeks; dose, interval and continuous administration time need appropriate adjustment according to patients' renal function and degree of drug tolerance. Maintenance dose is 90 ～ 120mg/kg a day, by 2-hour intravenous infusion. |
| 剂型、规格<br>Preparations | 　　注射液：每瓶 600mg（250ml）；1200mg（500ml）。<br>　　Injection: 600mg (250ml), 1200mg (500ml) per vial. |
| 药品名称 Drug Names | 去羟肌苷 Didanosine |
| 适应证<br>Indications | 　　用于Ⅰ型 HIV 感染，常与其他抗反转录酶药物联合应用（鸡尾酒疗法）。<br>　　It is intended to treat HIV infection Ⅰ , and often combined with other antiretroviral drugs (HAART). |
| 用法、用量<br>Dosage | 　　成人：体重≥60kg 者，一次 200mg，一日 2 次，或一日 400mg，一次顿服；体重 <60kg 者，一次 125mg，一日 2 次，或一日 250mg，一次顿服。儿童：120mg/m²，一日 2 次或一日 250mg，一次顿服。肾功能低下者应按肌酐清除率调整剂量。饭前 30 分钟服用，片剂应充分咀嚼或溶于 1 小杯水中、搅拌混匀后服用。<br>　　Adults: ≥ 60kg, give 200mg singly, 2 times a day or 400mg a day, at a draught; <60kg, give 125mg singly, 2 times a day or 250mg a day, at a draught. Children: give 120mg/ ㎡ , 2 times a day or 250mg a day, at a draught. Renal insufficiency patients need dose adjustment according to creatinine clearance. Taking medicine 30 minutes before meals; tablets should be fully chewed or dissolved in a glass of water and stirred for mixing. |
| 剂型、规格<br>Preparations | 　　片剂：50mg；100mg。<br>　　Tablets: 50mg, 100mg per tablet. |
| 药品名称 Drug Names | 茚地那韦 Indinavir |
| 适应证<br>Indications | 　　和其他抗反转录病毒药物联合使用，用于治疗成人及儿童 HIV-Ⅰ感染。<br>　　It is combined with other anti-retroviral drugs to treat HIV-Ⅰ infection of adults and children. |
| 用法、用量<br>Dosage | 　　推荐的开始剂量为 800mg，每 8 小时口服 1 次。与利福布汀联合治疗建议将利福布汀的剂量减半，而本药计量增加至每 8 小时 1g。与酮康唑合用，本药的剂量应减少至每 8 小时 600mg。肝功能不全患者，剂量应减至每 8 小时 600mg。3 岁以上（可口服胶囊的儿童）：本品的推荐剂量为每 8 小时口服 500mg/m²。儿童剂量不能超过成人剂量（即每 8 小时 800mg）。<br>　　It is recommended that the starting dose is 800mg, every eight hours, orally. If this drug is combined with rifabutin, it is recommended to halve the rifabutin dose and increase this drug's dose to 1g every 8 hours. If this drug is combined with ketoconazole, this drug's dose should be reduced to 600mg every 8 hours. Hepatic insufficiency patients: reduce the dose to every 600mg 8 hours. Children over the age of 3 (children who can take capsules): the recommended dose is 500mg/ ㎡ every 8 hours, orally. Children dose can not exceed adult dose ( 800mg every 8 hours). |
| 剂型、规格<br>Preparations | 　　胶囊剂：每粒 200mg。<br>　　Capsules: 200mg per capsule. |

**续　表**

| 药品名称 Drug Names | 金刚烷胺 Amantadine |
|---|---|
| 适应证<br>Indications | 用于亚洲 A-Ⅱ型流感染发热患者。常用于震颤麻痹。<br>It is use for febrile patients of Asian A-Ⅱ influenza infection. It is commonly used to treat Parkinsonism. |
| 用法、用量<br>Dosage | 流感 A 病毒感染：成人：一日 200mg，分 1～2 次服用；儿童：新生儿与 1 岁内婴儿不用；1～9 岁，一日 4.4～8.8mg/kg，1～2 次，每日最大剂量不超过 150mg，9～12 岁，100～200mg/d。<br>In treatment of Influenza A virus infection, Adults: give 200mg a day, in 1 to 2 divided doses; Children: newborns and infants within 1 year old do not use this drug; from 1 to 9 years old, give, 4.4～8.8mg/kg a day, 1～2 times a day, with maximum daily dose of 150mg; from 9 to 12 years old, give 100～200mg a day. |
| 剂型、规格<br>Preparations | 片（胶囊剂）：0.1g。<br>Tablets (capsules): 0.1g. |

## 7. 抗寄生虫病药 Antiparasitic drugs

### 7.1 抗疟药 Antimalarial drugs

| 药品名称 Drug Names | 氯喹 Chloroquine |
|---|---|
| 适应证<br>Indications | 主要用于治疗疟疾急性发作，控制疟疾症状，还可用于治疗肝阿米巴病、华支睾吸虫病、肺吸虫病、结缔组织病等。另可用于光敏性疾病，如日晒红斑症。<br>It is maily used in the treatment of acute attack of malaria, hepatic amebiasis, clonorchiasis, paragonimiasis and connective tissue disease, as well as in control malaria symptoms. It can also be used to treat photosensitivity diseases, such as sunburn erythema. |
| 用法、用量<br>Dosage | （1）控制疟疾发作：①口服：首剂 1g，6 小时后 0.5g，第 2、3 日各服 0.5g，如与伯氨喹合用，只需第 1 日服本品 1g。小儿首次 16mg/kg（高热者酌情减量，分次服），6～8 小时后及第 2～3 日各服 8mg/kg。②静脉滴注：恶性疟第 1 日 1.5g，第 2、3 日 0.5g。一般每 0.5～0.75g 氯喹用 5% 葡萄糖注射液或 0.9% 氯化钠注射液 500ml 稀释，静脉滴注速度为每分钟 12～20 滴，第 1 日量与 12 小时内全部输完。<br><br>（2）疟疾症状抑制性预防：每周服 1 次，每次 0.5g，小儿每周 8mg/kg。<br><br>（3）抗阿米巴肝脓肿：每 1、2 日一日 2～3 次，每次服 0.5g，以后一日 0.5g，连用 2～3 周。<br><br>（4）治疗结缔组织病：对盘状红斑狼疮及类风湿关节炎，开始剂量一日 1～2 次，每次 0.25g，经 2～3 周后，如症状得到控制，改为一日 2～3 次，每次量不宜超过 0.25g，长期维持。对系统性红斑狼疮，用皮质激素治疗症状缓解后，可加用氯喹以减少皮质激素用量。<br><br>(1) Malaria attack control: ① Oral medication: give first dose of 1g, 0.5g after 6 hours and 0.5g on the second and the third day; if combined with primaquine, only give1g of this drug on the first day; for children, give first dose of 16mg/kg (appropriate reduction for febrile children, in several divided doses), then 8mg/kg after 6 to 8 hours, on the second day and on the third day respectively. ② intravenous infusion: for falciparum malaria, give1.5g on the first day, and 0.5g on the second and the third day; generally, dilute every 0.5～0.75g of chloroquine with500ml of 5% dextrose injection or 0.9% sodium chloride injection, the infusion rate is 12 to 20 drip per minute, and the first day dose should finish within 12 hours.<br><br>(2) Inhibitory prevention of malaria symptoms: give 0.5g singly, once a week; give 8mg/kg a week for children.<br><br>(3) Anti-amebic hepatic abscess: give 0.5g singly, 2~3times a day, on the first and the second day, afterwards give 0.5g everyday, for 2 to 3 weeks.<br><br>(4) Connective tissue diseases: for discoid lupus erythematosus and rheumatoid arthritis, give the starting dose of 0.25g singly, 1 to 2 times a day, and 2 to 3 weeks later, as the symptoms are under control, give 2～3 times a day and single dose should not exceed 0.25g, for long-term maintenance; for systemic lupus erythematosus, start to give chloroquine for corticosteroids dose reduction after symptom remission showed in corticosteroids therapy . |
| 剂型、规格<br>Preparations | 片剂：每片含磷酸氯喹 0.075g；0.25g。<br>注射液：每支 129mg（盐基 80mg）（2ml）；250mg（盐基 155mg）（2ml）。<br>Tablets: 0.075g, 0.25g of chloroquine phosphate contained per tablet.<br>Injection: 129mg (base 80mg) (2ml), 250mg (base 155mg) (2ml) per vial. |

续 表

| 药品名称 Drug Names | 羟氯喹 Hydroxychloroquine |
|---|---|
| 适应证<br>Indications | 本品主要用于疟疾的预防和治疗，也用于类风湿关节炎和青少年类风湿关节炎，以及盘状红斑狼疮和系统性红斑狼疮的治疗。<br><br>It is mainly used in the prevention and treatment of malaria. It is also intended to treat rheumatoid arthritis and juvenile rheumatoid arthritis, as well as discoid lupus erythematosus and systemic lupus erythematosus. |
| 用法、用量<br>Dosage | 治疗急性疟疾：成人口服，首次 800mg，以后每 6 ~ 8 小时 400mg，然后每 2 日 400mg；儿童首剂量 10mg/kg，6 小时后第 2 次服药 5mg/kg，第 2、3 日，一日 1 次 5mg/kg。预防疟疾：在进入疟疾流行区前一周，服 400mg，以后每周 1 次 400mg；儿童 5mg/kg。治疗类风湿关节炎和红斑狼疮：成人开始每日 400mg，分次服，维持量一日 200 ~ 400mg，每日剂量不超过 6.5mg/kg。青少年患者治疗 6 个月无效即应停药。<br><br>Acute malaria: give adult first dose 800mg, afterwards 400mg 6 to 8 hours, then 400mg every two days; give children first dose of 10mg/kg and 5mg/kg 6 hours later, then give 5mg/kg on the second and the third day, once a day. Malaria prevention: in one week before entering malaria endemic areas, give 400mg, afterwards 400mg a week, once only; give children 5mg/kg. Rheumatoid arthritis and lupus erythematosus: in the beginning, give adults 400mg a day, in several divided doses; the maintenance dose is 200 ~ 400mg and daily dosage should not exceed 6.5mg/kg; if adolescent patients' treatment is effective for 6 months, stop the drug medication. |
| 剂型、规格<br>Preparations | 片剂：每片 100mg；200mg。<br>Tablets: 100mg; 200mg per tablet. |
| 药品名称 Drug Names | 青蒿素 Artemisinin |
| 适应证<br>Indications | 用于间日疟，恶性疟特别是抢救脑型疟有良效，其退热时间及疟原虫转阴时间都较氯喹短，对氯喹有耐药性的疟原虫，使用本品有效。<br><br>It is intended to treat vivax malaria and falciparum malaria. Especially, it has a good effect in rescuing cerebral malaria, during whose fever clearance time and plasmodium negative time is shorter than chloroquine, so the drug is effective at chloroquine-resistant plasmodium. |
| 用法、用量<br>Dosage | （1）口服：先服 1g，6 ~ 8 小时后再服 0.5g，第 2、3 日各服 0.5g，疗程为 3 日，总量为 2.5g。小儿总剂量 15mg/kg，按上述方法 3 日内服完。<br>（2）直肠给药：先服 0.6g，6 小时后再服 0.6g，第 2、3 日各服 0.4g。<br>（3）深部肌内注射：第 1 次 200mg，6 ~ 8 小时后再给 100mg，第 2、3 日各肌内注射 100mg，总剂量 500mg（个别重症第 4 日再给 100mg）。或连用 3 日，每日肌内注射 300mg，总量 900mg。小儿 15mg/kg，按上述方法 3 日内注完。<br><br>(1) Oral medication: give first dose of 1g and another 0.5g 6 ~ 8 hours later, then give0.5g on the second and the third day, with treatment course of 3 days and total dose of 2.5g; children's' total dose is 15mg/kg, the 3- day administration method is the same with above.<br>(2) Rectal administration: give first dose of 0.6g and another 0.6g 6 hours later, then give 0.4g on the second and the third day.<br>(3) Deep intramuscular injection: give the first dose of 200mg and 100mg 6 ~ 8 hours later, and give100mg on the second and the third day, with total dose of 500mg (give 100mg on the fourth day in severe case); or give300mg a day, for continuous 3 days, with total dose of 900mg; give 15mg/kg, the 3-day administration method is the same with the above. |
| 剂型、规格<br>Preparations | 油注射液：每支 50mg（2ml）；100mg（2ml）；200mg（2ml）；300mg（2ml）。<br>水混悬注射液：每支 300mg（2ml）。<br>片剂：每片 50mg；100mg。<br>栓剂：每粒 400mg；600mg。<br>Oil Injection: 50mg (2ml), 100mg (2ml), 200mg (2ml), 300mg (2ml) per bottle.<br>Water suspension injection: 300mg (2ml) per bottle.<br>Tablets: 50mg, 100mg per tablet.<br>Suppositories: 400mg, 600mg of each. |

**续　表**

| 药品名称 Drug Names | 青蒿素哌喹 Artemisinin and Piperaquine |
| --- | --- |
| 适应证<br>Indications | 用于恶性疟和间日疟。<br>It is intended to treat falciparum malaria and vivax malaria. |
| 用法、用量<br>Dosage | 口服，成人总剂量 8 片，每日早晚各一次，每次 2 片。<br>Oral medication: give adults 2 tablets singly, twice (in the morning and evening), with total dose of 8 tablets. |
| 剂型、规格<br>Preparations | 复方制剂，每片含青蒿素 6.25mg，哌喹 375mg。<br>Compound preparation: 6.25mg of artemisinin and 375mg of piperaquine contained per tablet. |
| 药品名称 Drug Names | 双氢青蒿素 Dihydroartemisinin |
| 适应证<br>Indications | 用于治疗各类疟疾，尤其适用于抗氯喹和哌喹的恶性疟和凶险型脑型疟疾的救治。<br>It is used in the treatment of various types of malaria, especially chloroquine-resistant and piperaquine resistant falciparum malaria and pernicious cerebral malaria. |
| 用法、用量<br>Dosage | 口服，一日 1 次，成人一日 60mg，首剂加倍；儿童按年龄递减；连用 5 ~ 7 日。<br>Oral medication: give adults 60mg a day, once a day and double the first dose; for children, reduce the dose by age, with continuous medication of 5 to 7 days. |
| 剂型、规格<br>Preparations | 片剂：每片 20mg。<br>复方制剂：每片含双氢青蒿素 40mg，磷酸氯喹 320mg。<br>Tablets: 20mg per tablet.<br>Compound Preparation: 40mg of Dihydroartemisinin and 320mg of chloroquine phosphate contained per tablet. |
| 药品名称 Drug Names | 双氢青蒿素磷酸哌喹 Dihydroartemisinin and Piperaquine Phosphate |
| 适应证<br>Indications | 用于恶性疟和间日疟。<br>It is intended to treat falciparum malaria and vivax malaria. |
| 用法、用量<br>Dosage | 口服，成人总剂量 8 片，每日早、晚各一次，每次 2 片。年龄 ≥16 岁者，首剂 2 片，第 6 ~ 8 小时服 2 片，第 24 小时服用 2 片，第 32 小时服用 2 片。年龄 11 ~ 15 岁者，首剂 1.5 片，第 6 ~ 8 小时服 1.5 片，第 24 小时服用 1.5 片，第 32 小时服用 1.5 片。年龄 7 ~ 10 岁者，首剂 1 片，第 6 ~ 8 小时服 1 片，第 24 小时服用 1 片，第 32 小时服用 1 片。<br>Oral medication: give adults 2 tablets singly, twice a day (in the morning and evening), with total dose of 8 tablets: for patients ≥ 16 years old, give first dose of 2 tablets and another 2 tablets on the sixth to eighth hour, then another 2 tablets singly on the twenty-fourth hour and the thirty-second hour; patients aging 11 to 15 years old, give the first dose of 1.5 tablets and another 1.5 tablets singly on the sixth hour, the eighth hour, the twenty-fourth hour and the thirty-second hour; patients aging 7 to 10 years old, give the first dose of 1 tablet and another 1 tablet on the sixth to eighth hour, then give 1 tablet singly on the twenty-fourth hour and the thirty-second hour . |
| 剂型、规格<br>Preparations | 复方制剂：每片含双氢青蒿素 40mg，磷酸哌喹 320mg。<br>Compound Preparation: 40mg of dihydroartemisinin and 320mg of piperaquine phosphate contained per tablet. |
| 药品名称 Drug Names | 蒿甲醚 Artemether |
| 适应证<br>Indications | 本品对恶性疟（包括抗氯喹恶性疟及凶险型疟）的疗效较佳，效果确切，显效迅速，近期疗效可达 100%。用药后 2 日内，多数病例血中原虫转阴并退热。复燃率 8%。较青蒿素低。与伯氨喹合用可进一步降低复燃率。<br>临床还适用于急性上呼吸道感染的高热患者，进行对症处理，取得较好疗效。退热效应一般在肌内注射后半小时即开始出现，体温呈梯形逐渐下降，4 ~ 6 小时再逐渐回升，无体温骤降的现象，退热作用稳定。本品肌内注射后，患者出汗少，不至引起老年人、儿童、虚弱患者发生虚脱等不良反应。<br>It is intended to treat falciparum malaria (including chloroquine-resistant falciparum malaria and pernicious malaria), with better, definite and quick effect; and the short-term efficacy can be 100%. 2 days after the medicaiotn, the blood plasmodium turns to negative and fever is done in most of the cases. The recrudescence rate is 8%, lower than artemisinin. It can further reduce the recrudescence rate when the drug is combined with primaquine. |

|  | It is clinically used for febrile patients with acute respiratory infection, and symptomatic treatment can achieve better results. Antipyretic effects usually shows half an hour after intramuscular injection: body temperature would have a gradually trapezoid drop, about 3 to 5 hours later it gradually rises; if there is no abrupt drop of body temperature, the effect is stable. After intramuscular injection of this drug, patients would sweat less, but it would not to cause prostration and other adverse reaction of the elderly, children and weak patients. |
|---|---|
| 用法、用量<br>Dosage | 抗疟：肌内注射，第 1 日 160mg，第 2～5 日各 80mg。小儿首剂量按 3.2mg/kg 计，以后按 1.6mg/kg 计。口服，首剂 160mg，第 2 日起每日一次，一次 80mg，连服 5～7 日。退热：肌内注射 160mg。<br><br>Anti-malaria: by intramuscular injection, give 160mg on the first day, then give 80mg singly on the second to the fifth day; for children, give first dose of 3.2mg/kg, then give 1.6mg/kg; by Oral medicaiton, give the first dose of 160mg and from the second day on, give 80mg singly, once a day, for continuous 5 to 7 days. Fever: by intramuscular injection, give 160mg. |
| 剂型、规格<br>Preparations | 油注射液：每支 80mg（1ml）。<br>胶囊：每胶囊 40mg。<br>片剂：每片 40mg。<br>复方制剂：每片含蒿甲醚 0.02g，本芴醇 0.12g。<br><br>Oil Injection: 80mg (1ml) per vial.<br>Capsules: 40mg per capsule.<br>Tablets: 40mg per tablet.<br>Compound Preparation: 0.02g of artemether and 0.12g of.lumefantrine contained per tablet. |
| 药品名称 Drug Names | 奎宁 Quinine |
| 适应证<br>Indications | 抑制或杀灭良性疟（间日疟、三日疟）及恶性疟原虫的红内期，能控制疟疾症状，有解热、收缩子宫的作用。<br><br>It is used to inhibit or kill benign malaria (vivax malaria and three-day malaria), as well as erythrocytic stage of falciparum malaria. It can control malaria symptoms, with antipyretic and uterine contraction effect. |
| 用法、用量<br>Dosage | 成人常用量：严重病例（如脑型）可采用二盐酸奎宁按体重 5～10mg/kg（最高量 500mg），加入氯化钠注射液 500ml 中静脉滴注，4 小时滴完，12 小时后重复一次，病情好转后改为口服。<br><br>Adults: for severe case (such as cerebral malaria), give quinine dihydrochloride 5～10mg/kg (maximum dose of 500mg), add it in 500ml of sodium chloride for 4-hour intravenous injection, ; then give the same dose after 12 hours; after the condition improved, change to oral medication. |
| 剂型、规格<br>Preparations | 硫酸奎宁片：0.3g。<br>盐酸奎宁片：0.33g；0.12g。<br>二盐酸奎宁注射液：0.25g（1ml）；0.5g（1ml）；0.25g（10ml）。<br>复方奎宁注射液：每支 2ml，含盐酸奎宁 0.136g，咖啡因 0.034g，乌拉坦 0.028g。<br><br>Quinine sulfate tablets: 0.3g.<br>Quinine hydrochloride tablets: 0.33g, 0.12g.<br>Quinine dihydrochloride injection: 0.25g (1ml), 0.5g (1ml), 0.25g (10ml).<br>Compound Quinine Injection: 2ml per bottle: 0.136g of quinine hydrochloride, 0.034g of caffeine and 0.028g of urethane contained. |
| 药品名称 Drug Names | 伯氨喹 Primaquine |
| 适应证<br>Indications | 主要用于根治间日疟和控制疟疾传播，常与氯喹或乙胺嘧啶合用，对红内期作用较弱，对恶性疟红内期则完全无效，不能作为控制症状的药物应用。对某些疟原虫的红前期也有影响，但因需用剂量较大，已接近极量，不够安全，故也不能作为病因预防药应用。<br><br>It is mainly used to cure vivax malaria and control the spread of malaria, and often used in combination with chloroquine or pyrimethamine. It has weak effect for erythrocytic stage and completely no effect for erythrocytic stage of falciparum malaria, so it can not be used in symptoms control. It may has effect for some plasmodium's early erythrocytic stage but the required dose is large, very close to the maximum dose, so it is not safe and can not be used in causal prophylaxis. |

续　表

| | |
|---|---|
| 用法、用量<br>Dosage | 　　成人常用量：口服，①根治间日疟：采用一次 13.2mg，一日 3 次，连服 7 日。②用于消灭恶性疟原虫配子体时采用一日 26.4mg，连服 3 日。<br>　　Usual dose for adults: by oral medicaiton, ① vivax malaria cure: give 13.2mg singly, 3 times a day, for 7 days; ② elimination of plasmodium falciparum gametocyte, give 26.4mg a day, for continuous 3 days. |
| 剂型、规格<br>Preparations | 　　片剂：每片含磷酸伯氨喹 13.2mg 或 26.4mg（相当于伯氨喹盐基 7.5mg 或 15mg）。<br>　　Tablets: 13.2mg or 26.4mg of primaquine phosphate contained per tablet (equivalent to 7.5mg or 15mg of primaquine base). |
| 药品名称 Drug Names | 乙胺嘧啶 Pyrimethamine |
| 适应证<br>Indications | 　　主要用于预防疟疾，也可用于治疗弓形虫病。最近发现本品有耐药性虫株产生，合并应用其他抗疟药及磺胺类药物等，可提高其抗疟效果。<br>　　It is mainly used in the prevention of malaria, as well as in the treatment of toxoplasmosis. Recently, it is discovered that it has drug-resistant gondii strains. Combined with other antimalarial drugs, such as sulfa drugs, can improve the antimalarial effect. |
| 用法、用量<br>Dosage | 　　(1) 预防疟疾：成人每次服 25mg，每周 1 次，小儿 0.9mg/kg，最高限于成人剂量。<br>　　(1) 抗复发治疗：成人每日服 25 ~ 50mg，连用 2 日，小儿酌减（多与伯氨喹合用）。<br>　　(3) 治疗弓形虫病：每日 50mg 顿服，共 1 ~ 3 日（视耐受力而定），以后每日 25mg，疗程为 4 ~ 6 周。小儿 1mg/kg，分 2 次服，1 ~ 3 日后 0.5mg/kg，分 2 次服，疗程为 4 ~ 6 周。必要时，可重复 1 ~ 2 个疗程。<br>　　(1) Malaria prevention: give adults orally 25mg singly, 1 times a week; give children orally 0.9mg/kg, and the maximum dose can not exceed adult dose.<br>　　(2) anti-retroviral therapy: give adults orally 25 ~ 50mg a day, for continuous 2 days; children dose need appropriate reduction (often combined with primaquine).<br>　　(3) Toxoplasmosis: give orally 50mg a day, at a draught, for 1 to 3 days (depending on the tolerance), afterwards 25mg a day, with treatment course of 4 to 6 weeks; give children 1mg/kg, in 2 divided doses, then 1 to 3 days later, give 0.5mg/kg, in 2 divided doses, with treatment course of 4 to 6 weeks. If necessary, repeat 1 to 2 courses. |
| 剂型、规格<br>Preparations | 　　片剂：每片 6.25mg。<br>　　膜剂：每格 6.25mg。<br>　　Tablets: 6.25mg per tablet.<br>　　Film formers: 6.25mg of each. |

## 7.2 抗阿米巴病药 AntiAmebicide drugs

| | |
|---|---|
| 药品名称 Drug Names | 双碘喹啉 Diiodohydroxyquinoline |
| 适应证<br>Indications | 　　用于治疗轻型或无明显症状的阿米巴痢疾。与依米丁、甲硝唑合用，治疗急性阿米巴痢疾及较顽固病例。对肠外阿米巴如肝脓肿无效。<br>　　It is used in treatment of mild amoebic dysentery amoebic dysentery without obvious symptoms. It is combined with emetine and metronidazole to treat acute amoebic dysentery and stubborn cases. It is ineffective at parenteral amebiasis, such as hepatic abscess. |
| 用法、用量<br>Dosage | 　　成人常规剂量：口服给药，一次 400 ~ 600mg，一日 3 次，连服 14 ~ 21 日，儿童常规剂量：口服给药，一次 5 ~ 10mg/kg，用法同成人，重复治疗需间隔 15 ~ 20 日。<br>　　Adult regular dose: by oral medication, give 400 ~ 600mg singly, 3 times a day, for14 to 21 days; Children regular dose: by oral medication, give 5 ~ 10mg/kg a day, 3 times a day, for14 to 21 days;, repeated treatment needs an interval of 15 to 20 days. |
| 剂型、规格<br>Preparations | 　　双碘喹啉片：每片 200mg。<br>　　Iodoquinol tablets: 200mg per tablet. |
| 药品名称 Drug Names | 依米丁 Emetine |
| 适应证<br>Indications | 　　适用于急性阿米巴痢疾急需控制症状者，肠外阿米巴病因其毒性大，已少用，由于消除急性症状效率较好，而根治作用低，故不适用于症状轻微的慢性阿米巴痢及无症状的带包囊者。此外，本品还可用于蝎子蜇伤。<br>　　It is used for acute amoebic dysentery patiens who urgently need symptoms control. It is seldom used in intestinal dysentery treatment because of its toxicity. Since its better effect in elimination of acute symptoms but lower effect for radical cure, it is not used for patients with mild symptoms of chronic amoebic dysentery and asymptomatic cysts. In addition, it also can be used to treat scorpion stings. |

续 表

| 用法、用量<br>Dosage | （1）治阿米巴痢：体重 60kg 以下按每日 1mg/kg 计（60kg 以上者，剂量仍按 60kg 计），一日 1 次或分 2 次做深部皮下注射，连用 6 ～ 10 日为 1 个疗程，如未愈，30 日后再用第二疗程。<br>（2）治蝎子蜇伤：以本品 3% ～ 6% 注射液少许注入蜇孔内即可。<br>（1）Amoebic dysentery: patients with body weight under 60kg, give 1mg/kg a day (above 60kg, give total dose of 60kg), in 1 or 2 divided doses, by deep subcutaneous injection, for a treatment course of continuously 6 to 10 days; if not healed, give use the second course after 30 days.<br>（2）Scorpion stings: give 3% to 6% of the injection, by a small injection into the sting. |
|---|---|
| 剂型、规格<br>Preparations | 注射液：每支 30mg（1ml）；60mg（1ml）。<br>Injection: 30mg (1ml), 60mg (1ml) per vial. |

## 7.3 抗滴虫病药 Antitrichomonal drug

| 药品名称 Drug Names | 甲硝唑 Metronidazole |
|---|---|
| 适应证<br>Indications | 用于治疗厌氧杆菌引起的产后盆腔炎、败血症、牙周炎等。还可用于治疗贾第鞭毛虫病、酒糟鼻。用于阑尾、结肠手术、妇产科手术，可降低或避免手术感染。也可用于治疗阿米巴痢和阿米巴肝脓肿，疗效与依米丁相仿。<br><br>It is used in the treatment of postpartum pelvic inflammation, septicemia and periodontitis caused by anaerobic bacilli. It can also be used to treat giardiasis and rosacea. It can reduce or avoid surgical infection when used in appendix and colon surgery, as well as gynecologic surgery . Besides, it can be used to treat amoebic dysentery and amoebic hepatic abscess, with similar effect with emetine. |
| 用法、用量<br>Dosage | （1）治滴虫病：成人一日 3 次，每次服 200mg，另每晚以 200mg 栓剂放入阴道内，连用 7 ～ 10 日，为保证疗效，需男女同治。<br>（2）治阿米巴病：成人一日 3 次，每次 400 ～ 800mg（大剂量宜慎用），5 ～ 7 日为 1 个疗程。<br>（3）治贾第鞭毛虫病：常用量每次 400mg，一日 3 次口服，疗程 5 ～ 7 日。<br>（4）治疗由厌氧菌引起的产后盆腔感染、败血症、骨髓炎等：一般口服 200 ～ 400mg，一日 600 ～ 1200mg，也可静脉滴注。<br>（5）治酒糟鼻：口服 200mg，一日 2 ～ 3 次，配合 2% 甲硝唑霜外搽，一日 3 次，1 个疗程为 3 周。<br><br>(1) Trichomoniasis: for adults, give 200mg singly, 3 times a day and another 200mg of suppository into vagina at night, for continuous 7 to 10 days; in order to ensure efficacy, men and women both need treatment.<br>(2) Amebiasis: give adults 400 ~ 800mg singly (megadose should be used with caution), 3 times a day, with a treatment course of 5 to 7 days.<br>(3) Giardiasis: give usual dose of 400mg singly, 3 times a day, orally, with treatment course for 5 to 7 days.<br>(4) Postpartum pelvic infections, septicemia, osteomyelitis, and etc caused by anaerobic bacteria: generally, give 200 ~ 400mg, 600 ~ 1200mg a day, by oral medication or intravenous infusion.<br>(5) Rosacea: give orally 200mg singly, 2 or 3 times a day, with 2% metronidazole cream for external use, 3 times a day; a course of treatment is three weeks. |
| 剂型、规格<br>Preparations | 片剂：每片 200mg。<br>阴道泡腾片：每片 200mg。<br>栓剂：每个 0.5g；1g。<br>注射液：50mg（10ml）；100mg（20ml）；500mg（100ml）；1.25g（250mg）；500mg（250ml）。<br>甲硝唑葡萄糖注射液：甲硝唑 0.5g+ 葡萄糖 12.5g（250ml）。<br><br>Tablets: 200mg per tablet.<br>Vaginal Effervescent Tablets: 200mg per tablet.<br>Suppositories: 0.5g, 1g of each.<br>Injection: 50mg (10ml), 100mg (20ml), 500mg (100ml), 1.25g (250mg), 500mg (250ml) Metronidazole glucose injection: 0.5g of metronidazole and 12.5g of glucose (250ml). |

**续　表**

### 7.4 抗血吸虫病药 Anti-Schistosmomicide drug

| 药品名称 Drug Names | 吡喹酮 Praziquantel |
|---|---|
| 适应证<br>Indications | 　　主要用于治疗血吸虫病。其特点为：剂量小（约为现用一般药物剂量的 1/10）、疗程短（从现用药物的 20 日或 10 日缩短为 1 ～ 2 日）、不良反应轻、由较高的近期疗效。血吸虫病患者经本品治疗后，半年粪检虫卵转阴率为 97.7% ～ 99.4%，由于本品对毛蚴、尾蚴也有杀灭效力，故也用于预防血吸虫感染。也有以本品治疗脑囊虫病。<br><br>　　It is used in treatment of schistosomiasis, with features of small dose (about1/10 of general drug doses), short course (shortened from 10 days or 20 days of currently used drug to 1 ~ 2 days), mild adverse reaction and better short-term curative effect. After receiving treatment, the egg negative rate would be 97.7% to 99.4% in stool exam of schistosomiasis patients in six months. Since this drug has elimination effect for miracidia and cercariae, it is also used in schistosomiasis infection prevention. Besides, it is also used in treatment of neurocysticercosis. |
| 用法、用量<br>Dosage | 　　口服治疗血吸虫病：一次 10mg/kg，一日 3 次，急性血吸虫病连服 4 日，慢性血吸虫病连服 2 日。皮肤涂搽 1% 浓度吡喹酮，12 小时内对血吸虫尾蚴有可靠的防护作用。治脑囊虫病，一日 20mg/kg，体重 >60kg 者，以 60kg 计量，分 3 次服，9 日为 1 个疗程，总量 180mg/kg，疗程间隔 3 ～ 4 个月。<br><br>　　Schistosomiasis: by oral medication, give10mg/kg a day, 3 times a day, continuing 4 days for acute schistosomiasis and 2 days for chronic schistosomiasis; smear1% praziquantel over skin, which has reliable protection to Schistosome cercariae within 12 hours. Neurocysticercosis: give 20mg/kg a day; body weight> 60kg, give the dose of 60kg, in 3 divided doses, with a treatment course of 9 days; the total dose is 180mg/kg and treatment interval is 3 to 4 months. |
| 剂型、规格<br>Preparations | 　　胶囊剂：每粒 25mg；50mg。<br>　　片剂：每片 25mg。<br>　　Capsules: 25mg; 50mg per capsule.<br>　　Tablets: 25mg per tablet. |

### 7.5 抗其他吸虫病药 Anti other fluke drug

| 药品名称 Drug Names | 硫氯酚 Bithionol |
|---|---|
| 适应证<br>Indications | 　　对肺吸虫囊蚴有明显杀灭作用，临床用于肺吸虫病、牛肉绦虫病、姜片虫病。<br>　　It has significant elimination effect to paragonimus metacercariae. It is clinically used to treat Paragonimiasis, beef tapeworm, and fasciolopsiasis. |
| 用法、用量<br>Dosage | 　　口服：每日 50 ～ 60mg/kg（成人与小儿同）。对肺吸虫病及华支睾吸虫病可将全日量分 3 次服，隔日服药，疗程总量 30 ～ 45g，对姜片虫病，可于睡前半空腹将 2 ～ 3g 药物 1 次服完；对牛肉绦虫病，可将总量（50mg/kg）分 2 次服，间隔半小时，服完第二次药后，3 ～ 4 小时服泻药。<br><br>　　Oral medicaiton: give 50 ~ 60mg/kg a day (adult and children are the same);.in paragonimiasis and clonorchiasis treatment, give the daily dose in 3 divided doses, every other day, with the total dose of 30 ~ 45g for a treatment course; in fasciolopsiasis treatment, give 2 ~ 3g, in 1 dose, on semi-empty stomach before sleep ; in beef tapeworm treatment, give total (50mg/kg) dose in 2 divided doses, with interval of half an hour, then give laxative 3 to 4 hours after the second dose. |
| 剂型、规格<br>Preparations | 　　片剂：每片 0.25g。<br>　　胶囊剂：每粒 0.5g。<br>　　Tablets: 0.25g per tablet.<br>　　Capsules: 0.5g per capsule. |

### 7.6 抗丝虫病药 Antifilarial drug

| 药品名称 Drug Names | 乙胺嗪 Diethylcarbamazine |
|---|---|
| 适应证<br>Indications | 　　用于马来丝虫病和斑氏丝虫病的治疗。<br>　　It is used in the treatment of malay filariasis and bancroft filariasis. |

续 表

| 用法、用量<br>Dosage | （1）口服：1 次 0.1 ~ 0.2g，一日 0.3 ~ 0.6g，分 2 ~ 3 次服用，7 ~ 14 日为 1 个疗程。<br>（2）大剂量短程疗法：治马来丝虫病可用本品 1.5g，一次顿服，或与一日内分 2 次服；治斑氏丝虫病总量 3g，于 2 ~ 3 日分服完，本方法不良反应较重。<br>（3）预防：于流行区按每日 5 ~ 6mg/kg 服药，服 6 ~ 7 日，或按上量每周或每月服一日，直至总量达 70 ~ 90mg/kg 为止。<br><br>(1) Oral medication: give 0.1 ~ 0.2g singly, 0.3 ~ 0.6g a day, in 2 to 3 times divided doses, with a treatment course of 7 to 14 days.<br>(2) Short-term therapy with large dose: in malay filariasis treatment, give 1.5g, at a draught or in 2 divided doses in a day ; in treating bancroft filariasis treatment, give total dose of 3g, within 2 to 3 days; this method have severe adverse reaction.<br>(3) Prevention: in endemic areas, give by 5 ~ 6mg/kg a day, for 6 to 7 days or give the above dose once a week or month, until the total dose comes to 70 ~ 90mg/kg. |
| --- | --- |
| 剂型、规格<br>Preparations | 片剂：每片 50mg；100mg。<br>Tablets: 50mg; 100mg per tablet. |

## 7.7 抗利什曼原虫药 Anti-Leishmanial drug

| 药品名称 Drug Names | 葡萄糖酸锑钠 Sodium Stibogluconate |
| --- | --- |
| 适应证<br>Indications | 用于黑热病病因治疗，近期疗效可达 99%，2 年复发率低于 10%，复发病例可再用本品治疗。<br>It is used in treatment of kala-azar, with 99% of short-term effect rate and less than 10% of 2-year recurrence rate. In recurrence case, it still can be used in treatment. |
| 用法、用量<br>Dosage | 肌内或静脉注射。<br>（1）一般成人 1 次 1.9g（6ml），一日 1 次，连用 6 ~ 10 日；或总剂量按体重 90 ~ 130mg/kg（以 50kg 为限），等分 6 ~ 10 次，一日 1 次。<br>（2）小儿总剂量按体重 150 ~ 200mg/kg，分为 6 次，一日 1 次。<br>（3）对敏感性较差的虫株感染者，可重复 1 ~ 2 个疗程，间隔 10 ~ 14 日。<br>（4）对全身情况较差者，可每周注射 2 次，疗程 3 周或更长。<br>（5）对近期曾接受锑剂治疗者，可减少剂量。<br><br>This drug is administered by intramuscular or intravenous injection.<br>(1) Generally, give adults 1.9g (6ml) singly, once a day, for 6 to 10 days; or give total dose of 90 ~ 130mg/kg ( 50kg as limit ), in 6 to 10 divided doses, once a day.<br>(2) For children, give total dose of 150 ~ 200mg/kg, in 6 divided doses, once a day.<br>(3) For patients infected by less sensitive insect strains, give repeated 1 to 2 treatment course, with interval of 10 to 14 days.<br>(4) For patients with poor condition, give injection twice a week, for three weeks or longer.<br>(5) If the patients recently received antimony preparations therapy, reduce the dose. |
| 剂型、规格<br>Preparations | 注射液：每支 6ml，含葡萄糖酸锑钠 1.9g，约相当于五价锑 0.6g。<br>Injection: 6ml per vial, 1.9g of sodium stibogluconate contained, equivalent to about 0.6g of pentavalent antimony. |

## 7.8 驱肠虫药 Intestinal anthelmintics

| 药品名称 Drug Names | 哌嗪 Piperazine |
| --- | --- |
| 适应证<br>Indications | 用于肠蛔虫病、蛔虫所致的不全性肠梗阻和胆道蛔虫病较痛的缓解期。此外亦可用于驱蛲虫。<br>It is used in treatment of intestinal ascariasis and incomplete intestinal obstruction caused by ascaris, as well as in the painful remission stage of biliary aascariasis. Besides, it can also be used to expelling pinworms. |
| 用法、用量<br>Dosage | （1）枸橼酸哌嗪：驱蛔虫，成人 3 ~ 3.5g，睡前一次服，连服 2 日，小儿每日 100 ~ 160mg/kg，一日量不得超过 3g，连服 2 日，一般不必服泻药；驱蛲虫，成人每次 1 ~ 1.2g，一日 2 ~ 2.5g，连服 7 ~ 10 日，小儿一日 60mg/kg，分 2 次服，每日总量不超过 2g，连服 7 ~ 10 日。<br>（2）磷酸哌嗪：驱蛔虫，一日 2.5 ~ 3g，睡前 1 次服，连服 2 日，小儿每日 80 ~ 130mg/kg，一日量不得超过 2.5g，连服 2 日；驱蛲虫，每次 0.8 ~ 1g，一日 1.5 ~ 2g，连服 7 ~ 10 日，小儿一日 50mg/kg，分 2 次服，一日总量不超过 2g，连服 7 ~ 10 日。 |

**续　表**

|  | (1) Piperazine citrate: for expelling ascarid, give adults $3 \sim 3.5g$ a day, once before bed, for 2 days; give children $100 \sim 160mg/kg$ a day, with daily maximum dose of 3g, for two days, generally without giving laxatives; for expelling pinworms, give adults $1 \sim 1.2g$ singly, $2 \sim 2.5g$ a day, for 7 to 10 days; give children 60mg/kg a day, in 2 divided doses, with daily maximum does of 2g, for 7 to 10 days.<br><br>(2) Piperazine phosphate: for expelling ascarid, give $2.5 \sim 3g$ a day, once before bedtime, for 2 days; give children $80 \sim 130mg/kg$ a day, with daily maximum dose of 2.5g, for 2 days; for expelling pinworms, give $0.8 \sim 1g$ singly, $1.5 \sim 2g$ a day, for 7 to 10 days; give children 50mg/kg a day, in 2 divided doses, with daily maximum does of 2g, for 7 to 10 days. |
|---|---|
| 剂型、规格<br>Preparations | 枸橼酸哌嗪片：每片 0.25g；0.5g。<br>枸橼酸哌嗪糖浆：每 100ml 含本品 16g。<br>磷酸哌嗪片：每片 0.2g；0.5g。<br><br>Piperazine citrate tablets: 0.25g, 0.5g per tablet.<br>Piperazine citrate syrup: 16g of this drug contained in every 100ml.<br>Piperazine phosphate tablets: 0.2g, 0.5g per tablet. |
| 药品名称 Drug Names | 左旋咪唑 Levamisole |
| 适应证<br>Indications | 主要用于驱蛔虫及钩虫。由于本品单剂量有效率较高，故适于集体治疗，可于噻嘧啶合用治疗严重钩虫感染；与噻苯唑或恩波吡维铵合用治疗肠线虫混合感染；与枸橼酸乙胺嗪先后序贯应用于抗丝虫感染。<br><br>It is mainly used for expelling ascarid and hookworm. Since the drug of single dose has a higher efficiency, it is intended to be used in combination. It can treat severe hookworm infection in combination with pyrantel and intestinal nematode mixed infection with thiabendazole or pyrvinium. Besides, it is used in anti-filarial infection in sequential combination with diethylcarbamazine citrate. |
| 用法、用量<br>Dosage | （1）驱虫病：口服，①成人 $1.5 \sim 2.5mg/kg$，空腹或睡前顿服；②小儿剂量为 $2 \sim 3mg/kg$。<br>（2）驱钩虫：口服，$1.5 \sim 2.5mg/kg$，每晚 1 次，连服 3 日。<br>（3）治疗丝虫病：$4 \sim 6mg/kg$，分 3 次服，连服 3 日。<br><br>(1) deworming disease: by oral medication, ① give adults $1.5 \sim 2.5mg/kg$, on an empty stomach or at a draught before sleep; ② give children $2 \sim 3mg/kg$.<br>(2) expelling hookworm: by oral medication, give $1.5 \sim 2.5mg/kg$, once at night, for 3 days.<br>(3) Filariasis: give $4 \sim 6mg/kg$, in 3 divided doses, for 3 days. |
| 剂型、规格<br>Preparations | 片剂：每片 25mg；50mg。<br>肠溶片：每片 25mg；50mg。<br>颗粒剂：每 1g 含盐酸左旋咪唑 5mg。<br>糖浆：0.8g（100ml）；4g（500ml）；16g（200ml）。<br>搽剂：为左旋咪唑的 0.7% 二甲亚砜溶液或其硼酸酒精溶液。<br><br>Tablets: 25mg, 50mg per tablet.<br>Enteric-coated tablets: 25mg, 50mg per tablet.<br>Granules: 1g containing 5mg of levamisole hydrochloride.<br>Syrup: 0.8g (100ml), 4g (500ml), 16g (200ml).<br>Liniment: 0.7% dimethyl sulfoxide or alcohol boric acid of levamisole. |
| 药品名称 Drug Names | 阿苯达唑 Albendazole |
| 适应证<br>Indications | 用于驱除蛔虫、蛲虫、钩虫、鞭虫，也可用于家畜的驱虫。<br><br>It is used in expelling ascarid, pinworm, hookworm, whipworm, as well as in deworming of livestock. |
| 用法、用量<br>Dosage | 口服，驱钩虫、蛔虫、蛲虫、鞭虫，0.4g 顿服。2 周岁以上小儿，单纯蛲虫、单纯蛔虫感染，0.2g 顿服。治疗囊虫病：每天 $15 \sim 20mg/kg$，分 2 次服用。10 日为 1 个疗程。停药 $15 \sim 20$ 日后，可进行第 2 疗程治疗。一般为 $2 \sim 3$ 个疗程。必要时可重复治疗。其他寄生虫如粪类圆线虫等，每日服 400mg，连服 6 日。必要时重复给药 1 次。12 岁以下儿童；用量减半，服法同成人或遵医嘱。<br><br>This drug is administered by oral medication. Expelling hookworm, ascarid, pinworm and whipworm: give 0.4g, at a draught; for children over the age of 2, in pure pinworm or ascarid infection treatment, give 0.2g, at a draught. Cysticercosis: give $15 \sim 20mg/kg$ a day, in 2 divided doses, with a |

| | treatment course of 10 days; receive second course of treatment after 15 to 20 days of drug withdrawal, generally for 2 to 3 courses; give repeated treatment if necessary. Other parasites such as Stercoralis: give 400mg a day, for 6 days; give repeated medication for once if necessary; for children under the age of 12, give half of the adult dose, with the same method as adult or following doctors' advice. |
|---|---|
| 剂型、规格<br>Preparations | 片（胶囊剂）：每片（粒）100mg；200mg。<br>干糖浆：每袋 200mg。<br>Tablets (capsules): 100mg; 200mg per tablet (capsule)<br>Dry Syrup: 200mg per bag. |

8. 主要作用于中枢神经系统的药物 Drugs mainly acting on the central nervous system

8.1　中枢神经系统兴奋药 Drugs exciting central nervous system

| 药品名称 Drug Names | 尼可刹米 Nikethamide |
|---|---|
| 适应证<br>Indications | 用于中枢性呼吸及循环衰竭、麻醉药及其中枢抑制药的中毒。<br>It is used to treat central respiratory and circulatory failure, anesthetics and central depressants poisoning. |
| 用法、用量<br>Dosage | 常用量：皮下注射、肌内注射或静脉注射，每次 0.25 ~ 0.5g。必要时 1 ~ 2 小时重复用药。极量：皮下注射、肌内注射或静脉注射，一次 1.25g。6 个月以下，婴儿每次 75mg，1 岁每次 125mg，4 ~ 7 岁每次 175mg。<br>The usual dose: by subcutaneous, intramuscular or intravenous injection, give 0.25 ~ 0.5g singly; repeat the medication within 1~2 hours if necessary. Maximum dose: by subcutaneous, intramuscular or intravenous injection, give 1.25g singly. Infants under 6 months, give 75 mg singly; with one-year old, give 125mg singly; with 4~7 years old, give175mg singly. |
| 剂型、规格<br>Preparations | 注射液：每支 0.375g（1.5ml）；0.5g（2ml）；0.25g（1ml）。<br>Injection: 0.375g (1.5ml), 0.5g (2ml), 0.25g (1ml) per vial. |
| 药品名称 Drug Names | 洛贝林 Lobeline |
| 适应证<br>Indications | 用于新生儿窒息、一氧化碳引起的窒息、吸入麻醉剂及其他中枢抑制药（如阿片、巴比妥类）的中毒及肺炎、白喉等疾病引起的呼吸衰竭。<br>It is used for neonatal asphyxia, carbon monoxide asphyxia and pensioning by anesthetics inhalation or other central nervous depressants (such as opioids, barbiturates), as well as respiratory failure caused by pneumonia, diphtheria and other diseases. |
| 用法、用量<br>Dosage | 皮下注射或肌内注射：常用量，成人 1 次 3 ~ 10mg（极量：1 次 20mg，1 日 50mg）；儿童 1 次 1 ~ 3mg。静脉注射：成人 1 次 3mg（极量：1 次 6mg，一日 20mg）；儿童 1 次 0.3 ~ 3mg。必要时每 30 分钟可重复 1 次。静脉注射需缓慢。新生儿窒息可注入脐静脉，用量为 3mg。<br>Usual dose by subcutaneous or intramuscular injection: give adults 3 ~ 10mg singly (maximum dose: 20mg singly, 50mg a day); give children 1 ~ 3mg singly. Intravenous injection: give adults 3mg singly (maximum dose: 6mg singly, 20mg a day); give children 0.3 ~ 3mg singly; repeat the medication once every 30 minutes if necessary; slow intravenous injection is needed. In neonatal asphyxia treatment, it can be injected into the umbilical vein, the dose is 3mg. |
| 剂型、规格<br>Preparations | 注射液：每支 3mg（1ml）；10mg（1ml）。<br>Injection: 3mg (1ml), 10mg (1ml) per vial. |
| 药品名称 Drug Names | 戊四氮 Pentetrazole |
| 适应证<br>Indications | 用于急性传染病、麻醉药及巴比妥类药物中毒时引起的呼吸抑制，急性循环衰竭。安全范围小，现已少用。<br>It is used in treatment of respiratory depression and acute circulatory failure caused by acute infectious diseases, anesthetics and barbiturate poisoning. It has been seldom used because of the narrow safe range. |

**续　表**

| 用法、用量<br>Dosage | 皮下注射、肌内注射、静脉注射，每次 0.05 ～ 0.1g，每 2 小时 1 次。极量 1 日 0.3g。<br>Subcutaneous injection, intramuscular injection or intravenous injection: 0.05 ～ 0.1g singly, once every 2 hours, with maximum daily dose of 0.3g |
|---|---|
| 剂型、规格<br>Preparations | 注射液：每支 0.1g（1ml）；0.3g（3ml）。<br>Injection: 0.1g (1ml), 0.3g (3ml) per vial. |
| **药品名称 Drug Names** | 贝美格 Bemegride |
| 适应证<br>Indications | 用于解救巴比妥类、格鲁米特、水合氯醛等药物的中毒。应用于加速硫喷妥钠麻醉后的恢复。<br>It is used in detoxication of barbiturates poisoning, glutethimide poisoning, chloral hydrate poisoning and other drugs' poisoning. It can be used to speed up the recovery after thiopental anesthesia. |
| 用法、用量<br>Dosage | 因本品作用迅速，多采用静脉滴注，作用维持 10 ～ 20 分钟。常用量 0.5%10ml（50mg），用 5% 葡萄糖注射液稀释静脉滴注。宜可静脉注射，每 3 ～ 5 分钟注射 50mg，治病情改善或出现中毒症状为止。<br>Because of the drug's quick effect, it is administered by intravenous infusion. The effect would maintain 10~20 minutes. The usual dose is 0.5% 10ml (50mg); dilute it with 5% glucose injection for intravenous drip. The drug can also be administered by intravenous injection, give 50mg every 3 to 5 minutes, until the patients' condition improves or symptoms of poisoning disappear. |
| 剂型、规格<br>Preparations | 注射液：每支 50mg（10ml）。<br>Injection: 50mg (10ml) per vial. |
| **药品名称 Drug Names** | 咖啡因 Caffeine |
| 适应证<br>Indications | （1）解救因急性感染中毒、催眠药、麻醉药、镇痛药中毒引起的呼吸、循环衰竭。<br>（2）与溴化物合用，使大脑皮质兴奋、抑制过程恢复平衡，用于神经官能症。<br>（3）与阿司匹林、对乙酰氨基酚制成复方制剂用于一般性头痛；与麦角胺合用治疗偏头痛。<br>（4）用于小儿多动症（注意力缺陷综合征）。<br>（5）治疗未成熟新生儿呼吸暂停或阵发性呼吸困难。<br>(1) It can be used in respiratory and circulatory failure caused by acute infection poisoning, hypnotics, anesthetics and analgesics poisoning.<br>(2) It is combined with bromides to treat neurosis because it can balance the cerebral cortex's excitatory and inhibitory process.<br>(3) It is associated with aspirin and compound preparations by acetaminophen to treat general headache, with ergotamine to treat migraine.<br>(4) It is also used to treat children's ADHD (Attention Deficit Syndrome).<br>(5) premature newborns' apnea or paroxysmal dyspnea. |
| 用法、用量<br>Dosage | （1）口服。常用量：1 次 0.1 ～ 0.3g，一日 0.3 ～ 1.0g；极量：1 次 0.4g，一日 1.5g。<br>（2）解救中枢抑制：肌内注射或皮下注射安钠咖注射液（详见制剂项下）。常用量：皮下注射或肌内注射，1 次 1 ～ 2ml，一日 2 ～ 4ml；极量皮下注射或肌内注射，1 次 3ml，一日 12ml。<br>（3）调节大脑皮质活动：口服咖溴合剂，一日 10 ～ 15ml，一日 3 次，餐后服。<br>(1) Oral medication: the usual dose is 0.1 ～ 0.3g singly, 0.3 ～ 1.0g a day; the maximum dose is 0.4g singly, 1.5g a day.<br>(2) Central inhibition: by intramuscular or subcutaneous injection of caffeine and sodium benzoate injection (see the preparations item). The usual dose is 1 ～ 2ml singly, 2 ～ 4ml a day; the maximum dose is 3ml singly, 12ml a day.<br>(3) Regulate cerebral cortex activity: give orally caffeine bromine mixture, 10 ～ 15ml a day, 3 times a day, after meals. |
| 剂型、规格<br>Preparations | 片剂：每片 30mg。<br>Tablets: 30mg per tablet. |

| 药品名称 Drug Names | 甲氯芬酯 Meclofenoxate |
|---|---|
| 适应证<br>Indications | 用于外伤性昏迷、新生儿缺氧、儿童遗尿症、意识障碍、老年性精神病、酒精中毒及某些中枢和周围神经症状。<br><br>It is used to treat traumatic coma, neonatal hypoxia, children enuresis, disturbance of unconsciousness, senile psychosis, alcoholism and some certain central and peripheral nervous symptoms. |
| 用法、用量<br>Dosage | （1）口服，成人1次0.1～0.3g，一日0.3～0.9g；最大剂量可达一日1.5g。儿童1次100mg，一日3次。<br>（2）肌内注射或静脉滴注：成人1次0.25g，一日1～3次。溶于5%葡萄糖溶液250～500ml中供静脉滴注。新生儿可注入脐静脉。小儿每次60～100mg，一日2次。新生儿缺氧症，一次0.06g，每2小时1次。<br><br>(1) Oral medication: give adults 0.1～0.3g singly, 0.3～0.9g a day, with maximum daily dose of 1.5g; give children 100mg singly, 3 times a day.<br>(2) Intramuscular injection or intravenous infusion: give adults 0.25g singly, 1 to 3 times a day; give children 60～100mg singly, twice a day; for Neonatal anoxia newborns, give. 0.06g singly, every two hours Dissolve the drug in 250～500ml of 5% glucose solution for intravenous infusion. It can be injected into the umbilical vein for newborns. |
| 剂型、规格<br>Preparations | 胶囊剂：每粒0.1g；注射用盐酸甲氯芬酯：每支0.1g；0.25g。<br>Capsules: 0.1g per capsules. Meclofenoxate hydrochloride for injection: 0.1g, 0.25g per vial. |
| 药品名称 Drug Names | 乙哌立松 Eperisone |
| 适应证<br>Indications | 可用于改善下列疾病的肌紧张状态：颈肩腕综合征，肩周炎，腰痛症；也可用于改善下列疾病所致的痉挛性麻痹：脑血管障碍，痉挛性脊髓麻痹，颈椎病，手术后遗症（包括脑、脊髓肿瘤），外伤后遗症（脊髓损伤、头部外伤），肌萎缩性侧索硬化症，婴儿大脑性轻瘫，脊髓小脑变性症，脊髓血管障碍，亚急性脊髓神经症（SMON）及其他脑脊髓疾病。<br><br>It can be used to improve muscle tension caused by the following disease: neck-shoulder-wrist syndrome, frozen shoulder, back pain. It can also be used to improve the spastic paralysis caused by the following disease: cerebrovascular disorders, spastic spinal paralysis, cervical spondylosis, operation sequela (including brain tumor and spinal cord tumor surgery), trauma sequela (including spinal cord injury and head injury), amyotrophic lateral sclerosis, infants cerebral paresis, spinocerebellar degeneration, spinal vascular disorders, subacute myelo-optico neuropoathy (SMON) and other brain spinal cord disease. |
| 用法、用量<br>Dosage | 餐后口服。通常成人一次50mg（1片），一日3次。<br>The drug is administered orally after meals. Give adults usually 50mg (1 tablet) singly, 3 times a day. |
| 剂型、规格<br>Preparations | 片剂：每片50mg。<br>Tablets: 50mg per tablet. |
| 药品名称 Drug Names | 细胞色素C　Cytochrome C |
| 适应证<br>Indications | 用于各种组织缺氧的急救或辅助治疗，如一氧化碳中毒、催眠药中毒、新生儿窒息、严重休克期缺氧、麻醉及肺部疾病引起的呼吸困难、高山缺氧、脑缺氧及心脏疾病引起的缺氧，但疗效有时不显著。<br><br>It is used in first aid or adjuvant therapy of a variety of hypoxia, such as carbon monoxide poisoning, hypnotic poisoning, neonatal asphyxia, anoxia in severe shock phase, breathing difficulties caused by anesthesia and lung disease, alpine hypoxia, cerebral anoxia and anoxia caused by heart disease, but the effect is not significant sometimes. |
| 用法、用量<br>Dosage | 静脉注射或滴注：成人每次15～30mg，一日30～60mg。儿童用量酌减。静脉注射时，加25%葡萄糖注射液20ml混匀后，缓慢注射。亦可用5%～10%葡萄糖注射液或生理盐水稀释后静脉滴注。粉针（冻干型）用25%葡萄糖注射液20ml或5%葡萄糖注射液或灭菌生理盐水溶解后滴注。<br><br>Intravenous injection or infusion: give adults 15～30mg singly, 30～60mg a day. Children need dose reduction. In intravenous injection, add 20ml of 25% glucose injection, then inject slowly after mixing. Or dilute with 5% to 10% glucose injection or saline infusion for injection. Powder for injection (lyophilized type) needs to be dissolved by 20ml of 25% glucose injection or 5% dextrose injection or sterile saline solution for infusion. |

**续　表**

| 剂型、规格<br>Preparations | 注射液：每支 15mg（2ml）。注射用细胞色素 C：每支 15mg。<br>Injection: 15mg (2ml) per vial. Cytochrome C for injection: 15mg per vial. |
|---|---|

## 8.2 镇痛药 Analgesics

| 药品名称 Drug Names | 吗啡 Morphine |
|---|---|
| 适应证<br>Indications | （1）镇痛：现仅用于创伤、手术、烧伤等引起的剧痛。<br>（2）心肌梗死。<br>（3）心源性哮喘。<br>（4）麻醉前给药。<br>(1) Analgesia: morphine is only used in severe pain caused by trauma, surgery and burns. It is also used in.<br>(2) Myocardial infarction.<br>(3) Cardiac asthma.<br>(4) Preanesthetic medication. |
| 用法、用量<br>Dosage | （1）常用量：口服，1 次 5 ~ 15mg，一日 15 ~ 60mg；皮下注射，1 次 5 ~ 15mg，一日 15 ~ 40mg；静脉注射，5 ~ 10mg。<br>（2）极量：口服，1 次 30mg，一日 100mg；皮下注射，1 次 20mg，1 日 60mg；硬膜外腔注射，一次极量 5mg，用于手术后镇痛。<br>(1) The usual dose: by oral medication, 5 ~ 15mg singly, 15 ~ 60mg a day; by subcutaneous injection, 5 ~ 15mg singly, 15 ~ 40mg a day; by intravenous injection, 5 ~ 10mg.<br>(2) Maximum dose: by oral medication, 30mg singly, 100mg a day; by subcutaneous injection, 20mg singly, 60mg a day; by epidural injection, 5mg singly, for post-operative analgesia. |
| 剂型、规格<br>Preparations | 注射液：每支 5mg（0.5ml）；10mg（1.0ml）。片剂：每片 5mg；10mg。<br>Injection: p5mg (0.5ml); 10mg (1.0ml) per vial. Tablets: 5mg, 10mg per tablet. |
| 药品名称 Drug Names | 哌替啶 Pethidine |
| 适应证<br>Indications | （1）各种剧痛，如创伤、烧伤、烫伤、术后疼痛等；<br>（2）心源性哮喘；<br>（3）麻醉前给药；<br>（4）内脏剧烈绞痛（胆绞痛、肾绞痛需与阿托品合用）；<br>（5）与氯丙嗪、异丙嗪等合用进行人工冬眠。<br>It can be used in<br>(1) all kinds of pain, such as trauma, burn, scald and postoperative pain, as well as<br>(2) cardiac asthma,<br>(3) preanesthetic medication and<br>(4) visceral severe colic (biliary colic, renal colic needs combination with atropine).<br>(5) It is combined with chlorpromazine or promethazine for artificial hibernation. |
| 用法、用量<br>Dosage | （1）口服：一次 25 ~ 100mg，一日 200 ~ 400mg；极量：1 次 150mg，一日 600mg。<br>（2）皮下注射或肌内注射：1 次 25 ~ 100mg，一日 100 ~ 400mg；极量：1 次 150mg，1 日 600mg。两次用药间隔不宜少于 4 小时。<br>（3）静脉注射：成人以每次 0.3mg/kg 为限。<br>（4）麻醉前肌内注射：成人以每千克体重 1.0mg，术前 30 ~ 60 分钟给予。麻醉过程中静脉滴注，成人以每千克体重 1.2 ~ 2.0mg 计算总量，配制成稀释液，以每分钟 1mg 静脉滴注，小儿滴速减慢。<br>（5）手术后镇痛及癌性镇痛：以每日 2.1 ~ 2.5mg/kg 计量为限，经硬膜外腔缓慢注入或泵入。<br>(1) Oral medication: give 25 ~ 100mg singly, 200 ~ 400mg a day, with maximum dose of 150mg singly, 600mg a day.<br>(2) Subcutaneous or intramuscular injection: give 25 ~ 100mg singly, 100 ~ 400mg a day, with maximum dose of 150mg singly, 600mg a day; the interval should be more than 4 hours.<br>(3) Intravenous injection: adults' limited dose is 0.3mg/kg singly.<br>(4) Intramuscular injection before anesthesia: give adults 1.0mg / kg, 30 to 60 minutes before surgery. Intravenous infusion during anesthesia: give adults 1.2 ~ 2.0mg/ kg; make diluted solution for intravenous infusion, with speed of 1mg per minute; children's drip rate should slow down.<br>(5) Post-operative analgesia and cancer analgesia: give 2.1 ~ 2.5mg/kg a day as limited daily dose, by slow epidural infusion or pumping . |

**续 表**

| | |
|---|---|
| 剂型、规格<br>Preparations | 片剂：每片 25mg；50mg。<br>注射液：每支 50mg（1ml）；100mg（2ml）。<br>Tablets: 25mg, 50mg per tablet.<br>Injection: 50mg (1ml), 100mg (2ml) per vial. |
| **药品名称 Drug Names** | 美沙酮 Methadone |
| 适应证<br>Indications | 适用于创伤性、癌症剧痛、外科手术后和慢性疼痛。也用于阿片、吗啡及海洛因成瘾者的脱毒治疗。<br><br>It is used for traumatic pain, cancer pain, postoperative pain and chronic pain. It is also used in the detoxification treatment of opium, morphine and heroin addicts. |
| 用法、用量<br>Dosage | （1）口服：成人每日 10～15mg；分 2～3 次服。儿童每日按 0.7mg/kg 计，分 4～6 次服。极量：1 次 10mg，一日 20mg。<br>（2）肌内注射或皮下注射：每次 2.5～5mg，一日 10～15mg。三角肌注射血浆峰值高，作用出现快，因此可采用三角肌注射。极量：1 次 10mg，一日 20mg。<br>(1) Oral medication: give adults 10～15mg a day, in 2~3 divided doses; give children 0.7mg/kg, in 4~6 divided doses. Maximum dose is 10mg singly, 20mg a day.<br>(2) Intramuscular injection or subcutaneous injection: give 2.5～5mg singly, 10mg～15mg a day. In deltoid injection is of high peak plasma and quick effect, so it can be used for deltoid injection. Maximum dose is 10mg singly, 20mg a day. |
| 剂型、规格<br>Preparations | 片剂：每片 2.5mg；7.5mg；10mg。<br>注射液：每支 5mg（1ml）7.5mg（2ml）。<br>Tablets: 2.5mg, 7.5mg, 10mg per tablet.<br>Injection: 5mg (1ml), 7.5mg (2ml) per vial. |
| **药品名称 Drug Names** | 芬太尼 Fentanyl |
| 适应证<br>Indications | 适用于各种疼痛及外科、妇科等手术后和手术过程中的镇痛；也用于防治或减轻手术后的谵妄；还可与麻醉药合用，作为麻醉辅助用药；与氟哌利多配伍制成"安定镇痛药"，用于大面积换药及进行小手术的镇痛。<br><br>It is intended to treat a variety of pain, as well as analgesia in or after the surgical operation, gynecological surgery and etc.. It is also used to prevent or alleviate delirium after surgery. It is combined with anesthetics to be used as an anesthetic adjuvant drug, with droperidol to be as "stability analgesic agent" for large-area dressing change and analgesia in minor surgery. |
| 用法、用量<br>Dosage | （1）麻醉前给药：0.05～0.1mg，于手术前 30～60 分钟肌内注射。<br>（2）诱导麻醉：静脉注射 0.05～0.1mg，间隔 2～3 分钟重复注射，直至达到要求；危重患者、年幼及年老患者的用量减小至 0.025～0.05mg。<br>（3）维持麻醉：当患者出现苏醒症状时，静脉注射或肌内注射 0.025～0.05mg。<br>（4）一般镇痛及术后镇痛：肌内注射 0.05～0.1mg。可控制手术后疼痛、烦躁和呼吸急迫，必要时可于 1～2 小时后重复给药。硬膜外腔注入镇痛，一般 4～10 分钟起效，20 分钟脑脊液浓度达峰值，作用持续 3～6 小时。<br>（5）贴片：每 3 天用 1 贴，贴于锁骨下胸部皮肤。<br>(1) Preanesthetic administration: 0.05～0.1mg, by intramuscular injection, 30 to 60 minutes before surgery.<br>(2) Induction of anesthesia: give 0.05～0.1mg, by intravenous injection, with intervals of 2 to 3 minutes for repeated injections, until meet the requirements; critically ill patients, children patients and elderly patients need dose reduction to 0.025～0.05mg.<br>(3) Maintenance of anesthesia: if patients appear awake state, give 0.025～0.05mg, by intravenous or intramuscular injection..<br>(4) General and postoperative analgesia: give 0.05～0.1mg, by intramuscular injection. It can control postoperative pain, dysphoria and urgent respiration; give repeated dose after 1 to 2 hours, if necessary. Analgesia by epidural injection usually takes effect within 4 to 10 minutes; the cerebrospinal fluid concentration reaches peak after 20 minutes, and the effect would last for 3 to 6 hours.<br>(5) Patch: give 1 patch every three days, on the skin chest under collarbone. |

**续　表**

| | |
|---|---|
| 剂型、规格<br>Preparations | 注射液：每支 0.1mg（2ml）。<br>贴片（多瑞吉）：每小时可释放芬太尼 25μg、50μg、75μg、100μg。<br>复方芬太尼注射液：每 1ml 含芬太尼 0.1mg，异丙嗪 25mg。<br>Injection: 0.1mg (2ml) per vial.<br>Patches (Durogesic): 25μg, 50μg, 75μg, 100μg of fentanyl released per hour.<br>Compound Fentanyl Injection: 0.1mg of fentanyl and25mg of promethazine contained in 1ml of injection. |
| **药品名称 Drug Names** | **阿芬太尼 Alfentanil** |
| 适应证<br>Indications | 用于麻醉前、中、后的镇静与镇痛，适用于心脏冠状动脉血管旁路术的麻醉。<br>It is used for sedation and analgesia before, during and after the anesthesia, as well as anesthesia in cardiac coronary artery bypass surgery. |
| 用法、用量<br>Dosage | 静脉注射：按手术长短而决定极量。手术 10 分钟以内完成者 7 ~ 15μg/kg；60 分钟手术，40 ~ 80μg/kg；手术超过 60 分钟者，可改为每分钟 1μg/kg，连续静脉滴注，至手术结束前 10 分钟停止给药。<br>Intravenous injection: the maximum dose is determined by the length of surgery; within 10 minutes, give 7 ~ 15μg/kg; of 60 minutes, give 40 ~ 80μg/kg; over 60 minutes, change to 1μg/kg/min, by continuous intravenous infusion until 10 minutes before the end of surgery. |
| 剂型、规格<br>Preparations | 注射液（盐酸盐）：每支 1mg（2ml）。<br>Injection (hydrochloride): 1mg (2ml) per vial. |
| **药品名称 Drug Names** | **舒芬太尼 Sufentanil** |
| 适应证<br>Indications | 用于麻醉前、中、后的镇静与镇痛，适用于冠状动脉旁路移植术的麻醉。<br>It is used for sedation and analgesia before, during and after the anesthesia, as well as anesthesia in cardiac coronary artery bypass surgery. |
| 用法、用量<br>Dosage | 麻醉时间长约 2 小时，总剂量 2μg/kg，维持量 10 ~ 25μg。麻醉时间为 2 ~ 8 小时，总剂量 2 ~ 8μg/kg，维持量 10 ~ 50μg。心血管手术麻醉，5μg/kg。<br>If the anesthesia lasts about 2 hours, give total dose of 2μg/kg and maintenance dose of 10 ~ 25μg; if The anesthesia lasts about 2 to 8 hours, give total dose of 2 ~ 8μg/kg and maintenance dose of 10 ~ 50μg. Cardiovascular anesthesia: 5μg/kg. |
| 剂型、规格<br>Preparations | 注射液：每支 50μg（2ml）；100μg（2ml）；250μg（2ml）。<br>Injection: 50μg (2ml), 100μg (2ml), 250μg (2ml) per vial. |
| **药品名称 Drug Names** | **瑞芬太尼 Remifentanil** |
| 适应证<br>Indications | 用于麻醉诱导和全麻中维持镇痛。<br>It is used for induction of anesthesia and maintaining analgesia during general. |
| 用法、用量<br>Dosage | 10mg 加入 200ml 生理盐水。用于静脉麻醉时，剂量为 0.25 ~ 2.0μg/（kg·min），或间断注射 0.25 ~ 1.0μg/kg。<br>10mg of the drug needs to add 200ml of the saline.. In intravenous anesthesia, give 0.25 ~ 2.0μg / (kg · min), or 0.25 ~ 1.0μg/kg by intermittent injection. |
| 剂型、规格<br>Preparations | 注射用瑞芬太尼：每支 1mg；2mg；5mg。<br>Remifentanil for injection: 1mg; 2mg; 5mg per vial. |
| **药品名称 Drug Names** | **布桂嗪 Bucinnazine** |
| 适应证<br>Indications | 临床上用于偏头痛、三叉神经痛、炎症性及外伤性疼痛、关节痛、痛经、癌症引起的疼痛等。<br>It is clinically used for migraine, trigeminal neuralgia, inflammatory and traumatic pain, joint pain, dysmenorrhea and pain caused by cancer etc. |
| 用法、用量<br>Dosage | （1）口服：成人 1 次 30 ~ 60mg，一日 90 ~ 180mg；小儿每次 1mg/kg。疼痛剧烈时用量可酌增。<br>（2）皮下或肌内注射：成人 1 次 50 ~ 100mg，一日 1 ~ 2 次。<br>(1) Oral medication: give adults 30 ~ 60mg singly, 90 ~ 180mg a day; give children 1mg/kg singly; the intense pain could appropriately increase dosage.<br>(2) Subcutaneous or intramuscular injection: give adults 50 ~ 100mg singly, 1~2 times a day. |

| | |
|---|---|
| 剂型、规格<br>Preparations | 片剂：每片 30mg；60mg。<br>注射液：每支 50mg（2ml）；100mg（2ml）。<br>Tablets: 30mg, 60mg per tablet.<br>Injection: 50mg (2ml), 100mg (2ml). |
| **药品名称 Drug Names** | 喷他佐辛 Pentazocine |
| 适应证<br>Indications | 适用于各种慢性剧痛。<br>It is intended to treat a variety of chronic intense pain. |
| 用法、用量<br>Dosage | 静脉注射、肌内注射或皮下注射，每次 30mg。口服，每次 25 ~ 50mg。必要时每 3 ~ 4 小时 1 次。<br>Intravenous, intramuscular or subcutaneous injection: 30mg singly Oral medication: 25 ~ 50mg singly; if necessary, once every 3 to 4 hours. |
| 剂型、规格<br>Preparations | 片剂：每片 25mg；50mg。注射液：每支 15mg（1ml）；30mg（1ml）。<br>Tablets: 25mg, 50mg per tablet. Injection: 15mg (1ml), 30mg (1ml) per vial. |
| **药品名称 Drug Names** | 羟考酮 Oxycodone |
| 适应证<br>Indications | 用于缓解中、重度疼痛。<br>It is used to relieve moderate and severe pain. |
| 用法、用量<br>Dosage | （1）一般阵痛，使用控释制剂，每 12 小时服用 1 次，用药剂量取决于患者的疼痛的严重程度和既往镇痛药用药史。首次服用阿片类或弱阿片类药物初始用药剂量一般为 5mg，每 12 小时服用 1 次。已接受口服吗啡治疗的患者，改用本品的每日用药剂量换算比例为：口服本品 10mg 相当于口服吗啡 20mg。应根据患者个体情况滴定用药剂量。调整剂量时，不改变用药次数，只调整每次剂量，调整幅度是在上次一次的用药剂量基础上增长 25% ~ 50%。大多数患者的最高用药剂量为每 12 小时服用 200mg，少数患者可能需要更高的剂量。控释制剂必须整片吞服，不得掰开、咀嚼或研磨。如果掰开、咀嚼或研磨药片，会导致羟考酮的快速释放与潜在致死量的吸收。<br>（2）术后疼痛：使用本药复方胶囊，每次 1 ~ 2 粒，间隔 4 ~ 6 小时可重复用药一次。<br>（3）癌症、慢性疼痛：使用本药复方胶囊，每次 1 ~ 2 粒，一日 3 次。儿童：口服，一次 0.05 ~ 0.15mg/kg，每 4 ~ 6 小时一次。一次用量最多 5mg。<br>(1) General pain: give controlled-release formulation, once every 12 hours; the dose depends on the severity of the pain and patients' previous history of analgesic medication . The initial dose of opioid or weak opioid is usually 5mg, once every 12 hours. For patients who have already received oral morphine treatment, there is a conversion ratio for daily dose: by oral medication, 10mg of the drug is equivalent to 20mg of morphine. The administration dose should be determined based on individual patient's condition. When make dose adjustment, change the single dose, rather than the frequency; increase 25% ~ 50% on the basisi of last dose. For most of the patients, maximum dose is to 200mg, singly, every 12 hours, but a minority of patients may need larger dose. Controlled release preparations must be swallowed in whole piece, no breaking apart, chewing or grinding, which can lead to rapid release of oxycodone and potential absorption lethal dose.<br>(2) Postoperative pain: give compound capsules, 1 ~ 2 capsule singly; repeat the dose with an interval of 4 ~ 6 hours.<br>(3) Cancer, chronic pain : give compound capsules, 1 ~ 2 capsule singly, 3 times a day; give children 0.05 ~ 0.15mg/kg singly, every 4 to 6 hours, by oral medication, with maximum single dose of 5mg. |
| 剂型、规格<br>Preparations | 片剂：5mg。控释片：5mg；10mg；20mg；40mg。复方胶囊剂：每粒含羟考酮 5mg、对乙酰氨基酚 500mg。<br>Tablets: 5mg. Controlled release tablets: 5mg, 10mg, 20mg, 40mg. Compound Capsules: 5mg of oxycodone and 500mg of paracetamol contained per capsule. |
| **药品名称 Drug Names** | 地佐辛 Dezocine |
| 适应证<br>Indications | 用于术后痛、内脏及癌性疼痛。<br>It is used for postoperative pain, visceral pain and cancer pain. |

**续　表**

| | |
|---|---|
| 用法、用量<br>Dosage | 　肌内注射：开始时 10mg，以后每隔 3～6 小时，2.5～10mg。静脉注射：开始 5mg，以后每隔 2～4 小时，2.5～10mg。<br>　Intramuscular injection: give starting dose of 10mg, afterwards 2.5～10mg every 3 to 6 hours. Intravenous injection: give starting dose of 5mg, afterwards 2.5～10mg every 2 to 4 hours. |
| 剂型、规格<br>Preparations | 　注射液：每支 5mg（1ml）；10mg（1ml）。<br>　Injection: 5mg (1ml), 10mg (1ml) per vial. |
| **药品名称 Drug Names** | 普瑞巴林 Pregabalin |
| 适应证<br>Indications | 　用于治疗外周神经痛及辅助性治疗局限性部分癫痫发作。我国批准的适应证为：用于治疗带状疱疹后神经痛。<br>　It is used in the treatment of peripheral neuropathic pain and adjuvant treatment localized seizures. The approved indication in China is post-herpetic neuralgia. |
| 用法、用量<br>Dosage | 　口服，每日剂量为 150～600mg，分 2～3 次给药。一般起始剂量为每次 75mg，一日 2 次。如果每日服用本品 300mg，2～4 周后疼痛仍未得到充分缓解、且可耐受本品的患者，剂量可增至每次 300mg，一日 2 次，或每次 200mg，一日 3 次（即 600mg/d）。由于不良反应呈剂量依赖性，且不良反应可导致更高的停药率，故剂量超过 300mg/d 仅应用于耐受 300mg/d 剂量的持续性疼痛患者。<br>　Oral medication: give daily dose of 150～600mg, in 2 to 3 divided does. Generally, start with 75mg singly, 2 times a day. If the patients receive medication of 300mg a day for 2～4 weeks but without fully relief of the pain and the patients can still tolerate the drug, increase the dose to 300mg singly, twice a day or 200mg singly, 3 times a day (i.e. 600mg a day ). Since the adverse reaction is dose-dependent and it can lead to higher drug withdrawal rate, so dose over300mg a day can only be administered to persistent pain patients whose drug tolerance is 300mg a day. |
| 剂型、规格<br>Preparations | 　胶囊：每粒 75mg；150mg。<br>　Capsules: 75mg, 150mg per capsule. |
| **药品名称 Drug Names** | 曲马多 Tramadol |
| 适应证<br>Indications | 　用于中、重度急慢性疼痛，服后 0.5 小时生效，持续 6 小时。亦用于术后痛、创伤痛、癌性痛、心脏病突发性痛、关节痛、神经痛及分娩痛。<br>　It is used for moderate and severe acute or chronic pain. It takes effect half an hour after administration, lasting 6 hours. It is also used for postoperative pain, trauma pain, cancer pain, heart attack pain, joint pain, neuralgia and childbirth pain. |
| 用法、用量<br>Dosage | 　成人：口服，每次量不超过 100mg，224 小时不超过 400mg，连续用药不超过 48 小时，累计用量不超过 800mg。静脉注射、皮下注射、肌内注射，每次 50～100mg，一日不超过 400mg。<br>　Oral medication: give adults no more than 100mg each time and no more than 400mg within 224; the continuous medication can not exceed 48 hours and the cumulative does can not exceed 800mg. Intravenous, subcutaneous and intramuscular injection: give 50～100mg singly; daily dose can not exceed 400mg. |
| 剂型、规格<br>Preparations | 　注射液：每支 50mg（2ml）；100mg（2ml）。<br>　胶囊剂：每粒 50mg。<br>　栓剂：每 1ml（40 滴）含药 100mg。<br>　缓释片：每片 100mg。<br>　Injection: 50mg (2ml), 100mg (2ml) per vial.<br>　Capsules: 50mg per capsule.<br>　Suppository: 100mg of drug contained in 1ml (40 drops).<br>　Sustained-release tablets: 100mg per tablet. |
| **药品名称 Drug Names** | 四氢帕马丁 Tetrahydropalmatine |
| 适应证<br>Indications | 　对胃肠、肝胆系统疾病的钝痛镇痛效果好，对外伤等剧痛效果差。亦用于分娩镇痛及痛经。催眠、镇静效果较好，治疗剂量无成瘾性。1 次服用 100mg，服后 20～30 分钟入睡，持续 5～6 小时，无后遗作用，故可用于暂时性失眠。 |

<table>
<tr>
<td colspan="2">It has a good effect on the analgesia for dull pain by gastrointestinal and hepatobiliary system diseases, but poor effect on traumatic pain. It is also used for labor analgesia and dysmenorrhea. The drug's effect on hypnosis and sedation is good, and the therapeutic dose is non-addictive. Take 100mg singly, and then fall asleep in 20 to 30 minutes; it lasts 5 to 6 hours without sequelae effect, so it can be used for temporary insomnia.</td>
</tr>
<tr>
<td>用法、用量<br>Dosage</td>
<td>（1）镇痛：口服，每次 100 ~ 150mg，一日 2 ~ 4 次；皮下注射，每次 60 ~ 100mg。痛经：口服每次 50mg。<br>（2）催眠：口服，每次 100 ~ 200mg。<br>(1) Analgesia: by oral medication, give 100 ~ 150mg singly, 2~4 times a day; by subcutaneous injection, give 60 ~ 100mg singly. Dysmenorrhea: give orally 50mg each time.<br>(2) Hypnosis: orally, 100 ~ 200mg each time.</td>
</tr>
<tr>
<td>剂型、规格<br>Preparations</td>
<td>片剂：每片 50mg。<br>注射液：每支 60mg（2ml）；100mg（2ml）。<br>Tablets: 50mg per tablet.<br>Injection: per 60mg (2ml), 100mg (2ml) per vial.</td>
</tr>
<tr>
<td>药品名称 Drug Names</td>
<td>罗通定 Rotundine</td>
</tr>
<tr>
<td>适应证<br>Indications</td>
<td>用于因疼痛而失眠的患者。亦可用于胃溃疡和十二指肠溃疡的疼痛、月经痛，分娩后宫缩痛、紧张性失眠、痉挛性咳嗽等。<br>It is used for patients who have insomnia caused by pain. It can also be used for pain by gastric ulcer and duodenal ulcer, menstrual pain, uterine contraction pain after childbirth, insomnia by tension and spasmodic cough.</td>
</tr>
<tr>
<td>用法、用量<br>Dosage</td>
<td>镇痛：口服，每次 60 ~ 120mg，一日 1 ~ 4 次；肌内注射，每次 60 ~ 90mg，一日 1 ~ 4 次。催眠：成人于睡前服 1 次 30 ~ 90mg。<br>Analgesia: by oral medication, give 60 ~ 120mg singly, 1~4 times a day; by intramuscular injection, give 60 ~ 90mg singly, 1~4 times a day. Hypnosis: give adults 30~90mg, once before sleep.</td>
</tr>
<tr>
<td>剂型、规格<br>Preparations</td>
<td>片剂：每片 30mg；60mg。注射液（硫酸罗通定）：每支 60mg（2ml）。<br>Tablets: 30mg, 60mg per tablet. Injection (sulfuric rotundine): 60mg (2ml) per vial.</td>
</tr>
<tr>
<td>药品名称 Drug Names</td>
<td>麦角胺 Ergotamine</td>
</tr>
<tr>
<td>适应证<br>Indications</td>
<td>主要用于偏头痛，可使头痛减轻，但不能预防和根治。亦用于其他神经性头痛。<br>The drug is mainly used for migraines; it can relieve the headache but can not prevent or give a radical cure for headache. It is also used for other nervous headache.</td>
</tr>
<tr>
<td>用法、用量<br>Dosage</td>
<td>（1）口服：每次 1 ~ 2mg，一日不超过 6mg，一周不超过 10mg。效果不及皮下注射。<br>（2）皮下注射：每次 0.25 ~ 0.5mg，24 小时内不超过 1mg，本品早期给药效果好，头痛发作时用药效果差。<br>(1) Oral medication: give 1 ~ 2mg singly; daily can not exceed 6mg and weekly can not exceed 10mg. Its effect is not as good as subcutaneous injection.<br>(2) Subcutaneous injection: give 0.25 ~ 0.5mg singly; the dose can not exceed 1mg within 24 hours. Early treatment has better effect but worse effect when headache occurs.</td>
</tr>
<tr>
<td>剂型、规格<br>Preparations</td>
<td>片剂：每片 0.5mg；1mg。注射液：每支 0.25mg（ml）；0.5mg（1ml）。<br>Tablets: 0.5mg, 1mg per tablet. Injection: 0.25mg (ml), 0.5mg (1ml) per vial.</td>
</tr>
<tr>
<td>药品名称 Drug Names</td>
<td>乙酰乌头碱 Acetylaconitine</td>
</tr>
<tr>
<td>适应证<br>Indications</td>
<td>用于各种中度程度疼痛、肩关节周围炎、颈椎病、肩臂痛、腰痛、关节扭伤、风湿性关节炎、类风湿关节炎、坐骨神经痛、带状疱疹、小手术后痛。<br>It is used for a variety of moderate pain, periarthritis, cervical spondylosis, shoulder and arm pain, lumbago, sprains, rheumatic arthritis, rheumatoid arthritis, sciatica, shingles and postoperative pain of minor surgery.</td>
</tr>
</table>

**续 表**

| | |
|---|---|
| 用法、用量<br>Dosage | 口服：每次 0.3mg，一日 1 ~ 2 次，餐后服。每次量不超过 0.3mg，每月不宜超过 2 次，服药间隔 6 小时。1 个疗程为 10 日，疗程间隔 3 ~ 5 日。<br>　　肌内注射：每次 0.3mg，一日 1 ~ 2 次，一注射用水稀释至 2ml 后注射。小儿或老年人每日或隔日 1 次。两个疗程宜间隔 3 ~ 5 日。<br>　　Oral medication: give 0.3mg singly, 1 or 2 times a day, after meals. Single dose can not exceed 0.3mg, the frequency can not exceed 2 times a month, with administration interval of 6 hours. A course of treatment is 10 days, with treatment interval of 3 to 5 days.<br>　　Intramuscular injection: give 0.3mg singly, 1 or 2 times a day; diluted it to 2ml for injection. Administration for children or elder patients is once a day or every other day. There should be an interval of 3 to 5 days between courses. |
| 剂型、规格<br>Preparations | 片剂：每片 0.3mg。<br>注射液：每支 0.3mg（1ml）。<br>Tablets: 0.3mg per tablet.<br>Injection: 0.3mg (1ml) per vial. |
| 药品名称 Drug Names | 洛美利嗪 Lomerizine |
| 适应证<br>Indications | 用于偏头痛的预防性治疗。<br>It is used for prophylactic treatment of migraine. |
| 用法、用量<br>Dosage | 成人 1 次 5mg，一日 2 次，早餐后及晚餐后或睡眠前服。根据症状适量增减，但 1 日剂量不超过 20mg。<br>Adults: give 5mg singly, twice a day, before sleep and after breakfast or after dinner; appropriately increase or reduce the dose according to patients' symptoms, but daily does can not exceed 20mg. |
| 剂型、规格<br>Preparations | 片剂（胶囊）：每片（粒）5mg。<br>Tablets (capsules): 5mg per tablet (capsule). |
| 药品名称 Drug Names | 齐考诺肽 Ziconotide |
| 适应证<br>Indications | 用于需要鞘内治疗且对其他镇痛治疗（如应用全身性镇痛药或鞘内注射吗啡等）不耐受或疗效差的严重慢性疼痛患者。<br>It is used for severe chronic pain patients who are required intrathecal therapy and intolerant to other analgesic therapy (such as systemic analgesics or intrathecal injection of morphine, etc.) or receive poor efficacy. |
| 用法、用量<br>Dosage | 鞘内输注给药。起始剂量不宜超过一日 2.4mg（或 1 小时 0.1mg）。宜缓慢增量，即每周增加剂量不超过 2 ~ 3 次，每次增量不超过一日 2.4mg（或 1 小时 0.1mg），直至第 21 日时达到最大推荐剂量一日 19.2mg（或 1 小时 0.8mg）。<br>Intrathecal infusion: starting dose should not exceed 2.4mg a day (or 0.1mg an hour); the dose should be increased gradually, it means every increasing dose can not exceed 2.4mg a day (or 0.1mg an hour) and its frequency is no more than 2 to 3 times until the 21st day when it treaches the maximum recommended dose:19.2mg a day (or 0.8mg an hour). |
| 剂型、规格<br>Preparations | 注射液：5ml:500μg(100μg/ml)；20ml:500μg(25μg/ml)。<br>Injection: 5ml:500μg(100μg/ml), 20ml:500μg(25μg/ml). |
| 药品名称 Drug Names | 他喷他多 Tapentadol |
| 适应证<br>Indications | 用于各种急性和慢性疼痛。<br>It is used for a variety of acute and chronic pain. |
| 用法、用量<br>Dosage | 口服，每 4 ~ 6 小时 1 次，每次 1 片。<br>Oral medication: 1 tablet singly, every 4 to 6 hours. |
| 剂型、规格<br>Preparations | 片剂：每片 50mg；75mg；100mg。<br>Tablets: 50mg, 75mg, 100mg per tablet. |
| 药品名称 Drug Names | 阿片全碱 Papaveretum |
| 适应证<br>Indications | 同吗啡。用于各种疼痛及止泻，药效持久。<br>It has the same indications with morphine: for a variety of pain and diarrhea, with long lasting effect. |

**续　表**

| | |
|---|---|
| 用法、用量<br>Dosage | 皮下注射，每次 6 ~ 12mg。口服，每次 5 ~ 15mg，一日 3 次。极量：1 次 30mg。<br>Subcutaneous injection: 6 ~ 12mg singly. Oral medication: 5 ~ 15mg singly, 3 times a day; maximum dose: 30mg singly. |
| 剂型、规格<br>Preparations | 片剂：每片 5mg。<br>注射液：20ml（1ml）。<br>栓剂：20mg。<br>Tablets: 5mg per tablet.<br>Injection: 20ml (1ml).<br>Suppository: 20mg. |
| 药品名称 Drug Names | 荷包牡丹碱 Dicentrine |
| 适应证<br>Indications | 有一定镇痛、镇静作用。用于头痛、腰痛、牙痛、小手术后疼痛及神经衰弱。<br>It has certain effect on analgesia and sedation. It is used for headache, lumbago, toothache, pain after minor surgery and neurasthenia. |
| 用法、用量<br>Dosage | 口服：1 次 20 ~ 60mg。<br>Oral medication: 20 ~ 60mg singly. |
| 剂型、规格<br>Preparations | 片剂：每片 20mg。<br>Tablets: 20mg per tablet. |
| 药品名称 Drug Names | 山豆碱 Total Alkaloids of Sophora Tonkinesis |
| 适应证<br>Indications | 用于慢性气管炎、哮喘、咽喉肿痛、关节痛等。<br>It is used for chronic bronchitis, asthma, sore throat, and joint pain, etc. |
| 用法、用量<br>Dosage | 肌内注射每次 2ml，一日 2 次。<br>Intramuscular injection: 2ml singly, twice a day. |
| 剂型、规格<br>Preparations | 注射液：10mg（2ml）。<br>Injection: 10mg (2ml). |
| 药品名称 Drug Names | 匹米诺定 Piminodine |
| 适应证<br>Indications | 用于术前给药，胆囊炎合并胆石、胰腺炎、癌症等引起的剧痛。<br>It is used for preoperative administration, and the severe pain caused by cholecystitis with gallstone, pancreatitis and cancer. |
| 用法、用量<br>Dosage | 皮下注射或肌内注射：1 次 10 ~ 20mg，必要时每 4 小时 1 次。口服：1 次 25 ~ 50mg。有成瘾性。<br>Subcutaneous or intramuscular injection: 10 ~ 20mg singly, if necessary, once every four hours. Oral medication: 25 ~ 50mg singly.The drugs have addictive nature. |
| 剂型、规格<br>Preparations | 片剂：每片 25mg；<br>注射液：10mg（1ml）。<br>Tablets: 25mg per tablet.<br>Injection: 10mg (1ml). |
| 药品名称 Drug Names | 西马嗪 Simazine |
| 适应证<br>Indications | 用于术后、外伤性疼痛。<br>It is used for postoperative pain and traumatic pain. |
| 用法、用量<br>Dosage | 口服：每次 0.4 ~ 0.8g。小儿酌减。<br>Oral medication: 0.4 ~ 0.8g singly. Children need appropriate dose reduction. |
| 剂型、规格<br>Preparations | 片剂：每片 0.4g。<br>Tablets: 0.4g per tablet. |

| 药品名称 Drug Names | 千金藤啶碱 Stepholidine |
|---|---|
| 适应证<br>Indications | 用于血管性头痛、偏头痛、多动性运动障碍、儿童多动秽语综合征。<br>It is used for vascular headache, migraine, hyperkinetic dyskinesia and children tourette syndrome. |
| 用法、用量<br>Dosage | 预防血管性头痛：1 次 25 ～ 75mg，一日 3 次，餐后服。治疗急性发作：1 次 15 ～ 100mg，顿服。治疗多动性运动障碍：25 ～ 100mg，一日 3 次，餐后服。儿童用量按成人量的 1/3 ～ 1/2 计量。<br>Vascular headache Prevention: 25 ～ 75mg singly, three times a day, after meals. Acute attack: 15 ～ 100mg singly, at a draught. Hyperactivity dyskinesia: 25 ～ 100mg singly, three times a day, after meals. Children dose is 1/3 to 1/2 of adult dose. |
| 剂型、规格<br>Preparations | 片剂：每片 25mg。<br>Tablets: 25mg per tablet. |
| 药品名称 Drug Names | 高乌甲素 Lappaconitine |
| 适应证<br>Indications | 用于中度以上疼痛、术后疼痛、坐骨神经痛。<br>It is used for moderate to severe pain, postoperative pain and sciatica. |
| 用法、用量<br>Dosage | 口服：每次 5 ～ 10mg，一日 1 ～ 3 次。肌内注射或静脉滴注，每次 4mg，一日 1 ～ 2 次。<br>Oral medication: 5 ～ 10mg singly, three times a day. Intramuscular injection or intravenous infusion: 4mg singly, 1~2 times a day. |
| 剂型、规格<br>Preparations | 片剂：每片 5mg。<br>注射液：4mg（2ml）。<br>Tablets: 5mg per tablet.<br>Injection: 4mg (2ml). |
| 药品名称 Drug Names | 美西麦角 Methysergide |
| 适应证<br>Indications | 用于预防反复发作的偏头痛。对急性头痛发作无效。<br>It is used for the prevention of recurrent migraine. And it has no effect on acute headache. |
| 用法、用量<br>Dosage | 起始剂量 1 ～ 2mg，一日 2 次；每 3 ～ 4 周增加 1 ～ 2mg；疗程不宜超过 6 个月。宜间断用药，每 6 个月停药 3 周以上。<br>The starting dose is 1 ～ 2mg, twice a day; increase 1 ～ 2mg every 3~4 weeks; the course of treatment should not exceed 6 months. It is appropriate to receive intermittent therapy, it needs withdrawal for over three weeks every six months. |
| 剂型、规格<br>Preparations | 片剂：每片 1mg。<br>Tablets: 1mg per tablet. |
| 药品名称 Drug Names | 氨酚氢可酮 Paracetamol and Hydrocodone Bitartrate |
| 适应证<br>Indications | 本品用于缓解中度到中重度头痛。<br>This drug is used to relieve moderate to severe headache. |
| 用法、用量<br>Dosage | 每 4 ～ 6 小时 1 ～ 2 片，24 小时的总用药量不应超过 5 片。<br>1~2 tablets singly, every 4~6 hours, with total dose of 5 tablets within 24hours. |
| 剂型、规格<br>Preparations | 片剂：每片含重酒石酸氢可酮 5mg、对乙酰氨基酚 500mg。<br>Tablets: 5mg of hydrocodone bitartrate and 500mg of acetaminophen contained per tablet. |

8.3　解热镇痛抗炎药 Nonsteroidal antiinflammatory drugs

| 药品名称 Drug Names | 阿司匹林 Aspirin |
|---|---|
| 适应证<br>Indications | （1）用于发热、头痛、神经痛、肌肉痛、风湿热、急性风湿性关节炎及类风湿关节炎等，为风湿热，风湿性关节炎及类风湿关节炎首选药，可迅速缓解急性风湿性关节炎的症状。对急性风湿热伴有心肌炎者，可合用皮质激素。<br>（2）用于痛风。<br>（3）预防心肌梗死、动脉血栓、动脉粥样硬化等。 |

|  |  |
|---|---|
|  | （4）用于治疗胆道蛔虫病（有效率 90% 以上）。<br><br>（5）粉剂外用可治足癣。<br><br>（6）儿科用于皮肤黏膜淋巴结综合征（川崎病）的治疗。<br><br>(1) It is used for fever, headache, neuralgia, muscle pain, rheumatic fever, acute rheumatic arthritis and rheumatoid arthritis. It is the prior choice for rheumatic fever, rheumatic arthritis and rheumatoid arthritis, because it can relieve symptoms of acute rheumatic arthritis quickly. For acute rheumatic fever patients with myocarditis, the drug should be combined with corticosteroids. It also can be used for.<br><br>(2) gout;<br><br>(3) prevention of myocardial infarction, arterial thrombosis, atherosclerosis and so on; and.treatment of<br><br>(4) biliary ascariasis (effect rate is more than 90%).<br><br>(5) External use of powder can cure tinea pedis.<br><br>(6) For children, it can be used in treatment of mucocutaneous lymph node syndrome (Kawasaki disease). |
| 用法、用量<br>Dosage | （1）解热阵痛：①口服，每次 0.3 ~ 0.6g，一日 3 次，或需要时服。②直肠给药：1 次 0.3 ~ 0.6g，一日 0.9 ~ 1.8g；儿童 1 ~ 3 岁，1 次 0.1g，一日 1 次；3 ~ 6 岁，1 次 0.1 ~ 0.15g，一日 1 ~ 2 次；6 岁以上，1 次 0.15 ~ 0.3g，一日 2 次。<br><br>（2）抗风湿：1 次 0.6 ~ 1g，一日 3 ~ 4g。服时宜嚼碎，并可与碳酸钙或氢氧化铝或复方氢氧化铝（胃舒平）合用以减少对胃的刺激。1 个疗程为 3 个月左右。小儿一日 0.1g/kg，分 3 次服，前 3 日先服半量以减少不良反应。<br><br>（3）抑制血小板聚集：预防心肌梗死、动脉血栓、动脉粥样硬化，一日 1 次，每次 75 ~ 150mg。<br><br>（4）治疗胆道蛔虫病：每次 1g，一日 2 ~ 3 次，连用 2 ~ 3 日。当阵发性绞痛停止 24 小时后即停药，然后再行常规驱虫。<br><br>（5）治疗 X 射线照射或放疗引起的腹泻：每次服 0.6 ~ 0.9g，一日 4 次。<br><br>（6）预防旁路移植术后再狭窄：每次服 50mg。<br><br>（7）治疗足癣：先用温开水或 1 ∶ 5000 的高锰酸钾溶液洗涤患处，然后用本品粉末撒布患处，一般 2 ~ 4 次可愈。<br><br>（8）用于小儿皮肤黏膜淋巴结综合征：开始每日按 80 ~ 100mg/kg，分 3 ~ 4 次服，热退 2 ~ 3 日后改为每日 30mg/kg，每 3 ~ 4 次服，连服 2 个月或更久。血小板增多、血液呈高凝状态期间，每日 5 ~ 10mg/kg，1 次顿服。<br><br>(1) Antipyresis and analgesia: ① by oral medication, give 0.3 ~ 0.6g singly, 3 times a day or give when necessary. ② by rectal administration : give 0.3 ~ 0.6g singly, 0.9 ~ 1.8g a day; for children from 1 to 3 years old, give 0.1g singly, once a day; from 3 to 6 years old, give 0.1 ~ 0.15g singly, 1~2 times a day; over 6 years old, give 0.15 ~ 0.3g singly, twice a day.<br><br>(2) Anti-rheumatism: give 0.6 ~ 1g singly, 3 ~ 4g a day; take this medicine need chewing; when take with calcium carbonate, aluminum hydroxide or aluminum hydroxide compound (gastropine ) can reduce stomach irritation. A course of treatment is about three months. For children, give 0.1g/kg a day, in 3 divided doses; in the first 3 days, give half dose to reduce adverse reaction.<br><br>(3) Platelet aggregation inhibition : for the prevention of myocardial infarction, arterial thrombosis and atherosclerosis, give 75 ~ 150mg singly, once a day.<br><br>(4) Biliary ascariasis: give 1g singly, 2~3 times a day, for continuous 2~3 days; drug withdrawal is required when paroxysmal pain stops after 24 hours, then receive routine deworming.<br><br>(5) Diarrhea by X -ray irradiation or radiotherapy: give 0.6 ~ 0.9g singly, 4 times a day.<br><br>(6) Prevention of restenosis after bypass : give 50mg singly.<br><br>(7) Tinea pedis: first wash the affected part with warm water or 1 ∶ 5000 potassium permanganate solution, and then use this powder smear over the affected part; usually 2~4 times of administration can be cured.<br><br>(8) Children's mucocutaneous lymph node syndrome: give starting dose of 80 ~ 100mg/kg a day, in 3~4 divided doses; 2~3 days after the fever reduction, change to 30mg/kg a day, in 3 ~4 divided doses, for two continuous months or longer . When thrombocyte increases or blood keeps hypercoagulability, give 5 ~ 10mg/kg a day, at a draught. |

续　表

| 剂型、规格<br>Preparations | 片剂：每片 0.05g；0.1g；0.2g；0.3g；0.5g。<br>泡腾片：每片 0.3g；0.5g。放于温水 150 ～ 250ml 中，溶化后饮下。<br>肠溶片（胶囊）：每片（粒）40mg；0.15g；0.3g；0.5g。对胃刺激小，适于长期大量服用。<br>散剂：每袋 0.1g；0.5g。<br>栓剂：每粒 0.1g；0.3g；0.45g；0.5g。<br>Tablets: 0.05g, 0.1g, 0.2g, 0.3g, 0.5g per tablet.<br>Effervescent tablets: 0.3g, 0.5g per tablet; put in 150 ～ 250ml of warm water and drink after melting.<br>Enteric-coated tablets (capsules): 40mg, 0.15g, 0.3g, 0.5g per tablet (capsule); it is suitable for large doses of long-term use because of its weak stimulation to stomach.<br>Powder: 0.1g, 0.5g per bag.<br>Suppositories: 0.1g, 0.3g, 0.45g, 0.5g of each. |
|---|---|
| 药品名称 Drug Names | 阿司匹林精氨酸盐 Aspirinarginine |
| 适应证<br>Indications | 主要用于发热、头痛、神经痛、牙痛、肌肉痛及活动性风湿病、类风湿关节炎、创伤及术后疼痛。<br>It is mainly used for fever, headache, neuralgia, toothache, muscle pain and active rheumatism, rheumatoid arthritis, traumatic pain and postoperative pain. |
| 用法、用量<br>Dosage | 肌内注射：成人每次 1g，一日 1 ～ 2 次，或依病情按医嘱用药，儿童 10 ～ 25mg/kg。临时用，每瓶内加入 0.9% 氯化钠生理盐水或加入灭菌注射用水 2 ～ 4ml，溶解后注入。<br>Intramuscular injection: give adults 1g singly, 1~2 times a day or follow doctors' advice based on patients' condition; give children 10 ～ 25mg/kg. For temporary use, add 2 ～ 4ml of 0.9% sodium chloride saline or sterile water for injection in one injection and make injection after dissolution. |
| 剂型、规格<br>Preparations | 注射用阿司匹林精氨酸盐：每瓶 0.5g（相当阿司匹林 0.25g）；1g（相当于阿司匹林 0.5g）。<br>Aspirin arginine for injection: 0.5g (equivalent to 0.25g of aspirin), 1g (equivalent to 0.5g of aspirin). |
| 药品名称 Drug Names | 阿司匹林赖氨酸盐 Aspirin-DL-lysine |
| 适应证<br>Indications | 主要用于发热及轻、中度的疼痛，如上呼吸道感染引起的发热、手术后痛、癌性疼痛、风湿痛、关节痛及神经痛等。<br>It is mainly used for fever, mild pain and moderate pain, such as fever caused by respiratory infection, postoperative pain, cancer pain, arthritis pain, joint pain and neuralgia. |
| 用法、用量<br>Dosage | 肌内注射或静脉滴注：每次 0.9 ～ 1.8g，一日 2 次；儿童 1 日 10 ～ 25mg/kg。以 0.9% 氯化钠注射液溶解后静脉滴注。<br>Intramuscular injection or intravenous infusion: give 0.9 ～ 1.8g singly, twice a day; give children 10 ～ 25mg/kg a day; dissolve the drug in 0.9% sodium chloride injection for intravenous infusion. |
| 剂型、规格<br>Preparations | 注射用阿司匹林赖氨酸盐：每瓶 0.9g（相当于阿司匹林 0.5g）；0.5g（相当于阿司匹林 0.28g）。<br>Aspirin-DL-lysine for injection: 0.9g (equivalent to 0.5g of aspirin); 0.5g (equivalent to 0.28g of aspirin). |
| 药品名称 Drug Names | 美沙拉秦 Mesalazine |
| 适应证<br>Indications | 适用于溃疡性结肠炎和克罗恩病。<br>It is intended to treat Crohn's disease and ulcerative colitis. |
| 用法、用量<br>Dosage | 口服：可用一杯水送服或在就餐时吞服。溃疡性结肠炎：急性期，每次 1 ～ 2 袋，一日 3 ～ 4 次（4g/d，8 袋）；缓解期，每次 1 袋，一日 3 ～ 4 次（2g/d，4 袋）。克罗恩病：缓解期，每次 1 袋，一日 3 ～ 4 次（2g/d，4 袋）。<br>Oral medication: it can be taken with a glass of water or swallowed during a meal. Ulcerative colitis: in acute phase, give 1 to 2 bags singly, 3 to 4 times a day (4g a day, 8 bags); in remission phase, give1 bag singly, 3 to 4 times a day (2g a day, 4 bags). Crohn's disease: in remission phase, give1 bag singly, 3 to 4 times a day (2g a day, 4 bags). |
| 剂型、规格<br>Preparations | 缓释颗粒剂：每袋 500mg。<br>Sustained-release granules: 500mg per bag. |

**续　表**

| 药品名称 Drug Names | 对乙酰氨基酚 Paracetamol |
|---|---|
| 适应证<br>Indications | 　　用于感冒发热、关节痛、神经痛及偏头痛、癌性痛及手术后镇痛。本品还可用于对阿司匹林过敏、不耐受或不适于应用阿司匹林的患者（水痘、血友病以及其他出血性疾病等）。<br><br>　　It is used for fever, joint pain, neuralgia, migraine, cancer pain and postoperative pain. It also can be used to patients who are allergic to, intolerance to or unsuitable for Aspirin (varicella, hemophilia and other bleeding disorders, etc.). |
| 用法、用量<br>Dosage | 　　口服：1 次 0.3 ~ 0.6g，一日 0.6 ~ 1.8g，一日量不宜超过 2g，1 个疗程不宜超过 10 日；儿童 12 岁以下按一日 1.5g/m² 分次服（如按年龄计：2 ~ 3 岁，一次 160mg；4 ~ 5 岁，一次 240mg；6 ~ 8 岁，一次 320mg；9 ~ 10 岁，一次 400mg；11 岁，一次 480mg。每 4 小时或必要时服一次）。肌内注射：1 次 0.15 ~ 0.25g。直肠给药：1 次 0.3 ~ 0.6g，一日 1 ~ 2 次。3 ~ 12 岁小儿，一次 0.15 ~ 0.3g，一日 1 次。<br><br>　　Oral medication: give0.3 ~ 0.6g singly, 0.6 ~ 1.8g a day; daily dose should not exceed 2g and a course of treatment should not exceed 10 days; for children under the age of 12, give 1.5g/m² a day, in several divided doses (for example, according to age: 2 to 3 years old, 160mg singly; 4 ~ 5 years old, 240mg singly; 6 ~ 8 years old, 320mg singly; 9 ~ 10 years old, 400mg singly; 11 years old, 480mg singly, every four hours or give once when necessary). Intramuscular injection: give 0.15 ~ 0.25g singly. Rectal administration: give 0.3 ~ 0.6g singly, 1 to 2 times a day; for children from 3 to 12 years old, give 0.15 ~ 0.3g a day, once a day. |
| 剂型、规格<br>Preparations | 　　片剂：每片 0.3g；0.5g。<br>　　胶囊剂：每粒 0.3g。<br>　　咀嚼片：每片 80mg。<br>　　泡腾冲剂：每袋 0.1g；0.5g。<br>　　口服液：每支 0.25g（10ml）。<br>　　栓剂：每粒 0.15g；0.3g；0.6g。<br>　　注射液：每支 0.075g（1ml）；0.25g（2ml）。<br>　　凝胶剂：每支 120mg（5g）。<br>Tablets: 0.3g, 0.5g per tablet.<br>Capsules: 0.3g per capsule.<br>Chewable Tablets: 80mg per tablet.<br>Effervescent granules: 0.1g, 0.5g per bag.<br>Oral liquid: 0.25g (10ml) of each.<br>Suppositories: 0.15g, 0.3g, 0.6g of each.<br>Injection: 0.075g (1ml), 0.25g (2ml) per vial.<br>Gel: 120mg (5g) of each. |
| 药品名称 Drug Names | 吲哚美辛 Indometacin |
| 适应证<br>Indications | 　　（1）急、慢性风湿性关节炎、痛风性关节炎及癌性疼痛。也可用于滑囊炎、腱鞘炎及关节囊炎等。还用于恶性肿瘤引起的发热或其他难以控制的发热。因本品不良反应较大，不宜作为治疗关节炎的首选药物，仅用于其他 NSAIDs 治疗无效的或不能耐受的患者。<br>　　（2）抗血小板聚集，可防止血栓形成，但疗效不如阿司匹林。<br>　　（3）治疗 Behcet 综合征，退热效果好；用于 Batter 综合征，效果尤其显著。<br>　　（4）用于胆绞痛、输尿管结石症引起的绞痛；对偏头痛也有一定的疗效，也可用于月经痛。<br>　　（5）本药滴眼液用于眼科手术及非手术因素引起的非感染性炎症。<br><br>　　(1) It can be used for acute and chronic rheumatic arthritis, gouty arthritis and cancer pain, as well as bursitis, tenosynovitis and capsulitis, etc.. It is also used to pyrexia caused by malignancy or pyrexia which is difficult to control. This drug has serious adverse reaction, so it is not the first choice in the treatment of arthritis and only used for patients who are resistant or intolerant to other NSAIDs therapy.<br>　　(2) It is used for anti-platelet aggregation and thrombosis prevention, but the effect is not as good as aspirin.<br>　　(3) It is intended to treat Behcet syndrome, with a good effect of fever reduction, and it has significant effect at Batter's syndrome.<br>　　(4) It is used for colic pain caused by ureteral lithiasis; it has a certain effect on migraine, as well as dysmenorrhea.<br>　　(5) The drug's eye drops is used for non-infectious inflammation caused by eye surgery or non-surgical factors. |

续　表

| 用法、用量<br>Dosage | 　　口服。开始时每次服25mg，一日2～3次，饭时或饭后立即服用（可减少胃肠道不良反应）。治疗风湿性关节炎等症时，如未见不良反应，可逐渐增至100～150mg，一日最大量不超过150mg，分3～4次服用，现已采用胶丸或栓剂剂型，使胃肠道不良反应发生率降低，栓剂且有维持药效较长的特点。直肠给药，1次50mg，一日50～100mg，一般连用10日为1个疗程。控释胶囊：一日1次，每次75mg，或1次25mg，一日2次。必要时1次75mg，一日2次。小儿口服常用量：每日按1.5～2.5mg/kg，分3～4次，有效后减至最低量。乳膏剂涂擦按摩患处，一日2～3次。经眼给药：眼科手术前：1次1滴，术前3、2、1和0.5小时各滴一次。眼科手术后：1次1滴，一日1～4次。其他非感染性炎症：1次1滴，一日4～6次。<br><br>　　Oral medication: in the beginning, give 25mg singly, 2 or 3 times a day, during meals or after meals immediately (to reduce gastrointestinal side effect). In treatment of rheumatic arthritis, if there is no adverse reaction, the dose can be gradually increased to 100～150mg, but the maximum dose should not exceed 150mg, in 3 to 4 divided doses. Now capsules or suppositories have been used in treatment, which can reduce the gastrointestinal adverse reaction and suppositories has longer pharmacodynamic effect. Rectal administration: give 50mg singly, 50～100mg a day; generally, a course of treatment is 10 days. Controlled Release Capsules: give 75mg singly, once day or 25mg singly, twice a day; give 75mg, twice a day, if necessary. Usual Oral dose for children: give 1.5～2.5mg/kg, in 3 to 4 divided doses; reduce to the minimum dose when the drug takes effect. Creams: smear over the affected area, 2 or 3 times a day. Ocular administration: 1 drop singly, 3 hours, 2 hours, 1 hour and half an hour before eye surgery respectively: 1 drop singly, 1 to 4 times a day, after eye surgery. Other non-infectious inflammation: 1 drop singly, 4 to 6 times a day. |
|---|---|
| 剂型、规格<br>Preparations | 肠溶片：每片25mg。<br>胶囊：25mg。<br>胶丸：每丸25mg。<br>控释胶囊：每粒25mg；75mg。<br>控释片：每片25mg；50mg；75mg。<br>贴片：每片12.5mg。<br>栓剂：每粒25mg；50mg；100mg。<br>乳膏剂：每支100mg（10g）。<br>滴眼液：8ml；40mg。<br>Enteric-coated tablets: 25mg per tablet.<br>Capsules: 25mg.<br>Gelatin pearl: 25mg of each.<br>Controlled Release Capsules: 25mg, 75mg per capsule.<br>Release tablets: 25mg, 50mg, 75mg per tablet.<br>Patch: 125mg of each.<br>Suppositories: 25mg, 50mg, 100mg of each.<br>Creams: 100mg (10g) of each.<br>Drops: 8ml: 40mg. |
| 药品名称 Drug Names | 双氯芬酸 Diclofenac |
| 适应证<br>Indications | 　　用于类风湿关节炎、神经炎、红斑狼疮及癌症、手术后疼痛，各种原因引起的发热。<br>　　It is used to treat rheumatoid arthritis, neuritis, lupus erythematosus, cancer pain, postoperative pain and fever caused by various reasons. |
| 用法、用量<br>Dosage | 　　口服：成人，每日剂量为100～150mg，分2～3次服用。对轻度患者以及14岁以上的青少年酌减。此药最好在餐前用水整片送下。肌内注射深部注射，1次50mg，一日1次，必要时数小时后再注射1次。外用：搽剂，根据疼痛部位大小，1～3ml均匀涂于患处，一日2～4次，一日总量不超过15ml。乳膏，根据疼痛部位大小，1次2～4g涂于患处，并轻轻按摩，一日3～4次，一日总量不超过30g。<br>　　Oral medication: for adults, give daily dose of 100mg～150mg, in 2~3 divided doses; for patients with mild disease and adolescents over the age of 14, reduce the dose appropriately. It had better swallow whole tablet with water before meals. Intramuscular deep injection: give 50mg singly, once a day; |

**续　表**

| | |
|---|---|
| | repeat the injection several hours later, if necessary. External use: by liniment, according to the size of the affected area, smear 1 ~ 3ml evenly to the affected area, 2~4 times a day; the total daily does can not exceed 15ml. Cream: according to the size of affected area, smear 2 ~ 4g over the affected area and give a massage gently, 3~4 times a day; the total daily does can not exceed 30g. |
| 剂型、规格<br>Preparations | 片剂：每片 25mg。<br>搽剂：20ml：200mg。<br>乳膏：25g：750mg。<br>注射液：50mg（2ml）。<br><br>Tablets: 25mg per tablet.<br>Liniment: 20ml: 200mg.<br>Cream: 25g: 750mg.<br>Injection: 50mg (2ml). |
| 药品名称 Drug Names | 萘普生 Naproxen |
| 适应证<br>Indications | 用于类风湿关节炎、骨关节炎、强直性脊柱炎、痛风、运动系统（如关节、肌肉及肌腱）的慢性变性疾病及轻、中度疼痛如痛经等。<br><br>It is used for rheumatoid arthritis, osteoarthritis, ankylosing spondylitis, gout and chronic degenerative diseases of locomotor system (such as joint, muscle and tendon), as well as mild pain and moderate pain, such as dysmenorrhea. |
| 用法、用量<br>Dosage | 口服，开始每日剂量 0.5 ~ 0.75g，维持量每日 0.375 ~ 0.75g，分早晨和傍晚 2 次服用。轻、中度疼痛或痛经时，开始用 0.5g，必需时 6 ~ 8 小时后再服 0.25g，日剂量不超过 1.25g。肌内注射，一次 100 ~ 200mg，一日 1 次。栓剂直肠给药，一次 0.25g，一日 0.5g。<br><br>Oral medication: begin with 0.5 ~ 0.75g a day; give maintenance dose of 0.375 ~ 0.75g, in two divided doses (in the morning and evening). For mild pain, moderate pain or dysmenorrhea, start with 0.5g and give another 0.25g 6~8 hours later, if necessary; the daily dose can not exceed 1.25g. Intramuscular injection: give 100 ~ 200mg singly, once a day. Rectal suppository administration: give 0.25g singly, 0.5g a day. |
| 剂型、规格<br>Preparations | 片（胶囊）剂：每片（粒）0.1g；0.125g；0.25g。<br>缓释胶囊（片）：每粒（片）0.25g。<br>注射液：每支 100mg（2ml）；200mg（2ml）。<br>栓剂：每粒 0.25g。<br><br>Tablets (capsules): 0.1g, 0.125g, 0.25g per tablet (capsule).<br>Release capsules (tablets): 0.25g per capsule (tablet).<br>Injection: 100mg (2ml), 200mg (2ml) per vial.<br>Suppositories: 0.25g of each. |
| 药品名称 Drug Names | 布洛芬 Ibuprofen |
| 适应证<br>Indications | 用于风湿性及类风湿关节炎，其抗炎、镇痛、解热作用与阿司匹林、保泰松相似，比对乙酰氨基酚好。在患者不能耐受阿司匹林、保泰松等时，可试用。<br><br>It is used for rheumatic and rheumatoid arthritis. In anti-inflammation, analgesia and antipyretic effect, it is similar with aspirin and phenylbutazone but better than acetaminophen. If patients are intolerant to aspirin and phenylbutazone, this drug can be used. |
| 用法、用量<br>Dosage | 抗风湿，一次 0.4 ~ 0.8g，一日 3 ~ 4 次。镇痛，一次 0.2 ~ 0.4g，每 4 ~ 6 小时一次。成人最大限量一日 2.4g。<br><br>Anti-rheumatism: give 0.4 ~ 0.8g singly, 3 to 4 times a day. Pain relief: give 0.2 ~ 0.4g singly, every 4 to 6 hours. The maximum dose for adult is 2.4g a day. |

续　表

| 剂型、规格<br>Preparations | 片剂（胶囊）：每片（粒）0.1g；0.2g；0.3g。缓释胶囊：每粒 0.3g。<br>颗粒剂：每袋 0.1g；0.2g。<br>干混悬剂：每瓶 1.2g（34g）。<br>糖浆剂：每支 0.2g（10ml）。<br>口服液：每支 0.1g（10ml）。<br>混悬剂：每瓶 2.0g（100ml）。<br>搽剂：每瓶 2.5g（50ml）。<br>栓剂：每粒 50mg；100mg。<br>Tablets (capsules): 0.1g, 0.2g, 0.3g per tablet (capsule).<br>Release capsules: 0.3g capsule.<br>Granules: 0.1g, 0.2g per bag.<br>Dry suspensions: 1.2g (34g) of each.<br>Syrup: 0.2g (10ml) of each.<br>Oral liquid: 0.1g (10ml) of each.<br>Suspension: 2.0g (100ml) of each.<br>Liniment: 2.5g (50ml) of each.<br>Suppositories: 50mg, 100mg of each. |
|---|---|
| 药品名称 Drug Names | 酮洛芬 Ketoprofen |
| 适应证<br>Indications | 用于类风湿关节炎、风湿性关节炎、骨关节炎、强直性脊柱炎及痛风等。本品治疗关节炎时，连续用药 2～3 周可达最佳疗效。<br>It is used for rheumatoid arthritis, rheumatic arthritis, osteoarthritis, ankylosing spondylitis and gout. It will achieve the best effect if it is continually used for 2~3 weeks in treatment of rheumatic arthritis. |
| 用法、用量<br>Dosage | 口服：每次 50mg，一日 150mg，分 3～4 次；每日最大用量 200mg，或每次 100mg，一日 2 次，为避免对胃肠道刺激，应餐后服用，整个胶囊吞服。<br>Oral medication: give 50mg singly, 150mg a day, in 3 to 4 divided doses; daily maximum dose is 200mg; or give 100mg singly, twice a day; in order to avoid gastrointestinal irritation, take after meals by swallowing the whole. |
| 剂型、规格<br>Preparations | 肠溶胶囊：每粒 20mg；50mg。<br>控释胶囊：每粒 20mg。<br>缓释片：每片 75mg。<br>搽剂：每支 0.3g（10ml）；0.9g（30ml）；1.5g（50ml）。<br>Enteric-coated capsules: 20mg, 50mg per capsule.<br>Controlled Release Capsules: 20mg per capsule.<br>Sustained-release tablets: 75mg per tablet.<br>Liniment: 0.3g (10ml), 0.9g (30ml), 1.5g (50ml) of each. |
| 药品名称 Drug Names | 芬布芬 Fenbufen |
| 适应证<br>Indications | 用于类风湿关节炎、风湿性关节炎、骨关节炎、强直性脊柱炎及痛风等。应用于牙痛、手术后疼痛、外伤疼痛等的镇痛。<br>It is used for rheumatoid arthritis, rheumatic arthritis, osteoarthritis, ankylosing spondylitis and gout. It is also used for toothache, postoperative pain and traumatic pain, etc. |
| 用法、用量<br>Dosage | 口服，成人一次 0.6～0.9g，一次或分次服用。多数患者晚上口服 0.6g 即可。分次服用时，每日总量不得超过 0.9g。<br>Oral medication: give adults 0.6～0.9g singly, in 1 dose or several divided doses; most patients only need orally 0.6g at night for once; when given in divided doses, the total dose can not exceed 0.9g. |
| 剂型、规格<br>Preparations | 片剂：每片 0.15g；0.3g。<br>胶囊剂：每粒 0.5g。<br>Tablets: 0.15g, 0.3g per tablet.<br>Capsules: 0.5g per capsule. |

**续　表**

| 药品名称 Drug Names | 吡洛芬 Pirprofen |
|---|---|
| 适应证<br>Indications | 用于风湿性关节炎、骨关节炎、强直性脊柱炎、非关节型风湿病、急性疼痛、术后痛及癌性痛等。<br><br>It is used for rheumatic arthritis, osteoarthritis, ankylosing spondylitis, non-articular rheumatism, acute pain, postoperative pain and cancer pain. |
| 用法、用量<br>Dosage | 开始口服，每日 800mg，一次 2 次分服。症状改善后，每日 600mg 维持。类风湿关节炎、强直性脊柱炎开始 1000mg/d，分 3 次服，持续 1～2 周。镇痛：每次 200～400mg，一日 1200mg。肌内注射每次 400mg。数小时后可重复使用。<br><br>Oral medication: start with 800mg a day, in 2 divided doses; give maintenance dose of 600mg a day when symptoms get improved.. In treatment of rheumatoid arthritis and ankylosing spondylitis, start with 1000mg a day, in 3 divided doses, for 1 to 2 weeks. In analgesia, give 200 to 400mg singly, 1200mg a day. Intramuscular injection: give 400mg singly; repeat the dose a few hours later. |
| 剂型、规格<br>Preparations | 片剂：每片 200mg。<br>Tablets: 200mg per tablet. |
| 药品名称 Drug Names | 阿明洛芬 Alminoprofen |
| 适应证<br>Indications | 用于风湿性和类风湿关节炎、神经根痛、肌腱炎、创伤（骨折、挫伤、扭伤）、痛经、产后子宫绞痛、牙痛、中耳炎等。<br><br>It is used to treat rheumatic and rheumatoid arthritis, nerve root pain, tendonitis, trauma (fractures, contusions and sprains), dysmenorrhea, postpartum uterine cramps, toothache and otitis media. |
| 用法、用量<br>Dosage | 口服，成人每次 300mg，一日 2～3 次，可根据疗效酌情减量。治疗子宫绞痛时，每日 300～600mg 分 2 次餐前服。<br><br>Oral medication: give adults 300mg singly, 2 to 3 times a day; reduce the dose according to curative effect. In treatment of uterine cramps, give 300～600mg a day, in 2 divided doses, before meals. |
| 剂型、规格<br>Preparations | 片剂：每片 150mg；300mg。<br>Tablets: 150mg, 300mg per tablet. |
| 药品名称 Drug Names | 洛索洛芬 Loxoprofen |
| 适应证<br>Indications | 用于类风湿关节炎、变形性关节炎、腰痛、关节周围炎、颈肩腕综合征，以及手术后、外伤后和拔牙后的镇痛抗炎，急性上呼吸道炎症和解热镇痛。<br><br>It is used to treat rheumatoid arthritis, deformed arthritis, lumbago, periarthritis, neck, shoulder and wrist syndrome, analgesia and anti-inflammation after surgery, trauma and tooth extraction; as well as acute upper respiratory tract inflammation and antipyretic pain. |
| 用法、用量<br>Dosage | 餐后服用。慢性炎症疼痛：成人一次 60mg，一日 3 次。急性炎症疼痛：顿服 60～120mg。可根据年龄、症状适当增减，一次最大剂量不超过 180mg。<br><br>Take the drug after meals. Chronic inflammatory pain: give adults 60mg 3 times a day. Acute inflammatory pain: give 60～120mg, at a draught. Make dose adjustment according to age and patients' condition. The single maximum dose can not exceed 180mg. |
| 剂型、规格<br>Preparations | 片剂：每片 60mg。<br>胶囊：每粒 60mg。<br>颗粒剂：2g：60mg。<br><br>Tablets: 60mg per tablet.<br>Capsules: 60mg per capsule.<br>Granules: 2g: 60mg. |
| 药品名称 Drug Names | 吡罗昔康 Piroxicam |
| 适应证<br>Indications | 用于治疗风湿性及类风湿关节炎。<br>It is intended to treat rheumatic and rheumatoid arthritis. |

续　表

| | |
|---|---|
| 用法、用量<br>Dosage | 口服：抗风湿，一日 20mg，一日 1 次；抗痛风，一日 40mg，一日 1 次，连续 4 ～ 6 日。<br>肌内注射：一次 10 ～ 20mg，一日 1 次。<br><br>Oral medication: in anti-rheumatism, give 20mg a day, once a day; in anti-gout, give 40mg a day, once a day, for 4 to 6 days. Intramuscular injection: give 10 ～ 20mg singly, once a day. |
| 剂型、规格<br>Preparations | 片（胶囊）剂：每片（粒）10mg；20mg。<br>注射液：每支 10mg（1ml）；20mg（2ml）。<br>凝胶剂：每支 50mg（10g）；60mg（12g）。<br>搽剂：每支 0.5g（50ml）。<br>软膏：每支 0.1g（10g）。<br><br>Tablets (capsules): 10mg, 20mg per tablet (capsule).<br>Injection: 10mg (1ml), 20mg (2ml) per vial.<br>Gel: 50mg (10g), 60mg (12g) of each.<br>Liniment: 0.5g (50ml) of each.<br>Ointment: 0.1g (10g) of each. |
| 药品名称 Drug Names | 美洛昔康 Meloxicam |
| 适应证<br>Indications | 用于类风湿关节炎和骨关节炎的对症治疗。<br>It is used in the symptomatic treatment of rheumatoid arthritis and osteoarthritis. |
| 用法、用量<br>Dosage | 类风湿骨关节炎：成人一日 15mg，一日 1 次，根据治疗后反应，剂量可减至 7.5mg/d。骨关节炎：7.5mg/d，如果需要，剂量可增至 15mg/d。严重肾衰竭者，剂量不应超过 7.5mg/d。<br><br>Rheumatoid osteoarthritis: give adults 15mg a day, only once; the dose can be reduced to 7.5mg a day according to the response to treatment. Osteoarthritis: give 7.5mg a day; if necessary, the dose can be increased to 15mg a day; for severe renal failure patients, the dose should not exceed 7.5mg a day. |
| 剂型、规格<br>Preparations | 片剂：每片 7.5mg；15mg。<br>Tablets: 7.5mg, 15mg per tablet. |
| 药品名称 Drug Names | 氯诺昔康 Lornoxicam |
| 适应证<br>Indications | 用于妇产科矫形手术后的急性疼痛，急性坐骨神经痛及腰痛。亦可用于慢性腰疼、关节炎、类风湿关节炎和强直性脊柱炎。<br><br>It is used for acute pain after orthopedic surgery in gynecology and obstetrics, acute sciatica and lumbago, as well as chronic lumbago, arthritis, rheumatoid arthritis and ankylosing spondylitis. |
| 用法、用量<br>Dosage | 急性轻度或中度疼痛：每日剂量为 8 ～ 16mg，分 2 ～ 3 次服用；每日最大剂量为 16mg。风湿性疾病引起的关节疼痛和炎症：每日剂量为 12mg，分 2 ～ 3 次服用；服用剂量不应超过 16mg。<br><br>Acute mild or moderate pain: give daily dose of 8 ～ 16mg, in 2~3 divided doses; the maximum daily dose is 16mg. Joint pain and inflammation caused by rheumatic disease: give daily dose of 12mg, in 2 to 3 divided doses; the maximum dose should not exceed 16mg. |
| 剂型、规格<br>Preparations | 片剂：4mg。<br>Tablets: 4mg. |
| 药品名称 Drug Names | 塞来昔布 Celecoxib |
| 适应证<br>Indications | 用于急、慢性骨关节炎和类风湿关节炎。<br>It is intended to treat acute and chronic osteoarthritis, as well as rheumatoid arthritis. |
| 用法、用量<br>Dosage | 治疗关节炎，一日 200mg，分 2 次服或顿服；用于类风湿关节炎，剂量为一日 100mg 或 200mg，一日 2 次。<br><br>Arthritis: 200mg a day, in 2 divided doses or at a draught. Rheumatoid arthritis: 100mg a day or 200mg a day, twice a day. |

| 剂型、规格<br>Preparations | 胶囊：每粒 100mg。<br>Capsules: 100mg per capsule. |
|---|---|
| 药品名称 Drug Names | 帕瑞昔布 Parecoxib |
| 适应证<br>Indications | 用于术后疼痛的短期治疗。<br>It used in the short-term treatment of postoperative pain. |
| 用法、用量<br>Dosage | 成人，每次 40mg，静注或深部肌内注射，随后视需要间隔 6 ～ 12 小时给药给予 20mg 或 40mg，总剂量不超过 80mg/d。<br>Adults: give 40mg singly,, by intravenous injection or deep intravenous injection, then give 20 or 40mg with interval of 6 to 12 hours if needed; the total daily dose can not exceed 80mg a day. |
| 剂型、规格<br>Preparations | 注射粉针：每瓶 20mg；40mg。<br>Powder for injection: 20mg, 40mg of each. |
| 药品名称 Drug Names | 尼美舒利 Nimesulide |
| 适应证<br>Indications | 主要用于类风湿关节炎和骨关节炎、痛经、手术后疼痛和发热等。<br>It is mainly used for rheumatoid arthritis, osteoarthritis, dysmenorrhea, postoperative pain and fever, etc. |
| 用法、用量<br>Dosage | 口服：成人，每次 100mg，一日 2 次，餐后服用。儿童常用剂量为 5mg/（kg·d），每 2 ～ 3 次服用。老年人不需要调整剂量。<br>Oral medication: give adults 100mg singly, twice a day, after meals; give children usual dose of 5mg / (kg·d), in 2 to 3 divided doses; elder patients do not need to dose adjustment. |
| 剂型、规格<br>Preparations | 片剂：每片 50mg；100mg。<br>Tablets: 50mg, 100mg per tablet. |
| 药品名称 Drug Names | 安乃近 Metamizole Sodium |
| 适应证<br>Indications | 主要用于解热、急性关节炎、头痛、风湿性痛、牙痛及肌肉痛等。<br>It is mainly used for fever, acute arthritis, headache, rheumatic pain, toothache and muscle pain. |
| 用法、用量<br>Dosage | 口服：一次 0.25 ～ 0.5g，一日 0.75 ～ 1.25g。滴鼻：小儿退热常以 10% ～ 20% 滴鼻，5 岁以下，每次每侧鼻孔 1 ～ 2 滴，必要时重复用一次；5 岁以上适当加量。深部肌内注射：每次 0.25 ～ 0.5g，小儿每次 5 ～ 10mg/kg。<br>Oral medicaiotn: 0.25 ～ 0.5g singly, 0.75 ～ 1.25g a day. Nasal drops: in children's antifebrile treatment, usually give 10% to 20% intranasally; under the age of 5, give 1 to 2 drops respectively on both sides of the nose, with repeated dose if necessary; over the age of 5, appropriately increase the dose. Deep intramuscular injection: give 0.25 ～ 0.5g singly; give children 5 ～ 10mg/kg singly. |
| 剂型、规格<br>Preparations | 片剂：每片 0.25g；0.5g。<br>滴液：1ml：200mg。<br>注射液：每支 0.25g（1ml）；0.5g（2ml）。<br>滴鼻剂：10% ～ 20%。<br>Tablets: 0.25g, 0.5g per tablet.<br>Drops: 1ml: 200mg.<br>Injection: 0.25g (1ml), 0.5g (2ml) per vial.<br>Nasal drops: 10% ~ 20%. |
| 药品名称 Drug Names | 保泰松 Phenylbutazone |
| 适应证<br>Indications | 用于类风湿关节炎、风湿性关节炎、强直性脊柱炎及急性痛风等。常需连续使用或与其他药物配合使用。亦用于丝虫病急性淋巴管炎。<br>It is used for rheumatoid arthritis, rheumatic arthritis, ankylosing spondylitis, acute gout and so on. It is often required continuous administration or to be used in conjunction with other drugs. It also can be used in filariasis acute lymphangitis. |

**续　表**

| | |
|---|---|
| 用法、用量<br>Dosage | （1）关节炎：开始一日量 0.3 ~ 0.6g，分 3 次餐后服用。一日量不宜超过 0.8g。1 周后如无不良反应，可继续服用递减至每日量 0.1 ~ 0.2g。<br>（2）丝虫病急性淋巴管炎：每次服 0.2g，一日 3 次，总量 1.2 ~ 3g，急性炎症控制后，再用抗丝虫药治疗。<br><br>(1) Arthritis: start with 0.3 ~ 0.6g, in 3 divided doses, after meals; the daily dose should not exceed 0.8g; if there is no adverse reaction after a week, continue the administration and gradually reduce dose to 0.1~0.2g a day.<br>(2) Filariasis acute lymphangitis: give 0.2g singly, 3 times a day, with total dose of 1.2 ~ 3g; when the acute inflammation is under control, take the anti-filarial drug medication. |
| 剂型、规格<br>Preparations | 片（胶囊）剂：每片（粒）0.1g；200mg。<br>栓剂：25mg。<br>注射液：600mg（3ml）。<br>Tablets (capsules): 0.1g, 200mg per tablet (capsule).<br>Suppository: 25mg.<br>Injection: 600mg (3ml). |
| 药品名称 Drug Names | 萘丁美酮 Nabumetone |
| 适应证<br>Indications | 本品用于急、慢性关节炎，以及运动性软组织损伤、扭伤和挫伤、术后疼痛、牙痛、痛经等。<br>It is used for acute and chronic arthritis, perpetual soft tissue injuries, sprains and contusions, post-operative pain, toothache and dysmenorrhea. |
| 用法、用量<br>Dosage | 口服，每次 1g，一日 1 次，睡前服。一次最大量为 2g。体重不足 50kg 的成人，可以一日 0.5g 起始，逐渐上调至有效剂量。<br>Oral medication: give 1g singly, once a day, before sleep; the maximum single dose is 2g, in two divided doses. For adults under 50kg, start with 0.5g a day, and gradually increase to the effective dose. |
| 剂型、规格<br>Preparations | 片剂：每片 0.25g；0.5g；0.75g。<br>胶囊剂：每粒 0.2g；0.25g。<br>分散片：每片 0.5g。<br>干混悬剂：0.5g。<br>Tablets: 0.25g, 0.5g, 0.75g per tablet.<br>Capsules: 0.2g, 0.25g per capsule.<br>Dispersible tablets: 0.5g per tablet.<br>Suspension: 0.5g. |
| 药品名称 Drug Names | 来氟米特 Leflunomide |
| 适应证<br>Indications | 用于成人风湿性关节炎的治疗。<br>It is used in the treatment of adults' rheumatic arthritis. |
| 用法、用量<br>Dosage | 由于半衰期较长建议间隔 24 小时给药。建议开始最初治疗的 3 日给予负荷量（50mg/d），之后给予维持剂量 20mg/d。<br>Because of the long half-life period, it is recommended to make administration with interval of 24 hours. In the first 3 days of the treatment, it is recommended to give loading dose of 50mg a day, then give maintaining dose of 20g a day. |
| 剂型、规格<br>Preparations | 片剂：每片 10mg；20mg；100mg。<br>Tablets: 10mg, 20mg, 100mg per tablet. |
| 药品名称 Drug Names | 复方骨肽注射液 Compound Ossotide |
| 适应证<br>Indications | 用于风湿性、类风湿关节炎、骨质疏松、颈椎病等疾病的症状改善。同时用于骨折或骨科手术后骨愈合，可促进骨愈合和骨新生。<br>It is used to improve the symptoms of rheumatic and rheumatoid arthritis, osteoporosis, cervical spondylosis and so on. The drug also can be used for fractures or orthopedic bone healing after orthopedic surgery, since it can promote bone healing and bone regeneration. |

续　表

| 用法、用量<br>Dosage | 肌内注射，一次 30 ～ 60mg，一日 1 次；静脉滴注，一次 60 ～ 150mg，一日 1 次，10 ～ 30 日为 1 个疗程或遵医嘱，亦可在痛点或穴位注射。<br>Intramuscular injection: 30 ～ 60mg singly, once a day. Intravenous infusion: 60 ～ 150mg singly, once a day, for 10 to 30 days as a course or following doctors' advice; or inject in the pain point or acupuncture point. |
|---|---|
| 剂型、规格<br>Preparations | 注射液：每支 30mg（2ml）；75mg（5ml）多肽物质。<br>Injection: 30mg (2ml), 75mg (5ml) per vial, polypeptide material. |
| **药品名称 Drug Names** | **硫辛酸 Thioctic Acid** |
| 适应证<br>Indications | 用于糖尿病周围神经病变引起的感觉异常。<br>It is used for paresthesia caused by diabetic peripheral neuropathy. |
| 用法、用量<br>Dosage | 静脉注射应缓慢，最大速度为每分钟 50mg（2ml）。本品也可加入生理盐水静脉滴注如 250 ～ 500mg（10 ～ 20ml）加入 100 ～ 250ml 生理盐水中，静脉滴注时间为 30 分钟。<br>The speed for intravenous injection should be slow, with maximal rate of 50mg (2ml)/min. The drug can also be added in normal saline for intravenous infusion, for example, 250~500mg (10~20ml) of the drug is added into 100~250ml of normal saline, and the infusion time lasts 30 minutes. |
| 剂型、规格<br>Preparations | 注射液：每支 0.6g（20ml）。<br>Injection: 0.6g (20ml) per vial. |
| **药品名称 Drug Names** | **氟比洛芬 Flurbiprofen** |
| 适应证<br>Indications | 主要用于风湿性关节炎。<br>It is mainly used for rheumatic arthritis. |
| 用法、用量<br>Dosage | 一日 150 ～ 200mg，分 2 次服。<br>150 ～ 200mg a day, in several divided doses. |
| 剂型、规格<br>Preparations | 片剂：每片 50mg；100mg。<br>Tablets: 50mg, 100mg per tablet. |
| **药品名称 Drug Names** | **醋氯芬酸 Aceclofenac** |
| 适应证<br>Indications | 用于类风湿关节炎及骨关节炎等。<br>It is used for rheumatoid arthritis, osteoarthritis and so on. |
| 用法、用量<br>Dosage | 每次 100mg，一日 2 次。<br>100mg singly, twice a day. |
| 剂型、规格<br>Preparations | 片剂：每片 100mg。<br>Tablets: 100mg per tablet. |

8.4　抗痛风药 Gout suppressants

| **药品名称 Drug Names** | **秋水仙碱 Colchicine** |
|---|---|
| 适应证<br>Indications | 用于痛风性关节炎的急性发作、预防复发性痛风性关节炎的急性发作、家族性地中海热。<br>It is used for acute attack of gouty arthritis, as well as prevents acute attack of recurrent gouty arthritis and familial Mediterranean fever. |
| 用法、用量<br>Dosage | （1）急性期治疗：①口服：成人常用量为每 1 ～ 2 小时服 0.5 ～ 1mg，至关节症状缓解或出现恶心、呕吐、腹泻等胃肠道不良反应时停用。一般需要 3 ～ 5mg，不宜超过 6mg，症状可在 6 ～ 12 小时减轻，24 ～ 48 小时控制，以后 48 小时不需服用本品。此后每次给 0.5mg，每日 2 ～ 3 次（0.5 ～ 1.5mg/d），共 7 日。②静脉注射：用于急性痛风发作和口服用药胃肠道反应过于剧烈者。可将此药 1mg 用 0.9% 氯化钠注射液 20ml 稀释，缓慢注射（20 ～ 30 分钟）。24 小时剂量不超过 2mg，但应注意勿使药物外漏，视病情需要 6 ～ 8 小时后可再次注射，有肾功能减退者 24 小时不超过 3mg。<br>（2）口服，口服每次 0.5 ～ 1mg，但疗程量酌定，要注意不良反应，出现即停药。 |

|  |  |
|---|---|
|  | (1) Treatment in acute phase: ① oral medication: give adults usual dose of 0.5~1mg singly, every 1~2 hours; make drug withdrawal when joints' symptoms get improved or there is gastrointestinal adverse reaction such as nausea, vomiting, diarrhea and so on. Generally, the dose is 3 ~ 5mg, no more than 6mg; it can alleviate symptoms in 6 to 12 hours, and control symptoms within 24 hours to 48 hours, so administration is not needed in the following 48 hours; then give 0.5mg singly, 2 to 3 times a day (0.5 ~ 1.5mg a day), for seven days. ② intravenous injection: it is used for patients who has acute gout attack or have severe gastrointestinal adverse reaction by oral medication. Dilute 1mg of this drug with 20ml of 0.9% sodium chloride injection for slow injection (20 to 30 minutes). The dose within 24 hours does not exceed 2mg, but attention should be paid to the drug leakage; repeat the injection after 6 to 8 hours depending on patients' condition. For insufficiency patients, the dose can not exceed 3mg.<br><br>(2) Oral medication: give 0.5 ~ 1mg singly, but the length of treatment course should depend on patients' condition; attention should be paid to adverse reaction, whose appearance lead to immediate drug withdrawal . |
| 剂型、规格<br>Preparations | 片剂：每片 0.5mg；1mg。<br>注射液：0.5mg/ml。<br>Tablets: 0.5mg, 1mg per tablet.<br>Injection: 0.5mg/ml. |
| 药品名称 Drug Names | 丙磺舒 Probenecid |
| 适应证<br>Indications | 用于慢性痛风的治疗。<br>It is used in the treatment of chronic gout. |
| 用法、用量<br>Dosage | （1）慢性痛风：口服每次 0.25g，一日 2 ~ 4 次，1 周后可增至每次 0.5 ~ 1g，一日 2 次。每日最大剂量不超过 2g。<br>（2）增强青霉素类的作用：每次 0.5g，一日 4 次。儿童：25mg/kg，每 3 ~ 9 小时 1 次。2 ~ 14 岁或体重在 50kg 以下儿童，首剂按体重 0.025g/kg，或按体表面积 0.7g/m²，以后每次 0.01g/kg 或按体表面积 0.3g/m²，一日 4 次。<br>(1) Chronic gout: by oral medication, give 0.25g singly, 2 to 4 times a day; a week later the dose can be increased to 0.5 ~ 1g singly, twice a day. The maximum daily dose can not exceed 2g.<br>(2) Penicillin enhancement: give 0.5g singly, 4 times a day; give children 25mg/kg, once every 3 to 9 hours; for children from 2 to 14 years old or weight under 50kg, give the first dose of 0.025g/kg, or 0.7g/m², afterwards 0.01g/kg or 0.3g/m², 4 times a day. |
| 剂型、规格<br>Preparations | 片剂：每片 0.25g；0.5g。<br>Tablets: 0.25g, 0.5g per tablet. |
| 药品名称 Drug Names | 苯溴马隆 Benzbromarone |
| 适应证<br>Indications | 用于反复发作的痛风性关节炎伴高尿酸血症即痛风患者。<br>It is used for recurrent gouty arthritis with hyperuricemia, which is? |
| 用法、用量<br>Dosage | 每次 25 ~ 100mg，一日 1 次，餐后服用，剂量逐渐增加，连用 3 ~ 6 个月。<br>Give 25 ~ 100mg singly, once a day, after meals; gradually increase the dose, for continuous 3 to 6 months. |
| 剂型、规格<br>Preparations | 片剂：每片 50mg。<br>Tablets: 50mg per tablet. |
| 药品名称 Drug Names | 别嘌醇 Allopurinol |
| 适应证<br>Indications | 用于慢性原发性或继发性痛风、痛风性肾病。<br>It is used for chronic primary or secondary gout and gouty nephropathy. |
| 用法、用量<br>Dosage | 用于降低血中尿酸浓度：开始每次 0.05g，一日 2 ~ 3 次，剂量渐增，2 ~ 3 周后增至每日 0.2 ~ 0.4g，分 2 ~ 3 次服，每日最大量不超过 0.6g。维持量：每次 0.1 ~ 0.2g，一日 2 ~ 3 次。儿童剂量每日 8mg/kg。<br>治疗尿酸结石：口服每次 0.1 ~ 0.2g，一日 1 ~ 4 次或 300mg，一日 1 次。 |

Reduction of uric acid concentration in blood: start with 0.05g singly, 2 to 3 times a day; 2~3 weeks later, increase the dose gradually to 0.2~0.4g a day, in 2~3 divided doses. The maximal daily can not exceed 0.6g. The maintenance dose is 0.1 ~ 0.2g singly, 2 to 3 times a day. Children's daily dose is 8mg/kg.

Uric acid stones: by oral medication, give 0.1 ~ 0.2g singly, 1 ~ 4 times a day or 300mg singly, once a day.

| 剂型、规格<br>Preparations | 片剂：每片 0.1g。<br>Tablets: 0.1g per tablet. |
|---|---|
| **药品名称 Drug Names** | 非布司他 Febuxostat |
| 适应证<br>Indications | 用于预防和治疗高尿酸血症及其引发的痛风。<br>It is used in the prevention and treatment of hyperuricemia and gout by hyperuricemia. |
| 用法、用量<br>Dosage | 本品服用剂量为一日 1 次 40mg 或 80mg，不推荐用于高尿酸血症的痛风患者。<br>Give 40mg or 80mg singly, once a day, which is not recommended for gout patients with hyperuricemia . |
| 剂型、规格<br>Preparations | 片剂：每片 80mg；120mg。<br>Tablets: 80mg, 120mg per tablet. |

### 8.5 抗癫痫药 Antiepileptics

| **药品名称 Drug Names** | 苯妥英钠 Phenytoin Sodium |
|---|---|
| 适应证<br>Indications | （1）主要用于复杂性癫痫发作、单纯部分性发作、全身强直阵挛性发作和癫痫持续状态。本品在脑组织中达有效浓度较慢，因此疗效出现缓慢，需要连续多次服药才有效。<br>（2）治疗三叉神经痛和坐骨神经痛、发作性舞蹈手足徐动症、发作性控制障碍、肌强直症及隐性营养不良性大疱性表皮松解。<br>（3）用于治疗室上性或室性期前收缩，室性心动过速，尤适用于强心苷中毒时的室性心动过速，室上性心动过速也可适用。<br>(1) It is mainly used for complex seizures, simple partial seizures, general tonic-clonic seizures and status epilepticus. It takes long time for the drug to reach effective concentration in brain tissue, administration repeatedly is needed.<br>(2) It is used in the treatment of trigeminal neuralgia, sciatica, paroxysmal choreoathetosis, paroxysmal control disorder, myotonia and recessive dystrophic epidermolysis bullosa.<br>(3) It is also used in the treatment of supraventricular or ventricular premature beats and ventricular tachycardia, especially the ventricular tachycardia caused by cardiac glycoside intoxication, as well as supraventricular tachycardia. |
| 用法、用量<br>Dosage | （1）口服抗癫痫：成人常用量，一次 50 ～ 100mg，一日 2 ～ 3 次，一日 100 ～ 200mg；极量：一次 300mg，一日 500mg。宜从小剂量开始，酌情增量，但需避免过量。体重在 30kg 以下的小儿，按每日 5mg/kg 给药，分 2 ～ 3 次服用，每日不宜超过 250mg。注射剂用于癫痫持续状态时，可用 150 ～ 250mg，加 5% 葡萄糖注射液 20 ～ 40ml，在 6 ～ 10 分钟缓慢静脉注射，每分钟不超过 50mg，必要时经 30 分钟在注射 100 ～ 150mg。<br>（2）治疗三叉神经痛：口服，每次 100 ～ 200mg，一日 2 ～ 3 次。<br>(1) Anti-epilepsy: by oral medication, give adults the usual dose of 50 ~ 100mg singly, 2 to 3 times a day, 100 ~ 200mg a day; the maximum dose is 300mg singly, 500mg a day. It had better start with small dose, then increase properly but avoid overdose; for children under 30kg, give5mg/kg a day, in 2 to 3 divided doses, with maximum daily dose of 250mg. The injection is used in treatment of status epilepticus; add 20 ~ 40ml of 150 ~ 250mg of 5% glucose injection, for slow injection lasting 6 to 10 minutes. The speed can not exceed 50mg per minute. If necessary, make another 100~150mg of injection after more than 30 minutes, .<br>(2) Trigeminal neuralgia: by oral medication, give 100 ~ 200mg singly, 2 to 3 times a day. |
| 剂型、规格<br>Preparations | 片剂：每片 50mg；100mg。<br>注射剂：每支 100mg；250mg。<br><br>Tablets: 50mg, 100mg per tablet.<br>Injection: per 100mg, 250mg. |

**续　表**

| 药品名称 Drug Names | 卡马西平 Carbamazepine |
|---|---|
| 适应证<br>Indications | （1）治疗癫痫：是单纯及复杂部分性发作的首选药，对复杂部分性发作疗效优于其他癫痫药。对典型或不典型失神发作、肌阵挛发作无效。<br>（2）抗外周神经痛：包括三叉神经痛、舌咽神经痛、多发性硬化、糖尿病性周围性神经痛及疱疹后神经痛。亦可用于三叉神经痛缓解后的长期预防用药。对三叉神经痛、舌咽神经痛疗效较苯妥英钠好，用药后 24 小时即可奏效。<br>（3）治疗神经源性尿崩症，可能是由于促进抗利尿激素的分泌有关。<br>（4）预防或治疗狂躁抑郁症：临床使用证明本药对狂躁症及抑郁症均有明显治疗作用，也能减轻或消除精神分裂症患者狂躁、妄想症状。<br>（5）抗心律失常作用：能对抗由地高辛中毒所致的心律失常。能使其完全或基本恢复正常心律。临床使用证明，对室性或室上性期前收缩均有效，可使症状消除，尤其是伴有慢性心功能不全者疗效更好。<br>（6）酒精戒断综合征。<br><br>(1) It is used in the treatment of epilepsy : it is the prior choice for simple and complex partial seizures. It has better effect on complex partial seizures than other antiepileptic drugs. It has no effect on typical or atypia absence seizures and myoclonic seizures.<br>(2) It is used in anti- peripheral neuropathic pain, including trigeminal neuralgia, glossopharyngeal neuralgia, multiple sclerosis, diabetic peripheral neuropathic pain and postherpetic neuralgia, as well as for long-term prophylaxis after trigeminal neuralgia get remission. This drug has better effect on trigeminal neuralgia and glossopharyngeal neuralgia than phenytoin, and it will take effect 24 hours after administration.<br>(3) It can treat neurogenic diabetes insipidus, probably because the drug can promote the secretion of antidiuretic hormone.<br>(4) It is used in prevention or treatment of manic depression. It is clinically proved that this drug has obvious effect on both mania and depression, and it also can relieve or eliminate schizophrenia patients' manic and delusional symptoms.<br>(5) It has antiarrhythmic effect: it can resist arrhythmia caused by digoxin poisoning and make heart rate back to normal completely or basically. It is clinically proved that it has effect on supraventricular or ventricular premature beats by eliminating the symptoms, and it has especially better effect on patients with chronic cardiac insufficiency.<br>(6) It also can be used in alcohol withdrawal syndrome. |
| 用法、用量<br>Dosage | （1）癫痫、三叉神经痛：口服，一日 300 ～ 1200mg，分 2 ～ 4 次服用。开始 1 次 100mg，一日 2 次，以后一日 3 次。个别三叉神经痛患者剂量可达每日 1000 ～ 1200mg。疗程最短 1 周，最长 2 ～ 3 个月。<br>（2）尿崩症：口服，一日 600 ～ 1200mg。<br>（3）抗躁狂症：口服，每日剂量为 300 ～ 600mg，分 2 ～ 3 次服，最大剂量每日 1200mg。<br>（4）心律失常：口服，每日 300 ～ 600mg，分 2 ～ 3 次服。<br>（5）酒精戒断综合征：口服，一次 200mg，一日 3 ～ 4 次。<br><br>(1) Epilepsy and trigeminal neuralgia: by oral medication, give 300 ～ 1200mg a day, in 2 to 4 divided doses; start with 100mg singly, twice a day, afterwards 3 times a day; for some individual trigeminal neuralgia patients, the dose can be 1000 ～ 1200mg a day. The course of treatment is at least one week, while 2 to 3 months at most.<br>(2) Diabetes insipidus: by oral medication, give 600 ～ 1200mg a day.<br>(3) Anti-mania: by oral medication, give 300 ～ 600mg a day, in 2~3 divided doses; the maximal daily dose is 1200mg.<br>(4) Arrhythmia: by oral medication, give 300 ～ 600mg a day, in 2 to 3 divided doses.<br>(5) Alcohol withdrawal syndrome: by oral medication, give 200mg singly, 3 to 4 times a day. |
| 剂型、规格<br>Preparations | 片剂：每片 100mg；200mg；400mg。<br>缓释片：每片 200mg；400mg。<br>咀嚼片：每片 100mg；200mg。<br>胶囊剂：每粒 200mg。<br>糖浆剂：20mg/ml。<br>栓剂：125mg；250mg。 |

| | Tablets: 100mg, 200mg, 400mg per tablet.<br>Release tablets: 200mg, 400mg per tablet.<br>Chewable Tablets: 100mg, 200mg per tablet.<br>Capsules: 200mg per capsule.<br>Syrup: 20mg/ml.<br>Suppositories: 125mg, 250mg. |
|---|---|
| 药品名称 Drug Names | 奥卡西平 Oxcarbazepine |
| 适应证<br>Indications | 用于复杂性部分发作、全身强直阵挛性发作的治疗，以及难治性癫痫的辅助治疗。本品的优点是没有自身诱导，可代替卡马西平，用于对后者有过敏反应者。<br><br>It is used in treatment of complex partial seizures and general tonic-clonic seizures, as well as in adjuvant treatment of refractory epilepsy. The advantage of this product is no self-induction, so it can be a substitution of carbamazepine for those who are allergic to carbamazepine . |
| 用法、用量<br>Dosage | 口服：开始剂量为 300mg/d，以后可逐渐增量至 600 ~ 2400mg/d，以达到满意的疗效。剂量超过 2400mg/d，神经系统不良反应增加。小儿从 8 ~ 10mg/（kg·d）开始，可逐渐增量至 600mg/d。以上每日剂量均应分 2 次服用。<br><br>Oral medication: start with 300mg a day, and gradually increase to 600~2400mg a day to achieve satisfactory effect. If the dose exceeds 2400mg a day, it will increase adverse reactions of nervous system. For children, start with 8~10mg/(kg·d), and gradually increase to 600~2400mg a day. The above daily dose should be administered in 2 divided doses. |
| 剂型、规格<br>Preparations | 片剂：每片 0.15g；0.3g；0.6g。<br>Tablets: 0.15g, 0.3g; 0.6g per tablet. |
| 药品名称 Drug Names | 托吡酯 Topiramate |
| 适应证<br>Indications | 主要作为其他抗癫痫药的辅助治疗，用于单纯部分性发作、复杂部分性发作和全身强直阵挛性发作，尤其对 Lennox-Gastaut 综合征和 West 综合征（婴儿痉挛症）的疗效较好。本品远期疗效好，无明显耐受性，大剂量可用作单药治疗。<br><br>It is mainly used as adjuvant therapy of other antiepileptic drugs for simple partial seizures, complex partial seizures and generalized tonic-clonic seizures. It especially has better effect on Lennox-Gastaut syntrome and West syndrome (infantile spasms). This drug's long-term effect is good, and it has no obvious tolerance, so large dose of this drug can be used as monotherapy. |
| 用法、用量<br>Dosage | 口服。成人：初始极量为每晚 25 ~ 50mg，然后每周增加 1 次，每次增加 25mg，直至症状控制为止。通常有效剂量为每日 200 ~ 300mg。2 岁以上儿童：初始剂量为每日 12.5 ~ 25mg，然后逐渐增加至 5 ~ 9mg/（kg·d），维持剂量为 100mg，分 2 次服。体重大于 43kg 的儿童，有效剂量范围与成人相当。<br><br>Oral medication: for adults, start with 25 ~ 50mg a night, then increased by 25mg once a week until symptoms get controlled; the effective dose is usually 200 ~ 300mg a day; for children over the age of 2, start with 12.5 ~ 25mg a day, and then gradually increase to 5 ~ 9mg/（kg·d）, with the maintenance dose of 100mg, in two divided doses; for children over 43kg, the range of effective dose is almost the same with adults. |
| 剂型、规格<br>Preparations | 片剂：每片 25mg；50mg；100mg。<br>Tablets: 25mg, 50mg, 100mg per tablet. |
| 药品名称 Drug Names | 乙琥胺 Ethosuximide |
| 适应证<br>Indications | 主要用于失神小发作，为首选药。<br>It is mainly used as the prior choice for absence petit mal. |
| 用法、用量<br>Dosage | 口服。剂量：开始量，3 ~ 6 岁为 1 次 250mg，一日 1 次。6 岁以上的儿童及成人，1 次 250mg，一日 2 次。以后可酌情增剂量。<br>最大剂量：6 岁以下最大剂量可增为 1 日 1g，6 岁以上儿童及成人可增加为 1.5g。一般是每 4 ~ 7 日增加 250mg，至满意控制症状而不良反应最小为止。<br><br>Starting dose: for children from 3 to 6 years old, give 250mg singly, once a day; for children over the age of 6 and adults, give 250mg singly, twice a day. Then the dose can be increased appropriately.<br>Maximum dose: for children under the age of 6, increase to 1g a day; for children over the age of 6 and adults, increase to 1.5g. Generally, the dose is increased by 250mg in 4 to 7 days, until the symptoms are under control and side effects keep minimal. |

续　表

| 剂型、规格<br>Preparations | 胶囊剂：每粒 0.25g。<br>糖浆剂：5g/100ml。<br>Capsules: 0.25g per capsule.<br>Syrup: 5g/100ml. |
|---|---|
| 药品名称 Drug Names | 丙戊酸钠 Sodium Valproate |
| 适应证<br>Indications | 主要用于单纯或复杂性失神发作、肌阵挛发作、全身强直阵挛发作（大发作，GTCS）的治疗。可使 90% 失神发作和全身强直阵挛发作得到良好控制，也用于单纯部分性发作、复杂部分性发作及部分性发作继发 GTCS。<br><br>It is mainly used in the treatment of simple or complex absence seizures, myoclonic seizures and generalized tonic-clonic seizures (grand mal seizures, GTCS). 90% of the absence seizures and generalized tonic-clonic seizures can be under well control by this drug. It is also used for simple partial seizures, complex partial seizures and partial seizures with secondary GTCS. |
| 用法、用量<br>Dosage | 口服：成人 1 次 200～400mg，一日 400～1200mg。儿童每日 20～30mg/kg，分 2～3 次服用。一般以从低剂量开始。如原服用其他抗癫痫药者，可合并应用，也可逐渐减少原药量，视情况而定。<br><br>Oral medication: give adults 200～400mg singly, 400～1200mg a day; give children 20 to 30mg/kg, in 2 to 3 divided doses. Generally, start from small dose. If the patients have been given other antiepileptic drugs before, combine with this drug or gradually reduce the dose of the original drug; either way depends on the circumstances. |
| 剂型、规格<br>Preparations | 片剂：每片 100mg；200mg。<br>胶囊剂：每粒 200mg；250mg。<br>肠溶片：每片 250mg；500mg。<br>缓释片：每片 500mg。<br>糖浆剂：200mg（5ml）；500mg（5ml）。<br>Tablets: 100mg, 200mg per tablet.<br>Capsules: 200mg, 250mg per capsule.<br>Enteric-coated tablets: 250mg, 500mg per tablet.<br>Sustained-release tablets: 500mg per tablet.<br>Syrup: 200mg (5ml), 500mg (5ml). |
| 药品名称 Drug Names | 拉莫三嗪 Lamotrigine |
| 适应证<br>Indications | 本品用于成人和 12 岁以上儿童复杂部分性发作或全身强直阵挛性癫痫发作的辅助治疗。作为辅助治疗用于难治性癫痫时，可用于 2 岁以上儿童及成人。<br><br>It is used in adjuvant therapy for complex partial seizures or generalized tonic-clonic seizures of adults and children over the age of 12. If it is used as an adjuvant therapy for intractable epilepsy, the patients should be children over the age of 2 and adults. |
| 用法、用量<br>Dosage | 口服。单独使用：成人初始剂量 25mg，一日 1 次；2 周后可增至 50mg，一日 1 次；在 2 周后，可酌情增加剂量，最大增加量为 50～100mg。此后，每隔 1～2 周，可增加剂量 1 次，直至达到最佳疗效，一般需经 6～8 周。通常有效维持量为 100～200mg/d，一次或分 2 次服用。儿童初始剂量 1mg/kg，维持剂量 3～6mg/kg。<br>与丙戊酸合用：成人和 12 岁以上儿童：初始剂量 25mg，隔日 1 次，每 3～4 周开始改为 25mg，一日 1 次，在 2 周后，酌情增加剂量，最大增量为 0.5～1mg/kg。此后，每隔 1～2 周，可增加剂量 1 次，直至达到最佳疗效，通常有效维持量为 1～2mg/（kg·d），一次或分 2 次服用。<br>与具诱导作用的抗癫痫药物合用：初始剂量 50mg，一日 1 次，服药 2 周后可增至 100mg/d，分 2 次服，在 2 周后，可酌情增加剂量，最大增加量为 100mg，此后，每隔 1～2 周，可增加剂量 1 次，直至达到最佳疗效。通常有效维持量为 200～400mg/d，分 2 次服用。2～12 岁儿童：初始剂量 2mg/（kg·d），分 2 次服，2 周后增至 5mg/（kg·d），分 2 次服，在 2 周后，可酌情增加剂量，最大增加量为，2～3mg/kg，此后，每隔 1～2 周，可增加剂量 1 次，直至达到最佳疗效。维持剂量 10mg/（kg·d），最大剂量为 400mg/d。 |

|  | The drug is administered by oral medication. Without combination with other drugs: for adults, start with 25mg once a day, then the dose can be increased to 50mg, once a day 2 weeks later; after another two weeks, make appropriate dose increase, the maximum increase is 50 ~ 100mg; afterwards make once or twice dose increase every 1 to 2 weeks until reach the best effect, which usually takes 6 to 8 weeks. Usually the effective maintenance dose is 100 ~ 200mg a day, in 1 or 2 divided doses. For children, give the starting dose of 1mg/kg and maintenance dose of 3 ~ 6mg/kg.<br><br>In combination with valproic acid: for adults and children over the age of 12, give the starting dose of 25mg, every other day; then every 3~4 weeks, change to 25mg, once a day; after two weeks, make appropriate dose increase and the maximum increase is 0.5 ~ 1mg/kg. Afterwards make once dose increase every 1 to 2 weeks until reach the best effect. Usually, the effective maintenance dose is 1 ~ 2mg / (kg·d), in 1 or 2 divided doses.<br><br>In combination with inducing anti-epileptic drugs: start with 50mg, once a day; after two weeks, increase to 100mg a day, in 2 divided doses; 2 more weeks later, make appropriate dose increase and the maximum increase is 100mg; afterwards make dose increase once every 1 to 2 weeks until reach the best effect. Usually, the effective maintenance dose is 200 ~ 400mg a day, in 2 divided doses. For children from 2 to 12 year old: start with 2mg / (kg·d), in 2 divided doses; two weeks later, increase to 5mg / (kg · d), in two divided doses; after another two weeks, make appropriate dose increase and the maximum increase is 2 ~ 3mg/kg; afterwards make dose increase once every 1 to 2 weeks until reach the best effect. The maintenance dose is 10mg / (kg · d) and the maximum dose is 400mg a day. |
|---|---|
| 剂型、规格<br>Preparations | 片剂：每片 25mg；100mg；150mg；200mg。<br>Tablets: 25mg, 100mg, 150mg, 200mg per tablet. |
| 药品名称 Drug Names | 加巴喷丁 Gabapentin |
| 适应证<br>Indications | 用于常规治疗无效的某些部分性癫痫辅助治疗，亦可用于治疗部分性癫痫发作继发全身性发作。<br><br>It is used in adjuvant treatment of some partial epilepsy which cannot be cured by conventional method, as well as in the treatment of partial seizures with secondary generalized seizures. |
| 用法、用量<br>Dosage | 口服，成人每天 300mg，睡前服；第 2 天 600mg，分 2 次服；第 3 天 900mg，分 3 次服。此剂量随疗效而定，多数患者在 900 ~ 1800mg 有效。肾功能不全者需要减少剂量。停药应缓停。<br><br>Oral medication: give adults 300mg a day, before sleep; on the second day, give 600mg, in 2 divided doses; on the third day, give 900mg, in 3 divided doses. The dose would changes according to the curative effect. For most of the patients, it will take effect when dose is between 900mg to 1800mg. Renal insufficiency patients need dose reduction. If drug withdrawal is required, stop the medication gradually |
| 剂型、规格<br>Preparations | 胶囊剂：每粒 100mg；300mg；400mg。<br>Capsules: 100mg, 300mg; 400mg per capsule. |
| 药品名称 Drug Names | 左乙拉西坦 Levetiracetam |
| 适应证<br>Indications | 用于成人及 4 岁以上儿童癫痫患者部分性发作的治疗。<br>It is used to treat partial epilepsy seizures of adults and children over the age of 4. |
| 用法、用量<br>Dosage | 口服：成人和青少年体重≥ 50kg，起始剂量为每次 500mg，一日 2 次，最多可增至每次 1500mg，一日 2 次，每 2 ~ 4 周增加或减少每次 500mg，一日 2 次。4 ~ 11 岁儿童和青少年体重 < 50kg，起始剂量为每次 10mg/kg，一日 2 次，最多可增至 30mg/kg，每 2 ~ 4 周增加或减少每次 10mg/kg，一日 2 次。<br><br>肾功能不全者，根据肌酐清除率调整剂量。<br><br>Oral medication: for adults and adolescents over 50kg, start with 500mg singly, 2 times a day; the dose can be increased at most to 1500mg singly, 2 times a day; make single dose increase or decrease of 500mg every 2~4 weeks, twice a day. For children from 4 to 11 years old and adolescents under 50kg, start with 10mg/kg, 2 times a day; the dose increase can be up to 30mg/kg; make dose increase or decrease of 10mg/kg every 2 to 4 weeks, twice a day.<br>Renal insufficiency patients need dose adjustment based on creatinine clearance. |
| 剂型、规格<br>Preparations | 片剂：每片 0.25g；0.5g；1.0g。<br>Tablets: 0.25g, 0.5g, 1.0g per tablet. |

续　表

| 药品名称 Drug Names | 扑米酮 Primidone |
| --- | --- |
| 适应证<br>Indications | 作用与苯巴比妥相似，但作用及毒性均较低。用于治疗癫痫大发作及精神运动性发作有效。<br>This drug has similar effect with barbiturates, but lower effect and toxicity. It is used in the treatment of grand mal seizures and psychomotor seizures. |
| 用法、用量<br>Dosage | 口服：开始每次 0.05g，1 周后逐渐增至每次 0.25g，一日 0.5 ~ 0.75g。极量一日 1.5g。儿童每日 12.5 ~ 25mg/kg。分 2 ~ 3 次服用，宜从小剂量开始，逐渐增量。<br>Oral medication: start with 0.05g singly, and one week later, increase to 0.25g singly, 0.5g to 0.75g a day, with maximum dose of 1.5g a day; for children, start with 12.5 ~ 25mg/kg, in 2 to 3 divided doses, it had better start with small dose and then make gradual dose increase. |
| 剂型、规格<br>Preparations | 片剂：0.25g。<br>Tablets: 0.25g. |

### 8.6 镇静药、催眠药和抗惊厥药 Sedative, hypnotics and anticonvulsants

| 药品名称 Drug Names | 咪达唑仑 Midazolam |
| --- | --- |
| 适应证<br>Indications | 用于治疗失眠症，亦可用于外科手术或诊断检查时作诱导睡眠用。<br>It is used in the treatment of insomnia, as well as for inducing sleep in surgery or diagnostic tests. |
| 用法、用量<br>Dosage | 口服：治疗失眠症，每次 15mg，睡前服。<br>肌内注射：术前 20 ~ 30 分钟注射，成人一般为 10 ~ 15mg（0.10 ~ 0.15mg/kg）。可单用，亦可与镇痛药合用。儿童剂量可稍高，为 0.15 ~ 0.2mg/kg。作儿童诱导麻醉时用本品 5 ~ 10mg（0.15 ~ 0.2mg/kg）与氯胺酮 50 ~ 100mg（8mg/kg）合用。<br>静脉注射：术前准备，术前 5 ~ 10 分钟注射 2.5 ~ 5mg（0.05 ~ 0.1mg/kg），可单用或与抗胆碱药合用。用于诱导麻醉，成人为 10 ~ 15mg（0.15 ~ 0.2mg/kg），儿童为 0.2mg/kg。用于维持麻醉，小剂量静脉注射，剂量和时间间隔视患者个体差异而定。<br>Oral medication: in the treatment of insomnia, give15mg singly, before sleep.<br>Intramuscular injection: usually give adults10 ~ 15mg (0.10 ~ 0.15mg/kg), 20 to 30 minutes before surgery; it can be used alone or with analgesic drugs. Children may need larger dose as 0.15 ~ 0.2mg/kg. In children's induction of anesthesia, give 5 ~ 10mg (0.15 ~ 0.2mg/kg)of this drug in combination with 50 ~ 100mg (8mg/kg) of ketamine.<br>Intravenous injection: in preoperative preparation, give2.5 ~ 5mg (0.05 ~ 0.1mg/kg), 5 to 10 minutes before surgery; it can be used alone or in combination with anticholinergic drugs. In induction of anesthesia, give adults 10 ~ 15mg (0.15 ~ 0.2mg/kg) and give children 0.2mg/kg. In anesthesia maintenance, give small dose of injection; and the dose and the time intervals depend on individual patient. |
| 剂型、规格<br>Preparations | 片剂：每片 15mg。<br>注射液：每支 5mg（1ml）；10mg（2ml）；15mg（3ml）。<br>Tablets: 15mg per tablet.<br>Injection: per 5mg (1ml), 10mg (2ml); 15mg (3ml). |

| 药品名称 Drug Names | 苯巴比妥 Phenobarbital |
| --- | --- |
| 适应证<br>Indications | 用于：①镇静：如焦虑不安、烦躁、甲状腺功能亢进、高血压、功能性恶心、小儿幽门痉挛症；②催眠：偶用于顽固性失眠症，但醒后往往有疲倦、嗜睡等后遗效应；③抗惊厥：常用其对抗中枢兴奋药中毒或高热、破伤风、脑炎、脑出血等病引起的惊厥；④抗癫痫：用于癫痫大发作和部分性发作的治疗，出现作用快，也可用于癫痫持续状态；⑤麻醉前给药；⑥与解热镇痛药配伍应用，以增强其作用；⑦治疗新生儿高胆红素血症。<br>It is used for ① sedation: such as anxiety, irritability, hyperthyroidism, hypertension, functional nausea and pediatric pyloric spasms; ② hypnosis: sometimes for intractable insomnia, but with aftermath effect of tiredness and lethargy, etc. ③ anticonvulsion: eg. convulsion caused by central stimulant drug intoxication, fever, tetanus, encephalitis, and cerebral hemorrhage, etc.; ④ anti-epilepsy: it has quick effect on grand mal seizures and partial seizures; it also can be used in status epilepticus; ⑤ administration before anesthesia; ⑥ effect enhancement in combination with antipyretic analgesics; ⑦ neonatal hyperbilirubinemia. |

续 表

| 用法、用量<br>Dosage | （1）口服：一般情况，常用量，1 次 15 ～ 150mg，一日 30 ～ 200mg；极量，1 次 250mg，一日 500mg。小儿，用于镇静每次 2mg/kg，用于惊厥每次 3 ～ 5mg/kg，用于抗高胆红素血症每日 5 ～ 8mg/kg，分次口服。<br>（2）皮下、肌内注射或缓慢静脉注射：常用量，1 次 0.1 ～ 0.2g，一日 1 ～ 2 次；极量，1 次 0.25g，一日 0.5g。<br>（3）镇静、抗癫痫：口服，每次 0.015 ～ 0.03g，一日 3 次。<br>（4）催眠：每次 0.03 ～ 0.09g，睡前口服 1 次。<br>（5）抗惊厥：肌内注射其钠盐，每次 0.1 ～ 0.2g，必要时 4 ～ 6 小时后重复一次。<br>（6）麻醉前给药：术前 0.5 ～ 1 小时肌内注射 0.1 ～ 0.2g。<br>（7）癫痫持续状态：肌内注射 1 次 0.1 ～ 0.2g。<br>(1) Oral medication: generally, give usual dose of 15 ～ 150mg singly, 30 ～ 200mg a day; the maximum dose is 250mg singly, 500mg a day; in children's sedation, give 2mg/kg singly; in children's convulsion, give 3 ～ 5mg/kg singly; in anti hyperbilirubinemia, give 5 ～ 8mg/kg a day, in several divided doses.<br>(2) Subcutaneous, intramuscular or slow intravenous injection: give the usual dose of 0.1 ～ 0.2g singly, 1 to 2 times a day; the maximum dose is 0.25g singly, 0.5g a day.<br>(3) Sedation and anticonvulsion: give 0.015 ～ 0.03g singly, 3 times a day.<br>(4) Hypnosis: by oral medication, give 0.03 ～ 0.09g singly, once before sleep.<br>(5) Anticonvulsion: by intramuscular injection of its sodium, give 0.1 ～ 0.2g singly; repeat the dose after 4 to 6 hours, if necessary.<br>(6) Administration before anesthesia: by intramuscular injection, give 0.1 ～ 0.2g, 0.5 to 1 hour before surgery.<br>(7) Status epilepticus: by intramuscular injection, give 0.1 ～ 0.2g singly. |
|---|---|
| 剂型、规格<br>Preparations | 片剂：每片 0.01g；0.015g；0.03g；0.1g。<br>注射用苯巴比妥：每支 0.05g；0.1g；0.2g。<br>鲁米托品片每片含苯巴比妥 15mg，硫酸阿托品 0.15mg。<br>用于神经功能失调所致头痛、呕吐、颤抖、胃肠道紊乱性腹痛等。每次 1 片，极量 1 次 5 片。<br>Tablets: 0.01g, 0.015g, 0.03g, 0.1g per tablet.<br>Phenobarbital for injection: per 0.05g, 0.1g, 0.2g.<br>Tab.Lumitropine: 15mg of phenobarbital contained per tablet; Tab. Atropine: 0.15mg.<br>It is used for headache, vomit, tremor and abdominal pain by gastrointestinal disorders caused by active and neurological dysfunction: give 1 tablet singly, with maximal single dose of 5 tablets. |
| 药品名称 Drug Names | 异戊巴比妥 Amobarbital |
| 适应证<br>Indications | 用于镇静、催眠、抗惊厥。<br>It is used for the sedation, hypnosis and anti-convulsion. |
| 用法、用量<br>Dosage | （1）口服：①成人，常用量：催眠，每次 0.1 ～ 0.2g，于睡前顿服，适用于难以入睡者；镇静，每次 0.02 ～ 0.04g，一日 2 ～ 3 次。极量：1 次 0.2g，一日 0.6g。老年人或体弱患者，即便是给予常用量也可产生兴奋、神经错乱或抑郁，须减量。②小儿，常用量：催眠，个体差异大；镇静，每次 2mg/kg（或 60mg/m2），一日 3 次。<br>（2）肌内或缓慢静脉注射：①成人，常用量：催眠，每次 0.1 ～ 0.2g；镇静，每次 0.03 ～ 0.05mg，一日 2 ～ 3 次；抗惊厥（癫痫持续状态），缓慢静脉注射 0.3 ～ 0.5g。极量：1 次 0.25g，一日 0.5g。②小儿，常用量：催眠（或抗惊厥），肌内注射每次 3 ～ 5mg/kg（或 125mg/ ）；镇静，每日 6mg/kg，一日 2 ～ 3 次。<br>(1) Oral medication: ① for adults, in hypnosis for those who have difficulties to fall asleep, give usual dose of 0.1 ～ 0.2g singly, at a draught, before sleep, ; in sedation, give usual dose of 0.02 ～ 0.04g singly, 2～3 times a day. The maximum dose is 0.2g singly, 0.6g a day. Elderly patients or weak patients need dose reduction because the usual dose would produce excitement, delirium or depression. ② for children, in hypnosis, the dose depend on individual differences; in sedation, give 2mg/kg (or 60mg/ $m^2$ ), 3 times a day.<br>(2) Intramuscular or slow intravenous injection: ① for adults, in hypnosis, give the usual dose of 0.1 ～ 0.2g singly; in sedation, give 0.03 ～ 0.05mg singly, 2～3 times a day; in anti-convulsion (status epilepticus), give 0.3 ～ 0.5g for slow intravenous injection. The maximum dose is 0.25g singly, 0.5g a day. ② for children, in hypnosis (or anti-convulsion), give the usual dose of 3 ～ 5mg/kg (or 125mg/ $m^2$ ) singly, by intramuscular injection; in sedation, give 6mg/kg a day, 2～ 3 times a day. |

**续　表**

| 剂型、规格<br>Preparations | 片剂：每片 0.1g 。<br>注射用异戊巴比妥钠：每支 0.1g；0.25g。<br>Tablets: 0.1g per tablet.<br>Amobarbital sodium for injection: 0.1g, 0.25g per vial. |
|---|---|
| **药品名称 Drug Names** | 司可巴比妥 Secobarbital |
| 适应证<br>Indications | 主要适用于不易入睡的患者。也可用于抗惊厥。<br>It is mainly used for patients who have difficulties to fall asleep. It can also be used in anti-convulsion. |
| 用法、用量<br>Dosage | 口服：成人常用量，催眠 0.1～0.2g，临睡前一次顿服；镇静 1 次 30～50mg，一日 3～4 次。成人极量 1 次 0.3g。尚可皮下注射（1 次量 0.1g）。<br>Oral medication: for adults, in hypnosis, give the usual dose of 0.1～0.2g singly, at a draught before sleep; in sedation, give 30～50mg singly, 3～4 times a day. Adults' maximum dose is 0.3g singly. Subcutaneous injection (0.1g singly) can also be used in administration. |
| 剂型、规格<br>Preparations | 胶囊剂：每粒 0.1g；<br>注射用司可巴比妥：每支 0.05g。<br>Capsules: 0.1g per capsule.<br>Secobarbital for injection: 0.05g per vial. |
| **药品名称 Drug Names** | 佐匹克隆 Zopiclone |
| 适应证<br>Indications | 用于各种原因引起的失眠症，尤其适用于不能耐受次晨残余作用的患者。<br>It is intended to treat insomnia caused by a variety of reasons. Especially, it has good effect on the patients who are intolerant to the residual effect of insomnia in the next morning. |
| 用法、用量<br>Dosage | 睡前服 7.5mg。老年人、肝功能不全者，睡前服 3.75mg，必要时可增加至 7.5mg。<br>Give 7.5mg, before sleep ; for elderly and liver dysfunction patients, give 3.75mg before sleep or increase to 7.5mg, if necessary. |
| 剂型、规格<br>Preparations | 片剂：每片 3.75mg；7.5mg。<br>Tablets: 3.75mg, 7.5mg per tablet. |
| **药品名称 Drug Names** | 唑吡坦 Zolpidem |
| 适应证<br>Indications | 用于治疗短暂性、偶发性失眠症或慢性失眠的短期治疗。<br>It is used in the treatment of transient and sporadic insomnia, as well as in short-term treatment of chronic insomnia. |
| 用法、用量<br>Dosage | 常用量为 10mg，睡前服。<br>偶发性失眠，一般用药 2～5 日。长期用药应不超过 4 周。老年人及肝功能不全者剂量减半，必要时可增至 10mg。<br>The usual dose is 10mg, before sleep.<br>Occasional insomnia: generally, the medication lasts from 2 to 5 days; the long-term medication should not exceed 4 weeks. For elderly patients and liver dysfunction patiens give half of the dose or increase to 10mg, if necessary. |
| 剂型、规格<br>Preparations | 片剂：每片 10mg ；5mg。<br>Tablets: 10mg, 5mg per tablet. |
| **药品名称 Drug Names** | 水合氯醛 Chloral Hydrate |
| 适应证<br>Indications | 用于神经性失眠、伴有显著兴奋的精神病及破伤风痉挛、士的宁中毒等。<br>It is used to treat neurological insomnia, psychosis with obvious excitment, tetanospasmin and strychnine poisoning, etc. |
| 用法、用量<br>Dosage | 口服或灌肠。常用量，一次 0.5～1.5g；极量，一次 2g，一日 4g。睡前 1 次。口服 10% 溶液 5～15ml（一般服 10ml），以多量水稀释并添加胶浆剂（掩盖其不良臭味，避免刺激）后服用，或服用其合剂（加有淀粉、糖浆剂）以减少刺激。抗惊厥：多用灌肠法给药，将 10% 溶液 15～20ml 稀释 1～2 倍后 1 次灌入。 |

| | Oral medication or enema: the usual dose is 0.5 ~ 1.5g singly; the maximum dose is 2g singly, 4g a day; Give once before sleep. Give 5 ~ 15ml (usually 10 ml), of 10% solution after diluting it with plenty of water and adding mucilage in it (to cover up the odor and avoid stimulation), or give the mixture (with starch, syrup) to reduce the stimulation. In anti-convulsion: enema is often used; dilute 15 ~ 20ml of 10% solution 1 to 2 times, and then give enema once. |
|---|---|
| 剂型、规格<br>Preparations | 水合氯醛合剂：有水合氯醛 65g，溴化钠 65g，淀粉 20g，枸橼酸 0.25g，薄荷水 0.5ml，琼脂糖浆 500ml，蒸馏水适量，共配成 1000ml。水合氯醛遇热易挥发分解，须调好其他成分防冷后再加入。如无琼脂糖浆时可用单糖浆代替。<br><br>Chloral Hydrate Mixture: 65g of chloral hydrate, 65g of sodium bromide, 20g of starch, 0.25g of citric acid, 0.5ml of mint water and 500ml of agarose syrup and appropriate amount of distilled water prepare 1000ml of mixture. Chloral hydrate is easy to volatile decompose by heat, so it must be added in anti-cold condition after other ingredients' preparation. When agarose syrup is not available, simple syrup can be a substitute. |
| **药品名称 Drug Names** | 扎来普隆 Zaleplon |
| 适应证<br>Indications | 用于入睡困难的失眠症的短期治疗。临床研究结果显示扎来普隆能缩短入睡时间，但还未见其能增加睡眠时间和减少清醒次数。<br><br>It is used in the short-term treatment of insomnia, in which people jave difficulties to fall asleep. Clinical research results have shown that zaleplon can shorten the time to fall asleep, but not reflected the frequency of extending sleep and reducing sober. |
| 用法、用量<br>Dosage | 口服，一次 5 ~ 10mg（1 ~ 2 粒），睡前服用或入睡困难时服用。与所有的镇静催眠药一样，当清醒时，服用会导致记忆损伤、幻觉、协调障碍、头晕。体重较轻的患者，推荐剂量为一次 5mg（1 粒）。老年患者、糖尿病患者和轻、中度肝功能不全患者，推荐剂量为一次 5mg（1 粒）。每晚只服用一次。持续用药时间限制在 7 ~ 10 日。如果服药 7 ~ 10 日后失眠仍未减轻，医生应对患者失眠的原因重新评估。<br><br>Oral medication: give 5 ~ 10mg (1 ~ 2 tablets) singly, before sleep or when there is difficulty to fall asleep. Like all sedative-hypnotics, it would lead to memory impairment, hallucinations, coordination disorders and dizziness when patients are sober. For patients with lighter weight, give the recommended dose of 5mg singly. For elderly patients, diabetic patients, and mild or moderate hepatic insufficiency patients, give the recommended dose of 5mg singly. Give only once every night. The continuous administration was limited within 7 to 10 days. If there is no any alleviation after receiving medication for 7 to 10 day, doctors need to reassess the reasons for patients' insomnia. |
| 剂型、规格<br>Preparations | 胶布剂：每粒 5mg。<br>片剂、分散片：片剂 5mg。<br>Tape agent: 5mg of each.<br>Tablets, dispersible tablets: 5mg. |
| **药品名称 Drug Names** | 艾司佐匹克隆 Eszopiclone |
| 适应证<br>Indications | 用于失眠的短期治疗。<br>It is used as a short-term treatment for insomnia. |
| 用法、用量<br>Dosage | 常用量为睡前口服 2mg，可逐渐增量至 3mg。对于入睡困难的老年患者起始剂量推荐为 1mg，可逐渐增量至 2mg。对于易醒的老年患者起始剂量为 2mg。<br><br>The usual dose is 2mg, orally, before sleep and it can be gradually increased to 3mg. For elderly patients who difficulties to fall asleep, it is recommended to start with 1mg and increase gradually to 2mg. For elderly patients who are easily wakened, the starting dose is 2mg. |
| 剂型、规格<br>Preparations | 片剂：2mg，3mg。<br>Tablets:2mg, 3mg. |
| **药品名称 Drug Names** | 溴化钾 Potassium Bromide |
| 适应证<br>Indications | 常用于神经衰弱。癔症、神经性失眠、精神兴奋状态。<br>It is commonly used to treat neurasthenia, hysteria, nervous insomnia, mental excitement. |

**续　表**

| | |
|---|---|
| 用法、用量<br>Dosage | 口服：10% 溶液 5 ～ 10ml，一日 3 次。饭后服。不宜空腹服用。<br>Oral medication: give 5 ~ 10ml of 10% solution, 3 times a day, after meals. It had better not give on an empty stomach. |
| 剂型、规格<br>Preparations | 溶液：10%。<br>Solution: 10%. |
| **药品名称 Drug Names** | 戊巴比妥钠 Pentobarbital Sodium |
| 适应证<br>Indications | 同异戊巴比妥，用于催眠、麻醉前给药。<br>It is used for hypnosis and preanesthetic administration, the same with amobarbital. |
| 用法、用量<br>Dosage | 催眠：0.1 ～ 0.2g；麻醉前给药：手术当日清晨服 0.1g，必要时术前半小时再服 0.1g。极量：1 次 0.2g，一日 0.6g。<br>Hypnosis: 0.1 ~ 0.2g. Preanesthetic administration: give 0.1g in the morning, on the surgery day; give another 0.1g half an hour before surgery, if necessary . The maximum dose is 0.2g singly, 0.6g a day. |
| 剂型、规格<br>Preparations | 片剂：0.05g；0.1g。<br>注射剂：0.1g；0.5g。<br>Tablets: 0.05g, 0.1g.<br>Injection: 0.1g, 0.5g. |
| 8.7 抗帕金森病药 Antiparkinsonian drugs | |
| **药品名称 Drug Names** | 左旋多巴 Levodopa |
| 适应证<br>Indications | 改善肌强直和运动迟缓效果明显，持续用药对震颤、流涎、姿势不稳及吞咽困难亦有效。①帕金森病（原发性震颤麻痹）；脑炎后或合并有脑动脉硬化以及中枢神经系统的一氧化碳与锰中毒后的症状性帕金森综合征（非药源性震颤麻痹综合征）。可减轻没震颤麻痹的症状，改善肌张力，使肢体活动更趋正常。对轻、中度病情者效果较好，重度或老年患者较差。②肝性脑病：可使患者清醒，症状改善。肝性脑病可能与中枢递质多巴胺异常有关，服用后，可改善中枢功能而奏效。亦有学者认为左旋多巴可提高大脑对氨的耐受性，但不能改善肝脏损伤和肝功能。③神经痛：早期服用可缓解神经痛。④高泌乳素血症：可抑制下丘脑的促甲状腺激素释放激素，兴奋泌乳素释放抑制因子，因而减少泌乳素的分泌，用于治疗高泌乳素血症，对乳溢症有一定疗效。⑤脱毛症：其机制可能是增加血液到组织的儿茶酚胺浓度，促进毛发生长。⑥促进小儿生长发育：可通过促进生长激素的分泌，加速小儿骨骼的生长发育。治疗垂体功能低下症。<br><br>It has obvious effect on improvement of the muscle rigidity and bradykinesia. Continuous medication would have effect on tremors, salivation, postural instability and dysphagia. ① Parkinson's disease ( primary paralysis agitans): for Symptomatic Parkinsonism (non- drug-induced Parkinsonism) after encephalitis, with cerebral arteriosclerosis and after carbon monoxide or manganese pensioning in central nervous system, it can alleviate the symptoms of paralysis agitans, improve muscular tension amd make physical activity become more normal. It has better effect on patients with mild or moderate condition, but worse effect on patients with severe condition and elderly patients. ② Hepatic encephalopathy: it can sober up the patient and improve the symptoms. Hepatic encephalopathy may be associated with the abnormalities of dopamine as central neurotransmitter so in the treatment, the drug would have effect by improving the function of central and work. It is also believed that levodopa may increase brain's tolerance to ammonia, but can not improve hepatic damage and function. ③ Neuralgia: give medication in early stage can alleviate the pain. ④ Hyperprolactinemia, it can inhibit the releasing of thyrotropin in hypothalamus and make prolactin release inhibitor, in order to reduce the secretion of prolactin; it is used in the treatment of hyperprolactinemia, as well as galactorrhea. ⑤ alopecia: it may increase the catecholamine concentrations from blood to the tissue, in order to promote hair growth. ⑥ Promotion for children's growth and development: it can accelerate the growth and development of children's bone by promoting the secretion of growth hormone. It is also used to treat hypopituitarism. |

**续 表**

| 用法、用量<br>Dosage | ①治疗震颤麻痹：口服，开始时一日 0.25 ~ 0.5g，分 2 ~ 3 次服用。每服 2 ~ 4 日后，每日量增加 0.125 ~ 0.5g。维持量 1 日 3 ~ 6g，分 4 ~ 6 次服，连续用药 2 ~ 3 周见效。在剂量递增过程中，如出现恶心等，应停止增量，带症状消失后在增量。②治疗肝性脑病：一日 0.3 ~ 0.4g，加入 5% 葡萄糖溶液 500ml 中静脉滴注，待完全清醒后，减量至 1 日 0.2g，继续 1 ~ 2 日后停药。或用本品 5g 加入生理盐水 100ml 中，鼻饲或灌肠。<br><br>① Parkinsonism: by oral medication, start with 0.25 ~ 0.5g a day, in 2 or 3 divided doses; increase by 0.125 ~ 0.5g a day after 2 to 4 days' medication. The maintenance dose is 3 to 6g a day, in 4~6 divided doses; it will take effect after continuous medication of 2 ~ 3 weeks. In the dose increase, if patients have nausea and etc., stop the increase; when symptoms disappear, recover the dose increase. ② Hepatic encephalopathy: give 0.3 ~ 0.4g a day; add it into 500ml of 5% glucose solution for intravenous infusion; after patients are fully awake, reduce the dose to 0.2g a day, for 1 ~ 2 days, and then make drug withdrawal. Or add 100ml of saline in 5g of the drug for nasal feeding or enema. |
|---|---|
| 剂型、规格<br>Preparations | 片剂：每片 50mg；100mg；250mg。胶囊剂：每粒 100mg；125mg；250mg。<br>Tablets: 50mg 100mg 250mg per tablet. Capsules: 100mg 125mg 250mg per capsule. |
| **药品名称 Drug Names** | 卡比多巴 Carbidopa |
| 适应证<br>Indications | ①主用与左旋多巴合用治疗各种原因引起的帕金森症，可获较好临床效果，但晚期重型患者的治疗较差。②本品与左旋多巴联合应用，治疗单眼弱视疗效好，尤其是对屈光参差性单眼弱视、弱视性质为中心注视的弱视。<br><br>① It is mainly used in combination with levodopa to treat Parkinson's disease caused by various reasons, and it can achieve better clinical effect. But for severe patients in advanced stage, the effect is worse. ② This drug is used in combination with levodopa, with good effect in monocular amblyopia treatment, especially the anisometropia monocular amblyopia and amblyopia with central fixation as amblyopia nature. |
| 用法、用量<br>Dosage | 首次剂量，卡比多巴 10mg，左旋多巴 100mg，一日 4 次；以后每隔 3 ~ 7 日每日增加卡比多巴 40mg，左旋多巴 400mg，直至每日量卡比多巴 200mg，左旋多巴 2g 为限。多采用其复方制剂如患者先用左旋多巴，需停药 8 小时以上才能在合用二药。<br><br>The first dose is 10mg of carbidopa and 100mg of levodopa, 4 times a day; then everyday increase by 40mg of carbidopa and 400mg of levodopa, every 3 ~ 7 days, until the dose reaches 200mg of carbidopa and 2g of levodopa, which is the limitation. It is often used the compound preparation; if the patients were given levodopa first, drug withdrawal is needed more than eight hours before the two drugs are given in combination. |
| 剂型、规格<br>Preparations | 片剂：每片 25mg。<br>Tablets: 25mg per tablet. |
| **药品名称 Drug Names** | 苄丝肼 Benserazide |
| 适应证<br>Indications | 一般苄丝肼与左旋多巴按 1：4 配伍应用，用于帕金森病和帕金森综合征，可减少左旋多巴的用量，增强其疗效并减其外周不良反应。对药物引起的帕金森症无效。<br><br>Generally, benserazide is used in combination with levodopa by 1：4 to treat Parkinson's disease and Parkinson's syndrome. The dose of levodopa can be reduced to enhance the effect and reduce adverse reaction of outer periphery. It has no effect on Parkinson's disease caused by drugs. |
| 用法、用量<br>Dosage | 多与左旋多巴合用，开始时 1 次，苄丝肼 25mg 以及左旋多巴 100ng，一日 2 次；然后每隔 1 周将苄丝肼增加 25mg/d 及左旋多巴 100mg/d，至每日剂量苄丝肼达 250mg 及左旋多巴达 100mg 为止。分 3 ~ 4 次服用。<br><br>In combination with levodopa: start with 25 mg of benserazide and100mg of levodopa, twice a day. Then increase by 25 mg of benserazide and 100 mg of levodopa a day, every other week until the daily dose is 250mg of benserazide and 100 mg of levodopa, in 3~4 divided doses. |
| 剂型、规格<br>Preparations | 多巴丝肼：每胶囊 125mg（含苄丝肼 25mg 及左旋多巴 100mg）；250mg（含苄丝肼 50mg 及左旋多巴 200mg）。<br>Capsules: 125 mg ( 25 mg of Benserazide and 100 mg of levodopa contained), 250 mg (50 mg of Benserazide and 200 mg of levodopa contained) per capsule. |

**续　表**

| 药品名称 Drug Names | 多巴丝肼 Levodopa and Benserazide |
|---|---|
| 适应证<br>Indications | 适用于原发性震颤麻痹（帕金森病）、脑炎后或合并有脑动脉硬化的症状性帕金森综合征。<br><br>It is used for primary paralysis agitans (Parkinson's disease), as well as Symptomatic Parkinsonism after encephalitis and with cerebral arteriosclerosis. |
| 用法、用量<br>Dosage | 口服，成人，第一周 1 次 125mg，2 次 / 日。以后每隔一周每日增加 125mg。一般日剂量不得超过 1g，分 3 ~ 4 次服用。<br><br>Oral medication: for adults, in the first week, give 125mg singly, twice a day; then increase by 125mg a day, every other week. Generally, the daily dose can not exceed 1g, in 3 or 4 divided doses. |
| 剂型、规格<br>Preparations | 胶囊剂、片剂：① 125mg：左旋多巴 100mg 和苄丝肼 25mg；② 250mg：左旋多巴 200mg 和苄丝肼 50mg。控释片：125mg。分散片：125mg。<br><br>Capsules, tablets: ① 125mg: 100mg of levodopa and 25mg of benserazide; ② 250mg: 200mg of levodopa and 50mg of benserazide. Controlled release tablet: 125mg. Dispersible tablets: 125mg. |
| 药品名称 Drug Names | 溴隐亭 Bromocriptine |
| 适应证<br>Indications | （1）抗震颤麻痹，疗效优于金刚烷胺及苯海索，对僵直、少动亦效果好，对重症患者亦效果好，常用于左旋多巴疗效不好或不能耐受患者，症状波动者，对左旋多巴复方制剂无效者。特点是显效快，持续时间长。<br>（2）治疗慢性精神分裂症和躁狂症，尤其是以阴性症状为主的精神病理基础，是多巴胺功能降低所致。治疗抑郁症，通过增强多巴胺能神经元的活性而对抑郁症有效。治疗抗精神病药恶性综合征。<br>（3）闭经或乳溢，用于各种原因所致催乳激素过高引起的闭经或乳溢，对垂体瘤诱发者，可作为手术或放射治疗的辅助治疗。<br>（4）抑制生理性泌乳。<br>（5）用于催乳激素过高的引起的经前期综合征，对周期性乳房痛和乳房结节，可使症状改善，但对非周期性乳房痛和月经正常几乎无效。<br>（6）用于肢端肥大症，无功能性垂体肿瘤，垂体性甲状腺功能亢进。治疗库欣病：大多数库欣病由皮质素瘤引起，少数为下丘脑分泌促甲状腺激素释放激素异常。溴隐亭可以降低促皮质素，故可以治疗库欣病。<br>（7）治疗女性不育症。<br>（8）治疗男性性功能减退，对男性乳腺发育、阳痿、精液不足等有一定疗效。<br>（9）治疗可卡因戒断综合征，可有效减轻可卡因的瘾欲和戒断的焦虑症状。<br>（10）可用于 Huntington 舞蹈症。<br><br>(1) Anti-parkinsonism: It has better than adamantane and benzhexol. It has good effect on spasticity and hypokinesia, as well as for patients with severe disease. It is often used for patients who receive worse effect by levodopa or are intolerant to levodopa, patients with symptoms' fluctuation, and patients who are resistant to levodopa compound preparations. The features are of quick effect and long duration.<br>(2) Chronic schizophrenia and mania: especially, the psychpathological basis with negative symptoms is caused by the reduction of dopamine function. So, depression can be treated by enhancing the activity of dopaminergic neurons. It is also used in treatment of psychiatric drug's malignant syndrome.<br>(3) Amenorrhea and galactorrhea: it is used to treat amenorrhea and galactorrhea by high prolactin, which ia induce by various reasons. For patients with pituitary tumor induction, it can be used as adjuvant therapy of surgery or radiation therapy.<br>(4) Physiological lactation inhibition.<br>(5) For premenstrual syndrome by high prolactin, cyclical mastodynia and breast nodules, it can make improvement on symptoms; but for aperiodic mastodynia and normal menstruation, it almost has no effect.<br>(6) It is used to treat acromegaly, non-functional pituitary tumor, pituitary hyperthyroidism. Most of the Cushing disease is caused by cortisol adenoma and only a minority is caused by the abnormal releasing of thyroid hormone secreted by hypothalamus, and Bromine can reduce corticotrophin, so it can be used to treat Cushing disease. |

**续 表**

| | |
|---|---|
| | (7) Female infertility.<br>(8) Male sexual dysfunction: it has certain effect on gynecomastia, impotence, insufficient semen.<br>(9) Cocaine withdrawal syndrome: it can effectively reduce the addiction of cocaine and anxiety symptoms by cocaine withdrawal.<br>(10) Huntington's Disease. |
| 用法、用量<br>Dosage | （1）震颤麻痹：开始每次 1.25mg，一日 2 次，2 周内逐渐加量，必要时每 2 ~ 4 周每日增加 2.5mg，以找到最佳治疗的最小剂量，每日剂量 20mg 为宜。<br>（2）用于闭经或溢乳、抑制泌乳、不育症、肢端肥大等。<br>(1) Parkinsonism: start with1.25mg singly, 2 times a day; gradually increase the dose in two weeks or increase 2.5mg everyday, every two to four weeks, if necessary, in order to find the minimum dose for the best treatment; the daily dose of 20mg is appropriate.<br>(2) amenorrhea or galactorrhea, lactation suppression, infertility, acromegaly, etc. |
| 剂型、规格<br>Preparations | 片剂：每片 2.5mg。<br>Tablets: 2.5mg per tablet. |
| **药品名称 Drug Names** | 普拉克索 Pramipexole |
| 适应证<br>Indications | 单独或与左旋多巴合用于治疗帕金森病，可明显减少静息时的震颤。晚期帕金森病用该药与左旋多巴共同的治疗时，可使患者对左旋多巴的治疗量减少 27% ~ 30%，并可延长症状最佳控制时间平均每天 2 小时。<br>It can be used alone or in combination with levodopa to treat Parkinson's disease. It can significantly reduce the tremor in resting. In treatment of advanced Parkinson's disease in combination with levodopa, reduce 27% to 30% of levodopa's therapeutic dose for patients and extend the optimal symptoms control time2 hours a day on average. |
| 用法、用量<br>Dosage | 按病情程度每次 1.5 ~ 4.5mg，一日 3 次。<br>Give 1.5 ~ 4.5mg singly according to patients' condition, 3 times a day. |
| 剂型、规格<br>Preparations | 片剂：0.125mg；0.25mg；0.5mg；1mg；1.5mg。<br>Tablets: 0.125mg; 0.25mg; 1mg; 1.5mg per tablet. |
| **药品名称 Drug Names** | 司来吉兰 Selegiline |
| 适应证<br>Indications | 适用于帕金森病，常作为左旋多巴、美多巴或信尼麦的辅助用药。<br>It is used in treatment of Parkinson's disease, often as the adjuvant drug for levodopa, Madopar or Sinemet . |
| 用法、用量<br>Dosage | 口服，每日 10mg，早晨 1 次顿服；或每次 5mg，早、晚 2 次服用。<br>Oral medication: 10mg a day, at a draught, in the morning or 5mg singly, 2 times a day (in the morning and evening). |
| 剂型、规格<br>Preparations | 片剂：每片 5mg。<br>Tablets: 5mg per tablet. |
| **药品名称 Drug Names** | 雷沙吉兰 Rasagiline |
| 适应证<br>Indications | 用于治疗帕金森病，可单用或作为左旋多巴的辅助用药。<br>It is used in the treatment of Parkinson's disease. It can be used alone or as an adjuvant drug for levodopa. |
| 用法、用量<br>Dosage | 单药治疗：每次 1mg，一日 1 次。与左旋多巴联合治疗：起始剂量每次 0.5mg，一日 1 次，维持剂量为 0.5 ~ 1mg，一日 1 次。老年患者需调整剂量。<br>Monotherapy: 1mg singly, once a day. In combination with levodopa: start with 0.5mg singly, once a day; the maintenance dose is 0.5 ~ 1mg, once a day. Elderly patients need dose adjustment. |
| 剂型、规格<br>Preparations | 片剂：0.5mg；1mg。<br>Tablets: 0.5mg, 1mg. |

续　表

| 药品名称 Drug Names | 苯海索 Trihexyphenidyl |
|---|---|
| 适应证<br>Indications | （1）临床用于震颤麻痹，脑炎后或动脉硬化引起的震颤麻痹，对改善流涎有效，对缓解僵直、运动迟缓疗效较差，改善震颤明显，但总的治疗效果不及左旋多巴、金刚烷胺。主要用于轻症及不耐受左旋多巴的患者。常与左旋多巴合用。<br>（2）药用利血平和吩噻嗪类引起的锥体外系反应。<br>（3）肝豆状核变性。<br>（4）畸形性肌张力障碍、癫痫、慢性精神分裂症、抗精神病药所致的静坐不能。<br>（1）It is clinically used in the treatment of parkinsonism or parkinsonism caused by encephalitis and atherosclerosis. It has effect on salivation and tremor improvement, but worse effect on relieving spasticity and bradykinesia. So the overall treatment effect is not as good as levodopa and amantadine. It is mainly for patients who have mild symptoms and are intolerant to levodopa. It is often used in combination with levodopa.<br>（2）It is used in treatment of extrapyramidal reactions caused by medicinal reserpine and phenothiazines,<br>（3）hepatolenticular degeneration, as well as.<br>（4）akathisia caused by dystonia musculorum deformans, epilepsy, chronic schizophrenia and antipsychotic drugs. |
| 用法、用量<br>Dosage | 常用量：口服，开始时一日 1～2mg，一日 2 次；逐日递增至一日 5～10mg，分次服用。对药物引起的锥体外系反应：口服开始第 1 日 1mg，并逐增剂量直至每日 5～10mg，1 日 2 次。口服，一日最多不超过 10mg。<br>Usual dose for oral medication: start with 1～2mg a day, 2 times a day; then increase day by day to 5～10mg a day, in several divided doses. Drug-induced extrapyramidal reactions: by oral medication, give 1 mg on the first day, and then gradually increase to 5～10mg a day, 2 times a day. The daily dose for oral medication is no more than 10mg. |
| 剂型、规格<br>Preparations | 片剂：每片 2mg。<br>胶囊剂：每粒 5mg。<br>Tablets: 2mg per tablet.<br>Capsules: 5mg per capsule. |
| 药品名称 Drug Names | 金刚烷胺 Amantadine |
| 适应证<br>Indications | ①用于不能耐受左旋多巴治疗的震颤麻痹患者；②亚洲 A-Ⅱ型流感、病毒性感染发热患者；③脑梗死所致的自发性意识低下。<br>It is used for ① parkinsonism patients who are intolerant to levodopa; ② Asian A-Ⅱ influenza, febrile patients by virus infection; ③ spontaneous low consciousness caused by cerebral infarction. |
| 用法、用量<br>Dosage | 口服：成人每次 100mg，早、晚各 1 次，最大剂量每日 400mg。小儿用量酌减，可连用 3～5 日，最多 10 日。1～9 岁小儿每日 3mg/kg，最大用量不超过 150mg/d。<br>Oral medication: for adults, give 100mg singly, twice a day (in the morning and evening); the maximum dose is 400mg everyday. For children, make appropriate dose reduction and give for continuous 3~5 days; the medication is at most 10 days; for children from 1 to 9 years old, give 3mg/kg a day; the maximum can not exceed 150mg a day. |
| 剂型、规格<br>Preparations | 片剂：每片 100mg。<br>胶囊剂：每粒 100mg。<br>糖浆剂：60ml：300mg。<br>颗粒剂：6g：60mg；12g：140mg。<br>Tablets: 100mg per tablet.<br>Capsules: 100mg per capsule.<br>Syrup: 60ml: 300mg.<br>Granules: 6g: 60mg, 12g, 140mg. |

**续 表**

| 药品名称 Drug Names | 美金刚 Memantine |
|---|---|
| 适应证<br>Indications | （1）用于震颤麻痹综合征。<br>（2）能够改善阿尔茨海默病患者的认知、行为、日常活动和临床症状，可用于重度患者。<br>(1) It is used in the treatment of parkinsonism.<br>(2) It can improve Alzheimer patients' cognition, behavior, daily activity and clinical symptoms . It can also be used for severe patients. |
| 用法、用量<br>Dosage | 口服或胃肠道给药，成人和 14 岁以上青年第 1 周，每日 10mg，分 2～3 次给药；以后每周增加 10mg/d。维持剂量：一次 10mg，一日 2～3 次。需要时还可增加。剂量因人而异。14 岁以下儿童的维持量为每日 0.5～1.0mg/kg。<br><br>Oral medication or gastrointestinal administration: for adults and young people over the age of 14: give 10mg a day in the first week, in 2 or 3 divided doses; afterwards increase by 10mg a day every week. The maintenance dose is 10mg singly, 2 or 3 times a day; dose can be increased if needed. The administration dose varies from patient to patient. For children under the age of 14, give maintenance doses of 0.5～1.0 mg/kg a day. |
| 剂型、规格<br>Preparations | 片剂：每片 10mg。<br>滴剂：10mg。<br>注射液：每支 10mg（2ml）。<br>Tablets: 10mg per tablet.<br>Drops: 10mg.<br>Injection: 10mg (2ml) per vial. |

8.8 抗精神病药 Anti-psychotic drugs

| 药品名称 Drug Names | 氯丙嗪 Chlorpromazine |
|---|---|
| 适应证<br>Indications | ①治疗精神病：用于控制精神分裂症或其他精神病的兴奋躁动、紧张不安、幻觉、妄想等症状，对忧郁症状及木僵症状的疗效较差。对Ⅱ型精神分裂症患者无效，甚至可以加重病情。②镇吐：几乎对各种原因引起的呕吐，如尿毒症、胃肠炎、癌症、妊娠及药物引起的呕吐均有效。也可治疗严重呃逆。但对晕动症呕吐无效。③低温麻醉剂人工冬眠：用于低温麻醉时可以防止休克发生。人工冬眠时，与哌替啶、异丙嗪配成冬眠合剂用于创伤性休克、中毒性休克、烧伤、高热及甲状腺危象的辅助治疗。④与镇痛药合用，治疗癌症晚期患者的剧痛。⑤治疗心力衰竭。⑥试用于治疗巨人症。<br><br>① Psychosis: it is used to control schizophrenia or psychotic agitation, nervousness, hallucination, delusion and so on. It has worse effect on depressive symptoms and symptoms of stupor. It has no effect on Type Ⅱ schizophrenia, sometimes even deteriorate the patients' condition.. ② Antiemetic effect: It has effect on vomiting by almost all kinds of causes, such as uremia, gastroenteritis, cancer, pregnancy and drugs. It also can be used to treat severe hiccups. But it has no effect on vomiting by motion sickness. ③ anesthesia under low temperature and artificial hibernation: In low temperature anesthesia, it can be used to prevent shock. In artificial hibernation, it is combined with meperidine and promethazine as lytic cocktail, which is used as adjuvant therapy in treatment of traumatic shock, toxic shock, burns, fever and thyroid crisis. ④ It is used in combination with analgesic to treat pain of advanced cancer patients. It is used in the ⑤ treatment of heart failure and ⑥ gigantism. |
| 用法、用量<br>Dosage | （1）口服：①用于呕吐，1 次 12.5～25mg，一日 2～3 次；②用于精神病，1 日 50～600mg。开始每日 25～50mg，分 2～3 次服，逐渐增加至每日 300～450mg，症状减轻后再减至一日 100～150mg。极量每次 150mg，每日 600mg。<br>（2）肌内或静脉注射：①用于呕吐，1 次 25～50mg；②用于神经病，1 次 25～100mg。目前多采用静脉注射。极量每次 100mg，一日 400mg。③治疗心力衰竭：肌内注射小剂量，每次 5～10mg，一日 1～2 次，也可静脉滴注，速度每分钟 0.5mg。<br><br>(1) Oral medication: ① in treatment of vomiting, give 12.5～25mg singly, 2 or 3 times a day; ② in treatment of psychosis, give 50～600mg a day: start with 25～50mg a day, in 2 or 3 divided doses and then gradually increase to 300～450mg a day; when symptoms get alleviated, reduced to 100～150mg a day. The maximum dose is 150mg singly, 600mg a day.<br>(2) Intramuscular or intravenous injection: ① in treatment of vomiting, give 25～50mg singly; ② in treatment of neuropathy, give 25～100mg singly, currently by intravenous injection; the maximum dose is 100mg singly, 400mg a day. ③ in treatment of heart failure: by intramuscular injection of small dose, give 5～10mg singly, 1 or 2 times a day or by intravenous infusion, with speed of 0.5mg per minute. |

**续　表**

| | |
|---|---|
| 剂型、规格<br>Preparations | 片剂：每片 5mg；12.5mg；25mg；50mg。<br>注射液：每支 10mg（1ml）；25g（1ml）；50mg（2ml）。<br>Tablets: 5mg 12.5mg 25mg 50mg per tablet.<br>Injection: 10mg (1ml) 25g (1ml) 50mg (2ml) per vial. |
| **药品名称 Drug Names** | 奋乃静 Perphenazine |
| 适应证<br>Indications | ①用于治疗偏执性精神病、反应性精神病、症状性精神病，单纯性及慢性精神分裂症。②用于治疗恶心、呕吐、呃逆等症，神经症具焦虑紧张症患者，亦可用小剂量配合其他药物治疗。<br>① It is used in the treatment of paranoid psychosis, reactive psychosis, symptomatic psychosis, simple schizophrenia and chronic schizophrenia. ② It is also used in the treatment of nausea, vomiting, hiccup and so on, as well as for neurosis patients with anxiety and catatonia. Its small dose can be used with other drugs in treatment. |
| 用法、用量<br>Dosage | 口服：用于呕吐、焦虑，1 次 2 ～ 4mg，一日 2 ～ 3 次；用于精神病，开始时一日 6 ～ 12mg，逐日增量至一日 30 ～ 60mg，分 3 次服。<br>肌内注射：用于精神病，一次 5 ～ 10mg，隔 6 小时 1 次或酌情调整；用于呕吐一次 5mg。<br>Oral medication: in vomiting by anxiety, give 2 ～ 4mg singly, 2 to 3 times a day; in treatment of psychosis, start with 6 ～ 12mg a day and gradually increase to 30 ～ 60mg a day, in 3 divided doses.<br>Intramuscular injection: in treatment of psychosis, give 5 ～ 10mg singly, every 6 hours or make appropriate dose adjustment; in treatment of vomit, give 5mg singly. |
| 剂型、规格<br>Preparations | 片剂：每片 2mg；4mg。<br>注射液：每支 5mg（2ml）；5mg（1ml）。<br>Tablets: 2mg, 4mg per tablet.<br>Injection: 5mg (2ml), 5mg (1ml) per vial. |
| **药品名称 Drug Names** | 氟奋乃静 Fluphenazine |
| 适应证<br>Indications | 用于妄想、紧张型精神分裂症、痴呆和中毒性精神病。亦可用于控制恶心呕吐。其癸酸酯注射液有长效作用。<br>It is used in the treatment of delusions, catatonic schizophrenia, dementia and toxic psychosis, as well as in control of nausea and vomiting. And the Fluphenazine Decanoate injection has long-lasting effect. |
| 用法、用量<br>Dosage | 口服：成人常用剂量 1 次 2mg，一日 1 ～ 2 次；逐渐递增，日服总量可达 20mg。<br>老年或体弱者从最小剂量开始，然后每日用量递增在 1 ～ 2mg。<br>Oral medication: give adults usual dose of 2mg singly, 1 or 2 times a day; gradually increase the dose and the total daily doses can be up to 20mg.<br>Elderly patients or weak patients should start with the smallest dose, and then gradually increase by 1 to 2mg a day. |
| 剂型、规格<br>Preparations | 片剂：1 片 2mg；5mg。<br>注射液：每支 2mg（1m）；5mg（1ml）；10mg（2ml）。<br>Tablet: 2mg 5mg per tablet.<br>Injection: 2mg (1m) 5mg (1ml) 10mg (2ml) per vial. |
| **药品名称 Drug Names** | 三氟拉嗪 Trifluoperazine |
| 适应证<br>Indications | ①主要用于治疗精神病，对急、慢性精神分裂症，尤其对妄想型与紧张型较好。②用于镇吐。<br>① It is mainly used in the treatment of psychosis, acute schizophrenia and chronic schizophrenia, especially with better effect for paranoid and catatonic type. ② It also can be used in anti-vomiting. |
| 用法、用量<br>Dosage | 口服，一次 5 ～ 10mg，一日 15 ～ 30mg。必要时可逐渐递增至每日 45mg。也用于镇吐，口服，一次 1 ～ 2mg，一日 2 ～ 4mg。<br>Oral medication: give 5 ～ 10mg singly, 15 ～ 30mg a day; gradually increase to 45mg a day, if necessary; in treatment of anti-vomiting, give1 ～ 2mg singly, 2 ～ 4mg a day. |
| 剂型、规格<br>Preparations | 片剂：每片 1mg；5mg。<br>Tablets: 1mg, 5mg per tablet. |

**续　表**

| 药品名称 Drug Names | 硫利达嗪 Thioridazine |
|---|---|
| 适应证<br>Indications | 主要用于治疗精神分裂症，适用于伴有激动、焦虑、紧张的精神分裂症、躁狂症、更年期精神病。亦用于儿童多动症及行为障碍。因锥体外系反应少而广泛应用。<br><br>It is mainly used in the treatment of schizophrenia, as well as schizophrenia with excitement, anxiety and tension, mania and menopause psychosis. It is also used in children's with ADHD and behavioral disorders. It is widely used because of its less extrapyramidal reactions. |
| 用法、用量<br>Dosage | 开始时口服每次 25 ~ 100mg，一日 3 次。然后根据病情及耐受情况逐渐递增至充分治疗剂量每次 100 ~ 200mg，一日 3 次。最多可达每日 800mg。老年或体质弱者，从小剂量开始逐渐增加，每日总量低于成年人。<br><br>By oral medication, start with 25 ~ 100mg singly, 3 times a day. Then according to patients' condition and the tolerance, gradually increase to full dose of 100 ~ 200mg singly, 3 times a day. The maximum daily dose can be 800mg. For elderly patients and weak patients, start with small dose and make gradual dose increase; the daily total dose should be less than adults' dose. |
| 剂型、规格<br>Preparations | 片剂：每片 10mg；25mg；50mg；100mg；200mg。<br>Tablets: 10mg 25mg 50mg 100mg 200mg per tablet. |
| 药品名称 Drug Names | 氟哌啶醇 Haloperidol |
| 适应证<br>Indications | 主要用于：①各种急、慢性精神分裂症。特别适合于急性青春型和伴有敌对情绪及攻击行动的偏执型精神分裂症，亦可用于对吩噻嗪类治疗无效的其他类型或慢性精神分裂症。②焦虑性神经症。③儿童抽动 - 秽语综合征，又称 Tourette 综合征（TS），小剂量本品治疗有效，能消除不自主的运动，又能减轻和消除伴存的精神症状。④呕吐及顽固性呃逆。<br><br>It is mainly used in treatment of ① all kinds of acute and chronic schizophrenia, especially acute hebephrenic schizophrenia and paranoia schizophrenia with hostility and aggressive behavior, as well as chronic or other types of schizophrenia which is resistant to phenothiazines . ② Anxiety neurosis. ③ Children's Tourette syndrome (TS): small doses of this drug has effect on eliminating involuntary movements and reducing or eliminating simultaneous mental symptoms. ④ Vomiting and intractable hiccups. |
| 用法、用量<br>Dosage | ①口服：用于精神病：成人开始剂量每次 2 ~ 4mg，一日 2 ~ 3 次；逐渐增至 8 ~ 12mg，一日 2 ~ 3 次。一般剂量每日 20 ~ 30mg。维持治疗每次 2 ~ 4mg，一日 2 ~ 3 次。儿童及老年人，剂量减半。用于呕吐和焦虑：一日 0.5 ~ 1.5mg。用于抽动 - 秽语综合征：一般剂量每次 1 ~ 2mg，一日 3 次。②肌内注射：每次 5 ~ 10mg，一日 2 ~ 3 次。③静脉注射：10 ~ 30mg 加入 25% 葡萄糖注射液在 1 ~ 2 分钟缓慢注入，每 8 小时 1 次。好转后可改口服。<br><br>① Oral medication: in treatment of psychosis, give adults starting dose of 2 ~ 4mg singly, 2 to 3 times a day; gradually increase to 8 ~ 12mg, 2 to 3 times a day. The average dose is 20 ~ 30mg a day; the maintenance dose is 2 ~ 4mg singly, 2 to 3 times a day. For children and the elderly patients, give the half dose. In treatment of vomiting and anxiety: give 0.5 ~ 1.5mg a day. In treatment of Tourette syndrome: give general dose of 1 ~ 2mg singly, 3 times a day. ② Intramuscular injection: give 5 ~ 10mg singly, 2 to 3 times a day. ③ Intravenous injection: add 25% glucose in 10 ~ 30mg of the drug for slow injection within 1 ~ 2 minutes, every 8 hours; when patients' condition get improvement, oral administration can be used. |
| 剂型、规格<br>Preparations | 片剂：每片 2mg；4mg；5mg。<br>注射液：每支 5mg（1ml）。<br>Tablets: 2mg 4mg 5mg per tablet.<br>Injection: 5mg (1ml) per vial. |
| 药品名称 Drug Names | 氟哌利多 Droperidol |
| 适应证<br>Indications | ①治疗精神分裂症的急性精神运动性兴奋躁狂状态。②神经安定镇痛术：利用本药的安定作用及增强镇痛作用的特点，将其与镇痛药芬太尼一起静脉注射，使患者产生一种特殊麻醉状态，用于烧伤大面积换药，各种内镜检查及造影等。③麻醉前给药，具有较好的抗精神紧张、镇吐、抗休克的作用等。<br><br>① It is used treat schizophrenia acute psychomotor state of excitement and mania. ② Neuroleptic analgesia: the drug has the effect of tranquillizing and enhancing analgesia, so when used with analgesic fentanyl for intravenous injection, it would produce a special anesthesia state, which can be used in large area dressing of burns and all kinds of endoscopy and radiography, etc. ③ Preanesthetic medication: it has better effect of anti-stress, anti-shock antiemetic, anti-vomiting and so on. |

**续　表**

| | |
|---|---|
| 用法、用量<br>Dosage | ①治疗精神分裂症：一日 10 ~ 30mg，分 1 ~ 2 次肌内注射。②神经安定镇痛术：每 5mg 加芬太尼 0.1mg，在 2 ~ 3 分钟缓慢静脉注射，5 ~ 6 分钟如未达一级麻醉状态，可追加 0.5 ~ 1 倍剂量。③麻醉前给药：手术前 0.5 小时肌内注射 2.5 ~ 5mg。<br><br>① Schizophrenia: give 10 ~ 30mg a day, in 1 to 2 divided doses of intramuscular injection. ② Neuroleptic analgesia: add 0.1mg of fentanyl into every 5mgof the drug, by slow intravenous injection within 2 to 3 minutes; if patients are not in first-grade anesthesia within 5 to 6 minutes, give another half times or doubled dose. ③ Preanesthetic medication: by intramuscular injection, give 2.5 ~ 5mg, 0.5 hour before surgery. |
| 剂型、规格<br>Preparations | 注射液：每支 5mg（1ml）。<br>Injection: 5mg (1ml) per vial. |
| 药品名称 Drug Names | 氯哌噻吨 Clopenthixol |
| 适应证<br>Indications | ①长期使用可预防精神分裂症复发，对慢性患者可改善症状；对幻觉、妄想、思维障碍、行为紊乱、兴奋躁动等效果较好。②对智力障碍伴精神运动性兴奋状态、儿童严重攻击性行为障碍、老年动脉硬化性痴呆疗效较好。<br><br>① Long-term medication can prevent recidivating of schizophrenia and improve symptoms of patients with chronic disease; it has better effect on hallucinations, delusions, thought disorder, behavioral disorder and excitement agitation. ② It has better effect on dysgnosia with psychomotor excitement, children's severe aggressive behavior disorder and elderly people's arteriosclerosis dementia. |
| 用法、用量<br>Dosage | 口服：开始剂量一日 10mg，一日 1 次，以后可逐渐增至每日 80mg，分 2 ~ 3 次服；维持剂量一日 10 ~ 40mg。速效针剂：深部肌内注射 50 ~ 100mg，一般 72 小时注射 1 次，累计总量不超过 400mg。癸酸酯长效针剂：一般 200mg 肌内注射，每 2 ~ 4 周一次，根据情况调整。<br><br>Oral medication: start with 10 mg a day, once a day; afterwards gradually increase to 80 mg a day, in 2 ~ 3 divided doses; the maintenance dose is 10 ~ 40 mg a day. Quick-acting injection: by deep intramuscular injection, give 50 ~ 100 mg, once every 72 hours; the cumulative total dose can not exceed 400 mg. Decanoate long-acting injection: by intramuscular injection, give 200 mg singly, every 2 ~ 4 weeks; make dose adjustment depending on patients' condition. |
| 剂型、规格<br>Preparations | 片剂：每片 10mg。<br>注射剂：速效针剂 50mg（1ml），长效针剂 200mg（1ml）。<br>Tablets: 10mg per tablet.<br>Injection: quick-acting injection 50mg (1ml), long-acting injection 200mg (1ml). |
| 药品名称 Drug Names | 氟哌噻吨 Flupentixol |
| 适应证<br>Indications | ①用于急、慢性精神分裂症，对淡漠，意志减退，违拗症状及分裂症后抑郁效果较好；长效制剂用于维持治疗和慢性精神分裂的治疗。②各种原因引起的抑郁或焦虑症状。③有癫痫、老年痴呆、精神发育迟滞以及酒、药依赖伴发的精神症状。<br><br>① It is used for acute and chronic schizophrenia, and has better effect on acedia, Hypobulia depression and postschizophrenic depression; long-acting preparation is used in maintenance therapy and in the treatment of chronic schizophrenia. ② It is used in treatment of depression symptoms or anxiety symptoms by various reasons. ③ It is also used in treatment of psychiatric symptoms caused by epilepsy, dementia, mental retardation, as well as alcohol and drug dependence. |
| 用法、用量<br>Dosage | ①用于精神病：口服，初始每次 5mg，一日 1 次，以后视情况可逐渐加量，必要时可增至每日 40mg；维持剂量每次 5 ~ 20mg，一日 1 次。深部肌内注射，起始剂量 10mg 注射一次，1 周后可酌情加量；治疗剂量每次 20 ~ 40mg，每 2 周注射一次；维持剂量每次 20mg，每 2 ~ 4 周注射一次。②用于治疗忧郁性神经症：口服，每次 1mg，一日 2 次。最大剂量为每日 3mg。<br><br>① Psychosis: by oral medication, start with 5mg singly, once a day; afterwards make dose increase gradually depending on patients; condition and if necessary, increase to 40mg a day; the maintenance dose is 5 ~ 20mg singly, once a day. By deep intramuscular injection, start with 10mg, only once; after a week, make appropriate dose increase depending on patients' condition; the therapeutic dose is 20 ~ 40mg singly, once every 2 weeks; the maintenance dose is 20mg singly, once every 2 to4 weeks. ② depressive neurosis: by oral medication, give 1mg singly, twice a day; the maximum dose is 3mg a day. |

| | |
|---|---|
| 剂型、规格<br>Preparations | 片剂：每片 0.5mg；3mg；5mg。癸酸酯注射剂：每支 20mg（1ml）。<br>Tablets: 0.5mg, 3mg, 5mg per tablet. Decanoate Injection: 20mg (1ml) per vial. |
| 药品名称 Drug Names | 氟哌噻吨美利曲辛 Flupentixol and Melitracen |
| 适应证<br>Indications | ①用于治疗神经症。治疗多种焦虑抑郁状态。②用于治疗神经性头痛、偏头痛、紧张性头痛，某些顽固性疼痛及慢性疼痛等。<br><br>① It is used in the treatment of neurosis and a variety of anxiety and depression, as well as ② nervous headache, migraine, tension headache, some intractable pain and chronic pain, etc. |
| 用法、用量<br>Dosage | 口服：一日 2 片，早晨单次顿服，或早晨、中午各服 1 片。严重者一日 3 片，早晨 2 片，中午 1 片。维持剂量为一日 1 片，早晨服。<br><br>Oral medication: give 2 tablets a day, at a draught, in the morning or 1 tablet singly, twice a day (in the morning and noon); in severe case, give 3 tablets a day (2 in the morning and 1 in the noon). The maintenance dose is 1 tablet a day, in the morning. |
| 剂型、规格<br>Preparations | 片剂：每片含哌噻吨 0.5mg 和美利曲辛 10mg。<br>Tablets: 0.5mg of Flupentixol and 10mg of melitracen contained per tablet. |
| 药品名称 Drug Names | 舒必利 Sulpiride |
| 适应证<br>Indications | ①对淡漠、退缩、木僵、抑郁、幻觉和妄想症状的效果较好,适用于精神分裂症单纯型、偏执型、紧张型及慢性精神分裂症的孤僻、退缩、淡漠症状；对抑郁症状有一定疗效。②用于治疗呕吐、酒精中毒性精神病、智力发育不全伴有人格障碍、胃及十二指肠溃疡等。<br><br>① It has better effect on symptoms of apathy, withdrawal, catalepsy, depression, hallucination and delusion. It is used in the treatment of simple schizophrenia, paranoid schizophrenia, catatonic schizophrenia and chronic schizophrenia, as well as the symptoms of unsociability, withdrawal and apathy. It also has curative effect on depressive symptoms. ② It is used in the treatment of vomiting, alcoholic psychosis, oligophrenia with personality disorder, gastric and duodenal ulcers and etc. |
| 用法、用量<br>Dosage | ①治疗精神病：口服，开始一日 300 ~ 600mg，可缓慢增至一日 600 ~ 1200mg；肌内注射，每日 200 ~ 600mg，分 2 次注射；静脉滴注，一日 300 ~ 600mg，稀释后缓慢滴注，滴注时间不少于 4 小时。一般以口服为主，对拒药者或治疗开始 1 ~ 2 周可用注射给药，以后改为口服。②治疗呕吐：口服，每次 100 ~ 200mg，一日 2 ~ 3 次。<br><br>① Psychosis: by oral medication, start with 300 ~ 600mg a day, and slowly increased to 600 ~ 1200mg a day; by intramuscular injection, give 200 ~ 600mg a day, in 2 divided doses of injection; by intravenous infusion, give 300 ~ 600 mg a day; give slow infusion after dilution; the infusion time is at least 4 hours. Generally give oral medication in priority; for patients who refuse the medicine or treatment, administer the drug by injection therapy in the first 1 to 2 weeks, and then change to oral medication. ② Vomiting: by oral medication, give 100 ~ 200mg singly, 2 to 3 times a day. |
| 剂型、规格<br>Preparations | 片剂：每片 10mg；50mg；100mg；200mg。<br>注射液：每支 50mg（2ml）；100mg（2ml）。<br><br>Tablets: 10mg 50mg 100mg 200mg per tablet.<br>Injection: 50mg (2ml) 100mg (2ml) per vial. |
| 药品名称 Drug Names | 氯氮平 Clozapine |
| 适应证<br>Indications | 对精神分裂症的阳性或阴性症状有较好的疗效，适用于急性和慢性精神分裂的各种亚型，对偏执型、青春型效果好。也可减轻与精神分裂症有关的感情症状（如抑郁、负罪感、焦虑）。本品也用于治疗躁狂症或其他精神障碍的兴奋躁动和幻觉、妄想，适用于难治性精神分裂症。因导致粒细胞减少症，一般不宜作为首选药，而用于患者经历了其他两种抗精神病药充分治疗无效或不耐受其他药物治疗时。<br><br>It has good curative effect on both positive and negative symptoms of schizophrenia. It is used in the treatment of various subtypes of acute and chronic schizophrenic, especially with better effect on paranoid type and youth type. It can reduce emotional symptoms associated with schizophrenia (such as depression, guilt and anxiety). This product is also used in the treatment of excitement agitation, hallucination and delusion by mania or other mental disorders, as well as refractory schizophrenia. Generally, it can not be the preferred drug because it would lead to granulocytopenia. However, it can be used for patients who have received adequate but ineffective treatment of two other antipsychotics or are intolerant to other medication. |

**续　表**

| | |
|---|---|
| 用法、用量<br>Dosage | 口服：开始一次 25mg，一日 1 ~ 2 次；然后每日增加 25 ~ 50mg，耐受性好，在开始治疗的两周末将一日总量增至 300 ~ 450mg，均为一日分 1 ~ 2 次服用。<br>肌内注射：每次 50 ~ 100mg，一日 2 次。<br>Oral medication: start with 25mg singly, 1 or 2 times a day; then increase by 25 ~ 50mg everyday; for patients with good tolerance, increase the dose to 300 ~ 450mg a day in the first two weekends of the treatment; give medicine in 2 divided doses.<br>Intramuscular injection: give 50 ~ 100mg singly, twice a day. |
| 剂型、规格<br>Preparations | 片剂：每片 25mg；50mg。<br>Tablets: 25mg, 50mg per tablet. |
| **药品名称 Drug Names** | 奥氮平 Olanzapine |
| 适应证<br>Indications | 用于治疗严重阳性症状或阴性症状的精神分裂症和其他精神病的急性期及维持期。亦可用于缓解精神分裂症及相关疾病常见的继发性感情症状。<br>It is used to treat schizophrenia with severe positive or negative symptoms, as well as in acute phase and maintenance phase of other psychosis. It can also be used to alleviate schizophrenia and secondary emotional symptoms of common related diseases. |
| 用法、用量<br>Dosage | 口服，每日 10 ~ 15mg。可根据病情调整剂量每日 5 ~ 20mg。老年人、女性、非吸烟者、有低血压倾向者、严重肾功能损害者或中度肝功能损伤者，起始剂量为每日 5mg，如需加量，剂递增为每次 5mg，递增一次间隔至少 1 周。<br>Oral medication: give 10 ~ 15mg a day; make dose adjustment from 5 to 20mg a day according to patients' condition. The elderly patients, women patients, non-smoker patients, patients with a tendency to low blood pressure, severe renal impairment patients and moderate hepatic injury patients, start with 5mg a day; if dose increase is needed, increase by 5mg every time, with interval of at least one week. |
| 剂型、规格<br>Preparations | 片剂：每片 2.5mg；5mg；7.5mg；10mg。<br>Tablets: 2.5mg 5mg 7.5mg 10mg per tablet. |
| **药品名称 Drug Names** | 喹硫平 Quetiapine |
| 适应证<br>Indications | ①用于各种精神分裂症，不仅对精神分裂症阳性症状有效，对阴性症状也有一定疗效。②也可以减轻与精神分裂症有关的感情症状如抑郁、焦虑及认知缺陷症状。<br>① It is used in the treatment of various schizophrenia; it has effect on not only the positive symptoms of schizophrenia, but also the negative symptoms. ② It can also alleviate emotional symptoms related to schizophrenia, such as depression, anxiety and cognitive defect. |
| 用法、用量<br>Dosage | 口服，成人：起始剂量为 1 次 25mg，一日 2 次。每隔 1 ~ 3 日增加 25mg，逐渐加量至一日 300 ~ 600mg，分 2 ~ 3 次服用。老年人：用本品应慎重，推荐起始剂量为每日 25mg。每日增加剂量幅度为 25 ~ 50mg，直至有效剂量，有效剂量可以较一般成人低。<br>Oral medication: for adults, start with 25mg singly, 2 times a day; increase by 25mg every 1 to 3 days and gradually increase to 300 ~ 600mg a day, in 2 to divided doses. For elderly patients, give medication with caution; it is recommended to start with 25mg a day and increase by 25 ~ 50mg a day until reach the effective dose; the effective dose can be smaller than average ad. |
| 剂型、规格<br>Preparations | 片剂：每片 25mg；100mg；200mg。<br>Tablets: 25mg 100mg 200mg per tablet. |
| **药品名称 Drug Names** | 利培酮 Risperidone |
| 适应证<br>Indications | 用于治疗急性和慢性精神分裂症。特别是对阳性及阴性症状及其伴发的情感症状（如焦虑、抑郁等）有较好的疗效。也可减轻与精神分裂症有关的情感症状。对于急性期治疗有效患者，维持期治疗中，本品可继续发挥临床效果。<br>It is used in the treatment of acute and chronic schizophrenia. It has good effect especially on the positive and negative symptoms, as well as its concurrent emotional symptoms (such as anxiety, depression, and etc.). It also can reduce emotional symptoms related to schizophrenia. For patients who received effective treatment in acute phase, the drug can still be clinically effective in the maintenance phase treatment. |

| 用法、用量<br>Dosage | 口服，宜从小剂量开始。初始剂量为每次 1mg，一日 2 次，剂量逐渐增至第 3 日为 3mg，以后每周调整一次剂量，最大疗效剂量为一日 4 ~ 6mg。<br>老年患者起始剂量为每次 0.5mg，一日 2 次。<br>Oral medication: it is recommended to start from small dose; give the starting dose of 1mg singly, 2 times a day and gradually increased to 3mg on the third day; afterwards make dose adjustment every week; the maximum effective dose is 4 ~ 6mg a day.<br>The starting dose for elderly patients is 0.5mg singly, twice a day. |
|---|---|
| 剂型、规格<br>Preparations | 片剂：每片 1mg；2mg。<br>Tablets: 1mg, 2mg per tablet. |
| **药品名称 Drug Names** | **帕潘立酮 Paliperidone** |
| 适应证<br>Indications | ①用于精神分裂症急性期治疗。②用于精神分裂症、双向情感障碍的躁狂期及孤独症的治疗。<br>① It is used to treat schizophrenia in acute phase. ② It is also be used to treat schizophrenia and autism, as well as in manic phase treatment of bipolar disorder . |
| 用法、用量<br>Dosage | 成人：口服，每次 6mg，一日 1 次，早晨服药。需要进行剂量增加时，推荐增量为每日增加 3mg。一日最大推荐剂量为 12mg。<br>Adults: by oral medication, give 6mg singly, once a day, in the morning; if dose increase is needed, increase recommended dose by 3mg a day; the maximum recommended dose is 12mg a day. |
| 剂型、规格<br>Preparations | 缓释片：3mg；6mg；9mg。<br>Release tablets: 3mg, 6mg, 9mg. |
| **药品名称 Drug Names** | **齐拉西酮 Ziprasidone** |
| 适应证<br>Indications | ①主要用于精神分裂症治疗。也能改善分裂症状伴发的抑郁症状。②可用于情感性障碍的狂躁期治疗。<br>① It is mainly used in the treatment of schizophrenia. It can also improve the depressive symptoms which is concurrent with schizophrenia. ② It can also be used in manic phase treatment of affective disorder. |
| 用法、用量<br>Dosage | 口服：初始治疗一日 2 次，每次 20mg，餐时口服。视病情可逐渐增加到一日 2 次，每次 80mg。调整剂量时间间隔一般应不少于 2 日。维持治疗一日 2 次，每次 20mg。肌内注射：用于精神分裂症患者的急性激越期治疗。每次 10 ~ 20mg，最大剂量为每日 40mg。如需长期使用，应改为口服。<br>Oral medication: in the beginning of the treatment, give 20mg singly, 2 times a day, during meals; make gradual dose increase to 80mg singly, 2 times a day depending on patients' condition, with interval of at least two days. In maintenance treatment, give 20mg singly, 2 times a day. Intramuscular injection: it is used in acute agitation treatment of schizophrenia; give 10 ~ 20mg singly, with the maximum dose of 40mg a day. If long- time medication is needed, injection should be replaced by oral medication. |
| 剂型、规格<br>Preparations | 片剂：20mg；60mg。<br>胶囊剂：20mg；40mg；60mg；80mg。<br>注射液：10mg（1ml）；20mg（1ml）。<br>Tablets: 20mg 60mg.<br>Capsules: 20mg 40mg 60mg 80mg.<br>Injection: 10mg (1ml) 20mg (1ml). |
| **药品名称 Drug Names** | **五氟利多 Penfluridol** |
| 适应证<br>Indications | 对精神分裂症各型和各病程均有疗效，控制幻觉、妄想及淡漠、退缩等症状疗效好。主要用于慢性精神分裂症患者的维持治疗，对急性患者也有效。<br>It is used in the treatment of schizophrenia with various types and in all phases. It has better effect on controlling hallucination, delusion and apathy, withdrawal and so on. It is mainly used in the maintenance treatment of chronic schizophrenia patients, as well as for acute patient. |

**续　表**

| | |
|---|---|
| 用法、用量<br>Dosage | 口服，每次 20 ～ 60mg，每周 1 次，重症或耐药患者可加至每周 120mg，1 次服或 2 次分服（一半在前半周，一半在后半周服）。<br><br>Oral medication: give 20 ~ 60mg singly, once a week' for severe or resistant patients, increase to 120mg a week, in 1 dose or 2 divided doses (one in the first half of the week, the other in latter half of the week). |
| 剂型、规格<br>Preparations | 片剂：每片 5mg；20mg。<br>Tablets: 5mg, 20mg per tablet. |
| **药品名称 Drug Names** | 阿立哌唑 Aripiprazole |
| 适应证<br>Indications | 用于治疗各类型的精神分裂症。国外临床试验表明，本品对精神分裂症的阳性和阴性症状均有明显疗效，也能改善伴发的情感症状，降低精神分裂症的复发率。<br><br>It is Uused to treat ment of various types of schizophrenia. In foreign clinical trials, it manifested that this drug have a significant effect on the positive and negative symptoms of schizophrenia and it also can improve the concurrent emotional symptoms and reduce the recidivating rate of schizophrenia. |
| 用法、用量<br>Dosage | 口服，一日 1 次。推荐用法为第 1 周起始剂量每日 5mg，第 2 周为每日 10mg，第 3 周为每日 15mg，之后可根据个体的疗效个耐受情况调整剂量。有效剂量范围每日 10 ～ 30mg，最大剂量不应超过每日 30mg。<br><br>Oral medication, give once a day. It is recommended to start with 5mg a day in the first week and give 10mg a day in the second week, 15mg a day in the third week, then make dose adjustment according to individual tolerance. The effective dose range is from 10 to 30mg a day and the maximum dose can not exceed 30mg a day. |
| 剂型、规格<br>Preparations | 片剂：每片 5mg；10mg。<br>Tablets: 5mg, 10mg per tablet. |
| **药品名称 Drug Names** | 曲美托嗪 Trimetozine |
| 适应证<br>Indications | 用于伴有恐惧、紧张和情绪激动的神经精神症状及儿童行为障碍；对于带有神经质综合征的患者，本品可有效地消除兴奋；在精神病的治疗上可作为一种维持治疗用药。<br><br>It is used in treatment of neuropsychiatric symptoms with fear, tension and emotional excitement, as well as children's behavioral disorder. For patients with neurotic syndrome, it can effectively eliminate excitement. In the treatment of psychosis, it can be used as maintenance therapy medication. |
| 用法、用量<br>Dosage | 每次口服 300mg，一日 3 ～ 6 次。<br>Oral medication: 300mg singly, 3 ~ 6 times a day. |
| 剂型、规格<br>Preparations | 片剂：每片 300mg。<br>Tablets: 300mg per tablet. |
| **药品名称 Drug Names** | 癸氟奋乃静 Fluphenazine Decanoate |
| 适应证<br>Indications | 应用同氟奋乃静。对幻觉、妄想、木僵、淡漠、孤独和紧张性兴奋有较好疗效。对兴奋躁动和焦虑紧张也有效。对慢性精神分裂症可使淡漠和退缩减轻，改善与环境接触的反应。也可用于精神分裂症缓解期的维持治疗。<br><br>It has the same usage with fluphenazine. It has good effect on excitement agitation and nervous anxiety, while better effect on hallucination, delusion, catalepsy, apathy, loneliness and catatonic. It can reduce symptoms of apathy and withdrawal in chronic schizophrenia and improve the reaction with the environment. It can also be used in maintenance treatment of schizophrenia in remission phase. |
| 用法、用量<br>Dosage | 深部肌内注射，开始剂量 12.5mg，以后每 2 周肌内注射 25mg。剂量宜从小剂量开始，以后酌情增加或减少。<br><br>Deep intramuscular injection: start with 12.5mg; afterwards give 25mg every two weeks. It is appropriate to start with small dose and make dose increase or reduction according to patients' condition. |

**续 表**

| 剂型、规格<br>Preparations | 注射液：每支 25mg（1ml）；25mg（2ml）。<br>Injection: 25mg (1ml), 25mg (2ml) per vial. |
|---|---|

## 8.9 抗焦虑药 Antianxietic drugs

| 药品名称 Drug Names | 地西泮 Diazepam |
|---|---|
| 适应证<br>Indications | ①焦虑症及各种功能性神经病。②失眠，尤其对焦虑性失眠疗效极佳。③癫痫：可与其他癫痫药合用，治疗癫痫大发作或小发作，控制癫痫持续状态时应静脉注射。④各种原因引起的惊厥，如癫痫、破伤风、小儿高热惊厥等。⑤脑血管意外或脊髓损伤性中枢性僵直或腰肌劳损、内镜检查等所致肌肉痉挛。⑥其他：偏头痛、肌紧张性头痛、呃逆、炎症引起的反射性肌肉痉挛、惊恐症、酒精戒断综合征，还可以治疗家族性、老年性和特发性震颤，可用于麻醉前给药。<br><br>① Anxiety disorder and various functional neuropathy' ② Insomnia, especially better effect on anxiety insomnia; ③ Epilepsy: it is used in combination with other drugs to treat epilepsy grand mal or petit mal; in status epilepticus control, intravenous injection should be used.. ④ Convulsion by a variety of causes, such as epilepsy, tetanus, children's high fever and etc. ⑤ muscle spasms caused by cerebrovascular accident, spinal cord injury rigidity, central rigidity, lumbar muscle strain and endoscopy, etc. ⑥ Others: it can be used in the treatment of migraine, muscle tension headache, hiccups, reflex muscle spasms caused by inflammation, panic disorder and alcohol withdrawal syndrome, as well as familial tremor, senile tremor and, essential tremor. It also can be used in preanesthetic medication. |
| 用法、用量<br>Dosage | （1）口服：①抗焦虑：每次 2.5～10mg，一日 3 次。②催眠：每次 5～10mg，睡前服用。③麻醉前给药：1 次 10mg。④抗惊厥：成人每次 2.5～10mg，一日 2～4 次。6 个月以上儿童，每次 0.1mg/kg，一日 3 次。⑤缓解肌肉阵挛：每次 2.5～5mg，一日 3～4 次。<br>（2）静脉注射：①成人基础麻醉：10～30mg。②癫痫持续状态：开始 5～10mg，每 5～10 分钟按需要重复，达 30mg 后必要时每 2～4 小时重复治疗。静脉注射要缓慢。<br><br>(1) Oral medication: ① anti-anxiety: give 2.5～10mg singly, 3 times a day. ② Hypnosis: give 5～10mg singly, before sleep. ③ preanesthetic medication: give 10mg singly. ④ anti-convulsion: for adults, give 2.5～10mg singly, 2 to 4 times a day; for vhildren over 6 months, give 0.1mg/kg singly, 3 times a day. ⑤ myoclonic remission: give 2.5～5mg singly, 3 to 4 times a day.<br>(2) Intravenous injection: ① adults' basic anesthesia: give 10～30mg. ② status epilepticus: start with 5～10mg and repeat the dose every 5 to 10 minutes as needed; if necessary, repeat treatment every 2 to 4 hours after total dose is up to 30mg. The intravenous injection should be slow. |
| 剂型、规格<br>Preparations | 片剂：每片 2.5mg；5mg。<br>胶囊剂：每粒 10mg。<br>注射液：每支 10mg（2ml）。<br>Tablets: 2.5mg, 5mg per tablet.<br>Capsules: 10mg per capsule.<br>Injection: 10mg (2ml) per vial. |
| 药品名称 Drug Names | 奥沙西泮 Oxazepam |
| 适应证<br>Indications | 用于焦虑障碍，伴有焦虑的失眠，并能缓解急性酒精戒断症状。<br>It is used in treatment of anxiety disorder and insomnia with anxiety. It can relieve the symptoms of acute alcohol withdrawal. |
| 用法、用量<br>Dosage | 口服。焦虑和戒酒症状：每次 15～30mg，一日 3～4 次；老年人应当适当减量。失眠：1 次 15mg，睡前服用。<br>The drug is administered by oral medication. Anxiety and alcohol withdrawal symptoms: give 15～30mg singly, 3 to 4 times a day; the elderly patients need appropriate dose reduction. Insomnia: give 15mg singly, before sleep. |
| 剂型、规格<br>Preparations | 片剂：每片 10mg；15mg；30mg。<br>Tablets: 10mg, 15mg, 30mg per tablet. |

**续　表**

| 药品名称 Drug Names | 硝西泮 Nitrazepam |
|---|---|
| 适应证<br>Indications | ①用于各种失眠的短期治疗，口服后 30 分钟左右起作用，维持睡眠 6 小时。②可用于治疗多种癫痫，尤其对阵挛性发作效果较好。<br><br>① It is used in short-term treatment of various insomnia. It would take effect about 30 minutes after oral medication, maintaining sleep for 6 hours. ② It also can be used to treat a variety of epilepsy, especially with better effect on clonic seizure. |
| 用法、用量<br>Dosage | 口服。催眠：成人 5 ~ 10mg，儿童 2.5 ~ 5mg，睡前 1 次服用；抗焦虑：每次 5mg，一日 2 ~ 3 次；抗癫痫：每次 5 ~ 30mg，1 日 3 次，可酌情增加。老年人、体弱者减半。<br><br>The drug is administered by oral medication.<br>Hypnosis: give adults 5 ~ 10mg and children 2.5 ~ 5mg, once before sleep.<br>Anti-anxiety: give 5mg singly, 3 times a day.<br>Anti-epilepsy: give 5 ~ 30mg singly, 3 times a day; dose increase can be made appropriately.. For elderly patients and weak patients, give half of the dose. |
| 剂型、规格<br>Preparations | 片剂：每片 5mg；10mg。<br>Tablets: 5mg, 10mg per tablet. |
| 药品名称 Drug Names | 氟西泮 Flurazepam |
| 适应证<br>Indications | 用于难以入睡、夜间屡醒及早醒的各种失眠。<br><br>It is used in treatment of various insomnia, in which patients have difficulties to fall asleep, wake up frequently at night and wake up early. |
| 用法、用量<br>Dosage | 口服：15 ~ 30mg，睡前 1 次服，年老体弱者开始时每次服用 15mg，根据反应适当加量。<br><br>Oral medication: give 15 ~ 30mg, once before sleep; for the elderly patients and weak patients, start with 15mg singly and make appropriate dose increase according to the reaction. |
| 剂型、规格<br>Preparations | 片剂：每片 15mg。<br>胶囊剂：每粒 5mg；15mg；30mg。<br><br>Tablets: 15mg per tablet.<br>Capsules: 5mg, 15mg, 30mg per capsule. |
| 药品名称 Drug Names | 氯硝西泮 Clonazepam |
| 适应证<br>Indications | ①主要用于治疗癫痫和惊厥，对各型癫痫均有效，尤以对小发作和肌阵挛发作疗效最佳。静脉注射治疗癫痫持续状态。②可用于治疗焦虑状态和失眠。③对舞蹈症亦有效。对药物引起的多动症、慢性多发性抽搐、僵人综合征、各类神经痛也有一定疗效。<br><br>① It is mainly used in the treatment of epilepsy and seizures. It has effect on all kinds of epilepsy and especially better effect on petit mal and myoclonic seizures. Intravenous injection can be used in the treatment of status epilepticus. ② It can be used to treat anxiety and insomnia. ③ It has effect on chorea, as well as drug-induced hyperactivity, chronic multiple tics, stiffman syndrome and various types of neuralgia. |
| 用法、用量<br>Dosage | ①口服：成人，初始剂量每天 1mg，2 ~ 4 周逐渐增加到每天 4 ~ 8mg，分 3 ~ 4 次服用；儿童，5 岁以下初始剂量每天 0.25mg，5 ~ 12 岁每天 0.5mg，分 3 ~ 4 次服用，逐渐增加剂量到每天 1 ~ 3mg（5 岁以下）和 3 ~ 6mg（5 ~ 12 岁）。②肌内注射：1 次 1 ~ 2mg，1 日 2 ~ 4mg。③静脉注射：癫痫持续状态，成人，一次 1 ~ 4mg；儿童，一次 0.01 ~ 0.1mg/kg，注射速度要缓慢。或将 4mg 溶于 500ml 生理盐水，以能够控制惊厥发作的速度而缓慢滴注。<br><br>① Oral medication: for adults, start with 1mg a day; gradually increase to 4 ~ 8mg a day within 2 to 4 weeks, in 3 to 4 divided doses; for children under the age of 5, start with 0.25mg a day, from 5 to 12 years old, give 0.5mg a day, in 3 to 4 divided doses; and then gradually increase the dose to 1 to 3mg (under the age of 5) and 3 to 6mg (5 to 12 years old) a day. ② Intramuscular injection: give 1 ~ 2mg singly, 2 ~ 4mg a day. ③ Intravenous injection: in treatment of status epilepticus, give adults 1 ~ 4mg and children 0.01 ~ 0.1mg/kg singly; the injection speed should be slow. Or dissolve 4mg of the drug in 500ml of saline for slow infusion by the speed which can control the seizures. |

**续　表**

| 剂型、规格<br>Preparations | 片剂：每片 0.5mg；1mg；2mg。<br>注射液：每支 1mg（1ml）；2mg（2ml）。<br>Tablets: 0.5mg 1mg 2mg per tablet.<br>Injection: 1mg (1ml) 2mg (2ml) per vial. |
| --- | --- |
| 药品名称 Drug Names | 劳拉西泮 Lorazepam |
| 适应证<br>Indications | ①主要用于严重焦虑症、焦虑状态及惊恐焦虑的急性期控制，适宜短期使用。可用于伴有精神抑郁的焦虑，但不推荐用于原发性抑郁症的患者。②失眠。③癫痫。④还可用于癌症化疗时止吐（限注射剂），治疗紧张性头痛，麻醉前及内镜检查前的辅助用药。<br><br>① It is mainly used in acute phase control of severe anxiety disorder, anxiety and panic anxiety. Short-term medication is more appropriate. It can be used for anxiety with depression, but it is not recommended to be used for primary depression. ② insomnia. ③ epilepsy. ④ It can also be used for anti-vomiting in cancer chemotherapy ( injection only) and tension headache, as well as adjuvant drug in before anesthesia and endoscopy. |
| 用法、用量<br>Dosage | ①焦虑症：口服，每次 1～2mg，一日 2～3 次。②失眠：睡前 1 小时一次服用 1～4mg。③麻醉前给药：术前 1～2 小时，口服 4mg 或肌内注射 2～4mg。④癫痫持续状态：肌内或静脉注射，1 次 1～4mg。⑤化疗止吐：在化疗前 30 分钟注射 1～2mg，预防呕吐发生。<br><br>① Anxiety disorder: by oral medication, give 1～2mg singly, 2 or 3 times a day. ② Insomnia: give 1～4mg an hour before sleep, once only. ③ Preanesthetic medication: give 4mg by oral medication or 2～4mg by intramuscular injection, 1 to 2 hours before surgery. ④ Status epilepticus: by intramuscular or intravenous injection, give 1～4mg singly. ⑤ Anti-vomiting in chemotherapy: give 1～2mg by injection, 30 minutes before chemotherapy to prevent vomiting. |
| 剂型、规格<br>Preparations | 片剂：每片 0.5mg；1mg；2mg。<br>注射液：每支 2mg（2ml）；4mg（2ml）。<br>Tablets: 0.5mg 1mg 2mg per tablet.<br>Injection: 2mg (2ml) 4mg (2ml) per vial. |
| 药品名称 Drug Names | 氟硝西泮 Flunitrazepam |
| 适应证<br>Indications | 用于催眠（主要用于严重失眠的短期治疗），麻醉前给药和诱导麻醉。<br><br>It is used for hypnosis (mainly in short-term treatment of severe insomnia), preanesthetic medication and induction of anesthesia. |
| 用法、用量<br>Dosage | 催眠：口服，1～2mg，睡前一次服。术前给药：肌内注射，1～2mg。诱导麻醉：缓慢静脉注射，1～2mg。<br><br>Hypnosis: by oral medication, give 1～2mg, at a draught, before sleep. Preoperative medication: by intramuscular injection, give 1～2mg. Induction of anesthesia: by slow intravenous injection, give 1～2mg. |
| 剂型、规格<br>Preparations | 片剂：每片 1mg；2mg。<br>注射液：每支 2mg（2ml）。<br>Tablets: 1mg, 2mg per tablet.<br>Injection: 2mg (2ml) per vial. |
| 药品名称 Drug Names | 艾司唑仑 Estazolam |
| 适应证<br>Indications | ①用于各种类型的失眠。催眠作用强，口服后 20～60 分钟可入睡，维持 5 小时。②用于焦虑、紧张、恐惧及癫痫大、小发作，亦可用于术前镇静。<br><br>① It is used for all types of insomnia. Its effect on Hypnotic is strong: patients can fall asleep 20 to 60 minutes after oral administration, keeping the effect for 5 hours. ② It is also used for anxiety, stress, fear, grand mal and petit mal epilepsy seizures, as well as for preoperative sedation. |

**续　表**

| 用法、用量<br>Dosage | 口服。镇静、抗焦虑：1 次 1 ～ 2mg，一日 3 次；催眠：1 次 1 ～ 2mg，睡前服；抗癫痫：1 次 2 ～ 4mg，一日 3 次；麻醉前给药：1 次 2 ～ 4mg，术前 1 小时服。<br><br>The drug is administered by oral medication. Sedation and anti-anxiety: 1 ～ 2mg, 3 times a day. Hypnosis: 1 ～ 2mg singly, before sleep. Anti-epilepsy: 2 ～ 4mg singly, 3 times a day. Preanesthetic medication: 2 ～ 4mg singly, an hour before surgery. |
| --- | --- |
| 剂型、规格<br>Preparations | 片剂：每片 1mg；2mg。<br>Tablets: 1mg, 2mg per tablet. |
| **药品名称 Drug Names** | 阿普唑仑 Alprazolam |
| 适应证<br>Indications | ①用于治疗焦虑症、抑郁症、失眠。可作为抗惊恐药。②能缓解急性酒精戒断症状。③对药源性顽固性呃逆有较好的治疗作用。<br><br>① It is used in the treatment of anxiety, depression and insomnia. It can be used as anti-panic drug. ② It can relieve the symptoms of acute alcoholic withdrawal. ③ It has a better therapeutic effect on drug-induced intractable hiccups. |
| 用法、用量<br>Dosage | 口服。抗焦虑：一次 0.4mg，一日 3 次，以后酌情增减，量大剂量每日 4mg。抗抑郁：一般为一次 0.8mg，一日 3 次，个别患者可增至每日 10mg。镇静、催眠：0.4 ～ 0.8mg，睡前顿服。抗惊恐：每次 0.4mg，一日 3 次，必要时可酌情增量。老年人：初始剂量每次 0.2mg，一日 3 次，根据病情和对药物反应酌情增量。<br><br>The drug is administered by oral medication. Anti-anxiety: give 0.4mg singly, 3 times a day and make dose increase or reduction appropriately; the maximum dose is 4mg a day. Anti-depression: generally, give 0.8mg singly, 3 times a day; for some individual patients, the dose can be increased to 10mg a day. Sedation and hypnosis: give 0.4 ～ 0.8mg, at a draught, before sleep. Anti-panic: give 0.4mg singly, 3 times a day; if necessary, make appropriate dose increase. For elderly patients, start with 0.2mg singly, 3 times a day and make dose increase according to patients' condition and response to drugs. |
| 剂型、规格<br>Preparations | 片剂：每片 0.25mg；0.4mg；0.5mg；1mg。<br>Tablets: 0.25mg, 0.4mg, 0.5mg, 1mg per tablet. |
| **药品名称 Drug Names** | 奥沙唑仑 Oxazolam |
| 适应证<br>Indications | 用于焦虑症、神经症的治疗。亦可用于麻醉前给药。<br>It is used to treat anxiety disorder and neurosis, and for dosing before anesthesia. |
| 用法、用量<br>Dosage | 口服。抗焦虑：每次 10 ～ 20mg，一日 3 次。镇静催眠：每次 15 ～ 30mg，睡前顿服。麻醉前给药：术前 1 小时给予 1 ～ 2mg/kg。<br><br>The drug is administered by oral. Antianxiety: 10 ～ 20mg, 3 times per day, Sedation and hypnosis: 15 ～ 30mg, at a draught, before sleep. Dosing before anesthesia: 1 ～ 2mg/kg, before the operation. |
| 剂型、规格<br>Preparations | 片剂：每片 5mg；10mg；20mg。<br>胶囊剂：每粒 10mg。<br>Tablets: 5mg, 10mg, 20mg per tablet.<br>Capsules: 10mg per capsule. |
| **药品名称 Drug Names** | 美沙唑仑 Mexazolam |
| 适应证<br>Indications | 可用于神经症、身心疾病，自主神经失调等疾病时的紧张、焦虑、抑郁、易疲劳、睡眠障碍等的治疗。<br><br>It is used in the treatment of tension, anxiety, depression, fatigue and sleep disorder in neurosis, physical and mental illness, autonomic imbalance and so on. |

| 用法、用量<br>Dosage | 口服，每日 1.5～3mg，分 3 次服，必要时根据年龄、症状适当调整剂量。老年人每日剂量为 1.5mg。<br>Oral medicaiton: give 1.5～3mg a day, in 3 divided doses; when necessary, make appropriate dose adjustment according to age and symptoms. Daily dose for elderly patients is 1.5mg. |
|---|---|
| 剂型、规格<br>Preparations | 片剂：每片 0.5mg；1mg。<br>Tablets: 0.5mg, 1mg per tablet. |
| 药品名称 Drug Names | 谷维素 Oryzanol |
| 适应证<br>Indications | 用于自主神经失调（包括胃肠、心血管神经症）、周期性精神病、脑震荡后遗症、精神分裂症和周期型、更年期综合征、月经前期紧张症等，但疗效不够明显。<br>It is used to treat autonomic imbalance (including gastrointestinal and cardiovascular neurosis), periodic psychosis, cerebral concussion sequelae and schizophrenia, as well as periodic catatonia, catatonia in menopausal syndrome and premenstrual catatonia, and etc, but with less obvious effect. |
| 用法、用量<br>Dosage | 口服：每次 10mg，一日 3 次。有时可用至每日 60mg。疗程一般 3 个月左右。<br>Oral medication: give 10mg singly, 3 times a day and sometimes 60mg a day, with treatment course of about 3 months. |
| 剂型、规格<br>Preparations | 片剂：每片 5mg；10mg。<br>Tablets: 5mg, 10mg per tablet. |

8.10 抗躁狂药 Antimanic drugs

| 药品名称 Drug Names | 碳酸锂 Lithium Carbonate |
|---|---|
| 适应证<br>Indications | ①主要用于治疗躁狂症，对躁狂和抑郁交替发作的双相情感性精神障碍有很好的治疗和预防复发作用，对反复发作的抑郁症也有预防发作作用。一般于用药后 6～7 日症状开始好转。因锂盐无镇静作用，一般主张对严重急性躁狂患者先与氯丙嗪或氟哌啶醇合用，急性症状控制后再单用碳酸锂维持。②还可用于治疗分裂 - 情感性精神病，粒细胞减少，再生障碍性贫血，月经过多症，急性菌痢。<br>① It is mainly used in the treatment of mania. It has good therapeutic and preventive effect on bipolar disorder, which has alternate manic and depressive episodes. It can well prevent the episodes of recurrent depression. Usually, symptoms get improvement within 6 to 7 days after medication. Since there is no sedation effect in lithium salt, it is generally recommended that the drug is used in combination with chlorpromazine or haloperidol for severe acute mania patients. After the acute symptom is under control, lithium carbonate can be used alone. ② It can also be used to treat schizophrenia, affective psychosis, granulocytopenia, aplastic anemia, menorrhagia and acute bacillary dysentery. |
| 用法、用量<br>Dosage | ①躁狂症：口服，一般以小剂量开始，每次 0.125～0.25g，一日 3 次。可逐渐加到每次 0.25～0.5g，一般不超过每日 1.5～2.0g。症状控制后维持量一般不超过每日 1g，分 3～4 次服。预防复发时，需持续用药 2～3 年。②粒细胞减少、再生障碍性贫血：口服 10 日，每次 0.3g。一日 3 次。③月经过多症：月经第 1 日服 0.6g，以后每日服 0.3g，均分为 3 次服，共服 3 日，总量 1.2g 为 1 个疗程。每一月经周期服 1 个疗程。④急性菌痢：每次 0.1g，一日 3 次，首剂加倍。少数症状较重者，头 1～3 日每次剂量均可加倍，至症状及粪便明显好转后，以原剂量维持 2～3 日，再递减剂量，3～4 日停药。<br>① Mania: usually start with small dose, by oral medicaiotn, give 0.125～0.25g singly, 3 times a day and make gradual dose increase to 0.25～0.5g singly; generally, the daily dose can not exceed 1.5～2.0g . When symptoms are under control, give maintenance dose; the maintenance dose generally can not exceed 1g a day, in 3 to 4 divided doses. In recidivation prevention, continuous medication for 2 to 3 years is needed. ② Granulocytopenia and aplastic anemia: by oral medication, give0.3g singly, 3 times a day, for 10 days. ③ Menorrhagia: give 0.6g on the first day of menstruation; afterwards give 0.3g a day, in 3 divided doses, for 3 days; the total dose of 1.2g is a course of treatment. Give one course of treatment in each menstrual cycle. ④ acute bacillary dysentery: give 0.1g singly, 3 times a day and double the first dose. For minority of patients with severe symptoms, double each single dose in the first 1 to 3 days until there is significant improvement in symptoms and excrement. Afterwards give the original dose for 2 to 3 days; then reduce dose gradually and make drug withdrawal after about 3 to 4 days. |

**续　表**

| 剂型、规格<br>Preparations | 片剂：每片 0.125g；0.25g；0.5g。<br>缓释片剂：每片 0.3g。<br>胶囊剂：每粒 0.25g；0.5g。<br>Tablets: 0.125g, 0.25g, 0.5g per tablet.<br>Release tablets: 0.3g per table.<br>Capsules: 0.25g; 0.5g per capsule. |
|---|---|
| **药品名称 Drug Names** | 卡马西平 Carbamazepine |
| 适应证<br>Indications | 可用于急性躁狂发作，抑郁发作以及双相情感性精神障碍的维持治疗。锂盐治疗无效或不能耐受时可考虑选用卡马西平代替。<br>It can be used in the maintenance treatment of acute manic episodes, depressive episodes and bipolar disorder. When lithium salt treatment is ineffective or patients are intolerant to lithium salt, consider the selection of carbamazepine as substitute. |
| 用法、用量<br>Dosage | 抗躁狂症：口服，成人开始每日 400mg，分 2 次服。以后隔 1 ~ 2 周每日量增加 200mg，分 3 ~ 4 次服。治疗量每日 600 ~ 1200mg，分 3 ~ 4 次服，与其他肝药酶诱导剂合用可达每日 1600mg。急性躁狂症，每日 600 ~ 1200mg，分 2 次服。<br>Anti-mania: by oral medication, give adults the starting dose of 400mg a day, in 2 divided doses; and then increase by 200mg a day, every 1 to 2 weeks, in 3 to 4 divided doses. The therapeutic dose is 600 ~ 1200mg a day, in 3 to 4 divided doses. When used in combination with other hepatic drug microsomal enzyme inducers, the dose can be 1600mg a day. Acute mania: give 600 ~ 1200mg a day, in 2 divided doses. |
| 剂型、规格<br>Preparations | 片剂：每片 100mg；200mg；400mg。<br>胶囊剂：每粒 200mg；300mg。<br>Tablets: 100mg, 200mg, 400mg per tablet.<br>Capsules: 200mg, 300mg per capsule. |
| **药品名称 Drug Names** | 丙戊酸钠 Sodium Valproate |
| 适应证<br>Indications | 可用于急性躁狂发作的治疗，长期服用对双相情感性神经障碍的反复发作具有预防作用。<br>It can be used to treat acute manic episodes. Long-term medication can prevent the recurrence of bipolar neurological disorders. |
| 用法、用量<br>Dosage | 治疗躁狂症：口服，小剂量开始，每次 200mg，一日 2 ~ 3 次，逐渐增加至每次 300 ~ 400mg，一日 2 ~ 3 次。最高剂量不超过每日 1600mg。6 岁以上儿童每日 20 ~ 30mg/kg，分 3 ~ 4 次服用。<br>Mania: by oral medication, start with the small dose of 200mg singly, 2 to 3 times a day and gradually increase to 300 ~ 400mg singly, 2 to 3 times a day. The maximum dose can not exceed 1600mg a day. For children over the age of 6, give 20 ~ 30mg/kg a day, in 3 to 4 divided doses. |
| 剂型、规格<br>Preparations | 片剂：每片 200mg。<br>Tablets: 200mg per tablet. |

8.11　抗抑郁药 Antidepressants

| **药品名称 Drug Names** | 丙米嗪 Imipramine |
|---|---|
| 适应证<br>Indications | ①用于各种类型的抑郁症治疗。对内源性抑郁症、反应性抑郁症及更年期抑郁症均有效，但疗效出现慢（多在 1 周后才出现效果）。对精神分裂症伴发的抑郁状态 则几乎无效或疗效差。②可用于惊恐发作的治疗，其疗效与 MAOIs 相当。③可用于小儿遗尿症。<br>① It is used in the treatment of various types of depression. It has effect on endogenous depression, reactive depression and involutional melancholia, but the effect appears slowly (more than a week after medication). It has worse or even no effect on the depressive state by schizophrenia. ② It can be used in the treatment panic attack, which has almost the same effect with MAOIs. ③ It also can be used to treat enuresis. |

| | |
|---|---|
| 用法、用量<br>Dosage | 　　口服。①治疗抑郁症、惊恐发作：成人每次 12.5 ~ 25mg，一日 3 次，老年体弱者一次量从 12.5mg 开始，逐渐增加剂量，极量 1 日 200 ~ 300mg。需根据耐受情况调整用量。②小儿遗尿：6 岁以上，每次 12.5 ~ 25mg，每晚 1 次。如在 1 周内未获满意效果，12 岁以下每日可增至 50mg，12 岁以上每日可增至 75mg。<br><br>　　① Depression and panic attack: for adults, give 12.5 ~ 25mg singly, 3 times a day; for elderly and weak patients, start from 12.5mg singly and gradually increase the dose, with the maximum dose of 200 ~ 300mg a day. Make dose adjustment according the tolerance. ② Enuresis: for children over the age of 6, give 12.5 ~ 25mg singly, once at night. If there is no satisfying results within a week, make dose increase to 50mg a day for children over the age of 12 and 75mg a day for children under the age of 12. |
| 剂型、规格<br>Preparations | 　　片剂：每片 10mg；25mg；50mg；75mg。<br>　　胶囊剂：每粒 75mg；100mg；125mg。<br>　　缓释胶囊：每粒 50mg。<br>　　注射剂：每支 25mg（2ml）。<br><br>　　Tablets: 10mg, 25mg, 50mg, 75mg per tablet.<br>　　Capsules: 75mg, 100mg, 125mg per capsule.<br>　　Release capsules: 50mg per capsule.<br>　　Injection: 25mg (2ml) per vial. |
| 药品名称 Drug Names | 氯米帕明 Clomipramine |
| 适应证<br>Indications | 　　①用于治疗内源性、反应性、神经性、隐匿性抑郁症及各种抑郁状态；伴有抑郁症的精神分裂症。②对强迫性神经症具有较好的疗效。③对恐怖症、惊恐发作、继发性焦虑、慢性疼痛综合征、神经性厌食及发作性睡病均有一定疗效。<br><br>　　① It is used in the treatment of different types of depression and depressive state, such as endogenous depression, reactive depression, neurological depression and masked depression, as well as schizophrenia with depression. ② It has good effect on obsessive-compulsive disorder. ③ It also has effect on phobias, panic attack, secondary anxiety to chronic pain syndrome, anorexia nervosa and narcolepsy. |
| 用法、用量<br>Dosage | 　　（1）治疗抑郁症、强迫症：①口服，成人初始每次 25mg，一日 3 次（或服缓释片，75mg，每晚一次），1 周内可见增至最适宜的治疗量。一日最大剂量为 250mg。症状好转后，改为维持量，每日 50 ~ 100mg（缓释片剂每日 75mg）。老年患者，开始每日 10mg，逐渐增加至 30 ~ 50mg（约 10 日），然后改维持量以每日不超过 75mg 为宜。②静脉滴注：开始每日剂量 25 ~ 50mg，用 250ml 葡萄糖注射液稀释，输入时间不低于 2 小时。通常剂量为每日 100mg。<br><br>　　（2）治疗慢性痛性疾病：每日 10 ~ 150mg，最好同时服用镇痛药。<br><br>　　(1) Depression and obsessive-compulsive disorder: ① by oral medication, for adults, start with 25mg singly, 3 times a day (or give sustained release tablet: 75mg, once at night) and make dose increase to the most appropriate therapeutic dose within a week. The maximum dose is 250mg a day. After the symptoms get improved, give maintenance dose of 50 ~ 100mg a day (or sustained-release tablet of 75mg a day). For elderly patients, start with 10mg a day and gradually increase to 30 ~ 50mg (about 10 days), then change to maintenance dose which can not exceed 75mg. ② by intravenous infusion: start with 25 ~ 50mg a day; dilute the drug with 250ml of glucose injection for infusion of at least two hours. The usual dose is 100mg a day.<br><br>　　(2) Chronic pain disorder: give approximately 10 ~ 150mg a day; it had better give with analgetic |
| 剂型、规格<br>Preparations | 　　片剂：每片 10mg；25mg；50mg。<br>　　缓释片：每片 75mg。<br>　　胶囊剂：每粒 25mg；50mg；75mg。<br>　　注射剂：每支 25mg（2ml）。<br><br>　　Tablets: 10mg 25mg, 50mg per tablet.<br>　　Sustained-release tablets: 75mg per tablet.<br>　　Capsules: 25mg, 50mg, 75mg per capsule.<br>　　Injection: 25mg (2ml) per vial. |

**续　表**

| 药品名称 Drug Names | 阿米替林 Amitriptyline |
|---|---|
| 适应证<br>Indications | ①用于治疗各型抑郁症或抑郁状态。对内因性抑郁症和更年期抑郁症疗效较好，对反应性抑郁症及神经官能症的抑郁状态亦有效。对兼有焦虑和抑郁症状的患者，疗效优于丙米嗪。与电休克联合使用于重症抑郁症，可减少电休克次数。②用于缓解慢性疼痛。③亦用于治疗小儿遗尿症、儿童多动症。<br><br>① It is used to treat various types of depression or depressive state. It has good effect on endogenous depression and involutional melancholia, as well as reactive depression and neurosis depression. For patients with both anxiety and depression symptoms, it has better effect than imipramine. It is used in treatment of severe depression when combined with electric shock, which can reduce the times of electric shock. ② It is used to relieve chronic pain. ③ It is also used in the treatment of enuresis and ADHD. |
| 用法、用量<br>Dosage | ①治疗抑郁症、慢性疼痛：口服，每次 25mg，一日 2～4 次，以后递增至每日 150～300mg，分次服。维持量每日 50～200mg。老年患者和青少年，每日 50mg，分次或夜间 1 次服。静脉注射或肌内注射，成人每次 20～30mg，一日 3～4 次。②治疗遗尿症：睡前 1 次口服，10～25mg。③治疗儿童多动症：7 岁以上儿童每次 10～25mg，一日 2～3 次。<br><br>① Depression and chronic pain: by oral medication, give 25mg singly, 2 to 4 times a day and increase to 150～300mg a day, in several divided doses; the maintenance dose is 50～200mg a day. For elderly and adolescent patients, give 50mg a day, in several divided doses or 1 dose at night. By intravenous or intramuscular injection, give adults 20～30mg singly, 3 or 4 times a day. ② Enuresis: by oral medication, give 10～25mg, once before sleep. ③ ADHD: for children over the age of 7, give 10～25mg singly, 2 to 3 times a day. |
| 剂型、规格<br>Preparations | 片剂：每片 10mg；25mg；50mg；75mg；100mg；150mg。<br>缓释胶囊剂：每粒 25mg；50mg；75mg。<br>注射剂：每支 20mg（2ml）；50mg（2ml）；100mg（10ml）。<br>Tablets: 10mg, 25mg, 50mg, 75mg, 100mg, 150mg per tablet.<br>Sustained-release capsules: 25mg, 50mg, 75mg per capsule.<br>Injection: 20mg (2ml), 50mg (2ml), 100mg (10ml) per vial. |

| 药品名称 Drug Names | 多塞平 Doxepin |
|---|---|
| 适应证<br>Indications | ①用于治疗抑郁症和各种焦虑抑郁为主的神经症，亦可用于更年期精神病，对抑郁和焦虑的躯体性疾病和慢性酒精性精神病也有效。也可用于镇静及催眠。②本品外用膏剂用于治疗慢性单纯性苔藓、湿疹、过敏性皮炎、特应性皮炎等。<br><br>① It is used to treat depression and anxiety and various neurosis with anxiety and depression as the dominated symptoms, as well as involutional psychosis. It has good effect on somatic disease with depression or anxiety and chronic alcoholic psychosis. It can also be used in sedation and hypnosis. ② The ointment of this drug can be used in the treatment of chronic lichen simplexchronicus, eczema, allergic dermatitis, atopic dermatitis and so on. |
| 用法、用量<br>Dosage | ①口服，初始剂量每次 25mg，一日 3 次，然后逐渐增至每日 150～300mg。宜在餐后服用，以减少胃部刺激。严重的焦虑性抑郁症可肌内注射，每次 25～50mg，一日 2 次。②局部外用：于患处涂布一薄层，一日 3 次，每次涂布面积不超过总面积的 5%，两次使用应间隔 4 小时。建议短期敷用，不超过 7～8 日。<br><br>① Oral medication: start with 25mg singly, 3 times a day and gradually increase to 150～300mg a day. It is appropriate to take medicine after meals, in order to reduce stomach's stimulation. In treatment of severe anxiety depression, give 25～50mg singly, twice a day, by intramuscular injection. ② Topical external use: smear on the affected area thinly, 3 times a day; the smeared area of each time can not exceed 5% of the total area; the interval is 4 hours. Short-term use is recommended, no more than 7～8 days. |
| 剂型、规格<br>Preparations | 片剂：每片 5mg；10mg；25mg；50mg；100mg。<br>胶囊剂：每粒 10mg；25mg；50mg；75mg；100mg；150mg。<br>注射剂：每支 25mg（1ml）；50mg（2ml）。<br>盐酸多塞平乳膏：每支 10g。<br>Tablet: 5mg, 10mg, 25mg, 50mg, 100mg, per tablet.<br>Capsules: 10mg, 25mg, 50mg, 75mg, 100mg, 150mg per capsule.<br>Injection: 25mg (1ml), 50mg (2ml) per vial.<br>Doxepin hydrochloride cream: 10g of each. |

| 药品名称 Drug Names | 吗氯贝胺 Moclobemide |
| --- | --- |
| 适应证<br>Indications | ①对双相、单相、激动型、阻滞型及各种亚型抑郁症均有效。对精神运动性阻滞和情绪抑郁症状的改善显著。用于对 TCAs 不适用或已不再有效的患者。②对睡眠障碍也有一定效果。<br><br>① It has effect on bipolar depression, unipolar depression, agitated depression, retardant depression, and various subtype depression. It can obviously improve the symptoms of psychomotor retardation and depression. It also can be used for patients who are not available for or are resistant to TCAs. ② It also have effect on sleep disorder. |
| 用法、用量<br>Dosage | 口服：每日 100 ~ 400mg，分次饭后服，可根据病情增减至每日 150 ~ 600mg。<br><br>Oral medication: give 100 ~ 400mg a day, in several divided doses, after meals and make dose reduction to 150 ~ 600 mg a day according to patients' condition. |
| 剂型、规格<br>Preparations | 片剂：每片 75mg；100mg；150mg；300mg。<br>胶囊剂：每粒 100mg。<br><br>Tablets: 75mg, 100mg, 150mg, 300mg per tablet.<br>Capsules: per 100mg. |

| 药品名称 Drug Names | 氟西汀 Fluoxetine |
| --- | --- |
| 适应证<br>Indications | ①用于治疗伴有焦虑的各种抑郁症，尤宜用于老年抑郁症。②用于治疗惊恐状态，对广泛性焦虑障碍也有一定疗效。③用于治疗强迫障碍，但药物剂量应相应加大。④适用于社交恐惧症、进食障碍。<br><br>① It is used to treat various kinds of depression with anxiety, especially senile depression. ② It is also used to treat panic state and has effect on generalized anxiety. ③ In treatment of obsessive-compulsive disorder, the dose should be increased accordingly. ④ It is intended to treat social phobia and eating disorder. |
| 用法、用量<br>Dosage | 口服。①治疗抑郁症：最初治疗建议每日 20mg，一般 4 周后才能显效。若未能控制症状，可考虑增加剂量，每日可增加 20mg。最大推荐剂量每日 80mg。维持治疗可以每日使用 20mg。②强迫症：建议初始剂量为每日晨 20mg，维持治疗可以每日 20 ~ 60mg。③暴食症：建议每日 60mg。④惊恐障碍：初始剂量每日 10mg，1 周后可逐渐增加至每日 20mg，如果症状没有有效控制，可适当增加剂量至每日 60mg。<br><br>The drug is administered orally. ① Depression: in the beginning of the treatment, it is recommended to give 20mg a day, and it would take effect generally excellent after 4 weeks. If it fails to control the symptoms, consider to make dose increase by 20mg a day. The maximum recommended dose is 80mg a day. In maintenance treatment, give 20mg a day. ② Obsessive-compulsive disorder: give recommended starting dose of 20mg a day, in the morning; in maintenance treatment, give 20 ~ 60mg a day. ③ Bulimia: give the recommended dose of 60mg a day. ④ Panic disorder: start with 10mg a day and gradually increase to 20mg a day after a week; if the symptoms can not be effectively controlled, make dose increase to 60mg a day. |
| 剂型、规格<br>Preparations | 片剂：每片 10mg；20mg。<br>肠溶片：90mg。<br>胶囊剂：每粒 5mg；10mg；20mg；40mg；60mg。<br><br>Tablets: 10mg, 20mg per tablet.<br>Enteric-coated tablets: 90mg.<br>Capsules: per 5mg, 10mg, 20mg, 40mg, 60mg. |

| 药品名称 Drug Names | 氟伏沙明 Fluvoxamine |
| --- | --- |
| 适应证<br>Indications | ①用于治疗各类抑郁症，特别是持久性抑郁症状及自杀风险大的患者。②还可治疗强迫症和心身性疾病。<br><br>① It is used to treat various types of depression, and especially has effect on patients with persistent depression symptoms and greater suicide risk. ② It also can treat obsessive-compulsive disorder and psychosomatic disorders. |

**续　表**

| 用法、用量<br>Dosage | 口服。① 抗抑郁：初始剂量每日 50 ～ 100mg，睡前服。每 4 ～ 7 日增加 50mg，剂量可视病情调整，剂量超过每日 150mg 时应分次服用，饭时或饭后服。维持期用药，以 1 日 50 ～ 100mg 为宜。② 强迫症：初始剂量每日 100 ～ 300mg。最大剂量为每日 300mg。<br><br>The drug is administered orally. ① Anti-depression: start with 50 ～ 100mg a day, before sleep and make dose increase by 50mg every 4 ～ 7 days; make dose adjustment depending on patients' condition; if the dose exceeds 150mg a day, take in divided doses, during or after meals. In maintenance treatment, it is appropriate to give 50 ～ 100mg a day. ② Obsessive-compulsive disorder: start with 100 ～ 300mg a day; the maximum dose is 300mg a day. |
|---|---|
| 剂型、规格<br>Preparations | 片剂：每片 50mg；100mg；200mg。<br>胶囊剂：每粒 20mg。<br>肠溶片：90mg。<br><br>Tablets: 50mg, 100mg, 200mg per tablet.<br>Capsules: 20mg per capsule.<br>Enteric-coated tablets: 90mg per tablet. |
| **药品名称 Drug Names** | 帕罗西汀 Paroxetine |
| 适应证<br>Indications | ①用于治疗抑郁症。适合治疗伴有焦虑症和抑郁症患者，作用比 TCAs 快，而且远期疗效比丙米嗪好。②亦可用于惊恐障碍、社交恐惧症及强迫症的治疗。<br><br>① It is used to treat depression. It is also intended to treat depression with anxiety and, with quicker effect than TCAs fast and better long-term effect than imipramine.　② Beside, it can be used in treatment of panic disorder, social phobia and obsessive-compulsive disorder. |
| 用法、用量<br>Dosage | 口服。通常一日剂量为 20 ～ 50mg，一般从 20mg 开始，一日 1 次，早餐时顿服。连续用药 3 周。以后根据临床反应增减剂量，每次增减 10mg，间隔不得少于 1 周。最大推荐剂量为每日 50mg（治疗强迫症可 60mg）。老年人或肝、肾功能不全者可从每日 10mg 开始，每日最高剂量不超过 40mg。对于肌酐清除率＜ 30ml/min 的患者，推荐剂量每日 20mg。<br><br>Oral medication: daily dose usually ranges from 20 tp 50mg; start from 20mg, once a day, at a draught, in breakfast, for continuous 3 weeks; and then make dose increase or reduction according to clinical response, increase or reduce by 10mg each time, with interval of at least one week. The maximum recommended dose is 50mg a day (in treatment of obsessive- compulsive disorder, it is 60mg a day). For elderly patients, hepatic dysfunction patients and renal insufficiency patients, start with 10mg a day, and the maximum daily dose can not exceed 40mg; for patients with creatinine clearance ＜ 30ml/min, give the recommended dose of 20mg a day. |
| 剂型、规格<br>Preparations | 片剂：每片 20mg；30mg。<br>Tablets: 20mg, 30mg per tablet. |
| **药品名称 Drug Names** | 舍曲林 Sertraline |
| 适应证<br>Indications | 用于治疗抑郁症、强迫症、心境恶劣、性欲倒错等。预防抑郁症复发。<br><br>It is used in the treatment of depression, obsessive-compulsive disorder, dysthymia, paraphilias and so on. It can also be used to prevent the recurrence of depression. |
| 用法、用量<br>Dosage | 口服。开始每日 50mg，一日 1 次，与食物同服，早晚均可。数周后增加 50mg。调整剂量时间间隔不能短于 1 周。常用剂量为每日 50 ～ 100mg，最大剂量为每日 200mg（此剂量不得连续服用超过 8 周以上）。需长期服用者，需用最低有效量。<br><br>Oral medication: start with 50mg a day, once a day, with food, in the morning or evening and make dose increase of 50mg a few weeks later. The interval for dose adjustment is at least one week. The usual dose is 50 ～ 100mg a day and the maximum dose is 200mg a day (this dose can not ne given for more than continuous 8 weeks). It patients need long-term medication, give the minimum effective dose. |
| 剂型、规格<br>Preparations | 片剂：每片 50mg；100mg。<br>胶囊剂：每粒 50mg；100mg。<br><br>Tablets: 50mg, 100mg per tablet.<br>Capsules: 50mg, 100mg per capsule. |

**续　表**

| 药品名称 Drug Names | 西酞普兰 Citalopram |
|---|---|
| 适应证<br>Indications | ①用于内源性或非内源性抑郁症。②焦虑性神经症、广场恐惧症、强迫症、经前期心境障碍神经症。③酒精依赖性行为障碍、痴呆的行为问题。④卒中后病理性哭泣。<br><br>① It is used in treatment of endogenous or non-endogenous depression, ② anxiety neurosis, agoraphobia, obsessive-compulsive disorder, premenstrual mood disorders neurosis, ③ alcohol dependent behavioral disorder, behavior problem of dementia and ④ post-stroke pathological crying. |
| 用法、用量<br>Dosage | 口服。每日 20 ~ 60mg，一日 1 次，晨起或晚间顿服。推荐初始剂量为每日 20mg，再根据患者症状控制情况酌情增减，逐渐达到稳定控制病情的最小有效剂量。剂量调整间隔时间不能少于 1 周，一般为 2 ~ 3 周。通常需要经过 2 ~ 3 周的治疗方可判定疗效。为防止复发，治疗至少持续 6 个月。肝功能不全及年龄超过 65 岁的老人：推荐剂量较常量减半。<br><br>Oral medication: give 20 ~ 60mg a day, once a day, at a draught, in the early morning or in the evening. It is recommended to give 20mg a day; make dose adjustment according to patients' symptom control and gradually reach the minimum effective dose .which can stably control the disease. The interval between dose adjustments is at least one week, usually 2 to 3 weeks. Usually it would take 2 to 3 week to determine the effect of the treatment. In order to prevent the recurrence, the treatment should last at least 6 months. For hepatic dysfunction patients and elder patients over the age of 65, it is recommended to give half of the usual dose. |
| 剂型、规格<br>Preparations | 片剂：每片 10mg；20mg；30mg；40mg。<br>口服液：每支 20mg（10ml）。<br><br>Tablets: 10mg, 20mg, 30mg, 40mg per tablet.<br>Oral liquid: 20mg (10ml) of each. |
| 药品名称 Drug Names | 艾司西酞普兰 Escitalopram |
| 适应证<br>Indications | ①用于内源性或非内源性抑郁症。②焦虑性神经症、广场恐惧症、强迫症、经前期心境障碍神经症。③酒精依赖性行为障碍、痴呆的行为问题。④卒中后病理性哭泣。<br><br>① It is used in treatment of endogenous or non-endogenous depression, ② anxiety neurosis, agoraphobia, obsessive-compulsive disorder, premenstrual mood disorders neurosis, ③ alcohol dependent behavioral disorder, behavior problem of dementia and ④ post-stroke pathological crying. |
| 用法、用量<br>Dosage | 口服。治疗抑郁症：每日 10mg，一日 1 次。根据患者的临床情况最大剂量可增至每日 20mg。通常 2 ~ 4 周可控制抑郁症状，症状缓解后需巩固维持治疗至少 6 个月。伴或不伴恐惧症的患者：初始剂量为每日 5mg，持续 1 周后可考虑增加至每日 10mg。根据患者的个体反应，剂量可增至每日 20mg。老年患者：推荐半量使用本品，最大剂量也不应超过每日 20mg。肝功能不全者或 CYP2C19 慢代谢者：建议起始剂量每日 5mg，持续 2 周后，可根据患者的个体反应，剂量增加至每日 10mg。<br><br>The drug is administered orally.<br>Depression: give 10mg a day, once a day and make dose increase according to patients' clinical condition; the maximum dose is 20mg a day. Usually it would take 2 to 4 weeks to control symptoms of depression; after symptomatic relief, patients need another 6 months of consolidation and maintenance therapy. For patients with or without phobia: start with 5mg a day and make dose increase to 10mg a day after a week; according to the individual response, the dose can be increased to 20mg a day. For elderly patients, it is recommended to give half of the dose; the maximum dose should not exceed 20mg a day. For hepatic dysfunction patients and poor CYP2C19 metabolizers, it is recommended to start with 5mg a day, for continuous 2 weeks, afterwards make dose increase to 10mg a day according to the individual response. |
| 剂型、规格<br>Preparations | 片剂：每片 5mg；10mg。<br>Tablets: 5mg, 10mg per tablet. |

### 8.12 抗脑血管病药 Anticerebrovascular disease drugs

| 药品名称 Drug Names | 尼莫地平 Nimodipine |
|---|---|
| 适应证<br>Indications | ①用于急性脑血管病恢复期的血液循环改善。各种原因的蛛网膜下腔出血后的脑血管痉挛及其所致的缺血性神经障碍高血压、偏头痛等。②也被用作缺血性神经元保护和血管性痴呆的治疗。③对突发性耳聋也有一定疗效。 |

**续　表**

① It is used to improve blood circulation in recovery phase of acute cerebrovascular disease. It is used in treatment of vasospasm after subarachnoid hemorrhage by various reasons, as well as high blood pressure and migraine headache of ischemic neurological deficit caused by vasospasm. ② It is also used in the prevention of ischemic neuronal protection and treatment of vascular dementia. ③ Besides, it has some effect on sudden deafness.

| 用法、用量<br>Dosage | 口服：①治疗缺血性脑血管病：片剂，每次 30 ～ 40mg，一日 3 次；缓释剂，每次从 60mg，一日 2 次。连用 1 个月。②治疗突发性耳聋：片剂，每次 10 ～ 20mg，一日 3 次；缓释剂，每次 60mg，一 1 次。5 日为 1 个疗程，可用 3 ～ 4 个疗程。③治疗轻、中度高血压：每次 40mg，一天 3 次。④治疗偏头痛：片剂，每次 40mg，一日 3 次；缓释剂，每次 60mg，一日 2 次，12 周为 1 疗程。⑤老年性认知功能减退或血管性痴呆：每次 30 ～ 40mg，一日 3 次，连服 2 个月。⑥蛛网膜下腔出血所致脑血管痉挛：片剂，每次 40 ～ 60mg，一日 2 ～ 3 次，发病当日即可服用；缓释剂每次 60mg，一日 2 次。连用 3 ～ 4 周为 1 个疗程。如需手术，术前停药，术后可继续服用。<br><br>静脉滴注：治疗蛛网膜下腔出血，滴速 0.5μg/（kg·min），随时检测血压，病情稳定后改口服，成人每次 20 ～ 30mg，一日 2 次。<br><br>The drug is administered orally. ① ischemic cerebrovascular disease: give tablets of 30 ～ 40mg singly, 3 times a day; give slow release formulation of 60mg singly, 2 times a day, for continuous one month. ② Sudden deafness: give tablets of 10 ～ 20mg singly, 3 times a day; give slow release formulation of 60mg, once a day; a course of treatment is 5 days, for 3 to 4 courses' medication. ③ Mild and moderate high blood pressure: give 40mg singly, 3 times a day. ④ Migraine: give tablets of 40mg singly, 3 times a day; give slow release formulation of 60mg, twice a day; a course of treatment is 12 weeks. ⑤ Senile cognitive dysfunction or vascular dementia: give 30 ～ 40mg singly, 3 times a day, for continuous 2 months. ⑥ vasospasm after subarachnoid hemorrhage: give slow release formulation of 60mg, twice a day; give tablets of 40 ～ 60mg singly, 2 to 3 times a day and patients can take it on the attack day. A treatment course of medication about 3 to 4 weeks is needed. If patients need surgery, make drug withdrawal before it and continue medication after it. The drug is administered by intravenous infusion.<br><br>Subarachnoid hemorrhage; the infusion speed is 0.5μg / (kg · min); monitor blood pressure at all times; change to oral medication when patients' in stable condition: 20 ～ 30mg, twice a day, for adults. |
| --- | --- |
| 剂型、规格<br>Preparations | 片剂：每片 10mg；20mg；30mg。<br>胶囊剂：20mg；30mg。<br>控释片：每片 60mg。<br>缓释片：每片 60mg。<br>缓释胶囊：每粒 60mg。<br>注射剂：每支 2mg（10ml）；4mg（20ml）；8mg（40ml）；10mg（50ml）；25mg（50ml）；20mg（100ml）。<br>Tablets: 10mg, 20mg, 30mg per tablet.<br>Capsules: 20mg, 30mg.<br>Release tablets: 60mg per tablet.<br>Sustained-release tablets: 60mg per tablet.<br>Release capsules: per 60mg.<br>Injection: per 2mg (10ml), 4mg (20ml), 8mg (40ml), 10mg (50ml), 25mg (50ml), 20mg (100ml). |
| 药品名称 Drug Names | 桂利嗪 Cinnarizine |
| 适应证<br>Indications | ①用于脑血栓形成、脑梗死、短暂性缺血发作、脑动脉硬化、脑出血恢复期、蛛网膜下腔出血恢复期、脑外伤后遗症、前庭性眩晕与平衡障碍（包括晕动病等）、冠状动脉硬化及供血障碍，以及由于末梢循环不良引起的疾病（如间歇性跛行及 Raynaud 病等）。②有文献报道，本品还可用于治疗慢性荨麻疹、老年性皮肤瘙痒等过敏性皮肤病。开可以治疗顽固性呃逆。<br><br>① It is used in treatment of cerebral thrombosis, cerebral infarction, transient ischemic attack, cerebral arteriosclerosis, sequelae of traumatic brain injury, vestibular vertigo, balance disorders (including motion sickness, etc.), coronary artery disease and blood disorder and diseases caused by poor peripheral circulation (such as intermittent claudication and Raynaud disease, etc.), as well as used in recovery phase of cerebral hemorrhage and subarachnoid hemorrhage. ② It is recorded in the literature that this drug can also be used to treat chronic urticaria, senile pruritus and other allergic dermatitis, as well as intractable hiccups. |

**续　表**

| 用法、用量<br>Dosage | 口服：一般每次 25 ~ 50mg，一日 3 次，饭后服。晕动病患者于乘车船前 1 ~ 2 小时，1 次服用 30mg；乘车船期间每 6 ~ 8 小时服用 1 次（根据头晕等症状情况）。静脉注射：1 次 20 ~ 40mg，缓慢注入。<br><br>Oral medication: generally give 25 ~ 50mg singly, 3 times a day, after meals. In motion sickness treatment, take 30mg, once only, 1 to 2 hours before taking ship or car, and then take medicine once every 6 to 8 hours during ride (depending on symptoms like dizziness, etc.). Intravenous: give 20 ~ 40mg singly, by slow injection. |
|---|---|
| 剂型、规格<br>Preparations | 片剂：每片 15mg；25mg。<br>胶囊剂：每粒 25mg；75mg。<br>注射剂：每支 20mg（20ml）。<br><br>Tablets: 15mg, 25mg per tablet.<br>Capsules: per 25mg, 75mg.<br>Injection: per 20mg (20ml). |
| 药品名称 Drug Names | 氟桂利嗪 Flunarizine |
| 适应证<br>Indications | ①脑动脉缺血性疾病，如脑动脉硬化、短暂性脑缺血发作、脑血栓形成、脑栓塞和脑血管痉挛。②有前庭刺激或脑缺血引起的头晕、耳鸣、眩晕。③血管性偏头痛的防治。④癫痫辅助治疗。⑤周围血管病：间歇性跛行、下肢静脉曲张及微循环障碍、足踝水肿等。<br><br>① It is intended to treat cerebral artery ischemic diseases, such as cerebral arteriosclerosis, transient ischemic attack, cerebral thrombosis, cerebral embolism and cerebral vasospasm. ② It is used to treat dizziness, tinnitus and vertigo caused by vestibular stimulation or cerebral ischemia. ③ It can both treat and prevent vascular migraine. ④ It also can be used in adjuvant treatment of epilepsy and in treatment of ⑤ peripheral vascular disease: intermittent claudication, varicose veins of lower limb and microcirculation disturbance, ankle edema and so on. |
| 用法、用量<br>Dosage | 口服。脑动脉硬化、脑梗死恢复期：每日 5 ~ 10mg，一日 1 次，睡前服用。中枢性和外周性眩晕者、椎动脉供血不足者：每日 10 ~ 30mg，2 ~ 8 周为 1 个疗程。特发性耳鸣者：每次 10mg，每晚一次，10 日为 1 个疗程。偏头痛预防：每次 5 ~ 10mg，一日 2 次。间歇性跛行：每日 10 ~ 20mg。<br><br>The drug is administered orally. Cerebral arteriosclerosis and in recovery phase of cerebral infarction: give 5 ~ 10mg a day, once a day, before sleep. Central vertigo and peripheral vertigo and vertebral artery insufficiency: give 10 ~ 30mg a day; a course of treatment is 2 to 8 weeks. Idiopathic tinnitus: give10mg singly, once at night; a course of treatment is 10 days. Migraine prevention: give 5 ~ 10mg singly, twice a day. Intermittent claudication: give 10 ~ 20mg a day. |
| 剂型、规格<br>Preparations | 片剂：每片 5mg。<br>胶囊剂：每粒 5mg。<br>滴丸：每丸 1.25mg。<br><br>Tablets: 5mg per tablet.<br>Capsules: 5mg per capsule.<br>Dripping Pills: 1.25mg per pill. |
| 药品名称 Drug Names | 降纤酶 Defibrase |
| 适应证<br>Indications | ①急性脑梗死，短暂性脑缺血发作（TIA），以及脑梗死再复发的预防。②心肌梗死，不稳定型心绞痛及心肌梗死再复发的预防。③四肢血管病，包括股动脉栓塞，血栓闭塞性脉管炎，雷诺病。④血液呈高黏状态、高凝状态、血栓前状态。⑤突发性耳聋。⑥肺栓塞。<br><br>① It is used to prevent acute cerebral infarction, transient ischemic attack (TIA), and recurrence of cerebral infarction. ② it can used for myocardial infarction, unstable angina and recurrence of myocardial infarction. ③ it is used for limb vascular disease, including the femoral artery embolism, thromboaangiitis obliterans and Raynaud's disease. ④ it is used for blood being high viscosity state, hypercoagulable state and prothrombotic state. ⑤ it is used for sudden deafness. ⑥ it is used for pulmonary embolism. |
| 用法、用量<br>Dosage | 静脉滴注：急性发作期，1 次 10U，一日 1 次，连用 3 ~ 4 日。非急性发作期，首次 10U，维持量 5 ~ 10U，每日或隔日 1 次，2 周为 1 个疗程。<br><br>Intravenous infusion: in the case of acute attack, the dose is10U once a day, used for continuous 3 to 4 days. In the case of non-acute attack, the first dose is 10U and the maintenance dose is 5 ~ 10U, once daily or every other day. Two weeks is a course of treatment. |

**续　表**

| | |
|---|---|
| 剂型、规格<br>Preparations | 注射剂（冻干制剂）：每支 5U；10U。<br>Injection (lyophilized preparation): 5U; 10U per vial. |
| **药品名称 Drug Names** | 巴曲酶 Batroxobin |
| 适应证<br>Indications | 用于急、慢性缺血性脑血管病（以急性效果明显），突发性耳聋，慢性动脉闭塞症，振动病，末梢循环障碍。也用于中、轻度高血压病。<br><br>It is used for acute and chronic ischemic cerebrovascular disease (acute effect is obvious), sudden deafness, chronic arterial occlusive disease, vibration disease, peripheral circulatory disorders. It can also be used in mild hypertension. |
| 用法、用量<br>Dosage | 静脉滴注：首次剂量 10BU，以后维持剂量为 5BU，隔日 1 次。用 100 ～ 250ml 生理盐水稀释，1 ～ 1.5 小时滴完。给药前血纤溶酶原超过 400mg/dl 或重度突发性耳聋患者剂量应加倍。通常治疗急性缺血性脑血管病 1 个疗程 3 次，治疗突发性耳聋必要时可延长至 3 周，治疗慢性动脉闭塞症可延长至 6 周，但在延长期每次剂量改为 5BU，隔日 1 次。<br><br>Intravenous infusion: the first dose is 10BU and later the maintenance dose is 5BU, once every other day. The drug is diluted by 100 ～ 250ml of saline and should be dripped off in1 to 1.5 hours. Before administration, if plasminogen is more than 400mg/dl or patients are those who have severe sudden deafness, the dose should be doubled. For acute ischemic cerebrovascular disease, the drug is generally used three times in a course of treatement. For sudden deafness, the treatment can be extended to three weeks when necessary. For chronic arterial occlusive disease, the treatment may be extended to six weeks, but over an extended period, the dose is 5BU once every other day. |
| 剂型、规格<br>Preparations | 注射剂：每支 5BU（0.5ml）；10BU（1ml）。<br>Injection: 5BU (0.5ml); 10BU (1ml) per vial. |
| **药品名称 Drug Names** | 倍他司汀 Betahistine |
| 适应证<br>Indications | 主要用于梅尼埃综合征、血管性头痛及脑动脉硬化，并可用于治疗急性缺血性脑血管疾病，如脑血栓、脑栓塞、一过性脑供血不足等；对高血压所致直立性眩晕、耳鸣等亦有效。<br><br>It is mainly used for Meniere's syndrome, vascular headache and cerebral arteriosclerosis. It can also be used for acute ischemic cerebrovascular disease, such as cerebral thrombosis, cerebral embolism, transient cerebral blood supply insufficiency, etc.; it is also effective for upright vertigo and tinnitus caused by hypertension. |
| 用法、用量<br>Dosage | 盐酸倍他司汀片：口服，成人每次 4 ～ 8mg，一日 2 ～ 4 次，最大日量不得超过 48mg。甲磺酸倍他司汀片：口服，成人每次 2 ～ 6mg，一日 3 次，餐后服用。盐酸倍他司汀注射液：肌内注射，每次 2 ～ 4mg，一日 2 次；静脉滴注，每次 20mg，一日 1 次。将本品溶于 2ml5% 葡萄糖溶液或 0.9% 氯化钠溶液中，在溶于静脉滴注液 500ml 中缓慢滴入。<br><br>Betahistine hydrochloride tablets: orally: for adults, the dose is 4 ～ 8mg per time, 2 to 4 times a day. The daily maximum dose should not exceed 48mg. Betahistine mesylate tablets: orally: for adults, the dose is 2 ～ 6mg per time, 3 times a day, taken after meals. Betahistine Hydrochloride Injection: intramuscular injection: the dose is 2 ～ 4mg per time, 2 times a day; intravenous infusion: the dose is 20mg per time, once a day. This product is first dissolved in 2ml of 5% glucose solution or 0.9% sodium chloride solution and then is dissolved in 500ml of intravenous fluid. |
| 剂型、规格<br>Preparations | 片剂（盐酸盐）：每片 4mg。<br>片剂（甲磺酸盐）：每片 6mg。<br>注射液：每支 2mg（2ml）；4mg（4ml）。<br>Tablets (hydrochloride): 4mg per tablet.<br>Tablets (mesylate): 6mg per tablet.<br>Injection: 2mg (2ml); 4mg (4ml) per vial. |
| **药品名称 Drug Names** | 罂粟碱 Papaverine |
| 适应证<br>Indications | 用于脑血栓形成、脑栓塞、肺栓塞、肢端动脉痉挛及动脉栓塞性疼痛。还可用于调节冠状动脉血流，缓解胃肠道痉挛和咳嗽治疗。海绵体注射用于勃起障碍治疗。<br><br>It is used for cerebral thrombosis, cerebral embolism, pulmonary embolism, peripheral arterial spasm and arterial embolism pain. It can also be used to adjust the coronary blood flow, relieve gastrointestinal cramps and treat cough. Its intracavernous injection is used for erectile dysfunction. |

**续 表**

| 用法、用量<br>Dosage | 成人常用量：口服，每次 30 ~ 60mg，一日 3 次。肌内注射，每次 30mg，一日 90 ~ 120mg。静脉注射，每次 30 ~ 120mg，3 小时 1 次，应缓慢注射，不少于 1 ~ 2 分钟，以免发生心律失常以及足以致命的窒息等。用于心脏停搏时，2 次给药要相隔 10 分钟。海绵体注射：推荐 1 次 30mg，每周连续 2 次或不超过 3 次。儿童：肌内注射或静脉注射，一次按体重 1.5mg/kg，一日 4 次。<br><br>Common dose for adults: orally: the dose is 30 ~ 60mg per time, 3 times a day. Intramuscular injection: the dose is 30mg per time, 90 ~ 120mg a day. Intravenous injection: the dose is 30 ~ 120mg per time, once 3 hours and it should be injected slowly, more than 1 to 2 minutes in order to avoid arrhythmia and lethal asphyxia. For cardiac arrest, the two doses should to be separated by 10 minutes. Intracavernous injection: the dose is recommended to be 30mg once, 2 times a week or no more than 3 times. For children: intramuscular or intravenous injection: the dose is 1.5mg/kg once, 4 times a day. |
|---|---|
| 剂型、规格<br>Preparations | 片剂：每片 30mg。<br>注射剂：每支 30mg（1ml）。<br>Tablets: 30mg per tablet.<br>Injection: 30mg (1ml) per vial. |
| 药品名称 Drug Names | 己酮可可碱 Pentoxifylline |
| 适应证<br>Indications | 用于脑血管障碍或脑卒中后引起的后遗症，伴有间歇性跛行的慢性闭塞性脉管炎，血管性头痛；也可用于血管性痴呆的预防和治疗（但目前国际上临床研究结论尚不肯定）。<br><br>It is used for sequelae caused by cerebrovascular disorders or post-stroke, chronic obliterans with intermittent claudication, vascular headache; it can also be used for prevention and treatment of vascular dementia (but now, clinical research conclusions haven't been reached internationally). |
| 用法、用量<br>Dosage | ①口服：每次 100 ~ 400mg，一日 3 次，建议餐后即时服用。控释片，每次 400mg，一日 1 次。口服用药治疗缺血性脑血管病后遗症或血管性痴呆等，需连续 2 ~ 8 周可产生治疗效果。②静脉滴注：每次 200 ~ 400mg，溶于 250 ~ 500ml 静脉滴注液中缓慢滴注，90 ~ 180 分钟滴完，每次 1 ~ 2 次。配制好的药物需在 24 小时内使用。<br><br>① orally: the dose is 100 ~ 400mg per time, 3 times a day. The drug is recommended to be taken immediately after meals. Controlled release tablet: the dose is 400mg per time, once a day. Oral medication of this drug can treat ischemic cerebrovascular disease sequelae or vascular dementia. The drug should be taken continuously for 2 to 8 weeks in order to work . ② intravenous infusion: the dose is 200 ~ 400mg per time, dissolved in 250 ~ 500ml infusion through slow drip and the drip should be finished within 90 to 180 minutes, 1 to 2 times per time. The well prepared drug should be used within 24 hours. |
| 剂型、规格<br>Preparations | 片剂（肠溶片）：每片 100mg。<br>控释片：每片 400mg。<br>注射液：每支 100mg（5ml）；300mg（15ml）。<br>Tablets (enteric-coated tablets): 100mg per tablet.<br>Release tablets: 400mg per tablet.<br>Injection: 100mg (5ml); 300mg (15ml) per vial. |
| 药品名称 Drug Names | 丁咯地尔 Buflomedil |
| 适应证<br>Indications | ①适用于慢性脑血管供血不足引起的症状：眩晕、耳鸣、智力减退、记忆力或注意力减退、定向障碍等。②外周性血管疾病：间歇性跛行、雷诺综合征、血栓闭塞性脉管炎等。<br><br>① It is used for the symptoms caused by chronic cerebrovascular insufficiency, including vertigo, tinnitus, mental deterioration, loss of memory or attention, disorientation, and so on. ② it can also be used for peripheral vascular disease: including intermittent claudication, Raynaud's syndrome, and thrombosis obliterans, etc. |
| 用法、用量<br>Dosage | 口服：片剂，每次 150 ~ 300mg，一日 2 ~ 3 次。每日最大剂量为 600mg；缓释片，每次 600mg，一日 1 次。肌内注射或静脉注射：每日 200 ~ 400mg。静脉滴注：每日 200 ~ 400mg，分 2 次，加于静脉滴注液 250 ~ 500ml 中缓慢滴注。轻中度肾功能不全者，用量减半，片剂，每次 150mg，一日 2 次，每日最大推荐剂量为 300mg；不推荐使用缓释片。肝功能不全者考虑减量使用。 |

**续　表**

| | |
|---|---|
| | Orally: tablets: the dose is 150 ~ 300mg per time, 2 to 3 times a day. The maximum dose is 600mg daily; sustained-release tablets: the dose is 600mg once a day. Intramuscular injection or intravenous injection: the dose is 200 ~ 400mg daily. Intravenous infusion: the dose is 200 ~ 400mg daily, divided into 2 doses, added into 250 ~ 500ml intravenous fluid through slow drip. For patients with mild and moderate renal insufficiency, the dosage should be half. The dose is150mg per time, 2 times a day. The maximum dose is recommended to be 300mg a day; Sustained-release tablets are not recommended. For patientswith liver dysfunction, the dose doesn't have to be half. |
| 剂型、规格<br>Preparations | 片剂：每片 150mg；300mg。<br>缓释片：600mg。<br>注射液：每支 50mg（5ml）；100mg（10ml）。<br>粉针剂：每支 50mg；100mg；200mg。<br>Tablets: 150mg; 300mg per tablet.<br>Release tablets: 600mg.<br>Injection: 50mg (5ml); 100mg (10ml) per vial.<br>Powder-iInjection: 50mg; 100mg; 200mg per vial. |
| 药品名称 Drug Names | 尼麦角林 Nicergoline |
| 适应证<br>Indications | 用于急、慢性脑血管疾病和代谢性脑供血不足，急、慢性外周血管障碍，老年性耳聋和视网膜疾病等。也用于血管性痴呆，尤其在早期治疗时对认知、记忆等有改善，并能减轻疾病严重程度。<br>It is used for acute and chronic cerebrovascular disease, metabolic cerebral insufficiency, acute, chronic peripheral vascular disorder, senile deafness and retinal diseases. It can alsio be used for vascular dementia. Especially in the early treatement, the drug can improve cognition, and memory and reduce the severity of disease. |
| 用法、用量<br>Dosage | 口服：每次 10 ~ 20mg，一日 3 次。片剂勿嚼服，可与食物同服。肌内注射：每次 2 ~ 4mg，一日 1 ~ 2 次。静脉注射：每次 2 ~ 4mg，溶于 100ml 的静脉滴注液中缓慢滴注，一日 1 ~ 2 次。<br>Orally: the dose is 10 ~ 20mg per time, 3 times a day. Do not chew the tablets and the drug can be served with food. Intramuscular injection: the dose is 2 ~ 4mg per time, 1 or 2 times a day. Intravenous injection: the dose is 2 ~ 4mg per time, dissolved in 100ml of intravenous fluid through slow drip, 1 ~ 2 times a day. |
| 剂型、规格<br>Preparations | 片剂：每片 10mg。<br>胶囊剂：每粒 15mg。<br>注射剂：2mg（1ml）；2.5mg（1ml）；4mg（2ml）；8mg（2ml）；8mg（5ml）。<br>Tablets: 10mg per tablet.<br>Capsules: per 15mg.<br>Injection: 2mg (1ml); 2.5mg (1ml); 4mg (2ml); 8mg (2ml); 8mg (5ml). |
| 药品名称 Drug Names | 川芎嗪 Ligustrazine |
| 适应证<br>Indications | 适用于脑供血不足、脑栓塞、脉管炎、冠心病、心绞痛、突发性耳聋等。<br>It is suitable for cerebral insufficiency, cerebral embolism, vasculitis, coronary heart disease, angina, sudden deafness. |
| 用法、用量<br>Dosage | 口服：每次 100mg，一日 3 次，30 日为 1 个疗程。肌内注射：每次 40 ~ 50mg，一天 1 ~ 2 次，缓慢推注，15 日为 1 个疗程。静脉滴注：每日 50 ~ 100mg，稀释于 250 ~ 500ml 静脉滴注液中缓慢滴注，15 日为 1 个疗程。<br>Orally: the dose is 100mg per time, 3 times a day and 30 days are a course of treatment. Intramuscular injection: the dose is 40 ~ 50mg per time, 1 ~ 2 times a day, through slow injection, and 15 days are a course of treatment. Intravenous infusion: the dose is 50 ~ 100mg every day, diluted in 250 ~ 500ml of liquid through slow drip, and 15 days are a course of treatment. |
| 剂型、规格<br>Preparations | 片剂：每片 50mg。<br>注射用川芎嗪（盐酸盐）：每支 40mg；<br>注射用川芎嗪（磷酸盐）：每支 50mg。<br>Tablets: 50mg per tablet.<br>Ligustrazine for injection (hydrochloride): 40mg per vial;<br>Ligustrazine for injection (phosphate): 50mg per vial. |

**续　表**

| 药品名称 Drug Names | 丁苯酞 Butylphthalide |
|---|---|
| 适应证<br>Indications | 适用于治疗轻、中度急性缺血性脑卒中及急性缺血性脑卒中患者神经功能缺损的改善。<br><br>It is used to treat mild and moderate acute ischemic stroke and improve neurological deficits of patients with acute ischemic stroke. |
| 用法、用量<br>Dosage | （1）可与复方丹参注射液联合使用。空腹口服。一次 2 粒（0.2g），一日 3 次，10 日为 1 个疗程。本品应在患者病发后 48 小时内开始服用。<br>（2）静脉滴注，一日 2 次，每次 25mg，每次滴注时间不少于 50 分钟；两次用药间隔不少于 6 小时，疗程为 14 日。<br><br>(1) It can be used with compound Danshen injection. The drug is taken on an empty stomach and the dose is two pills once (0.2g), three times a day. Ten days are a course of treatment. This product should be taken within 48 hours after patients start the disease.<br>(2) Intravenous injection: the dose is 25mg per time, twice a day. Infusion time is no less than 50 minutes every time; the interval between two times of infusion is not less than 6 hours and the course of treatment is 14 days. |
| 剂型、规格<br>Preparations | 胶囊：每粒 0.1g。<br>丁苯肽氯化钠注射：丁苯肽 25mg 与氯化钠 0.9g（100ml）。<br><br>Capsules: 0.1g per capsule.<br>Butylphthalide sodium chloride injection: 25mg of butylbenzene and 0.9g of sodium chloride (100ml). |
| 药品名称 Drug Names | 奥扎格雷 Ozagrel |
| 适应证<br>Indications | 用于缺血性脑卒中急性期，蛛网膜下腔出血术后的脑血管痉挛收缩和伴随的脑缺血症状。<br><br>It is used for the acute phase of ischemic stroke, cerebral vasospasm contraction after subarachnoid hemorrhage, and cerebral ischemia symptoms. |
| 用法、用量<br>Dosage | ①缺血性脑卒中急性期：每次 40～80mg，溶于 500ml 静脉滴注液中连续静脉滴注，每日 1～2 次，1～2 周为 1 个疗程。②蛛网膜下腔出血术后并发的脑血管痉挛及伴随而产生的脑缺血症状：每次 80mg，一日 1 次，溶于适量滴注液中，24 小时持续静脉滴注，可连续用药 2 周。<br><br>① acute phase of ischemic stroke: the dose is 40～80mg per time, dissolved in 500ml of infusion fluid through continuous intravenous infusion, 1 to 2 times a day, and 1 to 2 weeks is a course of treatment. ② cerebral vasospasm after subarachnoid hemorrhage and cerebral ischemic symptoms: the dose is 80mg per time, once a day, dissolved in an appropraite amount of infusion fluid, through 24-hour continuous intravenous infusion. The drug can be used continuously for 2 weeks. |
| 剂型、规格<br>Preparations | 注射用奥扎格雷：20mg（2ml）；40mg（2ml）。<br>奥扎格雷钠氯化钠（或葡萄糖）注射液：250ml（奥扎格雷钠 80mg）。<br><br>Ozagrel for injection: 20mg (2ml); 40mg (2ml).<br>sodium ozagrel common salt(or glucose) injection: 250ml (sodium ozagrel 80mg). |
| 药品名称 Drug Names | 曲克芦丁 Troxerutin |
| 适应证<br>Indications | 用于闭塞性脑血管病引起的偏瘫、失语、冠心病梗死前综合征、中心视网膜炎、血栓性静脉炎、静脉曲张、雷诺综合征、血管通透性升高引起的水肿、淋巴水肿、烧伤及创伤水肿、动脉硬化。<br><br>It is used for hemiplegia, aphasia, syndrome before coronary heart disease, central retinitis, thrombophlebitis, varicose veins and Raynaud's syndrome caused by occlusive cerebrovascular disease, and edema, lymphedema, burns, traumatic edema and atherosclerosis caused by increased vascular permeability. |
| 用法、用量<br>Dosage | 口服：每次 200～300mg，一日 3 次。肌内注射：每次 100～200mg，一日 2 次。静脉滴注：每次 400mg，一日 1 次，20 日为 1 个疗程，可用 1～3 个疗程，每疗程间隔 3～7 日。<br><br>Orally: the dose is 200～300mg per time, 3 times a day. Intramuscular injection: the dose is 100～200mg per time, 2 times a day. Intravenous infusion: the dose is 400mg per time, once a day and 20 days is a course of treatment. The drug can be used for 1～3 courses, and the interval between courses of treatment is 3 to 7 days. |
| 剂型、规格<br>Preparations | 片剂：每片 100mg。<br>注射液：每支 100mg（2ml）；200mg（2ml）。<br><br>Tablets: 100mg per tablet.<br>Injection: 100mg (2ml); 200mg (2ml) per vial. |

**续 表**

| 药品名称 Drug Names | 维生素 E 烟酸酯 Vitamin E Nicotinate |
|---|---|
| 适应证<br>Indications | 用于动脉硬化、脑震荡及轻微脑挫伤和脑外伤后遗症、头痛头晕，中心性视网膜炎等血管障碍性疾病，也可用于脂质代谢异常。<br><br>It is used for arteriosclerosis, cerebral concussion and mild cerebral concussion and post-traumatic brain syndrome, headache, dizziness, central retinitis and other vascular disorders. It can also be used for lipid metabolism. |
| 用法、用量<br>Dosage | 口服，每次 0.1 ~ 0.2g，一日 3 次，餐后服。老年人可做适当调整。<br><br>Orally: the dose is 0.1 ~ 0.2g per time, 3 times a day, taken after meals. For elder patients, the dose can be appropriately adjusted. |
| 剂型、规格<br>Preparations | 片剂：每片 0.1g。胶囊：每粒 0.1g。胶丸：每粒 0.1g。<br>Tablets: 0.1g per tablet. Capsules: 0.1g per capsule. Capsules: 0.1g per capsule. |
| 药品名称 Drug Names | 灯盏花素 Breviscapine |
| 适应证<br>Indications | ①用于缺血性脑血管病，如脑供血不足、椎基底动脉供血不足、脑出血后遗症。②亦用于冠心病、心绞痛、高血压、高黏滞血症等心血管疾病。<br><br>① it is used for ischemic cerebrovascular disease, such as cerebral blood supply insufficiency, vertebrobasilar insufficiency, cerebral hemorrhage sequela. ② it can also be used for coronary heart disease, angina, hypertension, hyperviscosity and other cardiovascular diseases. |
| 用法、用量<br>Dosage | 口服：每次 40mg，一日 3 次。肌内注射：每次 2ml，一日 2 次，15 日为 1 个疗程。静脉滴注：每次 4 ~ 8ml，一日 1 次，加入 500ml 静脉滴注液中稀释应用，10 日为 1 个疗程。<br><br>Orally: the dose is 40mg per time, 3 times a day. Intramuscular injection: the dose is 2ml twice a day, and 15 days are a course of treatment. Intravenous infusion: the dose is 4 ~ 8ml per time, once a day, diluted by 500ml of intravenous infusion, and 10 days are a course of treatment. |
| 剂型、规格<br>Preparations | 片剂：每片 20mg。<br>注射剂：每支 5mg（2ml）；20mg（5ml）。<br>Tablets: 20mg per tablet. Injection: 5mg (2ml); 20mg (5ml) per vial. |
| 药品名称 Drug Names | 地芬尼多 Difenidol |
| 适应证<br>Indications | 用于治疗各种原因引起的眩晕症（如椎基底动脉供血不足、梅尼埃病等）、恶心呕吐、自主神经功能紊乱、晕车晕船，运动病及外科麻醉手术后的呕吐等。<br><br>It is used for all kinds of vertigo (such as vertebrobasilar insufficiency, Meniere's disease, etc.), nausea, vomiting, autonomic dysfunction, motion sickness and vomiting after surgical anesthesia. |
| 用法、用量<br>Dosage | 口服：成人每次 25 ~ 50mg，一日 3 次；6 个月以上儿童，每次 0.9mg/kg，一日 3 次。肌内注射：每次 10 ~ 20mg，眩晕发作剧烈者可每次 20 ~ 40mg。<br><br>Orally: for adults, the dose is 25 ~ 50mg per time, 3 times a day; for children over 6 months, the dose is 0.9mg/kg per time, 3 times a day. Intramuscular injection: the dose is 10 ~ 20mg per time. For patients with severe vertigo, the dose can be 20 ~ 40mg per time. |
| 剂型、规格<br>Preparations | 片剂：每片 25mg。<br>注射液：每支 10mg（1ml）。<br>Tablets: 25mg per tablet.<br>Injection: 10mg (1ml) per vial. |
| 药品名称 Drug Names | 长春西汀 Vinpocetine |
| 适应证<br>Indications | ①用于改善脑梗死、脑出血后遗症及脑动脉硬化引起的各种症状，如记忆障碍、眩晕、头痛、失语、抑郁症等。②还可用于各种眼底血液循环不良所致的视力障碍；听力损伤、耳鸣前庭功能障碍。③各种颅脑手术后脑功能的康复治疗。<br><br>① it can be used to improve all kinds of symptoms caused by cerebral infarction, cerebral hemorrhage sequela and cerebral arteriosclerosis, such as memory impairment, dizziness, headache, aphasia, depression. ② it can be used for poor vision impairment caused by a variety of retinal blood circulation, hearing impairment, tinnitus and vestibular dysfunction. ③ it can be used for rehabilitation of brain function after a variety of brain surgery. |

| | |
|---|---|
| 用法、用量<br>Dosage | 　　口服：每次 5 ～ 10mg，一日 3 次，餐时口服。静脉滴注：起始剂量每日 20mg，一日 1 次；以后根据病情可增至每日 30mg，一日 1 次。<br><br>　　Orally: the dose is 5 ～ 10mg per time, 3 times a day, taken with meals. Intravenous infusion: the initial dose is 20mg once a day; later according to patients' conditons, the dose can be increased to 30mg once a day. |
| 剂型、规格<br>Preparations | 　　片剂：每片 5mg。<br>　　注射液：20mg（2ml）。<br>　　长春西汀葡萄糖注射液：100ml（长春西汀 10mg）；200ml（长春西汀 10mg）；250ml（长春西汀 10mg）。<br>　　Tablets: 5mg per tablet.<br>　　Injection: 20mg (2ml).<br>　　Vinpocetine glucose injection: 100ml (vinpocetine 10mg); 200ml (vinpocetine 10mg); 250ml (vinpocetine 10mg). |
| 药品名称 Drug Names | 依达拉奉 Edaravone |
| 适应证<br>Indications | 　　用于改善急性脑梗死所致的神经症状、日常生活活动能力和功能障碍。<br><br>　　It can be used to improve neurological symptoms caused by acute cerebral infarction, activities of daily living and dysfunction. |
| 用法、用量<br>Dosage | 　　静脉滴注：一次 30mg，加入适量生理盐水中稀释后静滴，30 分钟内滴完，一日 2 次，14 日为 1 个疗程。尽可能在发病 24 小时内开始给药。<br><br>　　Intravenous infusion: the dose is 30mg once, diluted by an appropriate amount of saline infusion, and the drip is finished within 30 minutes, 2 times a day. 14 days are a course of treatment. The drug should be used as soon as possible within 24 hours. |
| 剂型、规格<br>Preparations | 　　注射液：每支 10mg（5ml）；30mg（20ml）。<br>　　Injection: 10mg (5ml); 30mg (20ml) per vial. |
| 药品名称 Drug Names | 血塞通 Xuesaitong |
| 适应证<br>Indications | 　　①用于缺血性脑血管病、冠心病心绞痛，中医证见脑络瘀阻、中风偏瘫、心脉瘀阻、胸痹心痛。②还可用于治疗视网膜血管阻塞、眼前房出血、青光眼；急性黄疸型肝炎、病毒性肝炎；外伤、软组织损伤及骨折恢复期。<br><br>　　① It is used for ischemic cerebrovascular disease, coronary heart disease angina pectoris, cerebral collateral stasis Syndrome, hemiplegia, systolic blood stasis, chest stuffness and pains. ② it can also be used for retinal vascular occlusion, hyphema, glaucoma, acute jaundice hepatitis, viral hepatitis, trauma and fractures and soft tissue injury and recovery. |
| 用法、用量<br>Dosage | 　　口服：一次 50 ～ 100mg，一日 3 次。肌内注射：一次 100mg。一日 1 ～ 2 次。静脉滴注：一次 200 ～ 400mg，以 5% ～ 10% 葡萄糖注射液 250 ～ 500ml 稀释后缓缓滴注，一日 1 次。静脉注射：每次 200mg，以 25% ～ 50% 葡萄糖注射液 40 ～ 60ml 稀释后缓缓注射，一日 1 次。15 日为 1 个疗程。停药 1 ～ 3 日后可进行第 2 疗程。<br><br>　　Orally: the dose is 50 ～ 100mg once, three times a day. Intramuscular injection: the dose is 100mg per time. 1 to 2 times a day. Intravenous infusion: the dose is 200 ～ 400mg once, diluted by 250 ～ 500ml of 5% ～ 10% glouse injection through slow drip, once a day. Intravenous injection: the dose is 200mg per time, diluted by 40 ～ 60ml of 25% to 50% glucose injection through slow injection, once a day. 15 days are a course of treatemet. After 1 to 3 days of drug withdrawal, the second course of treatment can continue. |
| 剂型、规格<br>Preparations | 　　片剂：每片 50mg。<br>　　胶囊剂：每粒 60mg。<br>　　注射液：每支 100mg（2ml）。<br>　　Tablets: 50mg per tablet.<br>　　Capsules: 60mg per capsule.<br>　　Injection: 100mg (2ml) per vial. |
| 药品名称 Drug Names | 七叶皂苷钠 Sodium Aescinate |
| 适应证<br>Indications | 　　①用于各种病因引起的脑水肿、创伤或手术所致肿胀。②也可用于静脉回流障碍、下肢静脉曲张、血栓性静脉炎、慢性静脉功能不全，下肢动脉阻塞性疾病，运动系统创伤造成的软组织血肿、水肿。③用于周围神经言行疾病，如吉兰 - 巴雷综合征、多发性神经炎等。 |

续　表

| | |
|---|---|
| | ① it is used for cerebral edema, trauma caused by various reasons.or swelling caused by urgery ② it can also be used for venous return, lower limb varicose veins, thrombophlebitis, chronic venous insufficiency, lower extremity arterial occlusive disease, soft tissue hematoma and edema caused by the motion system trauma. ③ it is used for peripheral nerve diseases, such as Guillain - Barre syndrome, multiple neuritis. |
| 用法、用量<br>Dosage | ①静脉给药：一日 5 ~ 10mg 溶于 250ml 滴注液中静脉滴注；或 5 ~ 10ml 溶于 10 ~ 20ml 10% 葡萄糖溶液或 0.9% 氯化钠溶液中，静脉注射。儿童 3 岁以下一日 0.05 ~ 0.1mg/kg 体重；3 ~ 10 岁一日 0.1 ~ 0.2mg/kg 体重。重症患者可多次给药，但一日总量不得超过 20mg。疗程为 7 ~ 10 日。②口服：每次 30 ~ 60mg，一日 2 次，餐时或餐后口服，20 日为 1 个疗程。<br><br>① intravenous administration: the dose is 5 ~ 10mg a day, dissolved in 250ml of infusion solution, or 5 ~ 10mg of the drug can be dissolved in 10 ~ 20ml of 10% glucose solution or 0.9% NaCl solution. For children under 3 years old, the dose is 0.05 ~ 0.1mg per kg a day; for chidren at the age of 3 to 10 years old, the dose is 0.1 ~ 0.2mg per kg a day. Critically patients can be repeatedly administered, but the total dose may not exceed 20mg a day. 7 to 10 days are a course of treatment. ② Orally: the dose is 30 ~ 60mg twice a day, taken with meals or after meals. A course of treatment is 20 days. |
| 剂型、规格<br>Preparations | 片剂：每片 30mg。<br>注射剂：每支 5mg；10mg；25mg。<br>Tablets: 30mg per tablet.<br>Injection: 5mg; 10mg; 25mg per vial. |
| **药品名称 Drug Names** | 葛根素 Puerarin |
| 适应证<br>Indications | 可用于辅助治疗冠心病、心绞痛、心肌梗死，缺血性脑血管病，视网膜动、静脉阻塞，青光眼，突发性耳聋，小儿病毒性心肌炎、糖尿病。<br><br>It can be used for coronary heart disease, angina, myocardial infarction, ischemic cerebrovascular disease, retinal artery and vein occlusion, glaucoma, sudden deafness, children viral myocarditis and diabetes. |
| 用法、用量<br>Dosage | ①静脉滴注：每次 0.4 ~ 0.6g，一日 1 次，10 ~ 20 日为 1 个疗程，可连续使用 2 ~ 3 个疗程。最大用药剂量为 1.0g。②滴眼：一次 1 ~ 2 滴，闭目 3 ~ 5 分钟。首日 3 次，以后为每日 2 次。<br><br>① Intravenous infusion: the dose is 0.4 ~ 0.6g once a day, and 10 to 20 days are a course of treatment. The drug can be used continuously for 2 to 3 courses. The maximum dose is 1.0g. ② drops: Use 1 to 2 drops once and close eyes for 3 to 5 minutes. Take the drug 3 times on the first day, and later change to twice a day. |
| 剂型、规格<br>Preparations | 注射液：每支 100mg（2ml）；400mg（8ml）。<br>粉针剂：每支 200mg。<br>葛根素氯化钠注射液：100ml（葛根素 200mg）。<br>葛根素滴眼液：50mg（5ml）。<br><br>Injection: 100mg (2ml); 400mg (8ml) per vial.<br>Powder-injection: 200mg per vial.<br>Puerarin sodium chloride injection: 100ml (puerarin 200mg).<br>Puerarin eyedrops: 50mg (5ml). |

8.13 抗老年痴呆药和改善脑代谢药 Anti-senile dementia drugs and improving brain metabolic drugs

| | |
|---|---|
| **药品名称 Drug Names** | 加兰他敏 Galanthamine |
| 适应证<br>Indications | ①适用于治疗轻、中度阿尔茨海默病（AD），有效率 50% ~ 60%，疗效与他克林相当，但没有肝毒性。用药后 6 ~ 8 周治疗效果开始明显。②用于重症肌无力、脊髓灰质炎后遗症、儿童脑性麻痹、多发性神经炎、脊神经根炎及拮抗氯筒箭毒碱。<br><br>① it is used for mild and moderate Alzheimer's disease (AD). Its effect rate is 50% to 60% and its efficacy is equivalent to tacrine. And it has no liver toxicity. After 6 to 8 weeks, began treatment effect begins to become obvious. ② it is used for myasthenia gravis, polio sequelae, children with cerebral palsy, multiple neuritis, radiculitis and antagonize tubocurarine chloride. |
| 用法、用量<br>Dosage | 口服：每次 10 ~ 20mg，一日 3 次。小儿每日 0.5 ~ 1mg/kg，分 3 次服。皮下注射或肌内注射：每次 2.5 ~ 10mg，一日 1 次。小儿每次 0.05 ~ 0.1mg/kg，一日 1 次。每个疗程 8 ~ 10 周。用于抗氯筒箭毒碱时肌内注射起始剂量 5 ~ 10mg，5 分钟或 10 分钟后按需要可逐渐增加至每次 10 ~ 20mg。 |

| | |
|---|---|
| | Orally: the dose is 10 ~ 20mg per time, 3 times a day. For children, the dose is 0.5 ~ 1mg/kg a day, divided into 3 doses. Subcutaneous or intramuscular injection: the dose is 2.5 ~ 10mg once a day. For children, the dose is 0.05 ~ 0.1mg/kg per time, once a day. A course of treatment is 8 to 10 weeks. When it is used for antagonize tubocurarine chloride, the starting dose of intramuscular injection is 5 ~ 10mg. After 5 or 10 minutes, the dose can gradually be increased to 10 ~ 20mg per time according to needs. |
| 剂型、规格<br>Preparations | 口崩片：每片 5mg。<br>分散片：每片 2.5mg。<br>注射剂：每支 1mg（1ml）；2.5mg（1ml）；5mg（1ml）。<br>Orally disintegrating tablets: 5mg per tablet.<br>Dispersible tablets: 2.5mg per tablet.<br>Injection: 1mg (1ml); 2.5mg (1ml); 5mg (1ml) per vial. |
| 药品名称 Drug Names | 美金刚 Memantine |
| 适应证<br>Indications | 用于治疗中至重度的阿尔茨海默病（AD），以及震颤麻痹综合征的治疗。<br>It is used for moderate and severe Alzheimer's disease (AD), and parkinsonism syndrome. |
| 用法、用量<br>Dosage | 口服。成人或 14 岁以上青少年：在治疗的前 3 周按每周递增 5mg 的方法逐渐达到维持剂量，即治疗第 1 周每日 5mg（晨服），第 2 周每日 10mg，分 2 次服用；第 3 周每日 15mg（早上 10mg，下午 5mg）；第 4 周开始维持剂量每日 20mg，分 2 次服。片剂可空腹服用，也可随食物同服。14 岁以下小儿：维持量每日 0.55 ~ 1.0mg/kg。中度肾功能损害者，应将剂量减至每日 10mg；不推荐严重肾衰竭患者使用。<br>Orally: for adults or teenagers over the age of 14: in the first three weeks, the dose is progressively increased by 5mg every week till the maintenance dose, ie, in the first week, the dose is 5mg daily (taken in the morning). In the second week, the dose is 10mg daily, divided into 2 doses; in the third week, the dose is 15mg daily (10mg taken in the morning, 5mg taken in the afternoon); in the fourth week, the maintenance dose is 20mg daily, divided into 2 doses. Tablets can be taken on an empty stomach or with food. Children under 14 years of age: the maintenance dose is 0.55 ~ 1.0mg/kg daily. For patients with moderate renal impairment, the dose should be reduced to 10mg daily; the drug is not recommended to be used on patients with severe renal failure. |
| 剂型、规格<br>Preparations | 片剂：每片 5mg；10mg。<br>胶囊：每粒 10mg。<br>Tablets: 5mg; 10mg per tablet.<br>Capsules: 10mg per capsule. |
| 药品名称 Drug Names | 吡拉西坦 Piracetam |
| 适应证<br>Indications | 由衰老、脑血管病、脑外伤、CO 中毒等引起的记忆和轻中度脑功能障碍。亦可用于儿童发育迟缓。<br>It is used for memory and mild to moderate brain dysfunction caused by aging, cerebrovascular disease, brain trauma, and CO poisonin. It can also be used for children with developmental retardation. |
| 用法、用量<br>Dosage | ①口服：成人，每次 0.8 ~ 1.2g，一日 2 ~ 3 次，4 ~ 8 周为 1 个疗程。儿童、老年人，剂量酌减。②肌内注射：每次 1g，一日 2 ~ 3 次。③静脉注射：每次 4 ~ 6g，一日 2 次。④静脉滴注：用于改善脑代谢，每次 4 ~ 8g，用 250ml 滴注射液稀释后静脉滴注，一日 1 次。<br>① Orally: for adults, the doses is 0.8 ~ 1.2g per time, 2 to 3 times a day, and four to eight weeks are a course of treatment. For children and the elderly, the dose shoudle be reduced accroding to patients' conditons. ② intramuscular injection: the dose is 1g per time, 2 to 3 times a day. ③ intravenous injection: the dose is 4 ~ 6g twice a day. ④ intravenous infusion: to improve brain metabolism, the dose is 4 ~ 8g per time, diluted by 250ml of injection, once a day. |
| 剂型、规格<br>Preparations | 片剂：每片 0.4g。<br>分散片：每片 0.8g。<br>胶囊：每粒 0.2g；0.4g。<br>注射剂：每支 1g（5ml）；2g（10ml）；4g（20ml）。<br>氯化钠注射液：250ml（吡拉西坦 8g，氯化钠 2.25g）。<br>Tablets: 0.4g per tablet.<br>Dispersible tablet: 0.8g per tablet.<br>Capsules: 0.2g, 0.4g per capsule.<br>Injection: 1g (5ml); 2g (10ml); 4g (20ml) per vial.<br>Sodium Chloride Injection: 250ml (piracetam 8g, sodium chloride 2.25g). |

续　表

| 药品名称 Drug Names | 茴拉西坦 Aniracetam |
|---|---|
| 适应证<br>Indications | 用于治疗脑血管疾病后的记忆功能减退和血管性痴呆，中、老年记忆减退（健忘症），对帕金森病症状有改善作用，用于脑梗死后遗症的情绪不稳定和抑郁状态。<br><br>It is used for memory loss and vascular dementia after cerebrovascular disease, memory loss (amnesia) of the middle-aged and the aged. It could improve Parkinson's disease. It can also be used for emotional instability and depression of cerebral infarction sequelae. |
| 用法、用量<br>Dosage | 口服：每次 0.2g，一日 3 次。70 岁以上老年人，每次 0.1g，一日 3 次。1～2 个月为 1 个疗程。可根据病情调整用量和疗程。<br><br>Orally: the dose is 0.2g per time, three times a day. For patients more than 70 years old, the dose is 0.1g every time, 3 times a day. 1 to 2 months are a course of treatment. The dose and the course of treatment can be adjusted according to the disease. |
| 剂型、规格<br>Preparations | 胶囊：每粒 0.1g。<br>片剂：每片 0.05g。<br>Capsules: 0.1g per capsule.<br>Tablets: 0.05g per tablet. |
| 药品名称 Drug Names | 奥拉西坦 Oxiracetam |
| 适应证<br>Indications | 用于轻中度血管性痴呆、老年性痴呆及脑外伤等症引起的记忆与智能障碍、大脑功能不全。<br>It is used for memory and mental retardation, incomplete brain function caused by mild to moderate vascular dementia, Alzheimer's disease and brain trauma. |
| 用法、用量<br>Dosage | 口服：每次 0.8g，一日 2 次；重症每日 2～8g。静脉滴注：每次 4g，一日 1 次，可酌情减量，用前加入到 100～250ml 静脉滴注液中，摇匀。对功能缺失的治疗通常疗程为 2 周，对记忆与智能障碍的治疗通常疗程为 3 周。<br><br>Orally: the dose is 0.8g per time, twice a day; for severe case, the dose is 2～8g daily. Intravenous infusion: the dose is 4g once a day and it can be reduced accoriding to patients' conditions. The drug is added into 100～250ml of intravenous drip liquid, and should be shakenwell. The treatment course of the disfunction is usually two weeks, and the treatment course of memory and mental retardation is usually three weeks. |
| 剂型、规格<br>Preparations | 片剂：每片 0.4g。<br>注射液：每支 1g（5ml）。<br>Tablets: 0.4g per tablet.<br>Injection: 1g (5ml). per vial. |
| 药品名称 Drug Names | 银杏叶提取物 Ginkgo Biloba Leaf Extract |
| 适应证<br>Indications | 主要用于脑部、外周血管及冠状动脉血管障碍的患者，包括脑卒中、痴呆症、急慢性脑功能不全及其后遗症。对于阿尔茨海默病、血管性痴呆及缓和性痴呆等患者应用本品后，智力可有所提高，但对明显痴呆者作用仍不佳。<br><br>It is mainly used on patients within the brain, peripheral vascular and coronary vascular disorders, including stroke, Alzheimer's disease, acute and chronic brain dysfunction and its sequelae. AfterFor patients withafter Alzheimer's disease, vascular dementia and moderate dementia use the drug FDA should ease, their intelligence can be improved, but its efficacy is not so significant for patients with obviuous role in dementia still poor. |
| 用法、用量<br>Dosage | 口服：每次 1～2 片，一日 3 次。静脉滴注：1～2 支，加入 250ml 或 500ml 输液剂中静脉滴注，一日 1～2 次。本品不同厂家说明书所列剂量并不一致，主要成分的配比也不同，所以需要根据具体说明书使用药物。<br><br>Orally: the dose is 1 to 2 tablets every time, 3 times a day. Intravenous infusion: the dose is 1 to 2, added to 250ml or 500ml infusion, 1 or 2 times a day. The dose of this product can be different in various manufacturer's instructions, and the ratio of the main ingredients is also different. So you need to use the drug according to specific instructions. |

**续 表**

| 剂型、规格<br>Preparations | 片剂：每片 40mg。<br>注射剂：①金纳多：每支 5ml（含银杏叶提取物 17.5mg）。②舒血宁：2ml（含总黄酮醇苷 1.68mg；银杏内酯 A0.12mg）；5ml（含总黄酮醇苷 4.2mg；银杏内酯 A0.30mg）。<br>Tablets: 40mg per tablet.<br>Injection: ① ginaton: 5ml per vial (containing ginkgo biloba extract 17.5mg). ② Shuxuening: 2ml (including total flavonol glycosides 1.68mg; Ginkgolides A0.12mg); 5ml (including total flavonol glycosides 4.2mg; Ginkgolides A 0.30mg). |
|---|---|

| 药品名称 Drug Names | 阿米三嗪 / 萝巴新 Almitrine/Raubasine |
|---|---|
| 适应证<br>Indications | 用于治疗亚急性或慢性脑功能不全，如记忆力下降、缺血性听觉、前庭、视觉障碍；脑血管意外后的功能恢复。<br>It is used for subacute or chronic brain function insufficiency, such as memory loss; it can also be used for ischemic auditory, vestibular, visual disturbances and functional recovery after cerebrovascular accident. |
| 用法、用量<br>Dosage | 口服，每次 1 片，一日 2 次（早、晚服）。维持量一日一次，每次 1 片，餐后服。<br>Orally: the dose is one tablet per time, twice a day (taken in the morning and evening). The maintenance dose is 1 tablet once a day, taken after meals. |
| 剂型、规格<br>Preparations | 片剂：每片含二甲磺酸阿米三嗪 30mg，萝巴新 10mg。<br>Tablets: per tablet contains30mg of sulfonic acid dimethyl Almitrine, and 10mg of Raubasine. |

| 药品名称 Drug Names | 吡硫醇 Pyritinol |
|---|---|
| 适应证<br>Indications | 用于脑震荡综合征、脑外伤后遗症、脑炎及脑膜炎后遗症等引起的头痛、头晕、失眠、记忆力减退、注意力不集中、情绪变化等症状的改善，也可用于脑动脉硬化、老年痴呆等精神症状。<br>It is used for headaches dizziness, insomnia, memory loss, inability to concentrate, mood changes and other symptoms caused by cerebral concussion syndrome, brain trauma sequelae, encephalitis and meningitis sequelae. It can also be used for cerebral arteriosclerosis, senile dementia and other psychiatric symptoms. |
| 用法、用量<br>Dosage | 口服：成人每次 100 ~ 200mg，一日 3 次。小儿每次 50 ~ 100mg，一日 3 次。静脉滴注：每次 200 ~ 400mg，一日 1 次，用 250ml 静脉滴注液稀释后使用。<br>Orally: for adults, the dose is 100 ~ 200mg per time, 3 times a day. For children, the dose is 50 ~ 100mg per time, three times a day. Intravenous drip: the dose is 200 ~ 400mg once a day, diluted by 250 ml of intravenous drip liquid. |
| 剂型、规格<br>Preparations | 片剂：每片 100mg；200mg。<br>胶囊剂：每粒 100mg。<br>注射剂：每支 100mg（1ml）；200mg（2ml）。<br>盐酸吡硫醇葡萄糖注射液：250ml（盐酸吡硫醇 200mg，葡萄糖 5g）。<br>Tablets: 100mg; 200mg per tablet.<br>Capsules: 100mg per capsule.<br>Injection: 100mg (1ml); 200mg (2ml) per vial.<br>Pyritinol hydrochloride glucose injection: 250ml (HCl Pyritinol 200mg, glucose 5g). |

| 药品名称 Drug Names | 小牛血去蛋白提取物 Deprotenized Hemoderivative of Calf Blood |
|---|---|
| 适应证<br>Indications | ①用于脑卒中、脑外伤、周围血管病及腿部溃疡。②亦可用于皮移植术、烧伤、烫伤、糜烂、创伤、压疮的伤口愈合；放射所引起的皮肤、黏膜损伤。③各种病因引起的角膜溃疡，角膜损伤，酸或碱引起的角膜灼伤，大泡性角膜炎，神经麻痹性角膜炎，角膜和结膜变性等。<br>① It is used for brain stroke, brain trauma, peripheral vascular disease and leg ulcers. ② it can also be used for skin grafting, burns, burns, erosion, trauma, wound healing of pressure sore and skin, mucosal damage caused by radiation. ③ it is used for corneal ulcers caused by a variety of causes, corneal burns, corneal injury caused by acid or alkali, bullous keratitis, nerve palsy keratitis, corneal and conjunctival degeneration and so on. |
| 用法、用量<br>Dosage | 口服：每次 1 ~ 2 片，一日 3 次。整片吞服，1 个疗程 4 ~ 6 周。静脉注射或缓慢肌内注射：初期每天 10 ~ 20ml，进一步治疗剂量每天 5ml。静脉注射：10 ~ 50ml 加入静脉注射液 250ml 中滴注。皮肤外用：在保证创口或创面清洁的情况下外用。轻者可一日一次，涂于创面处；重者一日 2 ~ 6 次，或酌情增加次数。眼科外用：滴于眼部患处，每次 1 滴，一日 3 ~ 4 次，或视病情而定。口腔外用：涂抹于患处一日 3 ~ 5 次，其中 1 次在睡前使用。 |

续　表

<table>
<tr><td></td><td>Orally: the dose is 1 to 2 tablets per time, 3 times a day. Swallow the whole tablet. A course of treatment is four to six weeks. Intravenous or slow intramuscular injection: the initial dose is 10 ~ 20ml daily, and later the dose is 5ml per day. Intravenous injection: 10 ~ 50ml of the drug is added to 250ml of intravenous fluid infusion. Topical skin: use the drug if topical wound or wounds are clean. For mild case, use the drug on the wound once a day; for severe case, use the drug 2 to 6 times daily, or increase the times according to patients' conditions. Ophthalmic Topical: drip eye drops in the affected area, one drop per time, 3 to 4 times a day, or use the drug depending on the disease. Oral Topical: apply the drug to affected area 3 ~ 5 times a day, and one time, the drug is used before sleep.</td></tr>
<tr><td>剂型、规格<br>Preparations</td><td>片剂：每片 200mg。<br>注射剂：每支 80mg（2ml）；200mg（5ml）；400mg（10ml）。<br>软膏：10%（20g：2.0g）。<br>眼凝胶制剂：20%（5g：1g）。<br>口腔膏：5%（5g：0.25g）。<br>Tablets: 200mg per tablet.<br>Injection: 80mg (2ml); 200mg (5ml); 400mg (10ml) per vial.<br>Ointment: 10% (20g: 2.0g). Eye gel preparation: 20% (5g: 1g).<br>Oral cavity paste: 5% (5g: 0.25g).</td></tr>
<tr><td>药品名称 Drug Names</td><td>胞磷胆碱 Citicoline</td></tr>
<tr><td>适应证<br>Indications</td><td>主要用于急性颅脑外伤和脑手术所引起的意识障碍，以及脑卒中而致偏瘫的患者，也可用于耳鸣及神经性耳聋。对颅内出血引起意识障碍效果较差。<br>It is mainly used for acute craniocerebral trauma and disturbance of consciousness caused by brain surgery, and on patients with hemiplegia due to cerebral apoplexy. It can also be used for tinnitus and sensorineural deafness. Its efficacy for disturbance of consciousness caused by the intracranial hemorrhage is poorer.</td></tr>
<tr><td>用法、用量<br>Dosage</td><td>静脉滴注：一日 0.25 ~ 0.5g，用 5% 或 10% 葡萄糖注射液稀释后缓慢滴注，5 ~ 10 日为 1 个疗程。单纯静脉注射：每次 0.1 ~ 0.2g。肌内注射：一日 0.1 ~ 0.3g，分 1 ~ 2 次注射，脑出血急性期不宜大剂量应用。一般不采用肌内注射，若用时应经常更换注射部位。口服：每次 0.2g，一日 3 次。用于维持期治疗可为一次 0.1g，一日 3 次口服。<br>Intravenous drip: the dose is 0.25 g to 0.25 g a day, diluted by 5% or 10% glucose injection through slow drip, and 5 ~ 10 days are a course of treatment. Simple intravenous injection: the dose is 0.1 ~ 0.2 g per time. Intramuscular injection: the dose is 0.1 ~ 0.3 g a day, 1 ~ 2 times injection, and for acute phase of cerebral hemorrhage, high-dose applications are unfavorable. Generally the drug is given through intramuscular injection, and the injection site should be changed frequently. Orally: the dose is 0.2 g per time, 3 times a day. If the drug is used in the maintenance period, the dose is 0.1 g once, 3 times a day.</td></tr>
<tr><td>剂型、规格<br>Preparations</td><td>注射剂：每支 0.2g（2ml）；0.25g（2ml）。<br>片剂：每片 0.2g。<br>胶囊剂：每粒 0.1g。<br>Injection: 0.2g (2ml) 0.25g(2ml) per vial.<br>Tablets: 0.2g per tablet. Capsules: 0.1g per capsule.</td></tr>
<tr><td>药品名称 Drug Names</td><td>单唾液酸四己糖神经节苷脂 Monosialoteterahexosyl Ganglioside</td></tr>
<tr><td>适应证<br>Indications</td><td>用于脑脊髓创伤、脑血管意外，可用于帕金森病。<br>It is used for myelencephalon trauma, cerebral vascular accident, and Parkinson's disease.</td></tr>
<tr><td>用法、用量<br>Dosage</td><td>每日 20 ~ 40mg，一次或分次肌内注射或缓慢静脉注射。急性期：每日 100mg，静脉滴注；2 ~ 3 周后改为维持量，每日 20 ~ 40mg，一般 6 周。对帕金森病，首剂量 500 ~ 1000mg，静脉滴注；第 2 日起每日 200mg，皮下注射、肌内注射或静脉滴注，一般用至 18 周。<br>The dose is 20 ~ 40mg every day, taken once or several times through intramuscular injection or slow intravenous injection. Acute phase: the dose is100mg per day through intravenous drip; after 2 ~ 3 weeks, change to the maintenance dose, 20 to 40 mg daily, usually for six weeks. For Parkinson's disease, the first dose is 500 ~ 1000 mg through intravenous drip; from the second day, the dose is 200 mg per day, through subcutaneous and intramuscular injection or intravenous drip, commonly for 18 weeks.</td></tr>
</table>

**续 表**

| | |
|---|---|
| 剂型、规格<br>Preparations | 注射液：每支 20mg（2ml）；100mg（5ml）。粉针剂：每支 40mg；100mg。<br>Injection: 20mg (2ml) ;100mg (5ml) per vial. Powder- injection: per 40mg; 100mg. |
| **药品名称 Drug Names** | **脑蛋白水解物 Cerebroprotein Hydrolysate** |
| 适应证<br>Indications | 适用于尤以注意及记忆障碍的器质性脑病性综合征，原发性痴呆如老年性痴呆），血管性痴呆（如多发梗死性痴呆），混合性痴呆，卒中、颅脑手术后的脑功能障碍，神经衰弱及衰竭症状。<br><br>It applies to especially attention and memory disorder of organic brain syndrome, primary dementia like senile dementia, vascular dementia (like multi- infarct dementia), mixed dementia, stroke, brain dysfunction after craniocerebral surgery, neurasthenia and failure symptoms. |
| 用法、用量<br>Dosage | 成人常用 10～30ml 稀释于 5% 葡萄糖或生理盐水 250ml 中缓慢滴注，60～120 分钟滴完，一日 1 次，每疗程注射 10～20 次，依病情而定。轻微病例或经大剂量用药后为保持疗效者，可用于肌内注射、皮下注射或静脉注射，每次 1～5ml；皮下注射不超过每次 2ml，肌内注射不超过每次 5ml；静脉注射不超过每次 10ml。应用 10～20 次，以后每周 2～3 次，可重复几个疗程，直至临床表现不再改善为止。<br><br>For adults, the common dose is 10～30ml, diluted by 250ml of 5% dextrose or saline through slowdrip, finished within 60 to 120 minutes, once a day. In a course of treatment, give the drug 10 to 20 times, depending on the patients' conditions. For mild cases, after large doses of medication, in order to maintain the effects, the drug can be given through intramuscular, subcutaneous or intravenous injection and the dose is 1～5ml per time: for subcutaneous injection, the dose is no more than 2ml per time. For intramuscular injection, the dose is no more than 5ml per time; for intravenous injection, the dose does not exceed 10ml per time. Use the drug 10 to 20 times and later change to 2 to 3 times every week. The drug can be given for several treatment courses until clinical manifestations have no longer improved. |
| 剂型、规格<br>Preparations | 注射液：每支 2ml；5ml；10ml。<br>Injection: 2ml; 5ml; 10ml per vial. |
| **药品名称 Drug Names** | **赖氨酸 Lysine** |
| 适应证<br>Indications | ①用于颅脑损伤综合征、脑血管病、记忆力减退等。②赖氨酸缺乏引起的小儿食欲缺乏、营养不良及脑发育不全等。<br><br>① it is used for traumatic brain injury syndrome, cerebrovascular disease, memory loss, etc. ② it is used for children loss of appetite, malnutrition and cerebral hypoplasia caused by lysine deficiency. |
| 用法、用量<br>Dosage | 口服：每次 3g，一日 1 次，10～15 日为 1 个疗程。静脉滴注：一日 1 次，每次 3g，稀释于 250ml 静脉滴注液中缓慢滴注，20 次为 1 个疗程。<br><br>Orally: the dose is 3g once a day, and 10 to 15 days are a course of treatment. Intravenous drip: the dose is 3g once a day,, diluted by 250ml intravenous drip liquid and 20 times are a course of treatment. |
| 剂型、规格<br>Preparations | 散剂：每袋 3g。<br>注射液：每支 3g（10ml）。<br>Powder: 3g per bag.<br>Injection: 3g (10ml) per vial. |

### 8.14 麻醉药及其辅助用药 Anesthetics and their supplementary drugs

| | |
|---|---|
| **药品名称 Drug Names** | **恩氟烷 Enflurane** |
| 适应证<br>Indications | 应用于符合全身麻醉，（此时浓度 0.5% 即足够，3% 为极限），可与多种静脉全身麻醉药和全身麻醉辅助用药联用或合用。<br><br>It is used for general anesthesia, (the concentration of 0.5% is sufficient, and 3% is ultimate). It can be used with a variety of intravenous general anesthetic and general anesthesia adjuvant drugs. |
| 用法、用量<br>Dosage | 使用量应根据患者的具体情况而定。<br>The amount used should be determined according to the specific situation of the patient. |
| 剂型、规格<br>Preparations | 液体剂：每瓶 100ml；150ml；250ml。<br>Liquid agent: 100ml; 150ml; 250ml per bottle. |

**续　表**

| 药品名称 Drug Names | 异氟烷 Isoflurane |
|---|---|
| 适应证<br>Indications | 可用于各种手术的麻醉。<br>It can be used in a variety of surgical anesthesia. |
| 用法、用量<br>Dosage | 成人诱导麻醉时吸入气体内浓度一般为 1.5% ～ 3%；维持麻醉时气体内浓度为 1% ～ 1.5%。麻醉较深时对循环及呼吸系统均有抑制作用。骨骼肌松弛作用亦较好。<br><br>For adults, the suction gas concentration of the drug for induction of anesthesia is generally from 1.5% to 3%; for maintenance of anesthesia, the gas concentration is 1% ～ 1.5%. when anesthesia is deep, the circulatory and respiratory systems will be inhibited. Its efficacy for skeletal muscle relaxant is also good. |
| 剂型、规格<br>Preparations | 液体剂：每瓶 100ml，250ml。<br>Liquid agent: 100ml; 250ml per bottle. |
| 药品名称 Drug Names | 七氟烷 Sevoflurane |
| 适应证<br>Indications | 作为全身麻醉药应用。<br>It is used for general anesthesia |
| 用法、用量<br>Dosage | 麻醉诱导时，以 50% ～ 70% 氧化亚氮与本品 2.5% ～ 4% 吸入。使用睡眠量的静脉麻醉时，本品的诱导量通常为 0.5% ～ 5%。麻醉维持，应以最低有效浓度维持外科麻醉状态，常为 4% 以下。<br><br>For induction of anesthesia, 2.5% to 4% of the drug is inhaled with 50% ～ 70% of the nitrous oxide. When it is used for intravenous anesthesia to make patients sleep, the amount of this product is usually 0.5% ～ 5%. For maintenance of anesthesia, the minimal effective concentration of the drug should be used to maintain surgical anesthesia. The concentration is often less than 4%. |
| 剂型、规格<br>Preparations | 吸入用七氟烷：120ml；250ml。<br>Sevoflurane for inhalation: 120ml; 250ml. |
| 药品名称 Drug Names | 硫喷妥钠 Thiopental Sodium |
| 适应证<br>Indications | 常用于静脉麻醉、诱导麻醉、基础麻醉、抗惊厥及复合麻醉等。<br>It is commonly used for intravenous anesthesia, induction of anesthesia, basic anesthesia, anti-convulsion and combined anesthesia. |
| 用法、用量<br>Dosage | （1）静脉麻醉：一般多用 5% 或 2.5% 溶液，缓慢注入。成人，一次 4 ～ 8mg/kg，经 30 秒左右即进入麻醉，神志完全消失，但肌肉松弛不完全，也不能随意调节，麻醉深度，故多用于小手术。如患者有呼吸快、发声、移动等现象，即为苏醒的表现，可再注射少量以持续麻醉。极量：一次 1g（即 5% 溶液 20ml）。<br>（2）基础麻醉：用于小儿、甲状腺功能亢进症及精神紧张患者。成人，肌内注射，每次 0.5g，以 2.5% 溶液，做深部肌内注射。<br>（3）诱导麻醉：一般用 2.5% 溶液缓慢静脉注射，1 次 0.3g（1 次不超过 0.5g），继以乙醚吸入。<br>（4）抗惊厥：每次静脉注射 0.05 ～ 0.1g。<br><br>(1) intravenous anesthesia: 5% or 2.5% solution is often used through slow injection. For adults, the dose is 4 ～ 8 mg/kg at a time. After 30 seconds, anesthesia appears, and the patient's mind completely disappears. But if muscle relaxation is incomplete, the depth of anesthesia can not be adjusted at will. So the drug is often used for small surgery. If patients have fast breathing, voice and movement, which are the performance of awakening, a small amount of the drug can be given to maintain anesthesia. The maximum dose is 1 g every time (20 ml of 5% solution).<br>(2) basic anesthesia: it is used for children, and patients with hyperthyroidism and mental tension. For adults, the dose is 0.5 g per time, taking the form of 2.5% solution, through deep intramuscular injection.<br>(3) induction of anesthesia: 2.5% solution is generally used through slow intravenous injection. The dose is 0.3 g every time (the dose cannot exceed 0.5 g every tiem), followed by ether inhalation.<br>(4) Anti-convulsion: the dose is 0.05 ～ 0.1g per time through intravenous injection. |

**续 表**

| | |
|---|---|
| 剂型、规格<br>Preparations | 注射用硫喷妥钠：每支 0.5g；1g（含无水碳酸钠 6%）。<br>Thiopental for injection: 0.5g; 1g per vial (containing 6% of anhydrous sodium carbonate). |
| 药品名称 Drug Names | 氯胺酮 Ketamine |
| 适应证<br>Indications | 用于：①各种小手术或诊断操作时，可单独使用本品进行麻醉。对于需要肌肉松弛的手术，应加用肌肉松弛剂；对于内脏牵引较重的手术，应配合其他药物以减少牵引反应。②作为其他全身麻醉的诱导剂使用。③辅助麻醉性能较弱的麻醉剂进行麻醉，或与其他全身或局部麻醉剂复合使用。<br><br>① it is used for a variety of minor surgery or diagnostic operation, and it can be used alone for anesthesia. For muscle relaxation surgery, the drug should be combined with muscle relaxants; it should be compatible with other drugs to reduce the traction response for heavier traction visceral surgery. ② it can be used as other general anesthesia inductive agents. ③ it can assist anesthetic of which anesthesia performance is weak or be combined with other systemic or topical anesthetic. |
| 用法、用量<br>Dosage | （1）成人常用量：全身麻醉诱导，静脉注射 1～2mg/kg，注射应较慢（60 秒以上）。全身麻醉维持，一次静脉注射 0.5～1mg/kg。<br>（2）极量：静脉注射每分钟 4mg/kg；肌内注射，一次 13mg/kg。<br><br>(1) The usual dose for adults: induction of general anesthesia: the dose is 1～2mg/kg through intravenous injection, and the injection speed should be slow (60 seconds or more). Maintenance of anesthesia: the dose is 0.5～1mg/kg once through intravenous injection.<br>(2) the maximum dose: for intravenous injection, the dose is 4mg/kg per minute; for intramuscular injection, the dose is 13mg/kg once. |
| 剂型、规格<br>Preparations | 注射液：100mg（2ml）；100mg（1ml）；200mg（20ml）。<br>Injection: 100mg (2ml); 100mg (1ml); 200mg (20ml). |
| 药品名称 Drug Names | 依托咪酯 Etomidate |
| 适应证<br>Indications | 可用于诱导麻醉。<br>It can be used for induction of anesthesia. |
| 用法、用量<br>Dosage | 成人：0.3mg/kg，于 15～60 秒静脉注射完毕。<br>For adults: the dose is 0.3mg/kg, and the drug is given within 15~60 seconds through intravenous injection. |
| 剂型、规格<br>Preparations | 注射液：每支 20mg（10ml）。<br>Injection: 20mg (10ml) per vial. |
| 药品名称 Drug Names | 羟丁酸钠 Sodium Hydroxybutyrate |
| 适应证<br>Indications | 常用于全身麻醉或诱导麻醉，以及局部麻醉、腰麻的辅助用药，适用于老年人、儿童及脑、神经外科手术，外伤、烧伤患者的麻醉。<br><br>It is commonly used for induction of anesthesia or general anesthesia. It is also used as adjuvant drug for local anesthesia and lumbar anesthesia. It is suitable for the elderly, children, brain and neuro surgery, and patients with trauma and burns. |
| 用法、用量<br>Dosage | （1）诱导麻醉：一次静脉注射，成人 60mg/kg，注射速度 1g/min。<br>（2）维持麻醉：静脉注射，一次 12～80mg/kg。<br>（3）极量：一次总量 300mg/kg。<br><br>(1) Induction of anesthesia: intravenous injection: for adults, the dose is 60mg/kg once; and the injection speed is 1g/min.<br>(2) Maintenance of anesthesia: intravenous injection: the dose is 12～80mg/kg per time.<br>(3) Maximum dose: the total dose is 300mg/kg once. |
| 剂型、规格<br>Preparations | 注射液：每支 2.5g（10ml）。<br>Injection: 2.5g (10ml) per vial. |

**续　表**

| 药品名称 Drug Names | 丙泊酚 Propofol |
|---|---|
| 适应证<br>Indications | 用于全身麻醉的诱导和维持。常与硬膜外或脊髓麻醉同时应用，也常与镇痛药、肌松药及吸入性麻醉药同用。适用于门诊患者。<br><br>It can be used in general anesthesia induction and maintenance. It is often used with epidural or spinal anesthesia. It is also often used with pain relievers, muscle relaxant and inhaled anesthetics. It is suitable for outpatients. |
| 用法、用量<br>Dosage | 静脉注射。诱导麻醉：每 10 秒钟注射 40mg，直至产生麻醉。大多数成人用量为 2 ～ 2.5mg/kg。维持麻醉：常用量为每分钟 0.1 ～ 0.2mg/kg。<br><br>Intravenous injection: Induction of anesthesia: the dose is 40mg every 10 seconds, until anesthesia appears. The dosage is about 2 ～ 2.5mg/kg for most adults. Maintenance of anesthesia: the usual dose is 0.1 ～ 0.2mg/kg per minute. |
| 剂型、规格<br>Preparations | 注射液：每支 200mg（20ml）；500mg（50ml）；1g（100ml）。<br>丙泊酚中 / 长链脂肪乳注射液：200mg（20ml）。<br><br>Injection: 200mg (20ml); 500mg (50ml); 1g (100ml) per vial.<br>Propofol Medium and Long Chain Fat Emulsion injection: 200mg (20ml). |
| 药品名称 Drug Names | 普鲁卡因 Procaine |
| 适应证<br>Indications | 主要用于浸润麻醉、蛛网膜下腔阻滞麻醉、神经传导阻滞麻醉和用于治疗某些损伤和炎症，可使发炎损伤部位的症状得到一定的缓解（封闭疗法）。还可用于纠正四肢血管舒缩功能障碍。<br><br>It is mainly used for infiltration anesthesia, subarachnoid space block anesthesia, nerve conduction block anesthesia and certain injury and inflammation. It can remit symptoms of inflammation damage parts (block therapy). It can also be used to correct limbs vasomotor dysfunction. |
| 用法、用量<br>Dosage | （1）浸润麻醉，溶液浓度多为 0.25% ～ 0.5%（口腔科有时用其 4% 的溶液），每次用量 0.05 ～ 0.25g，每小时不可超过 1.5g。其麻醉时间短，可加入少量肾上腺素 [1：（100 000 ～ 200 000）] 以延长作用的时间。<br>（2）蛛网膜下隙阻滞麻醉，一次量不宜超过 0.15g，用 5% 溶液，约可麻醉 1 小时，主要用于腹部以下需时不长的手术。<br>（3）"封闭疗法"，将 0.25% ～ 0.5% 溶液注射于与病变有关的神经周围或病变部位 。<br><br>(1) Infiltration anesthesia, the solution concentration is usually 0.25% ～ 0.25% ( 4% solution for department of stomatology ). The dosage is 0.05 g ～ 0.25 g, and not more than 1.5 g per hour. Its anesthesia time is short, and can be used with a small amount of adrenaline [1：(10 0000 ～ 200 000)] in order to prolong the time of action.<br>(2) Subarachnoid block anesthesia: the dose should not be more than 0.15 g every time. Use its 5% solution for about 1 hour of anesthesia. It is mainly used for operations below abdomen which cannot take a long time.<br>(3) Block therapy: use 0.25% ～ 0.5% solution in the regions around the nerve associated with lesions or diseased regions. |
| 剂型、规格<br>Preparations | 注射液：每支 100mg（20ml）；50mg（20ml）；100mg（10ml）；40mg（2ml）。<br>注射用盐酸普鲁卡因：每支 150mg；1g。<br><br>Injection: 100mg (20ml); 50mg (20ml); 100mg (10ml); 40mg (2ml) per vial.<br>Procaine hydrochloride for injection: 150mg; 1g per vial. |
| 药品名称 Drug Names | 丁卡因 Tetracaine |
| 适应证<br>Indications | 用于黏膜表面麻醉、神经阻滞麻醉、硬膜外麻醉和蛛网膜下隙麻醉。<br><br>it can be used for mucosal surface anesthesia, nerve block anesthesia, epidural anesthesia and subarachnoid anesthesia. |
| 用法、用量<br>Dosage | （1）黏膜麻醉：眼科用 0.5% ～ 1% 溶液，鼻喉科用 1% ～ 2% 溶液，总量不得超过 20ml。应用时应于每 3ml 中加入 0.1% 盐酸肾上腺素溶液 1 滴。浸润麻醉 0.025% ～ 0.03% 溶液。<br>（2）神经阻滞用 0.1% ～ 0.3% 溶液。<br>（3）蛛网膜下隙麻醉时用 10 ～ 15ml 与 脑脊液混合后注入。<br>（4）硬膜外麻醉用 0.15% ～ 0.3% 溶液，与利多卡因合用时最高浓度为 0.3%。极量：浸润麻醉、神经传导阻滞，一次 0.1g。 |

**续　表**

| | |
|---|---|
| | (1) Mucosal anesthesia: for ophthalmology, its 0.5%~1% solution is used. For rhinology and Laryngology, its 1%~2% solution is used.The volume dose should not exceed 20ml. a drop of 0.1% adrenaline hydrochloric acid solution should be add in 3ml of the drug every time. Infiltration anesthesia uses its 0.025%~ 0.03% solutions.<br>(2) nerve block anesthesia uses its 0.1%~0.3%solution.<br>(3) Subarachnoid anesthesia uses 10 ~ 15ml of the drug mixed with cerebrospinal fluid.<br>(4) Epidural anesthesia uses its 0.15%~ 0.3% solution. When it is used with lidocaine, the highest concentration is 0.3%. Maximum dose: for infiltration anesthesia and nerve conduction block anesthesia, the dose is 0.1g once. |
| 剂型、规格<br>Preparations | 注射液：每支 50mg（5ml）。<br>注射用盐酸丁卡因：10mg；15mg；20mg；50mg。<br>盐酸丁卡因凝胶：1.5g：70mg。<br><br>Injection: 50mg (5ml) per vial<br>Tetracaine hydrochloride for injection: 10mg, 15mg, 20mg, 50mg<br>Tetracaine hydrochloride gel: 1.5g: 70mg. |
| 药品名称 Drug Names | 利多卡因 Lidocaine |
| 适应证<br>Indications | 主要用于阻滞麻醉及硬膜外麻醉。也用于室性心律失常，如室性心动过速及频发室性期前收缩。<br><br>It is mainly used for block anesthesia and epidural anesthesia. It can slso used for ventricular arrhythmia, such as ventricular tachycardia and frequent ventricular premature beat. |
| 用法、用量<br>Dosage | (1) 局部麻醉：阻滞麻醉用 1% ~ 2% 溶液，每次用量不宜超过 0.4g。表面麻醉用 2% ~ 4% 溶液，喷雾或蘸药贴敷，一次不超过 100mg，也可以 2% 胶浆剂抹于食管、咽喉气管或导尿管的外壁；妇女作阴道检查时可用棉签蘸 5 ~ 7ml 于局部。尿道扩张术或膀胱镜检查时用量 200 ~ 400mg。气雾剂或喷雾剂 2% ~ 4%，供做内镜检查用，每次 2%10 ~ 30ml，4%5 ~ 15ml。浸润麻醉用 0.25% ~ 0.5% 溶液，每小时用量不超过 0.4g。硬膜外麻醉用 1% ~ 2% 溶液，每次用量不超过 0.5g。<br>(2) 心律失常。<br><br>(1) Local anesthesia: block anesthesia uses 1%~ 2% solution and the dosage should not be more than 0.4g every time. Surface anesthesia uses 2% ~ 4% solution, through spray or applying patches. The dosage cannot exceed 100 mg every tiem. 2% mucilage agent can be used on esophagus, throat tracheal or catheter ektexine; for women vaginal examination, dip 5 ~ 7 ml and apply the drug on the local part with cotton swab. The dose for urethral dilatation or cystoscopy is 200 ~ 400 mg. Aerosol and sprays 2% ~ 4% are use for endoscopic examination. The dose is 2% 10 ~ 30 ml of 2%, and 5 ~ 15 ml of 4% every time. Infiltrating anesthesia uses 0.25% ~ 0.5% solution. The dosage is no more than 0.4 g per hour. Epidural anesthesia uses 1% ~ 2% solution. The dosage is not more than 0.5g every time.<br>(2) arrhythmia. |
| 剂型、规格<br>Preparations | 注射液：每支 0.1g（5ml）；0.4g（20ml）。<br>胶浆剂：2%。<br>盐酸利多卡因气雾剂：2%；4%。<br><br>Injection: 0.1g (5ml); 0.4g (20ml) per vial<br>Mucilage: 2%.<br>Lidocaine hydrochloride aerosol: 2%, 4%. |
| 药品名称 Drug Names | 布比卡因 Bupivacaine |
| 适应证<br>Indications | 浸润麻醉用；神经传导阻滞麻醉。<br>It is used for infiltration anesthesia and nerve conduction block anesthesia. |
| 用法、用量<br>Dosage | 浸润麻醉用 0.1% ~ 0.25% 溶液；神经传导阻滞用 0.5% ~ 0.75% 溶液。一次极量 200mg，一日极量 400mg。<br><br>Infiltration anesthesia uses 0.1%~0.25%solution ; Nerve conduction block uses 0.5%~0.75% solution. The maximum dose is 200mg once, and 400mg a day. |
| 剂型、规格<br>Preparations | 注射液：每支 12.5mg（5ml）；25mg（5ml）；37.5mg（5ml）。<br>Injection: 12.5mg (5ml), 25mg (5ml), 37.5mg (5ml) per vial. |

**续　表**

| 药品名称 Drug Names | 罗哌卡因 Ropivacaine |
|---|---|
| 适应证<br>Indications | 用于区域组织麻醉和硬膜外麻醉；也可用于区域组织镇痛，如硬膜外术后或分娩镇痛。<br>It is used for regional organizations anesthesia and epidural anesthesia; it can also used for pain relief of regional organizations, such as epidural postoperation or labor analgesia. |
| 用法、用量<br>Dosage | 区域组织麻醉和硬膜外麻醉：0.5% ～ 1% 溶液。一次最大剂量为 200mg。区域组织镇痛：0.2% 溶液。<br>Regional organizations anesthesia and epidural anesthesia uses 0.5%~1%solution. The maximum dose is 200mg every time. Regional organizations analgesia uses 0.2% solution. |
| 剂型、规格<br>Preparations | 注射液：20mg（10ml）；40mg（20ml）；75mg（10ml）；150mg（20ml）；100mg（10ml）；200mg（200ml）。<br>Injection: 20mg (10ml), 40mg (20ml), 75mg (10ml), 150mg (20ml), 100mg (10ml), 200mg (200ml). |
| 药品名称 Drug Names | 达克罗宁 Dyclonine |
| 适应证<br>Indications | 对黏膜穿透力强，作用迅速，可做表面麻醉。对皮肤有止痛、止痒及杀菌作用，可用于烧伤、擦伤、痒疹、虫咬伤、痔瘘、溃疡、压疮以及镜检前的准备。<br>The drug has strong mucous membrane penetrating power and acts very fast. It can be used for surface anesthesia. It can relieve pain and itching of skin and sterilize skin. It can be used for burns, abrasions, prurigo, insect bites, hemorrhoid and fistula, ulcers, bedsores and preparation before the microscopic examination. |
| 用法、用量<br>Dosage | 多制成 1% 的软膏、乳膏或 0.5% 的溶液供用。<br>The drug is often made into 1% ointment, emulsifiable paste, or 0.5% solution for use. |
| 剂型、规格<br>Preparations | 软膏：1%；乳膏 1%；溶液：0.5%。<br>Ointment: 1%; Cream: 1%; Solution: 0.5%. |
| 药品名称 Drug Names | 泮库溴铵 Pancuronium Bromide |
| 适应证<br>Indications | 主要用作外科手术麻醉的辅助用药（气管插管和肌松）。<br>It is mainly used as a surgical anesthetic adjuvant (endotracheal intubation and muscle relaxants). |
| 用法、用量<br>Dosage | 静脉注射。成人常用量 40 ～ 100μg/kg。与乙醚、氟烷合用时应酌减剂量。<br>Intravenous injection: Give adults the usual dose of 40 ～ 100μg/kg . Make appropriate dose reduction when combined with the ether and halothane. |
| 剂型、规格<br>Preparations | 注射液：每支 4mg（2ml）。<br>Injection: 4mg (2ml) per vial. |
| 药品名称 Drug Names | 罗库溴铵 Rocuronium Bromide |
| 适应证<br>Indications | 用于气管插管，也可用于各种手术中肌松的维持。<br>It is used for tracheal intubation, and for maintaining muscle relaxation in various surgical. |
| 用法、用量<br>Dosage | 插管：0.6mg/kg 单次静脉注射。<br>维持量：0.15mg/kg，单次静脉注射；每分钟 5 ～ 10μg/kg 连续静脉滴注。<br>吸入麻醉下应适当减量。<br>Intubation: the dose is 0.6mg/kg through single intravenous injection.<br>Maintenance dose: the dose is 0.15mg/kg throug single intravenous injection; continuous intravenous infusion 5 ～ 10μg/kg per minute.<br>Inhalation anesthesia should be decrement appropriately. |
| 剂型、规格<br>Preparations | 注射液：每支 50mg（5ml）；100mg（10ml）。<br>Injection: 50mg (5ml), 100mg (10ml) per vial. |
| 药品名称 Drug Names | 维库溴铵 Vecuronium Bromide |
| 适应证<br>Indications | 为中效非除极型肌松药。肌松效应及用途等均似于泮库溴铵，但稍强，持续时间为泮库溴铵的 1/3 ～ 1/2。<br>Vecuronium bromide is lente non-depolarizing muscle relaxants. Muscle relaxant effect and purpose are similar to pancuronium bromide, but stronger slightly. Its duration is 1/3~1/2 of pancuronium bromide. |

**续　表**

| 用法、用量<br>Dosage | 静脉注射，常用量为 70 ～ 100μg/kg。<br>Intravenous injection: the usual dose is 70 ～ 100μg/kg. |
|---|---|
| 剂型、规格<br>Preparations | 注射用维库溴铵：每支 4mg，以所附溶剂溶解后应用。<br>Vecuronium bromide for Injection: 4mg per vial, dissolved by the attached solvent for injection |
| 药品名称 Drug Names | 阿库氯铵 Alcuronium Chloride |
| 适应证<br>Indications | 为除极型肌松药，其特点与泮库溴铵相似，其效应比筒箭毒碱强 1.5 ～ 2 倍。静脉注射后肌松起效快（30 秒），2 ～ 3 分钟达高峰，维持 20 ～ 30 分钟。停药后恢复亦快。<br>It is a kind of depolarizing muscle relaxants and similar to pancuronium bromide. Its effects are 1.5 or 2 times stronger than those of tubocurarine. By intravenous injection, it can work very soon (30 seconds) and reach the strongest efficacy in 2 to 3 minutes, which can last 20 to 30 minutes. Recover very quickly after drug withdrawal. |
| 用法、用量<br>Dosage | 静脉注射：首次剂量为 150μg/kg，随后为 300μg/kg，间隔 15 ～ 25 分钟注射一次。<br>Intravenous injection: the first dose is 150μg/kg, and then 300μg/kg. Once every 15 to 25 minutes. |
| 剂型、规格<br>Preparations | 注射液：每支 10mg（2ml）。<br>Injection: 10mg (2ml) per vial. |
| 药品名称 Drug Names | 哌库溴铵 Pipecuronium Biomide |
| 适应证<br>Indications | 为长效非除极型肌松药，作用类似泮库溴铵，肌松持续时间为 20 分钟。也可用作外科手术麻醉的辅助用药。<br>It is depolarizing muscle relaxants. Its characteristics are similar to pancuronium bromide. After intravenous injection, the duration of the muscle relaxant was 20 minutes. |
| 用法、用量<br>Dosage | 气管插管在静脉注射后 3 分钟，用药量为静脉注射 0.08 ～ 0.1mg/kg；肾功能不全者用药量不超过 0.04mg/kg。<br>Intravenous injection: give first dose of 150μg/kg and then give 300μg/kg every15 to 25 minutes. |
| 剂型、规格<br>Preparations | 注射剂：每支 4mg（附有溶剂）。<br>Injection: 4mg per vial (attached solvent). |
| 药品名称 Drug Names | 阿曲库铵 Atracurium |
| 适应证<br>Indications | 为非除极型肌松药。作用与筒箭毒碱相同，起效快（1 分钟）、持续时间短（15 分钟）。大剂量可促使组胺释放。用于各种手术时需肌松或控制呼吸情况。<br>It is a kind of non-depolarizing muscle relaxants. It has the same effects as tubocurarine. It works very soon (1 minute) and with a short duration (15 minutes). Large doses can induce histamine release. It can be used for muscular flaccidity or breath control in a variety of surgeries. |
| 用法、用量<br>Dosage | 静脉注射起始剂量 0.3 ～ 0.6mg/kg，然后可以静脉滴注每分钟 5 ～ 10μg/kg 维持。<br>Its starting dose of intravenous injection is 0.3 ～ 0.6mg/kg and then the dosage can be maintained as 5 ～ 10μg/kg per minute through intravenous drip. |
| 剂型、规格<br>Preparations | 注射液：每支 25mg（2.5ml）；50mg（5ml）。<br>Injection: 25mg (2.5ml); 50mg (5ml) per vial. |
| 药品名称 Drug Names | 顺阿曲库铵 Cisatracurium |
| 适应证<br>Indications | ①其效能为阿曲库铵的 4 ～ 5 倍；②消除半衰期约为 24 分钟；③作用持续时间 45 ～ 75 分钟；④无组胺释放作用，无心血管不良反应。<br>① its potency is 4 to 5 times of the atracurium; ② its elimination half-life is approximately 24 minutes; ③ its duration of action is 45~75 minutes; ④ it has no effect on histamine release, and it cannot cause cardiovascular adverse reactions. |
| 用法、用量<br>Dosage | 成人用量为 0.05mg/kg，常用气管插管用量为 0.15 ～ 0.20mg/kg，插管时间在静脉注射后 150 秒左右。<br>For adults, the dosage is 0.05mg/kg. The commonly used dosage of endotracheal intubation is 0.15 ～ 0.20mg/kg. The intubation time is 150 seconds after the intravenous injection. |

**续　表**

| 剂型、规格<br>Preparations | 注射液：每支 10mg（5ml）；20mg（10ml）；40mg（20ml）。<br>Injection: 10mg (5ml); 20mg (10ml); 40mg (20ml) per vial. |
|---|---|
| **药品名称 Drug Names** | 琥珀胆碱 Succinylcholine |
| 适应证<br>Indications | 为速效肌肉松弛药；也用于需快速气管内插管。<br>Suxamethonium is quick-acting muscle relaxants and can also be used in rapid endotracheal intubation. |
| 用法、用量<br>Dosage | 成人静脉注射一次 1～2mg/kg。多用其 2%～5% 溶液。注射后 1 分钟即出现肌肉松弛，持续 2 分钟。如需继续维持其作用，可用其 0.1%～0.2% 溶液，以每分钟 2.5mg 的速度静脉注射；亦可静脉滴注，静脉滴注液可用生理盐水或 5% 葡萄糖液稀释至 0.1% 浓度。极量，静脉注射一次 250mg。<br>For adults, the dosage is 1~2mg/kg a time through intravenous injection. Its 2% to 5% solution is frequently used. Muscle relaxation appears one minute after injection and lasts for 2 minutes. To continue to maintain its effect, its 0.1%~0.2%solution can be used through intravenous injection at a speed of 2.5 mg per minute, or through intravenous drip. The intravenous drip fluid is diluted to 0.1% concentration by normal saline or 5% glucose solution. The maximum dose is 250mg once intravenously. |
| 剂型、规格<br>Preparations | 注射液：每支 50mg（1ml）；100mg（2ml）。<br>Injection: 50mg (1ml); 100mg (2ml) per vial. |

9. 作用于自主神经系统的药物 Drugs mainly acting on the autonomic nervous system

9.1 拟胆碱药和抗胆碱药 Cholinergic drugs and Anticholinergic drugs

| **药品名称 Drug Names** | 卡巴胆碱 Carbachol |
|---|---|
| 适应证<br>Indications | 主要用于治疗青光眼。<br>It is mainly used for glaucoma. |
| 用法、用量<br>Dosage | 局部用药。0.75%～3% 溶液滴眼，用于对毛果芸香碱无反应或不能耐受者。成人两眼分别滴入 1～2 滴，4～8 小时 1 次。给药后需用手指压迫内眦 1～2 分钟，以减少吸收，减少全身不良反应。在白内障手术时起缩瞳作用并减少后眼压上升，可用 0.01%0.5ml 滴眼。<br>It is suitable for local application. Its 0.75% to 3% solution can be used as eyedrops. It can be used for people who are unresponsive to pilocarpine or do not tolerate it. 1 to 2 drops were dropped into each of the adult's eyes, once every 4 to 8 hours. Inner canthus should be pressed by fingers in 1 to 2 minutes in order to reduce absorption, and systemic adverse reactions. In the cataract surgery, it can cause miosis and stop the intraocular pressure from increasing by using its 0.01% 0.5ml drops. |
| 剂型、规格<br>Preparations | 滴眼液：0.25%；1.5%；2.25%；3%。注射液：每支 0.1mg（1ml）。<br>Drops: 0.25%; 1.5%; 2.25%; 3%. Injection: 0.1mg (1ml) per vial. |
| **药品名称 Drug Names** | 毛果芸香碱 Pilocarpine |
| 适应证<br>Indications | 治疗原发性青光眼，包括开角型与闭角型青光眼。滴眼后，缩瞳作用于 10～30 分钟出现，维持 4～8 小时；最大降眼压作用约 75 分钟内出现，维持 4～14 小时；可缓解或消除青光眼症状。也可用于唾液腺功能。<br>It is used for primary glaucoma, including open-angle and angle-closure glaucoma. After using eyedrops, miotic effect appears within 10 to 30 minutes and lasts for 4 to 8 hours; The maximum effect of lowering intraocular pressure occurs in about 75 minutes and lasts for 4 to 14 hours; it can alleviate or eliminate symptoms of glaucoma and can also be used for salivary gland function. |
| 用法、用量<br>Dosage | 滴眼液配制成 0.5%～4% 毛果芸香碱（常用 1% 及 2%，增加浓度可增加药效，但超过 4% 时，药效无明显增加）。滴眼后 10～15 分钟开始缩瞳，30～50 分钟作用最强，约持续 24 小时，睫状肌痉挛作用约持续 2 小时。滴药后 10～15 分钟开始降眼压，持续 4～8 小时，故应每日滴眼 3～4 次。<br>The eyedrops are made of 0.5% to 4% pilocarpine (commonly 1% and 2%, increasing the concentration can increase efficacy, but more than 4%, no significant increase in efficacy). After 10 to 15 minutes, miosis starts. The strongest effect appears in 30 to 50 minutes and lasts about 24 hours. Ciliary muscle spasm lasts about two hours. After 10 to 15 minutes, intraocular pressure also decreases, which lasts for 4 to 8 hours. So, it should be used 3 to 4 times daily. |

**续 表**

| 剂型、规格<br>Preparations | 滴眼液：1%；2%。<br>片剂：（SALAGEN）：每片 5mg。<br>注射液：每支 10mg（1ml）。<br><br>Drops: 1%; 2%.<br>Tablets: (SALAGEN): 5mg per tablet.<br>Injection: 10mg (1ml) per vial. |
|---|---|
| **药品名称 Drug Names** | **毒扁豆碱 Physostigmine** |
| 适应证<br>Indications | 主要用其 0.2% ~ 0.5% 溶液点眼，用于治疗原发性闭角型青光眼，药效比毛果芸香碱强而持久。它对中枢神经系统的作用是小剂量时兴奋，大剂量时抑制，故已较少做全身给药，只用于眼科。<br><br>Its 0.2% to 0.5% solution is mainly used as eyedrops for the treatment of primary angle-closure glaucoma. Its efficacy is stronger and more durable than pilocarpine. Its effect on the central nervous system is that when a small dose used, excitement appears while when a large dose used, inhibition appears. So, it is seldom used for systemic administration, but only for ophthalmology. |
| 用法、用量<br>Dosage | 注射液，皮下注射或肌内注射，一次 0.5mg 或遵医嘱。眼膏，晚上临睡前点眼，涂于眼睑内，一般白天用毛果芸香碱，晚上用本品。或遵医嘱。<br><br>Injection can be used through subcutaneous or intramuscular injection, 0.5mg once or according to the doctor. Ointment is used inside the eyelid before going to sleep at night. During the day, pilocarpine is used and then in the evening, this product is used. Or you can use the drug by following the doctor's advice. |
| 剂型、规格<br>Preparations | 水杨酸毒扁豆碱滴眼剂：有水杨酸毒扁豆碱 0.25g，硼酸 1.8g，亚硫酸氢钠 0.1g，蒸馏水加至 100ml 配成；或由水杨酸毒扁豆碱 0.46g，氯化钠 0.8g，依地酸二钠 0.1g，尼泊金乙酯 0.03g（加热溶解），蒸馏水加至 100ml 配成。<br><br>Physostigmine salicylate eye drops: it includes 0.25g physostigmine salicylate, 1.8g acid, 0.1g sodium hydrogen sulfite, and distilled water which are mixed together into 100 ml; or it includes 0.46g physostigmine salicylate, 0.8g Sodium chloride, 0.1g disodium edetate, 0.03g ethyl paraben (heated to dissolve) and distilled water which are mixed together into 100ml. |
| **药品名称 Drug Names** | **新斯的明 Neostigmine** |
| 适应证<br>Indications | 多用于重症肌无力及腹部手术后的肠麻痹。<br>It is often used for myasthenia gravis and intestinal paralysis after abdominal surgery. |
| 用法、用量<br>Dosage | 口服其溴化物，一次 15mg，一日 45mg；极量：一次 30mg，一日 100mg。皮下注射、肌内注射其甲硫酸盐，一日 1 ~ 3 次，每次 0.25 ~ 1.0mg；极量：一次 1mg，一日 5mg。以 0.05% 眼药水用于青少年假性近视眼，一日 2 次，每次 1 ~ 2 滴，3 个月为 1 个疗程。<br><br>Its bromide is taken orally, 15mg once, 45mg one day; maximum dose: the dose is 30mg every time, 100mg one day. Its sulfate can be used through subcutaneous and intramuscular injection use, 0.25 ~ 1.0mg once, 1 to 3 times a day; maximum dose: the dose is 1mg once, 5mg one day. Its 0.05% eye drops can be used for teenager pseudo myopia, 1 to 2 drops every time, twice a day. A course of treatment lasts 3 months. |
| 剂型、规格<br>Preparations | 片剂：每片 15mg。<br>注射液：每支 0.5mg（1ml）；1mg（2ml）。<br>Tablet: 15mg per tablet.<br>Injection: 0.5mg (1ml), 1mg (2ml) per vial. |
| **药品名称 Drug Names** | **溴吡斯的明 Pyridostigmine Bromide** |
| 适应证<br>Indications | 用于重症肌无力；术后腹气胀或尿潴留；对抗非除极型肌松药的肌肉松弛作用。<br>It can be used for myasthenia gravis, postoperative abdominal bloating or urinary retention and against non-depolarizing muscle relaxants muscle relaxant effect. |

**续　表**

| 用法、用量<br>Dosage | （1）重症肌无力：口服，一次 60mg，一日 3 次；皮下注射或肌内注射，每日 1 ～ 5mg，或根据病情而定。<br>（2）术后腹气胀或尿潴留：肌内注射，一次 1 ～ 2mg。<br>（3）对抗非除极型肌松药的肌肉松弛：静脉注射，一次 2 ～ 5mg。<br>(1) Myasthenia gravis: orally: the dose is 60mg one time, 3 times a day; subcutaneous or intramuscular injection: the dose is 1 ~ 5mg every day, or according to the disease.<br>(2) Postoperative abdominal bloating or urinary retention: intramuscular injection, the dose is 1 ~ 2mg every time.<br>(3) Against non-depolarizing muscle relaxants muscle relaxants: intravenous injection: the dose is 2 ~ 5mg every time. |
|---|---|
| 剂型、规格<br>Preparations | 片剂：每片 60mg。<br>缓释片：180mg。<br>注射剂：每支 5mg（1ml）；10mg（2ml）。<br>Tablets: 60mg per tablet;<br>Sustained-release tablets: 180mg.<br>Injection: 5mg (1ml); 10mg (2ml) per vial. |
| 药品名称 Drug Names | 石杉碱甲 Huperzine A |
| 适应证<br>Indications | 可用于重症肌无力及良性记忆障碍。对阿尔茨海默病和脑器质性病变引起的记忆障碍也有所改善。<br>It can be used for myasthenia gravis and benign memory disorders. It can also work on Alzheimer's disease and memory disorders caused by organic brain disease. |
| 用法、用量<br>Dosage | （1）重症肌无力：肌内注射，每次 0.2 ～ 0.4mg，一日 1 ～ 2 次。<br>（2）记忆功能减退：口服，一次 0.1 ～ 0.2mg，一日 2 次。因个体差异，一般应从小剂量开始。每日最多不超过 0.45mg。<br>(1) Myasthenia gravis: intramuscular injection: the dose is 0.2 ~ 0.4mg every time, 1 or 2 times a day.<br>(2) Memory dysfunction: orally: the dose is 0.1 ~ 0.2mg every time, 2 times a day. Due to individual differences, it should generally be used from a small dose. The maximum dosage is less than 0.45mg daily. |
| 剂型、规格<br>Preparations | 片剂：每片 0.05mg。<br>Tablets: 0.05mg per tablet. |
| 药品名称 Drug Names | 多奈哌齐 Donepezil |
| 适应证<br>Indications | 可用轻、中度阿尔茨海默病的治疗。<br>It can be used for mild or moderate Alzheimer's disease. |
| 用法、用量<br>Dosage | 口服，一日 1 次，每次 5 ～ 10mg。<br>Orally: the dose is 5 ~ 10mg once a day. |
| 剂型、规格<br>Preparations | 片剂：每片 5mg；10mg。<br>Tablets: 5mg; 10mg per tablet. |
| 药品名称 Drug Names | 加兰他敏 Galanthamine |
| 适应证<br>Indications | 本品可用于重症肌无力，进行性肌营养不良，脊髓灰质炎后遗症，儿童脑型麻痹，因神经系统疾病所致感觉或运动障碍，多发性神经炎等。<br>This product can be used for myasthenia gravis, muscular dystrophy, polio sequelae, children cerebral palsy, sensory or motor disorders and multiple neuritis caused by neurological disorders. |
| 用法、用量<br>Dosage | （1）肌内注射或皮下注射：每次 2.5 ～ 10mg，小儿每次 0.05 ～ 0.1mg/kg，一日 1 次，1 个疗程 2 ～ 6 周。<br>（2）口服：每次 10mg，一日 3 次。小儿每日 0.5 ～ 1mg/kg，分 3 次服。<br>(1) Intramuscular injection or subcutaneous injection: the dose is 2.5 ~ 10mg every time. For children, the dose is 0.05 ~ 0.1mg/kg per time, once a day and a course of treatement is 2 to 6 weeks.<br>(2) Orally: the dose is 10mg every time, 3 times a day. For children, the dose is 0.5 ~ 1mg/kg every day, divided into 3 doses. |

**续 表**

| 剂型、规格<br>Preparations | 注射液：1mg（1ml）；2.5mg（1ml）；5mg（1ml）。<br>片剂：5mg。<br>Injection: 1mg (1ml); 2.5mg (1ml); 5mg (1ml).<br>Tablets: 5mg. |
|---|---|
| **药品名称 Drug Names** | 阿托品 Atropine |
| 适应证<br>Indications | 临床上的用途主要是：①抢救感染中毒性休克。②治疗锑剂引起的阿 - 斯综合征。③治疗有机磷农药中毒。④缓解内脏绞痛，包括胃肠痉挛引起的疼痛、肾绞痛、胆绞痛、胃及十二指肠溃疡。⑤用于麻醉前给药，可减少麻醉过程中支气管黏液分泌，预防术后引起肺炎，并可消除吗啡对呼吸的抑制。⑥眼科用药，用于角膜炎、虹膜睫状体炎。<br><br>The main clinical uses are: ① to rescue septic and toxic shock. ② to treat Adam-Stokes syndrome caused by antimony agents. ③ to treat organophosphorus pesticide poisoning. ④ to relieve colic organs, including pain, renal colic, biliary colic, gastric and duodenal ulcers caused by the gastrointestinal spasm. ⑤ to be used before anesthesia administered in order to reduce bronchial mucus secretion and prevent pneumonia after post-operation, and eliminate the inhibition of respiration of the morphine. ⑥ to be used as ophthalmic drugs for keratitis and iridocyclitis. |
| 用法、用量<br>Dosage | （1）感染中毒性休克：成人每次 1 ~ 2mg，小儿每次 0.03 ~ 0.05mg/kg，静脉注射，每 15 ~ 30 分钟 1 次，2 ~ 3 次后如情况不见好转可逐渐增加用量，至情况好转后即减量或停药。<br>（2）锑剂引起的阿 - 斯综合征：发现严重心律失常时，立即静脉注射 1 ~ 2mg（用 5% ~ 25% 葡萄糖液 10 ~ 20ml 稀释），同时肌内注射或皮下注射 1mg，15 ~ 30 分钟后再静脉注射 1mg。如患者无发作，可根据心律及心率情况改为每 3 ~ 4 小时 1 次皮下注射或肌内注射 1mg，48 小时后如不再发作，可逐渐减量，最后停药。<br>（3）有机磷农药中毒：①与碘解磷定等合用时：对中度中毒，每次皮下注射 0.5 ~ 1mg，隔 30 ~ 60 分钟 1 次；对严重中毒，每次静脉注射 1 ~ 2mg，隔 15 ~ 30 分钟 1 次，病情稳定后，逐渐减量并改用皮下注射。②单用时：对轻度中毒，每次皮下注射 0.5 ~ 1mg，隔 30 ~ 120 分钟 1 次；对中度中毒，每次皮下注射 1 ~ 2mg，隔 15 ~ 30 分钟 1 次；对重度中毒，即刻静脉注射 2 ~ 5mg，以后每次 1 ~ 2mg，隔 15 ~ 30 分钟 1 次，根据病情逐渐减量和延长间隔时间。<br>（4）缓解内脏绞痛：每次皮下注射 0.5mg。<br>（5）用于麻醉前给药：皮下注射：0.5mg。<br>（6）用于眼科：用 1% ~ 3% 眼药水滴眼或眼膏涂眼。滴时按住内眦部，以免流入鼻腔吸收中毒。<br><br>(1) septic and toxic shock: the dose is 1 ~ 2mg every time for adults and 0.03 ~ 0.05mg/kg every time for children through intravenous injection, once every 15 to 30 minutes. After 2 or 3 times, if the situation doesn't improve, the dosage can be gradually increased till the situation improves. And then reduce the dosage or stop the medicine.<br>(2) Adams Stokes syndrome caused by antimony agents: if severe arrhythmia is found, immediate intravenous injection of 1 ~ 2mg of this drug (diluted with 10 to 20 ml 5% to 25% glucose solution ) is needed. At the same time, intramuscular or subcutaneous injection of 1mg of this drug is also needed. After 15 ~ 30 minutes, intravenous injection of 1mg is taken again. If patients are without seizures, subcutaneous injection or intramuscular injection of 1mg can be taken once every 3 to 4 hours based on rhythm of the heart and heart rate. After 48 hours, if episodes stop, the drug can be decreased and finally discontinued.<br>(3) organophosphorus pesticide poisoning: ① When combined with pralidoxime iodide, etc.: for moderate intoxication, subcutaneous injection of 0.5 ~ 1mg every time can be taken, once every 30 to 60 minutes; for severe poisoning, intravenous injection of 1 ~ 2mg every time can be taken, once every 15 to 30 minutes. After stable condition, reduce the dosage and switch to subcutaneous injection. ② when it is used solely: for mild poisoning, subcutaneous injection of 0.5 ~ 1mg every time can be taken, once every 30 to 120 minutes; for moderate intoxication, subcutaneous injection of 1 ~ 2mg every time can be taken, once every 15 to 30 minutes; for severe poisoning, immediate intravenous injection of 2 ~ 5mg every time should be taken. Later, intravenous injection of 1 ~ 2mg every time are taken, once every 15 to 30 minutes. The dosage can be gradually reduced and the interval can be extended according to the disease.<br>(4) to alleviate visceral colic: subcutaneous injection of 0.5mg every time is taken .<br>(5) to be used before anesthesia administration: subcutaneous injection of 0.5mg every time is taken.<br>(6) ophthalmic: use1% ~ 3% eye drops or eye ointment . Hold down the canthus when taking the drops in order to stop them into the nasal cavity to avoid absorption of poisoning. |

| | |
|---|---|
| 剂型、规格<br>Preparations | 片剂：每片 0.3g。<br>注射液：每支 0.5mg（1ml）；1mg（2ml）；5mg（1ml）。<br>滴眼剂：取硫酸阿托品 1g，氯化钠 0.29g，无水磷酸二氢钠 0.4g，无水磷酸氢二钠 0.47g，羟胺乙酯 0.03g，蒸馏水加至 100ml 配成。<br><br>Tablets: 0 3g per tablet.<br>Injection: 0.5mg (1ml); 1mg (2ml); 5mg (1ml) per vial.<br>Eye drops: 1g atropine sulfate, 0.29g NaCl, 0.4g anhydrous sodium dihydrogen phosphate, 0.47g disodium hydrogen phosphate, 0.03g hydroxylamine ester, and distilled water are mixed together into 100ml. |
| 药品名称 Drug Names | 东莨菪碱 Scopolamine |
| 适应证<br>Indications | 临床用作镇静药，用于全身麻醉前给药、晕动病、震颤麻痹、狂躁性精神病、有机磷农药中毒等。由于本品既兴奋呼吸又对大脑皮质呈镇静作用，故用于抢救极重型流行性乙型脑炎呼吸衰竭（常伴有剧烈频繁的抽搐）亦有效。<br><br>Its clinical use is sedatives. It can used as the administration before general and for anesthesia, motion sickness, parkinsonism, manic psychosis, organic phosphorus pesticide poisoning. Since the product can both excite breathing and calm the brain cortex, it is used to rescue epidemic encephalitis respiratory failure(often accompanied by frequent violent convulsions). |
| 用法、用量<br>Dosage | 口服：一次 0.3 ～ 0.6mg，一日 0.6 ～ 1.2mg；极量一次 0.6mg，一日 1.8mg。皮下注射：一次 0.2 ～ 0.5mg；极量一次 0.5mg，一日 1.5mg。抢救乙型脑炎呼吸衰竭：以 1ml 含药 0.3mg 的注射液直接静脉注射或稀释于 10% 葡萄糖溶液 30ml 内做静脉注射，常用量为 0.02 ～ 0.04mg/kg，用药间歇时间一般为 20 ～ 30 分钟，用药总量最高达 6.3mg。<br><br>Orally: the dose is 0.3 ～ 0.6mg once, 0.6 ～ 1.2mg a day; the extreme amount is 0.6mg one time, 1.8mg one day. Subcutaneous injection: the dose is 0.2 ～ 0.5mg once; the extreme amount of one time is 0.5mg, 1.5mg one time. To rescue encephalitis respiratory failure: operate intravenous injection of 1ml injection containing 0.3mg of the drug or intravenous injection of 30 ml of the drug diluted by10% glucose solution . The usual dose is 0.02 ～ 0.04mg/kg, once every 20 to 30 minutes. The total amount of drug is up to 6.3mg. |
| 剂型、规格<br>Preparations | 片剂：每片 0.3mgg。<br>注射液：每支 0.3mg（1ml）；0.5mg（1ml）。<br>晕动片：每片含东莨菪碱 0.2mg、苯巴比妥钠 30mg、阿托品 0.15mg。<br><br>Tablets: 0.3mg per tablet.<br>Injection: 0.3mg (1ml); 0.5mg (1ml) per vial.<br>Motion sickness tablets: per tablet contains scopolamine 0.2mg, phenobarbital sodium 30mg, atropine 0.15mg. |
| 药品名称 Drug Names | 山莨菪碱 Anisodamine |
| 适应证<br>Indications | 适用于下列疾病：①感染中毒性休克：如暴发型流行性脑脊髓膜炎、中毒性痢疾等。②血管性疾病：脑血栓、脑栓塞、瘫痪、脑血管痉挛、血管神经性头痛、血栓闭塞性脉管炎等。③各种神经痛：如三叉神经痛、坐骨神经痛等。④平滑肌痉挛：胃、十二指肠溃疡，胆道痉挛等。⑤眩晕病。⑥眼底疾病：中心性视网膜炎、视网膜色素变性、视网膜动脉血栓等。⑦突发性耳聋：配合新针疗法可治疗其他耳聋。<br><br>It is available for the following diseases: ① septic and toxic shock: such as fulminant epidemic cerebrospinal meningitis, poisoning dysentery and so on. ② vascular disease: cerebral thrombosis, cerebral embolism, paralysis, cerebral vasospasm, angioneurotic headache, thrombosis obliterans. ③ various neuralgia: such as trigeminal neuralgia, sciatica. ④ smooth muscle spasm: stomach ulcer, biliary tract spasm. ⑤ vertigo. ⑥ fundus oculi diseases: central retinitis, retinitis pigmentosa, retinal artery thrombosis. ⑦ sudden deafness: combination with new acupuncture therapy to treat other kinds of epicophosis. |

**续 表**

| | |
|---|---|
| 用法、用量<br>Dosage | （1）肌内注射或静脉注射：成人一般一次 5 ～ 10mg，一日 1 ～ 2 次；也可经稀释后静脉注射。用于：①抢救感染中毒性休克：根据病情决定剂量。成人静脉注射每次 10 ～ 40mg；小儿 0.3 ～ 2mg/kg，需要时每隔 10 ～ 30 分钟可重复给药，情况不见好转可加量。病情好转可逐渐延长间隔时间，直至停药。②治疗脑血栓：加入 5% 葡萄糖液中静脉注射，每日 30 ～ 40mg。③一般慢性疾病：每次肌内注射 5 ～ 10mg，一日 1 ～ 2 次，可连用 1 个月以上。④治疗严重三叉神经痛：有时需加大剂量至每次 5 ～ 20mg，肌内注射。⑤治疗血栓闭塞性脉管炎：每次静脉注射 10 ～ 15mg，一日 1 次。<br><br>（2）口服：一日 3 次，一次 5 ～ 10mg。皮肤或黏膜局部使用，无刺激性。<br><br>(1) intramuscular injection or intravenous injection: the dose is generally 5 ～ 10mg every time for adults, 1 to 2 times a day; it can also be diluted and then used through intravenous injection. It can be used : ① to treat septic and toxic shock: the dosage is determined according to the disease. Intravenous injection of 10 ～ 40mg every time for adults and 0.3 ～ 2mg/kg for children are taken, once every 10 ～ 30 minutes. If the situation does not improve, the dosage can be increased. If the situation improves, the interval can be gradually extended until drug withdrawal. ② to treat thrombosis: operate intravenous injection of the drug mixed with 5% glucose solution, 30 ～ 40mg every day. ③ General Chronic Disease: operate intramuscular injection of 5 ～ 10mg every time, 2 times a day. It can be used successively in a month or more. ④ to treat severe trigeminal neuralgia: sometimes it needs to increase the dosage into 5 ～ 20mg every time through intramuscular injection. ⑤ to treat thrombosis obliterans:Operate intravenous injection of 10 ～ 15mg every time, once a day.<br><br>(2) Orally: The dose is 5 ～ 10mg every time three times a day. It is used on topical skin or mucous membranes and it's non-irritating. |
| 剂型、规格<br>Preparations | 氢溴酸山莨菪碱片剂：每片 5mg。<br>注射液：每支 1ml（10mg）；1ml（20mg）。<br>Mountain scopolamine hydrobromide tablets: 5mg per tablet.<br>Injection: 1ml (10mg); 1ml (20mg) per vial. |
| **药品名称 Drug Names** | 托吡卡胺 Tropicamide |
| 适应证<br>Indications | 散瞳药，主要用于散瞳检查眼底和散瞳验光。<br>It's a kind of mydriatic and mainly used for dilated fundus examination and dilated optometry. |
| 用法、用量<br>Dosage | 本品 0.5% 溶液滴眼 1 ～ 2 次，滴入结膜囊，一次一滴，间隔 5 分钟滴第二次，即可满足三通检查的需要。<br><br>Use its 0.5% solution as eyedrops for 1 ～ 2 times and drip them into the conjunctival sac, a drop every time with the interval of 5 minutes for the second time, which can meet the needs of the thee check. |
| 剂型、规格<br>Preparations | 滴眼液：每支 12.5mg（5ml）；25mg（5ml）；15mg（6ml）；30mg（6ml）。<br>Drops: 12.5mg (5ml); 25mg (5ml); 15mg (6ml); 30mg (6ml) per vial. |
| **药品名称 Drug Names** | 颠茄 Belladonna |
| 适应证<br>Indications | 用于胃及十二指肠溃疡、轻度胃肠、肾和胆绞痛等。<br>It is used for gastric and duodenal ulcers, mild gastrointestinal, renal and biliary colic. |
| 用法、用量<br>Dosage | （1）酊剂：每次服 0.3 ～ 1ml。极量：一次 1.5ml，一日 4.5ml。<br>（2）片剂：每次服 10 ～ 30mg，一日 30 ～ 90mg。极量：一次 50mg，一日 150mg。<br>(1) tincture: the dose is 0.3 ～ 1ml per time. Maximum dose: the does is 1.5ml per time, 4.5ml per day.<br>(2) tablets: the dose is10 ～ 30mg per time, 30 ～ 90mg a day. Maximum dose: the dose is 50mg once, 150mg a day. |
| 剂型、规格<br>Preparations | 酊剂：含生物碱 0.03%。<br>浸膏：含生物碱 1%。<br>片剂：每片含颠茄浸膏 10mg。<br>Tincture: it contains 0.03% alkaloids.<br>Extract: it contains 1% alkaloids.<br>Tablets: per tablet contains 10mg belladonna extract. |

**续　表**

| 药品名称 Drug Names | 后马托品 Homatropine |
|---|---|
| 适应证<br>Indications | 用于散瞳检查眼底和散瞳验光。也可用于弱视和斜视的压抑疗法。<br><br>It is used for inspection mydriatic fundus and specialized. It can also be used for depression therapy of amblyopia and strabismus . |
| 用法、用量<br>Dosage | 滴眼液滴入结膜囊，一次一滴。眼膏涂在结膜囊，一次少许。用药次数根据患者的年龄和使用目的以及瞳孔变化而决定。<br><br>Drip eye drops into the conjunctival sac, a drop at a time. Besmear eye ointment on the conjunctival sac, a little at a time. The frequency of drug administration is determined according to patients' age, purpose as well as the pupil change. |
| 剂型、规格<br>Preparations | 氢溴酸后马托品滴眼剂：1%～5%。<br>眼膏：2%。<br><br>Homatropine hydrobromide eye drops: 1% to 5%.<br>Ointment: 2%. |

9.2　拟肾上腺素药和抗肾上腺素药 Adrenergic drugs and Adrenoceptor Antagonists

| 药品名称 Drug Names | 萘甲唑啉 Naphazoline |
|---|---|
| 适应证<br>Indications | 用于过敏性及炎症性鼻充血、急慢性鼻炎、眼充血等，对细菌性，过敏性结膜炎也有效，并能减轻眼睑痉挛。对麻黄碱有耐受性者，可选用本品。<br><br>It is used for allergic and inflammatory nasal congestion, acute or chronic rhinitis, bloodshot eyes, and bacterial, allergic conjunctivitis. It can also reduce blepharospasm. For those who can tolerate ephedrine, they can use this product. |
| 用法、用量<br>Dosage | 治鼻充血，用其0.05%～0.1%溶液，每侧鼻孔滴2～3滴；治疗充血用其滴眼液，每次1～2滴。<br><br>Treat nasal congestion with its 0.05% to 0.1% solution, 2 to 3 drops on per side; treat bloodshot eyes with its eyedrops, 1 to 2 drops every time. |
| 剂型、规格<br>Preparations | 滴鼻剂：每瓶0.05%（10ml）；0.1%（10ml）。<br>盐酸萘甲唑啉滴眼液：1.2mg（10ml）。<br><br>Nose drops: a bottle of 0.05% (10 ml); 0.1% (10 ml).<br>Hydrochloric acid naphthyl methyl thiazole moiety eye drops: 1.2 mg (10 ml). |

| 药品名称 Drug Names | 米多君 Midodrine |
|---|---|
| 适应证<br>Indications | 主要用于各种原因引起的低血压，压力性尿失禁、射精功能障碍。<br><br>It is mainly used for all kinds of low blood pressure, stress urinary incontinence and ejaculatory dysfunction. |
| 用法、用量<br>Dosage | 口服：初剂量为1次2.5mg，一日2～3次。必要时可逐渐增加到一次10mg，一日3次的维持剂量。<br><br>Orally: Initial dose is 1 2.5mg every time, 2 or 3 times a day. If necessary, the dosage can be gradually increased to 10 mg per time, 3 times a day. |
| 剂型、规格<br>Preparations | 盐酸米多君片：2.5mg。<br><br>Tablets：2.5mg。 |

| 药品名称 Drug Names | 拉贝洛尔 Labetalol |
|---|---|
| 适应证<br>Indications | 用于治疗轻度和重度高血压和心绞痛。采用静脉注射能治疗高血压危象。<br><br>It is used for mild and severe hypertension and angina. It can treat hypertensive crisis through intravenous injection. |
| 用法、用量<br>Dosage | 口服：初剂量为1次100mg，一日2～3次。必要时可逐渐增加到一次200mg，一日3～4次。通常对轻、中、重度高血压患者的每日剂量相应为300～800mg、600～1200mg、1200～2400mg，加用利尿剂时可适当减量。静脉注射：一次100～200mg。<br><br>Orally: the initial dosage is 100 mg every time, 2 to 3 times a day. The dosage can be gradually increased to 200 mg every time time when necessary, 3～4 times a day. The daily dosage for patients with light, medium and severe high blood pressure is respectively 300～800 mg, 600～1200 mg, 1200～2400 mg. When it is combined with diuretics, the dosage can be appropriately reduced. Intravenous injection: 100～200 mg per time. |

续　表

| | |
|---|---|
| 剂型、规格<br>Preparations | 片剂：每片 100mg；200mg。<br>注射液：每支 50mg（5ml）。<br>Tablets: 100mg; 200mg per tablet.<br>Injection: 50mg (5ml) per vial. |
| 药品名称 Drug Names | 卡维地洛 Carvedilol |
| 适应证<br>Indications | 可用于原发性高血压及心绞痛。<br>It can be used for essential hypertension and angina. |
| 用法、用量<br>Dosage | 口服：初剂量为 25mg/d，一次服用；可根据需要逐渐增剂量至 50mg，分 1 ~ 2 次服下；最大日剂量不超过 100mg。<br>Orally: the initial dose is 25mg / d, taken at a time; the dose can be gradually increased to 50mg /d according to needs, divided into 1 to 2 doses; the daily maximum does not exceed 100mg. |
| 剂型、规格<br>Preparations | 片剂：每片 6.25mg；10mg；12.5mg；20mg。<br>胶囊：10mg。<br>Tablets: 6.25mg per tablet; 10mg; 12.5mg; 20mg.<br>Capsules: 10mg. |
| 药品名称 Drug Names | 酚妥拉明 Phentolamine |
| 适应证<br>Indications | 用于血管痉挛性疾病，如肢端动脉痉挛症（即雷诺病）、手足发绀症等、感染中毒性休克以及嗜铬细胞瘤的诊断试验等。用于室性早搏亦有效。<br>It is used for vascular spastic disease, such as limb artery spasm (i.e., Renault's disease), acrocyanosis disease, septic and toxic shock and diagnostic test of pheochromocytoma. It can also be used for ventricular premature beat. |
| 用法、用量<br>Dosage | （1）治疗血管痉挛性疾病：肌内注射或静脉注射。每次 5 ~ 10mg，20 ~ 30 分钟后按需要可重复给药。<br>（2）抗休克：以 0.3mg 每分钟的剂量进行静脉滴注。<br>（3）室性期前收缩：开始两日，每次口服 50mg，一日 4 次；如无效，则以后两日将剂量增加至每次 75mg，一日 4 次；如仍无效，可增至一日 400mg；如再无效，即应停用。无论何种剂量，一旦有效，就按该剂量继续服用 7 日。<br>（4）诊断嗜铬细胞瘤：静脉注射 5mg。注射后 30 分钟测血压一次，可连续测 10 分钟，如在 2 ~ 4 分钟血压降低 4.67/3.3ka（35/25mmHg）以上为阳性结果。<br>（5）做阴茎海绵体注射，可使阴茎海绵窦平滑肌松弛、扩张而勃起，可用于治疗勃起障碍，一次注射 1mg。<br>(1) To treat vascular spastic disease: intramuscular injection or intravenous injection: the dose is 5 ~ 10 mg per time. After 20 ~ 30 minutes, the drug can be used repeatedly as required.<br>(2) Anti-shock: the drug is taken through intravenous infusion with the dose of 0.3mg per minute.<br>(3) Ventricular premature beat: on the first two days, the drug is taken orally with 50 mg per time, 4 times a day. If invalid, the dose can be increased to 75 mg per time in the following two days, 4 times a day. If still invalid, the dose can be increased to 400 mg a day; if still invalid, the drug should be discontinued. Regardless of the dose, once it is effective, the drug should be taken for 7 days according to that dose.<br>(4) Diagnosis of pheochromocytoma: intravenous injection 5mg. After 30 minutes, the blood pressure can be measured and this measure can last for10 minutes. If the blood pressure decreases by 4.67/3.3kpa (35/25mmHg) in 2 to 4 minutes, the diagnosis is positive.<br>(5) To do the corpus cavernosum injection. The drug can make the penis cavernous sinus smooth muscle relax, expand and erect. It can be used to treat erectile dysfunction with the injection of 1 mg every time. |
| 剂型、规格<br>Preparations | 片剂：每片 25mg。<br>甲磺酸酚妥拉明注射液：每支 5mg（1ml）；10mg（1ml）。<br>Tablets: 25mg per tablet.<br>Phentolamine mesilate injection: 5mg (1ml); 10mg (1ml) per vial. |
| 药品名称 Drug Names | 妥拉唑林 Tolazoline |
| 适应证<br>Indications | 用于血管痉挛性疾病如肢端动脉痉挛症、手足发绀、闭塞性血栓静脉炎等。<br>It is used for vascular spastic disease such as raynaud's disease, acrocyanosis, occlusive thrombosis phlebitis, etc. |

| | |
|---|---|
| 用法、用量<br>Dosage | 口服，一次 15mg，一日 45 ～ 60mg；肌内注射或皮下注射，一次 25mg。<br>Orally: the dose is 15 mg every time, 45 ~ 60 mg a day; Intramuscular injection or hypodermic: the dose is 25 mg every time. |
| 剂型、规格<br>Preparations | 片剂：每片 25mg。<br>注射液：25mg（1ml）。<br>Tablets: 25 mg per tablet.<br>Injection: 25 mg (1 ml) |
| 药品名称 Drug Names | 酚苄明 Phenoxybenzamine |
| 适应证<br>Indications | 用于周围血管疾病，也可用于休克及嗜铬细胞瘤引起的高血压。早泄治疗。<br>It can be used for peripheral vascular disease and high blood pressure caused by pheochromocytoma and shock. It can also be used for premature ejaculation . |
| 用法、用量<br>Dosage | 口服：用于血管痉挛性疾病，开始每日 1 次，10mg，一日 2 次，隔日增 10mg；维持量一次 20mg，一日 2 次。用于早泄，一次 10mg，一日 3 次。静脉注射：每日 0.5 ～ 1mg/kg。静脉滴注（抗休克）：0.5 ～ 1mg/kg，加入 5% 葡萄糖液 250 ～ 500ml 中静脉滴注（2 小时滴完），一日总量不超过 2mg/kg。<br>Orally: it's used for vasospastic disorders. It's taken once a day at the beginning with10mg, twice a day. Every other day, the dosage increases by 10mg; the maintenance dose is 20mg once, 2 times a day. When it is used for premature ejaculation, it's taken with10mg once, 3 times a day. Intravenous injection: the dose is 0.5 ~ 1mg/kg every day. Intravenous infusion (anti-shock): the dose is 0.5 ~ 1mg/kg. The drug can be added into 250 ~ 500ml 5% glucose solution through intravenous infusion (drip finished in two hours). The total daily does cannot exceed 2mg/kg. |
| 剂型、规格<br>Preparations | 片剂：每片 5mg；10mg。<br>注射液：每支 10mg（1ml）。<br>Tablets: 5mg; 10mg per tablet.<br>Injection: 10mg (1ml) per vial. |
| 药品名称 Drug Names | 普萘洛尔 Propranolol |
| 适应证<br>Indications | 用于治疗多种原因所致的心律失常，如房性及室性期前收缩（效果较好）、窦性及室上性心动过速、心房颤动等，但室性心动过速应慎用。锑剂中毒引起的心律失常，当其他药物无效时可使用本品。此外也可用于心绞痛、高血压、嗜铬细胞瘤（术前准备）等。治疗心绞痛时，常与硝酸酯类合用，可提高疗效，互相抵消不良反应。对高血压有一定疗效，不易引起直立性低血压的影响的特点。<br>It can be used for cardiac arrhythmias caused by a variety of reasons, such as atrial and ventricular premature beats (with better effects), sinus and ventricular tachycardia, atrial fibrillation, but it should be used with caution for supraventricular tachycardia. It can be used for arrhythmias caused by Antimony agent poisoning when other medications fail. In addition, it can also be used for angina, hypertension, pheochromocytoma (preoperative preparation) and so on. When it is used for angina, it is often in combination with nitrates. The drug can improve the efficacy and offset adverse reactions each other. It has a certain effect on hypertension and is not easy to cause the orthostatic hypotension. |
| 用法、用量<br>Dosage | （1）口服：①心律失常：每日 10 ～ 30mg，分 3 次服，根据心律、心率及血压变化及时调整。②嗜铬细胞瘤：术前 3 日服，一日 60mg，分 3 次服。③心绞痛：每日 40 ～ 80mg，分 3 ～ 4 次服，从小剂量开始逐渐加至 80mg 以上。剂量过小常无效。④高血压：每次 5mg，一日 4 次，1 ～ 2 周后加 1/4 量，严密监控下可加至 1 日 100mg。<br>（2）静脉滴注：宜慎用。对麻醉中的心律失常以 1mg/min 的速度静脉滴注，一次 2.5 ～ 5mg，稀释于 5% ～ 10% 葡萄糖液 100ml 内滴注。严密监控血压、心律和、心率变化，随时调整速度。如心率转慢，立即停药。<br>(1) Orally: ① arrhythmia: the dose is 10 ~ 30mg a day, divided into 3 doses. It can be adjust based on heart rate and blood pressure changes. ② pheochromocytoma: it should be taken 3 days before operation with 60mg a day, divided into 3 doses. ③ angina: the dose is 40 ~ 80mg a day, divided into 3 to 4 doses. It starts with a small dose and gradually increases to 80mg or more. It's often ineffective if the dose is too small . ④ hypertension: the dose is 5mg per time, four times a day. Add 1/4 that dose after 1 or 2 weeks. It can be added to 100mg a day under strict surveillance. |

| | |
|---|---|
| | (2) Intravenous infusion: it should be used with caution. When it is used to treat anesthesia arrhythmias, it should be taken at the speed of 1mg/min through intravenous infusion with 2.5 ~ 5mg one time diluted in 100ml 5% to 10% glucose solution. Closely monitor the blood pressure, heart rate and heart rate changes and adjust the speed at any time. If heart rate turns slow, stop the medicine immediately. |
| 剂型、规格<br>Preparations | 片剂：每片 10mg。<br>注射液：每支 5mg（5ml）。<br>Tablets: 10mg per tablet.<br>Injection: 5mg (5ml) per vial. |
| 药品名称 Drug Names | 噻吗洛尔 Timolol |
| 适应证<br>Indications | 治疗高血压病、心绞痛、心动过速及青光眼。①对轻中度高血压疗效较好，无明显不良反应，可与利尿药合用。②心肌梗死患者长期服用本品可降低发病率和死亡率。对青光眼起效快，不良反应小、耐受性好。滴后 20 分钟，眼压下降，经 1 ~ 2 小时达最大效应，作用持续 24 小时。对瞳孔大小、对光反应及视力无影响。<br><br>It can be used for hypertension, angina pectoris, tachycardia and glaucoma. ① it has a better effect on mild and moderate hypertension. There are no significant adverse reactions and it can be used with diuretics. ② Taking this drug for a long term can reduce morbidity and mortality of patients with myocardial infarction. It has a quick effect on glaucoma with few side effects and good tolerance. After 20 minutes, intraocular pressure (IOP) decreases. It reaches the maximal effect in 1 to 2 hours, which lasts for 24 hours. It has no effect on pupil size, reaction to light and vision. |
| 用法、用量<br>Dosage | 口服：每次 5 ~ 10mg，一日 2 ~ 3 次。滴眼：0.25% 滴眼剂，每次 1 滴，一日 2 次。如效果不佳，可改用 5% 滴眼剂，每次 1 滴，一日 2 次。<br><br>Orally: the dose is5 ~ 10mg per time, 2 or 3 times a day. Drops: use 0.25% eye drops, 1 drop per time, 2 times a day. If the results are poor, you can switch to 5% eye drops with1 drop per time, 2 times a day. |
| 剂型、规格<br>Preparations | 片剂：每片 2.5mg；5mg。<br>滴眼剂：12.5mg（5ml）；25mg（5ml）。<br>Tablets: 2.5mg; 5mg per tablet.<br>Eye drops: 12.5mg (5ml); 25mg (5ml). |
| 药品名称 Drug Names | 索他洛尔 Sotalol |
| 适应证<br>Indications | 用于高血压，也可用于心绞痛、心律失常。<br>It is used for hypertension, angina pectoris and arrhythmia. |
| 用法、用量<br>Dosage | 高血压：初始 1 日 80mg，分 2 次服，需要时可加至一日 160 ~ 600mg。心绞痛和心律失常：口服，一日 160mg，一日 1 次（清晨）服用。<br><br>Hypertension: the initial dose is 80mg per day, divided into 2 doses. It can be added to 160 ~ 600mg per day if necessary. Angina and arrhythmia: orally: the dose is 160mg, once a day (in early morning). |
| 剂型、规格<br>Preparations | 片剂：每片 20mg；40mg；80mg；160mg；200mg。<br>Tablets: 20mg; 40mg; 80mg; 160mg; 200mg per tablet. |
| 药品名称 Drug Names | 阿替洛尔 Atenolol |
| 适应证<br>Indications | 用于高血压、心绞痛及心律失常。对青光眼有效。<br>It is used for hypertension, angina, arrhythmias and glaucoma. |
| 用法、用量<br>Dosage | 口服：一日 1 次 100mg 用于心绞痛，一日 1 次 100mg，或每次 25 ~ 50mg，一日 2 次。用于高血压每次 50 ~ 100mg，一日 1 ~ 2 次。青光眼用 4% 溶液滴剂。<br><br>Orally: for angina, the dose is 100mg once a day. The drug can be taken at a time or can be taken at 2 times a day with 25 to 50 mg every time. For high blood pressure, the dose is 50 ~ 100mg per time, 1 ~ 2 times a day. Glaucoma: use 4% solution eyedrops. |
| 剂型、规格<br>Preparations | 片剂：每片 12.5mg；25mg；50mg；100mg。<br>Tablets: 12.5mg; 25mg; 50mg; 100mg per tablet. |

**续　表**

| 药品名称 Drug Names | 美托洛尔 Metoprolol |
|---|---|
| 适应证<br>Indications | 用于各型高血压及心绞痛。静脉注射对心律失常、特别是室上性心律失常也有效。<br>It is used for various types of hypertension and angina. It is useful for arrhythmia, especially supraventricular arrhythmias through intravenous injection. |
| 用法、用量<br>Dosage | （1）口服：剂量需个体化。一般用于高血压，一日 1 次 100mg 维持量为一日 1 次，100 ～ 200mg，必要时加至每日 400mg，早晚分服。用于心绞痛，每日 100 ～ 150mg，分 2 ～ 3 次服，必要时加至每日 150 ～ 300mg。<br>（2）静脉注射：用于心律失常。开始为 5mg（每分钟 1 ～ 2mg）每隔 5 分钟重复注射，直至有效，一般总量为 10 ～ 15mg。<br>（1）Orally: the dosage depends on individuals. It is generally used for hypertension, with 100mg once a day. Its maintenance dose is 100 ～ 200mg once a day. If necessary, add to 400mg a day taken in the morning and evening. For angina, the dose is 100 ～ 150mg a day, divided into 2 ～ 3 doses. If necessary, add to 150 ～ 300mg a day.<br>（2）Intravenous injection: for arrhythmia: the initial dose is 5mg (1 ~ 2mg per minute) and the injection is repeated every 5 minutes until the drug is effective. The total amount is generally 10 ~ 15mg. |
| 剂型、规格<br>Preparations | 片剂：25mg；50mg；100mg。<br>胶囊剂：每粒 50mg。<br>缓释片：每片 100mg；200mg。<br>Tablets: 25mg; 50mg; 100mg.<br>Capsules: 50mg per capsule.<br>Sustained-release tablets: 100mg; 200mg per tablet. |
| 药品名称 Drug Names | 比索洛尔 Bisoprolol |
| 适应证<br>Indications | 用于高血压及心绞痛。<br>It is used for hypertension and angina. |
| 用法、用量<br>Dosage | 一日 5 ～ 20mg，一次口服。大多数一日口服 10mg 即可。<br>Orally: the dose is 5 ～ 20mg a day taken at a time. Most of the time 10mg one day is enough. |
| 剂型、规格<br>Preparations | 片剂：每片 2. 5mg；5mg。<br>胶囊：2.5mg；5mg；10mg。<br>Tablets: 2.5mg per tablet; 5mg.<br>Capsule: 2.5mg; 5mg; 10mg. |
| 药品名称 Drug Names | 倍他洛尔 Betaxolol |
| 适应证<br>Indications | 用于高血压、开角型青光眼的治疗。<br>It is used for hypertension and open-angle glaucoma. |
| 用法、用量<br>Dosage | 高血压：口服，一日 1 次 20mg，在 7 ～ 14 日达良效，如需要可加至一日 1 次 40mg。老年患者酌减。用于开角型青光眼：0.5% 滴眼剂一日 2 次。<br>Hypertension: Orally, the dose is 20mg one time a day. It can have a positive effect in 7 to 14 days. If needed, the dosage can be added to 40mg one time a day. According to the situation, the dosage for elderly patients can be reduced. Open-angle glaucoma: use 0.5% eye drops twice a day. |
| 剂型、规格<br>Preparations | 片剂：每片 20mg。<br>滴眼剂：0.25%；0.5%；1%。<br>Tablets: 20mg per tablet.<br>Eye drops: 0.25%; 0.5%; 1%. |
| 药品名称 Drug Names | 艾司洛尔 Esmolol |
| 适应证<br>Indications | 用于轻度高血压和心绞痛。<br>It is used for mild hypertension and angina. |
| 用法、用量<br>Dosage | 口服，一日 1 次，100 ～ 200mg。<br>Orally: 100 ～ 200mg once a day. |

**续 表**

| 剂型、规格<br>Preparations | 片剂：每片 200mg。<br>注射剂：每支 200mg（2ml）。<br>Tablet: 200mg, per tablet.<br>Injection: 200mg (2ml) per vial. |
|---|---|

### 10. 主要作用于心血管系统的药物 Drugs mainly acting on the cardiovascular system

#### 10.1 钙通道阻滞药 Calcium channel blockers

| 药品名称 Drug Names | 维拉帕米 Verapamil |
|---|---|
| 适应证<br>Indications | 用于抗心律失常和抗心绞痛。对于阵发性室上性心动过速最有效；对房室交界区心动过速疗效也很好；也可用于心房颤动、心房扑动、房性期前收缩。<br>It is used for anti-arrhythmia and anti-angina. It is the most effective for paroxysmal supraventricular tachycardia. It is useful for tachycardia atrioventricular junction. It can also be used for atrial fibrillation, atrial flutter, atrial premature. |
| 用法、用量<br>Dosage | 口服：一次 40 ～ 120mg，一日 3 ～ 4 次。维持剂量每一次 40mg，一日 3 次。稀释后缓慢静脉注射或静脉滴注，0.075 ～ 0.15mg/kg，症状控制后改用片剂口服维持。<br>Orally: the dose is 40 ～ 120mg one time, 3 to 4 times a day. The maintenance dose is 40mg every time, 3 times a day. After being diluted, it can be taken slowly through intravenous injection or intravenous infusion, and the dose is 0.075 ～ 0.15mg/kg. After the symptom is controlled, patients can take its tablets. |
| 剂型、规格<br>Preparations | 片剂：每片 40mg。<br>注射液：每支 5mg（2ml）<br>Tablets: 40mg per tablet.<br>Injection: 5mg (2ml) per vial |
| 药品名称 Drug Names | 硝苯地平 Nifedipine |
| 适应证<br>Indications | 用于预防和治疗冠心病和心绞痛，特别是变异型心绞痛和冠状动脉痉挛所致的心绞痛，对呼吸功能没有不良影响，故适用于患有呼吸道阻塞性疾病的心绞痛患者，其疗效优于 β 受体拮抗剂。还适用于各种类型的高血压，对顽固性、重度高血压也有较好疗效。由于能降低后负荷，对顽固性充血性心力衰竭亦有良好疗效，宜于长期服用。<br>It is used to prevent and treat coronary heart disease and angina, especially variant angina and angina caused by coronary spasm. It has no adverse effects on respiratory function. So it applies to patients with angina who are suffering from airway obstruction. Its efficacy is superior to β antagonists. It also applies to all types of hypertension. It has a better effect on intractable and severe high blood pressure. Because it can reduce the afterload, it can work well on intractable congestive heart failure and can be taken for a long time. |
| 用法、用量<br>Dosage | 口服：一次 5 ～ 10mg，一日 15 ～ 30mg。急用时可舌下含服。对慢性心力衰竭，每 6 小时 20mg，咽部喷药，每次 1.5 ～ 2mg（喷 3 ～ 4 次）。<br>Orally: the dose is 5 ～ 10mg one time, 15 ～ 30mg one day. It can be sublingual in emergency. For chronic heart failure, the dose is 20mg every six hours. Pharyngeal spray: the dose is 1.5 ～ 2mg one time (spray about 3 to 4 times). |
| 剂型、规格<br>Preparations | 片剂：普通片每片 5mg；10mg。<br>控释片：每片 20mg。<br>胶丸剂：每丸 5mg。<br>胶囊剂：每粒 5mg；10mg。<br>喷雾剂：每瓶 100mg。<br>Tablets: conventional tablet, 5mg ; 10mg per tablet.<br>Release tablets: 20mg per tablet.<br>Capsules: 5mg, 10mg per capsule.<br>Spray: per bottle 100mg. |
| 药品名称 Drug Names | 尼卡地平 Nicardipine |
| 适应证<br>Indications | 用于治疗高血压、脑血管疾病、脑血栓形成或脑出血后遗症及脑动脉硬化症等。<br>It is used for hypertension, cerebrovascular disease, cerebral thrombosis, cerebral hemorrhage sequelae and cerebral arteriosclerosis. |

**续 表**

| | |
|---|---|
| 用法、用量<br>Dosage | 口服：每次 20mg，一日 60mg。静脉滴注：高血压急症时以每分钟 0.5μg/kg 速度开始，根据血压监测调节滴速。<br>Orally: the dose is 20mg one time, 60mg a day. Intravenous drip: When hypertensive emergency appears, the drip starts with 0.5μg/kg per minute and the drip rate is adjusted according to blood pressure. |
| 剂型、规格<br>Preparations | 片剂：普通片每片 10mg；20mg；40mg。缓释片：每片 10mg。盐酸尼卡地平注射液：5ml：5mg（以尼卡地平计算）。<br>Tablet: ordinary tablets, 10mg per tablet; 20mg; 40mg. Sustained-release tablets: 10mg per tablet. Nicardipine hydrochloride injection: 5ml: 5mg (calculated according to nicardipine). |
| 药品名称 Drug Names | 尼群地平 Nitrendipine |
| 适应证<br>Indications | 用于冠心病及高血压，尤其是患有这两种疾病的患者，也可用于充血性心力衰竭。<br>It is used for coronary heart disease and hypertension, especially on patients suffering from these two diseases. It can also be used for congestive heart failure. |
| 用法、用量<br>Dosage | 口服，1 次 10mg，一日 30mg。<br>Orally: the dose is 10mg one time, 30mg a day. |
| 剂型、规格<br>Preparations | 片剂：每片 10mg。<br>Tablets: 10mg per tablet. |
| 药品名称 Drug Names | 尼莫地平 Nimodipine |
| 适应证<br>Indications | 用于脑血管疾病，如脑血管灌注不足、脑血管痉挛、蛛网膜下腔出血、脑卒中和偏头痛等。对突发性耳聋也有一定疗效。<br>It is used for cerebrovascular disorders, such as cerebral hypoperfusion, cerebral vasospasm, subarachnoid hemorrhage, brain stroke and migraine. It also has a certain effect on sudden deafness. |
| 用法、用量<br>Dosage | 口服：一日剂量 40 ~ 60mg，分 2 ~ 3 次服。<br>Orally: the dose is 40 ~ 60mg a day, divided into 2 to 3 doses. |
| 剂型、规格<br>Preparations | 片剂：20mg。<br>Tablets: 20mg. |
| 药品名称 Drug Names | 非洛地平 Felodipine |
| 适应证<br>Indications | 用于高血压病、缺血性心脏病和心力衰竭患者。<br>It is used for hypertension, ischemic heart disease and heart failure patients. |
| 用法、用量<br>Dosage | 一日剂量 20mg，分次服。<br>The dose is 20mg a day, divided doses. |
| 剂型、规格<br>Preparations | 片剂：每片 5mg；10mg。<br>Tablets: 5mg; 10mg per tablet. |
| 药品名称 Drug Names | 氨氯地平 Amlodipine |
| 适应证<br>Indications | 用于治疗高血压，单独应用或与其他抗高血压药合用均可；也可用于稳定型心绞痛患者，尤其是对硝酸盐和 β 受体拮抗剂无效者。<br>It is used for hypertension. It can be used alone or in combination with other anti-hypertensive drugs ; It may also be used on patients with stable angina, especially for patients for who ineffective nitrates and β receptor antagonists are ineffective . |
| 用法、用量<br>Dosage | 口服，开始时 1 次 5mg，一日 1 次，以后可根据患者的临床反应，可将剂量增加，最大可增至每日 10mg。<br>Orally: the initial dosage is 5mg once a day. Later according to the patients' clinical response, the dose may be increased to the maximum dose of 10mg every day. |
| 剂型、规格<br>Preparations | 片剂：每片 2.5mg；5mg；10mg。<br>Tablets: 2.5mg; 5mg; 10mg per tablet. |

| 药品名称 Drug Names | 左氨氯地平 Levamlodipine |
| --- | --- |
| 适应证<br>Indications | 用于治疗高血压，单独应用或与其他抗高血压药合用均可；也可用于稳定型心绞痛患者，尤其是对硝酸盐和β受体拮抗剂无效者。<br><br>It is used for hypertension. It can be used alone or in combination with other anti-hypertensive drugs ; It may also be used on patients with stable angina, especially for patients for who ineffective nitrates and β receptor antagonists are ineffective . |
| 用法、用量<br>Dosage | 口服，开始时 1 次 2.5mg，一日 1 次；根据患者的临床反应，可将剂量增加，最大可增至每日 5mg，一日 1 次。<br><br>Orally: The initial dose is 2.5mg, once a day; according to the patient's clinical response, the dose may be increased. The maximum dose is 5mg, once a day. |
| 剂型、规格<br>Preparations | 片剂：每片 2.5mg。<br>Tablets: 2.5mg per tablet |

| 药品名称 Drug Names | 西尼地平 Cilnidipine |
| --- | --- |
| 适应证<br>Indications | 用于治疗高血压，可单独应用，或与其他降压药合用。<br><br>It is used for high blood pressure. It can be used alone, or in combination with other antihypertensive drugs. |
| 用法、用量<br>Dosage | 口服：1 次 5 ~ 10mg，一日 1 次，必要时可增至 20mg，一日 1 次。早餐后服用。根据患者的临床反应，可将剂量增加，最大可增至每次 10mg。<br><br>Orally: the dose is 5 ~ 10mg, once a day. If necessary, the dose can be increased to 20mg, once a day. The drug should be taken after breakfast. According to the patient's clinical response, the dose may be increased and the maximum dose is 10mg every time. |
| 剂型、规格<br>Preparations | 片剂：每片 5mg。<br>Tablets: 5mg per tablet. |

| 药品名称 Drug Names | 拉西地平 Lacidipine |
| --- | --- |
| 适应证<br>Indications | 用于治疗高血压。<br>It is used for hypertension. |
| 用法、用量<br>Dosage | 开始时一日 1 次，每次 4mg，如效果不佳可增至一日 1 次，每次 6mg。肝功能不全患者，开始时需减半量。<br><br>At the beginning, the dose is 4mg, once a day. If it is not effective, the dose may be increased to 6mg once a day. For patients with liver dysfunction, the initial dose should be half. |
| 剂型、规格<br>Preparations | 片剂：每片 2mg；4mg。<br>Tablets: 2mg; 4mg per tablet. |

| 药品名称 Drug Names | 地尔硫䓬 Diltiazem |
| --- | --- |
| 适应证<br>Indications | 用于室上性心律失常、典型心绞痛、变异型心绞痛、老年人高血压等。<br>It is used for supraventricular arrhythmias, typical angina, variant angina, elder hypertension and so on. |
| 用法、用量<br>Dosage | 口服，常用量，1 次 30 ~ 60mg，一日 90 ~ 180mg。用于心律失常：口服，1 次 30 ~ 60mg，一日 4 次；起始剂量为 250μg/kg，于 2 分钟静脉注射；必要时 15 分钟后再给 350μg/kg。以后的剂量应根据患者的情况个体化制定。在心房颤动或心房扑动患者，最初输注速率 5 ~ 10mg/h，必要时可增至最大 15mg/h（增幅 5mg/h）。静脉输注最多可维持 24 小时。用于心绞痛：每 6 ~ 8 小时 30 ~ 60mg。用于高血压：一日剂量 120 ~ 240mg，分 3 ~ 4 次服。<br><br>Orally: the usual dose is 30 ~ 60mg one time, 90 ~ 180mg daily. For arrhythmias: orally, the dose is 30 ~ 60mg once, 4 times a day; the initial dose is 250μg/kg, taken in two minutes through intravenous injection; 15 minutes later, the dose of 350μg/kg should be given when necessary. Subsequent doses should be given according to the patient's condition. As for patients with atrial fibrillation or atrial flutter, the initial infusion rate is 5 ~ 10mg / h, when necessary, the rate can be increased to the maximum 15mg / h (increased by 5mg / h). Intravenous infusion can be maintained for up to 24 hours. For angina: the dose is 30 ~ 60mg every 6 to 8 hours. For hypertension: a daily dose is 120 ~ 240mg, divided into 3 to 4 doses. |

**续 表**

| | |
|---|---|
| 剂型、规格<br>Preparations | 片剂：普通片每片 30mg；60mg；90mg；缓释片：每片 30mg；60mg；90mg。<br>缓释胶囊：90mg。<br>注射用盐酸地尔硫䓬：10mg；50mg。<br>Tablet: Ordinary tablets, 30mg; 60mg; 90mg per tablet.<br>Sustained-release tablets: 30mg; 60mg; 90mg per tablet.<br>Release capsules: 90mg. Injection Diltiazem Hydrochloride: 10mg; 50mg. |
| 药品名称 Drug Names | 桂利嗪 Cinnarizine |
| 适应证<br>Indications | 用于脑血栓形成、脑栓塞、脑动脉硬化、脑出血恢复期、蛛网膜下腔出血恢复期、脑外伤后遗症、内耳眩晕症、冠状动脉粥样硬化、由于末梢循环不良引起的疾病等。<br>It is used for cerebral thrombosis, cerebral embolism, cerebral arteriosclerosis, cerebral hemorrhage recovery, recovery of subarachnoid hemorrhage, traumatic brain injury sequelae, inner ear vertigo, coronary atherosclerosis, diseases caused by poor peripheral circulation, etc. |
| 用法、用量<br>Dosage | 口服：每次 25 ～ 50mg，一日 3 次，餐后服。静脉注射：1 次 20 ～ 40mg，缓慢注入。<br>Orally: the dose is 25 ~ 50mg one time, 3 times a day, taken after meals. Intravenous injection: the dose is 20 ~ 40mg with slow injection. |
| 剂型、规格<br>Preparations | 片剂及胶囊剂：每片（粒）25mg。<br>注射液：每支 20mg（20ml）。<br>Tablets and capsules: 25mg per tablet (capsule).<br>Injection: 20mg (20ml) per vial. |
| 药品名称 Drug Names | 氟桂利嗪 Flunarizine |
| 适应证<br>Indications | 药理及应用同桂利嗪相似，有扩血管作用。此外，对注意力减弱、记忆力障碍、易激动以及平衡功能障碍、眩晕等均有一定疗效。用于老年患者。<br>Its efficacy is similar to cinnarizine and it can be used as vasodilator. In addition, it can be used for decreased attention, memory impairment, irritability and balance disorders, dizziness, etc. It applies to older patients. |
| 用法、用量<br>Dosage | 1 次 5 ～ 10mg，一日 10mg（以氟桂利嗪计），在一般情况下，可于晚上顿服。<br>The dose is 5 ~ 10mg once, 10mg a day (calculated by flunarizine ). The drug is usually taken at a time in the evening . |
| 剂型、规格<br>Preparations | 胶囊剂：每粒 5mg（以氟桂利嗪计）。<br>Capsules: 5mg per capsule (calculated by flunarizine). |
| 药品名称 Drug Names | 利多氟嗪 Lidoflazine |
| 适应证<br>Indications | 用于心绞痛。<br>It is used for angina. |
| 用法、用量<br>Dosage | 口服，1 次 60mg，一日 3 次。<br>Orally: the dose is 60mg one time, 3 times a day. |
| 剂型、规格<br>Preparations | 片剂：每片 60mg。<br>Tablets: 60mg per tablet. |
| 10.2 治疗慢性心功能不全的药物 Drugs treating chronic cardiac insufficiency | |
| 药品名称 Drug Names | 洋地黄毒苷 Digitoxin |
| 适应证<br>Indications | 用于维持治疗慢性心功能不全。<br>It is used for chronic cardiac insufficiency. |
| 用法、用量<br>Dosage | 主要采用口服，不宜口服者可以肌内注射，必要时静脉注射。全效量：成人 0.7 ～ 1.2mg；于 48 ～ 72 小时分次服用。小儿 2 岁以下 0.03 ～ 0.04mg/kg，2 岁以上 0.02 ～ 0.03mg/kg。维持量：成人每日 0.05 ～ 0.1mg，小儿为全效量的 1/10，一日 1 次。<br>The drug is usually taken orally. As for patients who are not suitable to take medicine orally, it can be taken through intramuscular injection, or through intravenous injection if necessary. Full effect amount: as for adults, it is 0.7 ~ 1.2mg, divided into several doses within 48 to 72 hours. As for children under 2 years old, the dose is 0.03 ~ 0.04mg/kg. As for children over 2 years old, the dose is 0.02 ~ 0.03mg/kg. Maintenance dose: as for adults, it's 0.05 ~ 0.1mg every day. As for children, it is 1/10 of full effective amount every day. |

**续　表**

| 剂型、规格<br>Preparations | 片剂：每片 0.1mg。注射液：每支 0.2mg（1ml）。<br>Tablets: 0.1mg per tablet. Injection: 0.2mg (1ml) per vial. |
|---|---|
| 药品名称 Drug Names | 地高辛 Digoxin |
| 适应证<br>Indications | 用于各种急性和慢性心功能不全和室上性心动过速、心房颤动和心房扑动等。<br>It is used for a variety of acute and chronic cardiac insufficiency, supraventricular tachycardia and atrial fibrillation and flutter, etc. |
| 用法、用量<br>Dosage | 全效量：成人口服 1 ～ 1.5mg；于 24 小时内分次服用。小儿 2 岁以下 0.06 ～ 0.08mg/kg，2 岁以上 0.04 ～ 0.06mg/kg。不宜口服者也可静脉注射，临用前以 10% 或 25% 葡萄糖注射液稀释后应用，常用量静脉注射 1 次 0.25 ～ 0.5mg；极量，1 次 1mg。维持量：成人每日 0.125 ～ 0.5mg，分 1 ～ 2 次服用；小儿为全效量的 1/4。<br>Full effect amount: as for adults, the oral dose is1 ～ 1.5mg divided into doses within 24 hours. As for children under 2 years, the dose is 0.06 ～ 0.08mg/kg. For children over 2 years old, the dose is 0.04 ～ 0.06mg/kg. For patients who are not suitable for oral administration, the drug can be taken through intravenous injection. It should be diluted by 10% or 25% glucose injection before its use. The usual dose of intravenous injection is 0.25 ～ 0.5mg one time; the extreme amount is 1mg one time. Maintenance dose: for adults, the daily dose is 0.125 ～ 0.5mg, divided into 1 to 2 doses; for children, the dose is 1/4 of full effective amount. |
| 剂型、规格<br>Preparations | 片剂：每片 0.25mg。注射液：0.5mg（2ml）。<br>Tablets: 0.25mg per tablet. Injection: 0.5mg (2ml). |
| 药品名称 Drug Names | 毛花苷 C  Lanatoside C |
| 适应证<br>Indications | 用于急性和慢性心力衰竭。<br>It is used for acute and chronic heart failure. |
| 用法、用量<br>Dosage | 缓慢全效量：口服，1 次 0.5mg，一日 4 次。维持量：一般为一日 1mg，以 2 次服用。静脉注射：成人常用量，全效量 1 ～ 1.2mg，首次剂量 0.4 ～ 0.6mg；2 ～ 4 小时后可再给予 0.2 ～ 0.4mg，用葡萄糖注射液稀释后缓慢注射。<br>Slow full effect amount: the oral dose is 0.5mg one time, 4 times a day. Maintenance dose: the dose is usually 1mg one day, divided into two doses. Intravenous injection: full effect amount for adults is usually 1~1.2 mg and the initial dose is 0.4 ～ 0.6mg; 2 ～ 4 hours later, the dose of 0.2 ～ 0.4mg can be given again, diluted by glucose injection through slow injection. |
| 剂型、规格<br>Preparations | 片剂：每片 0.5mg。注射液：0.4mg（2ml）。<br>Tablets: 0.5mg per tablet. Injection: 0.4mg (2ml). |
| 药品名称 Drug Names | 去乙酰毛花苷 Deslanoside |
| 适应证<br>Indications | 用于急性心力衰竭，以及心房颤动及心房扑动等。<br>It is used for acute heart failure and atrial fibrillation and atrial flutter etc. |
| 用法、用量<br>Dosage | 静脉注射成人常用量：用葡萄糖注射液稀释后缓慢注射，1 次 0.4 ～ 0.8mg。全效量 1 ～ 1.6mg，于 24 小时内分次注射。儿童每日 20 ～ 40μg/kg，分 1 ～ 2 次给药。然后改用口服毛花苷 C 维持治疗。<br>Intravenous injection: the usual dose for adults is 0.4 to 0.8 mg once, diluted by glucose injection through slow injection. Full effect amount is 1 to 1.6 mg, divided into doses within 24 hours. For children, the daily dose is 20 ～ 40μg/kg, divided into 1 to 2 doses. Then switch to oral administration of Lanatoside . |
| 剂型、规格<br>Preparations | 注射液：每支 0.2mg（1ml）；0.4mg（2ml）。<br>Injection: 0.2mg (1ml); 0.4mg (2ml) per vial. |

**续　表**

| 药品名称 Drug Names | 毒毛花苷 K　Strophanthin K |
|---|---|
| 适应证<br>Indications | 用于急性心力衰竭。动脉硬化性心脏病患者发生心力衰竭时，如心率不快可选用本品。<br>It is used for acute heart failure. When heart failure happens to patients with atherosclerotic heart disease, it can be used if heart rate is slow. |
| 用法、用量<br>Dosage | 静脉注射：首剂 0.125 ~ 0.25mg，加入等渗葡萄糖注射液 20 ~ 40ml 内缓慢注入（时间不少于 5 分钟），1 ~ 2 小时后重复 1 次，总量每日 0.25 ~ 0.5mg。病情转好后，可改用洋地黄苷口服制剂，给予适当的全效量。<br>Intravenous injection: the first dose is 0.125 ~ 0.25mg, added into 20 ~ 40ml isotonic glucose injection through slow injection (no less than 5 minutes). 1 to 2 hours later, the procedure is repeated once. The total daily dose is 0.25 ~ 0.5mg. After the condition improves, switch to oral administration of digitalis glycosides, appropriately with full effect amount. |
| 剂型、规格<br>Preparations | 注射液：每支 0.25mg（1ml）。<br>Injection: 0.25mg (1ml) per vial. |
| 药品名称 Drug Names | 氨力农 Amrinone |
| 适应证<br>Indications | 用于对洋地黄、利尿药、血管舒张药治疗无效或效果欠佳的各种原因引起的急性、慢性顽固性充血性心力衰竭的短期治疗。<br>It is used for acute and chronic intractable congestive heart failure in a short time caused by various reasons, to which digitalis, diuretics, vasodilators are ineffective. |
| 用法、用量<br>Dosage | 静脉注射负荷量：0.75mg/kg，2 ~ 3 分钟缓慢静脉注射，继之以每千克 5 ~ 10μg/min 维持静脉滴注，单次剂量最大不超过 2.5mg/kg。每日最大量 <10mg/kg。疗程不超过 2 周。<br>Intravenous injection loading dose: the dose is 0.75mg/kg through slow intravenous injection within 2 ~ 3 minutes. And the next step is 5 ~ 10μg/min per kg through intravenous infusion. The single dosage does not exceed the maximum 2.5mg/kg. The daily maximum amount is less than 10mg/kg. The course of treatment is no more than two weeks. |
| 剂型、规格<br>Preparations | 注射液：每支 50mg（2ml）；100mg（2ml）。<br>Injection: 50mg (2ml); 100mg (2ml) per vial. |
| 药品名称 Drug Names | 米力农 Milrinone |
| 适应证<br>Indications | 用于对洋地黄、利尿药、血管舒张药治疗无效或效果欠佳的各种原因引起的急性、慢性顽固性充血性心力衰竭的短期治疗。<br>It is used for acute and chronic intractable congestive heart failure in a short time caused by various reasons, to which digitalis, diuretics, vasodilators are ineffective. |
| 用法、用量<br>Dosage | 静脉滴注：每分钟 12.5 ~ 75μg/kg。一般开始 10 分钟以 50μg/kg，然后以每分钟 0.375 ~ 0.75μg/kg 维持。每日最大剂量不超过 1.13mg/kg。<br>Intravenous infusion: the dose is 12.5 ~ 75μg / kg per minute. The infusion generally begins with 50μg/kg every10 minutes and then maintains with 0.375 ~ 0.75μg / kg every minute. The daily maximum dose does not exceed 1.13mg / kg. |
| 剂型、规格<br>Preparations | 注射液：每支 10mg（10ml）。<br>Injection: 10mg (10ml) per vial. |

10.3 抗心律失常药 Anti-arrhythmics

| 药品名称 Drug Names | 奎尼丁 Quinidine |
|---|---|
| 适应证<br>Indications | 主要用于阵发性心动过速、心房颤动和期前收缩等。<br>It is mainly used for paroxysmal tachycardia, atrial fibrillation and premature and so on. |

| 用法、用量<br>Dosage | （1）口服：第 1 天，每次 0.2g，每 2 小时 1 次，连续 5 次；如无效而又无明显毒性反应，第 2 天增至每次 0.3g、第 3 天每次 0.4g，每 2 小时 1 次，连续 5 次。每日总量一般不宜超过 2g。恢复正常心律后，改维持量，每日 0.2 ~ 0.4g。若连服 3 ~ 4 日无效或有毒性反应者，应停药。<br>（2）静脉注射：在十分必要时采用静脉注射并须在心电图观察下进行。每次 0.25g，以 5% 葡萄糖液稀释至 50ml 缓慢静脉注射。<br>（1）orally: the first day, the dose is 0.2g once, every 2 hours, repeated 5 consecutive times; if it is invalid and has no apparent toxicity, the dose can be increased to 0.3g every time on the second day. On the third day of the dose can be 0.4g once, once every 2 hours, repeated five consecutive times. The daily total amount should not exceed 2g. After rhythm of the heart is normal, the dose can be changed to maintenance dose, 0.2 ~ 0.4g every day. If it is ineffective within 3 to 4 days or has toxic reactions, it should be discontinued.<br>（2）intravenous injection: when absolutely necessary, it can be taken through intravenous injection under observation of electrocardiogram. The dose is 0.25g, 5% every time, diluted by 5% glucose solution to 50ml through slow intravenous injection. |
|---|---|
| 剂型、规格<br>Preparations | 片剂：每片 0.2g。葡萄糖酸奎尼丁注射液：每支 0.5g（10ml）。<br>Tablets: 0.2g per tablet. Quinidine gluconate injection: 0.5g (10ml) per vial. |
| 药品名称 Drug Names | 普鲁卡因胺 Procainamide |
| 适应证<br>Indications | 用于阵发性心动过速、频发期前收缩（对室性期前收缩疗效较好）、心房颤动和心房扑动，常与奎尼丁交替使用。<br>It is used for paroxysmal tachycardia, frequent premature beats (it's better for ventricular premature beats), atrial fibrillation and atrial flutter. It is often used in combination with quinidine. |
| 用法、用量<br>Dosage | （1）口服：一日 3 ~ 4 次，每次 0.5 ~ 0.75g，心律正常后逐渐减至一日 2 ~ 6 次，每次 0.25g。<br>（2）静脉滴注：每次 0.5 ~ 1g，溶于 5% ~ 10% 葡萄糖溶液 100ml 内，开始 10 ~ 30 分钟，滴注速度可适当加快，于 1 小时内滴完。无效者，1 小时后再给一次，24 小时内总量不超过 2g。<br>（3）静脉注射：每次 0.1 ~ 0.2g。<br>（4）肌内注射：每次 0.25 ~ 0.5g。<br>(1) Orally: the dose is 0.5 ~ 0.75g every time, 3 to 4 times a day. After rhythm of the heart is normal, the dose can gradually be reduced to 0.25g every time, 2 to 6 times a day.<br>(2) Intravenous infusion: the dose is 0.5 ~ 1g every time, dissolved in 100ml 5% to 10% glucose solution. In the first 10 to 30 minutes, the infusion rate can appropriately be accelerated. The drop can be finished within one hour. If it is invalid, one hour later, the drug can be given again. The total dose within 24 hours does not exceed 2g.<br>(3) Intravenous injection: the dose is 0.1 ~ 0.2g every time.<br>(4) Intramuscular injection: the dose is 0.25 ~ 0.5g every time. |
| 剂型、规格<br>Preparations | 片剂：每片 0.125g；0.25g。<br>注射液：每支 0.1g（1ml）；0.2g（2ml）；0.5g（5ml）；1g（10ml）。<br>Tablets: 0.125g per tablet; 0.25g.<br>Injection: 0.1g (1ml); 0.2g (2ml); 0.5g (5ml); 1g (10ml) per vial. |
| 药品名称 Drug Names | 丙吡胺 Disopyramide |
| 适应证<br>Indications | 用于房性期前收缩、阵发性房性心动过速、心房颤动、室性期前收缩等，对室上性心律失常的疗效似较好。<br>It is used for atrial premature beats, paroxysmal atrial tachycardia, atrial fibrillation, ventricular premature beats. And it has a better effect on supraventricular arrhythmias . |
| 用法、用量<br>Dosage | 口服，每次 0.1 ~ 0.15g，一日 0.4 ~ 0.8g。最大剂量不超过 800mg/d。静脉注射，每次 1 ~ 2mg/kg，最大剂量每次不超过 150mg，用葡萄糖注射液 20ml 稀释后在 5 ~ 10 分钟注完。必要时，可在 20 分钟后重复一次。静脉滴注，每次 100 ~ 200mg，以 5% 葡萄糖注射液 500ml 稀释，一般滴注量为每小时 20 ~ 30mg。<br>Orally: the dose is 0.1 ~ 0.15g every time, 0.4 ~ 0.8g a day. The maximum dose does not exceed 800mg / d. Intravenous injection: the dose is 1 ~ 2mg/kg every time. The maximum dose is no more than150mg every time. The drug is diluted by 20ml glucose injection, and should be finished within 5 to 10 minutes. If necessary, do this again after 20 minutes. Intravenous drip: the dose is 100 ~ 200mg every time, diluted by 500ml 5% glucose injection. The drip amount is generally 20 ~ 30mg every hour. |

**续　表**

| | |
|---|---|
| 剂型、规格<br>Preparations | 片剂：每片 100mg。注射液：每支 50mg（2ml）；100mg（2ml）。<br>Tablets: 100mg per tablet. Injection: 50mg (2ml); 100mg (2ml) per vial. |
| 药品名称 Drug Names | 利多卡因 Lidocaine |
| 适应证<br>Indications | 本品适用于心肌梗死、洋地黄中毒、锑剂中毒、外科手术等所致的室性期前收缩、室性心动过速和心室颤动。<br>This product is suitable for ventricular premature beat, ventricular tachycardia and ventricular fibrillation caused by myocardial infarction, digitalis poisoning, antimony poisoning and surgery, etc. |
| 用法、用量<br>Dosage | 静脉注射，1 ~ 2mg/kg，继以 0.1% 溶液静脉滴注，每小时不超过 100mg。也可肌内注射，4 ~ 5mg/kg，60 ~ 90 分钟重复一次。<br>Intravenous injection: the dose is 1 ~ 2mg/kg. And then its 0.1% solution follows through intravenous drip. The dose cannot exceed 100mg every hour. The drug can also be taken through intramuscular injection. The dose is 4 ~ 5mg/kg. Do this again after 60 ~ 90 minutes. |
| 剂型、规格<br>Preparations | 注射液：每支 0.1g（5ml）；0.4g（20ml）。<br>Injection: 0.1g (5ml); 0.4g (20ml) per vial. |
| 药品名称 Drug Names | 苯妥英钠 Phenytoin Sodium |
| 适应证<br>Indications | 用于洋地黄中毒所引起的室上性和室性心律失常及对利多卡因无效的心律失常。<br>It is used for supraventricular and ventricular arrhythmias caused by digitalis intoxication and cardiac arrhythmias for which lidocaine is invalid. |
| 用法、用量<br>Dosage | 口服：每次 0.1 ~ 0.2g，一日 2 ~ 3 次。口服极量：每次 0.3g，一日 0.5g。静脉注射：每次 0.125 ~ 0.25g，缓慢注入，一日总量不超过 0.5g。<br>Orally: the dose is 0.1 ~ 0.2g every time, 2 or 3 times a day. The oral maximum dose is 0.3g every time, 0.5g a day. Intravenous injection: the dose is 0.125 ~ 0.25g every time through slow injection. The daily total amount does not exceed 0.5g. |
| 剂型、规格<br>Preparations | 片剂：每片 0.05g；0.1g。注射用苯妥英钠：每支 0.125g；0.25g。<br>Tablets: 0.05g; 0.1g per tablet. Phenytoin Injection: 0.125g; 0.25g per vial. |
| 药品名称 Drug Names | 美西律 Mexiletine |
| 适应证<br>Indications | 用于急、慢性室性心律失常，如室性期前收缩、室性心动过速、心室颤动及洋地黄中毒引起的心律失常。<br>It is used for acute and chronic ventricular arrhythmias, such as ventricular premature beat, ventricular tachycardia, ventricular fibrillation and cardiac arrhythmias caused digitalis poisoning. |
| 用法、用量<br>Dosage | （1）口服：每次 50 ~ 200mg，一日 150 ~ 600mg，或每 6 ~ 8 小时 1 次。以后可酌情减量维持。<br>（2）静脉注射、静脉滴注：开始量 100mg，加入 5% 葡萄糖注射液 20ml 中，缓慢静脉注射（3 ~ 5 分钟）。如无效，可在 5 ~ 10 分钟后再给 50 ~ 100mg1 次。然后以 1.5 ~ 2mg/min 的速度静脉滴注，3 ~ 4 小时后滴速减至 0.75 ~ 1mg/min，并维持 24 ~ 48 小时。<br>(1) Orally: the dose is 50 ~ 200mg every time, 150 ~ 600mg a day, or once every 6 to 8 hours. Later, the dose can be reduced according to patients' conditions.<br>(2) Intravenous injection, intravenous infusion: the initial dose is 100mg, added into 20ml 5% dextrose injection through slow intravenous injection (3 to 5 minutes). If invalid, the dose of 50 ~ 100mg can be given again after 5 to 10 minutes. And then intravenous infusion follows at the speed of 1.5 ~ 2mg/min. After 3 to 4 hours, the drip rate can be reduced to 0.75 ~ 1mg/min, and maintains for 24 to 48 hours. |
| 剂型、规格<br>Preparations | 片剂：每片 50mg；100mg；250mg。胶囊剂：每粒 50mg；100mg；400mg。注射液：100mg（2ml）。<br>Tablets: 50mg; 100mg; 250mg per tablet. Capsules: 50mg; 100mg; 400mg per capsule. Injection: 100mg (2ml). |

**续　表**

| 药品名称 Drug Names | 普罗帕酮 Propafenone |
| --- | --- |
| 适应证<br>Indications | 　　用于预防或治疗室性或室上性异位期前收缩，室性或室上性心动过速，预激综合征，电转复律后室颤发作等。经临床试用，疗效确切，起效迅速，作用时间持久，对冠心病、高血压所引起的心律失常有较好的疗效。<br><br>　　It is used to prevent or treat ventricular or supraventricular ectopic beats, ventricular or supraventricular tachycardia, WPW syndrome, ventricular fibrillation after electrical cardioversion. Based on clinical trial, its curative effect is accurate, rapid and lasting. It also has a better effect on arrhythmia caused by coronary heart disease and high blood pressure. |
| 用法、用量<br>Dosage | 　　口服：1 次 100 ~ 200mg，一日 3 ~ 4 次。治疗量，一日 300 ~ 900mg，分 4 ~ 6 次服用。维持量，一日 300 ~ 600mg，分 2 ~ 4 次服用。由于其局部麻醉作用，宜在饭后与饮料或食物同时吞服，不得嚼碎。必要时可在严密监护下缓慢静脉注射或滴注，1 次 70mg，每 8 小时 1 次。一日总量不超过 350mg。<br><br>　　Orally: the dose is 100 ~ 200mg every time, 3 to 4 times a day. Therapeutic dose: the dose is 300 ~ 900mg a day, divided into 5 to 6 doses. Maintenance dose: the dose is 300 ~ 600mg a day, divided into 2 to 4 doses. Because of its local anesthetic effect, it's better to be swallowed with drinks or food after meals. And it shouldn't be chewed. If necessary, the drug can be given through slow intravenous injection or infusion under close monitoring. The dose is 70mg every time, once every 8 hours. The daily total dose cannot exceed 350mg. |
| 剂型、规格<br>Preparations | 　　片剂：每片 50mg；100mg；150mg。注射液：每支 17.5mg（5ml）；35mg（10ml）。<br>Tablets: 50mg; 100mg; 150mg per tablet. Injection: 17.5mg (5ml); 35mg (10ml) per vial. |
| 药品名称 Drug Names | 恩卡尼 Encainide |
| 适应证<br>Indications | 　　用于室性期前收缩、室性心动过速及心室颤动。也可用于室上性心动过速，对折返性心动过速，尤其是预激综合征有效。<br><br>　　It is used for ventricular premature beat, ventricular tachycardia and ventricular fibrillation. It can also be used for supraventricular tachycardia and atrioventricular nodal reentry tachycardia, especially WPW syndrome. |
| 用法、用量<br>Dosage | 　　口服，每次 25 ~ 75mg，一日 3 ~ 4 次。静脉注射，以 0.5 ~ 1mg/kg，于 15 ~ 20 分钟注完。小儿口服一日剂量 60 ~ 120mg/m² 或 2 ~ 7.5mg/kg，分 3 ~ 4 次服。通常从小剂量开始，在严密观察下逐渐增量。<br><br>　　Orally: the dose is 25 ~ 75mg every time, 3 to 4 times a day. Intravenous injection: the dose is 0.5 ~ 1mg/kg, taken within 15 to 20 minutes. For children, the daily oral dose is 60 ~ 120mg/m² or 2 ~ 7.5mg/kg, divided into 3 to 4 doses. The dose usually starts with a small one and it can gradually be increased under close observation. |
| 剂型、规格<br>Preparations | 　　胶囊剂：每粒 25mg；35mg；50mg。注射液：25mg（1ml）；50mg（2ml）。<br>Capsules: 25mg; 35mg; 50mg per capsule. Injection: 25mg (1ml); 50mg (2ml). |
| 药品名称 Drug Names | 氟卡尼 Flecainide |
| 适应证<br>Indications | 　　用于室上性心动过速、房室结或房室折返心动过速、心房颤动、儿童顽固性交界性心动过速及伴有预激综合征患者。对其他抗心律失常药物无效的病例，氟卡尼常有效。<br><br>　　It is used for supraventricular tachycardia, atrioventricular node or atrioventricular nodal reentry tachycardia, atrial fibrillation, children intractable junctional tachycardia together with WPW syndrome. The drug is usually effective to cases when other antiarrhythmic drugs are invalid. |
| 用法、用量<br>Dosage | 　　口服：成人开始时每次 100mg，一日 2 次，然后每隔 4 日，每次增加 50mg，最大剂量每次 200mg，一日 2 次；儿童每次 50 ~ 100mg，一日 2 次。静脉滴注：成人 2mg/kg，于 15 分钟滴完；儿童 2mg/kg，于 10 分钟内滴完。<br><br>　　Orally: For adults, the initial dose is 100mg every time, 2 times a day, and then every 4 days, the dose is increased by 50 mg. The maximum dose is 200mg every day, 2 times a day; for children, the dose is 50 ~ 100mg every time, 2 times a day. Intravenous infusion: for adults, the dose is 2mg/kg, finished within 15 minutes; for children, the dose is 2mg/kg, finished within 10 minutes. |

续　表

| 剂型、规格<br>Preparations | 片剂：每片 100mg。注射液：50mg（5ml）；100mg（10ml）。<br>Tablets: 100mg per tablet. Injection: 50mg (5ml); 100mg (10ml). |
|---|---|
| **药品名称 Drug Names** | **胺碘酮 Amiodarone** |
| 适应证<br>Indications | 用于室性和室上性心动过速和期前收缩、阵发性心房扑动和心房颤动，预激综合征等。也可用于伴有充血性心力衰竭和急性心肌梗死的心律失常患者。对其他抗心律失常药物如丙吡胺、维拉帕米、奎尼丁、β 受体拮抗剂无效的顽固性阵发性心动过速常能奏效。此外，还用于慢性冠脉功能不全和心绞痛。<br><br>It is used for supraventricular, ventricular premature beats, atrial flutter and fibrillation and WPW syndrome. It can also be used on patients with arrhythmias who have congestive heart failure and acute myocardial infarction. It is useful for intractable paroxysmal tachycardia on which other anti-arrhythmic drugs such as disopyramide, verapamil, quinidine, β receptor antagonists are ineffective. Furthermore, it can be used for chronic coronary insufficiency and angina pectoris. |
| 用法、用量<br>Dosage | 口服：每次 0.1 ~ 0.2g，一日 1 ~ 4 次；或开始每次 0.2g，一日 3 次。餐后服。3 日后改用维持量，每次 0.2g，一日 1 ~ 2 次。<br><br>Orally: the dose is 0.1 ~ 0.2g every time, 1 to 4 times a day; or the initial dose is 0.2g every time, 3 times a day. The drug should be taken after meals. 3 days later, switch to maintenance dose, 0.2g every time, 1 to 2 times a day. |
| 剂型、规格<br>Preparations | 片剂：每片 0.2g。胶囊剂：每粒 0.1g；0.2g。注射液：150mg（3ml）。<br>Tablets: 0.2g per tablet. Capsules: 0.1g; 0.2g per capsule. Injection: 150mg (3ml). |
| **药品名称 Drug Names** | **依地酸二钠 Disodium Edetate** |
| 适应证<br>Indications | 常用于洋地黄中毒所致的心律失常。<br>It is commonly used for arrhythmia caused by moderate digitalis glycosides. |
| 用法、用量<br>Dosage | 静脉注射：每次 1 ~ 3g，以 50% 的葡萄糖注射液 20 ~ 40ml 稀释后注入。静脉滴注：每次 4 ~ 6g，用 5% ~ 10% 葡萄糖注射液 500ml 稀释后在 1 ~ 3 小时滴完。<br><br>Intravenous injection: the dose is 1 ~ 3g every time, diluted by 20 ~ 40ml 50% glucose injection. Intravenous infusion: the dose is 4 ~ 6g every time, diluted by 500ml 5% to 10% glucose injection, finished within 1 to 3 hours. |
| 剂型、规格<br>Preparations | 注射液：每支 1g（5ml）。<br>Injection: 1g (5ml) per vial. |
| **药品名称 Drug Names** | **门冬氨酸钾镁 Potassium Aspartate and Magnesium Aspartate** |
| 适应证<br>Indications | 用于期前收缩、阵发性心动过速、心绞痛、心力衰竭等。此外还可用于急性黄疸型肝炎、肝细胞功能不全、其他急慢性肝病、低钾血症等。<br><br>It is used for premature beats, paroxysmal tachycardia, angina and heart failure. It can also be used for acute jaundice hepatitis, hepatocellular dysfunction, other acute and chronic liver disease, hypokalemia, and so on. |
| 用法、用量<br>Dosage | 静脉滴注：一日量 10 ~ 20ml，用时以 10 倍量的输液稀释后缓慢滴注。<br>Intravenous drip: the daily dose is 10 ~ 20ml, diluted by 10 times of the dose fluid through slow drip. |
| 剂型、规格<br>Preparations | 注射液：每支 10ml，含钾盐及镁盐各 500mg。<br>Injection: 10ml per vial, containing 500 mg potassium salt and 500 mg magnesium salt. |

10.4　防治心绞痛药 Antianginal drugs

| **药品名称 Drug Names** | **硝酸甘油 Nitroglycerin** |
|---|---|
| 适应证<br>Indications | 用于防治心绞痛。<br>It is used for the prevention and treatment of angina. |

续 表

| 用法、用量<br>Dosage | 根据不同的临床需求，硝酸甘油可以通过舌下含服给药、黏膜给药、口服给药、透皮给药或静脉途径给药。<br><br>（1）用于治疗急性心绞痛：可给予硝酸甘油片舌下含服、舌下喷雾给药或黏膜给药。片剂（每片 0.3 ~ 0.6mg）置于舌下，必要时可重复含服。喷雾给药则可每次将 0.4 ~ 0.8mg（1 ~ 2 揿）喷至舌下，然后闭嘴，必要时可喷 3 次。硝酸甘油黏膜片应置于上唇和牙龈之间，1 次 1 ~ 2mg。<br><br>（2）用于稳定型心绞痛的长期治疗：通常以透皮剂的形式给予。将膜敷贴于皮肤上，药物以恒速进入皮肤。作用时间长，几乎可达 24 小时。<br><br>（3）用于控制性降压或治疗心力衰竭：静脉滴注，开始剂量按每分钟 5μg，可每 3 ~ 5 分钟增加 5μg/min 以达到满意效果。如在 20μg/min 时无效可以 10μg/min 递增，以后可 20μg/min，一俟有效则剂量渐减小和给药间期延长。<br><br>According to the clinical needs, sublingual nitroglycerin can be taken through sublingual administration, mucosal administration, oral administration, transdermal administration, or intravenous routes.<br><br>(1) to treat acute angina: it may be given through sublingual nitroglycerin tablets, sublingual spray administration or mucosal administration. Put the tablet (0.3 ~ 0.6mg per tablet) under the tongue. If necessary, do this repeatedly. Spray 0.4 ~ 0.8mg (1 ~ 2 press) every time under the tongue and then shut up. If necessary, spray the drug three times. Nitroglycerin tablets should be placed between the upper lip and gums, 1 ~ 2mg every time.<br><br>(2) to treat stable angina in a long time: the drug is usually given in the form of transdermal agent . The film is stuck on the skin and the drug permeates into the skin at a constant rate. The effect lasts for a long time, almost up to 24 hours.<br><br>(3) to control blood pressure or heart failure therapy: intravenous infusion, a starting dose is 5μg per minute, and it can be increased by 5μg/min every 3 to 5 minutes to achieve satisfactory results. If the dose of 20μg/min is invalid, it can be increased by10μg/min and later by 20μg/min. Once the drug works, the dose can gradually be reduced and the interval of administration should be prolonged. |
| --- | --- |
| 剂型、规格<br>Preparations | 片剂：每片 0.3mg；0.5mg；0.6mg。<br>缓释硝酸甘油片：每片含 2.5mg。<br>注射液：1mg（1ml）；2mg（1ml）；5mg（1ml）；10mg（1ml）。<br>硝酸甘油膜：每格含硝酸甘油 0.5mg。<br><br>Tablets: 0.3mg; 0.5mg; 0.6mg per tablet.<br>Sustained-release nitroglycerin tablets: 2.5mg per tablet.<br>Injection: 1mg (1ml); 2mg (1ml); 5mg (1ml); 10mg (1ml).<br>Nitroglycerin film: nitroglycerin 0.5mg per cell. |
| **药品名称 Drug Names** | 戊四硝酯 Pentaerythrityl Tetranitrate |
| 适应证<br>Indications | 用于预防心绞痛的发作。<br>It is used to prevent angina. |
| 用法、用量<br>Dosage | 口服：一日 3 ~ 4 次，每次 10 ~ 30mg。<br>Orally: the dose is 10 ~ 30mg every time, 3 to 4 times a day. |
| 剂型、规格<br>Preparations | 片剂：每片 10mg；20mg。复方制剂：每片含戊四硝醇 20mg、硝酸甘油 0.5mg。<br>Tablets: 10mg; 20mg per tablet. Compound preparation: 20mg alcohol pentaerythritol nitrate, 0.5mg nitroglycerin per tablet. |
| **药品名称 Drug Names** | 硝酸异山梨酯 Isosorbide Dinitrate |
| 适应证<br>Indications | 急性心绞痛发作的防治。<br>It is used for Prevention and treatment of acute attacks of angina. |
| 用法、用量<br>Dosage | 片剂：急性心绞痛发作时缓解心绞痛，舌下给药，1 次 5mg；预防心绞痛发作，口服，一日 2 ~ 3 次，1 次 5 ~ 10mg，一日 10 ~ 30mg；治疗心力衰竭，口服 1 次 5 ~ 20mg，6 ~ 8 小时一次。<br>外用乳膏：1 次 0.6g，均匀涂抹在心前区约 5cm×5cm，一日 1 次。缓释片：一日 2 次，1 次 1 片。<br>静脉滴注：每小时 2mg，剂量须根据患者反应而调节，且必须密切监测患者脉搏、心率及血压。<br>喷雾吸入：每次 1.25 ~ 3.75mg。 |

| | |
|---|---|
| | Tablets: when an attack of acute angina pectoris happens, the drug can relieve it. The drug is taken through sublingual administration, 5mg every time; it can also prevent angina pectoris, taken orally, 2 or 3 times a day, 5 ~ 10mg every time, 10 ~ 30mg a day; it can treat heart failure, taken orally, 5 ~ 20mg every time, once every 6 ~ 8 hours. Topical cream: the dose is 0.6g every time. The cream is smeared evenly on the praecordia with the area of 5cm × 5cm, once a day. Sustained-release tablets: the dose is one tablet every time, 2 times a day. Intravenous infusion: the dose is 2mg every hour. The dose must be adjusted according to the patients' response, and pulse, heart rate and blood pressure must be closely monitored. Spray Inhalation: 1.25 ~ 3.75mg every time. |
| 剂型、规格<br>Preparations | 普通片：每片 2.5mg；5mg；10mg。<br>缓释片：每片 20mg；40mg。<br>注射液：10mg（10ml）。<br>喷雾剂：250mg/200 次。<br>乳膏：1.5g（10g）。<br>Conventional tablets: 2.5mg; 5mg; 10mg per tablet.<br>Release tablets: 20mg; 40mg per tablet.<br>Injection: 10mg (10ml).<br>Sprays: 250mg/200 times.<br>Cream: 1.5g (10g). |
| 药品名称 Drug Names | 单硝酸异山梨酯 Isosorbide Mononitrate |
| 适应证<br>Indications | 用于冠心病的长期治疗和预防心绞痛发作，也用于心肌梗死后的治疗。<br>It is used for long-term treatment of coronary heart disease, and prevention of angina attack. It can also be used for post-myocardial infarction. |
| 用法、用量<br>Dosage | 口服，一日 20mg，一日 2 次，必要时可增至每日 3 次，饭后服。缓释片：1 次 1 片，一日 2 次，不宜嚼碎。<br>Orally: the dose is 20mg a day, 2 times a day. If necessary, the dose can be increased to three times a day. The drug is taken after meals. Release tablets: the dose is one tablet every time, 2 times a day. And the drug can't be chewed. |
| 剂型、规格<br>Preparations | 普通片：每片 20mg；40mg；60mg。<br>缓释片：每片 40mg。<br>Conventional tablets: 20mg; 40mg; 60mg per tablet. Sustained-release tablets: 40mg per tablet. |
| 药品名称 Drug Names | 曲美他嗪 Trimetazidine |
| 适应证<br>Indications | 用于冠状动脉功能不全、心绞痛、陈旧性心肌梗死等。对伴有严重心功能不全者，可与洋地黄苷并用。<br>It is used for coronary insufficiency, angina pectoris, and old myocardial infarction. For those with severe heart failure, the drug can be used with digitalis glycosides. |
| 用法、用量<br>Dosage | 口服：1 次 2 ~ 6mg，一日 3 次，饭后服；总剂量每日不超过 18mg。常用维持量为 1 次 1mg，一日 3 次。静脉注射：1 次 8 ~ 20mg，加于 25% 葡萄糖注射液 20ml 中。静脉滴注：8 ~ 20mg，加于 5% 葡萄糖注射液 500ml 中。<br>Orally: the dose is 2 ~ 6mg one time, three times a day and taken after meals; the daily total dose cannot exceed 18mg. Common maintenance dose is 1mg every time, three times a day. Intravenous injection: the dose is 8 ~ 20mg every time, added into 20ml 25% glucose injection. Intravenous drip: the dose is8 ~ 20mg, added into 500ml 5% glucose injection. |
| 剂型、规格<br>Preparations | 片剂：每片 2mg；3mg。注射液：每支 4mg（2ml）。<br>Tablets: 2mg; 3mg per tablet. Injection: 4mg (2ml) per vial. |
| 药品名称 Drug Names | 双嘧达莫 Dipyridamole |
| 适应证<br>Indications | 弥散性血管内凝血，血栓栓塞性疾病。防止冠心病发展。<br>It is used for disseminated intravascular coagulation disorders and thromboembolic disease. It can prevent the development of coronary heart disease. |
| 用法、用量<br>Dosage | 口服：每次 25 ~ 100mg，一日 3 次，饭前 1 小时服。在症状改善后，可改为每日 50 ~ 100mg，2 次分服。<br>Orally: the dose is 25 ~ 100mg every time, three times a day and taken one hour before meals. After symptoms are improved, the dose can be changed to 50 ~ 100mg every day, divided into 2 doses. |

**续　表**

| | |
|---|---|
| 剂型、规格<br>Preparations | 片剂：每片 25mg。<br>Tablets: 25mg per tablet. |
| 药品名称 Drug Names | 丹参酮Ⅱ A 磺酸钠 Sodium Tanshinon Ⅱ A sulfonate |
| 适应证<br>Indications | 用于冠心病心绞痛、胸闷及心肌梗死，对室性期前收缩也可使用。对冠心病患者的疗效与复方丹参注射液相似。<br><br>It is used for coronary heart disease angina pectoris, chest tightness, and myocardial infarction. It may be used for ventricular premature beats. The effect on coronary heart disease is similar to that of compound Danshen injection. |
| 用法、用量<br>Dosage | 肌内注射、静脉注射或静脉滴注：每日 1 次 40 ~ 80mg。注射用 25% 葡萄糖注射液 20ml 稀释，静脉滴注用 5% 葡萄糖注射液 250 ~ 500ml 稀释。<br><br>Intramuscular injection, intravenous injection or intravenous infusion: the dose is 40 ~ 80mg every day. When through injection, the drug should be diluted by 20ml 25% glucose injection. When through intravenous infusion, the drug should be diluted 250 ~ 500ml 5% glucose injection. |
| 剂型、规格<br>Preparations | 注射液：每支 10mg（2ml）。<br>Injection: 10mg (2ml) per vial. |
| 药品名称 Drug Names | 川芎嗪 Ligustrazine |
| 适应证<br>Indications | 适用于闭塞性血管疾病、脑血栓形成、脉管炎、冠心病、心绞痛等。对缺血性脑血管病的急性期、恢复期及其后遗症，如脑供血不足、脑血栓形成、脑栓塞、脑动脉硬化等均有较好疗效，能改善这些疾病引起的偏瘫、失语、吞咽困难、肢体麻木、无力、头痛、头晕、失眠、耳鸣、步态不稳、记忆力减退等症状。<br><br>It is intended to treat occlusive vascular disease, cerebral thrombosis, vasculitis, coronary heart disease and angina. It has a good effect on ischemic cerebrovascular disease acute phase, convalescence and its sequelae, such as cerebral ischemia, cerebral thrombosis, cerebral embolism, cerebral arteriosclerosis, etc. It can improve hemiplegia, aphasia, swallowing difficulties, numbness, weakness, headache, dizziness, insomnia, tinnitus, ataxia, memory loss and other symptoms caused by these diseases . |
| 用法、用量<br>Dosage | 口服：磷酸盐片剂每次 2 片，一日 3 次，1 个月为 1 个疗程。肌内注射：盐酸盐注射液，每次 2ml，一日 1 ~ 2 次。磷酸盐注射液，每次 2 ~ 4ml，一日 1 ~ 2 次，15 日为 1 个疗程，宜缓慢注射。静脉滴注：盐酸盐注射液，一日 1 次 2 ~ 4ml，或磷酸盐注射液一日 1 次 4 ~ 6ml，均稀释于 5% ~ 10% 葡萄糖注射液（或氯化钠注射液、低分子右旋糖酐注射液）250 ~ 500ml 中缓慢滴注，宜在 3 ~ 4 小时滴完，10 ~ 15 日为 1 个疗程。<br><br>Orally: phosphate tablets: the dose is 2 tablets once, three times a day. The course of treatment is a month. Intramuscular injection: hydrochloride injection: the dose is 2ml every time, 1 or 2 times a day. Phosphate injection: the dose is 2 ~ 4ml every time, 1 to 2 times a day. A course of treatment is 15 days. It should be slowly injected. Intravenous infusion: hydrochloride injection: the dose is 2 ~ 4ml once a day. Or phosphate injection: the dose is 4 ~ 6ml once a day. These two kinds of injection are diluted by 250 ~ 500ml 5% to 10% glucose injection (or Sodium Chloride Injection, low molecular dextran injection) through slow infusion. The infusion should be finished within 3 to 4 hours. A course of treatment is10 to 15 days. |
| 剂型、规格<br>Preparations | 片剂：每片含川芎嗪磷酸盐 50mg。<br>注射液：盐酸盐注射液，每支 40mg（2ml）；磷酸盐注射液，每支 50mg（2ml）。<br>Tablets: per tablet contains TMP phosphate 50mg.<br>Injection: hydrochloride injection, 40mg (2ml) per vial; phosphate injection, 50mg (2ml) per vial. |
| 药品名称 Drug Names | 葛根素 Puerarin |
| 适应证<br>Indications | 用于辅助治疗冠心病、心绞痛、心肌梗死，视网膜动、静脉阻塞、突发性耳聋、血性脑血管病、小儿病毒性心肌炎、糖尿病等。眼科用于原发性开角型青光眼、高眼压症、原发性闭角型青光眼、继发性青光眼。<br><br>It is used for the adjuvant treatment of coronary heart disease, angina, myocardial infarction, retinal artery and vein occlusion, sudden deafness, hemorrhagic cerebrovascular disease, children viral myocarditis, diabetes and so on. It can also be used for primary open-angle glaucoma, ocular hypertension, primary angle-closure glaucoma and secondary glaucoma. |

| 用法、用量<br>Dosage | 静脉滴注：每次 200 ～ 600mg，加入 5% 葡萄糖注射液 250 ～ 500ml 中静脉滴注，一日 1 次，10 ～ 20 日为 1 个疗程，可连续使用 2 ～ 3 个疗程。超过 65 岁的老年人连续使用总剂量不超过 5g。葛根素葡萄糖注射液：静脉滴注，每次 0.4 ～ 0.6g，一日 1 次，15 日为 1 个疗程。滴眼液：1%，一次 1 ～ 2 滴，滴入眼睑内，闭目 3 ～ 5 分钟。首日 3 次，以后一日 2 次，早晚各一次。偶有一过性异物感或刺激感。<br><br>Intravenous infusion: the dose is 200 ~ 600mg every time, added into 250 ~ 500ml 5% glucose injection through intravenous infusion, once a day. A course of treatment is10 to 20 days and the drug can be used continuously for 2 to 3 courses. For more than 65-year-old patients, the continuous total dose cannot exceed 5g. Purarin glucose injection: intravenous injection: the dose is 0.4 ~ 0.6g every time, once a day. A course of treatment is 15 days. Eyedrops: 1% drip 1 to 2 drops every time into eyelids and close eyes for 3 to 5 minutes. The first day is 3 times. After that, drip eyedrops twice a day in the morning and evening. Occasionally there is a transient foreign body sensation or irritation. |
|---|---|
| 剂型、规格<br>Preparations | 注射液：每支 100mg（2ml）；250mg（5ml）。<br>注射用葛根素：每支 0.1g。<br>葛根素葡萄糖注射液：每瓶 0.2g（100ml）；0.25g（100ml）；0.3g（150ml）；0.3g（250ml）；0.5g（250ml）。各种规格均含葡萄糖 5%。<br><br>Injection: 100mg (2ml); 250mg (5ml) per vial.<br>Puerarin Injection: 0.1g per vial. Purarin injection: 0.2 (100ml); 0.25 (100ml); 0.3 (150ml); 0.3 (250ml); 0.5 (250ml) per vial.<br>Various specifications include 5% glucose. |
| 药品名称 Drug Names | 愈风宁心片 Yufengningxin Tablets |
| 适应证<br>Indications | 具有增加脑血流量及冠脉血流量的作用。可用于缓解高血压症状（颈项强痛）、治疗心绞痛及突发性耳聋，有一定疗效。<br><br>It can increase coronary blood flow and cerebral blood flow. It can be used to relieve symptoms of hypertension (neck pain), treat angina and sudden deafness. |
| 用法、用量<br>Dosage | 每次 5 片，一日 3 次。<br>The dose is five tablets every time, three times a day. |
| 剂型、规格<br>Preparations | 片剂：每片含总黄酮 60mg。<br>Tablets: per tablet contains flavonoids 60mg. |
| 药品名称 Drug Names | 银杏叶提取物 Ginkgo Biloba Leaf Extract |
| 适应证<br>Indications | 用于治疗冠心病心绞痛、脑血管痉挛、脑供血不足、记忆力衰退等。也适用于支气管哮喘、老年性痴呆等。<br><br>It is used for coronary angina pectoris, cerebral vasospasm, cerebral blood supply insufficiency, memory loss, etc. It also applies to bronchial asthma, Alzheimer's disease and so on. |
| 用法、用量<br>Dosage | 口服：每次 20 ～ 40mg，一日 3 次。肌内注射：每次 7 ～ 15mg，一日 1 ～ 2 次。静脉滴注：每日 87.5 ～ 175mg。<br><br>Orally: the dose is 20 ~ 40mg every time, 3 times a day. Intramuscular injection: the dose is 7 ~ 15mg every time, 1 ~ 2 times a day. Intravenous infusion: the dose is 87.5 ~ 175mg every day. |
| 剂型、规格<br>Preparations | 常用的制剂有片剂、缓释糖衣片、口服液、强化滴剂、酊剂、注射液及静脉滴注剂等。<br>Common preparations include tablets, sustained release coated tablets, oral solution, strengthened drops, tinctures, injections and intravenous agents. |
| 药品名称 Drug Names | 地奥心血康 Diaoxinxuekang |
| 适应证<br>Indications | 用于冠心病、心绞痛，能改善症状。<br>It is used for coronary heart disease, angina pectoris and can improve the symptoms. |
| 用法、用量<br>Dosage | 口服，一次 0.2g，一日 3 次，有效后可改为 1 次 0.1g，一日 3 次。<br>Orally: the dose is 0.2g every time, 3 times a day. If the drug works, the dose can be changed to 0.1g every time, 3 times a day. |

| 剂型、规格<br>Preparations | 常用其胶囊、片剂、颗粒和软胶囊（均为 0.1g）。<br>口服液每支 0.1g（10ml）。<br>Its common preparations include capsules, tablets, granules, and capsules (all are 0.1g).<br>Oral solution: 0.1g (10ml) per vial. |
|---|---|
| 药品名称 Drug Names | 辅酶Ⅰ Coenzyme Ⅰ |
| 适应证<br>Indications | 用于冠心病，可改善冠心病的胸闷、心绞痛等症状。<br>It is used for coronary heart disease. It can improve chest tightness and angina of coronary heart disease. |
| 用法、用量<br>Dosage | 肌内注射：一日 1 次 5mg，溶于 0.9% 氯化钠注射液 2ml，14 日为 1 个疗程。大多应用 2 个疗程。<br>Intramuscular injection: the dose is 5mg once a day, dissolved in 2ml 0.9% sodium chloride injection. A course of treatment is 14 days. Use this drug for two courses. |
| 剂型、规格<br>Preparations | 注射用辅酶Ⅰ：每支 5mg。<br>Injection coenzyme Ⅰ : 5mg per vial. |

### 10.5 周围血管舒张药 Peripheral Vasodilators

| 药品名称 Drug Names | 二氢麦角碱 Dihydroergotoxine |
|---|---|
| 适应证<br>Indications | 主要与异丙嗪、哌替啶等配成冬眠合剂应用。也可用于动脉内膜炎、肢端动脉痉挛症、血管痉挛性偏头痛等。<br>It is mainly combined with promethazine and pethidine to make hibernation mixture.It can also be used for endarteritis, Reynaud's disease, and vascular spastic migraine. |
| 用法、用量<br>Dosage | 肌内注射或皮下注射，一日或隔日 1 次，每次 0.3 ~ 0.6mg；亦可舌下给药（含片），每 4 ~ 6 小时 1 次，每次 0.5 ~ 2mg。不宜口服。<br>Intramuscular or subcutaneous injection: the dose is 0.3 ~ 0.6mg every time, every day or two days; It can also be taken through sublingual administration (lozenge). The dose is 0.5 ~ 2mg every time, once every 4 to 6 hours. It should not be taken orally. |
| 剂型、规格<br>Preparations | 含片：每片 0.25mg；0.5mg。注射液：每支 0.3mg（1ml）。<br>Lozenge: 0.25mg; 0.5mg per tablet. Injection: 0.3mg (1ml) per vial. |
| 药品名称 Drug Names | 烟酸 Nicotinic Acid |
| 适应证<br>Indications | 烟酸可用于治疗糙皮病，但因易于产生面部潮红等不良反应，而烟酰胺则无，故一般选用后者。此外，烟酸还有较强的周围血管扩张作用，口服后数分钟即见效，可维持数分钟至 1 小时，用于治疗血管性偏头痛、头痛、脑动脉血栓形成、肺栓塞、内耳眩晕症、冻伤、中心性视网膜脉络膜炎等。大剂量（一日 2 ~ 6g）可降低血脂（主要是三酰甘油），适用于Ⅳ、Ⅲ、Ⅴ型高脂血症，亦可用于Ⅱ型患者。烟酰胺无扩张血管及降血脂作用。<br>Niacin can be used for pellagra, but it is prone to cause facial flushing and other adverse reactions while nicotinamide doesn't have these adverse reactions. So the latter is generally used. In addition, the drug can be used for peripheral vascular expansion and can work in several minutes after oral administration. Its efficacy can last for several minutes to 1 hour. It can be used for vascular migraine, headache, cerebral arterial thrombosis, pulmonary embolism, inner ear vertigo, frostbite, and central retinochoroiditis. The high dose (2 ~ 6 g a day) can reduce blood lipids (mainly triglycerides) and apply to Ⅳ, Ⅲ, Ⅴ hyperlipidemia. It can also be used in patients with type Ⅱ . Nicotinamide cannot expand blood vessels and lower blood pressure. |
| 用法、用量<br>Dosage | （1）口服：一次 50 ~ 200mg，一日 3 ~ 4 次，餐后服。用于降血脂，一日 3 ~ 6g，分 3 ~ 4 次于餐后服用。<br>（2）静脉注射或肌内注射：一次 10 ~ 50mg，一日 1 ~ 3 次。用于脑血管疾病：一次 50 ~ 200mg，加于 5% ~ 10% 葡萄糖注射液 100 ~ 200ml 中静脉滴注，一日 1 次。<br>(1) Orally: 50 ~ 200mg one time, 3 to 4 times one day, taken after meal. For lowering blood pressure, the dose is 3 ~ 6g a day, divided into 3 to 4 doses, taken after meals.<br>(2) intravenous or intramuscular injection: The dose is 10 ~ 50mg every time, 3 times a day 1. For cerebrovascular disease: the dose is 50 ~ 200mg every time, added into 100 ~ 200ml 5% to 10% glucose injection, once a day. |

**续　表**

| | |
|---|---|
| 剂型、规格<br>Preparations | 片剂：每片 50mg；100mg。<br>注射液：每支 20mg（2ml）；50mg（1ml）；100mg（2ml）；50mg（5ml）。<br>Tablets: 50mg, 100mg per tablet.<br>Injection: 20mg (2ml); 50mg (1ml); 100mg (2ml); 50mg (5ml)per vial |
| 药品名称 Drug Names | 烟酸肌醇酯 Inositol Nicotinate |
| 适应证<br>Indications | 用于高脂血症、冠心病、各种末梢血管障碍性疾病（如闭塞性动脉硬化症、肢端动脉痉挛症、冻伤、血管性偏头痛等）的辅助治疗。<br>It is used as adjuvant therapy for hyperlipidemia, coronary heart disease, a variety of peripheral vascular disorders (such as arteriosclerosis obliterans, Raynaud's disease, frostbite, vascular migraine, etc.). |
| 用法、用量<br>Dosage | 口服：每日 3 次，一次 0.2 ~ 0.6g。连续服用 1 ~ 3 个月。<br>Orally: the dose is 0.2 ~ 0.6g, 3 times a day, taken continuously for 1 to 3 months. |
| 剂型、规格<br>Preparations | 片剂：每片 0.2g。<br>Tablets: 0.2g per tablet. |
| 药品名称 Drug Names | 维生素 E 烟酸酯 Vitamin E Nicotinate |
| 适应证<br>Indications | 用于治疗脑动脉硬化、脑卒中、脑外伤后遗症、脂质代谢异常、高血压、冠心病及循环障碍引起的各种疾病。其不良反应小，无烟酸样面部潮红等不良反应。<br>It is used for cerebral arteriosclerosis, stroke, traumatic brain injury sequelae, abnormal lipid metabolism, hypertension, coronary heart disease and various diseases caused by circulatory disorders. Its adverse reactions are small and it has no niacin-like facial flushing or other adverse reactions. |
| 用法、用量<br>Dosage | 口服：每次 100 ~ 200mg，一日 3 次，餐后服用。<br>Orally: the dose is 100 ~ 200mg every time, 3 times a day, taken after meals. |
| 剂型、规格<br>Preparations | 胶囊剂：每粒 100mg。<br>Capsules: 100mg per capsule. |
| 药品名称 Drug Names | 罂粟碱 Papaverine |
| 适应证<br>Indications | 主要用于脑血栓形成、肺栓塞、肢端动脉痉挛症及动脉栓塞性疼痛等。对高血压、心绞痛、幽门痉挛、胆绞痛、肠绞痛、支气管哮喘等在一般剂量下疗效不显著。<br>It is mainly used for cerebral thrombosis, pulmonary embolism, Raynaud's disease, and arterial spasms and pain. It doesn't have an significant effect on hypertension, angina, pyloric spasm, biliary colic, colic, asthma if the common dose is taken. |
| 用法、用量<br>Dosage | 口服：常用量，每次 30 ~ 60mg，一日 3 次；极量，一次 200mg，一日 600mg。肌内注射或静脉滴注：每次 30mg，一日 90 ~ 120mg，一日量不宜超过 300mg。<br>Orally: The common dose is 30 ~ 60mg every time, 3 times a day; the maximum dose is 200mg once, 600mg a day. Intramuscular injection or intravenous infusion: the dose is 30mg every time, 90 ~ 120mg a day. The daily total dose should not exceed 300mg. |
| 剂型、规格<br>Preparations | 片剂：每片 30mg。<br>注射液：每支 30mg（1ml）。<br>Tablets: 30mg per tablet.<br>Injection: 30mg (1ml) per vial. |
| 药品名称 Drug Names | 西地那非 Sildenafil |
| 适应证<br>Indications | 用于治疗勃起功能障碍（ED）。<br>It is used for erectile dysfunction (ED). |
| 用法、用量<br>Dosage | 一般剂量为 50mg，在性活动前约 1 小时（或 0.5 ~ 4 小时）服用。基于药效和耐药性，剂量可增至 100mg（最大推荐剂量）或降至 25mg。每日最多服用 1 次。<br>The common dose is 50mg, taken about 1 hour (or 0.5 to 4 hours) before sexual activity taking. Based on efficacy and tolerability, the dose may be increased to 100mg (maximum recommended dose), or reduced to 25mg. The drug can be taken only once a day. |

| 剂型、规格<br>Preparations | 片剂：25mg；50mg；100mg。<br>Tablets: 25mg; 50mg; 100mg. |
|---|---|
| 药品名称 Drug Names | 环扁桃酯 Cyclandelate |
| 适应证<br>Indications | 用于脑血管意外及其后遗症、脑动脉硬化症、脑外伤后遗症、肢端动脉痉挛症、手足发绀、闭塞性动脉内膜炎、内耳眩晕症等。<br><br>It is used for cerebrovascular accident and its sequelae, cerebral arteriosclerosis, cerebral trauma sequelae, Raynaud's disease, acrocyanosis, endarteritis obliterans, and Meniere's syndrome.. |
| 用法、用量<br>Dosage | 一次服 100 ~ 200mg，一日 3 ~ 4 次。症状改善后，可减量至一日 300 ~ 400mg。对脑血管疾病一般每次服 200 ~ 400mg，一日 3 次。<br><br>The dose is 100 ~ 200mg every time, 3 to 4 times a day. After symptoms improve, you can reduce to 300 ~ 400mg a day. For cerebrovascular disease, the dose is generally 200 ~ 400mg every time, 3 times a day. |
| 剂型、规格<br>Preparations | 胶囊剂：每粒 100mg。<br>Capsules: 100mg per capsule. |
| 药品名称 Drug Names | 长春西汀 Vinpocetine |
| 适应证<br>Indications | 用于治疗由于大脑血液循环障碍引起的精神性或神经性症状如记忆力障碍、失语症、行动障碍、头晕、头痛等，高血压性脑病、大脑血管痉挛、大脑动脉内膜炎、进行性脑血管硬化。眼科用于因视网膜和脉络膜血管硬化及血管痉挛引起的斑点退化。耳科用于治疗老年性耳聋、眩晕等。<br><br>It is used for psychiatric or neurological symptoms caused by the brain blood circulation disorder, such as memory impairment, aphasia, mobility impairments, dizziness, headache, hypertensive encephalopathy, cerebral vasospasm, brain endarteritis, progressive cerebral atherosclerosis. It can also be used for spots degradation due to retinal and choroidal vascular sclerosis and vascular spasm. It can be used to treat age-related hearing loss and vertigo. |
| 用法、用量<br>Dosage | 急性病例可用注射剂，每次 10mg，一日 3 次，静脉滴注或静脉注射，用时以 0.9% 氯化钠注射液稀释到 5 倍体积。然后口服片剂，一日 3 次，每次 1 ~ 2 片。对慢性患者，一日 3 次，每次 1 ~ 2 片。维持剂量时一次 1 片，一日 3 次。<br><br>Acute cases can use injections. The dose is 10mg per time, 3 times a day. Intravenous infusion or intravenous injection: the drug should be diluted by 0.9% sodium chloride injection to 5 times of its volume. As for oral tablets, the dose is 1 to 2 tablet every time, 3 times a day. For chronic patients, the dose is 1 to 2 tablets every time, 3 times a day. The maintenance dose is one tablet every time, three times a day. |
| 剂型、规格<br>Preparations | 片剂：每片 5mg。注射液：每支 10mg（2ml）。<br>Tablets: 5mg per tablet. Injection: 10mg (2ml) per vial. |
| 药品名称 Drug Names | 倍他司汀 Betahistine |
| 适应证<br>Indications | 用于内耳眩晕症，对脑动脉硬化、缺血性脑血管病、头部外伤或高血压所致的体位性眩晕、耳鸣等亦可用。<br><br>It is used for Meniere's syndrome, cerebral arteriosclerosis, ischemic cerebrovascular disease, head trauma, and postural vertigo, tinnitus caused by high blood pressure. |
| 用法、用量<br>Dosage | 口服每次 4 ~ 8mg，一日 2 ~ 4 次。肌内注射一次 2 ~ 4mg，一日 2 次。<br>Orally: the dose is 4 ~ 8mg every time, 2 to 4 times a day. Intramuscular injection: the dose is 2 ~ 4mg once, 2 times a day. |
| 剂型、规格<br>Preparations | 片剂：每片 4mg；5mg。注射液：每支 2mg（2ml）；4mg（2ml）。<br>Tablets: 4mg per tablet; 5mg. Injection: 2mg (2ml); 4mg (2ml) per vial. |

续 表

| 药品名称 Drug Names | 地芬尼多 Difenidol |
|---|---|
| 适应证<br>Indications | 用于各种原因引起的眩晕症如椎基底动脉供血不全、梅尼埃病、自主神经功能紊乱、晕车晕船等。<br>It is used for vertigo caused by a variety of causes, such as vertebrobasilar insufficiency, Meniere's disease, autonomic dysfunction, and motion sickness and so on. |
| 用法、用量<br>Dosage | 口服：一日 3 次，每次 25 ~ 50mg。<br>Orally: the dose is 25 ~ 50mg every time, three times a day. |
| 剂型、规格<br>Preparations | 片剂：每片 25mg。<br>Tablets: 25mg per tablet. |
| 药品名称 Drug Names | 血管舒缓素 Kallidinogenase |
| 适应证<br>Indications | 用于脑动脉硬化症、闭塞性动脉内膜炎、闭塞性血管炎、四肢慢性溃疡、肢端动脉痉挛症、手足发绀、老年性四肢冷感、中央视网膜炎、眼底出血等。由于易被消化酶破坏，口服作用时间短，效力不及注射。<br>It is used for cerebral arteriosclerosis, endateritis bliterans, occlusive vasculitis, limbs chronic ulcer, Raynaud's disease, acrocyanosis, senile cold limbs, central retinitis, retinal bleeding.Because it is susceptible to the digestive enzymes, if it is taken orally, its efficacy lasts for a short time and weaker than injection. |
| 用法、用量<br>Dosage | (1) 口服，每次 1 片（含 10U），空腹时服。<br>(2) 注射临用时溶解（10U/1.5ml）后进行肌内注射或皮下注射，一次量 10 ~ 20U，一日 1 ~ 2 次。轻症每日 10U，以 3 周为 1 个疗程。眼科亦可作眼结膜下注射，每次 5U。<br>(1) Orally: the dose is one tablet one time (containing 10 units), taken on an empty stomach.<br>(2) intramuscular or subcutaneous injection: The dose is 10 to 20 units, 1 to 2 times a day, and the drug should be dissolved (10 units / 1.5ml) before its use. For patentis of mild symptom, the dose is10 units a day and three weeks are a course of treatment. The drug can also be given through eye subconjunctiva injection, with the dose of 5 units every time. |
| 剂型、规格<br>Preparations | 片剂：每片 10U。<br>注射用血管舒缓素：每支 10U。<br>Tablets: 10 U per tablet.<br>Kallikrein injection: 10 U per vial. |
| 药品名称 Drug Names | 二氢麦角胺 Dihydroergotamine |
| 适应证<br>Indications | 用于偏头痛急性发作及血管性头痛等。<br>It is used for acute attacks of and vascular headache. |
| 用法、用量<br>Dosage | 因口服吸收不好，治偏头痛多采用注射，肌内注射一次 1 ~ 2mg，一日 1 ~ 2 次。口服一次 1 ~ 3mg，一日 2 ~ 3 次。<br>Due to poor oral absorption, the drug is often given through injection for migraine. Intramuscular injection: the dose is1 ~ 2mg one time, 1 or 2 times a day. Orally: the dose is 1 ~ 3mg once, 2 or 3 times a day. |
| 剂型、规格<br>Preparations | 片剂：1mg。注射液：1mg（1ml）。<br>Tablets: 1mg. Injection: 1mg (1ml). |
| 药品名称 Drug Names | 尼麦角林 Nicergoline |
| 适应证<br>Indications | 用于脑血管疾病及下肢闭塞性动脉内膜炎等。<br>It is used for cerebrovascular disease and lower extremity occlusive endarteritis. |
| 用法、用量<br>Dosage | 口服：一次 5mg，一日 3 次；肌内注射或静脉注射：一次 2.5 ~ 5mg。<br>Orally: the dose is 5mg every time, 3 times a day; intramuscular injection or intravenous injection: the dose is 2.5 ~ 5mg everytime. |

| 剂型、规格<br>Preparations | 片剂：5mg。注射液：2.5mg（1ml）。<br>Tablets: 5mg. Injection: 2.5mg (1ml). |
|---|---|
| **药品名称 Drug Names** | **长春胺 Vincamine** |
| 适应证<br>Indications | 用于脑血管障碍、脑栓塞、脑血栓形成及出血后遗症等。对脑动脉硬化症的疗效比二氢麦角碱和罂粟碱强，需长期应用方见效。<br><br>It is used for cerebrovascular disorders, cerebral embolism, cerebral thrombosis and bleeding sequelae. Its efficacy for cerebral arteriosclerosis is stronger than Dihydroergotoxine and papaverine, but it takes a long time for the drug to work. |
| 用法、用量<br>Dosage | 口服：一次 5 ~ 20mg，一日 2 ~ 3 次；肌内注射：一次 5 ~ 15mg，一日 2 ~ 3 次。<br><br>Orally: the dose is 5 ~ 20mg every time, 2 or 3 times a day; intramuscular injection: the dose is 5 ~ 15mg every time, 2 or 3 times a day. |
| 剂型、规格<br>Preparations | 片剂：5mg。注射液：5mg（2ml）。<br>Tablets: 5mg. Injection: 5mg (2ml) |

## 10.6 抗高血压药 Antihypertensive Drugs

| **药品名称 Drug Names** | **可乐定 Clonidine** |
|---|---|
| 适应证<br>Indications | 本品预防偏头痛亦有效。亦能降低眼压，可用于治疗开角型青光眼。<br><br>This product is effective for prevention of migraine. It can reduce intraocular pressure and be used for open-angle glaucoma. |
| 用法、用量<br>Dosage | （1）治疗高血压：口服，常用量，每次服 0.075 ~ 0.15mg，一日 3 次。可逐渐增加剂量，通常维持剂量为每日 0.2 ~ 0.8mg。极量，一次 0.6mg。缓慢静脉注射：每次 0.15 ~ 0.3mg，加于 50% 葡萄糖注射液 20 ~ 40ml 中（多用于三期高血压及其他危重高血压病）注射。<br>（2）预防偏头痛：一日 0.1mg，分 2 次服，8 周为 1 个疗程（第 4 周以后，一日量可增至 0.15mg）。<br>（3）治青光眼：用 0.25% 液滴眼。低血压患者慎用。<br><br>(1) hypertension: orally: the common dose is 0.075 ~ 0.15mg every time, three times a day. The dose can gradually be increased. The maintenance dose is usually 0.2 ~ 0.8mg a day. The maximum dose is 0.6mg every time. Slow intravenous injection: the dose is 0.15 ~ 0.3mg every time, added into 20 ~ 40ml 50% glucose injection (often used for Phase III hypertension and other critical hypertension).<br>(2) migraine: the dose is 0.1mg a day, divided into 2 doses, and eight weeks are a course of treatment (after four weeks, the daily amount may be increased to 0.15mg).<br>(3) glaucoma: use 0.25% eye drops. For patients with hypotension, it should be used with caution. |
| 剂型、规格<br>Preparations | 片剂：每片 0.075mg；0.15mg。<br>贴片：每片 2mg。<br>注射液：每支 0.15mg（1ml）。<br>滴眼液：12.5mg（5ml）。<br><br>Tablets: 0.075mg per tablet; 0.15mg.<br>Paster: 2mg per tablet.<br>Injection: 0.15mg (1ml) per vial.<br>Drops: 12.5mg (5ml). |
| **药品名称 Drug Names** | **哌唑嗪 Prazosin** |
| 适应证<br>Indications | 用于治疗轻、中度高血压，常与 β 受体拮抗剂或利尿剂合用，降压效果更好。由于本品既能扩张容量血管，降低前负荷，又能扩张阻力血管，降低后负荷，可用于治疗中、重度慢性充血性心力衰竭及心肌梗死后心力衰竭。对常规疗法（洋地黄类、利尿剂）无效或效果不显著的心力衰竭患者也有效。<br><br>It is used for mild and moderate hypertension, and often used with β receptor antagonists or diuretics. The antihypertensive efficacy is better. Because the drug can expand the capacity of blood vessels, and reduce pre-load, ans also expand resistance vessels and reduce afterload, it can be used for moderate and severe chronic congestive heart failure and cardiac failure after myocardial infarction. It can be effective for heart failure patient for whom the conventional therapy (digitalis, diuretics) is invalid or dosen't have significant effect. |

| | |
|---|---|
| 用法、用量<br>Dosage | 口服：开始每次 0.5 ~ 1mg，一日 1.5 ~ 3mg，以后逐渐增至一日 6 ~ 15mg。对充血性心力衰竭，维持量通常为每日 4 ~ 20mg，分次服用。<br>Orally: the initial dose is 0.5 ~ 1mg every time, 1.5 ~ 3mg a day, and then the dose can gradually increased to 6 ~ 15mg a day. For congestive heart failure, the daily maintenance dose is usually 4 ~ 20mg, divided doses. |
| 剂型、规格<br>Preparations | 片剂：每片 0.5mg；1mg；2mg；5mg。<br>Tablets: 0.5mg; 1mg; 2mg; 5mg per tablet . |
| **药品名称 Drug Names** | 特拉唑嗪 Terazosin |
| 适应证<br>Indications | 用于高血压，也可用于良性前列腺增生。<br>It is used for hypertension and benign prostatic hyperplasia. |
| 用法、用量<br>Dosage | 口服：开始时，一次不超过 1mg，睡前服用，以后可根据情况逐渐增量，一般为一日 8 ~ 10mg，一日最大剂量 20mg。用于前列腺肥大，一日剂量为 5 ~ 10mg。<br>Orally: The initial dose is no more than 1mg every time, taken before bedtime. Later, the dose can begradually increased according to patients' conditions. The dose is usually 8 ~ 10mg a day; the daily maximum dose is 20mg. For an enlarged prostate, the dose is 5 ~ 10mg a day. |
| 剂型、规格<br>Preparations | 片剂：每片 0.5mg；1mg；2mg；5mg；10mg。<br>Tablets: 0.5mg; 1mg; 2mg; 5mg; 10mg per tablet. |
| **药品名称 Drug Names** | 多沙唑嗪 Doxazosin |
| 适应证<br>Indications | 用于高血压。<br>It is used for hypertension. |
| 用法、用量<br>Dosage | 开始时，口服一日 1 次 0.5mg，根据情况可每 1 ~ 2 周逐渐增加剂量至一日 2mg，然后再增量至一日 4 ~ 8mg。<br>Orally: the initial dose is 0.5mg once a day. According to patients' conditions, the dose can gradually be increased every 1 to 2 weeks and then to 2mg a day, and later increased to 1 4 ~ 8mg a day. |
| 剂型、规格<br>Preparations | 常用甲磺酸盐的片剂：每片 0.5mg；1mg；2mg；4mg；8mg。<br>Common mesylate tablets: 0.5mg; 1mg; 2mg; 4mg; 8mg per tablet. |
| **药品名称 Drug Names** | 乌拉地尔 Urapidil |
| 适应证<br>Indications | 用于各类型的高血压（口服）。可与利尿降压药、β 受体拮抗药合用；也用于高血压危象及手术前、中、后对高血压升高的控制性降压（静脉注射）。<br>It is used for various types of hypertension (orally). It can be used with diuretic antihypertensive drugs and β receptor antagonist drugs; it can be used for hypertensive crisis and is also used as controlled hypotension of high blood pressure rise before, during and after surgery (intravenous injection). |
| 用法、用量<br>Dosage | 口服：开始时一次 60mg，早、晚各服 1 次，如血压逐渐下降，可减量为每次 30mg。维持量一日 30 ~ 180mg。静脉注射：一般剂量为 25 ~ 50mg，如用 50mg，应分 2 次给药，其间隔为 5 分钟。静脉滴注：将 250mg 溶于输液 500ml 中，开始滴速为 6mg/min，维持剂量滴速平均为 120mg/h。<br>Orally: the initial dose is 60mg every time, twice a day and taken in the moring and evening. If blood pressure gradually decreases, the dose can be reduced to 30mg every time. The maintenance dose is 30 ~ 180mg a day. Intravenous injection: the common dose is 25 ~ 50mg. If the dose is 50mg, it should be divided into two doses, at intervals of five minutes. Intravenous infusion: Dissolve 250mg in 500ml injection. The inkection begins to drip at the speed of 6mg/min and the dripping speed shoule be maintained as 120mg / h. |
| 剂型、规格<br>Preparations | 缓释胶囊剂：每胶囊 30mg；60mg。<br>注射液：每支 25mg（5ml）；50mg（10ml）。<br>Sustained-release capsules: 30mg; 60mg per capsule.<br>Injection: 25mg (5ml); 50mg (10ml) per vial. |

| 药品名称 Drug Names | 利血平 Reserpine |
| --- | --- |
| 适应证<br>Indications | 对于轻度至中等度的早期高血压，疗效显著（精神紧张病例疗效尤好），长期应用小量，可将多数患者的血压稳定于正常范围内，但对严重和晚期病例，单用本品疗效较差，常与肼屈嗪、氢氯噻嗪等合用，以增加疗效。<br><br>It is used for mild and moderate early hypertension and the effect is significant (especially for mental stress cases). For a long-term use, the dose shoule be small. It can stabilize most patients' blood pressure within the normal range, but for the severe and advanced cases, if the drug is used alone, the efficacy is weak. So it is often used with hydralazine, hydrochlorothiazide in order to increase efficacy. |
| 用法、用量<br>Dosage | 作为降压药，每日服 0.25 ~ 0.5mg，一次顿服或 3 次分服。如长期应用，须酌减剂量只求维持药效即可。作为安定药，每日量 0.5 ~ 5mg。亦可肌内注射或静脉注射。<br><br>As antihypertensive drugs, the daily dose is 0.25 ~ 0.5mg, divided into one or three doses. If the drug is used for a long time, the dose should appropriately be reduced just for the purpose of maintaining efficacy. As antipsychotics, the daily dose is 0.5 ~ 5mg. It can be givcen through intramuscular injection or intravenous injection. |
| 剂型、规格<br>Preparations | 片剂：每片 0.25mg。注射液：每支 1mg（1ml）。<br>Tablets: 0.25mg per tablet. Injection: 1mg (1ml) per vial. |
| 药品名称 Drug Names | 肼屈嗪 Hydralazine |
| 适应证<br>Indications | 现多用于肾性高血压及舒张压较高的患者。单独使用效果不甚好，且易引起不良反应，故多与利血平、氢氯噻嗪、胍乙啶或普萘洛尔合用以增加疗效。<br><br>It is often used on patients with higher renal hypertension and diastolic blood pressure now. If the drug is used alone, the efficacy is not good, and it's easy to cause adverse reactions. So it is often used with reserpine, hydrochlorothiazide, guanethidine or propranolol in order to increase efficacy. |
| 用法、用量<br>Dosage | 口服或静脉注射、肌内注射。一般开始时用小量，每次 10mg，一日 3 ~ 4 次，用药 2 ~ 4 日。以后用量逐渐增加。维持量，一日 30 ~ 200mg，分次服用。<br><br>Orally or intravenous injection, intramuscular injection: The initial dose is usually small, with 10mg every time, 3 to 4 times a day, taken for 2 to 4 days. Later, the dose is gradually increased. The maintenance dose is 30 ~ 200mg a day, divided doses. |
| 剂型、规格<br>Preparations | 片剂：每片 10mg；25mg；50mg。<br>缓释片：每片 50mg。<br>注射液：每支 20mg（1ml）。<br>Tablets: 10mg; 25mg; 50mg per tablet.<br>Sustained-release tablets: 50mg per tablet.<br>Injection: 20mg (1ml) per vial. |
| 药品名称 Drug Names | 双肼屈嗪 Dihydralazine |
| 适应证<br>Indications | 现多用于肾性高血压及舒张压较高的患者。单独使用效果不甚好，且易引起不良反应，故多与利血平、氢氯噻嗪、胍乙啶或普萘洛尔合用以增加疗效。<br><br>It is often used on patients with higher renal hypertension and diastolic blood pressure now. If the drug is used alone, the efficacy is not good, and it's easy to cause adverse reactions. So it is often used with reserpine, hydrochlorothiazide, guanethidine or propranolol in order to increase efficacy. |
| 用法、用量<br>Dosage | 口服：一次 12.5 ~ 25mg，一日 25 ~ 50mg。发生耐受性后，可加大到每次 50mg，一日 3 次。<br><br>Oral medication: 12.5 ~ 25mg one time, 25 ~ 50mg a day. After the occurrence of tolerance, the dose can be increased to 50mg once, 3 times a day. |
| 剂型、规格<br>Preparations | 片剂：每片 12.5mg；25mg。注射用双肼屈嗪：25mg。<br>Tablets: 12.5mg or 25mg per tablet. Dihydralazine for Injection: 25mg. |

续　表

| 药品名称 Drug Names | 硝普钠 Sodium Nitroprusside |
|---|---|
| 适应证<br>Indications | 用于其他降压药无效的高血压危象，疗效可靠，且由于其作用持续时间较短，易于掌握。用于心力衰竭，能使衰竭的左心室排血量增加，心力衰竭症状得以缓解。<br><br>It's used to treat the hypertensive crisis that treatments by other antihypertensive drugs are ineffective. Being effective and reliable, it's easy to master because of its short effect duration. Besides, it's also used to treat heart failure, increasing cardiac output of the left ventricular, so as to relieve the heart failure symptoms. |
| 用法、用量<br>Dosage | 临用前，先用 5% 葡萄糖注射液溶解，再用 5% 葡萄糖注射液 250 ~ 1000ml 稀释。静脉滴注，每分钟 1 ~ 3μg/kg。开始时速度可略快，血压下降后可减慢。但用于心力衰竭、心源性休克时，开始宜缓慢，以 10 滴 / 分钟为宜，以后再酌情加快速度。用药不宜超过 72 小时。<br><br>Before usage, dissolve it with 5% glucose injection, then dilute the dissolved solution with another 250 ~ 1000ml 5% glucose injection .Intravenous infusion, 1 ~ 3μg/kg per minute. The injection speed can be slightly faster at the beginning, while slowing down after blood pressure drops. But for heart failure and cardiogenic shock, the injection speed should be slow at first, with 10 drops / minute being appropriate, later speeding up accordingly. However, the medication treatment should not exceed 72 hours. |
| 剂型、规格<br>Preparations | 注射用硝普钠：每支 50mg。<br>Sodium nitroprusside for injection: 50mg per vial. |

| 药品名称 Drug Names | 卡托普利 Captopril |
|---|---|
| 适应证<br>Indications | 用于治疗各种类型高血压，特别是常规疗法无效的高血压。由于本品通过降低血浆血管紧张素 Ⅱ 和醛固酮水平，而使心脏前、后负荷减轻，故可用于顽固性慢性心力衰竭，对洋地黄、利尿剂和血管扩张剂无效的心力衰竭患者也有效。<br><br>For the treatment of various types of hypertension, especially the hypertension that conventional therapy is ineffective. As this drug can reduce cardiac stress by decreasing the plasma angiotensin Ⅱ and aldosterone levels, it can be used for treating refractory chronic heart failure, besides, it's also effective for heart failure patients who cannot be treated by digitalis, diuretics and vasodilators. |
| 用法、用量<br>Dosage | 口服：一次 25 ~ 50mg，一日 75 ~ 150mg。开始时每次 25mg，一日 3 次（饭前服用）；渐增至每次 50mg，一日 3 次。每日最大剂量为 450mg。儿童，开始每日 1mg/kg，最大 6mg/kg，分 3 次服。<br><br>Oral medication: 25 ~ 50mg one time, 75 ~ 150mg a day. At the beginning, 25mg one time, 3 times a day (before meals); increasing to 50mg one time, 3 times a day. The maximum dose per day is 450mg. For children, 1mg/kg a day at the beginning, the maximum does is 6mg/kg, in 3 divided doses. |
| 剂型、规格<br>Preparations | 片剂：12.5mg；25mg；50mg；100mg。<br>复方卡托普利片：每片含卡托普利 10mg，氢氯噻嗪 6mg。<br>Tablets: 12.5mg; 25mg; 50mg; 100mg.<br>Compound Captopril Tablets: contains 10mg captopril per tablet, 6mg hydrochlorothiazide. |

| 药品名称 Drug Names | 依那普利 Enalapril |
|---|---|
| 适应证<br>Indications | 用于高血压及充血性心力衰竭的治疗。<br>For the treatment of hypertension and congestive heart failure. |
| 用法、用量<br>Dosage | 口服 10mg，日服 1 次，必要时也可静脉注射以加速起效。可根据患者情况增加至日剂量 40mg。<br><br>Oral medication: 10mg one time, once a day, taking intravenous injection to accelerate the onset if necessary. The dose can be increased to 40mg based on the patient's condition. |
| 剂型、规格<br>Preparations | 片剂：每片 5mg；10mg；20mg。<br>Tablets: 5mg; 10mg; 20mg per tablet. |

| 药品名称 Drug Names | 贝那普利 Benazepril |
|---|---|
| 适应证<br>Indications | 　　用于各型高血压和充血性心力衰竭患者。对正在服用地高辛和利尿药的充血性心力衰竭患者可使心排血量增加，全身和肺血管阻力、平均动脉压、肺动脉压及右心房压下降。<br><br>　　For all types of hypertension and congestive heart failure patients. For Congestive heart failure patients who are taking Digoxin and Diuretics, this dose can increase their cardiac output, meanwhile, reduce systemic and pulmonary vascular resistance, drop mean arterial pressure, pulmonary artery pressure and right atrial pressure. |
| 用法、用量<br>Dosage | 　　用于降压，口服，开始剂量为一日1次10mg，然后可根据病情渐增剂量至每日40mg，一次或分2次服用。严重肾功能不全者或心力衰竭患者或服用利尿药的患者，初始剂量为每日5mg，充血性心力衰竭患者，一日剂量为2.5～20mg。<br><br>　　For lowing blood pressure, the oral medication is 10mg once a day at the beginning. Then increase the dose according to the patient's condition to 40mg a day, in one dose or 2 divided doses. For patients who are with severe renal insufficiency, suffering heart failure, or taking diuretics, the initial dose is 5mg one day; and for congestive heart failure patients, the dose is 2.5～20mg one day. |
| 剂型、规格<br>Preparations | 　　片剂：每片5mg；10mg；20mg。<br>　　Tablets: 5mg; 10mg; 20mg per tablet. |
| 药品名称 Drug Names | 培哚普利 Perindopril |
| 适应证<br>Indications | 　　用于治疗高血压。<br>　　For the treatment of hypertension. |
| 用法、用量<br>Dosage | 　　口服，一日1次4mg，可根据病情增至一日8mg。老年患者及肾功能低下患者酌情减量。<br>　　Oral medication: 4mg once a day, which can be increased to 8mg a day according to the condition. Elderly patients and patients with renal dysfunction require appropriate reductions in their doses. |
| 剂型、规格<br>Preparations | 　　片剂：每片2mg；4mg。<br>　　Tablets: 2mg; 4mg per tablet. |
| 药品名称 Drug Names | 氯沙坦 Losartan |
| 适应证<br>Indications | 　　用于高血压和充血性心力衰竭的治疗。<br>　　For the treatment of hypertension and congestive heart failure. |
| 用法、用量<br>Dosage | 　　口服，一日1次，10～100mg；一般维持量一日1次50mg，剂量增加，抗高血压效果不再增加。<br>　　Oral medication: 10～100mg one time, once a day; General maintenance dose: 50mg once a day, in this period, though the dose increases, its antihypertensive effect will no longer increase. |
| 剂型、规格<br>Preparations | 　　氯沙坦钾，片剂：50mg；100mg。<br>　　胶囊：50mg。<br>　　Losartan potassium, tablets: 50mg, 100mg.<br>　　capsule: 50mg. |
| 药品名称 Drug Names | 缬沙坦 Valsartan |
| 适应证<br>Indications | 　　用于治疗高血压。<br>　　For the treatment of hypertension. |
| 用法、用量<br>Dosage | 　　常口服其胶囊剂，每粒含80mg或160mg，每次80mg，一日1次，亦可根据需要增加至每次160mg，或加用利尿药。也可与其他降压药合用。<br><br>　　Often, take its oral capsules, each one contains a dose of 80mg or 160mg; 80mg one time, once a day. The dose can be increased to 160mg one time as needed, or be combined with diuretics; it can also be used in combination with other antihypertensive drugs. |
| 剂型、规格<br>Preparations | 　　胶囊：80mg；160mg。<br>　　Capsules: 80mg; 160mg. |
| 药品名称 Drug Names | 厄贝沙坦 Irbesartan |
| 适应证<br>Indications | 　　用于治疗原发性高血压。<br>　　For the treatment of essential hypertension. |

**续　表**

| | |
|---|---|
| 用法、用量<br>Dosage | 口服每次 150mg，一日 1 次，对血压控制不佳者可加至 300mg 或合用小剂量噻嗪类利尿药。<br>Oral medication: 150mg one time, once a day, patients who are with a poor management of blood pressure can increase their doses to 300mg, or combine low-dose thiazide diuretics for treatment. |
| 剂型、规格<br>Preparations | 片剂：每片 150mg。<br>Tablets: 150mg per tablet. |
| 药品名称 Drug Names | 坎地沙坦 Candesartan |
| 适应证<br>Indications | 用于高血压治疗。<br>For the treatment of hypertension. |
| 用法、用量<br>Dosage | 口服，每次 8 ~ 16mg，一日 1 次。也可与氨氯地平、氢氯噻嗪合用。中、重度肝、肾功能不全患者应适当调整剂量。<br>Oral medication: 8 ~ 16mg one time, once a day. It also can be used with amlodipine and hydro-chlorothiazi de. Patients suffering moderate or severe liver and kidney dysfunctionhepatic should adjust their doses appropriately. |
| 剂型、规格<br>Preparations | 坎地沙坦酯，片剂：4mg；8mg。<br>胶囊：4mg；8mg。<br>分散片：4mg。<br>Tablet: 4mg; 8mg per tablet.<br>Capsule: 4mg; 8mg per capsule.<br>Dispersible tablet: 4mg pe tablet |
| 药品名称 Drug Names | 替米沙坦 Telmisartan |
| 适应证<br>Indications | 用于原发性高血压的治疗。<br>For the treatment of essential hypertension. |
| 用法、用量<br>Dosage | 一日 1 次，每次 1 片，40mg/ 片。<br>Once a day, one tablet one time, 40mg / tablet. |
| 剂型、规格<br>Preparations | 片剂：每片 40mg。<br>Tablets: 40mg per tablet. |
| 药品名称 Drug Names | 吲达帕胺 Indapamide |
| 适应证<br>Indications | 对轻、中度原发性高血压具有良好效果。单独服用降压效果显著，不必加用其他利尿剂。可与 β 受体拮抗剂合并应用。<br>It's quite effective for the treatment of mild and moderate essential hypertension. Significant effect can be achieved by taking this dose alone, so there is no need in using other diuretics. Besides, it can be used in combination with the β receptor antagonist. |
| 用法、用量<br>Dosage | 口服：一次 2.5mg，一日 1 次，维持量可 2 天一次 2.5mg。<br>Oral medication: 2.5mg one time, once a day; the maintenance dose can be 2.5mg one time, once in two days. |
| 剂型、规格<br>Preparations | 片剂：每片 2.5mg。<br>Tablets: 2.5mg per tablet. |
| 药品名称 Drug Names | 甲基多巴 Methyldopa |
| 适应证<br>Indications | 用于中、重度、恶性高血压。<br>For the treatment of moderate, severe, and malignant hypertension. |
| 用法、用量<br>Dosage | 每次服 250mg，一日 3 次。<br>Oral medication: 250mg once, 3 times a day. |
| 剂型、规格<br>Preparations | 片剂：250mg。<br>Tablets: 250mg per tablet. |

**续 表**

| 药品名称 Drug Names | 胍乙啶 Guanethidine |
|---|---|
| 适应证<br>Indications | 用于中、重度舒张压高的高血压。<br>For the treatment of moderate and severe diastolic high blood pressure. |
| 用法、用量<br>Dosage | 开始每日 10mg，以后视病情每隔 5 ~ 7 日递增 10mg，分次服用。一般一日不超过 100mg。<br>Oral medication: 10mg a day at the beginning, take 10mg more every 5 to 7 days in divided doses depending on the condition. Generally, the does must not exceed 100mg per day. |
| 剂型、规格<br>Preparations | 片剂：10mg；25mg。<br>Tablets: 10mg; 25mg per tablet. |
| 药品名称 Drug Names | 倍他尼定 Betanidine |
| 适应证<br>Indications | 用于中、重度舒张压高的高血压。<br>For the treatment of moderate and severe diastolic high blood pressure. |
| 用法、用量<br>Dosage | 开始：一次 10mg，一日 3 次；维持：20 ~ 200mg/d。<br>At the beginning: 10mg one time, 3 times a day; for maintenance: 20 ~ 200mg / d. |
| 剂型、规格<br>Preparations | 片剂：10mg；50mg。<br>Tablets: 10mg; 50mg per tablet. |
| 药品名称 Drug Names | 异喹胍 Debrisoquine |
| 适应证<br>Indications | 用于中、重度舒张压高的高血压。<br>For the treatment of moderate and severe diastolic high blood pressure. |
| 用法、用量<br>Dosage | 开始：一次 10mg，一日 1 ~ 2 次；维持：40 ~ 120mg/d。<br>At the beginning: 10mg one time, 1 or 2 times a day; for maintenance: 40 ~ 120mg / d. |
| 剂型、规格<br>Preparations | 片剂：10mg；20mg。<br>Tablets: 10mg; 20mg per tablet. |
| 药品名称 Drug Names | 西拉普利 Cilazapril |
| 适应证<br>Indications | 用于治疗各种程度原发性高血压和肾性高血压，也可与洋地黄和（或）利尿剂合用作为治疗慢性心力衰竭的辅助药物。<br>For the treatment of various degrees of essential hypertension and renal hypertension, but it can also be used with digitalis and (or) diuretics as an adjunct to treat chronic heart failure. |
| 用法、用量<br>Dosage | 口服：一日 1 次 2.5 ~ 5mg。<br>Oral medication: 2.5 ~ 5mg once a day. |
| 剂型、规格<br>Preparations | 片剂：2.5mg；5mg。<br>Tablets: 2.5mg; 5mg per tablet. |
| 药品名称 Drug Names | 喹那普利 Quinapril |
| 适应证<br>Indications | 高血压、充血性心力衰竭。<br>For the treatment of hypertension and congestive heart failure. |
| 用法、用量<br>Dosage | 口服：一日 10 ~ 80mg，1 次或分 2 次服。<br>Oral medication: 10 ~ 80mg a day, in 1 or 2 divided doses. |
| 剂型、规格<br>Preparations | 喹那普利片：10mg。<br>Tablet: 10mg per tablet. |
| 药品名称 Drug Names | 雷米普利 Ramipril |
| 适应证<br>Indications | 用于治疗原发性高血压。<br>For the treatment of essential hypertension. |

| 用法、用量<br>Dosage | 口服：一日 1 次 2.5 ～ 5mg。<br>Oral medication: 2.5 ～ 5mg, once a day. |
| --- | --- |
| 剂型、规格<br>Preparations | 片剂：1.25mg，2.5mg，5mg。<br>Tablet: 1.25mg, 2.5mg, 5mg per tablet. |

| 药品名称 Drug Names | 咪达普利 Imidapril |
| --- | --- |
| 适应证<br>Indications | （1）原发性高血压；<br>（2）肾实质性病变所致继发性高血压。<br>（1）For the treatment of essential hypertension;<br>（2）ssecondary hypertension caused by renal parenchymal lesions. |
| 用法、用量<br>Dosage | 口服：一日 1 次 5 ～ 10mg。<br>Oral medication: 5 ～ 10mg, once a day. |
| 剂型、规格<br>Preparations | 片剂：5mg；10mg。<br>Tablets: 5mg; 10mg per tablet. |

| 药品名称 Drug Names | 赖诺普利 Lisinopril |
| --- | --- |
| 适应证<br>Indications | 用于高血压和充血性心力衰竭。<br>For the treatment of hypertension and congestive heart failure. |
| 用法、用量<br>Dosage | 口服：一日 1 次 5 ～ 20mg。最多一日不超过 80mg。<br>Oral medication: 5 ～ 20mg, once a day. The maximum dose of one day must not exceed 80mg. |
| 剂型、规格<br>Preparations | 片剂：5mg；10mg；20mg。<br>Tablets: 5mg; 10mg; 20mg per tablet. |

| 药品名称 Drug Names | 福辛普利 Fosinopril |
| --- | --- |
| 适应证<br>Indications | 适用于治疗高血压和心力衰竭。治疗高血压时，可单独使用作为初始治疗药物，或与其他抗高血压药物联合使用。治疗心力衰竭时，可与利尿剂合用。<br>For the treatment of hypertension and heart failure. It can be used as initial therapy alone or in combination with other antihypertensive drugs to treat hypertension. Besides, it can be combined with diuretics to treat heart failure. |
| 用法、用量<br>Dosage | 口服：一日 1 次 5 ～ 40mg。最大剂量一日 80mg。<br>Oral medication: 5 ～ 40mg, once a day. The maximum dose of one day is 80mg. |
| 剂型、规格<br>Preparations | 片剂：10mg；20mg。<br>Tablets: 10mg; 20mg per tablet. |

10.7　抗休克的血管活性药 Antishock vasoactive drugs

| 药品名称 Drug Names | 去甲肾上腺素 Norepinephrine (Noradrenaline) |
| --- | --- |
| 适应证<br>Indications | 临床上主要用它的升压作用，静脉滴注用于各种休克（但出血性休克禁用），以升高血压，保证对重要器官（如脑）的血液供应。<br>Clinically, it's mainly used to increase blood pressure through intravenous infusion when a variety of shocks occurs (but prohibited for hemorrhagic shock), so as to ensure the blood supply to vital organs (such as the brain). |
| 用法、用量<br>Dosage | （1）静脉滴注：临用前稀释，每分钟滴入 4 ～ 10μg，根据病情调整剂量。可用 1 ～ 2mg 加入生理盐水或 5% 葡萄糖注射液 100ml 内静脉滴注，根据情况掌握滴注速度，待血压升至所需水平后，减慢滴速，以维持血压正常范围。如效果不好，应换用其他升压药。对危急病例可用 1 ～ 2mg 稀释到 10 ～ 20ml，徐徐注射入静脉，同时根据血压以调节其剂量，待血压回升后，再用滴注法维持。<br>（2）口服：治疗上消化道出血，每次服注射液 1 ～ 3ml（1 ～ 3mg），一日 3 次，加入适量冷盐水服下。 |

|  | (1) Intravenous infusion: dilute it before clinical usage, drip 4 ~ 10μg per minute, and adjust the dose according to the disease. Add 1 ~ 2mg into normal saline or 100ml 5% glucose injection for intravenous infusion, the infusion speed should be adjusted based on the condition; slow down the drip rate when blood pressure rises to the required level, so as to maintain the blood pressure in a normal range. If ineffective, it should be replaced by other vasopressors. For emergency cases, 1 ~ 2mg doses can be diluted to 10 ~ 20ml, then being slowly injected into the vein, at the same time, adjusting the dose according to blood pressure. Keep instilling after the blood pressure rises.<br><br>(2) Oral medication: for the treatment of gastrointestinal bleeding; adding the right amount of cold saline, 1 ~ 3ml (1 ~ 3mg) injection one time, three times a day. |
| --- | --- |
| 剂型、规格<br>Preparations | 注射液：每支 2mg（1ml）（以重酒石酸盐计）；10mg（2ml）（以重酒石酸盐计）。<br>Injection: 2mg (1ml) (measured by batartrate); 10mg (2ml) (measured by batartrate) per vial. |
| 药品名称 Drug Names | 去氧肾上腺素 Phenylephrine |
| 适应证<br>Indications | 用于感染中毒性及过敏性休克、室上性心动过速、防治全身麻醉及腰麻时的低血压。眼科用于散瞳检查，特点是作用时间短，不麻痹调节功能，不引起眼压升高。<br><br>For the treatment of septic and anaphylactic shock, ventricular tachycardia, preventing the hypotension caused by general anesthesia and lumbar anesthesia. In ophthalmology, it's used in dilated eye examination, which is characterized by short effect duration, no paralysis on adjustment function, and no increase of intraocular pressure. |
| 用法、用量<br>Dosage | （1）肌内注射或静脉滴注：①常用量：肌内注射，一次 2 ~ 5mg；静脉滴注，一次 10 ~ 20mg。稀释后缓慢滴注。②极量：肌内注射，一次 10mg；静脉滴注，每分钟 0.1mg。<br>（2）滴眼：用于散瞳检查，用 2% ~ 5% 溶液滴眼。<br><br>(1) Intramuscular injection or intravenous infusion: ① usual dose: for intramuscular injection, 2 ~ 5mg once; for intravenous infusion, 10 ~ 20mg once, requiring slow infusion after dilution. ② the maximum dose: for intramuscular injection, 10mg once; for intravenous infusion, 0.1mg per minute.<br>(2) eye drops: for the dilated eye examination, 2% to 5% solution drops. |
| 剂型、规格<br>Preparations | 注射液：每支 10mg（1ml）。滴眼剂：为 2% ~ 5% 溶液。<br>Injection: 10mg (1ml) per vial. Eye drops: 2% to 5% solution. |
| 药品名称 Drug Names | 甲氧胺 Methoxamine |
| 适应证<br>Indications | 用于外科手术，以维持或恢复动脉压，尤其适用于脊椎麻醉造成的血压降低。又用于大出血、创伤及外科手术所引起的低血压、心肌梗死所致休克以及室上性心动过速。<br><br>It's used in surgery, to maintain or restore arterial pressure, especially to relieve the low blood pressure caused by spinal anesthesia. It's also used to treat the hypotension caused by bleeding, trauma and surgery, shock due to myocardial infarction, and ventricular tachycardia. |
| 用法、用量<br>Dosage | （1）肌内注射、静脉注射或静脉滴注：①常用量：肌内注射，一次 10 ~ 20mg；静脉注射：一次 5 ~ 10mg；静脉滴注，一次 20 ~ 60mg，稀释后缓慢滴注。②极量：肌内注射，一次 20mg，一日 60mg；静脉注射：一次 10mg。<br>（2）对急症病例或收缩压降至 8kPa（60mmHg）甚至更低的病例，缓慢静脉注射 5 ~ 10mg，注射一次量不超过 10mg，并严密观察血压变动。静脉注射后，继续肌内注射 15mg，以维持较长药效。<br>（3）对室上性心动过速病例，用 10 ~ 20mg，以 5% 葡萄糖注射液 100ml 稀释，做静脉滴注。也可用 10mg 加入 5% ~ 10% 葡萄糖注射液 20ml 中缓缓静脉注射。注射时应观察心率及血压，当心率突然减慢时，应停注。<br>（4）对处理心肌梗死的休克病例，开始肌内注射 15mg，接着静脉滴注，静脉滴注液为 5% ~ 10% 葡萄糖注射液 500ml 内含本品 60mg，滴速应随血压反应而调整，每分钟不宜超过 20 滴。 |

续　表

| | |
|---|---|
| | (1) Intramuscular injection, intravenous injection or intravenous infusion: ① usual dose: for intramuscular injection, 10 ~ 20mg once; for intravenous injection: 5 ~ 10mg once; for intravenous infusion, 20 ~ 60mg once, requiring slow drip after dilution. ② the maximum dose: for intramuscular injection, 20mg one time, 60mg a day; for intravenous injection: 10mg once.<br><br>(2) For emergency cases, or patient whose systolic blood pressure has dropped to 8kPa (60mmHg) or even lower, a slow intravenous injection of 5 ~ 10mg is needed, the injection must not exceed 10mg one time, at the same time, closely observe changes of blood pressure. After intravenous injection, another 15mg intramuscular injection should be given, so as to maintain a longer efficacy.<br><br>(3) For supraventricular tachycardia cases, dilute 10 ~ 20mg solution with 100ml 5% glucose injection for intravenous infusion; or add 10mg into 20ml 5% to 10% glucose injection to do intravenous injection slowly. Heart rate and blood pressure should be observed during injection, when the heart rate suddenly slows down, you should stop injection.<br><br>(4) Cases of shock caused by myocardial infarction, first take 15mg for intramuscular injection, then begin intravenous infusion, the solution for intravenous infusion is 500ml 5% to 10% glucose injection containing 60mg dose of methoxamine; The drip rate should be adjusted with the blood pressure, not exceed 20 drops per minute. |
| 剂型、规格<br>Preparations | 注射液：每支 10mg（1ml）；20mg（1ml）。<br>Injection: 10mg (1ml); 20mg (1ml) per vial. |
| 药品名称 Drug Names | 间羟胺 Metaraminol |
| 适应证<br>Indications | 用于各种休克及手术时低血压。在一般用量下，不致引起心律失常，因此也可用于心肌梗死性休克。<br><br>For the treatment of shocks and hypotension caused by surgery . Since under normal usage, it will not cause arrhythmias, therefore, it can also be used for myocardial infarction shock. |
| 用法、用量<br>Dosage | （1）肌内注射或静脉滴注：① 常用量：肌内注射一次 10 ~ 20mg；静脉滴注，一次 10 ~ 40mg，稀释后缓慢滴注，如以 15 ~ 100mg 加入 0.9% 氯化钠注射液或 5% ~ 10% 葡萄糖注射液 250 ~ 500ml 中静脉滴注，每分钟 20 ~ 30 滴，用量及滴速随血压情况而定。② 极量：静脉滴注一次 100mg（每分钟 0.2 ~ 0.4mg）。<br><br>（2）局部鼻充血可用 0.25% ~ 0.5% 的等渗缓冲液（pH=6）每小时喷入或滴入 2 ~ 3 滴，每天不超过 4 次，1 个疗程为 7 日。<br><br>(1) Intramuscular injection or intravenous infusion: ① usual dose: for intramuscular injection, 10 ~ 20mg once; for intravenous infusion, 10 ~ 40mg once, requiring slow drip after dilution, for example, if you add 15 ~ 100mg into 0.9% sodium chloride injection or 250 ~ 500ml 5% to 10% glucose injection for intravenous infusion, 20 to 30 drops per minute, the dosage and drip should be adjusted with blood pressure conditions. ② the maximum dose: for intravenous infusion, 100mg once(0.2 ~ 0.4mg per minute).<br><br>(2) Topical nasal decongestants: 2 ~ 3 drops of 0.25% to 0.5% isotonic buffer (pH = 6) can be sprayed or dripped into nose per hour, no more than four times a day, a course of treatment is seven days. |
| 剂型、规格<br>Preparations | 注射液：每支 10mg（1ml）（以间羟胺计）；50mg（5ml）（以间羟胺计）。<br>Injection: 10mg (1ml) (measured by metaraminol); 50mg (5ml) (measured by metaraminol) per vial. |
| 药品名称 Drug Names | 肾上腺素 Epinephrine（Adrenaline） |
| 适应证<br>Indications | 用于抢救过敏性休克、心搏骤停、支气管哮喘急性发作。与局部麻醉药合用延长其药效。<br><br>For rescuing anaphylactic shock, cardiac arrest, acute exacerbation of bronchial asthma. Its efficacy can be extended by being combined with local anesthetics. |
| 用法、用量<br>Dosage | 常用量：皮下注射，一次 0.25 ~ 1mg；心室内注射，一次 0.25 ~ 1mg。极量：皮下注射，一次 1mg。<br><br>Usual dose: for subcutaneous injection, 0.25 ~ 1mg one time; for intraventricular injection, 0.25 ~ 1mg one time. Maximum dose: for subcutaneously, 1mg one time. |
| 剂型、规格<br>Preparations | 注射液：1mg（1ml）。<br>Injection: 1mg (1ml) per vial. |

**续　表**

| 药品名称 Drug Names | 多巴胺 Dopamine |
|---|---|
| 适应证<br>Indications | 用于各种类型休克，包括中毒性休克、心源性休克、出血性休克、中枢性休克，特别对伴有肾功能不全、心排血量降低、周围血管阻力增高而已补足血容量的患者更有意义。<br><br>For the treatment of all types of shocks, including toxic shock, cardiogenic shock, hemorrhagic shock and central shock. It's of particularly significance for patients with renal dysfunction, reduced cardiac output, and with increased peripheral vascular resistance while whose blood volumes have been made up. |
| 用法、用量<br>Dosage | 静脉注射，一次 20mg，稀释后缓慢滴注；极量，每分钟 20μg/kg。将 20mg 加入 5% 葡萄糖注射液 200 ～ 300ml 中静脉滴注，开始每分钟 20 滴左右（即每分钟滴入 75 ～ 100μg），以后根据血压情况，可加快速度或加大浓度。<br><br>For intravenous injection, 20mg once, requiring slow infusion after dilution; Maximum dose 20μg/kg per minute. Add 20mg into 200 ～ 300ml 5% glucose injection for intravenous infusion, about 20 drops per minute (ie drip 75 ～ 100μg per minute) at the beginning, later can speed up or increase the concentration according to blood pressure. |
| 剂型、规格<br>Preparations | 注射液：每支 20mg（2ml）。<br>Injection: per 20mg (2ml) per vial. |
| 药品名称 Drug Names | 多巴酚丁胺 Dobutamine |
| 适应证<br>Indications | 用于心排血量低和心率慢的心力衰竭患者，其改善左心室功能的作用优于多巴胺。<br><br>For heart failure patients with low cardiac output and slow heart rate, it works better than dopamine in improvement of left ventricular function. |
| 用法、用量<br>Dosage | 静脉滴注：250mg 加入 5% 葡萄糖注射液 250ml 或 500ml 中滴注，每分钟 2.5 ～ 10μg/kg。<br><br>For intravenous infusion: Add 250mg into 250 or 500ml 5% glucose injection for infusion, 2.5 ～ 10μg/kg per minute. |
| 剂型、规格<br>Preparations | 注射液：每支 20mg（按多巴酚丁胺计）（2ml）；200mg（按多巴酚丁胺计）（2ml）。<br>Injection: 20mg (measured by dobutamine) (2ml); 200mg (measured by dobutamine) (2ml) per vial. |
| 药品名称 Drug Names | 血管紧张素胺 Angiotensinamide |
| 适应证<br>Indications | 用于外伤或手术后休克和全身麻醉或腰椎麻醉时所致的低血压症等。<br><br>For the treatment of shocks caused by and trauma or surgery, and hypotension caused by general anesthesia or spinal anesthesia. |
| 用法、用量<br>Dosage | 静脉滴注：每次 1 ～ 1.25mg，溶解于 5% 葡萄糖或 0.9% 氯化钠注射液 500ml 中，滴速一般每分钟 3 ～ 10μg，应经常测定血压，随时调整滴速。<br><br>For Intravenous infusion: 1 ～ 1.25mg one time, dissolve it in 500ml 5% glucose or 0.9% sodium chloride injection, generally drip 3 ～ 10μg per minute, blood pressure should always be measured, adjust the drip rate at all times. |
| 剂型、规格<br>Preparations | 注射用血管紧张素胺：每支 1mg。<br>Angiotensinamine for injection: 1mg per vial. |

10.8 调节血脂药及抗动脉粥样硬化药 Blood lipid regulating drugs and antiatherosclerosis drugs

| 药品名称 Drug Names | 氯贝丁酯 Clofibrate |
|---|---|
| 适应证<br>Indications | 用于动脉粥样硬化及其继发症，如冠状动脉病、脑血管疾病、周围血管病及糖尿病所致动脉疾病等。<br><br>For the treatment of atherosclerosis and its secondary disease, such as coronary artery disease, cerebrovascular disease, peripheral vascular disease and diabetes-induced arterial disease. |
| 用法、用量<br>Dosage | 口服，一次 0.25 ～ 0.5g，一日 3 次，饭后服。<br>Oral medication: 0.25 ～ 0.5g once, 3 times a day, after meals. |
| 剂型、规格<br>Preparations | 胶囊剂：每粒 0.25g；0.5g。<br>Capsules: 0.25g; 0.5g per capsule. |

**续　表**

| 药品名称 Drug Names | 非诺贝特 Fenofibrate |
|---|---|
| 适应证 Indications | 用于高胆固醇血症、高三酰甘油血症及混合性高脂血症，疗效确切，且耐受性好。<br>For the treatment of hypercholesterolemia, hypertriglyceridemia, and mixed hyperlipidemia, it's effective and well tolerated. |
| 用法、用量 Dosage | 口服：一次 100mg，一日 2～3 次。<br>Oral medication: 100mg once, 2 to 3 times a day. |
| 剂型、规格 Preparations | 胶囊（片）剂；每粒（片）100mg；200mg；300mg。<br>Capsules (tablets): 100mg; 200mg; 300mg per capsule(tablet). |
| 药品名称 Drug Names | 洛伐他汀 Lovastatin |
| 适应证 Indications | 用于原发性高胆固醇血症（Ⅱa 及Ⅱb 型）。也用于合并有高胆固醇血症和高三酰甘油血症，而以高胆固醇血症为主的患者。<br>For the treatment of primary hypercholesterolemia (Ⅱa and Ⅱb type). It's also used to treat patients who are with both hypercholesterolemia and hypertriglyceridemia, while hypercholesterolemia being the main symptom. |
| 用法、用量 Dosage | 口服，开始剂量一日 1 次 20mg，晚餐时服用，必要时于 4 周内调整剂量，最大剂量一日 80mg，1 次或分 2 次服。<br>Oral medication: starting dose is 20mg, once a day, take at dinner; if necessary, adjust the dose in 4 weeks, the maximum dose is 80mg a day, in 1 time or 2 divided doses. |
| 剂型、规格 Preparations | 片剂：每片 10mg；20mg；40mg。<br>Tablets: 10mg; 20mg; 40mg per tablet. |
| 药品名称 Drug Names | 辛伐他汀 Simvastatin |
| 适应证 Indications | 用于原发性高胆固醇血症（Ⅱa 及Ⅱb 型）。也用于合并有高胆固醇血症和高三酰甘油血症，而以高胆固醇血症为主的患者。<br>For the treatment of primary hypercholesterolemia (Ⅱa and Ⅱb type). It's also used to treat patients who are with both hypercholesterolemia and hypertriglyceridemia, while hypercholesterolemia being the main symptom. |
| 用法、用量 Dosage | 口服，一日 1 次 10mg，晚餐时服，必要时于 4 周内增量至一日 1 次 40mg。<br>Oral medication: 10mg, once a day, take at dinner; when necessary, within 4 weeks increase the dose to 40mg, once a day. |
| 剂型、规格 Preparations | 片剂：每片 10mg；20mg。<br>Tablets: 10mg; 20mg per tablet. |
| 药品名称 Drug Names | 普伐他汀 Pravastatin |
| 适应证 Indications | 用于原发性高胆固醇血症（Ⅱa 及Ⅱb 型）。也用于合并有高胆固醇血症和高三酰甘油血症，而以高胆固醇血症为主的患者。<br>For the treatment of primary hypercholesterolemia (Ⅱa and Ⅱb type). It's also used to treat patients who are with both hypercholesterolemia and hypertriglyceridemia, while hypercholesterolemia being the main symptom. |
| 用法、用量 Dosage | 口服，一日 10mg，分 2 次服，可根据情况增量至一日 20mg。<br>Oral medication: 10mg a day, in 2 divided doses; the dose can be increased to 20mg a day according to conditions. |
| 剂型、规格 Preparations | 片剂：每片 5mg；10mg。<br>Tablets: 5mg; 10mg per tablet. |
| 药品名称 Drug Names | 氟伐他汀 Fluvastatin |
| 适应证 Indications | 用于饮食控制无效的高胆固醇血症。<br>For the treatment of hypercholesterolemia which cannot be relieved by diet control. |

**续　表**

| | |
|---|---|
| 用法、用量<br>Dosage | 用量：口服一日 1 次 20mg，晚间服用。<br>Dosage: oral medication, 20mg, once a day, take in the evening. |
| 剂型、规格<br>Preparations | 胶囊剂：每粒 20mg；40mg。<br>Capsules: 20mg; 40mg per capsule. |
| 药品名称 Drug Names | 阿托伐他汀 Atorvastatin |
| 适应证<br>Indications | 用于原发性高胆固醇血症、混合型高脂血症或饮食控制无效杂合子家族型高胆固醇血症患者。<br>For the treatment of patients with primary hypercholesterolemia, mixed hyperlipidemia, or patients with familial hypercholesterolemia that cannot be relieved by diet control. |
| 用法、用量<br>Dosage | 口服：每日 10mg，如需要，4 周后可增至每日 80mg。<br>Oral medication: 10mg a day, if necessary, increase the dose to 80mg a day after 4 weeks. |
| 剂型、规格<br>Preparations | 片剂：每片 10mg；20mg；40mg。<br>Tablets: 10mg; 20mg; 40mg per tablet. |
| 药品名称 Drug Names | 瑞舒伐他汀 Rosuvastatin |
| 适应证<br>Indications | 用于高脂血症和高胆固醇血症。<br>For the treatment of hyperlipidemia and hypercholesterolemia. |
| 用法、用量<br>Dosage | 口服，一日 5 ~ 40mg，开始治疗时应从 10mg 开始，需要时增至 20 ~ 40mg，不宜开始时直接用 40mg。<br>Oral medication: 5 ~ 40mg one day, starting dose is 10mg; if necessary, increase the dose to 20 ~ 40mg, do not use 40mg directly at the beginning. |
| 剂型、规格<br>Preparations | 片剂：每片 5mg；10mg；20mg。<br>Tablets: 5mg; 10mg; 20mg per tablet. |
| 药品名称 Drug Names | 普罗布考 Probucol |
| 适应证<br>Indications | 用于Ⅱa 型高脂血症，与其他降脂药物可用于Ⅱb 和Ⅲ、Ⅳ型高脂血症。<br>For the treatment of Ⅱa hyperlipidemia, and it can be used with other lipid-lowering drugs to treat Ⅱb and Ⅲ, Ⅳ hyperlipidemia. |
| 用法、用量<br>Dosage | 口服，每次 500mg，一日 2 次，早、晚餐时服用。<br>Oral medication: 500mg one time, 2 times a day, take at breakfast and at dinner. |
| 剂型、规格<br>Preparations | 片剂：每片 500mg。<br>Tablets: 500mg per tablet. |
| 药品名称 Drug Names | 考来烯胺 Colestyramine |
| 适应证<br>Indications | 用于Ⅱ型高脂血症、动脉粥样硬化以及肝硬化、胆石病引起的瘙痒。其缺点是用量大，约2% 的患者产生胃肠道反应。<br>For the treatment of itching caused by type Ⅱ hyperlipidemia, atherosclerosis, cirrhosis and cholelithiasis. The disadvantage is that it has to be used in a large amount, about 2% of the patients will have gastrointestinal reactions. |
| 用法、用量<br>Dosage | (1) 治疗动脉粥样硬化：一日 3 次，每次服粉剂 4 ~ 5g。<br>(2) 止痒：开始时一日量 6 ~ 10g，维持量每日 3g，分 3 次服。<br>(1) For the treatment of atherosclerosis: 3 times a day, 4 ~ 5g in powder once.<br>(2) Itching: starting dose is 6 ~ 10g a day; maintenance dose is 3g a day, in 3 divided doses. |
| 剂型、规格<br>Preparations | 散剂：每包 4g。<br>Powder: 4g per pack. |
| 药品名称 Drug Names | 依折麦布 Ezetimibe |
| 适应证<br>Indications | 治疗原发性高端固醇血症。<br>For the treatment of primary hypercholesterolemia. |

**续　表**

| | |
|---|---|
| 用法、用量<br>Dosage | 一日 1 次，每次 10mg，可单独服用或与他汀类联合应用。<br>10mg, once a day, it can be taken alone or in combination with statins. |
| 剂型、规格<br>Preparations | 片剂：每片 10mg。<br>Tablets: 10mg per tablet. |
| 药品名称 Drug Names | 血脂康 Xuezhikang |
| 适应证<br>Indications | 治疗动脉粥样硬化及原发性高脂血症。<br>For the treatment of atherosclerosis and primary hyperlipidemia. |
| 用法、用量<br>Dosage | 口服每次 2 粒，一日 2 次。<br>Oral medication: 2 tablets one time, 2 times a day. |
| 剂型、规格<br>Preparations | 胶囊（丸）：每粒 0.3g。<br>Capsules (pills): 0.3g per capsule. |
| 药品名称 Drug Names | 心脑康 Xinnaokang |
| 适应证<br>Indications | 用于治疗动脉粥样硬化、冠心病、心绞痛、高脂血症、高血压、脑动脉硬化、偏瘫（脑出血和脑血栓形成）等。亦可作为动脉粥样硬化症的预防用药。<br>For the treatment of atherosclerosis, coronary heart disease, angina, hyperlipidemia, hypertension, cerebral arteriosclerosis, hemiplegia (caused by cerebral hemorrhage and cerebral thrombosis) and so on. It can also be used as prophylaxis to treat atherosclerosis. |
| 用法、用量<br>Dosage | 口服：每次 2 粒，一日 3 次，饭后服用，1 个月为 1 个疗程，一般以连用 2～3 个疗程为宜。偏瘫患者每次 3 粒，一日 3 次，连服至症状好转或基本痊愈。<br>Oral medication: two pills one time, three times a day, take after meals; a course of treatment is one month, generally, two to three courses are appropriate. For hemiplegic patients, three pills one time, three times a day, insist taking until gaining improvement or basic recovery. |
| 剂型、规格<br>Preparations | 软胶囊剂：每粒 415mg。<br>Soft capsules: 415mg per capsule. |

11. 主要作用于呼吸系统的药物 Drugs mainly acting on the respiratory system

11.1 祛痰药 Expectorants

| | |
|---|---|
| 药品名称 Drug Names | 氯化铵 Ammonium Chloride |
| 适应证<br>Indications | 用于急性呼吸道炎症时痰黏稠不易咳出者。常与其他复方制剂合用。纠正代谢性碱中毒。其酸化尿液作用可使一些需要在酸性尿液中显效的药物产生作用。也可增加汞剂的利尿作用以及四环素和青霉素的抗菌作用；还可促进碱性药物的排泄。<br>It is used to treat patients with sputum ropy due to acute respiratory inflammation. Usually, it can be used in combination with other compound preparation, and relieve metabolic alkalosis. It can increase the diuretic effect of amalgam and the antibacterial effect of tetracycline and penicillin. It also can promote the excretion of alkaline drugs. |
| 用法、用量<br>Dosage | ①祛痰：口服，成人一次 0.3～0.6g，一日 3 次。②治疗代谢性碱中毒或酸化尿液：静脉滴注，每日 2～20g，每小时不超过 5g。<br>① Expelling phlegm: oral medication, 0.3~0.6g once for adults, 3 times a day. ② For treatment of metabolic alkalosis or acidification of urine: intravenous drip, 2～20g a day, less than 5g per hour. |
| 剂型、规格<br>Preparations | 片剂：每片 0.3mg。<br>注射液：每支 5g（500ml）。<br>Tablets: 0.3mg per tablet.<br>Injections: 5g (500ml) per vial. |
| 药品名称 Drug Names | 溴己新 Bromhexine |
| 适应证<br>Indications | 用于慢性支气管炎、哮喘、支气管扩张、矽肺等有白色痰液不易咳出的患者，脓性痰患者需加用抗生素控制感染。<br>It is used to treat patients with white sputum due to chronic bronchitis, asthma, bronchiectasis, and silicosis. Antibiotics should be added to control infection for patients with purulent sputum. |

**续 表**

| | |
|---|---|
| 用法、用量<br>Dosage | 口服：成人一次 8 ~ 16mg。肌内注射：一次 4 ~ 8mg，一日 2 次。静脉注射：一日 4 ~ 8mg，加入 5% 葡萄糖氯化钠溶液 500ml 中。气雾吸入：一次 2ml，一日 2 ~ 3 次。<br><br>Oral medication: 8 ~ 16mg once for adults, 2 times a day. Intramuscular injection: 4 ~ 8mg one time, 2 times a day. Intravenous injection: 4 ~ 8mg per day, dissolved in 500 ml 5% glucose saline. Inhalation: 2ml one time, 2 to 3 times a day. |
| 剂型、规格<br>Preparations | 片剂：每片 4mg；8mg。注射液：每支 0.2%，2mg（1ml）；4mg（2ml）。气雾剂：0.2% 溶液。<br><br>Tablets: 4 mg or 8 mg per tablet. Injections: 0.2%, 2mg (1ml);4mg (2ml) per vial. Aerosol: 0.2% solution. |
| 药品名称 Drug Names | 氨溴索 Ambroxol |
| 适应证<br>Indications | 用于急慢性支气管炎及支气管哮喘、支气管扩张、肺气肿、肺结核、肺尘埃沉着病、术后的咳痰困难等。注射药可用于术后肺部并发症的预防及早产儿、新生儿呼吸窘迫综合征的治疗。本品高剂量有降低血浆尿酸浓度和促进尿酸排泄的作用。可用于治疗痛风。<br><br>It is used to treat patients who have difficulty in expectoration due to acute and chronic bronchitis and bronchial asthma, bronchiectasis, emphysema, tuberculosis, pneumoconiosis, after operation. Injection drug can be used for the prevention of postoperative pulmonary complications, and the treatment of premature and neonatal respiratory distress syndrome. It can be used for the treatment of gout at a high dose due to reducing plasma uric acid concentrations and promoting uric acid excretion. |
| 用法、用量<br>Dosage | 口服：成人及 12 岁以上儿童，每次 30mg，一日 3 次。长期使用剂量可减半。静脉注射、肌内注射及皮下注射：成人每次 15mg，一日 2 次。亦可加入生理盐水或葡萄糖溶液中静脉滴注。<br><br>Oral medication: 30 mg once for adults and children over 12 years, 3 times a day. The dose can be halved for long-term use. Intravenous, intramuscular and subcutaneous injection: 15 mg once for adults, 2 times a day. It also can be dissolved in saline or glucose solution for intravenous injection. |
| 剂型、规格<br>Preparations | 片剂：每片 15mg；30mg。<br>胶囊剂：每粒 30mg。<br>缓释胶囊：每粒 75mg。<br>口服溶液剂：每支 15mg（5ml）；180mg（60ml）；300mg（100ml）；600mg（100ml）。<br>气雾剂：每瓶 15mg（2ml）。<br>注射液：每支 15mg（2ml）。<br><br>Tablets: 15 mg; 30 mg per tablet.<br>Capsules: 30 mg per capsule .<br>Release capsules: 75 mg per release capsules.<br>Oral solution: 15mg (5ml); 180mg (60ml); 300mg (100ml); 600mg (100ml) per bottle.<br>Aerosol: 15mg (2ml) per bottle. Injections: 15mg (2ml) per vial. |
| 药品名称 Drug Names | 乙酰半胱氨酸 Acetylcysteine |
| 适应证<br>Indications | ①用于术后、急慢性支气管炎、支气管扩张、肺结核、肺炎、肺气肿等引起的黏稠分泌物过多所致的咳痰困难。②用于对乙酰氨基酚中毒的解毒以及环磷酰胺引起的出血性膀胱炎的治疗。<br><br>① It is used to treat patients who have difficulty in expectoration for sticky excessive secretions due to afteroperation, acute and chronic bronchitis, bronchiectasis, tuberculosis, pneumonia, emphysema, etc. ② It can be used for detoxification of acetaminophen poisoning and the treatment of cyclophosphamide-induced hemorrhagic cystitis. |
| 用法、用量<br>Dosage | （1）喷雾吸入：仅用于非紧急情况下，临用下溶解于氯化钠液中成 10% 溶液，每次 1 ~ 3ml，一日 2 ~ 3 次。<br>（2）气管滴入：急救时 5% 溶液经气管插管或气管套管直接滴入，每次 0.5 ~ 2ml，一日 2 ~ 4 次。<br>（3）气管注入：急救时 5% 溶液用 1ml 注射器自自管的甲状软骨环骨膜处注入管腔内，每次 0.5 ~ 2ml（婴儿每次 0.5ml，儿童每次 1ml，成人每次 2ml）。<br>（4）口服：成人每次 200mg，一日 2 ~ 3 次。<br><br>(1) Spray inhalation: Only for non-emergency situations, dissolved in sodium chloride solution to make up a 10% solution under temporary use, 1 ~ 3ml one time, 2 to 3 times a day.<br>(2) Intratracheal instillation: direct instillation via intubation or tracheostomy tube with 5% solution in emergency circumstances, 0.5 ~ 2ml once, 2 to 4 times a day. |

续　表

|  | (3) Tracheal injection:1ml 5% solution in syringe is injected from the periosteum of the thyroid cartilage into the lumen in emergency circumstances. 0.5 ~ 2ml one time (0.5ml once for baby, 1ml once for children, 2ml once for adults).<br>(4) Oral medication: 200mg once for adults, 2 or 3 times a day. |
|---|---|
| 剂型、规格<br>Preparations | 片剂：每片 200mg；500mg。<br>喷雾剂：每瓶 0.5g；1g。<br>颗粒剂：每袋 100mg。<br>泡腾片：每片 600mg。<br>Tablets: 200mg or 500mg per tablet.<br>Spray: 0.5g or 1g per bottle.<br>Granules: 100mg per bag.<br>Effervescent tablets: 600mg per tablet. |
| 药品名称 Drug Names | 羧甲司坦 Carbocysteine |
| 适应证<br>Indications | 用于慢性支气管炎、支气管哮喘等引起的痰液黏稠、咳痰困难和痰阻气管等。亦可用于术后咳痰困难和肺炎合并症。用于小儿非化脓性中耳炎，有预防耳聋效果。<br>It is used to treat patients with ropy sputum, difficulty in expectoration, and stagnation of phlegm due to chronic bronchitis and bronchial asthma. It can also be used for treating difficult expectoration and postoperative pneumonia complications. And for non-suppurative otitis media in children, effective to prevent deafness. |
| 用法、用量<br>Dosage | 口服，成人每次 0.25 ~ 0.5g，一日 3 次。儿童 1 日 30mg/kg。<br>Oral medication: 0.25 ~ 0.5g once for adults, 3 times a day. 30mg/kg a day for children. |
| 剂型、规格<br>Preparations | 口服液：每支 0.2g（10ml）；0.5g（10ml）。<br>糖浆剂：2%（20mg/ml）。<br>片剂：每片 0.25g。<br>泡腾剂：每包 0.25g。<br>Oral solution: 0.2g (10ml) or 0.5g (10ml) of each.<br>Syrup: 2% (20mg/ml).<br>Tablets: 0.25g per tablet.<br>Effervescent: 0.25g per pack. |
| 药品名称 Drug Names | 标准桃金娘油 Gelomyrtol |
| 适应证<br>Indications | 用于急、慢性支气管炎、鼻窦炎、支气管扩张、肺结核、矽肺及各种原因引起的慢性阻塞性肺疾病。亦可用于支气管造影术后，可促进造影剂的排除。<br>For the treatment of chronic obstructive pulmonary disease (COPD) due to acute and chronic bronchitis, sinusitis, bronchiectasis, tuberculosis and silicosis etc. It also can be used for promoting the exclusion of contrast agents after bronchial angiography. |
| 用法、用量<br>Dosage | 口服。成人：每次 300mg，一日 2 ~ 3 次；4 ~ 10 岁儿童：每次 120mg，一日 2 次。<br>Oral medication: 300mg once for adults, 2 or 3 times a day; 120mg once for 4 to 10 years old children, 1 to 2 times a day. |
| 剂型、规格<br>Preparations | 胶囊剂：每粒 120mg；300mg。<br>Capsules: 120 mg or 300 mg per capsule. |
| 药品名称 Drug Names | 碘化钾 Potassium Iodide |
| 适应证<br>Indications | 为刺激性祛痰剂，可使痰液变稀，易于咳出，并可增加支气管分泌。配成含碘食盐制剂，预防地方性甲状腺肿。<br>It's worked as irritating expectorant for diluting sputum, and can increase bronchial secretion. It can be confected into iodized salt to prevent endemic goiter. |
| 用法、用量<br>Dosage | 口服：每次 6 ~ 10ml，一日 3 次。<br>Oral medication: 6~10 ml once, 3 times a day. |

**续　表**

| 剂型、规格<br>Preparations | 合剂：每 100ml 含碘化钾 5g。<br>Mixture: per 100ml solution contains 5g potassium iodide. |
|---|---|

| 药品名称 Drug Names | 美司钠 Mesna |
|---|---|
| 适应证<br>Indications | 用于慢性支气管炎、肺炎、肺癌患者痰液黏稠、术后肺不张等所致咳痰困难者。<br>For the treatment of patients with expectoration difficulties due to chronic bronchitis, pneumonia, lung cancer-induced sputum viscosity, and postoperative atelectasis etc. |
| 用法、用量<br>Dosage | 雾化吸入或气管内滴入，每次 20% 溶液 1～2ml。局部刺激作用，可引起咳嗽及支气管痉挛。不宜与红霉素、四环素、氨茶碱合用。<br>Inhalation or intratracheal instillation: 1～2ml 20% solution once. Its local irritation can cause coughing and bronchospasm, and it cannot be combined with erythromycin, tetracycline and theophylline. |
| 剂型、规格<br>Preparations | 气雾剂：0.2g/ml。溶液剂：10% 水溶液。<br>Aerosol: 0.2g/ml. Solutions: 10% aqueous solution. |

| 11.2 镇咳药 Antitussives |
|---|

| 药品名称 Drug Names | 可待因 Codeine |
|---|---|
| 适应证<br>Indications | ①各种原因引起的剧烈干咳和刺激性咳嗽，尤适用于伴有胸痛的剧烈咳嗽。由于本品能抑制呼吸道腺体分泌和纤毛运动，故对少量痰液的剧烈咳嗽，应与祛痰药并用。②用于中度疼痛的镇痛。③局部麻醉或全身麻醉时的辅助用药，具有镇静作用。<br>① For the treatment of severe cough and irritating cough caused by various reasons, especially for severe cough accompanied by chest pain. Since the product can inhibit glandular secretion and respiratory ciliary movement, so it should be combined with expectorants to treat severe cough with a small amount of sputum. ② As analgesia for moderate pain. ③ Adjuvant to local anesthesia or general anesthesia, having a sedative effect. |
| 用法、用量<br>Dosage | （1）成人：①常用量：口服或皮下注射，一次 15～30mg，一日 30～90mg。缓释片剂一次 1 片（45mg），一日 2 次，②极量：一次 100mg，一日 250mg。<br>（2）儿童：镇痛，口服，每次 0.5～1.0mg/kg，一日 3 次，或一日 3mg/kg；镇咳，为镇痛剂量的 1/3～1/2。<br>(1) Adult: ① usual dose: orally or subcutaneously, 15～30mg once, 30～90mg a day. For release tablets, (45mg) once, 2 times a day; ② maximum dose: 100mg once, 250mg a day.<br>(2) Children: analgesic, oral, 0.5～1.0mg/kg once, 3 times a day, or 3mg/kg a day; antitussive, 1/3 to 1/2 of analgesic doses. |
| 剂型、规格<br>Preparations | 片剂：每片 15mg；30mg。<br>缓释胶囊：每粒 45mg。<br>糖浆剂：0.5%，10ml，100ml。<br>注射液：每支 15mg（1ml）；30mg（1ml）。<br>Tablets: 15mg or 30 mg per tablet.<br>Release capsules: 45mg per capsule.<br>Syrup: 0.5%, 10ml, 100ml. Injections: 15mg (1ml); 30mg (1ml) per vial. |

| 药品名称 Drug Names | 福尔可定 Pholcodine |
|---|---|
| 适应证<br>Indications | 用于剧烈干咳和中等度疼痛。<br>For the treatment of severe dry cough and moderate pain. |
| 用法、用量<br>Dosage | 口服：常量，一次 5～10mg，一日 3～4 次；极量，一日 60mg。<br>Oral medication: usual dose, 5～10mg once, 3 to 4 times a day; maximum dose, 60mg a day. |
| 剂型、规格<br>Preparations | 片剂：每片 5mg；10mg；15mg；30mg。<br>Tablets: 5mg; 10mg; 15mg; 30mg per tablet. |

| 药品名称 Drug Names | 喷托维林 Pentoxyverine |
|---|---|
| 适应证<br>Indications | 用于上呼吸道感染引起的无痰干咳和百日咳等，对小儿疗效优于成人。<br>For the treatment of cough without phlegm and pertussis caused by upper respiratory tract infections, its efficacy in children is better than in adults. |

续　表

| 用法、用量<br>Dosage | 口服，成人，每次 25mg，一日 3 ～ 4 次。<br>Oral medication: 25mg once for adults, 3 to 4 times a day. |
|---|---|
| 剂型、规格<br>Preparations | 片剂：每片 25mg。<br>滴丸：每丸 25mg。<br>冲剂：每袋 10g。<br>糖浆剂：0.145%；0.2%；0.25%。<br>Tablets: 25mg per tablet.<br>Dripping Pills: 25mg per pill.<br>Granules: 10g per bag.<br>Syrups: 0.145%; 0.2%; 0.25%. |
| 药品名称 Drug Names | 右美沙芬 Dextromethorphan |
| 适应证<br>Indications | 用于干咳，适用于感冒、急慢性支气管炎、支气管哮喘、咽喉炎、肺结核以及其他上呼吸道感染时的咳嗽。<br>For the treatment of dry cough, and cough caused by colds, acute and chronic bronchitis, bronchial asthma, laryngitis, tuberculosis and other infections of the upper respiratory tract. |
| 用法、用量<br>Dosage | 口服，成人，每次 10 ～ 30mg，一日 3 次。一日最大剂量 120mg。<br>Oral medication: 10 ~ 30mg once for adults, 3 times a day. Maximum dose: 120mg a day. |
| 剂型、规格<br>Preparations | 片剂：每片 10mg；15mg。<br>分散片：每片 15mg；30mg。<br>胶囊剂：每粒 15mg。<br>颗粒剂：每袋 7.5mg；15mg。<br>糖浆剂：每瓶 15mg（20ml）；150mg（100ml）。<br>注射剂：每支 5mg。<br>Tablets: 10mg; 15mg per tablet.<br>Dispersible tablets: 15mg; 30mg per tablet.<br>Capsules: 15mg per capsule.<br>Granules: 7.5mg; 15mg per bag.<br>Syrups: 15mg (20ml); 150mg (100ml) per bottle.<br>Injection: 5mg per vial. |

## 11.3 平喘药 Antiasthmatics

| 药品名称 Drug Names | 麻黄碱 Ephedrine |
|---|---|
| 适应证<br>Indications | ①预防支气管哮喘发作和缓解轻度哮喘发作，对急性重度哮喘发作效果不佳。②用于蛛网膜下腔麻醉或硬膜外麻醉引起的低血压及慢性低血压。③治疗各种原因引起的鼻黏膜充血、肿胀引起的鼻塞。<br>① For prevention of bronchial asthma and the relief of mild asthma attacks, poor effect on acute severe asthma attack. ② For spinal anesthesia or epidural anesthesia-induced hypotension and chronic hypotension. ③ For the treatment of various nasal congestion and rhinocleisis due to swelling. |
| 用法、用量<br>Dosage | （1）支气管哮喘：口服：成人，常用量一次 15 ～ 30mg，一日 45 ～ 90mg；极量，一次 60mg，一日 150mg。皮下注射或肌内注射：成人，常用量一次 15 ～ 30mg，一日 45 ～ 60mg；极量，一次 60mg，一日 150mg。<br>（2）蛛网膜下隙麻醉或硬膜外麻醉时维持血压：麻醉前皮下注射或肌内注射 20 ～ 50mg。慢性低血压症，每次口服 20 ～ 50mg，一日 150mg。<br>（3）解除鼻黏膜充血、水肿：以 0.5% ～ 1% 溶液滴鼻。<br>(1) Bronchial asthma: Oral medication: the usual dose is 15 ~ 30mg once for adults, 45 ~ 90mg one day; the maximum dose is 60mg one time, 150mg one day. Subcutaneous or intramuscular injection: the usual dose is 15 ~ 30mg once for adults, 45 ~ 60mg one day; the maximum dose is 60mg once, and 150mg one day.<br>(2) Maintaining blood pressure while proceeding subarachnoid anesthesia or epidural anesthesia: subcutaneous or intramuscular injection before anesthesia at a dosage of 20 ~ 50mg. Chronic hypotension: oral medication, 20 ~ 50mg once, 150mg a day.<br>(3) Relieving nasal congestion and edema: drip 0.5% to 1%.solution into nose. |

| 剂型、规格<br>Preparations | 片剂：每片 15mg；25mg；30mg。注射液：每支 30mg（1ml）；50mg（1ml）。滴鼻剂：0.5%（小儿）；1%（成人）；2%（检查、手术或止血时用）。<br><br>Tablets: 15mg; 25mg; 30mg per tablet. Injection: 30mg (1ml); 50mg (1ml) of each. Nasal drops: 0.5% (for children); 1% (for adult); 2% (for checking, surgery or bleeding). |
|---|---|
| **药品名称 Drug Names** | 异丙肾上腺素 Isoprenaline |
| 适应证<br>Indications | （1）支气管哮喘：适用于控制哮喘发作，常气雾吸入给药，作用快而强，但持续时间短。<br>（2）心搏骤停：治疗各种原因及溺水、电击、手术意外和药物中毒等引起的心搏骤停。必要时可与肾上腺素和去甲肾上腺素配合使用。<br>（3）房室传导阻滞。<br>（4）抗休克：心源性休克和感染性休克。对中心静脉压高、心排血量低者，应在不足血容量的基础上使用本品。<br><br>(1) Bronchial asthma: for the treatment of controlling asthma, often aerosol inhalation, fast and strong effect, but of short duration.<br>(2) Cardiac arrest: for the treatment of cardiac arrest induced by various causes including drowning, electric shock, surgical accidents and poisoning, etc. In conjunction with epinephrine and norepinephrine if necessary.<br>(3)Atrioventricular block.<br>(4) Anti-shock: for the treatment of cardiogenic shock and septic shock. For patients with high central venous pressure and low cardiac output, it should be used on the basis of hypovolemia. |
| 用法、用量<br>Dosage | （1）支气管哮喘：舌下含服，成人常用量一次 10～15mg，一日 3 次；极量，一次 20mg，一日 60mg。气雾剂吸入，常用量，一次 0.1～0.4mg；极量，一次 0.4mg，一日 2.4mg。重复使用的间隔时间不宜少于 2 小时。<br>（2）心搏骤停：心腔内注射 0.5～1mg。<br>（3）房室传导阻滞：二度者采用舌下含服，每次 10mg，每 4 小时一次；三度者如心率低于 40 次 / 分时，可用 0.5～1mg 溶 5% 葡萄糖液 200～300ml 缓慢静脉滴入。<br>（4）抗休克：以 0.5～1mg 加入 5% 葡萄糖液 200ml 中，静脉滴注，滴速 0.5～2μg/min，根据心率调整滴速，使收缩压维持在 12kPa（90mmHg）脉压维持在 2.7kPa（20mmHg）以上，心率 120 次 / 分以下。<br><br>(1) Bronchial asthma: sublingual, usual dose for adults is 10 ~ 15mg once, 3 times a day; maximum dose is 20mg once, 60mg a day. Aerosol inhalation, usual dose is 0.1 ~ 0.4mg once; maximum dose is 0.4mg once, 2.4mg a day. Intervals of repeated use are not less than two hours.<br>(2) Cardiac arrest: intracardiac injection, 0.5 ~ 1mg.<br>(3) Atrioventricular block: sublingual for Ⅱ degree patients, 10mg once for every 4 hours; for degree Ⅲ patients, such as who are with the heart rate of less than 40 beats / min, dissolve 0.5 ~ 1mg in 200 ~ 300ml 5% glucose solution for slow intravenous infusion.<br>(4) Anti-shock: dissolve 0.5 ~ 1mg in 200 ml 5% glucose solution for intravenous infusion, drip 0.5 ~ 2μg / min, adjust drip speed according to heart rate to remain the systolic blood pressure at 12kpa(90mmHg), pulse pressure at above 2.7 kpa (20mmHg), and heart rate at 120 beats / min or less. |
| 剂型、规格<br>Preparations | 片剂：每片 10mg。<br>纸片：每片 5mg。<br>气雾剂：浓度为 0.25%，每瓶可喷吸 200 次左右，每揿约 0.175mg。注射液：每支 1mg（2ml）。<br>Tablets: 10mg per tablet.<br>Paper: 5mg per shift.<br>Aerosol: concentration of 0.25%, 200 times for ejection per bottle, 0.175mg per press. Injection: per 1mg (2ml) of each. |
| **药品名称 Drug Names** | 沙丁胺醇 Salbutamol |
| 适应证<br>Indications | 用于防治支气管哮喘，哮喘型支气管炎和肺气肿的支气管痉挛。制止发作多用气雾吸入，预防可用口服。<br><br>For the prevention and treatment of bronchial asthma, and bronchospasm accompanied with asthma and emphysema. Inhalation for stopping disease onset, oral medication for prevention. |

**续　表**

| | |
|---|---|
| 用法、用量<br>Dosage | 口服：成人，每次 2 ~ 4mg，一日 3 次。气雾吸入：每次 0.1 ~ 0.2mg，必要时每 4 小时重复一次，但 24 小时内不宜超过 8 次，粉雾吸入，成人每次吸入 0.4mg，一日 3 ~ 4 次。静脉注射：一次 0.4mg，用 5% 葡萄糖液 20ml 或氯化钠液 20ml 稀释后，缓慢注射。静脉滴注：一次 0.4mg，用 5% 葡萄糖液 100ml 稀释后滴入。肌内注射：一次 0.4mg，必要时可重复注射。<br><br>Oral medication: 2 ~ 4mg once for adult, 3 times a day. Inhalation: 0.1 ~ 0.2mg once, if necessary, repeat every four hours, but not more than 8 times within 24 hours. Powder inhalation: 0.4mg once for adult, 3 to 4 times a day. Intravenous injection: 0.4mg once, slow injection after being diluted with 20ml 5% glucose solution or 20ml sodium chloride solution. Intravenous infusion: 0.4mg once, diluted with 100ml 5% glucose solution for infusion. Intramuscular injection: 0.4mg once, repeat injections if necessary. |
| 剂型、规格<br>Preparations | 片（胶囊）剂：每片（粒）0.5mg；2mg。<br>缓释片（胶囊）剂：每粒 4mg；8mg。<br>气雾剂：溶液型 0.2%（g/g），每瓶 20mg（200 揿）每揿 0.1mg。<br>粉雾剂胶囊：每粒 0.2mg；0.4mg，用粉物吸入器吸入。<br>注射液：每支 0.4mg（2ml）。<br>糖浆剂：4mg（1ml）。<br><br>Tablets (capsules): 0.5mg; 2mg per tablet (capsule).<br>Release tablets (capsules): 4mg; 8mg per tablet (capsule).<br>Aerosol: 0.2% (g / g) solution, 20mg (200 presses) per bottle and 0.1mg per press.<br>Powder Inhalation Capsules: 0.2mg; 0.4mg per capsule, inhale with a powder inhaler.<br>Injection: 0.4mg (2ml) per vial.<br>Syrups: 4mg (1ml). |
| **药品名称 Drug Names** | 福莫特罗 Formoterol |
| 适应证<br>Indications | 用于慢性哮喘与慢性阻塞性肺疾病的维持治疗及预防发作，因其为长效制剂，特别适用于哮喘夜间发作患者，疗效尤佳。能有效预防运动型哮喘的发作。<br><br>For maintenance treatment and prevention of chronic asthma and chronic obstructive pulmonary disease. Being a long-acting formulation, it's especially effective for patients with nocturnal asthma. It can effectively prevent exercise-induced asthma. |
| 用法、用量<br>Dosage | 口服：成人每次 40 ~ 80μg，一日 2 次。气雾吸入：成人每次 4.5 ~ 9μg，一日 2 次。<br>Oral medication: 40 ~ 80μg once for adult, 2 times a day. Inhalation: 4.5 ~ 9μg once for adult, 2 times a day. |
| 剂型、规格<br>Preparations | 片剂：每片 20μg；40μg。<br>干糖浆：20mg（0.5g）。<br>气雾剂：每瓶 60 喷（每喷含本品 9μg）。<br>片剂：每片含本品 20μg。<br>干粉吸入剂：每瓶 60pen（每喷含本品 4.5μg）；每瓶 60 喷（每喷含本品 9μg）。<br><br>Tablets: 20μg ; 40μg per tablet.<br>Dry Syrup: 20mg (0.5g).<br>Aerosol: 60 sprays per bottle (per spray contains the product 9μg ).<br>Tablets: per tablet contains the product 20μg.<br>Dry powder inhalation: 60 sprays per bottle (per spray contains 4.5μg formoterol); 60 sprays per bottle (per spray contains 9μg formoterol. |
| **药品名称 Drug Names** | 丙卡特罗 Procaterol |
| 适应证<br>Indications | 用于防治支气管哮喘，喘息性支气管炎和慢性阻塞性肺疾病所致喘息症状。<br><br>For the prevention and treatment of wheezing due to bronchial asthma, asthmatic bronchitis and chronic obstructive pulmonary disease. |
| 用法、用量<br>Dosage | 口服，成人，每晚睡前一次服 50μg，或每次 25 ~ 50μg，早、晚（睡前）各服一次。<br>Oral medication: 50μg once every night before bedtime for adults, or 25 ~ 50μg once in the morning and before bedtime. |
| 剂型、规格<br>Preparations | 片剂（胶囊）剂：每片（粒）含本品 25μg；50μg。<br>口服液：0.15mg（30ml）。<br>气雾剂：2mg，每揿含 10μg。<br><br>Tablets (capsules): per tablet(capsule) contains the product 25μg or 50μg.<br>Oral liquid: 0.15mg (30ml).<br>Aerosol: 2mg, per press contains the product10μg . |

**续 表**

| 药品名称 Drug Names | 沙美特罗 Salmeterol |
|---|---|
| 适应证<br>Indications | 用于哮喘、喘息性支气管炎和可逆性气管阻塞。<br>For the treatment of asthma, asthmatic bronchitis and reversible airway obstruction. |
| 用法、用量<br>Dosage | 粉物吸入：成人，每次50μg，一日2次；儿童，每次25μg，一日2次。气雾吸入：剂量用法同上。<br>Powder inhalation: 50μg once, 2 times a day for adults; 25μg once, 2 times a day for children. Inhalation: the same as above. |
| 剂型、规格<br>Preparations | 粉雾剂胶囊：每粒含本品50μg。气雾剂：每喷含本品25μg。<br>Powder Capsules: per capsule contains the product 50μg. Aerosol: per spray contains the product 25μg. |
| 药品名称 Drug Names | 班布特罗 Bambuterol |
| 适应证<br>Indications | 用于支气管哮喘、慢性喘息性支气管炎、阻塞性肺气肿及其他伴有支气管痉挛的肺部疾病。<br>For the treatment of bronchial asthma, chronic asthmatic bronchitis, obstructive pulmonary emphysema and other lung diseases accompanied with bronchospasm. |
| 用法、用量<br>Dosage | 每晚睡前口服一次，成人10mg，12岁以下儿童5mg。<br>Oral medication: once every night before bedtime, 10mg for adults, 5mg for children under 12 years old. |
| 剂型、规格<br>Preparations | 片剂（胶囊）：每片（粒）10mg；20mg。<br>口服液：10mg（10ml）。<br>Tablets (capsules): 10mg; 20mg per tablet(capsule).<br>Oral medication: 10mg (10ml). |
| 药品名称 Drug Names | 异丙托溴铵 Ipratropium Bromide |
| 适应证<br>Indications | ①用于缓解慢性阻塞性肺疾病（COPD）引起的支气管痉挛、喘息症状。②防治哮喘、尤适用于因用β受体激动药产生肌肉震颤、心动过速而不能耐受此类药物的患者。<br>① It's used to relieve bronchospasm and wheezing due to chronic obstructive pulmonary disease (COPD). ② For the prevention and treatment of asthma, especially for patients with muscle tremors, agitation and tachycardia due to using β receptor agonists and can no longer tolerate this kind of drugs. |
| 用法、用量<br>Dosage | 气雾吸入：成人一次40～80μg，一日3～4次。雾化吸入：成人，一次100～500μg（14岁以下50～250μg），用生理盐水稀释到3～4ml，至雾化器中吸入。<br>Aerosol inhalation: 40～80μg once for adults, 3 to 4 times a day. Atomizing inhalation: 100～500μg once for adults (50～250μg once for children under 14 years old), diluted to 3～4ml with normal saline to the nebulizer for inhalation. |
| 剂型、规格<br>Preparations | 气雾剂：每喷20μg，40μg；每瓶200喷（10ml）。<br>吸入溶液剂：2ml：异丙托溴氨500μg。<br>雾化溶液剂：50μg（2ml）；250μg（2ml）；500μg（2ml）；500μg（20ml）。<br>Aerosol: 20μg or 40μg per spray, 200 sprays per bottle (10ml).<br>Inhalation solutions: 2ml: 500μg ipratropium bromide.<br>Atomizing solutions: 50μg (2ml); 250μg (2ml); 500μg (2ml); 500μg (20ml). |
| 药品名称 Drug Names | 噻托溴铵 Tiotropium Bromide |
| 适应证<br>Indications | 用于治疗慢性阻塞性肺疾病及支气管哮喘，对于急性哮喘发作无效。<br>For the treatment of chronic obstructive pulmonary disease and bronchial asthma, it is invalid for acute asthma. |
| 用法、用量<br>Dosage | 噻托溴铵粉吸入剂（胶囊）：每粒18μg，每次吸入1粒，一日1次。<br>Tiotropium ammonia inhalation powder (capsules): 18μg per capsule, 1 capsule per inhalation, once a day. |
| 剂型、规格<br>Preparations | 粉雾剂：18μg。<br>吸入剂：18μg。<br>Pink mist: 18μg.<br>Inhalant: 18μg. |

**续　表**

| 药品名称 Drug Names | 氨茶碱 Aminophylline |
|---|---|
| 适应证<br>Indications | 用于①支气管哮喘和喘息性支气管炎，与β受体激动剂合用可提高疗效。在哮喘持续状态，常选用本品与肾上腺皮质激素配伍进行治疗。②治疗急性心功能不全和心源性哮喘。③胆绞痛。<br><br>① For the treatment of bronchial asthma and asthmatic bronchitis, its efficacy can be improved in combination with β agonists. In status asthmaticus, the product is often used in combination with adrenal hormones for treatment; ② For the treatment of acute heart failure and cardiac asthma; ③ For the treatment of biliary colic. |
| 用法、用量<br>Dosage | 口服：成人，常用量，每次 0.1 ~ 0.2g，一日 0.3 ~ 0.6g；极量，一次 0.5g，一日 1g。肌内注射或静脉注射：成人，常用量，每次 0.25 ~ 0.5g，一日 0.5 ~ 1g；极量，一日 0.5g。以 50% 葡萄糖注射液 20 ~ 40mg 稀释后缓慢静脉注射（不少于 10 分钟）。静脉滴注：以 5% 葡萄糖注射液 500ml 稀释后滴注。直肠给药：栓剂或保留灌肠，每次 0.3 ~ 0.5g，一日 1 ~ 2 次。<br><br>Oral medication: for adults, usual dose, 0.1 ~ 0.2g once, 0.3 ~ 0.6g a day; maximum dose, 0.5g once, 1g a day. Intramuscular injection or intravenous injection: for adults, usual dose, 0.25 ~ 0.5g once, 0.5 ~ 1g a day; maximum dose, 0.5g a day. Slow intravenous injection is processed after being diluted with 20 ~ 40mg 50% glucose injection (not less than 10 minutes). Intravenous infusion: infusion after being diluted with 500ml 5% glucose injection. Rectal administration: suppositories or retention enemas, 0.3 ~ 0.5g once, 1 to 2 times a day. |
| 剂型、规格<br>Preparations | 片剂：每片 0.05g；0.1g；0.2g。<br>肠溶片：每片 0.05g；0.1g。<br>注射液：①肌内注射用每支 0.125g（2ml）；0.25g（2ml）；0.5g（2ml）。②静脉注射用每支 0.25g（10ml）。<br>栓剂：每粒 0.25g。<br>缓释片每片 0.15g；0.2g。<br>Tablets: 0.05g; 0.1g; 0.2g per tablet.<br>Enteric-coated tablets: 0.05g; 0.1g per tablet.<br>Injection: ① 0.125g (2ml); 0.25g (2ml); 0.5g (2ml) per vial for intramuscular injection. ② 0.25g (10ml) per vial for intravenous injection.<br>Suppositories: 0.25g per softgel.<br>Release tablets: 0.15g; 0.2g per tablet. |
| 药品名称 Drug Names | 多索茶碱 Doxofylline |
| 适应证<br>Indications | 适用于支气管哮喘、喘息性支气管炎及其他伴支气管痉挛的肺部疾病。<br>For the treatment of bronchial asthma, asthmatic bronchitis and other lung diseases accompanied with bronchospasm. |
| 用法、用量<br>Dosage | 口服：每日 2 片或每 12 小时 1 ~ 2 粒胶囊，或每日 1 ~ 3 包散剂冲服。急症可先注射 100mg，然后每 6 小时静脉注射一次，也可每日静脉滴注 300mg。<br><br>Oral medication: 2 tablets a day or 1 to 2 capsules every 12 hours, or 1 ~ 3 packs of powder after being infused in water a day. 100mg for injection in emergency, then give intravenous injection once every 6 hours; or 300mg a day for intravenous infusion. |
| 剂型、规格<br>Preparations | 片剂：每片 200mg；300mg；400mg。<br>胶囊剂：每粒 200mg；300mg。<br>散剂：每包 200mg。<br>注射液：每支 100mg（10ml）。<br>葡萄糖注射液：每瓶 0.3g 与葡萄糖 5g（100ml）。<br>Tablets: 200mg; 300mg; 400mg per tablet.<br>Capsules: 200mg; 300mg per capsule.<br>Powder: 200mg per pack. Injection:100mg (10ml) per bottle.<br>Glucose injection: 0.3g doxofylline and 5g glucose (100ml) per bottle. |
| 药品名称 Drug Names | 二羟丙茶碱 Diprophylline |
| 适应证<br>Indications | 用于支气管哮喘、喘息性支气管炎，尤适用于伴有心动过速的哮喘患者。亦可用于心源性肺水肿引起的喘息。<br><br>For the treatment of bronchial asthma, asthmatic bronchitis, especially for asthma patients with tachycardia. Also for the treatment of wheezing due to cardiogenic pulmonary edema. |

续 表

| | |
|---|---|
| 用法、用量<br>Dosage | 口服：每次 0.1 ~ 0.2g，一日 3 次。极量，一次 0.5g，一日 1.5g。肌内注射：每次 0.25 ~ 0.5g，静脉滴注：用于严重哮喘发作，每日 0.5 ~ 1g，加于 5% 葡萄糖液 1500 ~ 2000ml 中滴入。直肠给药：每次 0.25 ~ 0.5g。<br><br>Oral medication: 0.1 ~ 0.2g once, 3 times a day. Maximum dose, 0.5g once, 1.5g a day. Intramuscular injection: 0.25 ~ 0.5g once, intravenous infusion: for severe asthma attack, 0.5 ~ 1g a day, added into 1500 ~ 2000ml 5% glucose solution for infusion. Rectal administration: 0.25 ~ 0.5g once. |
| 剂型、规格<br>Preparations | 片剂：每片 0.1g；0.2g。<br>注射液：每支 0.25g（2ml）。<br>葡萄糖注射液：每瓶 0.25g 与葡萄糖 5g（100ml）。<br>栓剂：每粒 0.25g。<br><br>Tablets: 0.1g; 0.2g per tablet.<br>Injection: 0.25g (2ml) per vial.<br>Glucose injection: 0.25g diprophylline and 5g glucose (100ml) per bottle.<br>Suppositories: 0.25g per softgel. |
| 药品名称 Drug Names | 色甘酸钠 Sodium Cromoglicate |
| 适应证<br>Indications | ①支气管哮喘：可用于预防各型哮喘发作。对外源性哮喘疗效显著，特别是对已知抗原的年轻患者疗效更佳，对内源性哮喘和慢性哮喘亦有一定疗效，约 50% 患者的症状改善或完全控制。对依赖肾上腺皮质激素的哮喘患者，经本品治疗后可减少或完全停用肾上腺皮质激素。运动性哮喘患者预先给药几乎可防止全部病例发作。一般因于接触抗原前 1 周给药，但运动性哮喘可在运动前 15 分钟给药。β 肾上腺素受体激动剂合用可提高疗效。②过敏性鼻炎，季节性花粉症，春季角膜、结膜炎，过敏性湿疹及某些皮肤瘙痒症。③溃疡性结肠炎和直肠炎：本品灌肠后可改善症状，内镜检查和活检均可见炎症及损伤减轻。<br><br>① Bronchial asthma: For the prevention of various types of asthma attacks. Significant efficacy in exogenous asthma, especially having better efficacy in young patients with known antigens, having a certain effect on endogenous asthma and chronic asthma., these symptoms can be relieved or completely controlled for about half of the patients. For the asthma patients depending on adrenocorticotropic hormone, they can reduce the dose of or completely stopping using adrenocorticotropic hormone after taking the product. For patients with exercise-induced asthma, pre-administration can prevent almost all asthma attacks. Generally, administration should be processed a week before exposure to antigens, but which can be processed 15 minutes before exercise for exercise-induced asthma. Combined use with β-adrenergic agonists can increase the efficacy. ② Allergic rhinitis, seasonal hay fever, spring keratitis and conjunctivitis, atopic eczema and some pruritus. ③ Ulcerative colitis and proctitis: This product can help relieve symptoms after enema. Both inflammation and injury can be reduced by doing microscopic examination and biopsy. |
| 用法、用量<br>Dosage | （1）支气管哮喘：粉物吸入，每次 20mg，一日 4 次；症状减轻后，一日 40 ~ 60mg；维持量，一日 20mg。气雾吸入，每次 2.5 ~ 7mg，一日 3 ~ 4 次，每日最大剂量 32mg。<br>（2）过敏性鼻炎：干粉吸入或吹入鼻腔，每次 10mg，一日 4 次。<br>（3）季节性花粉症和春季角膜、结膜炎：滴眼，2% 溶液，每次 2 滴，一日数次。<br>（4）过敏性湿疹、皮肤瘙痒症：外用 5% ~ 10% 软膏。<br>（5）溃疡性结肠炎、直肠炎：灌肠，每次 200mg。<br><br>(1) Bronchial asthma: powder inhalation, 20mg once, 4 times a day; after symptom relief, 40 ~ 60mg a day; maintenance dose, 20mg a day. Aerosol inhalation, 2.5 ~ 7mg once, 3 to 4 times a day; maximum dose, 32mg a day.<br>(2) Allergic rhinitis: powder inhalation or blown into nasal cavity, 10mg once, 4 times a day.<br>(3) Seasonal hay fever, spring keratitis and conjunctivitis, : eye drops, 2% solution, 2 drops once, and several times a day.<br>(4) Atopic eczema, pruritus: 5% to 10% ointment for external use.<br>(5) Ulcerative colitis, proctitis: enema, 200mg once. |
| 剂型、规格<br>Preparations | 粉雾剂胶囊：每粒 20mg，装于专用喷雾器内吸入。<br>气雾剂：每瓶 700mg（200 揿），每揿 3.5mg。<br>软膏：5% ~ 10%。<br>滴眼剂：0.16g/8ml（2%）。<br><br>Powder Inhalation Capsules: 20mg per capsule, installed in a dedicated sprayer for inhalation. Aerosol: 700mg (200 presses) per bottle, 3.5mg per press.<br>Ointment: 5% ~ 10%.<br>Eye drops: 0.16g/8ml (2%). |

**续　表**

| 药品名称 Drug Names | 酮替芬 Ketotifen |
|---|---|
| 适应证<br>Indications | ①支气管哮喘，对过敏性、感染性和混合性哮喘均有预防发作效果。②哮喘性支气管炎、过敏性咳嗽。③过敏性鼻炎、过敏性结膜炎及过敏性皮炎。<br><br>① For the treatment of bronchial asthma, and for the prevention of allergic, infectious and mixed asthma. ② Asthmatic bronchitis, allergic cough. ③ Allergic rhinitis, allergic conjunctivitis and atopic dermatitis. |
| 用法、用量<br>Dosage | （1）口服：①片剂，成人及儿童均为每次 1mg，一日 2 次，早、晚服用；②小儿可服其口服溶液，一日 1 ～ 2 次（一次量：4 ～ 6 岁，2ml；6 ～ 9 岁，2.5ml；9 ～ 14 岁，3ml）。<br>（2）滴鼻：一次 1 ～ 2 滴，一日 1 ～ 3 次。<br>（3）滴眼：滴入结膜囊，一日 2 次，一次 1 滴，或每 8 ～ 12 小时滴 1 次。<br><br>(1) Oral medication: ① Tablets: 1mg once for both adults and children, 2 times a day, take in the morning and evening; ② Oral solution for children: 1 or 2 times a day (one dose: 4 to 6 years old, 2ml; 6 ~ 9 years old, 2.5ml; 9 ~ 14 years old, 3ml).<br>(2) Intranasal: 1 to 2 drops once, 1 ~ 3 times a day.<br>(3) Eye drops: drop into conjunctival sac, 2 times a day, one drop once; or one drop every 8 to 12 hours. |
| 剂型、规格<br>Preparations | 片剂：每片 0.5mg；1mg。胶囊剂：每粒 0.5mg；1mg。口服溶液：1mg（5ml）。滴鼻液：15mg（10ml）。滴眼液：2.5mg（5ml）。<br><br>Tablets: 0.5mg; 1mg per tablet. Capsules: 0.5mg; 1mg per capsule. Oral solution: 1mg (5ml). Nasal drops: 15mg (10ml). Eye Drops: 2.5mg (5ml). |
| 药品名称 Drug Names | 氮䓬斯汀 Azelastine |
| 适应证<br>Indications | 用于治疗支气管哮喘、过敏性鼻炎或过敏性结膜炎。<br>For the treatment of bronchial asthma, allergic rhinitis or allergic conjunctivitis. |
| 用法、用量<br>Dosage | 支气管哮喘：口服，成人每次 2 ～ 4mg，6 ～ 12 岁儿童每次 1mg，一日 2 次。过敏性鼻炎：口服，每次 1mg，一日 2 次，在早餐后及睡前各服 1 次；喷鼻，一次 1 喷，一日 2 ～ 4 次。过敏性结膜炎：滴眼，一次 1 滴，一日 2 ～ 4 次。<br><br>Bronchial Asthma: oral medication, 2 ~ 4mg once for adults, 1mg once for 6 ~ 12 years old children, 2 times a day. Allergic rhinitis: oral medication, 1mg once, 2 times a day, take once after breakfast and before bedtime; nasal spray, a spray once, 2 ~ 4 times a day. Allergic conjunctivitis: eye drops, one drop once, 2 ~ 4 times a day. |
| 剂型、规格<br>Preparations | 片剂：每片 1mg；2mg。颗粒剂：0.2%。喷鼻剂：10mg（10ml）。滴眼液：2.5mg（5ml）。<br><br>Tablets: 1mg; 2mg per tablet. Granules: 0.2%. Nasal Spray: 10mg (10ml). Eye Drops: 2.5mg (5ml). |
| 药品名称 Drug Names | 倍氯米松 Beclomethasone |
| 适应证<br>Indications | ①本品吸入给药可用于慢性哮喘患者；②鼻喷用于过敏性鼻炎；③外用治疗过敏所致炎症性皮肤病如湿疹、神经性或接触性皮炎、瘙痒症等。<br><br>① This product can be used for inhalation to treat patients with chronic asthma; ② Nasal spray for allergic rhinitis; ③ External treatment of inflammatory skin diseases caused by allergies such as eczema, neurological or contact dermatitis and pruritus. |
| 用法、用量<br>Dosage | 气雾吸入，成人开始剂量每次 50 ～ 200μg，一日 2 次或 3 次，每日最大剂量 1mg。儿童用量依年龄酌减，每日最大剂量 0.8mg。长期吸入的维持量应个体化，以减至最低剂量又能控制症状为准。粉雾吸入，成人每次 200μg，一日 3 ～ 4 次。儿童每次 100μg，一日 2 次或遵医嘱。<br><br>Inhalation, the starting dose for adults is 50 ~ 200μg once, 2 or 3 times a day, the maximum daily dose is 1mg. The amount is reduced according to children's age, the daily maximum dose is 0.8mg. Long-term maintenance dose for inhalation should be individualized, both minimize the dose and control symptoms. Powder inhalation, 200μg once for adults, 3 to 4 times a day. 100μg once for children, 2 times a day or as directed. |

**续　表**

| 剂型、规格<br>Preparations | 气雾剂：每瓶 200 喷（每喷 50μg；80μg；100μg；200μg；250μg）；每瓶 80 喷（每喷 250μg）。<br>粉雾剂胶囊：每粒 50μg；100μg；200μg。<br>喷鼻剂：每瓶 10mg（每喷 50μg）。<br>软膏剂：2.5mg/10g。<br>霜剂：2.5mg/10g。<br><br>Aerosols: 200 spray per bottle (50μg; 80μg; 100μg; 200μg; 250μg per spray ); 80 spray per bottle( 250μg per spray).<br>Powder Inhalation Capsules: 50μg; 100μg; 200μg per softgel.<br>Nasal spray: 10mg per bottle (50μg per spray ).<br>Ointment: 2.5mg/10g.<br>Cream: 2.5mg/10g. |
|---|---|
| **药品名称 Drug Names** | 布地奈德 Budesonide |
| 适应证<br>Indications | ①用于肾上腺皮质激素依赖性或非依赖性支气管哮喘及喘息性支气管炎患者，可有效地减少口服肾上腺皮质激素的用量，有助于减轻肾上腺皮质激素的不良反应。②用于慢性阻塞性肺病。<br><br>① For the treatment of patients with adrenocorticotropic hormone-dependent or non-dependent bronchial asthma, and patients with asthmatic bronchitis, which can effectively reduce the dose of oral glucocorticoid, helping mitigate the adverse reactions of adrenocorticotropic hormone.　② For chronic obstructive pulmonary disease. |
| 用法、用量<br>Dosage | 气雾吸入：成人，开始剂量每次 200 ~ 800μg，一日 2 次，维持量因人而异，通常为每次 200 ~ 400μg，一日 2 次；儿童，开始剂量每次 100 ~ 200μg，一日 2 次，维持量也应个体化，以减至最低剂量又能控制症状为准。<br><br>Aerosol Inhalation: for adults, the starting dose is 200 ~ 800μg once, 2 times a day, the maintenance dosage varies, usually 200 ~ 400μg once, 2 times a day; for children, the starting dose is 100 ~ 200μg once, 2 times a day, the maintenance dose should be individualized, but also aim to minimize the dose and control symptoms. |
| 剂型、规格<br>Preparations | 气雾剂：每瓶 10mg（100 喷，200 喷），每喷 100μg，50μg；每瓶 20mg（100 喷），每喷 200μg；每瓶 60mg（300 喷），每喷 200μg。<br>粉雾剂：每瓶 20mg；40mg，每喷 200μg。<br><br>Aerosol: 10mg per bottle (100 sprays; 200 sprays), 100μg or 50μg per spray; 20mg per bottle (100 sprays), 200μg per spray; 60mg per bottle (300 sprays), 200μg per spray.<br>Powder Inhalation: 20mg; 40mg per bottle, 200μg per spray. |
| **药品名称 Drug Names** | 氟替卡松 Fluticasone |
| 适应证<br>Indications | 雾化吸入用于慢性持续性哮喘的长期治疗，亦可治疗过敏性鼻炎。<br><br>Aerosol inhalation for the long-term treatment of chronic persistent asthma, and also for the treatment of allergic rhinitis. |
| 用法、用量<br>Dosage | （1）支气管哮喘：雾化吸入，成人和 16 岁以上青少年起始剂量：①轻度持续，一日 200 ~ 500μg，分 2 次给予；②中度持续，一日 500 ~ 1000μg，分 2 次给予；③重度持续，一日 1000 ~ 2000μg，分 2 次给予。16 岁以下儿童起始剂量，根据病情及身体发育情况酌情给予，一日 100 ~ 400μg；5 岁以下 1 日 100 ~ 200μg。维持量亦应个体化，以减至最低剂量又能控制症状为准。<br>（2）过敏性鼻炎：鼻喷，一次 50 ~ 200μg，一日 2 次。<br><br>(1) Bronchial asthma: Aerosol inhalation, the starting dose for adults and adolescents over 16 years old: ① mild persistent, 200 ~ 500μg a day, in 2 divided doses; ② moderate persistent, 500 ~ 1000μg a day, in 2 divided doses ③ severe persistent, 1000 ~ 2000μg a day, in 2 divided doses. The starting dose for children under 16 years is given according to their conditions and physical development, 100 ~ 400μg a day; for children less than 5 years old, 100 ~ 200μg a day. Maintenance dose should be individualized, also aim to minimize the dose and control symptoms.<br>(2) Allergic rhinitis: nasal spray, 50 ~ 200μg once, 2 times a day. |
| 剂型、规格<br>Preparations | 气雾剂：每瓶 60 喷；120 喷（每喷 25μg；50μg；125μg；250μg）。<br>喷鼻剂：每瓶 120 喷（每喷 50μg）。<br><br>Aerosol: 60 sprays per bottle; 120 sprays ( 25μg; 50μg; 125μg; 250μg per spray).<br>Nasal spray: 120 sprays per bottle( 50μg per spray). |

**续　表**

| 药品名称 Drug Names | 曲安奈德 Triamcinolone Acetonide |
|---|---|
| 适应证<br>Indications | 用于支气管哮喘。<br>For the treatment of bronchial asthma. |
| 用法、用量<br>Dosage | 常用气雾吸入：成人每日 0.8 ~ 1.0mg，儿童每日 0.4mg，分 4 次给药。<br>Usually in aerosol inhalation: 0.8 ~ 1.0mg a day for adults, 0.4mg a day for children, in 4 divided doses. |
| 剂型、规格<br>Preparations | 鼻喷雾剂：每支 6ml [6.6mg, 120 喷（55μg/ 喷）]。<br>Nasal spray: 6 ml [6.6 mg, 120 spray (55μg /spray)] per bottle.. |
| 药品名称 Drug Names | 糠酸莫米松 Mometasone Furoate |
| 适应证<br>Indications | 用于预防和治疗各种过敏性鼻炎，亦可试用于支气管哮喘。<br>For the prevention and treatment of various allergic rhinitis, also for bronchial asthma. |
| 用法、用量<br>Dosage | 成人常用量：每侧鼻孔 2 喷，每喷 50μg，一日 1 次，一日总量 200μg。症状控制后，剂量减至一日总量 100μg 以维持疗效。12 岁以下儿童：每侧鼻孔 1 喷，每喷 50μg，一日 1 次，一日总量 100μg。维持量酌减。<br>Usual dose for adults: 2 sprays on each side of the nose, 50μg per spray, once a day, the total dosage of a day is 200μg. Afte the symptom is controlled, the total dosage is reduced to 100μg a day to maintain efficacy.For children under 12 years old: 1 spray on each side of the nose, 50μg per spray, once a day, the total dosage of a day is 100μg. Maintenance dose should be reduced accordingly. |
| 剂型、规格<br>Preparations | 喷鼻剂：每支 60 喷，每喷 50μg。<br>Nasal spray: 60 sprays per bottle, 50μg per spray. |
| 药品名称 Drug Names | 扎鲁司特 Zafirlukast |
| 适应证<br>Indications | 用于①慢性轻至中度支气管哮喘的预防和治疗，尤其适用于对阿司匹林敏感或有阿司匹林哮喘的患者或伴有上呼吸道疾病（如鼻息肉、过敏性鼻炎）者，但不宜用于治疗急性哮喘；②激素抵抗型哮喘或拒绝使用激素的哮喘患者；③严重哮喘时加用本品以维持控制哮喘发作或用以减少激素用量。<br>① For the prevention and treatment of mild to moderate chronic bronchial asthma, especially suitable for patients sensitive to aspirin or with aspirin-induced asthma, and those with upper respiratory diseases (such as nasal polyps and allergic rhinitis), but not for the treatment of acute asthma; ② For the treatment of patients with steroid-resistant asthma or asthma patients who reject the use of hormones; ③ When severe asthma occurs, increase the dosage of this product in order to control asthma attacks, or to reduce the amount of hormones. |
| 用法、用量<br>Dosage | 口服：成人及 12 岁以上儿童，每次 20mg，一日 2 次，餐前 1 小时或餐后 2 小时服，用于预防哮喘时，应持续用药。<br>Oral medication: for adults and children over 12 years old, 20mg once, 2 times a day, take 1 hour before meals or 2 hours after meals, continue dosing when it is used to prevent asthma. |
| 剂型、规格<br>Preparations | 片剂：每片 20mg；40mg。<br>Tablets: 20mg ; 40mg per tablet. |
| 药品名称 Drug Names | 孟鲁司特钠 Montelukast Sodium |
| 适应证<br>Indications | 用于预防支气管哮喘和支气管哮喘的长期治疗。也用于治疗阿司匹林敏感的哮喘，预防运动性哮喘。对激素已耐药的患者本品亦有效。<br>For the prevention of bronchial asthma and long-term treatment of bronchial asthma. Also for the treatment of aspirin-sensitive asthma, and the prevention of exercise-induced asthma .This product is also effective for hormone-resistant patients. |
| 用法、用量<br>Dosage | 口服：成人 10mg，一日 1 次，每晚睡前服。6 ~ 14 岁儿童 5mg，一日 1 次。2 ~ 6 岁儿童 4mg，一日 1 次。<br>Oral medication: 10mg for adults, once a day, take every night before bedtime. 5mg for 6~14 years old children, once a day. 4mg for 2~6 years old children, once a day. |

**续　表**

| 剂型、规格<br>Preparations | 片剂：每片 4mg；5mg。包衣片：10mg。<br>Tablets: 4mg ; 5mg per tablet. Coated tablets: 10mg. |
| --- | --- |
| 药品名称 Drug Names | 普仑司特 Pranlukast |
| 适应证<br>Indications | 用于支气管哮喘的预防和治疗。<br>For the prevention and treatment of bronchial asthma. |
| 用法、用量<br>Dosage | 口服，成人一次 225mg，一日 2 次（餐后服）。<br>Oral medication: 225mg once for adults, 2 times a day (after meal). |
| 剂型、规格<br>Preparations | 胶囊剂：每粒 112.5mg。<br>Capsules: 112.5mg per capsule. |
| 药品名称 Drug Names | 吡嘧司特 Pemirolast |
| 适应证<br>Indications | 用于预防或减轻支气管哮喘发作，不能迅速缓解急性哮喘发作。<br>Used to prevent or alleviate bronchial asthma, it can not quickly relieve acute asthma attacks. |
| 用法、用量<br>Dosage | 口服：成人常用量每次 10mg，一日 2 次，早、午或临睡前服用。<br>Oral medication: usual dose for adults is 10mg once, 2 times a day, take in the morning, afternoon or before bedtime. |
| 剂型、规格<br>Preparations | 片剂：每片 10mg。<br>Tablets: 10mg per tablet. |
| 药品名称 Drug Names | 阿桔片 Compound Opioid and Platycodon grandiflorum Tablet |
| 适应证<br>Indications | 镇咳、祛痰<br>Relieving cough and reducing sputum. |
| 用法、用量<br>Dosage | 每次 3 ~ 4 片，一日 3 次。<br>3 ~ 4 tablets once, 3 times a day. |
| 剂型、规格<br>Preparations | 片剂：300mg。<br>Tablets: 300mg. |
| 药品名称 Drug Names | 川贝枇杷糖浆 ChuanBeiPiPa Syrup |
| 适应证<br>Indications | 化痰止咳<br>Relieving cough and reducing sputum. |
| 用法、用量<br>Dosage | 一次 10ml，一日 3 次。<br>10ml once, 3 times a day. |
| 剂型、规格<br>Preparations | 糖浆：100ml；120ml，150ml。<br>Syrup: 100ml, 120ml, 150ml. |
| 药品名称 Drug Names | 复方鲜竹沥液 FuFangXianZhuLi Oral Solution |
| 适应证<br>Indications | 清热化痰，止咳。<br>Clearing heat, relieving cough and reducing sputum. |
| 用法、用量<br>Dosage | 一次 20ml，一日 2 ~ 3 次。<br>20ml once, 2 to 3 times a day. |
| 剂型、规格<br>Preparations | 口服溶液：10ml；20ml；30ml。<br>Oral solution: 10ml, 20ml, 30ml. |
| 药品名称 Drug Names | 急支糖浆 Jizhi Syrup |
| 适应证<br>Indications | 清热化痰。用于外感风热咳嗽。<br>Clearing heat and reducing sputum. For the treatment of exogenous wind-heat cough. |

**续　表**

| | |
|---|---|
| 用法、用量<br>Dosage | 一次 20 ～ 30ml，一日 3 ～ 4 次。<br>20 ～ 30ml once, 3 to 4 times a day. |
| 剂型、规格<br>Preparations | 糖浆：100ml；200ml。<br>Syrup: 100ml, 200ml. |

| 12. 主要作用于消化系统的药物 Drugs mainly acting on the digestive system |
|---|

| 12.1　抗酸药 Antacids |
|---|

| 药品名称 Drug Names | 氢氧化铝 Aluminium Hydroxide |
|---|---|
| 适应证<br>Indications | 主要用于胃酸过多、胃及十二指肠溃疡、反流性食管炎及上消化道出血等。由于铝离子在肠内与磷酸盐结合成不溶解的磷酸铝自粪便排出，故尿毒症患者服用大剂量氢氧化铝后可减少磷酸盐的吸收，减轻酸血症（但同时应注意上述不良反应）。<br><br>Mainly used for hyperacidity, gastric and duodenal ulcers, reflux esophagitis and upper gastrointestinal bleeding. As the aluminum can react with phosphate in the intestine, forming insoluble aluminum phosphate that can be excreted in feces, so for uremic patients, taking large doses of aluminum hydroxide can help reduce the absorption of phosphate, and relieve acidosis (but above adverse reactions should be noted at the same time). |
| 用法、用量<br>Dosage | 口服，一次 0.6 ～ 0.9g，一日 1.8 ～ 2.7g。现多用氢氧化铝凝胶。治胃酸过多和溃疡病等，每次 4 ～ 8ml，一日 12 ～ 24ml，饭前 1 小时和睡前服；病情严重时剂量可加倍。<br><br>Oral medication: 0.6 ～ 0.9g once, 1.8 ～ 2.7g a day. Now aluminum hydroxide gel is more frequently used. For the treatment of hyperacidity and ulcer disease, 4 ～ 8ml once, 12 ～ 24ml a day, take 1 hour before meals and before bedtime; the dose can be doubled in serious condition. |
| 剂型、规格<br>Preparations | 片剂：每片 0.3g。<br>Tablets: 0.3g per tablet. |

| 药品名称 Drug Names | 铝碳酸镁 Hydrotalcite |
|---|---|
| 适应证<br>Indications | 主要用于胃及十二指肠溃疡、反流性食管炎、急慢性胃炎和十二指肠球炎等。也用于胃酸过多引起的胃部不适，如胃灼痛、胃灼热、反酸及腹胀、恶心、呕吐等的对症治疗。<br><br>Mainly used for gastric and duodenal ulcers, reflux esophagitis, acute and chronic gastritis and duodenal inflammation. Also used to treat stomach discomforts caused by hyperacidity, such as cardialgia, heartburn, acid reflux, bloating, nausea, vomiting and other symptoms. |
| 用法、用量<br>Dosage | 一般每日 3 次，每次 1.0g，餐后 1 小时服用。十二指肠球部溃疡 6 周为 1 个疗程，胃溃疡 8 周为 1 个疗程。<br><br>Usually 3 times a day, 1.0g once, take one hour after meals. For duodenal ulcer, one course of treatment is 6 weeks; for gastric ulcer, one course of treatment is 8 weeks. |
| 剂型、规格<br>Preparations | 片剂（咀嚼片）：每片 0.5g。<br>Tablet (chewable): 0.5g per tablet. |

| 药品名称 Drug Names | 碳酸钙 Calcium Carbonate |
|---|---|
| 适应证<br>Indications | 用于胃酸过多引起的反酸、胃灼热等症状。适用于胃、十二指肠溃疡及反流性食管炎的治疗。也用于补充机体钙缺乏，如各种机体对钙需求量增加的情况，可作为骨质疏松症的辅助治疗。另外，本品也用于治疗肾衰竭患者的高磷血症，同时纠正轻度代谢性酸中毒。作为磷酸盐结合剂，治疗继发性甲状旁腺功能亢进纤维性骨炎所致的高磷血症。<br><br>For the treatment of acid reflux, heartburn and other symptoms caused by hyperacidity. Suitable for treating stomach ulcer, duodenal ulcer, and reflux esophagitis. Also used for calcium deficiency supplement, for example, in the condition of increasing demand for calcium, the product can be used as adjuvant therapy for osteoporosis. In addition, the product is also used to treat hyperphosphatemia in patients with renal failure, while correct mild metabolic acidosis. As phosphate binder, it can be used to treat hyperphosphatemia caused by secondary hyperparathyroidism osteitis fibrosa. |

**续 表**

| | |
|---|---|
| 用法、用量<br>Dosage | 用于中和胃酸，每次 0.5 ~ 1g，一日 3 ~ 4 次，餐后 1 ~ 1.5 小时服用可维持缓冲时间长达 3 ~ 4 小时，如餐后即服，因随食物一起排空而失去作用。用于高磷血症，每日 1.5g，最高每日可用至 13g，进餐时服用或与氢氧化铝合用。用于补钙，每日 1 ~ 2g，分 2 ~ 3 次与食物同服，老年人可适当补充维生素 D。<br><br>Used to neutralize stomach acid, 0.5 ~ 1g once, 3 to 4 times a day, taking it 1 to 1.5 hours after meals can maintain the buffer time to 3 ~ 4 hours, if take after meals immediately, it will be useless for its being excreted along with food. For hyperphosphatemia, 1.5g a day, the maximum daily dose is 13g, take with meals or in combination with aluminum hydroxide. For calcium supplement, 1 ~ 2g a day, take with food in 2 to 3 divided doses, the elderly can appropriately add vitamin D supplement. |
| 剂型、规格<br>Preparations | 片剂：每片 0.5g（相当于元素钙 200mg）。<br>Tablets: 0.5g per tablet (equivalent to 200mg calcium) . |

## 12.2 胃酸分泌抑制剂 Inhibitors of gastric acid secretion

| 药品名称 Drug Names | 西咪替丁 Cimetidine |
|---|---|
| 适应证<br>Indications | 用于治疗十二指肠溃疡、胃溃疡、上消化道出血等。治疗十二指肠溃疡愈合率为 74%（对照组为 37%），愈合时间大多在 4 周左右。对胃溃疡疗效不及十二指肠溃疡。另据报道，还可用于治疗带状疱疹和包括生殖器在内的其他疱疹性感染。<br><br>For the treatment of duodenal ulcer, gastric ulcer, upper gastrointestinal bleeding etc. The healing rate of duodenal ulcer is 74% (37% in the contrast group), mostly the healing time is about 4 weeks. Less curative effects on gastric ulcer than duodenal ulcer. According to the report, it is also used to treat herpes zoster and other herpes infections, including genital herpes infection. |
| 用法、用量<br>Dosage | （1）口服，每次 200 ~ 400mg，一日 800 ~ 1600mg，一般于餐后及睡前各服一次，疗程一般为 4 ~ 6 周。亦有主张 1 次 400mg，一日 2 次的疗法。另外，也有报道夜间一次给予双倍剂量（800mg）的疗法。<br>（2）注射：用葡萄糖注射液或葡萄糖氯化钠注射液稀释后静脉滴注，每次 200 ~ 600mg；或用上述溶液 20ml 稀释后缓慢静脉注射，每次 200mg，4 ~ 6 小时一次。一日剂量不宜超过 2g。也可直接肌内注射。<br><br>(1) Oral medication, 200 ~ 400mg once, 800 ~ 1600mg a day, usually take both after meals and before bedtime, one course of treatment is usually 4 to 6 weeks. Or 400mg once, 2 times a day. Furthermore, it is also reported to give a double dose (800mg) at night for therapy.<br>(2) Injection: diluted with glucose injection or sodium chloride injection for intravenous infusion, 200 ~ 600mg once; or by slow intravenous injection after being diluted with 20ml above solution, 200mg once, 4 ~ 6 hours once. Daily dose should not exceed 2g. It can also be directly injected intramuscularly. |
| 剂型、规格<br>Preparations | 片剂：每片 0.2g；0.8g。胶囊剂：每粒 0.2g。注射液：每支 0.2g（2ml）。<br>Tablets: 0.2g; 0.8g per tablet. Capsules: 0.2g per capsule. Injection: 0.2g (2ml) per vial. |
| 药品名称 Drug Names | 雷尼替丁 Ranitidine |
| 适应证<br>Indications | 用于治疗十二指肠溃疡、良性胃溃疡、术后溃疡、反流性食管炎及卓 - 艾综合征等。静脉注射可用于上消化道出血。<br><br>For the treatment of duodenal ulcer, benign gastric ulcer, postoperative ulcer, reflux esophagitis and Zhuo-Ellison syndrome. Intravenous injection can be used for upper gastrointestinal bleeding. |
| 用法、用量<br>Dosage | 口服：一日 2 次，每次 150mg，早晚饭时服。维持剂量每日 150mg，于餐前顿服。用于反流性食管炎的治疗，一日 2 次，每次 150mg，共用 8 周。对卓 - 艾综合征，开始一日 3 次，每次 150mg，必要时剂量可加至每日 900mg。对慢性溃疡病有复发史患者，应在睡前给予维持剂量。治疗上消化道出血，可用本品 50mg 肌内注射或缓慢静脉注射（1 分钟以上），或以每小时 25mg 的速率间歇静脉滴注 2 小时。以上方法一般一日 2 次或每 6 ~ 8 小时 1 次。 |

| | Oral medication: 2 times a day, 150mg once, take at breakfast and at dinner. Daily maintenance dose is 150mg, take before meals. For reflux esophagitis treatment, 2 times a day, 150mg once, for eight weeks. For Zhuo - Ellison syndrome, three times a day at the beginning, 150mg once, if necessary, the daily dose can be increased to 900mg. For patients with chronic history of ulcer disease recurrence, the maintenance dose should be given before bedtime. For the treatment of gastrointestinal bleeding, 50mg of the product is for intramuscular injection or slow intravenous injection (more than 1 minute), or for intermittent intravenous infusion at a speed of 25mg per hour for 2 hours. The above methods are generally 2 times a day or once every 6 to 8 hours. |
|---|---|
| 剂型、规格<br>Preparations | 片（胶囊）剂：每片（粒）150mg。<br>泡腾颗粒：0.15g/1.5g。<br>糖浆剂：1.5g/100ml。<br>注射液：每支 50mg（2ml）；50mg（5ml）。<br>Tablets (capsules): 150mg per tablet (capsule).<br>Effervescent granules: 0.15g/1.5g.<br>Syrup: 1.5g/100ml.<br>Injection: 50mg (2ml); 50mg (5ml) per vial. |
| 药品名称 Drug Names | 枸橼酸铋雷尼替丁 Bismuth Citrate and Ranitidine |
| 适应证<br>Indications | 用于胃及十二指肠溃疡。与抗生素合用可协同根除幽门螺杆菌，预防十二指肠溃疡的复发。<br>For the treatment of gastric and duodenal ulcer. Combination with antibiotics can collaboratively eradicate helicobacter pylori, and prevent the recurrence of duodenal ulcer. |
| 用法、用量<br>Dosage | 成人每次 1 粒，一日 2 次，餐前服。治疗胃溃疡 8 周 1 个疗程，治疗十二指肠溃疡 4 周为 1 个疗程。轻至中度肾功能损害及肝功能不全者无须改变剂量。<br>1 capsule once, 2 times a day for adult, take before meals. The course of treatment is 8 weeks for gastric ulcer. The course of treatment is 4 weeks for duodenal ulcer. For patients with mild to moderate renal impairment or hepatic insufficiency, there is no need in changing the dose. |
| 剂型、规格<br>Preparations | 胶囊剂：每粒含枸橼酸铋雷尼替丁 350mg。<br>Capsules:350mg ranitidine bismuth per capsule. |
| 药品名称 Drug Names | 法莫替丁 Famotidine |
| 适应证<br>Indications | 口服用于胃及十二指肠溃疡、吻合口溃疡，反流性食管炎；口服或静脉注射用于上消化道出血（消化性溃疡、急性应激性溃疡，出血性胃炎所致），卓 - 艾综合征。<br>Oral medication for the treatment of gastric and duodenal ulcer, anastomotic ulcer, reflux esophagitis; Oral medication or intravenous injection for treating upper gastrointestinal bleeding (caused by peptic ulcer, acute stress ulcer, and hemorrhagic gastritis), Zhuo - Ellison syndrome. |
| 用法、用量<br>Dosage | 口服，每次 20mg，一日 2 次（早餐后，晚餐后或临睡前），4～6 周为 1 个疗程，溃疡愈合后维持量减半，睡前服。肾功能不全者应调整剂量。缓慢静脉注射或静脉滴注 20mg（溶于生理盐水或葡萄糖注射液 20ml 中），一日 2 次（间隔 12 小时），疗程为 5 日，一旦病情许可，应迅速将静脉给药改为口服给药。<br>Oral medication: 20mg once, 2 times a day (after breakfast, after dinner or before bedtime), 4～6 weeks for a course of treatment, maintenance dose can be halved after the ulcer heals, take before bedtime. The dose should be adjusted for patients with renal insufficiency. 20 mg for slow intravenous injection or intravenous infusion (dissolved in 20 ml saline or glucose injection), 2 times a day (12h intervals), the course of treatment is 5 days, once the condition permits, intravenous administration should be quickly changed to oral medication. |
| 剂型、规格<br>Preparations | 片剂：每片 10mg；20mg。<br>分散片：每片 20mg。<br>胶囊剂：每粒 20mg。<br>散剂：10%（100mg/g）。<br>注射液：每支 20mg（2ml）；每瓶 20mg/100ml。<br>Tablets: 10 mg; 20 mg per tablet.<br>Dispersible tablets: 20 mg per tablet.<br>Capsules: 20 mg per capsule.<br>Powder: 10% (100 mg/g).<br>Injection: 20 mg (2 ml) per vial; 20 mg / 100ml per bottle. |

**续 表**

| 药品名称 Drug Names | 奥美拉唑 Omeprazole |
|---|---|
| 适应证<br>Indications | 主要用于十二指肠溃疡和卓 - 艾综合征，也可用于胃溃疡和反流性食管炎；静脉注射可用于消化性溃疡急性出血的治疗。与阿莫西林和克拉霉素或与甲硝唑与克拉霉素合用，以杀灭幽门螺杆菌。<br><br>Mainly for duodenal ulcer and Zhuo - Ellison syndrome, also for gastric ulcer and reflux esophagitis; Intravenous injection can be used for acute peptic ulcer bleeding. Being used with amoxicillin and clarithromycin or with metronidazole and clarithromycin could kill helicobacter pylori. |
| 用法、用量<br>Dosage | 可口服或静脉给药。治疗十二指肠溃疡，一日 1 次，每次 20mg，疗程 2 ～ 4 周。治疗卓 - 艾综合征，初始剂量为每日 1 次，每次 60mg，90% 以上患者用每日 20 ～ 120mg 即可控制症状，如剂量大于每日 80mg，则应分 2 次给药，治疗反流性食管炎，剂量为每日 20 ～ 60mg，治疗消化性溃疡出血，静脉注射，一次 40mg，每 12 小时 1 次，连用 3 日。<br><br>Oral or intravenous.For duodenal ulcer, 1 time a day, 20 mg once, the treatment course lasts for 2 ～ 4 weeks. For Zhuo - Ellison syndrome, the initial dose is 60ml once, 1 times a day, more than 90% of the patients with 20 ～ 120 mg daily intaking can control symptoms, when the doses are greater than 80mg a day, it should be taken 2 times.For reflux esophagitis, the dose is 20 ～ 60 mg daily, for peptic ulcer bleeding, patients should have intravenous injection, 40 mg per time, once every 12 hours, stay for three days. |
| 剂型、规格<br>Preparations | 胶囊剂：每粒 20mg。<br>肠溶片：每片 20mg。<br>注射用奥美拉唑：每支 40mg。<br><br>Capsule: 20 mg per capsule.<br>Enteric-coated metformin hydrochloride: 20mg per tablet.<br>Injection with omeprazole: 40 mg per vial. |
| 药品名称 Drug Names | 兰索拉唑 Lansoprazole |
| 适应证<br>Indications | 用于胃溃疡、十二指肠溃疡、吻合口溃疡及反流性食管炎、卓 - 艾综合征等。<br>For gastric ulcer, duodenal ulcer, anastomotic ulcer and reflux esophagitis, Zhuo - Ellison syndrome, etc. |
| 用法、用量<br>Dosage | 成年人一般一日口服 1 次，每次 1 粒（片）。胃溃疡、吻合口溃疡、反流性食管炎 8 周为 1 个疗程。十二指肠溃疡 6 周为 1 个疗程。<br><br>Oral: 1 times a day for adults, 1 softgel(tablet) once . Treatment course for Gastric ulcer, anastomotic ulcer and reflux esophagitis lasts for 8 weeks . Treatment course for duodenal ulcer lasts for 6 weeks . |
| 剂型、规格<br>Preparations | 片（胶囊）剂：每片（粒）30mg。<br>Tablets (capsules): 30 mg per tablet (softgel). |
| 药品名称 Drug Names | 泮托拉唑 Pantoprazole |
| 适应证<br>Indications | 主要用于胃及十二指肠溃疡、胃 - 食管反流性疾病、卓 - 艾综合征等。<br>Mainly for gastric and duodenal ulcer, gastric, esophageal reflux disease, Zhuo - Ellison syndrome, etc. |
| 用法、用量<br>Dosage | 一般患者每日服用 1 片（40mg），早餐前或早餐间用少量水送服，不可嚼碎。个别对其他药物无反应的病例可每日服用 2 次；老年患者及肝功能受损者，每日剂量不得超过 40mg。十二指肠溃疡疗程 2 周，必要时再服 2 周；胃溃疡及反流性食管炎疗程 4 周，必要时再服 4 周。总疗程不超过 8 周。静脉滴注：一日 1 次 40mg，疗程依需要而定，但一般不超过 8 周。<br><br>Generally 1 tablet a day (40 mg), take it before breakfast or during breakfast with a small amount of water, do not chew.Take it 2 times a day for the cases having no respond to other drugs, ; For elderly patients and patient whose liver function is impaired, daily dose is no more than 40 mg. Duodenal ulcer treatment course lasts for 2 weeks, patients could take it 2 more weeks when it is necessary ; Gastric ulcer and reflux esophagitis's treatment course lasts for 4 weeks, patients could take it 4 more weeks when it is necessary The total course is should not more than eight weeks. Intravenous drip: 40mg once a day, the treatment course is depending on the need, but is generally not more than eight weeks. |

**续 表**

| | |
|---|---|
| 剂型、规格<br>Preparations | 片（肠溶）剂：每片 40mg。注射用泮托拉唑：每支 40mg。<br>Tablet(enteric): 40mg per tablet. Panxi tora azole for injection : 40 mg per vial. |
| **药品名称 Drug Names** | 雷贝拉唑 Rabeprazole |
| 适应证<br>Indications | 用于治疗活动性十二指肠溃疡、活动性良性胃溃疡、弥散性或溃疡性胃 - 食管反流症。<br>For active duodenal ulcer, active benign gastric ulcer, diffuse or ulcerative gastric - esophageal reflux disease. |
| 用法、用量<br>Dosage | 活动性十二指肠溃疡：每次 10 ～ 20mg，一日 1 次，连服 2 ～ 4 周；活动性良性胃溃疡：每次 20mg，一日 1 次，连服 4 ～ 6 周；胃 - 食管反流症：每次 20mg，一日 1 次，连服 6 ～ 10 周。均早晨服用，片剂必须整片吞服。<br>Active duodenal ulcer: 10 ～ 20mg once, 1 times a day, take for 2 ～ 4 weeks; Active benign gastric: 20mg once, 1 times a day, take for 4 ～ 6 weeks; Stomach - esophageal reflux disease: 20mg once, 1 times a day, take for 6 ～ 10 weeks. Take in the morning, must swallow for whole tablet. |
| 剂型、规格<br>Preparations | 片（肠溶）剂：每片 10mg；20mg。<br>Tablet(enteric): 10 mg; 20 mg per tablet |
| **药品名称 Drug Names** | 艾司奥美拉唑 Esomeprazole |
| 适应证<br>Indications | 用于食管反流性疾病。①治疗糜烂性反流性食管炎。②已经治愈的食管炎患者长期维持治疗，以防止复发。③为食管反流性疾病的症状控制。本品联合适当的抗菌疗法，用于根除幽门螺杆菌，使幽门螺杆菌感染相关的消化性溃疡愈合，并防止其复发。<br>For esophageal reflux disease. ① for treatment of erosive reflux esophagitis. ② for long-term maintenance treatment of the cured esophagitis patients, in order to prevent recurrence. ③ for disease control of esophageal reflux symptoms . Used with appropriate antimicrobial therapy, this product is for the trearment of helicobacter pylori eradication, helicobacter pylori infection related peptic ulcer, and prevents its recurrence. |
| 用法、用量<br>Dosage | （1）治疗糜烂性反流性食管炎：一次 40mg，一日 1 次，连服 4 周。对于食管炎未治愈或症状持续的患者，建议再治疗 4 周。<br>（2）已经治愈的食管炎患者长期维持治疗，以防止复发：一次 20mg，一日 1 次。<br>（3）胃食管反流性疾病的症状控制：无食管炎的患者一次 20mg，一日 1 次，如用药 4 周后症状未得到控制，应对患者做进一步检查，症状消除后，可采用即时疗法（即需要时口服 20mg，一日 1 次）。<br>（4）联合适当的抗菌疗法，用于根除幽门螺杆菌：采用联合用药方案，本品一次 20mg，阿莫西林一次 1g，克拉霉素一次 500mg，均为一日 2 次，共用 7 日。<br>老年人和轻度肾功能损害者，无须调整剂量；轻中度肝功能损害的患者无须调整剂量。严重肝功能损害的患者，一日用量为 20mg。<br>本品对酸不稳定，口服制剂均为肠溶制剂，服用时应整片（粒）吞服，不应嚼碎或压碎，至少应于餐前 1 小时服用。<br>(1)for erosive reflux esophagitis:40mg once, 1 time a day, it should be taken continuously for 4 weeks.For patients whose esophagitis has not bean cured or still have the symptoms, should take it for another 4 weeks.<br>(2) patients whose esophagitis has been cured, in order to get long-term maintenance treatment and prevent recurrence should take: 20mg once, 1 time a day.<br>(3) for the control for symptoms of gastroesophageal reflux disease : patients who does not have esophagitis should have 20 mg once, 1 time a day. If the symptoms is still out of control after four weeks, should do further examination for patients. After eliminate symptoms, can use instant therapy for patients (oral 20mg when patients need, once a day).<br>(4) Using with appropriate antimicrobial therapy for helicobacter pylori eradication: adopt combination scheme, take esomepr azole20 mg, amoxicillin 1g, clarithromycin 500mg per time, 2 times a day, take them continuously for 7 days.<br>No adjustment of dosage for the elderly and mild renal impairment, ; No adjustment of dosage for patients with mild-moderate donor liver damage. Patients with severe liver function damage, should take 20 mg a day.<br>The product is not stable for acid, oral preparations are enteric preparation, Patients should take the whole piece (tablet) to swallow, and should not chew or crush, should take it at least 1 hour before meal. |

续 表

| 剂型、规格<br>Preparations | 片（肠溶）剂：每片 20mg；40mg（以埃索美拉唑计）。<br>Tablets(enteric): 20mg per tablet; 40 mg (measured by esomeprazole). |
|---|---|
| **药品名称 Drug Names** | 丙谷胺 Proglumide |
| 适应证<br>Indications | 用于治疗胃溃疡和十二指肠溃疡、胃炎等。由于本品抑制胃酸分泌的作用较弱，临床已不再单独用于治疗溃疡病，但其利胆作用较受重视。也可用于非甾体抗炎药合用，预防后者对胃黏膜的损害。<br><br>Used for gastric and duodenal ulcer, gastritis, etc. Due to the weak role for inhibition of gastric acid secretion, clinically, this product is no longer used alone for the treatment of ulcers, but its cholagogic effect is valued. Used with non-steroidal anti-inflammatory drugs to prevent the latter damage of gastric mucosa. |
| 用法、用量<br>Dosage | 口服，每次 0.4g，一日 3 ～ 4 次，餐前 15 分钟给药，连续服 30 ～ 60 日（可根据胃镜或 X 线检查结果决定用药期限）。<br><br>Oral, 0.4g once, 3 ~ 4 times a day, 15 minutes before the meal, continuous taking about 30 ~ 60 days (according to the results of gastroscope or X-ray ). |
| 剂型、规格<br>Preparations | 片（胶囊）剂：每片（粒）0.2g。<br>Tablets (capsules): 0.2 g per tablet(softgel). |

12.3 胃黏膜保护剂 Gastric mucosal protectives

| **药品名称 Drug Names** | 枸橼酸铋钾 Bismuth Potassium Citrate |
|---|---|
| 适应证<br>Indications | 用于胃及十二指肠溃疡的治疗，也用于复合溃疡、多发溃疡、吻合口溃疡和糜烂性胃炎等。本品与抗生素合用，可根除幽门螺杆菌。用于幽门螺杆菌相关的胃、十二指肠溃疡及慢性胃炎、胃ＭＡＬＴ淋巴瘤、早期胃癌术后、胃食管反流病及功能性消化不良等。也可与抑制胃酸分泌药（质子泵抑制剂和 $H_2$ 受体拮抗剂）组成四联方案，作为根除幽门螺杆菌失败的补救治疗。<br><br>For gastric and duodenal ulcer, also for compound ulcer, multiple ulcers, anastomotic ulcer, erosive gastritis, etc. When this product is used with antibiotics, helicobacter pylori can be eradicated. For the stomach with helicobacter pylori and duodenum ulcer and chronic gastritis, gastric MALT lymphoma treatment, early postoperative gastric cancer, gastroesophageal reflux disease and functional dyspepsia. Can also be used with the inhibition of gastric acid secretion medicine (proton pump inhibitors and $H_2$ receptor antagonist) to unit a quadruple scheme, as the remedial treatment for the failure of eradication of helicobacter pylori. |
| 用法、用量<br>Dosage | 颗粒剂：一次一袋，一日 3 ～ 4 次，餐前半小时和睡前服用。片剂或胶囊剂：一次 2 片（粒），一日 2 次，早餐前半小时与睡前用温水送服，忌用含碳酸饮料（如啤酒等）；服药前、后半小时，不要喝牛奶或服用抗酸剂和其他碱性药物，疗程 4 ～ 8 周，然后停用含铋药物 4 ～ 8 周，如有必要，可再继续服用 4 ～ 8 周。<br><br>Granules: once a bag, 3 ~ 4 times a day, take it half an hour before meals and before bedtime. Tablet or capsule: 2 tablets (softgels)once, 2 times a day, take it with warm water half an hour before breakfast and before sleep, avoid taking it with carbonated beverages(such as beer, etc.); half an hour after or before taking the medicine, patients should not drink milk or antacids and other basic drugs. treatment lasts for 4 ~ 8 weeks, then patients stop using drugs containing bismuth for 4 ~ 8 weeks, if necessary, can continue to be taken for 4 ~ 8 weeks. |
| 剂型、规格<br>Preparations | 颗粒剂：每袋 1.2g，含本品 300mg。<br>片（胶囊）剂：每片（粒）120mg。<br>Granules: 1.2 g per bag, containing this product 300 mg.<br>Tablets (capsules): 120 mg per tablet(softgel). |
| **药品名称 Drug Names** | 胶体果胶铋 Colloidal Bismuth Pectin |
| 适应证<br>Indications | 用于胃及十二指肠溃疡，也可用于慢性浅表性胃炎、慢性萎缩性胃炎和消化道出血的治疗。本品与抗生素合用，可根除幽门螺杆菌。用于幽门螺杆菌相关的胃、十二指肠溃疡及慢性胃炎、胃 MALT 淋巴瘤、早期胃癌术后、胃食管反流病及功能性消化不良等。也可与抑制胃酸分泌药（质子泵抑制剂和 $H_2$ 受体拮抗药）组成四联方案，作为根除幽门螺杆菌失败的补救治疗。 |

| | For gastric and duodenal ulcer, also for compound ulcer, multiple ulcers, anastomotic ulcer, erosive gastritis, etc. When this product is used with antibiotics, helicobacter pylori can be eradicated. For the stomach with helicobacter pylori and duodenum ulcer and chronic gastritis, gastric MALT lymphoma treatment, early postoperative gastric cancer, gastroesophageal reflux disease and functional dyspepsia. Can also be used with the inhibition of gastric acid secretion medicine (proton pump inhibitors and $H_2$ receptor antagonist) to unit a quadruple scheme, as the remedial treatment for the failure of eradication of helicobacter pylori |
|---|---|
| 用法、用量<br>Dosage | 治疗消化性溃疡和慢性胃炎：每次 3 ~ 4 粒，一日 4 次，于三餐前半小时各服一次，睡前加服 1 次。疗程一般为 4 周。治疗消化道出血：将胶囊内药物倒出，用水冲开搅匀服用，日剂量一次服用，儿童用量酌减。<br><br>For Treatment of peptic ulcer and chronic gastritis: 3 ~ 4 softgels once, 4 times a day, take it half an hour before meals, add it 1 time before bedtime. Treatment usually lasts for 4 weeks.For gastrointestinal bleeding: pour out the drug from the capsulate, stir it evenly in water, take it once a day, children's dosage should be reduced. |
| 剂型、规格<br>Preparations | 胶囊剂：每粒 50mg。<br>Capsule:50 mg per softgel. |
| 药品名称 Drug Names | 胶体酒石酸铋 Colloidal Bismuth Tartrate |
| 适应证<br>Indications | 用于治疗慢性结肠炎、溃疡性结肠炎、肠功能紊乱及与幽门螺杆菌有关的消化性溃疡和慢性胃炎。<br><br>For chronic colitis, ulcerative colitis, bowel dysfunction, and peptic ulcer and chronic gastritis associated with helicobacter pylori . |
| 用法、用量<br>Dosage | 口服，每次 165mg（3 粒），一日 3 ~ 4 次，儿童用量酌减。一般 4 周为 1 个疗程。<br><br>Oral, 165 mg once (3 softgels), 3 ~ 4 times a day, children dosage should be reduced. The treatment course lasts for 4 weeks. |
| 剂型、规格<br>Preparations | 胶囊剂：每粒 55mg（以铋计）。<br>Capsule: 55mg per sotgel (measursed by bismuth). |
| 药品名称 Drug Names | 米索前列醇 Misoprostol |
| 适应证<br>Indications | 用于胃及十二指肠溃疡。对十二指肠溃疡，口服本品 200μg 一日 4 次，4 周后愈合率为 54%，对照组口服西咪替丁 300mg 一日 4 次，4 周后愈合率为 61%，疗效略低于西咪替丁，但本品在保护胃黏膜不受损伤方面比西咪替丁更为有效。<br><br>For gastric and duodenal ulcer. For duodenal ulcer, took 200ug 4 times a day.The healing rate was 54% after 4 weeks. The contast group took 300 mg cimetidine, 4 times a day, the healing rate was 61% after 4 weeks. Curative effect is slightly lower than cimetidine, but this product is more effective than cimetidine in protecting gastric mucosa from damage. |
| 用法、用量<br>Dosage | 每次 200μg，一日 4 次，于餐前和睡前口服。疗程为 4 ~ 8 周。<br>200ug once, 4 times a day, take before meals and before sleep. One course of treatment is 4 ~ 8 weeks. |
| 剂型、规格<br>Preparations | 片剂：每片 200μg。<br>Tablets:200ug per tablet. |
| 药品名称 Drug Names | 硫糖铝 Sucralfate |
| 适应证<br>Indications | 用于胃及十二指肠溃疡，也用于胃炎。<br>For gastric and duodenal ulcer, also for gastritis. |
| 用法、用量<br>Dosage | 口服，每次 1g，一日 3 ~ 4 次，餐前 1 小时及睡前服用。<br>Oral, 1g once, 3 ~ 4 times a day, take the pills 1 hour before meal or before bedtime. |
| 剂型、规格<br>Preparations | 片剂：每片 0.25g；0.5g。<br>分散片：每片 0.5g。<br>胶囊剂：每粒 0.25g。<br>悬胶剂：每袋 5ml（含硫糖铝 1g）。<br>Tablets: 0.25g per tablet ;0.5g.<br>Dispersible tablets: 0.5 g per tablet.<br>Capsule:0.25g per softgel.<br>Suspensoid agent: 5ml per bag (including 1g sucralfate). |

| 药品名称 Drug Names | 麦滋林 -S  Marzulene-S |
| --- | --- |
| 适应证<br>Indications | 用于胃炎、胃溃疡和十二指肠溃疡，可明显缓解临床症状，并有较好的预防溃疡复发的作用。<br>For gastritis, gastric and duodenal ulcer, it can obviously relieve the clinical symptoms, and it could prevent ulcer recurrence. |
| 用法、用量<br>Dosage | 成人一般每日 1.5 ~ 2.5g，分 3 ~ 4 次口服，剂量可随年龄与症状适当增减。<br>Oral: 1.5 ~ 2.5g, 3 ~ 4 times for adults/day, could be appropriately adjusted with different ages and symptoms. |
| 剂型、规格<br>Preparations | 颗粒剂：1g 内含水溶性　3mg 和 L- 谷酰胺 990mg。<br>Granules: 1 g contains 3 mg water-soluble azulene and 990mg L - l-glutamine . |
| 药品名称 Drug Names | 替普瑞酮 Teprenone |
| 适应证<br>Indications | 用于胃溃疡，也用于急性胃炎和慢性胃炎的急性加重期。<br>For gastric ulcer, also for acute gastritis and the acute aggravating period of chronic gastritis. |
| 用法、用量<br>Dosage | 餐后 30 分钟内口服，一日 3 次，每次 1 粒胶囊（50mg）或颗粒剂 0.5g（含本品 50mg）。<br>30mins after meal orally, 3 times a day, 1 capsules (50 mg) or 0.5 g granules (50 mg) once. |
| 剂型、规格<br>Preparations | 胶囊剂：每粒 50mg。颗粒剂：100mg（含本品）/g。<br>Capsules:50mg per softgel. Granules: 100 mg(incuding this product) /g. |
| 药品名称 Drug Names | 吉法酯 Gefarnate |
| 适应证<br>Indications | 用于治疗胃及十二指肠溃疡，急慢性胃炎，结肠炎，胃痉挛等。<br>For gastric and duodenal ulcers, acute or chronic gastritis and colitis, stomach cramps, etc. |
| 用法、用量<br>Dosage | 口服，对一般肠胃不适、胃酸过多、胃胀及消化不良等，可根据病情每次 1 ~ 2 片，一日 3 次。治疗消化性溃疡及急慢性胃炎，每次 2 片，一日 3 次，餐后服用；症状较轻者疗程 4 ~ 5 周，重症者疗程 2 ~ 3 个月。儿童剂量酌减。<br>Oral, for the average intestines and stomach discomfort, hyperacidity, stomach bilge and indigestion, according to the condition 1 ~ 2 tablets once, 3 times a day. For peptic ulcer and acute or chronic gastritis, 2 tablets once, 3 times a day, taking after the meal; For patients with light symptoms, the treatment course is 4 ~ 5 weeks, for patients with severe symptoms, the treatment course is 2 ~ 3 month. Children dose should be reduced accordingly. |
| 剂型、规格<br>Preparations | 片剂：每片 0.4g。<br>Tablets:0.4g per tablet. |
| 药品名称 Drug Names | 甘草锌 Licorzinc |
| 适应证<br>Indications | 用于口腔、胃、十二指肠及其他部位的溃疡症，还可用于促进刀口、创伤和烧伤的愈合。儿童厌食、异食癖、生长发育不良、肠病性肢端皮炎及其他儿童、成人锌缺乏症也可用本品治疗。本品还可用于青春期痤疮。<br>For the mouth, stomach, duodenum and other parts ulcer, can also be used to promote the healing of wound, trauma and burns.Can also for children anorexia, pica, growth stunted, enteropathy acrodermatitis, adults and children zinc deficiency. This product can also be used for adolescent acne. |
| 用法、用量<br>Dosage | （1）治疗消化性溃疡：片剂 1 次 0.5g，或颗粒剂 1 次 10g，一日 3 次，疗程为 4 ~ 6 周。必要时可减半再服 1 个疗程巩固疗效。<br>（2）治疗青春期痤疮，口腔溃疡及其他病症：片剂 1 次 0.25g，或颗粒剂 1 次 5g，一日 2 ~ 3 次。治疗青春期痤疮疗程为 4 ~ 6 周。愈后每日服药 1 次，片剂 0.25g，或颗粒剂 5g，服 4 ~ 6 周，以减少复发。<br>（3）保健营养性补锌，一日片剂 0.25g 即可，1 次或分 2 次服用；或颗粒剂 1 次 1.5g，一日 2 ~ 3 次。<br>（4）儿童用量每日按 0.5 ~ 1.5mg（以元素锌计）/kg 计算，分 3 次服用。 |

| | |
|---|---|
| | (1) treatment of peptic ulcer:0.5g tablets once or 10g granules once, 3 times a day, the course of treatment will last for 4 ~ 6 weeks. If necessary, patient could halve the dosage to consolidate the effect.<br><br>(2) treatment of adolescent acne, oral ulcer and other conditions:0.25g tablets once, or 5g granules once, 2 ~ 3 times a day. The course of adolescent acne treatment will last for 4 ~ 6 weeks. .After healing, take 0.25g tablet or 5g granules once a day for 4 ~ 6 weeks to prevent the recurrence.<br><br>(3) nutritional supplementation for zinc: 0.25g tablet a day, take 1 or 2 times; or1.5g granules once, 2 ~ 3 times a day.<br><br>(4) Dosage for children from 0.5 to 1.5mg(in element zinc)/kg, three times a day. |
| 剂型、规格<br>Preparations | 片剂：每片 0.25g（相当于含锌 12.5mg，甘草酸 87.5mg）。颗粒剂：每小袋 1.5g（相当于含元素锌 3.6 ~ 4.35mg）。<br><br>Tablets: 0.25 g per tablet (equivalent to 12.5 mg zinc, 87.5mg glycyrrhizic acid ). Granules: 1.5 g per pouch (equivalent to 3.6 ~ 4.35 mg elemental zinc ). |
| 药品名称 Drug Names | 瑞巴派特 Rebamipide |
| 适应证<br>Indications | 主要用于胃溃疡，但不宜单独用于 Hp 感染。也用于改善急性胃炎及慢性胃炎急性加重期的胃黏膜病变（如糜烂、出血、充血、水肿等）。<br><br>Mainly used for gastric ulcer, but should not be used for treating Hp infection alone. Also used to improve the acute gastritis and chronic gastritis with acute aggravating period of gastric mucosa lesions (such as erosion, hemorrhage, congestion and edema, etc.). |
| 用法、用量<br>Dosage | 口服，一般每次 0.1g，一日 3 次，早、晚及睡前服用。<br><br>Oral, 0.1g once, 3 times a day, take in the morning, evening and before bedtime. |
| 剂型、规格<br>Preparations | 片剂：每片 0.1g。<br><br>Tablets:0.1g per tablet. |
| 药品名称 Drug Names | 复方铝酸铋 Compound Bismuth Aluminate |
| 适应证<br>Indications | 用于胃及十二指肠溃疡、慢性浅表性胃炎、十二指肠球炎、胃酸过多症及功能性消化不良等。<br><br>For gastric and duodenal ulcer, chronic superficial gastritis, duodenal bulb inflammation, hyperacidity and functional dyspepsia. |
| 用法、用量<br>Dosage | 成人一日 3 次，每次 1 ~ 2 片，餐后嚼碎服。疗程为 1 ~ 3 个月；以后可减量维持防止复发。<br><br>3 times a day for adults, chew them after meals.The treatment course will last for 1 ~ 3months. Should reduce it gradually in case of relapse. |
| 剂型、规格<br>Preparations | 复方片剂，每片含铝酸铋 200mg、甘草浸膏粉 300mg、重质碳酸镁 400mg、碳酸氢钠 200mg、弗朗鼠李皮 25mg、茴香 10mg。<br><br>Compound tablets, per tablet contains bismuth aluminate 200 mg, licorice extract powder 300 mg, heavy magnesium carbonate 400 mg, sodium bicarbonate 200 mg, cortex frangulae 25 mg, fennel 10 mg. |

12.4 胃肠解痉药 Drugs relieving gastrointestinal spasm

| 药品名称 Drug Names | 丁溴东莨菪碱 Scopolamine Butylbromide |
|---|---|
| 适应证<br>Indications | （1）用于胃、十二指肠、结肠纤维内镜检查的术前准备，内镜逆行胰胆管造影和胃、十二指肠、结肠的气钡低张造影或计算机腹部体层扫描（CT 扫描）的术前准备，可有效减少或抑制胃肠道蠕动。<br><br>（2）用于治疗各种病因引起的胃肠道痉挛、胆绞痛、肾绞痛或胃肠道蠕动亢进等。<br><br>(1) For the preoperative preparation of stomach, duodenum and colon endoscopy examination, Endoscopic retrograde cholangiopancreatogra phyercp and Duodenum, colon barium contrast hypotonic or the preoperative preparation of Abdominal computer tomography (CT scan), which can effectively reduce or inhibit the gastrointestinal peristalsis.<br><br>(2) for the treatment for gastrointestinal tract spasm, biliary colic, renal colic and gastrointestinal peristalsis hyperfunction, which caused by various reasons. |

**续 表**

| 用法、用量 Dosage | 口服：1 次 10mg，一日 3 次。肌内注射、静脉注射或静脉滴注（溶于葡萄糖注射液、0.9% 氯化钠注射液中滴注）：每次 20 ~ 40mg；或 1 次 20mg，间隔 20 ~ 30 分钟后再用 20mg。<br><br>Oral:10mg once, 3 times a day.Intramuscular injection, intravenous injection or intravenous drip (dissolved in glucose injection, drip inject in 0.9% road warner): 20~40mg once or 20mg once and then intake 20mg after 20 to 30minutes. |
|---|---|
| 剂型、规格 Preparations | 注射液：每支 20mg（1ml）。<br>胶囊剂：每粒 10mg。<br>片剂：每片 10mg。<br><br>Injection: 20mg(1ml) per vial.<br>Capsules: 10mg per softgel.<br>Tablets: 10mg per tablet. |
| 药品名称 Drug Names | 曲美布汀 Trimebutine |
| 适应证 Indications | 用于慢性胃炎引起的胃肠道症状，如腹部胀满感、腹痛和嗳气等；也用于肠道易激综合征。<br><br>For gastrointestinal symptoms caused by chronic gastritis, such as abdominal fullness, abdominal pain and belching, etc.; Also for irritable bowel syndrome. |
| 用法、用量 Dosage | 治疗慢性胃炎，通常成人每次 100mg，一日 3 次。可根据年龄、症状适当增减剂量。治疗肠易激综合征，一般每次 100 ~ 200mg，一日 3 次。<br><br>For chronic gastritis, the adults usually take 100 mg once, 3 times a day. Patient could appropriate adjust the dose according to age and symptoms . For irritable bowel syndrome, 100 ~ 200 mg once, 3 times a day. |
| 剂型、规格 Preparations | 片剂：每片 100mg；200mg。<br>Tablets:100mg;200mg per tablet. |
| 药品名称 Drug Names | 溴丙胺太林 Propantheline Bromide |
| 适应证 Indications | 用于胃及十二指肠溃疡的辅助治疗，也用于胃炎、胰腺炎、胆汁排泄障碍、遗尿和多汗症。<br><br>For adjuvant therapy of gastric and duodenal ulcer, also used for gastritis, pancreatitis, bile excretion dysfunction, urinary incontinence, and hyperhidrosis. |
| 用法、用量 Dosage | 每次 15mg，一日 3 ~ 4 次，餐前服，睡前 30mg；治疗遗尿可于睡前口服 15 ~ 45mg。<br><br>15mg once, 3~4 times a day, take before meals with 30mg before going to bed;For urinary incontinence, could take 15 ~ 45 mg before bedtime. |
| 剂型、规格 Preparations | 片剂：15mg。<br>Tablets:15mg. |

12.5 助消化药 Digestants

| 药品名称 Drug Names | 多酶 Multienzyme |
|---|---|
| 适应证 Indications | 用于多种消化酶缺乏的消化不良症。<br>For indigestion due to a variety of digestive enzyme deficiency . |
| 用法、用量 Dosage | 口服，一次 1 ~ 2 片，一日 3 次，餐前服。<br>Oral, 1 to 2 tablets once, 3 times a day, take them before meals. |
| 剂型、规格 Preparations | 片剂：13mg（胃蛋白酶），300mg（胰酶）。<br>Tablets: 13mg (pepsin), 300mg (trypsin). |
| 药品名称 Drug Names | 复方慷彼申 Compound Combizym |
| 适应证 Indications | 用于各种原因所致的消化不良症。<br>For indigestion caused by a variety of factors. |
| 用法、用量 Dosage | 口服：每次 1 片，一日 3 次，饭时或餐后服用。<br>Oral: 1 tablet once, three times a day, take them during the meal or after meals. |

续　表

| 剂型、规格<br>Preparations | 肠溶片剂：24mg（米曲菌酶提取物）；220mg（胰酶）。<br>Enteric-coated tablets: 24mg (m aspergillosis enzyme extracts), 220mg (trypsin). |
|---|---|
| 药品名称 Drug Names | 干酵母 Dried Yeast |
| 适应证<br>Indications | 用于营养不良、消化不良、食欲缺乏、腹泻及胃肠胀气。<br>For malnutrition, indigestion, loss of appetite, diarrhea and flatulence. |
| 用法、用量<br>Dosage | 口服：每次 0.5 ~ 4g，嚼碎服。剂量过大可引起腹泻。<br>Oral: 0.5 ~ 4g once, take by chewing. Excessive doses can cause diarrhea. |
| 剂型、规格<br>Preparations | 片剂：每片 0.2g；0.3g；0.5g。<br>Tablets: 0.2g; 0.3g; 0.5g per tablet. |

12.6　促胃肠动力药 Gastrointestinal excitomotors

| 药品名称 Drug Names | 甲氧氯普胺 Metoclopramide |
|---|---|
| 适应证<br>Indications | （1）因脑部肿瘤手术、肿瘤放疗及化疗、脑外伤后遗症、急性颅脑损伤以及药物所引起的呕吐。<br>（2）胃胀气性消化不良、食欲缺乏、嗳气、恶心、呕吐。<br>（3）海空作业引起的呕吐及晕车。<br>（4）可增加食管括约肌压力，从而减少全身麻醉时胃肠道反流所致吸入性肺炎的发生率；可减轻钡剂检查时的恶心、呕吐反应，促进钡剂通过；十二指肠插管前服用，有助于顺利插管。<br>（5）对糖尿病性胃轻瘫，胃下垂等。<br>（6）可减轻偏头痛引起的恶心，并可能由于提高胃通过率而促进麦角胺的吸收。<br>（7）其催乳作用可试用于乳量严重不足的产妇。<br>（8）胆道疾病和慢性胰腺炎的辅助治疗。<br>(1) For vomiting caused by brain tumor surgery, radiotherapy and chemotherapy, sequelae of traumatic brain injury, acute brain injury and drugs .<br>(2) for Bloating dyspepsia, flatulence, loss of appetite, belching, nausea, and vomiting.<br>(3) for vomiting and motion sickness caused by sea and air operations.<br>(4) could increase esophageal sphincter pressure, thereby reducing the incidence of aspiration pneumonia during general anesthesia caused by gastrointestinal reflux; relieve nausea, and vomiting during barium meal examination, promote barium going through; take it before duodenal intubation would help intubation be smooth.<br>(5) diabetic gastroparesis, gastroptosis.<br>(6) relieve nausea caused by migraine, and promote absorption of ergotamine by increasing the rate of stomach throughout.<br>(7) its role of prolactin can be used for serious shortage of maternal milk.<br>(8) for adjuvant therapy of biliary tract disease and chronic pancreatitis. |
| 用法、用量<br>Dosage | （1）口服：一次 5 ~ 10mg，一日 10 ~ 30mg。餐前半小时服用。<br>（2）肌内注射：1 次 10 ~ 20mg。每日剂量一般不超过 0.5mg/kg，否则易引起锥体外系反应。<br>(1) Oral: 5 ~ 10mg once, 10 ~ 30mg a day. Take it half an hour before a meal.<br>(2) intramuscular injection: 10 ~ 20mg once. Daily dose should not exceed 0.5mg/kg, or would easily cause extrapyramidal reactions. |
| 剂型、规格<br>Preparations | 片剂：每片 5mg。注射液：每支 10mg（1ml）。<br>Tablets: 5mg per tablet. Injection: 10mg (1ml) per vial. |
| 药品名称 Drug Names | 多潘立酮 Domperidone |
| 适应证<br>Indications | （1）由胃排空延缓、反流性胃炎、慢性胃炎、反流性食管炎引起的消化不良症状；其他消化系统疾病引起的呕吐。<br>（2）胃轻瘫，尤其是糖尿病性胃轻瘫可缩短胃排空时间，使胃潴留症状消失。<br>（3）各种原因引起的恶心、呕吐；抗帕金森综合征药物引起的胃肠道症状及多巴胺受体激动药所致的恶心、呕吐。偏头痛、痛经、颅外伤及颅内病灶、放射治疗以及左旋多巴非甾体抗炎药等引起的恶心、呕吐。检查和治疗措施引起的恶心、呕吐；儿童因各种原因引起的急性和持续性呕吐等。对细胞毒性药物引起的呕吐只在不太严重时有效。<br>（4）可作为消化性溃疡的辅助治疗药物，用于消除胃窦部潴留。 |

续　表

| | |
|---|---|
| | (1) For dyspepsia symptms caused by delay of gastric emptying, reflux gastritis, chronic gastritis, indigestion reflux esophagitis-induced ; vomiting caused by other digestive diseases.<br><br>(2) gastroparesis, especially the gastric emptying time of diabetic gastroparesis can be shortened, so that gastric retention symptoms would disappear.<br><br>(3) nausea and vomiting caused by various reasons; anti-parkinsonism drug- induced gastrointestinal symptoms and dopamine receptor agonist-induced nausea and vomiting.Nausea and vomiting caused by migraine, dysmenorrhea, extracranial injuries intracranial lesions, radiation therapy and levodopa non-steroidal anti-inflammatory drugs. Examination and treatment-induced nausea and vomiting; acute and persistent vomiting due to various causes for children. Valid only when less severe cytotoxic drug-induced vomiting.<br><br>(4) can be used as an auxiliary treatment of peptic ulcer, for the elimination of the gastric antrum retention. |
| 用法、用量<br>Dosage | （1）肌内注射：每次 10mg，必要时可重复给药。<br><br>（2）口服：每次 10 ～ 20mg，一日 3 次，餐前服。<br><br>（3）直肠给药：每次 60mg，一日 2 ～ 3 次。栓剂最好在直肠空时插入。<br><br>(1) intramuscular injection:10mg once, repeated administration when necessary.<br>(2) oral: 10 ～ 20mg once, 3 times a day before meals.<br>(3) rectal administration: 60mg once, 2 to 3 times a day. It is better to insert it into the rectum when it is empty. |
| 剂型、规格<br>Preparations | 片剂：每片 10mg。<br><br>栓剂：每粒 60mg。<br><br>注射液：每支 10mg（2ml）。<br><br>滴剂：10mg/ml。<br><br>混悬液：1mg/ml。<br><br>Tablets: 10mg per tablet.<br>Suppositories:60mg per softgel.<br>Injection: 10mg (2ml) per vial.<br>Drops: 10mg/ml.<br>Suspension: 1mg/ml. |
| 药品名称 Drug Names | 西沙必利 Cisapride |
| 适应证<br>Indications | （1）可增加胃肠动力，用于胃轻瘫综合征，或上消化道不适，X 线、内镜检查阴性的症候群，特征为早饱、餐后饱胀、食量减低、胃胀、过多的嗳气、食欲缺乏、恶心、呕吐或类似溃疡的主诉（上腹部灼痛）。<br><br>（2）胃 - 食管反流：包括食管炎的治疗及维持治疗。<br><br>（3）与运动功能失调有关的假性肠梗阻导致的推进性蠕动不足和胃肠内容物滞留。<br><br>（4）可恢复结肠的推进性运动，作为慢性便秘患者的长期治疗。<br><br>(1) Could increase gastrointestinal motility, for the treatment of gastroparesis syndrome, or upper gastrointestinal discomfort, X-ray, endoscopy negative syndrome, it is characterized by early satiety, postprandial fullness, appetite reduced, bloating, excessive the belching, anorexia, nausea, vomiting, or similar ulcers(upper abdominal burning).<br>(2) stomach - esophageal reflux: including treatment and maintenance therapy of esophagitis .<br>(3) lack of propulsive motility and gastrointestinal contents stranded caused by intestinal pseudo-obstruction associated with movement disorders.<br>(4) it can restore the colonic propulsion movement, could be uesed as a long-term treatment for chronic constipation. |
| 用法、用量<br>Dosage | 口服，根据病情，一日总量为 15 ～ 40mg，分 2 ～ 4 次给药。食管炎的维持治疗：一次 10mg，一日 2 次，早餐前和睡前服用；或一次 20mg，一日 1 次，睡前服用。病情严重者剂量可加倍。<br><br>Oral, according to the disease, the total dosage of a day is 15 ～ 40mg, 2 to 4 doses. Maintening treatment of esophagitis:10mg once, 2 times a day, take it before breakfast and bedtime; or 20mg once, once a day, take it before bedtime. the dose could be doubled for severe cases. |
| 剂型、规格<br>Preparations | 片剂：每片 5mg；10mg。胶囊剂：每粒 5mg。干混悬剂：100mg。<br>Tablets: 5mg; 10mg per tablet . Capsules: 5mg per softgel. Suspension: 100mg. |

> 续　表

| 药品名称 Drug Names | 莫沙必利 Mosapride |
|---|---|
| 适应证<br>Indications | （1）慢性胃炎或功能性消化不良引起的消化道症状，如上腹部胀满感、腹胀、上腹部疼痛；嗳气、恶心、呕吐；胃烧灼感等。<br>（2）胃食管反流病和糖尿病胃轻瘫。<br>（3）胃大部切除术患者的胃功能障碍。<br>(1) For gastrointestinal symptoms caused by functional dyspepsia or chronic gastritis, such as abdominal fullness, bloating, abdominal pain; belching, nausea, vomiting; stomach burning sensation.<br>(2) For gastroesophageal reflux disease and diabetic gastroparesis.<br>(3) For gastrectomy in patients with gastric dysfunction. |
| 用法、用量<br>Dosage | 每次 5mg，一日 3 次，餐前服用。<br>5mg once, 3 times a day, before meals. |
| 剂型、规格<br>Preparations | 片剂：每片 5mg。<br>Tablets: 5mg per tablet . |

12.7　止吐药和催吐药 Antiemetics and emetics

| 药品名称 Drug Names | 昂丹司琼 Ondansetron |
|---|---|
| 适应证<br>Indications | 用于治疗由化疗和放疗引起的恶心、呕吐，也可用于预防和治疗手术后引起的恶心、呕吐。<br>For the treatment of chemotherapy and radiotherapy-induced nausea and vomiting, can also be used to prevent and treat nausea and vomiting caused by surgery. |
| 用法、用量<br>Dosage | （1）治疗由化疗和放疗引起的恶心、呕吐：①成人：给药途径和剂量应视患者情况因人而异，剂量一般为 8 ~ 32mg，为避免治疗 24 小时后出现恶心、呕吐，均应让患者持续服药，每次 8mg，一日 2 次，连服 5 日。②儿童：5mg/m$^2$ 静脉注射，12 小时后再口服 4mg，化疗后应持续给予患儿口服 4mg，一日 2 次，连服 5 日。③老年人：可依成年人给药法给药，一般不需要调整。<br>（2）预防或治疗手术后呕吐：①成人：一般可于麻醉诱导同时静脉滴注 4mg，或于麻醉前 1 小时口服 8mg，之后每隔 8 小时口服 8mg，共 2 次。已出现术后恶心、呕吐时，可缓慢静脉滴注 4mg 进行治疗。②肾衰竭患者：不需要调整剂量、用药次数或用药途径。③肝衰竭患者：由于主要自肝脏代谢，对中度或严重肝衰竭患者，每日用药剂量不应超过 8mg。<br>(1) treatment of chemotherapy and radiotherapy-induced nausea and vomiting: ① Adults: route of administration and dose should vary depending on the patient's condition, the dose is generally 8 ~ 32mg, to prevent nausea and vomiting after treatment of 24 hours, the patient should continue taking the medication, 8mg once, 2 times a day, continuously take it for 5 days. ② Children: 5mg/m$^2$ for intravenous injection, oral administration of 4mg after 12 hours, sick children should continue to be given 4mg orally after chemotherapy, 2 times a day, continuously take it for 5 days. ③ elderly: according to adult dosing method of administration, generally without adjustment.<br>(2) prevenation or treatment vomiting after surgery: ① Adults: Generally could do 4mg intravenous injection while doing anesthesia induced . or orally intake 8mg of the product within 1 hour before anesthesia, then every 8 hours for oral administration of 8mg, a total of 2 times. If postoperative nausea and vomiting was occurred, could do slow intravenous infusion for treatment. ② renal failure patients: No dose adjustment, no medication times adjustment or route of administration adjustment. ③ liver failure patients: As the produce mainly depends on hepatic metabolism, for moderate or severe liver failure patients, the daily dose should not exceed 8mg. |
| 剂型、规格<br>Preparations | 注射液：每支 4mg（1ml）；8mg（2ml）。片剂：每片 4mg；8mg。<br>Injection: 4mg (1ml); 8mg (2ml) per vial. Tablets: 4mg; 8mg per tablet. |

| 药品名称 Drug Names | 托烷司琼 Tropisetron |
|---|---|
| 适应证<br>Indications | 主要用于预防和治疗癌症化疗引起的恶心、呕吐。<br>Primarily used for the prevention and treatment of cancer chemotherapy-induced nausea and vomiting. |

**续 表**

| 用法、用量<br>Dosage | 每日 5mg，总疗程为 6 日。第 1 日，静脉给药，在化疗前将本品 5mg 溶于 100ml 生理盐水、林格液或 5% 葡萄糖注射液中静脉滴注或缓慢静脉注射，第 2 ～ 6 日，口服给药，一日一次，每次 1 粒胶囊（5mg），于进食前至少 1 小时服用，或于早上起床后立即用水送服。疗程为 2 ～ 6 日，轻症者可适当缩短疗程。<br><br>5mg a day, the total course is six days. The first day should have intravenous administration, make 5mg of the product dissolved in 100ml of saline, Ringer's solution or 5% glucose solution and then take intravenously or slow intravenous injection prior to chemotherapy. From the second day to 6th day, oral administration, once a day, one capsule (5mg) once, take it at least 1 hour before meals, or immediately take it with water after getting up in the morning. 2 to 6 days of treatment, mild patients could appropriatly shorten the course. |
|---|---|
| 剂型、规格<br>Preparations | 注射液：每支 5mg（1ml）。胶囊剂：每粒 5mg。<br>Injection: 5mg (1ml) per vail. Capsules: 5mg per softgel. |
| 药品名称 Drug Names | 格拉司琼 Granisetron |
| 适应证<br>Indications | 用于预防和治疗化疗、放疗及手术后引起的恶心和呕吐。<br>For the prevention and treatment of chemotherapy, radiotherapy-induced nausea and vomiting and post-operative nausea and vomiting . |
| 用法、用量<br>Dosage | 将本品以注射用生理盐水 20 ～ 50ml 稀释后，于化疗或放疗前每日 1 次静脉滴注，成人剂量每次 40μg/kg，或给予标准剂量 3mg，如症状未见改善，可再增补一次；对老年患者及肾功能不全患者一般不需要调整剂量。每 1 个疗程可连续使用 5 日。<br><br>Diluted it with 20 ～ 50ml of saline, intravenously infused before chemotherapy or radiotherapy once daily, 40μg/kg once for adult, or give the standard dose of 3mg, if the symptoms do not improve, you can then supplement one time; for elderly patients and the renal insufficiency patients, the dose does not need to be adjusted. per course can be used continuously for five days. |
| 剂型、规格<br>Preparations | 注射液：每支 3mg（3ml）。片（胶囊）剂：每片（粒）1mg。<br>Injection: 3mg (3ml) per vial. Tablets (capsules):(tablets) 1mg per tablet. |
| 药品名称 Drug Names | 阿扎司琼 Azasetron |
| 适应证<br>Indications | 用于化疗及放疗引起的消化系统症状，如恶心、呕吐等。<br>For chemotherapy and radiotherapy-induced gastrointestinal symptoms such as nausea and vomiting, etc. |
| 用法、用量<br>Dosage | 成人一般用量为 10mg，一日一次静脉注射。<br>Usual dosage is 10mg for adult, once daily for intravenous injection.. |
| 剂型、规格<br>Preparations | 注射剂：每支 10mg（2ml）。<br>Injection: 10mg (2ml) per vial. |
| 药品名称 Drug Names | 地芬尼多 Difenidol |
| 适应证<br>Indications | 用于各种原因引起的眩晕、恶心、呕吐等症状。<br>For dizziness, nausea, vomiting and other symptoms caused by various reasons. |
| 用法、用量<br>Dosage | 口服：每次 25 ～ 50mg，一日 3 次；肌内注射：每次 20 ～ 40mg，一日 4 次。儿童（6 个月以上）：每次 0.9mg/kg，一日 3 次。<br><br>Oral: 25 ～ 50mg once, 3 times a day; intramuscular injection: 20 ～ 40mg once, 4 times a day. For children (6 months or more): 0.9mg/kg once, three times a day. |
| 剂型、规格<br>Preparations | 片剂：25mg。注射液：10mg/1ml。<br>Tablets: 25mg. Injection: 10mg/1ml. |

**续　表**

| 12.8 泻药 Laxatives | |
|---|---|
| 药品名称 Drug Names | 硫酸镁 Magnesium Sulfate |
| 适应证<br>Indications | （1）导泻，肠内异常发酵，亦可与驱虫剂并用；与药用炭合用，可治疗食物或药物中毒。<br>（2）阻塞性黄疸及慢性胆囊炎。<br>（3）惊厥、子痫、尿毒症、破伤风、高血压脑病及急性肾性高血压危象等。<br>（4）也用于发作频繁而其他治疗效果不佳的心绞痛患者，对伴有高血压的患者效果较好。<br>（5）外用热敷消炎去肿。<br><br>(1) For catharsis, intestinal abnormal fermentation, also can be combined with insect repellent; combination with medicinal charcoal for treating food or drug poisoning.<br>(2) obstructive jaundice and chronic cholecystitis.<br>(3) convulsions, eclampsia, uremia, tetanus, hypertensive encephalopathy and acute renal hypertensive crisis and so on.<br>(4) also used for frequent seizures of angina and other poor treatment of angina, has good effect on patients with hypertension .<br>(5) hot topical anti-inflammatory to the swelling. |
| 用法、用量<br>Dosage | （1）导泻：每次口服 5 ～ 20g，清晨空腹服，同时饮 100 ～ 400ml 水，也可用水溶解后服用。<br>（2）利胆：每次 2 ～ 5g，一日 3 次，餐前或两餐间服。也可服用 33% 溶液，每次 10ml。<br>（3）抗惊厥、降血压等：肌内注射，一次 1g，10% 溶液，每次 10ml；静脉滴注，一次 1 ～ 2.5g，将 25% 溶液 10ml 用 5% 葡萄糖注射液稀释成 1% 浓度缓慢静脉滴注。<br><br>(1) catharsis: 5 ～ 20g once for oral, early in the morning with empty stomach and drink 100 ～ 400ml water, also it can be dissolved in water for intaking.<br>(2) gallbladder: 2 ～ 5g once, 3 times a day before meals or between two meals. 33% solution can be taken, 10ml once.<br>(3) anticonvulsants, hypotensive, etc.: intramuscular injection, 1g once, 10% solution, 10ml once; intravenous infusion, 1 ～ 2.5g once, slowly diluted 10ml 25% solution  to the 5% glucose injection to a concentration of 1%, then take intravenous drip. |
| 剂型、规格<br>Preparations | 注射液：每支 1g（10ml）；2.5g（10ml）。<br>Injection: 1g (10ml); 2.5g (10ml) per vial. |
| 药品名称 Drug Names | 甘油 Glycerol |
| 适应证<br>Indications | 用于便秘、降眼压和颅内压。<br>For constipation, lowering intraocular pressure and intracranial pressure. |
| 用法、用量<br>Dosage | （1）便秘：使用栓剂，每次 1 粒塞入肛门（成人用大号栓、小儿用小儿栓），对小儿及年老体弱者较为适宜。也可用本品 50% 溶液灌肠。<br>（2）降眼压和降颅内压：口服 50% 甘油溶液（含 0.9% 氯化钠），每次 200ml，日服 1 次，必要时日服 2 次，但要间隔 6 ～ 8 小时。<br><br>(1) constipation: using suppositories, inserting into the anus one softgel once (adult with a large bolt, children with pediatric suppository), it is appropriate for children and the elderly and infirm . 50% solution can be used for enema.<br>(2) lowering intraocular pressure and intracranial pressure: 50% glycerol solution (containing 0.9% sodium chloride) for oral, 200ml once, 1 time a day, 2 times at the necessary time, but there should be an interval of 6 to 8 hours. |
| 剂型、规格<br>Preparations | 栓剂：含甘油约 90%，大号每个约重 3g，小号每个约重 1.5g。甘油溶液：包括 10% 甘油生理盐水溶液、10% 甘油葡萄糖溶液、10% 甘油甘露醇溶液和 50% 甘油盐水溶液。<br><br>Suppository: containing about 90% of glycerol, the weight of per tuba is about 3g, the trumpet one is about 1.5g. Glycerol solution: contain 10% glycerol physiological saline solution, 10% glycerol glucose solution, 10% glycerol mannitol solution and 50% glycerol salt solution. |
| 药品名称 Drug Names | 开塞露 Enema Glycerini |
| 适应证<br>Indications | 本品为治疗便秘的直肠用溶液剂。<br>This product is used as rectal solutions for treating constipation. |

**续 表**

| | |
|---|---|
| 用法、用量<br>Dosage | 用时将容器顶端刺破，外面涂油脂少许，徐徐插入肛门，然后将药液挤入直肠内，引起排便。成人用量每次 20ml（1 支）。<br><br>Punctured the top of the container and grease the outside a little, slowly insert into the anus, and then squeeze the liquid inside the rectum to cause defecation. 20ml (1 bottle)once for adults. |
| 剂型、规格<br>Preparations | 每支 20ml。<br>20ml per bottle. |
| **药品名称 Drug Names** | **硫酸钠 Sodium Sulfate** |
| 适应证<br>Indications | 为容积性泻药。<br>Volume laxatives. |
| 用法、用量<br>Dosage | 散剂：一次 5 ~ 20g，溶于 250ml 水，清晨空腹服用；肠溶胶囊：一次 5g，一日 1 ~ 3 次。排便后即可停药，如 12 小时后未排便，可追加服药 1 ~ 2 次。<br><br>Powder: 5 ~ 20g once, dissolved in 250ml water, take in the morning on with an empty stomach; enteric-coated capsules: 5g once, 1 to 3 times a day. Can be discontinued after a bowel movement, if do not have defecation after taking it 12 hours, medication could be added 1 to 2 times. |
| 剂型、规格<br>Preparations | 散剂：500g。肠溶胶囊：1g/ 粒。<br>Powder: 500g. Enteric-coated capsules: 1g per softgel. |
| **药品名称 Drug Names** | **液状石蜡 Liquid Paraffin** |
| 适应证<br>Indications | 使粪便稀释变软，同时润滑肠壁，使粪便易于排出。<br>Diluting the stool softly, while lubricating the intestinal wall, so as to discharge the stool easily. |
| 用法、用量<br>Dosage | 每次 15 ~ 30ml，睡前服。<br>15 ~ 30ml once, take before bedtime. |
| 剂型、规格<br>Preparations | 原液：500ml。<br>Dope: 500ml. |

## 12.9 止泻药 Antidiarrheal drugs

| | |
|---|---|
| **药品名称 Drug Names** | **双八面体蒙脱石 Dioctahedral Smectite** |
| 适应证<br>Indications | 用于急慢性腹泻，尤以对儿童急性腹泻疗效为佳，但在必要时应同时治疗脱水，也用于食管炎及与胃、十二指肠、结肠疾病有关的疼痛的对症治疗。<br><br>For acute and chronic diarrhea, especially for children with acute diarrhea, but processing necessarily the treatment of dehydration at the same time, and also for the symptomatic treatment of pain caused by esophagitis and the stomach, duodenum, colon diseases . |
| 用法、用量<br>Dosage | 成人每次 1 袋，一日 3 次，治疗急性腹泻首剂应加倍。食管炎患者宜于餐后服用，其他患者于餐前服用，将本品溶于半杯温水中送服。<br><br>1 bag once for adults, 3 times a day, the first dose of the treatment of acute diarrhea should be doubled. Take after meals for patients with esophagitis, and take before meals for other patients, the product should be dissolved in half a glass of warm water for service. |
| 剂型、规格<br>Preparations | 散剂：每小袋内含双八面体蒙脱石 3g、葡萄糖 0.749g、糖精钠 0.007g、香兰素 0.004g。<br><br>Powder:containing 3g dioctahedral montmorillonite, 0.749g glucose, 0.007g sodium saccharin, 0.004g vanillin per pouch. |
| **药品名称 Drug Names** | **鞣酸蛋白 Tannalbin** |
| 适应证<br>Indications | 用于急性胃肠炎非细菌性腹泻。<br>For acute nonbacterial gastroenteritis diarrhea. |
| 用法、用量<br>Dosage | 一日 3 次，每次 1 ~ 2g，空腹服。<br>3 times a day, 1 ~ 2g once, take it with an empty stomach. |

**续　表**

| | |
|---|---|
| 剂型、规格<br>Preparations | 片剂：0.25g；0.5g。<br>Tablets: 0.25g;0.5g. |
| 药品名称 Drug Names | 碱式碳酸铋 Bismuth Subcarbonate |
| 适应证<br>Indications | 用于腹泻、慢性胃肠炎、胃及十二指肠溃疡。<br>For diarrhea, chronic gastroenteritis, gastric and duodenal ulcers. |
| 用法、用量<br>Dosage | 一日 3 次，每次 0.3 ~ 0.9g，餐前服。<br>3 times a day, 0.3 ~ 0.9g once, take it before the meal. |
| 剂型、规格<br>Preparations | 片剂：0.3g。<br>Tablets: 0.3g. |
| 12.10 微生态药物 Microecological drugs | |
| 药品名称 Drug Names | 地衣芽孢杆菌活菌 Live Bacillus Licheniformis |
| 适应证<br>Indications | 用于细菌与真菌引起的急慢性腹泻及各种原因所致的肠道菌群失调的防治。<br>For acute and chronic diarrhea caused by bacteria and fungi and the prevention of intestinal flora for variety of reasons. |
| 用法、用量<br>Dosage | 口服：每次 0.5g，一日 3 次，小儿减半或遵医嘱。<br>Oral: 0.5g once, 3 times a day, children should take it by half or as directed. |
| 剂型、规格<br>Preparations | 胶囊剂：每粒 0.25g。<br>Capsules: 0.25g per capsule. |
| 药品名称 Drug Names | 嗜酸乳杆菌 Lactobacillus LB |
| 适应证<br>Indications | 用于急慢性腹泻的对症治疗。<br>For the symptomatic treatment of acute and chronic diarrhea. |
| 用法、用量<br>Dosage | 胶囊剂：成人及儿童一日 2 次，每次 2 粒，成人首剂量加倍；婴儿一日 2 次，每次 1 ~ 2 粒，首剂量 2 粒。散剂：成人及儿童一日 2 次，每次 1 袋，成人首剂量加倍；婴儿一日 2 次，每次 1 袋。胶囊剂可用水吞服亦可倒出内容物混合于水中饮服。<br>Capsules: 2 times a day for adults and children, two softgels once, the first dose for adult doubles; 2 times a day for baby, 1 to 2 sofegels once, the first dose is 2 softgels. Powder: 2 times a day for adults and children, one bag once, the first dose for adult doubles; 2 times a day for baby, one bag once. Capsules can be swallowed with water, or pour out the contents and mix them with water for oral medication. |
| 剂型、规格<br>Preparations | 胶囊剂：每胶囊含灭活冻干的嗜酸乳杆菌 50 亿和中和后冻干的培养基 80mg。<br>散剂：每小袋含灭活冻干的嗜酸乳杆菌 50 亿和中和后冻干的培养基 160mg。<br>Capsules: containing 5 billion of inactivated lyophilized lactobacillus acidophilus and 80mg lyophilization medium after neutralize per capsule.<br>Powder: per sachet containing 5 billion of lyophilized inactivated lactobacillus acidophilus and 160mg lyophilization medium after neutralize . |
| 药品名称 Drug Names | 复合乳酸菌 Lactobacillus Complex |
| 适应证<br>Indications | 用于各种原因引起的肠道菌群紊乱、急慢性腹泻、肠易激综合征、抗生素相关性腹泻的治疗。亦可用于预防或减少抗生素及化疗药物所致的肠道菌群紊乱的辅助治疗。<br>Used for the treatment of intestinal flora disorder caused by various reasons, acute and chronic diarrhea, irritable bowel syndrome and antibiotic-associated diarrhea. And also used for adjuvant therapy of intestinal flora disorders caused by antibiotics and chemotherapy. |
| 用法、用量<br>Dosage | 口服：一次 1 ~ 2 粒，一日 1 ~ 3 次，根据病情和年龄可适当增减。<br>Oral: 1 to 2 softgels once, 1 to 3 times a day, patient could increase or decrease the dose according to the condition and age. |
| 剂型、规格<br>Preparations | 胶囊剂：每粒 0.33g（含活乳酸菌 2 万个以上）。<br>Capsules: 0.33g per softgel(containing 20, 000 live lactobacillus or more). |

**续 表**

| 药品名称 Drug Names | 双歧杆菌嗜酸乳杆菌肠球菌三联活菌 Live Combined Bifidobacterium, Lactobacillus and Enterococcus |
|---|---|
| 适应证<br>Indications | 用于肠道菌群失调引起的腹泻、腹胀等，也用于慢性腹泻和轻中型急性腹泻，以调节肠道功能；对缓解便秘也有较好疗效，还可作为肝硬化、急慢性肝炎及肿瘤化疗等的辅助用药。<br><br>For diarrhea and bloationg caused by intestinal flora, and also for chronic diarrhea and mild to moderate acute diarrhea, to regulate intestinal function; It also has a good effect on relieving constipation, and also be used as adjuvant chemotherapy of cirrhosis, acute and chronic hepatitis and cancer. |
| 用法、用量<br>Dosage | 口服：每次 420 ～ 630mg，一日 2 ～ 3 次，餐后服用。小于 1 岁儿童每次 105mg；1 ～ 6 岁每次 210mg；6 ～ 13 岁每次 210 ～ 420mg。婴幼儿可取胶囊内药粉用温开水调服。<br><br>Oral: 420 ～ 630mg once, 2 to 3 times a day, take it after meals. 105mg once for less than 1 year old child; 210mg once for 1 ～ 6 years old child; 210 ～ 420mg once for 6 ～ 13 years old. Infants could take the powder inside the capsule with warm water. |
| 剂型、规格<br>Preparations | 胶囊剂：每粒 210mg。散剂：每包 1g；2g。<br>Capsules: 210mg per softgel. Powder: 1g; 2g per package. |
| 药品名称 Drug Names | 枯草杆菌肠球菌二联活菌 Live Combined Bacillus Subtilis and Enterococcus |
| 适应证<br>Indications | 治疗和预防抗生素相关性腹泻、旅行者腹泻及其他腹泻；也可用于肠易激综合征（ＩＢＳ）及炎性肠病的辅助治疗。<br><br>For the treatment and prevention of antibiotic-associated diarrhea, traveler's diarrhea and other diarrhea; also be used for irritable bowel syndrome (IBS) and the adjuvant therapy of inflammatory bowel disease. |
| 用法、用量<br>Dosage | 12 岁以上儿童及成人：口服，每次 1 ～ 2 粒，一日 2 ～ 3 次。<br>Children over 12 years and adults : oral, 1 to 2 softgels once, 2 to 3 times a day. |
| 剂型、规格<br>Preparations | 胶囊（肠溶）剂：每粒 250mg。<br>Capsules (enteric) agent: 250mg per softgel. |
| 药品名称 Drug Names | 乳酶生 Lactasin |
| 适应证<br>Indications | 用于消化不良、肠发酵、小儿饮食不当引起的腹泻等。<br>For indigestion, intestinal fermentation, children's diarrhea caused by improper diet and so on. |
| 用法、用量<br>Dosage | 每次 0.3 ～ 1.0g，一日 3 次，餐前服。<br>0.3 ～ 1.0g once, 3 times a day, take it before meals. |
| 剂型、规格<br>Preparations | 片剂：0.15g；0.3g。<br>Tablets: 0.15g; 0.3g. |

### 12.11 治疗肝性脑病药 Drugs treating hepatic encephalopathy

| 药品名称 Drug Names | 乳果糖 Lactulose |
|---|---|
| 适应证<br>Indications | 用于肝性脑病的辅助治疗，也用于内毒素血症和治疗便秘。<br><br>For the adjuvant treatment of hepatic encephalopathy, also used for the treatment of endotoxemia and constipation. |
| 用法、用量<br>Dosage | 治疗肝性脑病和内毒素血症：开始每次 10 ～ 20mg，一日 2 次，后改为每次 3 ～ 5g，一日 2 ～ 3 次；以每日排软便 2 ～ 3 次为宜。治疗肝性脑病时可将本品 200g 加入 700ml 水或生理盐水中，保留灌肠 30 ～ 60 分钟，每 4 ～ 6 小时 1 次。本品与新霉素合用可提高对肝性脑病的疗效。治疗便秘：每次 5 ～ 10mg，一日 1 ～ 2 次，应根据个人反应调节，如 48 小时未见效果，可适当增加剂量。<br><br>Treatment of hepatic encephalopathy and endotoxemia: 10 ～ 20mg once at the beginning, 2 times a day, then changed 3 ～ 5g once later, 2 to 3 times a day; it would be better if patients discharge soft stools 2 ～ 3 times a day . For the treatment of hepatic encephalopathy, 200g of this product can be added to 700ml water or saline, take enema for 30 to 60 minutes, 4 to 6 hours once.The combination of this product and neomycin can improve the efficacy of hepatic encephalopathy. Treatment of constipation: 5 ～ 10mg once, 1 ～ 2 times a day, the dose is adjusted according to individual response, if it has no effect during 48 hours, the dose could be increased. |

**续　表**

| | |
|---|---|
| 剂型、规格<br>Preparations | 乳果糖粉：每袋 5g；100g；500g。<br>乳果糖颗粒：每袋 10g。<br>乳果糖口服液：5g（10ml）；50g（100ml）。<br>乳果糖糖浆：60%。<br>Lactulose powder: 5g; 100g; 500g per bag.<br>Lactulose particles: 10g per bag.<br>Oral lactulose: 5g (10ml); 50g (100ml).<br>Lactulose syrup: 60%. |
| 药品名称 Drug Names | 谷氨酸钠 Sodium Glutamate |
| 适应证<br>Indications | 用于肝性脑病及酸血症。<br>For hepatic encephalopathy and acidosis. |
| 用法、用量<br>Dosage | 肝性脑病：每次静脉滴注 11.5g，用 5% 葡萄糖注射液 750 ～ 1000ml 或 10% 葡萄糖注射液 250 ～ 500ml 稀释，于 1 ～ 4 小时滴完，滴注过快可引起流涎、潮红、呕吐等。必要时可于 8 ～ 12 小时后重复给药，一日量不宜超过 23g。酸血症：用量根据病情决定。<br>Hepatic encephalopathy: 11.5g once for infusion, diluted with 750 ～ 1000ml 5% glucose injection or 250 ～ 500ml 10% glucose injection, drop totally within 1 to 4 hours, excessive drip can cause salivation, flushing and vomiting. Repeated administration can be processed after 8 to 12 hours if necessary, the dose of a day should not exceed 23g. Acidosis: the dose is determined according to the condition. |
| 剂型、规格<br>Preparations | 注射液：每支 5.75g/20ml。<br>Injection: 5.75g/20ml per vial. |
| 药品名称 Drug Names | 支链氨基酸 Branched Amino Acid |
| 适应证<br>Indications | 支链氨基酸 3H 注射液、六合氨基酸注射液主要用于支 / 芳比失调引起的肝性脑病及各种肝病引起的氨基酸代谢紊乱。14 氨基酸 -800 主要用于肝功能不全合并蛋白营养缺乏症和肝性脑病。<br>Injection of 3H branched chain amino acids and amino acid injection are mainly used for hepatic encephalopathy caused by support / aromatic ratio imbalance and amino acid metabolism disorder caused by a variety of liver diseases. 14 amino acids -800 is mainly used for liver dysfunction combined with nutritional protein deficiencies and hepatic encephalopathy. |
| 用法、用量<br>Dosage | 静脉滴注：一日 2 次，每次 250ml，与等量 10% 葡萄糖注射液串联后做缓慢滴注（不宜超过 3ml/min）。如疗效显著者（完全清醒），后阶段剂量可减半。疗程一般为 10 ～ 15 日。中心静脉滴注：每日量以 0.68 ～ 0.87g/kg 计，成人剂量相当于每日 500 ～ 750ml，与 25% ～ 50% 高渗葡萄糖注射液等量混匀后，经中心静脉缓慢滴注，滴速不得超过 40 滴 / 分。<br>Intravenous infusion: 2 times a day, 250ml once, slow infusion with an equal amount of 10% glucose injection (not more than 3ml/min). If efficacy were significantly (fully awake), the dose can be halved at a later stage. Treatment course usually lasts for 10 to 15 days. Central venous infusion: Daily amount is of 0.68 ～ 0.87g/kg, adult dose is equivalent of 500 ～ 750ml a day, slow intravenous instilling from the central vein after mixed with equal amounts of 25% to 50% hypertonic glucose, the instilling speed should not exceed 40 drops / min. |
| 剂型、规格<br>Preparations | 注射液：250ml-10.65g（总氨基酸）。<br>Injection: 250ml-10.65g (total amino acids). |
| 药品名称 Drug Names | 谷氨酸钾 Potassium Glutamate |
| 适应证<br>Indications | 用于肝性脑病、酸血症，常与谷氨酸钠合用，以维持电解质平衡。<br>For hepatic encephalopathy, acidosis, often in combination with sodium glutamate to maintain electrolyte balance. |
| 用法、用量<br>Dosage | 静脉滴注：每次 6.3g，其余用法、注意同谷氨酸钠。<br>Intravenous infusion: 6.3g once, the rest usage and announcements are same as sodium glutamate. |
| 剂型、规格<br>Preparations | 注射液：6.3g（20ml）。<br>Injection: 6.3g (20ml). |

| 药品名称 Drug Names | 精氨酸 Arginine |
|---|---|
| 适应证<br>Indications | 用于肝性脑病，适用于忌钠患者。也适用于其他原因引起血氨过高所致的精神病症状。<br><br>For hepatic encephalopathy, applicable to patients who are forbidden to take sodium. Also applicable to high blood ammonia-induced psychotic state due to other reasons. |
| 用法、用量<br>Dosage | 静脉滴注：一次 15～20g，以5% 葡萄糖液 500～1000ml 稀释，滴注宜慢（每次4小时以上）。用其盐酸盐，可引起高氯性酸血症，肾功能不全者禁用。滴注太快可引起流涎、潮红、呕吐等。<br><br>Intravenous infusion: 15～20g once, diluted with 500～1000ml of 5% glucose solution, infusion should be slow (more than 4 hours once). With the hydrochloride salt, it can cause high chloride acidosis, so it is disabled for patients with renal insufficiency. Dripping too fast can cause salivation, flushing, vomiting. |
| 剂型、规格<br>Preparations | 注射液：5g（20ml）。<br>Injection: 5g (20ml). |

| 药品名称 Drug Names | 谷氨酸 Glutamic Acid |
|---|---|
| 适应证<br>Indications | 可预防肝性脑病；减少癫痫小发作发作次数；治疗胃酸不足。<br><br>Can prevent hepatic encephalopathy; reduce seizures episodes; for treatment of insufficient stomach acid. |
| 用法、用量<br>Dosage | 预防肝性脑病：每次 2.5～5g，一日4次；用于癫痫小发作：每次 2～3g，一日 3～4次；治疗胃酸不足：一次 0.3g，一日 3 次。肾功能不全或无尿患者慎用。不宜与碱性药物合用。与抗胆碱药合用有可能减弱后者的药效。<br><br>Prevention of hepatic encephalopathy: 2.5～5g once, 4 times a day; for seizures: 2～3g once, 3 to 4 times a day; treatment of gastric acid deficiency:0.3g once, 3 times a day. It must be used with caution for patients with renal insufficiency or no urine.It should not be combined with basic drugs. And used with anticholinergic drugs may weaken the latter's efficacy. |
| 剂型、规格<br>Preparations | 片剂：每片 0.3g；0.5g。<br>Tablets: 0.3g; 0.5g per tablet. |

## 12.12 治疗肝炎辅助用药 Adjuvant drugs treating hepatitis

| 药品名称 Drug Names | 联苯双酯 Bifendate |
|---|---|
| 适应证<br>Indications | 用于迁延性肝炎及长期单项丙氨酸氨基转移酶异常者。对肝炎主要症状如肝区痛、乏力、腹胀等的改善有一定疗效，但对肝脾大的改变无影响。<br><br>For persistent hepatitis and chronic single alanine aminotransferase abnormalities.It has a certain effect on improving the main symptoms of hepatitis, such as liver pain, fatigue, bloating, but had no effect on the changes in the liver and spleen enlargement. |
| 用法、用量<br>Dosage | 口服，一日量 75～150mg。多采用一日 3 次，每次服 25mg。<br>Oral, the dose of a day is 75～150mg. Ususlly three times a day, 25mg once. |
| 剂型、规格<br>Preparations | 片剂：每片 25mg。<br>滴丸：每丸 1.5mg，口服，一次 7.5～15mg，一日 22.5～45mg。<br>Tablets: 25mg per tablet.<br>Dripping Pills: 1.5mg per pill, oral, 7.5～15mg once, 22.5～45mg a day. |

| 药品名称 Drug Names | 门冬氨酸钾镁 Potassium Magnesium Aspartate |
|---|---|
| 适应证<br>Indications | 用于急性黄疸型肝炎、肝细胞功能不全，也可用于其他急慢性肝病。本品还可用于低钾血症、洋地黄中毒引起的心律失常、心肌炎后遗症、慢性心功能不全、冠心病等。<br><br>For acute jaundice hepatitis, hepatocellular dysfunction, can also be used for other acute and chronic liver disease. This product can also be used for arrhythmia, myocarditis sequelae, chronic heart failure, coronary heart disease etc. caused by hypokalemia, digitalis intoxication. |

**续　表**

| | |
|---|---|
| 用法、用量<br>Dosage | 注射液：一般为成人 10 ～ 20ml，加入 5% 或 10% 葡萄糖注射液 250 ～ 500ml 中缓慢静脉滴注，一日 1 次。儿童用量酌减。对重症黄疸患者，每日可用 2 次。对低血钾患者可适当加大剂量。口服：一般为一次 1 片，一日 3 次。由于各制品的含量有所不同，应用前须详阅产品说明书，并按其规定使用。<br><br>Injection: usually10 ～ 20ml for adults, adding 5% or 10% glucose injection into 250 ～ 500ml then take slow intravenous infusion, once a day. The dose is reduced for children. For patients with severe jaundice are available twice daily. Patients with hypokalemia could increase the dose rightly. Oral: usually 1 tablet once, three times a day. Since the content of per product is different, the product specification must be read before the application, and then use as its provisions. |
| 剂型、规格<br>Preparations | 片剂：含门冬氨酸 252mg，钾 36.1mg，镁 11.8mg。口服液：含无水 L- 门冬氨酸钾 451mg（钾 103mg），无水门冬氨酸镁 403.6mg（镁 34mg），按门冬氨酸计为 723mg，每支 5ml 或 10ml。门冬氨酸钾镁注射液：每支 10ml（每 1ml 含无水 L- 门冬氨酸 85mg、钾 11.4mg、镁 4.2mg）。注射用门冬氨酸钾镁：每瓶含无水 L- 门冬氨酸 850mg、钾 114mg、镁 42mg。<br><br>Tablets: containing aspartate of 252mg, Potassium of 36.1mg, magnesium of 11.8mg. Oral solution: containing anhydrous L-aspartate of 451mg (Potassium of 103mg), anhydrous magnesium aspartate of 403.6mg (magnesium of 34mg), according to aspartate, it should be counted as 723mg, 5ml or 10ml per vail. Potassium Magnesium Aspartate Injection: 10ml per vial (containing anhydrous L-aspartic acid of 85mg, potassium of 11.4mg, Magnesium of 4.2mg per 1ml). Injection of potassium magnesium aspartate: containing anhydrous L-aspartic acid of 850mg, Potassium of 114mg, Magnesium of 42mg per bottle. |
| **药品名称 Drug Names** | 水飞蓟宾 Silibinin |
| 适应证<br>Indications | 慢性迁延性肝炎、慢性活动性肝炎、初期肝硬化、中毒性肝损伤等。<br>Chronic persistent hepatitis, chronic active hepatitis, early cirrhosis, toxic liver damage. |
| 用法、用量<br>Dosage | 口服，每次 70 ～ 140mg，一日 3 次，餐后服。维持量可减半。<br>Oral, 70 ～ 140mg once, 3 times a day after meal. Maintenance dose may be halved. |
| 剂型、规格<br>Preparations | 水飞蓟宾片：35mg；38.5mg。水飞蓟宾胶囊剂：每粒 35mg；140mg。水飞蓟宾葡甲胺片：50mg（相当于水飞蓟宾 35.6mg）。<br><br>Silibinin tablets: 35mg, 38.5mg. Silibinin capsules: 35mg, 140mg per softgel. Silybin meglumine tablets: 50mg (equivalent to 35.6mg of silibinin ). |
| **药品名称 Drug Names** | 牛磺酸 Taurine |
| 适应证<br>Indications | 可用于急慢性肝炎、脂肪肝、胆囊炎等，也可用于支气管炎、扁桃体炎、眼炎等感染性疾病。感冒、乙醇戒断症状、关节炎、肌强直等可试用本品治疗。<br><br>Can be used for acute and chronic hepatitis, fatty liver, cholecystitis, etc., can also be used for bronchitis, tonsillitis, ophthalmia and other infectious diseases. Cold, alcohol withdrawal symptoms, arthritis, muscle rigidity, etc. can be tested by using this product. |
| 用法、用量<br>Dosage | 治疗急慢性肝炎，成人每次服 0.5g，一日 3 次；儿童每次 0.5g，一日 2 次。<br><br>For the treatment of acute and chronic hepatitis, 0.5g once for adults, 3 times a day; 0.5g once for children, 2 times a day. |
| 剂型、规格<br>Preparations | 片（胶囊）剂：每片（粒）0.5g。<br>冲剂：每袋含牛磺酸 0.5g。<br><br>Tablets (capsules): 0.5g per tablet(softgel).<br>Granules: containing 0.5g of taurine per bag. |
| **药品名称 Drug Names** | 促肝细胞生长因子 Hepatocyte Growth Promoting Factors |
| 适应证<br>Indications | 用于亚急性重型肝炎（病毒性；肝衰竭早期或中期）的辅助治疗。<br>For adjuvant therapy of sub-acute severe hepatitis (viral; early period or interim liver failure) . |

**续　表**

| 用法、用量 Dosage | 口服，每次 100 ~ 150mg，一日 3 次，疗程为 3 个月，可连续使用 2 ~ 4 个疗程；肌内注射，每次 40mg，一日 2 次；必要时也可将本品 80 ~ 120mg 加入 10% 葡萄糖注射液中静脉滴注，一日 1 次。疗程视病情而定，一般为 1 个月。<br><br>Oral, 100 ~ 150mg once, three times a day, the course lasts for 3 months, patients can continuously take it for 2 to 4 courses; intramuscular injection, 40mg once, 2 times a day; if necessary, 80 ~ 120mg of the product can be added into 10% glucose for intravenous injection, once a day. Treatment course is depending on the illness, it usually lasts a month. |
|---|---|
| 剂型、规格 Preparations | 颗粒剂：每袋 50mg。注射用促肝细胞生长素：20mg。<br>Granules: 50mg per bag. Injection PHGF: 20mg. |
| **药品名称 Drug Names** | 甘草酸二铵 Diammonium Glycyrrhizinate |
| 适应证 Indications | 用于伴有 ALT 升高的慢性肝炎。<br>For chronic hepatitis with elevated ALT. |
| 用法、用量 Dosage | 口服，每次 150mg，一日 3 次；静脉滴注，30ml 用 10% 葡萄糖注射液 250ml 稀释后缓慢静脉滴注，一日 1 次。<br><br>Oral, 150mg once, 3 times a day; intravenous infusion: slow intravenous infusion after 30ml produce being diluted with 250ml 10% glucose, once a day. |
| 剂型、规格 Preparations | 胶囊：每粒 50mg。注射液：每支 50mg（10ml）。<br>Capsules: 50mg per softgel. Injection: 50mg (10ml) per vial. |
| **药品名称 Drug Names** | 硫普罗宁 Tiopronin |
| 适应证 Indications | 用于：① 脂肪肝、早期肝硬化、急慢性肝炎、酒精及药物引起的肝炎。② 重金属中毒。③ 降低化疗及放疗的不良反应，升高白细胞，并可预防化疗、放疗所致二次肿瘤的发生。<br><br>Used for ① fatty liver, early cirrhosis, acute and chronic hepatitis, alcohol and drug-induced hepatitis. ② heavy metal poisoning. ③ reduce adverse effects of chemotherapy and radiotherapy, elevated white blood cell, and prevent chemotherapy, radiation therapy-induced secondary tumors. |
| 用法、用量 Dosage | （1）肝病治疗：餐后口服，每次 1 ~ 2 片，一日 3 次，连服 12 周，停药 3 个月后继续下 1 个疗程；急性病毒性肝炎初期每次 2 ~ 4 片，一日 3 次，连服 1 ~ 3 周，以后每次 1 ~ 2 片，一日 3 次。<br>（2）重金属中毒：每次 1 ~ 2 片，一日 2 次。<br>（3）化疗及放疗引起的白细胞减少症：餐后口服，化疗及放疗前 1 周开始服用，每次 2 ~ 4 片，一日 2 次，连服 3 周。<br><br>(1) liver disease: postprandial oral, 1 to 2 tablets once, 3 times a day, continuously take it for 12 weeks, continue the next course after three months of discontinuation; for early acute hepatitis, 2 to 4 tablets once, 3 times a day, continuously take it for 1 to 3 weeks, then take 1 to 2 tablets once, 3 times a day.<br>(2) heavy metal poisoning: 1 to 2 tablets once, 2 times a day.<br>(3) chemotherapy and radiotherapy-induced leukopenia: postprandial oral, take it a week ahead of chemotherapy and radiotherapy, 2 to 4 tablets once, 2 times a day for 3 weeks. |
| 剂型、规格 Preparations | 片剂：每片 0.1g。<br>Tablets: 0.1g per tablet. |
| **药品名称 Drug Names** | 葡醛内酯 Glucurolactone |
| 适应证 Indications | 用于急慢性肝炎、肝硬化；本品又有一定的解毒作用，可用于食物或药物中毒。<br>For acute and chronic hepatitis, liver cirrhosis; This product has a certain detoxification effect, it can be used for treating food or drugs detoxification. |
| 用法、用量 Dosage | 口服：一日 3 次，每次 0.1 ~ 0.2g。肌内或静脉注射：一日 1 ~ 2 次，每次 0.1 ~ 0.2g。<br>Oral: three times a day, 0.1 ~ 0.2g once. Intramuscular or intravenous injection: 1 or 2 times a day, 0.1 ~ 0.2g once. |

**续　表**

| | |
|---|---|
| 剂型、规格<br>Preparations | 片剂：0.05g；0.1g。<br>注射液：0.1g（2ml）。<br>Tablets: 0.05g; 0.1g.<br>Injection: 0.1g (2ml). |
| 药品名称 Drug Names | 辅酶 A　Coenzyme A |
| 适应证<br>Indications | 用于白细胞减少症、原发性血小板减少性紫癜、功能性低热等，对脂肪肝、肝性脑病、急慢性肝炎、冠脉硬化、慢性动脉炎、心肌梗死、慢性肾功能减退引起的肾病综合征、尿毒症等可作为辅助治疗药。<br>It is used in the treatment of leukopenia, idiopathic thrombocytopenic purpura, and functionality fever, fatty liver, etc. And it is used in the adjuvant therapy of nephrotic syndrome and uremia caused by fatty liver, hepatic encephalopathy, acute and chronic hepatitis, coronary sclerosis, chronic arteritis, myocardial infarction, chronic renal dysfunction. |
| 用法、用量<br>Dosage | 静脉滴注：一日 1 ～ 2 次或隔日 1 次，每次 50 ～ 100U；肌内注射：一日 1 次，每次 50 ～ 100U。一般以 7 ～ 14 日为 1 个疗程。<br>Intravenous drip: 1 or 2 times a day, or every other day, 50 to 100 units per time; intramuscular injection: 1 time a day, 50 to 100 units per time. Generally 7 to 14 day is a course of treatment. |
| 剂型、规格<br>Preparations | 注射用辅酶 A：50U；100U。<br>Injection coenzyme A: 50 units; 100 units. |

12.13 利胆药 Choleretic drug

| | |
|---|---|
| 药品名称 Drug Names | 熊去氧胆酸 Ursodeoxycholic Acid |
| 适应证<br>Indications | 用于不宜手术治疗的胆固醇型胆结石。应用时，仔细选择病例十分重要。对胆囊功能基本正常，结石直径在 5mm 以下，X 线能透过，非钙化型的浮动胆固醇型结石有较高的治愈率。结石的大小与溶石成功率密切相关，直径小于 5mm 者为 70%，5 ～ 10mm 者约为 50%。由于表面积 / 体积的比值较大，故较小的结石对治疗反应较好。本品不能溶解胆色素结石、混合结石及不透过 X 线的结石。对中毒性肝障碍、胆囊炎、胆道炎和胆汁性消化不良等也有一定的治疗效果。<br>It is used in the treatment of cholesterol gallstones that are not suitable for surgical treatment. It is very important to select patients in the application. It has a higher cure rate for non-calcified floating type of cholesterol calculus, the gallbladder of which is normal, stones of which is less than 5mm in diameter and is X-ray permeable. The success rate of dissolving stones is closely related to the size of the stone. The success rate is 70% for stones less than 5mm in diameter. The success rate is 50% for that of 5 ～ 10mm. Due to the large ratio of surface area / volume, the smaller stones have better response to the treatment. This product can not dissolve bile pigment stones, mixed stones and the stones that X-ray not penetrated. It also has a therapeutic effect on toxic liver disorder, cholecystitis, primary sclerosing cholangitis, biliary dyspepsia and so on. |
| 用法、用量<br>Dosage | 口服，利胆，1 次 50mg，一日 150mg。早、晚进餐时分次给予。疗程最短为 6 个月，6 个月后超声波检查及胆囊造影无改善者可停药；如结石已有部分溶解，则继续服药直至结石完全溶解。如治疗中有反复胆绞痛发作，症状无改善甚至加重，或出现明显结石钙化时，则宜终止治疗，并进行外科手术。溶胆石，一日 450 ～ 600mg，分 2 次服用。<br>Oral medication, cholagogue, 50mg per time, 150mg a day. The dose is given in breakfast and dinner seperately. The shortest course is six months. It can be discontinued if there is no improvement in ultrasound and gallbladder angiography after six months; if stones have been partially dissolved, then continue taking it until the stones are completely dissolved. If there are repeated episodes of biliary colic during the treament, or symptoms are not improved or even increased, or apparent calcified stones appear, it is desirable to terminate treatment, and have a surgery. Dissolve gallstones, 450 ～ 600mg a day, divided into 2 doses. |
| 剂型、规格<br>Preparations | 片剂：每片 50mg。<br>Tablets: 50mg per tablet. |

**续 表**

## 12.14 治疗炎性肠病药 Drugs treating inflammatory bowel disease

| 药品名称 Drug Names | 美沙拉秦 Mesalazine |
|---|---|
| 适应证<br>Indications | 用于治疗溃疡性结肠炎、克罗恩病（Crohn 病）；栓剂用于治疗溃疡性直肠炎。<br>For the treatment of ulcerative colitis, Crohn's disease; suppositories is used in the treatment of ulcerative proctitis. |
| 用法、用量<br>Dosage | （1）口服：溃疡性结肠炎急性发作，每次 1g，一日 4 次。维持治疗，每次 0.5g，一日 3 次。克罗恩病，每次 1g，一日 4 次。儿童及老年人用量应酌减。<br>（2）直肠给药：每次 1g，一日 1～2 次。<br>（1）Oral medication: acute attack of ulcerative colitis, 1g per time, 4 times a day. Maintenance treatment: 0.5g per time, 3 times a day. Crohn's disease, 1g per time, 4 times a day. The dosage for children and the elderly should be reduced.<br>（2）rectal administration: 1g per time, 1 to 2 times a day. |
| 剂型、规格<br>Preparations | 片剂：每片 0.25g；0.4g；0.5g。缓释片：每片 0.5g。缓释颗粒：每袋 0.5g。肠溶片：每片 0.5g。栓剂：每粒 1g。<br>Tablets: 0.25g; 0.4g; 0.5g per tablet. Sustained-release tablets: 0.5g per tablet. Release granules: 0.5g per bag. Enteric-coated tablets: 0.5g per tablet. Suppositories: 1g per softgel. |

| 药品名称 Drug Names | 柳氮磺吡啶 Sulfasalazine |
|---|---|
| 适应证<br>Indications | 主要用于炎性肠炎，即 Crohn 病和溃疡性结肠炎。<br>It is mainly used for the treatment of inflammatory bowel disease, that is Crohn's disease and ulcerative colitis. |
| 用法、用量<br>Dosage | 口服。成人常用量：初剂量为一日 2～3g，分 3～4 次口服，无明显不适，可渐增至一日 4～6g。待肠病症状缓解后逐渐减量至维持量，一日 1.5～2g。小儿初剂量为一日 40～60mg/kg，分 3～6 次口服，病情缓解后改为维持量一日 30mg/kg，分 3～4 次口服。<br>It is taken orally. Usual dose for adults: initial dose is 2～3g a day, divided into 3 to 4 times a day orally. Without obvious inappropriate reaction, the dosage can be gradually increased to 4～6g a day. After the symptoms of intestines is alleviated, the dose is decreased to a maintenance dose after, 1.5～2g a day. Pediatric dose for the first time is 40～60mg/kg a day, divided into 3 to 6 times a day orally. After the symptoms are alleviated, the dose is changed to the maintain dose: 30mg/kg a day, divided into 3 to 4 times a day orally. |
| 剂型、规格<br>Preparations | 片剂（胶囊剂）：每片（粒）0.25g。<br>栓剂：每粒 0.5g。<br>Tablets (capsules): 0.25g per tablet (softgel).<br>Suppositories: 0.5g per softgel. |

| 药品名称 Drug Names | 奥沙拉秦 Olsalazine |
|---|---|
| 适应证<br>Indications | 用于治疗急慢性溃疡性结肠炎与节段性回肠炎，并用于缓解期的长期维持治疗。<br>It is used in the treatment of acute and chronic ulcerative colitis and Crohn's disease, and is used for long-term maintenance therapy in remission. |
| 用法、用量<br>Dosage | 口服，治疗开始时每日 1g，分次服用，根据患者反应逐渐提高剂量至每日 3g，分 3～4 次服用。儿童为每日 20～40mg/kg。长期维持治疗，成人每日 1g，分 2 次服用；儿童每日 15～30mg/kg。本品随食物同服。<br>it is taken orally, 1g a day at the start of therapy in divided doses. The dose canbe increased gradually according to the patient's response to 3g per day, divided into three to four times. The dose is 20～40mg/kg a day for children. For long-term maintenance therapy, 1g a day for adults, in 2 divided doses; 15～30mg/kg a day for children. This product can be serviced with food. |
| 剂型、规格<br>Preparations | 胶囊剂：每粒 250mg。<br>Capsules: 250mg per softgel. |

**续　表**

## 12.15　其他消化系统用药 Other drugs of digestive system

| 药品名称 Drug Names | 奥曲肽 Octreotide |
|---|---|
| 适应证<br>Indications | 　　用于：①门静脉高压引起的食管静脉曲张破裂出血。②应激性溃疡及消化道出血。③重型胰腺炎及内镜逆行胰胆管造影（ＥＲＣＰ）术后急性胰腺炎并发症。④缓解由胃、肠及胰内分泌系统肿瘤所引起的症状。⑤突眼性甲状腺肿和肢端肥大症。⑥胃肠道瘘管。<br>　　Used for：① esophageal variceal bleeding caused by portal hypertension. ② stress ulcers and gastrointestinal bleeding. ③ severe acute pancreatitis and complication of acute pancreatitis after the surgery of endoscopic retrograde cholangiopancreatography(ERCP). ④ relieve symptoms caused by tumor in endocrine system of stomach, intestine and pancreas. ⑤ Graves' disease and acromegaly. ⑥ gastrointestinal fistula. |
| 用法、用量<br>Dosage | 　　(1) 预防胰腺手术后并发症：手术前 1 小时，0.1mg 皮下注射；以后 0.1mg 皮下注射，一日 3 次，连续 7 日。<br>　　(2) 治疗门脉高压引起的食管静脉曲张出血：静脉注射开始 0.1mg，以后 0.5mg，每 2 小时 1 次静脉滴注。<br>　　(3) 应激性溃疡及消化道出血：皮下注射 0.1mg，一日 3 次。<br>　　(4) 重型胰腺炎：皮下注射 0.1mg，一日 4 次，疗程为 3 ～ 7 日。<br>　　(5) 胃肠道瘘管和消化道内分泌系统肿瘤的辅助治疗：皮下注射 0.1mg，一日 3 次，疗程为 10 ～ 14 日。<br>　　(6) 突眼性甲状腺肿和肢端肥大症：皮下注射 0.1mg，一日 3 次；肢端肥大症疗程和剂量需视疗效而定，有时可长达数月。<br>　　(1) prevention of pancreatic surgery complications: the dose is 0.1mg in subcutaneous injection one hour before surgery; in the following days, 0.1mg injected subcutaneously, 3 times a day for 7 consecutive days.<br>　　(2) treatment for esophageal varices bleeding due to portal hypertension: intravenous injection is started at the dose of 0.1mg, 0.5mg later, once for every two hours by intravenous drip.<br>　　(3) stress ulcers and gastrointestinal bleeding: subcutaneous injection is started at the dose of 0.1mg, 3 times a day.<br>　　(4) severe pancreatitis: subcutaneous injection is started at the dose of 0.1mg, 4 times a day, 3 to 7 days for treatment.<br>　　(5) for adjuvant therapy of gastrointestinal fistula and tumor in endocrine system of digestive tract: subcutaneous injection is started at the dose of 0.1mg, 3 times a day, 10 to 14 days for treatment.<br>　　(6) Graves' disease and acromegaly: subcutaneous injection is started at the speed of of 0.1mg, 3 times a day; the course and dose of treatment of acromegaly depend on the curative effect, and sometimes up to several months. |
| 剂型、规格<br>Preparations | 　　注射液：每支 0.1mg（1ml）。<br>　　Injection: 0.1mg (1ml) per vial. |
| 药品名称 Drug Names | 生长抑素 Somatostatin |
| 适应证<br>Indications | 　　用于严重急性上消化道出血，如胃出血、十二指肠出血、胃和十二指肠溃疡出血、出血性胃炎、食管静脉曲张破裂出血等；预防胰腺术后及 ERCP 术后的并发症，急性胰腺炎，胰腺、胆囊和肠道瘘管的辅助性治疗；治疗类风湿关节炎引起的严重疼痛。<br>　　It is used in the treatment of severe acute upper gastrointestinal hemorrhage, such as Gastrorrhagia, duodenal bleeding, gastric and duodenal ulcers bleeding, hemorrhagic gastritis, esophageal variceal bleeding, etc; it is also used in the prevention of complications due to pancreatic surgery and post-ERCP. And it is also used in the adjuvant therapy of acute pancreatitis, pancreas, gallbladder and intestinal fistula; it is used in the treatment of severe pain caused by rheumatoid arthritis. |
|  | 　　(1) 治疗上消化道出血，以 3mg 溶于 500ml0.9% 氯化钠或 5% 葡萄糖注射液中，连续 12 小时静脉滴注。某些病例可在连续滴注前给予 250μg 缓慢（不少于 3 分钟）静脉注射。为避免再出血，在止血后用同一剂量维持治疗 48 ～ 72 小时，总疗程不应超过 120 小时，延长静脉滴注时间并不加强效果。<br>　　(2) 预防胰腺术后并发症，在手术开始时以 250μg/h 速度连续静脉滴注，术后连续静脉滴注 5 日。 |

| | |
|---|---|
| 用法、用量<br>Dosage | （3）预防 ERCP 术后并发症，术前 1 小时以 250μg/h 速度连续静脉滴注，持续 12 小时。<br>（4）急性胰腺炎：以 250μg/h 速度连续静脉滴注 5～7 日。<br>（5）胰腺、胆囊及肠道瘘管的辅助性治疗，以 250μg/h 速度连续静脉滴注，直到瘘管闭合之后 2 日，在此期间应结合全胃肠外营养治疗，疗程应不超过 20 日。<br>（6）治疗类风湿关节炎引起的严重疼痛，以 750μg 溶于 2ml0.9% 氯化钠注射液中做关节腔内注射，每隔 7 日或 15 日重复一次，连续 4～6 次。<br><br>(1) for the treatment of gastrointestinal bleeding: 3mg of this product is dissolved in 500ml of 0.9% sodium chloride or 5% of glucose injection. it is injected in intravenous injection for consecutive 12 hours . In some cases, the patient may be given 250μg in slow intravenous injection before continuous drip (not less than 3 minutes ). To prevent further bleeding, maintenance treatment should be given at the same dose for 48 to 72 hours, the total course should not exceed 120 hours. Prolonging intravenous drip time can not enhance the effect.<br>(2) for prevention of postoperative pancreatic complications: at the beginning of the surgery, continuous intravenous drip should be given at the speed of 250μg/h. After the surgery, the continuous intravenous drip last for 5 days.<br>(3) prevention of post-ERCP complications: continuous intravenous drip should be given one hour before the surgery at the speed of 250μg / h for 12 hours.<br>(4) acute pancreatitis: continuous intravenous drip should be given at the speed of 250μg/h for 5 to 7 days .<br>(5) for adjuvant therapy of pancreas, gallbladder and intestinal fistula: continuous intravenous drip should be given at the speed of 250μg/h, until 2 days after the fistula closes. During this period, it should be combined with total parenteral nutrition therapy. The course of treatment should not exceed 20 days.<br>(6) for treatment of severe pain caused by rheumatoid arthritis: 750μg of the product should be dissolved in 2ml of 0.9% sodium chloride injection for intra-articular injection. it should be repeated once every 7 days or 15 days, and 4 to 6 consecutive times. |
| 剂型、规格<br>Preparations | 注射用生长抑素：每支 250μg；750μg；3mg。<br>Somatostatin for injection: 250μg per vial; 750μg per vial; 3mg per vial. |
| 药品名称 Drug Names | 抑肽酶 Aprotinin |
| 适应证<br>Indications | 用于预防和治疗急性胰腺炎、纤维蛋白溶解所引起的出血、弥散性血管内凝血。也用于抗休克治疗。腹腔手术后，直接注入腹腔可预防术后肠粘连。<br><br>It is used in the treatment and prevention of bleeding and disseminated intravascular coagulation due to acute pancreatitis and fibrinolysis. It is also used in anti-shock therapy. After abdominal surgery, it can be injected directly into the abdominal cavity to prevent postoperative adhesions. |
| 用法、用量<br>Dosage | 第 1～2 日，每日 8 万～12 万 U，首剂用量应大些，缓慢静脉注射（每分钟不超过 2ml）。维持剂量宜采用静脉滴注，每日 2 万～4 万 U。由纤维蛋白溶解引起的出血，应立即静脉注射 8 万～12 万 U，以后每 2 小时 1 万 U，直至出血停止。预防剂量：手术前一日开始，每日 2 万 U，共 3 日。治疗肠瘘及连续渗血也可局部应用。预防术后肠粘连，在手术切口闭合前，腹腔直接注入 2 万～4 万 U，注意勿与伤口接触。<br><br>For the first and second day, the dose is 80, 000 to 120, 000U per day. The first dosage, which should be bigger, is injected in slow intravenous injection (no more than 2ml per minute). Maintenance dose should be injected intravenously, 20, 000 to 40, 000U per day. For the bleeding caused by fibrinolysis, you should immediately inject intravenously 80, 000 to 120, 000U, then 10, 000u for every two hours, until the bleeding stops. Prophylactic dose: the administration starts the day before surgery, 20, 000U a day, 3 days totally. In treatment for intestinal fistula and continuous bleeding, it can also be applied topically. For prevention of postoperative intestinal adhesion, inject 20, 000 to 40, 000U directly into the abdominal cavity before the incision closes. Be careful not to touch the wound. |
| 剂型、规格<br>Preparations | 注射抑肽酶：每支 1 万 U；5 万 U；10 万 U；50 万 U。<br>Aprotinin Injection: 10, 000U; 50, 000U; 100, 000U; 500, 000U per strip. |
| 药品名称 Drug Names | 加贝酯 Gabexate |
| 适应证<br>Indications | 用于急性轻型（水肿型）胰腺炎；也可用于急性出血性坏死型胰腺炎的辅助治疗。<br><br>It is used in the treatment of acute light (edematous) pancreatitis; may also be used to assist in the treatment of acute hemorrhagic necrotizing pancreatitis. |

| 用法、用量<br>Dosage | 仅供静脉滴注。每次 100mg，治疗开始 3 天，每日用量 300mg，症状减轻后改为每日 100mg，疗程为 6 ～ 10 日。先以 5ml 注射用水注入冻干粉针瓶内，待溶解后注入 5% 葡萄糖注射液或林格液 500ml 中，供静脉滴注用。滴注速度不宜过快，应控制在 1mg/（kg•h）以内，不宜超过 2.5mg/（kg•h）。<br><br>Only for intravenous injectin.100mg per time, three days after the treament, the daily dose is 300mg. The daily dose is changed to 100mg a day after symptoms are alleviated, with 6 to 10 days being a course of treatment. First, inject 5ml water for injection into the vial of freeze-dried powder. Then inject it into 5% Glucose Injection or 500ml Ringer's solution after dissolution for the use in intravenous drip. the speed of the drip should not be too fast and should be controlled at 1mg /（kg · h）or less, not more than 2.5mg /（kg · h）. |
| --- | --- |
| 剂型、规格<br>Preparations | 注射用加贝酯：每支 0.1g。<br>Injection Gabexate: 0.1g per vial |
| 药品名称 Drug Names | 二甲硅油 Dimethicone |
| 适应证<br>Indications | 用于胃肠道胀气及急性肺气肿。<br>For the treatment of gastrointestinal flatulence and acute emphysema. |
| 用法、用量<br>Dosage | （1）消胀气：一次 0.1 ～ 0.2g，一日 3 次，嚼碎服。<br>（2）抢救急性肺水肿：使用气雾剂，用时将瓶倒置，距患者口鼻约 15cm 处，揿压瓶帽，在吸气时（或呼气终末时）连续喷入或与给氧同时进行，直至泡沫减少、症状改善为止。必要时可反复使用。<br><br>(1) eliminate flatulence: 0.1 ~ 0.2g per time, 3 times a day, it should be taken after being chewed.<br>(2) treatment of acute pulmonary edema: use the aerosols, make the bottle upside down. When it is about 15cm away from mouth and nose of the patient, press the bottle cap, continuously spray it during the inspiration(or at the end Expiration) or spary it simultaneously with the inspiratory oxygen, until the foam reduces and the symptoms improve. It can be applied repeatedly, if necessary. |
| 剂型、规格<br>Preparations | 片剂：每片含二甲硅油 25mg 或 50mg，另含氢氧化铝 40mg 或 80mg，为分散剂。二甲硅油气雾剂：每瓶总量 18g，内含二甲硅油 0.15g，此外尚含适量薄荷脑及抛射剂氟利昂（F12）。二甲硅油散：含二甲硅油 6%，为抗泡沫药。<br><br>Tablets: per tablet contains 25mg or 50mg Dimethicone. Simethicone. And it contains 40mg or 80mg aluminum hydroxide, as a dispersant. Dimethicone Aerosol: a bottle contains 18g, with 0.15g dimethicone. In addition, it contains the right amount of menthol and propellant Freon (F12). Dimethicone powder: containing dimethicone 6%, as anti-foaming agents. |

13. 主要作用于血液和造血系统的药物 Drugs mainly acting on blood and hematopoietic system

13.1　促凝血药 Coagulants

| 药品名称 Drug Names | 亚硫酸氢钠甲萘醌 Menadione Sodium Bisulfite |
| --- | --- |
| 适应证<br>Indications | （1）止血：用于阻塞性黄疸、胆瘘、慢性腹泻、广泛性切除所致肠吸收功能不全者，早产儿、新生儿低凝血酶原血症，香豆素类或水杨酸类过量以及其他原因所致凝血酶原过低等引起的出血。亦可用于预防长期口服广谱抗生素类药物引起的维生素 K 缺乏症。<br>（2）镇痛：用于胆石症、胆道蛔虫病引起的胆绞痛。<br>（3）解救杀鼠药"敌鼠钠"（diphacin）中毒：此时宜用大剂量。<br><br>(1) Hemostasis: Menadione Sodium Bisulphite is used in the treatment of haemorrhage caused by deficiency in intestinal absorption associated with Obstructive Jaundice, Biliary Fistula, chronic diarrhea and wide excision, caused by hypoprothrombinemia of premature infant and newborns, caused by the overdose of Coumarin or sallcylic acid, or caused by low level of prothrombin induced by other reasons. It can also used in the prevention of deficiency of vitamin K caused by the oral medication of drugs like broad-spectrum antibiotics for a long time.<br>(2) Analgesia: Menadione Sodium Bisulphite is also used for the treatment of biliary colic induced by gallstones or biliary ascariasis.<br>(3) It is used in the treatment of the poisoning of rodenticide—diphacin. In this case, the dose should be given largely. |

**续　表**

| 用法、用量<br>Dosage | （1）止血：成人口服，一次 2 ～ 4mg，一日 6 ～ 20mg；肌内注射，每次 2 ～ 4mg，一日 4 ～ 8mg。防止新生儿出血，可在产前 1 周给妊娠期妇女肌内注射，每日 2 ～ 4mg。<br>（2）胆绞痛：肌内注射，每次 8 ～ 16mg。<br>(1) Hemostasis: oral medication for adults, 2mg to 4mg per time, 6mg to 20mg per day; Intramuscular injection: 2mg to 4 mg per time, 4mg to 8mg per day. For the prevention of haemorrhage of newborns, for intramuscular injection one week before the birth, with 2mg to 4mg per day.<br>(2) biliary colic: it should be given intramuscularly, 8mg to 16mg per time. |
|---|---|
| 剂型、规格<br>Preparations | 片剂：每片 2mg。注射液：每支 2mg（1ml）；4mg（1ml）。<br>Tablets: 2mg per tablet. Injections: 2mg(1ml) per vial；4mg(1ml) per vial. |
| 药品名称 Drug Names | 维生素 $K_1$ phytomenadione（Vitamin $K_1$） |
| 适应证<br>Indications | （1）止血：用于阻塞性黄疸、胆瘘、慢性腹泻、广泛性切除所致肠吸收功能不全者，早产儿、新生儿低凝血酶原血症，香豆素类或水杨酸类过量以及其他原因所致凝血酶原过低等引起的出血。亦可用于预防长期口服广谱抗生素类药物引起的维生素 K 缺乏症。<br>（2）镇痛：用于胆石症、胆道蛔虫病引起的胆绞痛。<br>（3）解救杀鼠药"敌鼠钠"（diphacin）中毒：此时宜用大剂量。<br>(1) Hemostasis: Menadione Sodium Bisulphite is used in the treatment of haemorrhage caused by deficiency in intestinal absorption associated with Obstructive Jaundice, Biliary Fistula, chronic diarrhea and wide excision, caused by hypoprothrombinemia of premature infant and newborns, caused by the overdose of Coumarin or sallcylic acid, or caused by low level of prothrombin induced by other reasons. It can also used in the prevention of deficiency of vitamin K caused by the oral medication of drugs like broad-spectrum antibiotics for a long time.<br>(2) Analgesia: Menadione Sodium Bisulphite is also used for the treatment of biliary colic induced by gallstones or biliary ascariasis.<br>(3) It is used in the treatment of the poisoning of rodenticide—diphacin. In this case, the dose should be given largely. |
| 用法、用量<br>Dosage | 肌内注射或静脉注射：每次 10mg，一日 1 ～ 2 次，或根据具体病情而定；口服：每次 10mg，一日 3 次。<br>For intramuscular injection or intravenous injection. the dose is 10mg per time, 1 to 2 times a day or it depends on the patient's condition; oral medication: 10mg per time, 3 times a day. |
| 剂型、规格<br>Preparations | 片剂：10mg。注射液：10mg（1ml）；2mg（1ml）。<br>Tablets: 10mg per tablet. Injections: 10mg(1ml) per vial；2mg(1ml) per vial. |
| 药品名称 Drug Names | 氨基己酸 Aminocaproic Acid |
| 适应证<br>Indications | 用于纤溶性出血、如脑、肺、子宫、前列腺、肾上腺、甲状腺等外伤或手术出血。术中早期用药或术前用药，可减少手术中渗血，并减少输血量。亦用于肺出血、肝硬化出血及上消化道出血。<br>Aminocaproic acid is used in the treatment of haemorrhage of fibrinolysis associated with trauma in brian, lung, uterine, prostate, adrenal gland, thyroid, etc or haemorrhage in surgery. Administration in early surgery or preoperative administration could reduce surgery bleeding during the surgery and reduce the blood transfusion. Aminocaproic acid is also used in the treatment of pulmonary hemorrhage, liver cirrhosis bleeding and upper gastrointestinal hemorrhage. |
| 用法、用量<br>Dosage | 静脉滴注，初用量 4 ～ 6g，以 5% ～ 10% 葡萄糖注射液或生理盐水 100ml 稀释，15 ～ 30 分钟滴完，维持量为每小时 1g，维持时间依病情而定，一日量不超过 20g，可连用 3 ～ 4 日。口服，成人，每次 2g，依病情服用 7 ～ 10 日或更久。<br>Intravenous drip: Aminocaproic acid may be given intravenously in an initial dose of 4 to 6g diluted with 100ml of 5% ～ 10% glucose injection or normal saline injection within 15 ～ 30 min. A continuous infusion of 1 hour should follow. The time for sustaining depends on the patients' condition. The maximum dose is not more than 20g. the administration could last for 3 to 4 day. It is taken orally for adults, 2g per time for 7 to 10 days or longer according to the patients' condition. |

**续　表**

| | |
|---|---|
| 剂型、规格<br>Preparations | 片剂：每片 0.5g。注射液：每支 1g（10ml）；2g（10ml）。<br>Tablets: 0.5g per tablet. Injections: 1g(10ml) per vial；2g(10ml) per vial. |
| 药品名称 Drug Names | 氨甲苯酸 Aminomethylbenzoic Acid |
| 适应证<br>Indications | 用于纤维蛋白溶解过程亢进所致的出血，如肺、肝、胰、前列腺、肾上腺等手术时的异常出血，妇产科和产后出血以及肺结核咳血或痰中带血、血尿、前列腺肥大出血、上消化道出血等，对一般慢性渗血效果较显著，但对癌症出血以及创伤出血无止血作用。此外，尚可用于链激酶或尿激酶过量引起的出血。<br><br>Aminomethylbenzoic acid is used in the treatment of bleeding during the course of fibrinolysis, like the abnormal bleeding in surgeries of lung, liver, pancreas prostate, adrenal, etc. it is also used in the treatment of obstetrics and gynecology, postpartum hemorrhage, hemoptysis in tuberculosis, blood-stained sputum, Hematuria, bleeding of hypertrophy of prostate, upper gastrointestinal hemorrhage, etc. Aminomethylbenzoic acid exhibits good effects on chronic bleeding, but has no effects on cancer or wound bleeding. Besides, Aminomethylbenzoic acid is also used in the in the treatment of haemorrhage induced by the overdose of streptokinase and urokinase. |
| 用法、用量<br>Dosage | 静脉注射，每次 0.1 ~ 0.3g，用 5% 葡萄糖注射液或 0.9% 氯化钠注射液 10 ~ 20ml 稀释后缓慢注射，一日最大用量 0.6g。<br><br>Aminomethylbenzoic acid may be given intravenously in a dose of 0.1g to 0.3g per time. It is diluted with 10 to 20ml of 5% glucose injection or 0.9% saline injection, and is injected slowly. The maximum dose is not more than 0.6 g per day. |
| 剂型、规格<br>Preparations | 片剂：每片 0.125g；0.25g。注射液：每支 0.05g（5ml）；0.1g（10ml）。<br>Tablets: 0.125g；0.25g per day. Injections: 0.05g(5ml)；0.1g(10ml) per vial. |
| 药品名称 Drug Names | 血凝酶 Hemocoagulase |
| 适应证<br>Indications | 可用于治疗和防治多种原因引起的出血。<br>Hemocoagulase is used in the treatment and prophylaxis of haemorrhage caused by various causes. |
| 用法、用量<br>Dosage | 静脉注射、肌内注射，也可局部使用。成人：每次 1.0 ~ 2.0kU，紧急情况下，立即静脉注射 1.0kU，同时肌内注射 1.0kU。各类外科手术：手术前 1 小时，肌内注射 1.0kU；或手术前 15 分钟，静脉注射 1.0kU。手术后每日肌内注射 1.0kU，连用 3 日，或遵医嘱。<br><br>1.0 to 2.0kU of Hemocoagulase may be given intravenously or intramuscularly to adults. It is also for topical use. In certain emergency situation, 1.0kU could be immediately injected by intravenous and intramuscular injection. For all kinds of surgeries, 1.0kU of hemocoagulase may be given intramuscularly 1h before surgery; or 1.0kU may be given intravenously 15min before surgery. After the surgery, a daily intramuscularly dose is 1.0kU for 3 consecutive days, or do as the doctor suggested. |
| 剂型、规格<br>Preparations | 注射用血凝酶（REPTILASE）每支 0.5kU；1kU；2kU。<br>Injection Thrombin(REPTILASE): 0.5kU per vial；1kU per vial；2kU per vial. |
| 药品名称 Drug Names | 酚磺乙胺 Etamsylate |
| 适应证<br>Indications | 用于预防和治疗外科手术出血过多，血小板减少性紫癜或过敏性紫癜以及其他原因引起的出血，如脑出血、胃肠道出血、泌尿道出血、眼底出血、牙龈出血、鼻出血和皮肤出血等。<br><br>Etamsylate is used in the treatment and prophylaxis of surgical haemorrhage or the haemorrhage caused by thrombocytopenic purpura, allergic purpura and other causes like cerebral hemorrhage, gastrointestinal bleeding, urinary tract bleeding, fundus hemorrhage, bleeding gums, Epistaxis, dermatorrhagia, etc. |
| 用法、用量<br>Dosage | （1）预防手术出血：术前 15 ~ 30 分钟静脉注射或肌内注射，一次 0.25 ~ 0.5g，必要时 2 小时后再注射 0.25g，一日 0.5 ~ 1.5g。<br>（2）治疗出血：成人，口服，每次 0.5 ~ 1g，一日 3 次。肌内注射或静脉注射每次 0.25 ~ 0.5g，一日 2 次或 3 次。也可与 5% 葡萄糖注射液或生理盐水混合静脉滴注，每次 0.25 ~ 0.75g，一日 2 次或 3 次，必要时可根据病情增加剂量。 |

**续 表**

|  | (1) For the prophylaxis of surgical haemorrhage: it should be given intravenously or intramuscularly 15 to 30 min before surgery, 0.25 to 0.5g per time. Further 0.25g may be given 2h later if necessary, up to a daily dose of 0.5 to 1.5g.<br>(2) For the treatment of haemorrhage, oral medication for the adults 0.5g to 1g per time, 3 times a day. the dose for intramuscular or intravenous injection is 0.25 to 0.5g two or three times a day. It could also be mixed with 5% glucose or 0.9% normal saline injection and be given intravenously, 0.25g to 0.75g per time, 2 or 3 times a day. The further doses may be given if necessary. |
|---|---|
| 剂型、规格<br>Preparations | 片剂：每片 0.25g；0.5g。注射液：每支 0.25g（2ml）；0.5g（5ml）；1.0g（5ml）。<br>Tablets: 0.25g per tablet；0.5g per tablet. Injections: 0.25g(2ml) per vial；0.5g(5ml) per vial；1.0g(5ml)per vial. |
| 药品名称 Drug Names | 卡巴克洛 Carbazochrome |
| 适应证<br>Indications | 用于毛细血管通透性增加所致的出血，如特发性紫癜、视网膜出血、慢性肺出血、肠胃出血、鼻出血、咯血、血尿、痔出血、子宫出血、脑出血等。<br>Carbazochrome is used in the treatment of haemorrhage induced by the increased capillary permeability, like idiopathic purpura, retinal hemorrhage, chronic pulmonary hemorrhage, gastrointestinal bleedings, Epistaxis, Hemoptysis, Hematuria, Bleeding hemorrhoid, metrorrhagia, cerebral hemorrhage, etc. |
| 用法、用量<br>Dosage | (1) 卡络柳钠片：口服，每次 2.5 ~ 5mg，一日 3 次。卡络柳钠注射液：肌内注射，每次 5 ~ 10mg，一日 2 ~ 3 次。不可静脉注射。<br>(2) 注射用卡络磺钠：肌内注射，每次 20mg，一日 2 次；静脉注射，每次 25 ~ 50mg，一日 1 次；静脉滴注，每次 60 ~ 80mg，加入输液中滴注。<br>(1) Carbazochrome salicylate tables: oral medication, 2.5 ~ 5mg per time, three times a day.<br>(2) The intramuscular injection dose of carbazochrome Salicylate is 5 to 10 mg for 2 or 3 times a day. It is forbidden for intravenous injection. 2. The intramuscular injection dose of Carbazochrome sodium sulfonate is 20mg per time, 2 times a day, it may be given in intravenous injection with 60mg to 80mg per time and put into the transfusion. |
| 剂型、规格<br>Preparations | 卡络柳钠片：每片 2.5mg；5mg。卡络柳钠注射液：每支 5mg（1ml）；10mg（2ml）。注射用卡络磺钠：20mg。<br>Carbazochrome Salicylate tablets: per containing 2.5mg；5mg per tablet.Carbazochrome Salicylate injections: 5mg(1ml) per vial；10mg(2ml) per vial.. Carbazochrome sodium sulfonate for injection: 20 mg per vial. |
| 药品名称 Drug Names | 重组人凝血因子Ⅷ Recombinant Human Coagulation Factor Ⅷ |
| 适应证<br>Indications | 用于纠正和预防凝血因子Ⅷ缺乏或因患获得性因子Ⅷ抑制物增多症而引起的出血。主要用于治疗甲型血友病。<br>Human Coagulation Factor Ⅷ is used in the rectification and prophylaxis of haemorrhage associated with Coagulation Factor Ⅷ deficiency or associated with increasing inhibitor caused by acquired coagulation Factor Ⅷ. It is mainly used in the treatment of Hemophilia A . |
| 用法、用量<br>Dosage | 静脉滴注：<br>(1) 轻度关节出血：一次 8 ~ 10U/kg，一日 1 ~ 2 次，连用 1 ~ 4 日；使 FⅧc 水平提高到正常水平的 15% ~ 20%。<br>(2) 中度关节、肌肉出血：一次 15U/kg，一日 2 次，需用 3 ~ 7 日，使 FⅧc 水平提高到正常水平的 30%。<br>(3) 大出血或严重外伤而无出血证据：一次 25U/kg，一日 2 次，至少用 7 日；使 FⅧc 水平提高到正常水平的 50%。<br>(4) 外科手术或严重外伤伴出血：40 ~ 50U/kg 于术前 1 小时开始输注，使 FⅧc 水平达到正常水平的 80 ~ 100%，随后使 FⅧc 水平维持在正常水平的 30% ~ 60%，10 ~ 14 日。<br>(5) 预防出血：体重大于 50kg，一日 500U；小于 50kg 者，一日 250u。使 FⅧc 水平达到到正常水平的 5% ~ 10%。 |

**续　表**

<table>
<tr>
<td></td>
<td>（6）抗 F Ⅷ c 抗体生成伴出血：首剂 5000 ～ 10，000U/h，维持剂量为 300 ～ 1000U/h，使体内 F Ⅷ c 水平维持在 30 ～ 50U/ml，如联合应用血浆交换术，宜追加本品 40U/kg，以增强疗效。<br><br>Intravenous drip:<br>（1）For the treatment of mild arthrorrhagia: the dose of Human Coagulation Factor Ⅷ is 8 to 10U/kg per time, 1to 2 times a day for 1 to 4 consecutive days; the F Ⅷ c level should be improved to 15% ～ 20% of the normal level.<br>（2）For the treatment of moderate arthrorrhagia and muscular hemorrhage: the dose of Human Coagulation Factor Ⅷ is 15U/kg per time, 2 times per day for 3 to 7 days to make the F Ⅷ c level reach 30% of the normal level;<br>（3）massive hemorrhage, or serious injury without evidence of hemorrhage: 25U/kg per time, 2 times per day for at least 7days; the F Ⅷ c level should be improved to 50% of the normal level.<br>（4）surgeries or serious injury with evidence of hemorrhage: 40 ～ 50U/kg should be infused 1 hour before the surgery to make the F Ⅷ c level reach 80% ～ 100% of the normal level. Later on, F Ⅷ c level should be sustained at 30% to 60% of the normal level for about 10 to 14 days.<br>（5）For the prophylaxis of hemorrhage: patients whose weight is over 50kg have 500U per day; patients whose weight is less than 50kg, have 250U per day. the F Ⅷ c level should be improved to 5% ～ 10% of the normal level.<br>（6）the generation of antibody for anti-F Ⅷ c with evidence of hemorrhage: the initial dose is 5000 ～ 10 000U/h, the followed dose should be sustained at 300 ～ 1000U/h to make F Ⅷ c level in vivo sustained at 30 ～ 50U/ml. If it used in combination with plasma exchange, there should be an additional dose of 40U/kg to enhance the effect.</td>
</tr>
<tr>
<td>剂型、规格<br>Preparations</td>
<td>人凝血因子Ⅷ：每瓶 100U；200U；250U；300U；400U；500U；750U；1000U。<br>Human Coagulation Factor Ⅷ : 100U per vial；200U per vial；250U per vial；300U per vial；400U per vial；500U per vial；750U per vial；1000U per vial.</td>
</tr>
<tr>
<td>药品名称 Drug Names</td>
<td>重组人血小板生成素 Recombinant Human Thrombopoietin</td>
</tr>
<tr>
<td>适应证<br>Indications</td>
<td>用于治疗实体瘤化疗后所致的血小板减少症，适用对象为血小板低于 $50×10^9$/L 且医师认为有必要升高血小板治疗的患者。<br><br>Recombinant Human Thrombopoietin is used in the treatment of thrombocytopenia after the chemotherapy for solid tumor. It is suitable for patients whose platelet level is lower than $50×10^9$/L and the patients have to be the ones that the doctors believe have the necessity to improve it at the same time.</td>
</tr>
<tr>
<td>用法、用量<br>Dosage</td>
<td>恶性实体肿瘤化疗时，可于给药结束后 6 ～ 24 小时皮下注射本品，剂量为每日 300U/kg，一日 1 次，连用 14 日。<br><br>In the chemotherapy for malignant solid tumor, a daily dose of 300U/kg Recombinant Human Thrombopoietin may be subcutaneously injected 6 to 24h after the administration, one time per day for continuous 14 days.</td>
</tr>
<tr>
<td>剂型、规格<br>Preparations</td>
<td>注射液：7500U（1ml）；15 000U（1ml）。<br>Injections: 7500U(1ml) per vial;15, 000U(1ml) per vial.</td>
</tr>
<tr>
<td>药品名称 Drug Names</td>
<td>重组人白细胞介素 -11 Recombinant Human Interleukin-11</td>
</tr>
<tr>
<td>适应证<br>Indications</td>
<td>用于实体瘤和白血病放、化疗后血小板减少症的预防和治疗及其他原因引起的血小板减少症的治疗。<br><br>Recombinant Human Interleukin-11 is used in the treatment and prophylaxis of thrombocytopenia caused by radiotherapy or chemotherapy for solid tumor and leukemia, and used in the treatment of thrombocytopenia induced by other causes.</td>
</tr>
<tr>
<td>用法、用量<br>Dosage</td>
<td>应用剂量为25μg/kg，于化疗结束后24 ～ 48小时或发生血小板减少症后皮下注射，一日一次，疗程一般为 7 ～ 14 日。血小板计数恢复后应及时停药。<br><br>The appropriate dose of 25μg/kg may be subcutaneously injected 24 to 48h after chemotherapy treatment or when the thrombocytopenia occurs. With the injection one time a day, 7 to 14 days are a course of treatment. As soon as the platelet count returns to normal, Recombinant Human Interleukin-11 is discontinued.</td>
</tr>
<tr>
<td>剂型、规格<br>Preparations</td>
<td>注射用重组人白细胞介素 -11：每支 1.5mg；3.0mg。<br>Recombinant Human Interleukin-11 for injection: 1.5mg per vial；3.0mg per vial</td>
</tr>
</table>

**续 表**

| 药品名称 Drug Names | 云南白药 Yunnan Baiyao |
|---|---|
| 适应证<br>Indications | 缩短凝血时间，具有止血作用。<br>Yunnan Baiyao could shorten clotting time and has the hemostatic effect . |
| 用法、用量<br>Dosage | 成人每次服 0.2～0.3g，重症可酌加，但一次不宜超过 0.5g，每隔 4 小时服 1 次。若初服无反应，可连续服用。小儿 2 岁以上者，每次服 0.03g；5 岁以上者，每次服 0.06g。<br><br>Adults: The usual dose is 0.2 to 0.3g per time. The dose could have considered additions if the patient is in severe condition. But the dose for one time should not exceed 0.5g, and it should be given at intervals of 4h. Without abnormal reaction, the treatment may be continued. The suggested doses for children who are older than 2 years oldare 0.03g per time, and the doses for children who are older than 5 years old are 0.06g |
| 剂型、规格<br>Preparations | 胶囊：250mg。<br>气雾剂：85g。<br>Capsule: 250mg per capsule.<br>Aerosol: 85g. |

| 药品名称 Drug Names | 氨甲环酸 Tranexamic Acid |
|---|---|
| 适应证<br>Indications | 用于各种出血性疾病、手术时异常出血等。<br>Tranexamic acid is used in the treatment of hemorrhagic disease, abnormal bleeding during surgery, etc. |
| 用法、用量<br>Dosage | 口服，每次 1.0～1.5g，一日 2～6g。静脉注射或静脉滴注：每次 0.25～0.5g，一日 0.75～2g。静脉注射以 25% 葡萄糖注射液稀释，静脉滴注液以 5%～10% 葡萄糖注射液稀释。<br><br>Oral medication：the doses are 1g to 1.5g per time, and 2 to 6g per day. Intravenous injection or drip: the doses are 0.25g to 0.5g per time and 0.75g to 2g per day. It should be diluted with 25% glucose injection in intravenous injection, and should be diluted with "5% to 10%" glucose injection in intravenous drip. |
| 剂型、规格<br>Preparations | 片剂：0.125g；0.25g。<br>胶囊：0.25g。<br>注射液：0.1g（2ml）；0.2g（2ml）；0.25g（5ml）；0.5g（5ml）；1.0g（10ml）。<br>注射用氨甲环酸：0.2g；0.4g；0.5g；1.0g。<br>Tablets: 0.125g per tablet; 0.25g per tablet.<br>Capsule: 0.25g per capsule.<br>Injections: 0.1g(2ml) pe vial；0.2g(2ml) per vial；0.25g(5ml) per vial；0.5g(5ml) per vial；1.0g(10ml)per vial.<br>Tranexamic Acid for injection: 0.2g per vial；0.4g per vial；0.5g per vial；1.0g per vial. |

| 药品名称 Drug Names | 鱼精蛋白 Protamine |
|---|---|
| 适应证<br>Indications | 用于因注射肝素过量而引起的出血，以及自发性出血，如咯血。<br>Protamine is used in the treatment of hemorrhage caused by the overdose injection of heparin and used in the treatment of spontaneous bleeding like hemoptysis. |
| 用法、用量<br>Dosage | ①抗肝素过量：静脉注射，用量应与最后一次作用肝素量相当（本品 1mg 中可中和肝素 100U），但一次不超过 50mg。②抗自发性出血：静脉滴注，每日 5～8mg/kg，分 2 次，间隔 6 小时。每次以生理盐水 300～500ml 稀释。连用不宜超过 3 日。注射宜缓慢（10 分钟内注入量以不超过 50mg 为度）。<br><br>① Overdose antiheparin: Intravenous injection. The dose is equivalent to the dose of heparin used for the last time (1mg of this product can neutralize 100 units of heparin), but the dose is not more than 50mg for one time. ② For the treatment of spontaneous bleeding: it should be given in intravenous drip, a daily dose of 5 to 8 mg/kg in 2 divided dosed with intervals of 6 h. It should be diluted with 300 to 500ml normal saline. The extent treatment is suggested to be controlled in 3 days and given by slow intravenous injection (the injection dose is not more than 50mg within 10 minutes). |
| 剂型、规格<br>Preparations | 硫酸鱼精蛋白注射液：50mg（5ml）；100mg（10ml）。<br>注射用硫酸鱼精蛋白：50mg。<br>Protamine Sulfate Injection: 50mg(5ml) per vial；100mg(10ml)per vial.<br>Protamine Sulfate for injection: 50 mg per vial. |

**续　表**

| 药品名称 Drug Names | 凝血酶 Thrombin |
|---|---|
| 适应证<br>Indications | 局部止血药。可用于局部出血及消化道出血。<br>Thrombin is used as local hemostatic. It can be used for local hemorrhage and gastrointestinal bleeding. |
| 用法、用量<br>Dosage | 局部出血：以干燥粉末或溶液（50 ～ 250U/ml）喷洒或喷雾于创伤表面。消化道出血：以溶液（10 ～ 100u/ml）口服或局部灌注。严禁注射。<br>Local hemorrhage: The dry powder or solution(50 ～ 250U/ml) is sprayed to the surface of trauma. Gastrointestinal haemorrhage: the solution(10 ～ 100U/ml) is given by oral or by regional perfusion. It is forbidded to inject Thrombin. |
| 剂型、规格<br>Preparations | 凝血酶冻干粉剂：200U；500U；1000U；2000U；5000U；10 000U。<br>Freeze-dried powder of thrombin: 200U per one; 500U per one; 1000U per one; 2000U per one; 5000U per one and 10 000U per one. |
| 药品名称 Drug Names | 凝血酶原复合物 Prothrombin Complex |
| 适应证<br>Indications | 用于手术、急性肝坏死、肝硬化等所致出血的防治。<br>Prothrombin Complex is used in the prophylaxis of haemorrhage result form sugery, acute hepatic necrosis or cirrhosis. |
| 用法、用量<br>Dosage | 本品仅供静脉滴注，且用前新鲜配制。每瓶加注射用水 25ml 使溶，按输血法过滤，滴速不超过 60 滴 / 分。<br>Prothrombin Complex is only used in intravenous drip and needs to be used immediately after prepared. Dissolved in 25ml of water for injection, Prothrombin Complex is filtered as hematometachysis and the drip speed is controlled within 60 drip/min. |
| 剂型、规格<br>Preparations | 注射剂（冻干粉）：200U；400U。<br>Injections (Freeze-dried powder): 200U per one; 400U per one. |
| 13.2 抗凝血药 Anticoagulants | |
| 药品名称 Drug Names | 枸橼酸钠 Sodium Citrate |
| 适应证<br>Indications | 仅用于体外抗凝血。<br>Sodium citrate is only used as an in vitro anticoagulant. |
| 用法、用量<br>Dosage | 输血时预防凝血，每 100ml 全血加入 2.5% 输血用枸橼酸钠注射液 10ml。<br>To prevent blood clotting during transfusion, 10ml of 2.5% sodium citrate injection for transfusion is added to every 100ml of whole blood. |
| 剂型、规格<br>Preparations | 输血用枸橼酸钠注射液：为枸橼酸钠的灭菌水溶液，含枸橼酸钠 2.35% ～ 2.65%。<br>Sodium Citrate injection for transfusion is sterile water solution of sodium citrate and contains 2.35% to 2.65% of Sodium Citrate. |
| 药品名称 Drug Names | 肝素钠 Heparin Sodium |
| 适应证<br>Indications | （1）预防血栓形成和栓塞，如深部静脉血栓、心肌梗死、肺栓塞、血栓静脉炎及术后血栓形成等。<br>（2）治疗各种原因引起的弥散性血管内凝血（DIC），如细菌性脓毒血症、胎盘早期剥离、恶性肿瘤细胞溶解所致的 DIC，但蛇咬伤所致的 DIC 除外。早期应用可防止纤维蛋白原和其他凝血因子的消耗。<br>（3）其他体外抗凝血，如心导管检查、心脏手术外循环、血液透析等。<br>(1) Heparin Sodium is used in the prophylaxis of thrombosis and thrombus, such as deep-vein thrombosis, myocardial infarction, pulmonary embolism, thrombophlebitis, post-operative thrombosis, etc.<br>(2) Heparin Sodium is also used in the treatment of disseminated intravascular coagulation (DIC), such as bacterial sepsis, premature separation of placenta, DIC caused by the lysis of malignant cell. but DIC caused by snake bites is not included. The early application of Heparin Sodium could avoid the consumption of fibrinogen and other coagulation factors.<br>(3) Besides, Heparin Sodium is used as an in vitro anticoagulant, like cardiac catheterization, extracorporeal circulation of cardiac surgery, hemodialysis, etc. |

**续　表**

| | |
|---|---|
| 用法、用量<br>Dosage | （1）静脉注射：成人首剂 5000U 加入 100ml 0.9% 氯化钠注射液中，在 30 ～ 60 分钟滴完。需要时可每隔 4 ～ 6 小时重复静脉滴注 1 次，每次 5000U，总量可达 25 000U/d。为维持恒定血药浓度，也可每 24 小时 10 000 ～ 20 000U 加入 1000ml 0.9% 氯化钠注射液中静脉滴注，速度 20 滴 / 分。用于体外循环时，375U/kg；体外循环超过 1 小时者，每 1kg 体重加 125U。<br><br>（2）静脉注射或深部肌内注射（或皮下注射）：每次 5000 ～ 10 000U。<br><br>（1）Intravenous injection: the initial dose for adults is 5000U diluted by 100ml of 0.9% sodium chloride injection and finished in 30 to 60 min. If necessary, an individual dose of 5000U for one time may be given every 4 to 6 h in intravenous drip, up to a total daily dose of 25 000U. To acquire a constant blood concentration, 10 000 ～ 20 000U diluted in 1000ml of 0.9% sodium chloride injection is given in ntravenous drip at the speed of 20 drip/min every 24 h. For cardiopulmonary bypass, the dose is 375U/kg; for patients who has cardiopulmonary bypass more than 1 h, the dose increases by 125 U/kg.<br><br>（2）Intravenous injection or deep-intramuscular injection (or subcutaneous injection): 5000 to 10 000U, per time. |
| 剂型、规格<br>Preparations | 注射液：每支 1000U（2ml）；5000U（2ml）；12 500U（2ml）。<br>Injections: 1000U(2ml) per vial; 5000U(2ml) per vial; 12500U(2ml) per vial. |
| 药品名称 Drug Names | 肝素钙 Heparin Calcium |
| 适应证<br>Indications | 用于预防和治疗血栓 - 栓塞性疾病及血栓形成。本品具有较明显的抗醛固酮活性，故亦适于人工肾、人工肝和体外循环使用。<br><br>Heparin Calcium is used for the prophylaxis and treatment of thromboembolic disease. This product, which has apparent anti-aldosterone activity, is suitable for artificial kidney, artificial liver and cardiopulmonary bypass. |
| 用法、用量<br>Dosage | （1）用于血栓 - 栓塞意外：皮下注射，首次 0.01ml/kg，5 ～ 7 小时后以 APTT 检测剂量是否合适，12 小时 1 次，每次注射后 5 ～ 7 小时进行新的检查，连续 3 ～ 4 日。<br><br>（2）用于内科预防：皮下注射，首剂 0.005ml/kg，注射后 5 ～ 7 小时以 APTT 检测调整合适剂量，一次 0.2ml，每日 2 ～ 3 次，或一次 0.3ml，一日 2 次。<br><br>（3）用于外科预防：皮下注射，术前 0.2ml，术后每 12 小时 0.2ml，至少持续 10 日。<br><br>（1）For the treatment of thromboembolism accident: an initial dose of 0.01 ml/kg is given in subcutaneous injection. Test if the dose is suitable with Activated Partial Thromboplastin Time (APTT) 5 to 7 hours later. Once every 12 hours. The new test should be done 5 to 7 hours every time after the injection for 3 to 4 consecutive days.<br><br>（2）For prophylaxis in internal medicine: an initial dose of 0.005 ml/kg is given hypodermic injection. Test and adjust the suitable dose with APTT 5 to 7 h after injection. 0.2ml per time, 2 to 3 times a day. Or 0.3ml per time, 2 times a day.<br><br>（3）For prophylaxis in surgery, 0.2ml is given in hypodermic injection pre-surgery. It should be given 0.2 ml post-surgery every 12 h for at least 10 days. |
| 剂型、规格<br>Preparations | 注射液：2500U（0.3ml）。<br>Injection: 2500U(0.3 ml). |
| 药品名称 Drug Names | 低分子量肝素 Low Molecular Weight Heparin |
| 适应证<br>Indications | （1）预防深部静脉血栓形成和肺栓塞。<br>（2）治疗已形成的急性深部静脉血栓。<br>（3）在血液透析或血液滤过时，防止体外循环系统中发生血栓或血液凝固。<br>（4）治疗不稳定型心绞痛及非 ST 段抬高心肌梗死。<br><br>（1）Low-molecular-weight-heparins are used in the prophylaxis of deep-vein thrombosis and pulmonary embolism.<br>（2）They are used in the treatment of acute deep-vein thrombosis.<br>（3）They are also used to prevent thrombosis and blood coagulation in the cardiopulmonary bypass system during hemodialysis and hemofiltration.<br>（4）They are also used in the treatment of unstable angina and Non-ST segment elevation myocardial infarction. |

**续　表**

| | |
|---|---|
| 用法、用量<br>Dosage | （1）本品给药途径为腹壁皮下注射或静脉注射或遵医嘱。<br>（2）血透时预防血凝块形成。<br>(1) The route of administration of this product is subcutaneous injection abdominal wall, or intravenous injection, or follows the doctors' advice.<br>(2) Prevent blood clot formation when doing hemodialysis. |
| 剂型、规格<br>Preparations | 针剂：5000U。<br>Injection:5000U per one. |
| **药品名称 Drug Names** | 华法林 Warfarin |
| 适应证<br>Indications | （1）防治血栓栓塞性疾病，可防止血栓形成与发展，如治疗血栓栓塞性静脉炎，降低肺栓塞的发病率和死亡率，减少外科大手术、风湿性心脏病、髋关节固定术、人工置换心脏瓣膜手术等的静脉血栓发生率。<br>（2）心肌梗死的治疗辅助用药。<br>(1) Warfarin is used for the prophylaxis of thromboembolic disease, and the formulation and development of thrombosis. Warfarin is used in the treatment of thromboembolic phlebitis, reducing the morbidity and mortality rate of pulmonary embolism, the incidence rate of vein thrombosis associated with surgery, rheumatic heart disease, hip fixation and heart valve replacement surgery.<br>(2) Warfarin is used as the adjuvant drug in the treatment of myocardial infarction. |
| 用法、用量<br>Dosage | 口服，第 1 日 5 ～ 20mg，次日起用维持量，一日 2.5 ～ 7.5mg。<br>Oral medication : its first day dose is 5 to 20 mg, followed by daily maintenance dose of 2.5 to 7.5 mg since the second day. |
| 剂型、规格<br>Preparations | 片剂：每片 2.5mg；5mg。<br>Tablets: 2.5 mg and 5 mg per tablet. |
| **药品名称 Drug Names** | 利伐沙班 Rivaroxaban |
| 适应证<br>Indications | 用于髋关节或膝关节置换手术成年患者，以预防静脉血栓形成（VTE）。<br>Rivaroxaban is used for the treatment of adult patients who have hip and knee replacements to prevent venous thrombus embolism(VTE). |
| 用法、用量<br>Dosage | 口服，10mg，一日 1 次。如伤口已止血，首次用药时间应于手术后 6 ～ 10 小时进行。<br>Oral medication: 10mg, once a day. If the wound has stopped bleeding, the time for initial dose should be between 6 to 10h after surgery. |
| 剂型、规格<br>Preparations | 片剂：每片 10mg。<br>Tablets: 10 mg per tablet. |
| **药品名称 Drug Names** | 重组链激酶 Recombinant Streptokinase |
| 适应证<br>Indications | 用于治疗血栓栓塞性疾病，如深静脉血栓、周围动脉栓塞、急性肺栓塞、血管外科手术后的血栓形成、导管给药所致血栓形成、新鲜心肌梗死、中央视网膜动静脉栓塞等。<br>Streptokinase is used in the treatment of thromboembolic disease, such as deep-vein thrombosis, peripheral arterial embolism symptoms, acute pulmonary embolism, the thrombosis after vascular surgery procedures, thrombosis caused by catheter administration, fresh myocardial infarction, central retinal artery or vein occlusion, etc |
| 用法、用量<br>Dosage | 一般推荐本品 150 万 U 溶解于 5% 葡萄糖 100ml，静脉滴注 1 小时。<br>The recommended dose is 1 500 000U dissolved in 100 ml of 5% glucose injection by intravenous drip for one hour. |
| 剂型、规格<br>Preparations | 注射用冻干链激酶：每支 10 万 U；15 万 U；20 万 U；25 万 U；30 万 U；50 万 U；75 万 U；150 万 U。<br>Freeze-dried streptokinase for injection: 100 000U per vial, 150 000U per vial, 200 000U per vial, 250 000U per vial, 300 000U per vial, 500 000U, 750 000U and 1 500 000U per vial. |

| 药品名称 Drug Names | 尿激酶 Urokinase |
|---|---|
| 适应证<br>Indications | 用于急性心肌梗死、肺栓塞、脑血管栓塞、周围动脉或静脉栓塞、视网膜动脉或静脉栓塞等。也可用于眼部炎症、外伤性组织水肿、血肿等。<br><br>Urokinase is used in the treatment of acute myocardial infarction, pulmonary embolism, cerebrovascular embolism, or cerebral embolism, peripheral arterial or venous embolism, retinal artery or vein occlusion and so on. Urokinase can also be used for the treatment of ocular inflammation, traumatic tissue edema, hematoma, etc. |
| 用法、用量<br>Dosage | ①肺栓塞：初次剂量 3 万～ 4 万 U，间隔 24 小时重复给药一次，最多使用 3 次。②心肌梗死：建议 0.9% 氯化钠注射液配制后，按 6000U/min 的给药速度冠状动脉内连续滴注 2 小时，滴注前应先行静脉给予肝素 2500 ～ 10 000U。<br><br>① For the treatment of pulmonary embolism: the initial dose is 30 000 to 40 000U. The dose is repeated at intervals. It can be used for at most three times. ② myocardial infarction: after it is prepared with recommended 0.9% sodium chloride injection, it should be given at the speed of 6000U per minute in coronary artery with continuous drip for 2 hours. Before the drip, the heparin of 2500 to 10 000U should be given by vein. |
| 剂型、规格<br>Preparations | 注射用尿激酶：每瓶 1 万 U；5 万 U；10 万 U；20 万 U；25 万 U；50 万 U；150 万 U；250 万 U。<br><br>Urokinase for injections: 10 000U per vial; 50 000U per vial; 100 000U pe vial; 200 000U per vial; 250 000U per vial; 500 000U per vial; 1 500 000U per vial; 2 500 000U per vial. |
| 药品名称 Drug Names | 阿替普酶 Alteplase |
| 适应证<br>Indications | 用于急性心肌梗死和肺栓塞的溶栓治疗。<br><br>Alteplase is used in the thrombolytic therapy for acute myocardial infarction and pulmonary embolism. |
| 用法、用量<br>Dosage | （1）静脉注射：将本品 50mg 溶于灭菌注射用水中，使溶液浓度为 1mg/ml，给予静脉注射。<br>（2）静脉滴注：将本品 100mg 溶于 0.9% 氯化钠注射液 500ml 中，在 3 小时内按以下方式滴完，即：前 2 分钟先注入 10mg，以后 60 分钟内滴入 50mg，最后剩余时间内滴完所余 40mg。<br><br>(1) Intravenous injection: Dissolve 50ml of this product in sterile water for injection until the solution concentrationis 1mg/ml and then infuse it by intravenous injection.<br>(2) Intravenous drip: Dissolve 100mg of this product in 9% sodium chloride injection of 500ml and finish the drip in the following way within 3 hours: 10 mg is finished in the first 2 min, 50 mg in the following 60 min and the last 40 mg in the rest time. |
| 剂型、规格<br>Preparations | 注射用：每瓶 20mg；50mg。<br><br>Injections: 20mg per vial; 50mg per vial. |
| 药品名称 Drug Names | 瑞替普酶 Reteplase |
| 适应证<br>Indications | 用于成人由冠状动脉梗死引起的急性心肌梗死的溶栓疗法，能改善心功能。<br><br>Reteplase is used in thrombolytic therapy for acute myocardial infarction induced by the coronary artery infarction and improves heart function. |
| 用法、用量<br>Dosage | 10MU 缓慢静脉注射 2 ～ 3 分钟以上，间隔 30 分钟后可重复给药（10MU）1 次，目前尚无 2 次以上重复给药的经验。<br><br>The average dose of Reteplase is 10 MU by slow intravenous injection over 2 to 3 min. The repeated dose may be given after 30 min. By now there is no experience in repeated administration over 2 times. |
| 剂型、规格<br>Preparations | 注射用：每支 5.0MU。<br><br>Injections: 5 MU pe vial. |
| 药品名称 Drug Names | 巴曲酶 Defibrin（Batroxobin） |
| 适应证<br>Indications | 用于急性缺血性脑血管病，突发性耳聋，慢性动脉闭塞症如闭塞性血栓脉管炎、闭塞性动脉硬化症和末梢循环障碍等。<br><br>Defibrin is used in the treatment of acute ischemic cerebrovascular disease, sudden deafness, and chronic arterial occlusive disease, such as thromboangiitis obliterans, arteriosclerosis obliterans, peripheral circulatory disturbance and so on. |

| | |
|---|---|
| 用法、用量<br>Dosage | 静脉滴注：成人首次巴曲霉 10 单位（BU），以后隔日 1 次，5BU。使用前用 100 ～ 200ml 的 0.9% 氯化钠注射液静脉滴注 1 小时以上。通常疗程为 1 周，必要时可增至 3 ～ 6 周。<br><br>Intravenous drip: The initial intravenous infusion dose for adults is 10 BU, once every other day in the following treatment with 5BU. 9% sodium chloride injection, which is about 100ml to 200ml, should be infused in intravenous drip. Usually, a course of treatment is 1 week, which could be extended to 3 to 6 weeks if necessary. |
| 剂型、规格<br>Preparations | 注射液：每支 10BU（1ml）；5BU（0.5ml）。<br>Injections: 10 BU(1ml) per vial; 5 BU(0.5ml) per vial. |
| 药品名称 Drug Names | 蚓激酶 Lumbrukinase |
| 适应证<br>Indications | 用于缺血性脑血管病中纤维蛋白原增高及血小板聚集率增高的患者。<br>Lumbrukinase is used to treat patients with higher fibrinogen levels in ischemic cerebrovascular disease and to treat patients with the increase of platelet aggregation rate. |
| 用法、用量<br>Dosage | 口服：一次 2 粒，一日 3 次，餐前半小时服用。3 ～ 4 周为 1 个疗程，也可连续服用。<br>Oral medication: 2 pills each time, three times a day, taken half an hour before meals. A course of treatment is 3 to 4 weeks. It can be taken continuously. |
| 剂型、规格<br>Preparations | 肠溶胶囊：每粒 30 万 U。<br>Enteric-coated capsules: per capsule contains 0.3 MU |

13.3　血浆代用品 Blood substitutes

| | |
|---|---|
| 药品名称 Drug Names | 右旋糖酐 40　Dextran 40 |
| 适应证<br>Indications | ①各种休克：用于失血、创伤、烧伤及中毒性休克，还可早期预防因休克引起的弥散性血管内凝血。②体外循环时，还可代替部分血液预充心肺机。③血栓性疾病如脑血栓形成、心绞痛和心肌梗死、血栓闭塞性脉管炎、视网膜动静脉血栓、皮肤缺血性溃疡等。④肢体再植和血管外科手术，可预防术后血栓形成，并可改善血液循环，提高再植成功率。<br><br>① Dextran 40 is used in the treatment of all kinds of shock, like hemorrhagic shock, traumatic shock, burn shock and toxic shock, and used in the early prevention of disseminated intravascular coagulation caused by shock. ② when dextran 40 is used in cardiopulmonary bypass, it could used to prime the heart-lung machine as the substitution of partial blodd. ③ It is also used in the treatment of thrombotic diseases, like cerebral thrombosis, angina pectoris and myocardial infarction, thromboangiitis obliterans, retinal arterial and venous thrombosis, ischemic ulcers of skin and so on. ④ Dextran 40 is used in the treatment of replantation of severed limb and vascular operation and used in the prophylaxis of postoperative thrombosis. It can also improve blood circulation and increase the odds of success of replantation. |
| 用法、用量<br>Dosage | 静脉滴注（10% 溶液），每次 250 ～ 500ml，成人和儿童每日不超过 20ml/kg。抗休克时滴注速度为 20 ～ 40ml/min，在 15 ～ 30 分钟注入 500ml。对冠心病和脑血栓患者应缓慢静脉滴注。疗程视病情而定，通常每日或隔日 1 次，7 ～ 14 次为 1 个疗程。<br><br>Intravenous drip: The average dose of 10% Dextran 40 solution is 250 to 500 ml, and the maximum daily dose for adults and children is not more than 20 ml/kg. In shock, the usual dose is 500ml infused at a speed of 20 to 40ml/minute, which is finished in 15 to 30 min. Dextran 40 may be given by slow intravenous drips to patients with coronary heart disease and cerebral thrombosis. The course of the treatment depends on the patients's condition. Usually, the treatment is conducted once a day or every other day, and 7 to 14 days is a course of treatment. |
| 剂型、规格<br>Preparations | 右旋糖酐 40（低分子右旋糖酐）葡萄糖注射液：每瓶 10g（100ml）；25g（250ml）；50g（500ml）；6g（100ml）；15g（250ml）；30g（500ml）。均含葡萄糖 5%。<br>右旋糖酐 40（低分子右旋糖酐）氯化钠注射液：每瓶 10g（100ml）；25g（250ml）；50g（500ml）；6g（100ml）；15g（250ml）；30g（500ml）。均含氯化钠 0.9%。<br><br>Dextran 40(dextran of low-molecular-weight): Glucose Injection: 10g(100ml) per bottle; 25g(250ml) per bottle; 50g(500ml) per bottle; 6g(100ml) per bottle; 15g(250ml) per bottle; 30g(500ml) per bottle. Each kind contains 5%.<br>Dextran 40(dextran of low-molecular-weight): Sodium Chloride Injection: 10g(100ml) per bottle; 25g(250ml) per bottle; 50g(500ml) per bottle; 6g(100ml) per bottle; 15g(250ml) per bottle;30g(500ml) per bottle. Each kind contains 0.9% sodium chloride. |

| 药品名称 Drug Names | 右旋糖酐 70 Dextran 70 |
| --- | --- |
| 适应证<br>Indications | 用于防治低血容量休克如出血性休克、手术中休克、烧伤性休克。也可用于预防手术后血栓形成和血栓性静脉炎。<br><br>Dextran 70 is used in the treatment of hypovolemic shock caused by hemorrhagic shock, shock during the surgery, burn shock and so on. Besides, Dextran 40 is used in the prophylaxis of postoperative thrombosis and thrombophlebitis. |
| 用法、用量<br>Dosage | 静脉滴注，每次 500ml，每分钟注入 20 ～ 40ml。每日最大量不超过 1000 ～ 1500ml。<br><br>Intravenous drip: The average dose is 500ml infused at a speed of 20 to 40ml/minute. And the daily maximum dose is 1000 to 1500 ml. |
| 剂型、规格<br>Preparations | 右旋糖酐 70（中分子右旋糖酐）葡萄糖注射液：每瓶 30g（500ml），含葡萄糖 5%。右旋糖酐 70（中分子右旋糖酐）氯化钠注射液：每瓶 30g（500ml），含氯化钠 0.9%。<br><br>Dextran 70(dextran of middle molecules): Glucose Injection: 30g(500ml) per bottle, containg 5 % glucose. Dextran 70(dextran of middle molecules): Sodium Chloride Injection: 30g(500ml) per bottle, containing 0.9% sodium chloride. |
| 药品名称 Drug Names | 右旋糖酐 10 Dextran 10 |
| 适应证<br>Indications | 用于急性失血性休克、创伤及烧伤性休克、急性心肌梗死、心绞痛、脑血栓形成、脑供血不足、血栓闭塞性脉管炎、雷诺病等。此外，术前有低血容量及硬膜外麻醉后所致的低血压者均可使用本品升压。<br><br>Dextran 10 is used in the treatment of acute hypovolaemic shock, trauma and burn shock, acute myocardial infarction, angina pectoris, cerebral thrombosis, cerebral vascular insufficiency, occlusive thrombotic vasculitis, Raynaud and so on. Moreover, patients who have hypovolemia before the operation and patients with hypotension caused by epidural anesthesia could use this product. |
| 用法、用量<br>Dosage | 静脉滴注：速度为 5 ～ 15ml/min，血压上升后，可酌情减慢。每次 500 ～ 1000ml（参见药品说明书）。<br><br>Intravenous drip: The average dose is 500 to 1000ml per time infused at a speed of 5 to 15 ml/minut. And the speed may be properly slowed down when the blood pressure rises(refer to the Medicine Specification). |
| 剂型、规格<br>Preparations | 右旋糖酐 10（小分子右旋糖酐）葡萄糖注射液：每瓶 30g（500ml）；50g（500ml），均含葡萄糖 5%。右旋糖酐 10（小分子右旋糖酐）氯化钠注射液：每瓶 30g（500ml）；50g（500ml），均含氯化钠 0.9%。<br><br>Dextran 10(dextran of small molecule): Glucose Injection: 30g(500ml) per bottle; 50g(500ml) per bottle. Both contain 5 % glucose. Dextran 10(dextran of small molecule): Sodium Chloride Injection: 30g(500ml) per bottle; 50g(500ml) per bottle. Both contain 0.9% sodium chloride. |
| 药品名称 Drug Names | 琥珀酰明胶 Succinylated Gelatin |
| 适应证<br>Indications | 用于各种原因引起的低血容量休克的早期治疗，如失血、创伤或手术、烧伤、败血症、腹膜炎、胰腺炎或挤压伤等引起的休克。也可用于体外循环或预防麻醉时出现的低血压。<br><br>Succinylated Gelatin is used in the early treatment of hypovolaemic shock induced by hemorrhage, trauma or surgery, burns, septicemia, peritonitis, pancreatitis, crush injury and so on. Succinylated Gelatin could also be used in the treatment of hypotension which occurs during cardiopulmonary bypass or anesthesia. |
| 用法、用量<br>Dosage | 静脉输入的剂量和速度取决于患者的实际情况。严重急性失血时可在 5 ～ 10 分钟输入 500ml，直至低血容量症状缓解。快速输入时应加温液体但不超过 37℃。大量输入时应确保维持血细胞比容不低于 25%。大出血者，本品可与血液同时使用。可经同一输液器输入本品和血液。成人少量出血，可在 1 ～ 3 小时输入 500 ～ 1000ml。<br><br>Doses and speed for intravenous infusions depend on the clinical condition of patients. For sever and acute hemorrhage, the usual dose is 500ml infused in 5 to 10 min, until the remission of symptoms of hypovolemia occurs. When rapidly infused, the liquid should be heated with the temperature below 37 ℃. When large amount is infused, the hematocrit should not be less than 25%. For sever hemorrhage, succinylated gelatin may be used together with blood. For minimal bleeding in adults, 500 to 1000 ml may be infused in 1 to 3 h. |

**续　表**

| 剂型、规格<br>Preparations | 注射液：每瓶 500ml。<br>Injections：500 ml per vial. |
|---|---|
| **药品名称 Drug Names** | 羟乙基淀粉 200/0.5 HydroxyethylStarch 200/0.5 |
| 适应证<br>Indications | 用于预防和治疗各种原因引起的血容量不足和休克，如手术、创伤、感染、烧伤等；急性等容血液稀释，减少手术中对供血的需要，节约用血；治疗性血液稀释，改善血液流变学指标，使红细胞聚集减少，血细胞和血液黏稠度下降，改善微循环。据报道，本品还有防止和堵塞毛细血管漏的作用，在毛细血管通透性增加的情况下使用本品，可减少白蛋白渗漏，减轻组织水肿，减少炎症介质产生，对危重患者更有利。<br><br>Hydroxyethyl Starch 200/0.5 is used in the treatment and prophylaxis of hypovolemia and shock induced by various reasons, such as surgery, trauma, infection, burn, etc; Hydroxyethyl Starch 200/0.5 is also used in acute normovolemic hemodilution, which could reduce the need for blood supply during the surgery and save the usage of blood; With the property of therapeutic hemodilution, it improves the hemodynamic indexes, decreases the aggregation of red blood cells, reduces blood cells and blood viscosity and improves. Hydroxyethyl Starch 200/0.5 is reported to have the effects of preventing and blocking capillary leak. In the case that capillary permeability is increased, the use of the product could reduce the leakage of albumin, tissue edema and the producing of inflammatory mediators, which is beneficial for critical patients. |
| 用法、用量<br>Dosage | 静脉滴注。由于能有过敏反应发生，开始的 10～20ml 应缓慢滴注，每日用量和滴注速度取决于失血量、血液浓缩程度，每日总量不应大于 33ml/kg（6% 浓度），在心肺功能正常的患者，其血细胞比容应不低于 30%。<br>（1）治疗和预防容量不足或休克（容量替代治疗）：使用不同浓度中分子羟乙基淀粉溶液最大剂量 6% 的为 33ml/kg，10% 的为 20ml/kg。<br>（2）急性等容血液稀释（ANH）：手术前即刻开展 ANH，按 1∶1 比例，每日剂量（2～3）×500ml（6%），采血量：（2～3）×500ml（自体血），输注速度 1000ml/（15～30min），采血速度 1000ml/（15～30min）。<br>（3）治疗性血液稀释：治疗可分为等容血液稀释（放血）和高容血液稀释（不放血），按药物不同浓度，给药剂量每日可分为低（250ml）、中（500ml）、高（1000ml）三种，滴注速度：0.5～2 小时 250ml，4～6 小时 500ml，8～24 小时 1000ml，建议治疗 10 日。<br><br>Intravenous drip, because of the possibilities that allergic reactions could happen, the starting dose of 10～20ml should be slowly infused. The daily dose and drip speed depend on the severity of hemorrhage and hemoconcentration. the maximum dose for one day should be not more than 33 ml/kg(the concentration of 6%). For patients with normal heart-lung function, the hematocrit should be controlled over 30%.<br>（1）For the treatment and prophylaxis of hypovolemia or shock(volume replacement), using as a plasma volume expander, the maximum dose of Hydroxyethyl Starch 200/0.5 solution is 33ml/kg for the concentration of 6% and the maximum dose of Hydroxyethyl Starch 200/0.5 solution is 20ml/kg for the concentration of 10%.<br>(2) acute normovolemic hemodilution (ANH) is conducted in the following way: 1000 to 1500 ml of 6% Hydroxyethyl Starch 200/0.5 is infused in a rate of 1000 ml finished in 15 to 30 min. The volume of blood collection: (2～3)×500ml(autologous blood) at the speed of 1000ml/(15～30min).<br>（3）Therapeutic hemodilution includes normovolemic and hypervolemic_hemodilution. According to the different kinds of concentration of drugs, the dosage for one day could be divided into 3 kinds: The low-dose, medium-dose and high-dose. The corresponding drip speed is 250ml for 0.5 to 2 h, 500ml for 4 to 6 h, 1000ml for 8 to 24 h in a day and the treatment is recommended for 10 days. |
| 剂型、规格<br>Preparations | 6% 中分子羟乙基淀粉 200/0.5 氯化钠注射液：每瓶 500ml。<br>10% 中分子羟乙基淀粉 200/0.5 氯化钠注射液：每瓶 500ml。<br><br>6% Hydroxyethyl Starch 200/0.5 sodium chloride injections: 500 ml per bottle.<br>10% Hydroxyethyl Starch 200/0.5 sodium chloride injections: 500ml per bottle. |
| **药品名称 Drug Names** | 羟乙基淀粉 130/0.4 Hydroxyethyl Starch 130/0.4 |
| 适应证<br>Indications | 用于治疗和预防血容量不足、急性等容血液稀释（ＡＮＨ）。<br><br>Hydroxyethyl Starch 130/0.4 is used in the treatment and prophylaxis of hypovolemia and acute normovolemic hemodilution (ANH). |

**续 表**

| 用法、用量<br>Dosage | 同中分子羟乙基淀粉 200/0.5，每日最大剂量按体重 33ml/kg，据患者需要可持续使用数日，治疗持续时间取决于低血容量程度及血流动力学参数和稀释效果。在欧洲已批准用于 0 ～ 2 岁儿童，每日最大剂量 50ml/kg。国内儿童用药正在研究中。<br><br>The same with Hydroxyethyl Starch 200/0.5, the maximum dose for one day of Hydroxyethyl Starch 130/0.4 is 33 ml/kg and may be continuously given for several days according to the need of patients. The duration of therapy depends on the degree of hypovolemia, hemodynamic parameters and the dilution effects. In European, it has been approved to be used in 0 to 2-year old children, with the maximum dose being 50 ml/kg. The study of its usage in domestic children is being researched. |
|---|---|
| 剂型、规格<br>Preparations | 6% 中分子羟乙基淀粉 130/0.4 氯化钠注射液：每瓶 250ml；500ml。<br>6% Hydroxyethyl Starch 130/0.4 in sodium chloride injection: each bottle is 250 ml, 500 ml. |
| 药品名称 Drug Names | 包醛氧淀粉 Coated Aldehyde Oxystarch |
| 适应证<br>Indications | 用于各种原因造成的氮质血症。<br>Coated Aldehyde Oxystarch is used in the treatment of azotemia induced by various causes. |
| 用法、用量<br>Dosage | 口服：餐后用温开水送福。一日 2 ～ 3 次，一次 5 ～ 10g，或遵医嘱。<br>Oral medication: taken after meals warm boiled water. The average dose is 5 to 10 g for one time, with 2 to 3 times a day, or or as directed by doctor by orally administration with with warm water after meals, or according to the doctors' prescription. |
| 剂型、规格<br>Preparations | 胶囊：每粒 0.625g。粉剂：每袋 5g。<br>Capsules: per softgel is 0.625 g. Powder: each bag is 5 g. |
| 药品名称 Drug Names | 聚维酮 Polyvidon |
| 适应证<br>Indications | 用于外伤性出血以及其他原因引起的血容量减少。<br>Povidone is used in the treatment of hypovolemia induced by traumatic hemorrhage and other causes. |
| 用法、用量<br>Dosage | 视病情而定，一般为 500 ～ 1000ml 静脉滴注。<br>The usual dose is 500 to 1000 ml in intravenous drip and adjusted according to the clinical condition. |
| 剂型、规格<br>Preparations | 注射液：3.5%（250ml）。<br>Injection: 3.5%(250ml) |
| 药品名称 Drug Names | 羟乙基淀粉 40　Hydroxyethyl Starch 40 |
| 适应证<br>Indications | 为血容量扩充剂。用于各种手术、外伤的失血，中毒性休克等的补液。<br>Hydroxyethyl Starch 40 is a kind of plasma volume expander used in the fluid replacement induced by all kinds of surgeries, blood loss by trauma, toxic shock and so on. |
| 用法、用量<br>Dosage | 视病情而定，一般为 500 ～ 1000ml 静脉滴注。<br>The usual dose is 500 to 1000 ml for intravenous infusion and adjusted according to the clinical condition. |
| 剂型、规格<br>Preparations | 注射液：6%（500ml）。<br>Injection: 6% (500ml). |
| 药品名称 Drug Names | 人血白蛋白 Human Albumin |
| 适应证<br>Indications | 用于失血性休克、脑水肿、流产等引起的白蛋白缺乏、肾病等。<br>Human Albumin is used for the treatment of hemorrhagic shock, cerebral edema, albumin deficiency caused by abortion, nephroma and so on. |
| 用法、用量<br>Dosage | 静脉注射或静脉滴注：用量视病情而定。<br>Human Albumin may be given by intravenous injection or intravenous drip. Its doses depend on the severity of patients' condition. |

**续　表**

| 剂型、规格<br>Preparations | 注射液：5%；10%；20%；25%。<br>冻干粉：5g；10g。<br>Injections: 5%, 10%, 20%, 25%.<br>Lyophilized powder: 5 g and 10 g. |
|---|---|

## 13.4 抗贫血药 Drugs treating anemia

| 药品名称 Drug Names | 硫酸亚铁 Ferrous Sulfate |
|---|---|
| 适应证<br>Indications | 用于慢性失血（月经过多、慢性消化道出血、子宫肌瘤出血、钩虫病失血等）、营养不良、妊娠、儿童发育期等引起的缺铁性贫血。用药后贫血症状迅速改善，用药 1 周左右即可见网织红细胞增多，血红蛋白每日可增加 0.1% ~ 0.3%，4 ~ 8 周可恢复至正常。<br>Ferrous Sulfate is used for the treatment of iron deficiency anemia caused by chronic blood loss (hypermenorrhea, chronic alimentary tract hemorrhage, bleeding of uterine fibroids, bleeding by ancylostomiasis, etc.), malnutrition, gravidity, children's growing period and so on. After medication the anaemic symptoms is improved quickly, with the number of reticulocyte increasing about one week later and hemoglobin increasing by 0.1% ~ 0.3% a day. The condition will come to normal in about 4 ~ 8 weeks. |
| 用法、用量<br>Dosage | 口服，成人，每次 0.3g，一日 3 次，餐后服用。<br>Oral medication for Adults: 0.3g per day for adults, three times a day after meals. |
| 剂型、规格<br>Preparations | 硫酸亚铁片：每片 0.3g。<br>硫酸亚铁缓释片：每片 0.25g；0.45g。<br>Ferrous Sulfate tablets: per tablet contains 0.3g.<br>Ferrous Sulfate Substained Release Tablets: per tablet contains 0.25g, 0.45g. |
| 药品名称 Drug Names | 葡萄糖酸亚铁 Ferrous Gluconate |
| 适应证<br>Indications | 用于各种原因引起的缺铁性贫血，如营养不良、慢性失血、月经过多、妊娠、儿童生长期等所致的缺铁性贫血。<br>Ferrous Gluconate is used for the treatment of iron deficiency anemia caused by various kinds of reasons, such as iron deficiency anemia caused by malnutrition, Chronic blood loss, menorrhagia, gravidity, children's growing period and so on. |
| 用法、用量<br>Dosage | 口服：预防，成人，每次 0.3g，一日 1 次；儿童：每次 0.1g，一日 2 次。治疗，成人，每次 0.3 ~ 0.6g，一日 3 次；儿童：每次 0.1 ~ 0.2g，一日 3 次。<br>Oral medication: for prophylaxis: 0.3g each time for adults, once a day; 0.1g each time for children, twice a day. For therapeutics: for adults it can be given orally in a dose of 0.3g to 0.6g each time for adults, three times a day; 0.1g to 0.2g each time for children, three times a day. |
| 剂型、规格<br>Preparations | 片剂（糖衣片）：每片 0.1g；0.3g。<br>胶囊剂：每粒 0.25g；0.3g；0.4g。<br>糖浆：每瓶 0.25g（10ml）；0.3g（10ml）。<br>Tablets (sugarcoated tablets): per tablet contains 0.1g and 0.3g.<br>Capsules: each one contains 0.25g, 0.3g, 0.4g.<br>Syrups: per bottle contains 0.25g (10ml)；0.3g(10ml). |
| 药品名称 Drug Names | 蔗糖铁 Iron Sucrese |
| 适应证<br>Indications | 主要用于治疗口服铁不能有效缓解的缺铁性贫血。<br>It is mainly used for the treatment of iron deficiency anaemia that cannot be eased by oral iron therapy effectively. |
| 用法、用量<br>Dosage | 本品只能与 0.9%w/v 生理盐水混合使用。应以滴注或缓慢注射的方式给药，或直接注射到透析器的静脉端给药。<br>This product can only be used when mixed with 0.9% normal saline. This product should be given in drip or slow injection method. Or it can be injected into the venous side of dialyzer directly. |
| 剂型、规格<br>Preparations | 蔗糖铁注射液：5ml：100mg（铁元素）。<br>Iron sucrose injections: per bottle contains 5ml：100mg (iron). |

| 药品名称 Drug Names | 叶酸 Folic Acid |
|---|---|
| 适应证<br>Indications | 　　巨幼红细胞性贫血，尤适用于营养不良或婴儿期、妊娠期叶酸需要增加所致的巨幼红细胞贫血。用于治疗恶性贫血时，虽可纠正异常血象，但不能改善神经损害症状，故应以维生素 $B_{12}$ 为主，叶酸为辅。也用于妊娠期和哺乳期妇女的预防用药。<br>　　Folic acid is used to treat megaloblastic anemia especially those induced by malnutrition and increasing requirement of folic acid in infancy and gestational period. Although it can redress anomaly hemogram treatment of malignant anemia, it is useless for nervous lesion. Therefore Vitamin $B_{12}$ should be used as a substitute while folic acid a supplement. It can also be used as prophylactic medicine for women in gestational and lactation period. |
| 用法、用量<br>Dosage | 　　口服：成人，每次 5 ～ 10mg，一日 5 ～ 30mg。肌内注射：每次 10 ～ 20mg。妊娠期和哺乳期妇女的预防用药：口服一次 0.4mg，一日 1 次。<br>　　Oral medication: for adults, 5mg to 30 mg a day and 5mg to 10mg a time. Intramuscular injection: 10mg to 20mg a time. Prophylactic medicine for women in gestational and lactation period: o.4mg singly and once a day. |
| 剂型、规格<br>Preparations | 　　叶酸片：每片 0.4mg；5mg。注射液：每支 15mg（1ml）。复方叶酸注射液：每支 1ml，含叶酸 5mg、维生素 $B_{12}$ 30μg。<br>　　Folic acid tablets: 0.4 mg, 0.5 mg per tablet. Injections: 15 mg per vial (1ml). Compound Folic Acid Injections: 1 ml per vial including 5 mg folic acid and 30μg vitamin $B_{12}$. |

| 药品名称 Drug Names | 氰钴胺（维生素 $B_{12}$）Cyanocobalamin （Vitamin $B_{12}$） |
|---|---|
| 适应证<br>Indications | 　　用于治疗恶性贫血，亦与叶酸合用用于治疗各种巨幼红细胞性贫血、抗叶酸药引起的贫血及脂肪泻、全胃切除或胃大部切除。尚用于神经系统疾病（如神经炎、神经萎缩等）、肝脏疾病（肝炎、肝硬化等）等。<br>　　It can not only be used to treat malignant anaemia, but also to treat megaloblastic anemia, anemia induced by atifolic, steatorrhea, total gastrectomy or part gastrectomy when used in combination with folic acid. Currently Vitamin $B_{12}$ is also uesd in the treatment of nervous system diseases, like neuritis, neuratrophy, and liver diseases like hepatitis, cirrhosis. |
| 用法、用量<br>Dosage | 　　肌内注射，成人，一日内 0.025 ～ 0.1mg 或隔日 0.05 ～ 0.2mg。用于神经系统疾病时，用量可酌增。<br>　　Intramuscular injection: for audlts, 0.025 mg to 0.1 mg a day or 0.05 mg to 0.2 mg per other day. Nervous System Diseases: dosage may reasonably increase accordingly. |
| 剂型、规格<br>Preparations | 　　注射液：每支 0.05mg（1ml）；0.1ng（1ml）；0.25mg（1ml）；0.5mg（1ml）；1mg（1ml）．<br>　　Injections: 0.05mg (1ml) per vial；0.1mg (1ml) per vial；0.25 mg (1ml) per vial；0.5 mg (1ml) per vial；1mg (1ml) per vial. |

| 药品名称 Drug Names | 腺苷钴胺 Cobamamide |
|---|---|
| 适应证<br>Indications | 　　主要用于巨幼红细胞型贫血、营养不良性贫血、妊娠期贫血，亦用于神经性疾患如多发性神经炎、神经根炎、三叉神经痛、坐骨神经痛、神经麻痹、营养性神经疾患以及放射线和药物引起的白细胞减少症。<br>　　It is mainly used to treat megaloblastic anemia, malnutritional anemia, gestational period anemia, as well as nervous system diseases like polyneuritis, neurodocitis, trifacial neuralgia, sciatica, nerve palsy, trophic nerve disease and leukopenia caused by radial line and drugs. |
| 用法、用量<br>Dosage | 　　口服，成人，每次 0.5 ～ 1.5mg，一日 1.5 ～ 4.5mg。肌内注射，每日 0.5 ～ 1mg。<br>　　Oral medication: 0.5 to 1.5 mg singly, 1.5 to 4.5 mg; Intramuscular injection: 0.5 to 1 mg a day. |
| 剂型、规格<br>Preparations | 　　片剂：每片 0.25mg。注射液：每支 0.5mg（1ml）。冻干粉针：0.5mg；1.0mg；1.5mg。<br>　　Tablets: 0.25 mg per tablet. Injections: 0.5 mg (1 ml) per vial. Freeze-dried powder injections: 0.5 mg, 1 mg, 1.5 mg per vial. |

续　表

| 药品名称 Drug Names | 甲钴胺 Mecobalamin |
|---|---|
| 适应证<br>Indications | 用于治疗缺乏维生素 $B_{12}$ 引起的巨幼细胞性贫血，也用于周围神经病。<br>It is used to treat megaloblastic anemia caused by vitamin $B_{12}$ deficiency, and peripheral nerve disease . |
| 用法、用量<br>Dosage | 肌内注射或静脉注射。成人巨红细胞性贫血：通常一次 500μg，一日 1 次，隔日 1 次。给药约 2 个月后，可维持治疗，一次 500μg，每 1～3 个月 1 次。周围神经病：通常，成人一次 500μg，一日 1 次，一周 3 次，可按年龄、症状酌情增减。<br><br>Intramuscular injections or intravenous infusions: For adult megaloblastic anemia, give 500μg singly, once every another day. Treatment could be continued, after 2 month administration, with 500μg singly, once every 1 to 3 month . For peripheral neuropathy, give adults 500μg singly, once a day and 3 times a week, the dosage may varied reasonably according to one's age and symptom. |
| 剂型、规格<br>Preparations | 注射液：1ml：500μg。<br>Injections: 500 ug (1 ml) per vial. |
| 药品名称 Drug Names | 重组人促红细胞生成素 Recombinant Human Erythropoietin |
| 适应证<br>Indications | 用于慢性肾衰竭和晚期肾病所致的贫血，也用于多发性骨髓瘤相关的贫血和骨髓增生异常综合征（MDS）及骨癌引起的贫血。对结缔组织病（类风湿关节炎和系统性红斑狼疮）所致的贫血也有效。<br><br>It is indicated used in the treatment of to treat anemia induced by end-stage renal disease, Chronic renal failure, as well as multiple myeloma related amenia, amenia caused by bone cancer and myelodysplastic syndrome (MDS). It is also active against connective tissue disease-dused anemia such as rheumatoid arthritis and systemic lupus erythematosus. |
| 用法、用量<br>Dosage | 可静脉注射或皮下注射，剂量应个体化，一般开始剂量为 50～150U/kg，每周 3 次。治疗过程中需视血细胞比容或血红蛋白水平调整剂量或调节维持量。建议以血细胞比容 30%～33% 或血红蛋白 100～120g/L 为指标，调节维持剂量。<br><br>Intravenous or subcutaneous injections with individualized amount: give first dose of 50 to 150 units / kg, 3 times a week. The intake dose or maintenance dose could be adjusted according to the level of hematocrit or hemoglobin. Adjustments is Ssuggested to made according to the index of 30% to 33% hematocrit or 100～120g / L hemoglobin . |
| 剂型、规格<br>Preparations | 重组人促红细胞生成素注射液（CHO 细胞）：每支 2000U（1ml）；4000U（1ml）；10 000U（1ml）。<br>注射用重组人促红细胞生成素（CHO 细胞）：每支 2000U；4000U；10 000U。<br>Recombinant human erythropoietin infusion: 2000 U1 (ml) per vial;4000 U1 (ml) per vial; 10 000 U1 (ml) per vial. |
| 药品名称 Drug Names | 琥珀酸亚铁 Ferrous Succinate |
| 适应证<br>Indications | 用于缺铁性贫血的预防和治疗。<br>It is used in the treatment and prophylaxis of iron deficiency anemia. |
| 用法、用量<br>Dosage | 预防：普通成人每日 0.1g；妊娠期妇女每日 0.2g；儿童每日 0.03～0.06g。治疗：成人一次 0.1～0.2g，一日 3 次；儿童一次 0.05～0.1g，一日 1～2 次餐后服。<br><br>Prophylaxis: for adults, give 0.1 g daily; for women in gestational period, 0.2g daily; for children, 0.03 g to 0.06 g daily . Treatment: for adults, 0.1 g to 0.2 g singly, 3 times a day; for children, 0.05 g to 0.1 g singly, 1 to 2 times a day after a meal. |
| 剂型、规格<br>Preparations | 片剂：0.1g。胶囊剂：0.1g。<br>Tablets: per containing 0.1 g. Capsules: per containing 0.1 g. |
| 药品名称 Drug Names | 富马酸亚铁 Ferrous Fumarate |
| 适应证<br>Indications | 用于治疗缺铁性贫血。<br>It is used to treat iron deficiency anemia. |

**续　表**

| 用法、用量<br>Dosage | 口服，一次 0.2 ～ 0.4g，一日 3 次，疗程：轻症 2 ～ 3 周，重症 3 ～ 4 周。<br>Oral medication: 0.2 g to 0.4 g singly, three times a day. The course of treatment is 2 to 3 weeks for miner ailment, 3 to 4 weeks for severe case. |
| --- | --- |
| 剂型、规格<br>Preparations | 片剂：0.2g；0.05g。胶囊剂：0.2g。<br>Tablets :0.2g, 0.05 per tablet; Capsules : 0.2 g per capsules . |
| **药品名称 Drug Names** | **枸橼酸铁铵 Ferric Ammonium Citrate** |
| 适应证<br>Indications | 适用于儿童及不能吞服药片的患者。由于含铁量低，不适于重症贫血病例。<br>It is intended for children and patients with dysphagia. Because of low iron content, it is not suitable to treat severe anemia |
| 用法、用量<br>Dosage | 口服，一次 0.5 ～ 2g，一日 3 次，餐后服。<br>Oral medication: 0.5g to 2g, three times a day after meals. |
| 剂型、规格<br>Preparations | 溶液：10%。<br>Solution: 10 % |
| **药品名称 Drug Names** | **右旋糖酐铁 Iron Dextran** |
| 适应证<br>Indications | 适用于不能耐受口服铁制剂的缺铁性贫血患者或者需要迅速纠正缺铁者。<br>It is intended for patients with iron deficiency anemia who are intolerant of oral iron preparation and those who need immediate iron deficiency treatment. |
| 用法、用量<br>Dosage | 深部肌内注射：每日 1ml。<br>Deep intramuscular injections: 1ml a day. |
| 剂型、规格<br>Preparations | 注射液：每毫升含元素铁 25mg。<br>Infusions: 25 mg iron /ml |
| **药品名称 Drug Names** | **山梨醇铁 Iron Sorbitex** |
| 适应证<br>Indications | 适用于不能耐受口服铁制剂的缺铁性贫血患者或需要迅速纠正缺铁者。<br>It is intended for patients with iron deficiency anemia who are intolerant of oral iron preparation and those who need immediate iron deficiency treatment. |
| 用法、用量<br>Dosage | 深部肌内注射，一次 1.5 ～ 2ml（相当于铁 75 ～ 100mg）。<br>Deep intramuscular injections: 1.5 to 2 ml singly (equivalent to 75 to 100 mg iron). |
| 剂型、规格<br>Preparations | 注射剂 2ml：50mg（以 Fe 计）<br>injections 2ml: 50mg (in terms of Fe) |
| **药品名称 Drug Names** | **亚叶酸钙 Calcium Folinate** |
| 适应证<br>Indications | 常用作氨蝶呤及甲氨蝶呤过量时的解毒剂。此外尚可用于巨幼红细胞性贫血以及白细胞减少症。<br>It is usually used as antidote of aminopterin methotrexate overdose. It can also be used to treat leukopenia and megaloblastic anemia. |
| 用法、用量<br>Dosage | 肌内注射：抗叶酸代谢药中度中毒，一次 6 ～ 12mg，每 6 小时 1 次，共 4 次。巨幼红细胞性贫血：一日 1mg，一日 1 次。白细胞减少症：每次 3 ～ 6mg，一日 1 次。静脉滴注：抗叶酸代谢药重度中毒：75mg 于 12 小时内滴注完毕，随后改为肌内注射。<br>Intramuscular injection: for the treatment of medium poisoning dused by antifolate metabolism, use 6 to 12 mg singly, every 6 hours a time ; for megaloblastic anemia, use 1 mg a day, once a day ; for leukopenia,   use 3 to 6 mg singly, once a day. Intravenous drip : for the treatment of severe poisoning dused by antifolate metabolism, first instill 75 mg in 12 hours, and then instill intramuscularly. |
| 剂型、规格<br>Preparations | 注射用冻干粉：3mg；5mg。<br>Freeze-dried powder injections: 3 mg, 5 mg per vial. |

**续　表**

### 13.5 促进白细胞增生药 Drugs promoting leukocytosis increase

| 药品名称 Drug Names | 腺嘌呤（维生素 $B_4$） Adenine (Vitamin $B_4$) |
| --- | --- |
| 适应证<br>Indications | 用于各种原因如放射治疗、苯中毒、抗肿瘤药和抗甲状腺药物等引起的白细胞减少症，也用于急性粒细胞减少症。<br>It is used to treat leukopenia caused by radiotherapeutics, benzolism, antineoplastic, antithyroid drug, as well as acute granulocytopenia. |
| 用法、用量<br>Dosage | 口服，成人，每次 10～20mg，一日 3 次。肌内注射或静脉注射，每日 20～30mg。<br>Oral medication: for adults, give10 to 20 mg singly, 3 times a day. Intramuscular or intravenous injections：20 mg to 30 mg a day . |
| 剂型、规格<br>Preparations | 片剂：每片 10mg；25mg。注射用维生素 $B_4$：每支 20mg。<br>Tablets: 10mg, 25mg per tablets. Injections: vitamin $B_4$, 20mg per vial. |
| 药品名称 Drug Names | 苦参总碱 Alkaloids Sophora |
| 适应证<br>Indications | 用于肿瘤放疗、化疗及其他原因引起的白细胞减少症（包括再生障碍性贫血、慢性放射病、慢性肝炎等）。<br>It is used to treat leukopenia ( including aplastic anemia, chronic radiation disease, chronic hepatitis etc.) caused by radiotherapeutics, chemotherapy etc. |
| 用法、用量<br>Dosage | 肌内注射，每次 0.2g，一日 2 次。<br>Intramuscular injections: 0.2g singly, twice a day. |
| 剂型、规格<br>Preparations | 注射液：0.2g（1ml）。<br>Infusions: 0.2 g (1 ml). |
| 药品名称 Drug Names | 鲨肝醇 Batilol |
| 适应证<br>Indications | 用于各种原因引起的粒细胞减少。<br>It is used to treat granulopenia caused by various reasons. |
| 用法、用量<br>Dosage | 一日 50～150mg，分 3 次口服。<br>Oral medication: 50 mg to 150 mg daily, in 3 divided doses. |
| 剂型、规格<br>Preparations | 片剂：25mg；50mg。<br>Tablets : 25 mg; 50 mg per tablet. |
| 药品名称 Drug Names | 利可君 Leucogen |
| 适应证<br>Indications | 用于防治各种原因引起的白细胞较少、再生障碍性贫血。<br>It could be used in the treatment and prophylaxis of leukopenia and aplastic anemia caused by carious reasons. |
| 用法、用量<br>Dosage | 口服，一次 20mg，一日 3 次。<br>Oral medication: 20 mg singly, 3 times a day. |
| 剂型、规格<br>Preparations | 片剂：10mg；20mg。<br>Tablets : 10 mg; 20 mg per tablet. |
| 药品名称 Drug Names | 肌苷 Inosine |
| 适应证<br>Indications | 用于治疗各种原因所致的白细胞较少、血小板减少等。<br>It is used to treat leukopenia, thrombocytopenia caused by various reasons. |
| 用法、用量<br>Dosage | 口服：一次 200～600mg，一日 3 次。静脉注射或静脉滴注：一次 200～600mg，一日 1～2 次。<br>Oral medication: 200 mg to 600 mg singly, 3 times a day. Intravenous injections and intravenous drips: 200 mg to 600 mg singly, once or twice a day. |

| 剂型、规格<br>Preparations | 片剂：每片 200mg。<br>注射液：100mg（2ml）；200mg（5ml）。<br>Tablet: 200mg per tablet.<br>Injections: 100mg (2 ml), 200mg(5ml)per vial. |
|---|---|
| **药品名称 Drug Names** | **氨肽素 Aminopolypeptide** |
| 适应证<br>Indications | 用于原发性血小板减少性紫癜、过敏性紫癜、白细胞减少症和再生障碍性贫血。<br>It is used to treat of thrombocytopenic purpura, allergic purpura, leukopenia and allergic purpura. |
| 用法、用量<br>Dosage | 口服：成人一次 1g，一日 3 次；小儿酌减。用药至少 4 周，有效者可连续服用。<br>Oral medication : for adults, give 1 g singly, 3 times a day; for children, give proportionally reduced doses. Patients are suggested to take the medicine for at least 4 weeks, if one's condition is improved, he/she may continously take it. |
| 剂型、规格<br>Preparations | 片剂：0.2g。<br>Tablets: 0.2g. |

## 13.6 抗血小板药物 Antiplatelet drugs

| **药品名称 Drug Names** | **阿司匹林 Aspirin** |
|---|---|
| 适应证<br>Indications | 可用于预防心、脑血管疾病的发作及人工心脏瓣膜或其他手术后的血栓形成。临床研究发现在男性患者预防脑卒中的效果似乎较女性患者为好，这可能与女性的血小板环氧酶对阿司匹林的耐受性较高有关。<br>It is used in the prophylaxis of cerebrovascular disorder and thrombopoiesis postoperative of Heart Valve Prosthesis. Clinical research discovered that male patients seem to have a higer rate in preventing cerebral apoplexy than females patients, this may be due to the fact that female platelet expoxidase have a higher tolerance to aspirin. |
| 用法、用量<br>Dosage | 用于防治短暂性脑缺血和卒中：成人常用量，每次 75 ～ 300mg，一日 1 次。预防用，一般一日 75 ～ 150mg；治疗用，一般一日 300mg。用于缺血性心脏病，可预防心肌梗死，减少心律失常的发生率和死亡率。<br>It is used for the treatment and prophylaxis of transient ischemic attack and apoplexia: for adults, give 75 mg to 300 mg singly as a general dose, once a day.Prophylaxis: generally 75 to 150mg a day. Treatment: 300 mg a day. |
| 剂型、规格<br>Preparations | 肠溶片：每片 25mg；40mg；100mg。<br>Enteric-coated tablets: 25 mg; 40mg; 100mg per tablet. |
| **药品名称 Drug Names** | **双嘧达莫 Dipyridamole** |
| 适应证<br>Indications | 用于血栓栓塞性疾病及缺血性心脏病。<br>It is used to treat thromboembolic disease and ischemic heart disease. |
| 用法、用量<br>Dosage | 单独应用疗效不及与阿司匹林合用者。单独应用时，每日口服 3 次，每次 25 ～ 100mg；与阿司匹林合用时其剂量可减少至每日 100 ～ 200mg。<br>It has better curative effect when used in combination with aspirin. Dipyridamole alone: 25mg to 100 mg singly, 3 times a day orally; if when used in combination with aspirin: the dosage could be reduced to 100 to 200 mg a day. |
| 剂型、规格<br>Preparations | 片剂：每片 25mg。<br>Tablets : 25 mg per tablet. |
| **药品名称 Drug Names** | **氯吡格雷 Clopidogrel** |
| 适应证<br>Indications | 用于预防和治疗因血小板高聚集引起的心、脑及其他动脉循环障碍疾病，如近期发作的脑卒中、心肌梗死和确诊的外周动脉疾病。<br>It is used in the treatment and prophylaxis of heart, brain and other artery circulatory disorder produced by platelet aggregation such as recent paroxysm of cerebral apoplexy, myocardial infarction, definite disease of periphery artery, |

**续　表**

| | |
|---|---|
| 用法、用量<br>Dosage | 一日一次，每次 75mg。<br>75 mg singly, once a day. |
| 剂型、规格<br>Preparations | 片剂：每片 25mg。<br>Tablets : 25 mg per tablet. |
| 药品名称 Drug Names | 替罗非班 Tirofiban |
| 适应证<br>Indications | 用于急性冠脉综合征、不稳定型心绞痛和非 Q 波心肌梗死、急性心肌梗死和急性缺血性心脏猝死等，包括可用药控制的患者和需做 PTCA、血管成形术或动脉粥样硬化血管切除术的患者。替罗非班可减少急性冠脉综合征和冠脉内介入治疗后冠心病事件发生率，改善患者症状和预后。<br><br>It is used to treat acute coronary syndrome, unstable angina pectoris, non-Q-wave myocardial infarction, acute myocardial infarction, acute ischemic sudden cardiac death and so on. It is used to treat patients whose condition could be controlled, those who need to have a PTCA operation or angioplasty or those who have had an atherosclerotic vascular surgery. It can reduce the incidence rate of acute coronary syndrome and coronary heart disease after interventional therapy to improve prognosis and symptom. |
| 用法、用量<br>Dosage | 与肝素合用，静脉给药。开始 30 分钟给药速度为 0.4μg/（kg·min），然后减为维持量 0.1μg/（kg·min），2 ~ 5 日为 1 个疗程。患者至少给药 48 小时，此期间不进行手术治疗（除非患者发病为顽固性心肌缺血或新的心肌梗死）。<br><br>Used in combination with hamocura, inject intravenously. The injection rate should be 0.4μg/(kg·min) in the first 30 minutes, then slow down to a stable 0.1μg/(kg·min). A course of treatment is 2 to 5 days. Administration should be continued at least 48 hours unless the patient is diagnosed as refractoriness myocardial ischemia or new myocardial infarction. |
| 剂型、规格<br>Preparations | 注射液：每瓶 5mg（100ml）。<br>Injections : 5 mg (100 ml) per bottle. |
| 药品名称 Drug Names | 奥扎格雷 Ozagrel |
| 适应证<br>Indications | 用于治疗急性血栓性脑梗死及伴发的运动障碍，改善蛛网膜下腔出血手术后血管痉挛及其并发的脑缺血症状。<br><br>It is useful in the treatment of acute thrombotic cerebral infarction and concomitant dyskinesia, and it is useful to mend vasospasm and cerebral ischemia after subarachnoid hemorrhage (SAH) surgery. |
| 用法、用量<br>Dosage | 常用制剂为奥扎格雷钠注射液，每支 20mg。以生理盐水或葡萄糖注射液稀释后静脉滴注，一日 80mg。如与其他抗血小板药合用时，本品剂量宜酌减。<br><br>Sodium ozagrel injection (20mg per vial) is used commonly in preparation. It is diluted with glucose or physiological saline in a daily dose of 80 mg given by intravenous drip. If using other antiplatelet drugs at the same time, the dosage should be reduced on the basis of patients' condition . |
| 剂型、规格<br>Preparations | 注射用奥扎格雷：20mg；40mg。奥扎格雷注射液：每支 20mg（1ml）；40mg（2ml）。<br>Ozagrel injection: 20 mg, 40 mg. Ozagrel infusion: 20 mg(1 ml) per vial, 40 mg(2 ml) per vial. |
| 药品名称 Drug Names | 曲克芦丁 Troxerutin |
| 适应证<br>Indications | 用于脑血栓形成和脑栓塞所致的偏瘫、失语以及心肌梗死前综合征、动脉硬化、中心性视网膜炎、血栓性静脉炎、静脉曲张、血管通透性高引起的水肿等。<br><br>It is useful in the treatment of hemiplegia and aphasia caused by cerebral thrombosis and cerebral embolism as well as the syndrome of myocardial infarction before death, atherosclerosis, central retinitis, thrombophlebitis, varicose veins, the edema-caused by high vascular permeability etc. |
| 用法、用量<br>Dosage | 口服：每次 300mg，一日 2 ~ 3 次。肌内注射：每次 100 ~ 200mg，一日 2 次，20 日为 1 个疗程，可用 1 ~ 3 个疗程，每疗程间隔 3 ~ 7 日。静脉滴注：每次 400mg，一日 1 次，用 5% ~ 10% 葡萄糖注射液稀释。<br><br>Oral medication: 2 to 3 times a day of 300mg. intramuscular injection: Twice a day of 100 to 200mg. 20 days for a course of treatment and take one to three of it. An interval of 3 to 7 days after each course. intravenous drips: Once a day of 400mg. Dilute with 5% to 10% glucose injection. |

**续　表**

| 剂型、规格<br>Preparations | 片剂：每片 100mg。注射液：每支 100mg（2ml）。<br>Tablets: 100 mg per tablet. Injection:100 mg (2ml) per vial. |
|---|---|
| 药品名称 Drug Names | 氯贝丁酯 Clofibrate |
| 适应证<br>Indications | 能降低血小板的黏附作用，它能降低血小板对 ADP 和肾上腺素导致聚集的敏感性，并可抑制 ADP 诱导的血小板聚集。它还可延长血小板寿命。可单独应用或与抗凝剂合用于缺血性心脏病的患者。<br><br>It can be used for reducing the adhesion of platelets, platelet sensitivity to ADP and epinephrine and inhibit ADP-induced platelet aggregation. It can also extend the lifetime of platelet. It can be used alone or simultaneously with anticoagulants for patients with ischemic heart disease. |
| 用法、用量<br>Dosage | 口服。一日 3 次，每次 0.25 ~ 0.5g。<br>Oral medication: Three times a day of 0.25g to 0.5g. |
| 剂型、规格<br>Preparations | 胶囊：0.25g；0.5g。<br>Capsules: 0.25 g;0.5 g. |

## 14. 主要作用于泌尿系统的药物 Drugs mainly acting on urinary system

### 14.1 利尿药 Diuretics

| 药品名称 Drug Names | 呋塞米 Furosemide |
|---|---|
| 适应证<br>Indications | （1）水肿性疾病：包括心脏性水肿、肾性水肿（肾炎、肾病及各种原因所致的急、慢性肾衰竭）、肝硬化腹水、功能障碍或血管障碍所引起的周围性水肿，尤其是应用其他利尿药效果不佳时，应用本品仍可能有效。静脉给药或与其他药物合用，可治疗急性肺水肿和急性脑水肿等。<br>（2）高血压：不作为原发性高血压的首选药，但当噻嗪类药物疗效不佳，尤其当伴有肾功能不全或出现高血压危象时，尤为适用。<br>（3）预防急性肾衰竭：用于各种原因导致的肾脏血流灌注不足，例如失水、休克、中毒、麻醉意外及循环功能不全等，及时应用可减少急性肾小管坏死的机会。<br>（4）高钾血症及高钙血症。<br>（5）抗利尿激素分泌过多症（SIADH）。<br>（6）稀释性低钠血症，尤其时当血钠浓度低于 120mmol/L 时。<br>（7）急性药物中毒：用本品可加速毒物排泄。<br><br>(1) Edema diseases include cardiac edema, renal edema (nephritis, kidney disease and acute and chronic renal failure caused by all kinds of reasons), liver cirrhosis with ascites, dysfunction or peripheral edema caused by vascular impairment, especially other diuretics with poor treatment, maybe it is still valid. Intravenous administration or in combination with other drugs can treat acute pulmonary edema and acute cerebral edema etc.<br>(2) hypertension: it is not the first choice for essential hypertension. But it applies to concomitant renal insufficiency or hypertensive crisis, especially when drugs of thiazine is not effective .<br>(3) prevention of acute renal failure: for all causes of renal blood flow hypoperfusion, such as dehydration, shock, poisoning, anesthesia accidents and circulatory insufficiency, timely application can reduce the chance of acute tubular necrosis.<br>(4) hyperkalemia and hypercalcemia.<br>(5) Syndrome of Inappropriate Antidiuretic Hormone (SIADH).<br>(6) dilutional hyponatremia, especially when serum sodium concentration is less than 120mmol / L.<br>(7) acute drug poisoning: it can accelerate excretion of toxins. |
| 用法、用量<br>Dosage | 成人：水肿<br>（1）口服，开始每日 20 ~ 40mg，一日 1 ~ 2 次，必要时 6 ~ 8 小时后追加 20 ~ 40mg，直至出现满意的利尿效果。最大剂量虽可达一日 600mg，但一般应控制在 100mg 以下，分 2 ~ 3 次服用。以防过度利尿和发生不良反应。部分患者剂量可减至 20 ~ 40mg，隔日 1 次，或 1 周中连续服药 2 ~ 4 日，一日 20 ~ 40mg。<br>（2）肌内注射或静脉注射，一次 20 ~ 40mg，隔日一次，根据需要亦可一日 1 ~ 2 次，必要时可每 2 小时追加剂量。一日量视需要可增至 120mg。静脉注射宜用氯化钠注射液稀释后缓慢注射，不宜与其他药物混合。 |

续　表

| | Adults edema:<br><br>(1) take orally, once or twice a day of 20mg to 40mg in the beginning, if necessary, add the same dose after 6 to 8 hours to reach a satisfactory diuretic effect. Although the maximum dose is up to 600mg a day, it should be controlled less than 100mg and be taken 2 to 3 times a day to prevent adverse reactions and excessive urination. The dose of some patients may be reduced to 20 to 40mg, every other day, or continuous medication of 2 to 4 days of 20 to 40mg.<br><br>(2) intramuscular injection or intravenous injection, once every other day of 20 to 40mg. Once or twice a day is feasible on the basis of patients' condition. If necessary, doses can be added every two hours. Daily dose can be increased as needed to 120mg.After diluted with sodium chloride injection, intravenous injection had better be slow and not be mixed with other drugs. |
|---|---|
| 剂型、规格<br>Preparations | 片剂：每片 20mg。注射液：每支 20mg（2ml）。<br>Tablets: 20mg per tablet. Injection: 20mg (2ml) per vial. |
| **药品名称 Drug Names** | **布美他尼 Bumetanide** |
| 适应证<br>Indications | （1）水肿性疾病：包括心脏性水肿、肾性水肿（肾炎、肾病及各种原因所致的急、慢性肾衰竭）、肝硬化腹水、功能障碍或血管障碍所引起的周围性水肿，尤其是应用其他利尿药效果不佳时，应用本品仍可能有效。静脉给药或与其他药物合用，可治疗急性肺水肿和急性脑水肿等。<br><br>（2）高血压：不作为原发性高血压的首选药，但当噻嗪类药物疗效不佳，尤其当伴有肾功能不全或出现高血压危象时，尤为适用。<br><br>（3）预防急性肾衰竭：用于各种原因导致的肾脏血流灌注不足，例如失水、休克、中毒、麻醉意外以及循环功能不全等，及时应用可减少急性肾小管坏死的机会。<br><br>（4）高钾血症及高钙血症。<br><br>（5）抗利尿激素分泌过多症（SIADH）。<br><br>（6）稀释性低钠血症，尤其时当血钠浓度低于 120mmol/L 时。<br><br>（7）急性药物中毒：用本品可加速毒物排泄。<br><br>(1) Edema diseases include cardiac edema, renal edema (nephritis, kidney disease and acute and chronic renal failure caused by all kinds of reasons), liver cirrhosis with ascites, dysfunction or peripheral edema caused by vascular impairment, especially other diuretics with poor treatment, maybe it is still valid. Intravenous administration or in combination with other drugs can treat acute pulmonary edema and acute cerebral edema etc.<br><br>(2) hypertension: it is not the first choice for essential hypertension. But it applies to concomitant renal insufficiency or hypertensive crisis, especially when drugs of thiazine is not effective .<br><br>(3) prevention of acute renal failure: for all causes of renal blood flow hypoperfusion, such as dehydration, shock, poisoning, anesthesia accidents and circulatory insufficiency, timely application can reduce the chance of acute tubular necrosis.<br><br>(4) hyperkalemia and hypercalcemia.<br><br>(5) Syndrome of Inappropriate Antidiuretic Hormone (SIADH).<br><br>(6) dilutional hyponatremia, especially when serum sodium concentration is less than 120mmol / L.<br><br>(7) acute drug poisoning: it can accelerate excretion of toxins. |
| 用法、用量<br>Dosage | （1）成人：①水肿：口服，一次 0.5 ~ 2mg，一日 1 次，必要时可一日 2 ~ 3 次，总量有时可高达一日 10mg；肌内注射或静脉注射，起始 0.5 ~ 1mg，必要时每隔 2 ~ 3 小时重复，最大剂量为一日 10mg。②急性肺水肿及左心衰竭：将本品 2 ~ 5mg 加入 500ml 氯化钠注射液中静脉滴注，30 ~ 60 分钟滴完。也可肌内注射或静脉注射，一次 1 ~ 2mg，必要时间隔 20 分钟再给药 1 次。<br><br>（2）儿童：口服，一次 0.01 ~ 0.02mg/kg，必要时 4 ~ 6 小时 1 次；肌内或静脉注射：剂量同口服。<br><br>(1) Adults: ① edema: take orally, once a time of 0.5mg to 2 mg if necessary, 2 or 3 times a day.Total dose is up to 10 mg a day. Intramuscular or intravenous injection starts from 0.5 to 1 mg, repeating every 2 or 3 hours when necessary. The maximum dose is 10 mg a day. ② acute pulmonary edema and left heart failure: add 2mg to 5 mg into 500 ml of sodium chloride injection and take intravenous drip, dripping off during 30 to 60 minutes. It can also be intramuscular or intravenous injection, 1 to 2 mg once giving another after 20 minutes when necessary.<br><br>(2) Children: take orally, 0.01 to 0.02mg/kg once once every 4 to 6 hours when necessary; the dose of intramuscular or intravenous injection is the same as taking orally. |

| 剂型、规格<br>Preparations | 片剂：每片 1mg。<br>注射液：每支 0.5mg（2ml）。<br>Tablets: 1 mg per tablet.<br>Injection: 0.5 mg (2 ml) per vial. |
|---|---|
| 药品名称 Drug Names | 托拉塞米 Torasemide |
| 适应证<br>Indications | ①各种原因所致水肿：如，由于原发或继发性肾脏疾病及何种原因所致急、慢性肾衰竭、充血性心力衰竭，以及肝硬化等所致的水肿；与其他药合用治疗急性脑水肿等。②急、慢性心力衰竭。③原发或继发性高血压。④急、慢性肾衰竭，本品可增加尿量，促进尿钠排出。⑤肝硬化腹水。⑥急性毒物或药物中毒。本品通过强效、迅速的利尿作用，配合充分的液体补充，不仅可以加速毒性物质和药物的排泄，而且由于其肾脏保护作用，还可减轻有毒物质对近曲小管上皮细胞的损害。<br><br>① edema caused by various reasons, such as acute and chronic renal failure and congestive heart failure caused by primary or secondary kidney disease and any other reason, and edema caused by cirrhosis of the liver, acute cerebral edema treated with other drugs etc. ② acute and chronic heart failure. ③ primary or secondary hypertension. ④ acute and chronic renal failure. It can increase urine and accelerate excretion of urine sodium . ⑤ cirrhosis ascites. ⑥ acute poison or drug poisoning. it can accelerate the excretion of toxic substances and drugs, and reduce damage of proximal convoluted tubule epithelial cell from toxic substances with the help of effective and quick diuresis and enough liquid supplyment. |
| 用法、用量<br>Dosage | （1）心力衰竭：口服或静脉注射（用 5% 葡萄糖注射液或氯化钠注射液稀释），初始剂量一般为一次 5 ～ 10mg，一日 1 次，递增至一次 10 ～ 20mg，一日 1 次。<br>（2）急性或慢性肾衰竭：口服，开始 5mg，可增加至 20mg，均为一日 1 次。需要时可静脉注射，一次 10 ～ 20mg，一日 1 次。必要时可由初始剂量逐渐增加为每日 100 ～ 200mg。<br>（3）肝硬化腹水：口服，开始 5 ～ 10mg，一日 1 次；以后可增加至一次 20mg，一日 1 次，但最多不超过 40mg。静脉注射同口服，一日剂量不超过 40mg。<br>（4）高血压：口服，开始每日 2.5mg 或 5mg，需要时可增至每日 10mg，单用或与其他降压药合用。<br><br>(1) heart failure:take orally or intravenous injection (dilute with 5% glucose injection or sodium chloride injection), the initial dose is usually once a day of 5 ～ 10 mg, increasing to once a day of 10 to 20 mg.<br>(2) acute or chronic renal failure: take orally, begins from 5 mg, and increases to 20 mg once a day. As needed, intravenous injection of 10 to 20 mg once a day. The initial dose is gradually increased to 100 ～ 200 mg a day when necessary .<br>(3) liver cirrhosis ascites: take orally, once a day of 5 ～ 10 mg at first, It can be increased to 20 mg, once a day, but not more than 40 mg. Intravenous injection is the same as taking orally.Daily dose is not more than 40 mg.<br>(4) Hypertension: take orally, 2.5 mg or 5 mg a day at first, when necessary, increased to 10 mg daily. It can be used alone or in combination with other antihypertensive agents. |
| 剂型、规格<br>Preparations | 片剂：每片 2.5mg；5mg；10mg；20mg。<br>注射液：每支 10mg（1ml）；20mg（2ml）。<br>Tablets: 2.5mg; 5 mg; 10 mg; 20 mg per tablet.<br>Injection: 10mg(1ml); 20mg(2ml); per vial. |
| 药品名称 Drug Names | 氢氯噻嗪 Hydrochlorothiazide |
| 适应证<br>Indications | （1）各种水肿性疾病：排泄体内过多的钠和水，减少细胞外液容量，消除水肿。常见的适应证包括充血性心力衰竭、肝硬化腹水、肾病综合征、急慢性肾炎水肿、慢性肾衰竭早期、肾上腺皮质激素和雌激素治疗所致的钠、水潴留。<br>（2）高血压：可单独或与其他降压药联合应用，主要用于治疗原发性高血压。<br>（3）肾性尿崩症、中枢性尿崩症：单独用于肾性尿崩症，与其他抗利尿剂联合亦可用于中枢性尿崩症。<br>（4）肾结石：主要用于预防含钙成分形成的结石。 |

**续　表**

| | |
|---|---|
| | (1) all kinds of edema diseases: discharge excessive sodium and water of your body, reduce the volume of extracellular fluid and eliminate edema. Common indications include congestive heart failure, liver cirrhosis ascites, nephrotic syndrome, acute or chronic nephritis edema, inchoate chronic renal failure, sodium and water retention caused by adrenal cortical hormone and estrogen.<br>(2) Hypertension: can be used alone or with other antihypertensive agents, mainly used in the treatment of essential hypertension.<br>(3) nephrogenic diabetes insipidus(NDI) and central diabetes insipidus: used alone in nephrogenic diabetes insipidus and associated with other diuretics can also be used in central diabetes insipidus.<br>(4) kidney stones: mainly used for the prevention of stone with calcium. |
| 用法、用量<br>Dosage | 成人口服：<br>（1）治疗水肿性疾病：一次 25～50mg，一日 1～2 次，或隔日治疗，或每周连服 3～5 日。为预防电解质紊乱及血容量骤降，宜从小剂量（12.5～25mg/d）用起，以后根据利尿情况逐渐加重。<br>（2）心源性水肿：开始用小剂量，一日 12.5～25mg，以免因盐及水分排泄过快而引起循环障碍或其他症状；同时注意调整洋地黄用量，以免由于钾的丢失而导致洋地黄中毒。<br>（3）肝性腹水：最好与螺内酯合用，以防血钾过低诱发肝性脑病。<br>（4）高血压：常与其他药合用，可减少后者剂量，减少不良反应。开始一日 50～100mg，分 1～2 次服用，并按降压效果调整剂量，1 周后为每日 25～50mg 的维持量。<br>（5）尿崩症：成人口服：一次 25mg，一日 3 次；或一次 50mg，一日 2 次。儿童口服：一日按体重 1～2mg/kg，或按体表面积 30～60mg/m²，分 1～2 次服用，并按疗效调整剂量。小于 6 个月的婴儿，剂量可达一日 3mg/kg。<br><br>Adults take orally:<br>(1) in treatment of edema diseases: once or twice a day of 25mg to50mg, or every other day therapy, or take 3 to 5 days a week. It is proper to begin from small dose (12.5~25mg/d) to prevent electrolyte disorders and plunging blood pressure. And it can be added gradually according to diuretic situation.<br>(2) cardiac edema: start with a small dose of 12.5 to 25 mg a day in order to avoid circulatory disturbance or other symptoms caused by excessive excretion of salt and water. At the same time, pay attention to adjust the dose of digitalis in order to avoid digitalis poisoning caused by loss of potassium.<br>(3) hepatic ascites: best used with spironolactone, in case of hepatic encephalopathy caused by hypokalemia.<br>(4) Hypertension: often used with other drugs, and it can reduce the latter dose and adverse reactions. 50 to 100 mg a day at first, and divide into1～2 times, and adjust the dose according to antihypertensive effect, keep 25 to 50 mg per day after a week.<br>(5) insipidus: adults po take orally: three times a day of 25mg or twice a day of 50mg. Children, take orally: according to the weight of 1～2 mg/kg, or according to the surface area of 30～60 mg/m², divide into 1 to 2 times, and adjust dosage according to curative effect. Infants less than 6 months take 3 mg/kg a day. |
| 剂型、规格<br>Preparations | 片剂：每片 10mg；25mg；50mg。<br>Tablets: 10 mg; 25 mg; 50 mg per tablet. |
| 药品名称 Drug Names | 吲达帕胺 Indapamide |
| 适应证<br>Indications | 作用与氢氯噻嗪相似，其利尿作用强 10 倍。可用于慢性肾衰竭。<br>Have the same effect as hydrochlorothiazide, its diuretic effect is 10 times more than hydrochlorothiazide. It can be used in the treatment of CRF(chronic renal failure) |
| 用法、用量<br>Dosage | 水肿，口服，一次 2.5mg，必要时 5mg，一日 1 次；降压，一次 2.5mg，一日 1 次，维持量可每 2 日 2.5～5mg。<br>Edema, take orally, once a day of 2.5mg, and of 5mg when necessary. Hypertension: once a day of 2.5mg, and, every two days of 2.5mg to 5mg as maintenance dose. |
| 剂型、规格<br>Preparations | 片剂：2.5mg。<br>Tablets: 2.5 mg |

**续 表**

| 药品名称 Drug Names | 螺内酯 Spironolactone |
|---|---|
| 适应证<br>Indications | ①治疗与醛固酮升高有关的顽固性水肿，故对肝硬化和肾病综合征的患者较有效，而对充血性心力衰竭效果较差（除因缺钠而引起的继发性醛固酮增多者外）。也可用于特发性水肿的治疗。单用本品时利尿效果往往较差，故常与噻嗪类、髓袢利尿药合用，既能增强利尿效果，又可防止低血钾。②治疗高血压，可作为原发性或继发性高血压的辅助用药，尤其是应用于有排钾离子作用的利尿药时。③原发性醛固酮增多症的诊断与治疗。④低钾血症的预防，与噻嗪类利尿药合用，增强利尿效果并预防低钾血症。<br><br>① It is used in the treatment of intractable edema associated with elevated aldosterone. Therefore, it is more effective for patients with cirrhosis of the liver and kidney disease syndrome, and less effective on congestive heart failure (except secondary aldosteronism-caused by lack of sodium).It can also be used in the treatment of idiopathic edema. Diuretic effect is not good when used alone, so it is often used with thiazide and loop diuretic. It can not only enhance diuretic effect, but also can prevent hypokalemia. ② treatment of hypertension: It can be used as the auxiliary medication of primary or secondary hypertension, especially applied to diuretic with the effect of excreting potassium . ③ diagnosis and treatment of primary aldosteronism.  ④ prevention of hypokalemia:It can be used with thiazide diuretic to enhance diuretic effect and to prevent hypokalemia. |
| 用法、用量<br>Dosage | （1）成人口服：①治疗水肿：一次 20 ～ 40mg，一日 3 次。用药 5 日后，如疗效满意，继续用原量。②治疗高血压：开始每日 40 ～ 80mg，分 2 ～ 4 次服用，至少 2 周，以后酌情调整剂量。本品不宜与血管紧张素转化酶抑制剂合用，以免增加发生高钾血症的机会。③治疗原发性醛固酮增多症：手术前患者一日用量 100 ～ 400mg，分 2 ～ 4 次服用。不宜手术的患者，则选用较小剂量维持。④诊断原发性醛固酮增多症：长期试验，一日 400mg，分 2 ～ 4 次服用，连续 3 ～ 4 周。短期试验，一日 400mg，分 2 ～ 4 次服用，连续 4 日。老年人对本药较敏感，开始用量宜偏小。<br><br>（2）儿童口服，治疗水肿性疾病，开始一日按体重 1 ～ 3mg/kg 或按体表面积 30 ～ 90mg/m²，单次或分 2 ～ 4 次服用，连用 5 日后酌情调整剂量。最大剂量一日 3 ～ 9mg/kg 或 90 ～ 270mg/m²。<br><br>(1)Adults take orally: ① in the treatment of edema: three times a day of 20mg to 40mg. After 5 days, keep the same dosage if curative effect is expected.  ② Treatment of hypertension: begins with 40 to 80 mg per day at first, divided into 2 to 4 times and take at least 2 weeks. Adjust the dosage on the basis of future situation. This product should not be used with angiotensin converting enzyme inhibitor, lest increase chance of hyperkalemia.  ③ treatment of primary aldosteronism: 100 to 400 mg a day before surgery, divided into 2 to 4 times. Patients who are not suitable to operation should choose a smaller dose.  ④ diagnosis of primary aldosteronism: long-term test, 400 mg a day, 2 to 4 times, 3 to 4 weeks. Short-term test, 400 mg a day, 2 to 4 times, 4 days in a row. The elderly is sensitive to it and should begin with a small dosage .<br><br>(2)Children take orally, treatment of edema diseases, begin with by the weight of 1 ～ 3 mg/kg or by the surface area of 30 ～ 90 mg/m², take once or 2 to 4 times, adjust the dosage after 5days. Maximal doses is 3 ～ 9 mg/kg or 90 ～ 270 mg/m² |
| 剂型、规格<br>Preparations | 片剂：每片20mg。胶囊剂：每粒20mg（微粒制剂20mg与普通制剂100mg的疗效相仿）。<br>Tablets: 20 mg per tablet.Capsules: 20 mg per capsule (20 mg of microcapsules has the same effect as 100mg of ordinary particles) |
| 药品名称 Drug Names | 氨苯蝶啶 Triamterene |
| 适应证<br>Indications | 用于治疗各类水肿，如心力衰竭、肝硬化及慢性肾炎引起的水肿或腹水，以及糖皮质激素治疗过程中发生的水钠潴留。常与排钾利尿药合用。亦用于对氢氯噻嗪或螺内酯无效的病例。<br><br>It is used to treat various types of edema, such as heart failure, cirrhosis of the liver and edema or ascites caused by chronic nephritis, and water- sodium retention by glucocorticoid treatment. It is often used with diuretic-which has the effect of excreting potassium. And it is also used to treat cases which are invalid to hydrochlorothiazide or spironolactone. |
| 用法、用量<br>Dosage | 口服，成人，开始一次 25 ～ 50mg，一日 2 次，餐后服，最大剂量每日不宜超过 300mg。维持阶段可改为隔日疗法。与其他利尿剂合用时，两者均应减量。儿童，开始一日按体重 2 ～ 4mg/kg 或按体表面积 120mg/m²，分 2 次服，每日或隔日疗法。以后酌情调整剂量。最大剂量不超过每日 6mg/kg 或 300mg/m²。 |

**续　表**

<table>
<tr><td></td><td>Adults take orally, twice a day of 25mg to50mg at first, take it after meals, and maximum dose should not be no more than 300 a day. Maintenance stage can be changed to alternate-day therapy. With other diuretics, both should be reduced. Children, start by the weight of 2 to 4mg/kg or by the surface area of $120mg/m^2$ and take it twice a day or twice every other day. Adjust it on the basis of future condition. Maximum daily dose is less than 6 mg/kg or $300 mg/m^2$ .</td></tr>
<tr><td>剂型、规格<br>Preparations</td><td>片剂：每片 50mg。<br>Tablets: 50 mg per tablet.</td></tr>
<tr><td>药品名称 Drug Names</td><td>阿米洛利 Amiloride</td></tr>
<tr><td>适应证<br>Indications</td><td>本品同氨苯蝶啶，主要用于治疗水肿性疾病，亦可用于难治性低钾血症的辅助治疗。氨苯蝶啶和螺内酯均大部分经肝脏代谢，当肝功能严重损害时，剂量不易控制，此时则可应用不经肝脏代谢的本品。另外，本品可增加氢氯噻嗪和利尿酸等利尿药的作用，并减少钾的丢失，故一般不单独应用。<br><br>It has the same effect as Triamterene and is mainly used to treat edema diseases . It can also be used as a supplement in the treatment of refractory hypokalemia. Much Ammonia benzene pteridine and spirono-lactone metabolize through liver, but when liver function is severely damaged, the dose is hard to control, so we can use it as a substitute. In addition, this product can increase the effect of the hydrochlorothiazide and uric acid diuretic, and reduce the loss of potassium, it is generally not used alone.</td></tr>
<tr><td>用法、用量<br>Dosage</td><td>口服：开始一次 2.5 ~ 5mg，一日 1 次；必要时可增加剂量，但每日不宜超过 20mg。<br>Oral medication: take 2.5 ~ 5 mg singly at the beginning, once a day. The dose could be increased when necessary, but it should not be more than 20 mg daily.</td></tr>
<tr><td>剂型、规格<br>Preparations</td><td>片剂：每片含 2.5mg；5mg。<br>Tablets: 2.5 mg ;5mg per tablet.</td></tr>
<tr><td>药品名称 Drug Names</td><td>乙酰唑胺 Acetazolamide</td></tr>
<tr><td>适应证<br>Indications</td><td>用于治疗青光眼、心脏性水肿、脑水肿，亦用于癫痫小发作。<br>It is used to treat glaucoma, cardiac edema, cerebral edema as well as petit mal epilepsy.</td></tr>
<tr><td>用法、用量<br>Dosage</td><td>（1）青光眼：一般口服给药，①开角型青光眼，首量 0.25g，一日 1 ~ 3 次。维持剂量根据患者对药物的反应而定，尽量适用较小剂量使眼压得到控制，一般 1 次 0.25g，一日 2 次就可使眼压控制在正常范围。②继发性青光眼和手术前降眼压，一次 0.25g，一般一日 2 ~ 3 次。③闭角型青光眼急性发作，首次 0.5g，以后一次 0.125 ~ 0.25g，一日 2 ~ 3 次维持。④青光眼急性发作时的抢救或某些恶心、呕吐不能口服的患者，可静脉或肌内注射本品。将本品 0.5g 溶于 5 ~ 10ml 灭菌注射用水静脉注射，或溶于 2.5ml 灭菌注射用水肌内注射；也可静脉注射 0.25g 或肌内注射 0.25g 交替使用。对于一些急性发作的青光眼患者，可在 2 ~ 4 小时重复上述剂量，但继续治疗应根据患者情况改为口服给药。<br>（2）脑水肿：口服，一次 0.25g，一日 2 ~ 3 次。<br>（3）心源性水肿：口服，一次 0.25 ~ 0.5g，一日 1 次，早餐后服用药效最佳。<br>（4）癫痫小发作：其作用可能与抑制脑组织中的碳酸酐酶有关。口服，一次 0.5 ~ 1g，一日 1 次。与其他药物合用时则不超过 0.25g。儿童：①青光眼：口服，一日 5 ~ 10mg/kg，分 2 ~ 3 次服用；②青光眼急性发作：静脉注射或肌内注射，一次 5 ~ 10mg/kg，每 6 小时 1 次。<br><br>(1) glaucoma: general oral medicine, ① primary open-angle glaucoma, give first dose of 0.25 g, 1 to 3 times a day. Maintenance dose should be determined according to the patients' response to drugs. Try to use smaller doses to get intraocular pressure under control, generally 0.25 g singly, use it twice a day could make a intraocular pressure in the normal range. ② secondary glaucoma and preoperative iop reduction, 0.25 g singly, generally 2 to 3 times a day. ③ acute angle-closure glaucoma, 0.5 g for the first time, after a 0.125 to 0.25 g singly, 2 to 3 times a day. ④ for the rescue of acute onset glauco-ma or certain patients who can not orally take the medicine because of nausea, vomiting, intravenous or intramuscular injection could be used . If adopt intravenous injection, make 0.5 g of this product soluble in 5 to10 ml sterilization injection water, If adopt intramuscular injection, make it soluble in 2.5 ml sterilizing water. Intravenous and intramuscular injection of 0.25 g could also be used interchange-ably. For some acute glaucoma patients, the above method can be used in 2 to 4 hours, but continuous treatment should be changed to oral medicine according to patients condition .<br>(2)cerebral edema: oral medication, 0.25 g singly, 2 to 3 times a day.</td></tr>
</table>

**续 表**

(3) cardiac edema: oral medication, 0.25 ~ 0.5 g singly, once a day, more effective if taken after breakfast.

(4) petit mal epilepsy: its role may be associated with inhibition of carbonic anhydrase in the brain tissue.Oral medication, 0.5g to 1g singly, once a day. When used in combination with other medicines, the dose should be no more than 0.25 g. Children: ① glaucoma: oral medication, 5 to 10 mg/kg a day, in 2 to 3 divided times; ② acute glaucoma: intravenous or intramuscular injection, 5 ~ 10 mg/kg singly, once every six hours .

| 剂型、规格<br>Preparations | 片剂：每片 0.25g。注射用乙酰唑胺：每支 500mg。<br>Tablets: 0.25 g per tablet. Acetazolamide for injection : 500 mg per vial. |
| --- | --- |

## 14.2 脱水药 Dehydrants

| 药品名称 Drug Names | 甘露醇 Mannitol |
| --- | --- |
| 适应证<br>Indications | ①治疗各种原因引起的脑水肿，降低颅内压，防止脑疝；②降低眼压：当在应用其他降眼压药无效或青光眼的术前准备时应用；③预防急性肾小管坏死：在大面积烧伤、严重创伤、广泛外科手术时，常因肾小球滤过率降低及血容量减少而出现少尿、无尿，极易发生肾衰竭，应及时用本品预防；④作为其他利尿药的辅助药，治疗某些伴有低钠血症的顽固性水肿（因本品排水多于排钠，故不适用于全身性水肿的治疗）；⑤鉴别肾前性因素或急性肾衰竭引起的少尿；⑥对于某些药物过量或毒物引起的重度，可促进上述物质的排泄，防止肾毒性；⑦术前肠道准备；⑧作清洗剂，应用于经尿道内做前列腺切除术。<br><br>① It is used to treat cerebral edema caused by various reasons, to reduce intracranial pressure, and prevent cerebral hernia; ② reduce intraocular pressure, adopted when the application of other intraocular pressure lowing drugs is invalid or as a preoperative preparation before glaucoma ; ③ it should be used to prevent kidney failure when oliguria, no urination appeared which usually caused by reduced glomerular filtration rate and hypovolemia in the operation of large area burns, severe trauma, surgical ; ④ as supplements of other diuretic drugs, it is used to treat some intractable edema accompanied by hyponatremia (because this product draine more water than sodium, it is not used in the treatment of systemic edema). ⑤ It is used to identify prerenal factors or less urination caused by acute renal failure ; ⑥ for poisoning caused by certain drugs overdose or poisons, the aforementioned product can be used to drain poisonous substances to prevent renal toxicity; ⑦ it could be used as an bowel preparation before operations; ⑧ as a cleaner, it is applicated in transurethral resection of the prostate. |
| 用法、用量<br>Dosage | （1）利尿：静脉滴注，按体重 1 ~ 2g/kg，一般为 20% 溶液 250 ~ 500ml，并调整剂量使尿量维持在每小时 30 ~ 50ml。<br><br>（2）脑水肿、颅内高压和青光眼：静脉滴注，按体重 1.5 ~ 2g/kg，配成 15% ~ 20% 浓度于 30 ~ 60 分钟滴完（当患者衰弱时，剂量可减为 0.5g/kg）。<br><br>（3）预防急性肾小管坏死：先给予 12.5 ~ 25g，10 分钟内静脉滴注，若无特殊情况，再给 50g，1 小时内静脉滴注，若尿量能维持在每小时 50ml 以上，则可继续应用 5% 溶液静脉滴注；若无效则立即停药。同时需注意补足血容量。<br><br>（4）鉴别肾前性少尿和肾性少尿：按体重 0.2g/kg，以 20% 浓度于 3 ~ 5 分钟静脉滴注。如用药 2 ~ 3 小时以后尿量仍低于 30 ~ 50ml/h，最多再试用一次，若仍无反应则应停药。心功能减退或心力衰竭者，慎用或不宜使用。<br><br>（5）药物或毒物中毒：50g 以 20% 溶液静脉滴注，调整剂量使尿量维持在每小时 100 ~ 500ml。<br><br>（6）术前肠道准备：口服，于术前 4 ~ 8 小时以 10% 溶液 1000ml 于 30 分钟内口服完毕。<br><br>(1) Diuretic: give intravenous injection according to the weight of 1 to 2 g/kg, generally use 250 ~ 500 ml 20% solution, and the doses should be adjusted to keep urine output at 30 to50 ml an hour.<br><br>(2)cerebral edema and intracranial pressure and glaucoma: give intravenous drip, according to the weight of 1.5 to 2 g/kg. Drip with a 15% ~ 20% dense in 30 to 60 minutes (when a patient is weak, the dose can be reduced to 0.5 g/kg).<br><br>(3) to prevent acute tubular necrosis: first give 12.5 to 25 g, intravenous drip in 10 minutes. If nothing special happens, give50 g, intravenous drip in 1 hour. If the amount of urination can remain above 50 ml per hour, 5% solution could be dripped continuously; If invalid, stopped the administration immediately. At the same time, pay attention to make up blood pressure. |

续　表

<table>
<tr><td></td><td>(4) Identification prerenal oliguria and renal oliguria: drip, with a 20% dense in 3 to 5 minutes according to the weight of 0.2 g/kg. If urineation output is still less than 30 to 50 ml/h after 2 to 3 hours of administration, the drug should be used up to once try again, .If still no response, the administration should be stopped. Those who have The reduced heart functions or heart failure, should use it careful or unfavorable use.<br><br>(5) drugs or toxic poisoning: 50 g intravenous drip with 20% solution, adjust the dose to keep of keeping urine output in 100 to 500 ml per hour.<br><br>(6) preoperative bowel preparation: oral, 4 to 8 hours before operation to 1000 ml of 10% solution in oral within 30 minutes to complete.</td></tr>
<tr><td>剂型、规格<br>Preparations</td><td>注射液：每瓶 10g（50ml）；20g（100ml）；50g（250ml）；100g（500ml）；150g（3000ml）。<br>Injection: 10g (50ml); 20g (100ml); 50g (250ml); 100g (500ml); 150g (3000ml) per bottle.</td></tr>
<tr><td>药品名称 Drug Names</td><td>甘油果糖氯化钠 Glycerin Fructose and Sodium Cloride</td></tr>
<tr><td>适应证<br>Indications</td><td>①由脑血管疾病、脑外伤、脑肿瘤、颅内炎症及其他原因引起的急、慢性颅内压增高，脑水肿症；②改善下列疾病的意识障碍、神经障碍和自觉症状，如脑梗死（脑栓死、脑血栓）、脑内出血、蛛网膜下腔出血、头部外伤、脑脊髓膜炎等；③脑外科手术术前缩小脑容积；④脑外科手术后降颅内压；⑤青光眼患者降低眼压或眼科手术缩小眼容积。<br><br>① It is used to treat acute and chronic increased intracranial pressure, cerebral edema disease caused by cerebrovascular disease, brain trauma, brain tumor, intracranial inflammation and other causes；② to improve the consciousness and neurological disorders, and self-conscious symptom of the following diseases, such as cerebral infarction (brain death, cerebral thrombosis), cerebral hemorrhage, subarachnoid hemorrhage, head trauma, cerebrospinal meningitis, etc；③ to narrow brain volume before cerebral surgery；④ to lower intracranial pressure after brain surgery；⑤ it will help glaucoma patients reduce intraocular pressure or eye eye surgery to reduce the volume.</td></tr>
<tr><td>用法、用量<br>Dosage</td><td>静脉滴注：<br>（1）治疗颅内压增高、脑水肿：成人一次 250～500ml，一日 1～2 次；儿童用量为 5～10ml/kg。每 500ml 需滴注 2～3 小时，连续给药 1～2 周。<br>（2）脑外科手术时缩小脑容积：每次 500ml，静脉滴注时间为 30 分钟。<br>（3）降低眼压或眼科手术时缩小眼容积：每次 250～500ml，静脉滴注时间为 45～90 分钟。<br><br>Intravenous drip:<br>(1) treatment of increased intracranial pressure, cerebral edema: for adult, give 250 to 500ml singly, once or twice a day; for children, give a dosage of 5 to 10 ml/kg. Every 500ml should be dripped in 2 to 3 hours, the administration should be continued for 1 to 2 weeks.<br>(2) to reduce brain volume in the brain surgery: 500 ml per time, intravenous drip for 30 minutes once.<br>(3) to reduce the intraocular pressure or the eye volume in the eye surgery: 250 to 500 ml per time, intravenous drip for 45 to 90 minutes once.</td></tr>
<tr><td>剂型、规格<br>Preparations</td><td>注射液：每瓶 250ml；500ml（每 1ml 中含甘油 100mg、果糖 50mg、氯化钠 9mg）。<br>Injection: 250 ml per bottle;500 ml (per 1 ml contains 100 mg of glycerin, fructose 50 mg, sodium chloride, 9 mg).</td></tr>
</table>

14.3　治疗尿崩症用药 Drugs treating diabetes insipidus

<table>
<tr><td>药品名称 Drug Names</td><td>鞣酸加压素 Vasopressin Tanate</td></tr>
<tr><td>适应证<br>Indications</td><td>①中枢性尿崩症、头部手术或外伤所致的暂时性尿崩症的治疗。②用于中枢性尿崩症、肾性尿崩症的鉴别诊断试验。③食管静脉曲张破裂出血及咯血。<br><br>① it is used to treat central diabetes insipidus, temporary diabetes insipidus caused by head surgery or trauma　② it is used to identify, diagnose and trial central diabetes insipidus, renal diabetes insipidus. ③ it is also used to treat esophageal variceal bleeding and hemoptysis.</td></tr>
<tr><td>用法、用量<br>Dosage</td><td>（1）中枢性尿崩症：①成人，加压素注射液 3mg 皮下注射或肌内注射，一日 2～3 次。②儿童，加压素注射液 1～1.5mg 皮下注射或肌内注射，一日 2～3 次。<br>（2）中枢性尿崩症的诊断：禁水 - 加压素试验时，皮下注射加压素注射液 3mg，继续禁水 2 小时测血和尿渗透压、尿量、尿比重、血压、脉率等。儿童酌情减量。<br>（3）食管静脉曲张破裂出血及咯血：加压素注射液 3mg 稀释后缓慢静脉注射，或 6～12mg 加入 200～500ml 的 5% 葡萄糖注射液中缓慢静脉滴注。</td></tr>
</table>

**续　表**

| | |
|---|---|
| | (1) central diabetes insipidus: ① for adults, give 3 mg vasopressin subcutaneous or intramuscular injection, 2 to 3 times a day. ② for children, give 1 to 1.5 mg vasopressin subcutaneous or intramuscular injection, 2 to 3 times a day.<br><br>(2) the diagnosis of central diabetes insipidus: in the test of water -deprivation vasopressin, give subcutaneous injection of 3 mg vasopressin injection, continue to ban water 2 hours blood and urine osmotic pressure measurement, and urine specific gravity of urine, blood pressure, pulse frequency, etc. For children, the dosage should be reduced proportionally.<br><br>(3) the esophagus varicosity burst hemorrhage and hemoptysis: slow intravenous injection of 3 mg after the vasopressin injection diluted, or put 6 to 12 mg in 200 ~ 500 ml of 5% glucose injection and intravenous drip slowly. |
| 剂型、规格<br>Preparations | 注射液：每支 6mg（1ml）；12mg（1ml）。<br>Injection: 6 mg (1ml) ;12 mg (1 ml) per vial. |
| **药品名称 Drug Names** | **垂体后叶粉 Powdered Posterior Pituitary** |
| 适应证<br>Indications | 治疗尿崩症。<br>It is used to treat diabetes insipidus. |
| 用法、用量<br>Dosage | 用特制小匙（每匙装量为 30 ~ 40mg）取出本品 1 小匙，用小指抹在鼻黏膜上；亦可将取出的粉剂倒在纸上，卷成卷，用左手压住左鼻孔，用右手将纸卷插入右鼻孔内，抬头轻轻将粉刺吸进鼻腔内。一日 3 ~ 4 次。<br><br>Use special spoon (per spoon has a filling quantity of about 30 to 40 mg) to remove 1 small spoon, put them on the nasal mucosa with a little finger wipe; the removed powder could be put on the paper, then roll the paper into a roll of paper. Pin left nostril with left hand, and insert paper roll into the right nostril, looking up and gently sucked the powder into the nasal cavity, 3 to 4 times a day. |
| 剂型、规格<br>Preparations | 鼻吸入粉剂：每瓶 1g（附小匙）。<br>Inhalation powder: 1g per bottle(attached tsp). |
| **药品名称 Drug Names** | **去氨加压素 Desmopressin** |
| 适应证<br>Indications | ①中枢性尿崩症及颅外伤或手术所致的暂时性尿崩症：用后可减少尿排出，增加尿渗透压，减低血浆渗透压，减少尿频和夜尿（一般对肾源性尿崩症无效）。②治疗 5 岁以上患有夜间遗尿症的患者。③肾尿液浓缩功能试验：有助于对肾功能的鉴别，对于诊断不同部位的尿道感染尤其有效。④对于轻度血友病及 I 型血管性血友病患者，在进行小型外科手术时可控制出血或预防出血。⑤因尿毒症、肝硬化以及先天的或用药诱发的血小板功能障碍而引起的出血时间过长和不明原因的出血，用本品可使出血时间缩短或恢复正常。<br><br>① It is used to treat central diabetes insipidus and temporary diabetes insipidus caused by cranial trauma or surgery: reduce the urine after using it, increase urine osmolality, decrease plasma osmolality, and reduce urinary frequency and nocturia (generally invalid to nephrogenic diabetes insipidus disease). ② to treat patients with nocturnal enuresis disease over the age of five. ③ the kidney urine concentration function test: aid in the identification of renal function, especially effective for the diagnosis of urinary tract infections from different parts. ④ for patients of mild hemophilia and type I von willebrand disease, control or prevent hemorrhage or bleeding in the small surgical prophylaxis. ⑤ bleeding time is too long and unexplained bleeding caused by uremia, cirrhosis of the liver and congenital or platelet dysfunction induced by drug, using this product can make the bleeding time shorten or return to normal. |
| 用法、用量<br>Dosage | （1）中枢性尿崩症①鼻腔给药：a. 鼻喷剂：成人开始 10μg，睡前喷鼻，以后根据尿量每晚递增 2.5μg，直至获得良好睡眠。b. 成人开始一次 10μg，逐渐调整到最适剂量，一日 3 ~ 4 次，儿童用量酌减。②口服：因人而异，区分调整。③静脉注射。<br>（2）夜间遗尿症：鼻腔给药或口服。<br>（3）肾尿液浓缩功能试验：鼻腔给药或肌内、皮下注射。<br>（4）治疗性控制出血或手术前预防出血：静脉滴注。 |

续 表

<table>
<tr>
<td colspan="2"></td>
<td>(1) central diabetes insipidus ① intranasal administration: a. nasal spray: for adults give 10μg at first, nasal spray before bedtime, increase 2.5μg every night according to the amount of urine, until get a good night's sleep. b. for adults, give 10μg at first, gradually adjust to the optimal dose, 3 to 4 times a day, reduce the amount for children. ② oral medication: vary and adjust according person ③ intravenous injection.<br>
(2) nocturnal enuresis: nasal or oral administration.<br>
(3) concentrated urine kidney function tests: intranasal administration or intramuscular, subcutaneous injection.<br>
(4) therapeuticly control bleeding or prevent bleeding before surgery: intravenous drip.</td>
</tr>
<tr>
<td colspan="2">剂型、规格<br>Preparations</td>
<td>片剂：每片 100μg；200μg。<br>
鼻喷雾剂：每支 250μg（2.5ml，每喷 0.1ml，含 10μg）。<br>
滴鼻液：每支 250μg（2.5ml）。<br>
注射液：每支 4μg（1ml）。<br><br>
Tablets: 100μg per tablet; 200μg.<br>
Nasal spray: 250μg (2.5 ml, 0.1 ml per spray, containing 10μg) per bottle.<br>
Nasal drops: 250μg(2.5 ml) per bottle.<br>
Injection: 4μg (1 ml) per bottle.</td>
</tr>
<tr>
<td colspan="3">15. 主要作用于生殖系统的药物 Drugs mainly acting on reproductive system</td>
</tr>
<tr>
<td colspan="3">15.1 子宫收缩药及引产药 Drugs that contractions the uterus and that induced labor</td>
</tr>
<tr>
<td colspan="2">药品名称 Drug Names</td>
<td>垂体后叶素 Pituitrin</td>
</tr>
<tr>
<td colspan="2">适应证<br>Indications</td>
<td>产后出血、产后子宫复原不全、促进宫缩引产（由于有升高血压作用，现产科已少用）、肺出血、食管及胃底静脉曲张破裂出血和尿崩症等。<br><br>
It is used to treat postpartum hemorrhage, incomplete postpartum uterus rehabilitation, promote the contractions induced labor (with elevated blood pressure effect, less use in maternity), pulmonary hemorrhage, ruptured esophageal and gastric varices bleeding and diabetes insipidus, etc.</td>
</tr>
<tr>
<td colspan="2">用法、用量<br>Dosage</td>
<td>（1）一般应用：肌内注射，每次 5 ~ 10U。<br>
（2）肺出血：可静脉注射或静脉滴注。<br>
（3）产后出血：必须在胎儿和胎盘均已分娩出之后方可肌内注射 10U，如作预防性应用，可在胎儿前肩娩出后立即静脉注射 10U。<br>
（4）临产阵缩弛缓不正常者（偶亦用于催生，但须谨慎）：将 5 ~ 10U 本品以 5% 葡萄糖注射液 500ml 稀释后缓慢静脉滴注，并严密观察宫缩情况，适时调整滴速。<br>
（5）尿崩症：肌内注射，常用量为每次 5U，一日 2 次。<br>
（6）消化道出血：可用本品静脉滴注，其用量和溶媒同肺出血，每分钟 0.1 ~ 0.5U。<br><br>
(1) general application: intramuscular injection, 5 ~ 10U singly.<br>
(2) pulmonary hemorrhage: intravenous injection or intravenous drip.<br>
(3) the postpartum hemorrhage: intramuscular inject 10U after the delivery of the fetus and placenta, such as preventive application, immediately intravenous inject 10U after the delivery of the front shoulder of the fetus.<br>
(4) abnormal person of labor matrix shrinkage relaxation (also used to produce, but with caution): dilute 5 ~ 10U of this product with 500 ml 5% glucose injection, then slowly intravenous drip, and closely observe the contractions, timely adjust dripping speed.<br>
(5) diabetes insipidus: intramuscular injection, often give 5u singly, twice a day.<br>
(6) Gastrointestinal bleeding: intravenous drip, the dosage and solvent with pulmonary hemorrhage, 0.1 ~ 0.5U per minute.</td>
</tr>
<tr>
<td colspan="2">剂型、规格<br>Preparations</td>
<td>注射液：每支 5U（1ml）；10U（1ml）。<br>
Injection:5U (1ml) ; 10U(1ml) per vial.</td>
</tr>
<tr>
<td colspan="2">药品名称 Drug Names</td>
<td>缩宫素 Oxytocin</td>
</tr>
<tr>
<td colspan="2">适应证<br>Indications</td>
<td>用于引产、催产、产后出血和子宫复原不全；滴鼻用于促排乳；催产素激惹试验。<br><br>
It is used for induced labor, oxytocin, postpartum hemorrhage and incomplete uterine recovery; Intranasal row is used to promote breast; Oxytocin irritability test.</td>
</tr>
</table>

**续 表**

| | |
|---|---|
| 用法、用量<br>Dosage | （1）引产或催产：静脉滴注。<br>（2）防治产后出血或促进子宫复原：将本品 5 ~ 10U 加于 5% 葡萄糖注射液中静脉滴注，每分钟滴注 0.02 ~ 0.04U，胎盘排出后可肌内注射 5 ~ 10U。<br>（3）子宫出血：肌内注射，1 次 5 ~ 10U。肌内注射极量，1 次 20U。<br>（4）催乳：在哺乳前 2 ~ 3 分钟，用滴鼻液，每次 3 滴或少量喷于一侧或双侧鼻孔内。<br>（5）催产素激惹试验：试验剂量同引产，用稀释后的缩宫素做静脉滴注，直到 10 分钟出现 3 次有效宫缩。<br>（1) induced labor or oxytocin.<br>（2) prevent and treat postpartum hemorrhage or promote uterine recovery: add 5 ~ 10U in 5% glucose injection intravenous drip, drip 0.02 ~ 0.04U per minute, intramuscular injection of 5 ~ 10U after the discharge of placenta.<br>（3)uterine bleeding: intramuscular injection, 5 ~ 10U singly.The intramuscular injection of Polaris, 20U singly.<br>（4)Lactation: 2 to 3 minutes before breastfeeding, using nasal drops, 3 drops singly or a small amount of spray on one side or double side nostrils.<br>（5)oxytocin irritability test: test dose with induced labor, using diluted oxytocin as intravenous drip, until3 times effective contractions occur after 10 minutes. |
| 剂型、规格<br>Preparations | 注射液：每支 2.5U（0.5ml）；5U（1ml）；10U（1ml）。滴鼻液：每支 40U（1ml）。鼻喷雾剂：每瓶 200U（5ml）（每喷 0.1ml，相当于 4U）。<br>Injection: 2.5U(0.5 ml)；5U (1ml);10U (1ml) per vial. Nasal drops: 40U (1ml) per bottle. Nasal spray: 200U(5ml) per bottle (0.1ml per spray, equivalent to 4U). |
| 药品名称 Drug Names | 米非司酮 Mifepristone |
| 适应证<br>Indications | 本品除用于抗早孕、催经止孕外，尚可用于中期妊娠引产（与前列腺素合用）、死胎引产、扩宫颈。<br>It is used to against early pregnant, push the stop pregnancy, as well as in mid pregnancy induced labor (share) and prostaglandin, stillbirth induced labor, and expanding cervix. |
| 用法、用量<br>Dosage | （1）中期妊娠引产（在妊娠 13 ~ 24 周用人工方法终止妊娠）：①与米索前列醇配伍；②与卡前列甲酯配伍。<br>（2）宫内死胎引产：口服，一次 200mg，一日 2 次或每日 1 次 400 ~ 600mg，连服 2 日，一般在 72 小时后排出死胎。<br>（3）扩宫颈：口服，1 次 100 ~ 200mg。宫内手术前软化和扩张宫颈：于术前 48 小时口服 600mg。<br>（1) the middle pregnancy induced labor (13 to 24 weeks of gestation) termination of pregnancy by artificial method ① with misoprostol compatibility; ② with methyl compatibility.<br>（2) intrauterine demise induced labor: oral medication, give 200mg singly, twice a day, or give 400 ~ 600mg daily, once a day, for 2 days, the stillbirth will be out after 72 hours generally.<br>（3) expanding cervix: oral medication, give 100 ~ 200 mg signly. oral medication: give 600mg, 48 hours before the intrauterine surgery to soften and expand the cervix. |
| 剂型、规格<br>Preparations | 片剂：每片 25mg；200mg。<br>Tablets: 25 mg;200 mg per tablet. |
| 药品名称 Drug Names | 地诺前列酮 Dinoprostone |
| 适应证<br>Indications | 可用于中期妊娠引产、足月妊娠引产和治疗性流产，对妊娠毒血症（先兆子痫、高血压）、妊娠合并肾病患者、过期妊娠、死胎不下、水泡状胎块、羊膜早破、高龄初产妇等均可应用。<br>It is used in the medium term pregnancy induced labor, full-term pregnancy induced labor and therapeutic abortion, for pre-eclampsia (preeclampsia, high blood pressure), as well as pregnancy with kidney disease patients, expired pregnancy, missed labor, bullate mole, premature rupture of amniotic membrane and elderly primipara. |

续　表

| 用法、用量<br>Dosage | （1）催产：普通阴道栓，一次 3mg，置于阴道后穹窿深处，6～8 小时后若产程无进展，可再放置一次。<br><br>（2）引产：①静脉滴注法；②宫腔内羊膜腔外注射法（中期妊娠引产）；③阴道内给药法；④宫颈内给药法。<br><br>（3）产后出血：将本品注射液 5mg 用所吸附的稀释液稀释后溶于氯化钠注射液中，缓慢静脉滴注（开始宜慢，以后可酌情加快）。<br><br>(1) OT: Normal vaginal suppository, give 3mg singly into the depths of the vault, if it is no use after 6 to 8 hours into the vagina, 3mg can be placed once again.<br><br>(2) abortion ① iv ② intravenous drip intrauterine amniotic injection method (trimester abortion) ③ Intravaginal drug delivery method ④ inner cervical vaginal administration method of administration law.<br><br>(3) postpartum hemorrhage: give 5mg of the dilution of the product into in sodium chloride injection, slow intravenous infusion (should be slow to start, after the discretion to accelerate). |
|---|---|
| 剂型、规格<br>Preparations | 注射液：每支 2mg（1ml）。阴道栓：每粒 3mg；20mg。控释阴道栓（普贝生）：每粒 10mg。凝胶剂：普比迪，每支 0.5mg/3g；普洛舒定，每支 1mg/3g；2mg/3g。<br><br>Injection: 2 mg (1ml) per bottle.Vaginal suppository: 3 mg;20 mg per capsule. Controlled release vaginal suppository (Pu Bei Sheng): 10 mg per capsule.Gels: biti, per 0.5 mg / 3 g per bottle;PuLuoShu, 1 mg / 3 g;2 mg / 3 g per bottle. |
| **药品名称 Drug Names** | 米索前列醇 Misoprostol |
| 适应证<br>Indications | 本品单于中期引产，效果不好，一般均与米非司酮联合应用，不良反应比卡前列甲酯栓轻。<br><br>If it is used for induced labor singly, the result is bad. It is generally used with mifepristone The adverse reaction lighter than methyl card top bolt. |
| 用法、用量<br>Dosage | 中期妊娠引产：①先顿服米非司酮 200mg，36 小时后在阴道后穹窿放置米索前列醇 3 片（600μg）。②在服用米非司酮 36～48 小时后，一次口服米索前列醇 500μg。<br><br>Mid pregnancy induced labor: ① give 200 mg of mifepristone, 36 hours later put 3 tablets (600μg) of misoprostol into the vaginal fomix. ② 36 to 48 hours after taking oral medication of mifepristone, take oral medication of 500μg misoprostol. |
| 剂型、规格<br>Preparations | 片剂：每片 200μg。<br><br>Tablets: 200μg per tablet. |
| **药品名称 Drug Names** | 依沙吖啶 Ethacridine |
| 适应证<br>Indications | ①中期妊娠引产，终止 12～26 周妊娠。②用于外科创伤、黏膜感染等消毒。<br><br>① It is used for mid-term gestation induced labor, 12～26 weeks of pregnancy termination. ② It is used for surgical trauma, and mucosal infection disinfection. |
| 用法、用量<br>Dosage | （1）羊膜腔内注射：由下腹壁向羊膜腔内注射本品 1% 溶液 5～10ml（含药 50～100mg）。每周用量不超过 100mg。妊娠在 20 周以内者用 50mg，在 20 周以上者用 100mg。<br><br>（2）羊膜腔外注射：先冲洗阴道，一日 1 次，冲洗 3 日。在消毒的情况下，将橡皮导尿管送入羊膜腔外，经导尿管注入药液 50ml（取本品 1% 的注射液 10ml，加注射用水 40ml，含药 100mg）。注药后将导尿管折叠结扎放入阴道，保留 24 小时后取出。(3)外用灭菌: 用 0.1%～0.2%（用片剂溶解配制而成）溶液，局部洗涤、湿敷。<br><br>(1) intra-amniotic injection: inject 1% solution 5~10ml (containing 50~100mg drug) into intra amniotic from abdominal wall. The amount of every week is not to exceed 100mg. 20 in less than 20 weeks gestation take 50mg, more than 20 weeks 100mg.<br><br>(2) amniotic injection: first wash the vagina once a day, for three days. Under sterile conditions, put the outer rubber catheter into the amniotic cavity, inject 50ml (take 10 ml of 1% of this injection, add 40ml water for injection, drug-containing 100mg) through the catheter. After injection, fold ligation catheter and put it into the vagina, keep it for 24 hours before take out.<br><br>(3) external sterilization: use 0.1 to 0.2% (by dissolving tablet preparation) to wash and wet compress . |

| 剂型、规格<br>Preparations | 片剂：每片 100mg。 |
| --- | --- |
| | 注射用依沙吖啶：每支 100mg。 |
| | Tablets: 100mg per tablet.<br>Ethacridine Injection: 100mg per bottle. |

15.2 退乳药物 A drug that inhibits lactation

| 药品名称 Drug Names | 溴隐亭 Bromocriptine |
| --- | --- |
| 适应证<br>Indications | ①分娩后、自发性、肿瘤性、药物等引起的闭经；②高泌乳素血症引起的月经紊乱、不孕、继发性闭经、排卵减少；③抑制泌乳，预防分娩后和早产后的泌乳；④产后的乳房充血、高泌乳素血症引起的特殊的乳房触痛、乳房胀痛和烦躁不安；⑤高泌乳素血症引起男性性功能低下（如阳痿和精子减少引起的不育）；⑥肢端肥大症的辅助治疗。<br><br>① It is used to treat amenorrhea caused by childbirth, spontaneity, tumor, drugs, etc; ② It is used to treat menstrual disorders, infertility, secondary amenorrhea, and reduction of ovulation caused by hyperprolactinemia; ③ It is used for inhibiting mammary, and preventing lactation after delivery and preterm birth; ④ It is used to treat special breast tenderness, breast tenderness, and restlessness caused by the postpartum breast engorgement and hyperprolactinemia; ⑤ It is used to treat low male sexual function (such as infertility caused by impotence and sperm decrease) caused by hyperprolactinemia; ⑥ It is used as aid in the treatment of acromegaly. |
| 用法、用量<br>Dosage | （1）产后回乳：口服，如为预防性用药，分娩后 4 小时开始服用 2.5mg，以后改为一日 2 次，1 次 2.5mg，连用 14 日；如已有乳汁分泌，则每日用 2.5mg，2～3 日后改为一日 2 次，一次 2.5mg，连用 14 日。<br>（2）高泌乳素血症引起的闭经溢乳、不孕症：口服，常用起始量为一次 1.25mg，一日 2～3 次；若症状未得到控制，可逐渐增量至一次 2.5mg，一日 2～3 次，餐后服用，直至月经恢复正常，再继续用药几周，完全停止则需 12～13 周，以防复发。<br>（3）产后乳房充血：轻者可口服，一次 2.5mg，如需要又没停止泌乳，则 6～12 小时后可重复一次。短时间用药不会抑制泌乳。<br>（4）男性高泌乳素血症引起的性功能低下：口服，1 次 1.25mg，一日 2～3 次，逐渐增加至一日 5～10mg，分 3 次服用。<br>（5）肢端肥大症：开始一日 2.5mg，经 7～14 日后根据临床反应可逐渐增至一日 10～20mg，分 4 次与食物同服。<br>（6）垂体泌乳素瘤：口服，起始量为每日 1.25mg，维持量为每日 5～7.5mg，最大量为每日 15mg。<br><br>(1) the postpartum breast back: oral medication, for example, serve as preventive medicine, give 2.5mg 4 hours after giving birth to a child, later change to twice a day, 2.5 mg singly, for 14 days of continuous treatment;With milk, give 2.5mg a day and change to twice a day, 2.5mg singly, for 14 days of continuous treatment.<br>(2)spilled milk, infertility caused by hyperprolactinemia amenorrhea: oral medication, give 1.25 mg singly, 2 to 3 times a day. If symptoms are not controlled, one can increase gradually to a 2.5 mg singly, 2 to 3 times a day, after the meal, until the period returns to normal menstruation, continue to use a few weeks, a complete stop after 12 to 13 weeks, to prevent recurrence.<br>(3) the postpartum breast engorgement: oral medication for light symptoms, 2.5 mg singly, if the lactation doesn't stop, then repeate after 6 to 12 hours when necessary. A short period of time will not inhibit lactation.<br>(4) male hyperprolactinemia caused by low sexual function: oral medication, 1.25 mg singly, 2 to 3 times a day, and gradually increased to 5～10 mg a day, in three divided times doses.<br>(5) acromegaly: 2.5 mg a day, after 7 to 14 days gradually increase to 10～20 mg a day according to the clinical response, in four divided doses with food.<br>(6) ituitary prolactin tumor: oral medication, the initial amount is 1.25 mg a day, maintain the quantity of 5～7.5 mg a day, the maximum is 15 mg a day. |
| 剂型、规格<br>Preparations | 片剂：每片 4mg。<br>Tablets: 4mg per tablet. |

**续　表**

| 16. 主要作用于内分泌系统药物 Drugs mainly acting on endocrine system |
|---|
| 16.1 肾上腺皮质激素和促肾上腺皮质激素 Adrenocortical hormones and adrenocorticotropic hormone |

| 药品名称 Drug Names | 氢化可的松 Hydrocortisone |
|---|---|
| 适应证<br>Indications | 　　用于结缔组织病、系统性红斑狼疮、严重的支气管哮喘、皮肌炎、血管炎等过敏性疾病、急性白血病、恶性淋巴瘤等病症。<br><br>　　It is used to treat connective tissue disease, systemic lupus erythematosus, severe bronchial asthma, dermatomyositis, vasculitis allergic diseases, acute leukemia, lymphoma and other diseases. |
| 用法、用量<br>Dosage | 　　氢化可的松注射液：每次 100 ~ 200mg，与 0.9% 氯化钠注射液或 5% 葡萄糖注射液 500ml 混合均匀后做静脉滴注。<br>　　注射用氢化可的松琥珀酸钠：50mg 或 100mg。临用时，以生理盐水或 5% 葡萄糖注射液稀释后静脉滴注或肌内注射。<br>　　醋酸氢化可的松片：一日 1 ~ 2 次，每次 1 片。<br>　　醋酸氢化可的松眼膏：一日 2 ~ 3 次。<br>　　醋酸氢化可的松滴眼液：用前摇匀。<br>　　Hydrocortisone injection: give 100 ~ 200 mg singly, mix with 0.9% sodium chloride injection or 500ml of 5% glucose injection as intravenous drip.<br>　　For injection hydrocortisone sodium succinate: 50 mg or 100 mg. intravenous drip or intramuscular injection after diluted with normal saline or 5% glucose injection.<br>　　Hydrocortisone acetate tablets: give 1 to 2 times a day, one tablet singly.<br>　　Hydrocortisone acetate eye ointment: 2 to 3 times a day.<br>　　Hydrocortisone acetate eye drops: shake well before use. |
| 剂型、规格<br>Preparations | 　　氢化可的松注射液：10mg（2ml）；25mg（5ml）；50mg（10ml）；100mg（20ml）（为氢化可的松的稀乙醇溶液）。<br>　　醋酸氢化可的松注射液：125mg（5ml）（为醋酸氢化可的松的无菌混悬液）。<br>　　注射用氢化可的松琥珀酸钠：50mg 或 100mg（按氢化可的松算）。<br>　　醋酸氢化可的松片：每片 20mg。<br>　　醋酸氢化可的松软膏：1%。<br>　　醋酸氢化可的松眼膏：0.5%。<br>　　醋酸氢化可的松滴眼液：3ml；15mg。<br>　　Hydrocortisone injection: 10mg (2ml); 25mg (5ml); 50mg (10ml); 100mg (20ml) (dilute ethanol solution as hydrocortisone).<br>　　Hydrocortisone Acetate Injection: 125mg (5ml) (hydrocortisone acetate sterile suspension).<br>　　Hydrocortisone sodium succinate for injection: 50mg or 100mg (calculated by hydrocortisone).<br>　　Hydrocortisone acetate tablets: 20mg per tablet.<br>　　Hydrocortisone acetate ointment: 1%.<br>　　Hydrocortisone acetate ointment: 0.5%.<br>　　Hydrocortisone acetate eye drops: 3ml: 15mg. |
| 药品名称 Drug Names | 泼尼松 Prednisone |
| 适应证<br>Indications | 　　用于结缔组织病、系统性红斑狼疮、严重的支气管哮喘、皮肌炎、血管炎等过敏性疾病、急性白血病、恶性淋巴瘤等病症。<br><br>　　It is used to treat connective tissue disease, systemic lupus erythematosus, severe bronchial asthma, dermatomyositis, vasculitis allergic diseases, acute leukemia, lymphoma and other diseases. |
| 用法、用量<br>Dosage | 　　（1）补充替代疗法口服，1 次 5 ~ 10mg，一日 10 ~ 60mg，早晨起床后服用 2/3，下午服用 1/3。<br>　　（2）抗炎口服，一日 5 ~ 60mg。<br>　　（3）自身免疫性疾病口服，每日 40 ~ 60mg，病情稳定后可逐渐减量。<br>　　（4）过敏性疾病，口服每日 20 ~ 40mg，病情症状减轻后减量，每隔 1 ~ 2 日减少 5mg。<br>　　（5）防止器官移植排异反应，一般在术前 1 ~ 2 日开始每日口服 100mg，术后 1 周改为每日 60mg，以后逐渐减量。<br>　　（6）治疗急性白血病、恶性肿瘤等，每日口服 60 ~ 80mg，症状缓解后减量。 |

|  | (1) oral medication as complementary and alternative therapies, 5 ~ 10mg singly, 10 ~ 60mg a day, give 2/3 in the morning, give 1/3 in the afternoon.<br>(2) oral medication as anti-inflammatory, 5 ~ 60mg a day.<br>(3) autoimmune diseases, oral medication, 40 ~ 60mg a day, if symptoms get well controlled, reduce the dose gradually.<br>(4) allergic diseases, oral medication, 20 ~ 40mg a day, if the symptoms get well controlled, reduce 5mg every 1 to 2 days .<br>(5) prevent organ transplant rejection, usually in 1 to 2 days before surgery 100mg a day for oral medication, after a week to daily 60mg, after tapering.<br>(6) It is used to treat acute leukemia, malignant tumors, 60 ~ 80mg a day for oral medication, reduce after symptoms get well controlled. |
|---|---|
| 剂型、规格<br>Preparations | 醋酸泼尼松片：每片 5mg。<br>醋酸泼尼松眼膏：0.5%。<br><br>Prednisone tablets: 5mg per tablet.<br>Prednisone ointment: 0.5%. |
| 药品名称 Drug Names | 泼尼松龙 Prednisolone |
| 适应证<br>Indications | 用于过敏性和自身免疫性疾病。<br>It is used to treat allergic and autoimmune diseases. |
| 用法、用量<br>Dosage | 口服：成人开始一日 15 ~ 40mg，需用时可用到 60mg 或每日 0.5 ~ 1mg/kg，发热患者分 3 次服用，体温正常者每日晨起一次顿服。病情稳定后应逐渐减量，维持量 5 ~ 10mg，视病情而定。小儿开始用量 1mg/kg。肌内注射：一日 10 ~ 30mg。静脉滴注：1 次 10 ~ 25mg，溶于 5% ~ 10% 葡萄糖溶液 500ml 中应用。关节腔或软组织内注射（混悬液）：1 次 5 ~ 50mg，用量依关节大小而定，应在无菌条件下操作，以防引起感染。滴眼：一次 1 ~ 2 滴，一日 2 ~ 4 次，治疗开始的 24 ~ 48 小时，剂量可酌情加大至每小时 2 滴，注意不宜过早停药。<br><br>Oral medication: for adults, 15 ~ 40mg a day at first, 60mg if necessary or 0.5 ~ 1mg/kg a day, give fever patients in three divided doses, the patients with nomal temperature take it in the morning. Reduce if the symptom gets well controlled, maintain the amount of 5 ~ 10mg, depending on the disease. Pediatric dosage is 1mg/kg at first. Intramuscular injection: 10 ~ 30mg a day. Intravenous infusion:10 ~ 25mg singly, application by dissolving it in 5% to 10% glucose solution 500ml. Soft tissue or articular injection (suspension): 1 5 ~ 50mg, the amount depending on the size of the joint, should operate under aseptic conditions to prevent infection. Drops: 1 to 2 drops singly, 2 to 4 times a day, 24 to 48 hours at the beginning of the treatment, the dose may be increased to 2 drops per hour, pay attention to premature withdrawal. |
| 剂型、规格<br>Preparations | 醋酸泼尼松龙片：每片 5mg。<br>醋酸泼尼松龙注射液（混悬液）：125mg（5ml）。<br>泼尼松龙磷酸钠注射液：20mg（1ml）。<br>泼尼松龙软膏：0.25% ~ 0.5%。<br>泼尼松龙眼膏：0.25%。<br>泼尼松龙滴眼液：1%。<br><br>Prednisolone acetate tablets: 5mg per tablet.<br>Prednisolone acetate injection (suspension): 125mg (5ml).<br>Prednisolone Sodium Phosphate Injection: 20mg (1ml).<br>Prednisolone ointment: 0.25% to 0.5%.<br>Prednisolone ointment: 0.25%.<br>Prednisolone drops: 1% |
| 药品名称 Drug Names | 甲泼尼龙 Methylprednisolone |
| 适应证<br>Indications | 用于抗炎治疗风湿性疾病、胶原疾病、皮肤疾病、过敏状态、眼部疾病、胃肠道疾病、呼吸道疾病、水肿状态；免疫抑制治疗、休克、内分泌失调等。<br><br>It is used as anti-inflammatory therapy for rheumatoid arthritis, muscle original diseases, skin diseases, allergic condition, eye disease, gastrointestinal disease, respiratory disease, edema, as well as immunosuppressive therapy, shock, endocrine disorders, etc. |

**续　表**

| | |
|---|---|
| 用法、用量<br>Dosage | 口服：开始一日 16 ~ 24mg，分 2 次，维持量一日 4 ~ 8mg。关节腔内及肌内注射：一次 10 ~ 40mg。用于危重病情作为辅助疗法时，推荐剂量时 30mg/kg 体重，将已溶解的药物与 5% 葡萄糖注射液、生理盐水注射液或者二者混合后至少静脉输注 30 分钟。此剂量可于 48 小时内，每 4 ~ 6 小时重复一次。冲击疗法：每日 1g，静脉注射，使用 1 ~ 4 日；或每月 1g，静脉注射，使用 6 个月。系统性红斑狼疮：每日 1g，静脉注射，使用 3 日。多发性硬化症：每日 1g，静脉注射，使用 3 日或 5 日。肾小球肾炎、狼疮性肾炎：每日 1g，静脉注射，使用 3 日、5 日或 7 日。<br><br>Oral medication: for adults, 15 ~ 40mg a day at first, 60mg if necessary or 0.5 ~ 1mg/kg a day, give fever patients in three divided doses, the patients with nomal temperature take it in the morning. Reduce if the symptom gets well controlled, maintain the amount of 5 ~ 10mg, depending on the disease. Pediatric dosage is 1mg/kg at first. Intramuscular injection: 10 ~ 30mg a day. Intravenous infusion:10 ~ 25mg singly, application by dissolving it in 5% to 10% glucose solution 500ml. Soft tissue or articular injection (suspension): 1 5 ~ 50mg, the amount depending on the size of the joint, should operate under aseptic conditions to prevent infection. Drops: 1 to 2 drops singly, 2 to 4 times a day, 24 to 48 hours at the beginning of the treatment, the dose may be increased to 2 drops per hour, pay attention to premature withdrawal. |
| 剂型、规格<br>Preparations | 片剂：每片 2mg；4mg。<br>注射液（混悬剂）：每支 20mg（1ml）；40mg（1ml）。<br>注射液：40mg；125mg；500mg。<br><br>Tablets: 2mg; 4mg per tablet.<br>Injection (suspension): 20mg (1ml); 40mg(1ml).<br>Injection: 40mg; 125mg; 500mg. |
| **药品名称 Drug Names** | 曲安西龙 Triamcinolone |
| 适应证<br>Indications | 用于类风湿关节炎、其他结缔组织炎症、支气管哮喘、过敏性皮炎、神经性皮炎、湿疹等，尤其适用于对皮质激素禁忌的伴有高血压或水肿的关节炎患者。<br><br>It is used to treat rheumatoid arthritis and other connective tissue inflammation, bronchial asthma, allergic dermatitis, neurodermatitis, eczema, etc., especially suitable for cortical hormone taboo arthritis patients with high blood pressure or edema. |
| 用法、用量<br>Dosage | （1）口服：开始时 1 次 4mg，每日 2 ~ 4 次。维持量为 1 次 1 ~ 4mg，一日 1 ~ 2 次，通常维持量不超过 8mg。<br>（2）肌内注射：每 1 ~ 4 周一次 40 ~ 80mg。<br>（3）皮下注射：一次 5 ~ 20mg。<br>（4）关节腔内注射：每 1 ~ 7 周一次 5 ~ 40mg。<br>(1) oral medication: at first 4 mg singly, 2 to 4 times a day. Maintain for 1 ~ 4 mg singly, 1 to 2 times a day, usually no more than 8 mg.<br>(2) intramuscular injection 40 ~ 80 mg per 1 to 4 times on Monday.<br>(3) subcutaneous injection: 5 ~ 20 mg singly.<br>(4) articular cavity injection every 1 to 7 weeks, 5 ~ 40 mg singly. |
| 剂型、规格<br>Preparations | 片剂：每片 1mg；2mg；4mg。<br>曲安西龙双醋酸酯混悬注射液：每支 125mg（5ml）；200mg（5ml）.<br><br>Tablets:1 mg per tablet:2mg; 4mg per tablet.<br>Triamcinolone diacetate suspension injection: 125 mg (5ml); 200 mg (5 ml). |
| **药品名称 Drug Names** | 曲安奈德 Triamcinolone Acetonide |
| 适应证<br>Indications | 用于各种皮肤病（如神经性皮炎、湿疹、牛皮癣等）、支气管哮喘、过敏性鼻炎、关节痛、肩周围炎、腱鞘炎、急性扭伤、慢性腰腿痛及眼科炎症等。鼻喷雾剂用于治疗常年性过敏性鼻炎或季节性过敏性鼻炎。<br><br>It is used for a variety of skin diseases (e.g., neurodermatitis, eczema, psoriasis, etc.), bronchial asthma, allergic rhinitis, joint pain, shoulder inflammation around, tenosynovitis, acute sprain, chronic lumbocrural pain and eye inflammation, etc.Nasal spray for the treatment of perennial allergic rhinitis or seasonal allergic rhinitis. |

续 表

| 用法、用量<br>Dosage | （1）支气管哮喘：肌内注射，成人每次 1ml（40mg），每 3 周 1 次，5 次为 1 个疗程，患者症状较重者可用 80mg；6 ～ 12 岁儿童减半，在必要时 3 ～ 6 岁幼儿可用成人剂量的 1/3。穴位或局部注射，成人每次 1ml（40mg），在扁桃体穴或颈前甲状软骨旁注射，每周 1 次，5 次为 1 个疗程，注射前先用少量普鲁卡因局部麻醉。<br>（2）过敏性鼻炎：肌内注射，每次 1ml（40mg），每 3 周 1 次，5 次为 1 个疗程；下鼻甲注射，鼻腔先喷 1% 利多卡因表面麻醉后，在双下鼻甲前端各注入本品 0.5ml，每周 1 次，4 ～ 5 次为 1 个疗程。<br>（3）各种关节病：每次 10 ～ 20mg，加 0.25% 利多卡因液 10 ～ 20ml，用 5 号针头，一次进针直至病灶，每周 2 ～ 3 次或隔日一次，症状好转后每周 1 ～ 2 次，4 ～ 5 次为 1 个疗程。<br>（4）皮肤病：直接注入皮损部分，通常每一部位用 0.2 ～ 0.3mg，视患部大小而定，每处每次不超过 0.5mg，必要时每隔 1 ～ 2 周重复使用。局部外用：一日 2 ～ 3 次，一般早、晚各一次。治疗皮炎、湿疹时，疗程为 2 ～ 4 周。<br>（5）鼻腔内用药：用前须振摇 5 次以上；12 岁以上的儿童、成人及老年人，推荐剂量为每鼻孔 2 喷（共 220μg），一日 1 次。症状得到控制时，可降低剂量至每鼻孔 1 喷（共 110μg），一日 1 次。如 3 周后症状无改善应看医师。<br><br>(1) bronchial asthma: intramuscular injection, for adults 1ml (40 mg) singly, once every three weeks, 5 times for a period of treatment, 80 mg if the symptom is serious; half the dosage for 6 to 12 years old children, 1/3 of the adult dosage for 3 to 6 years old preschool children when necessary, . Acupuncture point or local injections, for adults, 1 ml (40 mg) singly, inject in the amygdala hole or near the thyroid cartilage, once a week, five times for a period of treatment, use a small amount of procaine bureau before injection.<br>(2) allergic rhinitis: intramuscular injection, 1 ml (40 mg) singly, once every three weeks, 5 times for a period of treatment; Inferior turbinate injection, nasal spray surface of 1% lidocaine before anesthesia, inject 0.5ml of this product in double inferior turbinate front, once a week, 4 to 5 times for a period of treatment.<br>(3) all kinds of joint disease: 10 to 20 mg singly, 10 to 20 ml of 0.25% lidocaine fluid, with No.5 needles, until a needle into the lesions, 2 to 3 times a week or once every two days, 1 to 2 times per week if symptoms get well controlled r, 4 to 5 times for a period of treatment.<br>(4) skin disease: injected directly into the lesion part, usually per part with 0.2 ~ 0.3 mg, depending on the affected part size, not more than 0.5 mg singly, repeat every 1 to 2 weeks if necessary.Local external use: 2 to 3 times a day, usually in the morning and at night. When it is used to treat dermatitis, eczema, the treatment course 2 to 4 weeks.<br>(5) It is used in the nasal cavity, shake more than five times before giving; for children over the age of 12, adults and old men, the recommended dose is 2 sprays (200μg of total) per nostril, once a day. When symptoms get well controlled, reduce the dose to 1 spray (110μg) per nostril, once a day. Go to the doctor if there is no improvement three weeks later. |
|---|---|
| 剂型、规格<br>Preparations | 注射液（混悬剂）：每支 40mg（1ml）。<br>复方曲安奈德霜：每支 5g；10g；15g；20g。<br>鼻喷雾剂：每支 6ml [6.6mg，120 喷（55μg/ 喷）]。<br><br>Injection (suspension agent): 40 mg (1ml) per bottle.<br>Compound triamcinolone acetonide cream: 5 g per bottle; 10 g; 15 g; 20 g.<br>Nasal spray: 6 ml [6.6 mg, 120 spray (55μg /spray)] per bottle. |
| 药品名称 Drug Names | 布地奈德 Budesonide |
| 适应证<br>Indications | 用于支气管哮喘的症状和体征的长期控制。粉吸入剂用于需适用糖皮质激素维持治疗以控制基础炎症的支气管哮喘、慢性阻塞性肺疾病患者。鼻喷雾剂用于季节性和常年性过敏性鼻炎、血管运动性鼻炎；预防鼻息肉切除术后鼻息肉的再生，对症治疗鼻息肉。<br><br>It is used to long-term control the signs and symptoms of bronchial asthma. Powder inhaler is used to glucocorticoid therapy to control basic inflammation of bronchial asthma, chronic obstructive pulmonary disease patients.Nasal spray is used for seasonal and perennial allergic rhinitis . It is used to prevent nasal polyps regeneration after nasal polyps resection and to symptomaticly treat nasal polyps. |

**续　表**

| | |
|---|---|
| 用法、用量<br>Dosage | 剂量应个体化，成人初始剂量为 200 ～ 1600μg/d，分 2 ～ 4 次给药（较轻微的病例 200 ～ 800μg/d，较严重的 800 ～ 1600μg/d）。一般一次 200μg，早、晚各一次，病情严重时一日 4 次。7 岁以上儿童：200 ～ 800μg/d，分 2 ～ 4 次使用。2 ～ 7 岁儿童：200 ～ 400μg/d，分成 2 ～ 4 次使用。维持剂量成人一日 100 ～ 600μg，儿童 100 ～ 800μg；当哮喘控制后可减量至最低有效维持剂量。鼻喷，成人及 6 岁以上儿童，起始剂量为一日 256μg，次剂量可早晨一次喷入和早晚 2 次喷入（即早晨每个鼻孔内喷入 2 喷；或早晚 2 次，每个鼻孔内喷 1 喷）。<br><br>Dose should be individualized, for adults, the initial dose is 200 ～ 1600 μg /d, in 2 to 4 divided doses (mild cases of 200 ～ 800μg /d, serious 800 ～ 1600 μg /d).Generally 200 μg singly, once in the morning and once at night, when the symptom is severe, give 4 times a day. For childrenover the age of 200 ～ 800μg /d, give in 2 to 4 divided doses. For children aging 2 to 200 ～ 400μg /d, give 2 to 4 divide doses.Maintenance dose for adults, 100 ～ 1600μg a day, 100 ～ 800μg for children; After the asthma gets well controlled, reduce to the lowest effective maintenance dose. Nasal spray, for adults and children over the age of 6, 256μg at first, . 2 sprays per nostril in the morning; twice in the morning and evening 1 spray per nostril. |
| 剂型、规格<br>Preparations | 气雾剂：10ml：10mg（50μg/ 喷，200 喷 / 瓶）；10ml：20mg（100μg/ 喷，200 喷 / 瓶）；5ml：20mg（200μg/ 喷，100 喷 / 瓶）。<br>雷诺考特特鼻喷雾剂（白色或类白色黏稠混悬液）：64μg/ 喷（120 喷 / 支，药液浓度 1.28mg/ml）。<br>粉吸入剂：0.1mg/ 吸（200 吸 / 支）。<br>细微颗粒混悬液：0.5mg/2ml；1mg/2ml。<br>Aerosol: 10 ml: 10 mg (50μg /spray, 200 spray / bottle);10 ml: 20 mg (100μg /spray, 200 spray/ bottle);5 ml: 20 mg (200μg /spray, 100 spray / bottle).<br>Renault courtney nasal spray (white or kind of white sticky stiff suspension liquid) : 64μg /spray (120 spray / branch, 1.28 mg/ml of solution concentration).<br>The powder inhaler: 0.1 mg/vacuum suction/(200).<br>Fine particulate suspension liquid: 0.5 mg/2ml;1 mg/2ml. |
| **药品名称 Drug Names** | 氟替卡松 Fluticasone |
| 适应证<br>Indications | 用作持续性哮喘的长期治疗，季节性过敏性鼻炎（包括枯草热）和常年性过敏性鼻炎的预防和治疗。外用可缓解炎症性和瘙痒性皮肤病。吸入剂适用于 12 岁及以上患者预防用药维持治疗哮喘。<br><br>It is used for long-term treatment of persistent asthma, and the prevention and treatment of seasonal allergic rhinitis (hay fever) and perennial allergic rhinitis. External use can reduce inflammation and itching skin diseases. Inhalant applies to patients prevent drug maintenance treatment of asthma patients over the age of 12. |
| 用法、用量<br>Dosage | 成人，老年患者和 12 岁以上儿童：一日 1 次，每个鼻孔各 2 喷，以早晨用药为好，某些患者需每日 2 次，每个鼻孔各 2 喷。当症状得到控制时，维持剂量为一日 1 次，每个鼻孔各 1 喷。若症状复发，可相应增加剂量，每日最大剂量为每个鼻孔不超过 4 喷。4 ～ 11 岁儿童：一日 1 次，每个鼻孔各 1 喷。某些患者需每日 2 次，每个鼻孔各 1 喷，最大剂量为每个鼻孔不超过 2 喷。湿疹 / 皮炎：成人及 1 岁以上儿童，一日 1 次涂于患处。其他适应证，一日 2 次。吸入剂：轻度哮喘：100 ～ 250μg，一日 2 次；中度哮喘：250 ～ 500μg，一日 2 次；重度哮喘：500 ～ 1000μg，一日 2 次。<br><br>For adults, elderly patients and children over the age of 12: once a day, 2 sprays per nostril, better give in the morning, some patients need twice a day, 2 sprays per nostril. When symptoms get well controlled, maintaining dose for once a day, 1 spray per nostril. If symptoms relapse, increase the dose, the maximum daily dose is not more than 4 sprays per nostril. For children aging 4 to 11: once a day, 1 spray per nostril. Some patients need twice a day, 1 spray per nostril, the maximum dose is not more than 2 sprays per nostril. Eczema or dermatitis: for adults and children over the age of 1, apply to the affected part, once a day. Other indications, twice a day. Inhalation: mild asthma: 100 ～ 250μg, 2 times a day; Moderate asthma: 250 ～ 500μg, twice a day; Severe asthma: 500 ～ 1000 μg, twice a day. |

**续　表**

| 剂型、规格<br>Preparations | 鼻喷剂：50μg × 120 喷。吸入气雾剂：125μg × 60 喷 / 支，250μg × 60 泡 / 盒。乳膏：15g：7.5mg（0.05%）；30g：15mg（0.05%）。<br><br>Spray nasal spray: 50μg x 120 sprays. Inhaled aerosol spray 125μg x 60 spray/branch, 250μg x 60 bubble/box. Cream: 15 g: 7.5 mg (0.05%).30 g: 15 mg (0.05%). |
|---|---|
| **药品名称 Drug Names** | 莫米松 Mometasone |
| 适应证<br>Indications | 用于治疗成人及 12 岁以上儿童的季节性或常年性鼻炎。对于中至重度季节性过敏性鼻炎的患者，建议在花粉季节开始前 2 ～ 4 周使用本品作预防治疗。也用于对皮脂类固醇有效的皮肤病如异位性皮炎。<br><br>It is used for the treatment of seasonal or perennial rhinitis of adults and children over the age of 12. For patients with seasonal allergic rhinitis to severe, suggest to use this product as preventive treatment 2 ~ 4 weeks before the start of the season . It is also used for effective skin sebum steroids such as ectopic dermatitis. |
| 用法、用量<br>Dosage | 鼻喷剂：成人（包括老年患者）和 12 岁以上儿童，常用推荐剂量为每侧鼻孔 2 喷（每喷为 50μg），一日 1 次（总量为 200μg）。当症状被控制时，可减至每侧鼻孔 1 喷（总量为 100μg），如果症状未被有效控制，则可增至每侧鼻孔 4 喷（400μg），在症状控制后减少剂量。乳膏：一日 1 次，涂于患处。<br><br>Nasal spray: for adults (including elderly patients) and children over the age of 12, recommended dosage is commonly used for 2 sprays per nostril 50μg per spray), once a day ( 200μg of total).When symptoms are controlled, can be reduced to 1 per nostril spray (total of 100μg), if symptoms are not effectively controlled, increase to 4 sprays (400μg) of per nostril spray, reduce the dosage after the symptom get well controlled. Cream: 1 times a day, apply to affected area. |
| 剂型、规格<br>Preparations | 鼻喷剂：50μg × 60 揿 / 支；50μg × 120 揿 / 支。乳膏：5g：5mg。<br>Nasal spray: 50μg x 60 press/branch;50μg x 120 press/teams. Cream: 5 g: 5 mg. |
| **药品名称 Drug Names** | 地塞米松 Dexamethasone |
| 适应证<br>Indications | 用于过敏性与自身免疫性炎症性疾病。多用于结缔组织病、活动性风湿病、类风湿关节炎、红斑狼疮、严重支气管哮喘、严重皮炎、溃疡性结肠炎、急性白血病等，也用于某些严重感染及中毒、恶性淋巴瘤的综合治疗。片剂还用于某些肾上腺皮质疾病的诊断。<br><br>It is used to treat allergic and autoimmune inflammatory disease. It is often used in connective tissue diseases, more active rheumatism, rheumatoid arthritis, lupus erythematosus, serious bronchus asthma, serious dermatitis, ulcerative colitis, acute leukemia, etc, as well as in some severe infection and poisoning, comprehensive treatment of malignant lymphoma. Tablets are also used in some adrenocortical disease diagnosis. |
| 用法、用量<br>Dosage | 口服，每日 0.75 ～ 3mg，一日 2 ～ 4 次；维持剂量每日 0.75mg。一般剂量静脉注射每次 2 ～ 20mg；静脉滴注时，应以 5% 葡萄糖注射液稀释，可 2 ～ 6 小时重复给药至病情稳定，但大剂量连续给药一般不超过 72 小时。还可用于缓解恶性肿瘤所致的脑水肿，首剂静脉推注 10mg，随后每 6 小时肌内注射 4mg，一般 12 ～ 24 小时患者可有所好转，2 ～ 4 日后逐渐减量，5 ～ 7 日停药。对不宜手术的脑肿瘤，首剂可静脉推注 50mg，以后每 2 小时重复给予 8mg，数天后再减至每天 2mg，分 2 ～ 3 次静脉给予。用于鞘内注射每次 5mg，间隔 1 ～ 3 周注射一次；关节腔内注射一般每次 0.8 ～ 4mg，按关节腔大小而定。<br><br>Oral medication, 0.75 ~ 3 mg a day, 2 to 4 times a day; Maintain a dose of 0.75 mg a day. General 2 ~ 20 mg per time of intravenous injection; Intravenous drip, should be diluted with 5% glucose injection, can repeat giving medicine until a stable condition for 2 to 6 hours, but the big dose of continuous drug delivery is generally not more than 72 hours. It is used to relieve cerebral edema caused by malignant tumor, the first bottle of intravenous injection is 10 mg, afterwards intramuscular injection of 4 mg every 6 hours, then generally the patients can be improved in 12 to 24 hours, 2 to 4 days later gradually reduce the dose, 5 to 7 days later stop using the medicine. For unfavorable surgical brain tumors, the first bottle of intravenous injection is 50 mg, repeat giving 8 mg every 2 hours, reduce to 2 mg a day a few days later, give 2 to 3 divided doses of vein injection. Give intrathecal injection of 5 mg singly, give an injection at a interval of 1 to 3 weeks; Give articular cavity injection 0.8 ~ 4 mg singly, according to the size of joint cavity. |

**续　表**

| 剂型、规格<br>Preparations | 醋酸地塞米松片：每片 0.75mg。<br>地塞米松磷酸钠注射液：2mg（1ml）；5mg（1ml）。<br>Dexamethasone acetate tablets: 0.75 mg per tablet.<br>Dexamethasone sodium phosphate injection: 2 mg (1 ml);5 mg (1 ml). |
| --- | --- |
| 药品名称 Drug Names | 倍他米松 Betamethasone |
| 适应证<br>Indications | 用于治疗活动性风湿病、类风湿关节炎、红斑性狼疮、严重支气管哮喘、严重皮炎、急性白血病等，也可用于某些感染的综合治疗。<br><br>It is used to treat active rheumatism, rheumatoid arthritis, lupus erythematosus, serious bronchus asthma, serious dermatitis, acute leukemia, etc., as well as for comprehensive treatment of certain infections. |
| 用法、用量<br>Dosage | 口服：成人开始每日 0.5 ～ 2mg，分次服用。维持量为每日 0.5 ～ 1mg。肌内注射、静脉注射或静脉滴注用倍他米松磷酸钠：用于危急患者的抢救。<br><br>Oral medication: for adults, give 0.5 ～ 2 mg a day, in several divided doses. To maintain the amount of 0.5 ～ 1 mg a day. Intramuscular injection, intravenous injection or intravenous drip with betamethasone sodium phosphate: used to rescue critical patients. |
| 剂型、规格<br>Preparations | 片剂：每片 0.5mg。<br>倍他米松醋酸酯注射液：每支 1.5mg（1ml）。<br>Tablets: 0.5 mg per tablet.<br>Betamethasone acetate injection: 1.5 mg (1ml)per bottle. |
| 药品名称 Drug Names | 氟氢可的松 Fludrocortisone |
| 适应证<br>Indications | 可与糖皮质类固醇一起用于原发性肾上腺皮质功能减退症的替代治疗。也适用于低肾素低醛固酮综合征和自主神经病变所致直立性低血压等。因本品内服易致水肿，多供外用局部涂敷治疗皮脂溢性湿疹、接触性皮炎、肛门、阴部瘙痒等症。<br><br>It can be a replacement therapy for primary adrenal hypofunction with glucocorticoid steroids, as well as apply to low renin and low aldosterone syndrome caused by autonomic neuropathy orthostatic hypotension. This product is prone to cause edema due to oral medication, so it is used for topical application for the treatment of multiple seborrheic eczema, contact dermatitis, anal, genital itching embolism. |
| 用法、用量<br>Dosage | 替代治疗：成人口服，每日 0.1 ～ 0.2mg，分 2 次。局部皮肤涂敷一日 2 ～ 4 次。<br>Replacement therapy: for adults oral medication, 0.1 to 0.2 mg a day, in 2 divided doses. Apply to local skin, 2 to 4 times a day. |
| 剂型、规格<br>Preparations | 片剂：每片 0.1mg。<br>醋酸氟氢可的松软膏：0.025%。<br>Tablets: 0.1 mg per tablet .<br>Fludrocortisone acetate ointment: 0.025%. |
| 药品名称 Drug Names | 氯倍他索 Clobetasol |
| 适应证<br>Indications | 治疗皮肤炎症和瘙痒症，如神经性皮炎、接触性皮炎、脂溢性皮炎、湿疹、局限性瘙痒症、盘状红斑狼疮等。<br><br>It is used to treat skin inflammation and pruritus, such as neurodermatitis, contact dermatitis, seborrheic dermatitis, eczema, pruritus limitations, discoid lupus erythematosus. |
| 用法、用量<br>Dosage | 外用：涂患处，一日 2 ～ 3 次，待病情控制后，改为一日 1 次。<br>External use: apply to the affected part, 2 to 3 times a day, after controlling the disease, once a day. |
| 剂型、规格<br>Preparations | 软膏：0.05%。<br>霜剂：0.025%。<br>Ointment: 0.05%.<br>Cream: 0.025%. |

**续　表**

| 药品名称 Drug Names | 氟轻松 Fluocinolone |
|---|---|
| 适应证<br>Indications | 湿疹（特别是婴儿湿疹）、神经性皮炎、皮肤瘙痒症、接触性皮炎、牛皮癣、盘状红斑狼疮、扁平苔藓、外耳炎、日光性皮炎等。<br><br>It is used to treat eczema (especially infant eczema), neurodermatitis, itchy skin disease, contact dermatitis, psoriasis, discoid lupus erythematosus (sle), flat moss, otitis externa, solar dermatitis, and so on. |
| 用法、用量<br>Dosage | 皮肤洗净后局部外用，薄薄涂于患处，可轻揉促其渗入皮肤，一日 3 ～ 4 次。<br><br>Use it on partial skin after rinsing the skin, apply to the affected area, and gently rub to make it into the skin, 3 to 4 times a day. |
| 剂型、规格<br>Preparations | 醋酸氟轻松软膏、乳膏：0.025%。<br><br>Acetate fluocinolone ointment, cream: 0.025%. |
| 药品名称 Drug Names | 倍氯米松 Beclomethasone |
| 适应证<br>Indications | 外用可治疗各种炎症皮肤病如湿疹、过敏性皮炎、神经性皮炎、接触性皮炎、牛皮癣、瘙痒等。气雾剂可用于预防和治疗常年性及季节性的过敏性鼻炎和血管舒缩性鼻炎。<br><br>It is used for topical treatment of various inflammatory skin diseases such as eczema, allergic dermatitis, neurodermatitis, contact dermatitis, psoriasis, pruritus, etc. Aerosol can be used for the prevention and treatment of permanent and seasonal allergic rhinitis and vasomotor rhinitis. |
| 用法、用量<br>Dosage | 乳膏或软膏用于皮肤病：一日 2 ～ 3 次，涂于患处，必要时包扎之。气雾剂用于治疗哮喘：成人，一日 3 ～ 4 次，每次 2 揿，严重者每日 12 ～ 16 揿，根据病情好转情况逐渐减量；儿童，一日 2 ～ 4 次，每次 1 ～ 2 揿。鼻气雾剂，用于防止过敏性鼻炎，鼻腔喷雾给药，成人，一次每鼻孔 2 揿，一日 2 次，也可一次每鼻孔 1 揿（50μg），一日 3 ～ 4 次。一日总量不可超过 8 揿（400μg）。<br><br>Cream or ointment on skin: 2 to 3 times a day, apply to affected area, bind up when necessary. Aerosol is used in the treatment of asthma: for adults, 3 to 4 times a day, 2 press singly, 12 ～ 16 press a day if serious, reduce according to the improved situation; for children, 2 to 4 times a day, 1 ～ 2 press a day. Nasal aerosolis used to prevent allergic rhinitis, nasal spray, for adults, give 2 press per nostril singly, twice a day, or give 1 press (50μg) per nostril singly, 3 to 4 times a day. The daily amount shall not exceed 8 press ( 400μg). |
| 剂型、规格<br>Preparations | 软膏：0.025%。<br>鼻气雾剂、喷雾剂：50μg/ 揿（200 揿 / 支），250μg/ 揿（80 揿 / 支），50μg/ 揿（200 揿 / 支）。<br>Ointment: 0.025%.<br>Nasal aerosol and spray: 50μg /press (200 press /branch), 250μg /press (80 press /branch), 50μg / press( 200 press/branch). |
| 药品名称 Drug Names | 哈西奈德 Halcinonide |
| 适应证<br>Indications | 用于银屑病和湿疹性皮炎。用于银屑病，具有疗程短、不良反应少的特点。<br><br>It is used to treat psoriasis and eczema dermatitis. when used to treat psoriasis, the medicine has the characteristics of the short course, less adverse reaction. |
| 用法、用量<br>Dosage | 一日 2 ～ 3 次，涂于患处。<br><br>2 to 3 times a day, apply the medicine to affected area. |
| 剂型、规格<br>Preparations | 乳膏、软膏：0.1%。<br><br>Cream and ointment: 0.1%. |
| 药品名称 Drug Names | 可的松 Cortisone |
| 适应证<br>Indications | 主要用于肾上腺皮质功能减退症的替代治疗。<br><br>It is mainly used as a replacement therapy for adrenal cortex hypofunction. |
| 用法、用量<br>Dosage | 口服：成人，每日剂量 25 ～ 37.5mg，清晨服 2/3，午后服 1/3。当患者有应激状况时（如发热、感染）可适当加量，增到每日 100mg，肌内注射：每日 25mg，有应激状况适当加量，有严重应激时，应改用氢化可的松静脉滴注。<br><br>Oral medication: for adult, daily dose of 25 ～ 37.5 mg, take 2/3 in the early morning, 1/3 in the afternoon. Patients under stress conditions (such as fever, infection)can step up the quantity to a daily dose of 100 mg. Intramuscular injection: 25 mg a day, Patient under stress conditions can appropriately step up the quantity. Patient under severe stress conditions, should take hydrocortisone by intravenous infusion . |

**续　表**

| 剂型、规格<br>Preparations | 醋酸可的松注射液（混悬液）：每瓶 125mg（5ml）。<br>醋酸可的松片：每片 5mg；25mg。<br>Cortisone acetate injection (suspension): a bottle of 125mg (5ml).<br>Cortisone acetate tablets: 5mg per tablet; 25mg. |
|---|---|

## 16.2　雄激素及同化激素 Androgen and protein anabolic hormone

| 药品名称 Drug Names | 丙酸睾酮 Testosterone Propionate |
|---|---|
| 适应证<br>Indications | 原发性或继发性男性性功能减低，男性青春期发育迟缓；绝经期后女性晚期乳腺癌的姑息治疗等。<br>Primary or secondary decline of male sexual function, male adolescent developmental delays;Palliative treatment for advanced breast cancer of post-menopausal women, etc. |
| 用法、用量<br>Dosage | （1）成人常用量深部肌内注射，每次 25 ~ 50mg，每周 2 ~ 3 次。儿童常用量，每次 12.5 ~ 25mg，每周 2 ~ 3 次，疗程不超过 4 ~ 6 个月。<br>（2）功能性子宫出血，配合黄体酮肌内注射，每次 25 ~ 50mg，一日 1 次，共 3 ~ 4 次。<br>（3）绝经妇女晚期乳腺癌姑息性治疗，每次 50 ~ 100mg，每周 3 次，共用 2 ~ 3 个月。<br>(1) For adults, usual dose of deep intramuscular injection, 25 to 50 mg singly, 2 to 3 times a week. Usual dose for child, 12.5 ~ 25 mg singly, 2 to 3 times a week, with treatment course no more than 4 to 6 months.<br>(2) Functional uterine bleeding, with the use of intramuscular injections of progesterone, 25~50 mg singly, 1 times a day, a total of 3 to 4 times.<br>(3) palliative treatment for advanced breast cancer of post-menopausal women, 50 ~ 100 mg singly, three times a week, and the total treatment time within 2 to 3 months. |
| 剂型、规格<br>Preparations | 注射剂（油溶液）：每支 10mg（1ml）；25mg（1ml）；50mg（1ml）。<br>Injection (oil solution) : 10 mg (1 ml) ;25 mg (1 ml);50 mg (1 ml) per bottle. |
| 药品名称 Drug Names | 苯丙酸诺龙 Nandrolone Phenylpropionate |
| 适应证<br>Indications | 慢性消耗性疾病、严重灼伤、手术前后骨折不易愈合和骨质疏松症、早产儿、儿童发育不良等。尚可用于不可手术的乳腺癌、功能性子宫出血、子宫肌瘤等。<br>Chronic wasting disease, severe burns, before and after surgery, difficult to heal for bone fracture before and after surgery and osteoporosis, premature infants, stunted children, etc.It also can be used in treating inoperable diseases like breast cancer, functional uterine bleeding, uterine fibroids, etc. |
| 用法、用量<br>Dosage | 深部肌内注射：成人每次 25mg，每 1 ~ 2 周 1 次，儿童每次 10mg，婴儿每次 5mg。女性转移性乳腺癌姑息性治疗，每周 25 ~ 100mg，疗程的长短视疗效及不良反应而定。<br>Deep intramuscular injection: for adult, 25 mg singly, one time every 1 to 2 weeks; for children, give 10 mg singly; for baby, give 5 mg singly. Palliative treatment for women with metastatic breast cancer, 25 ~ 100 mg a week, the length of treatment course depends on efficacy and adverse reactions. |
| 剂型、规格<br>Preparations | 注射液（油溶液）：每支 10mg（1ml）；25mg（1ml）。<br>Injection (oil solution) : 10 mg (1 ml) ;25 mg (1 ml) per bottle. |
| 药品名称 Drug Names | 司坦唑醇 Stanozolol |
| 适应证<br>Indications | 预防和治疗遗传性血管神经性水肿、慢性消耗性疾病、重病及手术后体弱消瘦、年老体弱、骨质疏松症、小儿发育不良、再生障碍性贫血、白细胞减少症、血小板减少症、高脂血症等。还用于防治长期使用皮质激素引起的肾上腺皮质功能减退。<br>It is used to prevent and treat hereditary angioneurotic oedema, chronic wasting disease, serious illness, weakness and marasmus after the operation, weakness of old age, osteoporosis, infantile dysplasia, aplastic anemia, leukopenia, thrombocytopenia, hyperlipidemia, etc.It is also used to prevent and treat adrenocortical function caused by long-term use of hormone of fat loss. |
| 用法、用量<br>Dosage | 口服：成人，开始时每次 2mg，一日 2 ~ 3 次（女性酌减）。如治疗效果明显，可每隔 1 ~ 3 个月减量，直至每日 2mg 维持量。儿童，每日 1 ~ 2mg，仅在发作时应用。<br>Oral medication: for adults, at the beginning 2mg singly, 2 or 3 times a day(female dosage should be reduced accordingly ). If the treatment effect is obvious, then dosage should be reduced every 1 to 3 months until the maintenance dose of 2mg a day. For children, give daily dose of 1 ~ 2mg, applied only under seizures of disease. |

**续　表**

| 剂型、规格<br>Preparations | 片剂：每片 2mg。<br>Tablets: 2mg per tablet. |
|---|---|
| 药品名称 Drug Names | 达那唑 Danazol |
| 适应证<br>Indications | 治疗子宫内膜异位症，尚用于纤维性乳腺炎、男性乳房发育、乳腺痛、痛经、腹痛等，可使肿块消失、软化或缩小，使疼痛消失或减轻。还用于性早熟、自发性血小板减少性紫癜、血友病和 Christmas 病（凝血因子Ⅸ缺乏）、遗传性血管性水肿、系统性红斑狼疮等。<br><br>It is used to treat endometriosis, still used in fiber mastitis, gynecomastia, breast pain, dysmenorrhea, abdominal pain, It can make lumps disappear, softening or narrow, also make the pain disappear or reduce. It is also used to treat precocious puberty, idiopathic thrombocytopenic purpura, hemophilia and Christmas disease (lack of clotting factor Ⅸ ), hereditary angioedema, systemic lupus erythematosus, etc. |
| 用法、用量<br>Dosage | （1）子宫内膜异位症：口服，从月经周期第 1 ~ 3 日开始服用，一日 2 次，每次 200 ~ 400mg，总量一天不超过 800mg，连续 3 ~ 6 个月为 1 个疗程，必要时可继续到第 9 个月。<br>（2）纤维性乳腺炎：口服，每次 50 ~ 200mg，一日 2 次，连用 3 ~ 6 个月。<br>（3）男性乳房发育：口服，每日 200 ~ 600mg。<br>（4）性早熟：口服，每日 200 ~ 400mg。<br>（5）血小板减少性紫癜：口服，每次 200mg，一日 2 ~ 4 次。<br>（6）血友病：口服，每日 600mg，连用 14 天。<br>（7）遗传性血管性水肿：口服，开始每次 200mg，一日 2 ~ 3 次。急性发作时，剂量可提高到 200mg。<br>（8）红斑狼疮：每日 400 ~ 600mg。<br><br>(1) Endometriosis: oral medication, start to take it from the first to third day of menstrual cycle, 2 times a day, 200 ~ 400mg singly, daily dose does not exceed a total amount of 800mg, 3 to 6 consecutive months for a treatment course, and take it for nine consecutive months if necessary.<br>(2) Fiber mastitis: oral medication, 50 ~ 200mg singly, 2 times a day, for 3 to 6 months.<br>(3) Gynecomastia: oral medication, daily dose of 200 ~ 600mg.<br>(4) Precocious puberty: oral medication, daily dose of 200 ~ 400mg.<br>(5) Thrombocytopenic purpura: oral medication, 200mg singly, 2 to 4 times a day .<br>(6) Hemophilia: oral medication, daily dose of 600mg, for 14 days.<br>(7) Hereditary angioedema: oral medication, at the beginning 200mg singly, 2 to 3 times a day. When acute attack happens, the dose can be increased to 200mg.<br>(8) Erythematosus: 400 ~ 600mg a day. |
| 剂型、规格<br>Preparations | 胶囊剂：每粒 100mg；200mg。<br>Capsules: 100 mg;200 mg per capsule. |

## 16.3　雌激素及其类似合成药物 Estrogen and its similar synthetic drugs

| 药品名称 Drug Names | 雌二醇 Estradiol |
|---|---|
| 适应证<br>Indications | 卵巢功能不全或卵巢激素不足引起的各种症状，主要是功能性子宫出血、原发性闭经、绝经期综合征及前列腺癌等。<br><br>A variety of symptoms caused by ovarian dysfunction or ovarian hormone deficiency, mainly functional uterine bleeding, primary amenorrhea, menopause syndrome, prostate cancer, etc. |
| 用法、用量<br>Dosage | 肌内注射：每次 0.5 ~ 1.5mg，每周 2 ~ 3 次。口服，一日 1 片。<br>Intramuscular injection: 0.5 ~ 1.5 mg singly, 2 to 3 times a week.Oral medication, 1 time a day. |
| 剂型、规格<br>Preparations | 注射液：每支 2mg（1ml）。<br>凝胶：每支 80g；0.06%。<br>片剂：每片 1mg。<br>微粒化 17β 雌二醇片：每片 1mg；2mg。<br>控释贴片：周效片，每片 2.5mg；3 ~ 4 日效片：每片 4mg。<br><br>Injection: 2mg (1 ml)per bottle. Gel: 80g per bottle;0.06%. Tablets: 1mg per tablet. Micronized 17β estradiol tablets: 1mg; 2mg per tablet . Controlled-release patch: weekly patch, 2.5mg per patch; patch used every 3 to 4 days: 4mg per patch. |

**续　表**

| 药品名称 Drug Names | 苯甲酸雌二醇 Estradiol Benzoate |
|---|---|
| 适应证<br>Indications | 卵巢功能不全、闭经、绝经期综合征、退奶及前列腺癌等。<br>Ovarian dysfunction, menopause, menopausal syndrome, suppression of lactation and prostate cancer, etc. |
| 用法、用量<br>Dosage | （1）绝经期综合征：肌内注射，每次 1 ～ 2mg，每 3 日一次。<br>（2）子宫发育不良：肌内注射，每次 1 ～ 2mg，每 2 ～ 3 日一次。<br>（3）子宫出血：肌内注射，每次 1mg，一日 1 次，1 周后继续用黄体酮。<br>(1) Menopausal syndrome: intramuscular injection, 1 ～ 2 mg singly, once every 3 days.<br>(2) Uterine dysplasia: intramuscular injection, 1 ～ 2 mg singly, once every 2 to 3 days.<br>(3) Uterine bleeding: intramuscular injection, 1 mg singly, 1 time a day, after a week, continue to use progesterone. |
| 剂型、规格<br>Preparations | 注射液：每支 1mg（1ml）；2mg（1ml）。<br>Injection: 1 mg (1 ml);2 mg (1 ml)per bottle. |
| 药品名称 Drug Names | 戊酸雌二醇 Estradiol Valerate |
| 适应证<br>Indications | 口服缓解绝经后更年期症状、卵巢切除后及非癌性疾病、放疗性去势的雌激素缺乏引起的症状，外用于治疗扁平疣。<br>Oral medication can alleviate symptoms of menopause after menopause, symptoms caused by ovarian resection, non cancerous disease, and estrogen deficiency by radiotherapy of castration, external use of the drug can treat verruca plana. |
| 用法、用量<br>Dosage | 肌内注射：每次 5 ～ 10mg，每 1 ～ 2 周一次，平均替代治疗剂量为每 2 周 5 ～ 20mg，用于卵巢功能不全，每次 5 ～ 20mg，每月 1 次。口服，每日 1 ～ 2mg，连续 21 日，停服 1 周后开始下 1 个疗程。<br>Intramuscular injection: 5 ～ 10mg singly, once every 1 to 2 weeks, the average replacement therapy dose of 5 ～ 20mg, every 2 weeks, for ovarian disfunction, 5 ～ 20mg singly, 1 times a month.Oral medication, 1 ～ 2mg a day, for 21 days, continue the next course of treatment after stoping taking it for one week. |
| 剂型、规格<br>Preparations | 注射液：每支 5mg（1ml）；10mg（1ml）。<br>片剂：每片 0.5mg；1mg；2mg。<br>Injection: 5mg (1ml); 10mg (1ml) per bottle.<br>Tablets: 0.5mg; 1mg; 2mg per tablet. |
| 药品名称 Drug Names | 炔雌醇 Ethinylestradiol |
| 适应证<br>Indications | 月经紊乱，如闭经、月经过少、功能性子宫出血、绝经期综合征，子宫发育不全、前列腺癌等。也作为口服避孕药中常用的雌激素成分。<br>Menstrual disorders, such as amenorrhea, scanty menstrual flow, functional uterine bleeding, menopausal syndrome, uterus dysgenesis, prostate cancer, etc.It is also used commonly as estrogen component in oral contraceptives. |
| 用法、用量<br>Dosage | 口服：每次 0.012 5 ～ 0.05mg，每晚服用 1 次，用于前列腺癌每次 0.05 ～ 0.5mg，一日 3 次。<br>Oral medication: 0.012 5 ～ 0.05mg singly, take 1 time every night, when used to treat prostate cancer, take 0.05 ～ 0.5 mg singly, 3 times a day. |
| 剂型、规格<br>Preparations | 片剂：每片 5μg；12.5μg；50μg；500μg。<br>Tablets: 5μg; 12.5μg; 50μg; 500μg per tablet. |
| 药品名称 Drug Names | 雌三醇 Estriol |
| 适应证<br>Indications | 绝经后妇女因雌激素缺乏而引起的泌尿生殖道萎缩和萎缩性阴道炎（及老年性阴道炎），表现为外阴或阴道干燥、瘙痒、灼热、阴道分泌物异常及性交疼痛或尿频、尿急、尿失禁等症状。<br>Urogenital atrophy and atrophic vaginitis (and senile vaginitis) caused by estrogen deficiency after menopause, manifested by the vulva or vagina dry, itching, burning, abnormal vaginal discharge, pain during sexual intercourse, urinary frequency, urinary urgency, urinary incontinence, etc. |

| | |
|---|---|
| 用法、用量<br>Dosage | 阴道给药，常用剂量为一日 2mg，连续治疗 1 周，以后每周放置 1 粒维持或遵医嘱。绝经后妇女阴道手术前后，在手术前 2 周，每天使用 1 次 0.5g 软膏，术后 2 周内每周用药 2 次。可疑宫颈涂片辅助诊断检查前 1 周内，每 2 天用药 1 次，每次用 0.5g 乳膏。<br><br>Vaginal drug delivery, commonly used dose of 2 mg a day, continuous treatment for 1 week, afterwards place 1 grain into the vagina once a week or adhere to the instructions of the physician .To postmenopausal women with vaginal surgery, in the the two weeks before the surgery, use 0.5 g ointment, 1 time a day, in the two weeks after the surgery use the medicine two times a week.One week before inspection of S suspicious cervical smear auxiliary diagnosis medication use 1 time every 2 days, with 0.5 g cream singly . |
| 剂型、规格<br>Preparations | 栓剂：每枚 0.5mg；1mg；2mg。<br>乳膏：15g；15mg。<br><br>Suppositories: 0.5mg; 1mg; 2mg for each.<br>Cream: 15g: 15mg. |
| 药品名称 Drug Names | 尼尔雌醇 Nilestriol |
| 适应证<br>Indications | 用于雌激素缺乏引起的绝经期或更年期综合征，如潮热、出汗、头痛、目眩、疲劳、烦躁易怒、神经过敏、外阴干燥、老年性阴道炎等。<br><br>It is used to treat menopause or menopausal syndrome caused by lack of estrogen, such as hot flashes, sweating, headache, dizzy, fatigue, irritability, nervousness, vulva dry, senile vaginitis, etc. |
| 用法、用量<br>Dosage | 口服：一次 5mg，每月 1 次。症状改善后维持量为每次 1 ～ 2mg，每月 2 次，3 个月为 1 个疗程。<br><br>Oral medication: 5mg singly, 1 time a month. After symptoms improved maintain the dose of 1 ～ 2mg singly, 2 times a month, three months for a treatment course. |
| 剂型、规格<br>Preparations | 片剂：每片 1mg；2mg；5mg。<br>Tablets: 1mg; 2mg; 5mg per tablet. |
| 药品名称 Drug Names | 己烯雌酚 Diethylstilbestrol |
| 适应证<br>Indications | 卵巢功能不全或垂体功能异常引起的各种疾病、闭经、子宫发育不全、功能性子宫出血、绝经期综合征、老年性阴道炎等。也用于不能进行手术的晚期前列腺癌。<br><br>Various diseases, amenorrhea, uterine hypoplasia, dysfunctional uterine bleeding, menopausal syndrome, and senile vaginitis, etc.caused by ovarian dysfunction or pituitary dysfunction. It is also used to treat inoperable advanced prostate cancer. |
| 用法、用量<br>Dosage | （1）闭经：口服小剂量刺激垂体前叶分泌促性腺激素，每日不超过 0.25mg。<br>（2）用于人工月经周期：每日服 0.25mg，连用 20 日，待月经后再用同法治疗，共 3 个周期。<br>（3）用于月经周期延长及子宫发育不全：每日服 0.1 ～ 0.2mg，持续半年，经期停服。<br>（4）治疗功能性子宫出血：每晚服 0.5 ～ 1mg，连服 20 日。<br>（5）用于绝经期综合征：每日服 0.25mg，症状控制后改为每日 0.1mg。<br>（6）老年性阴道炎：阴道塞药，每晚塞入 0.2 ～ 0.4mg，共用 7 日。<br>（7）配合手术用于前列腺癌：每日 3mg，分 3 次服，连用 2 ～ 3 个月，维持量每日 1mg。<br>（8）用于因子宫发育不良及子宫颈分泌物黏稠所致不育症：以小剂量促使宫颈黏液稀薄，精子宜透入，于月经后每日服 0.1mg，共 15 日，疗程为 3 ～ 6 个月。<br>（9）用于稽留流产（妊娠 7 个月内死胎经 2 个月或以上仍未娩出）：每次服 5mg，一日 3 次，5 ～ 7 日为 1 个疗程，停药 5 日，如无效，可重复 1 个疗程。<br><br>(1) Amenorrhea : oral medication of low-dose stimulates pituitary front to secret gonadotropin. Daily dose does not exceed 0.25mg.<br>(2) It is used in artificial menstrual cycle : daily dose of 0.25mg, for consecutive 20 days, use the same method after menstruation, for a total of three cycles.<br>(3) It is used to treat prolonged menstrual cycle and uterine hypoplasia :0.1 ～ 0.2mg a day, for six months, stop taking it in menstruation .<br>(4) It is used to treat dysfunctional uterine bleeding : 0.5 ～ 1mg every evening, for 20 days .<br>(5) It is used to treat menopausal syndrome: 0.25mg a day, after symptoms controlled, change the daily dose to 0.1mg.<br>(6) Senile vaginitis : vaginal suppository, stuff 0.2 ～ 0.4mg every evening, for seven days . |

| | |
|---|---|
| | (7) Cooperate with surgery for prostate cancer : 3mg a day in 3 doses, for two to three months, a daily maintenance dose of 1mg.<br><br>(8) It is used to treat infertility caused by uterine hypoplasia and thick cervical secretions : small doses promote cervical mucus to be thin, and sperm penetration, after menstruation daily dose of 0.1mg, for 15 days, treatment course for 3 to 6 months .<br><br>(9) It is used to treat missed abortion ( pregnancy, stillbirth within seven months after two months or more have not delivered ) : 5mg singly, 3 times a day with treatment course of 5 to 7 days, afterwards stop taking it for five days, repeat a treatment course if there is no effect. |
| 剂型、规格<br>Preparations | 片剂：每片 0.5mg；1mg；2mg。<br>注射液：每支 0.5mg（1ml）；1mg（1ml）；2mg（1ml）。<br>Tablets: 0.5mg; 1mg; 2mg per tablet.<br>Injection: 0.5mg (1ml); 1mg (1ml); 2mg (1ml) per bottle. |

16.4 孕激素类 Progestogens

| 药品名称 Drug Names | 黄体酮 Progesterone |
|---|---|
| 适应证<br>Indications | 用于习惯性流产、痛经、经血过多或血崩症、闭经等。口服大剂量也用于黄体酮不足所致疾病，如经前综合征、排卵停止所致月经紊乱、良性乳腺病、围绝经期激素替代疗法。<br><br>It is used to treat habitual abortion, dysmenorrhea, hemorrhage or metrorrhagia, amenorrhea, etc. Oral medication of high dose also treat diseases caused by progesterone deficiency, such as menstrual disorders, benign breast disease caused by premenstrual syndrome, anovulation, and hormone replacement therapy in perimenopausal period. |
| 用法、用量<br>Dosage | （1）习惯性流产：肌内注射，一次 10 ~ 20mg，一日 1 次，或每周 2 ~ 3 次，一直用到妊娠第 4 个月。<br><br>（2）先兆流产：肌内注射，一般每日 20 ~ 50mg，待疼痛及出血停止后减为每日 10 ~ 20mg。<br><br>（3）痛经：在月经之前 6 ~ 8 日每天肌内注射 5 ~ 10mg，共 4 ~ 6 日，疗程可重复若干次，对子宫发育不全所致的痛经，可与雌激素配合使用。<br><br>（4）经血过多和血崩症：肌内注射，每日 10 ~ 20mg，5 ~ 7 日为 1 个疗程，可重复 3 ~ 4 个疗程，每疗程间隔 15 ~ 20 日。<br><br>（5）闭经：先肌内注射雌激素 2 ~ 3 周后，立即给予本品，每日肌内注射 3 ~ 5mg，6 ~ 8 日为 1 个疗程，总剂量不宜超过 300 ~ 350mg，疗程可重复 2 ~ 3 次。<br><br>（6）功能性出血：肌内注射，每日 5 ~ 10mg，连用 5 ~ 10 日，如在用药期间月经来潮，应立即停药。<br><br>(1) Habitual abortion: intramuscular injection, 10 ~ 20 mg singly, one times a day, or 2 to 3 times a week, use it to the fourth month of pregnancy.<br><br>(2) Threatened abortion: intramuscular injection, generally 20~50 mg a day, reduce to 10 ~ 20 mg a day after the stop of pain and bleeding.<br><br>(3) Dysmenorrhea: intramuscular injection of 5 ~ 10 mg a day for 6 to 8 days before menstruation, a total of 4 to 6 days, treatment course can be repeated for several times, to treat dysmenorrhea caused by the uterus dysgenesis, it can be used with estrogen.<br><br>(4) Hemorrhage and metrorrhagia: intramuscular injection, 10 ~ 20 mg a day, 5 to 7 days for a treatment course, repeat of 3 to 4 treatment courses is permitted, an interval of 15 to 20 days before the next treatment course.<br><br>(5) Amenorrhea: first intramuscular injection of estrogen for 2 ~ 3 weeks, afterwards use the medication immediately, intramuscular injection of 3 ~ 5 mg a day, 6 to 8 days, for a treatment course, the total dose should not be more than 300 ~ 350 mg, treatment course can be repeated for 2 to 3 times.<br><br>(6) Functional bleeding: intramuscular injection, 5 ~ 10 mg a day for 5 to 10 days, stop the medication immediately if menstrual cramps happens during the administration . |
| 剂型、规格<br>Preparations | 注射液：每支 10mg（1ml）；20mg（1ml）。<br>胶囊：每粒 100mg。<br>Injection: 10mg (1ml); 20mg (1ml)per bottle.<br>Capsules: 100mg per capsule. |

| 药品名称 Drug Names | 甲羟孕酮 Medroxyprogesterone |
|---|---|
| 适应证<br>Indications | 痛经、功能性闭经、功能性子宫出血、先兆流产或习惯性流产、子宫内膜异位症等。大剂量可用作长效避孕针，肌内注射 1 次 150mg，可避孕 3 个月。<br><br>Dysmenorrhea, functional sex amenorrhoea, functional uterine bleeding, threatened abortion, habitual abortion or endometriosis, etc.Large doses can be used as a long-acting contraceptive injections, intramuscular injection of 150 mg singly, can last the effect of contraception for 3 months. |
| 用法、用量<br>Dosage | （1）功能性闭经：每日口服 4 ~ 8mg，连用 5 ~ 10 日。<br>（2）子宫内膜癌或肾癌：口服，一次 100mg，一日 3 次，肌内注射，起始 0.4 ~ 1g，1 周后可重复一次，待病情改善或稳定后，剂量改为 400mg，每月 1 次。<br>（3）避孕：肌内注射，每 3 个月一次 150mg，于月经来潮第 2 ~ 7 日注射。<br><br>（1）Functional amenorrhea: oral medication of 4 ~ 8mg a day, for 5 to 10 days.<br>（2）Endometrial cancer or kidney cancer: oral medication, 100mg singly, 3 times a day, intramuscular injection, 0.4 ~ 1g at the beginning, the process can be repeated a week later. When disease to be improved or stable, change the dose to 400mg, 1 time every month .<br>（3）Contraception: intramuscular injection, take 150mg every three months, use the injection on the second to seventh day of menstruation. |
| 剂型、规格<br>Preparations | 片剂：每片 2mg；4mg；10mg。注射液：100mg；150mg。<br>Tablets: 2mg; 4mg; 10mg per tablet. Injection: 100mg; 150mg. |
| 药品名称 Drug Names | 炔孕酮 Ethisterone |
| 适应证<br>Indications | 功能性子宫出血、月经异常、闭经、痛经等。也用于防止先兆性流产和习惯性流产，但由于维持妊娠作用较弱，效果并不好。如与雌激素炔雌醇合用，则疗效较好。<br><br>Dysfunctional uterine bleeding, menstrual abnormalities, amenorrhea, dysmenorrhea, etc.It is also used to prevent threatened abortion and habitual abortion, due to the weak maintain pregnancy, the effect is not good.If the medication combine with estrogen ethinyl estradiol, the curative effect will be better. |
| 用法、用量<br>Dosage | 口服：一次 10mg，一日 3 次。舌下含服：一次 10 ~ 20mg，一日 2 ~ 3 次。<br>Oral medication: 10mg singly, 3 times a day. Sublingual administration: 10 ~ 20mg singly, 2 or 3 times a day. |
| 剂型、规格<br>Preparations | 片剂：每片 5mg；10mg；25mg。<br>Tablets: 5 mg ;10 mg; 25 mg per tablet. |
| 药品名称 Drug Names | 屈螺酮 Drospirenone |
| 适应证<br>Indications | 女性避孕。<br>Female contraceptive. |
| 用法、用量<br>Dosage | 必须按照包装所表明的顺序，每天约在同一时间用少量液体送服。每日 1 片，连服 21 日。停药 7 日后开始服用下一盒药，其间通常会出现撤退性出血。<br><br>You must follow the order indicated on the packaging that every day around the same time the medication is to be taken with a small amount of liquid. one tablet a day, for 21 successive days. After 7 days of medication withdrawal, began taking the next box of medicine, during which withdrawal bleeding usually occurs. |
| 剂型、规格<br>Preparations | 复方制剂（优思明）：每片含屈螺酮 3mg 和炔雌醇 0.03mg。<br>Compound preparations (Yasmin) : containing 3 mg of Drospirenone and 0.03 mg of ethinyl estradiol . |

## 16.5 促性腺激素 Gonadotrophin

| 药品名称 Drug Names | 绒毛膜促性腺激素 Chorionic Gonadotrophin |
|---|---|
| 适应证<br>Indications | （1）青春期隐睾症的诊断和治疗。<br>（2）垂体功能低下所致的男性不育。<br>（3）垂体促性腺激素不足所致的女性无排卵性不孕症。 |

续　表

| | |
|---|---|
| | （4）用于体外受精以获取多个卵母细胞。<br>（5）女性黄体功能不足、功能性子宫出血、妊娠早期先兆流产、习惯性流产。<br>(1) It is used to diagnosis and treat adolescent cryptorchidism.<br>(2) Male infertility caused by hypopituitarism .<br>(3) Women's anovulatory infertility caused by pituitary gonadotropin deficiency.<br>(4) It is used in vitro fertilization to obtain multiple oocytes.<br>(5) Female luteal insufficiency, dysfunctional uterine bleeding, threatened abortion in early pregnancy, habitual abortion. |
| 用法、用量<br>Dosage | （1）促排卵：于绝经后促性腺激素末次给药后一天或氯米芬末次给药后 5 ~ 7 日肌内注射一次 5000 ~ 10 000U，连续治疗 3 ~ 6 周期，如无效，应停药。<br>（2）黄体功能不足：于经期第 15 ~ 17 日排卵之日起，隔日注射一次 1500U，连用 5 次，剂量可根据患者的反应做调整，妊娠后需维持原剂量直至 7 ~ 10 孕周。<br>（3）功能性子宫出血：肌内注射一次 1000 ~ 3000 单位。<br>（4）青春期前隐睾症，肌内注射一次，1000 ~ 5000U，每周 2 ~ 3 次。<br>（5）男性性功能减退症：肌内注射一次 1000 ~ 4000U，每周 2 ~ 3 次，持续数周至数月。<br>（6）先兆流产或习惯性流产：肌内注射一次 1000 ~ 5000U。<br>(1) Ovulation: in postmenopausal, the day after the last administration of gonadotropin or 5 to 7 days after the last administration of clomiphene, intramuscular injection of 5000 ~10, 000U for once, continuous treatment for 3 to 6 cycles, if invalid, it should be discontinued.<br>(2) Luteal insufficiency: 15 to 17 days from the first day of menstruation in ovulation, 1500U is injected once every other day, for a total of five times, the dose may be adjusted according to the patient's response, after pregnancy, the original dose is required to maintain pregnancy for 7 to 10 weeks of gestation.<br>(3) Dysfunctional uterine bleeding: intramuscular injection of 1000 ~3000U singly.<br>(4) Prepubertal cryptorchidism, intramuscular injection, of 1000 ~5000U singly, two to three times a week.<br>(5)Male sexual dysfunction syndrome: intramuscular injection of 1000 ~ 4000U singly, 2 to 3 times a week, for several weeks to several months.<br>(6)Threatened abortion or habitual abortion: intramuscular injection of 1000 ~5000U singly. |
| 剂型、规格<br>Preparations | 注射用绒促性素：每支 500U；1000U；2000U；5000U。<br>HCG Injection: 500U; 1000U; 2000U; 5000U per bottle. |
| 药品名称 Drug Names | 尿促性素 Menotrophin |
| 适应证<br>Indications | ①与绒促性素或氯米芬配合使用以治疗无排卵性不孕症。②用于原发性或继发性闭经，男性精子缺乏症以及卵巢功能试验等。<br>① It is used in conjunction with HCG or clomiphene in treating anovulatory infertility.　② It is used to treat primary or secondary amenorrhea, male sperm deficiency and ovarian function tests, etc. |
| 用法、用量<br>Dosage | 肌内注射：用于诱导排卵，开始每天 75 ~ 150U，连用 7 ~ 12 日，至雌激素水平增高后，再肌内注射绒促性素，经 12 小时即排卵。用于男性性功能低下，开始 1 周给予 HCG 每次 2000U，共 2 ~ 3 次，以产生适当的男性特征。然后肌内注射本品，每次 75 ~ 150U，每周 3 次，同时给予 HCG 每次 2000U，每周 2 次。至少治疗 4 个月。<br>Intramuscular injection: It is used to induce ovulation, 75 ~150U a day at the beginning for 7 to12 successive days, after estrogen levels increase, then use intramuscular injection of hCG, 12 hours later ovulation will occur.It is also used to treat low male sexual function, use 2000 U of hCG, for a total of 2 to 3 times a week, to generate the appropriate masculinity .And use intramuscular injection of this product, 75 ~ 150 U singly, three times a week, with 2000U of hCG at the same time, 2 times a week, for at least 4 months. |
| 剂型、规格<br>Preparations | 注射用尿促性素：每支 75U；150U。<br>Injection of hMG: 75U; 150U per bottle. |
| 药品名称 Drug Names | 普罗瑞林 Protirelin |
| 适应证<br>Indications | 用于诊断 Graves 病、甲状腺功能减退症及促甲状腺素性突眼等。<br>It is used to diagnose Graves disease, hypothyroidism and thyrotropic exophthalmos, etc. |

| | |
|---|---|
| 用法、用量<br>Dosage | 静脉注射本品 200 ~ 500μg，观察血中促甲状腺激素水平的变化，正常人于注射后15 ~ 30分钟达峰值，为基础值的 2 ~ 3 倍以上。<br><br>Use intravenous injection of 200 ~ 500 μg of the drug, and observe changes in thyroid stimulating hormone levels in the blood, which peak for normal at 15 to 30 minutes after injection, 2 to 3 times of baseline. |
| 剂型、规格<br>Preparations | 注射用普罗瑞林：0.5mg。<br>Injection protirelin: 0.5mg. |
| 药品名称 Drug Names | 亮丙瑞林 Leuprorelin |
| 适应证<br>Indications | 子宫内膜异位症，对伴有月经过多、下腹痛、腰痛及贫血等的子宫肌瘤，可使肌瘤缩小和（或）症状改善，绝经前乳腺癌且雌激素受体阳性患者；前列腺癌、中枢性性早熟症。<br><br>Endometriosis, accompanied by menorrhagia, abdominal pain, waist pain and anemia, such as uterine fibroids, can narrow fibroids and (or) improve symptoms, premenopausal breast cancer and patients with estrogen receptor-positive; prostate cancer, central precocious puberty. |
| 用法、用量<br>Dosage | 前列腺癌、绝经前乳腺癌，皮下注射，每次 3.75mg，每 4 周 1 次。子宫内膜异位症：通常成人皮下注射，每次 3.75mg，每 4 周一次，对体重低于 50kg 时，可以使用 1.88mg 的制剂。初次给药于经期开始后的第 1 ~ 5 日。子宫肌瘤：通常成人皮下注射每次 1.88mg，每 4 周 1 次，对体重过重或子宫明显增大的患者，应注射 3.75mg。初次给药于经期开始后的 1 ~ 5 日。中枢性性早熟症：通常皮下注射 30μg/kg，每 4 周 1 次，根据患者症状可增量至 90μg/kg。<br><br>Prostate cancer, breast cancer before menopause, subcutaneous injection, 3.75 mg singly, once for every 4 weeks. Endometriosis: Usually adopt subcutaneous injection for adults, 3.75 mg singly, once for every 4 weeks, if the patient's weight is lower than 50 kg, 1.88 mg preparation may be used. The first drug delivery should be in the 1st to the 5th day during the period. .Uterine fibroids: adults usually receive subcutaneous injection of 1.88 mg singly, once for every 4 weeks, the overweight patients or those with obvious hysterauxesis should inject 3.75 mg. The first drug delivery should be in the 1st to the 5th day during the period .Central precocious puberty disease: 30 μg /kg, usually subcutaneously once for every 4 weeks, according to the symptoms can increase to 90 μg/kg. |
| 剂型、规格<br>Preparations | 注射用亮丙瑞林微球：3.75mg/ 瓶。<br>Leuprolide microspheres for Injection : 3.75mg / bottle. |
| 药品名称 Drug Names | 戈舍瑞林 Goserelin |
| 适应证<br>Indications | 前列腺癌：本品适用于可用激素治疗的前列腺癌。乳腺癌：适用于可用激素治疗的绝经前期及围绝经期妇女的乳腺癌。子宫内膜异位症：缓解症状包括减轻疼痛并减少子宫内膜损伤的大小和数目。<br><br>Prostate cancer: this product is suitable for prostate cancer which can be treated with hormone. Breast cancer: suitable for women with premenopausal or perimenopausal breast cancer which can be treated with hormone. Endometriosis: relieve symptoms, including relieving pain and reducing the size and number of endometrial lesions. |
| 用法、用量<br>Dosage | 腹部皮下注射植入剂：每 28 日一次，每次 3.6mg，如果必要可使用局部麻醉。子宫内膜异位症者治疗不应超过 6 个月。<br><br>Abdominal subcutaneous implantation dose: once every 28 days, 3.6 mg singly, can use local anesthesia if necessary. Endometriosis should not be treated more than 6 months. |
| 剂型、规格<br>Preparations | 缓释植入剂：每支 3.6mg。<br>Release implants: 3.6mg per vial. |
| 药品名称 Drug Names | 丙氨瑞林 Alarelin |
| 适应证<br>Indications | 子宫内膜异位症。<br>Endometriosis. |
| 用法、用量<br>Dosage | 皮下或肌内注射，从月经来潮的第 1 ~ 2 日开始治疗，每次 150μg，一日 1 次，或遵医嘱。制剂在临用前用 2ml 灭菌生理盐水溶解。对子宫内膜异位症，3 ~ 6 个月为 1 个疗程。<br><br>Subcutaneous or intramuscular injection, starting treatment from the 1st to the 2nd day of the menstrual period, 150μg singly, once a day, or as directed by the doctor's advice. Dissolve the preparation in 2 ml sterilization saline water before use. For endometriosis, a treatment course lasts 3 to 6 months. |

**续　表**

| 剂型、规格<br>Preparations | 注射用阿拉瑞林：每支 25μg；150μg。<br>Alarelin for Injection: 25μg per vial; 150μg. |
|---|---|
| **药品名称 Drug Names** | **曲普瑞林 Triptorelin** |
| 适应证<br>Indications | 临床主要用于前列腺癌，还用于促排卵，治疗妇女不育症。<br>Clinically, it is mainly used to treat prostate cancer, also to stimulate ovulation and treat women infertility. |
| 用法、用量<br>Dosage | 缓释剂型仅可肌内注射，一次 1 支，每 4 周 1 次。皮下注射：一日 1 次 0.1mg。用于促排卵：于月经周期第 2 日开始，一日 1 次，0.1mg，连续 10 ~ 12 日。<br>Sustained-release dosage form can only be injected intramuscularly, give one bottle singly, once for every 4 weeks. Subcutaneous injection: 0.1 mg singly, once a day. Used to stimulate ovulation: start from the 2nd day of the menstrual cycle, once a day, 0.1 mg, for 10 to12 days of continous treatment. |
| 剂型、规格<br>Preparations | 粉针剂：每支 0.1mg。<br>Powder-injection: 0.1mg per vial. |

16.6　短效口服避孕药 Short acting oral contraceptives

| **药品名称 Drug Names** | **炔诺酮 Norethindrone** |
|---|---|
| 适应证<br>Indications | 除作为口服避孕药外，还可用于功能性子宫出血、妇女不育症、痛经、闭经、子宫内膜异位症、子宫内膜增生过长等。<br>In addition to oral contraceptives, it can also be used to treat dysfunctional uterine bleeding, women infertility, dysmenorrhea, amenorrhea, endometriosis, endometrial hyperplasia, etc... |
| 用法、用量<br>Dosage | 口服，一次 1.25 ~ 5mg，一日 1 ~ 2 次。<br>Oral medication, 1.25 to 5mg singly, 1 to 2 times a day. |
| 剂型、规格<br>Preparations | 复方炔诺酮片（避孕片一号）：每片含炔诺酮 0.6mg 和炔雌醇 0.035mg。<br>Compound norethindrone contraceptive tablet (1) : containing 0.6 mg of norethindrone and 0.035 mg of ethinylestradiol per tablet. |
| **药品名称 Drug Names** | **甲地孕酮 Megestrol** |
| 适应证<br>Indications | 主要用作短效口服避孕药，也可作为肌内注射长效避孕药，还可用于治疗痛经、闭经、功能性子宫出血、子宫内膜异位症及子宫内膜腺癌等。由于其抗雌激素活性，亦用于乳腺癌的姑息治疗。<br>Mainly used as a short-acting oral contraceptives, but also as long-acting intramuscular injection, contraception, can also be used in the treatment of dysmenorrhea, amenorrhea, functional uterine bleeding, endometriosis, endometrial adenocarcinoma, and so on. Because of its anti estrogen activity, it is often used in the dividend treatment for breast cancer. |
| 用法、用量<br>Dosage | （1）用作短效口服避孕药：从月经周期第 5 日起，每天口服一片甲地孕酮片、膜或纸片，连服 22 日为 1 个周期，停药后 2 ~ 4 日来月经，然后于第 5 日继续服下一个月的药。<br>（2）治疗功能性子宫出血：口服甲地孕酮片、膜或纸片，每 8 小时一次，每次 2mg，然后将剂量每 3 天递减一次，直至维持量每天 4mg，连服 20 日，流血停止后，每天加服炔雌醇 0.05mg 或己烯雌酚 1mg，共 20 日。<br>（3）闭经：口服，每次一片甲地孕酮片，和炔雌醇 0.05mg，共 20 日，连服 3 个月。<br>（4）痛经和子宫内膜增生过长：于月经第 5 ~ 7 日开始，每天口服一片，共 20 日。<br>（5）子宫内膜异位症：每次一片，一日 2 次，共 7 日，然后每日 3 次，每次 1 片，共 7 天，再后，一日 2 次，每次 2 片，共 7 天，最后每天 20mg，共 6 周。<br>（6）子宫内膜癌：口服，一日 4 次，每次 10 ~ 80mg，连续 2 个月。<br>（7）乳腺癌：口服，一日 4 次，每次 40mg，连续 2 个月为 1 个疗程。<br>(1) used as short-acting oral contraceptives : From the 5th day of the menstrual cycle, take a daily pill of megestrol acetate orally, film or paper, at intervals of 22 days, menstruation comes 2 to 4 days after the discontinuation, then continue the drug dose for the next month from the 5th day. |

续 表

| | (2) treatment of dysfunctional uterine bleeding : take megestrol acetate orally, film or paper, once for every 8 hours, 2mg singly, then descending dose every 3 days until the maintenance dose of 4mg a day, and even served 20 days, after the bleeding stops, take a daily 0.05mg of ethinyl estradiol or 1mg of diethylstilbestrol besides for 20 successive days.<br><br>(3) amenorrhea : Oral medication, one megestrol acetate tablet and 0.05mg of ethinyl estradiol singly for 20 successive days, even served three months.<br><br>(4) dysmenorrhea and endometrial hyperplasia : begin from the 5th to 7th days of menstruation, take one tablet orally everyday, even served 20 days .<br><br>(5) Endometriosis :one tablet singly, twice daily for 7 days, then three times a day, one tablet singly, even served seven days, afterwards 2 times daily, two tablets for 7 days, at last 20mg daily for 6 weeks.<br><br>(6) endometrial cancer: take 4 times a day orally, 10 to 80mg singly, even served 2 months.<br><br>(7) breast cancer : take 4 times orally a day, 40mg singly, at intervals of 2 months. |
|---|---|
| 剂型、规格<br>Preparations | 片剂：每片 1mg；4mg。膜剂：每片 1mg；4mg。纸片：每片 1mg；4mg。<br>Tablets: 1mg per tablet; 4mg. Film formers: 1mg per tablet; 4mg. Paper: 1mg per tablet; 4mg. |
| **药品名称 Drug Names** | 炔诺孕酮 Norgestrel |
| 适应证<br>Indications | 主要以炔雌醇组成复方作为短效口服避孕药，也可通过剂型改变用作长效避孕药，还可用于治疗痛经、月经不调。<br><br>Mainly compound with ethinylestradiol compound as short-acting oral contraceptives, can also be used as long-acting contraception by changing dosage form, as well as in the treatment of dysmenorrheal and irregular menstruation. |
| 用法、用量<br>Dosage | （1）用作短效口服避孕药：口服复方炔诺孕酮一号片或滴丸，从月经第 5 日开始，每天服 1 片（丸），连服 22 日，不能间断，服完后 3～4 日即来月经，并于月经的第 5 日再服下一个月的药。<br><br>（2）用作探亲避孕药：于探亲当晚开始服炔诺孕酮探亲避孕药，一日 1 片，服法同炔诺酮。<br><br>（3）用作房事后避孕药：房事后 72 小时内口服 2 片事后避孕药，12 小时后再服 2 片。<br><br>(1)used as short-acting oral contraceptives: from the 5th day of menstruation, take one tablet or one dropping pill of compound norgestrel orally, 1 tablet(pill) a day, and even served 22 days without interruption, about 3 to 4 days later, the menstruation comes, in the 5th day afterwards, take another dose for a month again.<br><br>(2) used as norethisterone: begin to take norethindrone visiting pills on the evening of visiting relatives one tablet a day, administration as norethindrone.<br><br>(3) used as postcoital contraceptives: take two morning-after pills orally within 72 hours after sex, take another two pills 12 hours later. |
| 剂型、规格<br>Preparations | 复方炔诺酮一号片（复甲一号）：每片含炔诺孕酮 0.3mg 和炔雌醇 0.03mg。<br>Compound norethisterone No.1 tablets (complex No.1): contains 0.3mg norgestrel and 0.03mg ethinyl estradiol per tablet. |

16.7 抗早孕药 Anti-early pregnancy drug

| **药品名称 Drug Names** | 米非司酮 Mifepristone |
|---|---|
| 适应证<br>Indications | 除用于抗早孕、催经止孕、胎死宫内引产外，还用于妇科手术操作，如宫内节育器的放置和取出、取内膜标本、宫颈管发育异常的激光分离及宫颈扩张和刮宫术。<br><br>Except for anti-early pregnancy, inducing menstruation and terminating pregnancy, induction of labor after intrauterine fetal death, can also be used in gynecological surgery operation, such as the placement and remove of the intrauterine device extracting lining specimen, laser separation of cervical dysplasia, cervical dilation and curettage. |
| 用法、用量<br>Dosage | 停经 ≤ 49 日的健康早妊娠期妇女，于空腹或进食后 1 小时口服，①顿服 200mg；②每次 25mg，一日 2 次，连续 3 日，服药后禁食 1 小时。<br><br>Healthy women in early pregnancy whose menopause is less than 49 days should take the medicine on empty stomach or one hour after meals orally. ① take at a draught for 200mg; ② 25mg singly, 2 times a day for three days, one hour fasting after taking the medcine. |

**续 表**

| 剂型、规格<br>Preparations | 片剂：每片 25mg；200mg。<br>Tablets: 25 mg per tablet; 200 mg. |
|---|---|

## 16.8 高血糖素 Glucagon

| 药品名称 Drug Names | 高血糖素 Glucagon |
|---|---|
| 适应证<br>Indications | 用于低血糖症，在一时不能口服或静脉注射葡萄糖时特别有用。用于心源性休克有效。<br>Used for hypoglycemia when oral or intravenous glucose is not available. Used in cardiac shock effectively. |
| 用法、用量<br>Dosage | 肌内注射、皮下注射或静脉注射，用于低血糖症，每次 0.5 ~ 1.0mg，5 分钟左右即可见效。用于心源性休克，连续静脉滴注，每小时 1 ~ 12mg。<br>Intramuscular injection, subcutaneous injection or intravenous injection, used for hypoglycemia, 0.5 to 1.0 mg singly, the benefits can be seen about 5 minutes later . Used in cardiac shock, continuous intravenous drip, 1 to 12 mg per hour. |
| 剂型、规格<br>Preparations | 注射用高血糖素：每支 1mg；10mg。<br>Glucagon for Injection: 1 mg per vial; 10 mg. |

## 16.9 胰岛素 Insulin

| 药品名称 Drug Names | 胰岛素 Insulin |
|---|---|
| 适应证<br>Indications | 用于糖尿病患者，控制血糖，特别是餐后血糖。<br>For patients with diabetes, control blood sugar, especially the postprandial one. |
| 用法、用量<br>Dosage | 餐前 30 分钟皮下注射，用药后 30 分钟内须进食含糖类的食物，一日 3 ~ 4 次。<br>Subcutaneous injections 30 minutes before meal, patients should have food containing carbohydrates within 30 minutes after medication, 3 to 4 times a day. |
| 剂型、规格<br>Preparations | 注射液：重组人胰岛素注射液：每瓶 400U（10ml）。笔芯：300u（3ml）。生物合成人胰岛素注射液：每瓶 400U（10ml）。笔芯：300U（3ml）。胰岛素（猪）注射液：每瓶 400U（10ml）。<br>Injection: recombinant human insulin injection: 400 U (10 ml) per bottle. Penfill: 300U (3 ml).The biosynthetic human insulin injection: 400U (10 ml) per bottle. Penfill: 300U (3 ml).Insulin (pigs) injection: 400U(10ml) per bottle. |
| 药品名称 Drug Names | 门冬胰岛素 Insulin Aspart |
| 适应证<br>Indications | 用于控制餐后血糖，也可与中效胰岛素合用控制晚间或晨起高血糖。<br>Used to control the postprandial BG, can also be used to control high BGin the evening or morning with NPH. |
| 用法、用量<br>Dosage | 于 3 餐前 15 分钟至进餐开始时皮下注射一次，根据血糖情况调整剂量。<br>Subcutaneous injection within 15 minutes before meals, adjust doses according to the changes of BG. |
| 剂型、规格<br>Preparations | 注射液：300U（3ml）。<br>Injection: 300U (3ml). |
| 药品名称 Drug Names | 赖脯胰岛素 Insulin Lispro |
| 适应证<br>Indications | 用于控制餐后血糖，也可与中效胰岛素合用控制晚间或晨起高血糖。<br>Used to control the postprandial BG, can also be used to control high BGin the evening or morning with NPH. |
| 用法、用量<br>Dosage | 于 3 餐前 15 分钟至进餐开始时皮下注射一次，根据血糖情况调整剂量。<br>Subcutaneous injection within 15 minutes before meals, adjust doses according to the changes of BG. |

| 剂型、规格<br>Preparations | 注射液：300U（3ml）。<br>Injection: 300U (3ml). |
|---|---|
| **药品名称 Drug Names** | 低精蛋白锌胰岛素 Isophane Insulin |
| 适应证<br>Indications | 用于糖尿病控制血糖，一般与短效胰岛素配合使用，提供胰岛素的日基础用量。<br>For controlling diabetes BG, generally used with short-acting insulin, provide the basic daily dose of insulin. |
| 用法、用量<br>Dosage | 于睡前或早餐前每天一次给药或者早晚一日 2 次给药，以控制空腹血糖。<br>Dose once a day before breakfast or before going to bed or 2 times a day in the morning and evening, to control the BG on an empty stomach. |
| 剂型、规格<br>Preparations | 注射液：每瓶 400U（10ml）。笔芯：300U（3ml）。<br>Injection: 400U (10ml) per bottle. Penfill: 300U (3ml). |
| **药品名称 Drug Names** | 精蛋白锌胰岛素 Protamine Zinc Insulin |
| 适应证<br>Indications | 用于糖尿病控制血糖，一般与短效胰岛素配合使用，提供胰岛素的日基础用量。<br>For controlling diabetes BG, generally used with short-acting insulin, provide the basic daily dose of insulin. |
| 用法、用量<br>Dosage | 于早餐前 0.5 小时皮下注射一次，剂量根据病情而定，每日用量一般为 10 ~ 20U。<br>Give subcutaneous injection 0.5 hours before breakfast, dose according to condition, generally the daily dosage generally is 10 to 20U. |
| 剂型、规格<br>Preparations | 注射液：每瓶 400U（10ml）。<br>Injection: 400Uper bottle (10ml). |
| **药品名称 Drug Names** | 甘精胰岛素 Insulin Glargine |
| 适应证<br>Indications | 用于基础胰岛素替代治疗，一般也和短效胰岛素或口服降糖药配合使用。<br>Used for the replacement therapy of basic insulin, usually used with short-acting insulin or oral hypoglycemic drugs. |
| 用法、用量<br>Dosage | 每日傍晚注射一次，满足糖尿病患者的基础胰岛素需要量。<br>Give a daily injection in the evening, fulfill the basic insulin requirement for diabetic . |
| 剂型、规格<br>Preparations | 注射液：300U（3ml）。<br>Injection: 300U (3 ml). |
| **药品名称 Drug Names** | 地特胰岛素 Insulin Detemir |
| 适应证<br>Indications | 用于治疗糖尿病。<br>Used in the treatment of diabetes. |
| 用法、用量<br>Dosage | 与口服降糖药联合治疗：起始剂量为 10U 或 0.1 ~ 0.2U/kg，一天 1 次，皮下注射，以后根据早餐前平均自测血糖浓度进行个体化的调整。<br>Combination therapy with oral hypoglycemic agents: the starting dose is 10U or 0.1 to 0.2U/kg, once a day, subcutaneous injection, afterwards make individualized adjustments according to the average self-test blood glucose levels before breakfast. |
| 剂型、规格<br>Preparations | 注射液：300U（3ml）。<br>Injection: 300U (3ml). |
| **药品名称 Drug Names** | 预混胰岛素 Pre-mixed insulin |
| 适应证<br>Indications | 用于糖尿病控制血糖。<br>Used for controlling diabetes BG. |
| 用法、用量<br>Dosage | 于早餐前 0.5 小时皮下注射一次，剂量根据病情而定，每日用量一般为 10 ~ 20U。有时需要于晚餐前再注射一次。<br>Give subcutaneous injection 0.5 hours before breakfast, dose according to condition, generally the daily dosage is 10 to 20U. Sometimes need to inject again before dinner. |

**续　表**

| 剂型、规格<br>Preparations | 注射液：每瓶 400U（10ml）。<br>笔芯：300U（3ml）。<br>Injection: 400U (10ml) per bottle. Penfill: 300U (3ml). |
|---|---|

### 16.10 口服降糖药 Oral Anti- diabetics

| 药品名称 Drug Names | 甲苯磺丁脲 Tolbutamide |
|---|---|
| 适应证<br>Indications | 　　一般用于成年后发病，单用饮食控制无效而胰岛功能尚存的轻、中度糖尿病患者，对胰岛素抵抗患者，可加用本品。对胰岛素依赖型患者及酸中毒昏迷者无效，不能完全代替胰岛素。<br>　　Generally used for patients with light or moderate diabetes whose islets still function but the diabetes which attack after growing up cannot be controlled by diet alone, the product can also be used for patients with insulin resistance. But it is invalid for patients with insulin-dependent or acidosis coma, and can not completely replace insulin |
| 用法、用量<br>Dosage | 　　餐前服药效果较好，如有胃肠反应，进餐时服药可减少反应。口服，每日剂量 1 ~ 2g，分次服用，一日 2 ~ 3 次，从小剂量开始，每 1 ~ 2 周加量一次。<br>　　Dosing before meals can obtain better effect, if gastrointestinal reaction occurs, take drugs during meals can reduce the reaction. Oral medication, the daily dose is 1 to 2g, take by several times, 2 to 3 times a day, starting from small doses, then add dosage once every 1 to 2 weeks. |
| 剂型、规格<br>Preparations | 片剂：每片 0.5g。<br>Tablets: 0.5g per tablet. |
| 药品名称 Drug Names | 格列本脲 Glibenclamide |
| 适应证<br>Indications | 用于饮食不能控制的轻、中度 2 型糖尿病。<br>Used for the light, moderate type 2 diabetes which cannot be controlled by diet. |
| 用法、用量<br>Dosage | 　　开始时每日剂量 2.5 ~ 5mg，早餐前 1 次服，或一日 2 次，早晚餐前各一次，然后根据情况每周增加 2.5mg，一般每日量为 5 ~ 10mg，最大不超过 15mg。<br>　　The daily dosage is 2.5 to 5 mg at the beginning, dose once before breakfast or 2 times before breakfast and dinner, then increase 2.5 mg per week according to condition, the average daily dosage 5 to 10 mg, at most 15 mg. |
| 剂型、规格<br>Preparations | 片剂：每片 2.5mg。<br>Tablets: 2.5mg per tablet. |
| 药品名称 Drug Names | 格列吡嗪 Glipizide |
| 适应证<br>Indications | 　　本品主要用于单用饮食控制治疗未能达到良好控制的轻、中度非胰岛素依赖型患者；对胰岛素抵抗患者可加用本品，但用量应在 30 ~ 40U 以下者。<br>　　This product is mainly used for patients without insulin-dependent but with light or moderate diabetes which cannot be controlled well by diet alone; It can also be used for patients with insulin resistance, but the dosage should be within 30 to 40U. |
| 用法、用量<br>Dosage | 　　一般一日 2.5 ~ 20mg，先从小量 2.5 ~ 5mg 开始，餐前 30 分钟服用，一日剂量超过 15mg 时，应分成 2 ~ 3 次餐前服用。<br>　　Generally 2.5 to 20 mg a day, begin with a small amount of 2.5 to 5 mg, dose 30 minutes before meals, if a daily dose is more than 15 mg, it should be divided into 2 to 3 times. |
| 剂型、规格<br>Preparations | 片剂：每片 2.5mg；5mg。控释片：每片 5mg。<br>Tablets: 2.5mg per tablet; 5mg. Controlled-release Tablets 5mg per tablet. |
| 药品名称 Drug Names | 格列齐特 Gliclazide |
| 适应证<br>Indications | 成人 2 型糖尿病。<br>Type 2 Diabetes Mellitus |

**续 表**

| | |
|---|---|
| 用法、用量<br>Dosage | 开始时一日 2 次，一日 40～80mg，早晚 2 餐前服用；连服 2～3 周，然后根据血糖调整用量，一般剂量一日 80～240mg，最大日剂量不超过 240mg。<br><br>In the beginning, 2 times a day, 40～80mg a day, before breakfast and supper for 2~3 weeks of continuous treatment and adjust the dosage based on blood sugar. Generally, dosage is given 80～240mg single and the a day maximum dose does not exceed 240mg. |
| 剂型、规格<br>Preparations | 片剂：每片 80mg。缓释片：每片 30mg。<br>Tablets: 80mg per tablet. Sustained-release tablets: 30mg per tablet. |
| 药品名称 Drug Names | 格列喹酮 Gliquidone |
| 适应证<br>Indications | 2 型糖尿病合并轻至中度肾病者，但严重肾功能不全时应改用胰岛素治疗。<br><br>For treatment of mile or moderate Type 2 Diabetic Nephropathy, but patients with severe renal insufficiency should be treated by insulin. |
| 用法、用量<br>Dosage | 口服，开始时 15mg，应在餐前 30 分钟服用。1 周后按需调整，必要时逐步加量，一般日剂量为 15～20mg，日剂量为 30mg 以内者，可于早餐前一次服用，更大剂量应分 3 次，分别与 3 餐前服用，最大日剂量不超过 180mg。<br><br>Oral medication medication: In the beginning, 15mg a day, 30 minutes before meal. A week later adjust the dosage as required and gradually add quantity if necessary. Generally, a day dose is 15～20 mg. If the dosage is less than 30 mg, it can be taken at one time before breakfast, but larger dose should be in 3 divided doses, before three meals respectively and the maximum a day dose could not exceed 180 mg. |
| 剂型、规格<br>Preparations | 片剂：每片 30mg。<br>Tablets: 30mg per tablet. |
| 药品名称 Drug Names | 格列美脲 Glimepiride |
| 适应证<br>Indications | 成人 2 型糖尿病。<br>Type 2 Diabetes Mellitus |
| 用法、用量<br>Dosage | 开始用量一日 1mg，一次顿服，如不能满意控制血糖，每隔 1～2 周逐步增加剂量至每日 2mg、3mg、4mg，最大推荐剂量为每日 6mg。<br><br>In the beginning, 1 mg a day at one time. if blood sugar couldn't be controlled well, the dose could be added every 1～2 weeks to 2, 3, 4 mg. The maximum recommended dose is 6 mg per day. |
| 剂型、规格<br>Preparations | 片剂：每片 1mg；2mg。<br>Tablets: 1mg; 2mg per tablet. |
| 药品名称 Drug Names | 二甲双胍 Metformin |
| 适应证<br>Indications | （1）首选用于单纯饮食控制及体育锻炼治疗无效的 2 型糖尿病，特别是肥胖的 2 型糖尿病。<br>（2）与胰岛素合用可减少胰岛素用量，防止低血糖发生。<br>（3）与磺酰脲类降血糖药合用具协同作用。<br><br>(1) For the treatment of Type 2 Diabetes Mellitus, which has been ineffectively treated by diet control alone and physical exercise, especially for obese patients with type 2 diabetes.<br>(2) capable to reduce the dosage of insulin combined with Metformin and prevent the hypoglycemia.<br>(3) The hypoglycemic effect will be better when combined with Sulfonylurea hypolycemic agent. |
| 用法、用量<br>Dosage | （1）普通片：开始时一次 0.25g，一日 2～3 次，以后可根据病情调整剂量。口服，一次 0.5g，一日 1～1.5g，最大剂量不超过 2g。餐中服药可减轻胃肠反应。<br>（2）缓释片：开始时一日 1 次，每次 0.5g，晚餐时服用。后根据血糖调整剂量。日最大剂量不超过 2g。<br><br>(1) Ordinary piece: in the beginning 0.25g singly, 2 to 3 times a day, and adjust the dosage as the disease condition. Oral medication medication, 0.5g singly, 1～1.5g a day, and the maximum dose does not exceed 2g. If it is given when having meal, gastrointestinal reactions could lessen.<br>(2) release tablets: in the beginning, once a day, 0.5g singly at dinner time. Adjusting the dosage as blood glucose with the Maximum a day dose does not exceed 2g. |

**续　表**

| 剂型、规格<br>Preparations | 片剂：每片 0.25g；0.5g；0.85g。缓释片：0.5g。<br>Tablets: 0.25g; 0.5g; 0.85g per tablet. Release tablets: 0.5g. |
|---|---|
| **药品名称 Drug Names** | 苯乙双胍 Phenformin |
| 适应证<br>Indications | 用于单纯饮食控制不满意的 2 型糖尿患者，尤其是肥胖者和伴高胰岛素血症者。与磺酰脲类降血糖药合用具协同作用。<br><br>Patients with Type 2 Diabetes Mellitus, who are not satisfied by the treatment of diet control alone, especially for obese patients and those with hyperinsulinemia. The hypoglycemic effect will be better in combination with sulfonylurea hypolycemic agent. |
| 用法、用量<br>Dosage | 口服：成人开始时一次 25mg，一日 2 次，餐前服，数日后可再增加 25mg，但最多每日不超过 75mg。<br><br>Oral medication medication: for for adults, 25mg singly in the beginning, 2 times a day before meals. The dosage could increase by 25mg, but not more than a maximum of 75mg a day. |
| 剂型、规格<br>Preparations | 片剂：每片 25mg。<br>Tablets: 25mg per tablet. |
| **药品名称 Drug Names** | 瑞格列奈 Repaglinide |
| 适应证<br>Indications | 用于饮食控制、降低体重与运动不能有效控制高血糖的 2 型糖尿病。与二甲双胍合用对控制血糖有协同作用。<br><br>For the treatment of Type 2 Diabetes Mellitus, when diet control, weight loss or physical exercise cannot effectively solve the disease of hyperglycemia. |
| 用法、用量<br>Dosage | 服药时间应在餐前 30 分钟内服用，剂量依个人血糖而定。推荐起始剂量为 0.5mg，最大的推荐单次剂量为 4mg，但最大日剂量不应超过 16mg。<br><br>Medicine should be taken within 30 minutes before meal, when the dosage depends on individual blood sugar. Recommend starting dose is 0.5 mg, while the maximum single dose is 4 mg, but not more than 16 mg. |
| 剂型、规格<br>Preparations | 片剂：每片 0.5mg；1mg；2mg。<br>Tablets: 0.5mg; 1mg; 2mg per tablet. |
| **药品名称 Drug Names** | 那格列奈 Nateglinide |
| 适应证<br>Indications | 用于饮食控制、降低体重与运动不能有效控制高血糖的 2 型糖尿病。与二甲双胍合用对控制血糖有协同作用。<br><br>For the treatment of Type 2 Diabetes Mellitus, when diet control, weight loss or physical exercise cannot effectively solve the disease of hyperglycemia.Combined with metformin, it is better to control blood sugar. |
| 用法、用量<br>Dosage | 本品可单独应用，也可与二甲双胍合用，起始剂量一日 3 次，一次 60mg，餐前 15 分钟服药。常用剂量为餐前 60 ～ 120mg，并根据 HbA1c 检测结果调整剂量。<br><br>It can be used alone or in combination with metformin. The starting dose is three times a day, 60mg singly 15 minutes before meal. The usual dose is 60 ~ 120mg before meal, and adjust the dose as (HbAlc) test results. |
| 剂型、规格<br>Preparations | 片剂：每片 30mg；60mg；120mg。<br>Tablets: 30 mg;60 mg;120 mg per tablet. |
| **药品名称 Drug Names** | 罗格列酮 Rosiglitazone |
| 适应证<br>Indications | 本品仅适用于其他降糖药无法达到血糖控制目标的 2 型糖尿病患者。<br>It is only active against Type 2 Diabetes Mellitus patients unable to control blood sugar by other hypoglycemic drugs. |

**续　表**

| 用法、用量<br>Dosage | 单独用药：初始剂量为每日 4mg，单次或分 2 次口服，12 周后如空腹血糖下降不满意，剂量可加至每日 8mg，单次或分 2 次口服。<br><br>Monotherapy: In the beginning, 4mg a day in 1 or 3 divided doses with Oral medication medication. If the decline of fasting blood glucose is not satisfied 12 weeks later, the a day dose can be increased to 8mg a day in1 or 2 divided doses with Oral medication medication |
|---|---|
| 剂型、规格<br>Preparations | 片剂：每片 2mg；4mg；8mg。<br>Tablets: 2 mg;4 mg;8 mg per tablet. |
| **药品名称 Drug Names** | 吡格列酮 Pioglitazone |
| 适应证<br>Indications | 用于 2 型糖尿病，可于饮食控制和体育锻炼联合以改善血糖控制，可单独使用。当饮食控制、体育锻炼和单药治疗不能满意控制血糖时，也可与磺脲、二甲双胍或胰岛素合用。<br><br>For the treatment of Type 2 Diabetes Mellitus, capable to be used both together with diet control and physical exercise to improve blood sugar control and used alone. It is able to use combined with sulphonylurea, metformin or insulin when treatment is ineffective by methods of diet control, physical exercise and monotherapy to control blood sugar. |
| 用法、用量<br>Dosage | 口服，单药治疗初始剂量可为 15mg 或 30mg，一日 1 次；反应不佳时，可加量直至 45mg，一日 1 次。<br><br>Oral medication medication, when Monotherapy is applied, the initial dose may be 15mg or 30mg, once a day; If the performance is poor, you can increase the amount to the maximum of 45mg, once a day. |
| 剂型、规格<br>Preparations | 片剂：每片 15mg。<br>Tablets: 15 mg per tablet . |
| **药品名称 Drug Names** | 阿卡波糖 Acarbose |
| 适应证<br>Indications | 可与其他口服降血糖药或胰岛素联合应用于胰岛素依赖型或非胰岛素依赖型的糖尿病。<br><br>For the treatment of IDDM and NIDDM Diabetes, combined with use of other oral hypoglycemic agents or insulin. |
| 用法、用量<br>Dosage | 口服剂量需个体化。一般维持量为一次 50～100mg，一日 3 次，餐前即刻吞服，或与第一口主食一起咀嚼服用。开始时从小剂量 25mg，每日 3 次，6～8 周后加量至 50mg，必要时可加至 100mg，一日 3 次，一日量不宜超过 300mg。<br><br>Oral medication medication dose should be individualized. Generally 50～100 mg singly and three times a day before meal without water, or chewing with the first bite of staple food. In the beginning, a small dose of 25 mg, three times a day and increase the amount to 50 mg and 100 mg when necessary, three times a day, less than 300 mg a day is better. |
| 剂型、规格<br>Preparations | 片剂：每片 50mg；100mg。<br>Tablets: 50mg; 100mg per tablet. |
| **药品名称 Drug Names** | 伏格列波糖 Voglibose |
| 适应证<br>Indications | 改善糖尿病餐后高血糖。<br>Improve diabetics' postprandial hyperglycemia. |
| 用法、用量<br>Dosage | 口服，成人一次 200μg，一日 3 次，餐前服，疗效不明显时根据临床观察可将一次量增至 300μg。<br><br>Oral medication medication for adults, 200μg singly, three times a day before meal. If the curative effect is not obvious, the single dosage can amount to 300μg according to clinical observation. |
| 剂型、规格<br>Preparations | 片剂：每片 200μg。<br>Tablets: 200μg per tablet . |
| **药品名称 Drug Names** | 西格列汀 Sitagliptin |
| 适应证<br>Indications | 用于经生活方式干预无法达标的 2 型糖尿病患者。可采用单药治疗或与其他口服降糖药联合治疗。<br><br>For the treatment of Type 2 Diabetes Mellitus patients, who are unable to meet the treating target by lifestyle intervention. Monotherapy is available, when the alternative is to take other oral hypoglycemic agents together. |

**续　表**

| | |
|---|---|
| 用法、用量<br>Dosage | 本品单药治疗的推荐剂量为 100mg，一日 1 次。本品可与或不与食物同服。<br>This product monotherapy recommended dose of 100 mg, once a day.This product can be with or not with food and clothing. |
| 剂型、规格<br>Preparations | 每片 100mg。<br>100mg per tablet |

### 16.11 甲状腺激素类药物 Thyroid hormone drugs

| 药品名称 Drug Names | 左甲状腺素 Levothyroxine |
|---|---|
| 适应证<br>Indications | 适用于甲状腺激素缺乏的替代治疗。<br>It is administered in Thyroid Hormones Deficiency replacement therapy. |
| 用法、用量<br>Dosage | 口服一般开始剂量每日 25 ～ 50μg，每 2 周增加 25μg，直到 100 ～ 150μg，成人维持量为每日 75 ～ 125μg，高龄患者、心功能不全者及严重黏液性水肿患者开始剂量应减为每日 12.5 ～ 25μg，以后每 2 ～ 4 周递增 25μg，不必要求达到完全替代剂量，一般每日 75 ～ 100μg 即可。婴儿及儿童甲状腺功能减退症，每日完全替代剂量为：6 个月以内 6 ～ 8μg/kg；6 ～ 12 个月，6μg/kg；1 ～ 5 岁 5μg/kg，6 ～ 12 岁，4μg/kg。静脉注射适用于黏液性水肿昏迷，首次剂量宜较大，200 ～ 400μg，以后每日 50 ～ 100μg，直到患者清醒改为口服。<br>Oral medication medication, generally In the beginning, 25 ～ 50μg a day, an increase of 25μg every 2 weeks until the end of 100 ～ 150μg. For for adults, the maintenance dose is about 75 ～ 125μg per day. For elderly patients, the cardiac insufficiency and patients with severe myxedema, the starting dose should be reduced to 12.5 ～ 25μg per day with an increase of 25μg every 2 ～ 4 weeks. It is not necessary to reach the Dosage for Substitution completely, when 75 ～ 100 g is proper. For the treatment of hypothyroidism in Infant and children, the a day entire replacing dose is: 6 ～ 8μg/kg for less than 6-month infant;6 ～ 12 months, 6μg /kg; 1 ～ 5 year-old, 5μg /kg, 6 ～ 12 years old, 4μg/kg. Intravenous injection is active to myxedema coma, when the starting dose should be larger with 200 ～ 400μg, later 50 ～ 100μg per day is proper until the patient awake and then could changed into Oral medication medication |
| 剂型、规格<br>Preparations | 片剂：每片 25μg；50μg；100μg。注射液：每支 100μg（1ml）；200μg（2ml）；500μg（5ml）。<br>Tablets: 25μg; 50μg; 100μg per tablet. Injection: 100μg (1ml); 200μg (2ml); 500μg (5ml) per vial. |

| 药品名称 Drug Names | 甲状腺素 Thyroid Tablets |
|---|---|
| 适应证<br>Indications | 主要用甲状腺功能减退症的治疗。包括甲减引起的呆小病及黏液性水肿等。<br>It is mainly helpful in the treatment of hypothyroidism, including cretinism, myxedema, etc. caused by hypothyroidism. |
| 用法、用量<br>Dosage | 常用量开始时一日 10 ～ 20mg，逐渐加量，维持量一般为一日 40 ～ 80mg。<br>The common dose is 10 to 20 mg a day in the beginning, and gradually added to 40 ～ 80 mg a day. |
| 剂型、规格<br>Preparations | 片剂：每片 10mg；40mg；60mg。<br>Tablets: 10 mg;40 mg;60 mg per tablet. |

| 药品名称 Drug Names | 促甲状腺素 Thyrotrophin [Thyroid stimulating hormone（TSH）] |
|---|---|
| 适应证<br>Indications | 用于 TSH 试验及甲状腺癌诊断。<br>Used for TSH test and diagnosis of thyroid cancer. |
| 用法、用量<br>Dosage | ① TSH 试验：一日肌内注射 2 次，每次 10μg，共 3 日。②提高甲状腺癌转移病灶吸 [131]I：甲状腺全切除后。每日肌内注射 10μg，共 7 日。使转移病灶吸 [131]I 率提高后再给予治疗量碘。<br>① TSH test: intramuscular injection should be taken 2 times a day, 10μg singly for 3 days .<br>② To increase the absorption of [131]I in metastatic lesions of thyroid carcinoma: after a total excision of the thyroid gland, intramuscular injection should be given by 10μg a day for 7 days. After the absorption rate of [131]I by metastatic lesions improves, iodine of therapeutic dosecould be given. |
| 剂型、规格<br>Preparations | 注射液：每支 10μg（6ml）。<br>Injection: 10 mu g (6 ml) per vial. |

续 表

## 16.12 抗甲状腺药 Antithyroid drugs

| 药品名称 Drug Names | 丙硫氧嘧啶 Propylthiouracil |
|---|---|
| 适应证<br>Indications | ①甲状腺功能亢进症的内科治疗。②甲状腺危象的治疗。③术前准备。<br>① medical treatment of hyperthyroidism. ② treatment of thyroid storm. ③ preoperative preparation. |
| 用法、用量<br>Dosage | （1）成人甲状腺功能亢进症：口服常用量 300 ～ 450mg/d，分 3 次口服，极量一次 0.2g，一日 0.6g。小儿开始剂量每日按 4mg/kg 分次口服，维持量酌减。<br>（2）甲状腺危象：一日 0.4 ～ 0.8g，分 3 ～ 4 次服用，疗程不超过 1 周。<br>（3）甲状腺功能亢进症的术前准备：术前服用本品一次 100mg，一日 3 ～ 4 次，使甲状腺功能恢复到正常或接近正常，然后加服 2 周碘剂再进行手术。<br>(1) adult hyperthyroidism: Oral medication dosage is 300 ~ 450 mg/day in 3 divided doses, the smallest affective dose of 0.2 g singly and 0.6 g a day. For children, the starting dose is 4 mg/kg a day by divided doses and Oral medication. Besides, the maintenance dose should be reduced with discretion.<br>(2) thyroid crisis: 0.4 ~ 0.8 g a day, in 3 ~ 4 divided doses and not more than a week.<br>(3) preoperative preparation for hyperthyroidism: 100 mg singly before operation, 3 ~ 4 times a day. In this way, the thyroid function could recover to normal or close normal condition, and then iodine should be added for 2 weeks prior to surgery. |
| 剂型、规格<br>Preparations | 片剂：每片 50mg；100mg。<br>Tablets: 50mg; 100mg per tablet. |
| 药品名称 Drug Names | 甲巯咪唑 Thimazole |
| 适应证<br>Indications | ①甲状腺功能亢进症的内科治疗。②甲状腺危象的治疗。③术前准备<br>① medical treatment of hyperthyroidism. ② treatment of thyroid storm. ③ preoperative preparation. |
| 用法、用量<br>Dosage | 成人：开始时每天 30mg，可按病情轻重调节为每日 15 ～ 40mg，每日最大量 60mg，分次口服，病情控制后逐渐减量，维持量：一日 5 ～ 15mg，疗程一般 12 ～ 18 个月。小儿：开始剂量为每日 0.4mg/kg，分 3 次口服。维持量约减半或按病情轻重调节。<br>For For adults: in the beginning, 30mg a day and regulate dosage between 15 and 40mg according to disease condition, but the maximum amount is 60mg a day, in divided doses, gradually reducing dosage after disease condition is controlled. The maintenance dose: generally, 5 ~ 15mg a day for 12 to 18 months. For Pediatric: In the beginning, 0.4mg/kg a day, Oral medication in 3 diveded doses. The Maintainance dose could be approximately halved or regulated according to the disease condition. |
| 剂型、规格<br>Preparations | 片剂：每片 5mg。<br>Tablets: 5 mg per tablet. |

## 17. 主要影响变态反应和免疫功能的药物 Drugs mainly affecting allergy and immunologic function

### 17.1 抗变态反应药物 Antiallergic Drugs

| 药品名称 Drug Names | 苯海拉明 Diphenhydramine |
|---|---|
| 适应证<br>Indications | ①主要用于 I 型和 IV 型变态反应，对毛细血管通透性增加所致渗出、水肿、分泌物增多的疾病疗效较好，尤其适用于皮肤黏膜的过敏性疾病，如过敏性药疹、过敏性湿疹、血管神经水肿和荨麻疹等。对平滑肌痉挛所致支气管哮喘的效果较差，需与氨茶碱、麻黄碱等合用。②镇静催眠和手术前给药。③抗帕金森和药物所致锥体外系症状。④防晕止吐：可用于乘船乘车所致晕动病，以及放射病术后及药物引起的恶心呕吐。⑤乳膏外用，治虫咬、神经性皮炎、瘙痒症等。<br>① Mainly against I Type and IV Type allergic reaction, more effective for the treatment of exudation, edema and secretion increases after the increase of capillary permeability caused by increased secretions, especially for skin mucocutaneous allergic diseases, such as allergic epispasis, atopic eczema, angioneurotic edema, urticarial, etc. The effect is Poor in treating bronchial asthma caused by smooth muscle spasm, when combined with theophylline, ephedrine, etc is necessary. ② Hypnotic and sedative prior to surgery. ③ extrapyramidal symptoms by Parkinson's Drug. ④ Prevention of motion sickness and antiemetic function: motion sickness are resulted from traveling by boat or vehicles, while emesising are caused by postoperative radiotherapy and drugs. ⑤ creams for external use, for the treatment of insect bites, neurodermatitis, pruritus, etc. |

**续　表**

| | |
|---|---|
| 用法、用量<br>Dosage | 可口服、肌内注射及局部应用。不能皮下注射，因有刺激性。成人：口服，一次25～50mg，一日2～3次。饭后服。肌内注射，一次12.5～25mg，一日3～4次；或一日5mg/kg，分次给药；或一日150mg/m²，分次给药。<br><br>Oral medication or intramuscular injections and topical applications. No subcutaneous injection in fear of irritation. For For adults: Oral medication, 25～50mg singly, 2~3 times a day. After meals. Intramuscular injection, 12.5～25mg singly, 3~4 times a day; or 5mg/kg a day in divided doses; or 150mg / m² a day in divided doses. |
| 剂型、规格<br>Preparations | 片剂：每片25mg；50mg。注射液：每支20mg（1ml）。乳膏：每支20g。<br>Tablets: 25mg; 50mg per tablet. Injection: 20mg (1ml) per vial. Cream: 20g per strip. |
| 药品名称 Drug Names | 异丙嗪 Promethazine |
| 适应证<br>Indications | ①抗过敏：适用于各种过敏症（如哮喘、荨麻疹等）。②镇吐抗眩晕：可用于一些麻醉和手术后的恶心呕吐，乘车、船等引起的眩晕症等。③镇静催眠：可在外科手术和分娩时与哌替啶合用，缓解患者紧张情绪，或用于晚间催眠药。亦可与氯丙嗪等配成冬眠注射液用于人工冬眠。<br><br>① Anti-allergic effect: it is intended to Suitable for all kinds of allergies (such as asthma, urticaria, etc.). ② antiemetic and anti-vertigo effects: nausea and vomiting by anesthesia and operation, vertigo from traveling by vehicles and boat ③ sedative and hypnotic effects: in combination with pethidine, it helps to ease the tension of patients during surgery and parturition. Alternative uses are for hypnotic drugs for the evening and hibernation injection compounded with chlorpromazine for induced hibernation. |
| 用法、用量<br>Dosage | ①抗过敏：成人，口服，一次6.25～12.5mg，一日3次，饭后及睡前服用，必要时睡前25mg；儿童，口服，每次按体重0.125mg/kg或按体表面积7.5～15mg/m²，每4～6小时1次，或睡前按体重0.25～0.5mg/kg或按体表面积7.5～15mg/m²；按年龄计算，每日量5岁5～15mg，6岁以上10～15mg，可一日1次或分次服用。肌内注射，每次按体重0.125mg/kg或按体表面积3.75mg/m²，每4～6小时肌内注射1次。②止吐：成人，口服，开始时一次12.5～25mg，必要时可每4～6小时服12.5～25mg，通常24小时不超过100mg。③抗眩晕：成人，旅行前口服，一次12.5～25mg，必要时一日2次；儿童，口服，剂量减半。④镇静催眠：成人，口服，一次12.5～25mg，睡前服用。儿童，口服，5岁6.25mg，6～12岁6.25～12.5mg。<br><br>① anti-Allergy: for adults, Oral medication, 6.25～12.5mg singly, three times a day, after meals and at bedtime, 25mg before going to bed if necessary; for child, Oral medication, 0.125mg/kg according to body weight singly or 7.5～15mg/m² according to body surface area; one time every 4 to 6 hours or 0.25～0.5mg/kg at bedtime in terms of body weight or 7.5～15mg/m² according to body surface area; Measured by age, 5-year-old, 5～15mg singly, 6 years plus, 10～15mg singly in one or divided doses. Intramuscular injection, 0.125mg/kg singly according to the weight or 3.75mg/m² according to body surface area, one time every 4 to 6 hours ② antiemetic: for for adults, Oral medication, in the beginning, 12.5～25mg singly, 12.5～25mg every 4 to 6 hours if necessary and not exceeding 100mg within 24 hours ③ anti-vertigo: for adults, Oral medication before traveling, 12.5～25mg singly, 2 times a day if necessary; for child, Oral medication dose in half. ④ sedative and hypnotic: for for adults, Oral medication, 12.5～25mg singly, at bedtime. For Children, Oral medication, 5-year-old, 6.25mg, 6～12 year-old, 6.25～12.5mg. |
| 剂型、规格<br>Preparations | 片剂：每片12.5mg；25mg。注射液：每支25mg（1ml）；50mg（2ml）。<br>Tablets: 12.5mg; 25mg per tablet. Injection: 25mg (1ml); 50mg (2ml) per vial |
| 药品名称 Drug Names | 去氯羟嗪 Decloxizine |
| 适应证<br>Indications | 用于支气管哮喘、急慢性荨麻疹、皮肤划痕症、血管神经性水肿、接触性皮炎、光敏性皮炎、季节性花粉症、过敏性鼻炎及结膜炎等。<br><br>For the treatment of bronchial asthma, acute and chronic urticaria, Dermatographism, angioedema, contact dermatitis, photosensitivity dermatitis, seasonal hay fever, allergic rhinitis, conjunctivitis, etc. |
| 用法、用量<br>Dosage | 口服：一日3次，一次25～50mg。<br>Oral medication: three times a day, 25～50mg singly. |

| | |
|---|---|
| 剂型、规格<br>Preparations | 片剂：每片 25mg；50mg。<br>Tablets: 25mg; 50mg per tablet. |
| 药品名称 Drug Names | 阿伐斯汀 Acrivastine |
| 适应证<br>Indications | 用于过敏性鼻炎及荨麻疹等。<br>For the treatment of allergic rhinitis, urticarial, etc. |
| 用法、用量<br>Dosage | 成人及 12 岁以上儿童口服：1 次 8mg，一日不超过 3 次。<br>For For adults and children of 12 years plus: Oral medication, 8mg singly, no more than three times a day. |
| 剂型、规格<br>Preparations | 胶囊剂：每粒 8mg。<br>Capsules: 8mg per capsule |
| 药品名称 Drug Names | 左卡巴斯汀 Levocabastine |
| 适应证<br>Indications | 用于局部治疗的滴眼剂和喷鼻剂，缓解过敏性鼻炎，预防包括鼻炎及结膜炎在内的过敏反应。<br>It is eye drops and nasal spray for topical treatment to relieve allergic rhinitis and prevent allergic reactions, including rhinitis and conjunctivitis. |
| 用法、用量<br>Dosage | （1）喷鼻：成人及 12 岁以上儿童常用量为每个鼻孔喷 2 下，一日 2 次。必要时可增至每次喷 2 下，一日 3 ～ 4 次。连续用药直至症状消除。<br>（2）滴眼：每次 1 滴，一日 2 ～ 4 次。<br>(1) Nasal spray: for For adults and children 12 years plus, generally, 2 sprays per nostril, twice a day. if necessary, 2 sprays per nostril, 3 to 4 times a day with Continuous medication until the symptoms eliminate.<br>(2) eye Drops: 1 drop singly, 2 ～ 4 times a day. |
| 剂型、规格<br>Preparations | 喷鼻剂（微悬浮液）：每支 10ml（0.5g/ml）。滴眼剂：0.5mg/kg。<br>Nasal spray (micro-suspension): 10ml (0.5g/ml) per bottle. Eye drops: 0.5mg/kg. |
| 药品名称 Drug Names | 咪唑斯汀 Mizolastine |
| 适应证<br>Indications | 本品用于长效 $H_1$ 受体拮抗药，适用于季节性过敏性鼻炎、花粉症、常年性过敏性鼻炎及荨麻疹等皮肤过敏症状。<br>This product is used as long-acting $H_1$ receptor antagonist for seasonal allergic rhinitis, hay fever, perennial allergic rhinitis and urticaria and other skin allergies. |
| 用法、用量<br>Dosage | 口服，成人（包括老年人）和 12 岁以上儿童，推荐剂量为一次 10mg，一日 1 次。<br>Oral medication, for For adults (including the elderly) and children of 12 years plus, the recommended dose is 10mg singly, once a day. |
| 剂型、规格<br>Preparations | 片剂：每片 10mg。<br>Tablets: 10mg per tablet. |
| 药品名称 Drug Names | 赛庚啶 Cyproheptadine |
| 适应证<br>Indications | 用于荨麻疹、湿疹、过敏性和接触性皮炎、皮肤瘙痒、鼻炎、偏头痛、支气管哮喘等。皮肤瘙痒通常在服药后 2 ～ 3 日消失。对库欣病、肢端肥大症也有一定疗效。<br>For the treatment of urticaria, eczema, allergic dermatitis, contact dermatitis, pruritus, rhinitis, migraine, bronchial asthma, etc. Usually, Itching will disappear within 2~3 days after medication. It also can help treat Cushing's disease and acromegaly. |
| 用法、用量<br>Dosage | （1）口服，成人，一次 2 ～ 4mg，一日 3 次。儿童，口服，2 ～ 6 岁，一次 2mg，一日 2 ～ 3 次，7 ～ 14 岁，一次 4mg，一日 2 ～ 3 次，极量：一次 0.2mg/kg。作为食欲增进剂应用时，用药时间不超过 6 个月。<br>（2）乳膏外用。<br>(1) Oral medication, for for adults, 2 ～ 4mg singly, 3 times a day. For Children, Oral medication, 2 to 6 years old, 2mg singly, 2 or 3 times a day; 7 to 14 years old, 4mg singly, 2 or 3 times a day, the minmum dose: 0.2mg/kg singly. As an appetite enhancer, medication time should not be more than six months.<br>(2) Topical cream. |

**续　表**

| 剂型、规格<br>Preparations | 片剂：每片 2mg。<br>糖浆剂：4mg/kg。<br>霜剂：每支 10g（0.5%），20g（0.5%）。<br>乳膏剂：0.5%。<br>Tablets: 2mg per tablet.<br>Syrup: 4mg/kg.<br>Cream: 10g (0.5%), 20g (0.5%).<br>Creams: 0.5%. |
|---|---|
| **药品名称 Drug Names** | 氯雷他定 Loratadine |
| 适应证<br>Indications | 用于过敏性鼻炎、急性或慢性荨麻疹、过敏性结膜炎、花粉症及其他过敏性皮肤病。<br>For the treatment of allergic rhinitis, acute or chronic urticaria, allergic conjunctivitis, hay fever and other allergic skin diseases. |
| 用法、用量<br>Dosage | 口服，成人及 12 岁以上儿童，1 次 10mg，一日 1 次，空腹服用。日夜均有发作者，可一次 5mg，每日晨、晚各一次。儿童，口服，2 ~ 12 岁，体重大于 30kg 者，一次 5mg，一次 5mg，一日一次。复方氯雷他定片：成人及 12 岁以上儿童，一次 1 片，一日 2 次。<br>Oral medication, for for adults and children over 12 years, 10mg singly, once a day on an empty stomach. Patients who are uncomfortable day and night could have 5mg singly, once morning and evening. For Children, Oral medication, 2 to 12 years old, more than 30kg of weight, 5mg singly, once a day. Compound Loratadine tablets: for For adults and children over 12 years, once singly, two times a day. |
| 剂型、规格<br>Preparations | 片剂：每片 10mg。<br>胶囊剂：每粒 10mg。<br>颗粒剂：5mg。<br>糖浆剂：60mg/60ml。<br>Tablets: 10mg per tablet.<br>Capsules: 10mg per capsule.<br>Granules: 5mg.<br>Syrup: 60mg/60ml. |
| **药品名称 Drug Names** | 西替利嗪 Cetirizine |
| 适应证<br>Indications | 用于季节性和常年性过敏性鼻炎、结膜炎及过敏反应所致的瘙痒和荨麻疹。<br>For seasonal and perennial allergic rhinitis, conjunctivitis and itching and hives caused by allergic reactions. |
| 用法、用量<br>Dosage | 口服，成人及 12 岁以上儿童，1 次 10 ~ 20mg，一日 1 次，或早晚各服 5mg。肾功能损害者需减量。儿童，2 ~ 6 岁者，每日 5mg；7 ~ 11 岁者，每日 10mg。<br>Oral medication, for adults and children over 12 years, 10 ~ 20mg singly, once a day or 5mg for both morning and evening. Patients with Renal dysfunction require reductions. Children of 2 to 6 years of age, 5mg singly; 7 ~ 11 years of age, 10mg a day. |
| 剂型、规格<br>Preparations | 片剂：每片 10mg。<br>胶囊剂：每粒 10mg。<br>分散片：每片 10mg。<br>口服液：10mg/10ml。<br>Tablets: 10mg per tablet.<br>Capsules: 10mg per capsule.<br>Dispersible tablets: 10mg per tablet.<br>Oral liquid: 10mg/10ml. |
| **药品名称 Drug Names** | 依巴斯汀 Ebastine |
| 适应证<br>Indications | 用于季节性和常年性过敏性鼻炎和慢性荨麻疹、湿疹、皮炎、痒疹、皮肤瘙痒等。<br>For seasonal and perennial allergic rhinitis and chronic urticaria, eczema, dermatitis, rashes, itchying, etc. |

续 表

| | |
|---|---|
| 用法、用量<br>Dosage | （1）常年性过敏性鼻炎：成人，一日一次，每次 10mg；儿童（12～17 岁），一日 1 次，每次 5mg。<br><br>（2）季节性过敏性鼻炎：成人，一日 1 次，每次 10mg，早上服用效果更好。如严重过敏患者可日服 20mg，但应从小剂量开始。儿童（2～15 岁），一日 1 次，每次 2.5～5mg。<br><br>(1) Perennial allergic rhinitis: for adults, once a day, 10mg singly; for Children (12～17), once a day, 5mg singly.<br><br>(2) Seasonal allergic rhinitis: For adults, once a day, 10mg singly, morning taking is better. Patients with severe allergic patients can be served 20mg a day, but the starting dose should be small. Children (2～15 years old), once a day, 2.5～5mg singly. |
| 剂型、规格<br>Preparations | 片剂：每片 10mg。<br>Tablets: 10mg per tablet. |
| 药品名称 Drug Names | 地氯雷他定 Desloratadine |
| 适应证<br>Indications | 用于治疗慢性特发性荨麻疹、常年过敏性鼻炎及季节过敏性鼻炎。<br>For the treatment of chronic idiopathic urticaria, perennial allergic rhinitis and seasonal allergic rhinitis. |
| 用法、用量<br>Dosage | （1）慢性特发性荨麻疹、常年过敏性鼻炎及季节过敏性鼻炎：成人口服，一日 1 次，每次 5mg。<br><br>（2）慢性特发性荨麻疹、常年过敏性鼻炎：儿童，口服，12 岁以上，每次 5mg，一日 1 次；6～11 岁者，每次 2.5mg，一日一次；12 个月～5 岁者，每次 1.25mg，一日一次；6 个月～11 个月者，每次 1mg，一日 1 次。<br><br>（3）季节性过敏性鼻炎：儿童口服，12 岁以上者，每次 5mg，一日 1 次；6～11 岁者，每次 2.5mg，一日 1 次；2～5 岁者，每次 1.25mg，一日 1 次。<br><br>（4）肝、肾功能不全患者，在开始治疗时可隔日服用 5mg。<br><br>(1) Chronic idiopathic urticaria, perennial allergic rhinitis and seasonal allergic rhinitis: For adults, Oral medication, once a day, 5mg singly.<br><br>(2) Chronic idiopathic urticaria, perennial allergic rhinitis: for children, Oral medication, 12 years old or more, 5mg singly, once a day; 6 to 11 years of age, 2.5mg singly, once a day; 12-month to 5 years old of age, 1.25mg singly, once a day; 6 months to 11 months, 1mg singly, once per day.<br><br>(3) Seasonal allergic rhinitis: for Children, Oral medication, 12 years or more, 5mg singly, once per day; 6 to 11 years of age, 2.5mg singly, once per day; 2 to 5 years of age, 1.25mg singly, once a day.<br><br>(4) patients with liver and renal insufficiency can take 5mg every other day at the start of treatment. |
| 剂型、规格<br>Preparations | 片剂：每片 5mg。<br>Tablets: 5mg per tablet. |
| 药品名称 Drug Names | 氮䓬斯汀 Azelastine |
| 适应证<br>Indications | 口服或喷鼻可控制季节性或非季节性鼻炎及非过敏性血管收缩性鼻炎症状。滴眼剂可用于治疗过敏性结膜炎。<br>By means of oral or nasal spray, it is able to control seasonal or non-seasonal rhinitis and nonallergic vasomotor rhinitis. The kind of eye drops is for the treatment of allergic conjunctivitis. |
| 用法、用量<br>Dosage | （1）过敏性鼻炎（季节性或非季节性）：①成人及 12 岁以上儿童，经鼻给药：每次每鼻孔 1 喷（每喷 0.137mg），一天 2 次，作用持续时间 12 小时。在花粉季节连续用药对控制鼻部症状优于临时用药。对于非季节性过敏性鼻炎，可长期用药 6 个月，安全性和疗效良好。口服：每次 1～2mg，一日 2 次。或遵医嘱。②5～11 岁儿童，经鼻给药：每次每鼻孔 1 喷，一天 2 次。口服：6 岁以上儿童，每次 1～2mg，一天 2 次。或遵医嘱。<br><br>（2）血管收缩性鼻炎：成人及 12 岁以上患者，每次每鼻孔 1 喷（每喷 0.137mg），一天 2 次，或遵医嘱。<br><br>（3）过敏性结膜炎：成人滴患眼，每次 1 滴（0.05%），一天 2 次。有报道 1 个疗程可用 8 个月。儿童滴眼剂只能用于 3 岁以上儿童。每次 1 滴（0.05%），一天 2 次。有报道 1 个疗程可用至 8 个月。或遵医嘱。 |

续 表

<table>
<tr>
<td colspan="2"></td>
<td>
（4）治疗和预防哮喘：成人或 6 岁以上儿童，口服，每次 1 ~ 4mg，一天 2 次；或每次 8mg，一天 1 次，睡前服。睡前服可用于控制哮喘夜间和晨起发作。遵医嘱。

（5）肝功能不全和老年患者无须调整剂量。

(1) allergic rhinitis (seasonal and non- seasonal ): ① for adults and children over 12 years, nasal administration : 1 spray per nostril (0.137mg per spray), 2 times a day, 12 hours duration of action. Continuous medication on nasal symptoms during the pollen season is better than than temporary medication. Non- seasonal allergic rhinitis prefers long-term medication six months for good safety and efficacy . Oral medication: 1 ~ 2mg singly, 2 times a day or do as directed. ② 5 ~ 11 year-old children, nasal administration : 1 spray per nostril singly, twice a day . Oral medication: Children above 6 years ole of age, 1 ~ 2mg singly, 2 times a day or do as directed.

(2) vasomotor rhinitis : for adults and patients over the age of 12, 1 spray per nostril singly (0.137mg per spray), 2 times a day or do as directed.

(3) allergic conjunctivitis : For adults, eye dripping on the uncomfortable eye, one drop singly ( 0.05% ), 2 times a day. It is reported that one course of treatment is available for eight months. eye drops for Children can be used only for those over 3 years old . one drop singly ( 0.05% ), 2 times a day. It is reported that one course of treatment is available for eight months. Or doing as directed.

(4) for the treatment and prevention of asthma : for adults or children over 6 years, Oral medication, 1 ~ 4mg singly, 2 times a day ; or 8mg singly, onces a day at bedtime to control asthma attack at night and early morning . Do as doctor requires.

(5) hepatic dysfunction and elderly patients don't need dose adjustment
</td>
</tr>
<tr>
<td colspan="2">剂型、规格<br>Preparations</td>
<td>
片剂：每片 0.5mg；1mg。

颗粒剂：2mg/g。

喷鼻剂：10mg/10ml。

滴眼剂：2.5mg/5ml。

Tablets: 0.5mg; 1mg per tablet.<br>
Granules: 2mg / g.<br>
Nasal spray: 10mg/10ml.<br>
Eye drops: 2.5mg/5ml.
</td>
</tr>
<tr>
<td colspan="2">药品名称 Drug Names</td>
<td>溴苯那敏 Brompheniramine</td>
</tr>
<tr>
<td colspan="2">适应证<br>Indications</td>
<td>可用于慢性荨麻疹。<br>For the treatment of chronic urticaria.</td>
</tr>
<tr>
<td colspan="2">用法、用量<br>Dosage</td>
<td>口服：一日 3 ~ 4 次，一次 4 ~ 8mg。<br>Oral medication: 3 to 4 times a day, 4 ~ 8mg singly.</td>
</tr>
<tr>
<td colspan="2">剂型、规格<br>Preparations</td>
<td>片剂：4mg。<br>缓释片：12mg。<br>Tablets: 4mg.<br>sustained-release tablets: 12mg.</td>
</tr>
<tr>
<td colspan="2">药品名称 Drug Names</td>
<td>氯苯那敏 Chlorphenira- mine</td>
</tr>
<tr>
<td colspan="2">适应证<br>Indications</td>
<td>用于过敏性鼻炎、感冒和鼻窦炎及过敏性皮肤疾病如荨麻疹、过敏性药疹或湿疹、血管神经性水肿、虫咬所致皮肤瘙痒。<br><br>For the treatment of allergic rhinitis, colds and sinusitis and allergic skin disorders, such as urticaria, allergic epispasis or eczema, angioneurotic edema, skin itching caused by insect bites.</td>
</tr>
<tr>
<td colspan="2">用法、用量<br>Dosage</td>
<td>口服，成人一次量 4mg，一日 3 次。肌内注射，一次 5 ~ 20mg。<br>Oral medication, for aults, 4mg singly, 3 times a day. Intramuscular injection, 5 ~ 20mg singly.</td>
</tr>
<tr>
<td colspan="2">剂型、规格<br>Preparations</td>
<td>片剂：每片 4mg。<br>胶囊剂：每粒 8mg。<br>注射液：每支 10mg（1ml）；20mg（2ml）。<br>Tablets: 4mg per tablet.<br>Capsules: 8mg per capsule.<br>Injection: 10mg (1ml); 20mg (2ml) per vial.</td>
</tr>
</table>

| 药品名称 Drug Names | 茶苯海明 Dimenhydrinate |
|---|---|
| 适应证<br>Indications | 有镇吐、防晕作用、可用于妊娠、晕动症、放射线治疗及术后引起的恶心、呕吐。<br><br>It has antiemetic effect and have ability to prevent motion sickness, which is helpful for the treatment of nausea and vomiting cansed by pregnancy, motion sickness, radiation therapy and post-operation reactions. |
| 用法、用量<br>Dosage | 一次 25 ～ 50mg，一日 3 次。<br>25 ～ 50mg singly, 3 times a day. |
| 剂型、规格<br>Preparations | 片剂：25mg；50mg。<br>Tablets: 25mg; 50mg. |
| 药品名称 Drug Names | 色甘酸钠 Sodium Cromoglicate |
| 适应证<br>Indications | 用于预防过敏性哮喘的发作，改善主观症状，增加患者对运动的耐受能力，对于依赖皮质激素的患者，服用本品后可使之减量或完全缓解。患有慢性难治性哮喘的儿童应用本品大部分或完全缓解。与异丙肾上腺素合用，较单用时的效率显著增高。但本品起效较慢，需连续用药数天后才能见效。如已发病，用药多无效。对变态反应作用不明显的慢性哮喘也有疗效。用于过敏性鼻炎和季节性花粉症，能迅速控制症状。软膏外用于慢性过敏性湿疹及某些皮肤瘙痒症也有显著疗效。2% ～ 4% 滴眼液适用于花粉症、结膜炎和春季角膜炎结膜炎。<br><br>For the prevention of allergic asthma and the improvement of subjective symptoms and patients' resistence against exercise taking, especially for those dependent on corticosteroids whose can reduce the dosage and even completely recover after taking. Children with chronic refractory asthma could recover mostly or completely. Combined with isoproterenol, it is more effective than used alone. However, it will make effect so that continuous dosing for several days is necessary. If disease attacks, medication will not be effective. It is also intended to treat chronic allergic asthma which doesn't have obvious effect with allergic reaction. It can quickly control the symptoms of allergic rhinitis and seasonal hay fever. It is also active against Chronic allergic eczema and other pruritus by use of cream. The sort of 2% to 4% eye dropis intended for hay fever, conjunctivitis and vernal conjunctivitis and keratitis. |
| 用法、用量<br>Dosage | （1）支气管哮喘：干粉喷雾吸入：成人，一次 20mg，一日 4 次。症状减轻后，一日 2 ～ 3 次；维持量一日 20mg。5 岁以上儿童用量同成人。<br>（2）过敏性鼻炎：干粉鼻吸入：一次 10mg，一日 4 次；2% 或 4% 溶液滴鼻或喷雾，每次用药量约含色甘酸钠 5mg，一日 6 次。<br>（3）食物过敏：成人，一次 200mg，一日 4 次，饭前服。2 岁以上儿童，一次 100mg，一日 4 次。如 2 ～ 3 周效果不佳，剂量可增加，每日不超过 40mg/kg，症状控制后可减量。<br>（4）滴眼：2% 或 4% 滴眼剂滴眼，一日数次。<br>（5）外用：5% ～ 10% 软膏，涂患处，一日 2 次。<br><br>(1) Bronchial asthma: dry powder spray inhalation: for adult, 20mg singly, 4 times a day. After symptom relief, 2 or 3 times a day; maintenance dose is 20mg a day. Children under 5 years of age has the same dosage with adult.<br>(2) Allergic rhinitis: dry powder inhalation: 10mg singly, 4 times a day; 2% or 4% solution used as nasal drip or spray, 5mg cromolyn sodium singly, 6 times a day.<br>(3) Food allergies: for adults, 200mg singly, 4 times a day before meals. Children above 2 years old, 100mg singly, 4 times a day. If the effect is poor, 2 to 3 weeks for example, the dose can be increased, but not to exceed 40mg/kg a day. Dosage could be reduced for controlled symptoms.<br>(4) Eye Drops: 2% or 4% eye drops, several times a day.<br>(5) Topical: 5% to 10% ointment, coating the affected area for 2 times a day. |
| 剂型、规格<br>Preparations | 气雾剂：每瓶总量约 14g，内含色甘酸钠 0.7g，每揿含药量 3.5mg。<br>胶囊剂：每粒 20mg。<br>软膏：5% ～ 10%。<br>滴眼剂：2%（8ml）；4%（8ml）。<br><br>Aerosol: a total of about 14g per bottle, containing cromolyn sodium 0.7g, 3.5mg per press.<br>Capsules: 20mg per capsule.<br>Ointment: 5% ～ 10%.<br>Eye drops: 2% (8ml); 4% (8ml). |

续　表

| 药品名称 Drug Names | 酮替芬 Ketotifen |
|---|---|
| 适应证<br>Indications | （1）用于多种类型支气管哮喘，均有明显疗效，对过敏性哮喘疗效尤为明显，混合性次之，感染型约半数以上有效。对过敏性哮喘效果优于色甘酸钠。<br><br>（2）也可用于过敏性鼻炎、过敏性结膜炎、花粉症、急慢性荨麻疹、药物、食物或昆虫所致变态反应的预防和治疗。<br><br>(1) For the treatment of bronchial asthma of many types, allergic asthma in particular and then the mixed type. More than half of the infectious type will recover. Compared with cromolyn sodium, it is more effective on the treatment of allergic asthma.<br>(2) It can also be used for the treatment of allergic rhinitis, allergic conjunctivitis, hay fever, acute and chronic urticarial and prevention and treatment of allergic reaction caused by drugs, food or insect bites. |
| 用法、用量<br>Dosage | 口服：成人，一次 1mg，早、晚各服一次；若困意明显，可只在睡前服 1 次。<br>Oral medication: for adults, 1mg singly, once for morning and evening ; if one is extremely sleepy, once a day at bedtime is enough. |
| 剂型、规格<br>Preparations | 片剂：每片 1mg。<br>胶囊剂：每粒 1mg。<br>口服液：每支 1mg/5ml。<br>滴眼液：2.5mg/5ml。<br>滴鼻液：15mg/10ml。<br>分散片：每片 1mg。<br>鼻吸入粉雾剂：15.5mg/14g。<br>Tablets: 1mg per tablet.<br>Capsules: 1mg per capsule.<br>Oral liquid: 1mg/5ml per vial.<br>Drops: 2.5mg/5ml.<br>Nasal drip: 15mg/10ml.<br>dispersible tablet: 1mg per tablet.<br>Nasal powder for inhalation: 15.5mg/14g. |

## 17.2　免疫抑制药 Immunosuppressants

| 药品名称 Drug Names | 环孢素 Ciclosporin |
|---|---|
| 适应证<br>Indications | 主要用于肾、肝、心、肺、骨髓移植的抗排异反应，可与肾上腺皮质激素或其他免疫抑制剂合用，也可用于治疗类风湿关节炎、系统性红斑狼疮、肾病型慢性肾炎、自身免疫性溶血性贫血、银屑病、葡萄膜炎等自身免疫性疾病。<br><br>Mainly used as anti-rejection reaction drugs towards bone marrow transplant of kidney, liver, heart, lung. It can be used in combination with adrenal corticosteroids or other immunosuppressive agents. It is also effective to the treatment of autoimmune diseases, such as rheumatoid arthritis, systemic lupus erythematosus, chronic nephritis of nephrotic type, autoimmune hemolytic anemia, psoriasis, uveitis, etc. |
| 用法、用量<br>Dosage | （1）器官移植：①口服：于移植前 12 小时起每日服 8 ~ 10mg/kg，维持术后 1 ~ 2 周，根据血药浓度减至每日 2 ~ 6mg/kg，分 2 次服。②静脉注射：仅用于不能口服的患者，于移植前 4 ~ 12 小时每日给予 3 ~ 5mg/kg，以 5% 葡萄糖或生理盐水稀释至 1 ：20 至 1 ：100 的浓度于 2 ~ 6 小时缓慢滴注。<br><br>（2）自身免疫性疾病：口服，初始剂量为每日 2.5 ~ 5mg/kg，分 2 次服，症状缓解后改为最小剂量维持，但成人不应超过每日 5mg/kg，儿童不应超过 6mg/kg。<br><br>(1) Organ transplantation: ① Oral medication: 8 ~ 10mg/kg singly from 12 hours before transplantation and lasting till 1 to 2 weeks after surgery, make appropriate adjustment according to plasma concentration to reduce to 2 ~ 6mg/kg a day in 2 divided doses . ② intravenous injection: only for patients with Oral medication, 3 ~ 5mg/kg a day4 to 12 hours before transplantation, diluting with 5% dextrose or saline to a concentration of 1 ：20 to 1 ：100 and slow dripping within 2 to 6 hours.<br>(2) Autoimmune diseases: Oral medication, the initial dosage is 2.5 ~ 5mg/kg a day total in 2 divided doses. After symptom alleviation, it can be changed to the minimum dose for maintainance. The maximum dose for adults should not exceed the 5mg/kg a day, 6mg/kg for children. |

续　表

| 剂型、规格<br>Preparations | 胶囊剂：每粒 25mg；100mg。微乳化软胶囊：每粒 10mg；25mg；50mg；100mg。口服液：100mg/ml（50ml）。微乳化口服液：100mg/ml（50ml）。静脉滴注浓缩液：250mg/5ml；500mg/10ml。<br><br>Capsules: 25mg ;100mg per capsule. Microemulsifying soft capsules: 10mg; 25mg; 50mg; 100mg per capsule. Oral liquid: 100mg/ml (50ml). Oral microemulsion: 100mg/ml (50ml). Intravenous infusion concentrate: 250mg/5ml; 500mg/10ml. |
|---|---|
| **药品名称 Drug Names** | 他克莫司 Tacrolimus |
| 适应证<br>Indications | 主要用于器官移植的抗排异反应，尤其适用于肝移植，还可用于肾、心、肺、胰、骨髓及角膜移植等。<br><br>It is mainly used for anti-rejection of organ transplants, especially for liver transplantation, and for transplantation of kidney, heart, lung, pancreas, bone marrow and corneal. |
| 用法、用量<br>Dosage | 开始采用每日 0.05 ~ 0.1mg/kg（肾移植），或 0.01 ~ 0.05mg/kg（肝移植）持续静脉滴注。能进行口服时，改为口服胶囊，开始剂量为每日 0.15 ~ 0.3mg/kg，分 2 次服；在逐渐减至维持剂量，每日 0.1mg/kg，分 2 次服，亦可根据病情调整剂量，通常低于首次免疫抑制剂量。本品外用皮肤涂布可用于其他免疫抑制药疗效不佳或无法耐受的中重度特应性皮炎。<br><br>the initial dosage is 0.05 ~ 0.1mg/kg (kidney transplant) a day, or 0.01 ~ 0.05mg/kg (liver transplant) for continuous intravenous infusion. When Oral medication is available, change to Oral medication capsules with the starting dose of 0.15 ~ 0.3mg/kg a day in 2 divided doses and gradually reduce to a maintenance dose of 0.1mg/kg a day in 2 divided doses. Also, Dosage should be adapted to patients individually, which is less than the amount of the first immunosuppressant. This product is for external coating on atopic dermatitis intolerable or incurable against other immunosuppressive drugs. |
| 剂型、规格<br>Preparations | 胶囊剂：每粒 0.5mg；1mg；5mg。<br>注射液：每支 5mg（1ml），用时稀释在 5% 葡萄糖或生理盐水中缓慢静脉滴注。<br>外用软膏剂：3mg/10g；10mg/10g。<br>Capsules: 0.5mg; 1mg; 5mg per capsule.<br>Injection: 5mg (1ml) per vial, when diluted with 5% glucose or normal saline and slow intravenous infusion.<br>Topical ointment: 3mg/10g; 10mg/10g. |
| **药品名称 Drug Names** | 吗替麦考酚酯 Mycophenolate Mofetil |
| 适应证<br>Indications | 主要用于预防和治疗肾、肝、心脏及骨髓移植的排异反应。也可用于不能耐受其他免疫抑制剂或疗效不佳的类风湿关节炎、全身性红斑狼疮、原发性肾小球肾炎、牛皮癣等自身免疫性疾病。<br><br>It is mainly for the prevention and treatment of rejection of kidney, liver, heart and marrow. It is also for the treatment of autoimmune diseases, such as rheumatoid arthritis, systemic lupus erythematosus, primary glomerulonephritis, psoriasis, etc intolerant with other immunosuppressive agents or with poor efficacy. |
| 用法、用量<br>Dosage | 用于器官移植：空腹口服，成人每日 1.5 ~ 2.0g，小儿 30mg/kg，分 2 次服，首剂量应在器官移植后 72 小时内服用；静脉注射，主要用于口服不能耐受者，每次注射时间多于 2 小时。用于自身免疫病：成人每日 1.5 ~ 2.0g，维持量 0.25 ~ 0.5g，一日 2 次，空腹服用。<br><br>For organ transplantation: fasting and Oral medication, for adult, 1.5 ~ 2.0g a day, for children 30mg/kg in 2 divided doses, when the first dose should be taken within 72 hours after an organ transplant; Intravenous injection, mainly for those with Oral medication intolerance, more than 2 hours per injection time. For autoimmune disease: for adults, 1.5 ~ 2.0g a day, the maintenance dose of 0.25 ~ 0.5g, 2 times a day, taken on an empty stomach. |
| 剂型、规格<br>Preparations | 胶囊剂：每粒 250mg。片剂：每片 500mg。注射剂：每支 500mg。<br>Capsules: 250mg per capsule. Tablets: 500mg per tablet. Injection: 500mg per vial. |

续　表

| 药品名称 Drug Names | 来氟米特 Leflunomide |
| --- | --- |
| 适应证<br>Indications | 用于治疗风湿性关节炎、系统性红斑狼疮等自身免疫性疾病，亦可用于器官移植抗排异反应。<br>For the treatment of autoimmune diseases, such as rheumatoid arthritis, systemic lupus erythematosus, etc. and anti-rejection reactions of organ transplantation. |
| 用法、用量<br>Dosage | 口服，成人常用量：①类风湿关节炎、系统性红斑狼疮及银屑病关节炎，一次20mg，一日1次；病情控制后可以一日10～20mg维持。②韦格纳肉芽肿病，一日20～40mg维持。③器官移植，负荷剂量一日200mg，维持剂量一日40～60mg。<br>Oral medication, the usual dose for adults: ① rheumatoid arthritis, psoriatic arthritis and systemic lupus erythematosus, 20mg singly, once a day; the maintainance dose of 10～20mg after disease is control ② Wegener's granulomatosis, the maintainance dose of 20～40mg a day. ③ organ transplant, the loading dose of 200mg a day, the maintainance dose of 40～60mg a day. |
| 剂型、规格<br>Preparations | 片剂：每片10mg；20mg；100mg。<br>Tablets: 10mg; 20mg; 100mg per tablet |
| 药品名称 Drug Names | 泼尼松 Prednisone |
| 适应证<br>Indications | 糖皮质激素对Ⅰ、Ⅱ、Ⅲ、Ⅳ型变态反应性疾病具有程度不同的治疗效果。<br>（1）在Ⅰ型变态反应性疾病中，糖皮质激素应用广泛，可全身给药或局部给药，如用于过敏性鼻炎、异位性皮炎、过敏性哮喘等。<br>（2）糖皮质激素用于治疗Ⅱ型的自身免疫性疾病往往有效，是寻常性天疱疮、自身免疫性溶血性贫血的首选药物，如泼尼松可使60%～80%的自身免疫性溶血性贫血缓解。<br>（3）糖皮质激素广泛应用于治疗免疫复合物疾病（Ⅲ型变态反应性疾病），主要是依靠其抗炎作用，但仅仅可缓解症状，无消除病因作用。对系统性红斑狼疮，糖皮质激素往往可降低抗核抗体的浓度及减少狼疮红细胞的出现，而且某些证据表明，对肾损伤的患者应用大剂量的糖皮质激素能改善肾功能并延长患者生命。<br>（4）糖皮质激素是Ⅳ型变态反应性疾病的强力抑制剂，临床上用于移植器官或组织的排异反应、接触性皮炎等。<br>Glucocorticoids have varying efficacy on the treatment of Ⅰ, Ⅱ, Ⅲ and Ⅳ type allergic disease.<br>(1) In type Ⅰ allergic diseases, corticosteroids are widely used so as to be administered systemically or topically, such as allergic rhinitis, atopic dermatitis, allergic asthma, etc.<br>(2) Glucocorticoid is always effective on the treatment of II-type autoimmune diseases and is the first choice for the treatment of pemphigus vulgaris and autoimmune hemolytic anemia, when prednisone can be made up with 60%～80% proportion to remit autoimmune hemolytic anemia.<br>(3) It is widely used in the treatment of immune complex disease ( Ⅲ type allergic disease ), mainly anti-inflammatory function. However, it can only relieve symptoms without eliminating the cause completely . As to systemic lupus erythematosus, glucocorticoids can often reduce the concentration of antinuclear antibodies and red blood cells of lupus, and some evidence proves that large doses of glucocorticoid could improve renal function and prolong the lives of patients with kidney injury.<br>(4) It is a potent inhibitor to Ⅳ type allergic diseases, clinically used for the rejection of organ or tissue transplantation, contact dermatitis and the like. |
| 用法、用量<br>Dosage | 口服：一般每日20～60mg，如疗效不明显可逐渐增至每日100mg，维持量为每日10mg。用于肾、肝、心脏等器官移植：一般术后每日4mg/kg，加硫唑嘌呤每日5mg/kg；维持剂量每日10～20mg，加硫唑嘌呤每日1～2mg/kg。<br>Oral medication: generally, 20～60mg a day, gradually increase to 100mg a day when the efficacy is poor, the maintenance dose of 10mg a day. For kidney, liver, heart and other organ transplantation: generally postoperative patients should be given 4mg/kg a day, combined with azathioprine of 5mg/kg a day; the maintenance dose of 10～20mg a day, combined with azathioprine 1～2mg/kg a day. |
| 剂型、规格<br>Preparations | 片剂：每片5mg。<br>Tablets: 5mg per tablet. |

**续　表**

| 药品名称 Drug Names | 硫唑嘌呤 Azathioprine |
|---|---|
| 适应证<br>Indications | 　　主要用于器官移植时的排异反应，多与皮质激素并用，或加用淋巴细胞球蛋白（ALG），疗效好。也广泛用于类风湿关节炎、系统性红斑狼疮，自身免疫性溶血性贫血、特发性血小板减少性紫癜、活动性慢性肝炎、溃疡性结肠炎、重症肌无力、硬皮病等自身免疫性疾病。对慢性肾炎及肾病综合征，其疗效似不及环磷酰胺。由于其不良反应较多且严重，对上述疾病治疗不作为首选，通常是在单用糖皮质激素不能控制时才使用。<br><br>　　Mainly used for organ transplant rejection combined with corticosteroids and use, or antilymphocyte globulin (ALG) for better efficacy. It is also widely used in the treatment of rheumatoid arthritis, systemic lupus erythematosus, autoimmune hemolytic anemia, idiopathic thrombocytopenic purpura, chronic active hepatitis, ulcerative colitis, myasthenia gravis, scleroderma and other autoimmune diseases. As to chronic nephritis and nephrotic syndrome, its efficacy seems not better than that of cyclophosphamide. However, because of many severe adverse reactions, it is not the preferred treatment diseases mentioned above. Usually, it is used when corticosteroids couldnot control the patient's condition alone. |
| 用法、用量<br>Dosage | 　　口服：每日 1 ～ 3mg/kg，一般每日 100mg，一次服用，可连服数月。用于器官移植：每日 2 ～ 5mg/kg，维持量每日 0.5 ～ 3mg/kg。<br><br>　　Oral medication: 1 ～ 3mg/kg a day, generally, 100mg a day, taken in one time for a few months. For organ transplantation: 2 ～ 5mg/kg A day, the maintenance dose of 0.5 ～ 3mg/kg a day. |
| 剂型、规格<br>Preparations | 　　片剂：每片 25mg；50mg；100mg。<br>　　注射液：50mg（以硫唑嘌呤计量）。<br><br>　　Tablets: 25mg; 50mg; 100mg per tablet.<br>　　Injection: 50mg (measuring by azathioprine). |
| 药品名称 Drug Names | 羟基脲 Hydroxycarbamide |
| 适应证<br>Indications | 　　用于顽固性银屑病和脓疱性银屑病均有效，能减轻全身性脓疱性银屑病的脓疱、发热和中毒症状。短期用药，其毒性作用较甲氨蝶呤小，对有肝脏损伤不宜用甲氨蝶呤或用甲氨蝶呤无效的严重银屑病患者，可选用本品治疗。<br><br>　　For the treatment of stubborn psoriasis and pustular psoriasis, which can reduce pustules, fever and poisoning symptoms caused by systemic pustular psoriasis. Short-term medication has few toxic effects than methotrexate. Patients with liver damage or those with severe psoriasis but unsuitable or invalid to methotrexate could use Hydroxycarbamide for treatment. |
| 用法、用量<br>Dosage | 　　口服：每日 0.5 ～ 1.5g，4 ～ 8 周为 1 个疗程。<br>　　Oral medication: 0.5 ～ 1.5g A day, a course of treatment is 4 ～ 8 weeks. |
| 剂型、规格<br>Preparations | 　　片剂：每片 400mg；500mg。<br>　　胶囊剂：每粒 250mg；400mg；500mg。<br><br>　　Tablets: 400mg; 500mg per tablet.<br>　　Capsules: 250mg; 400mg; 500m g per capsule. |
| 药品名称 Drug Names | 甲氨蝶呤 Methotrexate |
| 适应证<br>Indications | 　　本品原为抗肿瘤药，经剂量、用法调整后用作免疫抑制药。主要用于类风湿关节炎、银屑病关节炎、红斑狼疮、脊柱关节病的周围关节炎、多肌炎、多发性肉芽肿等自身免疫性疾病。甲氨蝶呤间歇疗法治疗多发性肉芽肿起效较皮质激素、烷化剂或硫唑嘌呤迅速，故急性患者应首选本品。用于皮质激素无效的多肌炎、皮肌炎均见肌力改善、皮疹消退。根据报道甲氨蝶呤特别适用于顽固的进行性多发性肌炎和顽固的进行性眼色素层炎，治疗 1 ～ 2 周后可使麻痹或失明的患者恢复一定功能。其作用机制不明，可能与其抗炎作用有关。应用免疫抑制量的甲氨蝶呤后 24 小时内再给适量的甲酰四氢叶酸，可对抗甲氨蝶呤的毒性，但几乎不影响其免疫抑制作用。 |

**续　表**

<table>
<tr>
<td></td>
<td>This product was originally antineoplastic agents and then used as immunosuppressive drug after dose and usage adjustment. Mainly used for the treatment of rheumatoid arthritis, psoriatic arthritis, lupus, arthritis, spondyloarthropathy around, polymyositis, multiple granulomas and other auto-immune diseases. Methotrexate intermittent therapy will quickly treat intermittent onset compared corticosteroids, alkylating agents or azathioprine caused by multiple granulomas, so this product should be preferred in acute patients. For the treatment of polymyositis invalid for Corticosteroids and dermatomyositis will lessen by muscle strength improvement and subsiding skin rash. According to reports, methotrexate is especially for the treatment of stubborn progressive multiple polymyositis and stubborn progressive uveitis.Patients with paralysis or blindness can recover more or less after 1 to 2 weeks' treatment, but it's not clear about the mechanism of action. Maybe it is related to the anti-inflammatory effects. Appropriate amount of leucovorin should be administered 24 hours later after immunosuppressive amount of methotrexate to combat the toxicity of methotrexate, but hardly affect the immune inhibition.</td>
</tr>
<tr>
<td>用法、用量<br>Dosage</td>
<td>口服：初始剂量一次 7.5mg，一周 1 次；可酌情增加至 20mg，一周一次，分 2 次服。肌内注射：每次 10mg，一周一次。静脉注射：每次 10 ～ 15mg，一周 1 次。银屑病，口服，一次 0.25 ～ 5mg，一日 1 次，6 ～ 7 日为 1 个疗程。<br><br>Oral medication: the Initial dose is 7.5mg singly, a week singly; increase the drug dose to 20mg appropriately, in 2 divided doses and one time per week. Intramuscular injection: 10mg singly, once a week. Intravenous injection: 10 ～ 15mg singly, once a week. For Psoriasis, Oral medication, 0.25 ～ 5mg singly, once a day, 6 to 7 days for a course of treatment.</td>
</tr>
<tr>
<td>剂型、规格<br>Preparations</td>
<td>片剂：每片 2.5mg；5mg；10mg。注射液：每支 5mg；10mg；20mg；25mg；50mg；100mg。<br>Tablets: 2.5mg; 5mg; 10mg per tablet. Injection: 5mg; 10mg; 20mg; 25mg; 50mg; 100mg per vial.</td>
</tr>
<tr>
<td>药品名称 Drug Names</td>
<td>环磷酰胺 Cyclophosphamide</td>
</tr>
<tr>
<td>适应证<br>Indications</td>
<td>用于各种自身免疫性疾病，对严重类风湿关节炎及全身系统性红斑狼疮，大部分病例有效；对儿童肾病综合征，其疗效较硫唑嘌呤好，可长期缓解。可单独用药，但与质激素并用则疗效较佳，且不良反应较少。对多发性肉芽肿亦常用。与质激素并用则疗效较佳，且不良反应较少。与皮质激素并用于治疗天疱疮疗效也较好。此外，也用于治疗溃疡性结肠炎、特发性血小板减少性紫癜等自身免疫性疾病。也用于器官移植时抗排异反应，通常是与泼尼松、抗淋巴细胞球蛋白并用，其效果与硫唑嘌呤、泼尼松、抗淋巴细胞球蛋白的效果相似，且可避免硫唑嘌呤对肝脏可能产生的不良影响。<br><br>For the treatment of a variety of autoimmune diseases, severe rheumatoid arthritis and systemic lupus erythematosus and most cases are effectively treated; it can relieve nephrotic syndrome for children for a long time, better efficacy compared with azathioprine. Individually medication is available, but better with corticosteroids with fewer adverse reactions. Also used for multiple granulomas. Better treatment efficieny on pemphigus combined with corticosteroids with fewer adverse reactions. Also, for the treatment of ulcerative colitis, idiopathic thrombocytopenic purpura and other autoimmune diseases. Also used in treating organ transplant anti-rejection reaction, usually used with prednisone and anti-lymphocyte globulin, similar effect with azathioprine, prednisone, anti-lymphocyte globulin. It also can avoid the possible adverse effects on liver caused by Azathioprine.</td>
</tr>
<tr>
<td>用法、用量<br>Dosage</td>
<td>自身免疫性疾病：口服，一日 2 ～ 3mg/kg，一日 1 次或隔日一次，连用 4 ～ 6 周。器官移植：口服，一日 50 ～ 150mg；静脉注射，一次 0.2g，一日或隔日 1 次，总量 8 ～ 10g 为 1 个疗程。<br><br>Autoimmune diseases: Oral medication, 2 ～ 3mg/kg 1 day, once per day or every other day lasting for four to six weeks. Organ transplantation: Oral medication, 50 ～ 150mg a day; intravenous injection, 0.2g singly, once a day or every other day, the total amount of 8 ～ 10g is for a course.</td>
</tr>
<tr>
<td>剂型、规格<br>Preparations</td>
<td>片剂：50mg。<br>注射剂：100mg；200mg。<br>滴眼液：1%。<br>Tablets: 50mg.<br>Injection: 100mg; 200mg.<br>Eye drops: 1%.</td>
</tr>
</table>

| 药品名称 Drug Names | 苯丁酸氮芥 Chlorambucil |
|---|---|
| 适应证<br>Indications | 　　对于切特综合征、红斑狼疮病有较好疗效。尚用于治疗类风湿关节炎并发的脉管炎、伴有寒冷凝集素的自身免疫性溶血性贫血以及依赖皮质激素的肾病综合征，与泼尼松龙并用于频发的肾病综合征。用于硬皮病可迅速组织其发展，使皮肤溃疡痊愈，肺功能改善。<br><br>　　Better treating effect on Chet's syndrome, lupus disease. Still used in the treatment of rheumatoid arthritis complicated by vasculitis, autoimmune hemolytic anemia accompanied by cold coagulation factors and corticosteroid-dependent nephrotic syndrome, and frequent nephrotic syndrome combined with prednisolone. For the treatment of Scleroderma to quickly improve skin ulcers recovery and lung function. |
| 用法、用量<br>Dosage | 　　口服：每日 3 ~ 6mg，早饭前 1 小时或晚饭后 2 小时服用，连服数周，待疗效或骨髓抑制出现后减量，总量一般为 300 ~ 500mg。<br><br>　　Oral medication: 3 ~ 6mg A day, taken 1 hour before breakfast or two hours after dinner for continus weeks. The amount could be reduced when the efficacy is obvious or myelosuppression occurs and the total amount is generally 300 ~ 500mg. |
| 剂型、规格<br>Preparations | 　　片剂：每片 1mg；2mg。<br>　　纸型片：每格 2mg。<br><br>　　Tablets: 1mg per tablet; 2mg.<br>　　Matrix tablets: 2mg per cell. |

## 17.3　免疫增强药 Immunostimulants

| 药品名称 Drug Names | 香菇多糖 Lentinan |
|---|---|
| 适应证<br>Indications | 　　用于急慢性白血病、胃癌、肺癌、乳腺癌等肿瘤的辅助治疗，提高患者免疫功能，减轻放射治疗和化学治疗的副作用。亦可用于治疗乙型病毒性肝炎。<br><br>　　For adjuvant therapy of acute and chronic leukemia, stomach cancer, lung cancer and breast cancer to improve immune function and reduce side effects of radiation therapy and chemotherapy. It can also be used to treat virus hepatitis B. |
| 用法、用量<br>Dosage | 　　口服：成人每次 12.5mg，一日 2 次；儿童每次 5 ~ 7.5mg，一日 2 次。静脉注射或静脉滴注：一次 2mg，每周 1 次。一般 3 个月为 1 个疗程。<br><br>　　Oral medication: for adults, 12.5mg singly, 2 times a day; for children, 5 ~ 7.5mg singly, 2 times a day. Intravenous injection or intravenous infusion: 2mg singly, once a week. Generally, three months is for a course of treatment. |
| 剂型、规格<br>Preparations | 　　片剂：每片 2.5mg。<br>　　注射剂：每支 1mg。<br><br>　　Tablets: 2.5mg per tablet.<br>　　Injection: 1mg per vial |
| 药品名称 Drug Names | 重组人白细胞介素 -2 Recombinant HumanInterleukin-2 |
| 适应证<br>Indications | 　　用于肾细胞癌、黑色素瘤，控制癌性胸、腹水及其他晚期肿瘤；先天或后天免疫缺陷症，如艾滋病等；细菌、真菌及病毒感染，如慢性活动性乙型肝炎、慢性活动性 EB 病毒感染、麻风病、肺结核、白念珠菌感染等。<br><br>　　For renal cell carcinoma, melanoma, malig-nant pleural effusion and ascites, and other advanced tumors; congenital or acquired immunodeficiency syndrome, such as AIDS, etc.; bacterial, fungal and viral infections, such as chronic active hepatitis B, chronic active EB viral infections, leprosy, tuberculosis, Candida albicans infection. |
| 用法、用量<br>Dosage | 　　皮下注射：每日 20 万 ~ 40 万 $U/m^2$，加入无菌注射用水 2ml，一天 1 次，每周连用 4 日，4 周为 1 个疗程。肌内注射：慢性乙型肝炎每次 20 万 U，隔日一次。静脉滴注：20 万 ~ 40 万 $U/m^2$，加入生理盐水 500ml，一日一次，每周连用 4 日，4 周为 1 个疗程。腔内注射：癌性胸、腹水时先抽取胸腔内积液，再将本品 40 万 ~ 50 万 $U/m^2$ 加入生理盐水 20ml 注入，每周 1 ~ 2 次，3 ~ 4 周为 1 个疗程。瘤内或瘤周注射：10 万 ~ 30 万 $U/m^2$，加至 3 ~ 5ml 注射用生理盐水中，分多点注射到瘤内或瘤周。每周 2 次，连用 2 周为 1 个疗程。 |

续　表

| | |
|---|---|
| | Subcutaneous injection: 200,000 ~ 400,000U/m$^2$ a day added with 2ml sterile water for injection, once a day, 4 continous days a week and four weeks as a course. Intramuscular injection: for the treatment of chronic hepatitis B, 200, 000 U singly, once every other day. Intravenous infusion: 200,000 ~ 400,000U/m$^2$, added with normal saline 500ml, once a day, 4 continous days a week and four weeks as a course. Articular injection: for the treatment of cancer-related hydrothorax and ascites, pleural effusion should be extracted first from chest and inject 400,000 ~ 500,000U/m$^2$ Recombinant Human Interleukin with 20ml of saline, 1 ~ 2 times per week, 3 to 4 weeks as a course. Intratumoral or peritumoral injection: 100,000 ~ 300,000U/m$^2$, added with 3 ~ 5ml saline for injection, when intratumoral and peritumoral parts should be injected more, 2 times a week for two weeks continuously as a course. |
| 剂型、规格<br>Preparations | 注射剂：每支 2.5 万 U；5 万 U；10 万 U；20 万 U；50 万 U；100 万 U；200 万 U。<br>Injection: 25, 000 U; 50, 000 U; 100, 000 U; 200, 000 U; 500, 000 U; 1millon U; 2 millon U per vial. |
| 药品名称 Drug Names | 重组人白细胞介素 -11　Recombinant Human Interleukin-11 |
| 适应证<br>Indications | 用于实体瘤、非髓性白细胞病化疗后Ⅲ、Ⅳ度血小板减少症的治疗。<br>For the treatment of solid tumors, Ⅲ, Ⅳ type thrombocytopenia treatment after non-myeloid leukocytes disease chemotherapy. |
| 用法、用量<br>Dosage | 皮下注射，一次 25 ~ 50μg/kg（以 1ml 注射用水稀释），一日一次，7 ~ 14 日为 1 个疗程。于化疗结束后 24 ~ 48 小时开始或发生血小板减少症后给药，血小板计数恢复后应及时停药。<br>Subcutaneous injection: 25 ~ 50μg/kg singly (diluting with 1ml water for injection), once a day for 7 to 14 days as a course. 24 to 48 hours after chemotherapy or thrombocytopenia could administer the drug and promptly discontinue after platelet recovers . |
| 剂型、规格<br>Preparations | 注射用粉针剂：每支 0.75mg（600 万 U）；1.5mg（1200 万 U）；3mg（2400 万 U）。<br>Powder for injection: 0.75mg (6 millon U); 1.5mg (12 millon U); 3mg (24 millon U) per vial. |
| 药品名称 Drug Names | 重组人干扰素 Recombinant Human Interferon（rh IFN） |
| 适应证<br>Indications | 干扰素可用于肿瘤、病毒感染及慢性活动性乙型肝炎等。<br>Interferon can be used for cancer, viral infections and chronic active hepatitis B and so on. |
| 用法、用量<br>Dosage | 各种不同干扰素制剂的用法不同，简介于下，详见说明书。<br>Interferon of various kinds are different to use, profile are below and see in instructions. |
| 剂型、规格<br>Preparations | 详见下述干扰素 α、β、γ 各亚型内容。<br>See the following interferon α, β, γ subtypes content. |
| 药品名称 Drug Names | 重组人干扰素 α-2a　Recombinant Human Interferon α-2a（rh IFN α-2a） |
| 适应证<br>Indications | 用于治疗：①某些病毒性疾病：乙型肝炎、丙型肝炎、尖锐湿疣、带状疱疹、小儿病毒性肺炎和上呼吸道感染、慢性宫颈炎等。②某些恶性肿瘤：毛细胞白血病、慢性粒细胞白血病、多发性骨髓瘤、非霍奇金淋巴瘤、卡波西肉瘤、肾癌、喉乳头状瘤、黑色素瘤、蕈样肉芽肿、膀胱癌、基底细胞癌等。<br>For the treatment of: ① certain viral diseases: hepatitis B, hepatitis C, genital warts, herpes zoster, children with viral pneumonia and upper respiratory tract infection, chronic cervicitis. ② certain malignancies: hairy cell leukemia, chronic myelogenous leukemia, multiple myeloma, non-Hodgkin's lymphoma, Kaposi's sarcoma, kidney cancer, laryngeal papilloma, melanoma, mycosis fungoides, bladder carcinoma, basal cell carcinoma, etc. |
| 用法、用量<br>Dosage | 皮下或肌内注射给药，剂量和疗程如下：<br>（1）慢性活动性乙型肝炎：每次 500 万 U，一周 3 次，共用 6 个月。1 个月后病毒复制标志物如未见下降，剂量可增加至患者能耐受水平；如疗程 3 ~ 4 个月后症状未获改善，则应停止治疗。<br>（2）急、慢性丙型肝炎：起始剂量为一次 300 万 ~ 500 万 U，一周 3 次，持续 3 个月。对血清谷丙转氨酶（ALT）正常的患者给予维持治疗：一次 300 万 U，一周 3 次，持续 3 个月。ALT 异常者停止使用。 |

**续 表**

（3）多发性骨髓瘤：起始剂量为一次 300 万 U，一周 3 次，可根据患者的耐受性，逐周增加至最大耐受量（900 万～ 1800 万 U）。

（4）毛细胞白血病：起始剂量为一次 300 万 U，一日 1 次，持续 16 ～ 24 周。如患者难以忍受，则剂量减为一次 150 万 U，一周 3 次。

（5）慢性粒细胞白血病：采用逐渐增加剂量给药方案，即第 1 ～ 3 日，每日 300 万 U；第 4 ～ 6 日，每日 600 万 U；第 7 ～ 84 日，每日 900 万 U。治疗 8 ～ 12 周后，时视其疗效决定是否继续治疗。

（6）非霍奇金淋巴瘤：作为肿瘤化疗的辅助用药，推荐剂量为：一次 300 万 U，一周 3 次，至少持续 12 周。

（7）尖锐湿疣：皮下或肌内注射，一次 100 万～ 300 万 U，一周 3 次，使用 1 ～ 2 个月。

（8）宫颈糜烂：非月经期睡前用手指将一枚栓剂放入阴道贴近子宫颈处，隔日一次，9 次为 1 个疗程。

Subcutaneous or intramuscular injection, the dose and duration of treatment are as follows:

(1) Chronic active hepatitis B: 5 million U singly, three times a week for six months. If markers of viral replication don't decrease A month later, dose could be increased to the level of tolerant one for patient ;Treatment should be stopped if symptoms have not been improved 3 to 4 months after the course.

(2) Acute and chronic hepatitis C: the initial dose is 3 million to 5 million U singly, three times a week for 3 months continuously. patients reacted normally by Serum alanine aminotransferase (ALT) are given maintenance therapy: 3 million U singly, three times a week for 3 months continuously. ALT outlier should stop medication.

(3) Multiple myeloma: the starting dose of 3 million U singly, three times a week. It can be increased to the maximum tolerant dose week by week (900 million to 18 million U) according to the patient's tolerance.

(4) Hairy cell leukemia: the starting dose of 3 million U, once a day for 16 to 24 weeks. If the patient is unbearable, then the dose could be reduced to a 1.5 million U, three times a week.

(5) Chronic myeloid leukemia: A regimen to increase dosage gradually, ie. 1 to 3 days, the 3 million U a day for the first 3 days; 6 million U a day for the 4th to 6th day; 9 million U a day for the 7th to 8th day. 8 to 12 weeks after the treatment, whether to continue treatment depends on the efficacy.

(6) Non-Hodgkin's lymphoma: As the adjuvant chemotherapy, the recommended dose is: 1 ~ 3 million U singly, three times a week, for at least 12 weeks.

(7) Condyloma: subcutaneous or intramuscular injection, 1, 000, 000 ～ 3, 000, 000 U singly, three times a week for 1 to 2 months.

(8) Cervical erosion: during the Non-menstrual period, before going to bed, put a suppository into the vagina closer to the cervix with your fingers every other day, nine days is as a course of treatment.

| 剂型、规格 Preparations | 注射剂：每支 100 万 U；300 万 U；450 万 U；500 万 U；600 万 U；900 万 U；1800 万 U。栓剂：每支 6 万 U；50 万 U。<br><br>Injection: 1 million U; 3, 000, 000 U; 4, 500, 000 U; 5, 000, 000 U; 6, 000, 000 U; 9, 000, 000 U; 18, 000, 000 U per vial. Suppositories: 60, 000 U; 500, 000 U per vial. |
|---|---|
| 药品名称 Drug Names | 聚乙二醇干扰素 α -2a　Peginterferon alfa-2a |
| 适应证 Indications | 用于治疗慢性丙型肝炎，适用于无肝硬化和非肝硬化代偿期的患者。<br><br>For the treatment of chronic hepatitis C of patients without cirrhosis and decompensation. |
| 用法、用量 Dosage | 皮下注射，一次 180μg（1ml），每周 1 次，共 48 周。可根据发生的不良反应调整剂量，可减至 45 ～ 90μg 乃至 135μg，不良反应减轻后可增加或恢复之规定剂量。<br><br>Subcutaneous injection, 180μg (1ml) singly, once a week for 48 weeks. Dosage could be adapted according to the occurrence of adverse reactions, which can be reduced to 45 ~ 90μg and even 135μg. After adverse effects eases, the dosage could be increased or returned to the dose prescribed. |
| 剂型、规格 Preparations | 注射剂：每支 45ug/1ml；90ug/ml；135μg/1ml；180μg/1ml。注射剂（预充式注射器）：每支 135μg/0.5ml；180μg/0.5ml。<br><br>Injection: 45μg/ml; 90ug/ml; 135ug/1ml; 180ug/1ml per vial. Injection (prefilled syringe): 135ug/0.5ml; 180ug/0.5ml per vial. |

| 药品名称 Drug Names | 重组人干扰素 α-1b　Recombinant Human Interferon α-1b（rh IFN α-1b） |
| --- | --- |
| 适应证<br>Indications | 用于病毒性疾病和某些恶性肿瘤。①慢性乙型肝炎、丙型肝炎和毛细胞白血病。②带状疱疹、尖锐湿疣、流行性出血热和小儿呼吸道合胞病毒性肺炎等病毒性疾病，以及慢性粒细胞白血病、黑色素瘤、淋巴瘤、肝细胞瘤、肺癌、直肠癌、膀胱癌、多发性骨髓瘤等恶性肿瘤。③滴眼液可用于眼部病毒性疾病。<br><br>For the treatment of viral diseases and certain tumors. ① Chronic hepatitis B、hepatitis C and hair cell leukemia. ② Herpes zoster、acuteness wet wart epidemic hemorrhagic fever and respiratory syncytial virus pneumonia in children, as well as chronic myelogenous leukemia、melanoma、lymphoma、hepatoma、lung cancer、colorectal cancer、bladder cancer and multiple myeloma, etc. ③ Eye drops were used to treat viral disease of the eye. |
| 用法、用量<br>Dosage | 皮下或肌内注射给药，一次 30～50μg，隔日或每日 1 次，疗程不超过 6 个月或视病情而定。<br><br>Subcutaneous or intramuscular injection, 30～50ug singly, every other day or once a day, a course should not be more than six months or depended on the condition. |
| 剂型、规格<br>Preparations | 注射剂：每支 10μg（100 万 U）；20μg（200 万 U）；30μg（300 万 U）；50μg（500 万 U）。滴眼液：20 万 U/2ml。<br><br>Injection: 10μg (1000, 000 U), 20μg (2000, 000 U); 30μg (3000, 000 U); 50μg (5000, 000 U) per vial. Eye Drops: 200, 000 U/2ml. |
| 药品名称 Drug Names | 重组人干扰素 α-2b　Recombinant Human Interferon α-2b（rh IFN α-2b） |
| 适应证<br>Indications | 用于：①慢性活动性乙型、丙型、丁型病毒性肝炎、带状疱疹、尖锐湿疣等病毒性疾病；②毛细血管性白血病、慢性粒细胞性白血病、多发性骨髓瘤、非霍奇金淋巴瘤、艾滋病相关的喉乳头状瘤或卡波西肉瘤、肾细胞癌、卵巢癌、恶性黑色素瘤等恶性肿瘤。<br><br>Usages: ① chronic active hepatitis B, C, D viral hepatitis, herpes zoster, genital warts and other viral diseases; ② capillaries leukemia, chronic myelogenous leukemia, multiple myeloma, non-Hodgkin's lymphoma, AIDS-related Kaposi's sarcoma or laryngeal papilloma, renal cell carcinoma, ovarian cancer, malignant melanoma and other malignancies. |
| 用法、用量<br>Dosage | 推荐的给药途径、剂量及疗程如下：①慢性乙型、丙型肝炎：皮下注射，一次 300 万～500 万 U，每日或隔日 1 次，3～6 个月为 1 个疗程。②慢性丁型肝炎：皮下注射，一次 300 万 U，一周 3 次，至少使用 3～4 个月。③毛细胞性白血病或喉乳头状瘤：皮下注射，一次 300 万 U，一周 3 次（隔日 1 次）。④慢性粒细胞白血病：单药治疗：皮下注射，一次 400 万～500 万 U，一日 1 次，至白细胞计数得到控制后，给予最大耐受量维持治疗；与阿糖胞苷合用：先用本药一次 500 万 U，一日 1 次，2 周后加用阿糖胞苷。若以上方案 8～12 周未见效应停止治疗。⑤多发性骨髓瘤：皮下注射，一次 300 万～500 万 U，一周 3 次（隔日 1 次）。⑥非霍奇金淋巴瘤：皮下注射，一次 500 万 U，一周 3 次（隔日一次），与化疗药合用。⑦艾滋病相关的卡波西肉瘤：皮下注射，一次 300 万 U，一周 3～5 次，也可每天 100 万～1200 万 U。⑧肾细胞癌：皮下注射或静脉给药，单药治疗，一次 300 万～400 万 U，可以一周 3 次、5 次或一日一次。⑨转移性类癌瘤：皮下注射，一次 300 万 U，一周 3 次，每日或隔日 1 次。⑩恶性黑色素瘤：诱导治疗，可先静脉给药，剂量为一次 2000 万 U，一周 5 次，共 4 周，然后皮下注射，一次 1000 万 U，一周 3 次，共 48 周。⑪尖锐湿疣：皮下注射，一次 100 万～300 万 U，一周隔日注射 3 次，1～2 个月为 1 个疗程。<br><br>Recommended route of administration, dosage and treatment course as follows: ① chronic hepatitis B, hepatitis C: subcutaneous injection, 3 000 000U～5 000 000U singly, once a day or every other day, three to six months for a treatment course. ② chronic hepatitis D: subcutaneous injection, 3 million U singly, three times a week, at least 3 to 4 months. ③ hairy cell leukemia or laryngeal papilloma: subcutaneously, 3 million U singly, three times a week (every other day). ④ chronic myeloid leukemia: monotherapy: subcutaneously, 4, 000, 000～5, 000, 000 U singly, once a day. When the number of white blood cell is under control, it is allowed to give the maximum tolerated dose for maintenance therapy; In combination with cytarabine: firstly, 5, 000, 000 U of this product singly, once a day, plus cytarabine two weeks later. If the above scenario has no effect during 8 to 12 weeks, treatment should stop. ⑤ multiple myeloma: subcutaneously, 3 million to 5 million U singly, three times a week (every other day). ⑥ non-Hodgkin's lymphoma: subcutaneously, 5 million U singly, three times a week (every other day), used with chemotherapy drugs. ⑦ AIDS-related Kaposi's sarcoma: subcutaneously, 3, 000, 000 U singly, 3～5 times per week or 1 million～2 million U per day. ⑧ renal cell carcinoma: subcutaneous or intravenous administration, monotherapy, 3 million to 4 million U singly, three times or five times a week or once a day. ⑨ metastatic carcinoid tumors: subcutaneously, 3 million U singly, three times a week, once a day or every other day. ⑩ malignant melanoma: induction therapy can be administered firstly intravenous injection at a dose of 20 million U singly, 5 |

|  | times a week for 4 weeks, and then injected subcutaneously, 10 million U singly, three times a week for 48 weeks. ⑪ genital warts: subcutaneously, 1 million to 3 million U singly, three injections every other day for one week, 1 to 2 months for a treatment course. |
|---|---|
| 剂型、规格<br>Preparations | 注射用粉针剂：每支 100 万 U；300 万 U；500 万 U；1000 万 U；1800 万 U；3000 万 U。注射液（多剂量笔）：180 万 U/1（2）ml。栓剂：每支 50 万 U。<br><br>Powder for injection: 1 million U; 3 million U; 5millon U; 10millon U; 18millon U; 30millon U per vial. Injection (multi-dose pen): 1 800 000U / 1 (2) ml. Suppositories: 500 000U per vial. |
| 药品名称 Drug Names | 重组人干扰素 β Recombinant Human Interferon β（rh IFNβ） |
| 适应证<br>Indications | ①用于病毒性疾病的治疗，对 RNA、DNA 病毒均敏感，皮下或静脉注射给药用于治疗慢性活动性肝炎、新生儿巨细胞病毒性脑炎。外涂、滴鼻、病灶局部给药用于防治流感 A2 和 B 病毒、鼻病毒所致的感冒、带状疱疹、甚至起疱疹等。②用于多发性硬化疾病。③用于肿瘤性胸腔积液、毛细胞白血病、宫颈上皮肿瘤、或乳腺及子宫内膜肿瘤的甾体激素受体诱导治疗。<br><br>① For the treatment of viral diseases, such as RNA, DNA viruses. subcutaneous or intravenous injection types are for the treatment of chronic active hepatitis, neonatal cytomegalovirus encephalitis. Coated, nasal dripping and topical types are used to prevent and treat influenza A2 and B virus, rhinovirus, shingles and even herpes. ② For the treatment of multiple sclerosis disease. ③ For the treatment of cancer pleural effusion, hairy cell leukemia, cervical intraepithelial neoplasia, or breast and endometrial cancer steroid hormone receptor induction therapy. |
| 用法、用量<br>Dosage | ①多发性硬化疾病：皮下注射，每次 44μg，每周 3 次。②生殖器疱疹、带状疱疹：肌内注射，一次 200 万 U，一日 1 次，连续 10 日。③扁平或尖锐湿疣：皮下或病灶局部注射，每日 100 万 ~ 300 万 U，连用 5 日为 1 个疗程，每次 1 ~ 3 个疗程。或肌内注射，每日 200 万 U，连续 10 日。④慢性乙型肝炎：肌内注射，一次 500 万 U，每周 3 次，连续 6 个月。慢性丙型或丁型肝炎：前 2 个月每次 600 万 U，每周 3 次；后改为每次 300 万 U，每周 3 次，连续 3 ~ 6 个月。⑤宫颈上皮肿瘤：病灶内注射，300 万 U，一日 1 次，连续 5 日。后改为隔日一次，连续 2 周。⑥肿瘤性胸腔积液：胸穿后将 500 万 U 的本品注入胸膜腔。若 7 ~ 15 日后又出现胸腔积液，再次胸穿，注入本品 1000 万 U。若 15 日后再复发，用 50ml 生理盐水稀释 2000 万 U 药物注入胸腔。⑦毛细胞白血病：静脉内缓慢注入，诱导剂量每天 600 万 U，连续 7 日为 1 个疗程，共 3 周（隔周）。维持剂量 600 万 U，每周 2 次，连续 24 周。⑧乳腺肿瘤和子宫内膜肿瘤：肌内注射，每次 200 万 ~ 600 万 U，每周 3 次（隔天），共 2 周。此方案在激素治疗期每间隔 4 周可重复使用。<br><br>① Multiple sclerosis disease : subcutaneous injection, 44ug singly, three times a week . ② Genital herpes, herpes zoster : intramuscular injection, 2 million U singly, once a day for 10 consecutive days. ③ Flat or genital warts : subcutaneous injection or local lesions injection, 1 million to 3 million a day U, 5 consecutive days for a treatment course, 1 to 3 courses singly. Or intramuscular injection, 2 million U a day for 10 consecutive days. ④ Chronic hepatitis B : intramuscular injection, 5 million U singly, 3 times a week for six consecutive months. Chronic hepatitis C or hepatitis D : six million U singly for the first 2 months, 3 times a week ; later changed to 3 million U singly, 3 times a week for 3 to 6 consecutive months . ⑤ Cervical intraepithelial neoplasia : intralesional injection, 3 million U, once a day for 5 consecutive days. Later changed once every other day for 2 consecutive weeks. ⑥ Neoplastic pleural effusion : 5 000 000U injected after thoracentesis into the pleural cavity. If pleural effusion and thoracentesis occur 7 to 15 days later again, 10 million U should be injected. If relapsing 15 days later, 50ml saline should be diluted with 20 million U of drugs into the chest . ⑦ Hairy cell leukemia : a slow intravenous injection, 6 million U induction dose a day for seven consecutive days as a course, a total of 3 weeks (injecting every other week). Maintenance dose of 6 million U, 2 times a week for 24 consecutive weeks. ⑧ Breast cancer and endometrial cancer : intramuscular injection, 2 million to 6 million U singly, 3 times (every other day ) a week for two weeks . This method could be used 4 weeks at intervals repeatly during hormone therapy. |
| 剂型、规格<br>Preparations | 注射用冻干粉：每安瓿 11μg/2ml（300 万 U）。<br>注射液（预装式注射器）：22μg/0.5ml（600 万 U）；44μg/0.5ml（1200 万 U）。<br><br>Lyophilized powder for injection: 11ug/2ml (3millon U) per ampoule.<br>Injection (prefilled syringe): 22μg/0.5ml (6millon U); 44μg/0.5ml (12millon U). |

**续　表**

| 药品名称 Drug Names | 重组人干扰素 γ　Recombinant Human Interferon γ（rh IFN γ） |
|---|---|
| 适应证<br>Indications | 用于类风湿关节炎、迁延性肝病及肝纤维化的治疗。<br>For the treatment of rheumatoid arthritis, persistent hepatitis and hepatic fibrosis. |
| 用法、用量<br>Dosage | ①类风湿关节炎：皮下注射，初始剂量为一次 50 万 U，一日 1 次，连续 3～4 日，如无不良反应，将剂量加至每日 100 万 U；第 2 个月改为一次 150 万～200 万 U，隔日 1 次，总疗程为 3 个月。②肝纤维化：皮下注射，前 3 个月，一次 50 万 U，一日 1 次，后 6 个月，一次 100 万 U，隔日一次。<br>① Rheumatoid arthritis: subcutaneous injection, the initial dose of 500, 000 U singly, once a day for 3 to 4 days consecutively. If there is no adverse reaction, the dosecould be added to 1 million U a day; 1 500 000 to 2 000 000U singly in the second month, once every other day, the total course is three months. ② liver fibrosis: subcutaneous injection, the first three months, 500 000U singly, once a day; 6 months later, 1 million U singly, once every other day. |
| 剂型、规格<br>Preparations | 注射剂：每支 50 万 U；100 万 U；200 万 U。<br>Injection: 500 000U; 1 000 000 U; 2 000 000U per vial. |
| 药品名称 Drug Names | 人免疫球蛋白 Human Immunoglobulin |
| 适应证<br>Indications | 用于免疫缺陷疾病和传染性肝炎、麻疹、水痘、腮腺炎、带状疱疹等病毒感染和细菌感染的防治，也用于哮喘、过敏性鼻炎、湿疹等内源性过敏性疾病。<br>For the prevention and treatment of immunodeficiency diseases, infectious hepatitis, measles, chickenpox, mumps, herpes zoster, etc. and asthma, allergic rhinitis, eczema and other endogenous allergic diseases. |
| 用法、用量<br>Dosage | 肌内注射：①预防麻疹：0.05～0.15ml/kg 或儿童 5 岁以下 1.5～3ml，成人不超过 6ml，预防效果 1 个月。②预防甲型肝炎：0.05～0.15ml/kg 或儿童 1.5～3ml，成人每次 3ml，预防效果 1 个月。③预防乙型肝炎：成人一次 200U，儿童 100U，必要时隔 3～4 周再注射一次。母为乙肝表面抗原或核心抗原双阳者，婴儿出生 24 小时内注射 100U，阻断预防。<br>Intramuscular injection: ① for the prevention of measles: 0.05～0.15ml/kg or, 1.5～3ml singly for children under age 5, no more than 6ml for adults, one-month preventive effect. ② for the Prevention of hepatitis A: 0.05～0.15ml/kg or, 1.5～3ml singly for children under age 5, no more than 6ml for adults, one-month preventive effect. ③ for the prevention of hepatitis B: for adults, 200U singly, for children 100U singly, if necessary, reinjecting for another time three to four weeks later. When Mother has hepatitis B surface antigen or her core antigens are both positive, her newborn should be injected by 100U within 24 hours after birth to stop prevention. |
| 剂型、规格<br>Preparations | ①注射液（10%）：每支 150mg/1.5ml，300mg/3ml，500mg/5ml。②注射冻干粉：每支 150mg；300mg；500mg。③注射液：每支 100U；200U；400U。<br>① injection (10%): 150mg/1.5ml, 300mg/3ml, 500mg/5ml per vial. ② lyophilized powder for injection: 150mg; 300mg; 500mg per vial. ③ Injection: 100U; 200U; 400U per vial. |
| 药品名称 Drug Names | 静脉注射用人免疫球蛋白 Human immunoglobulin for Interavenous injection（IVIG） |
| 适应证<br>Indications | 用于原发性和继发性免疫球蛋白缺乏症如 X 连锁低免疫球蛋白血症、重症感染、艾滋病；自身免疫性疾病如原发性血小板减少性紫癜、川崎病、重症系统性红斑狼疮等。<br>For the treatment of primary and secondary immunoglobulin deficiency, such as X-linked Hypoimmunoglobulinia, severe infection, AIDS; autoimmune diseases such as idiopathic thrombocytopenic purpura, Kawasaki disease, severe systemic lupus erythematosus and so on. |
| 用法、用量<br>Dosage | （1）免疫球蛋白缺乏或低下症：按体重一日 400mg/kg，维持量为 200～400mg/kg，用药间隔视血清 IgG 水平定。<br>（2）特发性血小板减少性紫癜：开始一日 400mg/kg，连续 5 日，维持量一次 400mg/kg，每周一次或视血小板计数而定。<br>（3）川崎病：发病 10 日内使用。儿童一次 2.0g/kg，一次静脉滴注。<br>（4）严重感染：一日 200～400mg/kg，连续 3～5 日。<br>(1) immunoglobulin deficiency or Hypoimmunoglobulinia : 400mg/kg a day measured by weight, the maintenance dose of 200～400mg/kg, the dosing interval is determined by serum IgG levels. |

| | (2) idiopathic thrombocytopenic purpura: the initial dose is 400mg/kg for 5 consecutive days, when the maintenance dose is 400mg/kg, once a week or determined by platelet count.<br>(3) Kawasaki: it is used with 10 days after the onset of disease. Children are given 2.0g/kg singly by intravenous dripping.<br>(4) severe infection: 200 ~ 400mg/kg a day for 3 to 5 consecutive days. |
|---|---|
| 剂型、规格<br>Preparations | 注射液（PH4）每瓶 1g；1.25g；2.5g；4g。<br>Injection (PH4) 1g; 1.25g; 2.5g; 4g per vial. |
| **药品名称 Drug Names** | 乌苯美司 Ubenimex |
| 适应证<br>Indications | 竞争性抑制氨肽酶 B 及亮氨酸肽酶。可刺激骨髓细胞再生及分化。<br>Competitive inhibition of aminopeptidase B and leucine peptidase.used to stimulate cell regeneration and differentiation of bone marrow. |
| 用法、用量<br>Dosage | 口服，每日 30 ~ 100mg，1 次或分 2 次服。也可每周服 2 ~ 3 日，10 个月为 1 个疗程。<br>Oral medication, 30 ~ 100mg a day, in 1 or 2 divided doses or 2 to 3 days per week, 10 months as a course of treatment. |
| 剂型、规格<br>Preparations | 片剂：每片 10mg。<br>胶囊剂：每粒 10mg；30mg。<br>Tablets: 10mg per tablet.<br>Capsules: 10mg; 30mg per pill. |
| **药品名称 Drug Names** | 白芍总苷 Total Glucosides of Paeony |
| 适应证<br>Indications | 免疫调节药，改善类风湿关节炎患者症状。<br>Immunomodulatory agents to improve the symptoms of rheumatoid arthritis. |
| 用法、用量<br>Dosage | 口服，一次 300mg，一日 2 ~ 3 次。<br>Oral medication, 300mg singly, 2 or 3 times a day. |
| 剂型、规格<br>Preparations | 胶囊剂：每粒 300mg。<br>Capsules: 300mg per capsule. |

18. 维生素类、酶及其他生化制剂，调节水、电解质和酸碱平衡药物和营养支持药 Vitamins, enzymes and other biochemical preparation, drugs regulating balance of water electrolyte and acid-base, and nutritional support drugs

18.1 维生素类 Vitamins

| **药品名称 Drug Names** | 维生素 A Vitamin A（Retinol） |
|---|---|
| 适应证<br>Indications | 用于：①维生素 A 缺乏症：如夜盲症、眼干燥症、角膜软化症和皮肤粗糙等。②用于补充需要，如妊娠、哺乳期妇女和婴儿等。③有学者认为对预防上皮癌、食管癌的发生有一定意义。<br>Usages ① vitamin A deficiency: eg night blindness, dry eye syndrome, Keratomalacia and soften rough skin. ② used to supplement needs from pregnant, lactating women, infants and so on. ③ Perhaps for the prevention of epithelial cancer, esophageal cancer. |
| 用法、用量<br>Dosage | （1）严重维生素 A 缺乏症：口服，成人每日 10 万 U，3 日后改为每日 5 万 U，给药 2 周，然后每日 1 万 ~ 2 万 U，再用药 2 个月。吸收功能障碍或口服困难者可用肌内注射，成人每日 5 万 ~ 10 万 U，3 日后改为每日 5 万 U，给药 2 周；1 ~ 8 岁儿童，每日 0.5 万 ~ 1.5 万 U，给药 10 日；婴儿，每日 0.5 万 ~ 1 万 U，给药 10 日。<br>（2）轻度维生素 A 缺乏症：每日 1 万 ~ 2.5 万 U，分 2 ~ 3 次口服。<br>（3）补充需要：成人每日 5000U，哺乳期妇女每日 5000U，婴儿 每日 600 ~ 1500U，儿童每日 2000 ~ 3000U。<br>(1) Severe vitamin A deficiency: Oral medication, for adults, 100 000 U a day, 3 day later changing to 50 000U a day for two weeks, and then 12 000U a day for 2 months. For patients with Oral medication difficulty and absorption dysfunction, intramuscular injection is available; for adults, 50 000 to 100 000U a day, 3 day later changing to 50 000U a day for two weeks; for 1 to 8-year-old children, 5000 ~ 15 000U a day for 10 days; for infants, 5000 ~ 10 000U a day for 10 days.<br>(2) Mild vitamin A deficiency: 10 000 - 25 000 U A day in 2 to 3 divieded doses by Oral medication.<br>(3) Supplementary need: for adults, 5000U a day; for lactating women, 5000U a day; for baby, 600 ~ 1500U a day; for children, 2000 ~ 3000U a day. |

**续　表**

| 剂型、规格<br>Preparations | 胶丸剂：每丸 5000U；2.5 万 U。<br>Capsules: 5000U; 25 000U per pill. |
|---|---|
| **药品名称 Drug Names** | **维生素 D　Vitamin D** |
| 适应证<br>Indications | 维生素 D 缺乏，防治佝偻病、骨软化症和婴儿手足搐搦症。<br><br>For the treatment of Vitamin D deficiency and for the prevention and treatment of rickets, osteomalacia and baby tetany. |
| 用法、用量<br>Dosage | （1）治疗佝偻病：口服一日 2500 ~ 5000U，1 ~ 2 个月后待症状开始消失时即改用预防量。若不能口服者、重症的患者，肌内注射一次 30 万 ~ 60 万 U，如需要，1 个月后再肌内注射 1 次，两次总量不超过 90 万 U。用大剂量维生素 D 时如缺钙，应口服 10% 氯化钙，一次 5 ~ 10ml，一日 3 次，用 2 ~ 3 日。<br>（2）婴儿手足搐搦症：口服一日 2000 ~ 5000U，1 个月后改为每日 400U。<br>（3）预防维生素 D 缺乏症：用母乳喂养的婴儿 1 日 400U，妊娠期必要时 1 日 400U。<br><br>(1) for the treatment of rickets: Oral medication, 2500 ~ 5000U a day, 1 to 2 months later, if the symptoms began to disappear, the dosage could be switched to amount for prevention. For patients with Oral medication diffiiculty and severe symptoms, intramuscular injection is 300 000 to 600 000U singly, intramuscular injecting for another time one month later if necessary. The total amount should be less than 900 000U. When using large doses of vitamin D with a lack of calcium, patients should take 10% calcium chloride orally, 5 ~ 10ml singly, 3 times a day for 2 to 3 days.<br>(2) Baby tetany: Oral medication, 2000 ~ 5000U a day, a month later changing to 400U a day.<br>(3) for the prevention of vitamin D deficiency: for children breast-fed, 400U a day, when necessary, 400U a day in pregnancy. |
| 剂型、规格<br>Preparations | 维生素 $D_2$ 胶丸：每粒含 1 万 U。维生素 $D_2$ 片：每片 5000U；10 000U。维生素 $D_2$ 胶性钙注射液：每支 1ml；10ml。每 1ml 含 D25 万 U，胶性钙 0.5mg。维生素 D3 注射液：每支 15 万 U（0.5ml）；30 万 U（1ml）；60 万 U（1ml）。用前及用时需服钙剂。维生素 AD 胶丸：每粒含维生素 A 3000U，维生素 D 300U。浓维生素 AD 胶丸：每粒含维生素 A 1 万 U，维生素 D 1000U。维生素 AD 滴剂：每 1g 含维生素 A 5000U，维生素 D 500U；每 1g 含维生素 A 5 万 U，维生素 D 5000U；每 1g 含维生素 A 9000U，维生素 D 3000U。<br><br>Vitamin $D_2$ capsules: per capsule contains 10 000 U. Vitamin $D_2$ tablets: per tablet 5000U; 10000U. Vitamin $D_2$ glue calcium Injection: per 1ml; 10ml. Per 1ml D25 million U, gum, calcium 0.5mg. Vitamin $D_3$ Injection: per 150 000 U (0.5ml); 300 000 U (1ml); 600 000U (1ml). To be served before use and use when calcium. Vitamin AD capsules: per capsule contains vitamin A 3000U, vitamin D 300U. Concentrated vitamin capsules AD: per capsule contains Vitamin A 1 million U, vitamin D 1000U. Vitamin AD Drops: per 1g of vitamin A 5000U, vitamin D 500U; every 1g of vitamin A 5 million U, vitamin D 5000U; every 1g of vitamin A 9000U, vitamin D 3000U. |
| **药品名称 Drug Names** | **骨化三醇 Calcitriol** |
| 适应证<br>Indications | 应用于甲状腺功能低下症及血液透析患者的肾性营养不良，骨质疏松症，维生素 D 依赖性佝偻病（肾小管缺乏 1-α 羟化酶）。<br><br>For the treatment of renal malnutrition, osteoporosis, vitamin D-dependent rickets (1-α-hydroxylase deficiency tubules) which occur on patients with hypothyroidism and those who need hemodialysis patients with. |
| 用法、用量<br>Dosage | 口服剂量应根据患者的血钙浓度来决定。<br>（1）血液透析患者的肾性营养不良：如患者血钙浓度正常或略低，口服，一日 0.25μg。如 2 ~ 4 周生化指标及病情无明显改变，则一日剂量可达到 0.5μg。每周应测两次血钙浓度，随时调整剂量。大多数血透患者用量在一日 0.5 ~ 1μg。<br>（2）甲状腺功能低下：儿童 1 ~ 5 岁，一日 0.25 ~ 0.75μg；6 岁以上和成人，一日 0.5 ~ 2μg（用量须个体化）。<br><br>Oral medication dose should be based on the patient's serum calcium concentration.<br>(1) for the treatment of Hemodialysis patients' renal malnutrition: in the case of normal or slightly lower serum calcium concentration, Oral medication, 0.25μg a day. If biochemical markers and the disease doesn't improve in 2 to 4 weeks, the daily dose can be 0.5μg. serum calcium concentration should be measured twice a week and adjust the dose at any time. Most hemodialysis patients take Calcitriol 0.5 ~ 1μg a day. |

**续 表**

| | (2) Hypothyroidism: for Children of 1 to 5 years old, 0.25 ~ 0.75μg singly; for 6 years plus and adults, 0.5 ~ 2μg a day (dosage should be individually customized.). |
|---|---|
| 剂型、规格<br>Preparations | 胶囊剂：每粒 0.25μg；0.5μg。<br>Capsules: 0.25μg; 0.5μg per capsule. |
| 药品名称 Drug Names | 阿法骨化醇 Alfacalcidol |
| 适应证<br>Indications | 用于慢性肾衰合并骨质疏松症、甲状腺功能低下及抗维生素 D 的佝偻病患者。<br>For the treatment of chronic renal failure combined with osteoporosis, hypothyroidism and anti-vitamin D rickets patients. |
| 用法、用量<br>Dosage | （1）慢性肾衰竭合并骨质疏松：成人，口服，一次 0.5 ~ 1.0μg，一日 1 次。<br>（2）甲状腺功能低下和抗维生素 D 的佝偻病：成人，口服，一日 1.0 ~ 4.0μg，一日 2 ~ 3 次。<br>(1) Chronic renal failure with osteoporosis: for adults, Oral medication, 0.5 ~ 1.0μg singly, once a day.<br>(2) Hypothyroidism and anti-vitamin D rickets: for adults, Oral medication, 1.0 ~ 4.0μg a day, 2 or 3 times a day. |
| 剂型、规格<br>Preparations | 胶囊剂：每粒 0.25μg；0.5μg；1.0μg。<br>Capsules: 0.25μg; 0.5μg; 1.0μg per capsule. |
| 药品名称 Drug Names | 维生素 B₁ Vitamin B₁(Thiamine) |
| 适应证<br>Indications | 用于脚气病防治及各种疾病的辅助治疗（如全身感染、高热、糖尿病、多发性神经炎、小儿麻痹后遗症及小儿遗尿症、心肌炎、食欲缺乏、消化不良、甲状腺功能亢进和妊娠期等）。对解除某些药物如链霉素、庆大霉素等引起的听觉障碍有帮助。<br>For the prevention and treatment of beriberi and adjuvant treatment of various diseases (such as systemic infections, fever, diabetes, multiple neuritis, polio sequelae and pediatric enuresis, myocarditis, loss of appetite, indigestion, hyperthyroidism and pregnancy, etc.) . It can help the recovering of hearing impairment caused by certain drugs such as streptomycin, gentamicin, etc.. |
| 用法、用量<br>Dosage | 成人每日的最小必需量为 1mg，孕妇及小儿因发育关系需要较多。在治疗脚气病及消化不良时可根据病情调整。成人 1 次 10 ~ 20mg，一日 3 次，口服；或 1 次 50 ~ 100mg，一日 1 次，肌内注射。儿童 1 次 5 ~ 10mg，一日 3 次，口服；或 1 次 10 ~ 20mg，一日 1 次，肌内注射。不宜静脉注射。<br>The minimum required amount for adults is 1mg a day, more for pregnant women and children due to development. In the treatment of beriberi and indigestion, dosage can be adjusted to the disease. For Adults, 10 ~ 20mg singly, 3 times a day, Oral medication; or 50 ~ 100mg singly, once a day, intramuscular injection. For Children, 5 ~ 10mg singly, 3 times a day Oral medication; or 10 ~ 20mg singly, once a day, intramuscular injection. Intravenous injection is not recommended. |
| 剂型、规格<br>Preparations | 片剂：每片 5mg；10mg。<br>注射液：每支 10mg（1ml）；25mg（1ml）；50mg（2ml）；100mg（2ml）。<br>Tablets: 5mg; 10mg per tablet.<br>Injection: 10mg (1ml); 25mg (1ml); 50mg (2ml); 100mg (2ml) per vial. |
| 药品名称 Drug Names | 维生素 B₂ Vitamin B₂ (Riboflavin) |
| 适应证<br>Indications | 用于口角炎、唇炎、舌炎、眼结膜炎和阴囊炎等的防治。<br>For the prevention and treatment of angular cheilitis, cheilitis, glossitis, conjunctivitis and scrotitis, etc. |
| 用法、用量<br>Dosage | 成人每日的需要量为 2 ~ 3mg。治疗口角炎、舌炎、阴囊炎等时，一次可服 5 ~ 10mg，一日 3 次，或皮下注射或肌内注射 5 ~ 10mg，一日 1 次，连用数周，至病势减退为止。<br>For Adults, 2 ~ 3mg a day. For the Treatment of angular cheilitis, glossitis, scrotal, 5 ~ 10mg singly, 3 times a day, or subcutaneous or intramuscular injection, 5 ~ 10mg singly, once a day for continous weeks till illness diminishes. |
| 剂型、规格<br>Preparations | 片剂：每片 5mg；10mg。<br>注射液：每支 1mg（2ml）；5mg（2ml）；10mg（2ml）。<br>Tablets: 5mg; 10mg per tablet.<br>Injection: 1mg (2ml); 5mg (2ml); 10mg (2ml) per vial. |

**续　表**

| 药品名称 Drug Names | 烟酸 Nicotinic Acid |
| --- | --- |
| 适应证<br>Indications | 　　用于预防和治疗因烟酸缺乏引起的糙皮病等。也用作血管扩张药，及治疗高脂血症。对于严格控制或选择饮食或接受肠道外营养的患者，因营养不良体重骤减，妊娠期、哺乳期妇女，以及服用异烟肼者，严重烟瘾、酗酒、吸毒者，烟酸的需要量均需增加。<br>　　For the prevention and treatment of pellagra caused by niacin deficiency. Also used as a vasodilator and for the treatment of hyperlipidemia. For patients needed to strictly control diet or select diet or those receiving parenteral nutrition, patients with unexplained weight loss due to malnutrition, pregnancy, breastfeeding women and isoniazid people, people with severe addiction and alcoholism, drug addicts, niacin is required to increase. |
| 用法、用量<br>Dosage | 　　(1) 推荐膳食每日摄入量：出生至 3 岁 5 ~ 9mg，4 ~ 6 岁 12mg，7 ~ 10 岁 12mg，男性青少年及成人 15 ~ 20mg，女性青少年及成人 13 ~ 15mg，孕妇 17mg，哺乳期妇女 20mg。<br>　　(2) 糙皮病：成人口服：1 次 50 ~ 100mg，一日 5 次；静脉注射：1 次 25 ~ 100mg，一日 2 次或多次。儿童口服：1 次 25 ~ 50mg，一日 2 ~ 3 次；静脉缓慢注射：一日 300mg。<br>　　(3) 抗高血脂：成人口服，缓释片或缓释胶囊，推荐 1 ~ 4 周一次 0.5g，一日 1 次；5 ~ 8 周为一次 1g，一日 1 次；8 周后，根据患者的疗效和耐受性逐渐增加，如有必要，最大剂量可加至 2g。应在少量低脂肪饮食就睡前服用。须整片（粒）吞服。维持剂量：每日 1 ~ 2g。女性患者的剂量低于男性患者。<br>　　(1) Recommended daily dietary intake: from the birth to the age of 3, 5 ~ 9mg singly, the age of 4 ~ 6, 12mg singly, 7 ~ 10 years old, 12mg, male adolescents and adults, 15 ~ 20mg, female adolescents and adults, 13 ~ 15mg, pregnant women, 17mg, lactating women, 20mg.<br>　　(2) Pellagra: Oral medication for adults: 50 ~ 100mg singly, 5 times a day; Intravenous injection: 25 ~ 100mg singly, 2 times a day or more. Children oral medication: 25 ~ 50mg singly, 2~3 times a day ; slow intravenous injection: 300mg a day.<br>　　(3) Anti-high blood cholesterol: Oral medication for adults, sustained-release tablets or capsules, recommended 0.5g singly for the 1st-4st week as recommended, once a day; from 5 to 8 weeks, 1g singly, once a day; eight weeks later, according to efficacy and tolerability of the patient, dosage could be gradually increased. If necessary, the maximum dose could be increased to 2g. The whole capsule should be taken at bedtime, when having a small amount of low-fat diet . Maintenance dose: 1 ~ 2g a day. Female patients should have less dose than male patients. |
| 剂型、规格<br>Preparations | 　　片剂、胶囊剂：每片 50mg；100mg。注射液：50mg/ml；100mg/ml。<br>　　Tablets and capsules: 50mg; 100mg per pill. Injection: 50mg/ml; 100mg/ml. |
| 药品名称 Drug Names | 维生素 $B_6$　　Vitamin $B_6$ (Pyridoxine) |
| 适应证<br>Indications | 　　用于：①防治因大量或长期服用异烟肼、肼屈嗪等引起的周围神经炎、失眠、不安；减轻抗癌药和放射治疗引起恶心、呕吐或妊娠呕吐等。②治疗因而惊厥或给孕妇服用以预防婴儿惊厥。③白细胞减少症。④局部涂搽治疗痤疮、酒糟鼻、脂溢性湿疹等。<br>　　Usage: ① For the prevention and treatment of peripheral neuropathy, insomnia, restlessness caused by long-term or a large number of isoniazid, hydralazine, etc.; to alleviate nausea, vomiting or vomiting of pregnancy caused by anticancer drugs and radiation therapy. ② For the treatment of Convulsion or to treat pregnant women to prevent infant convulsions. ③ leukopenia. ④ topical application is for the treatment of acne, rosacea, seborrheic eczema, etc. |
| 用法、用量<br>Dosage | 　　口服：一次 10 ~ 20mg，一日 3 次（缓释片一次 50mg，一日 1 ~ 2 次）。皮下注射、肌内注射、静脉注射：一次 50mg，一日 1 ~ 2 次）。皮下注射、肌内注射、静脉注射：一次 50 ~ 100mg，一日 1 次。治疗白细胞减少症时，以 50 ~ 100mg，加入 5% 葡萄糖注射液 20ml 中，做静脉注射，一日 1 次。<br>　　Oral medication: 10 ~ 20mg singly, 3 times a day (for sustained-release tablets, 50mg singly, 1 or 2 times a day). Subcutaneous, intramuscular and intravenous injection: 50mg singly, 1 or 2 times a day). Subcutaneous, intramuscular and intravenous injection: 50 ~ 100mg singly, once a day. For The treatment of leukopenia: 50 ~ 100mg added to 20ml 5% dextrose injection for intravenous injection, once a day. |

| 剂型、规格<br>Preparations | 片剂：每片 10mg。维生素 B<sub>6</sub> 缓释片：每片 50mg。<br>注射液：每支 25mg（1ml）；50mg（1ml）；100mg（22ml）。<br>霜剂：每支含 12mg。<br><br>Tablets: 10mg per tablet. Vitamin $B_6$ release tablets: 50mg per tablet. Injection: 25mg (1ml); 50mg (1ml); 100mg (22ml) per vial. Cream: 12mg per strip. |
| --- | --- |
| 药品名称 Drug Names | 干酵母 Dried Yeast |
| 适应证<br>Indications | 用于：营养不良，消化不良，食欲降低及 B 族维生素缺乏症。<br>Used for: malnutrition, indigestion, loss of appetite and B vitamins deficiency. |
| 用法、用量<br>Dosage | 口服：成人，一次 0.5 ~ 4g；小儿，一次 0.3 ~ 0.9g；均为一日 3 次，嚼服。<br>Oral administration: adult, 0.5 ~ 4g; Children, 0.3 ~ 0.9g at a time; 3 times a day by chewing. |
| 剂型、规格<br>Preparations | 片剂：每片 0.2g，0.3g，0.5g（以干酵母计）<br>Tablet: 0.2g；0.3g; 0.5g. (In terms of dried yeast) |
| 药品名称 Drug Names | 维生素 C  Vitamin C (Ascorbic Acid) |
| 适应证<br>Indications | 用于：①维生素 C 缺乏症的防治。②急慢性传染病时的补充。③克山病患者出现心源性休克时，可用大剂量治疗。④用于肝硬化、急性肝炎和砷、汞、铅和苯等慢性中毒时的治疗。⑤其他：用于各种贫血、过敏性皮肤病、口疮、促进伤口愈合等。<br><br>For the treatment of  ① Prevention and treatment of scurvy  ② Vitamin C should be increased when acute and chronic infectious diseases occur and consumption increase, and so it is with patients in convalescence and those whose wound healing is poor. ③ Patients with Keshan disease should be administered by high-dose therapy in cardiogenic shock. ④ For the treatment of liver damage caused by cirrhosis, acute hepatitis and chronic toxicity of arsenic, mercury, lead, benzene, etc. ⑤ Other cases: For the treatment of all kinds of anemia, allergic skin diseases, mouth sores, and for wound healing, and so on. |
| 用法、用量<br>Dosage | （1）一般治疗：口服（饭后），一日 50 ~ 100mg；长期透析患者：一日 100 ~ 200mg；维生素 C 缺乏症患者：一次 100 ~ 200mg，一日 3 次，至少服用 2 周。静脉注射：维生素 C 缺乏症患者：一次 0.5 ~ 1g，5% 或 10% 葡萄糖注射液稀释后滴注。<br>（2）酸化尿液：口服，一日 4 ~ 12g，分次服用，每 4 小时一次。<br>（3）特发性高血红蛋白血症：一日 300 ~ 600mg，分次服用。<br>（4）克山病心源性休克：首剂 5 ~ 10g，25% 加入葡萄糖注射液，缓慢静脉注射。后视病情 2 ~ 4 小时重复一次，24 小时总量可达 15 ~ 30g。<br>（5）口疮：0.1g 压碎，撒于溃疡面上，一日 2 次。<br><br>(1) General treatment: orally (after meals) 50 ~ 100mg a day; Long-term dialysis patients: 100 ~ 200mg per day; Vitamin C deficiency patients: 100 ~ 200mg once, 3 times a day, at least 2 weeks. Intravenous injection: For patients with vitamin C deficiency: 0.5 ~ 1g at a time, diluted with 5% or 10% glucose injection and dripped.<br>(2) Acidified urine: take orally, 4 ~ 12g a day, in divided doses, every 4 hours.<br>(3) Idiopathic hyperhemoglobinemia: 300-600mg per day, divided doses.<br>(4) Cardiogenic shock of Keshan disease: the first dose was 5 ~ 10g, add it into 25% glucose injection, slowly inject it intravenously, repeat once 2 ~ 4 hours later depending on the condition, and the total amount within 24 hours can reach 15 ~ 30g.<br>(5) Mouth sore: crush 0.1g tablet and apply to ulcer surface, 2 times a day. |
| 剂型、规格<br>Preparations | 片剂：每片 20mg；25mg；50mg；100mg；250mg；<br>咀嚼片：每片 100mg。<br>泡腾片：每片 500mg。<br>颗粒剂：2g（含维生素 C 0.1g）。<br>注射剂：每支 100mg（2ml）；250mg（2ml）；500mg（5ml）；2.5g（20ml）。<br><br>Tablets: 20mg; 25mg; 50mg; 100mg; 250mg per tablet.<br>Chewable tablets: 100mg per tablet.<br>Effervescent tablets: 500mg per tablet.<br>Granules: 2g (contain 0.1g vitamin C).<br>Injection: 100mg (2ml); 250mg (2ml); 500mg (2 ml); 2.5g (20ml) per vial. |

**续　表**

| 药品名称 Drug Names | 维生素 E　　Vitamin E(Tocopherol) |
|---|---|
| 适应证<br>Indications | 用于：①未进食强化奶或有严重脂肪吸收不良母亲所生的新生儿、早产儿、低出生体重儿。②未成熟儿、低出生体重儿常规应用于预防维生素 E 缺乏。③进行性肌营养不良的辅助治疗。④维生素 E 需要量增加的情况，如甲状腺功能亢进、吸收功能不良综合征、肝胆系统疾病等。<br><br>For the treatment of ① newborns, premature child birth, low birth weight children without having fortified milk or those whose mother have severe fat malabsorption ② To immature child, low-birth-weight children, it is routinely used in the prevention of vitamin E deficiency. ③ For adjuvant treatment of muscular dystrophy. ④ In the case of requiring vitamin E increase, such as hyperthyroidism, absorption dysfunction syndrome, hepatobiliary diseases, etc. |
| 用法、用量<br>Dosage | 口服或肌内注射：一次 10 ~ 100mg，一日 1 ~ 3 次。<br>Oral medication or intramuscular injection: 10 ~ 100mg singly, 3 times a day. |
| 剂型、规格<br>Preparations | 片剂：每片 5mg；10mg；100mg。<br>胶丸：每丸 5mg；10mg；50mg；100mg；200mg。<br>粉剂：每克粉剂中含维生素 E0.5mg。<br>注射液：每支 5mg（1ml）；50mg（1ml）。<br>Tablets: 5mg; 10mg; 100mg per tablet.<br>Capsules: 5mg; 10mg; 50mg; 100mg; 200mg per pill.<br>Powder: vitamin E0.5mg per gram.<br>Injection: 5mg (1ml); 50mg (1ml) per vial. |

18.2　酶类和其他生化制剂 Enzymes and biochemical preparation

| 药品名称 Drug Names | 胰蛋白酶 Trypsin |
|---|---|
| 适应证<br>Indications | 临床上主要用于脓胸、血胸、外科炎症、溃疡、创伤性损伤、瘘管等所产生的局部水肿、血肿、脓肿等，虹膜睫状体炎、急性泪囊炎、视网膜周围炎、眼外伤等。喷雾吸入，用于呼吸道疾病。因对蛇毒蛋白（蛇毒的主要毒成分）有水解作用，故有将本品用于治疗毒蛇咬伤，曾试用于竹叶青、银环蛇、眼镜蛇、蝮蛇等毒蛇咬伤的各型病例。<br><br>Clinically mainly for the treatment of local edema, hematoma and abscess caused by empyema, hemothorax, surgical inflammation, ulcers, traumatic injuries, fistula arising, etc., iridocyclitis, acute dacryocystitis, retinal inflammation, the eye injury and so on. The spray type is for respiratory diseases. It has hydrolysis on venom proteins (mainly toxic components of snake venom), so it is used to treat snake bites and has been used in many snake biting cases like Trimeresurus, coral snake, cobra, viper snakebite and other various types of cases. |
| 用法、用量<br>Dosage | （1）一般应用：每次 5000U，一日 1 次，肌内注射，用量斟酌情况决定。为防止疼痛，可加适量普鲁卡因。局部用药视情况而定，可配成溶液剂（pH7.4 ~ 8.2，微碱性时活性最强）、喷雾剂、粉剂、软膏等，用于体腔内注射、患部注射、喷涂、湿敷、涂搽等。<br>（2）滴眼：0.25% 溶液，一日 4 ~ 6 次。冲洗泪道：0.25% ~ 0.5% 溶液（内加 2% 普鲁卡因少量），一日 1 次。眼浴 1：5000 ~ 1：10 000 溶液 10 ~ 20ml，1 次 10 ~ 20ml，一次 10 ~ 15 分钟，一日 1 次，或隔日 1 次。球后注射 1 次 1 ~ 2.5mg，隔日 1 次。肌内注射 1 次 2.5 ~ 5mg。一日 1 ~ 2 次。<br>（3）治蛇毒：取注射用结晶胰蛋白酶 2000 ~ 6000U，加 0.25% ~ 0.5% 盐酸普鲁卡因（或注射用水）4 ~ 20ml 稀释，以牙痕为中心，在伤口周围做浸润注射，或在肿胀部位上方作环状封闭 1 ~ 2 次。如病情需要，可重复使用。若伤肢肿胀明显，可于注射 30 分钟后，切开伤口排毒减压（严重出血者例外），也可在肿胀部位针刺排毒。如伤口已坏死、溃疡，可用其 0.1% 溶液湿敷患处。<br><br>(1) General application : 5000U singly, once a day, intramuscular injection, the amount is decided by current condition . To prevent the pain, you can add procaine of proper amount. Topical application depends on the disease condition. It can be made up as solutions (pH7.4 ~ 8.2, highest activie at the slight alkalinity property), sprays, powders, ointments and the like for body cavity injection, injection of the affected area, spraying, wetting, inunction and so on.<br>(2) eye Drops : 0.25% solution, 4 to 6 times a day . Lacrimal irrigation : 0.25% to 0.5 % solution ( a little 2% procaine is added), once a day. ophthalmic bath: 10 ~ 20ml solution of 1：5000 ~ 1：10 000, 10 ~ 20ml singly, 10 to 15 minutes singly, once a day or every other day. retrobulbar injection: 1 ~ 2.5mg singly, once every other day. Intramuscular injection : 2.5 ~ 5mg singly. 1 to 2 times a day. |

(3) for the treatment of Venom : Take 2000 ~ 6000U injectable crystalline trypsin, plus 4 ~ 20ml 0.25% to 0.5% procaine hydrochloride to dilute (or water for injection) . Take teeth marks as the center, infiltration injecting around the wound, or reloading and sealing for one or two times on the top of swelling. If necessary, it can be reused. If the injured limb swells significantly, incision wound could be cut open for detoxification and decompression 30 minutes after injection (except severe bleeding ones). Also, acupuncture is available for detoxification on the swelling . If the wound is necrotic or have ulcers, 0.1% solution is available to wet the surface of the skin.

| 剂型、规格<br>Preparations | 注射用胰蛋白酶：每支 1.25 万 U；2.5 万 U；5 万 U；10 万 U（附灭菌缓冲液 1 瓶）。<br><br>trypsin for Injection: 12, 500U; 25, 000U; 50, 000U; 100, 000U per vial (1 bottle of sterile buffer attached). |
|---|---|

**药品名称 Drug Names** 糜蛋白酶 Chymotrypsin

| 适应证<br>Indications | 主要用于创伤或手术后创口愈合、抗炎及防止局部水肿、积血、扭伤血肿、乳房手术后水肿、中耳炎、鼻炎、角膜溃疡、泪道疾病、眼外伤、眼睑水肿、出血和玻璃体积血、慢性支气管炎、支气管扩张、肺脓肿及毒蛇咬伤等。<br><br>Mainly used for wound healing, anti-inflammatory after trauma or surgery and preventing local edema, hemorrhage, hematoma sprains, edema after breast surgery, otitis media, rhinitis, corneal ulcers, lacrimal disease, ocular trauma, eyelid edema, hemorrhage and vitreous hemorrhage, chronic bronchitis, bronchiectasis, lung abscess and snakebite. |
|---|---|
| 用法、用量<br>Dosage | （1）肌内注射：以 0.9% 氯化钠注射液 5ml 溶解 4000U 后注射。<br>（2）经眼用药：本品对眼球睫状韧带有选择性松弛作用，故可用于白内障摘除，使晶状体比较容易移去。眼科注入后房，一次 800U，以 0.9% 氯化钠注射液配成 1 ∶ 5000 溶液，由瞳孔注入后房，经 2 ~ 3 分钟，在晶状体浮动后以生理盐水冲洗前后方中遗留的本品。<br>（3）喷雾吸入：每次 5mg，以 0.9%% 氯化钠注射液配成 0.5mg/ml 浓度溶液使用。<br>（4）用于处理软组织炎症或创伤，800U 糜蛋白酶溶于 1ml0.9% 氯化钠注射液注于创面。<br>（5）毒蛇咬伤：糜蛋白酶 10 ~ 20mg 用注射用水 4ml 稀释后，以蛇牙痕迹为中心区域向后行浸润注射，并在伤口中心区域注射 2 针，再在肿胀上方 3cm 做环状封闭 1 ~ 2 层，根据不同部位 0.3 ~ 0.7ml，至少 10 针，最多 26 针。<br><br>(1) Intramuscular injection: 4000U dissolved with 5ml 0.9% sodium chloride for injection<br>(2) ophthalmic medication: it has selective relaxation for ciliary ligament of eyeballs, so it can be used for cataract removal, easy to remove the lens. Injecting from posterior chamber: 800U singly added into 0.9% sodium chloride injection into 1 ∶ 5000 solution. Injecting to posterior chamber from pupil, 2 to 3 minutes later, flush the product left on anterior chamber and posterior chamber with saline after the lens floats.<br>(3) Spray Inhalation: 5mg singly added into 0.9% sodium chloride injection to make up a 0.5mg/ml solution.<br>(4) for the treatment of soft tissue inflammation or trauma, put 1ml 800U chymotrypsin soluble into 0.9% sodium chloride injection and inject it on the wound.<br>(5) snakebite: dilute 10 ~ 20mg chymotrypsin with 4ml water for injection, Take teeth marks as the center, infiltration injecting around the wound, inject 2 needles in the central area of the wound, and then make a a ring closure for 1~2 layers 3cm above the swelling. Different parts of the body should be sealed by 0.3~ 0.7ml, 10 needles at least, 26 needles at most. |
| 剂型、规格<br>Preparations | 注射用糜蛋白酶：每支 800U；4000U。<br>Chymotrypsin for injection: 800U; 4000U per vial. |

**药品名称 Drug Names** 抑肽酶 Aprotinin

| 适应证<br>Indications | 用于各型胰腺炎的治疗与预防；能抑制纤维蛋白溶酶，阻止胰腺中其他活性蛋白酶原的激活及胰蛋白酶原的活化，用于治疗和预防各种纤维蛋白溶解所引起的急性出血；能抑制血管舒张素，从而抑制其舒张血管、增加毛细血管通透性、降低血压的作用，用于各种严重休克状态。此外，在腹腔手术后直接注入腹腔，能预防肠粘连。<br><br>For treatment and prevention of pancreatitis of various types; for the inhibition of plasmin to prevent the activation of other active protease pancreas and trypsinogen; for the treatment and prevention of acute hemorrhagic caused by fibrinolysis ; it is to inhibit vasorelaxant, thereby inhibiting vasodilation, increasing the capillary permeability and lowering blood pressure; For the treatment of a variety of severe shock. In addition, after abdominal surgery it should be injected directly into the abdominal cavity to prevent intestinal adhesion. |
|---|---|

续　表

| 用法、用量<br>Dosage | （1）第 1、2 日每日注射 5 万～ 12 万 U，首剂用量应大一些，缓慢静脉注射（每分钟不超过 2ml）。维持剂量应采用静脉滴注，一般每日 4 次，每日总量 2 万～ 4 万 U。<br>（2）对由纤维蛋白溶解引起的急性出血，立即静脉注射 5 万～ 10 万 U，以后每 2 小时 1 万 U，直至出血停止。<br>（3）预防剂量：手术前 1 日开始，每日注射 2 万 U，共 3 日。治疗肠瘘及连续渗血也可局部使用。<br>（4）预防术后肠粘连：在手术切后闭合前，腹腔内直接注入 2 万～ 4 万 U，注意勿与伤口接触。<br>（5）用于体外循环心脏直视手术。<br><br>(1) 50, 000 to 120 000U a day in the 1st and 2nd day, the first dosage should be larger by slow intravenous injection (no more than 2ml per minute). The Maintenance dose should be injected intravenously, usually 4 times a day, a total 20, 000 to 40 000U generally.<br>(2) for Acute bleeding caused by the fibrinolysis, immediate intravenous injection is 5 million to 10 million U, and then 10000 U every two hours, until the bleeding stops.<br>(3) Prevention dose: Start 1 day prior to surgery, daily injection of 20 000U, 3 days in all. For the tropical Treatment of intestinal fistula and continuous bleeding.<br>(4) for The prevention of postoperative intestinal adhesion: Before or After surgical closure, directly inject 20 000 ~ 40 000U into the abdominal cavity and be careful not to touch the wound.<br>(5) For Open Heart Surgery under cardiopulmonary bypass. |
| --- | --- |
| 剂型、规格<br>Preparations | 注射液：每支 5 万 U（5ml）；10 万 U（5ml）；50 万 U（5ml）。<br>Injection: 50, 000 U (5ml); 100, 000 U (5ml); 500, 000 U (5ml) per vial. |
| 药品名称 Drug Names | 玻璃酸酶 Hyaluronidase |
| 适应证<br>Indications | 一些以缓慢速度进行静脉滴注的药物如各种氨基酸、水解蛋白等，在与本品合用的情况下可改为皮下注射或肌内注射，使吸收加快。<br><br>in combination with Hyaluronidase, some intravenous drugs dripped at a slow speed, such as amino acids of all types, hydrolyzed protein, etc, could be changed into subcutaneous or intramuscular injection to accelerate the absorption. |
| 用法、用量<br>Dosage | ①临用时将本品粉末溶于生理盐水中，常用量 50U 或 150U，配成每 ml 含 0.7U、1.5U 或 2.0U 的注射液，事先注射于灌注部位。②皮下注射大量的某些抗生素（如链霉素）或其他化疗药物（如异烟肼等）以及麦角制剂时，合用本品，可使扩散加速，减轻痛感。③以 150U 溶解在 25 ～ 50ml 局部麻醉药中，如加入肾上腺素，可加速麻醉，并减少麻醉药的用量。④与胰岛素合用，可防止注射局部浓度过高而出现的脂肪组织萎缩。胰岛素休克疗法中用本品 100 ～ 150U，促使胰岛素吸收量增加，注射较小量即可达血中有效浓度，因而减少其危险性。⑤球后注射促进玻璃体浑浊或出血的吸收，1 次 100 ～ 300U/ml，1 次 / 日。⑥结膜下注射促使秋后血肿的吸收，1 次 50 ～ 100U/0.5ml，一日或隔日 1 次。⑦滴眼预防结膜化学烧伤后睑球粘连，治疗外伤性眼眶出血、外伤性视网膜水肿，150U/ml，每 2 小时滴眼一次。⑧关节腔内注射，一次 2ml，一周 1 次，连续 3 ～ 5 周。<br><br>① For the temporary use, dissolve the powder in saline, the usual dose is 50 or 150 international U to make up the injection containing 0.7U, 1.5U or 2.0U, injected on perfusion part in advance. ② in the case of subcutaneous injection with large amounts of certain antibiotics ( such as streptomycin) or other chemotherapy drugs ( such as isoniazid, etc. ) and ergot preparations, this product could be used in combination to accelerate the proliferation and reduce pain. ③ dissolve 150U into dissolved in 25 ~ 50ml of local anesthetic, add epinephrine so that anesthesia can be accelerated and the amount of anesthetic can be reduced as an example. ④ in combination with insulin, adipose tissue atrophy caused by high local concentrations could be prevented. In insulin shock therapy, 100 ~ 150U should be used to prompt insulin absorption. a small amount of injection is available to reach effective blood concentration, thus reducing their risk . ⑤ retrobulbar injection is to promote the absorption of vitreous opacity or bleeding, 100 ~ 300U/ml singly, once per day. ⑥ subconjunctival injection promotes the absorption of hematoma after autumn, 50 ~ 100U/0.5ml singly, once a day or every other day. ⑦ instillation for the prevention of eyelid adhesions of conjunctiva after chemical burns, for the treatment of traumatic orbital hemorrhage and traumatic retinal edema, 150U/ml, eye dripping once every two hours . ⑧ intra-articular injection, 2ml singly, once a week for 3 to 5 weeks . |
| 剂型、规格<br>Preparations | 注射用玻璃酸酶：每支 150U；1500U。<br>Hyaluronidase for injection: 150U; 1500U per vial. |

**续 表**

| 药品名称 Drug Names | 三磷酸腺苷 Adenosine Triphosphate |
|---|---|
| 适应证<br>Indications | 　　用于心力衰竭、心肌炎、心肌梗死、脑动脉硬化、冠状动脉硬化、心绞痛、阵发性心动过速、急性脊髓灰质炎、进行性肌萎缩性疾病、肝炎、肾炎、视疲劳、眼肌麻痹、视网膜出血、中心性视网膜炎、视神经炎、视神经萎缩等。本品不易透过细胞膜，能否发挥其生理效应，值得怀疑。其能量注射液为本品与辅酶 A 等配制的复方注射液，用于肝炎、肾炎、心力衰竭等。<br><br>　　For the treatment of heart failure, myocarditis, myocardial infarction, cerebral arteriosclerosis, coronary artery disease, angina, paroxysmal tachycardia, acute poliomyelitis, progressive muscular atrophy disease, hepatitis, nephritis, visual fatigue, muscle paralysis, retinal hemorrhage, central retinitis, optic neuritis, optic atrophy, etc. This product is not easily to go through the cell membrane so that whether it could take physiological effect is questionable. The compound injection combined with energy-based Injection and coenzyme A is used for the treatment of hepatitis, nephritis, heart failure, etc. |
| 用法、用量<br>Dosage | 　　肌内注射或静脉注射，每次 20mg，一日 1 ~ 3 次。肌内注射多用注射液，静脉注射多用注射用三磷腺苷，另附有缓冲液溶解，再以 5% ~ 10% 葡萄糖注射液 10 ~ 20ml 稀释后缓慢静脉注射，也可用 5% ~ 10% 葡萄糖注射液稀释后静脉滴注。1% 生理盐水溶液滴眼，治疗弥漫性表层角膜炎和角膜外伤。<br><br>　　Intramuscular injection or intravenous injection, 20mg singly, 1 ~ 3 times a day. Injection liquid is mostly used in Intramuscular injection, adenosine triphosphate is mostly used in intravenous injection attached with buffer solution. Then 10 ~ 20ml of 5% to 10% glucose injection is diluted and intravenously and slowly injected. Also, intravenous infusion with 5% to 10% glucose diluted solution is available. Eye dripping with 1% saline solution for the treatment of diffuse superficial keratitis and corneal trauma. |
| 剂型、规格<br>Preparations | 　　注射液：每支 20mg（2ml）。<br>　　注射用三磷腺苷：每支 20mg；另附磷酸缓冲液 2ml。<br><br>Injection: 20mg (2ml) per vial.<br>Adenosine triphosphate for injection: 20mg per vial; combined with 2ml phosphate buffer. |

18.3 调节水、电解质和酸碱平衡药物 Drugs regulating balance of water electrolyte and acid-base

| 药品名称 Drug Names | 氯化钠 Sodium Chloride |
|---|---|
| 适应证<br>Indications | 　　氯化钠注射液可补充血容量和钠离子，用于各种缺盐性失水症（如大面积烧伤、严重吐泻、大量发汗、强利尿药、出血等引起）。在大量出血而又无法进行输血时，可输入氯化钠注射液以维持血容量进行急救。还用于慢性肾上腺皮质功能不全（艾迪生病）治疗过程中补充氯化钠，每日约 10g。此外，生理盐水可用于洗伤口、洗眼、洗鼻以及产科水囊引产等。<br><br>　　Sodium Chloride Injection is to supplement blood volume and sodium ions to treat salt depleting dehydration of all types caused by extensive burns, vomiting and diarrhea, mass sweating, strong diuretic, etc. When heavy bleeding but not for transfusion, enter sodium chloride injection is able to maintain blood volume for first aid, when patients bleed profusely without transfusion. It is for the treatment of chronic adrenal insufficiency (Addison's disease), when about 10g per day is appropriate during treatment. In addition, saline can be used to wash the wound, wash eyes, wash nasal and inducing abortion by water bag, etc. |
| 用法、用量<br>Dosage | 　　（1）口服：用于轻度急性胃肠患者恶心、呕吐不严重者。<br>　　（2）高渗性失水：高渗性失水时，患者脑细胞和脊髓液渗透浓度升高，若对其治疗则会使血浆和细胞外液钠浓度和渗透浓度下降过快，可致脑水肿。一般认为，在治疗开始的 48 小时内，血浆钠浓度每小时下降应不超过 0.5mmol/L。<br>　　（3）等渗性失水：原则给予等渗溶液，如 0.9% 氯化钠注射液或复方氯化钠注射液，但上述溶液氯浓度明显高于血浆，单独大量使用可致高氯血症，故可将 0.9% 氯化钠注射液和 1.25% 碳酸氢钠或 1.86%（1/6M）乳酸钠以 7∶3 的比例配制后补给。后者氯浓度为 107mmol/L，并可纠正代谢性酸中毒。 |

（4）低渗性失水：严重低渗性失水时，脑细胞内溶质减少以维持细胞容积。若治疗使血浆和细胞外液钠浓度和渗透浓度迅速回升，可致脑细胞损伤。一般认为，当血钠低于 120mmol/L 时，治疗使血钠上升速度在每小时 0.5mmol/L，不超过每小时 1.5mmol/L（稀释性低钠血症无须补钠）。当急性血钠低于 120mmol/L 或出现中枢神经系统症状时，可给予 3% 氯化钠注射液静脉滴注。一般要求在 6 小时内将血钠浓度提高至 120mmol/L 以上。参考补钠量为 3% 氯化钠 1ml/kg，可提高血钠 1mmol/L。待血钠回升至 120 ～ 125mmol/L 以上，可改用等渗溶液。慢性缺钠补钠速度要慢，剂量要少，使血钠浓度逐日回升至 130mmol/L。

（5）低氯性碱中毒：给予 0.9% 氯化钠注射液或复方氯化钠注射液（林格液）500 ～ 1000ml，以后根据碱中毒情况决定用量。

（6）外用：用生理氯化钠溶液洗涤伤口、冲洗眼部。

(1) Oral medication: for patients with nausea and vomiting caused by mild acute gastrointestis .

(2) Hypertonic dehydration : in case of hypertonic dehydration, if the brain cells and spinal fluid osmolality increase, the plasma and extracellular fluid sodium concentration and osmolality will decrease so fast with treatment as to cause cerebral edema. Generally, 48 hours before the treatment, plasma sodium concentration should not decrease at a speed of more than 0.5mmol / L.

(3) Isotonic dehydration : in principle, isotonic solution is required, such as 0.9% sodium chloride injection or compound sodium chloride injection, but the concentrations of chlorine in solution mentioned above is significantly higher than that in plasma, easy to cause hyperchloremia when using alone. Therefore, the compound of 0.9 % sodium chloride injection and 1.25 % sodium bicarbonate or 1.86% (1/6M) lactate with the ratio of 7 ： 3 is preferred for preparation replenishment . The latter chlorine concentration of 107mmol / L and is available for the correction of metabolic acidosis.

(4) Hypotonic dehydration : in the case of severe hypotonic dehydration, the brain cytosol will decrease to maintain cell volume. If the treatment quickly recovers the concentration and osmolality of plasma and extracellular fluid sodium, brain cell may have damage . Generally, when the serum sodium is less than 120mmol / L, the rate to increase serum sodium is 0.5mmol / L per hour, less than 1.5mmol / L per hour (sodium supplyment is not required in diluting hyponatremia) . When acute serum sodium is less than 120mmol / L or have central nervous system symptoms, 3% sodium chloride intravenous injectionmay be given. Generally, it is required to to raise serum sodium concentration to 120mmol / L or more within six hours. the reference amount of 3% sodium chloride 1ml/kg can increase sodium by 1mmol / L. When sodium recovers to 120 ~ 125mmol / L or more, it could be replaced by isotonic solution . Chronic sodium depletion should be supplemented slower and less to make sodium concentration rise to 130mmol / L.

(5) Low chlorine alkalosis poisoning: to give 500 ~ 1000ml 0.9% sodium chloride injection or compound sodium chloride injection ( Ringer ), and alkali poisoning condition determines the dosage.

(6) Topical usage: flushing the wound and eyes with physiological sodium chloride solution .

| 剂型、规格<br>Preparations | 注射液：为含 0.9% 氯化钠的灭菌水溶液。每支（瓶）2ml；10ml；250ml；500ml；1000ml。浓氯化钠注射液：每支 1g（1ml），0.3g（10ml）。临用前稀释。复方氯化钠注射液（林格液）：灭菌溶液，每 100ml 中含氯化钠 0.85g，氯化钾 0.03g，氯化钙 0.033g，比生理盐水成分完全，可替代生理盐水用。葡萄糖氯化钠注射液：每 1000ml 中含葡萄糖 5% 及氯化钠 0.9%。每瓶 250ml；500ml；1000ml。口服补液盐：①每包 14.75g（大包中含氯化钠 1.75g，葡萄糖 11g；小包中含氯化钾 0.75g，碳酸氢钠 1.25g）。②每包 13.95g（氯化钠 1.75g，葡萄糖 10g，枸橼酸钠 1.45g，氯化钾 0.75g）。治疗和预防轻度急性腹泻。<br><br>Injection: sterile aqueous solution containing 0.9% sodium chloride. 2ml;10ml; 250ml; 500ml; 1000ml per vial (bottle);. Concentrated Sodium Chloride Injection: 1g (1ml), 0.3g (10ml)per vial. Diluted before use. Compound Sodium Chloride Injection (Ringer): sterile solution containing 0.85g sodium, 0.03g potassium chloride and 0.033g calcium chloride per 100ml, where components are more complete than the saline and can replace the saline. Glucose and sodium chloride injection: 5% glucose and 0.9% sodium chloride per 1000ml. 250ml ; 500ml; 1000ml per Bottle. Oral rehydration salts: ① 14.75g per pack (in large package, there are 1.75g sodium chloride and 11g glucose; in small packet, there are 0.75gpotassium chloride and 1.25g sodium bicarbonate). ② 13.95g per pack (sodium chloride 1.75g, glucose 10g, sodium citrate 1.45g, potassium chloride 0.75g). For the treatment and prevention of mild acute diarrhea. |
| --- | --- |

**续　表**

| 药品名称 Drug Names | 氯化钾 Potassium Chloride |
|---|---|
| 适应证<br>Indications | 用于低钾血症（多由严重吐泻不能进食、长期应用排钾利尿剂或肾上腺皮质激素所引起）的防治，亦可用于强心苷中毒引起的阵发性心动过速或频发室性期外收缩。<br><br>For the prevention and treatment of hypokalemia caused by vomiting and diarrhea without eating, long-term use of potassium-sparing diuretics or adrenal hormones) and paroxysmal supraventricular tachycardia or frequent ventricular extrasystole caused by cardiac glycoside. |
| 用法、用量<br>Dosage | 补充钾盐大多采用口服，一次 1g，一日 3 次。血钾过低，病情危急或吐泻严重口服不易吸收时，可用静脉滴注，每次用 10% ～ 15% 液 10ml，用 5% ～ 10% 葡萄糖注射液 500ml 稀释或根据病情酌定用量。<br><br>potassium supplements is used by Oral medication, 1g singly, three times a day. In case of Hypokalemia, being in critical condition or vomiting and diarrhea, which lead to hard absorption by oral medication, intravenous injection is available, 10% to 15% solution, 10ml singly, using 500ml 5% to 10% glucose injection for dilution or deciding the dosage based on disease condition. |
| 剂型、规格<br>Preparations | 片剂：每片 0.25g；0.5g。控释片（SLOW-K）：每片 0.6g。微囊片（PEL-K）：每片 0.75g。氯化钾口服液：100ml：10g。注射液：：每支 1g（10ml）。复方氯化钾注射液：内含氯化钾 0.28%、氯化钠 0.42% 及乳酸钠 0.63%，可用于代谢性酸血症及低血钾。用量视病情而定，一般每日量 500 ～ 1000ml，静脉滴注。<br><br>Tablets: 0.25g; 0.5g per tablet. Adalat GITS (SLOW-K): 0.6g per tablet. Microcapsule sheet (PEL-K): 0.75g per tablet. Potassium chloride Oral liquid: 100ml: 10g. Injection : 1g (10ml) per vial. Injection of compound potassium chloride: containing 0.28% potassium chloride, sodium chloride, 0.42% and 0.63% sodium lactate, used for metabolic acidosis and hypokalemia. The amount depends on the condition of illness, generally daily amount of 500 ～ 1000ml, intravenous drip. |
| 药品名称 Drug Names | 门冬氨酸钾镁 Potassium Magnesium Aspartate |
| 适应证<br>Indications | 用于低钾血症、低钾及洋地黄中毒引起的心律失常、病毒性肝炎、肝硬化和肝性脑病的治疗。<br><br>For the treatment of cardiac arrhythmias, viral hepatitis, cirrhosis and hepatic encephalopathy induced by hypokalemia, potassium deficiency and digitalis poisoning, |
| 用法、用量<br>Dosage | 口服：每次 1 ～ 2 片，一日 3 次。静脉滴注：心律失常、心肌梗死，每次 10 ～ 20ml，加入 5% ～ 10% 葡萄糖液 50 ～ 100ml 中缓慢滴注，4 ～ 6 小时后有必要可重复。<br><br>Oral medication: 1~2 tables singly, 3 times a day. intravenous drip infusion: for the treatment of arrhythmia and myocardial infarction, 10 ～ 20ml singly, 50 ～ 100ml 5% to 10% glucose solution should be dripped slowly and should be rejected after 4 to 6 hours if necessary. |
| 剂型、规格<br>Preparations | 片剂：（钾 0.9mmol+ 镁 0.4mmol）；注射剂：（钾 2.7 ～ 3.1mmol+ 镁 1.5 ～ 1.9mmol）/10ml。<br><br>Tablet: (potassium 0.9mmol + Mg 0.4mmol); injection: (2.7 ～ 3.1mmol + Potassium Magnesium 1.5 ～ 1.9mmol) / 10ml. |
| 药品名称 Drug Names | 枸橼酸钾 Potassium Citrate |
| 适应证<br>Indications | 用于低钾血症。<br>For the treatment of hypokalemia. |
| 用法、用量<br>Dosage | 每次 10 ～ 20ml<br>10 ～ 20ml singly |
| 剂型、规格<br>Preparations | 10% 合剂口服。<br>10% mixture for oral treatment. |
| 药品名称 Drug Names | 氯化钙 Calcium Chloride |
| 适应证<br>Indications | 本品可用于血钙降低引起的手足搐搦症，以及肠绞痛、输尿管绞痛，荨麻疹、渗出性水肿、瘙痒性皮肤病，镁盐中毒，佝偻病、软骨病、孕妇及哺乳期妇女钙盐补充，高血钾等。<br><br>For the treatment of tetany and colic, ureteral colic, urticaria, exudative edema, itch Dermatoses, magnesium poisoning, rickets and osteomalacia caused by hypocalcemia and hyperkalemia, etc. For the supplement of calcium for pregnant and lactating women. |

**续 表**

| | |
|---|---|
| 用法、用量<br>Dosage | （1）成人：①治疗低钙血症，500 ~ 1000mg（含 Ca 离子 136 ~ 272mg）缓慢静脉注射，速度不超过每分钟 50mg，根据反应和血钙浓度，必要时 1 ~ 3 日后重复。②心脏复苏：静脉或心室腔内注射，每次 200 ~ 400mg。应避免注入心肌内。③治疗高钾血症：先静脉注射 500mg，每分钟速度不超过 100mg，以后酌情用药。<br><br>（2）小儿：①治疗低钙血症，按体重 25mg/kg（含 Ca 离子 6.8mg）缓慢静脉注射。但一般情况下本品不用于小儿，因刺激性较大。②心脏复苏心室内注射，一次 10mg/kg，间隔 10 分钟可重复注射。<br><br>(1) for adult: ① for the treatment of hypocalcemia, 500 ~ 1000mg (Ca ion 136 ~ 272mg), slow intravenous injection, speed does not exceed 50mg per minute. This process need to be repeated one to three days later if necessary, consideringthe calcium concentration and the reaction. ② cardiac resuscitation: intravenous injection or ventricular cavity injection, 200 ~ 400mg singly. Intramyocardial injection should be avoided. ③ for the treatment of hyperkalemia: 500mg of first intravenous injection, no more than 100mg per minute with appropriate medication in the future.<br><br>(2)for children: ① for the treatment of hypocalcemia, 25mg/kg measured by weight (containing 6.8mg Ca ions), slow intravenous injection. However, generally, the product is not used for children because of stronger irritation. ② CPR with intraventricular injection, 10mg/kg singly, repeated injections every 10 minutes. |
| 剂型、规格<br>Preparations | 注射液：每支 0.3g（10ml）；0.5g（10ml）；0.6g（20ml）；1g（20ml）。氯化钙葡萄糖注射液：为含氯化钙 5% 及葡萄糖 25% 的灭菌溶液，用于因血钙降低而至的手足搐搦、荨麻疹、血清反应等，1 次量 10 ~ 20ml，静脉注射，每日或隔日 1 次。禁用于进内注射，以免引起组织坏死。氯化钙溴化钠注射液：每支 5ml，含氯化钙 0.1g，溴化钠 0.25g。每次静脉注射 5ml（重症可用 10ml），一日 1 ~ 2 次。静脉注射时宜缓慢，以免引起全身发热反应。禁用于肌内注射。<br><br>Injection: 0.3g (10ml); 0.5g (10ml); 0.6g (20ml); 1g (20ml) per vial. Glucose injection with calcium chloride: sterile solution with calcium chloride 5% and 25% glucose for the treatment of tetany, urticaria, serum reactions due to the blood calcium decrease, 10 ~ 20ml per time, intravenous injection daily or every other day. intramuscular injection is not allowed to avoid tissue necrosis. Calcium chloride and sodium bromide Injection: 5ml per vial, containing calcium chloride 0.1g and sodium bromide 0.25g. intravenously injected for 5ml per time (10ml available for Severe case), 1 to 2 times a day. Intravenous injection should be slow, so as not to cause systemic febrile reaction. intramuscular injection is not allowed. |
| 药品名称 Drug Names | 碳酸钙 Calcium Carbonate |
| 适应证<br>Indications | 用于低钙血症和高磷血症。<br>For the treatment of hypocalcemia and hyperphosphatemia. |
| 用法、用量<br>Dosage | （1）低钙血症：成人口服，每次 1.25 ~ 1.5g，一日 1 ~ 3 次，近视时或进食后服用。尤其慢性肾衰竭患者伴高磷血症。<br><br>（2）制酸：成人口服：1 次 0.5 ~ 2g，一日 3 ~ 4 次。<br><br>（3）高磷血症：成人口服：一日 3 ~ 12g，分次在进食时服用。每日 2g 以上钙时即可发生高钙血症，故应密切监测血清钙浓度。<br><br>(1) Hypocalcemia: for adults, Oral medication, 1.25 ~ 1.5g singly, 1 to 3 times a day, taking at the time of or after meal. In particular, it is intended to patients with chronic renal failure accompanied by hyperphosphatemia.<br><br>(2) relieving hyperacidity:for Adults, Oral medication: 0.5 ~ 2g singly, 3 to 4 times a day.<br><br>(3)hyperphosphatemia: for adults, Oral medication: 3 ~ 12g A day in divided doses when eating meals. Hypercalcemia can occur when calcium is given by 2g and above a day, so close monitoring of serum calcium concentrations should made. |
| 剂型、规格<br>Preparations | 片剂：每片 0.5g（相当于元素钙 200mg）<br>Tabelts: 0.5g per tablet (equal to 200mg calcium). |
| 药品名称 Drug Names | 葡萄糖酸钙 Calcium Gluconate |
| 适应证<br>Indications | 本品可用于血钙降低引起的手足搐搦症，以及肠绞痛、输尿管绞痛，荨麻疹、渗出性水肿、瘙痒性皮肤病，镁盐中毒、佝偻病、软骨病、孕妇及哺乳期妇女钙盐补充，高血钾等。<br><br>For the treatment of tetany and colic, ureteral colic, urticaria, exudative edema, itch Dermatoses, magnesium poisoning, rickets and osteomalacia caused by hypocalcemia and hyperkalemia, etc. For the supplement of calcium for pregnant and lactating women. |

**续 表**

| 用法、用量<br>Dosage | (1) 口服：成人一次 0.5 ~ 2g，一日 3 次；儿童一次 0.5 ~ 1g，一日 3 次。<br>(2) 静脉注射：每次 10% 注射液 10 ~ 20ml（对小儿手足搐搦症，每次 5 ~ 10ml）。加等量 5% ~ 25% 葡萄糖注射液稀释后缓慢静脉注射（每分钟不超过 2ml）。<br><br>(1) Oral medication:0.5 ~ 2g singly for adults, 3 times a day; 0.5 ~ 1g singly for child, three times a day.<br>(2) Intravenous injection: 10 ~ 20ml 10% injection singly (for children's tetany, 5 ~ 10ml singly). Slow intravenous injection (no more than 2ml per minute) should be given after adding an equal amount of 5% to 25% glucose injection for dilution. |
|---|---|
| 剂型、规格<br>Preparations | 片剂：每片 0.1g；0.5g。含片：每片 0.1g；0.15g；0.2g。口服液：每支 1g（10ml）。注射液：每支 1g（10ml）。<br><br>Tablets: 0.1g; 0.5g per tablet. Tablets: 0.1g; 0.15g; 0.2g per tablet. Oral liquid: 1g (10ml) per vial. Injection: 1g (10ml) per vial. |
| 药品名称 Drug Names | 乳酸钙 Calcium Lactate |
| 适应证<br>Indications | 用于防治钙缺乏症如手足搐搦症、骨发育不全、佝偻病，以及结核病、妊娠和哺乳期妇女的钙盐补充。<br><br>For the prevention and treatment of calcium deficiency such as tetany, bone hypoplasia, rickets and calcium supplement for patients with tuberculosis, pregnant and lactating women. |
| 用法、用量<br>Dosage | 每 1g 乳酸钙含钙为 130mg。成人：口服，一日 1 ~ 2g，分 2 ~ 3 次口服。小儿：按体重一日 45 ~ 65mg/kg，分 2 ~ 3 次口服。<br><br>130mg calcium per gram of calcium lactate. For adults: Oral medication, 1 ~ 2g singly, in 2~ 3 divided doses a day by Oral medication. For Children: 45 ~ 65mg/kg measured by weight in 2 or 3 divided doses in a day by Oral medication. |
| 剂型、规格<br>Preparations | 片剂：每片 0.25g；0.5g。<br><br>Tablets: 0.25g; 0.5g per tablet. |
| 药品名称 Drug Names | 硫酸镁 Magnesium Sulfate |
| 适应证<br>Indications | (1) 可预防和治疗低镁血症，特别是急性低镁血症伴有肌肉痉挛、手足搐搦。<br>(2) 先兆子痫和子痫、早产子宫肌肉痉挛等。<br>(3) 导泻、利胆。<br><br>(1) For the Prevention and treatment of hypomagnesemia, especially for acute hypomagnesemia accompanied by muscle spasms, tetany.<br>(2) Pre-eclampsia and eclampsia, preterm uterine muscle spasms.<br>(3) catharsis purgation and cholagogue effect. |
| 用法、用量<br>Dosage | (1) 防止低镁血症：成人轻度镁缺乏，1g 硫酸镁，肌内注射或溶于 500ml5% 葡萄糖注射液内缓慢滴注，每日总量 2g。重度镁缺乏，一次按体重 0.25mmol/kg 硫酸镁，也可静脉滴注，将 2.5g 硫酸镁溶于 5% 葡萄糖注射液或氯化钠注射液 500ml 中，缓慢滴注 3 小时。严密观察呼吸等生命体征。<br>(2) 全静脉内营养，按体重每日 0.125 ~ 0.25mmol 镁 /kg 添加。儿童全静脉内营养，按体重每日 0.125mmol 镁 /kg 添加。<br>(3) 治疗先兆子痫和子痫，肌内注射：每次 1 ~ 2.5g 硫酸镁，根据病情决定剂量，最多每日肌注 6 次，并监测心电图、肌腱反射、呼吸和血压。静脉注射：将 1 ~ 2g 硫酸镁，以 5% 葡萄糖液稀释，推注速度每分钟不超过 150mg，静注硫酸镁可使血镁浓度突增至接近中毒浓度，必须严格掌握剂量，并严密观察呼吸、肌腱反射和心电图。静脉滴注：4g 硫酸镁加入 5% 葡萄糖注射液或氯化钠注射液 250ml 内，滴注速度每分钟不超过 4ml。<br>(4) 抗惊厥：儿童按体重 20 ~ 40mg/kg，配制成 20% 注射液肌内注射。慎用，不作为首选药物。<br>(5) 导泻：成人口服：1 次 5 ~ 20g，用水 200 ~ 400ml 溶解后顿服。 |

**续　表**

|  | （6）利胆：成人口服：1 次 2 ～ 5g，一日 3 次，用水配成 33% 溶液服用。 |
|  | (1) for the Prevention of hypomagnesemia : For adults with mild magnesium deficiency, 1g magnesium sulfate, intramuscular injection or slow infusion with 500ml 5% glucose injection, a total of 2g a day. For patients with Severe magnesium deficiency, 0.25mmol/kg magnesium sulfate singly measured by weight or intravenously dripping with 2.5g magnesium sulfate dissolved in 5% dextrose injection or sodium chloride injection of 500ml for three hours . Meanwhile, Close observation of breathing and other vital signs is needed. |
|  | (2) complete intravenous hyperalimentation, an increase of 0.125 ～ 0.25mmol / kg magnesium a day measured by weight . complete intravenous hyperalimentation for Children, an increase of 0.125mmol / kg magnesium a day measured by weight. |
|  | (3) for the treatment of pre-eclampsia and eclampsia, intramuscular injection : 1 ～ 2.5g magnesium sulfate singly which is decided by specific condition. The maximum intramuscular injection number is up to six times a day accompanied by monitoring of ECG, tendon reflexes, respiration and blood pressure. Intravenous injection: dilute 1 ～ 2g magnesium sulfate with 5% glucose solution, injection rate is no more than 150mg per minute. Intravenous injection could raise the magnesium concentration to that close to poisoning level suddenly, therefore a strict management to dasage and a close observation to breathing, tendon reflexes, and ECG is a must. Intravenous dripping : 4g magnesium sulfate was added into 5% dextrose injection or sodium chloride injection of 250ml, infusion rate is not allowed to exceed 4ml per minute. |
|  | (4) Anticonvulsant : for Children 20 ～ 40mg/kg measured by weight is made up to the 20% solution for intramuscular injection. |
|  | (5) catharsis: for Adults, Oral medication: 5 ～ 20g singly, diluted with 200 ～ 400ml water and administered at draught. |
|  | (6) gallbladder : for Adults, Oral medication: 2 ～ 5g singly, three times a day, made up to a 33% solution with water. |
| 剂型、规格<br>Preparations | 注射剂：1g/10ml；2.5g/10ml。口服粉剂，按需要取用，配制成溶液服用。<br>Injection: 1g/10ml; 2.5g/10ml. Oral powder, take as required in solution. |
| **药品名称 Drug Names** | **乳酸钠溶液 Sodium Lactate Solution** |
| 适应证<br>Indications | 可用于纠正代谢性酸血症。由于作用不及碳酸氢钠迅速，现已渐少用。但在高钾血症或普鲁卡因等引起的心律失常伴有酸血症者，仍以应用本品为宜。<br>Used to correct metabolic acidosis. It is not used as much as before for less effective than sodium bicarbonate. However, arrhythmias accompanied by acidosis caused by procaine or hyperkalemia should be treated by this product. |
| 用法、用量<br>Dosage | 静脉滴注：每次 11.2% 液 5 ～ 8ml/kg，先用半量，以后根据病情再给其余量。用时须以 5% ～ 10% 葡萄糖液 5 倍量稀释（陈给 1.87%，即 1/6 克分子溶液）后静脉滴注。成人每次量一般为 1.87% 液 500 ～ 2000ml。<br>Intravenous infusion: 5 ～ 8ml/kg 11.2% solution singly, first with half of the amount and give the rest amount based on the condition of patients. Diluting with 5 times the amount of 5% to 10% glucose solution and intravenously dripping(first 1.87%, equivalent to 1/6 molar solution) . Typically, adults should be given by 1.87% solution of 500 ～ 2000ml. |
| 剂型、规格<br>Preparations | 注射液：每支 1.12g（10ml）；2.24g（20ml）；5.6g（50ml）。<br>Injection: 1.12g (10ml); 2.24g (20ml); 5.6g (50ml) per vial. |
| **药品名称 Drug Names** | **葡萄糖 Glucose** |
| 适应证<br>Indications | 用于：①腹泻、呕吐、重伤大失血等，体内损失大量水分时，可静脉滴注含本品 5% ～ 10% 的溶液 200 ～ 1000ml，同时静脉滴注适宜生理盐水，以补充体液的损失及钠的不足。②不能摄取饮食物的重病患者，可注射本品或灌肠，以补助营养。③血糖过低症或胰岛素过量，静脉注射 50% 溶液 40 ～ 100ml，以保护肝脏。对糖尿病的酮中毒须与胰岛素同用。④降低眼压及因颅压增加引起的各种病症如脑出血、颅骨骨折、尿毒症等，25% ～ 50% 溶液静脉注射，因其高渗压作用，将组织（特别是脑组织）内液体进入循环系统内由肾排出。注射时切勿注于血管之外，以免刺激组织。⑤高钾血症。 |

**续 表**

| | |
|---|---|
| | For the treatment of ① diarrhea, vomiting, major blood loss injuries, etc. if a loss of large amounts of water occurs, the 5% to 10% solution of 200 ~ 1000ml could be dripped intravenously, appropriate to be combined with normal saline to supplement the loss of body fluids and sodium. ② It can be injected or used as an enema for seriously ill patients who can't eat food. ③ For patients with hypoglycemia or insulin overdose symptoms, the intravenous injection solution should be made up by 50% with the amount of 40 ~ 100ml in order to protect the liver. Diabetes ketoacidosis must be treated with the use of insulin at the same time. ④ For the treatment of diseases caused by intraocular pressure reduction and intracranial pressure increase, such as cerebral hemorrhage, skull fracture, uremia, etc. Here, a type of 25% to 50% solution should be injected intravenously. Because of the high osmotic pressure effect, fluid in tissues will enter the circulatory system and go out by renal excretion, especially for brain tissue. Avoid injecting outside the blood vessels, so as not to stimulate tissue. ⑤ For the treatment of hyperkalemia. |
| 用法、用量<br>Dosage | （1）补充热量：患者因为某些原因进食减少或不能进食，一般可予 10% ~ 25% 葡萄糖注射液静脉滴注，并同时补充体液。<br><br>（2）全静脉营养疗法：葡萄糖是此疗法中最重要的能量供给物质。在非蛋白质热能中，葡萄糖与脂肪供给热量之比为 2：1。<br><br>（3）低血糖症：轻者口服，重者可先给予 50% 葡萄糖注射液 20 ~ 40ml 静脉滴注。 （4）饥饿性酮症：轻者可先给予口服 5% ~ 25% 葡萄糖注射液静脉滴注，每日 100g 葡萄糖可基本控制病情。<br><br>（5）失水：等渗性失水给予 5% 葡萄糖注射液静脉滴注。<br><br>（6）高钾血症：应用 10% ~ 25% 注射液，每 2 ~ 4g 葡萄糖加正规胰岛素 1U，可降低血清钾浓度。但此疗法仅使细胞外钾离子进入细胞内，体内总钾含量不变。如不采取排钾措施，仍有再次出现高钾血症的可能。<br><br>（7）组织脱水：高渗溶液（一般采用 50% 注射液）快速静脉注射 20 ~ 50ml，但作用短暂。应注意防止高血糖，目前少用。用于调节腹膜透析液渗透压时，50% 葡萄糖注射液 20ml 即 10g 葡萄糖可使 1L 透析渗透压提高 55mOsm/（kg·$H_2O$）。<br><br>（8）葡萄糖耐量试验：空腹口服葡萄糖 1.75g/kg，于服后 0.5、1、2、3 小时抽血测血糖。血糖浓度正常上限分别为 6.9mmol/L、11.1mmol/L、10.5mmol/L、8.3mmol/L、6.9mmol/L。<br><br>(1) To supplement the heat : for the patients who can not eat or eat less for some reason, 10% to 25% glucose solution is dripped intravenously, when body fluid is replenished at the same time.<br><br>(2) Complete TPN : Glucose is the most important substance to supply energy. In the non-protein energy, the ratio of glucose and fat to supply energy is 2:1.<br><br>(3) Hypoglycemia : Oral medication for slight cases; for serious cases, intravenous dripping with 50% glucose injection of 20 ~ 40ml.<br><br>(4) Starvation ketosis : for slight cases, Oral medication and intravenously dripping with 5% to 25% glucose solution at the same time, 100g glucose a day is enough to control the disease .<br><br>(5) Dehydration : for isotonic dehydration, 5% glucose solution is dripped intravenously.<br><br>(6) Hyperkalemia : Apply 10% to 25 % injection, add one unit of regular insulin per 2 ~ 4g glucose to reduce serum potassium concentration. However, this therapy can make extracellular potassium ions go into the cell with the total body potassium content unchanged. Hyperkalemia may occur again without excretion of potassium without .<br><br>(7) tissue Dehydration : hypertonic solution ( generally using the injection with the concentration of 50% ) rapid intravenous injection with 20 ~ 50ml but the effect is short-lived. High blood sugar should be prevented, so the product should not be used frequently. For the adjustment of osmotic pressure regulated by peritoneal dialysis fluid, 20ml 50% glucose injection, equivalent to 10g glucose can increase 1L osmotic pressure of dialysis by 55mOsm/(kg·$H_2O$).<br><br>(8) Glucose tolerance test : Oral and fasting medication, 1.75g/kg glucose, blood glucose monitoring at the time of 0.5, 1, 2 and 3 hour later. Upper limit of normal blood glucose concentrations were 6.9mmol / L, 11.1mmol / L, 10.5mmol / L, 8.3mmol / L, 6.9mmol / L respectively. |
| 剂型、规格<br>Preparations | 粉剂：每袋 250g；500g。<br>注射液：每支（瓶）50g（1000ml）；100g（1000ml）；50g（500ml）；25g（500ml）；12.5g（250ml）；25g（250ml）；1g（20ml）；5g（20ml）；10g（20ml）；2g（10ml）；0.5g（10ml）。<br><br>Powder: 250g; 500g per bag.<br>Injection: (bottle) 50g (1000ml); 100g (1000ml); 50g (500ml); 25g (500ml); 12.5g (250ml); 25g (250ml); 1g (20ml); 5g (20ml); 10g (20ml); 2g (10ml); 0.5g (10ml) per vial. |

**续　表**

| 药品名称 Drug Names | 果糖 Fructose |
|---|---|
| 适应证<br>Indications | 对糖尿病、肝病患者供给能力、补充体液。此外,能加速乙醇代谢,用于急性中毒的辅助治疗。<br>Used for energy replenishment and rehydration to patients with diabetes and liver disease . In addition, it will accelerate alcohol metabolism for the adjuvant treatment of acute poisoning. |
| 用法、用量<br>Dosage | 用以静脉注射或静脉滴注,用量视病情而定。常用量为每次 500 ~ 1000ml。<br>For intravenous injection or intravenous infusion, the amount depends on the disease. Usual Amount is 500 ~ 1000ml singly. |
| 剂型、规格<br>Preparations | 注射液:每瓶 12.5g(250ml);25g(250ml;500ml);50g(500ml)。<br>Injection: 12.5g (250ml); 25g (250ml; 500ml); 50g (500ml) per bottle. |
| 药品名称 Drug Names | 口服补液盐 Oral Rehydration Salt |
| 适应证<br>Indications | 用于补充水、钠和钾丢失的失水。治疗急性腹泻。<br>Used to supplement water, sodium and potassium dehydration. For the Treatment of acute diarrhea. |
| 用法、用量<br>Dosage | 每份必须加水 500ml 溶解混匀后服用。<br>(1)预防和治疗因腹泻、呕吐、经皮肤和呼吸道等液体丢失引起的轻、中度失水,可补充水、钾和钠,重度失水需静脉补液。①轻度失水:成人口服:开始时 50ml/kg,4 ~ 6 小时饮完,以后酌情调整剂量。儿童口服:开始时 50ml/kg,4 小时内饮完,直至腹泻停止。②中度失水:成人口服:开始时 50ml/kg,6 小时内饮完,其余应以静脉补液。儿童应以静脉补液为主。<br>(2)急性腹泻:①轻度腹泻,口服:成人每日 50ml/kg。②重度腹泻,应以静脉滴注为主,直至腹泻停止。<br>500ml of water should be added to dissolve and mixed for each.<br>(1) for the Prevention and treatment of mild and moderate-induced fluid loss caused by diarrhea and vomiting, that is, fluid loss through skin and respiratory tract. Here, water, potassium and sodium is proper to supply. Severe dehydration require intravenous rehydration. ① mild dehydration: for Adults, Oral medication: in the beginning, 50ml/kg in 4 to 6 hours and adjust dosage appropriately. For Children, Oral medication: in the beginning, 50ml/kg within four hours until diarrhea stops. ② moderate dehydration: for Adults, Oral medication: in the beginning, 50ml/kg within six hours, the rest should adopt intravenous rehydration. Children should be given intravenous rehydration mainly.<br>(2) Acute diarrhea: ① mild diarrhea, Oral medication: for adults, 50ml/kg a day. ② severe diarrhea, mainly intravenous infusion until the diarrhea stops. |
| 剂型、规格<br>Preparations | 口服补液盐 I:口服补液盐:每包总重 14.75g(大包中含氯化钠 1.75g,葡萄糖 11g;小包中含氯化钾 0.75g,碳酸氢钠 1.25g)(为 500ml 用量)。口服补液盐 II,每包总重 13.95g(氯化钠 1.75g,葡萄糖 10g,枸橼酸钠 1.45g,氯化钾 0.75g)(为 500ml 用量)。<br>Oral rehydration salts I : oral rehydration salts: a total weight of 14.75g (large package containing sodium chloride 1.75g, glucose 11g; small packet containing potassium chloride 0.75g, sodium bicarbonate 1.25g) (the amount of 500ml) per package. ORS II , a total weight of 13.95g per package (sodium chloride 1.75g, Portugal, glucose 10g, sodium citrate 1.45g, potassium chloride 0.75g) (amount of 500ml). |
| 药品名称 Drug Names | 腹膜透析液 Peritoneal Dialysis Solution |
| 适应证<br>Indications | 腹膜透析液可用于:①急性或慢性肾衰竭;②药物中毒;③顽固性心力衰竭;④电解质紊乱和酸碱平衡失调;⑤急性出血性胰腺炎和广泛化脓性腹膜炎等。<br>Peritoneal dialysis solution is used for the treatment of : ① acute or chronic renal failure; ② intoxication; ③ refractory heart failure; ④ electrolyte imbalance and acid-base balance; ⑤ acute hemorrhagic pancreatitis and extensive purulent peritonitis. |
| 用法、用量<br>Dosage | (1)治疗急、慢性肾功能衰竭伴水潴留者,用间歇性腹膜透析每次 2L,留置 1 ~ 2 小时,每日交换 4 ~ 6 次。无水潴留者,用连续不卧床腹膜透析(CAPD),一般每日 4 次,每次 2L,日间每次间隔 4 ~ 5 小时,夜间一次留置 9 ~ 12 小时,以增加中分子尿毒症毒素清除。一般每日透析液量为 8L。<br>(2)治疗急性左心衰竭,酌情用 2.5% 或 4.25% 葡萄糖透析液 2L;后者留置 30 分钟,可脱水 300 ~ 500ml;前者留置 1 小时,可脱水 100 ~ 300ml。<br>(3)儿童:每次交换量一般为 50mg/kg 体重。 |

369

**续　表**

| | |
|---|---|
| | (1) for the treatment of acute and chronic renal failure with water retention, intermittent peritoneal dialysis is used by 2L singly and indwell it for 1 to 2 hours. Exchangement for 4~6 times a day. For patients with Anhydrous retention, continuous ambulatory peritoneal dialysis (CAPD), generally 4 times a day, 2L singly, 4~5 hours at daytime interval, 9 to 12 hours indwelling at one time at night. Our goal is to increase the removement of molecular uremic toxins. Generally, a day 8L dialysate a day.<br><br>(2) for The treatment of acute left ventricular failure, using 2.5% or 4.25% glucose dialysate of 2L appropriately; the latter is indwelled for 30 minutes which leads to dehydration of 300 ~ 500ml; the former is indwelled for 1 hour that will lead to dehydration of 100 ~ 300ml.<br><br>(3) for Children: exchange capacity is usually 50mg/kg body weight singly. |
| 剂型、规格<br>Preparations | (1) 腹膜透析液（乳酸盐）：①含 1.5% 葡萄糖（1L，1.5L，2L，2.5L，5L，6L）；②含 2.5% 葡萄糖（1L，1.5L，2L，2.5L，5L，6L）；③含 4.25% 葡萄糖（1L，1.5L，2L，2.5L，5L，6L）；④含葡萄糖 4.0%（1000ml）。<br><br>(2) 腹膜透析液（乳酸盐）（低钙）：①含葡萄糖 4.0%（2000ml）；②含葡萄糖 2.5%（1000ml）；③含葡萄糖 2.5%（2000ml）；④含葡萄糖 1.5%（2000ml）。<br><br>(1) the peritoneal dialysate (lactate): ① 1.5% glucose (1L, 1.5L, 2L, 2.5L, 5L, 6L); ② 2.5% glucose (1L, 1.5L, 2L, 2.5L, 5L, 6L); ③ containing 4.25% glucose (1L, 1.5L, 2L, 2.5L, 5L, 6L); ④ containing glucose 4.0% (1000ml).<br><br>(2) the peritoneal dialysate (lactate) (calcium): ① containing glucose 4.0% (2000ml); ② containing glucose 2.5% (1000ml); ③ containing glucose 2.5% (2000ml); ④ containing glucose 1.5% (2000ml ). |

## 18.4 营养药 Nutritional support drugs

| 药品名称 Drug Names | 安素 Ensure |
|---|---|
| 适应证<br>Indications | 用于乳糖不耐受患者，无法进固体饮食的外伤、慢性病、年老体弱、产妇、术前后及某些必须限制饮食的患者等。<br><br>For patients with lactose intolerance, For the treatment of trauma which leads to disability to intake solid food, chronic diseases, for the old, weak, the puerperal and preoperative and postoperative patients and patients needed to restrict diet. |
| 用法、用量<br>Dosage | 口服或鼻饲：取 5 量匙（约 55g）本品，加入开水溶解稀释至 250ml，按 1ml 标准稀释液提供 1cal 热量计算决定患者每日用量。<br><br>Oral medication or nasal feeding: Take 5 measuring spoons (about 55g) of this product, add boiling water to dissolve to 250ml. Daily dosage is depended on the result calculated by the standard that 1 ml Standard Diluent wiil provide 1ml calory. |
| 剂型、规格<br>Preparations | 粉剂：每罐 400g。<br>Powder: 400g per tank. |
| 药品名称 Drug Names | 肠内营养乳剂（TP）Enteral Nutritional Emulsion |
| 适应证<br>Indications | 用于有胃肠功能的营养不良或摄入障碍、重症或手术后需要补充营养的患者。<br><br>For patients with gastrointestinal malnutrition or disability of ingestion and those needed for nutritional supplement after surgery or severer ones. |
| 用法、用量<br>Dosage | 通过管饲或口服使用，应按照患者的体重和营养状况计算每日用量。<br>(1) 对作为唯一营养来源的患者：推荐剂量为一日 30ml/kg（30kcal/kg）。<br>(2) 作为补充营养的患者：根据患者需要推荐剂量为一日 500 ~ 1000ml。<br>(3) 管饲给药时，应逐渐增加给药速度，第一天的速度约为 20ml/h，以后每日逐增至最大滴速 150ml/h。通过重力或泵调整输注速度。<br><br>tube feed or Oral medication, daily dosage should be calculated according to body weight and nutritional status of the patient.<br>(1) as the sole source of nutrition : The recommended dose is 30ml/kg (30kCal/kg) a day.<br>(2) As nutritional supplement: the recommended dose based on patient needs is 500 ~ 1000ml a day.<br>(3) in use of tube feed, the rate of administration should be gradually increased with the speed of the first day is about 20ml / h and gradually increase to the maximum dripping pace of 150ml / h a day. Adjust the infusion rate by gravity or pump. |

**续　表**

| 剂型、规格<br>Preparations | 乳剂：500ml。<br>Emulsion: 500ml. |
|---|---|
| **药品名称 Drug Names** | **水解蛋白 Protein Hydrolysate** |
| 适应证<br>Indications | 用于各种原因的蛋白质缺乏和衰弱患者以及对一般蛋白质消化吸收障碍的病例。用量视病情酌定。<br><br>For patients with protein deficiency and weakness caused by a variety of reasons and patients with malabsorption of the general protein. The amount depends on the condition of the disease. |
| 用法、用量<br>Dosage | 口服：一次 1 ~ 5g/kg。静脉滴注：一般每次用 5% 溶液 500ml。<br>Oral medication: 1~ 5g/kg singly. Intravenous infusion: generally, 5% solution of 500ml singly. |
| 剂型、规格<br>Preparations | 注射用水解蛋白：每瓶 500g。注射液：每瓶 25g（500ml）。<br>hydrolyzed protein for Injection use: 500g per bottle. Injection: 25g (500ml) per bottle |
| **药品名称 Drug Names** | **复方氨基酸注射液（18AA）Compound Amino Acid Injection（18AA）** |
| 适应证<br>Indications | 用于营养不良或有发生营养不良危险的患者，分解代谢旺盛疾病的营养支持和蛋白质消耗或丢失过多或合成障碍引起的低蛋白血症。<br><br>For patients with malnutrition or who have risk of malnutrition, to provide nutritional support to patients with strong Catabolism and For the treatment of hypoalbuminemia caused by protein consumption, excessive loss or synthesis disorder of protein. |
| 用法、用量<br>Dosage | 静脉滴注，每次 250 ~ 500ml，1 ~ 4 次 / 日，滴速 40 ~ 50 滴 / 分。<br>Intravenous infusion, 250 ~ 500ml singly, 1 ~ 4 times/day, dropping speed is 40 to 50 drops/min. |
| 剂型、规格<br>Preparations | 250ml：12.5g（总氨基酸）；500ml：25g（总氨基酸）；500ml：60g（总氨基酸）。<br>250ml: 12.5g (total amino acids): 500ml: 25g (total amino acids); 500ml: 60g (total amino acid). |
| **药品名称 Drug Names** | **复方氨基酸注射液（9AA）Compound Amino Acid Injection（9AA）** |
| 适应证<br>Indications | 用于急性和慢性肾功能不全患者的肠道外支持；大手术、外伤或脓毒血症引起的严重肾衰竭。<br><br>To provide parenteral support for patients with acute and chronic renal insufficiency, severe renal failure caused by major surgery, trauma or sepsis. |
| 用法、用量<br>Dosage | 静脉滴注：成人一日 250 ~ 500ml，缓慢滴注。小儿用量遵医嘱。进行透析的急、慢性肾衰竭患者一日 1000ml，最大剂量不超过 1500ml。滴速不超过每分钟 15 滴。<br><br>Intravenous infusion: for Adults, 250 ~ 500ml a day, slow dripping. Pediatric dosage is prescribed. Dialysis for acute and chronic renal failure patients needs 1000ml a day, the maximum dosage should not exceed 1500ml. Dripping rate doesn't exceed 15 drops per minute. |
| 剂型、规格<br>Preparations | 注射液：每瓶 250ml。<br>Injection: 250ml per bottle. |
| **药品名称 Drug Names** | **复方 α- 酮酸 Compound α- Ketoacid** |
| 适应证<br>Indications | 配合低蛋白质和高热量饮食，预防和治疗因慢性肾功能不全而造成蛋白质代谢失调引起的损害，延缓肾脏病进展。<br><br>It is used combined with low protein and high calorie diet to prevent and treat damages caused by protein metabolism disorders led by chronic renal insufficiency and slow the progression of kidney disease. |
| 用法、用量<br>Dosage | 口服：慢性肾功能不全，一般每次 4 ~ 8 片，一日 3 次，饭时服用；代偿期：每次 4 ~ 6 片，一日 3 次，服药期间配合低蛋白、高热量饮食。蛋白质摄入量为一日 0.5 ~ 0.6g/kg，高热量饮食为一日 146.44 ~ 167.36kJ/kg；失代偿期：每次 4 ~ 8 片，一日 3 次，配合低蛋白、高热量饮食。蛋白质摄入量为一日 0.3 ~ 0.4g/kg，高热量饮食为 146.44 ~ 167.36kJ/kg。<br><br>Oral medication: chronic renal insufficiency, usually, 4 to 8 tables singly, 3 times a day, taking with each meal; compensated stage: 4 to 6 tablets singly, 3 times a day, taking with low-protein and high-calorie diet. Protein intake is 0.5 ~ 0.6g/kg a day, high-calorie diet is 146.44 ~ 167.36kJ/kg a day; decompensatory stage: 4 to 8 tablets singly, 3 times a day, taking with low-protein and high-calorie diet. Protein intake is 0.3 ~ 0.4g/kg a day, high-calorie diet is 146.44 ~ 167.36kJ/kg a day. |

| 剂型、规格<br>Preparations | 片剂：0.63g<br>Tablets: 0.63g per tablet |
|---|---|
| 药品名称 Drug Names | 复方氨基酸注射液（3AA）Compound Amino Acid Injection （3AA） |
| 适应证<br>Indications | 用于：①急性、亚急性、慢性重症肝炎及肝硬化、慢性活动肝炎等；②促进胰岛素的分泌；③胆固醇合成的前体；④供给合成蛋白质的必需氨基酸原料；⑤促进蛋白质的合成；⑥抑制蛋白质的分解。<br><br>① For the treatment of acute, subacute, and chronic severe hepatitis and cirrhosis, chronic active hepatitis; ② stimulate insulin secretion; ③ cholesterol synthesis precursors; ④ To supply essential amino acids for protein synthesis; ⑤ To promote protein synthesis; ⑥ inhibiting protein degradation. |
| 用法、用量<br>Dosage | 静脉滴注：一日 250～500ml，或用 5%～10% 葡萄糖注射液适量混合后，缓慢静脉滴注，每分钟不超过 40 滴。一般昏迷期可酌加量，疗程根据病情遵医嘱。<br><br>Intravenous infusion: 250～500ml per day, or mixed with 5% to 10% glucose injection for slow intravenous infusion, no more than 40 drops per minute. Generally, the dosage could be increased in coma stage and the course is prescribed by doctors who will make decision based on the condition. |
| 剂型、规格<br>Preparations | 注射液：每瓶 250ml。<br>Injection: 250ml per bottle. |
| 药品名称 Drug Names | 复方氨基酸注射液（15AA）Compound Amino Acid Injection （15AA） |
| 适应证<br>Indications | 用于大面积烧伤、创伤及严重感染等应激状态下肌肉分解代谢亢进、消化系统功能障碍、营养恶化及免疫功能下降的患者的营养支持，亦用于手术后患者，改善其营养状态。<br><br>It is to provide nutrition to patients with hypermetabolic muscle breakdown, deterioration of nutrition status and decrease of human immunologic function, when they are stressed due to extensive burns, trauma and stress of serious infections, but also for patients after surgery to improve their nutritional status. |
| 用法、用量<br>Dosage | 静脉滴注一日 250～500ml，用适量 5%～10% 葡萄糖注射液混合后缓慢滴注。滴速不宜超过每 1 分钟 20 滴。<br><br>Intravenous infusion, 250～500ml a day, mixed with 5% to 10% glucose injection and then dripping slowly. Dripping rate should not exceed 20 drops per minute. |
| 剂型、规格<br>Preparations | 每瓶 250ml（总氨基酸 20g）。<br>250ml (total amino acid 20g) per bottle. |
| 药品名称 Drug Names | 脂肪乳注射液 Fat Emulsion Injection |
| 适应证<br>Indications | 适用于需要高热量的患者（如肿瘤及其他恶性病）、肾损害、禁用蛋白质的患者和由于某种原因不能经胃肠道摄取营养的患者，以补充适当热量和必需脂肪酸。<br><br>For patients who need high calorie, such as those with cancer and other malignant diseases, patients with kidney damage, patients inhibited from protein and those who can't intake nutrition through gastrointestinal tract for some reason. It is for the supplement of proper calories and essential fatty acids. |
| 用法、用量<br>Dosage | 静脉滴注：第一日脂肪量不应超过 1g/kg，以后剂量可酌增，但脂肪量不得超过 2.5g/kg，静脉滴注速度度最初 10 分钟为 20 滴 / 分，如无不良反应出现，以后可逐渐增加，30 分钟后维持 40～60 滴 / 分。<br><br>Intravenous infusion: fat should not exceed 1g/kg in the first day, later the dose could increase at discretion, but the fat shall not exceed 2.5g/kg. the intravenous infusion rate initially is 20 drops / 10 minutes and could increase gradually, when no adverse reactions appears. After 30 minutes, the dose could be adjusted to 40～60 drops per minute as the maintainance dose. |
| 剂型、规格<br>Preparations | 注射乳剂：每瓶 100ml（10g）；100ml（20g）；100ml（30g）；250ml（25g）；250ml（50g）。<br>Emulsion for injection: 100ml (10g); 100ml (20g); 100ml (30g); 250ml (25g); 250ml (50g) per bottle. |

**续　表**

| 药品名称 Drug Names | ω-3 鱼油脂肪乳注射剂 ω-3 Fish Oil Emulsion Injection |
| --- | --- |
| 适应证<br>Indications | 用于全身炎症反应综合征较严重但又需要肠外营养的患者。<br>For patients with more severe systemic inflammatory response syndrome and parenteral nutrition requirement. |
| 用法、用量<br>Dosage | 按体重一日 1 ～ 2ml/kg，即按体重一日 0.1g ～ 0.2g 鱼油 /kg，70kg 患者每日用量不超过 140ml。最大输注速率按体重不超过每小时 0.5ml/kg。必须与其他类型脂肪乳剂同时输注时，推荐打的鱼油量应占其中的 10% ～ 20%。<br>1～ 2ml/kg singly measured by weight, 0.1g ～ 0.2g fish oil / kg measured by weight, patients of 70kg take no more than 140ml a day. The maximum infusion rate measured by weight is less than 0.5ml/kg per hour. In the case of using other types of fat emulsion infusion simultaneously with fish oil, it is recommended to give 10% to 20% fish oil. |
| 剂型、规格<br>Preparations | 注射剂：50ml；100ml。<br>Injection: 50ml; 100ml. |
| 药品名称 Drug Names | 多种微量元素注射液（Ⅰ）Multi -Trace Element Injection （Ⅰ） |
| 适应证<br>Indications | 本品用于新生儿和婴儿全肠外营养时补充电解质和微量元素日常需求。<br>This product is used to replenish daily electrolytes and trace elements to newborns and infants with total parenteral nutrition. |
| 用法、用量<br>Dosage | 新生儿和婴儿：一般每日用本品 4ml/kg，可根据病儿对电解质和微量元素需要的不同而调节用量。<br>For Newborns and infants: generally, 4ml/kg a day, dosage is adapted to the requirements of electrolytes and trace elements from sick children. |
| 剂型、规格<br>Preparations | 注射液：每支 10ml。<br>Injection: 10ml per vial. |
| 药品名称 Drug Names | 多种微量元素注射液（Ⅱ）Multi -Trace Element Injection （Ⅱ） |
| 适应证<br>Indications | 一般饮食摄入不会引起微量元素的缺乏和过量，但长期肠外营养，可造成微量元素摄入不足，本品可满足成人，每日对所含微量元素的生理需要。仅用于 15kg 以上儿童及成人长期肠外全营养时补充电解质和微量元素。妊娠期妇女对微量元素的需要量轻度增高，本品也适用于妊娠期妇女。<br>Genernally, normal dietary intake will not lead to a lack or excess of trace elements, but long-term parenteral nutrition can cause inadequate intake of trace elements. This product can meet the physiological needs of daily trace elements to adults. It is only employed to complement electrolytes and trace elements to children of more than 15kg weight and adults with long-term parenteral nutrition. Pregnant women need slightly high amount of trace elements, and this product is also suitable for pregnant women. |
| 用法、用量<br>Dosage | 成人推荐剂量为每日 10ml。加于复方氨基酸注射液或葡萄糖注射液 500ml 内滴注，滴注时间为 6 ～ 8 小时。配制好的输液必须在 24 小时内输注完毕，以免被污染。<br>Adults are recommended by 10ml a day. adding it to 500ml compound amino acid injection or glucose injection and dripping for 6 to 8 hours. The prepared infusion must be completed within 24 hours to avoid contamination. |
| 剂型、规格<br>Preparations | 注射液：每支 10ml。<br>Injection: 10ml per vial. |
| 药品名称 Drug Names | 脂溶性维生素注射液（Ⅰ）Fat-soluble Vitamin Injection （Ⅰ） |
| 适应证<br>Indications | 为长期肠外全营养患者补充需要的脂溶性维生素 A、维生素 D、维生素 E、维生素 K。<br>To supply long-term parenteralnutrition patients with fat-Soluble Vitamin A, D, E, K required. |
| 用法、用量<br>Dosage | 本品适用于 11 岁以下儿童及婴儿，每日 1ml/kg 体重，每日最大剂量 10ml。使用前在无菌条件下，将本品加入到脂肪乳注射液内（100ml 或以上量），轻轻摇匀后输注，并在 24 小时内用完。<br>This product is suitable for children and infants under the age of 11, 1ml/kg a day measured by weight, and the maximum dose is 10ml a day. Under sterile conditions prior to use, the goods will be added to the fat emulsion injection (100ml or more), within 24 hours. |

| 剂型、规格<br>Preparations | 注射液：每支 10ml。<br>Injection: 10ml per vial. |
|---|---|
| 药品名称 Drug Names | 脂溶性维生素注射液（Ⅱ）Fat-soluble Vitamin Injection （Ⅱ） |
| 适应证<br>Indications | 为长期肠外全营养患者补充需要量的脂溶性维生素 A、D、E、K。<br>To supply long-term parenteralnutrition patients with fat-Soluble Vitamin A, D, E, K required. |
| 用法、用量<br>Dosage | 静脉滴注：将本品 1 支（10ml）加到脂肪乳注射剂内，轻摇混合后输注。11 岁以上儿童及本人用成人注射液，每日 10ml。<br>Intravenous infusion: add one injection(10ml) to the fat emulsion injection, gently shaking and then infusing. For 11-year-old and plus children and adults, 10ml a day. |
| 剂型、规格<br>Preparations | 注射液：每支 10ml。<br>Injection: 10ml per vial. |
| 药品名称 Drug Names | 注射用水溶性维生素 Water-soluble Vitamin for Injection |
| 适应证<br>Indications | 用于长期肠外全营养患者补充水溶性维生素。<br>To supply long-term parenteralnutrition patients with fat-soluble vitamin required. |
| 用法、用量<br>Dosage | 10kg 以上儿童及成人，每日 1 瓶，10kg 以下儿童每日按每 kg 体重给予 1/10 瓶。本品用注射用水或葡萄糖注射液 10ml 溶解后再稀释于同一类型药液中静脉滴注。<br>For children of 10kg or more and adults, one bottle a day. For children below 10kg 1/10 bottles per kg of body weight and per day. This product is dissolved in 10ml water for injection or glucose injection and then diluted in the same type of liquid for intravenous injection. |
| 剂型、规格<br>Preparations | 冻干粉剂：每瓶含硝酸硫铵 3.1mg；核黄素磷酸钠 4.9mg；烟酰胺 40mg；盐酸吡多辛 4.9mg；泛酸钠 16.5mg，维生素 C 钠 113mg，生物素 60μg，叶酸 0.4mg，维生素 $B_{12}$ 5μg。<br>Freeze-dried powder: Sulfur ammonium nitrate 3.1mg, riboflavin sodium phosphate 4.9mg, nicotinamide 40mg, pydoxine hydrochloride 4.9mg, sodium pantothenate 16.5mg, vitamin C sodium 113mg, biotin 60μg, folic acid 0.4mg and vitamin $B_{12}$ 5μg. |

19. 专科用药 Special drugs

19.1 治疗骨质疏松、前列腺增生症及老年性白内障药物 Drugs for osteoporosis, prostatic hyperplasia and senile cataract

| 药品名称 Drug Names | 帕米膦酸二钠 Pamidronate Disodium |
|---|---|
| 适应证<br>Indications | （1）用于治疗恶性肿瘤患者骨转移疼痛和高钙血症。<br>（2）治疗骨质疏松症和骨质愈合不良。<br>（3）也用于甲状旁腺功能亢进症。<br>(1) For the treatment of painful bone metastases and hypercalcemia caused by malignancy<br>(2) For the treatment of osteoporosis and poor bone healing.<br>(3) For the treatment of hyperparathyroidism. |
| 用法、用量<br>Dosage | （1）用于治疗骨质疏松症：每月 1 次 30mg 静脉滴注，连续 6 个月，改为预防量；每 3 个月 1 次 30mg 静脉滴注，连续 2 年。<br>（2）治疗癌症骨转移性疼痛：一次用药 30～60mg，静脉缓慢滴注 4 小时以上，浓度不得超过 15mg/125ml，滴速不得大于 15～30mg/2h。<br>（3）治疗高钙血症：当血钙浓度 <3.0、3.0～3.5、3.5～4.0、>4.0mmol/L，或 <12.0、12.0～14.0、14.0～16.0、>16.0mg，用本品剂量为 15～30、30～60、60～90、90mg。<br>（4）治疗变形性骨炎及骨愈合不良：每日 30～60mg，连续 1～3 日；或每日 30mg，连续 6 周。<br>（5）预防癌症骨转移，每 4 周静滴 30～60mg。<br>(1)For the treatment of osteoporosis: 30mg for once per month by intravenous infusion for 6 consecutive months and then prevention volume; 30mg for once every 3 months by intravenous infusion for 2 years.<br>(2) for The treatment of metastatic bone cancer pain: 30～60mg singly, slow intravenous infusion for over four hours, the concentration should not exceed 15mg/125ml, drip rate not faster than 15～30mg / 2 hours. |

续　表

| | |
|---|---|
| | (3) for The treatment of hypercalcemia: in the case of the calcium concentration of < 3.0, 3.0 ~ 3.5, 3.5 ~ 4.0, > 4.0mmol / L, or <12.0, 12.0 ~ 14.0, 14.0 ~ 16.0, > 16.0mg, the dose should be 15 ~ 30, 30 ~ 60, 60 ~ 90, 90 mg respectively.<br>(4) for The treatment of Paget's disease of bone healing: 30 ~ 60mga day for 1 to 3 days consecutively; or 30mg a day for 6 consecutive weeks.<br>(5) for The prevention of cancer bone metastasis, intravenous infusing with 30 ~ 60mg every four weeks. |
| 剂型、规格<br>Preparations | 片剂：每片 150mg。注射液：每支 15mg（5ml）。<br>Tablets: 150mg per tablet. Injection: 15mg (5ml) per vial. |
| **药品名称 Drug Names** | 阿仑膦酸钠 Alendronate Sodium |
| 适应证<br>Indications | 用于治疗绝经后妇女骨质疏松症，预防髋部和脊柱骨折，也适用于男性骨质疏松症及增加骨质。<br>For the treatment of postmenopausal women's osteoporosis, for the prevention of hip and spine fractures, for the treatment of male osteoporosis and to increase sclerotin |
| 用法、用量<br>Dosage | 口服，一日 1 次 10mg，或每周一次 70mg，早餐前 30 分钟用至少 200ml 白开水送服，不要咀嚼或吮吸药片。<br>Oral medication, 10mg singly per day, or 70mg once a week, take it 30 minutes at least before breakfast with 200ml warm water at least without, chewing or sucking. |
| 剂型、规格<br>Preparations | 片剂：每片 10mg；70mg。<br>Tablets: 10mg; 70mg per tablet. |
| **药品名称 Drug Names** | 伊班膦酸钠 Ibandronate sodium |
| 适应证<br>Indications | 用于伴有或不伴有骨转移的恶性肿瘤引起的高钙血症。<br>For the treatment of hypercalcemia caused by malignancy with or without bone metastases. |
| 用法、用量<br>Dosage | 缓慢静脉滴注，滴注时间不得少于 2 小时。严格按照血钙浓度，治疗前适当给予 0.9% 氯化钠注射液进行水化治疗。中、重度单剂量给 2 ~ 4mg。<br>Slow intravenous drip, dripping time not less than two hours. hydration treatment with 0.9% sodium chloride injection before treatment and administering drug exactly as the calcium concentration . for Moderate and severe patients, single dose of 2 ~ 4mg. |
| 剂型、规格<br>Preparations | 注射液：每支 1mg（1ml）。<br>Injection: 1mg (1ml) per vial. |
| **药品名称 Drug Names** | 利塞膦酸钠 Risedronate Sodium |
| 适应证<br>Indications | （1）用于治疗绝经后妇女骨质疏松症，预防髋部和脊柱骨折，也适用于男性骨质疏松症，糖皮质激素诱导的骨质疏松症。<br>（2）治疗 Paget 病。<br>(1) For the treatment of postmenopausal women with osteoporosis, prevention of hip and spine fractures, but also for male osteoporosis, glucocorticoid-induced osteoporosis.<br>(2) The treatment of paget disease. |
| 用法、用量<br>Dosage | 口服，餐前 30 分钟直立服用，200ml 左右清水送服，服后 30 分钟内不应躺下。一日 1 次，一次 5mg。绝经后骨质疏松症：15mg/ 片，一日 1 次；35mg/ 片，一周 1 次；75mg/ 片，1 个月服 2 片；150mg/ 片，1 个月 1 次。治疗男性骨质疏松症：15mg/ 片，一日 1 次。治疗 Paget 病：30mg/ 片，一日 1 次，连服 2 个月。<br>Oral medication, stand upright and take it by 200ml water 30 minutes before meals. You should not lie down within 30 minutes after the service. 5mg singly, once a day. Postmenopausal osteoporosis: 15mg / tablet and once a day; 35mg / tablet and once a week; 75mg / tablets and 2 tables every month continuously; 150mg / tablet and once a month. Treatment of osteoporosis in men: 15mg / tablet and once a day. Treatment for paget disease: 30mg / tablet and once a day for 2 months continuously. |
| 剂型、规格<br>Preparations | 片剂：每片 5mg；15mg；30mg；35mg；75mg；150mg。<br>Tablets: 5mg ; 15mg; 30mg; 35mg; 75mg; 150mg per tablet. |

**续　表**

| 药品名称 Drug Names | 降钙素 Calcitonin |
|---|---|
| 适应证<br>Indications | （1）用于治疗绝经后妇女骨质疏松症，老年骨质疏松症。<br>（2）用于治疗恶性肿瘤患者骨转移疼痛和高钙血症。<br>（3）各种骨代谢疾病所致的骨痛。<br>（4）也用于甲状旁腺功能亢进症，缺乏动力或维生素 D 中毒导致的应变性骨炎。<br>（5）paget 病。<br>（6）高钙血症和高钙血症危象。<br><br>(1) For the treatment of postmenopausal women with osteoporosis and senile osteoporosis.<br>(2) For the treatment of bone metastases pain and hypercalcemia caused by malignant tumor.<br>(3) The pain caused by kinds of metabolic bone pain. (4) It is also used for the treatment of hyperparathyroidism and osteitis lack of motivation or that caused by vitamin D intoxication .<br>(5) Paget disease.<br>(6) Hypercalcemia and hypercalcemia crisis. |
| 用法、用量<br>Dosage | （1）绝经后或老年骨质疏松症：①皮下注射或肌内注射，每日 50～100U；或隔日 100U。②鼻内用药，每次 100U，一日 1～2 次；或每次 50IU，一日 2～4 次；或隔日 200U。12 周为 1 个疗程。治疗期间，应日服钙元素 0.5～1.0g，维生素 D400U。<br><br>（2）Paget 病：①皮下注射或肌内注射，每日 100U，改善后，隔日或每日注射 50U，必要时日剂量增至 200U。②鼻内用药：每次 100U，一日 2 次；或每次 50U，一日 4 次，少数病例可能需要每次 200IU，一日 2 次。<br><br>（3）高钙血症：危象紧急处理每日 5～10U/kg，溶于 500ml 生理盐水中，静脉滴注至少 6 小时或日剂量分 2～4 次缓慢静脉注射，同时补液。慢性症状每日 5～10U/kg，1 次或 2 次皮下注射或肌内注射。也可每日 200～400U，分数次鼻内给药。<br><br>（4）痛性神经营养不良症：①皮下注射或肌内注射，每日 100U，持续 2～4 周，然后每次 100U，每周 3 次，维持 6 周以上。②鼻内给药，每日 200U，分 2～4 次给药，持续 2～4 周，然后每次 200U，每周 3 次，持续 6 周以上。<br><br>(1) Postmenopausal or senile osteoporosis : ① subcutaneous or intramuscular injection, 50～100U a day or 100U every other day. ② intranasal administration, 100U singly, 1 to 2 times a day ; or 50U singly, 2 to 4 times a day ; or 200U every other day. 12 weeks for a treatment course. During the treatment, 0.5～1.0g and vitamin D400 units calcium a day.<br>(2) Paget disease: ① subcutaneous or intramuscular injection, 100U per day, after improvement, injection 50U every other day or a day, 200U of daily dosage if necessary. ② intranasal administration: 100U singly, 2 times a day ; or 50U singly, 4 times a day, a few cases may require 200U singly, 2 times a day .<br>(3)Hypercalcemia : for crisis emergency treatment, 5～10U/kg a day, dissolve it in 500ml saline and intravenous infusion for 6 hours at least or in 2 to 4 divided doses by slow intravenous injection accompanied by rehydration. Chronic symptoms: 5～10U/kg per day, subcutaneous or intramuscular injection for 1 or 2 times. 200～400U a day is also available in divided doses by fractional intranasal administration .<br>(4) Painful nerve dystrophy : ① subcutaneous or intramuscular injection for more than six weeks. ② intranasal administration, 200U a day in 2 to 4 divided doses, for 2 to 4 weeks, 200U singly, 3 times a week for more than six weeks . |
| 剂型、规格<br>Preparations | 注射液：每支 1ml；2ml。喷鼻剂：每瓶 2ml。<br>Injection: 1m l ; 2ml per vial. Nasal spray: 2ml per bottle. |
| 药品名称 Drug Names | 骨化三醇 Calcitriol |
| 适应证<br>Indications | （1）绝经后或老年骨质疏松症。<br>（2）肾性骨营养不良。<br>（3）特发性、假性或术后甲状旁腺功能低下。<br>（4）维生素 D 依赖型佝偻病，低血磷性抗维生素 D 型佝偻病。<br><br>(1) postmenopausal or senile osteoporosis.<br>(2) renal osteodystrophy.<br>(3) idiopathic, pseudo-or postoperative hypoparathyroidism.<br>(4) vitamin D-dependent rickets, hypophosphatemia vitamin D-resistant rickets. |

**续 表**

| 用法、用量<br>Dosage | ①绝经后或老年骨质疏松症：推荐剂量为每次 0.25μg，一日 2 次，最大剂量可至每次 0.5μg，一日 2 次。用药后第 1、3、6 个月应监测血钙及血肌酐，正常以后，可每 6 个月检测一次。调整剂量期间，需每周检测血钙。②肾性骨营养不良症：最初剂量为 0.25μg，每日口服一次，连服 2～4 周。对血清钙正常或偏低者，口服 0.25μg，每 2 日一次即可。注射剂的剂量为开始每次 0.5μg（0.01μg/kg），每周 3 次。如用药后 2～4 周患者时间骨化指标和临床症状无明显改善，可每隔 2～4 周将用量增高 0.25μg/d。在此期间，应每周监测血钙至少 2 次。③甲状旁腺功能低或佝偻病患者：初始剂量 0.25μg，每晨服用。如生化指标和临床症状无明显改善，可每隔 2～4 周提高药物剂量。<br><br>① post-menopause or senile osteoporosis: The recommended dose is 0.25μg singly, 2 times a day, the maximum dose can be 0.5μg singly, 2 times a day. At the 1st, 3th and 6th month after the treatment, serum calcium and serum creatinine should be monitored. When the indicators are normal, monitoring should be given once every six months. During dose adjustment, serum calcium is required to detect per week. ② Renal osteodystrophy: the initial dose is 0.25μg, Oral medication once a day for 2 to 4 weeks continuously. For patients with Normal or low serum calcium, Oral medication with 0.25μg, 2 times per day. In the beginning, 0.5μg (0.01μg/kg) per injection dose, 3 times a week. 2～4 weeks after the treatment, if time indicators and clinical symptoms have no significant improvement, the dosage could be increased to 0.25μg / d every 2 to 4 weeks. During this period, serum calcium should be monitored 2 times weekly at least. ③ patients with Low parathyroid function or rickets: the initial dose is 0.25μg taken every morning. if biochemical markers and clinical symptoms have no significant improvement, the dose can be increased every 2 to 4 weeks. |
| --- | --- |
| 剂型、规格<br>Preparations | 胶囊剂：每粒 0.25μg。注射剂：每支 1μg（1ml）；2μg（1ml）。<br>Capsules: 0.25μg per capsule. Injection: 1μg (1ml); 2μg (1ml) per vial. |
| **药品名称 Drug Names** | 阿法骨化醇 Alfacalcidol |
| 适应证<br>Indications | 用于：预防骨质疏松症、佝偻病和软骨病、肾源性骨病、甲状旁腺功能减退症。<br>For the prevention of osteoporosis, rickets and osteomalacia, Nephrogenic osteonosus and hypoparathyroidism. |
| 用法、用量<br>Dosage | 口服。骨质疏松症：成人，初始剂量每日 0.5μg，维持量为每日 0.25～0.5μg。其他指征患者：成人或体重 20kg 以上儿童初始剂量每日 1μg，老年人每日 0.5μg，维持剂量为每日 0.25～1μg。<br><br>Oral medication. Osteoporosis: for adults, the initial dose is 0.5μg a day, the maintenance dose is 0.25～0.5μg a day. patients with other indications: for adults or children weighing more than 20kg, the initial dose is 1μg a day; for elderly, 0.5μg per day, the maintainance dose is 0.25～1μg a day. |
| 剂型、规格<br>Preparations | 胶囊剂：每粒 0.25μg。片剂：每片 0.25μg；0.5μg。<br>Capsules: 0.25μg per capsule. Tablets: 0.25μg; 0.5μg per tablet. |
| **药品名称 Drug Names** | 碳酸钙 Calcium Carbonate |
| 适应证<br>Indications | 用于预防和治疗钙缺乏症，以及妊娠和哺乳期妇女、绝经期妇女钙的补充。<br>For the prevention and treatment of calcium deficiency and calcium supplement for pregnant and lactating women, postmenopausal women. |
| 用法、用量<br>Dosage | 口服，一日 1～3 次，分次服。可根据个人情况酌情进行补充。<br>Oral medication, 1～3 times a day in divided doses. It can be supplemented based on individual circumstances. |
| 剂型、规格<br>Preparations | 片剂：0.75g。咀嚼片：每片 1.25g。<br>Tablets: 0.75g. Chewable Tablets: 1.25g per tablet. |
| **药品名称 Drug Names** | 替勃龙 Tibolone |
| 适应证<br>Indications | 用于绝经后引起的多种症状。<br>For the treatment of a variety of symptoms caused by menopause. |

**续 表**

| 用法、用量<br>Dosage | 口服，一日一次 2.5mg，最好固定时间服用，症状消除后可每日服半量，连续服用 3 个月或更长时间。<br><br>Oral medication, 2.5mg singly and once a day, better at a fixed time. After the symptoms eliminate, take half the amount a day for three consecutive months or longer. |
|---|---|
| 剂型、规格<br>Preparations | 片剂：每片 2.5mg。<br>Tablets: 2.5mg per tablet. |

| 药品名称 Drug Names | 雌二醇 Estradiol |
|---|---|
| 适应证<br>Indications | 卵巢功能不全或卵巢激素不足引起的各种症状，主要是功能性子宫出血、原发性闭经、绝经期综合征及前列腺癌等。<br><br>A variety of symptoms caused by ovarian dysfunction or ovarian hormone deficiency, mainly functional uterine bleeding, primary amenorrhea, menopause syndrome, prostate cancer, etc. |
| 用法、用量<br>Dosage | 肌内注射：每次 0.5 ~ 1.5mg，每周 2 ~ 3 次。口服，一日 1 片。<br>Intramuscular injection: 0.5 ~ 1.5 mg singly, 2 to 3 times a week.Oral medication, 1 time a day. |
| 剂型、规格<br>Preparations | 注射液：每支 2mg（1ml）。<br>凝胶：每支 80g；0.06%。<br>片剂：每片 1mg。<br>微粒化 17β 雌二醇片：每片 1mg；2mg。<br>控释贴片：周效片，每片 2.5mg；3 ~ 4 日效片：每片 4mg。<br>Injection: 2mg (1 ml)per bottle.<br>Gel: 80g per bottle;0.06%.<br>Tablets: 1mg per tablet.<br>Micronized 17β estradiol tablets: 1mg; 2mg per tablet.<br>Controlled-release patch: weekly patch, 2.5mg per patch; patch used every 3 to 4 days: 4mg per patch. |

| 药品名称 Drug Names | 雷洛昔芬 Raloxifene |
|---|---|
| 适应证<br>Indications | 主要用于预防绝经后妇女的骨质疏松症。<br>Mainly used for the prevention of osteoporosis in postmenopausal women. |
| 用法、用量<br>Dosage | 口服，每日 60mg，不受仅是限制。老年人无须调整剂量。由于疾病的必然过程，本品需要长期使用。<br><br>Oral medication, 60mg per day. For Elderly, no need for dose adjustment. Due to the inevitable course of the disease, long-term use of this product is necessary. |
| 剂型、规格<br>Preparations | 片剂：每日 60mg。<br>Tablets: 60mg Daily. |

| 药品名称 Drug Names | 氨基葡萄糖 Glucosamine |
|---|---|
| 适应证<br>Indications | 用于治疗和预防全身部位的骨关节炎。可缓解和消除骨关节炎的疼痛、肿胀等症状，改善关节活动功能。<br><br>For the treatment and prevention of osteoarthritis of all parts of the body. It can alleviate and eliminate pain, swelling and other symptoms caused by Osteoarthritis and improve joint function. |
| 用法、用量<br>Dosage | 口服，每次 1 ~ 2 粒，一日 3 次，一般疗程 4 ~ 12 周，如有必要可延长服药时间。每年重复治疗 2 ~ 3 次。<br><br>Oral medication, 1 to 2 tables singly, 3 times a day, usually, 4 to 12 weeks is a treatment course, if necessary, extend the time for medication. Repeat the treatment 2 or 3 times every year. |
| 剂型、规格<br>Preparations | 胶囊剂：每粒 0.24mg。<br>Capsules: 0.24mg per capsule. |

**续　表**

| 药品名称 Drug Names | 酚苄明 Phenoxybenzamine |
|---|---|
| 适应证<br>Indications | （1）用于前列腺增生引起的尿潴留。<br>（2）嗜铬细胞瘤的治疗和术前准备。<br>（3）周围血管痉挛性疾病。<br><br>(1) For the treatment of urinary retention caused by prostatic hyperplasia.<br>(2) For the treatment of pheochromocytoma and preoperative preparation.<br>(3) Peripheral vascular spasm diseases. |
| 用法、用量<br>Dosage | 开始每次 10mg，一日 2 次，以后隔日加量 10mg，直至获得临床效果或出现轻微不良反应。以每次 20 ～ 40mg，一日 2 ～ 3 次维持。<br><br>In the Beginning, 10mg singly, 2 times a day, later an increase of 10mg every other day, until a clinical effect or mild adverse reactions. Later, 20 ～ 40mg singly, 2 to 3 times a day to maintain. |
| 剂型、规格<br>Preparations | 片剂：每片 10mg。<br>Tablets: 10mg per tablet. |
| 药品名称 Drug Names | 特拉唑嗪 Terazosin |
| 适应证<br>Indications | （1）用于改善良性前列腺增生患者的排尿症状。<br>（2）还用于治疗慢性、非细菌性前列腺炎和前列腺痛，女性膀胱颈梗阻，结肠手术拔出导尿管前服用，预防急性尿潴留的发生。<br>（3）用于治疗高血压，可单独使用或与其他药合用。<br><br>(1) It is used to improve urination symptoms in patients with benign prostatic hyperplasia.<br>(2) It is also used for the treatment of chronic non-bacterial prostatitis and prostate pain, female bladder neck obstruction. It should be used before catheter is pull out in colon surgery to avoid acute urinary retention.<br>(3) For the treatment of high blood pressure and used alone or in combination with other drugs. |
| 用法、用量<br>Dosage | （1）良性前列腺增生：口服，每次 2mg，一日一次，每晚睡前服用。<br>（2）高血压：初始剂量为睡前服用 1mg，且不应超过，以尽量减少首次低血压事件的发生。1 周后，每日单剂量可加倍以达到预期效果。常用维持剂量为一天 2 ～ 10mg。<br><br>(1) Benign prostatic hyperplasia: Oral medication, 2mg singly, once a day, every night at bedtime.<br>(2) Hypertension: the initial dose is 1mg at most taken at bedtime to minimize the occurrence of the first event of hypotension. A week later, doubled dosage single a day to achieve the desired results. the maintenance dose is 2 ～ 10mg a day. |
| 剂型、规格<br>Preparations | 片剂：每片 1mg；2mg；5mg。胶囊剂：每粒 2mg。<br>Tablets: 1mg /2mg/5mg per tablet. Capsules: 2mg per capsule. |
| 药品名称 Drug Names | 坦洛新 Tamsulosin |
| 适应证<br>Indications | 主要用于治疗前列腺增生而导致的异常排尿症状，适用于轻、中度患者及未导致排尿障碍者，如已发生严重尿潴留患者不宜单独服用此药。<br><br>For the treatment of abnormal urinary symptoms caused by prostatic hyperplasia. It is suitable for mild and moderate patients and those without voiding dysfunction. If severe urinary retention occurs, the patient should stop taking the drug alone. |
| 用法、用量<br>Dosage | 口服，每次 0.2mg，一日 1 次，餐后服。<br>Oral medication, 0.2mg singly, 1 times per day, after meal. |
| 剂型、规格<br>Preparations | 缓释胶囊剂：每粒 0.2mg。<br>Sustained-release capsules: 0.2mg per capsule. |
| 药品名称 Drug Names | 非那雄胺 Finasteride |
| 适应证<br>Indications | （1）用于治疗良性前列腺增生，使增大的前列腺缩小，其逆转过程需要 3 个月以上，可以改善排尿症状，使最大尿流率增加；减少发生尿潴留和手术概率。<br>（2）可以治疗男性秃发，能促进头发增长并防止继续脱发。 |

| | (1) For the treatment of benign prostatic hyperplasia, reducing the Magnitude of enlarged prostate, which needs more than three months; To improve urinary symptoms and increase the maximum flow rate; To reduce the incidence of urinary retention and surgery odds.<br>(2) To treat male baldness, promote hair growth and prevent further hair loss. |
|---|---|
| 用法、用量<br>Dosage | 口服。<br>（1）治疗良性前列腺增生：每次 5mg，一日 1 次，6 个月为 1 个疗程。空腹或与食物同时服用均可。肾功能不全者、老年人不需要调整剂量。<br>（2）治疗脱发：每次 1mg，一日 1 次，睡前服用。一般连续服用 3 个月或更长时间才能收到效果。<br>Oral medication.<br>(1) for The treatment of benign prostatic hyperplasia: 5mg singly, once a day, 6 months for a treatment course. Fasting and taking with food are both ok. Patients with renal dysfunction of degree and the elderly do not need to adjust the dose.<br>(2) for The treatment of hair loss: 1mg singly, once a day at bedtime. Generally take it for three consecutive months or longer could achieve the desired effect. |
| 剂型、规格<br>Preparations | 片剂：每片 1mg；5mg。<br>Tablets: 1mg/5mg per tablet. |
| 药品名称 Drug Names | 舍尼通 Cernilton |
| 适应证<br>Indications | 用于良性前列腺增生，慢性、非细菌性前列腺炎及前列腺疼痛等。<br>For the treatment of benign prostatic hyperplasia, chronic nonbacterial prostatitis and prostate pain. |
| 用法、用量<br>Dosage | 口服，一次 1 片，一日 2 次，早、晚各一片，疗程 3～6 个月。衰老或肾功能不全者无须改变剂量。<br>Oral medication, 1 tablet singly and 2 times a day, that is, morning and night for 3 to 6 months as a course. There is no need for Aging or renal dysfunction to chang the dose. |
| 剂型、规格<br>Preparations | 片剂：每片含 p5 70mg，E A10 4mg。<br>Tablets: p5 70mg and E A10 4mg per tablet. |
| 药品名称 Drug Names | 前列通 Qianlietong tablets |
| 适应证<br>Indications | 用于急性前列腺炎、前列腺增生引起的尿潴留、尿血、尿频等症。<br>For the treatment of acute prostatitis, urinary retention, hematuria, urinary frequency, etc. caused by benign prostatic hyperplasia. |
| 用法、用量<br>Dosage | 口服：大片每次服 4 片，或小片每次 6 片，一日 3 次。30～45 日为 1 个疗程。<br>Oral medication: 4 large or 6 small pieces singly, three times a day. 30 to 45 days as a course of treatment. |
| 剂型、规格<br>Preparations | 片剂：340mg。胶囊：250mg，380mg，400mg。<br>Tablet: 340mg. capsule: 250mg, 380mg, 400mg. |
| 药品名称 Drug Names | 谷丙甘氨酸 Glutamate Acid，Alanine and Glycine |
| 适应证<br>Indications | 用于治疗前列腺增生引起的尿频、排尿困难及尿潴留。尤适用于心肺功能不全和不宜手术的高龄患者。本品为氨基酸制剂，适合老年患者使用。<br>For the treatment of frequent urination, dysuria and urinary retention disease caused by prostatic hyperplasia. Especially for elderly patients with cardiopulmonary dysfunction and those unfitful for operation. This product is an amino acid formulations, suitable for elderly patients. |
| 用法、用量<br>Dosage | 口服，一次 2 片，一日 3 次，或根据病情适当增减。<br>Oral medication, 2 tables singly, 3 times a day, or be adjusted according to the condition. |
| 剂型、规格<br>Preparations | 片剂：每片 0.41g。<br>Tablets: 0.41g per tablet. |

**续　表**

| 药品名称 Drug Names | 吡诺克辛 Pirenoxine |
| --- | --- |
| 适应证<br>Indications | 用于治疗初期老年性白内障、轻度糖尿病性白内障或并发性白内障等。<br>For the treatment of senile cataract of incipient stage, mild diabetic cataract or complicated cataracts. |
| 用法、用量<br>Dosage | 滴眼，用前充分摇匀，每次 1 ～ 2 滴，一日 3 ～ 5 次。<br>Eye Drops, shake it well before use, 1 to 2 drops singly, 3 ～ 5 times a day. |
| 剂型、规格<br>Preparations | 滴眼剂：每瓶装有密封的药片 1 片；每瓶内装溶剂 15ml。<br>Eye drops: 1 sealed pills per bottle; 15ml solvent per bottle |

### 19.2　消毒防腐收敛药 Drugs for sterilizing, antisepsis and convergence

| 药品名称 Drug Names | 过氧乙酸 Peracetic Acid |
| --- | --- |
| 适应证<br>Indications | 用于空气、环境消毒和预防消毒。<br>For air sterilization, environmental disinfection and preventive disinfection. |
| 用法、用量<br>Dosage | 用前按比例稀释。最常用为稀释 500 倍，即用 20% 的本品 2ml 加水 998ml 制得，含过氧乙酸 0.04%。<br>　（1）空气消毒：1∶200 液对空气喷雾，每立方米空间含药 30ml。<br>　（2）预防性消毒：食具、毛巾、水果、蔬菜等用 1∶500 液洗刷浸泡，禽蛋用 1∶1000 液浸泡，时间为 5 分钟，密封 50 ～ 60 分钟。<br>Proportionately diluting before use. The most common use is to dilute 500 times as the original, that is 20% of the product of 2ml made up by water of 998ml, containing 0.04% peracetic acid.<br>(1) Air disinfection: 1∶200 liquid air spray to get 30ml peracetic acid per cubic meter of space.<br>(2) Preventive disinfection: for utensils, towels, fruit, vegetables, etc. soaking with 1:500 scrubbing liquid; for eggs, 1:1000 solution to soak for 5 minutes and sealing for 50 to 60 minutes. |
| 剂型、规格<br>Preparations | 溶液：16% ～ 20%。<br>Solution: 16% ～ 20%. |

| 药品名称 Drug Names | 聚维酮碘 Povidone Iodine |
| --- | --- |
| 适应证<br>Indications | 用于皮肤、黏膜的窗口消毒，也用于化脓性皮炎、皮肤真菌感染、小面积烧烫伤及念珠菌阴道炎、细菌性阴道炎、混合感染性阴道炎、老年性阴道炎等。<br>For skin and mucous membranes disinfection. For the treatment of suppurative dermatitis, fungal skin infections, a small area of burn and Candida vaginitis, bacterial vaginosis, mixed infection vaginitis, senile vaginitis, etc. |
| 用法、用量<br>Dosage | （1）外科手术消毒，0.5% 溶液刷洗 5 分钟。注射部位消毒，30 分钟以上。<br>（2）术野皮肤消毒，0.5% 溶液均匀涂抹 2 次。<br>（3）黏膜创伤或感染，用 0.1% ～ 0.025% 溶液冲洗或软膏涂抹病患部位。<br>（4）皮肤感染 0.5% 溶液局部涂擦或软膏涂抹患处。<br>（5）阴道或直肠给药，每晚睡前 1 次，一次 1 支软膏或 1 个栓剂，7 ～ 10 日为 1 个疗程。<br>(1) Surgical sterilization, scrub for 5 minutes with a solution of 0.5%. Disinfecting the injection site, 30 minutes or more.<br>(2) for The operative field skin disinfection, use 0.5% solution to smear evenly twice.<br>(3) for Mucosal trauma or infection, 0.1% to 0.025% solution or ointment on painful parts.<br>(4) for Skin infection, use 0.5% solution to smear topically or ointment to rub the affected area.<br>(5) Vaginal or rectal administration, once every night before going to bed, a cream or a suppository singly, 7 to 10 days for a treatment course. |
| 剂型、规格<br>Preparations | 溶液：0.5%；1%；5%。<br>软膏、乳膏或凝胶：10%。<br>栓剂：每个 0.29g。<br>Solution: 0.5%; 1%; 5%.<br>Ointments, creams or gels: 10%.<br>Suppositories: 0.29g per drug. |

**续 表**

| 药品名称 Drug Names | 氯己定 Chlorhexidine |
|---|---|
| 适应证<br>Indications | 　　用于皮肤、创面、妇产科、泌尿外科的消毒及卫生用品的消毒，也用于急性坏死性溃疡性牙龈炎、牙科术后口腔感染，预防和治疗癌肿和白血病患者的口腔感染、义齿引起的创伤性磨损继发细菌和真菌感染、滤泡性口炎等。<br><br>　　For the disinfection of skin, wound, obstetrics and urology. For the treatment of acute necrotizing and ulcerative gingivitis and oral infections after dental surgery. For the prevention and treatment of cancer and leukemia patients's oral infections, traumatic secondary bacterial and fungal infections caused by denture, follicular stomatitis, etc. |
| 用法、用量<br>Dosage | 　　(1) 手术消毒：以 1 ∶ 5000 水溶液泡手 3 分钟。<br>　　(2) 术野消毒：用 0.5% 乙醇（70%）溶液，其功效约与碘酊相当，但无皮肤刺激、亦不染色，因而特别适于面部、会阴部及儿童的术野消毒。<br>　　(3) 创伤伤口消毒：用 1 ∶ 2000 水溶液冲洗。<br>　　(4) 含漱：以 1 ∶ 5000 溶液漱口，对咽峡炎及口腔溃疡有效。<br>　　(5) 烧伤、烫伤：用 0.5% 乳膏或气雾剂。<br>　　(6) 分娩时产妇外阴及周围皮肤消毒，会阴镜检的润滑：用 1% 乳膏涂抹。<br>　　(7) 器械消毒：消毒用 1 ∶ 1000 水溶液，储存用 1 ∶ 5000 水溶液，加入 0.1% 亚硝酸钠浸泡，隔 2 周换一次。<br>　　(8) 房间、家具等消毒：用 0.02% 溶液膀胱冲洗。<br>　　(9) 滴眼液防腐：用 0.01% 溶液。<br>　　(10) 伤口护理：用贴剂，清洁患处后，将中间护创贴在创伤处，两端用胶带固定。<br><br>　　(1) Surgical sterilization: use 1 ∶ 5000 aqueous to foam hand for three minutes.<br>　　(2) Disinfection of the operative field: use 0.5% ethanol (70%) solution, ts efficacy approximately equivalent to that of iodine, but no skin irritation, nor stain, and thus particularly suitable for disinfection of the operative field on face, perineum and children's operative disinfection.<br>　　(3) Traumatic wound disinfection: use 1 ∶ 2000 solution to flush.<br>　　(4) gargling: use 1 ∶ 5000 solution to gargle for angina and mouth ulcers .<br>　　(5) Burns and scald: use 0.5% cream or aerosol.<br>　　(6) genital and its surrounding skin disinfection during delivery, lubrication for perineal examination: 1% cream to smear.<br>　　(7) Instrument disinfection: 1 ∶ 1000 solution for disinfection, 1 ∶ 5000 solution soked with 0.1% sodium nitrite for storage, once every two weeks.<br>　　(8) Urinary disinfection: 0.02% solution for bladder irrigation.<br>　　(9) The ophthalmic preservative: 0.01% solution.<br>　　(10) Wound Care: after cleaning the affected area, use the the middle of the patch to post on the trauma and fix it at both ends with tape. |
| 剂型、规格<br>Preparations | 　　制剂：葡萄糖酸氯己定含漱剂：0.016g（200ml）；0.04g（500ml）。葡萄糖酸氯己定溶液：50g（250ml）。稀葡萄糖酸氯己定溶液：12.5g（250ml）。醋酸氯己定片：每片 5mg。醋酸氯己定霜：1%。醋酸氯己定软膏：1%。<br><br>　　Preparation: Chlorhexidine Gluconate Gargle: 0.016g (200ml); 0.04g (500ml). Chlorhexidine gluconate solution: 50g (250ml). Dilute chlorhexidine gluconate solution: 12.5g (250ml). Chlorhexidine acetate tablets: 5mg per tablet. Chlorhexidine acetate cream: 1%. Chlorhexidine acetate ointment: 1%. |
| 药品名称 Drug Names | 戊二醛 Glutaraldehyde |
| 适应证<br>Indications | 　　用于器械消毒，也可用于治疗寻常疣、甲癣和多汗症。<br>　　For device disinfection and the treatment of warts, onychomycosis, and hyperhidrosis. |
| 用法、用量<br>Dosage | 　　(1) 碱性戊二醛水溶液或异丙醇溶液（浓度为 2%，pH 为 7.5～8.5）：对细菌繁殖体的作用时间为 10～20 分钟，对细菌芽孢为 4～12 小时。10% 溶液用于治疗寻常疣、甲癣和多汗症，局部涂搽，一日 1～2 次。配制好的 2% 碱性水溶液在室温下经 14 日后，杀菌作用即明显减退。 |

**续　表**

(2) 酸性强化戊二醛液：是在 2% 戊二醛溶液中加入某些非离子型化合物作为强化剂配制而成。所加强化剂有稳定作用，又有协同增效作用。国外商品名为 Sonacide。国内曾用 0.25% 聚氧乙烯脂肪醇醚作为强化剂配制。此溶液因仍保持酸性（pH3.4），故稳定，室温下放置 18 个月，杀菌效能不减。同时加强药物表面活性，协同增效。杀菌力与碱性戊二醛相似，用法也相同。唯一缺点易导致金属生锈。

(3) 人造心脏瓣膜消毒液：为其 0.65% 溶液，pH（7.4）与血液相似，系磷酸盐缓冲液。

(4) 戊二醛气体：用于密封空间内表面的熏蒸消毒，因其不易在物体表面聚合，故优于甲醛。

(1) Isopropyl or alkaline aqueous glutaraldehyde solution (concentration of 2%, pH 7.5 to 8.5 ): for the multiplication of bacteria, the disinfection time is 10 to 20 minutes, for the bacterial spores, 4 to 12 hours . 10% solution for the treatment of common warts, onychomycosis and hyperhidrosis. Tropically smearing for 1 or 2 times per day. The disinfection function of a well prepared 2% alkaline aqueous solution markedly diminishes after 14 days at room temperature.

(2) An acidic glutaraldehyde solution: it is made up by adding some non- ionic compound as a reinforcing agent preparation in 2% glutaraldehyde solution. The Added enhancer has a stabilizing effect and synergies . the Foreign trade name is Sonacide. In China, 0.25 % polyoxyethylene fatty alcohol ethers was used as enhancer formulation . This acidic solution was maintained by (pH3.4), so the sterilization performance never diminish and is stable at room temperature for 18 months. Strengthening the surface activity will help enhance the efficacy together. the sterilization performance is similar to that of alkaline glutaraldehyde. The only drawback is easy to cause metal to rust.

(3) Artificial heart valves disinfectant : 0.65% solution, pH (7.4), similar to the blood, phosphate buffer .

(4) Glutaraldehyde Gas: fumigation and sterilization for the surface of sealed space, because the surface is not easy for polymerization, then it is better than formaldehyde.

| 剂型、规格<br>Preparations | 溶液：20%；25%，稀释后使用。<br>Solution: 20%; 25% after dilution. |
|---|---|
| 药品名称 Drug Names | 洗消净 Sodium hypochlorite and sodium dodecyl sulfate |
| 适应证<br>Indications | 适用范围广泛，可供器械、用具、衣物及排泄物消毒。<br>It is widely used in the disinfection of devices, appliances, clothing and excreta. |
| 用法、用量<br>Dosage | 取本品 50ml，用 10kg 水稀释，将被洗涤物品放在其中刷洗，即可达到消毒洗净的目的。也可浸泡 3 ～ 5 分钟，然后再刷洗，配制本品可用自来水，最适水温为 40℃左右。<br><br>Take this product of 50ml diluted with 10kg water and flush items with it, you can achieve the purpose of disinfection and cleaning. the alternative is to soak for 3 to 5 minutes and then flush. The product can be formulated with tap water, and the optimum temperature is about 40 ℃ . |
| 剂型、规格<br>Preparations | 溶液。<br>solution. |
| 药品名称 Drug Names | 苯酚 Phenol |
| 适应证<br>Indications | 常用于消毒痰、脓、粪便和医疗器械。液化苯酚用于涂拭阑尾残端。<br>It is commonly used in the disinfection of sputum, pus, feces, and medical devices. Liquefied phenol is used for coating appendix stump. |
| 用法、用量<br>Dosage | 外用消毒防腐剂。本品对人有腐蚀性、毒性，可引起新生儿黄疸，不宜长期使用。<br>Antiseptic disinfectant for external use. This product is corrosive and toxic for people and can cause neonatal jaundice, thus inappropriate for long-term use. |
| 剂型、规格<br>Preparations | 1% ～ 5% 溶液。<br>1% to 5% solution. |
| 药品名称 Drug Names | 鱼石脂 Ichthammol |
| 适应证<br>Indications | 有抑菌、消炎、抑制分泌和消肿等作用，可用于疖肿及外耳道炎等。<br>It is used as antibacterial, anti-inflammatory, to inhibit the secretion and reduce the swelling on boils and otitis externa. |

**续　表**

| 用法、用量<br>Dosage | 外用涂擦，一日 2 次。滴耳，一日 3 次，一次 2 滴。<br>Inunction, 2 times a day. Ear drops, 3 times a day, 2 drops singly. |
|---|---|
| 剂型、规格<br>Preparations | 10% 软膏；鱼石脂甘油滴耳剂。<br>10% ointment; ichthyol glycerol eardrops. |

| 药品名称 Drug Names | 乙醇 Ethanol |
|---|---|
| 适应证<br>Indications | 75% 用于杀菌消毒。50% 用于防压疮。25% ~ 50% 擦浴用于高热患者物理退热。还可用于小面积烫伤的湿敷浸泡。在配制剂时用作溶剂。<br>75% for sterilization. 50% for bedsore. 25% to 50% for patients with physical febrifuge.It can be used for hydropathic compress and soaking on a small area of burns. It is used as a kind of solvent. |
| 用法、用量<br>Dosage | 用作消毒剂时注意浓度，过高或过低均影响杀菌效果。不宜用于伤口或破损的皮肤面。<br>As the sanitizer, if the concentration is too high or too low, sterilizing effect will be affected. Not suitable for skin surface of wounds or broken. |
| 剂型、规格<br>Preparations | 各种不同浓度的乙醇溶液。<br>Various concentrations of ethanol. |

| 药品名称 Drug Names | 甲紫 Methylrosanilinium |
|---|---|
| 适应证<br>Indications | 有较好的杀菌作用，且无刺激性。用于皮肤革兰阳性菌和皮肤黏膜念珠菌病。<br>Better bactericidal effect without irritation. For the treatment of Gram-positive bacteria skin and mucocutaneous candidiasis. |
| 用法、用量<br>Dosage | 外用涂搽。据报道，有一定致癌作用，故在伤口处禁用。<br>Inunction. it is reported there are certain carcinogenic effects, thus forbidden on the wound. |
| 剂型、规格<br>Preparations | 1% 溶液；1% 糊。<br>1% solution; 1% paste. |

| 药品名称 Drug Names | 依沙吖啶 Ethacridine |
|---|---|
| 适应证<br>Indications | 有消毒防腐作用，用于有感染及糜烂渗液的皮肤或创面。<br>Disinfection and antiseptic for skin or wound infected and with erosion and exudate. |
| 用法、用量<br>Dosage | 外用冲洗、湿敷。<br>Rinse and hydropathic compress for external use. |
| 剂型、规格<br>Preparations | 0.1% 溶液。<br>0.1% solution. |

| 药品名称 Drug Names | 高锰酸钾 Potassium Permanganate |
|---|---|
| 适应证<br>Indications | 有强氧化作用，可除臭消毒，但作用短暂表浅。冲洗感染创面及膀胱炎用 0.1% ~ 0.5% 溶液，清除皮损表面的脓性分泌物和恶臭、湿敷治疗湿疹 0.025% ~ 0.01% 溶液，眼科用 0.01% ~ 0.02% 溶液，洗胃 1：1000 ~ 1：5000，坐浴 0.02%，水果、食具消毒 0.1%。<br>It has strong oxidation for deodorizing and disinfecting, but the effect is transient on superficial skin. The 0.1% to 0.5% solution is for wound infections washing and cystitis treatment. The 0.025% to 0.01% solution is for the removing of purulent secretions and cacosmia from the wound and hydropathic compress to treat eczema. The 0.01% to 0.02% solution is used as ophthalmic solution, 1：1000~1：5000 for lavage, 0.02% for sitz bath, 0.1% for fruits and utensils disinfection. |
| 用法、用量<br>Dosage | 溶液应新配，久置或加热可迅速失效。其褐色斑可以用过氧化氢溶液或草酸溶液拭去。<br>The solution should be a new equipped one, for long-time placement or heating can quickly fail the efficacy. Brown spots can be wiped by hydrogen peroxide solution or a solution of oxalic acid. |
| 剂型、规格<br>Preparations | 外用片：100mg。<br>Topical tablets: 100mg. |

**续　表**

| 药品名称 Drug Names | 过氧化氢溶液 Hydrogen Peroxide Solution |
| --- | --- |
| 适应证<br>Indications | 　　为强氧化剂，具有消毒、防腐、除臭及清洁作用，用于清洗创面、溃疡、脓窦、耳内脓液；涂搽治疗面部褐斑；在换药时可以去痂皮和黏附在伤口的敷料；稀释至 1% 浓度用于扁桃体炎、口腔炎、白喉等含漱。<br>　　A strong oxidizing agent to disinfect, antisepticize, deodorizing and clean wounds, ulcers, pus sinus and ear pus; rubbing facial brown spots; to scratch crusta and dressing adhered to the wound; Type of 1% concentration is used to treat tonsillitis, stomatitis, diphtheria and other gargle. |
| 用法、用量<br>Dosage | 　　除用于恶臭不洁的创面外，尤适用于厌氧菌感染以及破损伤口、气性坏疽的创面，用 3% 溶液冲洗或湿敷，根据情况每日多次使用。<br>　　The stench and dirty wounds besides, it is especially for anaerobic infections and damage wounds and wounds by gas gangrene. wash or wet it with a 3% solution and use it for several times a day depending on the circumstances. |
| 剂型、规格<br>Preparations | 　　本品为过氧化氢的 3% 水溶液。<br>　　This product is a 3% hydrogen peroxide solution. |
| 药品名称 Drug Names | 呋喃西林 Nitrofural（Furacillin） |
| 适应证<br>Indications | 　　有广谱抗菌活性，但对假单胞菌属疗效甚微，对真菌和病毒无效。表面消毒用 0.001%～0.01% 水溶液，冲洗、湿敷患处，冲洗腔道或用于滴耳、滴鼻。<br>　　Broad-spectrum antibacterial activity, but less effective on Pseudomonas treatment and ineffective on fungi and viruses. When sterilizing on the surface, the 0.001% to 0.01% aqueous solution should be made up to rinse, put a wet compress round the wound, flush the cavitary mucosal or ear dropping and nasal dripping. |
| 用法、用量<br>Dosage | （1）对本品过敏者禁用。<br>（2）口服毒性较大，目前仅供外用。<br>(1) Allergic to the chemicals were banned.<br>(2) Oral medication has abundant toxicity, currently only for external use. |
| 剂型、规格<br>Preparations | 0.02% 溶液；0.2% 溶液。<br>0.02% solution; 0.2% solution. |
| 药品名称 Drug Names | 苯扎溴铵 Benzalkonium Bromide |
| 适应证<br>Indications | 　　阳离子活性的广谱杀菌剂，杀菌力强，对皮肤和局部组织无刺激性，对金属、橡胶制品无腐蚀作用。1∶1000～1∶2000 溶液广泛用于手、皮肤、黏膜、器械等的消毒。可长期保存效力不减。<br>　　Broad-spectrum fungicide of active Cationic type, strong bactericidal ability, no irritation to skin and local tissue and non-corrosion to metal and rubber. It is widely made up by a proportion of 1∶1000－1∶2000 to disinfect hands, skin, mucous membranes, equipment and the like with long-term effectiveness. |
| 用法、用量<br>Dosage | （1）不可与普通肥皂配伍。<br>（2）泡器械加 0.5% 亚硝酸钠。<br>（3）不适用于膀胱镜、眼科器械、橡胶、铝制品及排泄物消毒。<br>(1) It can not be compatible with ordinary soap.<br>(2) Foam the equipment plus 0.5% sodium nitrite.<br>(3) It does not apply to cystoscopy, ophthalmology equipment, rubber, aluminum and excreta disinfection. |
| 剂型、规格<br>Preparations | 1∶1000～1∶2000 溶液。<br>1:1000～1:2000 solution. |

**续 表**

### 19.3 皮肤科用药 Drugs for dermatology

| 药品名称 Drug Names | 莫匹罗星 Mupirocin |
|---|---|
| 适应证<br>Indications | 用于多种病菌引起的皮肤感染和湿疹、皮炎、糜烂、溃疡等继发性感染。有报道称，本品预防或治疗给药，对降低皮肤外科手术后伤口化脓十分有效。<br><br>For the treatment of a variety of skin infections caused by bacteria and eczema, dermatitis, erosions, ulcers and other secondary infections. It is reported to prevent and treat such diseases and is active against reducing post-surgical wounds festering. |
| 用法、用量<br>Dosage | 涂于患处，也可用敷料包扎或覆盖，一日 3 次，5 日为 1 个疗程。必要时可重复 1 个疗程。<br><br>Apply to affected area, dressing or coving three times a day, 5 days for a course of treatment. If necessary, repeat the treatment. |
| 剂型、规格<br>Preparations | 软膏：2%。<br>Ointment: 2%. |
| 药品名称 Drug Names | 夫西地酸 Fusidic acid |
| 适应证<br>Indications | 对与皮肤感染有关的革兰阳性球菌，尤其对葡萄球菌高度敏感，对耐药金葡菌也有效，对革兰阴性菌有一定作用。与其他抗生素无交叉耐药性。<br><br>Highly effective for Gram-positive cocci that results in skin infections, especially for Staphylococcus aureus. it is also effective against drug-resistant Staphylococcus aureus and Gram-negative bacteria . It is not cross-resistant with other antibiotics. |
| 用法、用量<br>Dosage | 涂于患处，并缓和摩擦。也可用敷料包扎，一日 2～3 次，7 日为 1 个疗程，必要时可重复 1 个疗程。<br><br>Apply to affected area and rubbing gently. Also available for dressing, 2 or 3 times a day, seven days for a course, repeat the treatment if necessary. |
| 剂型、规格<br>Preparations | 乳膏：2%。<br>Cream: 2%. |
| 药品名称 Drug Names | 环吡酮胺 Ciclopirox Olamine |
| 适应证<br>Indications | 外用于治疗各种皮肤浅表或黏膜的癣菌病。<br><br>for the treatment of ringworm on superficial skin or mucous membranes, which is used for external application. |
| 用法、用量<br>Dosage | 涂患处，一日 2 次，甲癣，先用温水泡软灰指甲，再削薄病甲，涂药包扎。疗程一般 1～4 周（甲癣 13 周）。阴道栓用于治疗阴道念珠菌感染。<br><br>Coating the affected area, 2 times a day. For onychomycosis, soak the nail fungus with warm water till soft, then thinning disease nail, coating and dressing. Treatment course is usually for 1 to 4 weeks (onychomycosis treatment needs 13 weeks). Vaginal suppository is for the treatment of vaginal candidiasis. |
| 剂型、规格<br>Preparations | 溶液或乳膏：均为 1%。<br>阴道栓：每个含药 50mg 或 100mg。<br>栓剂：1%。<br>洗剂：1%。<br>Solution or cream: 1%.<br>Vaginal suppository: 50mg or 100mg per drug.<br>Suppository: 1%.<br>lotion: 1%. |
| 药品名称 Drug Names | 联苯苄唑 Bifonazole |
| 适应证<br>Indications | 用于体癣、股癣、手足癣、花斑癣、红癣及皮肤念球菌病等表浅皮肤真菌感染及短小杆状菌引起的皮肤念球菌性外阴道炎。<br><br>For the treatment of Body ringworm, jock itch, tinea manus and pedis, tinea versicolor, erythrasma and superficial fungal infections caused by cutaneous moniliasis and candida vulvitis caused by short rod-shaped bacteria. |

**续　表**

| 用法、用量<br>Dosage | 涂患处，一日 1 次，2～4 周为 1 个疗程。阴道给药，于睡前将阴道片放入阴道深处，一日 1 次，一次 1 片。 |
| --- | --- |
| | Coating the wound, once per day, 2 to 4 weeks is a course of treatment. For Vaginal delivery, put the tablet into deep vagina at bedtime, once per day, 1 table singly. |
| 剂型、规格<br>Preparations | 溶液：1%。<br>乳膏：1%。<br>凝胶：1%。<br>阴道片：每片 100mg。<br>Solution: 1%.<br>Cream: 1%.<br>Gel: 1%.<br>Vaginal tablets: 100mg per tablet. |
| 药品名称 Drug Names | 酞丁安 Ftibamzone |
| 适应证<br>Indications | 用于带状疱疹、单纯疱疹、尖锐湿疣、浅部真菌感染及各型沙眼等。 |
| | For the treatment of herpes zoster, herpes simplex, genital warts, and the type of superficial fungal infections and trachoma of all types. |
| 用法、用量<br>Dosage | 涂患处，一日 2～3 次，体癣、股癣连用 3 周，手足癣连用 4 周；滴眼，一次 1～2 滴，一日 3～4 次，连用 4 周。 |
| | Coating the wound, 2 or 3 times a day, for body ringworm and jock itch needs three weeks, tineamanusandpedis needs four weeks; when dripping eyes, 1 to 2 drops singly, 3-4 times a day four consecutive weeks. |
| 剂型、规格<br>Preparations | 软膏或乳膏：1%。<br>搽剂：0.5%（5ml）。<br>滴眼液：0.1%。<br>Ointment or cream: 1%.<br>Liniment: 0.5% (5ml).<br>Eye Drops: 0.1%. |
| 药品名称 Drug Names | 克罗米通 Crotamiton |
| 适应证<br>Indications | 用于治疗疥疮、皮肤瘙痒及继发性皮肤感染。 |
| | For the treatment of scabies, skin itching and secondary skin infections. |
| 用法、用量<br>Dosage | （1）疥疮：治疗前应洗澡并擦干，将本品从颈部以下涂搽全身皮肤，特别应涂搽在手足、指（趾）间、腋下和腹股沟；24 小时后涂第 2 次，再隔 48 小时洗澡将药洗去，更换干净衣服和床单。必要时，1 周后重复 1 次；也可一日涂搽 1 次，连续 5～10 日。<br>（2）瘙痒症：局部涂于患处，一日 3 次。<br>（3）脓性皮肤病：将患处用浸渍本品的敷料覆盖。 |
| | (1) Scabies: bathe and dry before treatment.Use the cream to smear body skin form the neck down, the hand, foot, finger toes, armpits and groin specifically; 24 hours later for the second time, bathe to remove the drug after 48 hours, exchange clean clothes and bed sheet. If necessary, repeat once 1 week later; once per week for 5 to 10 days consecutively.<br>(2) for Pruritus: topically applied to the affected area three times a day.<br>(3) Purulent skin disease: The affected area is covered with dressings impregnated with this product. |
| 剂型、规格<br>Preparations | 片剂：每片 10mg；20mg。<br>乳膏或软膏：0.025%；0.05%；0.1%。<br>凝胶剂：0.05%。<br>乙醇溶液：0.05～0.1%。<br>Tablets: 10mg; 20mg per tablet.<br>Cream or ointment: 0.025%; 0.05%; 0.1%.<br>Gel: 0.05%.<br>Ethanol: 0.05 to 0.1%. |

| 药品名称 Drug Names | 维 A 酸 Tretinoin |
|---|---|
| 适应证<br>Indications | 适用于寻常痤疮、扁平苔藓、白斑、毛发红糠疹和面部单纯糠疹。还用作银屑病的辅助治疗，亦用于治疗多发性寻常疣及角化异常类的各种皮肤病如鱼鳞病、毛囊角化异常。<br>For the treatment of acne vulgaris, lichen planus, vitiligo, pityriasis rubra pilaris and facial Pityriasis simplex. Also used as adjuvant treatment of psoriasis, multiple skin warts and skin diseases with abnormal keratinization, such as ichthyosis, abnormal follicular keratosis. |
| 用法、用量<br>Dosage | 口服：一日 2～3 次，一次 10mg。外用 0.025% 乳膏或软膏治疗痤疮、单纯面部糠疹；0.1% 乳膏或软膏治疗扁平苔藓、毛发红糠疹、白斑等皮肤病，一日涂药 2 次，或遵医嘱。<br>Oral medication: 10mg singly, 2 or 3 times a day. 0.025% cream or ointment for external use for the treatment of acne, a simple facial rosea; 0.1% cream or ointment for the treatment of lichen planus, pityriasis rubra pilaris, vitiligo and other skin diseases, 2 times each day, or as directed. |
| 剂型、规格<br>Preparations | 片剂：每片 10mg；20mg。软膏或乳膏：0.025%；0.05%；0.1%。凝胶：0.05%。乙醇溶液：0.05%～0.1%。<br>Tablets: 10mg/20mg per tablet. Ointment or cream: 0.025%; 0.05%; 0.1%. Gel: 0.05%. Ethanol: 0.05% to 0.1%. |

| 药品名称 Drug Names | 异维 A 酸 Isotretinoin |
|---|---|
| 适应证<br>Indications | 用于其他药物治疗无效的严重痤疮，尤其是囊肿性痤疮及聚合性痤疮。<br>severe acne incurable by other medication, especially for cystic acne and acne conglobata. |
| 用法、用量<br>Dosage | 口服：开始量为每日 0.5mg/kg，4 周后改用维持量，按每日 0.1～1mg/kg 计，视患者耐受性决定，但最高每日不超过 1mg/kg。饭间或饭后服用，用量大时分次服用，一般 16 周为 1 个疗程。如需要，停药 8 周后再进行下 1 个疗程。局部外用：取适量涂于患处，每晚睡前涂一次。<br>Oral medication: the initial dose is 0.5mg/kg a day, 4 weeks later to switch to the maintenance dose--0.1～1mg/kg per day. The dose depends on patient tolerance, but does not exceed the maximum of 1mg/kg a day. Taking at the meal or after a meal. Larger dose should be in divided doses. 16 weeks is a treatment course. If necessary, withdrawal for eight weeks before the next course. Topical and external use: Applies onto the affected area, once painted every night before bed. |
| 剂型、规格<br>Preparations | 胶丸：每粒 5mg；10mg。凝胶：0.05%。<br>Capsules: 5mg/10mg per capsule;. Gel: 0.05%. |

| 药品名称 Drug Names | 糠酸莫米松 Mometasone Furoate |
|---|---|
| 适应证<br>Indications | 用于缓解对皮质激素有效的湿疹、接触性皮炎、特应性皮炎。神经性皮炎及皮肤瘙痒症等。<br>Used to treat skin disease curable by corticoid, such as eczema, contact dermatitis, atopic dermatitis. Neurodermatitis and itchy skin disorders. |
| 用法、用量<br>Dosage | 涂患处，一日 1 次，不应封闭敷裹。<br>coating the wound, once per day, no blocking or dressing. |
| 剂型、规格<br>Preparations | 乳膏或软膏：0.1%。<br>Cream or ointment: 0.1%. |

19.4 眼科用药 Drugs for ophthalmology

| 药品名称 Drug Names | 吡诺克辛 Pirenoxine |
|---|---|
| 适应证<br>Indications | 用于老年性白内障、外伤性白内障、轻度糖尿病性白内障、并发性白内障和先天性白内障。<br>For the treatment of senile cataract, traumatic cataract, mild diabetic cataract, complicated cataract and congenital cataracts. |
| 用法、用量<br>Dosage | 滴眼，用前摇匀，一日 3～5 次，一次 1～2 滴。<br>Eye Drops, shake well before use, 3 to 5 times a day, 1 to 2 drops singly. |

**续　表**

| 剂型、规格<br>Preparations | 滴眼液：含药片 7.5mg，溶剂 15ml 溶解药片后，浓度为 0.005%。<br>Eye Drops: 7.5mg tablets, 15ml of solvent, a concentration of 0.005% after dissolution. |
|---|---|
| **药品名称 Drug Names** | **布林佐胺 Brinzolamide** |
| 适应证<br>Indications | 用于治疗原发性及继发性开角型青光眼和高眼压症。也可用于防止激光手术后的眼压升高。<br>For the treatment of primary and secondary open-angle glaucoma and ocular hypertension. For the prevention of intraocular pressure increase after laser surgery. |
| 用法、用量<br>Dosage | 用前摇匀，滴眼，一日 2 ~ 3 次，一次 1 滴，滴于结膜囊内，滴后用手指压迫眦泪囊部 3 ~ 5 分钟。<br>Shake well before use, eye drops, 2 ~ 3 times a day, one drip singly, drip inside the conjunctiva, put pressure on the lacrimal sac canthus with finger for 3 to 5 minutes. |
| 剂型、规格<br>Preparations | 滴眼液：每支 1%（5ml）。<br>Eye Drops: 1% (5ml) per bottle. |
| **药品名称 Drug Names** | **拉坦前列腺素 Latanoprost** |
| 适应证<br>Indications | 用于治疗青光眼、高眼压症和其他各种眼压升高。<br>For the treatment of glaucoma, ocular hypertension and other intraocular pressure increase. |
| 用法、用量<br>Dosage | 滴眼，一日一次，一次 1 滴，最好在睡前用。<br>Eye Drops, once a day, one drop singly, it is best to use at bedtime. |
| 剂型、规格<br>Preparations | 滴眼液：每支 125μg（2.5ml）。<br>Eye Drops: 125μg (2.5ml) per bottle. |
| **药品名称 Drug Names** | **托吡卡胺 Tropicamide** |
| 适应证<br>Indications | 用于散瞳检查眼底和散瞳验光。<br>For dilated fundus examination and dilated optometry. |
| 用法、用量<br>Dosage | 滴眼，一次 1 滴，间隔 5 分钟滴第二次，即可满足散瞳检查之需。<br>Eye Drops, one drip singly, an interval of five minutes before the second time for dilating eyes and examination. |
| 剂型、规格<br>Preparations | 滴眼液：每支 0.25%（6ml）；0.5%（6ml）；1%（8ml）。<br>Eye Drops: 0.25% (6ml) / 0.5% (6ml) / 1% (8ml) per bottle. |
| **药品名称 Drug Names** | **玻璃酸钠 Sodium Hyaluronate** |
| 适应证<br>Indications | 滴眼用于防治干眼症、眼疲劳、斯 - 约综合征等内因性疾病和术后药物性、外伤、光线对眼造成的刺激及戴软性接触镜引起的外因性疾病。眼科手术用其注射液。<br>For the prevention and treatment of dry eye drops, eye fatigue, Steven-Johnson syndrome and other internal diseases, eye irritation by post-surgery drug, trauma and light, extrinsic disease by soft contact lens. When used in eye surgery, the injection-type is needed. |
| 用法、用量<br>Dosage | 前房内注射，一次 0.5 ~ 0.75ml。滴眼，一日 4 ~ 6 次，一次 1 ~ 2 滴。<br>Anterior chamber injection, 0.5 ~ 0.75ml singly. Eye Drops, 4 to 6 times per day, 1 to 2 drops singly. |
| 剂型、规格<br>Preparations | 注射液：每支 5mg（0.5ml）。滴眼液：每支 0.1%（5ml）。<br>Injection: 5mg (0.5ml) per vial. Eye Drops: 0.1% (5ml) . |
| 19.5　耳鼻喉科和口腔科用药 Drugs for otolaryngology and dental |  |
| **药品名称 Drug Names** | **羟甲唑啉 Oxymetazoline** |
| 适应证<br>Indications | 用于急性鼻炎、慢性单纯性鼻炎、慢性肥厚型鼻炎、变态反应性鼻炎（过敏性鼻炎）、鼻息肉、航空性鼻炎、航空性中耳炎、鼻出血、鼻阻塞性打喷嚏或其他鼻阻塞性疾病。<br>For the treatment of acute rhinitis, chronic simple rhinitis, chronic hypertrophic rhinitis, allergic rhinitis (allergic rhinitis), nasal polyps, rhinitis aviation, aviation otitis media, nasal bleeding, sneezing, nasal obstructive disorders or other nasal obstruction . |

**续　表**

| 用法、用量<br>Dosage | 每揿定量为 0.065ml。将 1/4 喷头伸入鼻孔内，揿压喷鼻。成人和 6 岁以上儿童，一次一侧 1 ~ 3 喷，早晨和睡前各一次；或滴鼻，一日 2 ~ 3 次，一次 1 ~ 2 滴。若需长期用药，可采用连续用药 7 日停药一段时间再用药的间歇用药方式。<br><br>0.065ml per press quantitative. put 1/4 nozzle insert into the nostril and press the nasal spray. For adults and children of 6 years of age and plus, once sprayed side 1 ~ 3 sprays for each side singly in the morning and before going to bed; intranasal dripping, 2 or 3 times a day, 1 to 2 drops singly. For long-term medication, it can be used continuously for seven days in a drug withdrawal period of intermittent mode of administration. |
|---|---|
| 剂型、规格<br>Preparations | 滴鼻剂：每支 1.5mg（3ml）；2.5mg（5ml）；5mg（10ml）。<br>喷雾剂：每支 2.5mg（5ml）；5mg（10ml）。<br>Nasal drop: 1.5mg(3ml) /2.5mg (5ml)/5mg (10ml) per vial;<br>Spray: 2.5mg (5ml) / 5mg (10ml) per vial. |
| 药品名称 Drug Names | 西地碘 Cydiodine |
| 适应证<br>Indications | 用于治疗慢性咽喉炎、白念珠菌性口炎、口腔溃疡、慢性牙龈炎及糜烂扁平苔藓等。<br>For the treatment of chronic pharyngitis, Candida albicans stomatitis, mouth ulcers, chronic gingivitis and anabrosis lichen planus, etc. |
| 用法、用量<br>Dosage | 含化，一次 1.5mg，一日 3 ~ 5 次。<br>(Sublingual). 1.5mg singly, 3 to 5 times per day. |
| 剂型、规格<br>Preparations | 含片：每片 1.5mg。<br>Tablets: 1.5mg per tablet. |
| 药品名称 Drug Names | 氯霉素滴耳液 Chloramphenicol Auristillae |
| 适应证<br>Indications | 用于外耳炎、中耳炎。<br>For otitis externa, otitis media. |
| 用法、用量<br>Dosage | 滴耳，一日 3 次。宜遮光保存。<br>Ear drops, 3 times a day. Keep away from sunlight. |
| 剂型、规格<br>Preparations | 氯霉素 2g，乙醇 16ml，甘油加至 100ml。<br>Chloramphenicol 2g, ethanol 16ml, glycerol was added when the amount reaches 100ml. |
| 药品名称 Drug Names | 氧氟沙星滴耳液 Ofloxacin Auristillae |
| 适应证<br>Indications | 用于化脓性中耳炎。<br>For suppurative otitis media. |
| 用法、用量<br>Dosage | 耳浴，一日 1 ~ 2 次。<br>Ear bath, 1 to 2 times a day. |
| 剂型、规格<br>Preparations | 氧氟沙星 0.3g，醋酸适量，甘油 20ml，乙醇（70%）加至 100ml。<br>Ofloxacin 0.3g, proper acetic acid, glycerol 20ml, ethanol (70%) was added when the amount reaches 100ml. |
| 药品名称 Drug Names | 酚甘油 Phenol glycerol Auristillae |
| 适应证<br>Indications | 有消炎杀菌及镇痛作用，用于急性及慢性中耳炎及外耳道炎。<br>Anti-inflammatory and analgesic for acute and chronic otitis media and otitis externa. |
| 用法、用量<br>Dosage | 滴耳，一日 3 次。<br>Ear drops, 3 times a day. |
| 剂型、规格<br>Preparations | 酚 2g，甘油加至 100ml。<br>Phenol 2g, glycerol was added when the amount reaches 100ml. |
| 药品名称 Drug Names | 硼酸滴耳液 Boric acid Auristillae |
| 适应证<br>Indications | 用于慢性化脓性中耳炎。<br>For chronic suppurative otitis media. |

**续　表**

| | |
|---|---|
| 用法、用量<br>Dosage | 滴耳，一日 3 次。<br>Ear drops, 3 times a day. |
| 剂型、规格<br>Preparations | 硼酸 2 ~ 3g，乙醇（70%）加至 100ml。<br>Acid 2 ~ 3g, ethanol (70%) was added when the amount reaches 100ml. |
| **药品名称 Drug Names** | 碳酸氢钠滴耳液（耵聍液）Sodium bicarbonate Auristillae （Earwax solution） |
| 适应证<br>Indications | 软化耵聍（耳垢）及冲洗耳道。<br>Softening cerumen (earwax) and flushing the ear canal. |
| 用法、用量<br>Dosage | 滴耳，一日 3 次。每次用量要大，应将药液充满耳内。<br>Ear drops, 3 times a day. the single dose should be larger and should be filled with the liquid inside the ear. |
| 剂型、规格<br>Preparations | 碳酸氢钠 5g，甘油 30ml，蒸馏水加至 100ml。<br>Sodium hydrogen carbonate 5g, Glycerol 30ml, distilled water was added when the amount reaches 100ml. |
| **药品名称 Drug Names** | 碘甘油 Iodine Glycerin |
| 适应证<br>Indications | 有防腐消毒作用，用于咽部慢性炎症及角化症，也可用于慢性萎缩性鼻炎。<br>Antiseptic and disinfectant for chronic throat inflammation and keratosis and chronic atrophic rhinitis. |
| 用法、用量<br>Dosage | 涂患处，一日 2 ~ 3 次。<br>smearing the affected area, 2 or 3 times a day. |
| 剂型、规格<br>Preparations | 碘 2g，碘化钾 1g，甘油加至 100ml。<br>Iodine 2g, potassium 1g, glycerol was added when the amount reaches 100ml. |
| **药品名称 Drug Names** | 呋麻滴鼻液 Furacilin/ Ephedrine Naristillae |
| 适应证<br>Indications | 用于鼻炎或鼻黏膜肿胀。<br>For the treatment of rhinitis or nasal swelling. |
| 用法、用量<br>Dosage | 滴鼻，一日 3 次，遮光保存。<br>Intranasally, three times a day, Keep away from sunlight. |
| 剂型、规格<br>Preparations | 盐酸麻黄碱 10g，羟苯乙酯 0.3g，0.01% 呋喃西林溶液加至 1000ml。<br>Ephedrine hydrochloride 10g, Ethylparaben 0.3g, 0.01% nitrofurazone solution was added when the amount reaches 1000ml. |
| **药品名称 Drug Names** | 复方薄荷滴鼻液 Compound Mint Naristillae |
| 适应证<br>Indications | 用于干燥性鼻炎、萎缩性鼻炎、鼻出血，有除臭及滋养黏膜的作用。<br>It is deodorant and nourishing to mucosa for rhinitis sicca, atrophic rhinitis, atrophic rhinitis and epistaxis. |
| 用法、用量<br>Dosage | 滴鼻或涂鼻。<br>Intranasally or smearing nose. |
| 剂型、规格<br>Preparations | 薄荷脑 1g，樟脑 1g，液状石蜡加至 100ml。<br>Menthol 1g, camphor 1g, liquid paraffin was added when the amount reaches 100ml. |
| **药品名称 Drug Names** | 盐酸麻黄碱滴鼻液 Ephedrine Hydrochloride Naristillae |
| 适应证<br>Indications | 有收缩血管作用，用于急性鼻炎、鼻窦炎、慢性肥大性鼻炎。<br>It can contract the blood vessels to treat acute rhinitis, sinusitis, chronic hypertrophic rhinitis. |
| 用法、用量<br>Dosage | 滴鼻，一日 3 次。<br>Intranasally, three times a day. |

| 剂型、规格<br>Preparations | 盐酸麻黄碱 10g，氯化钠 0.6g，羟苯乙酯 0.03g，蒸馏水加至 1000ml。<br>Ephedrine hydrochloride 10g, sodium chloride 0.6g, Ethylparaben 0.03g, distilled water was added when the amount reaches 100ml. |
|---|---|
| 药品名称 Drug Names | 复方硼砂片（漱口）Compound borax tablet（for Gargle） |
| 适应证<br>Indications | 用于口腔炎、咽喉炎及扁桃体炎等。<br>For the treatment of stomatitis, pharyngitis and tonsillitis. |
| 用法、用量<br>Dosage | 一片加温开水一杯（60～90ml）溶后含漱，一日数次。<br>One tablet with a cup of warm water (60~90ml) to gargle, several times a day. |
| 剂型、规格<br>Preparations | 每片含：硼砂 0.324g，碳酸氢钠 0.162g，氯化钠 0.162g，麝香草酚 0.003 2g。<br>per tablet contains: borax 0.324g, sodium bicarbonate 0.162g, sodium chloride 0.162g, thymol 0.003 2g. |

## 20. 其他类药物 Other drugs

### 20.1 妇产科外用药 Drug for Gynaecology(for external use)

| 药品名称 Drug Names | 硝呋太尔制霉素（阴道用）Nifuratel/Nysfungin（Used in the vagina） |
|---|---|
| 适应证<br>Indications | 硝呋太尔制霉素在体外具有抗真菌、抗滴虫、抗细菌的广谱活性。用于细菌性阴道病、滴虫阴道炎、念珠菌性外阴阴道炎、阴道混合感染。<br>In vitro, it is anti-fungal, anti-trichomoniasis and anti-bacterial. It is active agaaingst bacterial vaginosis, trichomoniasis vaginitis, vulvovaginal candidiasis and vaginal mixed infections. |
| 用法、用量<br>Dosage | 阴道给药，每晚一粒，连用 6 日。亦可遵医嘱调整。<br>Vaginal delivery, one table a night for six consecutive days. Also available as doctor's directions. |
| 剂型、规格<br>Preparations | 每粒含硝呋太尔 0.5g，制霉素 20 万 U。<br>0.5g Nifuratel and 200, 000 units of nystatin per capsule. |

### 20.2 解毒药 Alexipharmacons

| 药品名称 Drug Names | 谷胱甘肽 Glutathione |
|---|---|
| 适应证<br>Indications | 临床上用于①解毒：对丙烯腈、氟化物、一氧化碳、重金属及有机溶剂等的中毒均有解毒作用。对红细胞膜有保护作用，故防止溶血，从而减少高铁血红蛋白。②对某些损伤的保护作用：由于放射线治疗、放射性药物或由于使用肿瘤药物所引起白细胞减少症以及由于放射线引起的骨髓组织炎症，本品均可改善其症状。③保护肝脏：能抑制脂肪肝的形成，也能改善中毒性肝炎和感染性肝炎的症状。④抗过敏：能纠正乙酰胆碱、胆碱酯酶的不平衡，从而消除由于 这种不平衡所引起的过敏症状。⑤改善某些疾病的症状：对缺氧血症的不适、恶心、呕吐、瘙痒等症状以及由于肝脏疾病引起的其他症状，均有改善作用。⑥防止皮肤色素沉着：可防止新的黑色素形成并减少其氧化。⑦眼科疾病：可抑制晶体蛋白质巯基的不稳定，因而可以抑制进行性白内障及控制角膜及视网膜疾病的发展等。<br><br>Clinically : ① for the detoxification of acrylonitrile poisoning, fluoride, carbon monoxide, heavy metals and organic solvents. For the protection of Red cell membrane from hemolysis, thereby reducing methemoglobin . ② for the protection from some damage and improvement of symptoms: leukopenia, caused by radiation therapy, radioactive drugs or cancer drugs and radiation-induced bone myelosis inflammation, this product can improve their symptoms. ③ to protect the liver :it can inhibit the development of fatty liver and improve the symptoms of toxic hepatitis and infectious hepatitis. ④ Antiallergy : to correct the imbalance between acetylcholine esterase, thereby eliminating allergy caused by this imbalance . ⑤ improve the symptoms of certain diseases : discomfort, nausea, vomiting, itching, and other symptoms caused by hypoxia and ischemia and other symptoms caused by liver disease ⑥ To prevent skin pigmentation : to prevent the formation of new melanin and reduce oxidation . ⑦ Eye diseases: for the suppression of unstable crystal protein sulfhydryl groups, thus controlling the Deterioration of cataract and corneal and retinal disease and the like . |

**续　表**

| 用法、用量<br>Dosage | 肌内或静脉注射，将本品注射剂用所附的 2ml 维生素 C 注射液溶解后使用。肝脏患者一般 30 日为 1 个疗程，其他情况根据病情决定。滴眼，一次 1～2 滴，一日 4～8 次。<br>Intramuscular or intravenous injection, the use of this product after injection with vitamin C attached 2ml injection dissolved. Liver patients are generally 30 days for a course, other cases decided according to the disease. Drops, 1 to 2 drops singly, 4～8 times a day. |
|---|---|
| 剂型、规格<br>Preparations | 注射剂：每支 300mg；600mg。<br>Injection: 300mg; 600mg per vial. |
| **药品名称 Drug Names** | **二巯丙醇 Dimercaprol** |
| 适应证<br>Indications | 对砷、汞及金的中毒有解救作用，但治疗慢性汞中毒效果差。对锑中毒的作用因锑化合物的不同而异，它能够减轻酒石酸锑钾的毒性而能增加锑波芬与新斯锑波散等的毒性。能减轻镉对肺的损害，故使用时要注意掌握。它还能减轻发泡性砷化合物战争毒气所引起的损害。<br>For the treatment of Arsenic, mercury and gold poisoning, but poor performance for chronic mercury poisoning. The effect on treating antimony poisoning varies according to the amount of antimony compounds, which reduces the toxicity of antimony potassium tartrate and increases the toxicity of stibophen. It is able to reduce lung damage caused by Cadmium, so pay attention to the amount. It can also reduce the damage caused by toxic arsenic compounds war foaming. |
| 用法、用量<br>Dosage | 成人，肌内注射，按体重 2～3mg/kg，最初 2 日，每 4 小时注射 1 次。第 3 日，每 6 小时注射 1 次，以后每 12 小时注射 1 次，一个疗程为 10 日。小儿用量同成人。治疗小儿铅脑病，与依地酸钙钠同用。<br>For adults, intramuscular injection, 2～3mg/kg measured by weight, the first 2 days, one injection every 4 hours. In the third day, one injection every six hours, later one injection every 12 hours, a course of 10 days. The amount for children is the same as that for adults. For the Treatment of children with lead encephalopathy, used with EDTA. |
| 剂型、规格<br>Preparations | 注射液：每支 0.1g/1ml，0.2g/ml。<br>Injection: 0.1g/1ml, 0.2g/ml per vial. |
| **药品名称 Drug Names** | **二巯丁二钠 Sodium Dimercaptosuccinate** |
| 适应证<br>Indications | 用于治疗锑、铅、汞、砷、铜的中毒（治疗汞中毒的效果不如二巯丙磺钠）及预防镉、钴、镍中毒，对肝豆状核变性病有驱铜及减轻症状的作用。<br>For the treatment of antimony, lead, mercury, arsenic and copper poisoning (The treatment effect on mercury poisoning is not as good as DMPS), the prevention of cadmium, cobalt and nickel poisoning and copper removing and alleviation of Hepatolenticular degeneration. |
| 用法、用量<br>Dosage | （1）成人解毒：1g，临用时配成 10% 溶液，立即缓慢静脉注射，10～15 分钟注射完毕。<br>（2）急性锑中毒引起的心律失常：本品首次剂量为 2g，用 5% 葡萄糖液 20ml 溶解后，静脉缓慢注射。以后每小时 1g，共 4～5 次。用于亚急性金属中毒：每次 1g，每日 2～3 次，共用 3～5 日。用于慢性中毒，每日 1g，共 5～7 日，或每日 1g，连续 3 日，停药 4 日为 1 个疗程，按病情可用 2～4 个疗程。<br>（3）小儿常用量：按体重 20mg/kg。<br>(1) for adult detoxification: 1g to make up a 10% temporary solution for immediate slow intravenous injection, completed within 10 to 15 minutes. (2) cardiac arrhythmia caused by acute Antimony poisoning : the first dose is 2g, dissolved in 20ml 5% glucose solution, slow intravenous injection. later using 1g per hour in 4 to 5 divided doses. For sub-acute metal poisoning: 1g singly, 2 to 3 times a day for 3 to 5 days. For chronic poisoning, 1g a day, 5 to 7 days, or 1g a day for 3 consecutive days and then stop for 4 days as a course, 2 to 4 courses is preferred according to the condition. (3) the common dose for children: 20mg/kg measured by weight. |
| 剂型、规格<br>Preparations | 注射剂：每支 0.5g；1g。<br>Injection: 0.5g ; 1g per vial. |

**续表**

| | |
|---|---|
| 药品名称 Drug Names | 去铁胺 Deferoxamine |
| 适应证<br>Indications | 　　本品主要用于急性铁中毒和海洋性贫血、铁粒幼细胞贫血、溶血性贫血、再生障碍性贫血或其他慢性贫血，因反复输血引起的继发性含铁血黄素沉着症；亦用于特发性血色病有放血禁忌证者。对慢性肾衰竭伴有铝过量负荷引起的脑病、骨病和贫血，在进行透析过程中亦可应用。本品还可用作铁负荷试验。<br><br>　　For the treatment of acute iron poisoning and thalassemia, sideroblastic anemia, hemolytic anemia, aplastic anemia or other chronic anemia, secondary hemosiderosis disease caused by repeated blood transfusions; idiopathic hemochromatosis with contraindications to Bloodletting. It is available for encephalopathy, bone disease and anemia caused by chronic renal failure with excessive aluminum and so it is available during dialysis. This product is also used iron load test. |
| 用法、用量<br>Dosage | 　　(1) 成人：①急性铁中毒：肌内注射，首次 0.5～1g，隔 4 小时 0.5g，共 2 次，以后根据病情 4～12 小时 1 次，24 小时总量不超过 6g。静脉滴注，一次 0.5g，加入 5%～10% 葡萄糖注射液 50～500ml 中滴注，滴注速度，按体重 1 小时不超过 15mg/kg，24 小时总量不超过 90mg/kg。②慢性铁负荷过量，肌内注射，一日 0.5～1g。腹壁皮下注射，按体重 20～40mg/kg，8～24 小时，以微型泵作动力。<br><br>　　(2) 小儿：①急性铁中毒：按体重一次 20mg/kg。②慢性铁负荷过量，按体重一日 10mg/kg，腹壁皮下注射，8～12 小时或 24 小时，用微型泵作动力。③慢性肾衰伴铁负荷过量：按体重 20mg/kg，一周 1～2 次，在透析初 2 小时通过动脉导管滴注，一周总量一般不超过 6g。铁负荷试验：成人肌内注射本品 0.5g。注射前，排空膀胱内剩余尿，注射后留 6 小时尿。尿铁超过 1mg，提示有过量铁负荷；超过 1.5mg，对机体可引起病理性损害。<br><br>　　(1) for adults: ① acute iron poisoning: intramuscular injection, for the first time, 0.5～1g singly, 0.5g every four hours for a total of 2 times and once every 4 to 12 hours according to the disease condition. However, the total dosage couldn't exceed 6g within 24 hours. Intravenously, 0.5g singly, adding 5% to 10% glucose injection into 50～500ml for infusion, infusion rate could not exceed 15mg/kg measured by weight and the total dosage couldn't exceed 90mg/kg within 24 hours measured by weight. ② chronic iron overload, intramuscular injection, 0.5～1g a day. Abdominal subcutaneous, 20～40mg/kg measured by weight for 8～24 hours powered by the micropump.<br><br>　　(2) for Children: ① acute iron poisoning: 20mg/kg singly measured by body weight. ② chronic iron overload, 10mg/kg a day measured by weight, abdominal subcutaneous injection for 8 to 12 hours or 24 hours, using a micro-powered pump. ③ iron overloaded chronic renal failure: 20mg/kg measured by body weight, 1 or 2 times per week. At the first 2 hours of dialysis, infusing through through artery catheter, the total amount is not more than 6g within a week. Iron overload test: for Adults, intramuscular injection by 0.5g. Before injection, emptying residual urine of the bladder, and leaving urine for six hours after injection. If Urinary iron exceeds 1mg, it is a signal of an excess of iron overload; when exceeding 1.5mg, there will be pathological damages. |
| 剂型、规格<br>Preparations | 注射剂：0.5g。<br>Injection: 0.5g. |
| 药品名称 Drug Names | 碘解磷定 Pralidoxime Iodide |
| 适应证<br>Indications | 有机磷中毒。<br>For the treatment of organophosphate poisoning. |
| 用法、用量<br>Dosage | 　　(1) 治疗轻度中毒：成人每次 0.4～0.8g，以葡萄糖液或生理盐水稀释后静脉滴注或缓慢静脉注射，必要时 2～4 小时重复一次。小儿 1 次 15mg/kg。<br><br>　　(2) 治疗中度中毒：成人首次 0.8～1.6g，缓慢静注，以后每 1 小时重复 0.4～0.8g，肌颤缓解和血液胆碱酯酶活性恢复至正常的 60% 以上后酌情减量或停药。或以静脉滴注给药维持，每小时给 0.4g，共 4～6 次。小儿 1 次 20～30mg/kg。<br><br>　　(3) 治疗重度中毒：成人首次用 1.6～2.4g，缓慢静脉注射，以后每小时重复 0.8～1.6g，肌颤缓解和血液胆碱酯酶活性恢复至正常以后的 60% 以上后酌情减量或停药。小儿 1 次 30mg/kg。<br><br>　　(1) for The treatment of mild poisoning: for Adults, 0.4～0.8g / time, diluting with glucose solution or saline infusion or slow intravenous injection, repeat every 2 to 4 hours if necessary. For Children, 15mg/kg singly. |

|  | (2) for The treatment of moderate poisoning: for adults, the first time is 0.8 ~ 1.6g, slow intravenous injection, every one hour after repeated 0.4 ~ 0.8g, When twitch disappears or cholinesterase activity recovers to more than 60% of normal level, the dose could be adapted at discretion, reduction or withdrawal. Or by intravenous infusion to maintain, 0.4g per hour, a total of 4 to 6 times. For Children, 20 ~ 30mg/kg singly.<br><br>(3) for The treatment of severe poisoning : for adults, for the first time with 1.6 ~ 2.4g, slow intravenous injection, later administing repeatedly 0.8 ~ 1.6g hourly, When twitch disappears or cholinesterase activity recovers to more than 60% of normal level, the dose could be adapted at discretion, reduction or withdrawal. For Children 30mg/kg singly. |
|---|---|
| 剂型、规格<br>Preparations | 注射剂：每支 0.4g。<br>注射液 0.4g/10ml。<br>Injection: 0.4g per vial;<br>injection 0.4g/10ml. |
| 药品名称 Drug Names | 氯解磷定 Pralidoxime Chloride |
| 适应证<br>Indications | 有机磷中毒。<br>For the treatment of organophosphate poisoning. |
| 用法、用量<br>Dosage | （1）成人：①轻度中毒：0.5 ~ 0.75g 肌内注射，必要时 1 小时后重复一次。②中度中毒：首次 0.75 ~ 1.5g，肌内注射或稀释后缓慢静脉注射，以后每小时重复 0.5 ~ 1.0g，肌颤消失或胆碱酯酶活性恢复至正常的 60% 以上后酌情减量或停药。③重度中毒：成人首次用 1.5 ~ 2.5g 分两处肌内注射或稀释后缓慢静脉注射，以后每 0.5 ~ 1 小时重复 1.0 ~ 1.5g，肌颤消失或血液胆碱酯酶活性恢复至正常以后的 60% 以上后酌情减量或停药。<br><br>（2）小儿：用法与成人同，①轻度中毒：按体重 15 ~ 20mg/kg；②中度中毒：按体重 20 ~ 30mg/kg；③重度中毒：按体重 30mg/kg。<br><br>(1) for Adults: ① mild poisoning: 0.5 ~ 0.75g intramuscular injection,, repeat an hour later if necessary. ② moderate poisoning: the initial dosage is 0.75 ~ 1.5g, slow intravenous injection after intramuscular injection or dilution, later repeat with 0.5 ~ 1.0g per hour. When twitch disappears or cholinesterase activity recovers to more than 60% of normal level, the dose could be adapted at discretion, reduction or withdrawal. ③ for the treatment of severe poisoning: for Adults, for the first time, 1.5 ~ 2.5g intramuscular injection at two body positions or slow intravenous injection after diluting. Later, repeated 1.0 ~ 1.5g per 0.5 to 1 hour. When twitch disappears or cholinesterase activity recovers to more than 60% of normal level, the dose could be adapted at discretion, reduction or withdrawal.<br><br>(2) for Children: the Usage is the same as that for adults, ① mild poisoning: 15 ~ 20mg/kg measured by body weight; ② moderate poisoning: 20 ~ 30mg/kg measured by body weight; ③ severe poisoning: 30mg/kg measured by body weight. |
| 剂型、规格<br>Preparations | 注射液：0.5g/2ml。<br>Injection: 0.5g/2ml. |
| 药品名称 Drug Names | 阿托品 Atropine |
| 适应证<br>Indications | 做解毒药使用时：①治疗有机磷类（包括有机磷农药及军用神经性毒剂）与氨基甲酸酯类农药中毒。应与胆碱酯酶复活剂合用，单独使用效果差（除西维因中毒外）。②治疗胃肠型毒蕈（如捕蝇蕈）中毒。③治疗中药乌头中毒。④治疗锑剂中毒引起的心律失常与钙通道阻滞剂引起的心动过缓。<br><br>When used as antidotes: ① For the treatment of intoxication of organophosphate (including organophosphate pesticides and military nerve agents) and carbamate pesticide poisoning, and it should be used in combination with cholinesterase Resurrection agent, for the effect will be poor when used alone ( carbaryl poisoning not included). ② For the treatment of gastrointestinal-type muscarinic (eg Amanitaceae) poisoning. ③ For the treatment of herb poisoning. ④ For the treatment of arrhythmia caused by Antimonial intoxication and bradycardia caused by calcium channel blockers. |

**续 表**

| 用法、用量<br>Dosage | 静脉注射或静脉滴注。<br>（1）成人：①治疗有机磷中毒：首次，轻度中毒，2.0 ~ 4.0mg；中度中毒，4.0 ~ 10mg；重度中毒，10 ~ 20mg。重复用药剂量为其半数，重复的次数依病情而异，达到阿托品化后减量或改用维持量。②治疗氨基甲酸酯类农药中毒，根据病情给药，首次应给足量，用量范围为 0.5 ~ 3.0mg，经口严重中毒可用 5mg；如毒蕈碱症状未消失，可重复给 0.5 ~ 1mg，除经口严重中毒外，一般不需要达到阿托品化。③治疗锑剂中毒引起的阿 - 斯综合征，立即静脉注射 1.0 ~ 2.0mg，15 ~ 30 分钟后在注射 1mg。④治疗乌头中毒及钙拮抗剂过量，按消化系统用药的用量给药，一次 0.5 ~ 1mg，肌内注射，1 ~ 4 小时一次，至中毒症状缓解为止。<br>（2）小儿：用量可根据体重折算，用法与成人同。<br><br>Intravenous injection or intravenous drip. (1) for Adults: ① for the treatment of organophosphate poisoning: the first dose for mild poisoning is 2.0 ~ 4.0mg; moderate poisoning, 4.0 ~ 10mg; severe poisoning, 10 ~ 20mg. Repeated dose is half of the initial amount. repetition times varies by the condition and then reduce the dosage until post-atropinization or switch to the maintenance dosage. ② for the treatment of carbamate pesticide poisoning, administered by condition, the first dosage should be sufficient in the range of 0.5 ~ 3.0mg and 5mg for severe oral poisoners. if muscarinic symptoms do not disappear, administer 0.5 ~ 1mg repeatedly. In addition to severe poisoning by mouth, post-atropinization is not needed. ③ for the treatment of Adam-Stoke syndrome caused by antimony poisoning, give an immediate intravenous injection of 1.0 ~ 2.0mg, injecting 1mg 15 ~ 30 minutes later ④ for the treatment of calcium antagonist overdose and aconite poisoning, the amount of drug administered by the digestive system, 0.5 ~ 1mg singly, intramuscular injection, once 1 to 4 hours, until poisoning symptoms remit.<br>(2) for children: dosage could be calculated by body weight conversion, while the usage is the same as the adults. |
| --- | --- |
| 剂型、规格<br>Preparations | 注射液：每支 0.5mg/1ml；1mg/2ml；5mg/1ml。<br>Injection: 0.5mg/1ml ; 1mg/2ml; 5mg/1ml per vial. |
| **药品名称 Drug Names** | 东莨菪碱 Scopolamine |
| 适应证<br>Indications | 有机磷农药类中毒的治疗。<br>For the treatment of organophosphorus pesticide poisoning |
| 用法、用量<br>Dosage | 成人首次为：轻度中毒：0.3 ~ 0.5mg；中度中毒：0.5 ~ 1.0mg；重度中毒：2.0 ~ 4.0mg。重复用药量 0.3 ~ 0.6mg。<br><br>For Adults initial dose, mild poisoning: 0.3 ~ 0.5mg; moderate poisoning: 0.5 ~ 1.0mg; severe poisoning: 2.0 ~ 4.0mg. Repeated dosage of 0.3 ~ 0.6mg. |
| 剂型、规格<br>Preparations | 注射液：1ml：0.3mg；1mg：0.5mg。<br>Injection: 1ml: 0.3mg; 1mg: 0.5mg. |
| **药品名称 Drug Names** | 亚甲蓝 Methylthioninium Chloride |
| 适应证<br>Indications | （1）治疗亚硝酸盐及苯胺类引起的中毒。<br>（2）治疗氰化物中毒。<br><br>(1) For the treatment of nitrite and aniline-induced intoxication.<br>(2) For the treatment of cyanide poisoning. |
| 用法、用量<br>Dosage | （1）治疗亚硝酸盐中毒：用 1% 溶液 5 ~ 10ml（1 ~ 2mg/kg），稀释于 25% 葡萄糖溶液 20 ~ 40ml 中，缓慢静脉注射（10 分钟注完）。若注射后 30 ~ 60 分钟发绀不消退，可重复注射首次剂量。3 ~ 4 小时后，根据病情还可注射半量。若口服本品，可用 150 ~ 250mg，每 4 小时 1 次。<br>（2）治疗氰化物中毒（用 1% 溶液 50 ~ 100ml（5 ~ 10mg/kg），以 25% 葡萄糖溶液稀释后缓慢注射，尔后，再注入 25% 硫代硫酸钠 20 ~ 40ml。严重者二者交替使用。<br><br>(1) for the Treatment of nitrite poisoning: 1% solution of 5 ~ 10ml (1 ~ 2mg/kg), dilute it in 20 ~ 40ml 25% glucose solution for slow intravenous injection (10 minutes to finish injection). If cyanosis does not subside after 30 to 60 minutes, the first dose should be repeated. It is capable to inject half the amount 3 to 4 hours later according to the condition. Oral medication needs 150 ~ 250mg and once every four hours.<br>(2) for The treatment of cyanide poisoning (with a 1% solution of 50 ~ 100ml (5 ~ 10mg/kg), diluting with 25% glucose solution for slow injection, and then adding into 25% sodium thiosulfate of 20 ~ 40ml. For Severe patients, the tow products should be used interchangeably. |

续　表

| 剂型、规格<br>Preparations | 注射液：20mg/2ml。<br>Injection: 20mg/2ml. |
|---|---|
| 药品名称 Drug Names | 硫代硫酸钠 Sodium Thiosulfate |
| 适应证<br>Indications | ①抢救氰化物中毒。②抗过敏。③治疗降压药硝普钠过量中毒。④治疗可溶性钡盐（如硝酸钡）中毒。⑤治疗砷、汞、铋、铅等金属中毒。<br><br>① To rescue cyanide poisoning. ② Antiallergy. ③ For the treatment of overdose intoxation of antihypertensive drug of sodium nitroprusside. ④ For the treatment of soluble barium salt (e.g., barium nitrate) poisoning. ⑤ For the treatment of arsenic, mercury, bismuth, lead and other metal poisoning |
| 用法、用量<br>Dosage | （1）成人：①抢救氰化物中毒：由于本品解毒作用较慢，须先用作用迅速的亚硝酸钠、亚硝酸异戊酯或亚甲蓝，然后缓慢静脉注射 10 ～ 30g（25% ～ 50% 溶液 40 ～ 60ml），每分钟 5ml 以下。必要时，1 小时后再与高铁血红蛋白形成剂合用半量至全量。口服中毒者，还须用 5% 溶液洗胃，洗后留本品溶液适量于胃内。②硝普钠过量中毒：单独使用 25% 溶液 20 ～ 40ml，缓慢静脉注射。③可溶性钡盐中毒：缓慢静脉注射 25% 溶液 20 ～ 40ml。④治疗砷、汞铋。铅等金属中毒：静脉注射，每次 0.5 ～ 1.0g。⑤抗过敏：0.5 ～ 1.0g（5%10 ～ 20ml）静脉注射，一日一次，10 ～ 14 日为 1 个疗程。<br><br>（2）小儿：按体重计算，25% 溶液 1.0 ～ 1.5ml/kg（250 ～ 375mg/kg）。<br><br>(1) for Adults: ① to rescue cyanide poisoning: due to a slow detoxification, it is needed to use sodium nitrite, amyl nitrite or methylene blue which get effect quickly first, and then take a slow intravenous injection with 10 ～ 30g (25% ～ 50% solution of 40 ～ 60ml), 5ml below per minute or less. If necessary, using combined with methemoglobin of half or full amount one hour later. For Oral medication poisoners, it is needed to use 5% solution for Gastric lavage and to leave a certain amount of solution in the stomach. ② overdose SNP: 20 ～ 40ml 25% solution alone for slow intravenous injection. ③ soluble barium salt poisoning: slow intravenous injection with 20 ～ 40ml 25% solution. ④ for the treatment of arsenic, mercury, bismuth and lead poisoning: intravenous injection, 0.5 ～ 1.0g / time. ⑤ anti-Allergy: 0.5 ～ 1.0g (5% 10 ～ 20ml) intravenous injection for once a day, 10 to 14 days for a treatment course. (2) for children: 25% solution, 1.0 ～ 1.5ml/kg (250 ～ 375mg/kg), measured by weight. |
| 剂型、规格<br>Preparations | 注射用硫代硫酸钠：有无水物 0.32g（相当于含结晶水者 0.5g），无水物 0.64g（相当于含结晶水者 1.0g）；注射液：每支 0.5g/10ml，1.0g/20ml。<br><br>Injection type : Anhydrous type, 0.32g (equivalent with 0.5g crystal water), anhydrous type, 0.64g (equivalent with 1.0g crystal water); Injection: 0.5g/10ml per vial, 1.0g/20ml per vial. |
| 药品名称 Drug Names | 亚硝酸钠 Sodium Nitrite |
| 适应证<br>Indications | 治疗氰化物中毒及硫化氢中毒。<br>For the treatment of cyanide poisoning and hydrogen sulfide poisoning. |
| 用法、用量<br>Dosage | （1）成人，静脉注射：每次 3% 溶液 10 ～ 15ml（或 6 ～ 12mg/kg），注射速度宜慢（按 2ml/mim）。和用氯化钠注射液稀释至 100ml 后静脉注射（5 ～ 20 分钟），随后静脉注射 25% 硫代硫酸钠 40ml（硫化氢中毒不需要注射硫代硫酸钠）。必要时，0.5 ～ 1 小时后可重复给半量或全量。<br><br>（2）小儿：按体重 3% 溶液 0.15 ～ 0.3mg/kg。本品 3% 溶液，仅供静脉注射用，每次 10 ～ 20ml，每分钟注射 2 ～ 3ml；需要时在 1 小时后重复半量或全量。<br><br>(1) For adults, intravenous injection: 10 ～ 15ml (or 6 ～ 12mg/kg) of 3% solution singly, injection speed should be slow (by 2ml/mim). And diluting with sodium chloride injection fluid until 100ml for intravenous injection (5 to 20 minutes). Next, intravenous injection with 40ml 25% sodium thiosulfate (in the case of hydrogen sulfide poisoning, it does not require sodium thiosulfate). When necessary, repeated medication is available with half or full quantity 0.5 to 1 hour later.<br><br>(2) for Children: 3% solution of 0.15 ～ 0.3mg/kg measured by weight. This 3% solution is only for intravenous use, 10 ～ 20ml singly, 2 ～ 3ml per minute; repeated medication is available with half or full quantity 1 hour later if needed. |
| 剂型、规格<br>Preparations | 注射液：0.3g/10ml。<br>Injection: 0.3g/10ml. |

续 表

| 药品名称 Drug Names | 氟马西尼 Flumazenil |
| --- | --- |
| 适应证<br>Indications | 苯二氮䓬类药物之中毒解救。也可用于乙醇中毒之解救。<br>For the treatment of Benzodiazepine drugs intoxation and ethanol poisoning. |
| 用法、用量<br>Dosage | 成人常用量 0.5 ~ 2mg，静脉注射。小儿常用量：0.01mg/kg，静脉注射。最大剂量 1mg。<br>（1）麻醉后：因苯二氮䓬类常用于术前的麻醉诱导和术中的麻醉维持。本药则于术后使用，以终止 BZD 类的镇静作用。开始用量是 15 秒内缓慢静脉注射 0.2mg，如 30 秒内尚未清醒，可再注射 0.1 ~ 0.3mg，必要时，60 秒重复一次，直至总量达 3mg 为止。通常使用 0.3 ~ 0.6mg 即可。<br>（2）急救：对原因不明的神志丧失患者，可用本品来鉴别是否为苯二氮䓬类所致，如反复给药也不能使意识或呼吸功能改善，则可判定为非苯二氮䓬所致。开始用量是 0.2mg，以氯化钠注射液或 5% 葡萄糖注射液稀释后静脉注射；重复给药每次增加 0.1mg，或每小时 0.1 ~ 0.4mg/h，滴速个体化，直至清醒为止。<br>For Adults, the usual dose is 0.5 ~ 2mg with intravenous injection. Pediatric usual dose: 0.01mg/kg, intravenous injection with the maximum dose of 1mg.<br>(1) After anesthesia: benzodiazepine class is commonly used in the preoperative induction of anesthesia and intranperative maintenance of anesthesia. This product is used after surgery to terminate the sedation of BZD class. The initial dose is slow intravenous injection with 0.2mg within 15 seconds. If the patientdoesn't regain consciousness after 30 seconds, reinject 0.1 ~ 0.3mg and once per 60 seconds when necessary but less than a total amount of 3mg. Usually, 0.3 ~ 0.6mg is appropriate.<br>(2) for First Aid: for patients with unexplained loss of consciousness, it can be used to identify whether it is caused by benzodiazepine class. If repeated administration does not make sense or improve respiratory function, we can determine that a non-benzodiazepine-induced condition. The initial dosage is 0.2mg, diluting with sodium chloride injection or 5% dextrose injection for intravenous injection; repeated dosing with anincrement of 0.1mg singly, or 0.1 ~ 0.4mg / h hourly.The speed of dripping is individualized until refreshment. |
| 剂型、规格<br>Preparations | 注射液：每支 0.5mg/5ml；1mg/10ml。<br>Injection: 0.5mg/5ml per vial, 1mg/10ml per vial. |
| 药品名称 Drug Names | 纳洛酮 Naloxone |
| 适应证<br>Indications | ①治疗阿片类药物及其他麻醉性镇痛药（如哌替啶、阿法罗定、美沙酮、芬太尼、二氢埃托啡、依托尼嗪等）中毒，②治疗镇静催眠药与急性酒精中毒。③阿片类及其他麻醉性镇痛药依赖性的诊断。<br>① For the treatment of intoxication of opioid drugs and other narcotic analgesics (eg, meperidine, A Faluo be, methadone, fentanyl, Dihydroetorphine, Etonitazene, etc.) ② For the treatment of intoxication of sedative hypnotics and acute alcohol poisoning. ③ For diagnosis of pharmacological dependence of opioid drugs and other narcotic analgesics. |
| 用法、用量<br>Dosage | 成人：静脉注射 0.4 ~ 0.8mg（小儿用量与成人同）。治疗阿片类。镇静催眠药类与急性酒精中毒，首剂 0.4 ~ 0.8mg，无效时可重复一次。因纳洛酮的作用只能持续 45 ~ 90 分钟，以后必须根据病情重复用药，以巩固疗效。<br>For adults: intravenous injection of 0.4 ~ 0.8mg (the same amount as adults'for children ). For the Treatment of opioid. Sedative hypnotics class and acute alcoholism, the first dose is 0.4 ~ 0.8mg, repeated medication for once if invalid. The function of Naloxone only lasts for 45 to 90 minutes, so repeated medication is a must based on the condition to consolidate the curative effect. |
| 剂型、规格<br>Preparations | 注射液：0.4mg/1ml。<br>Injection: 0.4mg/1ml. |
| 药品名称 Drug Names | 乙酰半胱氨酸 Acetylcysteine |
| 适应证<br>Indications | 对乙酰氨基酚中毒。<br>For the treatment of Acetaminophen poisoning. |

**续　表**

| 用法、用量<br>Dosage | 5% 乙酰半胱氨酸（痰易净）水溶液加果汁内服，如服后 1 小时呕吐，可在补服一次，如连续呕吐可下胃管将药液直接导入十二指肠内。用量：140mg/kg 为起始量，70mg/kg 为后续量，每 4 小时一次，17 次可达解救的负荷量。静脉滴注：成人，第 1 阶段，140mg/kg 加入葡萄糖液 200ml 中，静脉滴注 15 ～ 20 分钟。第二阶段，70mg/kg 加入 5% 葡萄糖液 500ml 中静脉滴注。每 4 小时 1 次，共给 17 次。儿童，根据患儿的年龄和体重调整用量，解毒剂量同成人，但需按体重折算（将成人剂量按 50 ～ 69kg 折算成每千克的剂量）。<br><br>5% acetylcysteine (sputum easy to clean) queous solution plus juice for oral medication. In the case of vomiting one hour after taking, another time of medication is preferred. In the case of continuous vomiting can lower the liquid directly into the duodenum by stomach tube. Dosage: 140mg/kg as the starting amount, 70mg/kg for subsequent volume, once every 4 hours, a total of 17 times could meet the load capacity to rescue. Intravenous infusion: for adults, stage 1, 140mg/kg is added to 200ml glucose solution and then take intravenous infusion for 15 to 20 minutes. The second phase, 70mg/kg is added to 500ml 5% glucose solution for intravenous infusion. Once Every four hours, for a total of 17 times. For Children, Dosage should be adapted according to the children's age and weight. The dosage for detoxification is equivalent to adults', but should be converted by weight (Converting adult dose by 50 ~ 69kg into that of per kilogram dose). |
| :--- | :--- |
| 剂型、规格<br>Preparations | 颗粒剂：100mg。<br>泡腾片：600mg。<br>Granules: 100mg.<br>Effervescent tablets: 600mg. |
| **药品名称 Drug Names** | 亚叶酸钙 Calcium Folinate |
| 适应证<br>Indications | 用于抗叶酸代谢药过量中毒和甲醇中毒。<br>For the treatment of intoxication of anti-metabolite and methanol poisoning. |
| 用法、用量<br>Dosage | （1）抗叶酸代谢药过量中毒：用量相当于抗叶酸代谢药的剂量（15 ～ 100mg），静脉注射。以后，如为甲氨蝶呤过量中毒，每 3 ～ 6 小时再注射或口服 15mg，共 8 次；如为甲氧苄啶过量中毒，口服 15mg，一日 1 次，共 5 ～ 7 日。<br>（2）甲醇中毒：亚叶酸钙 50mg，静脉注射，每 4 小时 1 次，共 2 日。<br><br>(1) anti-drug overdose of folate metabolism: the amount is equivalent to that to anti-folate metabolism drugs (15 ~ 100mg), intravenous injection. Later, in the case of methotrexate overdose, 15mg of injection or Oral medication every 3 to 6 hours, 8 times in total; in the case of trimethoprim overdose, 15mg of Oral medication, once a day, 5 to 7 days in total.<br>(2) Methanol poisoning: 50mg leucovorin, intravenous injection, once every 4 hours for two days. |
| 剂型、规格<br>Preparations | 片剂：5mg；15mg；25mg。<br>注射液：50mg；100mg；300mg。<br>胶囊：25mg。<br>Tablets: 5mg, 15mg, 25mg.<br>Injection: 50mg, 100mg, 300mg.<br>Capsule: 25mg. |

20.3 诊断用药 Drugs for Diagnosis

| **药品名称 Drug Names** | 碘海醇 Iohexol |
| :--- | :--- |
| 适应证<br>Indications | 心血管造影、冠状动脉造影、尿路造影、CT 增强扫描及脊髓造影等。<br>For angiography, coronary angiography, urography, CT enhancement scanning and spinal angiography. |
| 用法、用量<br>Dosage | ①脊髓造影：腰穿注入造影剂 7 ～ 10ml。②泌尿系造影（300mg/ml）：成人，静脉注射 40 ～ 80ml；儿童，<7kg，3ml/kg；>7kg，2ml/kg（最高 40ml）。③主动脉血管造影：每次注射 30 ～ 40ml。④ CT 增强扫描（300mg/ml）：成人，100 ～ 180ml 静脉注射；儿童，按 1.5 ～ 2mg/kg 体重计。<br><br>① Myelography: 7 ~ 10ml lumbar puncture contrast agent. ② Urography (300mg/ml): for adults, intravenous injection of 40 ~ 80ml; children, <7kg, 3ml/kg;> 7kg, 2ml/kg (the maximum amount is 40ml). ③ Aortic angiography: injection of 30 ~ 40ml / times. ④ CT enhanced scan (300mg/ml): for adult, 100 ~ 180ml intravenous injection; for Children, by 1.5 ~ 2mg/kg body weight. |

**续　表**

| 剂型、规格<br>Preparations | 注射液：每支 20ml。<br>Injection: 20ml per vial. |
|---|---|
| **药品名称 Drug Names** | 碘佛醇 Ioversol |
| 适应证<br>Indications | 心血管造影、冠状动脉造影、尿路造影、CT 增强扫描及脊髓造影等。<br>For angiography, coronary angiography, urography, CT enhancement scanning and spinal angiography. |
| 用法、用量<br>Dosage | ①脊髓造影：腰穿注入造影剂 7 ～ 10ml。②泌尿系造影（300mgI/ml）：成人，静脉注射 40 ～ 80ml；儿童，<7kg，3ml/kg；>7kg，2ml/kg（最高 40ml）。③主动脉血管造影：每次注射 30 ～ 40ml。④ CT 增强扫描（300mgI/ml）：成人，100 ～ 180ml 静脉注射；儿童，按 1.5 ～ 2mg/kg 体重计。<br>① Myelography: 7 ~ 10ml lumbar puncture contrast agent. ② Urography (300mgI/ml): for adults, intravenous injection of 40 ~ 80ml; children, <7kg, 3ml/kg;> 7kg, 2ml/kg (the maximum amount is 40ml). ③ Aortic angiography: injection of 30 ~ 40ml / times. ④ CT enhanced scan (300mgI/ml): for adult, 100 ~ 180ml intravenous injection; for Children, by 1.5 ~ 2mg/kg body weight. |
| 剂型、规格<br>Preparations | 注射液：20ml；50ml；100ml。<br>Injection: 20ml/50ml/100ml per vial. |
| **药品名称 Drug Names** | 碘帕醇 Iopamidol |
| 适应证<br>Indications | 主要适用于腰、胸及颈段脊髓造影，脑血管造影，周围动、静脉造影，心血管造影，冠状动脉造影，尿路、关节造影及 CT 增强扫描等。<br>Mainly used for CTM of the waist, chest and cervical parts, cerebral angiography, peripheral arterial and venous angiography, cardiac angiography, coronary angiography, IVU, arthrography and CT Evaluation of enhanced. |
| 用法、用量<br>Dosage | 脊髓造影，成人用浓度为 200 ～ 300mg/ml 溶液 5 ～ 15ml。大脑血管造影用 300mg/ml 溶液 5 ～ 10ml（成人）。3 ～ 7ml（儿童）。周围动静脉造影用 300mg/ml 溶液 20 ～ 50ml（成人）。冠状动脉造影用 370mg/ml 溶液 4 ～ 8ml（成人）。主动脉造影（逆行）用 370mg/ml 溶液 50 ～ 80ml（成人）。尿路造影用 300 ～ 370mg/ml 溶液 20 ～ 50ml（成人），1 ～ 2.5ml（儿童）。CT 扫描用 300 ～ 370mg/ml 溶液 50 ～ 100ml（成人）等。<br>Myelography, for adults, 5 ~ 15ml solution with a concentration of 200 ~ 300mg/ml . Cerebral angiography, with 5 ~ 10ml 300mg/ml solution (for adults). 3 ~ 7ml (children). Arteriovenous contrast: 20 ~ 50ml 300mg/ml solution (for adults). Coronary angiography: 4 ~ 8ml 370mg/ml solution (adult). Angiography (retrograde) : 50 ~ 80ml 370mg/ml solution (for adults). Urography : 20 ~ 50ml 300~ 370mg/ml solution (for adults), 1 ~ 2.5ml (children). CT scanning : 50 ~ 100ml 300 ~ 370mg/ml solution (for adults) and the like. |
| 剂型、规格<br>Preparations | 注射液：每支 20ml，50ml，100ml。<br>Injection: 20ml/50ml/100ml per vial. |
| **药品名称 Drug Names** | 碘克沙醇 Iodixanol |
| 适应证<br>Indications | 成人的心、脑血管造影（常规的与 i.a.DSA）、外周动脉造影（常规的与 i.a.DSA）腹部血管造影（i.a.DSA）尿路造影、静脉造影以及 CT 增强检查。<br>For adult angiocardiography and cerebral angiography (conventional ones and i. a. DSA), peripheral arterial angiography (conventional and i. a. DSA) abdominal angiography (i. a. DSA) urography, venography and CT Evaluation of enhanced. |
| 用法、用量<br>Dosage | 用药剂量取决于检查类型、年龄、体重、心排血量和患者全身情况及所使用的技术。<br>The dosage depends on the examination type, age, weight, cardiac output and general condition of patients, and the technology used. |
| 剂型、规格<br>Preparations | 注射液：150mg/ml（50ml；200ml）；270mg/ml（20ml；50ml；100ml）；320mg/ml（20ml；50ml；100ml）。<br>Injection: 150mg/ml (50ml; 200ml); 270mg/ml (20ml; 50ml; 100ml); 320mg/ml (20ml; 50ml; 100ml). |

续　表

| 药品名称 Drug Names | 硫酸钡 Barium Sulfate |
| --- | --- |
| 适应证<br>Indications | 适用于上、下消化道造影。<br>For upper and lower gastrointestinal contrast. |
| 用法、用量<br>Dosage | （1）上消化道造影，根据检查部位和检查方法不同，加适量水调成不同浓度的混悬液，通常成人使用量食管：检查方法：经口，浓度为 100% ～ 180%（w/v），用量为 50 ～ 150ml；胃、十二指肠：检查方法：经口，浓度为 100% ～ 180%（w/v），用量为 50 ～ 150ml。<br>（2）下消化道造影：经肛门灌入肠内。灌前准备：按常规肠清洗（控制饮食、大量饮水、加用泻剂），肌注解痉灵（可根据医院临床经验及习惯选择）。使用前，加适量水调成 180%（w/v）浓度混悬液，按照自动灌肠机操作程序进行，每次 250 ～ 300ml。<br><br>(1) Upper gastrointestinal contrast, according to the inspection site and checking methods, add appropriate amount of water to make suspension of different concentrations, usually through esophagus for adults: inspection methods: oral, concentration of 100% ～ 180% (w / v), in an amount of 50 ～ 150ml; gastroduodenal: inspection methods: orally, at a concentration of 100% ～ 180% (w / v), in an amount of 50 ～ 150ml.<br>(2) Lower gastrointestinal contrast: poured into the intestine through the anus. Irrigation preparation: intestinal cleansing by conventional (control diet, drink lots of water, plus laxatives). Inject antispasmodics intramuscularly (can choose the dosage based on the hospital clinical experience and habits). Before use, add appropriate amount of water to make the suspension of 180% (w / v) concentration, in accordance with operating procedures of the automatic eneme machine, 250 ～ 300ml once. |
| 剂型、规格<br>Preparations | 混悬液：（w/v）100%，120%，130%，140%。<br>Suspension: (w / v) 100%, 120%, 130%, 140%. |

| 药品名称 Drug Names | 碘化油 Iodinated Oil |
| --- | --- |
| 适应证<br>Indications | 主要用于支气管及子宫、输卵管、瘘管、腔道等的造影检查，亦用于肝癌的栓塞治疗及地方性甲状腺肿。<br>Mainly used for bronchial angiography and contrast examination of uterus, fallopian tubes, fistula, cavity, etc. and treatment of embolization of liver cancer and endemic goiter. |
| 用法、用量<br>Dosage | ①支气管造影：经气管导管直接注入气管或支气管腔内。成人单侧 15 ～ 20ml（40%），双侧 30 ～ 40ml；小儿酌减。注入应缓慢，采用体位使各叶支气管充盈。②子宫输卵管造影：经宫颈管直接注入子宫腔内，5 ～ 12ml（40%）。③各种腔室（如鼻旁窦、腮腺管、泪腺管等）和窦道、瘘管造影：依据病灶大小酌量直接注入。④肝癌栓塞治疗：先做选择性或超选择性肝动脉插管造影，将与抗癌药混合的碘化油 5 ～ 10ml 注入肿瘤供血动脉内。⑤预防地方甲状腺肿：多用肌内注射，亦可口服（应用其胶丸剂）。肌内注射：学龄前儿童 1 次剂量 0.5ml，学龄期儿童或成人 1 次量 1ml，每 2 ～ 3 年注射 1 次；口服，学龄前儿童每次服 0.2 ～ 0.3g，学龄期至成人服 0.4 ～ 0.6g，每 1 ～ 2 年服 1 次。<br><br>① Bronchography: directly injected into the trachea or bronchial lumen through endotracheal tube . For adult, unilateral, 15 ～ 20ml (40%); bilateral, 30 ～ 40ml; Dose for children should be reduced accordingly. Injection should be slow, changing positions to make per lobe bronchus filling. ② HSG: directly injected into the uterine cavity through cervical canal, 5 ～ 12ml (40%). ③ various chambers (such as the paranasal sinuses, parotid gland, lacrimal duct, etc.) and sinus, fistula angiography: direct injection proportionally based on lesion size. ④ embolization of liver cancer: First make selective or super-selective hepatic artery angiography, inject 5 ～ 10ml mixture solution comprising iodized oil and the anti-cancer drug into the tumor feeding artery. ⑤ prevent goiter place: more intramuscular injections, but also orally (take capsules). Intramuscular injection: for preschoolers, a dose is 0.5ml. for school-age children or adults, a dose is 1ml, 1 injection every 2 to 3 years. Oral medication: for preschoolers, 0.2 ～ 0.3g once; for school-age children to adults, 0.4 ～ 0.6g one time, once every 1 to 2 years. |
| 剂型、规格<br>Preparations | 油注射液：每支 10ml（含碘 40%）。<br>胶丸剂：每丸 0.1g；0.2g。<br>Oil Injection: 10ml (iodine 40%) per vial.<br>Capsules: 0.1g, 0.2g per pill. |

| 药品名称 Drug Names | 复方泛影葡胺 Compoud Meglumine Diatrizoate |
|---|---|
| 适应证<br>Indications | 常用于尿路造影，也可用于肾上腺肾盂、心、脑血管等的造影。<br>It is used for urography, adrenal pelvis, heart, and cerebrovascular arteriography. |
| 用法、用量<br>Dosage | ①逆行肾盂造影：20%，6～10ml。②尿路造影50%，20～30ml。③脑血管造影：45%以下溶液，10ml。④心脏大血管造影：50%，40ml。<br><br>① retrograde pyelography: 20%, 6～10ml. ② IVU: 50%, 20～30ml. ③ cerebral angiography: the concentration of 45% or less of the solution, 10ml. ④ heart MR angiography: 50%, 40ml. |
| 剂型、规格<br>Preparations | 注射液：60%20ml；76%20ml。<br>Injection: 60% 20ml; 76% 20ml. |
| 药品名称 Drug Names | 钆喷酸葡胺 Gadopentetate Dimethyl Meglumine |
| 适应证<br>Indications | 本品适用于中枢神经（脑脊髓）、腹、盆腔、四肢等人体脏器和组织的磁共振成像。还可替代 X 线含碘造影剂，用于不能使用者。<br><br>This product is used for magnetic resonance imaging of central nervous system (marrowbrain), abdomen, pelvis, limbs and other body organs and tissues of. For patients who can't use X-rays iodine contrast agent. |
| 用法、用量<br>Dosage | （1）静脉注射：成人及 2 岁以上儿童，按体重一次 0.2ml/kg（或 0.1mmol/kg），最大用量为按体重一次 0.4ml/kg。颅脑及脊髓磁共振成像：为获得充分的强化，可按体重一次 0.4ml/kg 给药。最佳强化时间，一般在注射后数分钟之内（不超过 45 分钟）。<br><br>（2）将 1ml 钆喷酸葡胺（相当于 2mmol/L GD-DTPA）加 2449ml 氯化钠注射液或用 1mlGD-DTPA 加 49ml 氯化钠注射液稀释后，可直接用于体腔的造影，如关节造影或腹腔造影等。<br><br>（3）将 1ml 钆喷酸葡胺 +15g/L 甘露醇和 25mmol/L 缓冲剂枸橼酸钠配合，有较佳效果，胃肠涂布穿透力强，不易产生腔内浓缩的胃肠道阳性磁共振造影剂。尽管钆喷酸葡胺在大鼠脑池内注射的神经毒性，低于泛影葡胺及优维显等含碘造影剂，但目前仍不主张将它用于直接鞘内注射造影。<br><br>（4）利用钆喷酸葡胺中 Gd 元素原子序数高（157.3）有吸收 X 线的特点，可用于碘过敏患者的肾动脉 X 线造影或肾排泄性造影（即代替 X 线含碘造影剂）。<br><br>(1) Intravenous injection: Adults and children over 2 years old, 0.2ml/kg per time according to the body weight ( or 0.1mmol/kg), the maximum amount of dose is once 0.4ml/kg according to the body weight. magnetic resonance imaging of brain and spinal: In order to obtain the full strengthening, according to body weight the administration can be 0.4ml/kg per time. Best time to strengthen is usually within minutes after injection (no more than 45 minutes).<br>(2) add 1ml GD-DTPA( equivalent to 2mmol / L GD-DTPA) to 2449ml sodium chloride injection or 1mlGD-DTPA injection is diluted with sodium chloride injection, the solution can be used for the Radiography of pelvic cavity, like arthrography, peritoneography and so on.<br>(3) if 1ml GD-DTPA+15 g / L mannitol is used in combination with 25mmol / L sodium citrate buffer fit, the effects will be better. The gastrointestinal coating penetration is stronger, and it is not easy to produce concentrated gastrointestinal lumen positive MRI contrast agents. Although the neurotoxicity of GD-DTPA injected in rats' intracisternal is less than Urografin, Ultravist and other iodine contrast medium, it is still not advocated for direct intrathecal injection arteriography.<br>(4) element Gd ( 157.3 )with high atomic number in gadolinium –DTPA has the character of X-ray absorption and can be used for patients allergic to iodine X -ray contrast renal artery or renal excretion of contrast media ( replace X-ray contrast agents containing iodine ) . |
| 剂型、规格<br>Preparations | 注射液：每支 7.42g（20ml）；5.57g（15ml）；3.71g（10ml）。<br>Injection: 7.42g (20ml) per vial; 5.57g (15ml) per vial; 3.71g (10ml) per vial. |
| 药品名称 Drug Names | 吲哚菁绿 Indocyanine Green |
| 适应证<br>Indications | 本品用于诊断肝硬化、肝纤维化、韧性肝炎，对职业和药物中毒性肝病的诊断极有价值。也可用于循环系统功能（心排血量、平均循环时间或异常血流量）的检查测定。<br><br>This product is used for the diagnosis of cirrhosis, liver fibrosis, hepatitis toughness and is extremely valuable on treating occupational poisoning drug toxic hepatic damage. For check and measurement of circulation system function (cardiac output, average circulation-time or abnormal blood flow). |

**续　表**

| | |
|---|---|
| 用法、用量<br>Dosage | 静脉注射：①血浆消失率及血中停滞率的测定：0.5mg/kg，用蒸馏水稀释为 5mg/ml 浓度，在 30 秒从肘静脉慢慢注入。②肝血流量的测定：将本品 25mg 用少量蒸馏水溶解后，稀释成 2.5～5.90mg/ml 浓度，开始时，注射相当于 3mg 的此浓度溶液，以后再 50 分钟内慢慢静滴至采血完毕。③用于循环功能检查：通常从前臂静脉注入，成人 1 次量 5～10mg，小儿按体重酌减。<br><br>Intravenous injection: ① The measurement of blood plasma disappearance rate and the blood retention rate: 0.5mg/kg, diluted with distilled water to the concentration of 5mg/ml and then get injected gently in the cubital vein in 30 seconds. ② The measurement of hepatic blood flow: Dissolve 25mg of this product with a small amount of distilled water, dilute it to concentration of 2.5～5.90mg/ml. at the beginning, inject what is equivalent to 3mg with this concentration, then the rest is in intravenous drip till it is finished within 50 minutes. ③ it is used for the checking of circulation: usually it is injected in the forearm vein, 5～10mg per adult for one time. Dosage for children should be reduced according to their weights. |
| 剂型、规格<br>Preparations | 注射剂：每支 25mg（附注射用水 10ml）。<br>Injection: 25mg per bottle(notions: WFI is 10ml). |
| **药品名称 Drug Names** | 荧光素钠 Fluorescein Sodium |
| 适应证<br>Indications | ①滴眼液用于眼科诊断，正常角膜不显色，异常角膜显色。②针剂用于测血液循环时间，静脉注射后，在紫外线灯下观察，以 10～15 秒唇部黏膜能见到黄绿色荧光为正常。<br><br>① Eyedrop type is used to ophthalmic diagnose, when the color is not normal cornea, corneal abnormal color. ② Type of injection is for measuring blood circulation time: when yellow-green fluorescence is seen on lip mucosa within 10 to 15 seconds through ultraviolet light observation after intravenous injection, it is a normal situation. |
| 用法、用量<br>Dosage | ①滴眼后于角膜显微镜下观察颜色。②测血循环时间，于臂静脉注 2ml，每次用量 0.4～0.8g（2～4ml）。<br><br>① Observe the color with the corneal microscope after the eye drops. ② measuring the time of blood circulation. Inject 2ml in vena brachialis, with 0.4～0.8g (2～4ml) for each time. |
| 剂型、规格<br>Preparations | 滴眼液：2% 注射液：0.4g（2ml）。<br>Eye drops: 2% injection: 0.4g (2ml). |

### 20.4　生物制品 Biological Products

| | |
|---|---|
| **药品名称 Drug Names** | 人用狂犬病疫苗（vero 细胞）Rabies Vaccine for Human Use（vero cell） |
| 适应证<br>Indications | 用于预防狂犬病。凡被狂犬或其他疯动物咬伤、抓伤时，不分年龄、性别均应立即处理局部伤口（用清水或肥皂水反复冲洗后，再用碘酊或酒精消毒数次），并及时按暴露后免疫程序注射本疫苗；凡有接触狂犬病病毒危险的人员（如兽医、动物饲养员、林业从业人员、屠宰厂工人、狂犬病实验人员等），按暴露前免疫程序预防接种。<br><br>For the prevention of rabies. Anyone bitten or scratched by crazy animals, regardless of age and gender should deal with local wound immediately (repeated washing with water or soapy water and repeated disinfecting with tinctures or alcohol) and should receive Rabies Vaccine according to the post-exposure immunization program; Anyone exposed to rabies (such as veterinarians, animal breeders, forestry personnel, abattoir workers, rabies experimenters, etc.) should receive injection according to pre-exposure immunization program. |
| | （1）于上臂三角肌处肌内注射，幼儿可在大腿前外侧区肌内注射。<br>（2）暴露后免疫程序：一般咬伤者于 0 日（第 1 日，当天）、3 日（第 4 日，以下类推）7 日、14 日和 28 日各注射本疫苗 1 剂，全程免疫共注射 5 剂，儿童用量相同。对有下列情况之一的，建议首剂狂犬疫苗剂量加倍给予：①注射疫苗前一天或更早一些时间内，注射过狂犬病人免疫球蛋白或狂犬病血清的慢性患者。②先天性或获得性免疫缺陷患者。③接受免疫抑制剂（包括抗疟疾药物）治疗的患者。④老年人。⑤于暴露后 48 小时或更长时间后才注射狂犬病疫苗的人员。⑥暴露后免疫程序按下述伤及程度分级处理：Ⅰ级暴露：触摸动物，被动物舔及无破损皮肤，一般不需要处理，不必注射狂犬疫苗。Ⅱ级暴露：未出血的皮肤咬伤、抓伤，应按暴露后免疫程序接种狂犬病疫苗。Ⅲ级暴露：一处或多处皮肤出血性咬伤或被抓伤出血，可疑或确诊的疯动物唾液污染黏膜，破损的皮肤被舔，应按暴露后程序立即接种狂犬病疫苗 |

| 用法、用量<br>Dosage | 和抗狂犬病血清或抗狂犬病人免疫球蛋白按 20U/kg 给予。将尽可能多的抗狂犬病血清或抗狂犬病人免疫球蛋白做咬伤局部浸润注射，剩余部分做肌内注射，抗狂犬病血清或抗狂犬病人免疫球蛋白仅为单次应用。<br>　　（3）暴露前免疫程序：按 0 日、7 日、21 日或 28 日各注射 1 剂，全程免疫共注射 3 剂。<br>　　（4）对曾经接种过狂犬病疫苗的一般患者，再需接种疫苗的建议：① 1 年内进行过全程免疫，被可疑疯动物咬伤者，应于 0 天或 3 天各注射 1 剂疫苗。② 1 年前进行过全程免疫，被可疑疯动物咬伤者，则应全程接种疫苗。③ 3 年内进行过全程免疫，并且进行过加强免疫，被可疑疯动物咬伤者，应于 0 日或 3 日各注射 1 剂疫苗。④ 3 年前进行过全程免疫，并且进行过加强免疫，被可疑疯动物咬伤者，应全程接种疫苗。<br><br>　　(1) The intramuscular injection is taken in the deltoid of the upper arm. For infants, the intramuscular injection can be taken in the lateral zone of the thigh.<br>　　(2) Post-exposure immunization program : Generally people who are bitten should get one injection of vaccine at day 0 (day 1, day), days 3 (day 4, the rest can be done in the same manner), days 7, days 14, and days 28. The total number of injections for full-access immunization of is 5. Children take the same amount. For any of the following circumstances, the first dose of rabies vaccine is recommended to double: ① people with chronic disease who have been injected human rabies immunoglobulin or rabies antiserum the day before vaccination or some time earlier ② patients who have congenital or acquired immune deficiency ③ patients who received the treatment of immunosuppressive (including anti-malarial drugs). ④ the elderly. ⑤ people who get the rabies vaccine within 48 hours or longer after exposure. ⑥ After exposure immunization programs are dealt with according to the extent of injuries and its treatment is graded: Ⅰ level exposure : people who touch animals, are licked by animals and have no damaged skin, do not need treatment or injection of rabies vaccine. Ⅱ level exposure : People whose skin is bitten, scratched but has no bleeding should be injected rabies vaccine according to the immunization program after exposure . Ⅲ level exposure: if one spot or multiple spots are bitten or scratched with bleeding, if mucous membranes is polluted by the suspected or confirmed rabid animals' saliva contaminatio, and if the damaged skin is licked, the injury one should be injected rabies vaccine and rabies antiserum, or human rabies immunoglobulin the dosage of which is 20IU/kg . Inject as much rabies antiserum or human rabies immunoglobulin as possible in syringe-infiltrating. Inject the remaining part in intramuscular injection. Rabies antiserum and human rabies immunoglobulin is only used only for one time.<br>　　(3) Pre-exposure immunization program : People should have one injection in days 0, days 7, days 21 ordays 28. The total number of injections for full-access immunization of is 3.<br>　　(4)For general patients who have been vaccinated against rabies, there are following recommendations for getting vaccination again: ① full immunization is within one year. If the patient is bitten by suspect rabid animal, he should get one injection of the vaccine at day 0 and at days 3. ② If the full immunization is taken 1 year ago, patient who is bitten by suspect rabid animals should be vaccinated during the whole course. ③ If the full immunization is taken within three years, the booster immunization has also been taken, patient who is bitten by suspect rabid animal should be should get one injection of the vaccine at day 0 and at days 3. ④ If the full immunization is taken 3 years ago, the booster immunization has also been taken, patient who is bitten by suspect rabid animals should be vaccinated during the whole course. |
|---|---|
| 剂型、规格<br>Preparations | 注射液：每瓶 1ml，每人 1 次用量为 1ml。狂犬病疫苗效价应不低于 2.5U。<br><br>Injection: each bottle is 1ml. the dosage per person for one time is 1ml. The titer of rabies vaccine is not less than 2.5U. |
| 药品名称 Drug Names | 破伤风抗毒素 Tetanus Antitoxin |
| 适应证<br>Indications | 本品用于预防和治疗破伤风。已出现破伤风或可疑症状时，应在进行外科处理及其他疗法的同时，及时使用抗毒素治疗。开放性外伤（特别是伤口深、污染严重者）有感染破伤风的危险时，应注射抗毒素进行紧急预防。凡已接受过破伤风的危险时，应在再受伤后，再注射 1 剂疫苗，以加强免疫，不必注射抗毒素；如受伤者未接受过破伤风疫苗免疫或免疫史不清者，须注射抗毒素预防，但也应同时开始疫苗预防注射，以获得持久免疫。<br><br>This product is used for the prevention and treatment of tetanus. When tetanus or suspicious symptoms occur, anti-toxin treatment should be promptly taken combined with surgical treatment and other therapies. When open trauma (especially for deep and severely affected wounds) may be affected into tetanus, antitoxin should be injected for emergency prevention. If one has been affected by tetanus, another vaccination to enhance immunity, not needed to inject antitoxin; If the injured never receive any tetanus vaccine or doesn't have a clear immunization history, he must be injected by antitoxin combined with tetanus vaccine at the same time to realize a long-lasting immunity. |

**续　表**

| 用法、用量<br>Dosage | （1）预防用：皮下注射或肌内注射，一次 1500 ~ 3000U，儿童与成人用量相同；伤势严重者可增加用量 1 ~ 2 倍。经 5 ~ 6 日，如破伤风感染危险还未消除，应重复注射。<br><br>（2）治疗用：肌内注射或静脉注射，第 1 次肌内或静脉注射 50 000 ~ 200 000U，儿童与成人用量相同；以后视病情决定注射剂量和间隔时间，同时还可将适量的抗毒素注射于伤口周围的组织中。初生儿破伤风，24 小时内分次或 1 次肌内或静脉注射 20 000 ~ 100 000U。皮下注射应在上臂三角肌处，同时注射疫苗时，注射部位应分开。肌内注射应在上臂三角肌处或臀部。只有经过皮下或肌内注射未发生异常反应者，方可做静脉注射。静脉注射应缓慢，开始每分钟不超过 1ml，以后每分钟亦不宜超过 4ml。一次静脉注射总量不应超过 40ml。儿童每千克体重不宜超过 0.8ml。亦可将抗毒素加入葡萄糖注射液或氯化钠注射液等溶液中静脉滴注。静脉注射前应将安瓿置温水浴中加温至接近体温，注射中如发现异常反应，应立即停止。<br><br>(1)For prevention : subcutaneous or intramuscular injection, with 1500 ~ 3000U for one time. the dosage for children and adults are the same; people who are seriously injuried can increase the dosage for 1 to 2 times. If the risk of tetanus infection has not been eliminated after 5 to 6 days, the injections should be repeated.<br><br>(2) For treatment: intramuscular injection or intravenous injection, with 50 000~200 000U for the first time. The dosage for children and adults are the same; the dosage and intervals for injections is dependent on the patient's condition. And the adequate amount of antitoxin can be injected into the tissues around the wound. If the newborn child gets tetanus, the injection of 20 000 ~ 100 000U should be injected in intramuscular injection or intravenous injection within 24 hours for one time or more times. Subcutaneous injection should be injected in deltoid of the upper arm. Whern it was injected with the vaccine at the same time, the injection sites should be separated. Intramuscular injection should be injected in the deltoid of the upper arm or buttocks. Only people who have no abnormal reaction to subcutaneous or intramuscular injection can have the intravenous injection. The intravenous injection should be taken gently, no more than 1ml per minute at the beginning, then no more than 4ml per minute. The total amount the intravenous injection for one time should not exceed 40ml. The amount for Children should not exceed 0.8ml per kilogram according to their weight. The dextrose injection or sodium chloride injection can be added to the Antitoxin during the intravenous drip. Before the intravenous injection, the ampoules should be set in the warm water until it is heated to the approach the body temperature. If there is any abnormal reaction during the injection, it should be immediately stopped. |
| --- | --- |
| 剂型、规格<br>Preparations | 750μl：1.5mu，2.5ml：1wu<br>750μl：1.5mu，2.5ml：1wu |
| **药品名称 Drug Names** | 抗蛇毒血清 Antivenin |
| 适应证<br>Indications | 用于毒蛇咬伤中毒。<br>For the treatment of snakebite poisoning. |
| 用法、用量<br>Dosage | 稀释后静脉注射湖静脉滴注，也可肌内注射或皮下注射。用量根据被咬伤者的受毒量及血清效价而定。以下为中和一条毒蛇的剂量：<br><br>（1）抗蝮蛇毒血清：主要用于蝮蛇咬伤的治疗，对竹叶青和烙铁头毒蛇也有交叉中和作用。一次用 6000 ~ 16 000U，以氯化钠或 25% 葡萄糖注射液稀释 1 倍，缓慢静脉注射。<br><br>（2）抗五步蛇毒血清：主要用于五步蛇咬伤的治疗，对蝮蛇蛇毒也有交叉中和作用。每次用 8000U，以氯化钠注射液稀释 1 倍，缓慢静脉注射。<br><br>（3）抗银环蛇毒血清：主要用于银环蛇咬伤的治疗，一次用 10 000U，缓慢静脉注射。<br><br>（4）抗眼镜蛇毒血清：主要用于眼镜蛇咬伤的治疗，对其他科的毒蛇蛇毒也有交叉中和作用。一次用 2500 ~ 10 000U，缓慢静脉注射。<br><br>After being diluted, it can be injected in intravenous therapy or intravenous infusion. It can also be injected in intramuscular or subcutaneous injection. The dosage is decided by the degree of toxicity and serum titer. The following is the dosage that is needed to neutralize the toxicity of a venomous snake:<br><br>(1) Agkistrodon Halys Antivenin: it is mainly used for the treatment of viper bites and has the cross-neutralization effect on Trimeresurus stejnegeri and ovophis. With 6000 ~ 16 000U for one time, it should be diluted with sodium chloride or 25% glucose injection to 1 time and be injected in intravenous injection gently. |

续　表

| | |
|---|---|
| | (2) Agkistrodon Acutus Snake Antivenin: it is mainly used for the treatment of agkistrodon acutus bites and has cross-neutralization effect on viper bites. With 8000U for one tiem, it should be diluted to 1 time with sodium chloride injection and be injected in intravenous injection gently. <br><br> (3) Bungarus multicnctus Antivenin: it is mainly used for the treatment of bungarus multicinctus bites. With 10 000U for one time, it should be injected in intravenous injection gently. <br><br> (4) Naja Antivenin: it is mainly used for the treatment of cobra bites, and has cross-neutralization effect on venom of other kinds of venomous snakes. With 2500 ~ 10 000U for one time, for slow intravenous injection. |
| 剂型、规格 <br> Preparations | 注射液： <br> （1）抗蝮蛇蛇毒血清：每瓶含抗蝮蛇毒血清 6000U。 <br> （2）抗五步蛇毒血清：每瓶含抗眼镜蛇毒血清：2000U。 <br> （3）抗银环蛇毒血清：每瓶含抗银环蛇毒血清：10 000U。 <br> （4）抗眼镜蛇毒血清：每瓶含抗眼镜蛇毒血清：1000U。 <br><br> Injection: <br> (1) Agkistrodon Halys Antivenin: every bottle contains 6000U agkistrodon halys antivenin. <br> (2) Agkistrodon Acutus Snake Antivenin: every bottle contains 2000U agkistrodon acutus snake antivenin. <br> (3) Bungarus multicnctus Antivenin: every bottle contains 10 000U bungarus multicnctus antivenin. <br> (4) Naja Antivenin: every bottle contains 1000U naja antivenin. |
| 药品名称 Drug Names | 人血白蛋白 Human Albumin |
| 适应证 <br> Indications | 用于治疗因失血、创伤及烧伤等引起的休克，脑水肿及大脑损伤所致的脑压增高，防治低蛋白血症以及肝硬化或肾病引起的水肿和腹水，有较好的疗效。 <br><br> For the treatment of shock caused by blood loss, trauma and burns, etc. cerebral edema and increased intracranial pressure by brain damage. For the prevention and treatment of edema and ascites caused by hypoalbuminemia and cirrhosis or kidney disease |
| 用法、用量 <br> Dosage | 静脉滴注，用量由医师酌定。一般因严重烧伤或失血等所致的休克可直接注射本品 5 ~ 10g，隔 4 ~ 6 小时重复注射一次。在治疗肾病及肝硬化等慢性白蛋白缺乏症时，可每日注射本品 5 ~ 10g，直至水肿消失、血清白蛋白恢复正常为止。 <br><br> The dosage of intravenous infusion is decided by the physicians. Generally the shock due to severe burns or blood loss can be treated with the injection of this product of 5 ~ 10g directly. The injections should be repeated every 4 to 6 hours. In the treatment of chronic albumin deficiency, such as kidney disease, cirrhosis and so on, this product could be injected with 5 ~ 10g everyday till edema disappears and serum albumin restores to normal. |
| 剂型、规格 <br> Preparations | 注射液：1g（10ml）；2g（10ml）；2.5g（10ml）；5g（10ml）；10g（50ml）；12.5g（50ml）；25g（125ml）。 <br><br> 冻干品：10g；20g。 <br><br> Injection: 1g (10ml), 2g (10ml), 2.5g (10ml), 5g (10ml), 10g (50ml), 12.5g (50ml), 25g (125ml). <br> Lyophilized: 10g, 20g |
| 药品名称 Drug Names | 人免疫球蛋白 Human Immunoglobulin |
| 适应证 <br> Indications | 主要用于预防麻疹和甲型肝炎等病毒性感染。 <br> Mainly used for the prevention of viral infections of measles and hepatitis A. |
| 用法、用量 <br> Dosage | （1）预防麻疹：0.05 ~ 0.15ml/kg 或 5 岁以内儿童注射 1.5 ~ 3ml，成人不得超过 6ml，预防效果为 1 个月。 <br><br> （2）预防甲型肝炎：按每千克体重注射 0.05 ~ 0.1ml/kg 或儿童每次注射 1.5 ~ 3ml，成人每次注射 3ml。1 次注射，预防效果为 1 个月。 <br><br> (1) Prevention of measles: 0.05 ~ 0.15ml/kg for injection. Children less than 5 years old can have the injection of 1.5 ~ 3ml or, the dosage for adults is not more than 6ml. The results of the prevention last for one month. <br><br> (2) Prevention of Hepatitis A: the injection is 0.05 ~ 0.1ml/kg according to the body weight. Children have the injection of 1.5 ~ 3ml for each time, while adults have the injection of 3ml for each time. The results of the prevention last for one month per injection. |

**续 表**

| | |
|---|---|
| 剂型、规格<br>Preparations | 注射液：10%/1.5ml（150mg）；10%/3ml（300mg）。<br>Injection: 10% / 1.5ml (150mg), 10% / 3ml (300mg). |
| 药品名称 Drug Names | 乙型肝炎人免疫球蛋白 Human Hepatitis B Immunoglobulin |
| 适应证<br>Indications | 用于乙型肝炎的预防。主要适用于：①乙型肝炎表面抗原阳性母亲的新生儿。②预防意外感染人群，如血友病患者、肾透析患者、医务人员或皮肤破损被乙型肝炎表面抗原阳性的血液或分泌物污染的人员等。③与乙型肝炎患者或携带者密切接触的易感人群。<br><br>For hepatitis B prevention. Mainly used by: ① newborns whose mother is HBsAg positive. ② accidental infected people, such as patients with hemophilia, kidney dialysis patients, medical personnel or people with skin damage which is affected by blood or secretions when Hepatitis B surface is antigen-positive. ③ susceptible populations who have close contact with patients with hepatitis B or carriers . |
| 用法、用量<br>Dosage | （1）母婴阻断：乙型肝炎表面抗原阳性母亲的婴儿出生24小时内，肌内注射100～200U，同时联合乙型肝炎疫苗，按乙型肝炎疫苗注射程序全程注射（按照0个月、1个月、6个月或医生推荐的适宜方案）；亦可在婴儿出生24小时内肌内注射100～200U，1个月时在注射一次，同时按乙型肝炎疫苗注射程序全程注射。单独使用乙型肝炎免疫球蛋白很少获得满意结果，如果单独使用应多次注射，每3～4周1次，每次肌内注射100～200U。<br>（2）乙型肝炎预防：用于预防意外暴露时，注射越早越好，一般应在24小时内进行肌内注射，最迟不超过7日。一次注射量，儿童为100U，成人为200U，必要时剂量可加倍，每3～4周再注射1次，必要时按注射程序全程注射乙型肝炎疫苗。<br><br>(1) PMTCT: babies, whose mothers are hepatitis B surface antigen-positive, should be injected 100～200U in intramuscular injection within the 24 hours following their birth, in combination with the full-course injection of hepatitis B vaccine according to the injection procedure (in accordance with appropriate solutions of 0, 1, 6 months or with what doctors recommend); babies can also be injected 100～200U in intramuscular injection within the 24 hours following their birth, and then can be injected with full-course injection one more time when they are one month old according to the injection procedure of hepatitis B vaccine. The single use of hepatitis B immune globulin rarely obtains satisfactory results. If used alone, it should be injected for multiple times. It is usually injected once every 3 to 4 weeks with 100～200U in intramuscular injection.<br>(2) Prevention of Hepatitis B: it is used for the prevention of accidental exposure. The sooner the injection starts, the better the results will be. It is usually injected within 24 hours in intramuscular injection. It can be injected no later than 7 days. The dosage of one injection for children is 100U, and for adults is 200U. If necessary, the dose may be doubled and may be injected once again every 3 to 4 weeks. If necessary, hepatitis B vaccine can be injected with the full-course injection according to the injection procedure. |
| 剂型、规格<br>Preparations | 注射液（冻干）：乙型肝炎免疫球蛋白 100U；200U；400U。<br>Injection (lyophilized): Hepatitis B immunoglobulin 100U, 200U, 400U. |
| 药品名称 Drug Names | 破伤风人免疫球蛋白 Human Tetanus Immunoglobulin |
| 适应证<br>Indications | 用于预防和治疗破伤风，尤其适用于对破伤风抗毒素（TAT）有过敏反应的患者。<br><br>For the prophylaxis and treatment of tetanus, especially for patients with allergic reactions of tetanus antitoxin (TAT). |
| 用法、用量<br>Dosage | 肌内注射。①预防用：儿童、成人一次用量均为250U。创面严重或创面严重和感染严重者可加倍注射。②治疗用：3000～6000U。可多点注射。<br><br>Intramuscular injection: ① preventive: the dosage for one time is 250U for both children and adults, . For people whose wound is serious and people whose wound is with serious infections, the dosage for injection should double. ② for treatment: 3000～6000U. Multi-point injection is feasible. |
| 剂型、规格<br>Preparations | 注射液：100U；200U；250U。<br>注射剂（冻干品）：100U；200U；250U。<br><br>Injection: 100U, 200U, 250U.<br>Injection (lyophilized product): 100U, 200U, 250U. |

**续 表**

| 药品名称 Drug Names | 狂犬病人免疫球蛋白 Human Rabies Immunoglobulin |
|---|---|
| 适应证<br>Indications | 　　本品主要配合狂犬病疫苗使用，当被狂犬或其他疯动物严重咬伤者，进行狂犬病疫苗预防注射的同时，配合使用本品，对狂犬病做紧急的被动免疫，以提高预防性治疗效果。<br><br>　　This product is mainly used together with the rabies vaccine. If One is bitten by rabid animals, it is better to take rabies vaccine injections together with Human Rabies Immunoglobulin, which helps to improve the prophylactic treatment when doing passive immunotherapy. |
| 用法、用量<br>Dosage | 　　肌内注射：动物咬伤部位及时清创后，于受伤部位用本品总剂量的 1/2 做皮下浸润注射，余下制剂进行肌内注射（头部咬伤者可于背部肌内注射），按体重每千克 20U（或遵医嘱），一次注射，如所需剂量大于 10ml，可于 1～2 日分次注射。同时或随后即可进行狂犬病疫苗注射，但两种制品的注射部位和器具应严格分开。<br><br>　　Intramuscular injection: after the animal bite is treated timely with debridement, 1/2 of this total dose is used in the injured area with subcutaneous infiltration injection, while the remaining preparations is used with intramuscular injection of (for people whose heads are bitten, the intramuscular injection on the back is available), 20U per kilogram of body weight (or as professionally prescribed). If the total dose for one injection is greater than 10ml, the injections can be finished within 1 to 2 days. The injection of rabies vaccine can be done simultaneously or subsequently, but the injection site and utensils of the two products should be strictly separated. |
| 剂型、规格<br>Preparations | 　　注射液：100U；200U；500U。注射剂（冻干品）：100U；200U；500U。<br>　　Injection: 100U, 200U, 500U. Injection (lyophilized product): 100U, 200U, 500U. |
| 药品名称 Drug Names | 人纤维蛋白原 Human Fibrinogen |
| 适应证<br>Indications | 　　①遗传性纤维蛋白原减少症，包括遗传性异常纤维蛋白原血症或遗传性纤维蛋白原缺乏症。②获得性纤维蛋白原减少症，主要见于严重肝脏损害所致的纤维蛋白原合成不足及局部或弥散性血管内凝血导致纤维蛋白原消耗量增加。<br><br>　　① For the treatment of fibrinogen decrease, including genetic or dysfibrinogenemia or hereditary fibrinogen. ② For the treatment of acquired fibrinogen deficiency, mainly including deficiency in fibrinogen synthesis caused by severe liver damage caused and increase to consumption of fibrinogen caused by local or disseminated intravascular coagulation. |
| 用法、用量<br>Dosage | 　　静脉注射：其用量视血浆纤维蛋白原水平及要达到止血所学的纤维蛋白原水平（1g/L）而定。由于纤维蛋白原的生物半衰期长达 96～144 小时，故开始每 1～2 日，以后每 3～4 日，滴注 1 次即可。能够按每 2g 纤维蛋白原可使血浆纤维蛋白原水平升至 0.5g/L 的原则推算所需剂量，一般首次用量 1～2g，必要时可加量。大出血时应立即给予 4～8g。<br><br>　　Intravenous injection: the dosage depends on and plasma fibrinogen levels and the fibrinogen levels (1g / L) needed for hemostasis. As the biological half-life of fibrinogen is as long as 96 to 144 hours, there is only 1 drip needed every 1 to 2 days at the beginning, then also one drip every 3 to 4 days in the following days. The dosage can be calculated according to the principle that every 2g fibrinogen can make plasma fibrinogen levels rise to 0.5g / L. Generally the initial dose is 1 ~ 2g and can be increased if necessary. 4g to 8g should be given immediately if there is massive hemorrhage. |
| 剂型、规格<br>Preparations | 　　注射剂（冻干品）：每支 0.5g。<br>　　Injection (lyophilized product): 0.5g per vial. |
| 药品名称 Drug Names | 重组人干扰素 α-1b　Recombinant Human Interferon α-1b |
| 适应证<br>Indications | 　　用于病毒性疾病和某些恶性肿瘤。①已批准用于治疗慢性乙型肝炎、丙型肝炎和毛细胞白血病。②已有临床试验结果或文献报道，用于病毒性疾病，如带状疱疹、尖锐湿疣、流行性出血热和小儿呼吸道合胞病毒肺炎等。③用于治疗恶性肿瘤，如慢性粒细胞白血病、黑色素瘤、淋巴瘤等。④滴眼液，可用于眼部病毒性疾病。<br><br>　　For the treatment of viral diseases and certain malignancy ① It has been approved for the treatment of chronic hepatitis B, hepatitis C and hairy cell hemophilia. ② Clinical trial and documents have been ready to prove that it can be used to treat viral diseases, such as herpes zoster, Condyloma acuminatum, epidemic hemorrhagic fever and pediatric respiratory syncytial virus pneumonia, etc. ③ For the treatment of malignant tumors, such as chronic myelogenous leukemia, melanoma, lymphoma, etc. ④ The sort of eye drop can be used for ocular viral diseases. |

续　表

| 用法、用量<br>Dosage | （1）慢性乙型肝炎：一次 30 ~ 50µg，隔日一次，疗程为 4 ~ 6 个月，可根据病情延长疗程至一年，也可进行诱导治疗，即在治疗开始时，每天用药 1 次，0.5 ~ 1 个月后改为每周 3 次，直到疗程结束。<br><br>（2）慢性丙型肝炎：一次 30 ~ 50µg，隔日一次，疗程 4 ~ 6 个月，无效者停用。有效者可继续治疗至 12 个月。根据病情需要，可延长至 18 个月。在治疗的第 1 个月，一日 1 次。疗程结束后随访 6 ~ 12 个月。急性丙型肝炎，应及早使用本品治疗，可减少慢性化。<br><br>（3）慢性粒细胞白血病：一次 30 ~ 50µg，一日 1 次，连续用药 6 个月以上。可根据病情适当调整，缓解后可改为隔日注射。<br><br>（4）肿瘤：视病情可延长疗程。如患者未出现病情恶化或严重不良反应，应当在适当剂量下继续用药。<br><br>(1) Chronic hepatitis B: 30 ~ 50µg for each time, once every other day, 4 to 6 months is a course of treatment. The course of treatment may be extended to one year of according to the severity of patient's conditon. Induction therapy is also possible, one time a day at the starting of treatment, then three times a week 0.5 ~ 1 month later till the end of treatment<br><br>(2) chronic hepatitis C: 30 ~ 50µgµ for each time, once every other day, four to six months is a course of treatment. People, for whom the treatment is ineffective, should stop it. People, for whom the treatment is effective, can continue the treatment for 12 months. According to the severity of patient's condition, the treatment may be extended to 18 months. People can take it 1 time a day in the first month of treatment. After the treatment is finished, a following-up visit of 6 to 12 months should be done. People with acute hepatitis C should start the treatment early, which can reduce chronicity.<br><br>(3) chronic myeloid leukemia: 30 ~ 50µg for each time, once a day, there should be more than six months of continuous medication. It can be adjusted according to the severity of patien's condition. The treatment can be changed to once every other day until the patient is in remission.<br><br>(4) tumors: the treatment can be extended depending on the severity of patient's conditon. If the patient;s condition doesn't worsen or doesn't have severe adverse reactions, the treatment should continue in appropriate doses. |
| --- | --- |
| 剂型、规格<br>Preparations | 注射剂（冻干品）：10µg（10 万 U）；20µg（20 万 U）；30µg（30 万 U）；50µg（50 万 U）。<br>Injection (lyophilized): 10µg (100, 000U); 20µg (200, 000U); 30µg (300, 000U); 50µg (500, 000U). |
| **药品名称 Drug Names** | 重组人白细胞介素 -2　Recombinant Human Interleukin-2 |
| 适应证<br>Indications | ①用于肾细胞癌、黑色素瘤，用于控制晚期腹水及其他晚期肿瘤。②用于先天或后天免疫缺陷症，如艾滋病等。③对某些病毒性、细菌性疾病、胞内寄生感染性疾病，如乙型肝炎、麻风病、肺结核、白念珠菌感染等，有一定作用。<br><br>① For the treatment of renal cell carcinoma, melanoma and management of advanced ascites and other advanced cancer. ② For the treatment of congenital or acquired immunodeficiency syndrome, such as AIDS. ③ Limited effect on the treatment of viral diseases, bacterial diseases and intracellular parasitic infections, such as hepatitis B, leprosy, tuberculosis, candida albicans, etc. |
| 用法、用量<br>Dosage | 皮下注射：20 万 ~ 40 万 U/m$^2$ 加入灭菌注射用水 2ml，一日 1 次，每周注射 4 日，4 周为 1 个疗程。肌内注射：慢性乙型肝炎，一次 20 万 U，隔日 1 次。静脉滴注：20 万 ~ 40 万 U/m$^2$，加入注射用生理盐水 500ml，一日 1 次，每周连用 4 日，4 周为 1 个疗程。腔内注射：先抽去腔内积液，再将本品 40 万 ~ 50 万 U/m$^2$ 加入注射用生理盐水 20ml 注入，1 周 1 ~ 2 次，3 ~ 4 周为 1 疗程。瘤内、瘤周注射：10 万 ~ 30 万 U 加入注射用生理盐水 3 ~ 5ml，分多点注射到瘤内或瘤周，一周 2 次，连用 2 周为 1 个疗程。<br><br>Subcutaneous injection: Add 2ml sterile water for injection into 200, 000 ~ 400, 000U/m$^2$. Once a day and four days a week for injection. 4 weeks can be a course of treatment. Intramuscular injection: chronic hepatitis B, once every other day with 200, 000U. Intravenous infusion: Add 500ml saline for injection into 200, 000 ~ 400, 000U/m$^2$, 1 time per day, four consecutive days in a week, 4 weeks can be a course of treatment. Intrapleural injection: first remove the effusion in the intracvitary, then inject the product 400 000 ~ 500 000U/m$^2$ with 20ml saline 1 or 2 times a week, 3 to 4 weeks as a course of treatment. Intratumoral peritumoral injection: 100, 000 to 300, 000U injected with 3 ~ 5ml saline for injection. Put most of the injection into the intratumoral and peritumoral area. Twice a week, 2 consecutive weeks is a course of treatment. |

**续 表**

| 剂型、规格<br>Preparations | 注射剂（冻干品）：每支 50 万 U；100 万 U；200 万 U；1800 万 U。<br>Injection (lyophilized): 500, 000U; 1 millon U; 2 millon U; 18 millon U per vial. |
|---|---|
| **药品名称 Drug Names** | 结核菌素纯蛋白衍生物 Purified Protein Derivative of Tuberculin（TB-PPD） |
| 适应证<br>Indications | 本品 5U 用于结核病的临床诊断，卡介苗接种对象的选择及卡介苗接种后机体免疫反应的监测。2U 制品用于临床诊断及流行病学监测。<br><br>This product 5U is used for clinical diagnosis of tuberculosis, choice of BCG vaccination and monitoring of immune response after BCG vaccination and. The 2U product is used for clinical diagnosis and epidemiological surveillance. |
| 用法、用量<br>Dosage | ①婴儿、儿童及成人均可用。②皮内注射，吸取本品 0.1ml（5U），皮内注射于前臂掌侧，于注射后 48 ～ 72 小时检查注射部位反应。测量应以硬结的横径及其垂直径的毫米数记录。5U 制品反应平均直径应不低于 5mm 为阳性反应。凡有水疱、坏死、淋巴管炎者均属阳性反应，应详细注明。<br><br>① infants, children and adults are all suitable for it. ② the intradermal injection: draw the product 0.1ml (5U) and inject it in the forearm palm-side. Test the response of the injection site 48 to 72 hours after the injection. Records should be measured in mm of diameter and vertical diameter of the induration. The average diameter of the 5U that is not less than 5mm in the reaction is positive. Any case with blisters, necrosis, lymphangitis are positive and should be specified in detail. |
| 剂型、规格<br>Preparations | 注射剂：每瓶 1ml；2ml。①每 1 次人用剂量为 0.1ml 含 5UTB-PPD。②每 1 次人用剂量为 0.1ml 含 2U TB-PPD。<br><br>Injection: 1ml; 2ml per vial. ① the dose for one person is 0.1ml containing 5UTB-PPD. ② the dose for one person is 0.1ml containing 2U TB-PPD. |
| **药品名称 Drug Names** | 布氏菌纯蛋白衍生物 Purified Protein Derivative of Brucellin（BR-PPD） |
| 适应证<br>Indications | 可用于布氏疫苗接种对象的选择及布氏疫苗接种后机体免疫反应的监测和布氏菌的临床诊断与流行病学调查。<br><br>It can be used as vaccination of Brucellin to monitor the immune response after Brucella vaccination and to carry out epidemiological investigation and Clinical diagnosis of Brucellin. |
| 用法、用量<br>Dosage | 用药途径：吸取本品 0.1ml（1U）皮内注射于前臂掌侧。于注射后 48 ～ 72 小时的检查注射部位反应，测量时应以硬节的横径及其垂直径的毫米数记录之。反应平均直径应不低于 5mm 为阳性。凡有水疱、坏死、淋巴管炎者均属阳性反应，应详细注明。<br><br>Route of administration: draw this product 0.1ml (1U) and inject it into forearm palm-side in intradermal injection. After the injection of 48 to 72 hours, check the injection site reactions. The record should be measured in millimeters of diameter and vertical diameter of the induration. The average diameter that is not less than 5mm in the reaction is positive. Any case with blisters, necrosis and lymphangitis are positive and should be specified in detail. |
| 剂型、规格<br>Preparations | 注射液：每支 1ml；2ml。每人用量为 0.1ml 含 1U UBR-PPD。<br><br>Injection: 1ml per vial; 2ml per vial. Dosage for one person is 0.1ml including 1U UBR-PPD. |

# 第3章

# 中文—法文对照药品临床使用说明

Instructions pour l'application clinique du médicament(Chinois – Français)

| 1. 抗生素 Antibiotiques | |
|---|---|
| 1.1　青霉素类 Pénicillines | |
| 药品名称 Drug Names | 青霉素 Pénicilline |
| 适应证<br>Les indications | 　　青霉素用于敏感菌所致的急性感染，如菌血症、败血症、猩红热、丹毒、肺炎、脓胸、扁桃体炎、中耳炎、蜂窝织炎、疖、痈、急性乳腺炎、心内膜炎、骨髓炎、流行性脑膜炎（流脑）、钩端螺旋体病（对本病早期疗效较好），奋森咽峡炎、创伤感染、回归热、气性坏疽、炭疽、淋病、放线菌病等。治疗破伤风、白喉宜与相应的抗毒素联用。<br>　　普鲁卡因青霉素吸收缓慢，肌内注射 30 万 U，血药浓度峰值约 2U/ml，24 小时仍可测得。适用于梅毒和一些敏感菌所致的慢性感染。<br>　　苄星青霉素吸收极缓慢，血药浓度低，适用于需长期使用青霉素预防的患者，如慢性风湿性心脏病患者。<br>　　Les pénicillines sont utilisées dans le traitement d'infections bactériennes, telles que la bactériémie, la septicémie, la scarlatine, l'érésipèle, la pneumonie, l'empyème, l'amygdalite, l'otite moyenne, la cellulite, le furoncle, la mammite aiguë, l'endocardite, l'ostéomyélite, la méningite cérébro spinale, la leptospirose (efficace au stade précoce), l'angine de Vincent, l'infection des plaies, la fièvre récurrente, la gangrène gazeuse, l'anthrax, la blennorragie, l'actinomycose, etc. Quand il s'agit du traitement du tétanos et de la diphtérie, il vaut mieux utiliser la pénicilline en association avec l'antitoxine concernée.<br>　　La résorption de la procaïne pénicilline G est lente. L'administration intramusculaire de 300 000 unités de pénicilline G chez des adultes engendre des concentrations sanguines maximales d'environ 2 unités par mL, ce qui est testé en 24 heures. Elle sert contre la syphilis et des infections bactériennes chroniques.<br>　　lpénicilline est extrêmement lente. Ses concentrations sanguines sont basses. Elle est utilisée dans le traitement des patients qui utilisent pour une longue durée la pénicilline pour la prévention, tels que les malades atteints de cardiopathie rhumatismale chronique. |
| 用法、用量<br>Les modes d'emploi et la posologie | 　　青霉素钠常用于肌内注射或静脉滴注。肌内注射成人一日量为 80 万～ 320 万 U，儿童一日量为 3 万～ 5 万 U/kg，分为 2 ～ 4 次给予。静脉滴注适用于重病，如感染性心内膜炎、化脓性脑膜炎患者。成人一日量为 240 万～ 2000 万 U，儿童一日量为 20 万～ 40 万 U/kg，分 4 ～ 6 次加至少量输液中做间歇快速滴注。输液的青霉素（钠盐）浓度一般为 1 万～ 4 万 U/ml。本品溶液（20 万～ 40 万 U/2 ～ 4ml）可用于气雾吸入，一日 2 次。<br>　　青霉素钾通常用于肌内注射，由于注射局部较痛，可以用 0.25% 利多卡因注射液作为溶剂（2% 苯甲醇注射液已不用），钾盐也可静脉滴注，但必须注意患者体内血钾浓度和输液的钾含量（每 100 万 U 青霉素 G 钾中含钾量为 65mg，与氯化钾 125mg 中的含钾量相近），并注意滴注速度不可太快。<br>　　普鲁卡因青霉素仅供肌内注射，1 次量 40 万～ 80 万 U，每日 1 次。<br>　　苄星青霉素仅供肌内注射，1 次 60 万 U，10 ～ 14 日 1 次；1 次 120 万 U，14 ～ 21 日 1 次。 |

|  | Lapénicilline sodiqueest souvent administrée par voie intramusculaire (IM) ou en perfusion. Chez des adultes, 800 000 à 3,2 millions d'unités/jour par voie IM ; chez des enfants, 30 000 à 50 000 unités/kg/jour, à travers deux à quatre fois par jour. L'administration en perfusion est réservée aux patients gravement malades, tels que les patients atteints d'endocardite infectieuse ou de méningite purulente. Chez des adultes, 2,4 millions à 20 millions d'unités/jour ; chez des enfants, 200 000 à 400 000 unités/kg/jour, à travers quatre à six fois en perfusion rapide intermittente. La concentration de la pénicilline sodique est d'ordre de 10 000 à 40 000 unités/ml. Ce produit sous forme de solution (200 000 à 400 000 unités/2à 4 ml) peut être utilisé par l'inhalation d'aérosol, deux fois par jour.

La pénicilline de potassium est souvent administrée par voie IM.Il est recommandé d'y inclure 0,25 % d'injection de lidocaïne pour soulager la douleur (2 % d'injection de l'alcool benzylique ne sert plus). Ce produit peut être aussi administré par voie IV en perfusion, mais il faut faire attention à la concentration sanguine en potassium et à la teneur en potassium de l'injection (1 million d'unités de pénicilline G de potassium contient 65 mg de potassium, avec une teneur en potassium similaire à celle de 125 mg de chlorure de potassium). La perfusion ne doit pas être trop rapide.

La procaïne pénicilline G ne peut être administrée que par voie IM. 400 000 à 800 000 unités par fois, une fois par jour.

La benzylpénicillinene peut être administrée que par voie IM. 600 000 unités par fois, tous les 10 à 14 jours ; 1,2 million d'unités par fois, tous les 14 à 21 jours. |
|---|---|
| 剂型、规格<br>Les formes pharmaceutiques et les spécifications | 注射用青霉素钠：每支（瓶）0.24g（40 万 U）、0.48g（80 万 U）或 0.6g（100 万 U）。<br>注射用青霉素钾：每支 0.25g（40 万 U）。<br>注射用普鲁卡因青霉素：每瓶 40 万 U 者，含普鲁卡因青霉素 30 万 U 及青霉素钾盐或钠盐 10 万 U；每瓶 80 万 U 者其含量加倍。既有长效，又有速效作用。每次肌内注射 40 万～80 万 U，每日 1 次。<br>注射用苄星青霉素（长效青霉素，长效西林）：每瓶 120 万 U，肌内注射。<br>La pénicilline sodique pour injection : 0,24 g (400 000 unités) par flacon, 0,48 g (800 000 unités) par flacon ou 0,6 g (1 million d'unités) par flacon.<br>La pénicilline de potassium pour injection : 0,25 g (400 000 unités) par flacon.<br>La procaïne pénicilline G pour injection : celle qui contient 400 000 unités par flacon est composée de 300 000 unités de procaïne pénicilline G et de 100 000 unités de pénicilline de sodium ou de potassium ; celle qui contient 800 000 unités par flacon est composée de 600 000 unités de procaïne pénicilline G et de 200 000 unités de pénicilline de sodium ou de potassium. Son action peut être brève ou prolongée. L'administration par voie IM : 400 000 à 800 000 unités par fois, une fois par jour.<br>La benzylpénicilline pour injection (la pénicilline à action prolongée) : 1,2 million d'unités par flacon, l'administration par voie IM. |
| 药品名称 Drug Names | 青霉素 V Phénoxyméthylpénicilline |
| 适应证<br>Les indications | 青霉素用于敏感菌所致的急性感染，如菌血症、败血症、猩红热、丹毒、肺炎、脓胸、扁桃体炎、中耳炎、蜂窝织炎、疖、痈、急性乳腺炎、心内膜炎、骨髓炎、流行性脑膜炎（流脑）、钩端螺旋体病（对本病早期疗效较好）、奋森咽峡炎、创伤感染、回归热、气性坏疽、炭疽、淋病、放线菌病等。治疗破伤风、白喉宜与相应的抗毒素联用。<br>普鲁卡因青霉素吸收缓慢，肌内注射 30 万 U，血药浓度峰值约 2U/ml，24 小时仍可测得。适用于梅毒和一些敏感菌所致的慢性感染。<br>苄星青霉素吸收极缓慢，血药浓度低，适用于需长期使用青霉素预防的患者，如慢性风湿性心脏病患者。<br>Les pénicillines sont utilisées dans le traitement d'infections bactériennes, telles que la bactériémie, la septicémie, la scarlatine, l'érésipèle, la pneumonie, l'empyème, l'amygdalite, l'otite moyenne, la cellulite, le furoncle, la mammite aiguë, l'endocardite, l'ostéomyélite, la méningite cérébro spinale, la leptospirose (efficace au stade précoce), l'angine de Vincent, l'infection des plaies, la fièvre récurrente, la gangrène gazeuse, l'anthrax, la blennorragie, l'actinomycose, etc. Quand il s'agit du traitement du tétanos et de la diphtérie, il vaut mieux utiliser la pénicilline en association avec l'antitoxine concernée.<br>La résorption de la procaïne pénicilline G est lente. L'administration intramusculaire de 300 000 unités de pénicilline G chez des adultes engendre des concentrations sanguines maximales d'environ 2 unités par mL, ce qui est testé en 24 heures. Elle sert contre la syphilis et des infections bactériennes chroniques.<br>Lpénicilline est extrêmement lente. Ses concentrations sanguines sont basses. Elle est utilisée dans le traitement des patients qui utilisent pour une longue durée la pénicilline pour la prévention, tels que les malades atteints de cardiopathie rhumatismale chronique. |

续　表

| | |
|---|---|
| 用法、用量<br>Les modes d'emploi et la posologie | 口服。成人：125 ～ 500mg（20 万～ 80 万 U）/ 次，每 6 ～ 8 小时 1 次。儿童：每日 15 ～ 50mg/kg，分 3 ～ 6 次服用。<br><br>L'administration par voie orale. Chez des adultes : 125 à 500 mg (200 000 à 800 000 unités) par fois, toutes les 6 à 8 heures. Chez des enfants : 15 à 50 mg par kg, à travers 3 à 6 fois. |
| 剂型、规格<br>Les formes pharmaceutiques et les spécifications | 片剂、胶囊剂：每片或粒 125mg（20 万 U）；250mg（40 万 U）；500mg（80 万 U）。还有颗粒剂或口服干糖浆。<br><br>Comprimés et capsules : 125 mg (200 000 unités),250 mg (400 000 unités)ou 500 mg (800 000 unités) par comprimé ou par capsule. Ce produit sous forme de granule et de sirop sec oral est aussi disponible. |
| 药品名称 Drug Names | 苯唑西林钠 Oxacilline sodique |
| 适应证<br>Les indications | 本品主要用于产酶的金黄色葡萄球菌和表皮葡萄球菌的周围感染，包括内脏、皮肤和软组织等部位的感染，但对耐甲氧西林金黄色葡萄球菌（MSRA）感染无效。对中枢感染不适用。<br><br>L'oxacilline sodique est utilisée comme traitement des infections causées par des staphylocoques dorésproducteurs de pénicillinase et des staphylococcus epidermidis, y compris des infections viscérales, cutanées et des tissus mous. Mais ce produit est inutile dans le traitement des staphylococcus aureus résistant à la méticilline (SARM). Il n'est pas applicable dans le traitement de l'infection du système nerveux central. |
| 用法、用量<br>Les modes d'emploi et la posologie | 静脉滴注：1 次 1 ～ 2g，必要时可用到 3g，溶于 100ml 输液内滴注 0.5 ～ 1 小时，一日 3 ～ 4 次。小儿每日用量 50 ～ 100mg/kg，分次给予。肌内注射：1 次 1g，一日 3 ～ 4 次。口服、肌内注射均较少用。肾功能轻中度不足者可按正常用量，重度不足者应适当减量。<br><br>L'administration par voie IV en perfusion : 1 à 2 g par fois, 3 g le cas échéant, dissoudre dans 100ml d'infusion pour la perfusion pendant 0,5 à 1h, 3 à 4 fois par jour. Chez des enfants, 50 à 100 mg/kg/jour, à plusieurs reprises. L'administration par voie IM : 1 g par fois, 3 à 4 fois par jour. L'administration par voie orale et par voie IM est relativement rarement pratiquée. Les patients insuffisants rénaux chroniques peuvent prendre la dose usuelle, alors que les patients insuffisants rénaux aigues doivent diminuer la dose. |
| 剂型、规格<br>Les formes pharmaceutiques et les spécifications | 注射用苯唑西林钠：每瓶 0.5g；1g（效价）。<br>L'oxacilline sodique pour injection : 0,5 g ou 1 g par flacon (titre). |
| 药品名称 Drug Names | 氯唑西林钠 Cloxacilline sodique |
| 适应证<br>Les indications | 主要用于产酶金黄色葡萄球菌或不产酶葡萄球菌所致的败血症、肺炎、心内膜炎、骨髓炎或皮肤软组织感染等。但对耐甲氧西林金黄色葡萄球菌（MSRA）感染无效。<br><br>La cloxacilline de sodium est utilisée comme traitement des infections causées par des staphylocoques dorés producteurs de pénicillinase ou des staphylocoquesnon producteurs de pénicillinase, y compris la septicémie, la pneumonie, l'endocardite, l'ostéomyélite et les infections de la peau et des tissus mous. Mais ce produit est inutile dans le traitement des staphylococcus aureus résistant à la méticilline (SARM). |
| 用法、用量<br>Les modes d'emploi et la posologie | 肌内注射：1 次 0.5 ～ 1g，一日 3 ～ 4 次。静脉滴注：一次 1 ～ 2g，溶于 100ml 输液中，滴注 0.5 ～ 1 小时，一日 3 ～ 4 次。小儿每日用量 30 ～ 50mg/kg，分次给予。口服剂量：每次 0.25 ～ 0.5g，一日 4 次，空腹服用。<br><br>L'administration par voie IM : 0,5 à 1 g par fois, 3 à 4 fois par jour.L'administration par voie IV en perfusion : 1 à 2 g par fois, plus 100 ml d'eau pour injection de 0,5 à 1 h, 3 à 4 fois par jour.Chez des enfants, 30 à 50 mg/kg/jour, à travers plusieurs fois.L'administration par voie orale : 0,25 à 0,5 g par fois, 4 fois par jour, l'estomac vide. |
| 剂型、规格<br>Les formes pharmaceutiques et les spécifications | 注射用氯唑西林钠：每瓶 0.5g（效价）。<br>胶囊剂：每胶囊 0.125g；0.25g；0.5g。<br>颗粒剂：50mg。<br><br>La cloxacilline de sodium pour injection : 0,5 g par flacon.<br>Comprimés : 0,125g, 0,25g ou 0,5 g par comprimé.<br>Granules : 50 mg. |

**续 表**

| 药品名称 Drug Names | 氟氯西林 Flucloxacilline |
|---|---|
| 适应证<br>Les indications | 主要应用于葡萄球菌所致的各种周围感染，但对耐甲氧西林金黄色葡萄球菌（MSRA）感染无效。<br><br>La flucloxacilline est utilisée comme traitement des infections causées par des staphylocoques, mais ce produit est inutile dans le traitement des staphylococcus aureus résistant à la méticilline (SARM). |
| 用法、用量<br>Les modes d'emploi et la posologie | 口服（用游离酸）：常用量为每次 250mg，一日 3 次；重症用量为每次 500mg，一日 4 次，于食前 0.5 ～ 1 小时空腹服用。肌内注射：常用量为每次 250mg，一日 3 次；重症用量为每次 500mg，一日 4 次。静脉注射：每次 500mg，一日 4 次，将药物溶于 10 ～ 20ml 注射用水或葡萄糖输液中使用，每 4 ～ 6 小时 1 次。一日量不超过 8g。儿童：2 岁以下按成人量的 1/4；2 ～ 10 岁按成人量的 1/2，根据体重适当调整。也可按照每日 25 ～ 50mg/kg，分次给予。<br><br>L'administration par voie orale (avec acide libre) : dose usuelle : 250 mg par fois, 3 fois par jour ; dose pour les patients gravement malades : 500 mg par fois, 4 fois par jour, 0,5 à 1 h avant le repas, l'estomac vide. L'administration par voie IM : dose usuelle : 250 mg par fois, 3 fois par jour ; dose pour les patients gravement malades : 500 mg par fois, 4 fois par jour. L'administration par voie IV : 500 mg par fois, 4 fois par jour, dissoudre dans 10 à 20 ml d'eau pour injection ou de solution de glucose, toutes les 4 à 6 heures, ne pas dépasser 8 g par jour. Chez des enfants : mois de 2 ans, 1/4 de la dosechez l'adulte ; de 2 à 10 ans, 1/2 de la dosechez l'adulte, ajuster la dose en fonction du poids. Il est aussi possible de prendre 25 à 50 mg/kg/jour, à travers plusieurs fois. |
| 剂型、规格<br>Les formes pharmaceutiques et les spécifications | 片剂（游离酸）：每片 125mg。<br>注射用氟氯西林钠：每瓶 500mg；1000mg。<br>Comprimés (avec acide libre) : 125 mg par comprimé.<br>La flucloxacilline pour injection : 500 mg ou 1 000 mg par flacon. |
| 药品名称 Drug Names | 氨苄西林 Ampicilline |
| 适应证<br>Les indications | 本品主要用于敏感菌所致的泌尿系统、呼吸系统、胆道、肠道感染以及脑膜炎、心内膜炎等。<br><br>L'ampicilline est utilisée comme traitement des infections causées par des staphylocoques, telles que les infections urinaires, respiratoires, des voies biliaires et intestinales, ainsi que le traitement de la méningite et de l'endocardite. |
| 用法、用量<br>Les modes d'emploi et la posologie | 口服：一日 50 ～ 100mg/kg，分成 4 次空腹服用；儿童一日 50 ～ 100mg/kg，分成 4 次。肌内注射：1 次 0.5 ～ 1g，一日 4 次；儿童一日 50 ～ 100mg/kg，分成 4 次。静脉滴注：1 次 1 ～ 2g，必要时可用到 3g，溶于 100ml 输液中，滴注 0.5 ～ 1 小时，一日 2 ～ 4 次，必要时每 4 小时 1 次；儿童一日 100 ～ 150mg/kg，分 4 次给予。<br><br>L'administration par voie orale : 50 à 100 mg/kg/jour, à travers 4 fois, l'estomac vide ; chez des enfants, 50 à 100 mg/kg/jour, à travers 4 fois. L'administration par voie IM : 0,5 à 1 g par fois, 4 fois par jour ; chez des enfants, 50 à 100 mg/kg/jour, à travers 4 fois. L'administration par voie IV en perfusion : 1 à 2 g par fois, 3 g le cas échéant,dissoudre dans 100ml d'infusion, la perfusion pendant 0,5 à 1h, 2 à 4 fois par jour, s'il est nécessaire, toutes les 4 heures ; chez des enfants, 100 à 150 mg/kg/jour, à travers 4 fois. |
| 剂型、规格<br>Les formes pharmaceutiques et les spécifications | 胶囊剂：每胶囊 0.25g。<br>注射用氨苄西林钠：每瓶 0.5g；1.0g。<br>Capsules: 0,25 g par capsule.<br>L'ampicilline pour injection : 0,5 g ou 1,0 g par flacon. |
| 药品名称 Drug Names | 阿莫西林 Amoxicilline |
| 适应证<br>Les indications | 常用于敏感菌所致的呼吸道、尿路和胆道感染及伤寒等。<br><br>L'ampicilline est utilisée comme traitement des infections causées par des staphylocoques, telles que les infections respiratoires, urinaires et des voies biliaires, ainsi que le traitement dela typhoïde. |

| | |
|---|---|
| 用法、用量<br>Les modes d'emploi et la posologie | 口服：成人每日 1 ～ 4g，分 3 ～ 4 次服。儿童每日 50 ～ 100mg/kg，分 3 ～ 4 次服。肾功能严重不足者，应延长用药间隔时间；肾小球滤过率（GFR）为 10 ～ 15ml/min 者，8 ～ 12 小时给药 1 次；＜ 10ml/min 者，12 ～ 16 小时给药 1 次。<br>　　L'administration par voie orale : chez des adultes, 1 à 4 g/jour, à travers 3 à 4 fois ; chez des enfants, 50 à 100 mg/kg/jour, à travers 3 à 4 fois.Les patients insuffisants rénaux aigues doivent prolonger l'intervalle de dosage.Pour ceux dont le débit de filtration glomérulaire (DFG) est de 10 à 15 ml/min, une administration toutes les 8 à 12 heures, alors que ceux dont le DFG est inférieur à 10 ml/min, une administration toutes les 12 à 16 heures. |
| 剂型、规格<br>Les formes pharmaceutiques et les spécifications | 片剂（胶囊）：每片（粒）0.125g；0.25g（效价）。<br>Comprimés (capsules) : 0,125 g ou 0,25 g par comprimé ou par capsule (titre). |
| 药品名称 Drug Names | 哌拉西林钠 Pipéracilline sodique |
| 适应证<br>Les indications | 临床上用于上述敏感菌中所引起的感染（对中枢感染疗效不确切）。<br>　　La pipéracilline sodiqueest utilisée dans les cliniques comme traitement des infections causées par des staphylocoques mentionnées précédemment. Mais son efficacité dans le traitement de l'infection du système nerveux central n'est pas certaine. |
| 用法、用量<br>Les modes d'emploi et la posologie | 尿路感染，1 次 1g，一日 4 次，肌内注射或静脉注射。其他部位（呼吸道、腹腔、胆道等）感染：一日 4 ～ 12g，分 3 ～ 4 次静脉注射或静脉滴注。严重感染一日可用 10 ～ 24g。<br>　　Pour les infections urinaires, 1 g par fois, 4 fois par jour, l'administration par voie IM ou IV. Pour les infections respiratoires, des voies biliaires et abdominales, 4 à 12 g par jour, à travers 3 à 4 fois, l'administration par voie IV ou par voie IV en perfusion. Pour les les infections graves, 10 à 24 g par jour. |
| 剂型、规格<br>Les formes pharmaceutiques et les spécifications | 注射用哌拉西林钠：每瓶 0.5g；1.0g（效价）。<br>La pipéracilline sodique pour injection : 0,5 g ou 1,0 g par flacon (titre). |
| 药品名称 Drug Names | 替卡西林 Ticarcilline |
| 适应证<br>Les indications | 主要用于革兰阴性菌感染，包括变形杆菌、大肠埃希菌、肠杆菌属、淋球菌、流感杆菌等所致全身感染，对尿路感染的效果好。对于铜绿假单胞菌感染，常需与氨基糖苷类抗生素联合应用。本品不耐酶，对 MRSA 也无效。<br>　　La ticarcilline est efficace dans le traitement de certaines bactéries à Gram négatif, y compris l'infection systémique causée par le proteus, le colibacille, l'enterobacter, le gonocoque et l'haemophilusinfluenzae. Elle est efficace dans le traitement des infections urinaires. Pour traiter l'infection à pseudomonasaeruginosa, il faut utiliser à la fois la ticarcilline et les aminosides. Ce produit est résistant aux enzymatique, il est inutile dans le traitement des SARM. |
| 用法、用量<br>Les modes d'emploi et la posologie | 成人一日 200 ～ 300mg/kg，分次给予或 1 次 3g，根据病情，每 3、4 或 6 小时 1 次。按每 1g 药物用 4ml 溶剂溶解后缓缓静脉注射或加入适量溶剂中静脉滴注 0.5 ～ 1 小时。泌尿系统感染可肌内注射给药，1 次 1g，每日 4 次，用 0.25% ～ 0.5% 利多卡因注射液 2 ～ 3ml 溶解后深部肌内注射。<br>　　儿童一日为 200 ～ 300mg/kg。婴儿一日为 225mg/kg，7 日龄以下婴儿则一日 150mg/kg，均分 3 次给予。<br>　　Chez des adultes, 200 à 300 mg/kg/jour, à travers plusieurs fois, ou 3g par fois, une administration toutes les 3, 4 ou 6 heures selon les cas. Pour 1g de ticarcilline, dissoudre 1g de ticarcilline dans 4ml de solvant, pour l'injection IV lente ou pour la perfusion pendant 0,5 à 1 h. Pour traiter les infections urinaires, on peut l'administrer par voie IM, 1 g par fois, 4 fois par jour, utiliser 2 à 3 ml d'injection de lidocaïne à0,25 % à 0,5 % pour la dissoudre avant de l'administrer par voie IM.<br>　　Chez des enfants, 200 à 300mg/kg/jour. Chez des bébés, 225 mg/kg/jour. Chez des bébés âgés moins de 7 jours, 150 mg/kg/jour, à travers 3 fois. |

**续 表**

| 剂型、规格<br>Les formes pharmaceutiques et les spécifications | 注射用替卡西林钠：每瓶 1g；3g；6g（效价）。<br>La ticarcilline sodique pour injection : 1 g, 3 g ou 6 g par flacon (titre). |
| --- | --- |
| 药品名称 Drug Names | 美洛西林钠 Mézlocilline sodique |
| 适应证<br>Les indications | 　　本品主要用于一些革兰阴性病原菌，如假单胞菌、克雷伯菌、肠杆菌属、沙雷菌、变形杆菌、大肠埃希菌、嗜血杆菌，以及拟杆菌和其他一些厌氧菌（包括革兰阳性的粪链球菌）所致的下呼吸道、腹腔、胆道、尿路、妇科、皮肤及软组织部位感染及败血症。<br>　　Ce produit est utilisé comme traitement des infections causées par des bactéries à Gram négatif (le pseudomonas, le klebsiella, l'enterobacter, le marcescens, le proteus, le colibacille, l'haemophilus, le bacteroides et des anaérobies), telles que les infections respiratoires, abdominales, des voies biliaires, urinaires, gynécologiques, cutanées et des tissus mous, ainsi que le traitement de la septicémie. |
| 用法、用量<br>Les modes d'emploi et la posologie | 　　用氯化钠液、葡萄糖液或乳酸钠林格液溶解后静脉注射或静脉滴注，也可肌内注射给药。成人一般感染每日 150～200mg/kg，或每次 2～3g，每 6 小时 1 次；重症感染每日 200～300mg/kg，或每次 3g，每 4 小时 1 次；极重感染可用到每日 24g 分 6 次用；淋球菌尿道炎，1～2g，只用 1 次，用前 0.5 小时服用丙磺舒 1g。<br>　　新生儿用量：≤ 7 日龄者，每日 150mg/kg 或 75mg/kg，每 12 小时 1 次。＞ 7 日龄者，根据体重不同可按每日 225～300mg/kg，或每次 75mg/kg，一日 3～4 次。肾功能受损者：肌酐清除率＞ 30ml/min 者，可按正常用量；10～30ml/min 者，按疾病轻重用每次 1.5～3g，每 8 小时一次；＜ 10ml/min 者，用 1.5g，每 8 小时 1 次，重症可用到 2g，每 8 小时 1 次。<br>　　手术预防感染给药：每次 4g，与术前 1 小时及术后 6～12 小时各给药 1 次。<br>　　Dissoudre le produit dans la solution de chlorure de sodium, la solution de glucose ou le liquide de Ringer avant de l'administrer par voie IV, par voie IV en perfusion ou par voie IM. Chez des adultes pour une dose usuelle, 150 à 200 mg/kg/jour, ou 2 à 3 g par fois, une administration toutes les 6 heures ; pour traiter des infections graves, 200 à 300 mg/kg/jour, ou 3 g par fois, une administration toutes les 4 heures ; pour traiter des infections extrêmement graves, 24 g par jour, à travers 6 fois ; pour traiter l'urétrite gonococcique, 1 à 2 g, seulement 1 fois, prendre 1 g de probénécide 0,5 h avant l'administration.<br>　　Chez des nouveau-nés moins de 7 jours, 150 mg/kg/jour ou 75 mg/kg/jour, une administration toutes les 12 heures. Chez des nouveau-nés plus de 7 jours, 225 à 300 mg/kg/jour en fonction du poids, ou 75 mg/kg/fois, 3 à 4 fois par jour. Chez des patients insuffisants rénaux : ceux dont la clairance de la créatinine est supérieure à 30 ml/min, utiliser une dose usuelle ; ceux dont la clairance de la créatinine est de 10 à 30 ml/min, utiliser 1,5 à 3 g par fois, une administration toutes les 8 heures ; ceux dont la clairance de la créatinine est inférieure à 10 ml/min, utiliser 1,5 g par fois, une administration toutes les 8 heures ; pour les patients gravement malades, 2 g, toutes les 8 heures.<br>　　L'administration de la prévention de l'infection chirurgicale : 4 g par fois, une administration 1h avant l'opération chirurgicale et une administration 6 à 12 h après l'opération. |
| 剂型、规格<br>Les formes pharmaceutiques et les spécifications | 粉针剂：每瓶 1g。<br>Poudre : 1g par flacon. |
| 药品名称 Drug Names | 阿洛西林钠 Azlocilline sodique |
| 适应证<br>Les indications | 　　主要用于铜绿假单胞菌与其他革兰阴性菌所致的系统感染，如败血症、脑膜炎、肺炎及尿路和软组织感染。必要时可与氨基糖苷类联合以加强抗铜绿假单胞菌的作用。<br>　　Ce produit est utilisé comme traitement des infections causées par le bacille pyocyanique et d'autres bactéries à Gram négatif, telles que la septicémie, la méningite, la pneumonie et des infections urinaires et des tissus mous. Le cas échéant, on peut utiliser à la fois ce produit et l'aminoglycoside pour combattre le bacille pyocyanique. |

续　表

| | |
|---|---|
| 用法、用量<br>Les modes d'emploi et la posologie | 尿路感染：每日 50 ～ 100mg/kg；重症感染，成人每日 200 ～ 250mg/kg，儿童每日 50 ～ 150mg/kg。以上量分 4 次，静脉注射或静脉滴注，也可肌内注射给予。可用氯化钠注射液、葡萄糖液或乳酸钠林格液溶解后给予，也可加入墨菲管中，随输液进入（但要掌握速度，不宜过快）。<br><br>Les infections urinaires : 50 à 100 mg/kg/jour ; les infections graves : chez des adultes, 200 à 250 mg/kg/jour, chez des enfants, 50 à 150 mg/kg/jour, à travers 4 fois, par voie IV, en perfusion ou par voie IM. Utiliser une solution de chlorure de sodium, une solution de glucose ou le liquide de Ringer pour la dissoudre avant de l'administrer, ou l'inclure dans un tube à perfusion Murphy, mais le débit ne doit pas être trop vite. |
| 剂型、规格<br>Les formes pharmaceutiques et les spécifications | 粉针剂：每支 2g；3g；4g。<br>Poudre : 2 g, 3 g ou 4 g par pièce. |
| 药品名称 Drug Names | 磺苄西林钠 Sulbénicilline sodique |
| 适应证<br>Les indications | 临床上用于敏感的铜绿假单胞菌、某些变形杆菌属及其他敏感革兰阴性菌所致肺炎、尿路感染、复杂性皮肤软组织感染和败血症等。对本品敏感菌所致腹腔感染、盆腔感染宜与抗厌氧菌药物联合应用。<br><br>Ce produit est utilisé dans les cliniques comme traitement des infections causées par le bacille pyocyanique et d'autres bactéries à Gram négatif, telles que la septicémie, la méningite, la pneumonie et des infections urinaires et des tissus mous. |
| 用法、用量<br>Les modes d'emploi et la posologie | 中度感染，成人一日 8g，重症感染或铜绿假单胞菌感染时剂量需增至一日 20g，分 4 次静脉滴注或可静脉注射；儿童根据病情每日剂量按体重 80 ～ 300mg/kg，分 4 次给药。<br><br>Pour des infections modérées, chez des adultes, 8 g par jour, pour des infections graves ou des infections causées par le bacille pyocyanique, 20 g par jour, à travers 4 fois, en perfusion ou par voie IV; chez des enfants, 80 à 300 mg/kg/jour en fonction du poids, à travers 4 fois. |
| 剂型、规格<br>Les formes pharmaceutiques et les spécifications | 注射用磺苄西林钠：每瓶 1.0g；2g；4g。<br>La sulbénicilline de sodium pour injection : 1 g, 2 g ou 4 g par flacon. |
| 药品名称 Drug Names | 阿帕西林钠 Apalcilline sodique |
| 适应证<br>Les indications | 临床可用于敏感革兰阳性或阴性菌感染，如呼吸道、尿路、胆道、妇科感染，也可用于术后感染和五官科感染的治疗。<br><br>Ce produit peut être utilisé dans les cliniques dans le traitement des infections causées par les bactéries à Gram négatif et positif, telles que les infections respiratoires, urinaires, des voies biliaires et gynécologiques. Il peut être aussi utilisé après l'opération chirurgicale. |
| 用法、用量<br>Les modes d'emploi et la posologie | 成人 1 次 2 ～ 3g，一日 3 次，肌内或静脉给药。10 岁以下儿童，一日 60 ～ 220mg/kg，分 3 ～ 4 次静脉滴注。10 岁以上儿童剂量同成人。<br><br>Chez des adultes, 2 à 3g par fois, 3 fois par jour, par voie IM ou IV. Chez des enfants moins de 10 ans, 60 à 220 mg/kg par jour, à travers 3 à 4 fois en perfusion. Chez des enfants âgés de plus de 10 ans, la même dose que chez les adultes. |
| 剂型、规格<br>Les formes pharmaceutiques et les spécifications | 注射用阿帕西林钠：每瓶 1g；3g。<br>L'amoxicilline de sodium pour injection : 1g ou 3g par flacon. |

续 表

| 1.2 头孢菌素类 Céphalosporines | |
|---|---|
| 药品名称 Drug Names | 头孢氨苄 Céfalexine |
| 适应证<br>Les indications | 用于敏感菌所致的呼吸道、泌尿道、皮肤和软组织、生殖器官（包括前列腺）等部位的感染，也常用于中耳炎。<br>Ce produit est utilisé dans le traitement des infections causées par des bactéries, telles que les infections respiratoires, urinaires, cutanées, des tissus mous, génitales. Il sert souvent contre l'otite moyenne. |
| 用法、用量<br>Les modes d'emploi et la posologie | 成人：一日 1～2g，分 3～4 次服用，空腹服用。小儿：一日 25～50mg/kg，分 3～4 次服用。<br>Chez des adultes : 1 à 2g par jour, à travers 3 à 4 fois, l'estomac vide. Chez des enfants : 25 à 50 mg/kg par jour, à travers 3 à 4 fois. |
| 剂型、规格<br>Les formes pharmaceutiques et les spécifications | 片（胶囊）剂：每片（粒）0.125g；0.25g。<br>颗粒剂：1g 含药 50mg。<br>Comprimés (capsules) : 0,125g ou 0,25g par comprimé ou par capsule.<br>Granules : 1g contenant 50 mg de céfalexine. |
| 药品名称 Drug Names | 头孢唑林钠 Céfazoline sodique |
| 适应证<br>Les indications | 用于敏感菌所致的呼吸道、泌尿生殖系、皮肤软组织、骨和关节、胆道等感染，也可用于心内膜炎、败血症、咽和耳部感染。<br>Ce produit est utilisé dans le traitement des infections causées par des bactéries, telles que les infections respiratoires, urinaires, cutanées, des tissus mous, articulaires et des voies biliaires. Il est ainsi applicable dans le traitement de l'endocardite, de la septicémie, de l'infection pharyngée et de l'infection de l'oreille. |
| 用法、用量<br>Les modes d'emploi et la posologie | 肌内或静脉注射，1 次 0.5～1g，一日 3～4 次。革兰阳性菌所致轻度感染一日 0.5g，一日 2～3 次；中度或重症感染：1 次 0.5～1g，一日 3～4 次；极重感染：1 次 1～1.5g，一日 4 次。泌尿系感染：1 次 1g，一日 2 次。儿童一日量为：20～40mg/kg，分 3～4 次给予；重症可用到一日 100mg/kg。新生儿 1 次不超过 20mg/kg，一日 2 次。<br>Administration par voie IM ou IV, 0,5g à 1g par fois, 3 à 4 fois par jour. Pour l'infection bénigne causée par les bactéries à Gram positif, 0,5g par jour, 2 à 3 fois par jour ; pour l'infection modérée ou grave, 0,5 à 1g par fois, 3 à 4 fois par jour ; pour l'infection extrêmement grave, 1 à 1,5g par fois, 4 fois par jour. Pour des infections urinaires, 1g par fois, 2 fois par jour. Chez des enfants, 20 à 40 mg/kg par jour, à travers 3 à 4 fois ; pour des patients gravement malades, 100 mg/kg par jour. Chez des nouveau-nés, ne pas dépasser 20 mg/kg par fois, 2 fois par jour. |
| 剂型、规格<br>Les formes pharmaceutiques et les spécifications | 注射用头孢唑林钠：每瓶 0.5g；1g；2g。<br>La céfazoline de sodium pour injection : 0,5g, 1g ou 2g par flacon. |
| 药品名称 Drug Names | 头孢羟氨苄 Céfadroxil |
| 适应证<br>Les indications | 用于呼吸道、泌尿道、咽部、皮肤等部位敏感菌感染。<br>Ce produit est utilisé dans le traitement des infections causées par des bactéries, telles que les infections respiratoires, urinaires, pharyngées et cutanées. |
| 用法、用量<br>Les modes d'emploi et la posologie | 成人平均用量：一日 1～2g，分 2～3 次口服，泌尿道感染时，也可 1 次服下。小儿一日量 50mg/kg，分 2 次服用。肾功能不全者，首次服 1g，以后按肌酐清除率制订给药方案：肌酐清除率为 25～50ml/min 者，每 12 小时服 0.5g；10～25ml/min 者，每 24 小时服 0.5g；＜10ml/min 者，每 36 小时服 0.5g。<br>Chez des adultes : 1 à2g par jour, à travers 2 à 3 fois, par voie orale, en cas d'infections urinaires, aussi possible de prendre le médicament en une seule fois. Chez des enfants : 50 mg/kg par jour, à travers 2 fois. Chez des patients insuffisants rénaux, 1g pour la première fois, et ensuite élaborer des schémas posologiques en fonction de la clairance de la créatinine : ceux dont la clairance de la créatinine est de 25 à 50 ml/min, utiliser 0,5 g toutes les 12 h ; ceux dont la clairance de la créatinine est de 10 à 25 ml/min, 0,5g toutes les 24 h ; ceux dont la clairance de la créatinine est inférieure à 10 ml/min, 0,5g toutes les 36 heures. |

**续　表**

| 剂型、规格<br>Les formes pharmaceutiques et les spécifications | 片剂（胶囊剂）：每片（粒）0.125g；0.25g。<br>Comprimés (capsules) : 0,125g ou 0,25g par comprimé ou par capsule. |
|---|---|
| **药品名称 Drug Names** | 头孢拉定 Céfradine |
| 适应证<br>Les indications | 用于呼吸道、泌尿道、咽部、皮肤等部位的敏感菌感染，注射剂也可用于败血症和骨感染。<br>Ce produit est utilisé dans le traitement des infections causées par des bactéries, telles que les infections respiratoires, urinaires, pharyngées et cutanées.Son injection sert aussi à traiter la septicémie et l'infection osseuse. |
| 用法、用量<br>Les modes d'emploi et la posologie | 口服：成人一日 1～2g，分 3～4 次服用。小儿每日 25～50mg/kg，分 3～4 次服用。肌内注射、静脉注射或滴注：成人一日 2～4g，分 4 次注射。小儿每日 50～100mg/kg，分 4 次注射。肾功能不全者患者肌酐清除率制订给药方案：肌酐清除率为＞20ml/min 者，每 6 小时服 500mg；15～20ml/min 者，每 6 小时服 250mg；＜15ml/min 者，每 12 小时服 250mg。<br>Administration par voie orale : chez des adultes, 1 à 2g par jour, à travers 3 à 4 fois ; chez des enfants, 25 à 50 mg/kg par jour, à travers 3 à 4 fois. Administration par voie IM, par voie IV ou par voie IV en perfusion : chez des adultes, 2 à 4g par jour, à travers 4 fois ; chez des enfants, 50 à 100 mg/kg par jour, à travers 4 fois.Chez des patients insuffisants rénaux,élaborer des schémas posologiques en fonction de leur clairance de la créatinine : ceux dont la clairance de la créatinine est supérieure à 20 ml/min, utiliser 500 mg toutes les 6 h ; ceux dont la clairance de la créatinine est de 15 à 20 ml/min, 250mg toutes les 6 h ; ceux dont la clairance de la créatinine est inférieure à 15 ml/min, 250mg toutes les 12 h. |
| 剂型、规格<br>Les formes pharmaceutiques et les spécifications | 胶囊剂：每粒 0.25g；0.5g。<br>干混悬剂：0.125g；0.25g。<br>注射用头孢拉定（添加碳酸钠）：每瓶 0.5g；1g。<br>注射用头孢拉定 A（添加精氨酸）：每瓶 0.5g；1g。<br>Capsules : 0,25g ou 0,5g par capsule.<br>Suspension : 0,125g ou 0,25g.<br>La céfradine pour injection (y compris le carbonate de sodium) : 0,5 g ou 1g par flacon.<br>La céfradine A pour injection (y compris l'arginine) : 0,5 g ou 1g par flacon. |
| **药品名称 Drug Names** | 头孢呋辛钠 Céfuroxime sodique |
| 适应证<br>Les indications | 临床应用于敏感的革兰阴性菌所致的下呼吸道、泌尿系、皮肤和软组织、骨和关节、女性生殖器等部位的感染。对败血症、脑膜炎也有效。<br>Ce produit est utilisé dans les cliniques comme traitement des infections causées par des bactéries à Gram négatif, telles que les infections respiratoires, urinaires, cutanées, des tissus mous, articulaires et gynécologiques, ainsi que le traitement de la septicémie et de la méningite. |
| 用法、用量<br>Les modes d'emploi et la posologie | 肌内注射或静脉注射，成人：1 次 750～1500mg，一日 3 次；对严重感染，可按 1 次 1500mg，一日 4 次。应用于脑膜炎，一日剂量在 9g 以下。儿童：平均一日量为 60mg/kg，严重感染可用到 100mg/kg，分 3～4 次给予。肾功能不全者按患者肌酐清除率制订给药方案：肌酐清除率为＞20ml/min 者，一日 3 次，每次 0.75～1.5g；10～20ml/min 者，每次 0.75g，一日 2 次；＜10ml/min 者，每次 0.75g，一日 1 次。<br>肌内注射：1 次用 0.75g，加注射用水 3ml，振摇使成混悬液，用粗针头做深部肌内注射。静脉给药：每 0.75g 本品，用注射用水约 10ml，使溶解成澄明溶液，缓慢静脉注射或加到墨菲管中随输液滴入。<br>Administration par voie IM ou IV, chez des adultes, 750 à 1500mg par fois, 3 fois par jour. Pour l'infection grave, 1500mg par fois, 4 fois par jour. Pour traiter la méningite, ne pas dépasser 9g par jour. Chez des enfants, 60mg/kg par jour, pour l'infection grave, 100 mg/kg par jour, à travers 3 à 4 fois.Chez des patients insuffisants rénaux, élaborer des schémas posologiques en fonction de leur clairance de la créatinine : ceux dont la clairance de la créatinine est supérieure à 20 ml/min, 0,75 à 1,5g par fois, 3 fois par jour ; ceux dont la clairance de la créatinine est de 10 à 20 ml/min, 0,75g par fois, 2 fois par jour ; ceux dont la clairance de la créatinine est inférieure à 10 ml/min, 0,75g par fois, 1 fois par jour.<br>Administration par voie IM : 0,75g par fois, ajouter 3ml d'eau pour injection, l'agiter pour qu'il devienne la suspension, utiliser l'aiguille grossière pour une injection intramusculaire profonde. Administration par voie IV : pour 0,75g de produit, utiliser 10 ml d'eau pour injection pour qu'il devienne une solution claire. Administrer lentement le produit par voie IV ou l'inclure dans un tube à perfusion Murphy avant de l'administrer par voie IV en perfusion. |

**续 表**

| | |
|---|---|
| 剂型、规格<br>Les formes pharmaceutiques et les spécifications | 注射用头孢呋辛钠：每瓶 0.75g；1.5g。<br>La céfuroxime sodique pour injection : 0,75 g ou 1,5 g par flacon. |
| **药品名称 Drug Names** | 头孢呋辛酯 Céfuroxime axétil |
| 适应证<br>Les indications | 临床用于敏感菌所致的上、下呼吸道及泌尿系统、皮肤和软组织等部位的感染。<br>Ce produit est utilisé dans les cliniques comme traitement des infections causées par des bactéries, telles que les infections des voies respiratoires inférieures et supérieures, des voies urinaires, cutanées et des tissus mous. |
| 用法、用量<br>Les modes d'emploi et la posologie | 成人每次口服 250mg，一日 2 次，重症可服到每次 500mg。儿童每次 125mg，一日 2 次。一般疗程为 7 日。<br>Chez des adultes : par voie orale, 250 mg par jour, 2 fois par jour, pour l'infection grave, 500mg par fois. Chez des enfants : 125mg par fois, 2 fois par jour. Administration pendant 7 jours. |
| 剂型、规格<br>Les formes pharmaceutiques et les spécifications | 片剂（薄膜衣片）：每片 125mg；250mg。<br>Comprimés (comprimés pelliculés) : 125mg ou 250mg par comprimé. |
| **药品名称 Drug Names** | 头孢克洛 Céfaclor |
| 适应证<br>Les indications | 用于上述敏感菌所致的呼吸道、泌尿道和皮肤、软组织感染，以及中耳炎等。<br>Ce produit est utilisé comme traitement des infections causées par des bactéries, telles que les infections des voies respiratoires, des voies urinaires, cutanées et des tissus mous, ainsi que l'otite moyenne. |
| 用法、用量<br>Les modes d'emploi et la posologie | 成人口服常用量为 250mg，每 8 小时 1 次。重病或微生物敏感性较差时，剂量可加倍，但一日量不可超过 4g。儿童：一日口服剂量为 20mg/kg，分 3 次（每 8 小时 1 次）；重症可按一日 40mg/kg 给予，但一日量不超过 1g。<br>Chez des adultes, par voie orale, dose usuelle, 250mg, toutes les 8h. Pour l'infection grave, doubler la dose, mais ne pas dépasser 4g par jour. Chez des enfants : par voie orale, 20 mg/kg par jour, à travers 3 fois, toutes les 8h ; pour l'infection grave, 40 mg/kg par jour, mais ne pas dépasser 1g par jour. |
| 剂型、规格<br>Les formes pharmaceutiques et les spécifications | 胶囊剂（片剂）：每粒（片）0.125g；0.25g。<br>干混悬剂：0.125g；1.5g。<br>Capsules (comprimés) : 0,125g ou 0,25g par capsule ou par comprimé.<br>Suspension : 0,125g ou 1,5g. |
| **药品名称 Drug Names** | 头孢噻肟钠 Céfotaxime sodique |
| 适应证<br>Les indications | 用于敏感菌所致的呼吸道、泌尿道、骨和关节、皮肤和软组织、腹腔、胆道、消化道、五官、生殖器等部位的感染，对烧伤、外伤引起的感染及败血症、中枢感染也有效。<br>Ce produit est utilisé comme traitement des infections causées par des bactéries, telles que les infections des voies respiratoires, des voies urinaires, osseuses, articulaires, cutanées et des tissus mous,abdominales, des voies biliaires,gastro-intestinales, les infections liés aux traits du visage, ainsi que les infections génitales. Il est aussi utile dans le traitement des infections causées par la brûlure et le traumatisme ainsi que dans le traitement de la septicémie et de l'infection du système nerveux central. |
| 用法、用量<br>Les modes d'emploi et la posologie | 临用前，加灭菌注射用水使其溶解，溶解后立即使用。成人：肌内或静脉注射，1 次 0.5～1g，一日 2～4 次。一般感染用 2g/d，分成 2 次肌内注射或静脉注射；中等或较重感染 3～6g/d，分为 3 次肌内注射或静脉注射；败血症等 6～8g/d，分为 3～4 次静脉给药；极重感染一日不超过 12g，分为 6 次静脉给药；淋病用 1g 肌内注射（单次给药已足）。静脉滴注，2～3g/d。小儿：肌内注射或静脉注射一日量为 50～100mg/kg，分成 2～3 次给予。婴幼儿不能肌内注射。<br>Dissoudre dans l'eau stérile pour injection avant d'administrer immédiatement. Chez des adultes : par voie IM ou IV, 0,5 à 1g par fois, 2 à 4 fois par jour. Pour l'infection générale, 2g/jour, à travers 2 fois, par voie IM ou IV ; pour l'infection modérée ou grave, 3à 6g/jour, à travers 3 fois, par voie IM ou IV ; pour la septicémie, 6 à 8g/jour, à travers 3 à 4 fois, par voie IV ; pour l'infection extrêmement grave, ne pas dépasser 12g par jour, à travers 6 fois, par voie IV ; pour la blennorragie, 1g par voie IM, 1 fois seulement. Par voie IV en perfusion, 2 à 3 g/jour. Chez des enfants : par voie IM ou IV, 50 à 100 mg/kg par jour, à travers 2 à 3 fois. Chez des bébés, interdit de l'administrer par voie IM. |

**续　表**

| 剂型、规格<br>Les formes pharmaceutiques et les spécifications | 注射用头孢噻肟钠：每瓶 0.5g；1g；2g。<br>La céfotaxime sodique pour injection : 0,5g, 1g ou 2g par flacon. |
|---|---|
| **药品名称 Drug Names** | 头孢匹胺钠 Céfpiramide sodique |
| 适应证<br>Les indications | 用于敏感菌所致的下呼吸道、胆道、泌尿道、生殖系统、皮肤和软组织等部位的感染及败血症，腹腔炎时与甲硝唑或克林霉素合用。<br>Ce produit est utilisé comme traitement des infections causées par des bactéries, telles que les infections des voies respiratoires, des voies biliaires, des voies urinaires, les infections génitales, cutanées et des tissus mous, ainsi que la septicémie. Quand il s'agit de l'inflammation abdominale, il est recommandé de l'utiliser en association avec le métronidazole et la clindamycine. |
| 用法、用量<br>Les modes d'emploi et la posologie | 成人：轻中度感染，口服，一日 1～2g，分 2 次给予；肌内注射，用 0.5%～1% 利多卡因注射液作溶剂，进行深部肌内注射；静脉注射，溶于 5% 的葡萄糖注射液或 0.9% 氯化钠注射液中，缓慢滴注 30～60 分钟。重度感染，一日剂量 4g，用法同上。<br>儿童：静脉给药，轻中度感染，一日 20～80mg/kg，分成 2～3 次给予；重度感染，一日剂量增至 150mg/kg，分 2～3 次缓慢静脉注射或静脉滴注。<br>Chez des adultes : pour l'infection bénigne et modérée, par voie orale, 1 à 2 g par jour, à travers 2 fois ; par voie IM, utiliser l'injection de lidocaine à 0,5 % à 1 % comme solvant, pour l'injection IM profonde ; par voie IV, utiliser la solution de glucose à 5 % ou l'injection de chlorure de sodium à 0,9 %, perfusion lente pendant 30 à 60 minutes. Pour l'infection grave, 4g par jour, le même mode d'emploi mentionné précédemment. Chez des enfants : par voie IV, pour l'infection bénigne ou modérée, 20 à 80 mg/kg par jour, à travers 2 à 3 fois ; pour l'infection grave, 150 mg/kg par jour, à travers 2 à 3 fois, par voie IV lente ou en perfusion. |
| 剂型、规格<br>Les formes pharmaceutiques et les spécifications | 注射用头孢匹胺钠：每瓶 0.5g；1g。<br>La céfpiramide sodique pour injection : 0,5g ou 1g par flacon. |
| **药品名称 Drug Names** | 头孢曲松钠 Céftriaxone sodique |
| 适应证<br>Les indications | 对罗氏芬敏感的致病菌引起的感染，如脓毒血症，脑膜炎，播散性莱姆病（早、晚期），腹部感染（腹膜炎、胆道及胃肠道感染），骨、关节、软组织、皮肤及伤口感染，免疫机制低下患者之感染，肾脏及泌尿道感染，呼吸道感染，尤其是肺炎、耳鼻喉感染，生殖系统感染，包括淋病，术前预防感染。<br>Ce produit est utilisé comme traitement des infections causées par des bactéries sensibles àRocephin, telles que la toxémie, la méningite, la maladie de Lyme disséminée (au stade précoce et avancé), les infections abdominales (l'inflammation abdominale), les infections osseuses, articulaires, cutanées, des tissus mous et de plaies, du rein, des voies urinaires, des voies respiratoires, surtout la pneumonie, les infections liées à l'oreille et au nez, les infections génitales, y compris la blennorragie et la prévention des infections avant l'opération. |
| 用法、用量<br>Les modes d'emploi et la posologie | 一般感染，每日 1g，1 次肌内注射或静脉注射。严重感染，每日 2g，分 2 次给予。脑膜炎，可按一日 100mg/kg（但总量不超过 4g），分 2 次给予。淋病，单次用药 250mg 即足。儿童用量一般按成人量的 1/2 给予。肌内注射：将 1 次药量溶于适量 0.5% 盐酸利多卡因注射液，做深部肌内注射。静脉注射：按 1g 药物用 10ml 灭菌注射用水溶解，缓缓注入，历时 2～4 分钟。静脉滴注：成人 1 次量 1g 或一日量 2g，溶于等渗氯化钠注射液或 5%～10% 葡萄糖液 50～100ml 中，于 0.5～1 小时滴入。<br>Pour l'infection générale, 1g par jour, une fois, par voie IM ou IV. Pour l'infection grave, 2g par jour, à travers 2 fois. Pour la méningite, 100 mg/kg par jour, mais ne pas dépasser 4g par jour, à travers 2 fois. Pour la blennorragie, 250 mg, une fois seulement. Chez des enfants, 1/2 de la dose chez des adultes. Par voie IM : pour une dose de medicament, utiliser l'injection de lidocaïne de chlorhydrate à 0,5 % comme solvant, injection IM profonde. Par voie IV : dissoudre 1g de médicament dans 10 ml d'eau stérile pour injection, injection lente, pendant 2 à 4 minutes. Par voie IV en perfusion : chez des adultes, 1g par fois ou 2g par jour, dissoudre dans 50 à 100 ml de solution isotonique de chlorure de sodium ou de solution de glucose à 5 % à 10 %, perfusion pendant 0,5 à 1h. |

**续 表**

| | |
|---|---|
| 剂型、规格<br>Les formes pharmaceutiques et les spécifications | 注射用头孢曲松钠：每瓶 0.5g；1g；2g。<br>La céftriaxone sodique pour injection : 0,5g, 1g ou 2g par flacon. |
| 药品名称 Drug Names | 头孢哌酮钠 Céfoperazone sodique |
| 适应证<br>Les indications | 用于各种敏感菌所致的呼吸道、泌尿道、腹膜、胸膜、皮肤和软组织、骨和关节、五官等部位的感染，还可用于败血症和脑膜炎等。<br>Ce produit est utilisé comme traitement des infections causées par des bactéries, telles que les infections respiratoires, urinaires, péritonéales, pleurales, cutanées, des tissus mous, articulaires et du visage, ainsi que le traitement de la septicémie et de la méningite. |
| 用法、用量<br>Les modes d'emploi et la posologie | 肌内或静脉注射，成人 1 次 1～2g，一日 2～4g。严重感染，1 次 2～4g，一日 6～8g。小儿每日 50～100mg/kg，分 2～4 次注射。<br>Administration par voie IM ou IV, chez des adultes, 1 à 2g par fois, 2 à 4 g par jour. Pour l'infection grave, 2 à 4 g par fois, 6 à 8 g par jour.Chez des enfants, 50 à 100 mg/kg par jour, à travers 2 à 4 fois. |
| 剂型、规格<br>Les formes pharmaceutiques et les spécifications | 注射用头孢哌酮钠：每瓶 0.5g；1g；2g。<br>注射用头孢哌酮钠/舒巴坦（1：1；2：1；4：1；8：1）。<br>La céfoperazone de sodium pour injection : 0,5g, 1g, ou 2g par flacon.<br>La céfoperazone de sodium pour injection ou sulbactam(1：1；2：1；4：1；8：1). |
| 药品名称 Drug Names | 头孢他啶 Céftazidime |
| 适应证<br>Les indications | 用于革兰阴性菌的敏感菌株所致的下呼吸道、皮肤和软组织、骨和关节、胸腔、腹腔、泌尿生殖系及中枢等部位感染，也用于败血症。<br>Ce produit est utilisé dans les cliniques comme traitement des infections causées par des bactéries à Gram négatif, telles que les infections respiratoires, cutanées, des tissus mous, articulaires, péritonéales, abdominales, urinaires et de l'infection du système nerveux central, ainsi que le traitement de la septicémie. |
| 用法、用量<br>Les modes d'emploi et la posologie | 轻症一日剂量为 1g，分 2 次肌内注射。中度感染一次 1g，一日 2～3 次肌内注射或静脉注射；重症一次 2g，一日 2～3 次，肌内注射或静脉注射。本品可加入氯化钠注射液、5%～10%葡萄糖注射液、含乳酸钠的输液、右旋糖酐输液中。<br>Pour l'infection bénigne,1g par jour, à travers 2 fois par voie IM ; pour l'infection modérée, 1g par fois, à travers 2 à 3 fois par voie IM ou IV ; pour l'infection grave, 2g par fois, 2 à 3 fois par jour par voie IM ou IV. Aussi possible de dissoudre le produit dans la solution de chlorure de sodium, la solution de glucose à 5 % à 10 %, l'infusion contenant du lactate de sodium ou l'infusion de dextran. |
| 剂型、规格<br>Les formes pharmaceutiques et les spécifications | 注射用头孢他啶：每瓶 1g；2g。<br>La céftazidime pour injection : 1g ou 2g par flacon. |
| 药品名称 Drug Names | 头孢美唑 Cefmétazole |
| 适应证<br>Les indications | 用于葡萄球菌、大肠埃希菌、克雷伯杆菌、吲哚阴性和阳性杆菌、拟杆菌等微生物的敏感菌株所致的肺炎、支气管炎、胆道感染、腹膜炎、泌尿系统感染、子宫及附件感染等。<br>Ce produit est utilisé comme traitement des infections causées par des bactéries (le staphylocoques, le colibacille, le klebsiella, les bactéries négatives et positives indoliques, le bacteroides), telles que la pneumonie, la bronchite, l'infection des voies biliaires, la péritonite, l'infections urinaire, et l'infection de l'utérus et des accessoires. |
| 用法、用量<br>Les modes d'emploi et la posologie | 成人，一日 1～2g，分 2 次静脉注射或静脉滴注。小儿，一日 25～100mg/kg，分 2～4次静脉注射或者静脉滴注。重症或顽症时，成人可用到一日 4g，儿童可用到一日 150mg/kg。溶剂可选用等渗氯化钠注射液或 5% 葡萄糖液，静脉注射时还可用灭菌注射用水（但不可用于滴注，因渗透压过低）。<br>Administration par voie IV ou par voie IV en perfusion, chez des adultes, 1 à 2g par jour, à travers 2fois. Chez des enfants, 25 à 100 mg/kg par jour, à travers 2 à 4 fois. Pour l'infection grave ou réfractaire, chez des adultes, 4 g par jour, chez des enfants, 150 mg/kg par jour. C'est possible d'utiliser l'injection de chlorure de sodium isotonique ou la solution de glucose à 5%. L'eau stérile pour injection est aussi utilisable pour l'injection IV, mais pas pour l'injection en perfusion, car la pression osmotique est trop faible. |

续　表

| | |
|---|---|
| 剂型、规格<br>Les formes pharmaceutiques et les spécifications | 注射用头孢美唑钠：每瓶 0.25g；0.5g；1g；2g（效价）。<br>La cefmétazole de sodium pour injection : 0,25g, 0,5g, 1g ou 2g par flacon (titre). |
| **药品名称 Drug Names** | 头孢克肟 Céfixime |
| 适应证<br>Les indications | 用于上述敏感菌所引起的肺炎、支气管炎、泌尿道炎、淋病、胆囊炎、胆管炎、猩红热、中耳炎、副鼻窦炎。<br>Ce produit est utilisé comme traitement des infections causées par des bactéries mentionnées précédemment, telles que la pneumonie, la bronchite, l'urétrite, la blennorragie, la cholécystite, la cholangite, la scarlatine, l'otite moyenne et la sinusite. |
| 用法、用量<br>Les modes d'emploi et la posologie | 成人及体重为 30kg 以上的儿童：1 次 50 ～ 100mg，一日 2 次；重症 1 次口服量可增至 200mg。体重为 30kg 以下的儿童：1 次 1.5 ～ 3mg/kg，一日 2 次；重症 1 次量可增至 6mg/kg。<br>Chez des adultes et des enfants plus de 30kg, 50 à 100 mg par fois, 2 fois par jour ; pour l'infection grave, administration par voie orale, 200mg. Chez des enfants moins de 30 kg, 1,5 à 3 mg/kg par fois, 2 fois par jour, pour l'infection grave, 6mg/kg par fois. |
| 剂型、规格<br>Les formes pharmaceutiques et les spécifications | 胶囊剂：每粒 50mg 或 100mg；<br>颗粒：每 1g 中含本品 50mg（效价）。<br>Capsules : 50mg ou 100mg par capsule.<br>Granules : 1g contenant 50 mg de céfixime (titre). |
| **药品名称 Drug Names** | 头孢西丁钠 Céfoxitine sodique |
| 适应证<br>Les indications | 临床应用于敏感的革兰阴性菌或厌氧菌所致的下呼吸道、泌尿生殖系、腹腔、骨和关节、皮肤和软组织等部位感染，也可用于败血症。<br>Ce produit est utilisé dans les cliniques comme traitement des infections causées par des bactéries à Gram négatif ou des anaérobies, telles que les infections respiratoires, urinaires, abdominales, articulaires, cutanées, des tissus mous, ainsi que le traitement de la septicémie. |
| 用法、用量<br>Les modes d'emploi et la posologie | 成人：1 次 1 ～ 2g，一日 3 ～ 4 次。肾功能不全者按患者肌酐清除率制订给药方案：肌酐清除率为 30 ～ 50mg/min 者，每 8 ～ 12 小时用 1 ～ 2g；10 ～ 29ml/min 者，每 12 ～ 24 小时用 1 ～ 2g；5 ～ 9ml/min 者，每 12 ～ 24 小时用 0.5 ～ 1g；< 5ml/min 者，每 24 ～ 48 小时用 0.5 ～ 1g。<br>Chez des adultes : 1 à 2 g par fois, 3 à 4 fois par jour. Chez des patients insuffisants rénaux,élaborer des schémas posologiques en fonction de leur clairance de la créatinine : ceux dont la clairance de la créatinine est de 30 à 50 ml/min, 1 à 2g toutes les 8 à 12 h ; ceux dont la clairance de la créatinine est de 10 à 29 ml/min, 1 à 2g toutes les 12 à 24 h ; ceux dont la clairance de la créatinine est de 5 à 9 ml/min, 0,5 à 1 g toutes les 12 à 24 h ; ceux dont la clairance de la créatinine est inférieure à 5 ml/min, 0,5 à 1 g toutes les 24 à 48 h. |
| 剂型、规格<br>Les formes pharmaceutiques et les spécifications | 注射用头孢西丁钠：每瓶 1g。<br>La céfoxitine sodique pour injection : 1g par flacon. |
| **药品名称 Drug Names** | 头孢米诺钠 Cefminox sodique |
| 适应证<br>Les indications | 用于上述敏感菌所致的扁桃体、呼吸道、泌尿道、胆道、腹腔、子宫等部位的感染，也可用于败血症。<br>Ce produit est utilisécomme traitement des infections causées par des bactéries mentionnées précédemment, telles que les infections amygdales, respiratoires, urinaires, biliaires, abdominales et utérines, ainsi que le traitement de la septicémie. |

**续　表**

| | |
|---|---|
| 用法、用量<br>Les modes d'emploi et la posologie | 静脉注射或静脉滴注。成人每次 1g，一日 2 次；儿童每次 20mg/kg，一日 3～4 次。败血症时，成人一日可用到 6g，分 3～4 次给予。本品静脉注射，每 1g 药物用 20ml 注射用水、5%～10% 葡萄糖液或 0.9% 氯化钠液溶解。滴注时，每 1g 药物溶于输液 100～200ml 中，滴注 1～2 小时。<br><br>Administration par voie IV ou par voie IV en perfusion. Chez des adultes, 1g par fois, 2 fois par jour ; chez des enfants, 20mg/kg par fois, 3 à 4 fois par jour. Pour traiter la septicémie, chez des adultes, 6g par jour, à travers 3 à 4 fois. Par voie IV, pour 1g de produit, utiliser 20ml d'eau pour injection, de solution de glucose à 5 % à 10 % ou desolution de chlorure de sodium à 0,9 % pour le dissoudre. Par voie IV en perfusion, pour 1g de produit, utiliser 100 à 200 ml d'infusion pour le dissoudre, la perfusion pendant 1 à 2 h. |
| 剂型、规格<br>Les formes pharmaceutiques et les spécifications | 注射用头孢米诺钠：每瓶 0.5g；1g（效价）。<br>Le cefminox de sodium pour injection : 0,5 g ou 1g par flacon (titre). |
| **药品名称 Drug Names** | 头孢吡肟 Céfepime |
| 适应证<br>Les indications | 用于敏感菌所致的下呼吸道、皮肤和骨组织、泌尿系、妇科和腹腔感染及菌血症等。<br><br>Ce produit est utilisé comme traitement des infections causées par des bactéries, telles que les infections respiratoires, de la peau et du tissu osseux, des voies urinaires, les infections gynécologiques et abdominales, ainsi que le traitement de la bactériémie. |
| 用法、用量<br>Les modes d'emploi et la posologie | 常用剂量每日 2～4g，分 2 次给予。治疗泌尿系感染每日 1g。极严重感染每日 6g，分 3 次给予。可用 0.9% 氯化钠、5%～10% 葡萄糖、0.16mol/L 乳酸钠、林格液等溶解。溶解液在室温 24 小时内应用。<br><br>Dose usuelle : 2 à 4 g par jour, à travers 2 fois. Pour traiter l'infection urinaire, 1 g par jour. Pour l'infection extrêmement grave, 6 g par jour, à travers 3 fois. Utiliser la solution de chlorure de sodium à 0,9 %, la solution de glucose à 5 % à 10 %, le lactate de sodium à 0,16mol/L ou le liquide de Ringer pour dissoudre ce produit. La solution est utilisable en 24 h à la température ambiante. |
| 剂型、规格<br>Les formes pharmaceutiques et les spécifications | 粉针剂：每瓶 0.5g；1g；2g。<br>Poudre : 0,5 g, 1g ou 2 g par flacon. |
| **药品名称 Drug Names** | 头孢布烯 Céftibutene |
| 适应证<br>Les indications | 主要用于上述敏感菌所致的呼吸道感染，如慢性气管炎急性发作、咽炎、扁桃体炎、泌尿道感染等。<br><br>Ce produit est utilisé comme traitement des infections causées par des bactéries, telles que une exacerbation aiguë de bronchite chronique, la pharyngite, l'amygdalite, les infections des voies urinaires. |
| 用法、用量<br>Les modes d'emploi et la posologie | 成人和体重 45kg 以上儿童：每日 1 次 400mg。儿童：体重 10kg 服 90mg，20kg 服 180mg，40kg 服 360mg。服用混悬剂必须避开进食（食前 1 小时或食后 2 小时服用）；胶囊剂则无碍。肾功能不全者，肌酐清除率 > 50ml/min 者，可按正常剂量服用（9mg/kg 或 400mg/QD）；肌酐清除率 30～49ml/min 者，照上量减半；肌酐清除率为 5～29ml/min 者，给上量 1/4。<br><br>Chez des adultes et des enfants plus de 45 kg, 400mg par fois par jour. Chez enfants de 10kg, 90mg, enfants de 20kg, 180mg, enfants de 40 kg, 360 mg. Administrer le céftibuten en suspension 1 h avant le repas ou 2 h après le repas. La nourriture ne pose pas de problème pour les capsules. Chez des patients insuffisants rénaux, élaborer des schémas posologiques en fonction de leur clairance de la créatinine : ceux dont la clairance de la créatinine est supérieure à 50 ml/min, une dose usuelle (9mg/kg ou 400mg/QD) ; ceux dont la clairance de la créatinine est de 30 à 49 ml/min, 1/2 de la dose usuelle ; ceux dont la clairance de la créatinine est de 5 à 29 ml/min, 1/4 de la dose usuelle. |
| 剂型、规格<br>Les formes pharmaceutiques et les spécifications | 胶囊剂：每粒 200mg，400mg。<br>混悬剂：90mg/5ml、180mg/5ml，每瓶 30ml、60ml、120ml。<br>Capsules : 200mg ou 400mg par capsule.<br>Suspension : 90mg/5ml ou 180mg/5ml, 30ml, 60ml ou 120ml par flacon. |

**续　表**

| 药品名称 Drug Names | 头孢丙烯 Céfprozil |
|---|---|
| 适应证<br>Les indications | 用于敏感菌所致上呼吸道、下呼吸道、中耳、皮肤和皮肤组织、尿路等部位感染。<br>Ce produit est utilisé comme traitement des infections causées par des bactéries, telles que les infections des voies respiratoires supérieures, des voies respiratoires inférieures, de l'otite moyenne, de la peau et des tissus, et des voies urinaires. |
| 用法、用量<br>Les modes d'emploi et la posologie | 成人（含 13 岁以上）：上呼吸道感染，每次 500mg，一日 1 次；下呼吸道感染，每次 500mg，一日 2 次；皮肤感染，250mg，一日 1 次（重症一日 2 次）。儿童（2～12 岁）：上呼吸道感染，每次 7.5mg/kg，一日 2 次；皮肤感染，每次 20mg/kg，一日 2 次；中耳炎，每次 15mg/kg，一日 2 次。肾功能不全：肌酐清除率小于 30mg/min 者，用量减半。<br>Chez des adultes (plus de 13 ans) : pour traiter l'infection des voies respiratoires supérieures, 500mg par fois, 1 fois par jour ; pour l'infectiondes voies respiratoires inférieures, 500mg par fois, 2 fois par jour ; pour l'infection de la peau, 250mg, 1 fois par jour (l'infection grave, 2 fois par jour). Chez des enfants (2 à 12 ans) : pour traiter l'infection des voies respiratoires supérieures, 7.5mg/kg par fois, 2 fois par jour ; pour l'infection de la peau, 20mg/kg par fois, 2 fois par jour ; pour l'otite moyenne, 15mg/kg par fois, 2 fois par jour. Chez des patients insuffisants rénaux, dont la clairance de la créatinine est inférieure à 30 ml/min, 1/2 de la dose usuelle. |
| 剂型、规格<br>Les formes pharmaceutiques et les spécifications | 片剂：每片 250mg；500mg。<br>干混悬剂：每瓶 2.5g、5g，加水后成为 125mg/5ml 和 250mg/5ml。<br>Comprimés : 250mg ou 500mg par comprimé.<br>Suspension : 2,5g ou 5g par flacon, avec l'eau, devenir 125mg/5ml et 250mg/5ml. |
| 药品名称 Drug Names | 头孢泊肟酯 Céfpodoxime pivoxil |
| 适应证<br>Les indications | 用于敏感菌所致支气管炎、肺炎、泌尿系统、皮肤组织、中耳、扁桃体等部位的感染。<br>Ce produit est utilisé comme traitement des infections causées par des bactéries, telles que la bronchite, la pneumonie, les infections des voies urinaires, de la peau, et amygdales, ainsi que le traitement de l'otite moyenne. |
| 用法、用量<br>Les modes d'emploi et la posologie | 成人（或大于 12 岁儿童）用量：一般感染，每日 200mg；重度感染，每日 400mg；皮肤及皮肤组织感染，每日 800mg，以上均分为 2 次服用。妇女淋球菌感染，服用单剂量 200mg。儿童：每日 10mg/kg，一般分为 2 次给予（单次剂量不超过 400mg）。肾功能严重不足（肌酐清除率 < 30ml/min）者给药间隔延长至 24 小时（按以上每日剂量的 1/2），透析患者于透析后每日给药 3 次。<br>Chez des adultes (ou plus de 12 ans) : l'infection générale, 200mg par jour ; l'infection grave, 400mg par jour ; l'infection de la peau et des tissus cutanés, 800mg par jour, à travers 2 fois. L'infection gonococcique chez des femmes, dose unique, 200mg. Chez des enfants : 10 mg par kg par jour, à travers 2 fois (la dose ne dépasse pas 400mg par fois). Chez des patients insuffisants rénaux, dont la clairance de la créatinine est inférieure à 30 ml/min, prolonger l'intervalle de la dose à 24 h (1/2 de la dose usuelle). Chez des patients dialysés, 3 fois par jour après la dialyse. |
| 剂型、规格<br>Les formes pharmaceutiques et les spécifications | 片剂：每片 100mg；200mg。<br>干混悬剂：每瓶 1000mg，加水至 100ml，得 50mg/5ml 混悬剂。<br>Comprimés : 100mg ou 200mg par comprimé.<br>Suspension : 1000mg par flacon, avec 100ml d'eau, obtenir 50mg/5ml de suspension. |
| 药品名称 Drug Names | 头孢托仑匹酯 Céfditorène pivoxil |
| 适应证<br>Les indications | 临床用于敏感菌引起的皮肤感染、乳腺炎、肛周脓肿、泌尿生殖系统感染、胆囊炎、胆管炎、中耳炎、鼻窦炎、牙周炎、睑腺炎、泪囊炎、咽喉炎、扁桃体炎、急慢性支气管炎。<br>Ce produit est utilisé dans les cliniques comme traitement des infections causées par des bactéries, telles que les infections de la peau, la mastite, l'abcès, les infections urogénitales, la cholécystite, la cholangite, l'otite moyenne, la sinusite, la parodontite, l'orgelet, la dacryocystite,la pharyngite, l'amygdalite, la bronchite aiguë et chronique. |

**续 表**

| 用法、用量 Les modes d'emploi et la posologie | 口服：成人每次 200 ～ 400mg，一日 2 次，连续用药 10 ～ 14 日。肾功能不全者，肌酐清除率＜ 30ml/min 者，每次用量不应超过 200mg，一日 1 次，肌酐清除率为 30 ～ 49ml/min 者，每次用量不应超过 200mg，一日 2 次。<br><br>Par voie orale : chez des adultes, 200mg à 400mg par fois, 2 fois par jour, 10 à 14 jours consécutifs. Chez des patients insuffisants rénaux, dont la clairance de la créatinine est inférieure à 30 ml/min, ne pas dépasser 200 mg par fois, 1 fois par jour ; ceux dont le taux de clairance de la créatinine est de 30 à 49ml/min, ne pas dépasser 200 mg par fois, 2 fois par jour. |
|---|---|
| 剂型、规格 Les formes pharmaceutiques et les spécifications | 片剂：每片 100mg；200mg。<br>Comprimés : 100mg ou 200mg par comprimé. |
| **药品名称 Drug Names** | 头孢地嗪 Céfodizime |
| 适应证 Les indications | 临床用于敏感菌所致的下呼吸道、泌尿系感染。<br><br>Ce produit est utilisé comme traitement des infections causées par des bactéries, telles que les infections des voies respiratoires inférieures et des voies urinaires. |
| 用法、用量 Les modes d'emploi et la posologie | 成人：每次 1g（重症可用到 2g），溶于注射用水 10ml，再加入其他输液中，使其成 50 ～ 100ml，静脉滴注，一日 2 次。肌内注射：用注射用水 4ml 溶解，也可用 0.5% ～ 1% 利多卡因注射液溶解，以减轻疼痛。淋病的治疗只注射 1 次，用量 0.5g。<br><br>Chez des adultes : 1g par fois (l'infection grave, 2g), utiliser 10ml d'eau pour injection et d'autres infusions pour former 50 à 100ml de solution, administration par voie IV en perfusion, 2 fois par jour. Voie IM : utiliser 4ml d'eau pour injection ou l'injection de lidocaïne à 0,5 % à 1 % pour soulager la douleur. Pour traiter la blennorragie, une injection seulement, 0,5g. |
| 剂型、规格 Les formes pharmaceutiques et les spécifications | 粉针剂：每瓶 1g；2g。<br>Poudre : 1g ou 2g par flacon. |
| **药品名称 Drug Names** | 头孢硫脒 Céfathiamidine |
| 适应证 Les indications | 用于上述敏感菌所致的呼吸道、泌尿道、胆道、皮肤及软组织感染，对心内膜炎、败血症也有较好疗效。<br><br>Ce produit est utilisé comme traitement des infections causées par des bactéries, telles queles infections des voies respiratoires, des voies urinaires, des voies biliaires, de la peau et des tissus mous, ainsi que le traitement de l'endocardite et de la septicémie. |
| 用法、用量 Les modes d'emploi et la posologie | 成人：一日 2 ～ 4g，分 2 ～ 4 次给药，肌内注射或静脉滴注，严重者可增至一日 8g。儿童：一日 50 ～ 100mg/kg，分 2 ～ 4 次给药，肌内注射或静脉滴注。先用生理盐水或注射用水溶解后，再用生理盐水或 5% 葡萄糖注射液 250ml 稀释。<br><br>Chez des adultes : 2 à 4 g par jour, à travers 2 à 4 fois, par voie IM ou par IV en perfusion, pour l'infection grave, 8g par jour. Chez des enfants, 50 à 100mg/kg par jour, à travers 2 à 4 fois, par voie IM ou par IV en perfusion. Utiliser la solutionsaline ou l'eau pour injection pour dissoudre le produit avant d'utiliser 250ml de solution saline ou de solution de glucose à 5 % pour le diluer. |
| 剂型、规格 Les formes pharmaceutiques et les spécifications | 注射用头孢硫脒：每瓶 0.5g；1g。<br>La céfathiamidine pour injection : 0,5g ou 1g par flacon. |
| **药品名称 Drug Names** | 头孢替安 Céfotiam |
| 适应证 Les indications | 用于敏感菌所致的术后感染、烧伤感染、皮肤软组织感染、骨及关节感染、呼吸系统扁桃体炎、肺炎、支气管炎、泌尿道炎、前列腺炎、胆囊炎、胆管炎，以及子宫内膜炎、盆腔炎。<br><br>Ce produit est utilisé comme traitement des infections causées par des bactéries, telles que les infections postopératoires, des brûlures infectées, les infections de la peau, des tissus mous et ostéo-articulaires, l'amygdalite du système respiratoire, la pneumonie, la bronchite, l'urétrite, la prostatite, la cholécystite, la cholangite, l'endométrite, ainsi que la maladie inflammatoire pelvienne. |

**续 表**

| | |
|---|---|
| 用法、用量<br>Les modes d'emploi et la posologie | 成人：静脉给药，一日 1～2g，2～4 次缓慢静脉注射或静脉滴注；严重感染增至一日 4g。儿童：一日 40～80mg/kg，分 3～4 次静脉给药；重症时剂量可增至一日 160mg/kg。<br>Chez des adultes : 1 à 2 g par jour, à travers 2 à 4 fois, injection IV lente ou en perfusion ; pour l'infection grave, 4g par jour. Chez des enfants, 40 à 80mg/kg par jour, à travers 3 à 4 fois, par voie IV ; pour l'infection grave, 160mg/kg par jour. |
| 剂型、规格<br>Les formes pharmaceutiques et les spécifications | 注射用盐酸头孢替安：每瓶 0.25g；0.5g；1g。<br>Le chlorhydrate de céfotiam pour injection : 0,25g, 0,5g ou 1g par flacon. |
| **药品名称 Drug Names** | 头孢替坦 Céfotetan |
| 适应证<br>Les indications | 用于敏感菌所致的呼吸道、肺部感染、腹部感染、尿路感染、妇科感染及皮肤软组织感染。<br>Ce produit est utilisé comme traitement des infections causées par des bactéries, telles que les infections respiratoires, pulmonaires, abdominales, urinaire, gynécologiques, cutanées et des tissus mous. |
| 用法、用量<br>Les modes d'emploi et la posologie | 深部肌内注射、静脉注射或静脉滴注。成人：常用量每次 1～2g，每 12 小时 1 次，每日最大剂量不超过 6g。儿童：每日 40～60mg/kg，病情严重者可增至 100mg/kg，分 2～3 次。<br>Injection IM profonde, IV ou en perfusion. Chez des adultes, la dose usuelle est de 1 à 2g par fois, toutes les 12 h, ne pas dépasser 6g par jour. Chez des enfants, 40 à 60 mg/kg par jour, pour l'infection grave, 100 mg/kg par jour, à travers 2 à 3 fois. |
| 剂型、规格<br>Les formes pharmaceutiques et les spécifications | 注射用头孢替坦二钠：每瓶 1g；2g；10g。<br>Le céfotetan disodique pour injection : 1g, 2g ou 10g par flacon. |
| **药品名称 Drug Names** | 头孢唑肟 Céftizoxime |
| 适应证<br>Les indications | 敏感菌所致的下呼吸道感染、尿路感染、腹腔感染、盆腔感染、败血症、皮肤软组织感染、骨和关节感染、肺炎链球菌或流感嗜血杆菌所致脑膜炎和单纯性淋病。<br>Ce produit est utilisé comme traitement des infections causées par des bactéries, telles que les infections des voies respiratoires inférieures, les infections des voies urinaires, les infections intra-abdominales, les infections pelviennes, la septicémie, les infections cutanées et des tissus mous, les infections osseuses et articulaires, ainsi que la méningite et la gonorrhée causée par le streptococcus pneumoniae ou l'haemophilus influenzae. |
| 用法、用量<br>Les modes d'emploi et la posologie | 静脉滴注或静脉注射。成人：1 次 1～2g，每 8～12 小时 1 次；严重感染者的剂量可增至 1 次 3～4g，每 8 小时 1 次；治疗非复杂性尿路感染时，1 次 0.5g，每 12 小时 1 次。6 个月及 6 个月以上的婴儿及儿童常用量：按体重 1 次 50mg/kg，每 6～8 小时 1 次。<br>Administration par voie IV en perfusion ou par voie IV. Chez des adultes : 1 à 2 g par fois, toutes les 8 à 12 h ; pour l'infection grave, 3 à 4 g par fois, toutes les 8 h ; pour traiter les infections des voies urinaires non complexe, 0,5g par fois, toutes les 12h. Chez des bébés de 6 mois ou plus ou des enfants, dose usuelle : 50 mg/kg par fois en fonction du poids, toutes les 6 à 8h. |
| 剂型、规格<br>Les formes pharmaceutiques et les spécifications | 注射用头孢唑肟钠：每瓶 0.5g；1g。<br>Le céftizoxime sodique pour injection : 0,5g ou 1g par flacon. |
| **药品名称 Drug Names** | 头孢孟多 Céfamandol |
| 适应证<br>Les indications | 临床应用于敏感的革兰阴性菌所致的呼吸道、泌尿生殖系、皮肤和软组织、骨和关节、咽耳鼻喉等部位感染以及腹膜炎、败血症等。对胆道和肠道感染有较好疗效。<br>Ce produit est utilisé dans les cliniques comme traitement des infections causées par des bactéries à Gram négatif, telles que les infections respiratoires, génito-urinaires, cutanées et des tissus mous, osseuses et articulaires, les infections à propos de l'ORL, du pharynx et de la gorge, ainsi que la péritonite et la septicémie. Il est aussi utile dans le traitement des infections biliaires et intestinales. |

**续　表**

| 用法、用量<br>Les modes d'emploi et la posologie | 静脉注射或静脉滴注。成人，一般感染 1 次 0.5 ～ 1g，一日 4 次；较重感染 1 次 1g，一日 6 次；极严重感染一日可用到 12g。儿童，一日剂量为 50 ～ 100mg/kg；极重感染可用到 150mg/kg，分 3 ～ 4 次给予。<br>Administration par voie IV en perfusion ou par voie IV. Chez des adultes : pour l'infection générale, 0,5 à 1 g par fois, 4 fois par jour ; pour l'infection grave, 1g par fois, 6 fois par jour ; pour l'infection extrêmement grave, 12g par jour. Chez des enfants, 50 à 100 mg/kg par jour, pour l'infection extrêmement grave, 150 mg/kg par jour, à travers 3 à 4 fois. |
|---|---|
| 剂型、规格<br>Les formes pharmaceutiques et les spécifications | 注射用头孢孟多甲酸酯钠：每瓶 0.5g、1g。每 1g 药物添加碳酸钠 63mg。<br>La formiate de céfamandole sodique pour injection : 0,5g ou 1g par flacon. 1g de médicament contient 63mg de carbonate de sodium. |
| 药品名称 Drug Names | 头孢尼西 Céfonicide |
| 适应证<br>Les indications | 用于上述敏感菌所致的下呼吸道感染、尿路感染、败血症、皮肤软组织感染、骨和关节感染。也可用于手术预防感染。<br>Ce produit est utilisé comme traitement des infections causées par des bactéries, telles que les infections des voies respiratoires inférieures, les infections des voies urinaires, la septicémie, les infections cutanées et des tissus mous, ainsi que les infections ostéo-articulaires. Il est aussi applicable dans la prévention des infections chirurgicales. |
| 用法、用量<br>Les modes d'emploi et la posologie | 一般轻度至中度感染成人每日剂量为 1g，一日 1 次；在严重感染或危及生命的感染中，可每日 2g，每 24 小时给药 1 次；无并发症的尿路感染：每日 0.5g，每 24 小时 1 次；手术预防感染：手术前 1 小时单剂量给药 1g，术中和术后没有必要再用。必要时如关节成形手术或开胸手术可重复给药 2 天；剖宫产手术中，应在脐带结扎后才给予本品。<br>Pour l'infection bénigne et modérée, chez des adultes, 1g par jour, 1 fois par jour ; pour l'infection extrêmement grave, 2g par jour, toutes les 24h ; pour l'infection des voies urinaires sans complication, 0,5g par jour, toutes les 24h ; pour la prévention des infections chirurgicales, 1g 1h avant l'opération chirurgicale, il n'est pas nécessaire de l'utiliser pendant et après l'opération. Le cas échéant, en cas d'arthroplastie ou de thoracotomie par exemple, il est permissible de l'administrer pendant 2 jours ; dans le cas de césarienne, il faut l'utiliser après la ligature du cordon ombilical. |
| 剂型、规格<br>Les formes pharmaceutiques et les spécifications | 注射用头孢尼西钠：每瓶 0.5g；1g；2g。<br>La céfonicide sodique pour injection : 0,5g, 1g ou 2g par flacon. |
| 药品名称 Drug Names | 拉氧头孢钠 Latamoxef sodique |
| 适应证<br>Les indications | 用于上述敏感菌所致肺炎、气管炎、胸膜炎、腹膜炎，以及皮肤和软组织、骨和关节、五官、创面等部位的感染，还可用于败血症和脑膜炎。<br>Ce produit est utilisé comme traitement des infections causées par des bactéries, telles que la pneumonie, la bronchite, la pleurésie, la péritonite, les infections cutanées et des tissus mous, osseuses et articulaires, ainsi que les infections à propos des traits du visage et de plaies. Il est aussi utile dans le traitement de la septicémie et de la méningite. |
| 用法、用量<br>Les modes d'emploi et la posologie | 肌内注射：1 次 0.5 ～ 1g，一日 2 次，用 0.5% 利多卡因注射液溶解，做深部肌内注射。静脉注射：1 次 1g，一日 2 次，溶解于 10 ～ 20ml 液体中，缓缓注入。静脉滴注：1 次 1g，一日 2 次，溶于液体 100ml 中滴入，重症可加倍量给予。儿童用量：一日 40 ～ 80mg/kg，分 2 ～ 4 次。<br>静脉注射和静脉滴注可用等渗氯化钠溶液或 5% ～ 10% 葡萄糖注射液、灭菌注射用水、低分子右旋糖酐注射液等作溶剂，但不得与甘露醇注射液配伍。<br>Administration par voie IM : 0,5 à 1g par fois, 2 fois par jour, injection de lidocaïne à 0,5% pour la dissolution, injection IM profonde. Administration par voie IV : 1 g par fois, 2 fois par jour, dissoudre dans 10 à 20ml d'eau pour injection. En perfusion : 1g par fois, 2 fois par jour, dissoudre dans 100ml d'eau pour injection avant d'administrer en perfusion, pour l'infection grave, doubler la dose usuelle. Chez des enfants : 40 à 80 mg/kg par jour, à travers 2 à 4 fois, en cas d'injection par voie IV ou IV en perfusion, il est permissible d'utiliser la solution de chlorure de sodium isotonique, l'injection de glucose à 5% à 10%, l'eau stérile pour injection, l'injection de dextrane à bas poids moléculaire comme solvant. Mais il est interdit de l'utiliser en association avec l'injection de mannitol. |

**续 表**

| | |
|---|---|
| 剂型、规格<br>Les formes pharmaceutiques et les spécifications | 注射用拉氧头孢钠：每瓶 0.25g；0.5g；1g。<br>Le latamoxef de sodium pour injection : 0,25g, 0,5g ou 1g par flacon. |
| 药品名称 Drug Names | 氟氧头孢钠 Flomoxef sodique |
| 适应证<br>Les indications | 用于上述敏感菌所致的咽炎、扁桃体炎、支气管炎、肺炎、肾盂肾炎、膀胱炎、前列腺炎、胆道感染、腹膜炎、盆腔炎、子宫及附属组织炎症、中耳炎、创口感染、心内膜炎及败血症等。<br>Ce produit est utilisé comme traitement des infections causées par des bactéries, telles que la pharyngite, l'amygdalite, la bronchite, la pneumonie, la pyélonéphrite, la cystite, la prostatite, les infections des voies biliaires, la péritonite, la pelvipéritonite, la métrite, l'otite moyenne, les infections de plaies, l'endocardite et la septicémie. |
| 用法、用量<br>Les modes d'emploi et la posologie | 轻症：成人一日量 1 ～ 2g，分成 2 次静脉注射；儿童一日 60 ～ 80mg/kg，分 2 次静脉注射或静脉滴注。重症：成人一日 4g，分 2 ～ 4 次用；儿童一日 150mg/kg，分 3 ～ 4 次用。<br>Pour l'infection bénigne : chez des adultes, 1 à 2 g par jour, à travers 2 fois, par voie IV ; chez des enfants, 60 à 80 mg/kg par jour, à travers 2 fois, par voie IV ou par IV en perfusion. Pour l'injection grave : chez des adultes, 4g par jour, à travers 2 à 4 fois ; chez des enfants, 150 mg/kg par jour, à travers 3 à 4 fois. |
| 剂型、规格<br>Les formes pharmaceutiques et les spécifications | 注射用氟氧头孢钠：每瓶 0.5g；1g；2g。<br>Le flomoxef de sodium pour injection : 0,5g, 1g ou 2g par flacon. |

1.3　β-内酰胺酶抑制剂及其与 β-内酰胺类抗生素配伍的复方制剂
Inhibiteur de la bêta-lactamase et préparations composées associées à des antibiotiques du groupe du bêta-lactama

| | |
|---|---|
| 药品名称 Drug Names | 克拉维酸钾 Clavulanate de potassium |
| 适应证<br>Les indications | 与 β-内酰胺类抗生素联用于敏感菌所致的下呼吸道感染、耳鼻喉科感染、尿路感染、腹腔感染、盆腔感染、骨和关节感染、皮肤软组织感染、血流感染及败血症等<br>Et lactamines ß combinés avec, pour le traitement des infections des voies respiratoires inférieures causées par des souches sensibles, les infections ORL, infections des voies urinaires, des infections abdominales, infections pelviennes, infections osseuses et articulaires, la peau et les infections des tissus mous, les infections sanguines et septicémie. |
| 用法、用量<br>Les modes d'emploi et la posologie | 本药单用无效，常与 β-内酰胺类抗生素组成复方制剂应用。各复方制剂的具体用法与用量参见"阿莫西林克拉维酸钾""替卡西林钠克拉维酸钾"。<br>Le médicament seul inefficaces, souvent avec la composition de lactamines β- applications de préparation de composé. Utilisation spécifique et le montant de chaque préparation de composé Voir "amoxicilline et clavulanate de potassium", "Ticarcilline clavulanate de sodium potassium" . |
| 剂型、规格<br>Les formes pharmaceutiques et les spécifications | 参见"阿莫西林克拉维酸钾""替卡西林钠克拉维酸钾"的相关项。<br>Voir "amoxicilline et clavulanate de potassium", "Ticarcilline clavulanate de potassium de sodium" articles connexes. |
| 药品名称 Drug Names | 舒巴坦钠 Sulbactam Sodique |
| 适应证<br>Les indications | 与青霉素类或头孢菌素类药联用于治疗敏感菌所致的败血症、尿路感染、肺部感染、支气管感染、胆道感染、腹腔感染、盆腔感染、皮肤软组织感染及耳、鼻、喉部感染等。<br>Les médicaments et les pénicillines ou les céphalosporines combinés avec, pour le traitement de la septicémie provoquée par des souches sensibles, les infections des voies urinaires, des infections pulmonaires, infections bronchiques, infections des voies biliaires, infections intra-abdominales, infections pelviennes, la peau et les infections des tissus mous et des oreilles, du nez , infections de la gorge. |
| 用法、用量<br>Les modes d'emploi et la posologie | 静脉滴注：与氨苄西林联用，本药一日 1 ～ 2g，氨苄西林一日 2 ～ 4g，分 2 ～ 3 次给药。<br>Perfusion intraveineuse, et l'ampicilline en conjonction avec, le jour de la drogue 1 à 2g, jour ampicilline 2 à 4g, 2 à 3 doses. |

**续　表**

| | |
|---|---|
| 剂型、规格<br>Les formes pharmaceutiques et les spécifications | 注射用舒巴坦钠：0.5g；1g。<br>Le sulbactam de sodium pour injection : 0,5g ou 1g. |
| **药品名称 Drug Names** | **他唑巴坦 Tazobactam** |
| 适应证<br>Les indications | 参见"哌拉西林钠 - 他唑巴坦钠"的相关项。<br>Éléments - "tazobactam de sodium pipéracilline de sodium" liée Voir. |
| 用法、用量<br>Les modes d'emploi et la posologie | 参见"哌拉西林钠 - 他唑巴坦钠"的相关项。<br>Éléments - "tazobactam de sodium pipéracilline de sodium" liée Voir. |
| 剂型、规格<br>Les formes pharmaceutiques et les spécifications | 参见"哌拉西林钠 - 他唑巴坦钠"的相关项。<br>Éléments - "tazobactam de sodium pipéracilline de sodium" liée Voir. |
| **药品名称 Drug Names** | **阿莫西林 - 克拉维酸钾 Amoxiciline et Clavulanate de potassium** |
| 适应证<br>Les indications | 用于上述敏感菌所致的下呼吸道、中耳、鼻窦、皮肤组织、尿路等部位感染。对肠杆菌属尿路感染也可有效。<br>Ce produit est utilisé comme traitement des infections causées par des bactéries, telles que les infections des voies respiratoires inférieures, l'otite moyenne, la sinusite, les infections cutanées et urinaires. Il est aussi utile dans le traitement des infections des voies urinaires d'enterobacter. |
| 用法、用量<br>Les modes d'emploi et la posologie | 一般感染：用 2∶1 比例片，每次 1 片，每 8 小时 1 次。重症或呼吸道感染，用 4∶1 比例片，每次 1 片，每 6～8 小时 1 次。注射应用见阿莫西林。<br>Pour l'infection générale : comprimés avec un ratio de 2∶1, un comprimé par fois, toutes les 8h. L'infection grave ou l'infection respiratoire : comprimés avec un ratio de 4∶1, un comprimé par fois, toutes les 6 à 8 h. Le mode d'emploi pour injection, voir l'amoxicilline. |
| 剂型、规格<br>Les formes pharmaceutiques et les spécifications | 片剂：0.375g（2∶1）；0.625g（4∶1）；0.3125g（4∶1）；0.475g（7∶1）；1.0g（7∶1）。<br>注射用阿莫西林钠 - 克拉维酸钾：1.2g/ 瓶（5∶1）。<br>Comprimés：0.375g(2∶1)；0.625g(4∶1)；0.3125g(4∶1)；0.475g(7∶1)；1.0g(7∶1).<br>L'amoxicilline et clavulanate de potassium pour injection : 1,2g par flacon (5∶1). |
| **药品名称 Drug Names** | **替卡西林钠 - 克拉维酸钾 Ticarcilline de sodium et clavulanate de potassium** |
| 适应证<br>Les indications | 本品适用于上述敏感菌引起的呼吸道、骨和关节、皮肤组织、尿路等部位的感染以及败血症、骨髓炎和各种手术后感染。<br>Ce produit est utilisé comme traitement des infections causées par des bactéries, telles que les infections des voies respiratoires inférieures, osseuses et articulaires, cutanées et urinaires, ainsi que dans le traitement de la septicémie, l'ostéomyélite et des infections survenues après l'opération chirurgicale. |
| 用法、用量<br>Les modes d'emploi et la posologie | 每次注射 3g，每 4～6 小时 1 次，溶于 13ml 等渗盐水或灭菌注射用水中，缓缓静脉推注，或溶于适量溶剂中静脉滴注，30 分钟内滴完。<br>3g par injection, toutes les 4 à 6 h, dissoudre dans 13ml d'eau salée isotonique ou d'eau stérile pour injection, injecter lentement. Ou par voie IV en perfusion, en 30 minutes. |
| 剂型、规格<br>Les formes pharmaceutiques et les spécifications | 注射用替卡西林钠 - 克拉维酸钾：3g（3∶0.1）；3g（3∶0.2）。<br>La ticarcilline de sodium et la clavulanate de potassium pour injection : 3g(3∶0.1)ou 3g(3∶0.2). |
| **药品名称 Drug Names** | **氨苄西林钠 - 舒巴坦钠 Ampicilline de sodium et sulbactam de sodium** |
| 适应证<br>Les indications | 可用于治疗上述敏感菌所致的下呼吸道、泌尿道、胆道、皮肤和软组织、中耳、鼻窦等部位感染。<br>Ce produit est utilisés comme traitement des infections causées par des bactéries, telles que les infections des voies respiratoires inférieures, des voies urinaires, des voies biliaires, de la peau et des tissus mous, l'otite moyenne ainsi que la sinusite. |

续　表

| | |
|---|---|
| 用法、用量<br>Les modes d'emploi et la posologie | 氨苄西林和舒巴坦钠以 2 ∶ 1（效价）的比率联合应用。肌内注射：一次 0.75g（氨苄西林 0.5g 和舒巴坦钠 0.25g），一日 2～4 次。静脉注射或静脉滴注：1 次 1.5g，一日 2～4 次。静脉滴注时以 100ml 等渗氯化钠液或注射用水溶解，滴注 0.5～1 小时。<br>Utiliser l'ampicilline et le sulbactame avec un ratio de 2 ∶ 1 (titre). Par voie IM : 0,75g par fois (0,5g d'ampicilline et 0,25g de sulbactame), 2 à 4 fois par jour. Par voie IV ou par voie IV en perfusion : 1,5g par jour, 2 à 4 fois par jour. En cas d'injection par voie IV en pefusion, dissoudre le produit dans 100ml de solutionde chlorure de sodium isotonique ou d'eau stérile pour injection, perfusion pendant 0,5 à 1h. |
| 剂型、规格<br>Les formes pharmaceutiques et les spécifications | 注射用氨苄西林钠 - 舒巴坦钠：0.75g；1.5g［含氨苄西林钠和舒巴坦钠（重量效价比）2 ∶ 1］。<br>L'ampicilline de sodium et le sulbactam de sodium pour injection : 0,75g ou 1,5g (l'ampicilline et le sulbactame avec un ratio de titre 2 ∶ 1). |
| **药品名称 Drug Names** | 舒他西林 Sultamicilline |
| 适应证<br>Les indications | 用于治疗敏感细菌引起的下列感染：①上呼吸道感染：鼻窦炎、中耳炎、扁桃体炎等。②下呼吸道感染：支气管炎、肺炎等。③泌尿道感染及肾盂肾炎。④皮肤、软组织感染。⑤淋病。<br>Pour le traitement des infections suivantes causées par des bactéries sensibles: ① Infections des voies respiratoires supérieures: la sinusite, l'otite moyenne, l'amygdalite. ② Infections des voies respiratoires inférieures: bronchite, la pneumonie. ③ Les infections urinaires et pyélonéphrite. ④ Des infections cutanées et des tissus mous. ⑤ La gonorrhée |
| 用法、用量<br>Les modes d'emploi et la posologie | 1 次 375mg，一日 2～4 次，在餐前 1 小时或餐后 2 小时服用。<br>375mg par fois, 2 à 4 fois par jour, 1h avant le repas ou 2h après le repas. |
| 剂型、规格<br>Les formes pharmaceutiques et les spécifications | 片剂：375mg（效价）。<br>Comprimés : 375mg (titre). |
| **药品名称 Drug Names** | 哌拉西林钠 - 他唑巴坦钠 Pipéracilline de sodium et tazobactam de sodium |
| 适应证<br>Les indications | 临床主要用于敏感菌所致下呼吸道、腹腔、妇科、泌尿、骨及关节、皮肤组织等部位感染和败血症。也可用于多种细菌的混合感染和患中性粒细胞缺乏者的感染。<br>Ce produit est utilisé comme traitement des infections causées par des bactéries, telles que les infections des voies respiratoires inférieures, abdominales, gynécologiques, urologiques, osseuses,articulaires, cutanées ainsi que la septicémie. Il peut être également utilisé dans le traitement des infections bactériennes mixtes et des infections des patients neutropéniques. |
| 用法、用量<br>Les modes d'emploi et la posologie | 成人和 12 岁以上儿童的常用量为：每次 4.5g，一日 3 次静脉滴注（滴注 30 分钟），也可静脉注射。<br>Chez des adultes ou des enfants plus de 12 ans, dose usuelle : 4,5g par fois, 3 fois par jour, en perfusion (30 minutes), c'est aussi possible par voie IV. |
| 剂型、规格<br>Les formes pharmaceutiques et les spécifications | 注射用哌拉西林钠 - 他唑巴坦：2.25g（8 ∶ 1）；4.5g（8 ∶ 1）。<br>La pipéracilline de sodium et le tazobactam pour injection : 2.25g(8 ∶ 1) ou 4.5g(8 ∶ 1). |

1.4　碳青霉烯类和其他 β - 内酰胺类 Carbapénèmes et autres β –lactames

| | |
|---|---|
| **药品名称 Drug Names** | 亚胺培南 - 西司他汀钠 Imipénème et cilastatine sodique |
| 适应证<br>Les indications | 用于敏感菌所致的腹膜炎、肝胆感染、腹腔内脓肿、阑尾炎、妇科感染、下呼吸道感染、皮肤和软组织感染、尿路感染、骨和关节感染及败血症等。<br>Ce produit est utilisés comme traitement des infections causées par des bactéries, telles que la péritonite, les infections hépatobiliaires, les abcès intra-abdominaux, l'appendicite, les infections gynécologiques, les infections des voies respiratoires inférieures, cutanées, des tissus mous, des voies urinaires, osseuses, articulaires ainsi que la septicémie. |

| 续 表 | |
|---|---|
| 用法、用量<br>Les modes d'emploi et la posologie | 静脉滴注或肌内注射。用量以亚胺培南计，根据病情，一次 0.25 ～ 1g，一日 2 ～ 4 次，对中度感染一般可按 1 次 1g，一日 2 次给予。静脉滴注可选用等渗氯化钠注射液、5% ～ 10% 葡萄糖液作溶剂。每 0.5g 药物用 100ml 溶剂，制成 5mg/ml 液体，缓缓滴入。肌内注射用 1% 利多卡因注射液为溶剂，以减轻疼痛。<br><br>对肾功能不全者应按肌酐清除率调整剂量：肌酐清除率为 31 ～ 70ml/min 的患者，每 6 ～ 8 小时用 0.5g，每日最高剂量为 1.5 ～ 2g；肌酐清除率为 21 ～ 30ml/min 的患者，每 8 ～ 12 小时用 0.5g，每日最高剂量为 1 ～ 1.5g；肌酐清除率为 < 20ml/min 的患者，每 12 小时用 0.25 ～ 0.5g，每日最高剂量为 0.5 ～ 1g。<br><br>Administration par voie IV en perfusion ou par voie IM. La dose est mesurée en imipénème, selon les cas, 0,25 à 1g par fois, 2 à 4 fois par jour, pour l'injection modérée, 1g par fois, 2 fois par jour. En perfusion, utiliser une solution de chlorure de sodium ou une solution de glucose à 5 % à 10 % comme solvant. Pour 0,5g de médicament, utiliser 100ml de solvant pour le transformer en 5 mg/ml de liquide, injecter lentement. En cas d'injection par voie IM, utiliser injection de lidocaïne à 1 % comme solvant, afin de soulager la douleur.<br><br>Chez des patients insuffisants rénaux : ceux dont la clairance de la créatinine est de 31 à 70 ml/min, 0,5g toutes les 6 à 8 h, ne pas dépasser 1,5 à 2 g par jour ; ceux dont la clairance de la créatinine est de 21 à 30 ml/min, 0,5g toutes les 8 à 12h, ne pas dépasser 1 à 1,5g par jour ; ceux dont la clairance de la créatinine est inférieure à 20 ml/min, 0,25 à 0,5g toutes les 12h, ne pas dépasser 0,5 à 1g par jour. |
| 剂型、规格<br>Les formes pharmaceutiques et les spécifications | 注射用亚胺培南 - 西司他汀：每支 0.25g；0.5g；1g（以亚胺培南计量）。其中含有等量的西司他汀钠。<br><br>L'imipénème et la cilastatine pour injection : 0,25g, 0,5g ou 1g par pièce (mesuré en imipénème). Elle contient la même dose de cilastatine sodique. |
| 药品名称 Drug Names | 美罗培南 Méropénème |
| 适应证<br>Les indications | 用于敏感菌所致的呼吸道、尿路、肝胆、外科、骨科、妇科、五官科感染及腹膜炎、皮肤化脓性疾病等。本品可适用于敏感菌所致脑膜炎。<br><br>Ce produit est utilisé comme traitement des infections causées par des bactéries, telles que les infections des voies respiratoires, des voies urinaires, hépatobiliaires, chirurgicales, osseuses, gynécologiques, les infections à propros de l'ORL, ainsi que la péritonite et les infections purulentes. Il est aussi applicable dans le traitement de la méningite. |
| 用法、用量<br>Les modes d'emploi et la posologie | 成人每日 0.5 ～ 1g，分为 2 ～ 3 次，稀释后静脉滴注每次 30 分钟。重症每日剂量可增至 2g。连续应用不超过 2 周。本品每 0.5g 用生理盐水约 100ml 溶解，不可用注射用水。<br>儿童 (3 月龄以上) 推荐用量：周围感染 20mg/kg，每 8 小时 1 次，脑膜炎 40mg/kg，每 8 小时 1 次。<br>肾功能减退者应按肌酐清除率调整剂量：肌酐清除率为 26 ～ 50ml/min 的患者，每 12 小时用 1g；肌酐清除率为 10 ～ 25ml/min 的患者，每 12 小时用 0.5g；肌酐清除率为 < 10/min 的患者，每 24 小时用 0.5g。<br><br>Chez des adultes, 0,5 à 1g par jour, à travers 2 à 3 fois, après la dilution, en perfusion pendant 30 minutes. Pour traiter des cas graves, 2g par jour. Ne pas l'utiliser pendant plus de 2 semaines consécutives. Pour 0,5g de médicament, il faut utiliser 100ml de solution saline comme solvant, ne pas utiliser d'eau pour injection.<br><br>Chez des enfants (plus de 3 mois), dose recommandée : pour l'infection entourante, 20 mg/kg, toutes les 8 h ; pour la méningite, 40 mg/kg, toutes les 8h.<br><br>Chez des patients insuffisants rénaux : ceux dont la clairance de la créatinine est de 26 à 50 ml/min, 1 g toutes les 12 h ; ceux dont la clairance de la créatinine est de 10 à 25 ml/min, 0,5g toutes les 12h ; ceux dont la clairance de la créatinine est inférieure à 10 ml/min, 0,5g toutes les 24h. |
| 剂型、规格<br>Les formes pharmaceutiques et les spécifications | 粉针剂：每瓶 0.5g；1g。<br>Poudre, 0,5g ou 1g par flacon. |

**续　表**

| 药品名称 Drug Names | 帕尼培南 - 倍他米隆 Panipénem-bétamipron |
|---|---|
| 适应证<br>Les indications | 用于治疗敏感菌引起的呼吸系统、泌尿生殖系统、腹内、眼科、皮肤及软组织、骨及关节的感染。如急慢性支气管炎、肺炎、肺脓肿、胆囊炎、腹膜炎、肝脓肿，肾盂肾炎、前列腺炎、子宫内感染，角膜溃疡、眼球炎、丹毒、蜂窝织炎、骨髓炎、关节炎等。还可用于败血症、感染性心内膜炎等严重感染。<br><br>Ce produit est utilisé comme traitement des infections causées par des bactéries, telles que les infections respiratoires, urinaires, intra-abdominales, des yeux, cutanées et des tissus mous, ainsi que osseuses et articulaires. Par exemple, la bronchite aiguë et chronique , la pneumonie, les abcès du poumon, la cholécystite , la péritonite, les abcès du foie, la pyélonéphrite, la prostatite, les infections intra-utérines, les ulcères de la cornée, une inflammation de l'œil , l'érysipèle, la cellulite, l'ostéomyélite ainsi que l'arthrite. Il est aussi applicable dans le traitement de la septicémie et de l'endocardite infectieuse. |
| 用法、用量<br>Les modes d'emploi et la posologie | 静脉滴注：成人，一般感染，每次 0.5g，一日 2 次，用不少于 100ml 的生理盐水或 5% 葡萄糖注射液溶解后，于 30 ～ 60 分钟滴注；重症或顽固性感染，剂量为每次 1g，一日 2 次，静脉滴注时间不少于 1 小时。儿童，每日 30 ～ 60mg/kg，分 2 ～ 3 次，每次 30min 静脉滴注；严重感染可增加至每日 100mg/kg，分 3 ～ 4 次。<br><br>En perfusion : chez des adultes, pour l'infection générale, 0,5g par fois, 2 fois par jour, utiliser plus de 100ml de solution saline ou de solution de glucose à 5 % comme solvant, la perfusion pendant 30 à 60 minutes ; pour l'infection grave ou réfractaire, 1g par fois, 2 fois par jour, la perfusion pendant 1h au moins. Chez des enfants, 30 à 60 mg/kg par jour, à travers 2 à 3 fois, pendant 30 minutes en perfusion ; pour l'infection grave, 100 mg/kg par jour, à travers 3 à 4 fois. |
| 剂型、规格<br>Les formes pharmaceutiques et les spécifications | 注射用帕尼培南 - 倍他米隆：250mg/ 瓶；500mg/ 瓶。帕尼培南与等量倍他米隆配伍，以帕尼培南含量计。<br><br>Le panipénem/bétamipron pour injection : 250 mg ou 500mg par flacon. Utiliser la même dose de panipénème que le bétamipron, mesurée en panipénème. |
| 药品名称 Drug Names | 厄他培南 Ertapénème |
| 适应证<br>Les indications | 用于治疗敏感菌引起的呼吸系统、泌尿生殖系统、腹腔、皮肤及软组织、盆腔等部位的感染。<br><br>Ce produit est utilisé comme traitement des infections causées par des bactéries, telles que les infections respiratoires, génito-urinaires, abdominales, cutanées, des tissus mous ainsi que les infections pelviennes. |
| 用法、用量<br>Les modes d'emploi et la posologie | 静脉滴注：成人，每日 1g，用不少于 100ml 的生理盐水稀释。肾功能不全者，肌酐清除率＜ 30ml/min，每天剂量 0.5g。3 个月及以上的儿童每日 2 次按 15mg/kg 给予肌内注射或静脉滴注，日剂量不超过 1g。<br><br>En perfusion, chez des adultes, 1g par jour, utiliser plus de 100ml de solution saline pour la dilution. Chez des patients insuffisants rénaux dont la clairance de la créatinine est inférieure à 30 ml/min, 0,5g par jour. Chez des enfants plus de 3 mois, 15 mg/kg par fois, 2 fois par jour, par voie IM ou par voie IV en perfusion, ne pas dépasser 1g par jour. |
| 剂型、规格<br>Les formes pharmaceutiques et les spécifications | 注射用厄他培南：每支 1g。<br><br>L'ertapénème pour injection : 1g par injection. |
| 药品名称 Drug Names | 比阿培南 Biapénème |
| 适应证<br>Les indications | 用于肠杆菌属、假单胞属、不动杆菌、枸橼酸杆菌、脆弱拟杆菌所致慢性呼吸道感染急性发作、肺炎、肺脓肿、腹膜炎、复杂性膀胱炎、女性生殖器感染。对某些革兰阳性菌也有效。<br><br>Ce produit est utilisé comme traitement des infections causées par l'Enterobacter, le Pseudomonas, l'Acinetobacter,le Citrobacter et les Bacteroides fragilis, telles que l'exacerbation aiguë de l'infection chronique des voies respiratoires, la pneumonie, les abcès du poumon, la péritonite, la cystite compliquée, les infections génitales féminines. Il est utile dans le traitement de certaines bactéries à Gram positif. |

| 续　表 | |
|---|---|
| 用法、用量<br>Les modes d'emploi et la posologie | 静脉滴注：成人一般感染，每次 0.3g，一日 2 次。可根据病情增加剂量，但每日不可超过 1.2g。用 0.9% 的生理盐水或 5% 葡萄糖注射液稀释。<br>En perfusion : chez des adultes, pour l'infection générale, 0,3g par fois, 2 fois par jour. Selon les cas, il est permissible de doubler la dose, mais ne pas dépasser 1,2 g par jour. Utiliser la solution saline à 0,9 % ou la solution de glucose à 5 % pour la dilution. |
| 剂型、规格<br>Les formes pharmaceutiques et les spécifications | 注射用比阿培南：每支 300mg。<br>Le biapénème pour injection, 300mg par injection. |
| 药品名称 Drug Names | 法罗培南钠 Faropénème sodique |
| 适应证<br>Les indications | 用于皮肤及软组织、呼吸系统、泌尿生殖系统及眼、耳、鼻、喉、口腔等部位的敏感菌感染。<br>Ce produit est utilisé comme traitement des infections causées par des bactéries, telles que les infections cutanées et des tissus mous, des voies respiratoires, urinaires ainsi que des infections à propos des yeux, des orielles, du nez, de la gorge et de la bouche. |
| 用法、用量<br>Les modes d'emploi et la posologie | 口服：成人常用量每次 150 ～ 200mg，一日 3 次。重症每次 200 ～ 300mg，一日 3 次。<br>Administration par voie orale : chez des adultes, dose usuelle, 150 à 200mg par fois, 3 fois par jour. Pour l'infection grave, 200 à 300 mg par fois, 3 fois par jour. |
| 剂型、规格<br>Les formes pharmaceutiques et les spécifications | 片剂：每片 150mg；300mg。<br>Comprimés : 150mg ou 300mg par comprimé. |
| 药品名称 Drug Names | 氨曲南 Aztréonam |
| 适应证<br>Les indications | 用于敏感的革兰阴性菌所致的感染，包括肺炎、胸膜炎、腹腔感染、胆道感染、骨和关节感染、皮肤和软组织炎症，尤适用于尿路感染，也用于败血症。由于本品有较好的耐酶性能，因此，当细菌对青霉素类、头孢菌素类、氨基糖苷类等药物不敏感时，可试用本品。<br>Ce produit est utilisé comme traitement des infections causées par des bactéries à Gram négatif, telles que la pneumonie, la pleurésie, les infections intra-abdominales, les infections des voies biliaires, les infections osseuses et articulaires, cutanées et des tissus mous, en particulier pour les infections des voies urinaires, ainsi que pour la septicémie. Comme ce produit est bien résistant à l'enzyme, il est permissible de l'utiliser quand les bactéries ne sont pas sensibles aux pénicillines, aux céphalosporines, ni aux aminosides. |
| 用法、用量<br>Les modes d'emploi et la posologie | 肌内注射、静脉注射、静脉滴注。成人，一般感染，3 ～ 4g/d，分 2 ～ 3 次给予；严重感染，1 次 2g，一日 3 ～ 4 次，一日最大剂量为 8g；无其他并发症的尿路感染，只需用 1g，分 1 ～ 2 次给予。儿童，每次 30mg/kg，一日 3 次，重症感染可增加至一日 4 次给药，一日最大剂量为 120mg/kg。肌内注射：每 1g 药物，加液体 3 ～ 4ml 溶解。静脉注射：每 1g 药物，加液体 10ml 溶解，缓慢注射。静脉滴注：每 1g 药物，加液体 50ml 以上溶解（浓度不超过 2%），滴注时间 20 ～ 60 分钟。注射时，下列药液可用作本品的溶解 - 稀释液：灭菌注射用水、等渗氯化钠注射液、林格液、乳酸钠林格液、5% ～ 10% 葡萄糖液、葡萄糖氯化钠注射液等。用于肌内注射时，还可用含苯甲醇的氯化钠注射液作溶剂。<br>Par voie IM, par voie IV ou IV en perfusion. Chez des adultes, pour l'infection générale, 3 à 4g/jour, à travers 2 à 3 fois ; pour l'infection grave, 2g par fois, 3 à 4 fois par jour, ne pas dépasser 8g par jour ; pour l'infection urinaire sans complication, 1g seulement, à travers 1 à 2 fois. Chez des enfants, 30 mg/kg par fois, 3 fois par jour, pour l'infection grave, 4 fois par jour, ne pas dépasser 120 mg/kg par jour. Par voie IM : pour 1g de médicament, utiliser 3 à 4ml de liquide pour la dissolution. Injection IV : pour 1g de médicament, utiliser 10ml ou plus de liquide pour la dissolution, injection lente. Par voie IV en perfusion : pour 1g de médicament, utiliser plus de 50ml de solution (la concentration ne dépasse pas 2 %), pendant 20 à 60 minutes. Les liquides suivantes peuvent être les solutions pour ce médicament : l'eau stérile pour injection, l'injection de chlorure de sodium isotonique, la solution de Ringer, le lactate de sodium de Ringer, la solution de glucose à 5% à 10 % ainsi que l'injection de glucose de chlorure de sodium. En cas d'injection par voie IM, il est possible d'utiliser l'injection de chlorure de sodium contenant le benzène méthanol comme solvant. |

**续　表**

| 剂型、规格<br>Les formes pharmaceutiques et les spécifications | 注射用氨曲南：每天 1g( 效价 )。内含精氨酸 0.78g( 稳定、助溶用 )。<br>L'aztréonam pour injection : 1g par jour (titre). Il contient 0,78g d'arginie (pour la stabilisation et la solubilisation). |
| --- | --- |

### 1.5　氨基糖苷类 Aminoglycosides

| 药品名称 Drug Names | 卡那霉素 Kanamycine |
| --- | --- |
| 适应证<br>Les indications | 口服用于治疗敏感菌所致的肠道感染及用作肠道手术前准备，并有减少肠道细菌产生氨的作用，对肝硬化消化道出血患者的肝性脑病有一定防治作用。<br>肌内注射用于敏感菌所致的系统感染，如肺炎、败血症、尿路感染等，常与其他抗菌药物联合应用。<br>Par voie orale : il est utilisé comme traitement des infections causées par des bactéries, telles que les infections intestinales, ainsi que dans la préparation avant l'opération chirurgicale intestinale. Il peut aussi servir à réduire l'ammoniac produit par les bactéries intestinales, et à prévenir l'encéphalopathie hépatiquechez les patients atteints de saignements gastro-intestinaux.<br>Par voie IM : il est utilisé comme traitement des infections causées pas des bactéroes, telles que la pneumonie, la septémie, les infections urinaires. il est souvent utilisé avec d'autres médicaments servant à réduire l'ammoniac produit par les bactéries intestinales. |
| 用法、用量<br>Les modes d'emploi et la posologie | 肌内注射或静脉滴注：1 次 0.5g，一日 1 ～ 1.2g；小儿每日 15 ～ 25mg/kg，分 2 次给予。静脉滴注时应将一次用量以输液约 100ml 稀释，滴入时间为 30 ～ 60 分钟，切勿过速。口服：用于防治肝性脑病，一日 4g，分次给予。腹部手术前准备：每小时 1g，连续 4 次 ( 常与甲硝唑联合应用 ) 后，改为每 6 小时 1 次，连服 36 ～ 72 小时。<br>Par voie IM ou par voie IV en perfusion : 0,5g par fois, 1 à 1,2g par jour ; chez des enfants, 15 à 25 mg/kg par jour, à travers 2 fois. En cas d'injection par voie IV en perfusion, pour une dose de médicament, utiliser 100ml d'infusion comme solvant, la perfusion pendant 30 à 60 minutes, ne pas trop vite.<br>Par voie orale : pour prévenir l'encéphalopathie hépatique, 4g par jour, à travers plusieurs fois. Pour la préparation avant l'opération chirurgicale intestinale, 1g par heure, 4 fois consécutives (souvent utilisé en association avec le métronidazole), et puis toutes les 6h, pendant 36 à 72 heures consécutives. |
| 剂型、规格<br>Les formes pharmaceutiques et les spécifications | 注射用硫酸卡那霉素：每瓶 0.5g；1g。<br>注射液 ( 含单硫酸卡那霉素 )：每支 500mg(2ml)。<br>滴眼液：8ml(40mg)。<br>Sulfate de kanamycinepour injection : 0,5g ou 1g par flacon.<br>Injection (contient lemonosulfate de kanamycine) : 500 mg (2ml) par injection.<br>Gouttes pour les yeux : 8ml (40mg). |
| 药品名称 Drug Names | 阿米卡星 Amikacine |
| 适应证<br>Les indications | 临床主要用于对卡那霉素或庆大霉素耐药的革兰阴性杆菌所致的尿路、下呼吸道、腹腔、软组织、骨和关节、生殖系统等部位的感染，以及败血症等。<br>Ce produit est utilisé dans les cliniques comme traitement des infections causées par des bactéries à Gram négatif résistant à la kalamycine ou à la gentamicine, telles que les infections des voies urinaires, des voies respiratoires inférieures, adominales, des tissus mous, osseuses, articulaires et l'appareil reproducteur, ainsi que dans le traitement de la septicémie. |
| 用法、用量<br>Les modes d'emploi et la posologie | 肌内注射或静脉滴注：成人 7.5mg/kg，每 12 小时 1 次，每日总量不超过 1.5g，可用 7 ～ 10 日；无并发症的尿路感染，每次 0.2g，每 12 小时 1 次：小儿，开始用 10mg/kg，以后 7.5mg/kg，每 12 小时 1 次；较大儿童可按成人用量。<br>给药途径以肌内注射为主，也可用 100 ～ 200ml 输液稀释后静脉滴注，30 ～ 60 分钟进入体内，儿童则为 1 ～ 2 小时。疗程一般不超过 10 日。<br>肾功能不全者首次剂量 7.5mg/kg，以后则调整使血药峰浓度为 25μg/ml，谷浓度 5 ～ 8μg/ml。 |

**续　表**

| | |
|---|---|
| | Par voie IM ou IV en perfusion : chez des adultes, 7,5 mg/kg, toutes les 12 h, ne pas dépasser 1,5g par jour, utilisable pendant 7 à 10 jours ; pour l'infection des voies urinaires sans complication, 0,2g par fois, toutes les 12h. Chez des petits enfants, comencer par 10 mg/kg et puis 7,5 mg/kg, toutes les 12h. Chez des enfants plus âgés, la même dose que chez les adultes.<br><br>Principalement par voie IM, c'est aussi permissible d'injecter par voie IV en perfusion après la dilution par 100 à 200 d'infusion, la perfusion pendant 30 à 60 minutes. Chez des enfants, 1 à 2 h. Ne pas dépasser 10 jours comme un traitement medical.<br><br>La première dose administrée aux patients souffrant d'insuffisance rénale est de 7.5 mg/kg, ensuite, ajuster la dose administrée jusgu'à ce que la concentration du pic sauguin soit de 25μg/ml, La concentration en vallées est de 5～8μg/ml. |
| 剂型、规格<br>Les formes pharmaceutiques et les spécifications | 注射液：每支 0.1g(1ml)；0.2g(2ml)。<br>注射用硫酸阿米卡星：每瓶：0.2g。<br>Injection : 0,1g (1ml) ou 0,2g (2ml) par injection.<br>Sulfate d'amikacine pour injection : 0,2g par flacon. |
| 药品名称 Drug Names | 妥布霉素 Tobramycine |
| 适应证<br>Les indications | 临床主要用于铜绿假单胞菌感染。如烧伤、败血症等。对其他敏感革兰阴性杆菌所致的感染也可应用。与庆大霉素间存在较密切的交叉耐药性。<br><br>Ce produit est utilisé dans les cliniques comme traitement des infections à bactérie pseudomonas aeruginosa, telles que la brûlure et la septicémie. Il est aussi applicable dans le traitement des infections causées par des bactéries à Gram négatif. Il y a une résistance croisée assez étroite entre la tobramycine et la gentamicine. |
| 用法、用量<br>Les modes d'emploi et la posologie | 肌内注射或静脉滴注，一日 4.5mg/kg，分为 2 次给予，一日剂量不可超过 5mg/kg。静脉滴注时 1 次量用输液 100ml 稀释，于 30 分钟左右滴入。新生儿一日量 4mg/kg，分为 2 次给予。一般用药不超过 7～10 日。<br><br>Injection par voie IM ou par voie IV en perfusion, 4,5 mg/kg par jour, à travers 2 fois, ne pas dépasser 5 mg/kg par jour. En cas d'injection par voie IV en perfusion, pour une dose de ce produit, utiliser 100ml d'infusion pour la dilution, la perfusion pendant 30 minutes. Chez des nouveau-nés, 4 mg/kg par jour, à travers 2 fois. Ne pas dépasser 7 à 10 jours. |
| 剂型、规格<br>Les formes pharmaceutiques et les spécifications | 注射液：每支 80mg(2ml)。<br>Injection : 80mg (2ml) par injection. |
| 药品名称 Drug Names | 庆大霉素 Gentamicine |
| 适应证<br>Les indications | 临床主要用于大肠埃希菌、痢疾杆菌、克雷伯肺炎杆菌、变形杆菌、铜绿假单胞菌等革兰阴性菌引起的系统或局部感染（对中枢感染无效）。<br><br>Ce produit est utilisé dans les cliniques comme traitement des infections locales ou systématiques causées par des bactéries à Gram négatif, y comrpis Escherichia coli, bacille dysentérique, Klebsiella pneumoniae, Proteus et Pseudomonas aeruginosa (Il est inutile dans le traitement de l'infection du système nerveux central). |
| 用法、用量<br>Les modes d'emploi et la posologie | 肌内注射或静脉滴注，一次 80mg，一日 2～3 次（间隔 8 小时）。对于革兰阴性杆菌所致重症感染或铜绿假单胞菌全身感染，一日量可用到 5mg/kg。静脉滴注给药可将 1 次量（80mg），用输液 100ml 稀释，于 30 分钟左右滴入。小儿一日 3～5mg/kg，分 2～3 次给予。<br>口服：一次 80～160mg，一日 3～4 次。小儿每日 10～15mg/kg，分 3～4 次服，用于肠道感染或术前准备。<br><br>Injection par voie IM ou par voie IV en perfusion, 80mg par fois, 2 à 3 fois par jour (toutes les 8h). Pour traiter l'infection grave causée par des bactéries à Gram négatif ou traiter l'infection systémique à bactéries Pseudomonas aeruginosa, 5 mg/kg par jour. En cas d'injection par voie IV en perfusion, 80mg par fois, utiliser 100ml d'infusion pour la dilution, la perfusion pendant 30 minutes. Chez des enfants, 3 à 5 mg par kg par jour, à travers 2 à 3 fois.<br>Par voie orale : 80 à 160 mg, à travers 3 à 4 fois par jour. Chez des enfants, 10 à 15 mg/kg par jour, à travers 3 à 4 fois, pour traiter l'infection intestinale ou la préparation préopératoire. |

续　表

| 剂型、规格<br>Les formes pharmaceutiques et les spécifications | 注射液：每支 20mg(1ml)；40mg(1ml)；80mg(2ml)。<br>片剂：每片 40mg。<br>滴眼液：8ml(40mg)。<br>Injection : 20mg (1ml), 40mg (1ml) ou 80 mg (2ml) par injeciton.<br>Comprimés : 40mg par comprimé.<br>Gouttes pour les yeux : 8ml (40mg). |
|---|---|
| **药品名称 Drug Names** | 西索米星 Sisomicine |
| 适应证<br>Les indications | 临床主要用于大肠埃希菌、痢疾杆菌、克雷伯杆菌、变形杆菌等革兰阴性菌引起的局部或系统感染（对中枢感染无效），对尿路感染作用尤佳。<br>　　Ce produit est utilisé dans les cliniques comme traitement des infections locales ou systématiques causées par des bactéries à Gram négatif, y comrpis Escherichia coli, bacille dysentérique, Klebsiella pneumoniae et Proteus (Il est inutile dans le traitement de l'infection du système nerveux central). Il est extrêmement utile dans le traitement des infections des voies urinaires. |
| 用法、用量<br>Les modes d'emploi et la posologie | 成人一日量 3mg/kg，分为 3 次，肌内注射。疗程不超过 7 ～ 10 日。<br>　　Chez des adultes, 3 mg/kg par jour, à travers 3 fois, par voie IM, ne pas dépasser 7 à 10 jours. |
| 剂型、规格<br>Les formes pharmaceutiques et les spécifications | 注射液：每支 75mg(1.5ml)；100mg(2ml)。<br>Injection : 75mg (1,5 ml) ou 100 mg (2ml) par injection. |
| **药品名称 Drug Names** | 奈替米星 Nétilmicine |
| 适应证<br>Les indications | 临床主要用于大肠埃希菌、克雷伯杆菌、变形杆菌、肠杆菌属、枸橼酸杆菌、沙雷杆菌、流感嗜血杆菌、沙门杆菌、志贺杆菌、奈瑟球菌等革兰阴性菌所致呼吸道、消化道、泌尿生殖系，皮肤和软组织、骨和关节、腹腔、创伤等部位的感染，也适用于败血症。<br>　　Ce produit est utilisé dans les cliniques comme traitement des infections (infections des voies respiratoires, gastro-intestinales, génito-urinaires, cutanées et des tissus mous, osseuses et articulaires, abdominal et le traumatisme) causées par des bactéries à Gram négatif, y compris Escherichia coli, Klebsiella pneumoniae, Proteus, des Enterobacteriaceae, Al-Shara bacilles, Haemophilus influenzae, Bactérie Salmonella, Shigella et Neisseria. Il est aussi applicable dans le traitement de la septicémie. |
| 用法、用量<br>Les modes d'emploi et la posologie | 单纯泌尿系感染：成人一日量为 3 ～ 4mg/kg，分为 2 次。较严重的系统感染：成人一日量为 4 ～ 6.5mg/kg，分为 2 ～ 3 次给予；新生儿（6 周龄以内）：一日 4 ～ 6.5mg/kg；婴儿和儿童：一日 5 ～ 8mg/kg，分为 2 ～ 3 次给予，肌内注射给药。如必须静脉滴注，则将 1 次药量加入 50 ～ 200ml 输液中，缓慢滴入。有报道，本品一日按 4.5 ～ 6mg/kg 量，1 次肌内注射，效果好，且不良反应少。<br>　　Pour l'infection des voies urinaires simplexe : chez des adultes, 3 à 4 mg/kg par jour, à travers 2 fois. Pour l'injection systématique assez grave : chez des adultes, 4 à 6,5 mg/kg par jour, à travers 2 à 3 fois ; chez des nouveau-nés (moins de 6 semaines), 4 à 6,5 mg/kg par jour ; chez des bébés et des enfants : 5 à 8 mg/kg par jour, à travers 2 à 3 fois, par voie IM. En cas d'injection par voie IM en perfusion, pour une dose de médicament, utiliser 50 à 200 ml d'infusion pour la dilution, la perfusion lente. Selon des rapports, il est bon d'administrer ce produit par voie IM, 4,5 à 6 mg/kg par jour, une fois par jour, avec peu de réactions indésirables. |
| 剂型、规格<br>Les formes pharmaceutiques et les spécifications | 注射液：每支 150mg(1.5ml)。<br>Injectin : 150 mg (1,5 ml) par injection. |
| **药品名称 Drug Names** | 小诺米星 Micronomicine |
| 适应证<br>Les indications | 临床主要用于大肠埃希菌、克雷伯杆菌、变形杆菌、肠杆菌属、沙雷杆菌、铜绿假单胞菌等革兰阴性杆菌引起的呼吸道、泌尿道、腹腔及外伤感染，也适用于败血症。<br>　　Ce produit est utilisé dans les cliniques comme traitement des bactéries à Gram négatif (le colibacille, le klebsiella, le proteus, l'enterobacter,le marcescens, le pseudomonas aeruginosa), telles que les infections respiratoires, uriniares, abdominiales et les infections liées au traumatisme, ainsi que le traitement de la septicémie. |

**续 表**

| 用法、用量<br>Les modes d'emploi et la posologie | 泌尿道感染：1 次 120mg，肌内注射，一日 2 次。其他感染：1 次 60mg，一日 2 ～ 3 次，肌内注射。用药疗程一般不超过 2 周。<br>Pour l'infection des voies urinaires : 120mg par fois, par voie IM, 2 fois par jour. Pour d'autres infections : 60mg par fois, 2 à 3 fois par jour, par voie IM. Le traitement médical ne dépasse pas généralement 2 semaines. |
|---|---|
| 剂型、规格<br>Les formes pharmaceutiques et les spécifications | 注射液：每支 60mg(2ml)。<br>Injection : 60mg (2ml) par injection. |

| 药品名称 Drug Names | 异帕米星 Isépamicine |
|---|---|
| 适应证<br>Les indications | 临床适用于上述敏感菌所致外伤或烧伤创口感染、肺炎、支气管炎、肾盂肾炎、膀胱炎、腹膜炎及败血症。<br>Ce produit est utilisé dans les cliniques comme traitement des bactéries, telles que les infections liées à la brûlure ou au traumatisme, la pneumonie, la bronchite, la pyélonéphrite, la cystite, l'inflammtion abdominale et la septicémie. |
| 用法、用量<br>Les modes d'emploi et la posologie | 成人一日量 400mg，通常分为 2 次（或一日 1 次）肌内注射或静脉滴注。静脉滴注速度控制 0.5 ～ 1 小时滴毕，按年龄、体质和症状适当调整。<br>Chez des adultes, 400mg par jour, à travers 2 fois ou 1 fois par jour, par voie IM ou par voie IV en perfusion. En cas de perfusion, finir en 0,5 à 1 h, ajuster le débit de la perfusion en fonction de l'âge et de la maladie. |
| 剂型、规格<br>Les formes pharmaceutiques et les spécifications | 注射液：每支 200mg(2ml)。<br>Injection : 200mg (2ml) par injection. |

| 药品名称 Drug Names | 依替米星 Etimicine |
|---|---|
| 适应证<br>Les indications | 临床主要用于革兰阴性杆菌、大肠埃希菌、肺炎克雷伯菌、沙雷菌属、奇异变形杆菌、沙门菌属、流感嗜血杆菌等敏感菌株所引起的呼吸道、泌尿生殖系统、腹腔、皮肤和软组织等部位的感染及败血症。<br>Ce produit est utilisé dans les cliniques comme traitement des infections causées par des bactéries (les bactéries à Gram négatif, le colibacille, le klebsiella, le serratia, le proteus, le salmonella et l'haemophilus influenzae), telles ques les infections respiratoires, urinaires, génitales, abdominales, cutanées et des tissus mous ainsi que la septicémie. |
| 用法、用量<br>Les modes d'emploi et la posologie | 成人量每日 200mg，一次加入输液 (0.9% 氯化钠液或 5% 葡萄糖液)100ml 中，静脉滴注 1 小时，每日只用 1 次，连用 3 ～ 7 日。<br>Chez des adultes, 200mg par jour, utiliser 100ml d'infusion (solution de chlorure à 0,9 % ou solution de glucose à 5 %), en perfusion pendant 1h, 1 fois par jour, 3 à 7 jours consécutifs. |
| 剂型、规格<br>Les formes pharmaceutiques et les spécifications | 注射用粉针：每支 50mg；100mg。<br>注射液：50mg(1ml)；100mg(2ml)。<br>Poudre pour injection : 50 mg ou 100 mg par injection.<br>Injection : 50mg (1ml) ou 100mg (2ml). |

| 药品名称 Drug Names | 大观霉素 Spectinomycine |
|---|---|
| 适应证<br>Les indications | 临床主要应用于淋球菌所引起的泌尿系感染，适用于对青霉素、四环素等耐药的病例。<br>Ce produit est utilisé dans les cliniques comme traitement des infections urinaires causées par le neisseria gonorrhoeae. Il est aussi applicable dans le traitement des maladies résistant à la pénicilline et à la tétracycline. |

续　表

| | |
|---|---|
| 用法、用量<br>Les modes d'emploi et la posologie | 1 次肌内注射 2g。将特殊稀释液 (0.9% 苯甲醇溶液 )3.2ml 注入药瓶中，猛力振摇，使成混悬液 ( 约 5ml)，用粗针头注入臀上部外侧深部肌肉内。一般只用 1 次即可。对于使用其他抗生素治疗而迁延未愈的患者，可按 4g 剂量给药，即 1 次用药 4g，分注于两侧臀上外侧肌内，或 1 次肌内注射 2g，一日内用药 2 次。<br>2g par fois, par voie IM. Dissoudre le produit dans 3,2 ml de solution d'alcool benzylique à 0,9 %, agiter pour obtenir 5ml de solution en suspension. Injecter profondément dans le muscle externe sur les fesses hautes. 1 fois suffit en général. Pour des patients ayant utilisé d'autres anti-biotiques sans résultat, 4g par fois, injecter dans le muscle externe sur les fesses à deux côtés, ou 2g par fois, injection IM, 2 fois par jour. |
| 剂型、规格<br>Les formes pharmaceuti-ques et les spécifications | 注射用盐酸大观霉素：每支 2g；4g( 附 0.9% 苯甲醇注射液 1 支 )。<br>Le chlorhydrate de spectinomycine pour injection : 2g ou 4g par injection (y compris une injection d'alcool benzylique à 0,9 %). |

1.6　四环素类 Tétracyclines

| 药品名称 Drug Names | 四环素 Tétracycline |
|---|---|
| 适应证<br>Les indications | 现主要用于立克次体病、布氏杆菌病、淋巴肉芽肿、支原体肺炎、螺旋体病、衣原体病，也可用于敏感的革兰阳性球菌或革兰阴性杆菌所引起的轻症感染。<br>Ce produit est principalement utilisé comme traitement de la rickettsiose, de la brucellose, de la lymphogranulomatose vénérienne, de la pneumonie à mycoplasme, de la leptospirose et de la chlamydiose. Il est aussi applicable dans le traitement des infections bénignes causées par des bacté-ries à Gram négatif ou positif. |
| 用法、用量<br>Les modes d'emploi et la posologie | 口服：成人一日 3 ～ 4 次，1 次 0.5g；8 岁以上小儿一日 30 ～ 40mg/kg，分 3 ～ 4 次用。<br>Par voie orale : chez des adultes, 3 à 4 fois par jour, 0,5g par fois ; chez des enfants plus de 8 ans, 30 à 40 mg/kg par jour, à travers 3 à 4 fois. |
| 剂型、规格<br>Les formes pharmaceutiques et les spécifications | 片剂：每片 0.125g；0.25g。<br>胶囊剂：每粒 0.25g。<br>Comprimés : 0,125g ou 0,25g par comprimé.<br>Capsules : 0,25g par capsule. |
| 药品名称 Drug Names | 土霉素 Oxytetracycline |
| 适应证<br>Les indications | 现主要用于立克次体病、布氏杆菌病、淋巴肉芽肿、支原体肺炎、螺旋体病、衣原体病，也可用于敏感的革兰阳性球菌或革兰阴性杆菌所引起的轻症感染。<br>Ce produit est principalement utilisé comme traitement de la rickettsiose, de la brucellose, de la lymphogranulomatose vénérienne, de la pneumonie à mycoplasme, de la leptospirose et de la chlamydiose. Il est aussi applicable dans le traitement des infections bénignes causées par des bactéries à Gram négatif ou positif. |
| 用法、用量<br>Les modes d'emploi et la posologie | 口服：1 次 0.5g，一日 3 ～ 4 次。8 岁以上小儿每日 30 ～ 40mg/kg，分 3 ～ 4 次服。<br>Par voie orale : 0,5g par fois, 3 à 4 fois par jour. Chez des enfants plus de 8 ans, 30 à 40 mg/kg par jour, à travers 3 à 4 fois. |
| 剂型、规格<br>Les formes pharmaceutiques et les spécifications | 片剂：每片 0.125g；0.25g(1mg= 盐酸土霉素 1000U)。<br>Copriés : 0,125g ou 0,25g par comprimé (1mg = 1000 unités de chlorhydrate d'oxytétracycline). |
| 药品名称 Drug Names | 多西环素 Doxycycline |
| 适应证<br>Les indications | 临床主要用于敏感的革兰阳性球菌和革兰阴性杆菌所致的上呼吸道感染、扁桃体炎、胆道感染、淋巴结炎、蜂窝织炎、老年慢性支气管炎等，也用于斑疹伤寒、恙虫病、支原体肺炎等。尚可用于治疗霍乱，也可用于预防恶性疟疾和钩端螺旋体感染。<br>Ce produit est principalement utilisé dans les cliniques comme traitement des infections causées par des bactéries à Gram positif et négatif, telles que les infections respiratoires, intestinales, l'amygdalite, la lymphadénite, la cellulite et la bronchite chronique. Il est aussi applicable dans le traitement du typhus, du typhus des broussailles, et de la pneumonie mycoplasme. Il est aussi utile pour traiter le choléraat prévenir le paludisme à falciparum et la leptospirose. |

**续 表**

| | |
|---|---|
| 用法、用量<br>Les modes d'emploi et la posologie | 口服，首次 0.2g，以后每次 0.1g，一日 1～2 次。8 岁以上儿童，首次 4mg/kg，以后每次 2～4mg/kg，一日 1～2 次。一般疗程为 3～7 日。预防恶性疟：每周 0.1g；预防钩端螺旋体病：每周 2 次，每次 0.1g。<br><br>Par voie orale : la première fois, 0,2g, ensuite, 0,1g par fois, 1 à 2 fois par jour. Chez des enfants plus de 8 ans, la première fois, 4 mg/kg, ensuite 2 à 4 mg/kg par fois, 1 à 2 fois par jour. Le traitement médical : 3 à 7 jours. Pour la prévention du paludisme à falciparum, 0,1g par semaine ; pour la prévention de la leptospirose, 2 fois par semaine, 0,1g par fois. |
| 剂型、规格<br>Les formes pharmaceutiques et les spécifications | 片剂：每片 0.05g；0.1g。<br>胶囊剂：每粒 0.1g(1mg= 盐酸多西环素 1000U)。<br>Comprimés : 0,05g ou 0,1g par comprimé.<br>Capsules : 0,1g par capsule (1mg = 1 000 unites de chlorhydrate de doxycycline). |
| 药品名称 Drug Names | 米诺环素 Minocycline |
| 适应证<br>Les indications | 临床主要用于立克次体病、支原体肺炎、淋巴肉芽肿、下疳、鼠疫、霍乱、布氏杆菌病（与链霉素联合应用）等引起的泌尿系、呼吸道、胆道、乳腺及皮肤软组织感染。<br><br>Ce produit est principalement utilisé dans les cliniques comme traitement des infections causées par des bactéries(y comrpis la rickettsiose, la pneumonie à mycoplasme, la lymphogranulomatose vénérienne, la chancre, la peste, le choléra et la brucellose (avec la streptomycine), telles que les infections urinaires, respiratoires, des voies biliaires, du sein, cutanées et des tissus mous. |
| 用法、用量<br>Les modes d'emploi et la posologie | 成人一般首次量 200mg，以后每 12 小时服 100mg。或在首次量后，每 6 小时服用 50mg。<br>Chez des adultes, pour la première fois, 200mg, ensuite, 100mg toutes les 12h, ou après la première fois, 50 mg toutes les 6 h. |
| 剂型、规格<br>Les formes pharmaceutiques et les spécifications | 片剂：每片 0.1g( 效价 )。<br>Comprimés : 0,1g par comprimé (titre). |

## 1.7 林可霉素类 Lincomycines

| | |
|---|---|
| 药品名称 Drug Names | 氯霉素 Chloramphénicol |
| 适应证<br>Les indications | 临床主要用于伤寒、副伤寒和其他沙门菌、脆弱拟杆菌感染。与氨苄西林合用于流感嗜血杆菌性脑膜炎。由脑膜炎球菌或肺炎链球菌引起的脑膜炎，在患者不宜用青霉素时，也可用本品。外用治疗沙眼或化脓菌感染。<br><br>Ce produit est principalement utilisé dans les cliniques comme traitement de la typhoïde, de la paratyphoïde, des salmonelles et d'autres bactéries. Avec l'ampicilline, il peut être applicable dans le traitement de la méningite à haemophilus. En cas de méningite causée par le méningocoques ou le streptococcus pneumoniae, chez des patients résistant à la pénicilline, il est aussi possible d'utiliser ce produit. Il est également utile dans le traitement topique du chlamydia trachomatis ou de l'infection à bactéries pyogènes. |
| 用法、用量<br>Les modes d'emploi et la posologie | 口服：成人 1 次 0.25～0.5g，一日 1～2g；小儿每日 25～50mg/kg，分 3～4 次服；新生儿每日不超过 25mg/kg。<br>静脉滴注：一日量为 1～2g，分 2 次注射。以输液稀释，1 支氯霉素 (250mg) 至少用稀释液 100ml。氯霉素注射液 ( 含乙醇、甘油或丙二醇等溶媒 )，宜用干燥注射器抽取，边稀释边振荡，防止析出结晶。症状消退后应酌情减量或停药。<br><br>Par voie orale : chez des adultes, 0,25g à 0,5g par fois, 1 à 2 g par jour ; chez des enfants, 25 à 50 mg/kg par jour, à travers 3 à 4 fois ; chez des nouveau-nés, ne pas dépasser 25 mg/kg par jour.<br><br>Par voie IV en perfusion : 1 à 2 g par jour, à travers 2 fois. Pour 250g de chloramphénicol, utiliser au moins 100ml d'infusion pour la dilution. Pour l'injection de chloramphénicol (y compris l'éthanol, la glycérine ou le propylène glycol), il vaut mieux utiliser la seringue sèche, en agitant, de manière à éviter la précipitation de cristallisation. Après la disparition des symptômes, le cas échéant, réduire la dose ou arrêter le traitement médical. |

**续　表**

| 剂型、规格<br>Les formes pharmaceutiques et les spécifications | 片（胶囊剂）：每片（粒）0.25g。<br>注射液：每支 0.25g(2ml)。<br>滴眼液：8ml(20mg)。<br>滴耳液：10ml(0.25g)。<br>眼膏：1%；3%。<br>Comprimés (capsules) : 0,25g par comprimé (capsule).<br>Injection : 0,25g (2 ml) par injection.<br>Gouttes pour les yeux : 8ml (20mg).<br>Gouttes pour les oreilles : 10ml (0,25g).<br>Pommade ophtalmique : 1 % ou 3 %. |
|---|---|
| **药品名称 Drug Names** | 林可霉素 Lincomycine |
| 适应证<br>Les indications | 用于葡萄球菌、链球菌、肺炎链球菌引起的呼吸道感染、骨髓炎、关节和软组织感染及胆道感染。对一些厌氧菌感染也可应用。外用治疗革兰阳性菌化脓性感染。<br>Ce produit est utilisé comme traitement de l'ostéomyélite, des infections respiratoires, articulaires, des tissus mous, des voies biliaires, causées par le staphylococcus aureus et le streptococcus pneumoniae. Il est aussi applicable dans le traitement des infections anaérobies, ainsi que le traitement des infections pyogènes caussées par des bactéries à Gram positif. |
| 用法、用量<br>Les modes d'emploi et la posologie | 口服（空腹）：成人，1 次 0.25 ～ 0.5g( 活性 )，一日 3 ～ 4 次；小儿一日 30 ～ 50mg( 活性 )/kg，分 3 ～ 4 次服用。肌内注射：成人 1 次 0.6g( 活性 )，一日 2 ～ 3 次；小儿一日 10 ～ 20mg( 活性 )/kg，分 2 ～ 3 次给药。静脉滴注：成人 1 次 0.6g( 活性 )，溶于 100 ～ 200ml 输液内，滴注 1 ～ 2 小时，每 8 ～ 12 小时 1 次。<br>Par voie orale (l'estomac vide) : chez des adultes, 0,25 à 0,5g par fois (actif), 3 à 4 fois par jour ; chez des enfants, 30 à 50 mg/kg (actif) par jour, à travers 3 à 4 fois. Par voie IM : chez des adultes, 0,6g par fois (actif), 2 à 3 fois par jour ; chez des enfants, 10 à 20 mg /kg par jour, à travers 2 à 3 fois. Par voie IV en perfusion : chez des adultes, 0.6g par fois, utiliser 100 à 200 ml d'eau pour injection, perfusion pendant 1 à 2 h, toutes les 8 à 12h. |
| 剂型、规格<br>Les formes pharmaceutiques et les spécifications | 片（胶囊）剂：每片（粒）0.25g( 活性 )；0.5g( 活性 )。<br>注射液：每支 0.2g( 活性 )(1ml)；0.6g( 活性 )(2ml)。<br>滴眼液：每支 3%(8ml)。<br>Comprimés (capsules) : 0,25g ou 0,5g (actif) par comprimé ou par capsule.<br>Injection : 0,2g (1ml) ou 0,6g (2ml) (actif) par injection.<br>Gouttes pour les yeux : 3 % (8 ml) par injection. |
| **药品名称 Drug Names** | 克林霉素 Clindamycine |
| 适应证<br>Les indications | 主要用于厌氧菌（包括脆弱拟杆菌、产气荚膜杆菌、放线菌等）引起的腹腔和妇科感染（常需与氨基糖苷类联合以消除需氧病原菌）。还用于敏感的革兰阳性菌引起的呼吸道、关节和软组织、骨组织、胆道等感染及败血症、心内膜炎等。本品是金黄色葡萄球菌骨髓炎的首选治疗药物。<br>Ce produit est souvent utilisé comme traitement des infections abdominales et gynécologiques, causées par les bactéries anaérobies (y compris Bacteroides fragilis, Clostridium perfringens, les actinomycètes). Il faut souvent recourir à la fois à la clindamycine et à l'aminoglycoside pour l'élimination des bactéries aérobies. Ce produit est aussi applicable dans le traitement des infections respiratoires, articulaires, des tissus mous, osseuses, des voies biliaires, la septicémie, l'endocardite, causées par des bactéries à Gram positif. Il est également le favori dans le traitement de l'ostéomyélite causée par le staphylococcus aureus. |
| 用法、用量<br>Les modes d'emploi et la posologie | 盐酸盐口服：成人，一次 0.15 ～ 0.3g( 活性 )，一日 3 ～ 4 次；小儿，一日 10 ～ 20mg( 活性 )/kg，分 3 ～ 4 次给予。棕榈酸酯盐酸盐（供儿童应用）：一日 8 ～ 12mg/kg，极严重时可增至 20 ～ 25mg/kg，分为 3 ～ 4 次给予；10kg 以下体重的婴儿可按一日 8 ～ 12mg/kg 用药，分为 3 次给予；磷酸酯（注射剂）：成人革兰阳性需氧菌感染，一日 600 ～ 1200mg，分为 2 ～ 4 次肌内注射或静脉滴注；厌氧菌感染，一般用一日 1200 ～ 2700mg，极严重感染可用到 4800mg/d。儿童 (1 月龄以上 )，重症感染一日量 15 ～ 25mg/kg，极严重可按 25 ～ 40mg/kg，均分为 3 ～ 4 次应用。<br>肌内注射量一次不超过 600mg，超过此量应静脉给予。静脉滴注前应先将药物用输液稀释，600mg 药物应加入不少于 100ml 输液中，至少输注 20 分钟。1 小时输注的药量不应超过 1200mg。 |

续　表

|  | Le chlorhydrate de clindamycine administré par voie orale : chez des adultes, 0,15 à 0,3g par fois (actif), 3 à 4 fois par jour ; chez des enfants, 10 à 20 mg/kg par jour (actif), à travers 3 à 4 fois. Le chlorhydrate de palmitate de clindamycine, réservé aux enfants : 8 à 12 mg/kg par jour, pour l'infection extrêmement grave, 20 à 25 mg/kg par jour, à travers 3 à 4 fois ; chez des enfants moins de 10kg, 8 à 12 mg/kg par jour, à travers 3 fois. Le phosphate de clindamycine (injection) : chez des adultes atteints d'infections causées par des bactéries à Gram positif, 600 à 1200 mg par jour, à travers 2 à 4 fois, par voie IM ou IV en perfusion. En cas d'infections causées par des anaérobies, 1200 à 2700mg par jour, pour l'infection extrêmement grave, 4 800 mg/jour. <br><br> Chez des enfants (plus de 1 mois), pour l'infection grave, 15 à 25 mg/kg par jour, pour l'infection extrêmement grave, 25 à 40 mg/kg par jour, à travers 3 à 4 fois. En cas d'injection par voie IM, ne pas dépasser 600mg par fois. Pour plus de 600mg, il faut administrer par voie IV. En cas de perfusion, pour 600mg de médicament, il faut utiliser au moins 100ml d'infusion, perfusion pendant au moins 20 minutes, avec un débit de 1 200mg par h au plus. |
|---|---|
| 剂型、规格 <br> Les formes pharmaceutiques et les spécifications | 盐酸克林霉素胶囊剂：每胶囊 75mg( 活性 )；150mg( 活性 )。<br> 盐酸克林霉素注射液：每支 150mg(2ml)；300mg(2ml)；600mg(4ml)。<br> Le chlorhydrate de clindamycine en capsules : 75mg ou 150mg par capsule (activé). <br> Injection de chlorhydrate de clindamycine : 150mg (2ml), 300mg (2ml) ou 600mg (4ml) par injection. |
| 药品名称 Drug Names | 甲砜霉素 Thiamphénicol |
| 适应证 <br> Les indications | 临床主要用于伤寒、副伤寒和其他沙门菌感染，也用于敏感菌所致的呼吸道、胆道、尿路感染。<br> Ce produit est principalement utilisé dans les cliniques comme traitement des infections respiratoires, biliaires et urinaires causées par la typhoïde, la paratyphoïde ou d'autres salmonelles. |
| 用法、用量 <br> Les modes d'emploi et la posologie | 1 次 0.25 ～ 0.5g，一日 3 ～ 4 次。<br> 0,25 à 0,5g par fois, 3 à 4 fois par jour. |
| 剂型、规格 <br> Les formes pharmaceutiques et les spécifications | 片剂 / 胶囊剂：0.125g；0.25g。<br> Comprimés ou capsules : 0,125g ou 0,25g. |

1.8　大环内酯类 Macrolides

| 药品名称 Drug Names | 红霉素 Erythromycine |
|---|---|
| 适应证 <br> Les indications | 临床主要应用于链球菌引起的扁桃体炎、猩红热、白喉及带菌者、淋病、李斯特菌病、肺炎链球菌下呼吸道感染 ( 以上适用于不耐青霉素的患者 )。对于军团菌肺炎和支原体肺炎，本品可作为首选药应用。尚可应用于流感杆菌引起的上呼吸道感染、金黄色葡萄球菌皮肤及软组织感染、梅毒、肠道阿米巴病等。<br><br> Ce produit est principalement utilisé dans les cliniques comme traitementdes infections causées par le streptocoque, telles que l'amygdalite, la scarlatine, la diphtérie et les transporteurs, la gonorrhée, la listériose ainsi que lesinfections respiratoires causées par le streptococcus pneumoniaes (applicable pour le traitement des patients résistant à la pénicilline). Pour traiter la pneumonie de Legionella et la pneumonie de Mycoplasma, ce produit peut être un premier choix. Il est aussi permissible de l'utiliser dans le traitement des infections respiratoires causées par l'haemophilus influenzae, des infections cutanées et des tissus mous causées par le staphylococcus aureus ainsi que dans le traitement du syphilis, et de l'amibiase intestinale. |
| 用法、用量 <br> Les modes d'emploi et la posologie | 口服：成人一日 1 ～ 2g，分 3 ～ 4 次服用，整片吞服；小儿，每日 30 ～ 50mg/kg，分 3 ～ 4 次服用。静脉滴注：成人一日 1 ～ 2g，分 3 ～ 4 次滴注；小儿每日 30 ～ 50mg/kg，分 3 ～ 4 次滴注。用时，将乳糖酸红霉素溶于 10ml 灭菌注射用水中，再添加到输液 500ml 中，缓慢滴入 ( 最后稀释浓度一般小于 0.1%)。不能直接用含盐输液溶解。<br><br> Par voie orale : chez des adultes, 1 à 2 g par jour, à travers 3 à 4 fois, avaler en entier ; chez des petits enfants, 30 à 50 mg/kg par jour, à travers 3 à 4 fois. Par voie IV en perfusion : chez des adultes, 1 à 2 g par jour, à travers 3 à 4 fois ; chez des enfants, 30 à 50 mg/kg par jour, à travers 3 à 4 fois. Utiliser 10ml d'eau stérile comme solvant de l'érythromycine lactobionate, ajouter ensuite 500ml d'eau stérile pour injection, perfusion lente (avec la concentration diluée inférieure à 0,1 %). Il est interdit d'utiliser seulement l'infusion saline pour la dissolution. |

| 续　表 | |
| --- | --- |
| 剂型、规格<br>Les formes pharmaceutiques et les spécifications | 片剂 ( 肠溶 )：每片 0.1g(10 万 U)；0.125g(12.5 万 U)；0.25g(25 万 U)。<br>注射用乳糖酸红霉素：每瓶 0.25g(25 万 U)；0.3g(30 万 U)。<br>红霉素软膏：1%。<br>红霉素眼膏：0.5%。<br>Comprimé (à enrobage entérique): 0,1g (100 000 unités), 0,125g (125 000 unités) ou 0,25g (250 000 unités) par comprimé.<br>Le lactobionate d'érythromycine pour injection : 0,25g (250 000 unités) ou 0,3g (300 000 unités) par.<br>Onguent d'érythromycine: 1%.<br>Érythromycine crème pour les yeux: 0.5% . |
| 药品名称 Drug Names | 琥乙红霉素 Ethylsuccinate Erythromycine |
| 适应证<br>Les indications | 临床主要应用于链球菌引起的扁桃体炎、猩红热、白喉及带菌者、淋病、李斯特菌病、肺炎链球菌下呼吸道感染 ( 以上适用于不耐青霉素的患者 )。对于军团菌肺炎和支原体肺炎，本品可作为首选药应用。尚可应用于流感杆菌引起的上呼吸道感染、金黄色葡萄球菌皮肤及软组织感染、梅毒、肠道阿米巴病等。<br>Ce produit est principalement utilisé dans les cliniques comme traitementdes infections causées par le streptocoque, telles que l'amygdalite, la scarlatine, la diphtérie et les transporteurs, la gonorrhée, la listériose ainsi que lesinfections respiratoires causées par le streptococcus pneumoniaes (applicable pour le traitement des patients résistant à la pénicilline). Pour traiter la pneumonie de Legionella et la pneumonie de Mycoplasma, ce produit peut être un premier choix. Il est aussi permissible de l'utiliser dans le traitement des infections respiratoires causées par l'haemophilus influenzae, des infections cutanées et des tissus mous causées par le staphylococcus aureus ainsi que dans le traitement du syphilis, et de l'amibiase intestinale. |
| 用法、用量<br>Les modes d'emploi et la posologie | 口服：成人一次 0.25 ～ 0.5g，一日 3 ～ 4 次；小儿一日量 30 ～ 50mg/kg，分 3 ～ 4 次用。或按下列方案应用：体重＜ 5kg 者，1 次 40mg/kg，一日 4 次；5 ～ 7kg 者，1 次 50mg，一日 4 次；7 ～ 11kg 者，1 次 100mg，一日 4 次；11 ～ 23kg 者，1 次 200mg，一日 4 次；23 ～ 45kg 者，1 次 300mg，一日 4 次；＞ 45kg 者，按成人量给予。<br>Par voie orale : chez des adultes, 0,25 à 0,5g par fois, 3 à 4 fois par jour ; chez des enfants, 30 à 50 mg/kg par jour, à travers 3 à 4 fois. Ou comme la posologie suivante : pour moins de 5kg, 40 mg/kg par fois, 4 fois par jour ; pour 5 à 7kg, 50 mg par fois, 4 fois par jour ; pour 7 à 11kg, 100mg par fois, 4 fois par jour ; pour 11 à 23kg, 200mg par fois, 4 fois par jour ; pour 23 à 45 kg, 300mg par fois, 4 fois par jour ; pour plus de 45 kg, la même dose que chez des adultes. |
| 剂型、规格<br>Les formes pharmaceutiques et les spécifications | 片剂：每片 0.1g；0.125g( 按红霉素计 )。<br>颗粒剂：每袋 0.05g；0.1g；0.125g；0.25g( 按红霉素计 )。<br>Comprimés : 0,1g ou 0,125g par comprimé (mesuré en érythromycine).<br>Granules : 0,05g, 0,1g, 0,125g ou 0,25g par sachet (mesuré en érythromycine). |
| 药品名称 Drug Names | 罗红霉素 Roxithromycine |
| 适应证<br>Les indications | 临床应用于上述敏感菌所致的呼吸道、泌尿道、皮肤和软组织、五官科感染。<br>Ce produit est principalement utilisé dans les cliniques comme traitementdes infections causées par des bactéries, telles que les infections des voies respiratoires, des voies urinaires, cutanées, des tissus mous et des traits du visage. |
| 用法、用量<br>Les modes d'emploi et la posologie | 成人 一次 150mg，一日 2 次，餐前服。幼儿：每次 2.5 ～ 5mg/kg，一日 2 次。老年人与肾功能一般减退者不需调整剂量。严重肝硬化者，每日 150mg。<br>Chez des adultes, 150mg par fois, 2 fois par jour, avant le repas. Chez des petits enfants, 2,5 à 5 mg/kg par fois, 2 fois par jour. Chez des personnes âgées et des patients insuffisants rénaux, pas nécessaire d'ajuster la dose. Chez des patients atteints de cirrhose grave, 150mg par jour. |
| 剂型、规格<br>Les formes pharmaceutiques et les spécifications | 片剂：每片 150mg；250mg；300mg。<br>Comprimés : 150mg, 250mg ou 300mg par comprimé. |

| 药品名称 Drug Names | 克拉霉素 Clarithromycine |
|---|---|
| 适应证<br>Les indications | 临床用于化脓性链球菌所致的咽炎和扁桃体炎，肺炎链球菌所致的急性中耳炎、肺炎和支气管炎，流感嗜血杆菌、卡他球菌所致支气管炎，支原体肺炎以及葡萄球菌、链球菌所致皮肤及软组织感染。 |
| | Ce produit est utilsé dans les cliniques comme traitement des infections suivantes : la pharyngite et l'amygdalitecausées par le streptococcus pyogenes ; l'otite moyenne aiguë, la pneumonie et la bronchite causées par le streptococcus pneumoniae; labronchite et la pneumonie à mycoplasmecausées par l'haemophilus influenzae et lecocci catarrhal, ainsi que les infections cutanées et des tissus mous causées par le staphylocoques et le streptocoques. |
| 用法、用量<br>Les modes d'emploi et la posologie | 轻症：每次 250mg，重症每次 500mg，均为 12 小时 1 次口服，疗程 7 ～ 14 日。12 岁以上儿童按成人量。6 个月以上小儿至 12 岁以下儿童用量每日 15mg/kg，分为 2 次；或按以下方法口服给药：8 ～ 11kg 体重每次 62.5mg，12 ～ 19kg 体重每次 125mg，20 ～ 29kg 体重每次 187.5mg，30 ～ 40kg 体重每次 250mg，按上量每日用药 2 次。 |
| | Pour l'infection bénigne, 250mg par fois, pour l'infection grave, 500mg par fois, toutes les 12h, le traitement médical dure de 7 à 14 jours. Chez plus de 12ans, la même dose que chez des adultes. Chez des petits enfants de 6 mois à 12 ans, 15 mg/kg par jour, à travers 2 fois ; ou comme la posologie suivante : pour 8 à 11kg, 62,5mg par fois, pour 12 à 19 kg, 125mg par fois, pour 20 à 29kg, 187.5mg par fois, pour 30 à 40kg, 250mg par fois. Dans tous les cas précédents, 2 fois par jour. |
| 剂型、规格<br>Les formes pharmaceutiques et les spécifications | 片剂：每片 250mg 或 500mg。 |
| | Comprimés : 250mg ou 500mg par comprimé. |
| 药品名称 Drug Names | 阿奇霉素 Azithromycine |
| 适应证<br>Les indications | 临床应用于敏感微生物所致的呼吸道、皮肤和软组织感染。 |
| | Ce produit est utilisé dans les cliniques comme traitement des infections causées par des micro-organismes sensibles, telles que les infections respiratoires, cutanées et des tissus mous. |
| 用法、用量<br>Les modes d'emploi et la posologie | 每日只需服 1 次，成人 500mg；儿童 10mg/kg，连用 3 日。 |
| | 重症可注射给药，一日 1 次，每次 500mg，以注射用水 5ml 溶解后，加入 0.9% 氯化钠液或 5% 葡萄糖液中使成 1 ～ 2mg/ml 浓度，静脉滴注 1 ～ 2 小时，约 2 日症状控制后改成口服巩固疗效。 |
| | 1 fois par jour seulement, chez les adultes, 500mg ; chez des enfants, 10 mg/kg, pendant trois jours consécutifs. |
| | Pour l'infection grave, possible d'administration en perfusion, 1 fois par jour, 500mg par fois, utiliser 5m d'eau pour injection pour la dissolution, ensuite ajouter la solution de chlorure de sodium à 0,9 % ou la solution de glucose à 5 % pour former une solution à 1 à 2mg/ml, perfusion pendant 1 à 2 h, 2 jours après, quand les symtômes se contrôlent, administration par voie orale. |
| 剂型、规格<br>Les formes pharmaceutiques et les spécifications | 片剂（胶囊）：每粒 250mg 或 500mg。<br>乳糖酸阿奇霉素（冻干粉针）：每支 500mg。 |
| | Comprimés (capsules) : 250m g ou 500mg par comprimé.<br>Le lactobionate d'azithromycine (poudre lyophilisée) : 500mg par injection. |
| 药品名称 Drug Names | 泰利霉素 Télithromycine |
| 适应证<br>Les indications | 临床主要用于敏感菌所致的呼吸道感染，包括社区获得性肺炎、慢性支气管炎、急性上颌窦咽炎及扁桃体炎。 |
| | Ce produit est utilisé dans les cliniques comme traitement des infections causées par des bactéries, telles que les infections repiratoires, y compris la pneumonie, la bronchite chronique, la pharyngite maxillaire aiguë et l'amygdalite. |
| 用法、用量<br>Les modes d'emploi et la posologie | 口服，一日 1 次 800mg，疗程 5 ～ 10 日。 |
| | Par voie orale, 800mg par fois par jour, pendant 5 à 10 jours. |

续　表

| | |
|---|---|
| 剂型、规格<br>Les formes pharmaceutiques et les spécifications | 片剂：400mg；800mg。<br>Comprimés : 400mg ou 800mg. |
| 药品名称 Drug Names | 地红霉素 Dirithromycine |
| 适应证<br>Les indications | 本品适用于敏感菌所致的轻、中度感染，慢性支气管炎 ( 包括急性发作 )、社区获得性肺炎、咽炎、扁桃体炎等。<br>Ce produit est utilisé comme traitement des infections bénignes ou modérées, de la bronchite chronique (y compris une exacerbation aiguë), la pneumonie, la pharyngite et l'amygdalite causées par des bactéries. |
| 用法、用量<br>Les modes d'emploi et la posologie | 每次 500mg，一日 1 次，餐时服用，疗程根据病情为 7 ～ 14 日。<br>500mg par fois, 1 fois par jour, durant le repas, pendant 7 à 14 jours selon les cas. |
| 剂型、规格<br>Les formes pharmaceutiques et les spécifications | 片剂 ( 肠溶衣片 )：每片 250mg。<br>Comprimés (Comprimés à enrobage entérique) : 250mg par comprimé. |
| 药品名称 Drug Names | 吉他霉素 Kitasamycine |
| 适应证<br>Les indications | 可作为红霉素的替代品，用于上述敏感菌所致的口咽部、呼吸道、皮肤和软组织、胆道等感染。<br>Comme alternative de l'érythromycine, ce produit est utilisé comme traitement des infections oropharyngées, respiratoires, cutanées, des tissus mous et biliaires causées par des bactéries. |
| 用法、用量<br>Les modes d'emploi et la posologie | 口服：每次 0.3 ～ 0.4g，每日 3 ～ 4 次。静脉注射：1 次 0.2 ～ 0.4g，一日 2 ～ 3 次，将 1 次用量溶于 20ml 氯化钠注射液或葡萄糖液中，缓慢注射。<br>Par voie orale : 0,3 à 0,4g par fois, 3 à 4 fois par jour. Par voie IV : 0,2 à 0,4g par fois, 2 à 3 fois par jour, utiliser 20ml de solution de chlorure de sodium ou de glucose comme solvant, injection lente. |
| 剂型、规格<br>Les formes pharmaceutiques et les spécifications | 片剂：每片 0.1g。<br>注射用酒石酸吉他霉素：每瓶 0.2g。<br>Comprimés : 0,1g par comprimé.<br>Le tartrate de kitasamycine pour injection : 0,2g par flacon. |
| 药品名称 Drug Names | 麦迪霉素 Midécamycine |
| 适应证<br>Les indications | 可作为红霉素的替代品，用于上述敏感菌所致的口咽部、呼吸道、皮肤和软组织、胆道等感染。<br>Comme alternative de l'érythromycine, ce produit est utilisé comme traitement des infections oropharyngées, respiratoires, cutanées, des tissus mous et biliaires causées par des bactéries. |
| 用法、用量<br>Les modes d'emploi et la posologie | 口服，成人一日量 0.8 ～ 1.2g，分 3 ～ 4 次用。儿童一日量 30mg/kg，分 3 ～ 4 次给予。<br>Par voie orale : chez des adultes, 0,8 à 1,2 g par jour, à travers 3 à 4 fois, chez des enfants, 30 mg/kg par jour, à travers 3 à 4 fois. |
| 剂型、规格<br>Les formes pharmaceutiques et les spécifications | 麦迪霉素片：每片 0.1g。<br>Comprimés de midécamycine : 0,1g par comprimé. |
| 药品名称 Drug Names | 乙酰麦迪霉素 Acétylmidécamycine |
| 适应证<br>Les indications | 主要适用于金黄色葡萄球菌、溶血性链球菌、肺炎球菌等所致的呼吸道感染及皮肤、软组织感染，也可用于支原体肺炎。<br>Principalement applicable aux infections des voies respiratoires et la peau et les infections des tissus mous par Staphylococcus aureus, Streptococcus hémolytiques bactéries pneumoniae causés, peuvent également être utilisés pour Mycoplasma pneumoniae. |

**续　表**

| | |
|---|---|
| 用法、用量<br>Les modes d'emploi et la posologie | 成人：一日 300 ～ 900mg，分 3 ～ 4 次服。儿童：一日 15 ～ 30mg/kg，分 3 ～ 4 次给予。<br>Chez des adultes : 300 à 900mg par jour, à travers 3 à 4 fois. Chez des enfants : 15 à 30 mg/kg par jour, à travers 3 à 4 fois. |
| 剂型、规格<br>Les formes pharmaceutiques et les spécifications | 醋酸乙酰麦迪霉素颗粒剂：1.0g：0.2g；干混悬剂：0.1g<br>Acétyl acétate midécamycine granulés: 1,0 g: 0,2 g; suspension sèche: 0,1g. |
| 药品名称 Drug Names | 交沙霉素 Josamycine |
| 适应证<br>Les indications | 临床应用于敏感菌所致的口咽部、呼吸道、肺、鼻窦、中耳、皮肤及软组织、胆道等部位的感染。<br>Ce produit est utilisé comme traitement des infections oropharyngées, respiratoires, cutanées, des tissus mous et biliaires ainsi que la pneumonie, la sinusite, l'otite moyenne causées par des bactéries. |
| 用法、用量<br>Les modes d'emploi et la posologie | 成人：一日量 0.8 ～ 1.2g，分 3 ～ 4 次应用。儿童：一日量为 30mg/kg，分 3 ～ 4 次给予。<br>空腹服用吸收好。<br>Chez des adultes : 0,8 à 1,2g par jour, à travers 3 à 4 fois. Chez des enfants : 30 mg/kg par jour, à travers 3 à 4 fois. L'estomac vide. |
| 剂型、规格<br>Les formes pharmaceutiques et les spécifications | 交沙霉素片剂：每片 0.1g。<br>丙酸交沙霉素散剂：每包含药 0.1g( 效价 )。<br>Comprimés : 0,1g par comprimé.<br>La josamycine de propionate en poudre : chaque sachet contient 0,1g de médicament (titre). |
| 药品名称 Drug Names | 麦白霉素 Méleumycine |
| 适应证<br>Les indications | 用于敏感菌所致的呼吸道感染、皮肤感染、软组织感染、胆道感染、支原体性肺炎等。<br>Infections des voies respiratoires, des infections cutanées, infections des tissus mous, l'infection des voies biliaires, la pneumonie à mycoplasme, causées par les souches sensibles. |
| 用法、用量<br>Les modes d'emploi et la posologie | 成人一日量 0.8 ～ 1.2g，分 3 ～ 4 次服。儿童一日量 30mg/kg，分 3 ～ 4 次服。<br>Chez des adultes : 0,8 à 1,2g par jour, à travers 3 à 4 fois. Chez des enfants : 30 mg/kg par jour, à travers 3 à 4 fois. |
| 剂型、规格<br>Les formes pharmaceutiques et les spécifications | 片剂：每片 0.1g。<br>Comprimés : 0,1g par comprimé. |
| 药品名称 Drug Names | 罗他霉素 Rokitamycine |
| 适应证<br>Les indications | 临床应用于上述敏感菌所致的咽、扁桃体、支气管、肺、中耳、鼻旁窦、牙周、皮肤及软组织等部位的感染。<br>Ce produit est utilisé dans les cliniques comme traitement de la pharyngite, de l'amygdalite, de la bronchite, de la pneumonie, de l'otite moyenne, de la sinusite, dela parodontite et des infections cutanées et des tissus mous causées par des bactéries. |
| 用法、用量<br>Les modes d'emploi et la posologie | 口服，成人每次 200mg，一日 3 次。儿童：一日量 20 ～ 30mg/kg，分 3 次服。<br>Par voie orale, chez des adultes, 200mg par fois, 3 fois par jour. Chez des enfants, 20 à 30 mg/kg par jour, à travers 3 fois. |
| 剂型、规格<br>Les formes pharmaceutiques et les spécifications | 片剂：每片 100mg。<br>Comprimés : 100mg par comprimé. |

**续 表**

| 药品名称 Drug Names | 乙酰螺旋霉素 Acetylspiramycine |
|---|---|
| 适应证<br>Les indications | 适用于上述敏感菌所致的扁桃体炎、支气管炎、肺炎、咽炎、中耳炎、皮肤和软组织感染、乳腺炎、胆囊炎、猩红热、牙科和眼科感染等。<br><br>Ce produit est utilisé comme traitement de la pharyngite, de l'amygdalite, de la bronchite, de la pneumonie, de l'otite moyenne, de lamammite, de la cholécystite, de la scarlatine, des infections dentaires, oculaires, cutanées et des tissus mous causées par des bactéries. |
| 用法、用量<br>Les modes d'emploi et la posologie | 成人一次 0.2g，一日 4～6 次。重症一日可用至 1.6～2g。儿童一日量 30mg/kg，分 4 次给予。<br>Chez des adutes, 0,2 g par fois, 4 à 6 fois par jour. Pour l'infection grave, 1,6 à 2g par jour. Chez des enfants, 30 mg/kg par jour, à travers 4 fois. |
| 剂型、规格<br>Les formes pharmaceutiques et les spécifications | 乙酰螺旋霉素片（肠溶）剂：每片 0.1g（效价）。<br>Comprimés (Comprimés à enrobage entérique) : 0,1g par comprimé (titre). |

## 1.9　糖肽类 Glycopeptides

| 药品名称 Drug Names | 去甲万古霉素 Norvancomycine |
|---|---|
| 适应证<br>Les indications | 主要用于葡萄球菌（包括产酶株和耐甲氧西林株）、肠球菌（耐氨苄西林株）、难辨梭状芽孢杆菌等所致的系统感染和肠道感染，如心内膜炎、败血症，以及假膜性肠炎等。<br><br>Ce produit est utilisé comme traitement des infections systématiques et intestinales, y compris l'endocardite, la septicémie et la colite pseudomembraneuse, causées par le staphylococcus aureus (y compris les souches productrices et les souches résistantes à la méthicilline), l'entérocoque (souches résistantes à l'ampicilline) ainsi que le clostridium difficile. |
| 用法、用量<br>Les modes d'emploi et la posologie | 口服：成人一次 0.4g，每 6 小时 1 次，每日量不可超过 4g；儿童酌减。静脉滴注：成人一日量 0.8～1.6g，1 次或分次给予；小儿一日量 16～24mg/kg，1 次或分次给予。一般将 1 次量的药物先用 10ml 灭菌注射用水溶解，再加入到适量等渗氯化钠注射液或葡萄糖输液中，缓慢滴注。如采取连续滴注给药，则可将一日量药物加到 24 小时内所用的输液中给予。<br><br>Par voie orale: chez des adultes,7.5mg/Kg toutes les 6h, pas plus de 4g par jour, réduction de la dose chez les enfants.Par voie Ⅳ en perfusion: chez des adultes, 0.8～1.6g par jour, administration unique ou fractionnée; chez des enfants, 16～24mg/Kg par jour, administration unique ou fractionnée. Généralement, après avoir dissous 1 dose administrée du médicament dans 10ml d'eau stérilisée pour injections, ajouter à la quantité appropriée de solution saline ou d'injection de glucose goutte lente. Si l'administration est effectuée par goutte à goutte continue, Une dose journalière peut être ajoutée à l'infusion dans les 24 heures. |
| 剂型、规格<br>Les formes pharmaceutiques et les spécifications | 注射用盐酸去甲万古霉素：每瓶 0.4g(40 万 U)［相当万古霉素约 0.5g(50 万 U)］。<br>Le chlorhydrate de norvancomycine pour injection : 0,4g (400 000 unités) par flacon [équivalent à 0,5 g de vancomycine (500 000 unités)]. |
| 药品名称 Drug Names | 万古霉素 Vancomycine |
| 适应证<br>Les indications | 临床用于革兰阳性菌严重感染，尤其是对其他抗菌药耐药的耐甲氧西林菌株。血液透析患者发生葡萄球菌属所致的动静脉分流感染。口服用于对甲硝唑无效的假膜性结肠炎或多重耐药葡萄球菌小肠结肠炎。<br><br>Ce produit est utilisé dans les cliniques comme traitement des infections graves causées par les bactéries à Gram positif, en particulier les souches résistantes à la méthicilline, qui sont résistantes aux autres agents antimicrobiens. Il est aussi applicable dans le traitement de l'infection de shunt artério-veineuse causéee par le staphylococcus chez des patients faisant l'objet d'hémodialyse. En cas d'administration par voie orale, il sert aussi à traiter la colite pseudomembraneuse résistante à la métronidazole ou l'entérocolite à staphylocoque multirésistant. |

**续　表**

| | |
|---|---|
| 用法、用量<br>Les modes d'emploi et la posologie | 口服：每次 125 ~ 500mg，每 6 小时 1 次，每日剂量不宜超过 4g，疗程 5 ~ 10 日；小儿 1 次 10mg/kg，每 6 小时 1 次，疗程 5 ~ 10 日。静脉滴注：全身感染，成人每 6 小时 7.5mg/kg，或每 12 小时 15mg/kg。严重感染，可一日 3 ~ 4g 短期应用；新生儿（0 ~ 7 日）首次 15mg/kg，以后 10mg/kg，每 12 小时给药 1 次；婴儿（7 日至 1 个月）首次 15mg/kg，以后 10mg/kg，每 8 小时给药 1 次；儿童每次 10mg/kg，每 6 小时给药 1 次，或每次 20mg/kg，每 12 小时 1 次。<br><br>Par voie orale : 125 à 500 mg par fois, toutes les 6h, ne pas dépasser 4g par jour, pendant 5 à 10 jours ; chez des enfants, 10 mg/kg par fois, toutes les 6h, pendant 5 à 10 jours.Par voie IV en perfusion : pour l'infection systématique, chez des adultes, 7,5 mg/kg toutes les 6h, ou 15 mg/kg toutes les 12h. Pour l'infection grave, 3 à 4g par jour, pour une courte durée ; chez des nouveau-nés (0 à 7 jours), pour la première fois, 15 mg/kg, ensuite, 10 mg/kg, toutes les 12h ; chez des bébés (7 jours à 1 mois), première fois, 15 mg/kg, ensuite, 10 mg/kg, toutes les 8h ; chez des enfants, 10 mg/kg par fois, toutes les 6h, ou 20 mg/kg par fois, toutes les 12h. |
| 剂型、规格<br>Les formes pharmaceutiques et les spécifications | 胶囊：每粒 20mg；250mg。<br>注射用盐酸万古霉素：每支 0.5g；1.0g。<br>Capsules : 20mg ou 250mg par capsule.<br>Le chlorhydrate de vancomycine pour injection : 0,5g ou 1,0g par injection. |

| 药品名称 Drug Names | 替考拉宁 Tèicoplanine |
|---|---|
| 适应证<br>Les indications | 临床用于耐甲氧西林金黄色葡萄球菌和耐氨苄西林肠球菌所致的系统感染（对中枢感染无效）。本类药物（万古霉素与本品）现用于上述适应证，其目的是防止过度应用（即用于其他抗生素能控制的一些病原菌感染而造成耐药菌滋长）。<br><br>Ce produit est utilisé dans les cliniques comme traitement des infections graves causées par le staphylococcus aureus résistant à l'ampicilline et l'entérocoquerésistant à la méthicilline (il ne sert pas à traiter les infections liées aux cathéters veineux centraux). L'utilisation de la teicoplanine et de la vancomycine dans le traitement des maladies précédentes a pour objectif d'éviter l'applicastion excessive. |
| 用法、用量<br>Les modes d'emploi et la posologie | 首剂（第一日）400mg，次日开始每日 200mg，静脉注射或肌内注射；严重感染，每次 400mg，一日 2 次，3 日后减为一日 200 ~ 400mg。<br>用前以注射用水溶解，静脉注射应不少于 1 分钟。若采取静脉滴注，则将药物加入 0.9% 氯化钠溶液中，静脉滴注不少于 30 分钟。也可采用肌内注射。<br><br>Pour la première fois (le premier jour), 400mg, à partir du deuxième jour, 200mg par jour, par voie IV ou par voie IM ; pour l'infection grave, 400mg par fois, 2 fois par jour, 3 jours après, 200 à 400mg par jour.<br>Utiliser l'eau pour injection comme solvant, injection IV pendant au moins 1 minute. En cas d'administration par voie IV en perfusion, utiliser la solution de chlorure de sodium à 0,9 % pour la dissolution, perfusion pendant au moins 30 minutes. Par voie IM aussi possible. |
| 剂型、规格<br>Les formes pharmaceutiques et les spécifications | 粉针：每支 200mg；400mg。<br>Poudre : 200mg ou 400 mg par injection. |

### 1.10　其他抗菌抗生素 Autres antibiotiques

| 药品名称 Drug Names | 磷霉素 Fosfomycine |
|---|---|
| 适应证<br>Les indications | 临床主要用于敏感菌引起的尿路、皮肤及软组织、肠道等部位感染。对肺部、脑膜感染和败血症也可考虑应用。可与其他抗生素联合治疗由敏感菌所致重症感染。也可与万古霉素合用治疗 MRSA 感染。<br><br>Il est utilisé dans les cliniques comme traitement des infections urinaires, cutanées, des tissus mous et intestinales, causées par des bactéries sensibles. Il est aussi possible de l'utiliser dans le traitement de la pneumonie, de la méningite et de la septicémie. Il est recommandé de l'utiliser la fosfomycine avec d'autres anti-biotiques pour traiter les infections graves bactériennes. Il sert aussi à traiter les staphylococcus aureus résistant à la méticilline (SARM) avec la vancomycine. |

**续　表**

| | |
|---|---|
| 用法、用量<br>Les modes d'emploi et la posologie | 口服磷霉素钙，适用于尿路感染及轻症感染，成人 2～4g/d，儿童一日量为 50～100mg/kg，分 3～4 次服用。静脉注射或静脉滴注磷霉素钠，用于中度或重度系统感染，成人 4～12g/d，重症可用到 16g/d；儿童一日量为 100～300mg/kg，均分为 2～4 次给予。1g 药物至少应用 10ml 溶剂，如一次用数克，则应按每 1g 药物用 25ml 溶剂的比率进行溶解，予以静脉滴注或缓慢静脉注射。适用的溶剂有：灭菌注射用水、5%～10% 葡萄糖液、0.9% 氯化钠注射液、含乳酸钠的输液等。<br>La fosfomycine de calcium, administrée par voie orale, applicable dans le traitement des infections urinaires et des infections bénignes, chez des adultes, 2 à 4 g/jour, chez des enfants, 50 à 100 mg/kg par jour, à travers 3 à 4 fois. La fosfomycine de sodium, administrée par voie IV ou par voie IV en perfusion, applicable dans le traitement des infections systématiques modérées ou graves, chez des adultes, 4 à 12 g/jour, pour l'infection extrêmement grave, 16g/jour ; chez des enfants, 100 à 300 mg/kg par jour, à travers 2 à 4 fois. Pour 1g de médicament, utiliser au moins 10 ml de solvant, pour plus de 1g de médiciament, utiliser 25ml de solvant pour dissoudre 1g de médicament, pour la perfusion ou l'injection lente. Les solvants permissibles : l'eau stérile pour injection, la solution de glucose à 5 % à 10 %, la solution de chlorure de sodium à 0,9 %, l'infusion contenant du lactate de sodium. |
| 剂型、规格<br>Les formes pharmaceutiques et les spécifications | 磷霉素钙胶囊：每粒 0.1g；0.2g；0.5g。<br>注射用磷霉素钠：每瓶 1g；4g。<br>La fosfomycine de calcium en capsules : 0,1g, 0,2g ou 0,5g par capsule.<br>La fosfomycine sodique pour injection : 1g ou 4g par flacon. |
| **药品名称 Drug Names** | 达托霉素 Daptomycine |
| 适应证<br>Les indications | 临床用于复杂性皮肤及皮肤软组织感染。<br>Il est utilisé dans les cliniques comme traitement des infections cutanées et des tissus mous difficiles. |
| 用法、用量<br>Les modes d'emploi et la posologie | 静脉注射：每次 4mg/kg，一日 1 次，连续用药 7～14 日。肌酐清除率低于 30ml/min 者，每次 4mg/kg，每 2 日 1 次。<br>Par voie IV : 4 mg/kg par fois, 1 fois par jour, pendant 7 à 14 jours consécutifs. Chez des patients dont la clairance de la créatinine est inférieure à 30ml/min, 4 mg/kg par fois, tous les 2 jours. |
| 剂型、规格<br>Les formes pharmaceutiques et les spécifications | 注射用达托霉素：每支 250mg；500mg。<br>La daptomycine pour injection : 250 mg ou 500mg par injection. |
| **药品名称 Drug Names** | 利福昔明 Rifaximine |
| 适应证<br>Les indications | 临床用于敏感菌所致的肠道感染，预防胃肠道围术期感染性并发症，也可用于高氨血症的辅助治疗。<br>Il est utilisé dans les cliniques comme traitement des infections bactériennes, telles que les infections intestinales. Il sert aussi à prévenir les complications infectieuses périopératoires gastro-intestinales. Il est aussi possible de l'utiliser dans le traitement adjuvant de l'hyperammoniémie. |
| 用法、用量<br>Les modes d'emploi et la posologie | 口服，肠道感染：成人每次 200mg，一日 4 次，连续使用 5～7 日。6～12 岁儿童，每次 100～200mg，一日 4 次。手术前后预防感染：成人每次 400mg，6～12 岁儿童每次 200～400mg，一日 2 次，在手术前 3 日给药。高氨血症的辅助治疗：成人每次 400mg，疗程 7～21 日。6～12 岁儿童每次 200～300mg，一日 3 次。<br>Par voie orale, pour l'infection intestinale : chez des adultes, 200mg par fois, 4 fois par jour, pendant 5 à 7 jours consécutifs. Chez des enfants de 6 à 12ans, 100 à 200 mg par fois, 4 fois par jour. Pour la prévention des infections avant et après l'opération chirurgicale, chez des adultes, 400mg par fois, chez des enfants de 6 à 12ans, 200 à 400mg par fois, 2 fois par jour, prendre le médicament 3 jours avant l'opération. Pour le traitement adjuvant de l'hyperammoniémie : chez des adultes, 400mg par fois, pendant 7 à 21 jours. Chez des enfants de 6 à 12 ans, 200 à 300 mg par fois, 3 fois par jour. |
| 剂型、规格<br>Les formes pharmaceutiques et les spécifications | 片剂（胶囊剂）：每片（粒）200mg。<br>Comprimés (capsules) : 200mg par comprimé ou par capsule. |

| 药品名称 Drug Names | 多黏菌素 B Polymyxine B |
| --- | --- |
| 适应证<br>Les indications | 　　临床主要应用于铜绿假单胞菌及其他假单胞菌引起的创面、尿路以及眼、耳、气管等部位感染，也可用于败血症。鞘内注射用于铜绿假单胞菌脑膜炎。<br>　　Ce produit est utilisé dans les cliniques dans le traitement des infections à propos du traumatisme, des voies urinaires, des yeux, des oreilles, des voies respiratoires, ainsi que de la septicémie, causées par les pseudomonas aeruginosa. L'injection intrathécale de ce produit est applicable dans le traitement de la méningite causée par lepseudomonas aeruginosa. |
| 用法、用量<br>Les modes d'emploi et la posologie | 　　静脉滴注：成人及儿童肾功能正常者一日 1.5～2.5mg/kg(一般不超过 2.5mg/kg)，分 2 次给予，每 12 小时滴注 1 次。每 50mg 本品，以 5% 葡萄糖液 500ml 稀释后滴入。婴儿肾功能正常者可耐受一日 4mg/kg 的用量。肌内注射：成人及儿童一日 2.5～3mg/kg，分次给予，每 4～6 小时用药 1 次。婴儿一日量可用到 4mg/kg，新生儿可用到 4.5mg/kg，滴眼液浓度 1～2.5mg/ml。<br>　　Par voie IV en perfuion : chez des adultes et des enfants dont la fonction rénale est normale, 1,5 à 2,5 mg/kg par jour, ne pas dépasser 2,5 mg/kg par jour, à travers 2 fois, toutes les 12h. Pour 50 mg de polymyxine B, utiliser 500ml de solution de glucose à 5 % pour la dilution. Chez des bébés dont la fonction rénale est normale, 4 mg/kg par jour. Par voie IM : chez des adultes et des enfants, 2,5 à 3 mg/kg par jour, à travers plusieurs fois, toutes les 4 à 6h. Chez des bébés, 4 mg/kg par jour, chez des nouveau-nés, 4,5 mg/kg par jour. La concentration des gouttes pour les yeux est de 1 à 2,5 mg/ml. |
| 剂型、规格<br>Les formes pharmaceutiques et les spécifications | 　　注射用硫酸多黏菌素 B：每瓶 50mg(1mg=10 000U)。<br>　　Le sulfate de polymyxine B pour injection : 50mg (1mg = 10 000 unités) par flacon. |
| 药品名称 Drug Names | 黏菌素 Colistine |
| 适应证<br>Les indications | 　　用于治疗大肠埃希菌性肠炎和对其他药物耐药的菌痢。外用于烧伤和外伤引起的铜绿假单胞菌局部感染和耳、咽等部位敏感菌感染。<br>　　Ce produit sert à traiter l'entérite causée par le colibacille et la dysenterie résistant à d'autres médicaments. En cas d'usage externe, il sert aussi à traiter les infections à pseudomonas aeruginosa causées par la brûlure et le traumatisme, et à traiter les infections batériennes liées aux oreilles et la pharyngée. |
| 用法、用量<br>Les modes d'emploi et la posologie | 　　口服：成人一日 150 万～300 万 U，分 3 次服。儿童 1 次量 25 万～50 万 U，一日 3～4 次。重症时上述剂量可加倍。外用：溶液剂 1 万～5 万 U/ml，氯化钠注射液溶解。<br>　　Par voie orale : chez des adultes, 1,5 million à 3 millions d'unités par jour, à travers 3 fois. Chez des enfants, 250 000 à 500 000 unités par fois, 3 à 4 fois par jour. Pour l'infection grave, possible de doubler la dose. Pour l'usage externe : 10 000 à 50 000 unités /ml injectables, la solution de chlorure de sodium comme solvant. |
| 剂型、规格<br>Les formes pharmaceutiques et les spécifications | 　　片剂：每片 50 万 U；100 万 U；300 万 U。<br>　　灭菌粉剂：每瓶 100 万 U，供制备溶液用 (1mg=6500U)。<br>　　Comprimés : 500 000 unités, 1 million d'unités ou 3 millions d'unités par comprimé.<br>　　Poudre stérile : 1 million d'unités par flacon, destinée pour la préparation de la solution (1mg = 6500 unités). |
| 药品名称 Drug Names | 夫西地酸钠 Fusidate sodique |
| 适应证<br>Les indications | 　　主治由各种敏感细菌，尤其是葡萄球菌引起的各种感染，如骨髓炎、败血症、心内膜炎，反复感染的囊型纤维化、肺炎、皮肤及软组织感染，外科及创伤性感染等。<br>　　Ce produit est principalement utilisé comme traitement des infections bactériennes, en particulier des infections causées par infections intra-auriculaire, telles que l'ostéomyélite, la septicémie, l'encocardite, les infections répétées de la fibrose kystique,la pneumonie, les infections cutanées et des tissus mous, chirurgicales et les infections liées au traumatisme. |

**续　表**

| | |
|---|---|
| 用法、用量<br>Les modes d'emploi et la posologie | 口服：每 8 小时 500mg，重症感染可加倍服用；儿童 1 岁以下，每日 50mg/kg，分次给予；1～5 岁，每次 250mg，一日 3 次；5～12 岁，可按成人量给予。静脉滴注：成人每次 500mg，每天 3 次；儿童及婴儿每日 20mg/kg，分 3 次给药。将本品 500mg 溶于 10ml 所附的无菌缓冲溶液中，然后用氯化钠注射液或 5% 葡萄糖注射液稀释至 250～500ml 静脉输注。若葡萄糖注射液过酸，溶液会呈乳状，如出现此情况即不能使用。输注时间不应少于 2～4 小时。<br><br>Par voie orale : 500mg, toutes les 8h, pour l'infection grave, possible de doubler la dose ; chez des enfants moins de 1 an, 50 mg/kg par jour, à travers plusieurs fois ; chez 1 à 5 ans, 250mg par fois, 3 fois par jour ; chez 5 à 12 ans, la même dose que chez des adultes. Par voie IV en perfusion : chez des adultes, 500mg par fois, 3 fois par jour ; chez des enfants et des bébés, 20 mg/kg par jour, à travers 3 fois. Dissoudre 500mg de médicament dans 10 ml de tampon stérile fourni, puis le diluer dans l'injection de chlorure de sodium ou l'injection de glucose à 5 % pour former une solution de 250 à 500 ml, perfusion. Si l'injection de glucose est trop acide, la solution sera lactée. Dans ce cas-là, ne plus l'utiliser. Perfuion pendant au moins 2 à 4 h. |
| 剂型、规格<br>Les formes pharmaceutiques et les spécifications | 片剂：每片 250mg。<br>注射用夫西地酸：每瓶 500mg( 钠盐 )；580mg( 二乙醇胺盐 )。<br>Comprimés : 250mg par comprimé.<br>La fusidate pour injection : 500mg (sodium) par flacon ; 580mg (diéthanolamine) par flacon. |

**2. 化学合成的抗菌药 Anti-microbiens de synthèse chimique**

**2.1　磺胺类 Sulfamides**

| 药品名称 Drug Names | 磺胺嘧啶 Sulfadiazine |
|---|---|
| 适应证<br>Les indications | 防治敏感脑膜炎球菌所致的流行性脑膜炎。<br>Ce produit sert à prévenir et à traiter la méningite à méningocoques. |
| 用法、用量<br>Les modes d'emploi et la posologie | 口服：成人：预防脑膜炎，1 次 1g，一日 2g；治疗脑膜炎：1 次 1g，一日 4g。儿童：一般感染，可按一日 50～75mg/kg，分为 2 次用；流脑：则按一日 100～150mg/kg 应用。<br>缓慢静脉注射或静脉滴注：治疗严重感染，成人 1 次 1～1.5g，一日 3～4.5g。本品注射液为钠盐，需用灭菌注射用水或等渗氯化钠注射液稀释，静脉注射时浓度应低于 5%；静脉滴注时浓度约为 1%( 稀释 20 倍 )，混匀后应用。<br><br>Par voie orale : chez des adultes, pour la prévention de la méningite, 1g par fois, 2g par jour ; pour le traitement de la méningite, 1g par fois, 4g par jour. Chez des enfants : pour l'infection générale, 50 à 75 mg/kg par jour, à travers 2 fois ; pour la méningite à méningocoques, 100 à 150 mg/kg par jour. Injection lente par voie IV ou par voie IV en perfusion : pour l'infection grave, chez des adultes, 1 à 1,5g par fois, 3 à 4,5 g par jour. Pour l'injection de sodium, utiliser l'eau stérile pour injection ou l'injection de chlorure de sodium pour la dilution. En cas d'injection par voie IV, la concentration doit être inférieure à 5 % ; en cas de perfusion, la concentration est de 1 % (dilué 20 fois). Application après le mélange. |
| 剂型、规格<br>Les formes pharmaceutiques et les spécifications | 片剂：每片 0.5g。<br>磺胺嘧啶混悬液：10%(g/ml)。<br>磺胺嘧啶钠注射液：每支 0.4g(2ml);1g(5ml)。<br>注射用磺胺嘧啶钠：每瓶 0.4g;1g。<br>复方磺胺嘧啶( 双嘧啶，SD-TMP) 片：每片含磺胺嘧啶 (SD)400mg 和甲氧苄啶 (TMP)50mg。本品的治疗效果约与复方磺胺甲噁唑 (SMZ-TMP) 片相近。<br>Comprimé : 0,5g par comprimé.<br>La sulfadiazine en suspension : 10% (g par ml).<br>Injection de sulfadiazine sodique : 0,4g (2ml) ou 1g (5ml) par injection.<br>La sulfadiazine sodique pour injection : 0,4g ou 1g par flacon.<br>Les comprimés composés de sulfadiazin (Bispyrimidine, SD-TMP) : 400mg de sulfadiazine (SD) et 50mg de triméthoprime (TMP) par comprimé.<br>Ce produit a un effet similaire au comprimé composé de sulfaméthoxazole (SMZ-TMP). |

| 药品名称 Drug Names | 磺胺甲噁唑 Sulfaméthoxazole |
|---|---|
| 适应证<br>Les indications | 用于急性支气管炎、肺部感染、尿路感染、伤寒、布氏杆菌病、菌痢等，疗效与氨苄西林、氯霉素、四环素等相近。<br><br>Ce produit sert à traiter la bronchite aigue, les infections pulmonaires et uriniaires, ainsi que la fièvre typhoïde, la brucellose et la dysenterie. Son efficacité est similaire à celle de l'ampicilline, du chloramphénicol et de la tétracycline. |
| 用法、用量<br>Les modes d'emploi et la posologie | 一日 2 次，每次服 1g。<br>2 fois par jour, 1g par fois. |
| 剂型、规格<br>Les formes pharmaceutiques et les spécifications | 片剂：每片 0.5g。<br>复方磺胺甲噁唑 ( 复方新诺明，SMZ-TMP) 片：每片含 SMZ0.4g、TMP0.08g。<br>联磺甲氧苄啶片 ( 增效联磺片 )：每片含 SMZ0.2g、SD0.2g、TMP0.08g。<br>复方磺胺甲噁唑 ( 复方新诺明；SMZ-TMP) 注射液：每支 2ml，含 SMZ0.4g、TMP0.08g。<br>Comprimés : 0,5g par comprimé.<br>Composé sulfaméthoxazole (SMZ-TMP) en comprimés : 0,4g de SMZ et 0,08g de TMP par comprimé.<br>Comprimés triméthoprime sulfaméthoxazole : 0,2g de SMZ et 0,2g de SD et 0,08g de TMP par comprimé.<br>Injection de composé sulfaméthoxazole (SMZ-TMP) : 2ml par injection qui contient 0,4g de SMZ et 0,08g de TMP. |
| 药品名称 Drug Names | 柳氮磺吡啶 Sulfasalazine |
| 适应证<br>Les indications | 用于治疗轻中度溃疡性结肠炎，活动期的克罗恩病，类风湿关节炎。<br>Ce produit sert à traiter la colite ulcéreuse bénigne et modérée, la maladie de Crohn active, ainsi que la polyarthrite rhumatoïde. |
| 用法、用量<br>Les modes d'emploi et la posologie | 口服：治疗溃疡性结肠炎，1 次 0.5 ~ 1g，一日 2 ~ 4g。如需要可逐渐增量至一日 4 ~ 6g，好转后减量为一日 1.5g，直至症状消失。也可用于灌肠，每日 2g，混悬于生理盐水 20 ~ 50ml 中，作保留灌肠，也可添加白及粉以增大药液黏滞度。<br>治疗类风湿关节炎：用肠溶片，每次 1g(4 片 )，一日 2 次。<br>直肠给药：重症患者，1 次 0.5g，早、中、晚各 1 次。轻、中度患者，早、晚各 0.5g。症状明显改善后，每晚或隔日睡前 0.5g。用药后需侧卧半小时。<br><br>Par voie orale : pour traiter la colite ulcéreuse, 0,5 à 1g par fois, 2 à 4g par jour ; s'il est nécessaire, 4 à 6 g par jour, avec le soulagement des symptômes, 1,5g par jour jusqu'à la disparition des symptômes.<br><br>Applicable dans le lavement : 2g par jour, en suspension dans 20 à 50 ml de solution saline pour effectuer le lavement à garder, aussi possible d'ajouter le rhizoma Bletillae en poudre pous augmenter la viscosité de la solution.<br><br>Pour traiter la polyarthrite rhumatoide : en comprimé à enrobage entérique, 1g par fois (4 comprimés), 2 fois par jour. Administration rectale : pour l'infection grave, 0,5 par fois, trois fois par jour ; pour l'infection bénigne et modérée, 0,5g le matin et le soir. Avec le soulagement des symptômes, 0,5g avant le repos chaque soir ou tous les deux soirs. Après l'administration, il faut se reposer sur le côté pendant une demi-heure. |
| 剂型、规格<br>Les formes pharmaceutiques et les spécifications | 片剂：每片 0.25g。<br>栓剂：每个 0.5g。<br>肠溶片：每片 0.25g。<br>Comprimés : 0,25g par comprimé.<br>Suppositoires : 0,5g par suppositoire.<br>Comprimé à enrobage entérique : 0,25g par comprimé. |

**续　表**

2.2　甲氧苄啶类 Triméthoprimes

| 药品名称 Drug Names | 甲氧苄啶 Triméthoprime |
| --- | --- |
| 适应证<br>Les indications | 常与磺胺药合用（多应用复方制剂）于治疗肺部感染、急慢性支气管炎、菌痢、尿路感染、肾盂肾炎、肠炎、伤寒、疟疾等，也与多种抗生素合用。本品单独可应用于大肠埃希菌、奇异变形杆菌、肺炎克雷伯杆菌、肠杆菌属、凝固酶阴性的金黄色葡萄球菌所致单纯性尿路感染。本品单用易引起细菌耐药，故不宜单独用。<br><br>Souvent associée à des sulfamides (en particulier applicalbe dans la préparation complexe), la triméthoprime sert, avec une variété d'antibiotiques, à traiter la pneumonie, la bronchite chronique et aigue, la dysenterie, les infections urinaies, la pyélonéphrite, l'entérite,la typhoide et le paludisme. Ce produit seul peut être utilisé comme traitement du colibacille, du proteus, du klebsiella, de l'enterobacter, ainsi que des infections urinaires causées par le staphylococcus aureus à coagulase négative. Comme l'utilisation unique de ce produitpeut entraîner une résistance bactérienne, il vaut mieux éviter de l'utiliser seul. |
| 用法、用量<br>Les modes d'emploi et la posologie | 口服，每次 0.1～0.2g，一日 0.2～0.4g。<br>Par voie orale : 0,1 à 0,2g par fois, 0,2 à 0,4g par jour. |
| 剂型、规格<br>Les formes pharmaceutiques et les spécifications | 片剂：每片 0.1g。<br>Comprimés : 0,1g par comprimé. |

2.3　硝基呋喃类 Nitrofuranes

| 药品名称 Drug Names | 呋喃妥因 Nitrofurantoïne |
| --- | --- |
| 适应证<br>Les indications | 本品主要应用于敏感菌所致的泌尿系统感染。一般地说，微生物对本品不易耐药，如停药后重新用药，仍可有效。但近年来耐药菌株有一定程度发展。必要时可与其他药物（如 TMP）联合应用以提高疗效。<br><br>Ce produit sert à traiter les infections bactériennes urinaires. En général, le micro-organisme n'est pas résistant à ce produit. Celui-ci reste donc efficace lorsqu'on le reprend après l'arrêt de l'administration.Mais ces dernières années, on assiste au développement des souches résistantes. Le cas échéant, on peut l'utiliser avec d'autres médicaments, tels que TMP, pour améliorer son efficacité. |
| 用法、用量<br>Les modes d'emploi et la posologie | 每次 0.1g，一日 0.2～0.4g，至尿内检菌阴性再继续用 3 日。但连续应用不宜超过 14 日。<br>0,1g par fois, 0,2 à 0,4g par jour, jusqu'à trois jours après le résultat négatif de l'examen urinaire des bactéries. Ne pas l'administrer pendant plus de 14 jours consécutifs. |
| 剂型、规格<br>Les formes pharmaceutiques et les spécifications | 肠溶片：每片 0.05g；0.1g。<br>Comprimé à enrobage entérique : 0,05g ou 0,1g par comprimé. |

| 药品名称 Drug Names | 呋喃唑酮 Furazolidone |
| --- | --- |
| 适应证<br>Les indications | 主要用于菌痢、肠炎，也可用于伤寒、副伤寒、梨形鞭毛虫病和阴道滴虫病。<br>Ce produit sert à traiter la dysenterie, l'entérite, la typhoide, la paratyphoïde, le giardiase en forme de poire et la trichomonase vaginale. |
| 用法、用量<br>Les modes d'emploi et la posologie | 常用量 1 次 0.1g，一日 3～4 次，症状消失后再服 2 日。梨形鞭毛虫病疗程为 7～10 日。<br>Dose usuelle, 0,1g par fois, 3 à 4 fois par jour, jusqu'à 2 jours après la disparition des symptômes. Le traitement médical dure 7 à 10 jours pour le giardiase en forme de poire. |
| 剂型、规格<br>Les formes pharmaceutiques et les spécifications | 片剂：每片 0.1g。<br>Comprimés : 0,1g par comprimé. |

**续　表**

### 2.4　喹诺酮类 4-Quinolones

| 药品名称 Drug Names | 吡哌酸 Acide pipémidique |
| --- | --- |
| 适应证<br>Les indications | 临床主要应用于敏感革兰阴性杆菌和葡萄球菌所致尿路、肠道和耳道感染，如尿道炎、膀胱炎、菌痢、肠炎、中耳炎等。<br>Ce produit est souvent utilisé dans les cliniques comme traitement des infections urinaiers, intestinales et intra-auriculaire causées par les bactéries à Gram négatif et le staphylococcus, telles que l'urétrite, la cystite, la dysenterie, l'entérite et l'otite moyenne. |
| 用法、用量<br>Les modes d'emploi et la posologie | 成人口服：1 次 0.5g，一日 1.5 ～ 2g，分次给予，一般不超过 10 日。<br>Chez des adultes, par voie orale : 0,5g par fois, 1,5 à 2g par jour, à travers plusieurs fois, ne pas dépasser 10 jours. |
| 剂型、规格<br>Les formes pharmaceutiques et les spécifications | 片剂：每片 0.25g;0.5g。<br>胶囊剂：每胶囊 0.25g。<br>Comprimés : 0,25g ou 0,5g par comprimé.<br>Capsules : 0,25g par capsule. |
| 药品名称 Drug Names | 诺氟沙星 Norfloxacine |
| 适应证<br>Les indications | 本品应用于敏感菌所致泌尿道、肠道、耳鼻喉科、妇科、外科和皮肤科等感染性疾病。<br>Ce produit sert à traiter les infections bactériennes liées aux voies urinaires, aux voies biliaires, au nez, aux oreilles, à la gorge, à la gynécologie, à la chirurgie et à la dermatologie. |
| 用法、用量<br>Les modes d'emploi et la posologie | 口服，成人 1 次 0.1 ～ 0.2g，一日 3 ～ 4 次。空腹服药吸收较好。一般疗程为 3 ～ 8 日，少数病例可达 3 周。对于慢性泌尿道感染病例，可先用一般量 2 周，再减量为 200mg/d，睡前服用，持续数月。严重病例及不能口服者静脉滴注。用量：每次 200 ～ 400mg，每 12 小时 1 次。将一次量加于输液中，滴注 1 小时。<br>Par voie orale, chez des adultes, 0,1g à 0,2g par fois, 3 à 4 fois par jour, l'estomac vide. Pendant 3 à 8 jours, dans certains cas, jusqu'à 3 semaines. Pour traiter l'infection chronique des voies urinaires, appliquer d'abord la dose usuelle pendant 2 semaines, ensuite,200 mg/jour, avant le sommeil, pendant plusieurs mois. Pour l'infection grave et pour ceux qui ne peuvent pas l'administrer par voie orale, essayer l'injection par voie IV en perfusion : 200 à 400 mg par fois, toutes les 12h, inclure un dosage dans l'infusion, la perfusion pendant 1h. |
| 剂型、规格<br>Les formes pharmaceutiques et les spécifications | 胶囊：每粒 100mg。<br>输液：每瓶 200mg/100ml( 尚有其他规格 )。<br>滴眼液：8ml(24mg)。<br>软膏：1%。<br>Capsules : 100mg par capsule.<br>Infusion : 200mg/100ml par flacon (il y a encore d'autres spécifications).<br>Gouttes pour les yeux : 8ml (24mg).<br>Pommade : 1 %. |
| 药品名称 Drug Names | 氧氟沙星 Ofloxacine |
| 适应证<br>Les indications | 主要用于上述革兰阴性菌所致的呼吸道、咽喉、扁桃体、泌尿道( 包括前列腺 )、皮肤及软组织、胆囊及胆管、中耳、鼻窦、泪囊、肠道等部位的急、慢性感染。<br>Ce produit sert à traiter les infections aigues et chroniques causées par des bactéries à Gram négatif, telles que les infections respiratoires, pharyngée, urinaires (y compris la prostatite), intestinales, cutanées, des tissus mous, des voies biliaires, l'amygdalite, l'otite moyenne ainsi que le lacrymal. |
| 用法、用量<br>Les modes d'emploi et la posologie | 口服：每日 200 ～ 600mg，分 2 次服。根据病情适当调整剂量。抗结核用量为每日 0.3g，顿服。控制伤寒反复感染：每日 50mg，连用 3 ～ 6 个月。<br>滴注给药：每次 200 ～ 400mg，每 12 小时 1 次，以适量输液稀释，滴注 1 小时。<br>Par voie orale : 200 à 600mg par jour, à travers 2 fois, en fonction de la maladie. Pour traiter la tuberculose, 0,3g par jour, une fois par jour. Pour contrôler l'infection par typhoïde récurrente : 50mg par jour, pendant 3 à 6 mois consécutifs.<br>Perfusion : 200 à 400 mg par fois, toutes les 12h, perfusion après dilution pendant 1h. |

续　表

| | |
|---|---|
| 剂型、规格<br>Les formes pharmaceutiques et les spécifications | 片剂：每片 100mg。<br>注射液：每支 400mg/10ml( 用前需稀释 )。<br>输液：每瓶 400mg/100ml( 可直接输注 )。<br>Comprimés : 100mg par comprimé.<br>Solution injectable : 400mg/10ml par injection (il faut la dilution avant de l'utiliser).<br>Perfusion : 400mg/100ml par flacon (applicable directement). |
| 药品名称 Drug Names | 左氧氟沙星 Lévofloxacine |
| 适应证<br>Les indications | 主要用于上述革兰阴性菌所致的呼吸道、咽喉、扁桃体、泌尿道 ( 包括前列腺 )、皮肤及软组织、胆囊及胆管、中耳、鼻窦、泪囊、肠道等部位的急、慢性感染。<br>Ce produit sert à traiter les infections aigues et chroniques causées par des bactéries à Gram négatif, telles que les infections respiratoires, pharyngée, urinaires (y compris la prostatite), intestinales, cutanées, des tissus mous, des voies biliaires, l'amygdalite, l'otite moyenne ainsi que le lacrymal. |
| 用法、用量<br>Les modes d'emploi et la posologie | 口服：每次 100mg，一日 2 次，根据感染严重程度可增量，最多每次 200mg，一日 3 次。静脉滴注，一日 200 ～ 600mg，分 1 ～ 2 次静脉滴注。<br>Par voie orale : 100mg par fois, 2 fois par jour, en fonction de la maladie, 200mg par fois, 3 fois par jour au plus.En perfusion, 200 à 600 mg par jour, à travers 1 à 2 fois. |
| 剂型、规格<br>Les formes pharmaceutiques et les spécifications | 片剂：每片 100mg；200mg；500mg。<br>注射液：200mg(100ml)；300mg(100ml)；500mg(100ml)。<br>Comprimés : 100mg, 200mg ou 500mg par comprimé.<br>Injection : 200mg (100ml), 300mg (100ml) ou 500mg (100ml). |
| 药品名称 Drug Names | 依诺沙星 Enoxacine |
| 适应证<br>Les indications | 用于敏感菌所致的咽喉、支气管、肺、尿路、前列腺、胆囊、肠道、中耳、鼻旁窦等部位感染，也可用于脓皮病及软组织感染。<br>Ce produit sert à traiter les infections bactériennes, telles que la pharyngite, la bronchite, la pneumonie, les infections des voies urinaiers, la prostatite, la cholécystite, les infections des voies intestinales, l'otite moyenne, la sinusite. Il est aussi applicable dans le traitement du pyoderma et des infections des tissus mous. |
| 用法、用量<br>Les modes d'emploi et la posologie | 成人常用量一日 400 ～ 600mg( 按无水物计量 )。分 2 次给予。<br>Chez des adultes, dose usuelle, 400 à 600mg par jour (quantité mesurée enmédicament andydre), à travers 2 fois. |
| 剂型、规格<br>Les formes pharmaceutiques et les spécifications | 片剂：每片 100mg( 标示量以无水物计，相当于含水物 108.5mg)；200mg( 相当于含水物 217mg)。<br>Comprimés : 100mg par comprimé (quantité mesurée enmédicament andydre, équivalent à 108.5mg de dydrate) ou 200mg par comprimé (équivalent à 217mg de dydrate). |
| 药品名称 Drug Names | 环丙沙星 Ciprofloxacine |
| 适应证<br>Les indications | 适用于敏感菌所致的呼吸道、尿道、消化道、胆道、皮肤和软组织、盆腔、眼、耳、鼻、咽喉等部位的感染。<br>Ce produit sert à traiter les infections bactériennes, telles que les infections respiratoires, urinaires, gastro-intestinales, biliaires, cutanées, des tissus mous, pelviennes, ainsi que les infections liées aux yeux, aux oreilles, au nez et à la gorge. |
| 用法、用量<br>Les modes d'emploi et la posologie | 口服：成人 1 次 250mg，一日 2 次，重症者可加倍量。但一日最高量不可超过 1500mg。肾功能不全者 ( 肌酐清除率低于 30ml/min) 应减少服量。<br>静脉滴注：1 次 100 ～ 200mg，一日 2 次，预先用等渗氯化钠或葡萄糖注射液稀释，滴注时间不少于 30 分钟。<br>Par voie orale : chez des adultes, 250mg par fois, 2 fois par jour, doubler la dose chez des patients gravement malades. Ne pas dépaser 1500mg par jour. chez des patients insuffisants rénaux (Taux d'élimination de la créatinine inférieur à30ml/min), il faut diminuer la dose.<br>En perfusion : 100 à 200mg par fois, 2 fois par jour, utiliser la solution isotonique de chlorure de sodium ou la solution de glucose pour la dilution, perfusion pendant 30 minutes au moins. |

**续 表**

| 剂型、规格<br>Les formes pharmaceutiques et les spécifications | 片剂：每片 ( 标示量按环丙沙星计算 ) 为 250mg；500mg；750mg( 含盐酸盐一水合物量分别为 291mg、582mg 和 873mg)。<br>注射液：每支 100mg(50ml)；200mg(100ml)( 含乳酸盐分别为 127.2mg 和 254.4mg)。<br>Comprimés : 250mg ou 500mg ou 750mg par comprimé (quantité calculée en ciprofloxacine), qui contient respectivement 291mg, 582mg et 873mg de monohydrates de chlorhydrate.<br>Injection : 100mg (50ml), 200mg (100ml) par solution, qui contient respectivement 127,2mg et 254,4mg de lactate. |
|---|---|
| **药品名称 Drug Names** | 洛美沙星 Lomefloxacine |
| 适应证<br>Les indications | 应用于上述敏感菌所致的下呼吸道、尿道感染。本品对链球菌、肺炎链球菌、洋葱假单胞菌、支原体和厌氧菌均无效。<br>Ce produit sert à traiter les infections bactériennes, telles que les infections respiratoires et urinaires. Il est inutile dans le traitement des infections causées par le streptococcus, le streptococcus pneumoniae, le pseudomonas cepacia, les mycoplasmes et les anaérobies. |
| 用法、用量<br>Les modes d'emploi et la posologie | 口服：每日 1 次 400mg，疗程 10～14 日。手术感染的预防，手术前 2～6 小时，1 次服 400mg。静脉滴注：每次 200mg，一日 2 次，或每次 400mg，一日 1 次。每 100mg 药物需用 5% 葡萄糖液或 0.9% 氯化钠液 60～100ml 稀释后缓慢滴注。肾功能不全者的用量，按血清肌酐值，依下式计算：男性： [ 体重 (kg)×(140- 年龄 )] / [72× 血清肌酐值 (mg/dl)] 女性：按男性结果 ×0.85.<br>Par voie orale : 400mg par fois par jour, pendant 10 à 14jours. Pour la prévention de l'infection chirurgicale, 2 à 6 h avant la chirurgie, 400mg par fois.<br>En perfusion : 200mg par fois, 2 fois par jour, ou 400mg par fois, 1 fois par jour.<br>Pour 100mg de médicament, utiliser 60 à 100ml de solution de glucose à 5 % ou de solution de chlorure de sodium à 0,9 % pour la dilution, et puis, perfusion lente.<br>Chez des patients insuffisants rénaux : chez les hommes : [poids (kg)×(140 -âge)]/[72×la créatinine sérique (mg /dl)] ; chez les femmes : le résultat chez les hommes ×0,85. |
| 剂型、规格<br>Les formes pharmaceutiques et les spécifications | 薄膜衣片：每片 400mg。<br>注射液 ( 盐酸盐或天冬氨酸盐 )：每支 100mg/2ml；每瓶 200mg/100ml、400mg/250ml。<br>Comprimés pelliculés : 400mg par comprimé.<br>Injection (chlorhydrate ou aspartate): 100mg/2ml par solution ; 200mg/100ml par flacon ou 400mg/250ml par flacon. |
| **药品名称 Drug Names** | 培氟沙星 Péfloxacine |
| 适应证<br>Les indications | 用于治疗革兰阴性菌和金黄色葡萄球菌引起的中度或重度感染。如泌尿系统、呼吸道、耳鼻喉、生殖系统、腹部和肝、胆系统感染、脑膜炎、骨和关节感染、败血症和心内膜炎。<br>Ce produit sert à traiter des infections modérées et graves causées par les bactéries à Gram négatif et le staphylococcus aureus, telles que les infections des voies urinaires, respiratoires, génitales, abdominales, hépatobiliaires, osseuses, articulaires, ORL, ainsi que la méningite, la septicémie et l'endocardite. |
| 用法、用量<br>Les modes d'emploi et la posologie | 口服：成人每日 400～800mg，分 2 次给予。静脉滴注：一次 0.4g，加入 5% 葡萄糖注射液 250ml 中，缓慢滴入，滴注时间不少于 60 分钟，每 12 小时 1 次。<br>Par voie orale : chez des adultes, 400 à 800mg par jour, à travers 2 fois. (En perfusion : 0,4g par fois, dissoudre le produit dans 250 ml de solution de glucose à 5 %, perfusion lente, pendant 60 minutes au moins, toutes les 12h.) |
| 剂型、规格<br>Les formes pharmaceutiques et les spécifications | 片剂：每片 200mg。<br>注射液 ( 甲磺酸盐 )：每支 400mg(5ml)。<br>Comprimés : 200mg par comprimé.<br>Injection (mésylate) : 400mg (5ml) par solution. |

**续　表**

| 药品名称 Drug Names | 芦氟沙星 Rufloxacine |
|---|---|
| 适应证<br>Les indications | 临床用于敏感菌引起的下呼吸道及尿道感染。如肺炎、急慢性支气管炎、急慢性肾盂肾炎、急性膀胱炎、尿道炎及皮肤软组织化脓性感染。<br><br>Ce produit est utilisé dans les cliniques comme traitement des infections des voies respiratoires inférieures et des voies urinaires causées pas des bactéries sensibles. Par exemple, la pneumonie, la bronchite aigue et chronique, la pyélonéphrite aigue et chronique, la cystite aigue, l'urétrite ainsi que l'infection purulente cutanée et des tissus mous. |
| 用法、用量<br>Les modes d'emploi et la posologie | 成人一日 1 次，每次 200mg，早餐后服。5 ～ 10 日为 1 个疗程。前列腺炎的疗程可达 4 周。<br>Chez des adultes, 1 fois par jour, 200mg par fois, après le petit déjeuner, pendant 5 à 10jour. Pour traiter la prostatite, traitement pendant 4 semaines. |
| 剂型、规格<br>Les formes pharmaceutiques et les spécifications | 片剂：每片 200mg。<br>胶囊剂：每粒 100mg。<br>Comprimés : 200mg par comprimé.<br>Capsules : 100mg par capsule. |
| 药品名称 Drug Names | 司帕沙星 Sparfloxacine |
| 适应证<br>Les indications | 临床用于敏感菌所致的咽喉、扁桃体、支气管、肺、胆囊、尿道、前列腺、肠道、子宫、中耳、鼻旁窦等部位感染，还可用于皮肤、软组织感染及牙周组织炎。<br><br>Ce produit est utilisé dans les cliniques comme traitement des infections bactériennes, telles que les infections dans les parties du corp suivantes : la gorge, les amygdales, la bronche, le poumon, la vésicule biliaire, l'urètre, la prostate, l'intestin, l'utérus, l'oreille moyenne etle sinus. Il est aussi applicalbe dans les infections cutanées, des tissus mous et l'inflammation du tissu parodontal. |
| 用法、用量<br>Les modes d'emploi et la posologie | 口服：成人每次 100 ～ 300mg，最多不超过 400mg，一日 1 次。疗程一般为 5 ～ 10 日。<br>Par voie orale : chez des adultes, 100 à 300mg par fois, ne pas dépasser 400mg, 1 fois par jour, pendant 5 à 10 jours. |
| 剂型、规格<br>Les formes pharmaceutiques et les spécifications | 胶囊剂：每粒 100mg。<br>Capsules : 100mg par capsule. |
| 药品名称 Drug Names | 氟罗沙星 Fleroxacine |
| 适应证<br>Les indications | 用于敏感菌所致的呼吸系统、泌尿生殖系统、消化系统的感染，以及皮肤软组织、骨、关节、耳鼻喉、腹腔、盆腔感染。<br><br>Ce produit sert à traiter les infections respiratoires, urinaires et gestro-intestinales, ainsi que les infections cutanées, des tissus mous, osseuses, articulaires, ORL, abdominales et pelviennes. |
| 用法、用量<br>Les modes d'emploi et la posologie | 口服：每日 0.4g，一次顿服。疗程视感染不同而定：复杂性尿路感染 1 ～ 2 周；呼吸道感染 1 ～ 3 周；皮肤、软组织感染 4 日～ 3 周；骨髓炎、化脓性关节炎 2 ～ 12 周；伤寒 1 ～ 2 周；沙眼衣原体尿道炎 5 日；单纯性尿路感染、细菌性痢疾、淋球菌尿道炎（宫颈炎）只用 1 次。<br>静脉滴注：一次 200 ～ 400mg，一日 1 次，加入 5% 葡萄糖注射液 250ml 中，避光缓慢滴注（每 100ml 滴注至少 45 ～ 60 分钟）。<br><br>Par voie orale, 0,4g par jour, 1 fois par jour. La durée du traitement en fonction des infections : pour l'infection des voies urinaires complexe, pendant 1 à 2 semaines ; pour l'infection des voies respiratoires, pendant 1 à 3 semianes ; pour l'infection cutanée et des tissus mous, pendant 4 jours à 3 semaines ; pour l'ostéomyélite et l'arthrite septique, pendant 2 à 12semaines ; pour la typhoide, pendant 1 à 2 semaines ; pour l'urétrite à chlamydia trachomati, pendant 5 jours ; pour l'infection urinaire simple, la dysenterie bacillaire, l'urétrite non-gonococcique (cervicite), une fois seulement. En perfusion : 200 à 400 mg par fois, 1 fois par jour, dissoudre le produit dans 250 ml de solution de glucose à 5 %, perfusion lente, abri de la lumière (pour 100ml, perfusion pendant 45 à 60 minutes au moins). |

| 剂型、规格<br>Les formes pharmaceutiques et les spécifications | 胶囊剂：每粒 200mg；400mg。<br>Capsules : 200mg ou 400mg par capsule. |
|---|---|
| **药品名称 Drug Names** | **莫西沙星 Moxifloxacine** |
| 适应证<br>Les indications | 适用于敏感菌所致的呼吸道感染，包括慢性支气管炎急性发作，轻度或中度的社区获得性肺炎，急性鼻窦炎等。<br>Ce produit sert à traiter les infections respiratoirse causées par des bactéries sensibles, y compris l'exacerbation aiguë de bronchite chronique, la pneumonie légère ou modérée, et la sinusite aigue. |
| 用法、用量<br>Les modes d'emploi et la posologie | 成人每日 1 次 400mg，连用 5～10 日，口服或静脉滴注。滴注时间为 90 分钟。<br>Chez des adultes, 400mg par fois par jour, pendant 5 à 10 jours consécutifs, par voie orale ou IV en perfusion. Perfusion pendant 90 minutes. |
| 剂型、规格<br>Les formes pharmaceutiques et les spécifications | 片剂 400mg。<br>注射液 250ml( 莫西沙星 0.4g)。<br>Comprimés : 400mg.<br>Injection : 250ml (0,4g de moxifloxacine). |
| **药品名称 Drug Names** | **加替沙星 Gatifloxacine** |
| 适应证<br>Les indications | 用于敏感菌所致的慢性支气管炎急性发作、急性鼻窦炎、社区获得性肺炎、尿路感染、急性肾盂肾炎、女性淋球菌性宫颈感染。<br>Ce produit sert à traiter les infections bactériennes, telles que l'exacerbation aiguë de bronchite chronique, la pneumonie, la sinusite aigue, les infections des voies urinaires, la pyélonéphrite aigue et L'infection gonococcique féminie de l'utérus. |
| 用法、用量<br>Les modes d'emploi et la posologie | 静脉给药：成人每次 200～400mg，一日 1 次，疗程一般 5～10 日。治疗中由静脉给药改为口服给药时，无须调整剂量。治疗非复杂性淋球菌尿路或直肠感染和女性淋球菌性宫颈感染，400mg 单次给药。中度肝功能不全者，无须调整剂量；中、重度肾功能不全者，应减量使用。<br>Administration par voie IV : chez des adultes, 200 à 400mg par fois, 1 fois par jour, pendant 5 à 10 jours consécutifs. S'il on remplace l'administration par voie IV par l'administration par voie orale, la même dose qu'autrefois. Pour traiter les infections des voies urinaires gonococciques simples ou les infections rectales ainsi que l'infection gonococcique féminie de l'utérus, prendre 400mg par fois. Chez des patients insuffisans hépatiques modérés, pas nécessaire d'ajuster la dose ; chez des patients insuffisans rénaux modérés et graves, diminuer la dose. |
| 剂型、规格<br>Les formes pharmaceutiques et les spécifications | 片剂：每片 100mg；200mg；400mg。<br>注射液：100mg(100ml)；200mg(100ml)； 400mg(40ml)。<br>Comprimés : 100mg, 200mg ou 400mg par comprimé.<br>Injection : 100mg (100ml), 200mg (100ml) ou 400mg (40ml). |
| **药品名称 Drug Names** | **帕珠沙星 Pazufloxacine** |
| 适应证<br>Les indications | 用于敏感菌所致的呼吸道感染、泌尿道感染，妇科、外科、耳鼻喉科和皮肤科等感染性疾病。<br>Ce produit sert à traiter les infections bactériennes liées aux voies urinaires, aux voies respiratoires, à ORL, à la gynécologie, à la chirurgie et à la dermatologie. |
| 用法、用量<br>Les modes d'emploi et la posologie | 静脉滴注，每次 300mg，滴注时间为 30～60 分钟，一日 2 次，疗程 7～14 日。肾功能不全者应调整剂量：肾清除率＞ 44.7ml/min，每次 300mg，一日 2 次；肾清除率为 13.6～44.7ml/min，每次 300mg，一日 1 次；透析患者用量为每次 300mg，每 3 日 1 次。<br>En perfusion : 300mg par fois, pendant 30 à 60 minutes, 2 fois par jour, pendant 7 à 14 jours. Chez des patients insuffisans rénaux, ajuster la dose : pour ceux dont la clairance rénale est supérieure à 44,7ml/min, 300mg par fois, 2 fois par jour ; chez ceux dont la clairance rénale est de 13,6 à 44,7 ml/min, 300mg par fois, 1 fois par jour ; chez des patients de dialyse, 300mg par fois, 1 fois tous les 3 jours. |

**续　表**

| 剂型、规格<br>Les formes pharmaceutiques et les spécifications | 甲磺酸帕珠沙星注射液：100mg(10ml)；150mg(10ml)；200mg(100ml)；300mg(100ml)。<br>Injection de mésylate de pazufloxacine : 100mg (10ml), 150mg (10ml), 200mg (100ml) ou 300mg (100ml). |
|---|---|

| 药品名称 Drug Names | 托氟沙星 Tosufloxacine |
|---|---|

| 适应证<br>Les indications | 临床用于敏感菌引起的呼吸系统、泌尿系统、胃肠道、皮肤软组织感染，以及中耳炎、牙周炎、眼睑炎等。<br>Ce produit est utilisé dans les cliniques comme traitement des infections respiratoires, urinaires, gastro-intestinales, cutanées et des tissus mous, ainsi que l'otite moyenne, la parodontite et la blépharite. |
|---|---|
| 用法、用量<br>Les modes d'emploi et la posologie | 口服每次 75 ～ 150mg，一日 2 ～ 3 次，一般疗程 3 ～ 7 日；最多每日剂量 600mg，分 2 ～ 3 次服用，疗程 14 日。<br>Par voie orale, 75 à 150mg par fois, 2 à 3 fois par jour, pendant 3 à 7 jours ; dose maximale, 600mg par jour, à travers 2 à 3 fois, pendant 14 jours. |
| 剂型、规格<br>Les formes pharmaceutiques et les spécifications | 片剂：每片 150mg。<br>Comprimés: 150mg par comprimé. |

## 2.5　硝咪唑类 Nitroimidazoles

| 药品名称 Drug Names | 甲硝唑 Métronidazole |
|---|---|

| 适应证<br>Les indications | 主要用于治疗或预防上述厌氧菌引起的系统或局部感染，如腹腔、消化道、女性生殖系、下呼吸道、皮肤及软组织、骨和关节等部位的厌氧菌感染，对败血症、心内膜炎、脑膜感染及使用抗生素引起的结肠炎也有效。治疗破伤风常与破伤风抗毒素 (TAT) 联用。还可用于口腔厌氧菌感染。<br>Ce produit sert à prévenir et à traiter les infections systématiques ou locales, causées par des anaérobies, telles que les infections abdominales, gastro-intestinales, génitales, des voies respiratoires inférieures, cutanées, des tissus mous, osseuses, articulaires, ainsi que la septicémie, l'endocardite, la méningite et la colite provoquée par l'utilisation des antibiotiques. En cas de traitement du tétanos, il est souvent associé à TAT. Il est aussi applicable dans le traitement des infections buccales causées par des anaérobies. |
|---|---|
| 用法、用量<br>Les modes d'emploi et la posologie | 厌氧菌感染：口服，1 次 0.2 ～ 0.4g，一日 0.6 ～ 1.2g；静脉滴注，1 次 500mg，8 小时 1 次，每次滴注 1 小时。一个疗程 7 日。预防用药：用于腹部或妇科手术前一天开始服药，1 次 0.25 ～ 0.5g，一日 3 次。治疗破伤风：1 个日量 2.5g，分次口服或滴注。<br>Pour traiter les infection causée par des anaérobies : par voie orale, 0,2 à 0,4g ar fois, 0,6 à 1,2g par jour ; en perfusion, 500mg par fois, une toutes les 8h, perfusion pendant 1h. Un traitement médical dure 7 jours. Pour la prévention : un jour avant la chirurgie abdominale ou gynécologique, 0,25 à 0,5g par fois, 3 fois par jour. Pour traiter le tétanos : 2,5g par jour, à travers plusieurs fois, administré par voie orale ou en perfusion. |
| 剂型、规格<br>Les formes pharmaceutiques et les spécifications | 片剂：每片 0.2g。<br>注射液：50mg(10ml)；100mg(20ml)；500mg(100ml)；1.25g(250ml)；500mg(250ml)。<br>甲硝唑葡萄糖注射液：250ml，含甲硝唑 0.5g 及葡萄糖 12.5g。<br>栓剂：每个 0.5g；1g。<br>甲硝唑阴道泡腾片：每片 0.2g。<br>Comprimés : 0,2g par comprimé.<br>Injection : 50mg (10ml), 100mg (20ml), 500mg (100ml), 1,25g (250ml) ou 500mg (250ml).<br>Injection de glucose de métronidazole : 250ml, qui contient 0,5g de métronidazole et 12,5g de glucose.<br>Suppositoires : 0,5g ou 1g par suppositoire.<br>Comprimés effervescents vaginaux de métronidazole : 0,2g par comprimé. |

**续　表**

| 药品名称 Drug Names | 替硝唑 Tinidazole |
|---|---|
| 适应证<br>Les indications | 　　用于厌氧菌的系统与局部感染，如腹腔、妇科、手术创口、皮肤软组织、肺、胸腔等部位感染，以及败血症、肠道或泌尿生殖道毛滴虫病、梨形鞭毛虫病及肠道和肝阿米巴病。<br>　　Ce produit sert à traiter les infections systématiques ou locales causées par des anaérobies, telles que les infections abdominales, gynécologiques, des plaies chirurgicales, cutanées, des tissus mous, pulmonaires, ainsi que la septicémie, la trichomonase intestinale et urogénitale, le giardiasis en forme de poire et l'amibiase intestinale et hépatique. |
| 用法、用量<br>Les modes d'emploi et la posologie | 　　厌氧菌系统感染：口服每日 2g；重症可静脉滴注，每日 1.6g，1 次或分为 2 次给予。手术感染的预防：术前 12 小时服 2g，手术间或结束后输注 1.6g( 或口服 2g)。非特异性阴道炎：每日 2g，连服 2 日。急性牙龈炎：1 次口服 2g。泌尿生殖道毛滴虫病：1 次口服 2g，必要时重复 1 次；或每次 0.15g，一日 3 次，连用 5 日。需男女同治以防再次感染。儿童 1 次 50 ～ 75mg/kg，必要时重复 1 次。合并白念珠菌感染者须同时进行抗真菌治疗。梨形鞭毛虫病：1 次 2g。肠阿米巴病：每日 2g，服 2 ～ 3 日。儿童每日 50 ～ 60mg，连用 5 日。肝阿米巴病：每日 1.5 ～ 2g，连用 3 日，必要时可延长至 5 ～ 10 日。应同时排出脓液。口服片剂应于餐间或餐后服用。静脉滴注每 400mg(200ml) 应不少于 20 分钟。<br>　　Pour traiter infections causées par des anaérobies : par voie orale, 2g par jour ; chez des patients gravement malades, en perfusion, 1,6g par our, à travers 1 ou 2 fois. Pour la prévention des infections chirurgicales : 12h avant la chirurgie prendre 2g, durant ou après la chirurgie, administrer 1,6g par voie IV en perfusion ou 2g par voie orale. Pour traiter la viginite non spécifique : 2g par jour, pendant 2 jours consécutifs.Pour traiter la gingivite aigue : 2g, une fois en voie orale. Pour traiter la trichomonase urogénitale : 2g, une fois en voie orale, s'il est nécessaire, reprendre 1 fois ; ou 0,15g par fois, 3 fois par jour, pendant 5 jours consécutifs. Les couples doivent prendre le médicament en même temps pour éviter la récurrence. Chez des enfants, 50 à 75 mg/kg, une seule fois, s'il est nécessaire, reprendre une fois. Chez des patients atteints d'infection à Candida albicans, il faut appliquer le traitement antifongique en même temps. Pour traiter le giardiasis en forme de poire : 2g par fois. Pour traiter l'amibiase intestinale : 2g par jour, pendant 2 à 3 jours. Chez des enfants, 50 à 60mg par jour, pendant 5 jours consécutifs. Pour traiter l'amibiase hépatique : 1,5 à 2g par jour, pendant 3 jours consécutifs, s'il est nécessaire, pendant 5 à 10 jours. Il faut décharger le pus en même temps. Pour l'administratin par voie orale, administrer durant ou après le repas. Pour l'administration de 400mg (200ml) en perfusion pendant 20 minutes au moins. |
| 剂型、规格<br>Les formes pharmaceutiques et les spécifications | 　　片剂：每片 0.25g；0.5g。<br>　　注射液：每瓶 400mg/200ml 或 800mg/400ml( 含葡萄糖 5.5%)。<br>　　栓剂：每个 0.2g。<br>　　Comprimés : 0,25g ou 0,5g par comprimé.<br>　　Injection : 400mg/200ml ou 800mg/400ml (y compris la glucose à 5,5 %) par flacon.<br>　　Suppositoires : 0,2g par suppositoire. |
| 药品名称 Drug Names | 奥硝唑 Ornidazole |
| 适应证<br>Les indications | 　　用于由厌氧菌感染引起的多种疾病。男女泌尿生殖道毛滴虫、贾第鞭毛虫感染引起的疾病。还用于肠、肝阿米巴病。<br>　　Ce produit sert à traiter des maladies causées pas des anaérobies, telles que la trichomonase génito-urinaire masculine et féminine, l'infection à Giardia lamblia, ainsi que l'amibiase intestinale et hépatique. |
| 用法、用量<br>Les modes d'emploi et la posologie | 　　口服：预防术后厌氧菌感染，术前 12 小时服用 1500mg，以后每次 500mg，一日 2 次，至术后 3 ～ 5 日；治疗厌氧菌感染，每次 500mg，一日 2 次；急性毛滴虫病，于夜间单次服用 1500mg；慢性毛滴虫病，1 次 500mg，一日 2 次，共用 5 日；贾第鞭毛虫病，于夜间顿服 1500mg，用药 1 ～ 2 日；阿米巴痢疾，于夜间顿服 1500mg，用药 3 日；其他阿米巴病，1 次 500mg，一日 2 次。静脉滴注：预防术后厌氧菌感染，术前 1 ～ 2 小时给药 1000mg，术后 12 小时给药 500mg，24 小时再给药 500mg；治疗厌氧菌感染，初始剂量为 500 ～ 1000mg，以后每 12 小时 500mg，疗程 3 ～ 6 日。 |

**续　表**

| | |
|---|---|
| | Par voie orale : pour la prévention des infections causées par des anaérobies après l'opération, 1500mg 12h avant l'opération, ensuite, 500mg par fois, 2 fois par jour, jusqu'à 3 à 5 jours après l'opération ; pour traiter les infections causées par des anaérobies, 500mg par fois, 2 fois par jour ; pour la trichomonase aigue, 1500mg, dose unique la nuit ; pour la trichomonase chronique, 500mg par fois, 2 fois par jour, 5 jours consécutifs ; pour traiter l'infection à Giardia lamblia, 1500mg la nuit, pendant 1 à 2 jours ; pour traiter la dysenterie amibienne, 1500mg la nuit, pendant 3 jours ; pour d'autres amibiases, 500mg par fois, 2 fois par jour. Par voie IV en perfusion : pour la prévention des infections causées par des anaérobies après l'opération, 1000mg 1 à 2 h avant l'opération, 500mg 12h après l'opération, 500mg 24h après ; pour le traitement des infections causées par des anaérobies, pour la première fois, 500 à 1000 mg, ensuite, 500mg toutes les 12h, pendant 3 à 6 jours consécutifs. |
| 剂型、规格<br>Les formes pharmaceutiques et les spécifications | 片剂（胶囊剂）：每片（粒）0.25g。<br>注射液：0.25g(5ml)。<br>奥硝唑氯化钠（葡萄糖）注射液：0.25g(100ml)；0.5g(100ml)。<br>Comprimés (capsules) : 0,25g par comprimé ou par capsule.<br>Injection : 0,25g (5ml).<br>Injection de chlorure de sodium (glucose) d'ornidazole : 0,25g (100ml) ou 0,5g (100ml). |
| **药品名称 Drug Names** | 塞克硝唑 Secnidazole |
| 适应证<br>Les indications | 主要用于由阴道毛滴虫引起的尿道炎和阴道炎，肠阿米巴病，肝阿米巴病及贾第鞭毛虫病。<br>Ce produit sert à traiter l'urétrite et la vaginite causées par le trichomonas vaginalis, l'amibiase intestinale et hépatique ainsi que la giardiase. |
| 用法、用量<br>Les modes d'emploi et la posologie | 口服，成人 2g，单次服用。治疗阴道滴虫病和尿道滴虫病，配偶应同时服用。肠阿米巴病：有症状的急性阿米巴病，成人 2g，单次服用；儿童 30mg/kg，单次服用；无症状的急性阿米巴病，成人一次 2g，一日 1 次，连服 3 日；儿童一次 30mg/kg，一日 1 次，连服 3 日。肝脏阿米巴病：成人一日 1.5g，一次或分次口服，连服 5 日；儿童一次 30mg/kg，一次或分次口服，连服 5 日。贾第鞭毛虫病：儿童 30mg/kg，单次服用。<br>Par voie orale, chez des adultes, 2g, dose unique. Pour traiter le trichomonas vaginalis et le trichomonase urétral, les couples doivent prendre des médicaments en même temps. Pour l'amibiase intestinale : en cas d'amibiase aigue avec des symptômes, chez des adultes, 2g, dose unique, chez des enfants, 30mg/kg, dose unique ; en cas d'amibiase aigue sans symptômes, chez des adultes, 2g, 1 fois par jour, pendant 3 jours consécutifs, chez des enfants, 30 mg/kg par fois, 1 fois par jour, pendant 3 jours consécutifs. Pour traiter l'amibiase hépatique : chez des adultes, 1,5g par jour, à travers une fois ou plusieurs fois, pendant 5 jours consécutifs ; chez des enfants, 30 mg/kg par fois, à travers une ou plusieurs fois, pendant 5 jours consécutifs. Pour la giardiase, chez des enfants, 30 mg/kg, dose unique. |
| 剂型、规格<br>Les formes pharmaceutiques et les spécifications | 片剂（胶囊）：每片 / 粒 0.25g；0.5g。<br>Comprimés (capsules) : 0,25g ou 0,5g par comprimé ou par capsule. |

2.6　噁唑烷酮类 Oxazolidinones

| | |
|---|---|
| **药品名称 Drug Names** | 利奈唑胺 Linézolide |
| 适应证<br>Les indications | 主要用于控制耐万古霉素粪肠球菌所致的系统感染，包括败血症、肺炎及复杂性皮肤和皮肤组织感染等。<br>Ce produit sert à traiter des infections systématiques causées par les excréments d'entérocoques résistant à la vancomycine, y comrpis la septicémie, la pneumonie et les infections cutanées et des tissus mous difficiles. |
| 用法、用量<br>Les modes d'emploi et la posologie | 口服与静脉滴注剂量相同。成人和超过 12 岁儿童，每次 600mg，每 12 小时 1 次。治疗耐万古霉素肠球菌感染疗程 14～28 日。肺炎、菌血症及皮肤软组织感染疗程 10～14 日。儿童（出生至 11 岁者），每次 10mg/kg，每 12 小时 1 次，疗效欠佳可增至每 8 小时 1 次，口服或静脉给药。<br>La même dose tant par voie orale que par voie IV en perfusion. Chez des adultes et des enfants de plus de 12 ans, 600mg par fois, toutes les 12h. Pour traiter des infections systématiques causées par les excréments d'entérocoques résistant à la vancomycine, le traitement médical dure 14 à 28 jours. Pour traiter bactériémie et des infections cutanées ou des tissus mous, 10 à 14 jours. Chez des enfants ( 0 à 11 ans), 10 mg/kg par fois, toutes les 12h, en cas de mauvaise efficacité, toutes les 8h, administratio par voie orale ou par voie IV. |

续 表

| 剂型、规格<br>Les formes pharmaceutiques et les spécifications | 片剂：每片 600mg。<br>注射液：600mg(300ml)。<br>Comprimés : 600mg par comprimé.<br>Injection : 600mg (300ml). |
|---|---|

### 3. 抗结核药 Antituberculose

| 药品名称 Drug Names | 异烟肼 Isoniazide |
|---|---|
| 适应证<br>Les indications | 主要用于各型肺结核的进展期、溶解播散期、吸收好转期，尚可用于结核性脑膜炎和其他肺外结核等。本品常需和其他抗结核病药联合应用，以增强疗效和克服耐药菌。此外，对痢疾、百日咳、麦粒肿等也有一定疗效。<br><br>Ce produit est principalement utilisé dans le traitement de différentes tuberculoses au stade actif, au stade de dissolution et de diffusion et au stade d'amélioration. Il est aussi applicable dans le traitement de la méningite tuberculeuse et de la tuberculose extrapulmonaire. Il faut souvent prescrire en même temps plusieurs antibiotiques antituberculeux pour améliorer leur efficacité dans la lutte contre les bactéries résistant aux médicaments.Il est aussi utile dans le traitement de la dysenterie, de la coqueluche, et de la porcherie. |
| 用法、用量<br>Les modes d'emploi et la posologie | 口服：成人 1 次 0.3g，1 次顿服；对急性粟粒性肺结核或结核性脑膜炎，1 次 0.2 ～ 0.3g，一日 3 次。静脉注射或静脉滴注：对较重度浸润结核，肺外活动结核等，1 次 0.3 ～ 0.6g，加 5% 葡萄糖注射液或等渗氯化钠注射液 20 ～ 40ml，缓慢推注；或加入输液 250 ～ 500ml 中静脉滴注。百日咳：一日按 10 ～ 15mg/kg，分为 3 次服。麦粒肿：一日按 4 ～ 10mg/kg，分为 3 次服。局部（胸腔内注射治疗局灶性结核等）：1 次 50 ～ 200mg。<br><br>Par voie orale : chez des adultes, 0,3g par fois, une fois par jour ; pour traiter la tuberculose miliaire aiguë, 0,2 à 0,3 g par fois, 3 fois par jour. Par voie IV ou en perfuion : pour l'infiltration tuberculeuse et la tuberculose extrapulmonaire, 0,3 à 0,6g par fois, inclure 20 à 40ml d'injection de glucose à 5 % ou d'injection de chlorure de sodium, injection lente ; ou inclure 250 à 500 ml d'eau pour injection, perfusion. Pour la cqueluche, 10 à 15 mg/kg par jour, à travers 3 fois. Pour traiter la porcherie, 4 à 10 mg/kg par jour, à travers 3 fois. Injection topique (injection intra-thoracique sur la zone touchée) : 50 à 200mg par fois. |
| 剂型、规格<br>Les formes pharmaceutiques et les spécifications | 片剂：每片 0.05g；0.1g；0.3g。<br>注射液：每支 0.1g(2ml)。<br>Comprimés : 0,05g, 0,1g ou 0,3g par comprimé.<br>Injection : 0,1g (2ml) par solution. |
| 药品名称 Drug Names | 对氨基水杨酸钠 Aminosalicylate de sodium |
| 适应证<br>Les indications | 本品很少单独应用，常配合异烟肼、链霉素等应用，以增强疗效并避免细菌产生耐药性。也可用于甲状腺功能亢进症。对于甲亢合并结核患者较适用，在用碘剂无效而影响手术时，可短期服用本品为手术创造条件。本品尚有较强的降血脂作用。<br><br>Ce produit est souvent utilisé avec l'isoniazide et la streptomycine, pour renforcer son effciacité et éviter la résistance bactérienne. Il est aussi applicable dans le traitement de l'hyperthyroïdie. Chez les patients attients de la tuberculose thyroïdienne, ce produit peut être administré pour une courte durée pour préparer l'opération, lorsque l'iode est inutile et affecte l'opération.Il a également un effet hypolipidémiant. |
| 用法、用量<br>Les modes d'emploi et la posologie | 口服：每次 2 ～ 3g，一日 8 ～ 12g，饭后服。小儿每日 200 ～ 300mg/kg，分 4 次服。静脉滴注：每日 4 ～ 12g（先从小剂量开始），以等渗氯化钠注射液或 5% 葡萄糖液溶解后，配成 3% ～ 4% 浓度滴注。小儿每日 200 ～ 300mg/kg。胸腔内注射：每次 10% ～ 20% 溶液 10 ～ 20ml（用等渗氯化钠注射液溶解）。甲亢手术前：一日 8 ～ 12g，分 4 次服，同时服用维生素 B、维生素 C。服药时间不可过长，以防毒性反应出现。<br><br>Par voie orale : 2 à 3g par fois, 8 à 12g par jour, après le repas. Chez des enfants, 200 à 300 mg/kg par jour, à travers 4 fois. En perfusion : 4 à 12g par jour (commencer par une dose mineure), dissoudre dans la solution de chlorure de sodium ou la solution de glucose à 5 % isotonique, avant d'obtenir une injection à 3 % à 4 % pour la perfusion. Chez des enfants, 200 à 300 mg/kg par jour. Injection intra-thoracique : 10 à 20ml de solution à 10% à 20 % (utiliser la solution de chlorure de sodium isotonique pour la dilution). Avant la chirurgie de l'hyperthyroïdie : 8 à 12g par jour, à travers 4 fois, prendre la vitamine B et C en même temps. Ne pas l'administrer pour une durée trop longue afin d'éviter des réactions toxiques. |

续　表

| | |
|---|---|
| 剂型、规格<br>Les formes pharmaceutiques et les spécifications | 片剂：每片 0.5g。<br>注射用对氨基水杨酸钠：每瓶 2g；4g；6g。<br>Comprimés : 0,5g par comprimé.<br>L'aminosalicylate de sodium pour injection : 2g ou 4g par flacon. |
| 药品名称 Drug Names | 利福平 Rifampicine |
| 适应证<br>Les indications | 主要应用于肺结核和其他结核病，也可用于麻风病的治疗。此外也可考虑用于耐甲氧西林金黄色葡萄球菌（MRSA）所致的感染。抗结核治疗时应与其他抗结核药联合应用。<br>Il sert à lutter contre la tuberculose pulmonaire, d'autres tuberculoses et la lèpre. Il peut aussi être applicable dans le traitement des infections causées parles staphylococcus aureus résistant à la méticilline. Il faut prescrire en même temps plusieurs antibiotiques antituberculeux. |
| 用法、用量<br>Les modes d'emploi et la posologie | 肺结核及其他结核病：成人，口服，1 次 0.45 ～ 0.6g，一日 1 次，于早饭前服，疗程半年左右；1 ～ 12 岁儿童 1 次量为 10mg/kg，一日 2 次；新生儿 1 次 5mg/kg，一日 2 次。其他感染：一日量 0.6 ～ 1g，分 2 ～ 3 次给予，饭前 1 小时服用。沙眼及结膜炎：用 0.1% 滴眼剂，一日 4 ～ 6 次。治疗沙眼的疗程为 6 周。<br>Pour traiter la tuberculose pulmonaire et d'autres tuberculoses : chez des adultes, par voie orale, 0,45 à 0,6g par fois, 1 fois par jour, avant le petit-déjeuner, pendant 6 mois ; chez des enfants de 1 à 12 ans, 10 mg/kg par fois, 2 fois par jour ; chez des nouveau-nés, 5 mg/kg par fois, 2 fois par jour. Pour traiter d'autres infections : 0,6 à 1g par jour, à travers 2 à 3 fois, 1h avant le repas. Pour traiter le trachome et la conjonctivite : des gouttes pour les yeux à 0,1 %, 4 à 6 fois par jour. Le traitement médical pour le trachome dure 6 semaines. |
| 剂型、规格<br>Les formes pharmaceutiques et les spécifications | 片（胶囊）剂：每片（粒）0.15g；0.3g；0.45g；0.6g。口服混悬液：20mg/ml。<br>复方制剂：RIMACTAZIDE（含利福平及异烟肼）；RIMATAZIDE+Z（含利福平、异烟肼及吡嗪酰胺）。<br>Comprimés (capsules) : 0,15g, 0,3g, 0,45g ou 0,6g par comprimé ou par capsule. Suspension buccale : 20mg/ml.<br>La préparation de composés : RIMACTAZIDE (y compris la rifampicine et l'isoniazide) ou RIMATAZIDE +Z (y compris la rifampicine, l'isoniazide et le pyrazinamide). |
| 药品名称 Drug Names | 利福定 Rifandine |
| 适应证<br>Les indications | 用于各型肺结核和其他结核病，包括对多种抗结核药物已产生耐药性患者。亦用于麻风病及敏感菌感染性皮肤病等。<br>Il est utilisé dans le traitement des tuberculoses pulmonaires de toutes sortes et d'autres types de tuberculose, y compris dans le traitement des patients résistants aux médicaments antituberculeux. Il sert aussi à lutter contre la lèpre et des affections cutanées. |
| 用法、用量<br>Les modes d'emploi et la posologie | 成人每日 150 ～ 200mg，早晨空腹一次服用。儿童按 3 ～ 4mg/kg，一次服用。治疗肺结核病的疗程为半年～ 1 年。眼部感染采取局部用药（滴眼剂浓度 0.05%）。<br>Chez des adultes, 150 à 200mg par jour, une seule fois le petit matin, l'estomac vide. Chez des enfants, 3 à 4 mg/kg, une seule fois. Pour traiter la tuberculose pulmonaire, le traitement dure 6 mois à 1an. Pour traiter les infections oculaires, utiliser la topique (les gouttes pour les yeux à 0,05 %). |
| 剂型、规格<br>Les formes pharmaceutiques et les spécifications | 胶囊：每粒 75mg；150mg。<br>Capsules : 75mg ou 150 mg par capsule. |
| 药品名称 Drug Names | 利福喷丁 Rifapentine |
| 适应证<br>Les indications | 主要用于治疗结核病（常与其他抗结核药联合应用）。<br>Il sert à combattre les tuberculoses. Il faut prescrire en même temps plusieurs médicaments antituberculeux. |
| 用法、用量<br>Les modes d'emploi et la posologie | 1 次 600mg，每周只用 1 次（其作用约相当于利福平 600mg，一日 1 次）。必要时可按上量，每周 2 次。<br>600mg par fois, 1 fois par semaine (son effet est similaire à 600mg de lifampicine, 1 fois par jour). S'il est nécessaire, prendre 2 fois par semaine. |

| | |
|---|---|
| 剂型、规格<br>Les formes pharmaceutiques et les spécifications | 片（胶囊）剂：每片（粒）150mg；300mg。<br>Comprimés (capsules) : 150mg ou 300mg par comprimé ou par capsule. |
| 药品名称 Drug Names | 利福霉素钠 Rifamycine de sodium |
| 适应证<br>Les indications | 用于不能口服用药的结核患者和耐甲氧西林金葡菌（MRSA）感染，以及难治性军团菌病。<br>　　Il sert à traiter les patients atteints de tuberculose qui ne peuvent pas administrer les médicaments par voie orale. Il est aussi applicable dans le traitement des infections causées par les staphylococcus aureus résistant à la méticilline et la maladie des légionnaires difficile. |
| 用法、用量<br>Les modes d'emploi et la posologie | 肌内注射：成人 1 次 250mg，每 8 ～ 12 小时 1 次。静脉注射（缓慢注射）：1 次 500mg，一日 2 ～ 3 次；小儿一日量 10 ～ 30mg/kg。此外亦可稀释至一定浓度局部应用或雾化吸入。重症患者宜先静脉滴注，待病情好转后改肌内注射。用于治疗肾盂肾炎时，每日剂量在 750mg 以上。对于严重感染，开始剂量可酌增到一日 1000mg。<br>　　Injection par voie IM : chez des adultes, 250mg par fois, une fois toutes les 8 à 12h. Injection par voie IV (injection lente) : 500mg par fois, 2 à 3 fois par jour ; chez des enfants, 10 à 30 mg/kg par jour. Il est aussi possible de diluer ce produit avant de l'appliquer en topique ou de l'administrer par l'inhalationd'aérosol. Chez des patients gravement malades, il vaut mieux commencer par la perfusion avant de l'administrer par voie IM selon les cas. Pour traiter la pyélonéphrite, 750mg par jour au moins. Pour l'infection grave, prendre 1000mg par jour au début. |
| 剂型、规格<br>Les formes pharmaceutiques et les spécifications | 注射用利福霉素钠：每瓶 250mg。<br>注射液：每支 0.25g（5ml）（供静脉滴注用）；0.125g（2ml）（供肌内注射用）。<br>La rifamycine de sodium par injection : 250 mg par flacon.<br>Injection : 0,25g (5ml) par solution (réservé à la perfusion) ou 0,125g (2ml) par solution (réservé à l'administration par voie IM). |
| 药品名称 Drug Names | 链霉素 Streptomycine |
| 适应证<br>Les indications | 主要用于结核杆菌感染，也用于布氏杆菌病、鼠疫及其他敏感菌所致的感染。<br>　　Ce produit sert à traiter l'infection à mycobacterium tuberculosis, la maladie de Brucella et d'autres infections bactériennes. |
| 用法、用量<br>Les modes d'emploi et la posologie | 口服不吸收，只对肠道感染有效，现已少用。系统治疗需肌内注射，一般应用 1 次 0.5g，一日 2 次，或 1 次 0.75g，一日 1 次，1 ～ 2 周为 1 个疗程。用于结核病，一日剂量为 0.75 ～ 1g，1 次或分成 2 次肌内注射。儿童一般一日 15 ～ 25mg/kg，分 2 次给予；结核病治疗则一日 20mg/kg，隔日用药。新生儿一日 10 ～ 20mg/kg。<br>用于治疗结核病时，常与异烟肼或其他抗结核药联合应用，以避免耐药菌株的产生。<br>　　Ce produit ne s'absorbe pas par voie orale. Il n'est efficace que dans le traitement des infections des voies intestinales. Il est donc peu appliqué à l'heure actuelle. Pour le traitement systématique, il faut l'injection par voie IM, 0,5g par fois, 2 fois par jour, ou 0,75g par fois, 1 fois par jour, pendant 1 à 2 semaines. Pour traiter la tuberculose, 0,75 à 1g par jour, à travers 1 à 2 fois, injection par voie IM. Chez des enfants, 15 à 25 mg/kg par jour, à travers 2 fois ; pour traiter la tuberculose, 20 mg/kg par jour, une fois tous les 2 jours. Chez des nouveau-nés, 10 à 20 mg/kg par jour.<br>　　Pour traiter la tuberculose, il est souvent utilisé en association avec l'isoniazide ou d'autres médicaments anti-tuberculeux, pour éviter l'apparition des souches résistantes. |
| 剂型、规格<br>Les formes pharmaceutiques et les spécifications | 注射用硫酸链霉素：每瓶 0.75g；1g；2g；5g。<br>Le sulfate de streptomycine pour injection : 0,75g, 1g, 2g ou 5g par flacon. |
| 药品名称 Drug Names | 乙胺丁醇 Ethambutol |
| 适应证<br>Les indications | 为二线抗结核药，可用于经其他抗结核药治疗无效的病例，应与其他抗结核药联合应用。以增强疗效并延缓细菌耐药性的产生。<br>　　Ce produit fait partie des médicaments antituberculeux de seconde ligne. Il sert à traiter des cas résistants aux autres médicaments antituberculeux, et doit être prescrit avec d'autres médicaments antituberculeux pour renforcer son efficacité et ralentir la résistance bactérienne. |

**续　表**

| | |
|---|---|
| 用法、用量<br>Les modes d'emploi et la posologie | 结核初治：一日15mg/kg，顿服；或每周3次，每次25～30mg/kg（不超过2.5g）；或每周2次，每次50mg/kg（不超过2.5g）。结核复治，每次25mg/kg，每日一次顿服，连续60日，继而按每次15mg/kg，每日1次顿服。非典型分枝杆菌感染，按每次15～25mg/kg，一日1次顿服。<br>Le traitement initial de la tuberculose : 15 mg/kg par jour, une fois par jour ; ou 3 fois par semaine, 25 à 30 mg/kg par fois (ne pas dépasser 2,5g) ; ou 2 fois par semaine, 50 mg/kg par fois (ne pas dépasser 2,5g). Le retraitement de la tuberculose : 25 mg/kg par fois, une fois par jour, pendant 60 jours consécutifs, ensuite, 15 mg/kg par fois, 1 fois par jour. Pour traiter l'infection mycobactérienne atypique, 15 à 25 mg/kg par fois, une fois par jour. |
| 剂型、规格<br>Les formes pharmaceutiques et les spécifications | 片剂：每片0.25g。<br>Comprimés : 0,25g par comprimé. |
| **药品名称 Drug Names** | 乙硫异烟胺 Ethionamide |
| 适应证<br>Les indications | 单独应用少，常与其他抗结核病药联合应用以增强疗效和避免病菌产生耐药性。<br>Il doit être toujours precrit avec d'autres médicaments antituberculeux pour renforcer son efficacité et ralentir la résistance bactérienne. |
| 用法、用量<br>Les modes d'emploi et la posologie | 一日量0.5～0.8g，一次服用或分次服（以一次服效果为好），必要时也可从小剂量（0.3g/d）开始。<br>0,5 à 0,8g par jour, à travers 1 ou plusieurs fois (il faut mieux le prendre en une fois), en cas de besoin, commencer par une dose mineure (0,3g par jour). |
| 剂型、规格<br>Les formes pharmaceutiques et les spécifications | 肠溶片：每片0.1g。<br>Comprimés à enrobage entérique : 0,1g par comprimé. |
| **药品名称 Drug Names** | 丙硫异烟胺 Protionamide |
| 适应证<br>Les indications | 本品仅对分枝杆菌有效，与其他抗结核药联合用于结核病经一线药物（如链霉素、异烟肼、利福平和乙胺丁醇）治疗无效者。<br>Ce produit n'est utile que dans le traitement des mycobactéries. Il sert à traiter des cas résistants aux médicaments antituberculeux de première ligne (la streptomycine, l'isoniazide, la rifampicine et l'éthambutol) avec d'autres médicaments antituberculeux. |
| 用法、用量<br>Les modes d'emploi et la posologie | 口服，成人常用量，与其他抗结核药物合用，一次250mg，一日2～3次。小儿常用量，与其他抗结核药合用，一次按体重口服4～5mg/kg，一日3次。<br>Par voie orale, chez des adultes, dose usuelle, utilisé en association avec d'autres médicament anti-tuberculeux, 250 mg par fois, 2 à 3 fois par jour. Chez des enfants, utilisé en association avec d'autres médicament anti-tuberculeux, 4 à 5 mg/kg par fois, par voie orale, 3 fois par jour. |
| 剂型、规格<br>Les formes pharmaceutiques et les spécifications | 肠溶片：每片0.1g。<br>Comprimés à enrobage entérique : 0,1g par comprimé. |
| **药品名称 Drug Names** | 吡嗪酰胺 Pyrazinamide |
| 适应证<br>Les indications | 与其他抗结核药联合用于经一线抗结核药（如链霉素、异烟肼、利福平和乙胺丁醇）治疗无效的结核病。本品仅对分枝杆菌有效。<br>Il sert à traiter des cas résistants aux médicaments antituberculeux de première ligne (la streptomycine, l'isoniazide, la rifampicine et l'éthambutol) avec d'autres médicaments antituberculeux. Ce produit n'est utile que dans le traitement des mycobactéries. |
| 用法、用量<br>Les modes d'emploi et la posologie | 口服。成人常用量，与其他抗结核药联合，每6小时按体重5～8.75mg/kg，或每8小时按体重6.7～11.7mg/kg给予，最高每日3g。治疗异烟肼耐药菌感染时可增加至每日60mg/kg。<br>Par voie orale. Chez des adultes, utilisé en association avec d'autres médicament anti-tuberculeux, 5 à 8,75 mg/kg par fois, une fois toutes les 6h, ou 6,7 à 11,7 mg/kg par fois, une fois toutes les 8h, ne pas dépasser 3g par jour. Pour traiter les infections résistantes à l'isoniazide, 60 mg/kg par jour. |

**续 表**

| 剂型、规格<br>Les formes pharmaceutiques et les spécifications | 肠溶片：每片 0.25g；0.5g。<br>Comprimés à enrobage entérique : 0,25g ou 0,5g par comprimé. |
|---|---|

### 4. 抗麻风病药及抗麻风病反应药 Médicaments anti-lépreux et médicaments anti-réactions lépreuses

| 药品名称 Drug Names | 氨苯砜 Dapsone |
|---|---|
| 适应证<br>Les indications | 主要用于治疗各型麻风。近年试用本品治疗系统性红斑狼疮、痤疮、银屑病、带状疱疹等。<br>Ce produit sert principalement à traiter les lèpres de toutes sortes. Ces dernières années, on le prescrit pour lutter contre le lupus érythémateux, l'acné, le psoriasis et l'herpès zoster. |
| 用法、用量<br>Les modes d'emploi et la posologie | 治疗麻风病，口服，1 次 50～100mg，一日 100～200mg。可于开始每日 12.5～25mg，以后逐渐加量到每日 100mg。由于本品有蓄积作用，故每服药 6 日后停药一日，每服 10 周停药 2 周。必要时，可与利福平每日 600mg 联合应用。儿童剂量一日 1.4mg/kg。治疗红斑狼疮，一日 100mg，连用 3～6 个月；痤疮，一日 50mg；银屑病或变应性血管炎一日 100～150mg；带状疱疹，一日 3 次，1 次 25mg，连服 3～14 日；糜烂性扁平苔藓，一日 50mg，连用 3 个月。以上治疗中，均遵循服药 6 日，停药一日的原则。<br><br>Pour traiter les lèpres, par voie orale, 50 à 100mg par fois, 100 à 200 mg par jour. Ou commencer par prendre 12,5 à 25mg par jour avant d'augmenter la dose pour atteindre 100mg par jour. Comme ce produit a des effets cumulatifs, il faut arrêter l'administration pendant 1 jour après 6 jours d'administration, arrêter l'administration pendant 2 semaines après 10 semaines d'administration. En cas de besoin, utilisé en association avec la rifampicine, 600mg par jour. Ches des endants, 1,4 mg/kg par jour. Pour traiter le lupus érythémateux, 100mg par jour, pendant 3 à 6 mois ; pour traiter l'acné, 50mg par jour ; pour traiter le psoriasis ou la vascularite allergique, 100 à 150 mg par jour ; pour traiter l'herpès zoster, 3 fois par jour, 25mg par fois, pendant 3 à 14 jours consécutifs. Pour tous les traitements cités auparavant, il faut arrêter l'administration pendant 1 jour après 6 jours d'administration. |
| 剂型、规格<br>Les formes pharmaceutiques et les spécifications | 片剂：每片 50mg；100mg。<br>Comprimés：50mg ou 100mg par comprimé. |
| 药品名称 Drug Names | 醋氨苯砜 Acédapsone |
| 适应证<br>Les indications | 用于各型麻风病。<br>Ce produit sert à traiter les lèpres de toutes sortes. |
| 用法、用量<br>Les modes d'emploi et la posologie | 肌内注射，1 次 0.225g，隔 60～75 日注射 1 次，疗程长达数年。为了防止长期单用本品导致细菌产生耐药性，可在用药期间加服氨苯砜 0.1～0.15g，每周 2 次。<br>Injection par voie IM, 0,225g par fois, une fois tous les 60 à 75 jours, pendant plusieurs années. Pour éviter l'apprition de souches résistantes, il faut prendre la dapsone en même temps, 0,1 à 0,15g, 2 fois par semaine. |
| 剂型、规格<br>Les formes pharmaceutiques et les spécifications | 油注射液：每支 225mg（1.5ml）；450mg（3ml）；900mg（6ml）。为 40% 苯甲酸苄酯及 60% 蓖麻油的混悬剂。用前振摇均匀，用粗针头吸出，注入臀肌。<br>Injection d'huile : 225mg (1,5ml), 450 mg (3ml) ou 900mg (6ml) par solution. Il s'agit de suspension composée de 40% de Benzoate de benzyle et de 60% d'huile de ricin. Agiter avant de l'utiliser, prendre le produit avec une aiguille grossière pour l'injecter dans le fessier. |
| 药品名称 Drug Names | 苯丙砜 Solasulfone |
| 适应证<br>Les indications | 主要用于治疗各型麻风。近年试用本品治疗系统性红斑狼疮、痤疮、银屑病、带状疱疹等。<br>Ce produit sert principalement à traiter les lèpres de toutes sortes. Ces dernières années, on le prescrit pour lutter contre le lupus érythémateux, l'acné, le psoriasis et l'herpès zoster. |

**续　表**

| | |
|---|---|
| 用法、用量<br>Les modes d'emploi et la posologie | 肌内注射：每周 2 次，第 1 ～ 2 周每次 100 ～ 200mg，以后每 2 周递增 100mg/ 次，至第 14 ～ 16 周，每次量为 800mg，继续维持，每用药 10 周后，停药 2 周。<br>口服：300mg/d，逐渐增量至 3g。每服药 10 周，停药 2 周。<br>　　Injection par voie IM : 2 fois par semaine, pour la première et la deuxième semaine, 100 à 200mg par fois, ensuite, augmenter 100mg par fois toutes les 2 semaines, pour atteindre 800mg par fois de la 14ème à la 16ème semaine, et maintenir cette dose. Arrêter l'administration pendant 2 semaines après 10 semaines d'administration.<br>　　Par voie orale : 300mg par jour, augmenter la dose pour atteindre 3g. Arrêter l'administration pendant 2 semaines après 10 semaines d'administration. |
| 剂型、规格<br>Les formes pharmaceutiques et les spécifications | 注射液：每支 2g（5ml）；4g（10ml）。<br>片剂：每片 0.5g。<br>Injection : 2g (5ml) ou 4g (10ml) par solution.<br>Comprimés : 0,5g par comprimé. |
| 药品名称 Drug Names | 氯法齐明 Clofazimine |
| 适应证<br>Les indications | 对于瘤型麻风和其他型麻风均有一定疗效，对耐砜类药物麻风杆菌感染也有效。可用于因用其他药物而引起急性麻风反应的病例。<br>　　Il peut être applicable dans le traitement de la lèpre lépromateuse et d'autres genres de lèpres. Il sert aussi à traiter les infections de la lèpre résistant aux médicaments sulfone. Il est aussi utilisé comme traitement des réactions lépreuses aigues causeés par l'administration des autres médicaments. |
| 用法、用量<br>Les modes d'emploi et la posologie | 口服。对麻风病，每日 100mg；对麻风反应，一日 200 ～ 400mg，麻风反应控制后，逐渐减量至每日 100mg。<br>　　Par voie orale. Pour traiter la lèpre, 100mg par jour ; pour traiter les réactions lépreuses, 200 à 400mg par jour, dès le contrôle de ces réactions, diminuer la dose pour atteindre 100mg par jour. |
| 剂型、规格<br>Les formes pharmaceutiques et les spécifications | 胶囊：每粒 50mg；100mg。<br>胶丸（油蜡或聚乙二醇基质）：每丸 50mg。<br>Capsules : 50mg ou 100mg par capsule.<br>Pilules (huile-cire oumatrice de polyéthylène glycol) : 50mg par pilule. |
| 药品名称 Drug Names | 沙利度胺 Thalidomide |
| 适应证<br>Les indications | 用于麻风结节性红斑。在 2006 年美国 FDA 批准用于治疗多发性骨髓瘤。中华医学会认可：除了可以治疗麻风结节性红斑外，在《临床诊疗指南·血液学分册》中沙利度胺可以治疗多发性骨髓瘤；在《临床诊疗指南·风湿学分册》中沙利度胺可以治疗强直性脊柱炎和白塞病。<br>　　Applicable dans le traitement de l'érythème noueux lépreux. Il a été autorisé en 2006 par la FDA (autorité sanitaire américaine) pour traiter le myélome multiple. Selon l'Association médicale chinoise, la thalidomide est non seulement applicable dans le traitement de l'érythème noueux lépreux, elle peut aussi traiter le myélom multiple, ce qui est reconnu dans le document de référence appelé Le volume d'hématologie des indications pour la pratique clinique, elle peut aussi traiter la spondylarthrite ankylosante et la maladie de Behcet, ce qui est reconnu dans le même document appelé Le volume de rhumatologie des indications pour la pratique clinique. |
| 用法、用量<br>Les modes d'emploi et la posologie | 口服每日 100 ～ 200mg，分 4 次服。对严重反应，可增至 300 ～ 400mg（反应得到控制即逐渐减量）。对长期反应者，需要较长期服药，每日或隔日服 25 ～ 50mg。<br>移植后用药：一日 800 ～ 1600mg，分 4 次服，治疗可持续 2 ～ 700 日（平均为 240 日）。治疗完全有效的患者，再持续 3 个月以后逐渐减量（每 2 周减少 25%）；部分有效的患者，再观察到最大效应后还应再治疗 6 个月。<br>　　Par voie orale, 100 à 200mg par jour, à travers 4 fois. Chez des patients dont les réactions sont graves, 300 à 400mg (diminuer la dose dès le contrôle des réactions). Chez des patients dont les réactions sont chroniques, il faut prendre le médicament pour une longue durée, 25 à 50mg tous les jours ou tous les 2 jours.<br>　　L'administration après la greffe : 800 à 1 600 mg par jour, à travers 4 fois, pendant 2 à 700 jours onsécutifs (en moyenne, 240 jours). Chez des patients dont le traitement est parfaitement efficace, diminuer progressivement la dose 3 mois après (diminuer de 25 % toutes les 2 semaines) ; chez des patients dont le traitment est partiellement efficace, observer l'effet maximal avant de continuer le traitement pendant 6 mois. |

**续 表**

| 剂型、规格<br>Les formes pharmaceutiques et les spécifications | 片剂：每片 25mg；50mg。<br>Comprimés : 25mg ou 50mg par comprimé. |
|---|---|

## 5. 抗真菌药 Médicaments Antifongiques

| 药品名称 Drug Names | 两性霉素 B Amphotericine B |
|---|---|
| 适应证<br>Les indications | 用于隐球菌、球孢子菌、荚膜组织胞浆菌、芽生菌、孢子丝菌、念珠菌、毛霉、曲霉等引起的内脏或全身感染。<br>Ce produit sert à traiter les infections viscérales ou systémiques causées par la cryptococcose, le coccidioidomycosis, l'histoplasma capsulatum, le blastomyces, le sporothrix, la candidose, l'enzyme velu et l'aspergillus. |
| 用法、用量<br>Les modes d'emploi et la posologie | 临用前加灭菌注射用水适量使溶解（不可用氯化钠注射液溶解与稀释），再加入 5% 葡萄糖注射液（pH > 4.2）中浓度每 1ml 不超过 1mg。静脉滴注：开始用小剂量 1～2mg，逐日递增到一日 1mg/kg。每日给药一次，滴注速度通常为每分钟 1～1.5ml。疗程总量：白念珠菌感染约 1g，隐球菌脑膜炎约 3g。<br>鞘内注射：对隐球菌脑膜炎，除静脉滴注外尚需鞘内给药。每次从 0.05～0.1mg 开始，逐渐递增至 0.5～1mg（浓度为 0.1～0.25mg/ml）。溶于注射用水 0.5～1ml 中，按鞘内注射法常规操作，共约 30 次，必要时可酌加地塞米松注射液以减轻反应。雾化吸入：适用于肺及支气管感染病例。一日量 5～10mg，溶于注射用水 100～200ml 中，分 4 次用。局部病灶注射：浓度 1～3mg/ml，3～7 日用 1 次，必要时可加普鲁卡因注射液少量；对真菌性脓胸和关节炎，可局部抽脓后，注入药 5～10mg，每周 1～3 次。局部外用：浓度 2.5～5mg/ml。腔道用药：栓剂 25mg。眼部用药：眼药水 0.25%；眼药膏 1%。口服：对肠道真菌感染一日 0.5～2g，分 2～4 次服。<br>Utiliser l'eau stérile pour préparations injectables pour dissoudre le médicament (interdit d'utiliser la solution de chlorure de sodium pour la dilution), ajouter ensuite la solution de glucose à 5 % (PH > 4.2), pour que la concentration ne dépasse pas 1mg par 1ml. En perfusion : commencer par une dose mineure, 1 à 2 mg, avant d'augmenter tous les jours la dose avant d'attendre 1mg/kg par jour. Administration une fois par jour, la vitesse de la perfusion : 1 à 1,5ml par minute. La dose totale pour un traitement médical : pour traiter l'injection à Candida albicans, il faut 1g ; pour traiter la méningite cryptococcique, il faut 3g.<br>Injection intrathécale : pour traiter la méningite cryptococcique, il faut appliquer à la fois la perfusion et l'injection intrathécale. Commencer par 0,05 à 0,1 mg par fois avant d'augmenter la dose pour atteindre 0,5 à 1mg (la concentration est de 0.1 à 0.25mg/ml). Dissoudre le produit dans 0,5 à 1ml d'eau pou préparations injectables, en suivant le fonctionnement normal de l'injection intrathécale, il faut au total 30 fois. S'il est nécessaire, ajouter l'injection de Dexaméthasone pour réduire les réactions indésirables. L'inhalationd'aérosol : utilisée pour traiter les infections pulmonaires et bronchiques. 5 à 10mg par jour, dissoudre le produit dans 100 à 200mg d'eau pour préparations injectables, à travers 4 fois.Injection topique sur la zone touchée : la concentration, 1 à 3 mg/ml, une fois tous les 3 à 7 jours, en cas de besoin, ajouter une dose mineure de solution de procaine ; pour traiter l'empyème et l'arthrite fongiques, après le retrait du pus, injecter 5 à10mg, 1 à 3 fois par semaine. Pour un usage externe tropique : la concentration, 2,5 à 5 mg/ml. L'administration par la cavité : suppositoires, 25mg. Les médicaments pour les yeux : collyres à 0,25 % ; pommades pour les yeux à 1 %. Par voie orale : pour traiter les infections fongiques intestinales, 0,5 à 2 g par jour, à travers 2 à 4 fois. |
| 剂型、规格<br>Les formes pharmaceutiques et les spécifications | 注射用两性霉素 B（脱氧胆酸钠复合物）：每支 5mg；25mg；50mg。<br>L'amphotericine B pour injection (Complexes de désoxycholate de sodium) : 5mg, 25mg ou 50mg par solution. |
| 药品名称 Drug Names | 伊曲康唑 Itraconazole |
| 适应证<br>Les indications | 主要应用于深部真菌所引起的系统感染如类球孢子菌病、组织胞浆菌病、芽生菌病、着色真菌病、孢子丝菌病等。也可用于念珠菌病和曲霉病。<br>Il sert à traiter les infections systématiques fongiques, telles que la coccidioïdomycose, l'histoplasmose, la blastomycose, la maladie fongique de couleur et la sporotrichose. Il est aussi applicable dans el traitement de la candidose et de l'aspergillose. |

**续　表**

| | |
|---|---|
| 用法、用量<br>Les modes d'emploi et la posologie | 一般为一日 100 ～ 200mg，顿服，一般疗程为 3 个月，个别情况下疗程延长到 6 个月。短程间歇疗法：1 次 200mg，一日 2 次，连服 7 日为 1 个疗程。停药 2 日，开始第 2 疗程，指甲癣服 2 个疗程，趾甲癣服 3 个疗程，治愈率分别为 97% 和 69.4%。<br><br>En général, 100 à 200mg par jour, une fois par jour, pendant 3 mois, dans certains cas, pendant 6 mois. Pour le traitement intermittent à court terme : 200mg par fois, 2 fois par jour, pendant 7 jours consécutifs comme un traitement médical. Arrêter l'administration pendant 2 jours et puis, commencer le deuxième traitement. Pour traiter la teigne des ongles, 2 traitements médicaux, pour la teigne des ongles d'orteil, 3 traitements médicaux, avec un taux de guérison respectivement de 97 % et de 69,4 %. |
| 剂型、规格<br>Les formes pharmaceutiques et les spécifications | 片剂：每片 100mg；200mg。<br>注射液：25ml：250mg。<br>Comprimés : 100mg ou 200mg par comprimé.<br>Injection : 25ml : 250mg. |
| 药品名称 Drug Names | 氟康唑 Fluconazole |
| 适应证<br>Les indications | 应用于敏感菌所致的各种真菌感染，如隐球菌性脑膜炎、复发性口咽念珠菌病等。<br>Ce produit sert à traiter des infections fongiques, telles que la méningite cryptococcique et la candidose oropharyngée récurrente. |
| 用法、用量<br>Les modes d'emploi et la posologie | 念珠菌性口咽炎或食管炎：第 1 天口服 200mg，以后每日服 100mg，疗程 2 ～ 3 周（症状消失仍需用药），以免复发。念珠菌系统感染：第 1 天 400mg，以后每天 200mg。疗程 4 周或症状消失后再用 2 周。隐球菌性脑膜炎第 1 天 400mg，以后每天 200mg。如患者反应正常，也可用每日 1 次 400mg，至脑脊液细菌培养阴性后 10 ～ 12 周。肾功能不全者，减少用量。肌酐清除率＞ 50ml/min 者用正常量；肌酐清除率为 21 ～ 50ml/min 者用 1/2 量；肌酐清除率为 11% ～ 20%ml/min 者用 1/4 量。口服和静脉输注用量相同。静脉滴注速度约为 200mg/h。可加入到葡萄糖液、生理氯化钠液、乳酸钠林格液中滴注。<br><br>Pour traiter la pharygite ou l'oesophagiteà Candida : le premier jour, 200mg par voie orale, ensuite, 100mg par jour, pendant 2 à 3 semaines (l'administration continue même après la disparition des symptômes pour éviter la récurrence). Les infections systématiques à Candida : le premier jour, 400mg, ensuite, 200mg par jour, pendant 4 semaines ou jusqu'à 2 semaines après la disparition des symptômes. Pour traiter la méningite cryptococcique, le premier jour, 400mg, ensuite, 200mg par jour. Si les réactions des patients sont normales, il est aussi possible de prendre 400mg par fois par jour, jusqu'à 10 à 12 semaines après la culture négative des bactéries du liquide céphalo-rachidien. Chez des patients insuffisants rénaux, diminuer la dose. Chez les patients dont la clairance de la créatinine est supréreire à 50 ml/min, la dose usuelle ; de 21 à 50 ml/min, la moitié de la dose usuelle ; de 11 à 20 ml/min, le quart de la dose usuelle. La même dose par voie orale et en perfusion. La vitesse de la perfusion est de 200 mg par heure. Possible d'introduire le produit dans la solution de glucose, la solution de chlorure de sodium ou la solution de Ringer pour la perfusion. |
| 剂型、规格<br>Les formes pharmaceutiques et les spécifications | 片剂（胶囊）：每片（粒）50mg；100mg；150mg 或 200mg。<br>注射剂：每瓶 200mg/100ml。<br>Comprimés (capsules) : 50mg, 100mg, 150mg ou 200mg par comprimé ou par capsule.<br>Injection : 200mg /100ml par flacon. |
| 药品名称 Drug Names | 伏立康唑 Voriconazole |
| 适应证<br>Les indications | 用于治疗侵入性曲霉病，以及对氟康唑耐药的严重进入性念珠菌病感染及由足放线病菌属和镰刀菌属引起的严重真菌感染。主要用于进行性、致命危险的免疫系统受损的 2 岁以上患者。<br>Ce produit sert à traiter l'aspergillose invasive, l'infection grave à candidose envahissante résistant à la fluconazole, ainsi que l'infection fongique grave causée par le genre fusarium et l'actinomycète. Il est utilisé dans le traitement des patients plus de 2 ans atteints de dommages progressifs et fatals du système immunitaire. |

**续 表**

| | |
|---|---|
| 用法、用量<br>Les modes d'emploi et la posologie | 负荷剂量：第 1 天静脉滴注 6mg/kg/ 次，12 小时 1 次；口服 400mg/ 次（体重≥ 40kg）或 200mg/ 次（体重< 40kg），每 12 小时 1 次。<br>维持剂量：第 2 天起静脉滴注 4mg/kg 一日 2 次，或 200mg 一日 2 次（体重≥ 40kg），或 100mg 一日 2 次（体重< 40kg）。均为 12 小时 1 次。治疗口咽、食管、白念珠菌病：口服，每次 200mg，一日 2 次；静脉注射，每次 3 ～ 6mg/kg，12 小时 1 次。<br>La dose de charge : le premier jour, en perfusion, 6 mg/kg par fois, une fois toutes les 12h. par voie orale, 400mg par fois (chez des patients de 40kg ou plus) ou 200mg par fois (chez des patients moins de 40kg), une fois toutes les 12h. La dose d'entretien : à partir du deuxième jour, en perfusion, 4 mg/kg, 2 fois par jour, ou 200mg, 2 fois par jour (chez des patients de 40kg ou plus), ou 100mg, 2 fois par jour (chez des patients moinsde 40kg). Une fois toutes les 12h.<br>Pour traiter les candidoses oropharyngée etoesophagienne：par voie orale,  200mg par fois, 2 fois par jour；par voie IV,  3 à 6 mg/kg par fois,  une fois toutes les 12h. |
| 剂型、规格<br>Les formes pharmaceutiques et les spécifications | 片剂：每片 50mg；200mg。<br>注射用伏立康唑：每支 200mg。<br>Comprimés : 50mg ou 200mg par comprimé.<br>Le voriconazole pour injection : 200mg par solution. |
| 药品名称 Drug Names | 氟胞嘧啶 Flucytosine |
| 适应证<br>Les indications | 用于念珠菌和隐球菌感染，单用效果不如两性霉素 B，可与两性霉素 B 合用，以增疗效（协同作用）。<br>Il sert à traiter les infections cauées par la candidose et la cryptococcose. Il vaut mieux l'utiliser en combinaison avec l'amphotericine B pour améliorer leur efficacité. |
| 用法、用量<br>Les modes d'emploi et la posologie | 口服：一日 4 ～ 6g，分 4 次服，疗程自数周至数月。静脉注射，一日 50 ～ 150mg/kg，分 2 ～ 3 次。单用本品时真菌易产生耐药性，宜与两性霉素 B 合用。<br>Par voie orale : 4 à 6g par jour, à travers 4 fois, la durée du traitement médical varie de quelques semaines à quelques mois. En perfusion, 50 à 150 mg/kg par jour, à travers 2 à 3 fois. L'utilisation unique de la flucytosine peut entraîner la résistance du champignon pathogène, il vaut mieux donc l'utiliser en association avec l'amphotericine B. |
| 剂型、规格<br>Les formes pharmaceutiques et les spécifications | 片剂：每片 250mg；500mg。<br>注射液：2.5g（250ml）。<br>Comprimés : 250mg ou 500mg par comprimé.<br>Injection : 2,5g (250ml). |
| 药品名称 Drug Names | 特比萘芬 Terbinafine |
| 适应证<br>Les indications | 用于浅表真菌引起的皮肤、指甲感染，如毛癣菌、狗、小孢子菌、絮状表皮癣菌等引起的体癣、股癣、足癣、甲癣及皮肤白念珠菌感染。<br>Ce produit sert à traiter des infections fongiques superficielles liées à la peau et aux ongles, telles que le tinea corporal, le tinea cruris, le tinea pedis, le tinea unguium ainsi que les infections de la peau par Candida albicans causées par le trichophyton, les chiens, les petites spores et l'épidermophyton floccosum. |
| 用法、用量<br>Les modes d'emploi et la posologie | 口服，每日 1 次 250mg，足癣、体癣、股癣服用 1 周；皮肤念珠菌病 1 ～ 2 周；指甲癣 4 ～ 6 周，趾甲癣 12 周（口服对花斑癣无效）。外用（1% 霜剂）用于体癣、股癣、皮肤念珠菌病、花斑癣等，每日涂抹 1 ～ 2 次，疗程不定（1 ～ 2 周）。<br>Par voie orale, 250mg par fois par jour, pour traiter le tinea pedis, le tinea corporal et le tinea cruris, administrer pendant 1 semaine ; pour traiter la candidose cutanée, 1 à 2 semaines ; pour traiter la teigne des ongles, 4 à 6 semaines, pour traiter la teigne des ongles d'orteil, 12 semaines (l'administration par voie orale est inutile dans le traitement du tinea versicolor). Un usage externe (crème à 1 %) pour traiter le tinea corporal, le tinea cruris, la candidose cutanée et le tinea versicolor, essuyer 1 à 2 fois par jour, le traitement médical n'est pas fixé (environ 1 à 2 semaines). |

续　表

| | |
|---|---|
| 剂型、规格<br>Les formes pharmaceutiques et les spécifications | 片剂：每片 125mg 或 250mg。<br>霜剂：1%。<br>Comprimés : 125mg ou 250 mg par comprimé.<br>Crème : 1 %. |
| **药品名称 Drug Names** | 美帕曲星 Mépartricine |
| 适应证<br>Les indications | 用于白念珠菌阴道炎和肠道念珠菌病，也可用于阴道或肠道滴虫病。本品在肠道内与甾醇类物质结合成不吸收的物质，可用于治疗良性前列腺肿大。<br>Ce produit sert à traiter la vaginite à Candida albicans et la candidose intestinale, ainsi que la trichomonase vaginale ou intestinale.Combiné avec les stérols dans les voies intestinales en matériau non résorbable, il est utilisé dans le traitement de l'hypertrophie bénigne de la prostate. |
| 用法、用量<br>Les modes d'emploi et la posologie | 阴道或肠道念珠菌感染或滴虫病（用含十二烷基硫酸钠的复合片）：1 次 100 000U（2 片），每 12 小时 1 次，连用 3 日为 1 个疗程。对于复杂性病例，疗程可酌情延长。宜食后服用。治疗前列腺肿大或肠道念珠菌病、滴虫病（用不含十二烷基硫酸钠的片剂）：一日 1 次，每次 100 000U。<br>Pour traiter la candidose ou la trichomonase vaginale ou intestinale (utiliser les composés contenant le dodécyl sulfate de sodium) : 100 000 unités (2 comprimés) par fois, une fois toutes les 12h, pendant 3 jours consécutifs comme un traitement médical. Pour les cas complexes, prolonger le traitement médical. Administration après le repas. Pour traiter l'hypertrophie de la prostate ou la candidose, la trichomonase intestinales (sans utiliser les comprimés contenant le dodécyl sulfate de sodium) : 1 fois pr jour, 100 000 unités par fois. |
| 剂型、规格<br>Les formes pharmaceutiques et les spécifications | 肠溶片：每片 50 000U。<br>阴道片：每片 25 000U。<br>乳膏：供黏膜用。<br>Comprimés à enrobage entérique : 50 000 unités par comprimé.<br>Comprimés viginaux : 25 000 unités par comprimé.<br>Crème : utilisée pour la muqueuse. |
| **药品名称 Drug Names** | 阿莫罗芬 Amorolfine |
| 适应证<br>Les indications | 用于治疗皮肤及黏膜浅表真菌感染，如体癣、手癣、足癣、甲真菌病及阴道白念珠菌病等。<br>Ce produit sert à traiter les infections fongiques superficielles muqueuse et cutanées, tellse que le tinea corporal, le tinea manuum, le tinea pedis, l'onychomycose et les infections vaginales par Candida albicans. |
| 用法、用量<br>Les modes d'emploi et la posologie | 甲真菌病：锉光病甲后将擦剂均匀涂抹于患处，每周 1～2 次。指甲感染一般连续用药 6 个月，趾甲感染持续用药 9～12 个月。皮肤浅表真菌感染：用 0.25% 乳膏局部涂抹，一日 1 次，至临床症状消失后继续治疗 3～5 日。阴道念珠菌病：先用温开水或 0.02% 高锰酸钾无菌溶液冲洗阴道或坐浴，再将一枚栓剂置于阴道深处。<br>Pour traiter l'onychomycose : après avoir coupé les ongles malades, essuyer la zone touchée avec le liniment, 1 à 2 fois par semaine. Pour traiter les infections des ongles, l'administration pendant 6 mois consécutifs, pour traiter les infections des ongles d'orteil, pendant 9 à 12 mois consécutifs. Pour traiter les infections fongiques superficielle cutanées : essuyer la zone touchée avec la crème à 0,25 %, 1 fois par jour, jusqu'à 3 à 5 jours après la disparition des symptômes cliniques. Pour traiter les infections vaginales par Candia albicans : les douches vaginales ou le bain de siège avec l'eau chaude ou une solution stérile de permanganate de potassium à 0,02 %, ensuite, placer un suppositoire au fond du vagin. |
| 剂型、规格<br>Les formes pharmaceutiques et les spécifications | 擦剂：每瓶 125mg（2.5ml）。<br>乳膏剂：每支 0.25%（5g）。<br>栓剂：每枚 25mg；50mg。<br>Liniment : 125mg (2,5ml) par flacon.<br>Crème : 0,25 % (5g) par pièce.<br>Suppositoire : 25mg ou 50mg par suppositoire. |

**续　表**

| 药品名称 Drug Names | 醋酸卡泊芬净 Acétate de caspofungine |
|---|---|
| 适应证<br>Les indications | 　　用于治疗对其他治疗无效或不能耐受的侵袭性曲霉菌病；对疑似真菌感染的粒缺伴发热患者的经验治疗；口咽及食管念珠菌病。侵袭性念珠菌病，包括中性粒细胞减少症及非中性粒细胞减少症患者的念珠菌血症。<br>　　Le produit sert à traiter l'aspergillose invasive résistant à d'autres traitements médicaux. Il est utilisé dans le traitement empirique des patients neutropéniques avec fièvre attients d'infections fongiques présumées. Il sert également à traiter la candidose oropharyngée et oesophagienne. L'aspergillose invasive comporte la candiose chez les patients atteints de neutropénie et non neutropénie. |
| 用法、用量<br>Les modes d'emploi et la posologie | 　　第 1 天给予单次 70mg 负荷剂量，随后每天给予 50mg 的剂量。本品约需要 1 小时经静脉缓慢输注给药。疗程取决于患者疾病的严重程度、被抑制的免疫功能恢复情况以及对治疗的临床反应。对于治疗无临床反应而对本品耐受性良好的患者可以考虑将每日剂量加大到 70mg。<br>　　Le premier jour, 70mg comme dose de charge, une fois, ensuite, 50mg par jour. Il faut l'administrer par voie IV lentement pendant 1h. La durée du traitement médical dépend de la gravité de la maladie, de la récupération de la fonction immunitaire et des réactions cliniques au traitement. Chez des patients qui n'ont pas de réactions cliniques et qui tolèrent bien ce produit, augmenter la dose pour atteindre 70mg par jour. |
| 剂型、规格<br>Les formes pharmaceutiques et les spécifications | 　　注射用醋酸卡泊芬净：50mg；70mg（以卡泊芬净计）。<br>　　L'acétate de caspofungine pour injection : 50mg ou 70mg (quantité mesurée en caspofungine). |
| 药品名称 Drug Names | 米卡芬净 Micafungine |
| 适应证<br>Les indications | 　　用于治疗食管念珠菌感染，预防造血干细胞移植患者的念珠菌感染。<br>　　Le produit sert à traiter les infections causées par la candidose oesophagienne, et à prévenir les infections à Candida chez des patients recevant une greffe de cellules souches hématopoïétiques. |
| 用法、用量<br>Les modes d'emploi et la posologie | 　　治疗食管念珠菌病的推荐剂量为 150mg/d，预防造血干细胞移植患者的念珠菌感染的推荐剂量为 50mg/d。平均疗程分别为 15 日和 19 日。只能用生理盐水（可用 5% 葡萄糖注射液代替）配制和稀释。每 50mg 米卡芬净钠先加入 5ml 生理盐水溶解。为减少泡沫的产生，须轻轻转动玻璃瓶，不可用力振摇。随后将已溶解好的米卡芬净钠溶液加入到 100ml 生理盐水中滴注给药，给药时间至少 1 小时。<br>　　Pour traiter la candidose oesophagienne, la dose recommandée, 150mg par jour, chez des patients recevant une greffe de cellules souches hématopoïétiques, pour prévenir les infections à Candida, la dose recommandée, 500mg par jour. Leur traitement médical dure respectivement 15 jours et 19 jours. Il faut utiliser la solution saline (ou la solution de glucose à 5 %) pour la dilution. Pour diluer 50mg de micafungine, il faut 5ml de solution saline. Pour réduire les mousses, il faut tourner doucement le flacon, au lieu de l'agiter fortement. Ensuite, introduire la solution dissoute de micafungine dans 100ml de solution saline, en perfusion pendant 1h au moins. |
| 剂型、规格<br>Les formes pharmaceutiques et les spécifications | 　　米卡芬净钠冻干粉针：每瓶 50mg；100mg。<br>　　La micafungine sodique en poudre lyophilisée : 50mg ou 100mg par flacon. |
| 药品名称 Drug Names | 阿尼芬净 Anidulafungine |
| 适应证<br>Les indications | 　　用于治疗食管念珠菌感染，念珠菌性败血症，念珠菌引起的腹腔脓肿及念珠菌性腹膜炎。<br>　　Le produit sert à traiter les infections causées par la candidose oesophagienne, la septicémie à Candida, les abcès abdominaux à Candida et la péritonite à Candida. |

**续　表**

| | |
|---|---|
| 用法、用量<br>Les modes d'emploi et la posologie | 静脉给药：食管性念珠菌病，第 1 天 100mg，随后每天 50mg 疗程至少 14 日，且至少持续至症状消失后 7 日。念珠菌性败血症等，第 1 天 200mg，随后每天 100mg，疗程持续至最后一次阴性培养后至少 14 日。<br><br>Par voie IV : pour traiter la candidose oesophagienne, le premier jour, 100mg, ensuite, 50mg par jour, pendant 14 jours au moins, et maintenir l'administration jusqu'à 7 jours après la disparition des symptômes. Pour traiter la septicémie à Candida, le premier jour, 200mg, ensuite, 100mg par jour, maintenir le traitement jusqu'à 14 jours après la dernière culture négative au moins. |
| 剂型、规格<br>Les formes pharmaceutiques et les spécifications | 注射用阿尼芬净：每瓶 50mg；100mg。<br>L'anidulafungine pour injection : 50mg ou 100mg par flacon. |
| 药品名称 Drug Names | 制霉菌素 Nystatine |
| 适应证<br>Les indications | 口服用于治疗消化道念珠菌病。<br>Ce produit est adminitré par voie orale pour traiter la candidose gastro-intestinale. |
| 用法、用量<br>Les modes d'emploi et la posologie | 消化道念珠菌病：口服，成人 1 次 50 万～ 100 万 U，一日 3 次。小儿每日按体重 5 万～ 10 万 U/kg，分 3 ～ 4 次服。<br><br>Pour traiter la candidose gastro-intestinale : par voie orale, chez des adultes, 500 000 à 1 million d'unités par fois, 3 fois par jour. Chez des enfants, 50 000 à 100 000 unités par kg par jour, à travers 3 à 4 fois. |
| 剂型、规格<br>Les formes pharmaceutiques et les spécifications | 片剂：50 万 U。<br>软膏：每克 10 万 U。<br>栓剂：每枚 10 万 U。<br>Comprimés : 500 000 unités.<br>Pommade : 100 000 unités par g.<br>Suppositoires : 100 000unités par suppositoire. |
| 药品名称 Drug Names | 咪康唑 Miconazole |
| 适应证<br>Les indications | 局部治疗念珠菌性外阴阴道病和革兰阳性细菌引起的双重感染。<br>Il s'agit d'une thérapie locale de la maladie vulvo-vaginale à Candida et de la double infection causée par les bactéries à Gram positif. |
| 用法、用量<br>Les modes d'emploi et la posologie | 静脉给药：治疗深部真菌病一日常用量为 600 ～ 1800mg，分 3 次给予。局部用药：常作为全身用药的补充。<br><br>Par voie IV : pour traiter la mycose profonde, dose usuelle, 600 à 1 800 mg par jour, à travers 3 fois. Pour le topique, il sert de médicament adjuvant à l'administration systématique. |
| 剂型、规格<br>Les formes pharmaceutiques et les spécifications | 注射液：200mg。<br>栓剂：100mg。<br>霜剂：15g。<br>Injection : 200mg.<br>Suppositoires : 100mg.<br>Crème : 15g. |
| 6. 抗病毒药 Médicaments Antiviraux | |
| 药品名称 Drug Names | 阿昔洛韦 Aciclovir |
| 适应证<br>Les indications | 用于防治单纯疱疹病毒 HSV1 和 HSV2 的皮肤或黏膜感染，还可用于带状疱疹病毒感染。<br>Ce produit sert à prévenir et à traiter les infections cutanées ou mugueuses causées par les virus de l'herpès simplex HSV1 et HSV2. Il est aussi applicable dans le traitement de l'infection par le virus de zona. |

**续　表**

| | |
|---|---|
| 用法、用量<br>Les modes d'emploi et la posologie | 口服：1 次 200mg，每 4 小时 1 次或一日 1g，分次给予。疗程根据病情不同，短则几天，长者可达半年。肾功能不全者酌情减量。静脉滴注：1 次用量 5mg/kg，加入输液中，滴注时间为 1 小时，每 8 小时 1 次，连续 7 日。12 岁以下儿童 1 次按 250mg/m² 用量给予。急性或慢性肾功能不全者，不宜用本品静脉滴注，因为滴速过快时可引起肾衰竭。国内治疗乙型肝炎的用法为 1 次滴注 7.5mg/kg，一日 2 次，溶于适量输液，维持滴注时间约 2 小时，连续应用 10～30 日。<br><br>治疗生殖器疱疹，1 次 0.2g，一日 4 次，连用 5～10 日。<br><br>Par voie orale : 200mg par fois, toutes les 4h, ou 1g par jour, à travers plusieurs fois. La durée du traitement médical varie de quelques jours à 6 mois, selon les cas. Chez des patients insuffisants rénaux, diminuer la dose. En perfusion : 5 mg/kg par fois, introduire le médicament dans l'infusion, en perfusion pendant 1h, une fois toutes les 8h, pendant 7 jours consécutifs. Chez des enfants moins de 12 ans, 250 mg/m² par fois. Chez des patients insuffisants rénaux chroniques ou aigus, ne pas administrer ce produit en perfusion, car la vitesse excessive de la perfusion pourrait conduire à l'insuffisance rénale. Le traitement de l'hépatite B pratiquée en Chine : en perfusion, 7,5 mg/kg par fois, 2 fois par jour, introduire le produit dans l'infusion, perfusion pendant 2 h, durant 10 à 30 jours consécutifs.<br><br>Pour traiter l'herpès génital, 0,2g par fois, 4 fois par jour, pendant 5 à 10 jours consécutifs. |
| 剂型、规格<br>Les formes pharmaceutiques et les spécifications | 胶囊剂：每粒 200mg。<br>注射用阿昔洛韦（冻干制剂）：每瓶 500mg（标示量，含钠盐 549mg，折合纯品 500mg）。<br>滴眼液：0.1%。<br>眼膏：3%。<br>霜膏剂：5%。<br><br>Capsules : 200mg par capsule.<br>L'aciclovir pour injection (préparation lyophilisée) : 500mg par flacon (quantitié marquée, qui contient 549mg d'aciclovirde sodium, équivalant à 500mg de produit pur).<br>Les gouttes pour les yeux : 0,1 %.<br>Pommade ophtalmique : 3 %.<br>Crème pommade : 5 %. |
| **药品名称 Drug Names** | 更昔洛韦 Ganciclovir |
| 适应证<br>Les indications | 用于巨细胞病毒感染的治疗和预防，也可适用于单纯疱疹病毒感染。<br><br>Ce produit sert à traiter et à prévenir l'infection à cytomégalovirus. Il est aussi applicable dans le traitement de l'infection par les virus de l'herpès simplex. |
| 用法、用量<br>Les modes d'emploi et la posologie | 诱导治疗：静脉滴注 5mg/kg（历时至少 1 小时），每 12 小时 1 次，连用 14～21 日（预防用药则为 7～14 日）。维持治疗：静脉滴注，5mg/kg，一日 1 次，每周用药 7 日；或 6mg/kg，一日 1 次，每周用药 5 日。口服，每次 1g，一日 3 次，与食物同服，可根据病情选用其中之一。输液配制：将 500mg 药物（钠盐），加 10ml 注射用水振摇，使其溶解，液体应澄明无色，此溶液在室温时稳定 12 小时，切勿冷藏。进一步可用 0.9% 氯化钠、5% 葡萄糖、林格或乳酸钠林格等输液稀释至含药量低于 10mg/ml，供静脉滴注 1 小时。<br><br>Pour l'induction du traitement : en perfusion, 5 mg/kg (pendant au moins 1h), 1 fois toutes les 12h, pendant 14 à 21 jours (pour la prévention, pendant 7 à 14 jours) ; pour le traitement d'entretien: en perfusion, 5 mg/kg, 1 fois par jour, 7 jours par semaine ; ou 6 mg/kg, 1 fois par jour, 5 jours par semaine. Par voie orale, 1g par fois, 3 fois par jour, durant le repas, choisir ces deux doses selon les cas. En perfusion : ajouter 500mg de médicament (sodium) dans 10ml d'eau pour injection, agiter pour le dissoudre, la liquide doit être claire et incolore, placer la solution à la température ambiante pendant 12h, non congelée. Ensuite, utiliser la solution de chlorure de sodium, de glucose à 5 %, de Ringer ou de lactate de Ringer pour la dilution. La concentration doit être inférieure à 10mg/ml. Perfusion pendant 1h. |
| 剂型、规格<br>Les formes pharmaceutiques et les spécifications | 胶囊剂：每粒 250mg。<br>注射剂（冻干粉针）：每瓶 500mg。<br>Capsules : 250mg par capsule.<br>Injection (poudre lyophilisée) : 500mg par flacon. |

**续　表**

| 药品名称 Drug Names | 伐昔洛韦 Valaciclovir |
| --- | --- |
| 适应证<br>Les indications | 本品主要应用于治疗带状疱疹，也可用于治疗 HSV1 和 HSV2 感染。<br>Ce produit sert à lutter contre le zona et les infections par HSV1 et HSV2. |
| 用法、用量<br>Les modes d'emploi et la posologie | 口服，成人每日 0.6g，分 2 次服，疗程 7 ～ 10 日。<br>Par voie orale, chez des adultes, 0,6g par jour, à travers 2 fois, pendant 7 à 10 jours. |
| 剂型、规格<br>Les formes pharmaceutiques et les spécifications | 片剂：每片 200mg；300mg。<br>Comprimés : 200mg ou 300mg par comprimé. |
| 药品名称 Drug Names | 泛昔洛韦 Famciclovir |
| 适应证<br>Les indications | 用于治疗带状疱疹和原发性生殖器疱疹。<br>Ce produit est utilisé comme traitement du zona et de l'herpès génital primaire. |
| 用法、用量<br>Les modes d'emploi et la posologie | 口服，成人一次 0.25g，每 8 小时 1 次，治疗带状疱疹的疗程为 7 日，治疗原发性生殖器疱疹的疗程为 5 日。<br>Par voir orale, chez des adultes, 0,25g par fois, une fois toutes les 8h, pour traiter le zona, pendant 7 jours, pour traiter l'herpès génital primaire, pendant 5 jours. |
| 剂型、规格<br>Les formes pharmaceutiques et les spécifications | 片剂：每片 125mg；250mg；500mg。<br>Comprimés : 125mg, 250mg ou 500mg par comprimé. |
| 药品名称 Drug Names | 奥司他韦 Oseltamivir |
| 适应证<br>Les indications | 用于成人和 1 岁及 1 岁以上儿童的甲型和乙型流感的治疗（磷酸奥司他韦能够有效治疗甲型和乙型流感，但是乙型流感的临床应用数据尚不多）。用于成人和 13 岁及 13 岁以上青少年的甲型和乙型流感的预防。<br>Il sert à traiter la grippe A et B chez des adultes et des enfants plus de 1 an (Le phosphate d'oseltamivir peut traiter efficacement la grippe A et B, mais les données de son application clinique dans la lutte contre la grippe B sont assez limitées). Il est aussi utilisé comme prévention de la grippe A et B chez des adultes et des enfants plus de 13 ans. |
| 用法、用量<br>Les modes d'emploi et la posologie | 成人推荐量，每次 75mg，一日 2 次，共 5 日。肾功能不全者：肌酐清除率＜ 30ml/min 者每日 75mg，共 5 日。肌酐清除率＜ 10ml/min 者尚无研究资料，应慎重使用。<br>Chez des adulte, dose recommandée, 75mg par fois, 2 fois par jour, pendant 5 jours. Chez des patients insuffisants rénaux : dont la clairance de cléatinine est moins de 30 ml/min, 75mg par jour, pendant 5 jours ; dont la clairance de cléatinine est moins de 10 ml/min, sans document de référence, soyez prudent. |
| 剂型、规格<br>Les formes pharmaceutiques et les spécifications | 胶囊剂：每粒 75mg（以游离碱计）。<br>Capsules : 75mg par capsule (mesuré en oseltamivir base libre). |
| 药品名称 Drug Names | 扎那米韦 Zanamivir |
| 适应证<br>Les indications | 用于治疗流感病毒感染及季节性预防社区内 A 和 B 型流感。<br>Il sert à lutter contre les virus de la grippe et à prévenir la grippe saisonnière A et B. |
| 用法、用量<br>Les modes d'emploi et la posologie | 成人和 12 岁以上的青少年，一日 2 次，间隔约 12 小时。每日 10mg，分 2 次吸入，一次 5mg，经口吸入给药，连用 5 日。随后数日，两次的服药时间尽可能保持一致，剂量间隔 12 小时。季节性预防社区内 A 和 B 型流感：成人 10mg，一日 1 次，28 日，在流感暴发 5 日内开始治疗。<br>Chez des adultes et des adolescents plus de 12 ans, 2 fois par jour, un intervalle de 12h, 10mg par jour, à travers 2 fois, 5 mg par fois, administré par l'inhalation orale, pendant 5 jours consécutifs. Pendant les quelques jours suivants, l'intervalle entre deux administrations est de 12h. Pour prévenir la grippe saisonnière A et B dans les communautés : chez des adultes, 10mg, 1 fois par jour, pendant 28 jours, commencer le traitement dans les 5 jours suivant la crise de la grippe. |

**续　表**

| 剂型、规格<br>Les formes pharmaceutiques et les spécifications | 吸入粉雾剂：每个泡囊含扎那米韦（5mg）和乳糖（20mg）的混合粉末。<br>poudre pour inhalation : chaque vésicule contient 5mg de zanamivir et 20mg de lactose. |
|---|---|
| **药品名称 Drug Names** | **阿巴卡韦 Abacavir** |
| 适应证<br>Les indications | 本品常与其他药物联合用于艾滋病的治疗。<br>Ce produit est souvent utilisé en combinaison avec d'autres médicaments dans le traitement du sida. |
| 用法、用量<br>Les modes d'emploi et la posologie | 与其他抗反转录酶药物合用。成人：一次 300mg，一日 2 次。3 月龄至 16 岁儿童：一次 8mg/kg，一日 2 次。<br>Utilisé en combinaison avec d'autres médicaments antirétroviraux. Chez des adultes : 300mg par fois, 2 fois par jour. Chez des enfants de 3 mois à 16 ans : 8 mg/kg par fois, 2 fois par jour. |
| 剂型、规格<br>Les formes pharmaceutiques et les spécifications | 片剂：300mg（以盐基计）。<br>口服液：20mg/ml。<br>Compriés : 300mg (l'abacavir de base).<br>La solution buccale : 20mg par ml. |
| **药品名称 Drug Names** | **阿糖腺苷 Vidarabine** |
| 适应证<br>Les indications | 有抗单纯疱疹病毒 HSV1 和 HSV2 作用，用以治疗单纯疱疹病毒性脑炎，也用以治疗免疫抑制患者的带状疱疹和水痘感染。但对巨细胞病毒则无效。本品的单磷酸酯有抑制乙肝病毒复制的作用。<br>Ce produit est efficace dans la lutte contre les virus de l'herpès simplex HSV1 et HSV2, dans le traitement de l'encéphalite à virus herpès simplex, ainsi que dans le traitement du zona et de l'infection de la varicelle chez les patients immunodéprimés. Mais il est inutile dans la lutte contre le cytomégalovirus. Lemonophosphate de vidarabine est à supprimer la réplication du virus de l'hépatite B. |
| 用法、用量<br>Les modes d'emploi et la posologie | 单纯疱疹病毒性脑炎：一日量为 15mg/kg，按 200g 药物、500ml 输液（预热至 35～40℃）的比率配液，做连续静脉滴注，疗程为 10 日。带状疱疹：10mg/kg 连用 5 日，用法同上。<br>Pour traiter l'encéphalite à virus herpès simplex : 15 mg/kg par jour, dissourdre 200g de médicament dans 500ml d'infusion (35 à 40℃), en perfusion continue, pendant 10 jours. Pour traiter le zona, 10 mg/kg, pendant 5 jours consécutifs, mêmes indications. |
| 剂型、规格<br>Les formes pharmaceutiques et les spécifications | 注射液（混悬液）：200mg（1ml）；1000mg（5ml）。加入输液中滴注用。<br>注射用单磷酸阿糖腺苷：每瓶 200mg。<br>Injection (en suspension): 200mg (1ml) ou 1 000mg (5ml). Dissourdre dans l'infusion pour la perfusion.<br>Le monophosphate de vidarabine pour injection : 200mg par flacon. |
| **药品名称 Drug Names** | **利巴韦林 Ribavirine** |
| 适应证<br>Les indications | 用于呼吸道合胞病毒引起的病毒性肺炎与支气管炎，皮肤疱疹病毒感染。<br>Ce produit sert à traiter la pneumonie et la bronchite virales causées par le virus respiratoire syncytial, ainsi que l'infection cutanée par le virus de l'herpès. |
| 用法、用量<br>Les modes d'emploi et la posologie | 口服：一日 0.8～1g，分 3～4 次服用。肌内注射或静脉滴注：一日 10～15mg/kg，分 2 次，静脉滴注宜缓慢。用于早期出血热，每日 1g，加入输液 500～1000ml 中静脉滴注，连续应用 3～5 日。<br>滴鼻：用于防治流感，用 0.5% 溶液（以等渗氯化钠溶液配制），每 1 小时 1 次。<br>滴眼：治疗疱疹感染，浓度 0.1%，一日数次。<br>Par voie orale : 0,8 à 1g par jour, à travers 3 à 4 fois. Injection par voie IM ou en perfusion : 10 à 15 mg/kg par jour, à travers 2 fois, perfusion lente. Pour traiter la fièvre hémorragique au stade précoce, 1g par jour, dissourdre dans 500 à 1 000ml d'infusion, en perfusion, pendant 3 à 5 jours consécutifs.<br>Les gouttes nasales : pour prévenir la grippe, utiliser la solution à 0,5 % (utiliser la solution de chlorure de sodium isotonique), une fois par heure.<br>Les gouttes pour les yeux : pour traiter l'infection par le virus de l'herpès, la concentration est de 0,1 %, plusieurs fois par jour. |

续　表

| 剂型、规格<br>Les formes pharmaceutiques et les spécifications | 片剂：每片 50mg；100mg。<br>颗粒剂：每袋 50mg；100mg。<br>注射液：100mg（1ml）；250mg（2ml）。<br>Comprimés : 50mg ou 100mg par comprimé.<br>Granules : 50mg ou 100mg par sachet.<br>Injection : 100mg (1ml) ou 250 mg (2ml). |
|---|---|
| **药品名称 Drug Names** | 齐多夫定 Zidovudine |
| 适应证<br>Les indications | 用于治疗获得性免疫缺陷综合征（AIDS）。患者有并发症（卡氏肺囊虫病或其他感染）时尚需应用对症的其他药物联合治疗。<br>Ce produit sert à traiter le sida. Lorsque les patients ont des applications (le pneumocystis carinii ou d'autres sortes d'infections), il est souvent utilisé en association avec d'autres médicaments. |
| 用法、用量<br>Les modes d'emploi et la posologie | 成人常用量：1 次 200mg，每 4 小时 1 次，按时间给药。有贫血的患者：可按 1 次 100mg 给药。<br>Chez des adultes, la dose usuelle : 200mg par fois, une fois toutes les 4h. Chez des patients atteints d'anémie : 100mg par fois. |
| 剂型、规格<br>Les formes pharmaceutiques et les spécifications | 胶囊剂：每粒 100mg。<br>Capsules : 100mg par capsule. |
| **药品名称 Drug Names** | 拉米夫定 Lamivudine |
| 适应证<br>Les indications | 用于乙型肝炎病毒所致的慢性乙型肝炎，与其他抗反转录病毒药连用于治疗人类免疫缺陷病毒感染。<br>Ce produit sert à traiter l'hépatite chronique provoquée par le virus de l'hépatite B. Il est utilisé en combinaison avec d'autres médicaments anti –rétroviraux pour traiter les infections par le virus de l'immunodéficience humaine. |
| 用法、用量<br>Les modes d'emploi et la posologie | 成人：慢性乙型肝炎，一日 1 次，100mg 口服；HIV 感染，推荐剂量一次 150mg，一日 2 次，或一次 300mg；一日 1 次。<br>Chez des adultes : pour traiter l'hépatite B chronique, 1 fois par jour, 100mg, par voie orale ; pour traiter les infections par le VIL, la dose recommandée, 150 mg par fois, 2 fois par jour, ou 300mg par fois, 1 fois par jour. |
| 剂型、规格<br>Les formes pharmaceutiques et les spécifications | 片剂：每片 100mg；150mg。<br>Comprimés : 100mg ou 150mg par comprimé. |
| **药品名称 Drug Names** | 阿德福韦酯 Adéfovir dipivoxil |
| 适应证<br>Les indications | 用于乙型肝炎病毒感染，人类免疫缺陷病毒感染。<br>Ce produit sert à traiter l'infection par le virus de l'hépatite B et l'infection par le virus de l'immunodéficience humaine. |
| 用法、用量<br>Les modes d'emploi et la posologie | 成人口服：慢性乙型肝炎，一日 1 次，每次 10mg；HIV 感染，一日 1 次，每次 125mg，疗程 12 周。静脉滴注：HIV 感染，每次 1～3mg/kg，每日 1 次或每周 3 次，每次给药时间不少于 30 分钟。皮下注射剂量同静脉滴注。<br>Chez des adultes par voie orale : pour traiter l'hépatite B chronique, 1 fois par jour, 10mg par fois ; pour traiter les infections par le VIH, 1 fois par jour, 125mg par fois, pendant 12 semaines comme un traitement médical. En perfusion : pour traiter les infections par le VIH, 1 à 3 mg/kg par fois, 1 fois par jour ou 3 fois par semaine, perfusion pendant 30 minutes au moins. L'injection sous-cutanée, la même dose pour la perfusion. |
| 剂型、规格<br>Les formes pharmaceutiques et les spécifications | 阿德福韦酯片（胶囊）：每片（粒）10mg。<br>Comprimés d'adéfovir dipivoxil (capsules) : 10mg par comprimé ou par capsule. |

**续　表**

| 药品名称 Drug Names | 恩替卡韦 Entecavir |
|---|---|
| 适应证<br>Les indications | 用于病毒复制活跃，血清转氨酶 ALT 持续升高或肝脏组织学显示有活动性病变的慢性成人乙型肝炎的治疗。<br><br>Ce produit sert à traiter l'hépatite B chronique chez des adultesayant des symptômes suivants : la réplication virale active, l'élévation persistante des transaminases sériques, oudes lésions actives montrées par l'histologie hépatique. |
| 用法、用量<br>Les modes d'emploi et la posologie | 口服，一日 1 次，每次 0.5mg。拉米夫定治疗时发生病毒血症或出现拉米夫定耐药突变的患者推荐剂量为一日 1 次，每次 1.0mg，空腹服用。<br><br>Par voie orale, 1 fois par jour, 0,5mg par fois. Chez des patients dont le traitement avec lalamivudine a conduit à la virémie ou chez des patients présentant des mutations de résistantce à la lamivudine, il est recommandé de prendre ce produit 1 fois par jour, 1,0 mg par fois, l'estomac vide. |
| 剂型、规格<br>Les formes pharmaceutiques et les spécifications | 片剂：每片 0.5mg。<br>Comprimés : 0,5mg par comprimé. |
| 药品名称 Drug Names | 替比夫定 Telbivudine |
| 适应证<br>Les indications | 用于有病毒复制证据，血清转氨酶（ALT 或 AST）持续升高或肝组织学显示有活动性病变的慢性成人乙型肝炎的成人患者。<br><br>Ce produit sert à traiter l'hépatite B chronique chez des adultes ayant des symptômes suivants : la réplication virale active, l'élévation persistante des transaminases sériques, ou des lésions actives montrées par l'histologie hépatique. |
| 用法、用量<br>Les modes d'emploi et la posologie | 成人和青少年（≥ 16 岁）推荐剂量为 600mg，一日 1 次口服，餐前或餐后均可，不受进食影响。<br><br>Chez des adultes et des adolescents (16 ans et plus), la dose recommandée, 600mg, une fois par jour, par voie orale, avant ou après le repas. |
| 剂型、规格<br>Les formes pharmaceutiques et les spécifications | 片剂：每片 600mg。<br>Comprimés : 600mg par comprimé. |
| 药品名称 Drug Names | 聚乙二醇干扰素α-2a　Interféron pégylé alfa-2a |
| 适应证<br>Les indications | 用于肝硬化代偿期或无肝硬化的慢性乙型或丙型肝炎的治疗。<br><br>Ce produit est utilisé comme traitement de l'hépatite B ou C sous forme de cirrhose décompensée ou sans cirrhose. |
| 用法、用量<br>Les modes d'emploi et la posologie | 皮下注射，推荐剂量为一次 180μg，每周 1 次，共用 48 周。发生中度和重度不良反应的患者，应调整剂量，初始剂量一般减至 135μg，有些病例需减至 90μg 或 45μg。随不良反应的减轻，逐渐增加或恢复至常规剂量。<br><br>Injection sous-cutanée, la dose recommandée, 180μg par fois, une fois par semaine, pendant 48 semaines. Chez des patients qui ont des réactions indésirables modérées et graves, il faut ajuster la dose, diminuer la dose pour la première fois jusqu'à 135μg, chez certains patients, il faut diminuer jusqu'à 90 ou 45μg. Avec la réduction des réactions indésirables, augmenter progressivement la dose ou reprendre la dose usuelle. |
| 剂型、规格<br>Les formes pharmaceutiques et les spécifications | 注射液：每支 180μg（1ml）；135μg（1ml）。<br>Injection : 180μg (1ml) ou 135μg (1ml) par solution. |

**续　表**

| 药品名称 Drug Names | 奈韦拉平 Nevirapine |
| --- | --- |
| 适应证<br>Les indications | 常与其他药物联合应用于治疗 I 型 HIV 感染。单独用本品则病毒可迅速产生耐药性。<br><br>Ce produit est souvent utilisé en combinaison avec d'autres médicaments comme traitement de l'infection par le VIH de type A. Son utilisation unique peut entraîner rapidement la résistance du virus. |
| 用法、用量<br>Les modes d'emploi et la posologie | 成人：先导期剂量，一日 1 次 200mg，用药 14 日（以减少皮疹发生）；以后一日 2 次，每次 200mg。儿童：2 个月～8 岁，一日一次 4mg/kg，用药 14 日，以后一日 2 次，每次 7mg/kg；儿童：8 岁以上，一日 1 次 4mg/kg，用药 14 日，以后一日 2 次，每次 4mg/kg。所有患者的用量每日不超过 400mg。<br><br>Chez des adultes : la dose initiale est de 200mg par fois par jour, pendant 14 jours (pour éviter l'éruption) ; ensuite, 2 fois par jour, 200mg par fois. Chez des enfants : chez de 2 mois à 8 ans, 4 mg/kg par fois par jour, pendant 14 jours, ensuite, 2 fois par jour, 7 mg/kg par fois ; chez des enfants plus de 8 ans, 4 mg/kg par fois par jour, pendant 14 jours, ensuite, 2 fois par jour, 4 mg/kg par fois. Pour tous les patients, ne pas dépasser 400mg par jour. |
| 剂型、规格<br>Les formes pharmaceutiques et les spécifications | 片剂（胶囊剂）：每片（粒）200mg。<br>Comprimés (capsules) : 200mg par comprimé ou par capsule. |
| 药品名称 Drug Names | 司他夫定 Stavudine |
| 适应证<br>Les indications | 用于治疗 I 型 HIV 感染。<br>Ce produit sert à traiter l'infection par le HIV de type A. |
| 用法、用量<br>Les modes d'emploi et la posologie | 成人：体重≥60kg 者，口服一次 40mg，一日 2 次（相隔 12 小时）；体重＜60kg 者，口服一次 30mg，一日 2 次。儿童：体重≥30kg 者，按成人剂量；体重＜30kg 者，一次 1mg/kg，一日 2 次。肾功能低下者，需根据其肌酐清除率调整剂量。<br><br>Chez des adultes : chez des patients de 60kg ou plus, 40mg par fois, par voie orale, 2 fois par jour (un intervalle de 12h) ; chez des patients moins de 60kg, 30mg par fois, par voie orale, 2 fois par jour. Chez des enfants : chez des enfants de 30kg ou plus, la même dose que chez des adultes ; chez des enfants moins de 30kg, 1 mg/kg par fois, 2 fois par jour. Chez des patients insuffisants rénaux, ajuster la dose en fonction de la clairance de la créatinine. |
| 剂型、规格<br>Les formes pharmaceutiques et les spécifications | 胶囊剂：每粒 20mg；30mg；40mg。<br>Capsules : 20mg, 30mg ou 40mg par capsule. |
| 药品名称 Drug Names | 利托那韦 Ritonavir |
| 适应证<br>Les indications | 单独使用或与其他反转录酶抑制药联合用于治疗 HIV 感染。<br><br>Ce produit peut être utilisé seul ou en association avec d'autres médicaments anti-rétroviraux comme traitement de l'infection par le HIV. |
| 用法、用量<br>Les modes d'emploi et la posologie | 口服：成人初始剂量一次 300mg，一日 2 次，之后每 2～3 日每次用量增加 100mg，直至达推荐剂量每次 600mg，一日 2 次。2 岁以上儿童初始剂量一次 250mg/m²，一日 2 次，之后每 2～3 日每次用量增加 50mg/m²，直至达推荐剂量每次 400mg/m²，一日 2 次。最大剂量不超过每次 600mg，一日 2 次。<br><br>Par voie orale : chez des adults, commencer par prendre 300mg par fois, 2 fois par jour, ensuite, augmenter 100mg par fois tous les 2 à 3 jours pour atteindre la dose recommandée, soit 600mg par fois, 2 fois par jour. Chez des enfants plus de 2 ans, commencer par prendre 250 mg/m² par fois, 2 fois par jour, ensuite, augmenter 50 mg/m² par fois tous les 2 à 3 jours pour atteindre la dose recommandée, soit 400 mg/m² par fois, 2 fois par jour. Ne pas dépasser 600mg par fois, 2 fois par jour. |
| 剂型、规格<br>Les formes pharmaceutiques et les spécifications | 软胶囊：每粒 100mg。<br>Capsules : 100mg par capsule. |

| 药品名称 Drug Names | 膦甲酸钠 Foscarnet de sodium |
|---|---|
| 适应证<br>Les indications | 主要用于免疫缺陷者（如艾滋病患者）发生的巨细胞病毒性视网膜炎的治疗。也可用于对阿昔洛韦耐药的免疫缺陷者（如 HIV 感染患者）的皮肤黏膜单纯疱疹病毒感染或带状疱疹病毒感染。<br><br>Ce produit sert à traiter les rétinites à cytomégalovirus chez des immunodéprimés (par exemple le malade du sida). Il est aussi applicable dans le traitement des infections cutanéo-muqueuses par le virus d'herpès simplex et des infections par le virus de l'herpès chez des immunodéprimés résistant à l'acyclovir (par exemple le patient atteint du HIV). |
| 用法、用量<br>Les modes d'emploi et la posologie | 静脉滴注：初始剂量 60mg/kg，每 8 小时 1 次，至少需 1 小时恒速滴入，用 2～3 周；剂量、给药间隔、连续应用时间须根据患者的肾功能与用药耐受程度予以调节。维持量为每日 90～120mg/kg，静脉滴注 2 小时。<br><br>En perfusion : au début, 60 mg/kg, une fois toutes les 8h, perfusion à débit constant pendant au moins 1h, pendant 2 à 3 semaines ; ajuster la dose, l'intervalle et la durée de l'administration continue en fonction de le fonction rénale et de la résistance au médicament chez les patients. La dose d'entretien, 90 à 120 mg/kg par jour, perfusion pendant 2h. |
| 剂型、规格<br>Les formes pharmaceutiques et les spécifications | 注射液：每瓶 600mg（250ml）；1200mg（500ml）。<br>Injection : 600mg (250ml) ou 1 200mg (500ml) par flacon. |

| 药品名称 Drug Names | 去羟肌苷 Didanosine |
|---|---|
| 适应证<br>Les indications | 用于 I 型 HIV 感染，常与其他抗反转录酶药物联合应用（鸡尾酒疗法）。<br>Ce produit sert à lutter contre l'infection par le HIV de type I. Il est souvent utilsé en combinaison avec d'autres médicaments anti-rétroviraux (HAART). |
| 用法、用量<br>Les modes d'emploi et la posologie | 成人：体重≥ 60kg 者，一次 200mg，一日 2 次，或一日 400mg，一次顿服；体重＜ 60kg 者，一次 125mg，一日 2 次，或一日 250mg，一次顿服。儿童：120mg/m²，一日 2 次或一日 250mg，一次顿服。肾功能低下者应按肌酐清除率调整剂量。饭前 30 分钟服用，片剂应充分咀嚼或溶于 1 小杯水中、搅拌混匀后服用。<br><br>Chez des adultes : chez des patients de 60kg ou plus, 200mg par fois, 2 fois par jour, ou 400mg par jour, une fois par jour ; chez des patients moins de 60kg, 125mg par fois, 2 fois par jour, ou 250 mg par jour, une fois par jour. Chez des enfants : 120 mg/m², 2 fois par jour ou 250mg par jour, une fois par jour. Chez des patiens insuffisants rénaux, ajuster la dose en fonction de la clairance de la créatinine. 30 minutes avant le repas, des comprimés doivent être pleinement mâchés ou être dissolus dans un verre d'eau, mélangés avant d'être administrés. |
| 剂型、规格<br>Les formes pharmaceutiques et les spécifications | 片剂：50mg；100mg。<br>Comprimés : 50mg ou 100mg. |

| 药品名称 Drug Names | 茚地那韦 Indinavir |
|---|---|
| 适应证<br>Les indications | 和其他抗反转录病毒药物联合使用，用于治疗成人及儿童 HIV-1 感染。<br>Ce produit sert, en association avec d'autres médicaments anti-rétroviraux, à lutter contre l'infection par le VIH -1 chez des adultes et des enfants. |
| 用法、用量<br>Les modes d'emploi et la posologie | 推荐的开始剂量为 800mg，每 8 小时口服 1 次。与利福布汀联合治疗建议将利福布汀的剂量减半，而本药剂量增加至每 8 小时 1g。与酮康唑合用，本药的剂量应减少至每 8 小时 600mg。肝功能不全患者，剂量应减至每 8 小时 600mg。3 岁以上（可口服胶囊的儿童）：本品的推荐剂量为每 8 小时口服 500mg/m²。儿童剂量不能超过成人剂量（即每 8 小时 800mg）。 |

续 表

| | |
|---|---|
| | Il est recommandé de commencer par 800mg, une fois toutes les 8h, par voie orale. Si ce produit est utilisé en association avec la rifabutine, diminuer de moitié la dose de la rifabutine tout en augmentant la dose de l'indinavir pour atteindre 1g toutes les 8h. Si ce produit est utilisé en combinaison avec le kétoconazole, il faut diminuer la dose de l'indinavir jusqu'à 600mg toutes les 8h. Chez des patients insuffisants hépatiques, diminuer la dose pour atteindre 600mg toutes les 8h. Chez des enfants plus de 3 ans (des enfants capables d'administrer les capsules par voie orale) : la dose recommandée, 500 mg/m$^2$ par voie orale, toutes les 8h. La dose chez des enfants ne doit pas dépasser la dose chez des adultes (à savoir 800mg toutes les 8h). |
| 剂型、规格<br>Les formes pharmaceutiques et les spécifications | 胶囊剂：每粒 200mg。<br>Capsules : 200mg par capsule. |
| **药品名称 Drug Names** | 金刚烷胺 Amantadine |
| 适应证<br>Les indications | 用于亚洲 A- Ⅱ 型流感感染发热患者。常用于震颤麻痹。<br>Ce produit sert à traiter les infections par la grippe asiatique de type A-II chez des patients atteints de fièvre. Il est souvent utilisé dans le traitement du parkinsonisme. |
| 用法、用量<br>Les modes d'emploi et la posologie | 流感A病毒感染：成人：每日200mg，分1～2次服用；儿童：新生儿与1岁内婴儿不用；1～9岁，每日4.4～8.8mg/kg，1～2次，每日最大剂量不超过150mg，9～12岁，100～200mg/d。<br>Pour traiter les infections par la grippe de type A : chez des adultes : 200mg par jour, à travers 1 à 2 fois ; chez des enfants : chez des nouveau-nés et moins de 1 an, ne pas prendre le médicament ; chez de 1 à 9 ans, 4,4 à 8,8 mg/kg par jour, 1 à 2 fois, ne pas dépasser 150mg par jour ; chez de 9 à 12 ans, 100 à 200 mg par jour. |
| 剂型、规格<br>Les formes pharmaceutiques et les spécifications | 片（胶囊剂）：0.1g。<br>Comprimés (capsules) : 0,1g. |

7. 抗寄生虫病药 Médicaments antiparasites

7.1 抗疟药 Antipaludiques

| | |
|---|---|
| **药品名称 Drug Names** | 氯喹 Chloroquine |
| 适应证<br>Les indications | 主要用于治疗疟疾急性发作，控制疟疾症状，还可用于治疗肝阿米巴病、华支睾吸虫病、肺吸虫病、结缔组织病等。另可用于光敏性疾病，如日晒红斑症。<br>Ce produit sert à traiter la crise aiguë du paludisme, les symtômes du paludisme, l'amibiase hépatique, la clonorchiase, la paragonimose et la maladie liée au tissu conjonctif. Il est aussi applicable dans le traitement des maladies liées à la photosensibilité, telles que l'érythème solaire. |
| 用法、用量<br>Les modes d'emploi et la posologie | （1）控制疟疾发作：①口服：首剂1g，6小时后0.5g，第2、3日各服0.5g，如与伯氨喹合用，只需第一日服本品1g。小儿首次16mg/kg（高热其酌情减量，分次服），6～8小时后及第2～3日各服8mg/kg。②静脉滴注：恶性疟第1日1.5g，第2、3日0.5g。一般每0.5～0.75g氯喹用5%葡萄糖注射液或 0.9% 氯化钠注射液 500ml 稀释，静脉滴注速度为每分钟12～20滴，第1日量与12小时内全部输完。<br>（2）疟疾症状抑制性预防：每周服1次，每次0.5g，小儿每周8mg/kg。<br>（3）抗阿米巴肝脓肿：每1、2日每日2～3次，每次服0.5g，以后每日0.5g，连用2～3周。<br>（4）治疗结缔组织病：对盘状红斑狼疮及类风湿关节炎，开始剂量一日1～2次，每次0.25g，经2～3周后，如症状得到控制，改为一日2～3次，每次量不宜超过0.25g，长期维持。对系统性红斑狼疮，用皮质激素治疗症状缓解后，可加用氯喹以减少皮质激素用量。 |

续　表

|  |  |
|---|---|
|  | (1) Pour contrôler la crise du paludisme : a) Par voie orale, pour la première fois, prendre 1g, 6 h après, reprendre 0,5g, pour le deuxième et le troisième jour, prendre 0,5g respectivement. Si le produit est utilisé en association avec la primaquine, il faut seulement prendre 1g de chloroquine le premier jour. chez des enfants, pour la première fois, 16 mg/kg (en cas de fièvre, diminuer la dose selon les cas, à travers plusieurs fois), 6 à 8 h après, prendre 8 mg/kg, pour le deuxième et le troisième jour, reprendre 8mg/kg respectivement. b) En perfusion : pour traiter le paludisme à falciparum, 1,5g pour le premier jour, 0,5g pour le deuxième et troisième jour. En général, dissouddre 0,5 à 0,75g de chloroquine dans 500ml de solution de glucose à 5 % ou de solution de chlorure de sodium à 0,9 %, perfusion (12 à 20 gouttes par minute). Injecter en perfusion la dose pour le premier jour en 12h.<br><br>(2) Pour la prévention des symptômes du paludisme : 1 fois par semaine, 0,5g par fois, chez des enfants, 8 mg/kg par fois par semaine.<br><br>(3) Pour lutter contre l'abcès du fois amibien : 0,5g par fois, 2 à 3 fois par jour, tous les 1 à 2 jours, ensuite, 0,5g par jour, pendant 2 à 3 semaines consecutives.<br><br>(4) Pour traiter la maladie liée au tissu conjonctif : pour traiter le lupus érythémateux discoïde et la polyarthrite rhumatoïde, au début, 1 à 2 fois par jour, 0,25g par fois, 2 à 3 semaines après, s'il l'on contrôle les symptômes, 2 à 3 fois par jour, ne pas dépasser 0,25g par fois, maintenir la dose. Pour traiter le lupus érythémateux systématique, après l'amélioration des symptômes consécutive au traitement avec des corticostéroïdes, il est possible d'utiliser en même temps la chloroquine pour éviter l'utilisation excessive des corticostéroïdes. |
| 剂型、规格<br>Les formes pharmaceutiques et les spécifications | 片剂：每片含磷酸氯喹 0.075g；0.25g。<br>注射液：每支 129mg（盐基 80mg）（2ml）；250mg（盐基 155mg）（2ml）。<br>Comprimés : chaque comprimé contient 0,075g ou 0,25g de phosphate de chloroquine.<br>Injection : 129mg (80mg de chloroquine base) (2ml) ou 250mg (155mg de chloroquine base) (2ml) par solution. |

**药品名称 Drug Names**　羟氯喹 Hydroxychloroquine

|  |  |
|---|---|
| 适应证<br>Les indications | 本品主要用于疟疾的预防和治疗，也用于类风湿关节炎和青少年类风湿关节炎，以及盘状红斑狼疮和系统性红斑狼疮的治疗。<br><br>Ce produit sert à prévenir et à traiter le paludisme. Il est aussi utilisé comme traitement de la polyarthrite rhumatoïde, de l'arthrite rhumatoïde juvénile, ainsi que du lupus érythémateux discoïde et du lupus érythémateux systématique. |
| 用法、用量<br>Les modes d'emploi et la posologie | 治疗急性疟疾：成人口服，首次 800mg，以后每 6～8 小时 400mg，然后每 2 日 400mg；儿童首剂量 10mg/kg，6 小时后第 2 次服药 5mg/kg，第 2、3 日，每日 1 次 5mg/kg。预防疟疾：在进入疟疾流行区前 1 周，服 400mg，以后每周 1 次 400mg；儿童 5mg/kg。治疗风湿性关节炎和红斑狼疮：成人开始每日 400mg，分次服，维持量每日 200～400mg，每日剂量不超过 6.5mg/kg。青少年患者治疗 6 个月无效即应停药。<br><br>Pour traiter le paludisme aigu : chez des adultes, par voie orale, pour la première fois, 800mg, ensuite, 400mg toutes les 6 à 8h, ensuite, 400mg tous les deux jours ; chez des enfants, 10 mg/kg pour la première fois, 6 h après prendre 5 mg/kg, le 2ème et le 3ème jour, prendre 5 mg/kg par jour. Pour prévenir le paludisme : une semaine avant d'entrer dans les zones d'endémie, prendre 400mg, ensuite, 400mg toutes les semaines ; chez des enfants, 5 mg/kg. Pour traiter l'arthrite rhumatismal et le lupus érythémateux : chez des adultes, au début, 400mg par jour, à travers plusieurs fois, la dose d'entretien, 200 à 400mg par jour, ne pas dépasser 6,5 mg/kg. Chez des patients jeunes, s'il n'est pas efficace en 6 mois, il faut arrêter l'administration. |
| 剂型、规格<br>Les formes pharmaceutiques et les spécifications | 片剂：每片 100mg；200mg。<br>Comprimés : 100mg ou 200mg par comprimé. |

**药品名称 Drug Names**　青蒿素 Artémisinine

|  |  |
|---|---|
| 适应证<br>Les indications | 用于间日疟，恶性疟特别是抢救脑型疟有良效，其退热时间及疟原虫转阴时间都较氯喹短，对氯喹有抗药性的疟原虫，使用本品有效。<br><br>Ce produit est efficace dans le traitement du paludisme à vivax, du paludisme à falciparum et surtout dans la sauvegarde du paludime cérabral.Son temps de refroidissement et son temps nécessaire pour la clairance parasitaire sont tous plus courts que la chloroquine et Il est utile dans le traitement du plasmodium résistant à la chloroquine. |

**续　表**

| | |
|---|---|
| 用法、用量<br>Les modes d'emploi et la posologie | （1）口服：先服 1g，6～8 小时后再服 0.5g，第 2、3 日各服 0.5g，疗程 3 日，总量为 2.5g。小儿总剂量 15mg/kg，按上述方法 3 日内服完。<br>（2）直肠给药：先服 0.6g，6 小时后再服 0.6g，第 2、3 日各服 0.4g。<br>（3）深部肌内注射：第 1 次 200mg，6～8 小时后再给 100mg，第 2、3 日各肌内注射 100mg，总剂量 500mg（个别重症第 4 日再给 100mg）。或连用 3 日，每日肌内注射 300mg，总量 900mg。小儿 15mg/kg，按上述方法 3 日内注完。<br><br>(1) Par voie orale : pour la première fois, 1g, 6 à 8 h après, reprendre 0,5g, le 2ème et le 3ème jour, prendre 0,5g par jour, pendant 3 jours, la dose totale : 2,5g. Chez des enfants, la dose totale, 15 mg/kg, les mêmes indications, administrer en 3 jours.<br>(2) L'administration par voie rectale : pour la première fois, 0,6g, 6 h après, reprendre 0,6g, le 2ème et le 3ème jour, prendre 0,4g par jour.<br>(3) Injection par voie IM profonde : pour la première fois, 200mg, 6 à 8 h après, reprendre 100mg, le 2ème et le 3ème jour, prendre 100mg par jour, la dose totale : 500mg (chez certains patients gravement malades, reprendre 100mg pour le 4ème jour). Ou pendant 3 jours consécutifs, injecter par voie IM 300mg par jour, la dose totale : 900mg. Chez des enfants, 15 mg/kg, les mêmes indications, injecter en 3 jours. |
| 剂型、规格<br>Les formes pharmaceutiques et les spécifications | 油注射液：每支 50mg（2ml）；100mg（2ml）；200mg（2ml）；300mg（2ml）。<br>水混悬注射液：每支 300mg（2ml）。<br>片剂：每片 50mg；100mg。<br>栓剂：每粒 400mg；600mg。<br><br>L'injection d'huile : 50mg (2ml), 100mg (2ml), 200mg (2ml) ou 300mg (2ml) par solution.<br>Injection en suspension : 300mg (2ml) par pièce.<br>Comprimés : 50mg ou 100mg par comprimé.<br>Suppositoires : 400mg ou 600mg par suppositoire. |
| 药品名称 Drug Names | 青蒿素哌喹 Artemisinine et piperaquine |
| 适应证<br>Les indications | 用于恶性疟和间日疟。<br>Ce produit sert à traiter le paludisme à falciparum et le paludisme à vivax. |
| 用法、用量<br>Les modes d'emploi et la posologie | 口服，成人总剂量 8 片，每日早、晚各一次，每次 2 片。<br>Par voie orale, chez des adultes, la dose totale, 8 comprimés, 2 comprimés par fois, 2 fois par jour, le petit matin et le soir. |
| 剂型、规格<br>Les formes pharmaceutiques et les spécifications | 复方制剂，每片含青蒿素 6.25mg，哌喹 375mg。<br>La préparation de composés : chaque comprimé contient 6,25mg d'artemisinine et 375mg de piperaquine. |
| 药品名称 Drug Names | 双氢青蒿素 Dihydroartémisinine |
| 适应证<br>Les indications | 用于治疗各类疟疾，尤其适用于抗氯喹和哌喹的恶性疟和凶险型脑型疟疾的救治。<br>Ce produit sert à traiter toutes sortes de paludisme, surtout le paludisme à falciparum et le paludisme cérébral dangereux résistant à la chloroquine et à la piperaquine. |
| 用法、用量<br>Les modes d'emploi et la posologie | 口服，一日 1 次，成人一日 60mg，首剂加倍；儿童按年龄递减；连用 5～7 日。<br>Par voie orale, 1 fois par jour, chez des adultes, 60mg par jour, doubler la dose pour la première fois ; chez des enfants, diminuer la dose en fonction des âges ; pendant 5 à 7 jours consécutifs. |
| 剂型、规格<br>Les formes pharmaceutiques et les spécifications | 片剂：每片 20mg。<br>复方制剂：每片含双氢青蒿素 40mg，磷酸氯喹 320mg。<br>Comprimés : 20mg par comprimé.<br>La préparation de composés : chaque comprimé contient 40mg de dihydroartémisinine et 320mg de phosphate de chloroquine. |

**续 表**

| 药品名称 Drug Names | 双氢青蒿素磷酸哌喹 Dihydroartémisinine et Phosphate de piperaquine |
|---|---|
| 适应证<br>Les indications | 用于恶性疟和间日疟。<br><br>Ce produit sert à traiter le paludisme à falciparum et le paludisme à vivax. |
| 用法、用量<br>Les modes d'emploi et la posologie | 口服，成人总剂量8片，每日早、晚各一次，每次2片。年龄≥16岁者，首剂2片，第6～8小时服2片，第24小时服用2片，第32小时服用2片。年龄11～15岁者，首剂1.5片，第6～8小时服1.5片，第24小时服用1.5片，第32小时服用1.5片。年龄7～10岁者，首剂1片，第6～8小时服1片，第24小时服用1片，第32小时服用1片。<br><br>Par voie orale, chez des adultes, la dose totale : 8 comprimés, 2 comprimés par fois, 2 fois par jour, le petit matin et le soir. Chez des patients plus de 16 ans, pour la première fois, 2 comprimés, la 6ème à 8ème h, prendre 2 comprimés, la 24ème h, 2 comprimés, la 32èmeh, 2 comprimés. Chez des patients de 11 à 15 ans, pour la première fois, 1,5 comprimés, la 6ème à 8ème h, prendre 1,5 comprimés, la 24ème h, 1,5 comprimés, la 32èmeh, 1 comprimé. Chez des patients de 7 à 10 ans, pour la première fois, 1 comprimé, de la 6ème à la 8ème h, prendre 1 comprimé, la 24ème h, 1 comprimé, la 32èmeh, 1 comprimé. |
| 剂型、规格<br>Les formes pharmaceutiques et les spécifications | 复方制剂：每片含双氢青蒿素 40mg，磷酸哌喹 320mg。<br><br>La préparation de composés : chaque comprimé contient 40mg de dihydroartémisinine et 320mg de phosphate de piperaquine. |
| 药品名称 Drug Names | 蒿甲醚 Artéméther |
| 适应证<br>Les indications | 本品对恶性疟（包括抗氯喹恶性疟及凶险型疟）的疗效较佳，效果确切，显效迅速，近期疗效可达100%。用药后2日内，多数病例血中原虫转阴并退热。复燃率8%。较青蒿素低。与伯氨喹合用可进一步降低复燃率。临床还适用于急性上呼吸道感染的高热患者，进行对症处理，取得较好疗效。退热效应一般在肌内注射后半小时即开始出现，体温呈梯形逐渐下降，4～6小时再逐渐回升，无体温骤降的现象，退热作用稳定。本品肌内注射后，患者出汗少，不致引起老人、儿童、虚弱患者发生虚脱等不良反应。<br><br>Ce produit est utilisé dans le traitement du paludisme à falciparum (y compris le paludisme à falciparum résistant à la chloroquine) avec un effet exact et rapide, et un taux de réussite à 100 % enregistré ces derniers temps. 2 jours après l'administration, le parasite dans le sang s'élimine et la fièvre tombe. Le taux de recrudescence est de 8 %, soit un niveau inférieur à l'artémisinine. Utilisé en combinaison avec la primaquine, il peut réduire le taux de recrudescence. Il est aussi applicable dans les cliniques comme traitement des infections aigues des voies respiratoires supérieures chez des patients avec fièvre. L'abaissement de la fièvre se produit une demi-heure après l'injection par voie IM. 4 à 6 h après, on assistera à l'élévation de la température du corp, sans la chute de la température. Après l'administration de ce produit, les patients ont peu de tranpiration, ce qui permet d'éviter les effets indésirables tels la prostation chez des personnes âgées, des enfants ou des patients faibles. |
| 用法、用量<br>Les modes d'emploi et la posologie | 抗疟：肌内注射，第1日160mg，第2～5日各80mg。小儿首剂量按3.2mg/kg计，以后按1.6mg/kg计。口服，首剂160mg，第2日起一日一次，一次80mg，连服5～7日。退热：肌内注射160mg。<br><br>Pour la lutte contre le paludisme : injection par voie IM, pour le premier jour, 160mg, du 2ème au 5ème jour, 80mg par jour. Chez des enfants, au début, 3,2 mg/kg, ensuite, 1,6mg/kg.Par voie orale, au début, 160mg, à partir du 2ème jour, 1 fois par jour, 80mg par fois, pendant 5 à 7 jours consécutifs. Pour l'abaissement de la fièvre : injection par voie IM, 160mg. |
| 剂型、规格<br>Les formes pharmaceutiques et les spécifications | 油注射液：每支80mg（1ml）。<br>胶囊：每胶囊40mg。<br>片剂：每片40mg。<br>复方制剂：每片含蒿甲醚0.02g，本芴醇0.12g。<br><br>Injection d'huile : 80mg (1ml) par solution.<br>Capsules : 40mg par capsule.<br>Comprimés : 40mg par comprimé.<br>La préparation de composés : chaque comprimé contient 0,02g d'artéméther et 0,12g de luméfantrine. |

**续 表**

| 药品名称 Drug Names | 奎宁 Quinine |
|---|---|
| 适应证<br>Les indications | 抑制或杀灭良性疟（间日疟、三日疟）及恶性疟原虫的红内期，能控制疟疾症状，有解热、子宫收缩的作用。<br><br>Ce produit sert à inhiber ou tuer le paludisme bénin (le paludisme à vivax et le paludisme à malariae) ou le paludisme à falciparum au stade érythrocytaire. Il peut aussi traiter les symptômes du paludisme. Il a un effet antipyrétiqueet peut provoquer des contractions utérines. |
| 用法、用量<br>Les modes d'emploi et la posologie | 成人常用量：严重病例（如脑型）可采用二盐酸奎宁按体重 5～10mg/kg（最高量 500mg），加入氯化钠注射液 500ml 中静脉滴注，4 小时滴完，12 小时后重复一次，病情好转后改为口服。<br><br>Chez des adultes, dose usuelle : pour les cas graves (tels que le paludisem cérébral), prendre 5 à 10 mg/kg de dichlorhydrate de quinine en fonction du poids (dose maximale : 500mg), dissoudre dans 500ml de solution de chlorure de sodium, en perfusion pendant 4 h, répéter 12h après. Avec l'amélioration des symptômes, administrer par voie orale. |
| 剂型、规格<br>Les formes pharmaceutiques et les spécifications | 硫酸奎宁片：0.3g。<br>盐酸奎宁片：0.33g；0.12g。<br>二盐酸奎宁注射液：0.25g（1ml）；0.5g（1ml）；0.25g（10ml）。<br>复方奎宁注射液：每支 2ml，含盐酸奎宁 0.136g，咖啡因 0.034g，乌拉坦 0.028g。<br>Comprimés de sulfate de quinine : 0,3g.<br>Comprimés de chlorhydrate de quinine : 0,33g ou 0,12g.<br>Injection de dichlorhydrate de quinine : 0,25g (1ml), 0,5g (1ml) ou 0,25g (10ml).<br>Injection de composés de quinine : une solution de 2ml contient 0,136g de chlorhydrate de quinine, 0,034g de caféine et 0,028g d'uréthane. |
| 药品名称 Drug Names | 伯氨喹 Primaquine |
| 适应证<br>Les indications | 主要用于根治间日疟和控制疟疾传播，常与氯喹或乙胺嘧啶合用，对红内期作用较弱，对恶性疟红内期则完全无效，不能作为控制症状的药物应用。对某些疟原虫的红前期也有影响，但因需用剂量较大，已接近极量，不够安全，故也不能作为病因预防药应用。<br><br>Ce produit est utilisé dans le traitement radical du paludisme à vivax et dans le contrôle de la transmission du paludisme. Souvent utilisé en combinaison avec la chloroquine ou la pyriméthamine, il est peu efficace dans le traitement du paludisme au stade érythrocytaire, et complètement inefficace dans la lutte contre le paludisme à falciparum au stade érythrocytaire. Il ne peut pas être employé dans le contrôle des symptômes du paludisme. Bien qu'il soit un peu efficace dans la lutte contre le plasmodium au stade précoce, il ne peut pas être utilisé comme prévention du paludime, car cela nécessite une dose assez importante de sa part et que cela n'est pas sûr. |
| 用法、用量<br>Les modes d'emploi et la posologie | 成人常用量：口服，①根治间日疟：采用一次 13.2mg，一日 3 次，连服 7 日。②用于消灭恶性疟原虫配子体时采用一日 26.4mg，连服 3 日。<br><br>Chez des adultse, dose usuelle : par voie orale, ① pour le traitement radical du paludisme à vivax : 13,2mg par fois, 3 fois par jour, pendant 7 jours consécutifs.<br>② pour l'élimination des gamétocytes de plasmodium falciparum, 26,4mg par jour, pendant 3 jours consécutifs. |
| 剂型、规格<br>Les formes pharmaceutiques et les spécifications | 片剂：每片含磷酸伯氨喹 13.2mg 或 26.4mg（相当于伯氨喹盐基 7.5mg 或 15mg）。<br>Comprimés : 13,2mg ou 26,4mg de phosphate de primaquine par comprimé (équivalant à 7,5mg ou 15mg de primaquine base). |
| 药品名称 Drug Names | 乙胺嘧啶 Pyriméthamine |
| 适应证<br>Les indications | 主要用于预防疟疾，也可用于治疗弓形虫病，最近发现本品有抗药性虫株产生，合并应用其他抗疟药及磺胺类药物等，可提高其抗疟效果。<br><br>Ce produit est utilisé comme prévention du paludisme et comme traitement de la toxoplasmose. Récemment, on a déouvert des souches gondii résistant à la pyriméthamine. Il vaut mieux donc utiliser en même temps ce produit et d'autres médicaments antipaludiques et des sulfamides pour renforcer son efficacité. |

续 表

| 用法、用量<br>Les modes d'emploi et la posologie | ①预防疟疾：成人每次服25mg，每周1次，小儿0.9mg/kg，最高限于成人剂量。②抗复发治疗：成人每日服25～50mg，连用2日，小儿酌减（多与伯氨喹合用）。③治疗弓形虫病：每日50mg顿服，共1～3日（视耐受力而定），以后每日25mg，疗程4～6周。小儿1mg/kg，分2次服，1～3日后0.5mg/kg，分2次服，疗程4～6周。必要时，可重复1～2个疗程。<br><br>① Pour le prévention du paludisme : chez des adultes, 25mg par fois, 1 fois par semaine, chez des enfants, 0.9mg/kg, ne pas dépasser la dose chez des adultes. ② Pour La thérapie anti – rétrovirale : chez des adultes, 25 à 50 mg par jour, pendant 2 jours consécutifs, chez des enfants, diminuer la dose (utilisé souvent en association avec la primaquine). ③ Pour traiter la toxoplasmose : 50mg par jour, une fois par jour, pendant 1 à 3 jours (selon les cas), ensuite, 25mg par jour, pendant 4 à 6 semaines comme un traitement médical. Chez des enfants, 1 mg/kg, à travers 2 fois, 1 à 3 jours après, 0,5 mg/kg, à travers 2 fois, pendant 4 à 6 semines comme un traitement médical. S'il est nécessaire, reprendre 1 à 2 traitements médicaux. |
|---|---|
| 剂型、规格<br>Les formes pharmaceutiques et les spécifications | 片剂：每片6.25mg。<br>膜剂：每格6.25mg。<br><br>Comprimés : 6,25mg par comprimé.<br>Les filmogènes : 6,25mg par grille. |

7.2 抗阿米巴病药 Médicaments anti-amibiens

| 药品名称 Drug Names | 双碘喹啉 Diiodohydroxyquinoline |
|---|---|
| 适应证<br>Les indications | 用于治疗轻型或无明显症状的阿米巴痢疾。与依米丁、甲硝唑合用，治疗急性阿米巴痢疾及较顽固病例。对肠外阿米巴如肝脓肿无效。<br><br>Ce produit sert à traiter la dysenterie amibienne bénigne ou sans symptômes. Utilisé en assocation avec l'émétine et le métronidazole, il sert à traiter la dysenterie amibienne aigue et des cas difficiles. Il est inefficace dans la lutte contre l'amibe parentérale telle que les abcès du foie. |
| 用法、用量<br>Les modes d'emploi et la posologie | 成人常规剂量：口服给药，一次400～600mg，一日3次，连服14～21日，儿童常规剂量：口服给药，一次5～10mg/kg，用法同成人，重复治疗需间隔15～20日。<br><br>Chez des adultes, dose usuelle : par voie orale, 400 à 600 mg par fois, 3 fois par jour, pendant 14 à 21 jours consécutifs.Chez des enfants : par voie orale, 5 à 10 mg/kg par fois, les mêmes indications que chez des adultes, un intervalle de 15 à 20 jours entre deux traitements médicaux. |
| 剂型、规格<br>Les formes pharmaceutiques et les spécifications | 双碘喹啉片：每片200mg。<br><br>Comprimés : 200mg par comprimé. |

| 药品名称 Drug Names | 依米丁 Emétine |
|---|---|
| 适应证<br>Les indications | 适用于急性阿米巴痢疾急需控制症状者，肠外阿米巴病因其毒性大，已少用，由于消除急性症状效率较好，而根治作用低，故不适用于症状轻微的慢性阿米巴痢及无症状的带包囊者。此外，本品还可用于蝎子蜇伤。<br><br>Ce produit est applicable dans le contrôle des symptômes de la dysenterie amibienne aigue. Comme sa toxicité est importante, il est rarement employé dans le traitement de l'amibe parentérale. Compte tenu du fait qu'il est efficace dans l'élimination des symptômes aigus et peu efficace dans le traitement radical, il est peu applicable dans le traitement de la dysenterie amibienne chronique avec des symptômes bénins et des kystes asymptomatiques. En outre, ce produit peut être employé dans le traitement des piqûres de scorpion. |
| 用法、用量<br>Les modes d'emploi et la posologie | (1) 治阿米巴痢：体重60kg以下按每日1mg/kg计（60kg以上者，剂量仍按60kg计），每日1次或分2次做深部皮下注射，连用6～10日为1个疗程，如未愈，30日后再用第二疗程。<br>(2) 治蝎子蜇伤：以本品3%～6%注射液少许注入蜇孔内即可。<br><br>(1) Pour traiter l'amibiase : chez des patients moins de 60kg, 1 mg/kg par jour (chez des patients plus de 60kg, prendre la même dose que chez des patients de 60kg), injection sous-cutanée profonde, 1 à 2 fois par jour, pendant 6 à 10 jours comme un traitement médical. S'il le patient ne se guérit pas, 30 jours après, continuer le deuxième traitement médical.<br>(2) Pour traiter les piqûres de scorpion : injecter un peu de solution d'émétine à 3 % à 6 % dans le trou de piqûre. |

**续　表**

| 剂型、规格<br>Les formes pharmaceutiques et les spécifications | 注射液：每支 30mg（1ml）；60mg（1ml）。<br>Injection : 30mg (1ml) ou 60mg (1ml) par solution. |
| --- | --- |

### 7.3　抗滴虫病药 Médicaments anti-trichomonase

| 药品名称 Drug Names | 甲硝唑 Métronidazole |
| --- | --- |
| 适应证<br>Les indications | 用于治疗厌氧杆菌引起的产后盆腔炎、败血症、牙周炎等。还可用于治疗贾第鞭毛虫病、酒糟鼻。用于阑尾、结肠手术、妇产科手术，可降低或避免手术感染。也可用于治疗阿米巴痢和阿米巴肝脓肿，疗效与依米丁相仿。<br><br>Ce produit sert à traiter l'inflammation pelvienne post-partum, la septicémie et la parodontite causées par les bactéries anaérobies.Il est aussi applicable dans le traitement de la giardiase et de la rosacée.Appliqué dans l'opération chirurgicale sur l'appendice, le côlon et la chirurgie gynécologique, il permet de réduire ou d'éliminer le risque de l'infection. Il peut être aussi utilisé comme traitement dela dysenterie amibienne et des abcès du foie amibiens, avec un effet similaire à l'émétine. |
| 用法、用量<br>Les modes d'emploi et la posologie | ①治滴虫病：成人一日 3 次，每次服200mg，另每晚以200mg栓剂放入阴道内，连用 7～10 日，为保证疗效，需男女同治。②治阿米巴病：成人一日 3 次，每次 400～800mg（大剂量宜慎用），5～7 日为 1 个疗程。③治贾第鞭毛虫病：常用量每次400mg，一日 3 次口服，疗程 5～7 日。④治疗由厌氧菌引起的产后盆腔感染、败血症、骨髓炎等：一般口服 200～400mg，一日 600～1200mg，也可静脉滴注。⑤治酒糟鼻：口服200mg，一日 2～3 次，配合 2% 甲硝唑霜外擦，一日 3 次，一疗程 3 周。<br><br>① Pour traiter la trichomonase : chez des adultes, 3 fois par jour, 200mg par fois, mettre autre 200mg en suppositoire dans le vagin le soir, pendant 7 à 10 jours consécutifs pour assurer l'efficacité. Il faut que les couples prennent en même temps les médicaments. ② Pour traiter l'amibiase : chez des adultes, 3 fois par jour, 400 à 800 mg par fois (soyez prudent avec la dose importante), pendant 5 à 7 jours comme un traitement médical. ③ Pour traiter la giardiase : dose usuelle, 400mg par fois, 3 fois par jour, par voie orale, pendant 5 à 7 jours comme un traitement médical. ④ Pour traiter l'inflammation pelvienne post-partum, la septicémie et l'ostéomyélite causées par les bactéries anaérobies : 200 à 400mg par voie orale, 600 à 1 200mg par jour, ou en perfusion. ⑤ Pour traiter la rosacée : 200mg par voie orale, 2 à 3 fois par jour, frotter de crème de métronidazole à 2 % pour un usage externe, 3 fois par jour, pendant 3 semaines comme un traitement. |
| 剂型、规格<br>Les formes pharmaceutiques et les spécifications | 片剂：每片 200mg。<br>阴道泡腾片：每片 200mg。<br>栓剂：每个 0.5g；1g。<br>注射液：50mg（10ml）；100mg（20ml）；500mg（100ml）；1.25g（250mg）；500mg（250ml）。<br>甲硝唑葡萄糖注射液：甲硝唑 0.5g+ 葡萄糖 12.5g（250ml）。<br><br>Comprimés : 200mg par comprimé.<br>Comprimés effervescents vaginaux : 200mg par comprimé.<br>Suppositoires : 0,5g ou 1g par suppositoire.<br>Injection : 50mg (10ml), 100mg (20ml), 500mg (100ml), 1,25g (250mg) ou 500mg (250ml).<br>Injection de glucose de métronidazole : 0,5g de métronidazole + 12,5g de glucose (250ml). |

### 7.4　抗血吸虫病药 Médicaments anti-schistosomiase

| 药品名称 Drug Names | 吡喹酮 Praziquantel |
| --- | --- |
| 适应证<br>Les indications | 主要用于治疗血吸虫病。其特点为：剂量小（约为现用一般药物剂量的1/10），疗程短（从现用药物的 20 日或 10 日缩短为 1～2 日）、不良反应轻、由较高的近期疗效。血吸虫病患者经本品治疗后，半年粪检虫卵转阴率为97.7%～99.4%,由于本品对毛蚴、尾蚴也有杀灭效力，故也用于预防血吸虫感染。也有以本品治疗脑囊虫病。<br><br>Ce produit sert souvent à traiter la schistosomiase. Ses avantages : dose peu importante (1/10 de la dose usuelle d'autres médicaments), cours abrégé (1 à 2 jours contre 10 à 20 jours pour des médicaments en usage), peu d'effets indésirables, belle performance enregistrée ces derniers jours. Chez des patients atteints de schistosomiase, le taux de guérison est de 97,7% à 99,4% après six mois de traitement. Comme il est efficace dans la lutte contre les miracidiums et les cercaires, il est aussi appliqué dans la prévention de la schistosomiase. Il sert aussi à traiter la neurocysticercose. |

**续　表**

| | |
|---|---|
| 用法、用量<br>Les modes d'emploi et la posologie | 口服治疗血吸虫病：一次10mg/kg，一日3次，急性血吸虫病连服4日，慢性血吸虫病连服2日。皮肤涂擦1%浓度吡喹酮，12小时内对血吸虫尾蚴有可靠的防护作用。治脑囊虫病，每日20mg/kg，体重＞60kg者，以60kg计量，分3次服，9日为1个疗程，总量180mg/kg，疗程间隔3～4个月。<br><br>Par voie orale, pour traiter la schistosomiase : 10 mg/kg par fois, 3 fois par jour, pour la schistosomiase aigue, pendant 4 jours consécutifs, pour la schistosomiase chronique, pendant 2 jours consécutifs. Frotter la peau de praziquantel à 1 %, ce qui permet de se défendre de cercaires de schistosome pendant 12h. Pour traiter la neurocysticercose, 20 mg/kg par jour, chez des patients plus de 60kg, prendre la même dose que chez des patients de 60kg, à travers 3 fois, pendant 9 jours comme un traitement médical, la dose totale : 180 mg/kg. L'intervalle entre deux traitements : 3 à 4 mois. |
| 剂型、规格<br>Les formes pharmaceutiques et les spécifications | 胶囊剂：每粒25mg；50mg。<br>片剂：每片25mg。<br>Capsules : 25mg ou 50mg par capsule.<br>Comprimés : 25mg par comprimé. |

### 7.5　抗其他吸虫病 Médicaments autres aitiparasites

| 药品名称 Drug Names | 硫氯酚 Bithionol |
|---|---|
| 适应证<br>Les indications | 对肺吸虫囊蚴有明显杀灭作用，临床用于肺吸虫病、牛肉绦虫病、姜片虫病。<br>Ce produit est très efficace dans la lutte contre les paragonimus métacercaires. Il est utilisé dans les cliniques comme traitement de la paragonimose, du ténia saginata et du fasciolopsiasis. |
| 用法、用量<br>Les modes d'emploi et la posologie | 口服：每日50～60mg/kg（成人与小儿同）。对肺吸虫病及华支睾吸虫病可将全日量分3次服，隔日服药，疗程总量30～45g，对姜片虫病，可于睡前半空腹将2～3g药物1次服完；对牛肉绦虫病，可将总量（50mg/kg）分2次服，间隔半小时，服完第二次药后，3～4小时服泻药。<br><br>Par voie orale : 50 à 60 mg/kg par jour, tant chez des adultes que chez des enfants. Pour traiter la paragonimose et la clonorchiase, administrer la même dose à travers 3 fois, tous les 2 jours, la dose totale : 30 à 45g. Pour traiter le fasciolopsiasis, prendre 2 à 3g, une seule fois, avant le sommeil, semi- jeûne ; pour taiter le ténia saginata, prendre 50 mg/kg à travers 2 fois, avec un intervalle de 30 minutes, 3 à 4 h après la deuxième administration, prendre le laxatif. |
| 剂型、规格<br>Les formes pharmaceutiques et les spécifications | 片剂：每片0.25g。<br>胶囊剂：每粒0.5g。<br>Comprimés : 0,25g par comprimé.<br>Capsules : 0,5g par capsule. |

### 7.6　抗丝虫病 Anti-filarial

| 药品名称 Drug Names | 乙胺嗪 Diethylcarbamazine |
|---|---|
| 适应证<br>Les indications | 用于马来丝虫病和斑氏丝虫病的治疗。<br>Ce produit sert à traiter la filariose de Malaisie et la filariose de Bancroft. |
| 用法、用量<br>Les modes d'emploi et la posologie | ①口服：1次0.1～0.2g，一日0.3～0.6g，分2～3次服用，7～14日为1个疗程。②大剂量短程疗法：治马来丝虫病可用本品1.5g，一次顿服，或与一日内分2次服；治斑氏丝虫病总量3g，与2～3日分服完，本法不良反应较重。③预防：于流行区按每日5～6mg/kg服药，服6～7日，或按上量每周或每个月服一日，直至总量达70～90mg/kg为止。<br><br>① Par voie orale : 0,1 à 0,2g par fois, 0,3 à 0,6 g par jour, à travers 2 à 3 fois, pendant 7 à 14 jours comme un traitement médical. ② La thérapie à court terme avec une dose importante : Pour traiter la filariose de Malaisie, 1,5g, une fois par jour, ou à travers 2 fois ; pour traiter la filariose de Bancroft, 3g, en 2 à 3 jours, à travers plusieurs fois, cette thérapie a un effet indésirable évident. ③ Pour la prévention : dans les zones d'endémie, 5 à 6 mg/kg par jour, pendant 6 à 7 jours consécutifs, ou la même dose, administrée une fois toutes les semines ou tous les mois, pour atteindre 70 à 90 mg/kg au total. |

**续　表**

| 剂型、规格<br>Les formes pharmaceutiques et les spécifications | 片剂：每片 50mg；100mg。<br>Comprimés : 50mg ou 100mg par comprimé. |
|---|---|

## 7.7　抗利什曼原虫药 Médicaments anti-Leishmania

| 药品名称 Drug Names | 葡萄糖酸锑钠 Stibogluconate sodique |
|---|---|
| 适应证<br>Les indications | 用于黑热病病因治疗，近期疗效可达99%，2年复发率低于10%，复发病例可再用本品治疗。<br>Ce produit est utilsé comme traitement dukala-azar, avec un taux de réussite à 99 % et un taux de récurrence de 2 ans à moins de 10%. Il est encore applicable dans le traitement de la récurrence. |
| 用法、用量<br>Les modes d'emploi et la posologie | 肌内或静脉注射。①一般成人 1 次 1.9g（6ml），一日 1 次，连用 6～10 日；或总剂量按体重 90～130mg/kg（以 50kg 为限），等分 6～10 次，一日 1 次。②小儿总剂量按体重 150～200mg/kg，分为 6 次，一日 1 次。③对敏感性较差的虫株感染者，可重复 1～2 个疗程，间隔 10～14 日。④对全身情况较差者，可每周注射 2 次，疗程 3 周或更长。⑤对近期曾接受锑剂治疗者，可减少剂量。<br>Injection par voie IM ou IV.<br>① Chez des adultes, 1,9g (6ml) par fois, 1 fois par jour, pendant 6 à 10 jours consécutifs ; ou la dose totale administrée en fonction du poids : 90 à 130 mg/kg (50kg comme la limite), à travers 6 à 10 fois, une fois par jour. ② Chez des enfants, la dose totale administrée en fonction du poids : 150 à 200 mg/kg, à travers 6 fois, une fois par jour. ③ Pour traiter les infections causées par des souches d'insectes moins sensibles, reprendre 1 à 2 traitements médicaux, avec un intervalle de 10 à 14 jours. ④ Chez des patients systématiquement pauvres, injection 2 fois par semaine, pendant 3 semaines ou plus. ⑤ Chez des patients ayant réçu récemment le traitement de l'antimoine, diminuer la dose. |
| 剂型、规格<br>Les formes pharmaceutiques et les spécifications | 注射液：每支 6ml，含葡萄糖酸锑钠 1.9g，约相当于五价锑 0.6g。<br>Injection : 6ml par solution, qui contient 1,9g de gluconate d'antimoine sodique, équivalant à 0,6g d'antimoine pentavalent. |

## 7.8　驱肠虫药 Anthelminthiques

| 药品名称 Drug Names | 哌嗪 Pipérazine |
|---|---|
| 适应证<br>Les indications | 用于肠蛔虫病、蛔虫所致的不全性肠梗阻和胆道蛔虫病较痛的缓解期。此外亦可用于驱蛲虫。<br>Ce produit est utilisé comme traitemetn de l'ascaris intestinal, de l'obstruction intestinale incomplète causée par les ascaris, et de l'ascaris des voies biliaires au stade de rémission. Il sert aussi à traiter les oxyures. |
| 用法、用量<br>Les modes d'emploi et la posologie | （1）枸橼酸哌嗪：驱蛔虫，成人 3～3.5g，睡前一次服，连服 2 日，小儿每日 100～160mg/kg，一日量不得超过 3g，连服 2 日，一般不必服泻药；驱蛲虫，成人每次 1～1.2g，一日 2～2.5g，连服 7～10 日，小儿一日 60mg/kg，分 2 次服，每日总量不超过 2g，连服 7～10 日。<br>（2）磷酸哌嗪：驱蛔虫，一日 2.5～3g，睡前 1 次服，连服 2 日，小儿每日 80～130mg/kg，一日量不得超过 2.5g，连服 2 日；驱蛲虫，每次 0.8～1g，一日 1.5～2g，连服 7～10 日，小儿一日 50mg/kg，分 2 次服，一日总量不超过 2g，连服 7～10 日。<br>(1) Le citrate de pipérazine : pour lutter contre les ascaris, chez des adultes, 3 à 3,5g, une fois avant le sommeil, pendant 2 jours consécutifs, chez des enfants, 100 à 160 mg/kg par jour, ne pas dépasser 3g par jour, pendant 2 jours consécutifs, généralement, il n'est pas nécessaire de prendre le laxatif.<br>Pour lutter contre oxyures, chez des adultes, 1 à 1,2 g par fois, 2 à 2,5g par jour, pendant 7 à 10 jours consécutifs, chez des enfants, 60 mg/kg par jour, à travers 2 fois, ne pas dépasser 2g par jour, pendant 7 à 10 jours consécutifs.<br>(2) Le phosphate de pipérazine : pour lutter contre les ascaris, 2,5 à 3g par jour, une fois avant le sommeil, pendant 2 jours consécutifs, chez des enfants, 80 à 130 mg/kg par jour, ne pas dépasser 2,5g par jour, pendant 2 jours consécutifs ; pour lutter contre les oxyures, 0,8 à 1g par fois, 1,5 à 2g par jour, pendant 7 à 10 jours consécutifs, chez des enfants, 50 mg/kg par jour, à travers 2 fois, ne pas dépasser 2g par jour, pendant 7 à 10 jours consécutifs. |

续　表

| 剂型、规格<br>Les formes pharmaceutiques et les spécifications | 枸橼酸哌嗪片：每片 0.25g；0.5g。<br>枸橼酸哌嗪糖浆：每 100ml 含本品 16g。<br>磷酸哌嗪片：每片 0.2g；0.5g。<br><br>Comprimés de citrate de pipérazine : 0,25g ou 0,5g par comprimé.<br>Sirops de citrate de pipérazine : 16g de produit par 100ml.<br>Comprimés de phosphate de pipérazine : 0,2g ou 0,5g par comprimé. |
|---|---|
| **药品名称 Drug Names** | 左旋咪唑 Lévamisole |
| 适应证<br>Les indications | 主要用于驱蛔虫及钩虫。由于本品单剂量有效率较高，故适于集体治疗，可于噻嘧啶合用治疗严重钩虫感染；与噻苯唑或恩波吡维铵合用治疗肠线虫混合感染；与枸橼酸乙胺嗪先后序贯应用于抗丝虫感染。<br><br>Ce produit sert à lutter contre les ascaris et les ankylostomes. Comme il est hautement efficace avec une dose unique, il est applicable dans la thérapie de groupe. Utilisé en combinaison avec le pyrante, il sert à traiter l'infection grave par l'ankylostome ; utilisé en association avec le thiabendazole, il sert à lutter contre l'infection intestinale mixte parles nématodes ; utilisé en combinaison avec la diethylcarbamazine citrate, il sert à lutter contre l'infection par la filariose. |
| 用法、用量<br>Les modes d'emploi et la posologie | ①驱虫病：口服，a. 成人 1.5 ～ 2.5mg/kg，空腹或睡前顿服；b. 小儿剂量为 2 ～ 3mg/kg。②驱钩虫：口服，1.5 ～ 2.5mg/kg，每晚 1 次，连服 3 日。③治疗丝虫病：4 ～ 6mg/kg，分 3 次服，连服 3 日。<br><br>① Pour le déparasitage : par voie orale, chez des adultes, 1,5 à 2,5 mg/kg, l'estomac vide ou avant le sommeil, une fois par jour ; chez des enfants, 2 à 3 mg/kg. ② Pour lutter contre les ankylostomes : par voie orale, 1,5 à 2,5 mg/kg, 1 fois par soir, pendant 3 jours consécutifs. ③ Pour lutter contre la filariose : 4 à 6 mg/kg, à travers 3 fois, pendant 3 jours consécutifs. |
| 剂型、规格<br>Les formes pharmaceutiques et les spécifications | 片剂：每片 25mg；50mg。<br>肠溶片：每片 25mg；50mg。<br>颗粒剂：每 1g 含盐酸左旋咪唑 5mg。<br>糖浆：0.8g（100ml）；4g（500ml）；16g（200ml）。<br>搽剂：为左旋咪唑的 0.7% 二甲亚砜溶液或其硼酸酒精溶液。<br><br>Comprimés : 25mg ou 50mg par comprimé.<br>Comprimés à enrobage entérique : 25mg ou 50mg par comprimé.<br>Granules : 1g de produit contient 5mg de chlorhydrate de lévamisole.<br>Sirops : 0,8g (100ml), 4g (500ml) ou 16g (200ml).<br>Liniment : la solution de sulfoxyde de dimé de lévamisole à 0,7 % ou la solution d'alcool de l'acide borique de lévamisole. |
| **药品名称 Drug Names** | 阿苯达唑 Albendazole |
| 适应证<br>Les indications | 用于驱除蛔虫、蛲虫、钩虫、鞭虫，也可用于家畜的驱虫。<br><br>Ce produit sert à lutter contre les ascaris, les oxyures, les ankylostomes et les trichures. Il est aussi applicable dans le déparasitage chez le bétail. |
| 用法、用量<br>Les modes d'emploi et la posologie | 口服，驱钩虫、蛔虫、蛲虫、鞭虫，0.4g 顿服。2 周岁以上小儿，单纯蛲虫、单纯蛔虫感染，0.2g 顿服。治疗囊虫病：每天 15 ～ 20mg/kg，分 2 次服用。10 日为 1 个疗程。停药 15 ～ 20 日后，可进行第 2 疗程治疗。一般为 2 ～ 3 疗程。必要时可重复治疗。其他寄生虫如粪类圆线虫等，每日服 400mg，连服 6 日。必要时重复给药 1 次。12 岁以下儿童，用量减半，服法同成人或遵医嘱。<br><br>Par voie orale, pour lutter contre les ascaris, les oxyures, les ankylostomes et les trichures, 0,4g, une fois par jour. Chez des enfants plus de 2 ans, pour les infections simples causées par les oxyures et les ascaris, 0,2g, une fois par jour. Pour traiter la cysticercose : 15 à 20 mg/kg par jour, à travers 2 fois. Un traitement médical dure 10 jours. 15 à 20 jours après l'arrêt de l'administration, on peut continuer le deuxième traitement médical. En général, il faut 2 à 3 traitements médicaux. En cas besoin, il est permissible de reprendre le traitement. Pour lutter contre d'autres parasites tels que les stercoralis, 400mg par jour, pendant 6 jours consécutifs. S'il est nécessaire, l'administration répétée pour une fois. Chez des enfants moins de 12 ans, diminuer de moitié la dose, mêmes indications que chez des adultes ou suivre les ordonnances. |

**续　表**

| 剂型、规格<br>Les formes pharmaceutiques et les spécifications | 片（胶囊剂）：每片（粒）100mg；200mg。<br>干糖浆：每袋 200mg。<br>Comprimés (capsules) : 100mg ou 200mg par comprimé ou par capsule.<br>Sirops secs : 200mg par sachet. |
|---|---|

### 8. 主要作用于中枢神经系统的药物 Médicaments Action Principale Système Nerveux Central

#### 8.1　中枢神经系统兴奋药 Médicaments excitation du système nerveux central

| 药品名称 Drug Names | 尼可刹米 Nicéthamide |
|---|---|
| 适应证<br>Les indications | 用于中枢性呼吸及循环衰竭、麻醉药及其中枢抑制药的中毒。<br>Ce produit sert à traiter l'insuffisance respiratoire et circulatoire centrale ainsi que l'intoxication par lenarcotiqueet l'inhibiteur du système nerveux central. |
| 用法、用量<br>Les modes d'emploi et la posologie | 常用量：皮下注射、肌内或静脉注射，每次 0.25～0.5g。必要时 1～2 小时重复用药。极量：皮下、肌内或静脉注射，一次 1.25g。6 个月以下，婴儿 75mg/ 次，一岁 125mg/ 次，4～7 岁 175mg/ 次。<br>Dose usuelle : injection sous-cutanée, IM ou IV, 0,25 à 0,5g par fois. En cas de besoin, encore une fois toutes les 1 à 2h. Dose maximale : injeciton sous-cutanée, IM ou IV, 1,25g par fois. Chez des bébés moins de 6 mois, 75mg par fois, chez 1an, 125mg par fois, chez de 4 à 7 ans, 175 mg par fois. |
| 剂型、规格<br>Les formes pharmaceutiques et les spécifications | 注射液：每支 0.375g（1.5ml）；0.5g（2ml）；0.25g（1ml）。<br>Injection : 0,375g (1,5ml), 0,5g (2ml) ou 0,25g (1ml) par solution. |

| 药品名称 Drug Names | 洛贝林 Lobéline |
|---|---|
| 适应证<br>Les indications | 用于新生儿窒息、一氧化碳引起的窒息、吸入麻醉剂及其他中枢抑制药（如阿片、巴比妥类）的中毒及肺炎、白喉等疾病引起的呼吸衰竭。<br>Ce produit sert à traiter l'asphyxie des nouveau-nés, la suffocation causée par le monoxyde de carbone, l'intoxication par le narcotique et l'inhibiteur du système nerveux central (tel que les opiacés et les barbituriques), ainsi que l'insuffisance respiratoire causée par la pneumonie et la diphtérie. |
| 用法、用量<br>Les modes d'emploi et la posologie | 皮下注射或肌内注射：常用量，成人 1 次 3～10mg（极量：1 次 20mg，1 日 50mg）；儿童 1 次 1～3mg。静脉注射：成人 1 次 3mg（极量：1 次 6mg，1 日 20mg）；儿童 1 次 0.3～3mg。必要时每 30 分钟可重复 1 次。静脉注射需缓慢。新生儿窒息可注入脐静脉，用量为 3mg。<br>Injection par voie sous-cutanée ou IM : dose usuelle, chez des adultes, 3 à 10mg par fois, (dose maximale, 20mg par fois, 50mg par jour) ; chez des enfants, 1 à 3mg par fois. Administratio par voie IV : 3mg par fois chez des adultes (dose maximale, 6mg par fois, 20mg par jour) ; chez des enfants, 0,3 à 3mg par fois. En cas de besoin, toutes les 30minutes. Injection par voie IV lente. En cas d'asphyxie des nouveau-nés, permissible d'injecter dans la voie veine ombilicale, 3mg. |
| 剂型、规格<br>Les formes pharmaceutiques et les spécifications | 注射液：每支 3mg（1ml）；10mg（1ml）。<br>Injection : 3mg (1ml) ou 10mg (1ml) par solution. |

| 药品名称 Drug Names | 戊四氮 Pentétrazole |
|---|---|
| 适应证<br>Les indications | 用于急性传染病、麻醉药及巴比妥类药物中毒时引起的呼吸抑制，急性循环衰竭。安全范围小，现已少用。<br>Ce produit sert à traiter la dépression respiratoire causée par les maladies infectueuses aigues et par l'intexication du narcotique et des barbituriques. Il est aussi applicable dans le traitement de l'insuffisance respiratoire aigue. Il est rarement utilisé aujourd'hui. |
| 用法、用量<br>Les modes d'emploi et la posologie | 皮下注射、肌内注射、静脉注射，每次 0.05～0.1g，每 2 小时 1 次。极量 1 日 0.3g。<br>Injection par voie sous-cutanée, IM ou IV, 0,05 à 0,1g par fois, toutes les 2h. Ne pas dépasser 0,3g par jour. |

**续 表**

| 剂型、规格<br>Les formes pharmaceutiques et les spécifications | 注射液：每支 0.1g（1ml）；0.3g（3ml）。<br>Injection : 0,1g (1ml) ou 0,3g (3ml) par solution. |
|---|---|
| **药品名称 Drug Names** | 贝美格 Bémégride |
| 适应证<br>Les indications | 用于解救巴比妥类、格鲁米特、水合氯醛等药物的中毒。应用于加速硫喷妥钠麻醉后的恢复。<br>Ce produit est utilisé dans le sauvetage de l'intoxication par les barbituriques, la glutéthimide et l'hydrate de chloral. Il est aussi applicable dans l'accélécation de la récupération après l'anesthésie par thiopental. |
| 用法、用量<br>Les modes d'emploi et la posologie | 因本品作用迅速，多采用静脉滴注，作用维持 10～20 分钟。常用量 0.5%10ml（50mg），用 5% 葡萄糖注射液稀释静脉滴注。宜可静脉注射，每 3～5 分钟注射 50mg，治病情改善或出现中毒症状为止。<br>Comme ce produit a un effet rapide, on l'administre souvent en perfusion, pendant 10 à 20 miniutes. Dose usuelle, 10ml (50mg) à 0,5 %, utiliser la solution de glucose à 5 % pour la dilution. Aussi possible de l'administer par voie IV, 50mg toutes les 3 à 5 minutes, jusqu'au soulagement des symptômes ou à la parition des symtômes d'intoxication. |
| 剂型、规格<br>Les formes pharmaceutiques et les spécifications | 注射液：每支 50mg（10ml）。<br>Injection : 50mg (10ml) par solution. |
| **药品名称 Drug Names** | 咖啡因 Caféine |
| 适应证<br>Les indications | （1）解救因急性感染中毒、催眠药、麻醉药、镇痛药中毒引起的呼吸、循环衰竭。<br>（2）与溴化物合用，使大脑皮质兴奋、抑制过程恢复平衡，用于神经官能症。<br>（3）与阿司匹林、对乙酰氨基酚制成复方制剂用于一般性头痛；与麦角胺合用治疗偏头痛。<br>（4）用于小儿多动症（注意力缺陷综合征）。<br>（5）治疗未成熟新生儿呼吸暂停或阵发性呼吸困难。<br>(1) Sauver l'insuffisance respiratoire et circulatoire causée par l'intoxication de l'infection aigue, du narcotique, des hypnotiques et des analgésiques.<br>(2) Utilisé en association avec le bromure, il sert à traiter la névrose, à rétablir l'équilibre entre l'excitabilité corticale et son inhibition.<br>(3) Utilisé en combinaison avec l'aspirine et l'acétaminophène pour devenir la préparation complexe, il sert à traiter céphalée générale ; en association avec l'ergotamine, il sert à traiter la migraine.<br>(4) Traiter le trouble du déficit de l'attention avec ou sans hyperactivité (TDAH)<br>(5) Traiter l'apnée ou la dyspnée paroxystique chez des nouveau-nés. |
| 用法、用量<br>Les modes d'emploi et la posologie | ①口服。常用量：一次 0.1～0.3g，一日 0.3～1.0g；极量：一次 0.4g，一日 1.5g。②解救中枢抑制：肌内注射或皮下注射安钠咖注射液（详见制剂项下）。常用量：皮下或肌内注射，1 次 1～2ml，一日 2～4ml；极量皮下或肌内注射，1 次 3ml，一日 12ml。③调节大脑皮质活动：口服咖溴合剂，每日 10～15ml，一日 3 次，餐后服。<br>① Par voie orale. Dose usuelle : 0,1 à 0,3g par fois, 0,3 à 1,0g par jour ; dose maximale : 0,4g par fois, 1,5g par jour. ② Pour sauver inhibition centrale : injection de caféine-sodium benzoate par voie IM ou sous-cutanée, (cf. préparations). Dose usuelle : injection sous-cutanée ou IM, 1 à 2 ml par fois, 2 à 4 ml par jour ; dose maximale, 3 ml par fois, 12ml par jour. ③ Pour le réglage de l'activité du cortex cérébral, prendre le bromure de caféine par voie orale, 10 à 15ml par jour, 3 fois par jour, après le repas. |
| 剂型、规格<br>Les formes pharmaceutiques et les spécifications | 片剂：每片 30mg。<br>Comprimés : 30mg par comprimé. |

**续　表**

| 药品名称 Drug Names | 甲氯芬酯 Méclofénoxate |
|---|---|
| 适应证<br>Les indications | 　用于外伤性昏迷、新生儿缺氧、儿童遗尿症、意识障碍、老年性精神病、酒精中毒及某些中枢和周围神经症状。<br><br>　Ce produit sert à traiter le coma traumatique, l'hypoxie néonatale, l'énurésie des enfants, l'inconscience, la psychose sénile, l'alcoolisme et certains symptômes des nerveux centraux et périphériques. |
| 用法、用量<br>Les modes d'emploi et la posologie | 　① 口服，成人 1 次 0.1～0.3g，1 日 0.3～0.9g；最大剂量可达一日 1.5g。儿童 1 次 100mg，一日 3 次。② 肌内注射或静脉滴注：成人 1 次 0.25g，一日 1～3 次。溶于 5% 葡萄糖溶液 250～500ml 中供静脉滴注。新生儿可注入脐静脉。小儿每次 60～100mg，一日 2 次。新生儿缺氧症，一次 0.06g，每 2 小时 1 次。<br><br>　① Par voie orale : chez des adultes, 0,1 à 0,3g par fois, 0,3 à 0,9 g par jour ; dose maximale, 1,5g par jour. Chez des adultes, 100mg par fois, 3 fois par jour. ② Par voie IM ou par voie IV en perfusion : chez des adultes, 0,25g par fois, 1 à 3 fois par jour. Dissoudre le produit dans 250 à 500ml de solution de glucose à 5 %. Chez des nouveaunés, possible d'injecter dans la voie veine ombilicale. Chez des enfants, 60 à 100mg par fois, 2 fois par jour. En cas d'hypoxie néonatale, 0,06g par fois, toutes les 2h. |
| 剂型、规格<br>Les formes pharmaceutiques et les spécifications | 　胶囊剂：每粒 0.1g；注射用盐酸甲氯芬酯：每支 0.1g；0.25g。<br>Capsules : 0,1g par capsule.<br>Méclofenoxate d'acide chlorhydrique pour injection : 0,1g ou 0,25g par solution. |
| 药品名称 Drug Names | 乙哌立松 Epérisone |
| 适应证<br>Les indications | 　可用于改善下列疾病的肌紧张状态：颈肩腕综合征，肩周炎，腰痛症；也可用于改善下列疾病所致的痉挛性麻痹：脑血管障碍，痉挛性脊髓麻痹，颈椎病，手术后遗症（包括脑、脊髓肿瘤），外伤后遗症（脊髓损伤、头部外伤），肌萎缩性侧索硬化症，婴儿大脑性轻瘫，脊髓小脑变性症，脊髓血管障碍，亚急性脊髓神经症（SMON）及其他脑脊髓疾病。<br><br>　Ce produit sert à soulager la tension musculaire de ces maladies suivantes : TMS des membres supérieurs (cou, épaule, coude, poignet, main), lapériarthrite de l'épaule, la lombalgie. Il sert à traiter la paralysie spastique causée par des maladies suivantes : les troubles cérébro-vasculaires, la paralysie spinale spasmodique, l'arthrose cervicale, les complications chirurgicales (y compris les tumeurs cérébrales et les tumeurs de la moelle épinière), les complications des traumatismes séquelles ( les lésions de la moelle épinière et les traumatismes crâniens), la sclérose latérale amyotrophique, la parésie cérébrale infantile, la dégénérescence spino-cérébelleuse, les troubles vasculaires de la colonne vertébrale, la myélo-optico-neuropathie subaiguë (S.M.O.N.) et d'autre troubles de la moelle épinière. |
| 用法、用量<br>Les modes d'emploi et la posologie | 　餐后口服。通常成人一次 50mg（1 片），一日 3 次。<br>Après le repas. En général, chez des adultes, 50mg (1 comprimé) par fois, 3 fois par jour. |
| 剂型、规格<br>Les formes pharmaceutiques et les spécifications | 　片剂：每片 50mg。<br>Comprimés : 50mg par comprimé. |
| 药品名称 Drug Names | 细胞色素 C　Cytochrome C |
| 适应证<br>Les indications | 　用于各种组织缺氧的急救或辅助治疗，如一氧化碳中毒、催眠药中毒、新生儿窒息、严重休克期缺氧、麻醉及肺部疾病引起的呼吸困难、高山缺氧、脑缺氧及心脏疾病引起的缺氧，但疗效有时不显著。<br><br>　Ce produit est utilisé dans les premiers soins ou le traitement adjuvant de l'hypoxie tissulaire, y compris l'empoisonnement au monoxyde de carbone, l'intoxication hypnotique, l'asphyxie néonatale, l'hypoxie de choc grave, la dyspnée provoquée par l'anesthésie et des maladies pulmonaires, l'hypoxie alpine, l'hypoxie cérébrale et l'anoxie causée par la cardiopathie. Mais il n'est pas toujours efficace. |

| 用法、用量<br>Les modes d'emploi et la posologie | 静脉注射或滴注：成人每次 15～30mg，每日 30～60mg。儿童用量酌减。静脉注射时，加 25% 葡萄糖注射液 20ml 混匀后，缓慢注射。亦可用 5%～10% 葡萄糖注射液或生理盐水稀释后静脉滴注。粉针（冻干型）用 25% 葡萄糖注射液 20ml 或 5% 葡萄糖注射液或灭菌生理盐水溶解后滴注。<br><br>Administration par voie IV ou par voie IV en perfusion : chez des adultes, 15 à 30 mg par fois, 30 à 60 mg par jour. chez des enfants, dose moins importante. Injection par voie IV, ajouter 20ml de solution de glucose à 25 %, injection lente. En perfusion, utiliser la solution de glucose de 5 % à 10 % ou la solution saline pour la dilution. En poudre (lyophilisation), utiliser 20ml de solution de glucose à 25 %, la solution de glucose à 5 % ou la solution saline pour la dilution. |
|---|---|
| 剂型、规格<br>Les formes pharmaceutiques et les spécifications | 注射液：每支 15mg（2ml）。<br>注射用细胞色素 C：每支 15mg。<br>Injection : 15mg (2ml) par solution.<br>Le cytochrome C pour injection : 15mg par solution. |

### 8.2　镇痛药 Analgésiques

| 药品名称 Drug Names | 吗啡 Morphine |
|---|---|
| 适应证<br>Les indications | ①镇痛：现仅用于创伤、手术、烧伤等引起的剧痛。②心肌梗死。③心源性哮喘。④麻醉前给药。<br>① L'analgésique : seulement utilisée dans la douleur provoquée par un traumatisme, une chirurgie, des brûlures. ② L'infarctus du myocarde. ③ L'asthme cardiaque. ④ L'administration avant l'anesthésie. |
| 用法、用量<br>Les modes d'emploi et la posologie | （1）常用量：口服，1 次 5～15mg，1 日 15～60mg；皮下注射，1 次 5～15mg，1 日 15～40mg；静脉注射，5～10mg。<br>（2）极量：口服，1 次 30mg，1 日 100mg；皮下注射，1 次 20mg，1 日 60mg；硬膜外腔注射，一次极量 5mg，用于手术后镇痛。<br>(1) Dose usuelle : par voie orale, 5 à 15mg par fois, 15 à 60mg par jour ; injection sous-cutanée, 5 à 15mg par fois, 15 à 40 mg par jour ; injection par voie IV, 5 à 10mg.<br>(2) Dose maximale : par voie orale, 30mg par fois, 100mg par jour ; injection sous-cutanée, 20mg par fois, 60mg par jour ; injection épidurale, 5mg par fois, pour l'analgésique postopératoire. |
| 剂型、规格<br>Les formes pharmaceutiques et les spécifications | 注射液：每支 5mg（0.5ml）；10mg（1.0ml）。<br>片剂：每片 5mg；10mg。<br>Injection : 5mg (0,5ml) ou 10mg (1,0ml) par solution.<br>Comprimés : 5mg ou 10mg par comprimé. |
| 药品名称 Drug Names | 哌替啶 Péthidine |
| 适应证<br>Les indications | ①各种剧痛，如创伤、烧伤、烫伤、术后疼痛等；②心源性哮喘；③麻醉前给药；④内脏剧烈绞痛（胆绞痛、肾绞痛需与阿托品合用）；⑤与氯丙嗪、异丙嗪等合用进行人工冬眠。<br>① Les douleurs provoquées par un traumatisme, une chirurgie, des brûlures. ② L'asthme cardiaque. ③ L'administration avant l'anesthésie. ④ Les coliques viscérales (en cas de colique biliaire et néphrétique, il faut utiliser ce produit et l'atropine en même temps.). ⑤ L'hibernation artificielle, en association avec la chlorpromazine et la prométhazine. |
| 用法、用量<br>Les modes d'emploi et la posologie | ①口服：一次 25～100mg，1 日 200～400mg；极量：1 次 150mg，1 日 600mg。②皮下注射或肌内注射：1 次 25～100mg，1 日 100～400mg；极量：1 次 150mg，1 日 600mg。两次用要间隔不宜少于 4 小时。③静脉注射：成人以每次 0.3mg/kg 为限。④麻醉前肌内注射：成人以每 1kg 体重 1.0mg，术前 30～60 分钟给予。麻醉过程中静脉滴注，成人以每 1kg 体重 1.2～2.0mg 计算总量，配成稀释液，以每分钟 1mg 静脉滴注，小儿滴速减慢。⑤手术后镇痛及癌性镇痛：以每日 2.1～2.5mg/kg 剂量为限，经硬膜外腔缓慢注入或泵入。 |

续　表

<table>
<tr>
<td></td>
<td>① Par voie orale : 25 à 100mg par fois, 200 à 400 mg par jour ; dose maximale, 150mg par jour, 600mg par jour.　② Injection sous-cutanée ou par voie IM : 25 à 100mg par fois, 100 à 400mg par jour ; dose maximale : 150mg par fois, 600mg par jour. Un intervalle de 4h au moins entre les deux administrations.　③ Injection par voie IV : chez des adultes, 0,3 mg/kg au plus.　④ Injection par voie IM avant l'anesthésie : chez des adultes, 1,0 mg par kg, 30 à 60 minutes avant la chirurgie. Perfusion durant l'anesthésie, chez des adultes, 1,2 à 2,0 mg par kg, la dilution, perfusion avec 1mg par minute, plus lente chez des enfants.　⑤ Pour l'analgésique postopératoire et le soulagement des douleurs canceuses : 2,1 à 2,5 mg/kg par jour au plus, injection épidurale ou pompée lente.</td>
</tr>
<tr>
<td>剂型、规格<br>Les formes pharmaceutiques et les spécifications</td>
<td>片剂：每片 25mg；50mg。<br>注射液：每支 50mg（1ml）；100mg（2ml）。<br>Comprimés : 25mg ou 50mg par comprimé.<br>Injection : 50mg (1ml) ou 100mg (2ml) par solution.</td>
</tr>
<tr>
<td>药品名称 Drug Names</td>
<td>美沙酮 Méthadone</td>
</tr>
<tr>
<td>适应证<br>Les indications</td>
<td>适用于创伤性、癌症剧痛、外科手术后和慢性疼痛。也用于阿片、吗啡及海洛因成瘾者的脱毒治疗。<br><br>Ce produit est applicable dans l'atténuation de ladouleur traumatique, de la douleur cancéreuse, de la douleur chronique et de la douleur après la chirurgie. Il est aussi applicable dans la désintoxication des toxicomanes de l'opium, de la morphine et de l'héroïne.</td>
</tr>
<tr>
<td>用法、用量<br>Les modes d'emploi et la posologie</td>
<td>（1）口服：成人每日 10 ～ 15mg；分 2 ～ 3 次服。儿童每日按 0.7mg/kg 计，分 4 ～ 6 次服。极量：1 次 10mg，1 日 20mg。<br>（2）肌内注射或皮下注射：每次 2.5 ～ 5mg，1 日 10 ～ 15mg。三角肌注射血浆峰值高，作用出现快，因此可采用三角肌注射。极量：1 次 10mg，1 日 20mg。<br><br>(1) Par voie orale : chez des adultes, 10 à 15mg par jour, à travers 2 à 3 fois. Chez des enfants, 0,7 mg/kg par jour, à travers 4 à 6 fois. Dose maximale : 10mg par fois, 20mg par jour.<br>(2) Injection par voie IM ou sous-cutanée : 2,5 à 5mg par fois, 10 à 15mg par jour. En cas d'injection deltoide, le pic plasmatique est élevé, avec un effet rapide, en conséquence, possible de l'administrer en injection deltoide. Dose maximale :</td>
</tr>
<tr>
<td>剂型、规格<br>Les formes pharmaceutiques et les spécifications</td>
<td>片剂：每片 2.5mg；7.5mg；10mg。<br>注射液：每支 5mg（1ml）7.5mg（2ml）。<br>Comprimés : 2,5mg, 7,5mg ou 10mg par comprimé.<br>Injection : 5mg (1ml) ou 7,5mg (2ml) par solution.</td>
</tr>
<tr>
<td>药品名称 Drug Names</td>
<td>芬太尼 Fentanyl</td>
</tr>
<tr>
<td>适应证<br>Les indications</td>
<td>适用于各种疼痛及外科、妇科等手术后和手术过程中的镇痛；也用于防止或减轻手术后的谵妄；还可与麻醉药合用，作为麻醉辅助用药；与氟哌利多配伍制成"镇静镇痛药"，用于大面积换药及进行小手术的镇痛。<br><br>Ce produit est utilisé dans le soulagement de toutes sortes de douleurs et l'atténuation des douleurs durant et après l'opération chirurgicale et la chirurgie gynécologique. Il sert aussi à atténuer ou à prévenir le délire après l'opération chirurgicale. Il peut être utilisé comme adjuvant à l'anesthésie. Utilisé en association avec le dropéridol pour devenir l'analgésique, il est utilisé comme analgésique dans le changement de pansement étendu et une petite opération chirurgicale.</td>
</tr>
<tr>
<td>用法、用量<br>Les modes d'emploi et la posologie</td>
<td>（1）麻醉前给药：0.05 ～ 0.1mg，于手术前 30 ～ 60 分钟肌内注射。<br>（2）诱导麻醉：静脉注射 0.05 ～ 0.1mg，间隔 2 ～ 3 分钟重复注射，直至达到要求；危重患者、年幼及年老患者的用量减小至 0.025 ～ 0.05mg。<br>（3）维持麻醉：当患者出现苏醒症状时，静脉注射或肌内注射 0.025 ～ 0.05mg。<br>（4）一般镇痛及术后镇痛：肌内注射 0.05 ～ 0.1mg。可控制手术后疼痛、烦躁和呼吸急迫，必要时可于 1 ～ 2 小时后重复给药。硬膜外腔注入镇痛，一般 4 ～ 10 分钟起效，20 分钟脑脊液浓度达峰值，作用持续 3 ～ 6 小时。<br>（5）贴片：每 3 日用 1 贴，贴于锁骨下胸部皮肤。</td>
</tr>
</table>

续　表

|  | (1) Avant l'anesthésie, 0,05 à 0,1mg, 30 à 60 minutes avant la chirurgie en voie IM.<br>(2) Induction de l'anesthésie : 0,05 à 0,1mg, par voie IV, toutes les 2 à 3 minutes, jusqu'à la satisfaction des besoins ; chez des patients extrêmement malades, des enfants et des personnes âgées, 0,025 à 0,05mg.<br>(3) Entretien de l'anesthésie : quand les patients se réveillent, 0,025 à 0,05mg par voie IV ou IM.<br>(4) Pour l'analgésique générale et postopératoire : 0,05 à 0,1mg par voie IM. Possible de contrôler les douleurs et l'irritabilité postopératoires, en cas de besoin, administration toutes les 1 à 2h. Pour l'analgésique péridural, commencer à prendre effet 4 à 10 minutes après l'administration, le pic des concentrationsdans le liquide céphalorachidienapparaît 20 minutes après l'administration, efficace pendant 3 à 6 h.<br>(5) Patch : un patch tous les 3 jours, apposer sur la peau de la poitrine sous la clavicule. |
| 剂型、规格<br>Les formes pharmaceutiques et les spécifications | 注射液：每支 0.1mg（2ml）。<br>贴片（多瑞吉）：每小时可释放芬太尼 25μg、50μg、75μg、100μg。<br>复方芬太尼注射液：每 1ml 含芬太尼 0.1mg，异丙嗪 25mg。<br>Injection : 0,1mg (2ml) par solution.<br>Patch : capable de libérer 25μg, 50μg, 75μg ou 100μg de fentanyl par h.<br>Injection de fentanyl de composés : 0,1mg de fentanyl et 25mg de prométhazine par 1ml. |
| 药品名称 Drug Names | 阿芬太尼 Alfentanil |
| 适应证<br>Les indications | 用于麻醉前、中、后的镇静与镇痛，适用于心脏冠状动脉血管旁路术的麻醉。<br>Ce produit sert de sédation et d'analgésie avant, durant et après l'anesthésie. Il est aussi applicable dans l'anesthésie du pontage aortocoronarien. |
| 用法、用量<br>Les modes d'emploi et la posologie | 静脉注射：按手术长短而决定极量。手术 10 分钟以内完成者 7 ～ 15μg/kg；60 分钟手术，40 ～ 80μg/kg；手术超过 60 分钟者，可改为每分钟 1μg/kg，连续静脉滴注，至手术结束前 10 分钟停止给药。<br>Injection par voie IV : ajuster la dose en fonction de la durée de la chirurgie. En 10 minutes, 7~15µg/kg ; en 60 minutes, 40~80µg/kg ; plus de 60minutes, 1µg/kg par minute, perfusion continue, jusqu'à 10 minutes avant la fin de la chirurgie. |
| 剂型、规格<br>Les formes pharmaceutiques et les spécifications | 注射液（盐酸盐）：每支 1mg（2ml）。<br>Injeciton (chlorhydrate d'alfentanil) : 1mg (2ml) par solution. |
| 药品名称 Drug Names | 舒芬太尼 Sufentanil |
| 适应证<br>Les indications | 用于麻醉前、中、后的镇静与镇痛，适用于心脏冠状动脉血管旁路术的麻醉。<br>Ce produit sert de sédation et d'analgésie avant, durant et après l'anesthésie. Il est aussi applicable dans l'anesthésie du pontage aortocoronarien. |
| 用法、用量<br>Les modes d'emploi et la posologie | 麻醉时间长约 2 小时，总剂量 2μg/kg，维持量 10 ～ 25μg。麻醉时间长 2 ～ 8 小时，总剂量 2 ～ 8μg/kg，维持量 10 ～ 50μg。心血管手术麻醉，5μg/kg。<br>Quand l'analgésie dure 2 h, la dose totale, 2µg/kg, la dose maintenue, 10 à 25µg. Quand l'analgésie dure 2 à 8h, la dose totale, 2 à 8 µg/kg, la dose maintenue, 10 à 50µg. Pour l'analgésie de la chirurgie cardiovasculaire, 5µg/kg |
| 剂型、规格<br>Les formes pharmaceutiques et les spécifications | 注射液：每支 50μg（2ml）；100μg（2ml）；250μg（2ml）。<br>Injection : 50µg(2ml), 100µg(2ml)ou 250µg(2ml)par solution. |
| 药品名称 Drug Names | 瑞芬太尼 Rémifentanil |
| 适应证<br>Les indications | 用于麻醉诱导和全麻中维持镇痛。<br>Ce produit est utilisé comme analgésie durant l'induction de l'anesthésie et l'anesthésie générale. |

续　表

| 用法、用量<br>Les modes d'emploi et la posologie | 10mg 加入 200ml 生理盐水。用于静脉麻醉时，剂量为 0.25 ～ 2.0μg/（kg·min），或间断注射 0.25 ～ 1.0μg/kg。<br><br>Pour 10mg de rémifentanil, ajouter 200ml de solution saline. En cas de anesthésie intraveineus, 0.25 à 2.0μg/(kg•min)ou injection intermittente 0.25 à 1.0μg/kg. |
|---|---|
| 剂型、规格<br>Les formes pharmaceutiques et les spécifications | 注射用瑞芬太尼：每支 1mg；2mg；5mg。<br>Le rémifentanil pour injection : 1mg, 2mg ou 5mg par solution. |
| **药品名称 Drug Names** | 布桂嗪 Bucinnazine |
| 适应证<br>Les indications | 临床上用于偏头痛、三叉神经痛、炎症性及外伤性疼痛、关节痛、痛经、癌症引起的疼痛等。<br>Ce produit est utilisé dans les cliniques pour traiter la migraine, la névralgie du trijumeau, lesdouleurs inflammatoires et traumatiques, les douleurs articulaires, la dysménorrhée et la douleur causée par le cancer. |
| 用法、用量<br>Les modes d'emploi et la posologie | （1）口服：成人 1 次 30 ～ 60mg，1 日 90 ～ 180mg；小儿每次 1mg/kg。疼痛剧烈时用量可酌增。<br>　（2）皮下或肌内注射：成人 1 次 50 ～ 100mg，一日 1 ～ 2 次。<br>　(1) Par voie orale : 30 à 60 mg par fois, 90 à 180 mg par jour ; chez des enfants, 1 mg/kg par fois. En cas de douleurs sévères, augmenter la dose.<br>　(2) Injection par voie sous-cutanée ou IM : chez des adultes, 50 à 100mg par fois, 1 à 2 fois par jour. |
| 剂型、规格<br>Les formes pharmaceutiques et les spécifications | 片剂：每片 30mg；60mg。<br>注射液：每支 50mg（2ml）；100mg（2ml）。<br>Comprimés : 30mg ou 60 mg par comprimé.<br>Injection : 50mg (2ml) par solution. |
| **药品名称 Drug Names** | 喷他佐辛 Pentazocine |
| 适应证<br>Les indications | 适用于各种慢性剧痛。<br>Ce produit s'utilise dans le traitement de toutes sortes de douleurs chroniques. |
| 用法、用量<br>Les modes d'emploi et la posologie | 静脉注射、肌内注射或皮下注射，每次 30mg。口服，每次 25 ～ 50mg。必要时每 3 ～ 4 小时 1 次。<br>Injection par voie IV, IM ou sous-cutanée, 30mg par fois. Par voie orale, 25 à 50 mg par fois. En cas de besoin, toutes les 3 à 4h. |
| 剂型、规格<br>Les formes pharmaceutiques et les spécifications | 片剂：每片 25mg；50mg。<br>注射液：每支 15mg（1ml）；30mg（1ml）。<br>Comprimés : 25mg ou 50mg par comprimé.<br>Injection : 15 mg (1ml) ou 30mg (1ml) par solution. |
| **药品名称 Drug Names** | 羟考酮 Oxycodone |
| 适应证<br>Les indications | 用于缓解中、重度疼痛。<br>Ce produit sert à soulager la douleur modérée et sévère. |
| 用法、用量<br>Les modes d'emploi et la posologie | （1）一般镇痛，使用控释制剂，每 12 小时服用 1 次，用药剂量取决于患者的疼痛的严重程度和既往镇痛药用药史。首次服用阿片类或弱阿片类药物初始用药剂量一般为 5mg，每 12 小时服用 1 次。已接受口服吗啡治疗的患者，改用本品的每日用药剂量换算比例为：口服本品 10mg 相当于口服吗啡 20mg。应根据患者个体情况滴定用药剂量。调整剂量时，不改变用药次数，只调整每次剂量，调整幅度是在上次一次的用药剂量基础上增长 25% ～ 50%。大多数患者的最高用药剂量为每 12 小时服用 200mg，少数患者可能需要更高的剂量。控释制剂必须整片吞服，不得掰开、咀嚼或研磨。如果掰开、咀嚼或研磨药片，会导致羟考酮的快速释放与潜在致死量的吸收。<br>　（2）术后疼痛：使用本药复方胶囊，每次 1 ～ 2 粒，间隔 4 ～ 6 小时可重复用药一次。<br>　（3）癌症、慢性疼痛：使用本药复方胶囊，每次 1 ～ 2 粒，一日 3 次。<br>　儿童：口服，一次 0.05 ～ 0.15mg/kg，每 4 ～ 6 小时一次。一次用量最多 5mg。 |

|  | (1) Pour adoucir les douleurs générales, prendre les comprimés à libération contrôlée, toutes les 12h, dose en fonction des douleurs et des antécédents de médicament analgésique. L'administration des opioïdes faibles ou opioïdes pour la première fois, au début, 5mg, toutes les 12h. Pour ceux qui ont pris la morphine par voie orale et veulent prendre l'oxycodone : 10mg d'oxycodone équivaut à 20mg de morphine. Ajuster la dose en fonction des patients. En cas d'ajustement de la dose, ne pas changer le nombre d'administrations, mais la dose par fois, à savoir augmenter 25 % à 50 % par fois à partir du niveau précédent. Pour la plupart des patients, ne pas dépasser 200mg toutes les 12h, pour les autres patients, une dose plus importante. Pour prendre les comprimés à libération contrôlée, il faut l'avaler en entier, interdit de le briser, de le mâcher ni de le broyer. Sinon, l'oxycodone risquerait d'être libérée rapidement et on risquerait d'absorber une dose potientiellement mortelle.<br>(2) Pour adourcir les douleurs postopératoires : prendre les capsules de composés, 1 à 2 capsules par fois, toutes les 4 à 6h.<br>(3) Pour les douleurs canceuses ou chroniques : prendre les capsules de composés, 1 à 2 capsules par fois, 3 fois par jour. chez des enfants : par voie orale, 0,05 à 0,15 mg/kg par fois, toutes les 4 à 6h. Ne pas dépaser 5mg par fois. |
|---|---|
| 剂型、规格<br>Les formes pharmaceutiques et les spécifications | 片剂：5mg。<br>控释片：5mg；10mg；20mg；40mg。<br>复方胶囊剂：每粒含羟考酮5mg、对乙酰氨基酚500mg。<br>Comprimés : 5mg.<br>Comprimés à libération contrôlée : 5mg, 10mg, 20mg ou 40mg.<br>Capsules de composés : 5mg d'oxycodone et 500mg d'acétaminophène par capsule. |
| **药品名称 Drug Names** | 地佐辛 Dézocine |
| 适应证<br>Les indications | 用于术后痛、内脏及癌性疼痛。<br>Ce produit sert à atténuer la douleur postopératoire, la douleur viscérale et la douleur cancéreuse. |
| 用法、用量<br>Les modes d'emploi et la posologie | 肌内注射：开始时10mg，以后每隔3～6小时，2.5～10mg。<br>静脉注射：开始5mg，以后每隔2～4小时，2.5～10mg。<br>Injection par voie IM : au début, 10mg, ensuite, 2,5 à 10mg toutes les 3 à 6h.<br>Par voie IV : au début, 5mg, ensuite, 2,5 à 10mg toutes les 2 à 4h. |
| 剂型、规格<br>Les formes pharmaceutiques et les spécifications | 注射液：每支5mg（1ml）；10mg（1ml）。<br>Injection : 5mg (1ml) ou 10mg (1ml) par solution. |
| **药品名称 Drug Names** | 普瑞巴林 Prégabaline |
| 适应证<br>Les indications | 用于治疗外周神经痛及辅助性治疗局限性部分癫痫发作。我国批准的适应证为：用于治疗带状疱疹后神经痛。<br><br>Ce produit est utilisé comme traitement de la douleur neuropathique périphérique ainsi que comme thérapie adjuvante de la crise de l'épilepsie partielle. Les indications approuvées par la Chine : utilisé comme traitement de la névralgie post-herpétique. |
| 用法、用量<br>Les modes d'emploi et la posologie | 口服，每日剂量为150～600mg，分2～3次给药。一般起始剂量为每次75mg，一日2次。如果每日服用本品300mg，2～4周后疼痛仍未得到充分缓解、且可耐受本品的患者，剂量可增至每次300mg，一日2次，或每次200mg，一日3次（即600mg/d）。由于不良反应呈剂量依赖性，且不良反应可导致更高的停药率，故剂量超过300mg/d仅应用于耐受300mg/d剂量的持续性疼痛患者。<br><br>Par voie orale, 150 à 600 mg par jour, à travers 2 à 3 fois. Au début, 75mg par fois, 2 fois par jour. Si on prend 300mg par jour, pendant 2 à 4 semaines, sans soulagement des symptômes, prendre 300mg par fois, 2 fois par jour, ou 200mg par fois, 3 fois par jour, à savoir 600mg par jour. Comme les effets indésirables sont dépendants de la dose, et que les effets indésirables peuvent conduire à un taux de discontinuité plus élevé, appliquer plus de 300mg par jour seulement chez des patients avec une douleur persistante tolérant 300mg par jour. |

**续　表**

| 剂型、规格<br>Les formes pharmaceutiques et les spécifications | 胶囊：每粒 75mg；150mg。<br>Capsules : 75mg ou 150mg par capsule. |
|---|---|
| 药品名称 Drug Names | 曲马多 Tramadol |
| 适应证<br>Les indications | 用于中、重度急慢性疼痛，服后 0.5 小时生效，持续 6 小时。亦用于术后痛、创伤痛、癌性痛、心脏病突发性痛、关节痛、神经痛及分娩痛。<br><br>Ce produit est utilisé pour soulager la douleur aigue ou chronique, médérée ou sévère. Il sera efficace 0,5h après l'administration, pendant 6h. Il est également appliqué pour atténuer la douleur postopératoire, la douleur traumatique, la douleur cancéreuse, la douleur cardiaque soudaine, les douleurs articulaires, les névralgies et la douleur de l'accouchement. |
| 用法、用量<br>Les modes d'emploi et la posologie | 成人：口服，每次量不超过 100mg，224 小时不超过 400mg，连续用药不超过 48 小时，累计用量不超过 800mg。静脉、皮下、肌内注射，每次 50～100mg，1 日不超过 400mg。<br><br>Chez des adultes : par voie orale, ne pas dépasser 100mg par fois, 400mg par jour au plus. Le traitement continu ne dépasse pas 48h, 800mg au plus. Injection par voie IV, sous-cutanée ou IM, 50 à 100 mg par fois, ne pas dépasser 400mg par jour. |
| 剂型、规格<br>Les formes pharmaceutiques et les spécifications | 注射液：每支 50mg（2ml）；100mg（2ml）。<br>胶囊剂：每粒 50mg。<br>栓剂：每 1ml（40 滴）含药 100mg。<br>缓释片：每片 100mg。<br><br>Injection : 50mg (2ml) ou 100mg (2ml) par solution.<br>Capsules : 50mg par capsule.<br>Suppositoires : 100mg par 1ml (40 gouttes).<br>Comprimés à libération prolongée : 100mg par comprimé. |
| 药品名称 Drug Names | 四氢帕马丁 Tétrahydropalmatine |
| 适应证<br>Les indications | 对胃肠、肝胆系统疾病的钝痛镇痛效果好，对外伤等剧痛效果差。以用于分娩镇痛及痛经。催眠、镇静效果较好，治疗剂量无成瘾性。1 次服用 100mg，服后 20～30 分钟入睡，持续 5～6 小时，无后遗作用，故可用于暂时性失眠。<br><br>Ce produit est efficace dans l'atténuation de la douleur sourde des maladies gastro-intestinales et hépato-biliaires. Mais il est peu efficace dans le soulagement de la douleur traumatique. Il sert aussi à atténuer la douler de l'accouchement et la dysménorrhée. Son effet hypnotique et sédatif est très bien, sans dépendance de médicaments. 100mg par fois, s'endormir 20 à 30 minutes après l'administration, pendant 5 à 6h, sans séquelles, applicable dans le traitement de l'insomnie temporaire. |
| 用法、用量<br>Les modes d'emploi et la posologie | ①镇痛：口服，每次 100～150mg，一日 2～4 次；皮下注射，每次 60～100mg。痛经：口服每次 50mg。②催眠：口服，每次 100～200mg。<br><br>① Pour l'analgésique : par voie orale, 100 à 150 mg par fois, 2 à 4 fois par jour ; injection par voie sous cutanée, 60 à 100 mg par fois. ② Pour la dysménorrhée, par voie orale, 50mg par fois. Pour l'hypnose : chez des adultes, 100 à 200 mg par fois, par voie orale. |
| 剂型、规格<br>Les formes pharmaceutiques et les spécifications | 片剂：每片 50mg。注射液：每支 60mg（2ml）；100mg（2ml）。<br>Comprimés : 50mg par comprimé.<br>Injection : 60mg (2ml) ou 100 mg (2ml) par solution. |
| 药品名称 Drug Names | 罗通定 Rotundine |
| 适应证<br>Les indications | 用于因疼痛而失眠的患者。亦可用于为胃溃疡和十二指肠溃疡的疼痛、月经痛，分娩后宫缩痛、紧张性失眠、痉挛性咳嗽等。<br><br>Applicable dans le traitement des patients souffrant d'insomnie causée par la douleur. Aussi applicable pour soulager les douleurs dues à l'ulcère gastrique et à l'ulcère duodénal, les douleurs menstruelles, la douleur après les contractions de l'accouchement, l'insomnie nerveuse ainsi que les toux spasmodiques. |

**续 表**

| 用法、用量<br>Les modes d'emploi et la posologie | 镇痛：口服，每次 60～120mg，一日 1～4 次；肌内注射，每次 60～90mg，一日 1～4 次。<br>催眠：成人于睡前服 1 次 30～90mg。<br><br>Pour l'analgésique : par voie orale, 60 à 120 mg par fois, 1 à 4 fois par jour ; injection par voie IM, 60 à 90 mg par fois, 1 à 4 fois par jour. Pour l'hypnose : chez des adultes, 30 à 90 mg par fois avant le sommeil. |
| --- | --- |
| 剂型、规格<br>Les formes pharmaceutiques et les spécifications | 片剂：每片 30mg；60mg。<br>注射液（硫酸罗通定）：每支 60mg（2ml）。<br><br>Comprimés : 30mg ou 60mg par comprimé.<br>Injection (rotundine sulfurique) : 60mg (2ml) par solution. |
| **药品名称 Drug Names** | 麦角胺 Ergotamine |
| 适应证<br>Les indications | 主要用于偏头痛，可是头痛减轻，但不能预防和根治。以用于其他神经性头痛。<br><br>Il sert à traiter la migraine, à soulager la douler au lieu de la prévenir ou la guérir. Aussi applicable dans le traitement d'autres maux de tête par tension nerveuse. |
| 用法、用量<br>Les modes d'emploi et la posologie | ①口服：每次 1～2mg，1 日不超过 6mg，一周不超过 10mg。效果不及皮下注射。②皮下注射：每次 0.25～0.5mg，24 小时内不超过 1mg，本品早期给药效果好，头痛发作时用药效果差。<br><br>① Par voie orale : 1 à 2 mg par fois, ne pas dépasser 6mg par jour, 10mg par semaine au plus. Moins efficace que l'injection sous-cutanée. ② Injection sous-cutanée : 0,25 à 0,5 mg par fois, ne pas dépasser 1mg par jour, efficace au stade précoce, moins efficace en cas de céphlalgie. |
| 剂型、规格<br>Les formes pharmaceutiques et les spécifications | 片剂：每片 0.5mg；1mg。<br>注射液：每支 0.25mg（ml）；0.5mg（1ml）。<br><br>Comprimés : 0,5mg ou 1mg par comprimé.<br>Injection : 0,25mg (ml) par solution. |
| **药品名称 Drug Names** | 乙酰乌头碱 Acetylaconitine |
| 适应证<br>Les indications | 用于各种中度程度疼痛、肩关节周围炎、颈椎病、肩臂痛、腰痛、关节扭伤、风湿性关节炎、类风湿关节炎、坐骨神经痛、带状疱疹、小手术术后痛。<br><br>Il sert à traiter des douleurs modérées, la périarthrite, l'arthrose cervicale, les maux d'épaule, de bras et de dos, les entorses, l'arthrite rhumatoïde, l'arthrite rhumatoïde, la sciatique, le zona ainsi que la douleur postopératoire mineure. |
| 用法、用量<br>Les modes d'emploi et la posologie | 口服：每次 0.3mg，一日 1～2 次，餐后服。每次量不超过 0.3mg，每月不宜超过 2 次，服药间隔 6 小时。1 个疗程 10 日，疗程间隔 3～5 日。肌内注射：每次 0.3mg，一日 1～2 次，注射用水稀释至 2ml 后注射。小儿或老人每日或隔日 1 次。两个疗程宜间隔 3～5 日。<br><br>Par voie orale : 0,3mg par fois, 1 à 2 fois par jour, après le repas. Ne pas dépasser 0,3mg par fois, 2 fois par jour au plus, toutes les 6. Un traitement médical dure 10 jours, unintervalle de 3 à 5 jours entre des traitements. Injection par voie IM : 0,3mg par fois, 1 à 2 fois par jour, utiliser 2ml d'eau pour injection pour la dilution. Chez des enfants et des personnes âgées, 1 fois par jour ou tous les deux jours. Un intervalle de 3 à 5 jours entre deux traitements. |
| 剂型、规格<br>Les formes pharmaceutiques et les spécifications | 片剂：每片 0.3mg。<br>注射液：每支 0.3mg（1ml）。<br><br>Comprimés : 0,3mg par comprimé.<br>Injection : 0,3mg (1ml) par solution. |
| **药品名称 Drug Names** | 洛美利嗪 Lomérizine |
| 适应证<br>Les indications | 用于偏头痛的预防性治疗。<br>Ce produit sert à prévenir la migraine. |
| 用法、用量<br>Les modes d'emploi et la posologie | 成人 1 次 5mg，一日 2 次，早餐后及晚餐后或睡眠前服用。根据症状适量增减，但 1 日剂量不超过 20mg。<br><br>Chez des adultes, 5mg par fois, 2 fois par jour, après le petit-déjeuner et après le diner ou avant le sommeil. Ajuster la dose en fonction des symptômes, mais ne pas dépasser 20mg par jour. |

**续　表**

| | |
|---|---|
| 剂型、规格<br>Les formes pharmaceutiques et les spécifications | 片剂（胶囊）：每片（粒）5mg。<br>Comprimés (capsules) : 5mg par comprimé ou par capsule. |
| **药品名称 Drug Names** | 齐考诺肽 Ziconotide |
| 适应证<br>Les indications | 用于需要鞘内治疗且对其他镇痛治疗（如应用全身性镇痛药或鞘内注射吗啡等）不耐受或疗效差的严重慢性疼痛患者。<br>Ce produit est applicable dans le traitement des patients souffrant de douleur chronique sévère, qui ont besoin de thérapie intrathécale et qui sont cependant résistants à d'autres traitements antalgiques (tels que l'application des analgésiques systémiques ou l'injfection de la morphine intrathécale). |
| 用法、用量<br>Les modes d'emploi et la posologie | 鞘内输注给药。起始剂量不宜超过 1 日 2.4mg（或 1 小时 0.1mg）。宜缓慢增量，即每周增加剂量不超过 2 ～ 3 次，每次增量不超过 1 日 2.4mg（或 1 小时 0.1mg），直至第 21 日时达到最大推荐剂量 1 日 19.2mg（或 1 小时 0.8mg）。<br>Perfusion intrathécale. Au début, ne pas dépasser 2,4mg par jour ou 0,1mg par h. augmenter lentement la dose : 2 à 3 fois de plus par semaine, augmenter 2,4mg par jour ou 0,1mg par h au plus, jusqu'à la dose la plus importante à la 21ème journée, soit 19,2mg par jour ou 0,8mg par h. |
| 剂型、规格<br>Les formes pharmaceutiques et les spécifications | 注射液：5ml:500μg(100μg/ml)；20ml:500μg(25μg/ml)。<br>Injection: 5ml:500μg(100μg/ml)；20ml:500μg(25μg/ml). |
| **药品名称 Drug Names** | 他喷他多 Tapentadol |
| 适应证<br>Les indications | 用于各种急性和慢性疼痛。<br>Ce produit est applicable dans l'atténuation de toutes sortes de douleurs aigues et chroniques. |
| 用法、用量<br>Les modes d'emploi et la posologie | 口服，每 4 ～ 6 小时 1 次，每次 1 片。<br>Par voie orale : 1 fois toutes les 4 à 6h, 1 comprimé par fois. |
| 剂型、规格<br>Les formes pharmaceutiques et les spécifications | 片剂：每片 50mg；75mg；100mg。<br>Comprimées : 50mg, 75mg ou 100mg par comprimé. |
| **药品名称 Drug Names** | 阿片全碱 Papaveretum |
| 适应证<br>Les indications | 同吗啡。用于各种疼痛及止泻，药效持久。<br>c.f. La morphine. Il est applicable dans le traitement de toutes sortes de douleurs et dans l'antidiarrhéique avec un effet durable. |
| 用法、用量<br>Les modes d'emploi et la posologie | 皮下注射，每次 6 ～ 12mg。<br>口服，每次 5 ～ 15mg，一日 3 次。<br>极量：1 次 30mg。<br>Injection sous cutanée : 6 à 12mg par fois.<br>Par voie orale : 5 à 15mg par fois, 3 fois par jour.<br>Ne pas dépasser 30mg par fois. |
| 剂型、规格<br>Les formes pharmaceutiques et les spécifications | 片剂：每片 5mg。<br>注射液：20ml（1ml）。<br>栓剂：20mg。<br>Comprimés : 5mg par comprimé.<br>Injection : 20ml (1ml).<br>Suppositoires : 20mg. |

**续 表**

| 药品名称 Drug Names | 荷包牡丹碱 Dicentrine |
| --- | --- |
| 适应证<br>Les indications | 有一定镇痛、镇静作用。用于头痛、腰痛、牙痛、小手术后疼痛及神经衰弱。<br>Ce produit a un effet analgésique et sédatif. Il sert à supprimer ou à atténuer la céphalalgie, le mal de dos, le mal de dents, la douleur après la chirurgie mineure et à traiter la neurasthénie. |
| 用法、用量<br>Les modes d'emploi et la posologie | 口服：1 次 20 ～ 60mg。<br>Par voie orale : 20 à 60mg par fois. |
| 剂型、规格<br>Les formes pharmaceutiques et les spécifications | 片剂：每片 20mg。<br>Comprimés : 20mg par comprimé. |

| 药品名称 Drug Names | 山豆碱 Total Alcaloïdes de Sophora Tonkinese |
| --- | --- |
| 适应证<br>Les indications | 用于慢性气管炎、哮喘、咽喉肿痛的、关节痛等。<br>Ce produit sert à traiter la bronchite chronique, l'asthme, les maux de gorge et les douleurs articulaires. |
| 用法、用量<br>Les modes d'emploi et la posologie | 肌内注射每次 2ml，一日 2 次。<br>Injection par voie IM, 2ml par fois, 2 fois par jour. |
| 剂型、规格<br>Les formes pharmaceutiques et les spécifications | 注射液：10mg（2ml）。<br>Injection : 10mg (2ml). |

| 药品名称 Drug Names | 匹米诺定 Piminodine |
| --- | --- |
| 适应证<br>Les indications | 用于术前给药，胆囊炎合并胆石、胰腺炎、癌症等引起的剧痛。<br>Ce produit est utilisé pour l'administration préopératoire et pour supprimer ou atténuer les douleurs causées par la lithiase de la vésicule biliaire, la pancréatite et le cancer. |
| 用法、用量<br>Les modes d'emploi et la posologie | 皮下注射或肌内注射：1 次 10 ～ 20mg，必要时每 4 小时 1 次。口服：1 次 25 ～ 50mg。有成瘾性。<br>Injection par voie sous-cutanée ou par voie IM : 10 à 20mg par fois, en cas de besoin, 1 fois toutes les 4h. Par voie orale : 25 à 50 mg par fois. Ce produit est toxicomaniaque. |
| 剂型、规格<br>Les formes pharmaceutiques et les spécifications | 片剂：每片 25mg。<br>注射液：10mg（1ml）。<br>Comprimés : 25mg par comprimé.<br>Injection : 10mg (1ml). |

| 药品名称 Drug Names | 西马嗪 Simazine |
| --- | --- |
| 适应证<br>Les indications | 用于术后、外伤性疼痛。<br>Ce produit sert à soulager ou à supprimer les douleurs postopératoires et traumatiques. |
| 用法、用量<br>Les modes d'emploi et la posologie | 口服：每次 0.4 ～ 0.8g。小儿酌减。<br>Par voie orale, 0,4 à 0,8 g par fois. Chez des enfants, diminuer la dose en cas de besoin. |
| 剂型、规格<br>Les formes pharmaceutiques et les spécifications | 片剂：每片 0.4g。<br>Comprimés : 0,4g par comprimé. |

**续　表**

| 药品名称 Drug Names | 千金藤啶碱 Stepholidine |
| --- | --- |
| 适应证<br>Les indications | 用于血管性头痛、偏头痛、多动性运动障碍、儿童多动秽语综合征。<br>Applicable dans le traitement de la céphalée vasculaire, la migraine, les troubles hyperkinétiques et le syndrome de Gilles de la Tourette (SGT) chez des enfants. |
| 用法、用量<br>Les modes d'emploi et la posologie | 预防血管性头痛：1 次 25～75mg，一日 3 次，餐后服。治疗急性发作：1 次 15～100mg，顿服。治疗多动性运动障碍：25～100mg，一日 3 次，餐后服。儿童用量按成人量的 1/3～1/2 计量。<br>Pour prévenir la céphalée vasculaire : 25 à 75mg par fois, 3 fois par jour, après le repas. Pour traiter la crise aigue : 15 à 100mg par fois, une fois par jour. Pour traiter les troubles hyperkinétiques, 25 à 100mg, 3 fois par jour, après le repas. Chez des enfants, 1/3 à 1/2 de la dose chez des adultes. |
| 剂型、规格<br>Les formes pharmaceutiques et les spécifications | 片剂：每片 25mg。<br>Comprimés : 25mg par comprimé. |

| 药品名称 Drug Names | 高乌甲素 Lappaconitine |
| --- | --- |
| 适应证<br>Les indications | 用于中度以上疼痛、术后疼痛、坐骨神经痛。<br>Applicable dans le soulagement des douleurs modérées et sévères, de la douleur postopératoire et de la sciatique. |
| 用法、用量<br>Les modes d'emploi et la posologie | 口服：每次 5～10mg，一日 1～3 次。<br>肌内注射或静脉滴注，每次 4mg，一日 1～2 次。<br>Par voie orale : 5 à 10 mg par fois, 1 à 3 fois par jour.<br>Injection par voie IM ou par voie IV en perfusion : 4mg par fois, 1 à 2 fois par jour. |
| 剂型、规格<br>Les formes pharmaceutiques et les spécifications | 片剂：每片 5mg。<br>注射液：4mg（2ml）。<br>Comprimés : 5mg par comprimé.<br>Injection : 4mg (2ml). |

| 药品名称 Drug Names | 美西麦角 Méthysergide |
| --- | --- |
| 适应证<br>Les indications | 用于预防反复发作的偏头痛。对急性头痛发作无效。<br>Ce produit sert à prévenir la migraine récurrente. Il est inefficace dans le traitement de la crise de la céphalée aigue. |
| 用法、用量<br>Les modes d'emploi et la posologie | 起始剂量 1～2mg，一日 2 次；每 3～4 周增加 1～2mg；疗程不宜超过 6 个月。宜间断用药，每半年停药 3 周以上。<br>Au début, 1 à 2 mg, 2 fois par jour ; augmenter 1 à 2mg toutes les 3 à 4 semaines ; ne pas dépasser 6 mois. Il vaut mieux prendre le médicament de manière intermittente, arrêter l'administration pendant plus de 3 semaines tous les six mois. |
| 剂型、规格<br>Les formes pharmaceutiques et les spécifications | 片剂：每片 1mg。<br>Comprimés : 1mg par comprimé. |

| 药品名称 Drug Names | 氨酚氢可酮 Paracétamol et Hydrocodone Bitartrate |
| --- | --- |
| 适应证<br>Les indications | 本品用于缓解中度到中重度头痛。<br>Ce produit sert à atténuer la céphalée modérée et grave. |
| 用法、用量<br>Les modes d'emploi et la posologie | 每 4～6 小时 1～2 片，24 小时的总用药量不应超过 5 片。<br>1 à 2 comprimés toutes les 4 à 6h, ne pas dépasser 5 comprimés par jour. |

**续 表**

| 剂型、规格<br>Les formes pharmaceutiques et les spécifications | 片剂：每片含重酒石酸氢可酮 5mg、对乙酰氨基酚 500mg。<br><br>Comprimés : chaque comprimé contient 5mg de bitartrate d'hydrocodone et 500mg d'acétaminophène. |
| --- | --- |

8.3　解热镇痛抗炎药 Médicaments non-steroidens antiinflammatoires

| 药品名称 Drug Names | 阿司匹林 Aspirine |
| --- | --- |
| 适应证<br>Les indications | （1）用于发热、头痛、神经痛、肌肉痛、风湿热、急性风湿性关节炎及类风湿关节炎等，为风湿热，风湿性关节炎及类风湿关节炎首选药，可迅速缓解急性风湿性关节炎的症状。对急性风湿热伴有心肌炎者，可合用糖皮质激素。（2）用于痛风。（3）预防心肌梗死、动脉血栓、动脉粥样硬化等。（4）用于治疗胆道蛔虫病（有效率 90% 以上）。（5）粉剂外用可治足癣。（6）儿科用于皮肤黏膜淋巴结综合征（川崎病）的治疗。<br><br>(1) Ce produit sert à traiter la fièvre, la céphalée, la névralgie, les douleurs masculaires, le rhumatisme articulaire aigu, la polyarthrite rhumatoide aigue, et l'arthrite rhumatismale aigue. Il s'agit de médicament de choix dans le traitement du rhumatisme articulaire aigu, de la polyarthrite rhumatoide et de l'arthrite rhumatismale. Il peut soulager rapidemen les symptômes de l'arthrite rhumatismale aigue. Pour traiter les patients atteints de myocardite rhumatismale aigue, il vaut mieux l'utiliser en association avec les corticostéroïdes.<br>(2) Applicable dans le traitement de la goutte.<br>(3) Il sert à prévenir l'infarctus du myocarde, la thrombose artérielle et l'athérosclérose.<br>(4) Applicable dans le traitement de l'ascaridiose biliaire avec un taux de réussite supérieur à 90 %.<br>(5) L'aspirine en poudre pour l'usage externe peut traiter le tinea pedis.<br>(6) Il sert à traiter le syndrome des ganglions lymphatiques cutanéo-muqueuse (maladie de Kawasaki) chez des enfants. |
| 用法、用量<br>Les modes d'emploi et la posologie | （1）解热镇痛：①口服，每次 0.3～0.6g，一日 3 次，或需要时服。②直肠给药：1 次 0.3～0.6g，一日 0.9～1.8g；儿童 1～3 岁，1 次 0.1g，一日 1 次；3～6 岁，1 次 0.1～0.15g，一日 1～2 次；6 岁以上，1 次 0.15～0.3g，一日 2 次。<br>（2）抗风湿：1 次 0.6～1g，一日 3～4g。服时宜嚼碎，并可与碳酸钙或氢氧化铝或复方氢氧化铝（胃舒平）合用以减少对胃刺激。一疗程 3 个月左右。小儿 1 日 0.1g/kg，分 3 次服，前 3 日先服半量以减少不良反应。<br>（3）抑制血小板聚集：预防心肌梗死、动脉血栓、动脉粥样硬化，一日 1 次，每次 75～150mg。<br>（4）治疗胆道蛔虫病：每次 1g，一日 2～3 次，连用 2～3 日。当阵发性绞痛停止 24 小时后即停药，然后再行常规驱虫。<br>（5）治疗 X 射线照射或放疗引起的腹泻：每次服 0.6～0.9g，一日 4 次。<br>（6）预防搭桥术后再狭窄：每次服 50mg。<br>（7）治疗足癣：先用温开水或 1 ：5000 的高锰酸钾溶液洗涤患处，然后用本品粉末撒布患处，一般 2～4 次可愈。<br>（8）用于小儿皮肤黏淋巴结综合征：开始每日按 80～100mg/kg，分 3～4 次服，热退 2～3 日后改为每日 30mg/kg，每 3～4 次服，连服 2 个月或更久。血小板增多、血液呈高凝状态期间，每日 5～10mg/kg，1 次顿服。<br><br>(1) Pour l'analgésique et l'antipyrétique : par voie orale, 0,3 à 0,6g par fois, 3 fois par jour, ou en cas de besoin ; l'administration rectale, 0,3 à 0,6 g par fois, 0,9 à 1,8 g par jour, chez des enfants de 1 à 3 ans, 0,1 g par fois, 1 fois par jour, chez de 3 à 6 ans, 0,1 à 0,15g par fois, 1 à 2 fois par jour, chez plus de 6 ans, 0.15 à 0,3g par fois, 2 fois par jour.<br>(2) Pour lutter contre l'arthrite : 0,6 à 1g par fois, 3 à 4 g par jour. il vaut mieux l'administrer en association avec le carbonate de calcium ou l'hydroxyde d'aluminium ou un composé d'hydroxyde d'aluminium, pour diminuer l'effet indésirable gastro-intestinal. Pendant 3 mois.<br>Chez des enfants, 0,1g/kg par jour, à travers 3 fois, pendant les 3 premiers jours, prendre la moitié de la dose usuelle pour éviter les effets indésirables.<br>(3) Pour prévenir l'infarctus du myocarde, la thrombose artérielle et l'athérosclérose : 1 fois par jour, 75 à 150mg par fois. |

**续　表**

| | |
|---|---|
| | (4) Pour traiter l'ascaridiose biliaire : 1g par fois, 2 à 3 fois par jour, pendant 2 à 3 jours consécutifs. Arrêter l'administration immédiatement 24 h après la disparition de la douleur paroxystique, ensuite, prendre des médicaments usuels pour lutter contre l'ascaridiosc.<br>(5) Pour traiter la diarrhée causée par l'irradiation aux rayons X ou la radiothérapie, 0,6 à 0,9 g par fois, 4 fois par jour.<br>(6) Pour la prévention de la resténose après le pontage aorto-coronarien, 50mg par fois.<br>(7) Pour traiter le tinea pedis : laver la zone touchée avec l'eau chaude ou lasolution de permanganate de potassium à 1 : 5000, ensuite, appliquer l'aspirine en poudre à la zone touchée, 2 à 4 fois avant la guérison.<br>(8) Pour traiter le syndrome des ganglions lymphatiques cutanéo-muqueuse (maladie de Kawasaki) chez des enfants : au début, 80 à 100 mg/kg par jour, à travers 3 à 4 fois, 2 à 3 jours après avoir fait tombé la fièvre, 30 mg/kg par jour, à travers 3 à 4 fois, pendant 2 mois ou plus. En cas de thrombocytose et d'hypercoagulation sanguine, 5 à 10 mg/kg par jour, 1 fois par jour. |
| 剂型、规格<br>Les formes pharmaceutiques et les spécifications | 片剂：每片 0.05g；0.1g；0.2g；0.3g；0.5g。泡腾片：每片 0.3g；0.5g。放于温水 150～250ml 中，溶化后饮下。肠溶片（胶囊）：每片（粒）40mg；0.15g；0.3g；0.5g。对胃刺激小，适于长期大量服用。散剂：每袋 0.1g；0.5g。栓剂：每粒 0.1g；0.3g；0.45g；0.5g。<br>Comprimés : 0,05g, 0,1g, 0,2g, 0,3g, 0,5g par comprimé. Comprimés effervescents : 0,3g ou 0,5g par comprimé. Le mettre dans 150 à 250 ml d'eau, le boire après la dissolution. Comprimés ou capsules à enrobage entérique : 40mg, 0,15g, 0,3g ou 0,5g par comprimés ou par capsule. Peu d'effet indésirable gastro-intestinal, possible de l'administrer pour une longue durée. Poudre : 0,1g ou 0,5g par sachet. Suppositoires : 0,1g, 0,3g, 0,45g ou 0,5g par suppositoire |
| **药品名称 Drug Names** | 阿司匹林精氨酸盐 Aspirine arginine |
| 适应证<br>Les indications | 主要用于发热、头痛、神经痛、牙痛、肌肉痛及活动性风湿病、类风湿关节炎、创伤及术后疼痛。<br>Ce produit sert à traiter la fièvre, la céphalée, lanévralgie, l'odontalgie, les douleurs masculaires, le rhumatisme actif, la polyarthrite rhumatoïde et les douleurs traumatiques et postopératoires. |
| 用法、用量<br>Les modes d'emploi et la posologie | 肌内注射：成人每次 1g，一日 1～2 次，或依病情按医嘱用药；儿童 10～25mg/kg。临时用，每瓶内加入 0.9% 氯化钠生理盐水或加入灭菌注射用水 2～4ml，溶解后注入。<br>Injection par voie IM : chez des adultes, 1g par fois, 1 à 2 fois par jour, ou en suivant les ordonnances ; chez des enfants, 10 à 25 mg/kg. Avant de l'utiliser, ajouter 2 à 4ml de solution saline de chlorure de sodium à 0,9 % ou d'injection stérile pour la dilution, puis l'injection. |
| 剂型、规格<br>Les formes pharmaceutiques et les spécifications | 注射用阿司匹林精氨酸盐：每瓶 0.5g（相当阿司匹林 0.25g）；1g（相当于阿司匹林 0.5g）。<br>L'aspirine arginine pour injection : 0,5g par flacon (équivalent à 0,25g d'aspirine), ou 1g par flacon (équivalent à 0,5g d'aspirine). |
| **药品名称 Drug Names** | 阿司匹林赖氨酸盐 Aspirine-DL-lysine |
| 适应证<br>Les indications | 主要用于发热及轻、中度的疼痛，如上呼吸道感染引起的发热、手术后痛、癌性疼痛、风湿痛、关节痛及神经痛等。<br>Ce produit sert à traiter la fièvre et les douleurs bénignes et modérées, telles que la fièvre causée par l'infection des voies respiratoires supérieures, la douleur postopératoire, la douleur canceuse, le rhumatisme, l'arthralgie et la névralgie. |
| 用法、用量<br>Les modes d'emploi et la posologie | 肌内注射或静脉滴注：每次 0.9～1.8g，一日 2 次；儿童 1 日 10～25mg/kg。以 0.9% 氯化钠注射液溶解后静脉滴注。<br>Injection par voie IM ou par voie IV en perfusion : 0,9 à 1,8g par fois, 2 fois par jour ; chez des enfents, 10 à 25 mg/kg par jour. Utiliser la solution de chlorure de sodium à 0,9 % pour la dilution, puis la perfusion. |
| 剂型、规格<br>Les formes pharmaceutiques et les spécifications | 注射用阿司匹林赖氨酸盐：每瓶 0.9g（相当于阿司匹林 0.5g）；0.5g（相当于阿司匹林 0.28g）。<br>La lysine d'aspirine pour injection : 0,9g par flacon (équivalent à 0,5g d'aspirine), ou 0,5g par flacon (équivalent à 0,28g d'aspirine). |

**续　表**

| 药品名称 Drug Names | 美沙拉秦 Mésalazine |
|---|---|
| 适应证<br>Les indications | 适用于溃疡性结肠炎和克罗恩病。<br>Ce produit sert à traiter la colite ulcéreuse et la maladie de Crohn. |
| 用法、用量<br>Les modes d'emploi et la posologie | 口服：可用一杯水漱服或在就餐时吞服。溃疡性结肠炎：急性期，每次 1 ～ 2 袋，一日 3 ～ 4 次（4g/d，8 袋）；缓解期，每次 1 袋，一日 3 ～ 4 次（2g/d，4 袋）。克罗恩病：缓解期，每次 1 袋，一日 3 ～ 4 次（2g/d，4 袋）。<br><br>Par voie orale : prendre avec de l'eau ou avaler avec des aliments. Pour traiter la colite ulcéreuse : au stade aigu, 1 à 2 sachet par fois, 3 à 4 fois par jour (4g par jour, 8 sachets) ; au stade de rémission, 1 sachet par fois, 3 à 4 fois par jour (2g par jour, 4 sachets). Pour traiter la maladie de Crohn : au stade de rémission, 1 sachet par fois, 3 à 4 fois par jour (2g par jour, 4 sachets). |
| 剂型、规格<br>Les formes pharmaceutiques et les spécifications | 缓释颗粒剂：每袋 500mg。<br>Granules à libération prolongée : 500mg par sachet. |
| 药品名称 Drug Names | 对乙酰氨基酚 Paracetamol |
| 适应证<br>Les indications | 用于感冒发热、关节痛、神经痛及偏头痛、癌性痛及手术后镇痛。本品还可用于对阿司匹林过敏、不耐受或不适于应用阿司匹林的患者（水痘、血友病及其他出血性疾病等）。<br><br>Il sert à traiter la fièvre, l'arthralgie, la névralgie, la migraine, les douleurs canceuses et postopératoires. Il est aussi applicable dans le traitement des patients allergiques ou résistant à l'aspirine (La varicelle, l'hémophilie et d'autres maladies hémorragiques). |
| 用法、用量<br>Les modes d'emploi et la posologie | 口服：1 次 0.3 ～ 0.6g，1 日 0.6 ～ 1.8g，一日量不宜超过 2g，一疗程不宜超过 10 日；儿童 12 岁以下按每日 $1.5g/m^2$ 分次服（如按年龄计：2 ～ 3 岁，一次 160mg；4 ～ 5 岁，一次 240mg；6 ～ 8 岁，一次 320mg；9 ～ 10 岁，一次 400mg；11 岁，一次 480mg。每 4 小时或必要时服一次）。肌内注射：1 次 0.15 ～ 0.25g。直肠给药：1 次 0.3 ～ 0.6g，一日 1 ～ 2 次。3 ～ 12 岁小儿，一次 0.15 ～ 0.3g，一日 1 次。<br><br>Par voie orale : 0,3 à 0,6g par fois, 0,6 à 1,8g par jour, ne pas dépasser 2g par jour, pendant 10 jours consécutifs au plus ; chez des enfants moins de 12ans, $1.5g/m^2$ par jour, à travers plusieurs fois (en fonction de l'âge : 2 à 3 ans, 160 mg par fois ; 4 à 5 ans, 240mg par fois ; 6 à 8 ans, 320 mg par fois ; 9 à 10 ans, 400mg par fois ; 11ans, 480 mg par fois. Toutes les 4 h ou le cas échéant.). Injection par voie IM : 0,15 à 0,25g par fois. Administration rectale : 0,3 à 0,6g par fois, 1 à 2 fois par jour. Chez des enfants de 3 à 12 ans, 0,15 à 0,3g par fois, 1 fois par jour. |
| 剂型、规格<br>Les formes pharmaceutiques et les spécifications | 片剂：每片 0.3g；0.5g。<br>胶囊剂：每粒 0.3g。<br>咀嚼片：每片 80mg。<br>泡腾冲剂：每袋 0.1g；0.5g。<br>口服液：每支 0.25g（10ml）。<br>栓剂：每粒 0.15g；0.3g；0.6g。<br>注射液：每支 0.075g（1ml）；0.25g（2ml）。<br>凝胶剂：每支 120mg（5g）。<br>Comprimés : 0,3g ou 0,5g par comprimé.<br>Capsules : 0,3g par capsule.<br>Les comprimés à mâcher : 80mg par comprimé.<br>Granules effervescents : 0,1g ou 0,5g par sachet.<br>La solution buccale : 0,25g (10ml) par solution.<br>Suppositoires : 0,15g, 0,3g ou 0,6g par suppositoire.<br>Injection : 0,075g (1ml), 0,25g (2ml) par injection.<br>Gels : 120mg (5g) par pièce. |

| 药品名称 Drug Names | 吲哚美辛 Indométacine |
|---|---|
| 适应证<br>Les indications | （1）急、慢性风湿性关节炎、痛风性关节炎及癌性疼痛。也可用于滑囊炎、腱鞘炎及关节囊炎等。还用于恶性肿瘤引起的发热或其他难以控制的发热。因本品不良反应较大，不宜作为治疗关节炎的首选药物，仅用于其他 NSAIDs 治疗无效的或不能耐受的患者。<br>（2）抗血小板聚集，可防止血栓形成，但疗效不如阿司匹林。<br>（3）治疗 Behcet 综合征，退热效果好；用于 Batter 综合征，效果尤其显著。<br>（4）用于胆绞痛、输尿管结石症引起的绞痛；对偏头痛也有一定的疗效，也可用于月经痛。<br>（5）本药滴眼液用于眼科手术及非手术因素引起的非感染性炎症。<br><br>(1) Applicable dans le traitement de l'arthrite rhumatismale, de l'arthrite goutteuse et des douleurs canceuses. Il s'utilise également pour traiter la bursite, la capsulite et la ténosynovite. Il sert aussi à traiter la fièvre causée par le cancer et d'autres fièvres difficilement contrôlées. Comme ce produit a des effets indésirables assez importants, il n'est pas un médicament de premier choix pour le traitement de l'arthrite. Il n'est utilisé que pour traiter les patients résistant aux AINS.<br>(2) Il s'utilise pour lutter contre l'agrégation plaquettaire et pour prévenir la thrombose, mais il est moins efficace que l'aspirine.<br>(3) Il est utilisé dans le traitement du syndrome de Behcet, efficce pour faire tomber la fièvre ; très efficace dans le traitement du syndrome de Batter.<br>(4) Il sert à traiter la colique biliaire et la colique causée par la lithiase urétérale ; également applicable dans le traitement de la migraine et de la dysménorrhée.<br>(5) Les gouttes pour les yeux de l'indométacine peuvent traiter l'inflammation non infectieuse causée par la chirurgie ophtalmique et les facteurs non – chirurgicaux. |
| 用法、用量<br>Les modes d'emploi et la posologie | 口服。开始时每次服 25mg，一日 2～3 次，饭时或饭后立即服用（可减少胃肠道不良反应）。治疗风湿性关节炎等症时，如未见不良反应，可逐渐增至 100～150mg，1 日最大量不超过 150mg，分 3～4 次服用，现已采用胶丸或栓剂剂型，使胃肠道不良反应发生率降低，栓剂且有维持药效较长的特点。直肠给药，1 次 50mg，1 日 50～100mg，一般连用 10 日为 1 个疗程。控释胶囊：一日 1 次，每次 75mg，或 1 次 25mg，一日 2 次。必要时 1 次 75mg，一日 2 次。小儿口服常用量：每日按 1.5～2.5mg/kg，分 3～4 次，有效后减至最低量。乳膏剂涂擦按摩患处，一日 2～3 次。经眼给药：眼科手术前：1 次 1 滴，术前 3、2、1 和 0.5 小时各滴一次。眼科手术后：1 次 1 滴，一日 1～4 次。其他非感染性炎症：1 次 1 滴，一日 4～6 次。<br><br>Par voie orale : au début, 25mg par fois, 2 à 3 fois par jour, durant ou immédiatement après le repas (pour éviter les effets indésirables gastro-intestinaux). Pour traiter l'arthrite rhumatismale, s'il n'y a pas d'effets indésirables, 100 à 150mg, ne pas dépasser 150mg par jour, à travers 3 à 4 fois. Aujourd'hui, les pilules et les suppositoires sont disponibles, ce qui permet de diminuer les effets indésirables gastro-intestinaux. L'administration rectale, 50mg par fois, 50 à 100mg par jour, pendant 10 jours consécutifs. Capsules à libération contrôlée : 1 fois par jour, 75mg par fois, ou 25mg par fois, 2 fois par jour. La dose usuelle en voie orale chez des enfants : 1,5 à 2,5 mg/kg par jour, à travers 3 à 4 fois, après le soulagement des symptômes, diminuer la dose. Pommades avec massage, 2 à 3 fois par jour. Gouttes pour les yeux : avant la chirurgie ophtalmique, 1 goutte par fois, respectivement 3, 2, 1, 0,5h avant la chirurgie ; après la chirurgie ophtalmique, 1 goutte par fois, 1 à 4 fois par jour. Pour d'autres inflammations non infectieuses, 1 goutte par fois, 4 à 6 fois par jour. |
| 剂型、规格<br>Les formes pharmaceutiques et les spécifications | 肠溶片：每片 25mg。胶囊：25mg。胶丸：每丸 25mg。控释胶囊每粒 25mg；75mg。控释片：每片 25mg；50mg；75mg。贴片：每片 12.5mg。栓剂：每粒 25mg；50mg；100mg。乳膏剂：每支 100mg（10g）。滴眼液：8ml；40mg。<br><br>comprimés à enrobage entérique : 25mg par comprimé.Capsules : 25mg. Pilules : 25mg par pilule. Capsules à libération contrôlée : 25mg ou 75mg par capsule. Comprimés à libération contrôlée : 25mg, 50mg ou 75mg par comprimé. Patch : 12,5mg par pièce. Suppositoires : 25mg, 50mg ou 100mg par suppositoire. Pommades : 100mg (10g) par pommade. Gouttes pour les yeux : 8ml : 40mg. |
| 药品名称 Drug Names | 双氯芬酸 Diclofénac |
| 适应证<br>Les indications | 用于类风湿关节炎、神经炎、红斑狼疮及癌症、手术后疼痛，各种原因引起的发热。<br>　　Ce produit sert à traiter la polyarthrite rhumatoide, la névrite, le lupus érythémateux, des douleurs canceuses et postopératoires ainsi que la fièvre. |

**续　表**

| 用法、用量<br>Les modes d'emploi et la posologie | 口服：成人，每日剂量为 100 ～ 150mg，分 2 ～ 3 次服用。对轻度患者及 14 岁以上的青少年酌减。此药最好在餐前用水整片送下。肌内注射深部注射，1 次 50mg，一日 1 次，必要时数小时在注射 1 次。外用：擦剂，根据疼痛部位大小，1 ～ 3ml 均匀涂于患处，一日 2 ～ 4 次，一日总量不超过 15ml。乳膏，根据疼痛部位大小，1 次 2 ～ 4g 涂于患处，并轻轻按摩，一日 3 ～ 4 次，一日总量不超过 30g。<br><br>Par voie orale : chez des adultes, 100 à 150mg par jour, à travers 2 à 3 fois. Chez des patients bénins et des enfants plus de 14ans, diminuer un peu la dose. Il vaut mieux l'avaler tout entier avant le repas. Injection par voie IM profonde : 50mg par fois, 1 fois par jour, le cas échéant, plusieurs heures après, encore une injection. Pour l'usage externe : comme liniment, 1 à 3ml par fois, 2 à 4 fois par jour, ne pas dépasser 15ml par jour. Comme crème, 2 à 4g par fois, masser doucement, 3 à 4 fois par jour, ne pas dépasser 30g par jour. |
| :-- | :-- |
| 剂型、规格<br>Les formes pharmaceutiques et les spécifications | 片剂：每片 25mg。擦剂：20ml：200mg。乳膏：25g：750mg。注射液：50mg（2ml）。<br><br>Comprimés : 25mg par comprimé. Liniment : 20ml : 200mg. Crème : 25g : 750mg. Injection : 50mg (2ml). |
| 药品名称 Drug Names | 萘普生 Naproxène |
| 适应证<br>Les indications | 用于类风湿关节炎、骨关节炎、强直性脊柱炎、痛风、运动系统（如关节、肌肉及肌腱）的慢性变性疾病及轻、中度疼痛如痛经等。<br><br>Ce produit sert à traiter la polyarthrite rhumatoide, l'arthrose, la spondylarthrite ankylosante, la goutte, les maladies dégénératives chroniques du système locomoteur (tel que les articulations, les muscles et les tendons), ainsi que les douleurs bénignes et modérées telles que la dysménorrhée. |
| 用法、用量<br>Les modes d'emploi et la posologie | 口服，开始每日剂量 0.5 ～ 0.75g，维持量每日 0.375 ～ 0.75g，分早晨和傍晚 2 次服用。轻、中度疼痛或痛经时，开始用 0.5g，必需时 6 ～ 8 小时在服 0.25g，日剂量不超过 1.25g。肌内注射，一次 100 ～ 200mg，一日一次。栓剂直肠给药，一次 0.25g，一日 0.5g。<br><br>Par voie orale, au début, 0,5 à 0,75g par jour, ensuite, maintenir 0,375 à 0,75g par jour, 2 fois par jour (le petit matin et le coucher du soleil). Pour traiter les douleurs bénignes, modérées ou la dysménorrhée, au début, 0,5g, s'il est nécessaire, 6 à 8 h après, encore 0,25g, ne pas dépasser 1,25g par jour. Injection par voie IM, 100 à 200 mg par fois, 1 fois par jour. Pour les suppositoires, 0,25g par fois, 0,5g fois par jour. |
| 剂型、规格<br>Les formes pharmaceutiques et les spécifications | 片（胶囊）剂：每片（粒）0.1g；0.125g；0.25g。缓释胶囊（片）：每粒（片）0.25g。注射液：每支 100mg（2ml）；200mg（2ml）。栓剂：每粒 0.25g。<br><br>Comprimés (capsules) : 0,1g, 0,125g ou 0,25g par comprimé ou par capsule. Capsules (comprimés) à libération prolongée : 0,25g par capsule ou par comprimé.Injection : 100mg (2ml) ou 200mg (2ml) par solution.Suppositoires : 0,25g par suppositoire. |
| 药品名称 Drug Names | 布洛芬 Ibuprofène |
| 适应证<br>Les indications | 用于风湿性及类风湿关节炎，以及抗炎、镇痛、解热作用与阿司匹林、保泰松相似，比对乙酰氨基酚好。在患者不能耐受阿司匹林、保泰松等时，可试用。<br><br>Ce produit sert à traiter la polyarthrite rhumatoide, l'arthrite rhumatismale et a un effet analgésique, antipyrétique et anti-inflammatoire. Il est similaire à l'aspirine, à la phénylbutazone et meilleur à l'acétaminophène en termes d'efficacité. Il est applicable dans le traitemetn des patients résistant à l'aspirine et à la phénylbutazone. |
| 用法、用量<br>Les modes d'emploi et la posologie | 抗风湿，一次 0.4 ～ 0.8g，一日 3 ～ 4 次。镇痛，一次 0.2 ～ 0.4g，每 4 ～ 6 小时 1 次。成人最大限量每日 2.4g。<br><br>Pour lutter contre l'arthrite, 0,4 à 0,8g par fois, 3 à 4 fois par jour. pour l'analgésique, 0,2 à 0,4g par fois, toutes les 4 à 6h. chez des adultes, ne pas dépasser 2,4g par jour. |
| 剂型、规格<br>Les formes pharmaceutiques et les spécifications | 片剂（胶囊）：每片（粒）0.1g；0.2g；0.3g。缓释胶囊：每粒 0.3g。颗粒剂：每袋 0.1g；0.2g。干混悬剂：每瓶 1.2g（34g）。糖浆剂：每支 0.2g（10ml）。口服液：每支 0.1g（10ml）。混悬剂：每瓶 2.0g（100ml）。擦剂：每瓶 2.5g（50ml）。栓剂：每粒 50mg；100mg。<br><br>Comprimés (capsules) : 0,1g, 0,2g ou 0,3g par comprimé ou par capsule. Capsules à libération prolongée : 0,3g par capsule. Granules : 0,1g ou 0,2g par sachet. Suspension sèche : 1,2g (34g) par flacon. Sirops : 0,2g (10ml) par solution. Solution buccale : 0,1g (10ml) par pièce. Suspension : 2,0g (100ml) par flacon. Liniment : 2,5g (50ml) par flacon. Suppositoires : 50 mg ou 100mg par suppositoire. |

**续　表**

| 药品名称 Drug Names | 酮洛芬 Kétoprofène |
|---|---|
| 适应证<br>Les indications | 用于类风湿关节炎、风湿性关节炎、骨关节炎、强直性脊柱炎及痛风等。本品治疗关节炎时，连续用药 2～3 周可达最佳疗效。<br><br>Ce produit sert à traiter la polyarthrite rhumatoide, l'arthrite rhumatismale, l'arthrose, la spondylarthrite ankylosante et la goutte. En cas de traitement de l'arthrite, il faut prendre ce médicament pendant 2 à 3 semaines pour obtenir un effet désirable. |
| 用法、用量<br>Les modes d'emploi et la posologie | 口服：每次 50mg，一日 150mg，分 3～4 次；每日最大用量 200mg，或每次 100mg，一日 2 次，为避免对胃肠道刺激，应餐后服用，整个胶囊吞服。<br><br>Par voie orale : 50mg par fois, 150 mg par jour, à travers 3 à 4 fois ; ne pas dépasser 200mg par jour. Ou 100mg par fois, 2 fois par jour. Pour éviter l'irritation gastro-intestinale, il faut le prendre après le repas en avalant la capsule en entier. |
| 剂型、规格<br>Les formes pharmaceutiques et les spécifications | 肠溶胶囊：每粒 20mg；50mg。控释胶囊：每粒 20mg。缓释片：每片 75mg。搽剂：每支 0.3g（10ml）；0.9g（30ml）；1.5g（50ml）。<br><br>Capsules à enrobage entérique : 20mg ou 50 mg par capsule. Capsules à libération contrôlée : 20mg par capsule. Comprimés à libération prolongée : 75mg par comprimé. Liniments : 0,3g (10ml), 0,9g (30ml) ou 1,5g (50ml) par liniment. |
| 药品名称 Drug Names | 芬布芬 Fenbufène |
| 适应证<br>Les indications | 用于类风湿关节炎、风湿性关节炎、骨关节炎、强直性脊柱炎及痛风等。应用于牙痛、手术后疼痛、外伤疼痛等的镇痛。<br><br>Ce produit sert à traiter la polyarthrite rhumatoide, l'arthrite rhumatismale, l'arthrose, la spondylarthrite ankylosante et la goutte. Il est aussi applicable dans le traitement de l'odontalgie, des douleurs postopératoires et traumatiques. |
| 用法、用量<br>Les modes d'emploi et la posologie | 口服，成人一次 0.6～0.9g，一次或分次服用。多数患者晚上口服 0.6g 即可。分次服用时，每日总量不得超过 0.9g。<br><br>Par voie orale, chez des adultes, 0,6 à 0,9 g par fois, à travers 1 ou plusieurs fois. Pour la plupart des patients, il suffit de prendre 0,6g par voie orale le soir. En cas d'administration à travers plusieurs fois, ne pas dépasser 0,9g par jour. |
| 剂型、规格<br>Les formes pharmaceutiques et les spécifications | 片剂：每片 0.15g；0.3g。<br>胶囊剂：每粒 0.5g。<br>Comprimés : 0,15g ou 0,3g par comprimé.<br>Capsules : 0,5g par capsule. |
| 药品名称 Drug Names | 吡洛芬 Pirprofène |
| 适应证<br>Les indications | 用于风湿性关节炎、骨关节炎、强直性脊柱炎、非关节型风湿病、急性疼痛、术后痛及癌性痛等。<br><br>Ce produit sert à traiter l'arthrite rhumatismale, l'arthrose, la spondylarthrite ankylosante, le rhumatisme non articulaire, les douleurs aigues, les douleurs postopératoires et la douleur canceuse. |
| 用法、用量<br>Les modes d'emploi et la posologie | 开始口服，每日 800mg，一日 2 次分服。症状改善后，每日 600mg 维持。类风湿关节炎、强直性脊柱炎开始 1000mg/d，分 3 次服，持续 1～2 周。镇痛：每次 200～400mg，每日 1200mg。肌内注射每次 400mg。数小时后可重复使用。<br><br>Par voie orale, 800 mg par jour, 2 fois par jour. Avec l'amélioration des symptômes, 600mg par jour. Pour taiter la polyarthrite rhumatoide, la spondylarthrite ankylosante, au début, 1000 mg par jour, à travers 3 fois, pendant 1 à 2 semaines. Pour l'analgésique, 200 à 400 mg par fois, 1200 mg par jour. Injection par voie IM, 400mg par fois. Quelques heures après, possible de le réutiliser. |
| 剂型、规格<br>Les formes pharmaceutiques et les spécifications | 片剂：每片 200mg。<br>Comprimés : 200mg par comprimé. |

**续 表**

| 药品名称 Drug Names | 阿明洛芬 Alminoprofène |
|---|---|
| 适应证<br>Les indications | 用于风湿性和类风湿关节炎、神经根痛、肌腱炎、创伤（骨折、挫伤、扭伤）、痛经、产后子宫绞痛、牙痛、中耳炎等。<br><br>Ce produit sert à traiter l'arthrite rhumatismale et la polyarthrite rhumatoide, la douleur radiculaire, les tendinites, les traumatismes (fractures, contusions, entorses), la dysménorrhée, les crampes utérines post-partum, l'odontalgie ainsi que l'otite moyenne. |
| 用法、用量<br>Les modes d'emploi et la posologie | 口服，成人每次300mg，一日2～3次，可根据疗效酌情减量。治疗子宫绞痛时，每日300～600mg分2次餐前服。<br><br>Par voie orale, 300mg par fois chez des adultes, 2 à 3 fois par jour, ajuster la dose en fonction des maladies. Pour traiter les crampes utérines post-partum, 300 à 600 mg par jour, à travers 2 fois, avant le repas. |
| 剂型、规格<br>Les formes pharmaceutiques et les spécifications | 片剂：每片150mg；300mg。<br>Comprimés : 150 mg ou 300mg par comprimé. |

| 药品名称 Drug Names | 洛索洛芬 Loxoprofene |
|---|---|
| 适应证<br>Les indications | 用于类风湿关节炎、变形性关节炎、腰痛、关节周围炎、颈肩腕综合征，以及手术后、外伤后和拔牙后的镇痛抗炎，急性上呼吸道炎症和解热镇痛。<br><br>Il s'utilise dans le traiment de l'arthrose, de la lombalgie, l'arthrite périphérique,TMS des membres supérieurs (cou, épaule, coude, poignet, main). Il sert aussi d'analgésique postopératoire, traumatique et après l'extraction dentaire. Il est également utilisé dans le traitement de l'inflammation des voies respiratoires supérieures et dans l'antipyrétique. |
| 用法、用量<br>Les modes d'emploi et la posologie | 餐后服用。慢性炎症疼痛：成人一次60mg，一日3次。急性炎症疼痛：顿服60～120mg。可根据年龄、症状适当增减，一次最大剂量不超过180mg。<br><br>Administration après le repas. Pour traiter les douleurs inflammatoires chroniques : 60mg par fois chez des adultes, 3 fois par jour. Pour traiter les douleurs inflammatoires aigues, 60 à 120 mg, 1 fois par jour. possible d'ajuster la dose en fonction de l'âge et des maladies, ne pas dépasser 180mg par fois. |
| 剂型、规格<br>Les formes pharmaceutiques et les spécifications | 片剂：每片60mg。<br>胶囊：每粒60mg。<br>颗粒剂：2g：60mg。<br>Comprimés : 60mg par comprimé.<br>Capsules : 60mg par capsule.<br>Granules : 2g : 60mg. |

| 药品名称 Drug Names | 吡罗昔康 Piroxicam |
|---|---|
| 适应证<br>Les indications | 用于治疗风湿性及类风湿关节炎。<br>Ce produit sert à traiter l'arthrite rhumatismale et la polyarthrite rhumatoide. |
| 用法、用量<br>Les modes d'emploi et la posologie | 口服：抗风湿，一日20mg，一日1次；抗痛风，一日40mg，一日1次，连续4～6日。肌内注射：一次10～20mg，一日1次。<br><br>Par voie orale : pour traiter le rhumatisme, 20mg par jour, 1 fois par jour ; pour traiter la goutte, 40mg par jour, 1 fois par four, pendant 4 à 6 jours consécutifs. Injection par voie IM : 10 à 20 mg par fois, 1 fois par jour. |
| 剂型、规格<br>Les formes pharmaceutiques et les spécifications | 片（胶囊）剂：每片（粒）10mg；20mg。注射液：每支10mg（1ml）；20mg（2ml）。凝胶剂：每支50mg（10g）；60mg（12g）。搽剂：每支0.5mg（50ml）。软膏：每支0.1g（10g）。<br><br>Comprimés (capsules) : 10mg ou 20mg par comprimé ou par capsule. Injection : 10mg (1ml) ou 20mg (2ml) par injection. Gels : 50mg (10g) ou 60mg (12g) par gel. Liniment : 0,5 g (50ml) par liniment. Pommade : 0,1g (10g) par pommade. |

**续　表**

| 药品名称 Drug Names | 美洛昔康 Méloxicam |
|---|---|
| 适应证<br>Les indications | 用于类风湿关节炎和骨关节炎的对症治疗。<br>Ce produit sert à traiter la polyarthrite rhumatoide et l'arthrose. |
| 用法、用量<br>Les modes d'emploi et la posologie | 类风湿骨关节炎：成人一日 15mg，一日 1 次，根据治疗后反应，剂量可减至 7.5mg/d。骨关节炎：7.5mg/d，如果需要，剂量可增至 15mg/d。严重肾衰竭者，剂量不应超过 7.5mg/d。<br>Pour traiter la polyarthrite rhumatoide : chez des adultes, 15mg par jour, 1 fois par jour, ensuite, en fonction de l'effet du traitement, 7,5 mg par jour. Pour traiter l'arthrose : 7,5 mg par jour, s'il est nécessaire, 15 mg par jour. Chez des patients insuffisants rénaux sévères, ne pas dépasser 7,5 mg par jour. |
| 剂型、规格<br>Les formes pharmaceutiques et les spécifications | 片剂：每片 7.5mg；15mg。<br>Comprimés : 7,5 mg ou 15mg par comprimé. |
| 药品名称 Drug Names | 氯诺昔康 Lornoxicam |
| 适应证<br>Les indications | 用于妇产科矫形手术后的急性疼痛，急性坐骨神经痛及腰痛。亦可用于慢性腰痛、关节炎、类风湿关节炎和强直性脊柱炎。<br>Ce produit sert à traiter les douleurs aigues après la chirurgie orthopédique obstétrique, la sciatique et le lumbago. Il est également applicable dans le traitement du lumbago chronique, de l'arthrite, de la polyarthrite rhumatoide et de la spondylarthrite ankylosante. |
| 用法、用量<br>Les modes d'emploi et la posologie | 急性轻度或中度疼痛：每日剂量为 8～16mg，分 2～3 次服用；每日最大剂量为 16mg。风湿性疾病引起的关节疼痛和炎症：每日剂量为 12mg，分 2～3 次服用；服用剂量不应超过 16mg。<br>Pour traiter des douleurs aigues bénignes ou modérées : 8 à 16mg par jour, à travers 2 à 3 fois, ne pas dépaser 16 mg par jour. Pour traiter la douleur et l'inflammation articulaires causées par les maladies rhumatismales : 12mg par jour, à travers 2 à 3 fois, ne pas dépasser 16mg par jour. |
| 剂型、规格<br>Les formes pharmaceutiques et les spécifications | 片剂：4mg。<br>Comprimés : 4mg. |
| 药品名称 Drug Names | 塞来昔布 Célécoxib |
| 适应证<br>Les indications | 用于急、慢性骨关节炎和类风湿关节炎。<br>Applicable dans le traitement de l'arthrose aigue et chronique, ainsi que de la polyarthrite rhumatoide. |
| 用法、用量<br>Les modes d'emploi et la posologie | 治疗关节炎，一日 200mg，分 2 次服或顿服；用于类风湿关节炎，剂量为一日 100mg 或 200mg，一日 2 次。<br>Pour traiter l'arthrite, 200mg par jour, à travers 2 fois ou 1 fois seulement. Pour traiter la polyarthrite rhumatoide, 100mg ou 200mg par jour, 2 fois par jour. |
| 剂型、规格<br>Les formes pharmaceutiques et les spécifications | 胶囊：每粒 100mg。<br>Capsules : 100mg par capsule. |
| 药品名称 Drug Names | 帕瑞昔布 Parécoxib |
| 适应证<br>Les indications | 用于术后疼痛的短期治疗。<br>Capsules : 100mg par capsule. |
| 用法、用量<br>Les modes d'emploi et la posologie | 成人，40mg/ 次，静脉注射或深部肌内注射，随后视需要间隔 6～12 小时给药给予 20mg 或 40mg，总剂量不超过 80mg/d。<br>Chez des adultes, 40 mg par fois, administration par voie IV ou injection par voie IM profonde, ensuite, 20mg ou 40 mg toutes les 6 à 12h, ne pas dépasser 80 mg par jour. |

**续 表**

| 剂型、规格<br>Les formes pharmaceutiques et les spécifications | 注射粉针：每瓶 20mg；40mg。<br>Poudre pour injection : 20mg pou 40mg par flacon. |
|---|---|
| **药品名称 Drug Names** | 尼美舒利 Nimésulide |
| 适应证<br>Les indications | 主要用于类风湿关节炎和骨关节炎、痛经、手术后疼和发热等。<br>Ce produit sert à traiter la polyarthrite rhumatoïde, l'arthrose, la dysménorrhée, les douleurs postopératoires et la fièvre. |
| 用法、用量<br>Les modes d'emploi et la posologie | 口服：成人，每次 100mg，一日 2 次，餐后服用。儿童常用剂量为 5mg/（kg·d），每 2～3 次服用。老年人无须调整剂量。<br>Par voie orale : chez des adultes, 100mg par fois, 2 fois par jour, après le rapas. Chez des enfants, dose usuelle, 5 mg/kg par jour, à travers 2 à 3 fois. Pas nécessaire d'ajuster la dose chez des personnes âgées. |
| 剂型、规格<br>Les formes pharmaceutiques et les spécifications | 片剂：每片 50mg；100mg。<br>Comprimés : 50mg pou 100mg par comprimé. |
| **药品名称 Drug Names** | 安乃近 Métamizole sodique |
| 适应证<br>Les indications | 主要用于解热、急性关节炎、头痛、风湿性痛、牙痛及肌肉痛等。<br>Ce produit s'utilise comme antipyrétique et comme traitement de l'arthrite aigue, des douleurs rhumatismales et masculaires, de l'odontalgie et de la céphalée. |
| 用法、用量<br>Les modes d'emploi et la posologie | 口服：一次 0.25～0.5g，一日 0.75～1.25g。滴鼻：小儿退热常以 10%～20% 滴鼻，5 岁以下，每次每侧鼻孔 1～2 滴，必要时重复用一次；5 岁以上适当加量。深部肌内注射：每次 0.25～0.5g；小儿每次 5～10mg/kg。<br>Par voie orale : 0,25 à 0,5 g par fois, 0,75 à 1,25g par jour. Gouttes nasales : pour faire tomber la fièvre chez des enfants, gouttes nasales de 10 % à 20 %, chez moins de 5 ans, 1 à 2 gouttes par narine par fois, le cas échéant, encore une fois ; chez plus de 5 ans, augmenter la dose. Injection par voie IM profonde : 0,25 à 0,5 g par fois ; chez des enfants, 5 à 10 mg/kg par fois. |
| 剂型、规格<br>Les formes pharmaceutiques et les spécifications | 片剂：每片 0.25g；0.5g。滴液：1ml；200mg。注射液：每支 0.25g（1ml）；0.5g（2ml）。滴鼻剂：10%～20%。<br>Comprimés : 0,25g ou 0,5g par comprimé. Gouttes : 1ml : 200mg. Injection : 0,25g (1ml) ou 0,5g (2ml) par injection. Gouttes nasales : 10 % à 20 %. |
| **药品名称 Drug Names** | 保泰松 Phénylbutazone |
| 适应证<br>Les indications | 用于类风湿关节炎、风湿性关节炎、强直性脊柱炎及急性痛风等。常需连续使用或与其他药物配合使用。亦用于丝虫病急性淋巴管炎。<br>Ce produit sert à traiter la polyarthrite rhumatoïde, la polyarthrite rhumatoïde, la spondylarthrite obligatoire et la goutte aiguë. Il faut toujours l'utiliser pour une longue durée ou avec d'autres médicaments. Il est aussi applicable dans le traitement de la lymphangite filarienne aiguë. |
| 用法、用量<br>Les modes d'emploi et la posologie | （1）关节炎：开始一日量 0.3～0.6g，分 3 次餐后服用。一日量不宜超过 0.8g。一周后如无不良反应，可继续服用递减至每日量 0.1～0.2g。<br>（2）丝虫病急性淋巴管炎：每次服 0.2g，一日 3 次，总量 1.2～3g，急性炎症控制后，再用抗丝虫药治疗。<br>(1) Pour traiter l'arthrite : au début, 0,3 à 0,6 g par jour, trois fois par jour. Ne pas dépasser 0,8g par jour. S'il n'y pas d'effets indésirables une semaine après, 0,1 à 0,2g par jour.<br>(2) Pour traite la lymphangite filarienne aigue : 0,2g par fois, 3 fois par jour, 1,2 à 3 g au total. Après le contrôle de l'inflammation aigue, prendre des médicaments antifilariens. |

| 续　表 | |
|---|---|
| 剂型、规格<br>Les formes pharmaceutiques et les spécifications | 片（胶囊）剂：每片（粒）0.1g；200mg。<br>栓剂：25mg。<br>注射液：600mg（3ml）。<br>Comprimés (capsules) : 0,1g ou 200mg par comprimé ou par capsule.<br>Suppositoires : 25mg.<br>Injection : 600mg (3ml). |
| 药品名称 Drug Names | 萘丁美酮 Nabumétone |
| 适应证<br>Les indications | 本品用于急、慢性关节炎及永动性软组织损伤、扭伤和挫伤、术后疼痛、牙痛、痛经等。<br>Ce produit sert à traiter l'arthrite chronique et aigue, les blessures perpétuelles des tissus mous, les entorses, les contusions, la douleur postopératoire, l'odontalgie ainsi que la dysménorrhée. |
| 用法、用量<br>Les modes d'emploi et la posologie | 口服，每次 1g，一日 1 次，睡前服。一次最大量为 2g。一日 2 次服。体重不足 50kg 的成人，可以每日 0.5g 起始，逐渐上调至有效剂量。<br>Par voie orale, 1g par fois, 1 fois par jour, avant le sommeil. Ne pas dépasser 2g par fois. Chez des adultes moins de 50kg, commencer par prendre 0,5g par jour avant de renforcer le dosage pour atteindre la dose efficace. |
| 剂型、规格<br>Les formes pharmaceutiques et les spécifications | 片剂：每片 0.25g；0.5g；0.75g。胶囊剂：每粒 0.2g；0.25g。分散片：每片 0.5g。干混悬剂：0.5g。<br>Comprimés : 0,25g, 0,5g ou 0,75g par comprimé. Capsules : 0,2g ou 0,25g par capsule. Comprimés dispersibles : 0,5g par comprimé. Suspension sèche : 0,5g. |
| 药品名称 Drug Names | 来氟米特 Léflunomide |
| 适应证<br>Les indications | 用于成人风湿性关节炎的治疗。<br>Ce produit sert à traiter la polyarthrite rhumatoïde. |
| 用法、用量<br>Les modes d'emploi et la posologie | 由于半衰期较长建议间隔 24 小时给药。建议开始最初治疗的 3 日给予负荷量（50mg/d），之后给予维持剂量 20mg/d。<br>Comme sa demi-vie est longue, il est recommandé de l'administrer toutes les 24h. Il vaut mieux prendre 50 mg par jour pendant les trois premiers jours avant de maintenir 20 mg par jour. |
| 剂型、规格<br>Les formes pharmaceutiques et les spécifications | 片剂：每片 10mg；20mg；100mg。<br>Comprimés : 10mg, 20mg ou 100mg par comprimé. |
| 药品名称 Drug Names | 复方骨肽 Composée Ossotide |
| 适应证<br>Les indications | 用于风湿性关节炎、类风湿关节炎、骨质疏松、颈椎病等疾病的症状改善。同时用于骨折或骨科手术后骨愈合，可促进骨愈合和骨新生。<br>Ce produit sert à traiter le rhumatisme, l'arthrite rhumatoïde, l'ostéoporose, l'arthrose cervicale. Il est aussi applicable dans la consolidation osseuse après la fracture ou une chirurgie orthopédique. Il favoriser la guérison osseuse. |
| 用法、用量<br>Les modes d'emploi et la posologie | 肌内注射，一次 30～60mg，一日 1 次；静脉滴注，一次 60～150mg，一日 1 次，10～30 日为 1 个疗程或遵医嘱，亦可在痛点或穴位注射。<br>Injection par voie IV, 30 à 60 mg par fois, 1 fois par jour; Perfusion, 60 à 150 mg par fois, 1 fois par jour, pendant 10 à 30 jours comme un traitement médical ou en suivant les ordonnances. Aussi possible de l'injecter au point de douleur ou au point d'acupuncture. |
| 剂型、规格<br>Les formes pharmaceutiques et les spécifications | 注射液：每支 30mg（2ml）；75mg（5ml）多肽物质。<br>Injection : 30mg (2ml) ou 75mg (5ml) de peptide par injection. |

**续 表**

| 药品名称 Drug Names | 硫辛酸 Acide Lipoique |
|---|---|
| 适应证<br>Les indications | 用于糖尿病周围神经病变引起的感觉异常。<br>Ce produit sert à traiter la paresthésie causée par la neuropathie diabétique périphérique. |
| 用法、用量<br>Les modes d'emploi et la posologie | 静脉注射应缓慢，最大速度为每分钟 50mg（2ml）。本品也可加入生理盐水静脉滴注如 250～500mg（10～20ml）加入 100～250ml 生理盐水中、静脉滴注时间为 30 分钟。<br>Injection lente par voie IV, ne pas dépasser 50 mg (2ml) par minute. En perfusion avec la solution saline, par exemple, pour 250 à 500 mg (10 à 20ml) de ce produit, ajouter 100 à 250 ml de solution saline, perfusion pendant 30 minutes. |
| 剂型、规格<br>Les formes pharmaceutiques et les spécifications | 注射液：每支 0.6g（20ml）。<br>Injection : 0,6g (20ml) par injection. |
| 药品名称 Drug Names | 氟比洛芬 Flurbiprofène |
| 适应证<br>Les indications | 主要用于风湿性关节炎。<br>Ce produit sert à traiter la polyarthrite rhumatoïde. |
| 用法、用量<br>Les modes d'emploi et la posologie | 一日 150～200mg，分次服。<br>100 à 200 mg par jour, à travers plusieurs fois. |
| 剂型、规格<br>Les formes pharmaceutiques et les spécifications | 片剂：每片 50mg；100mg。<br>Comprimés : 50mg ou 100mg par comprimé. |
| 药品名称 Drug Names | 醋氯芬酸 Acéclofénac |
| 适应证<br>Les indications | 用于类风湿关节炎及骨关节炎等症状。<br>Ce produit sert à traiter la polyarthrite rhumatoïde et l'arthrose. |
| 用法、用量<br>Les modes d'emploi et la posologie | 每次 100mg，一日 2 次。<br>100mg par fois, 2 fois par jour. |
| 剂型、规格<br>Les formes pharmaceutiques et les spécifications | 片剂：每片 100mg。<br>Comprimés : 100mg par comprimé. |

8.4 抗痛风药 Médicaments anti-goutte

| 药品名称 Drug Names | 秋水仙碱 Colchicine |
|---|---|
| 适应证<br>Les indications | 用于痛风性关节炎的急性发作、预防复发性痛风性关节炎的急性发作、家族性地中海热。<br>Ce produit sert à traiter la crise aiguë de l'arthrite goutteuse, à prévenir la crise aigue de l'arthrite goutteuse récurrente età traiter la fièvre méditerranéenne familiale. |
| 用法、用量<br>Les modes d'emploi et la posologie | （1）急性期治疗：①口服：成人常用量为每 1～2 小时服 0.5～1mg，至关节症状缓解或出现恶心、呕吐、腹泻等胃肠道不良反应时停用。一般需要 3～5mg，不宜超过 6mg，症状可在 6～12 小时减轻，24～48 小时控制，以后 48 小时不需要服用本品。此后每次给 0.5mg，一日 2～3 次（0.5～1.5mg/d），共 7 日。②静脉注射：用于急性痛风发作和口服用药胃肠道反应过于剧烈者。可将此药 1mg 用 0.9% 氯化钠注射液 20ml 稀释，缓慢注射（20～30 分钟）。24 小时剂量不超过 2mg，但应注意勿使药物外漏，视病情需要 6～8 小时后可再注射，有肾功能减退者 24 小时不超过 3mg。 |

**续　表**

| | |
|---|---|
| | （2）口服，口服每次 0.5～1mg，但疗程量酌定，要注意不良反应的出现，出现即停药。<br><br>（1) Pour le traitement au stade aigu : ① Par voie orale : chez des adultes, dose usuelle, 0,5 à 1mg toutes les 1 à 2h, arrêter l'administration quand les symptômes articulaires s'améliorent ou quand se produisent des réactions indésirables gastro-intestinales, telles que la nausée, le vomissement ou la diarrhée. En général, il faut 3 à 5mg, et 6mg au plus, pour réduire les symptômes en 6 à 12h, contrôler la maladie en 24 à 48h. Durant les 48h suivantes, il n'est pas nécessaire de prendre le médicament. Après, 0,5mg par fois, 2 à 3 fois par jour (0,5 à 1,5 mg par jour), pendant 7 jours. ② Injection par voie IV : pour traiter la crise aigue de la goutte et les patients dont la réaction indésirable gastro-intestinale est trop importante en cas d'administration par voie orale. Dissoudre 1mg de ce produit dans 20ml de solution de chlorure de sodium à 0,9 %, injection lente pendant 20 à 30 minutes. Ne pas dépasser 2mg par jour. Veiller à ce que le médicament ne fuit pas. Selon les cas, possible d'injecter encore une fois 6 à 8 h après. Ne pas dépaser 3mg par jour chez des patients insuffisants rénaux.<br><br>(2) Par voie orale, 0,5 à 1mg par fois selon les cas. Arrêter l'administration du médicament une fois qu'il y a des réactions indésirables. |
| 剂型、规格<br>Les formes pharmaceutiques et les spécifications | 片剂：每片 0.5mg；1mg。<br>注射液：0.5mg/ml。<br>Comprimés : 0,5mg ou 1mg par comprimé.<br>Injection : 0,5mg/ml. |
| 药品名称 Drug Names | 丙磺舒 Probénécide |
| 适应证<br>Les indications | 用于慢性痛风的治疗。<br>Ce produit sert à traiter la goutte chronique. |
| 用法、用量<br>Les modes d'emploi et la posologie | （1）慢性痛风：口服每次 0.25g，一日 2～4 次，一周后可增至每次 0.5～1g，一日 2 次。每日最大剂量不超过 2g。<br>（2）增强青霉素类的作用：每次 0.5g，一日 4 次。儿童：25mg/kg，每 3～9 小时 1 次。2～14 岁或体重在 50kg 以下儿童，首剂按体重 0.025g/kg，或按体表面积 0.7g/m²，以后每次 0.01g/kg 或按体表面积 0.3g/m²，一日 4 次。<br><br>(1) Pour traiter la goutte chronique : par voie orale, 0,25g par fois, 2 à 4 fois par jour, une semaine après, augmenter la dose pour atteindre 0,5 à 1 g par fois, 2 fois par jour. Ne pas dépasser 2g par jour.<br>(2) Pour renforer le rôle de la pénicilline : 0,5g par fois, 4 fois par jour. Chez des enfants : 25 mg/kg, toutes les 3 à 9 h. chez de 2 à 14ans ou des enfants moins de 50kg, au début, 0,025g/kg en fonction du poids ou 0,7g/m² en fonction de la surface corporelle, ensuite, 0,01g/kg ou 0,3 g/m², 4 fois par jour. |
| 剂型、规格<br>Les formes pharmaceutiques et les spécifications | 片剂：每片 0.25g；0.5g。<br>Comprimés : 0,25g ou 0,5g par comprimé. |
| 药品名称 Drug Names | 苯溴马隆 Benzbromarone |
| 适应证<br>Les indications | 用于反复发作的痛风性关节炎伴高尿酸血症即痛风湿患者。<br>Il sert à traiter l'arthrite goutteuse récurrente et l'hyperuricémie, à savoir la goutte humide. |
| 用法、用量<br>Les modes d'emploi et la posologie | 每次 25～100mg，一日 1 次，餐后服用，剂量逐渐增加，连用 3～6 个月。<br>25 à 100mg par fois, 1 fois par jour, après le repas, augmenter progressivement la dose, pendant 3 à 6 mois consécutifs. |
| 剂型、规格<br>Les formes pharmaceutiques et les spécifications | 片剂：每片 50mg。<br>Comprimés : 50mg par comprimé. |
| 药品名称 Drug Names | 别嘌醇 Allopurinol |
| 适应证<br>Les indications | 用于慢性原发性或继发性痛风、痛风性肾病。<br>Ce produit sert à traiter la goutte primaire ou secondaire chronique ainsi que la néphropathie goutteuse. |

**续 表**

| | |
|---|---|
| 用法、用量<br>Les modes d'emploi et la posologie | 用于降低血中尿酸浓度：开始每次 0.05g，一日 2～3 次，剂量渐增，2～3 周后增至每日 0.2～0.4g，分 2～3 次服，每日最大量不超过 0.6g。维持量：每次 0.1～0.2g，一日 2～3 次。儿童剂量每日 8mg/kg。治疗尿酸结石：口服每次 0.1～0.2g，每日 1～4 次或 300mg，一日 1 次。<br><br>Pour la réduction de la concentration d'acide urique dans le sang : au début, 0,05g par fois, 2 à 3 fois par jour, augmenter progressivement la dose pour atteindre 0,2 à 0,4g par jour 2 à 3 semaines après, à travers 2 à 3 fois. Ne pas dépasser 0,6g par jour. La dose d'entretien : 0,1 à 0,2g par fois, 2 à 3 fois par jour. La dose chez des enfants : 8mg/kg par jour. Pour traiter les pierres d'acide urique : par voie orale, 0,1 à 0,2g par fois, 1 à 4 fois par jour, ou 300mg, 1 fois par jour. |
| 剂型、规格<br>Les formes pharmaceutiques et les spécifications | 片剂：每片 0.1g。<br><br>Comprimés : 0,1g par comprimé. |
| **药品名称 Drug Names** | 非布司他 Febuxostat |
| 适应证<br>Les indications | 用于预防和治疗高尿酸血症及其引发的痛风。<br><br>Ce produit sert à prévenir et à traiter l'hyperuricémie ainsi que la goutte provoquée par l'hyperuricémie. |
| 用法、用量<br>Les modes d'emploi et la posologie | 本品服用剂量为一日 1 次 40mg 或 80mg，不推荐用于高尿酸血症的痛风患者。<br><br>40mg ou 80mg par fois, une fois par jour. Il n'est pas recommandé de l'appliquer chez les patients atteints de goutte accompagnée de l'hyperuricémie. |
| 剂型、规格<br>Les formes pharmaceutiques et les spécifications | 片剂：每片 80mg；120mg。<br><br>Comprimés : 80mg ou 120mg par comprimé. |

8.5　抗癫痫药 Médicaments anti-épileptiques

| | |
|---|---|
| **药品名称 Drug Names** | 苯妥英钠 Phénytoïne sodium |
| 适应证<br>Les indications | ①主要用于复杂性癫痫发作、单纯部分性发作、全身强直阵挛性发作和癫痫持续状态。本品在脑组织中达有效浓度较慢，因此疗效出现缓慢，需要连续多次服药才有效。②治疗三叉神经痛和坐骨神经痛、发作性舞蹈手足徐动症、发作性控制障碍、肌强直症及隐性营养不良性大疱性表皮松解。③用于治疗室上性或室性早搏、室性心动过速，尤适用于强心苷中毒时的室性心动过速，室上性心动过速也可适用。<br><br>① Ce produit sert à traiter la crise d'épilepsie complexe, sa crise partielle simple, sa crise tonico-clonique généralisée et l'état maintenu de l'épilepsie. Comme il prend effet lentement, il faut prendre des médicaments de manière continue. ② Il sert à traiter la névralgie du trijumeau, la sciatique,le syndrome de choréoathétose paroxystique,la trouble du contrôle paroxystique, la myotonie et l'épidermolyse bulleuse invisible dystrophique. ③ Il sert aussi à traiter les extrasystoles supraventriculaires ou ventriculaires, la tachycardie ventriculaire, surtout la tachycardie ventriculaire provoquée par l'intoxication par les glycosides cardiaques. Aussi applicable dans le traitement de la tachycardie supraventriculaire. |
| 用法、用量<br>Les modes d'emploi et la posologie | ①口服抗癫痫：成人常用量，一次 50～100mg，一日 2～3 次，一日 100～200mg；极量：一次 300mg，一日 500mg。宜从小剂量开始，酌情增量，但需避免过量。体重在 30kg 以下的小儿，按每日 5mg/kg 给药，分 2～3 次服用，每日不宜超过 250mg。注射剂用于癫痫持续状态时，可用 150～250mg，加 5% 葡萄糖注射液 20～40ml，在 6～10 分钟缓慢静脉注射，每分钟不超过 50mg，必要时经 30 分钟再注射 100～150mg。②治疗三叉神经痛：口服，每次 100～200mg，一日 2～3 次。<br><br>① Par voie orale, pour l'antiépileptique : chez des adultes, dose usuelle, 50 à 100mg par fois, 2 à 3 fois par jour, 100 à 200mg par jour ; dose maximale : 300mg par fois, 500mg par jour. Il vaut mieux commencer par une dose mineure, augmenter la dose selon les cas, mais éviter la dose trop importante. Chez des enfants moins de 30kg, 5 mg/kg par jour, à travers 2 à 3 fois, ne pas dépasser 250mg par jour. L'injection utilisée dans le traitement de l'état de mal épileptique, dissoudre 150 à 250 mg de produit dans 20 à 40 ml de solution de glucose à 5 %, injection lente par voie IV pendant 6 à 10 minutes, ne pas dépasser 50mg par minute, en cas de besoin, injecter de nouveau 100 à 150mg pendant 30 minutes. ② Pour traiter la névralgie du trijumeau : par voie orale, 100 à 200mg par fois, 2 à 3 fois par jour. |

续　表

| | |
|---|---|
| 剂型、规格<br>Les formes pharmaceutiques et les spécifications | 片剂：每片 50mg；100mg。<br>注射剂：每支 100mg；250mg。<br>Comprimés : 50mg ou 100mg par comprimé.<br>Injection : 100mg ou 250mg par solution. |
| 药品名称 Drug Names | 卡马西平 Carbamazépine |
| 适应证<br>Les indications | （1）治疗癫痫：是单纯及复杂部分性发作的首选药，对复杂部分性发作疗效优于其他癫痫药。对典型或不典型失神发作、肌阵挛发作无效。<br>（2）抗外周神经痛：包括三叉神经痛、舌咽神经痛、多发性硬化、糖尿病性周围性神经痛及疱疹后神经痛。亦可用于三叉神经痛缓解后的长期预防用药。对三叉神经痛、舌咽神经痛疗效较苯妥英钠好，用药后 24 小时即可奏效。<br>（3）治疗神经源性尿崩症，可能是由于促进抗利尿激素的分泌有关。<br>（4）预防或治疗狂躁抑郁症：临床使用证明本药对狂躁症及抑郁症均有明显治疗作用，也能减轻或消除精神分裂症患者狂躁、妄想症状。<br>（5）抗心律失常作用：能对抗由地高辛中毒所致的心律失常。能使其完全或基本恢复正常心律。临床使用证明，对室性或室上性早搏均有效，可使症状消除，尤其是伴有慢性心功能不全者疗效更好。<br>（6）酒精戒断综合征。<br><br>(1) Ce produit sert à traiter l'épilepsie : il s'agit d'un médicament de choix dans le traitement de sa crise partielle simple et complexe. Il est plus efficace dans le traitement de sa crise partielle complexe que d'autres médicaments anti-épileptiques. Il est inutile dans le traitement de sa crise myoclonique et de sa crise d'absence typique ou atypique.<br>(2) Il sert à lutter contre la douleur neuropathique périphérique : la névralgie du trijumeau, la névralgie du glossopharyngien, la sclérose en plaques, les douleurs neuropathiques périphériques diabétiques et la névralgie post-herpétique. Aussi applicable dans la prévention à long terme après la rémission de la névralgie du trijumeau. Il est plus efficace dans le traitement de la névralgie du trijumeau et de la névralgie du glossopharyngien que la phénytoïne de sodium. Il prend effet 24 h après l'administration.<br>(3) Il sert à traiter le diabète neurogène. Cela s'explique peut-être par le fait qu'il favoriser la sécrétion de l'hormone antidiurétique.<br>(4) Il sert à prévenir et à traiterla maniaco-dépression : l'utilisation clinique a prouvé que ce produit était efficace dans le traitement de la manie et de la dépression. Aussi applicable dans la réduction et l'élimination de la schizophrénie maniaque et délirante.<br>(5) Il a un effet antiarythmique : il sert à lutter contre l'arythmie provoquée par l'empoisonnement de la digoxine. Il permet de rétablir complètement ou presque le rythme cardiaque normal. L'utilisation clinique a prouvé qu'il était efficace dans le traitement des extrasystoles supraventriculaires ou ventriculaires. Il est surtout efficace chez les patients insuffisants cardiaques chroniques.<br>(6) Il est également utilisé dans le traitement du syndrome de sevrage de l'alcool. |
| 用法、用量<br>Les modes d'emploi et la posologie | ①癫痫、三叉神经痛：口服，1 日 300～1200mg，分 2～4 次服用。开始 1 次 100mg，一日 2 次，以后一日 3 次。个别三叉神经痛患者剂量可达每日 1000～1200mg。疗程最短 1 周，最长 2～3 个月。②尿崩症：口服，每日 600～1200mg。③抗躁狂症：口服，每日剂量为 300～600mg，分 2～3 次服，最大剂量每日 1200mg。④心律失常：口服，每日 300～600mg，分 2～3 次服。⑤酒精戒断综合征：口服，一次 200mg，一日 3～4 次。<br><br>① Pour traiter l'épilepsie et la névralgie du trijumeau : par voie orale, 300 à 1 200mg par jour, à travers 2 à 4 fois. Au début, 100mg par fois, 2 fois par jour, ensuite, 3 fois par jour. Chez certains patients souffrant de névralgie du trijumeau, 1 000 à 1 200mg par jour. Un traitement médical varie de 1 semaine à 2 ou 3 mois. ② Pour traiter le diabète : par voie orale, 600 à 1 200mg par jour. ③ Pour traiter la manie : par voie orale, 300 à 600mg par jour, à travers 2 à 3 fois, ne pas dépasser 1 200mg par jour. ④ Pour traiter l'arythmie : par voie orale, 300 à 600mg par jour, à travers 2 à 3 fois. ⑤ Pour traiter le syndrome de sevrage de l'alcool : par voie orale, 200mg par fois, 3 à 4 fois par jour. |
| 剂型、规格<br>Les formes pharmaceutiques et les spécifications | 片剂：每片 100mg；200mg；400mg。缓释片：每片 200mg；400mg。咀嚼片：每片 100mg；200mg。胶囊剂：每粒 200mg。糖浆剂：20mg/ml。栓剂：125mg；250mg。<br><br>Comprimés : 100mg, 200mg ou 400mg par comprimé. Comprimés à libération prolongée : 200mg ou 400mg par comprimé. Comprimés à croquer : 100mg ou 200mg par comprimé. Capsules : 200mg par capsule. Sirops : 20mg/ml. Suppositoires : 125 mg ou 250 mg. |

**续 表**

| 药品名称 Drug Names | 奥卡西平 Oxcarbazépine |
|---|---|
| 适应证<br>Les indications | 　　用于复杂性部分发作、全身强直阵挛性发作的但要治疗以及难治性癫痫的辅助治疗。本品的优点是没有自身诱导，可代替卡马西平，用于对后者有过敏反应者。<br><br>　　Ce produit sert de traitement adjuvant de la crise partielle complexe et de la crise tonico-clonique de l'épilepsie réfractaire. Il peut remplacer la carbamazépine chez des patients allergiques à celle-ci. |
| 用法、用量<br>Les modes d'emploi et la posologie | 　　口服：开始剂量为 300mg/d，以后可逐渐增量至 600～2400mg/d，以达到满意的疗效。剂量超过 2400mg/d，神经系统不良反应增加。小儿从 8～10mg/（kg·d）开始，可逐渐增量至 600mg/d。以上每日剂量均应分 2 次服用。<br><br>　　Par voie orale : au début, 300mg par jour, ensuite, augmenter progressivement la dose pour atteindre 600 à 2400 mg par jour. Ne pas dépasser 2 400mg par jour, car les réactions du système nerveux augmentent en même temps. Chez des enfants, au début, 8 à 10mg/(kg·jour), augmenter pour atteindre 600mg par jour. Pour toutes les doses citées, 2 fois par jour. |
| 剂型、规格<br>Les formes pharmaceutiques et les spécifications | 　　片剂：每片 0.15g；0.3g；0.6g。<br>　　Comprimés : 0,15g, 0,3g ou 0,6g par comprimé. |

| 药品名称 Drug Names | 托吡酯 Topiramate |
|---|---|
| 适应证<br>Les indications | 　　主要作为其他抗癫痫药的辅助治疗，用于单纯部分性发作、复杂部分性发作和全身强直阵挛性发作，尤其对 Lennox-Gastaut 综合征和 West 综合征（婴儿痉挛症）的疗效较好。本品远期疗效好，无明显耐受性，大剂量可用作单药治疗。<br><br>　　Ce produit sert de traitement adjuvant pour d'autres médicaments anti-épilepsiques. Il est utilisé comme traitement de la crise partielle simple, de la crise partielle complexe et de la crise tonico-clonique de l'épilepsie, il est surtout efficace dans le traitement du syndrome de Lennox-Gastaut et du syndrome de West (les spasmes infantiles). Son effet à long terme est très bien, sans tolérance importante. Avec une forte dose, il peut être utilsé en monothérapie. |
| 用法、用量<br>Les modes d'emploi et la posologie | 　　口服。成人：初始极量为每晚 25～50mg，然后每周增加 1 次，每次增加 25mg，直至症状控制为止。通常有效剂量为每日 200～300mg。2 岁以上儿童：初始剂量为每日 12.5～25mg，然后逐渐增加至 5～9mg/（kg·d），维持剂量为 100mg，分 2 次服。体重大于 43kg 的儿童，有效剂量范围与成人相当。<br><br>　　Par voie orale. Chez des adultes : au début, la dose maximale, 25 à 50mg par soir, ensuite, augmenter 25mg par semaine pour contrôler les symptômes. La dose usuelle efficace, 200 à 300mg par jour. Chez des enfants plus de 2 ans : au début, 12,5 à 25mg par jour, augmenter progressivement pour atteindre 5 à 9mg/ (kg·jour), la dose d'entretien, 100mg, à travers 2 fois. Chez des enfants plus de 43kg, la même dose efficace que chez des adultes. |
| 剂型、规格<br>Les formes pharmaceutiques et les spécifications | 　　片剂：每片 25mg；50mg；100mg。<br>　　Comprimés : 25mg, 50mg ou 100mg par comprimé. |

| 药品名称 Drug Names | 乙琥胺 Ethosuximide |
|---|---|
| 适应证<br>Les indications | 　　主要用于失神小发作，为首选药。<br>　　Ce produit sert de médicament de choix dans le traitement des crises d'absence. |
| 用法、用量<br>Les modes d'emploi et la posologie | 　　口服。剂量：开始量，3～6 岁为 1 次 250mg，一日 1 次。6 岁以上的儿童及成人，1 次 250mg，一日 2 次。以后可酌情增剂量。最大剂量：6 岁以下最大剂量可增为 1 日 1g，6 岁以上儿童及成人可增加为 1.5g。一般是每 4～7 日增加 250mg，至满意控制症状而不良反应最小为止。<br><br>　　Par voie orale. Au début, chez des enfants de 3 à 6 ans, 250mg par fois, 1 fois par jour ; chez des enfants plus de 6ans et des adultes, 250 mg par fois, 2 fois par jour. Ensuite, augmenter la dose selon les cas. La dose maximale : chez des enfants moins de 6 ans, 1g par jour, chez des enfants plus de 6 ans et des adultes, 1,5g par jour. En général, augmenter 250mg tous les 4 à 7 jours jusqu'au contrôle des symptômes alors que les réactions indésirables sont les moins importantes. |

续 表

| 剂型、规格<br>Les formes pharmaceutiques et les spécifications | 胶囊剂：每粒 0.25g。<br>糖浆剂：5g/100ml。<br>Capsules : 0,25g par capsule.<br>Sirops : 5g/100ml. |
| --- | --- |
| 药品名称 Drug Names | 丙戊酸钠 Valproate sodium |
| 适应证<br>Les indications | 主要用于单纯或复杂性失神发作、肌阵挛发作、全身强直阵挛发作（大发作，GTCS）的治疗。可使 90% 失神发作和全身强直阵挛发作得到良好控制，也用于单纯部分性发作、复杂部分性发作及部分性发作继发 GTCS。<br>Ce produit sert à traiter les crises d'absence simples ou complexes, la crise myoclonique ainsi que la crise tonico-clonique généralisée (GTCS). Il peut contrôler la crise d'absence et la crise tonico-clonique généralisée avec un taux de réussite de 90 %. Il est aussi applicable dans le traitement de la crise partielle simple et complexe et de la crise partielle avec GTCS secondaire. |
| 用法、用量<br>Les modes d'emploi et la posologie | 口服：成人 1 次 200～400mg，一日 400～1200mg。儿童每日 20～30mg/kg，分 2～3 次服用。一般以从低剂量开始。如原服用其他抗癫痫药者，可合并应用，也可逐减少原药量，视情况而定。<br>Par voie orale : chez des adultes, 200 à 400mg par fois, 400 à 1 200mg par jour. Chez des enfants, 20 à 30 mg/kg par jour, à travers 2 à 3 fois. Il vaut mieux commencer par une dose mineure. Si le patient utilise d'autres antiépileptiques, il est permissible d'utiliser ce produit en même temps ou de diminuer l'ancienne dose selon les cas. |
| 剂型、规格<br>Les formes pharmaceutiques et les spécifications | 片剂：每片 100mg；200mg。胶囊剂：每粒 200mg；250mg。肠溶片：每片 250mg；500mg。缓释片：每片 500mg。糖浆剂：200mg（5ml）；500mg（5ml）。<br>Comprimés : 100mg ou 200mg par comprimé. Capsules : 200mg ou 250mg par capsule. Comprimés à enrobage entérique : 250mg ou 500mg par comprimé. Comprimés à libération prolongée : 500mg par comprimé. Sirops : 200mg (5ml) ou 500mg (5ml). |
| 药品名称 Drug Names | 拉莫三嗪 Lamotrigine |
| 适应证<br>Les indications | 本品用于成人和 12 岁以上儿童复杂部分性发作或全身强直阵挛性癫痫发作的辅助治疗。作为辅助治疗用于难治性癫痫时，可用于 2 岁以上儿童及成人。<br>Ce produit sert de traitement adjuvant de la crise partielle complexe et de la crise tonico-clonique généralisée de l'épilepsie chez des adultes et des enfants plus de 12 ans. Quand il sert de traitement adjuvant de l'épilepsie réfractaire, il peut être appliqué chez des enfants plus de 2 ans et des adultes. |
| 用法、用量<br>Les modes d'emploi et la posologie | 口服。单独使用：成人初始剂量 25mg，一日 1 次；2 周后可增至 50mg，一日 1 次；在 2 周后，可酌情增加剂量，最大增加量为 50～100mg。此后，每隔 1～2 周，可增加剂量 1 次，直至达到最佳疗效，一般需经 6～8 周。通常有效维持量为 100～200mg/d，一次或分 2 次服用。儿童初始剂量 1mg/kg，维持剂量 3～6mg/kg。与丙戊酸合用：成人和 12 岁以上儿童：初始剂量 25mg，隔日 1 次，每 3～4 周开始改为 25mg，一日 1 次，在 2 周后，酌情增加剂量，最大增加为 0.5～1mg/kg。此后，每隔 1～2 周，可增加剂量 1 次，直至达到最佳疗效，通常有效维持量为 1～2mg/（kg·d），一次或分 2 次服用。与具诱导作用的抗癫痫药物合用：初始剂量 50mg，一日 1 次，服药 2 周后可增至 100mg/d，分 2 次服，在 2 周后，可酌情增加剂量，最大增加量为 100mg，此后，每隔 1～2 周，可增加剂量 1 次，直至达到最佳疗效。通常有效维持量为 200～400mg/d，分 2 次服用。2～12 岁儿童：初始剂量 2mg/（kg·d），分 2 次服，2 周后增至 5mg/（kgd），分 2 次服，在 2 周后，可酌情增加剂量，最大增加量为 2～3mg/kg，此后，每隔 1～2 周，可增加剂量 1 次，直至达到最佳疗效。维持剂量 10mg/（kg·d），最大剂量为 400mg/d。 |

**续 表**

| | |
|---|---|
| | Par voie orale. En monothérapie : chez des adultes, au début, 25mg, 1 fois par jour ; 2 semaines après, augmenter pour atteindre 50mg, 1 fois par jour ; 2 semaines après, augmenter 50 à 100mg au plus selon les cas. Ensuite, augmenter la dose une fois toutes les 1 à 2 semaines jusqu'à la dose la plus efficace. Cela nécessite généralement 6 à 8 semaines. La dose d'entretien efficace, 100 à 200 mg par jour, à travers 1 à 2 fois. Chez des enfants : au début 1mg/kg, la dose d'entretien, 3 à 6mg/kg. Utilisé en association avec l'acide valproïque : chez des adultes et des enfants plus de 12 ans : au début, 25mg, une fois tous les 2 jours, 3 à 4 semaines après, 25mg, 1 fois par jour, 2 semaines après, augmenter 0,5 à 1 mg/kg au plus. Ensuite, augmenter la dose une fois tous les 1 à 2 semaines jusqu'à la dose la plus efficace. La dose d'entretien efficace, 1 à 2 mg/(kg·jour), à travers 1 à 2 fois. Utilisé en combinaison avec les antiépileptiques inducteurs : au début, 50mg, 1 fois par jour, 2 semaines après l'administration, 100mg par jour, à travers 2 fois, après 2 semaines, augmenter 100mg au plus. Ensuite, augmenter la dose une fois toutes les 1 à 2 semaines jusqu'à la dose la plus efficace. La dose d'entretien efficace, 200 à 400 mg par jour, à travers 2 fois. Chez des enfants de 2 à 12 ans : au début, 2mg/(kg·jour), à travers 2 fois, 2 semaines après, 5mg/(kg·jour), à travers 2 fois, 2 semaines après augmenter 2 à 3 mg par kg au plus. Ensuite, augmenter la dose une fois toutes les 1 à 2 semaines jusqu'à la dose la plus efficace. La dose d'entretien, 10 mg/(kg·jour), la dose maximale, 400mg par jour. |
| 剂型、规格<br>Les formes pharmaceutiques et les spécifications | 片剂：每片 25mg；100mg；150mg；200mg。<br>Comprimés : 25mg, 100mg, 150mg ou 200mg par comprimé. |
| 药品名称 Drug Names | 加巴喷丁 Gabapentine |
| 适应证<br>Les indications | 用于常规治疗无效的某些部分性癫痫辅助治疗，亦可用于治疗部分性癫痫发作继发全身性发作。<br>Ce produit sert de traitement adjuvant de certaines épilepsies partielles résistantes à la thérapie usuelle. Il est aussi applicable dans le traitement de la crise systématique secondaire de la crise partielle de l'épilepsie. |
| 用法、用量<br>Les modes d'emploi et la posologie | 口服，成人每天 300mg，睡前服；第 2 日 600mg，分 2 次服；第 3 日 900mg，分 3 次服。此剂量随疗效而定，多数患者在 900～1800mg 有效。肾功能不全者需要减少剂量。停药应缓停。<br>Par voie orale, chez des adultes, 300mg par jour, avant le sommeil ; pour le deuxième jour, 600mg, à travers 2 fois ; le troisième jour, 900 mg, à travers 3 fois. Ajuster la dose en fonction de l'efficacité, chez la plupart des patients, la dose efficace, 900 à 1 800mg. Chez des patients insuffisants rénaux, diminuer la dose. Il faut arrêter doucement l'administration des médicaments. |
| 剂型、规格<br>Les formes pharmaceutiques et les spécifications | 胶囊剂：每粒 100mg；300mg；400mg。<br>Capsules : 100mg, 300mg ou 400mg par capsule. |
| 药品名称 Drug Names | 左乙拉西坦 Lévétiracétam |
| 适应证<br>Les indications | 用于成人及 4 岁以上儿童癫痫患者部分性发作的治疗。<br>Ce produit sert à traiter la crise partielle de l'épilepsie chez des adultes et des enfants plus de 4 ans. |
| 用法、用量<br>Les modes d'emploi et la posologie | 口服：成人和青少年体重≥50kg，起始剂量为每次 500mg，一日 2 次，最多可增至每次 1500mg，一日 2 次，每 2～4 周增加或减少每次 500mg，一日 2 次。4～11 岁儿童和青少年体重＜50kg，起始剂量为每次 10mg/kg，一日 2 次，最多可增至 30mg/kg，每 2～4 周增加或减少每次 10mg/kg，一日 2 次。肾功能不全者，根据肌酐清除率调整剂量。<br>Par voie orale : chez des adultes et des enfants plus de 50 kg, au début, 500mg par fois, 2 fois par jour, ensuite, augmenter la dose pour atteindre 1 500mg au plus, 2 fois par jour. Augmenter ou diminuer de 500mg toutes les 2 à 4 semaines, 2 fois par jour. Chez des enfants de 4 à 11 ans ou des adolescents moins de 50kg, au début, 10 mg/kg par fois, 2 fois par jour, ensuite, augmenter la dose pour atteindre 30 mg/kg par fois au plus, 2 fois par jour. Augmenter ou diminuer de 10 mg/kg par fois toutes les 2 à 4 semaines, 2 fois par jour. Chez des patients insuffisants rénaux, ajuster la dose en fonction de la clairance de la créatinine. |

| 续　表 | |
|---|---|
| 剂型、规格<br>Les formes pharmaceutiques et les spécifications | 片剂：每片 0.25g；0.5g；1.0g。<br>Comprimés : 0,25g, 0,5g ou 1,0g par comprimé. |
| 药品名称 Drug Names | 扑米酮 Primidone |
| 适应证<br>Les indications | 作用于苯巴比妥相似，但作用及毒性均较低。用于治疗癫痫大发作及精神运动性发作有效。<br>Son effet est similaire au phénobarbital, mais moins efficace et moins toxique. Il est applicable dans le traitement des crises tonico-cloniques généralisées de l'épilepsie et ses crises psychomotrices. |
| 用法、用量<br>Les modes d'emploi et la posologie | 口服：开始每次 0.05g，1 周后逐渐增至每次 0.25g，1 日 0.5～0.75g。极量一日 1.5g。儿童每日 12.5～25mg/kg。分 2～3 次服用，宜从小剂量开始，逐渐增量。<br>Par voie orale : au début, 0,05g par fois, 1 semaine après, augmenter progressivement pour atteindre 0,25g par fois, 0,5 à 0,75g par jour. La dose maximale : 1,5g par jour. Chez des enfants, 12,5 à 25 mg/kg par jour. À travers 2 à 3 fois, commencer par une dose mineure et augmenter progressivement la dose. |
| 剂型、规格<br>Les formes pharmaceutiques et les spécifications | 片剂：0.25g。<br>Comprimés : 0,25g. |

8.6　镇静药、催眠药和抗惊厥药 Sédatifs, hypnotiques et anticonvulsifs

| 药品名称 Drug Names | 咪达唑仑 Midazolam |
|---|---|
| 适应证<br>Les indications | 用于治疗失眠症，亦可用于外科手术或诊断检查时作诱导睡眠用。<br>Il sert à traiter l'insomnie. Il sert aussi à induire le sommeil lors de la chirurgie et du diagnostic. |
| 用法、用量<br>Les modes d'emploi et la posologie | 口服：治疗失眠症，每次 15mg，睡前服。肌内注射：术前 20～30 分钟注射，成人一般为 10～15mg（0.10～0.15mg/kg）。可单用，亦可与镇痛药合用。儿童剂量可稍高，为 0.15～0.2mg/kg。作儿童诱导麻醉时，用本品 5～10mg（0.15～0.2mg/kg）与氯胺酮 50～100mg（8mg/kg）合用。静脉注射：术前准备，术前 5～10 分钟注射 2.5～5mg（0.05～0.1mg/kg），可单用或与抗胆碱药合用。用于诱导麻醉，成人为 10～15mg（0.15～0.2mg/kg），儿童为 0.2mg/kg。用于维持麻醉，小剂量静脉注射，剂量和时间间隔视患者个体差异而定。<br>Par voie orale : pour traiter l'insomnie, 15mg par fois, avant le sommeil. Injection par voie IM : 20 à 30 minutes avant la chirurgie, chez des adultes, 10 à 15mg (0.10 à 0.15mg/kg). Il peut être utilisé seul ou en association avec d'autres analgésiques. Pour l'induction de l'anesthésie chez des enfants, utiliser 5 à 10mg (0.15 à 0.2mg/kg) de midazolam et 50 à 100mg(8mg/kg) de kétamine. Injection par voie IV : 5 à 10 minutes avant la chirurgie, 2.5 à 5mg (0.05 à 0.1mg/kg), utilisé seul ou association avec des anticholinergiques. Pour l'induction de l'anesthésie, chez des adultes, 10 à 15mg (0.15 à 0.2mg/kg), chez des enfants, 0.2mg/kg. Pour le maintien de l'anesthésie, injection par voie IV avec une dose mineure, ajuster la dose et l'intervalle en fonction des patients. |
| 剂型、规格<br>Les formes pharmaceutiques et les spécifications | 片剂：每片 15mg。<br>注射液：每支 5mg（1ml）；10mg（2ml）；15mg（3ml）。<br>Comprimés : 15mg par comprimé.<br>Injection : 5mg (1ml), 10mg (2ml) ou 15mg (3ml) par solution. |
| 药品名称 Drug Names | 苯巴比妥 Phénobarbital |
| 适应证<br>Les indications | 用于：①镇静：如焦虑不安、烦躁、甲状腺功能亢进、高血压、功能性恶心、小儿幽门痉挛症；②催眠：偶用于顽固性失眠症，但醒后往往有疲倦、嗜睡等后遗效应；③抗惊厥：常用其对抗中枢兴奋药中毒或高热、破伤风、脑炎、脑出血等病引起的惊厥；④抗癫痫：用于癫痫大发作和部分性发作的治疗，出现作用快，也可用于癫痫持续状态；⑤麻醉前给药；⑥与解热镇痛药配伍应用，以增强其作用；⑦治疗新生儿高胆红素血症。 |

续 表

| | |
|---|---|
| | ① La sédation : l'anxiété, l'irritabilité, l'hyperthyroïdie, l'hypertension artérielle, des nausées fonctionnelles et des spasmes pyloriques chez les enfants. ② L'hypnotique : il sert parfois à traiter l'insomnie réfractaire, mais avec des effets indésirables, tels que la fatigue et la somnolence. ③ L'anticonvulsivant : il sert à traiter le convulsivant causé par l'intoxication par le stimulant central, la fièvre, le tétanos, l'encéphalite ou l'hémorragie cérébrale. ④ L'antiépileptique : il sert à traiter les crises tonico-cloniques généralisées et les crises partielles de l'épileptie, avec un effet rapide. Aussi applicable dans le traitement de l'état de mal épileptique. ⑤ L'administration avant l'anesthésie. ⑥ Utilisé en association avec les analgésiques et les antipyrétiques, pour renforcer son efficacité. ⑦ Traiter l'hyperbilirubinémie néonatale. |
| 用法、用量<br>Les modes d'emploi et la posologie | ①口服：一般情况，常用量，1 次 15 ～ 150mg，1 日 30 ～ 200mg；极量，1 次 250mg，1 日 500mg。小儿，用于镇静每次 2mg/kg，用于惊厥每次 3 ～ 5mg/kg，用于抗高胆红素血症每日 5 ～ 8mg/kg，分次口服。②皮下、肌内注射或缓慢静脉注射：常用量，1 次 0.1 ～ 0.2g，一日 1 ～ 2 次；极量，1 次 0.25g，1 日 0.5g。③镇静、抗癫痫：口服，每次 0.015 ～ 0.03g，一日 3 次。④催眠：每次 0.03 ～ 0.09g，睡前口服 1 次。⑤抗惊厥：肌内注射其钠盐，每次 0.1 ～ 0.2g，必要时 4 ～ 6 小时后重复一次。⑥麻醉前给药：术前 0.5 ～ 1 小时肌内注射 0.1 ～ 0.2g。⑦癫痫持续状态：肌内注射 1 次 0.1 ～ 0.2g。<br><br>① Par voie orale : la dose usuelle, 15 à 150 mg par fois, 30 à 200mg par jour ; dose maximale, 250 mg par fois, 500mg par jour. Chez des enfants, pour la sédation, 2 mg/kg par fois, pour l'anticonvulsivant, 3 à 5 mg/kg par fois, pour traiter l'hyperbilirubinémie, 5 à 8 mg/kg par jour, à travers plusieurs fois. ② Injection par voie sous-cutanée, IM ou IV lente : dose usuelle, 0,1 à 0,2 g par fois, 1 à 2 fois par jour ; dose maximale, 0,25g par fois, 0,5g par jour. ③ Pour la sédation et l'antiépileptique : par voie orale, 0,015 à 0,03g par fois, 3 fois par jour. ④ Pour l'hypnose : 0,03 à 0,09g par fois, une fois avant le sommeil par voie orale. ⑤ Pour l'anticonvulsivant : injecter par voie IM le phénobarbital de sodium, 0,1 à 0,2g par fois, s'il est nécessaire, reprendre 4 à 6h après. ⑥ Pour l'administration avant l'anesthésie : 0,5 à 1h avant la chirurgie, injecter par voie IM 0,1 à 0,2g. ⑦ Pour traiter l'état de mal épileptique : 0,1 à 0,2g par fois, injection par voie IM. |
| 剂型、规格<br>Les formes pharmaceutiques et les spécifications | 片剂：每片 0.01g；0.015g；0.03g；0.1g。注射用苯巴比妥：每支 0.05g；0.1g；0.2g。鲁米托品片每片含苯巴比妥 15mg，硫酸阿托品 0.15mg。用于主动和神经功能失调所致头痛、呕吐、颤抖、胃肠道紊乱性腹痛等。每次 1 片，极量 1 次 5 片。<br><br>Comprimés : 0,01g, 0,015g, 0,03g ou 0,1g par comprimé. Le phénobarbital pour injection : 0,05g, 0,1g ou 0,2g par solution. Les comprimés de Lumitropine : contenant 15mg de phénobarbital et 0,15mg desulfate d'atropine. Utilisé pour tratier la céphalée, la nausée, le tremblement, la colique liée aux affections gastro-intestinales causées par les troubles neurologiques actifs. 1 comprié par fois, la dose maximale, 5 comprimés par fois. |
| 药品名称 Drug Names | 异戊巴比妥 Amobarbital |
| 适应证<br>Les indications | 用于镇静、催眠、抗惊厥。<br>Ce produit est utilisé pour la sédation, l'hyphotique et l'anticonvulsivant. |
| 用法、用量<br>Les modes d'emploi et la posologie | (1) 口服：①成人，常用量：催眠，每次 0.1 ～ 0.2g，于睡前顿服，适用于难入睡者；镇静，每次 0.02 ～ 0.04g，一日 2 ～ 3 次。极量：1 次 0.2g，1 日 0.6g。老年人或体弱患者，即便是给予常用量也可产生兴奋、神经错乱或抑郁，须减量。②小儿，常用量：催眠，个体差异大；镇静，每次 2mg/kg（或 60mg/m²），一日 3 次。<br>(2)肌内或缓慢静脉注射：①成人，常用量：催眠，每次 0.1 ～ 0.2g；镇静，每次 0.03 ～ 0.05mg，一日 2 ～ 3 次；抗惊厥（癫痫持续状态），缓慢静脉注射 0.3 ～ 0.5g。极量：1 次 0.25g，1 日 0.5g。②小儿，常用量：催眠（或抗惊厥），肌内注射每次 3 ～ 5mg/kg（或 125mg/m²）；镇静，每日 6mg/kg，一日 2 ～ 3 次。 |

**续　表**

<table>
<tr><td></td><td>(1) Par voie orale : ① Chez des adultes, dose usuelle : pour l'hypnose, 0,1 à 0,2g par fois, une fois avant le sommeil, réservé à ceux souffrant d'endormissement difficile ; pour la sédation, 0,02 à 0,04g par fois, 2 à 3 fois par jour. La dose maximale : 0,2 g par fois, 0,6g par jour. Chez des personnes âgées ou des faibles, la dose usuelle peut entraîner l'excitation, les troubles nerveux ou la dépression, il faut diminuer la dose. ② Chez des enfants, dose usuelle : pour l'hypnose, en fonction des patients ; pour la sédation, 2mg/kg(ou 60mg/m$^2$), 3 fois par jour.<br><br>(2) Injection par voie IM ou IV : ① Chez des adultes, dose usuelle : pour l'hypnose, 0,1 à 0,2 g par fois ; pour la sédation, 0,03 à 0,05mg par fois, 2 à 3 fois par jour ; pour l'anticonvulsivant (pour traiter l'état de mal épileptique), injecter lentement 0,3 à 0,5g par voie IV. Dose maximale : 0,25g par fois, 0,5g par jour. ② Chez des enfants, dose usuelle : pour l'hypnose (ou l'anticonvulsivant), injecter par voie IM 3~5mg/kg(ou 125mg/ ㎡ ) par fois ; pour la sédation, 6 mg/kg par jour, 2 à 3 fois par jour.</td></tr>
<tr><td>剂型、规格<br>Les formes pharmaceutiques et les spécifications</td><td>片剂：每片 0.1g。<br>注射用异戊巴比妥钠：每支 0.1g；0.25g。<br>Comprimés : 0,1g par comprimé.<br>L'amobarbital de sodium pour injection : 0,1g ou 0,25g par solution.</td></tr>
<tr><td>药品名称 Drug Names</td><td>司可巴比妥 Sécobarbital</td></tr>
<tr><td>适应证<br>Les indications</td><td>主要适用于不易入睡的患者。也可用于抗惊厥。<br>Ce produit est applicable dans le traitement des patients qui ont difficulté à s'endormir. Il sert aussi d'anticonvulsivant.</td></tr>
<tr><td>用法、用量<br>Les modes d'emploi et la posologie</td><td>口服：成人常用量，催眠 0.1～0.2g，临睡前一次顿服；镇静 1 次 30～50mg，一日 3～4 次。成人极量 1 次 0.3g。尚可皮下注射（1 次量 0.1g）。<br>Par voie orale: Doses administrées couramment chez les adultes, pour l'hypnose, 0.1～0.2g, prendre une fois avant le coucher; pour la sédation, 30～50mg par dose, 3～4 fois par jour. Dose maximale à administrer aux adultes, 0.3g une fois. Peut être injecté sous la peau(0.1g une fois).</td></tr>
<tr><td>剂型、规格<br>Les formes pharmaceutiques et les spécifications</td><td>胶囊剂：每粒 0.1g。<br>注射用司可巴比妥：每支 0.05g。<br>Capsules : 0,1g par capsule.<br>Le secobarbital pour injection : 0,05g par solution.</td></tr>
<tr><td>药品名称 Drug Names</td><td>佐匹克隆 Zopiclone</td></tr>
<tr><td>适应证<br>Les indications</td><td>用于各种原因引起的失眠症，尤其适用于不能耐受次晨残余作用的患者。<br>Ce produit sert à traiter l'insomnie de toutes sortes, surtout applicable dans le traitement des patients qui ne peuvent pas tolérer l'effet résiduel du lendemain matin.</td></tr>
<tr><td>用法、用量<br>Les modes d'emploi et la posologie</td><td>睡前服 7.5mg。老年人、肝功能不全者，睡前服 3.75mg，必要时可增加至 7.5mg。<br>7,5mg avant le sommeil. Chez des personnes âgées et des patients insuffisants rénaux, 3,75mg avant le sommeil, s'il est nécessaire, augmenter pour atteindre 7,5mg.</td></tr>
<tr><td>剂型、规格<br>Les formes pharmaceutiques et les spécifications</td><td>片剂：每片 3.75mg；7.5mg。<br>Comprimés : 3,75mg ou 7,5mg par comprimé.</td></tr>
<tr><td>药品名称 Drug Names</td><td>唑吡坦 Zolpidém</td></tr>
<tr><td>适应证<br>Les indications</td><td>用于治疗短暂性、偶发性失眠症或慢性失眠的短期治疗。<br>Il sert à traiter l'insomnie provisoire ou occasionnelle. Il sert aussi de traitement à court terme de l'insomnie chronique.</td></tr>
<tr><td>用法、用量<br>Les modes d'emploi et la posologie</td><td>常用量为 10mg，睡前服。偶发性失眠，一般用药 2～5 日。长期用药应不超过 4 周。老年人及肝功能不全者剂量减半，必要时可增至 10mg。<br>Dose usuelle, 10mg, avant le sommeil. Pour traiter l'insomnie occasionnelle, administrer pendant 2 à 5 jours. Pour un traitement à long terme, ne pas dépasser 4 semaines. Chez des personnes âgées et des patients insuffisants rénaux, diminuer de moitié la dose usuelle, s'il est nécessaire, augmenter la dose pour atteindre 10mg.</td></tr>
</table>

续　表

| 剂型、规格<br>Les formes pharmaceutiques et les spécifications | 片剂：每片 10mg；5mg。<br>Comprimés : 10mg ou 5mg par comprimé. |
|---|---|
| **药品名称 Drug Names** | 水合氯醛 Hydrate de chloral |
| 适应证<br>Les indications | 用于神经性失眠、伴有显著兴奋的精神病及破伤风痉挛、士的宁中毒等。<br>Ce produit sert à traiter l'insomnie nerveuse, les troubles mentaux accompagnés d'une excitation importante, la tétanospasmine et l'intoxication de la strychnine. |
| 用法、用量<br>Les modes d'emploi et la posologie | 口服或灌肠。常用量，一次 0.5 ～ 1.5g；极量，一次 2g，一日 4g。睡前 1 次。口服 10% 溶液 5 ～ 15ml（一般服 10ml），以多量水稀释并添加胶浆剂（掩盖其不良臭味，避免刺激）后服用，或服其合剂（加有淀粉、糖浆剂）以减少刺激。抗惊厥：多用灌肠法给药，将 10% 溶液 15 ～ 20ml 稀释 1 ～ 2 倍后 1 次灌入。<br><br>Par voie orale ou par le lavement. Dose usuelle, 0,5 à 1,5g par fois ; dose maximale, 2g par fois, 4g par jour. Une fois avant le sommeil. Administrer par voie orale 5 à 15ml de solution à 10 % (10ml généralement), utiliser beaucoup d'eau pour la dilution et ajouter des mucilages (pour cacher des mauvaises odeurs) avant de l'administrer, ou prendre la préparation de composés (des fécules et des sirops) pour réduire l'irritation. Pour l'anticonvulsivant : administré souvent par voie de lavement. Dissoudre 15 à 20 ml de solution à 10 % de 1 à 2 fois avant le lavement. |
| 剂型、规格<br>Les formes pharmaceutiques et les spécifications | 水合氯醛合剂：有水合氯醛 65g，溴化钠 65g，淀粉 20g，枸橼酸 0.25g，薄荷水 0.5ml，琼脂糖浆 500ml，蒸馏水适量，共配成 1000ml。水合氯醛遇热易挥发分解，须调好其他成分防冷后再加入。如无琼脂糖浆时可用单糖浆代替。<br><br>Composé de l'hydrate de chloral : 65g d'hydrate de chloral, 65g de bromure de sodium, 20g de fécule, 0,25g de citrate, 0,5ml d'eau de menthe, 500ml de suspension d'agarose et de l'eau distillée, pour former 1 000ml. Comme l'hydrate de chloral se volatilise losqu'il est exposé à la chaleur, il faut préparer d'autres ingrédients avant de l'ajouter. S'il n'y a pas de sirop d'agar, possible d'utiliser le sirop simple. |
| **药品名称 Drug Names** | 扎来普隆 Zaleplon |
| 适应证<br>Les indications | 用于入睡困难的失眠症的短期治疗。临床研究结果显示扎来普隆能缩短入睡时间，但还未见其能增加睡眠时间和减少清醒次数。<br><br>Ce produit sert de traitement à court terme des patients qui ont difficulté à s'endormir. Les recherches cliniques montrent que le zaleplon peut faciliter l'endormissement, mais qu'il ne peut pas aider à augmenter la durée du sommeil ni à réduire le nombre de réveils. |
| 用法、用量<br>Les modes d'emploi et la posologie | 口服，一次 5 ～ 10mg（1 ～ 2 粒），睡前服用或入睡困难时服用。与所有的镇静催眠药一样，当清醒时，服用会导致记忆损伤、幻觉、协调障碍、头晕。体重较轻的患者，推荐剂量为一次 5mg（1 粒）。老年患者、糖尿病患者和轻、中度肝功能不全患者，推荐剂量为一次 5mg（1 粒）。每晚只服用一次。持续用药时间限制在 7 ～ 10 日。如果服药 7 ～ 10 日后失眠仍未减轻，医师应对患者失眠的原因重新评估。<br><br>Par voie orale, 5 à 10mg (1 à 2 granules) par fois, avant le sommeil ou en cas d'endormissement difficile. Comme tous les sédatifs et les hyptoniques, l'administration du zaleplon lors de l'éveil peut entraîner des troubles de la mémoire, des hallucinations, des troubles de la coordination et des vertiges. Chez des patients légers, il est recommandé de prendre 5mg par fois (1 granule). Chez des personnes âgées, des diabétiques, des patients insuffisants hépatiques bénins et modérés, il est recommandé de prendre 5mg (1 granule) par fois. Une fois par soir. Pendant 7 à 10 jours consécutifs au plus. S'il ne prend effet 7 à 10 jours depuis l'administration, le docteur doit réexaminer la cause de l'insomnie du patient. |
| 剂型、规格<br>Les formes pharmaceutiques et les spécifications | 胶布剂：每粒 5mg。<br>片剂、分散片：片剂 5mg。<br><br>Les bandes : 5mg par pièce.<br>Comprimés ou comprimés dispersibles : 5mg par comprimé. |

续 表

| 药品名称 Drug Names | 艾司佐匹克隆 Eszopiclone |
|---|---|
| 适应证<br>Les indications | 用于失眠的短期治疗。<br>Ce produit sert de traitement à court terme de l'insomnie. |
| 用法、用量<br>Les modes d'emploi et la posologie | 常用量为睡前口服 2mg，可逐渐增至 3mg。对于入睡困难的老年患者起始剂量推荐为 1mg，可逐渐增至 2mg。对于易醒的老年患者起始剂量为 2mg。<br>Dose usuelle, 2mg avant le sommeil, augmenter progressivement pour atteindre 3mg. Chez des personnes âgées souffrant d'endormissement difficile, il est recommandé de prendre 1mg au début avant d'augmenter la doser pour atteindre 2 mg. Chez des personnes âgées souffrant de trop de réveils, prendre 2mg au début. |
| 剂型、规格<br>Les formes pharmaceutiques et les spécifications | 片剂：2mg，3mg。<br>Comprimés:2mg,3mg. |
| 药品名称 Drug Names | 溴化钾 Bromure de potassium |
| 适应证<br>Les indications | 常用于神经衰弱。癔症、神经性失眠、精神兴奋状态。<br>Ce produit sert à traiter la neurasthénie. Aussi applicable dans le traitement de l'hystérie, de l'insomnie nerveuse et de l'excitation. |
| 用法、用量<br>Les modes d'emploi et la posologie | 口服：10% 溶液 5～10ml，一日 3 次。饭后服。不宜空腹服用。<br>Par voie orale : 5 à 10ml de solution à 10 %, 3 fois par jour, après le repas, éviter l'estomac vide. |
| 剂型、规格<br>Les formes pharmaceutiques et les spécifications | 溶液：10%。<br>Solution : 10 %. |
| 药品名称 Drug Names | 戊巴比妥钠 Pentobarbital sodique |
| 适应证<br>Les indications | 同异戊巴比妥，用于催眠、麻醉前给药。<br>c.f. à l'amobarbital, il sert de sédation et d'administration avant l'anesthésie. |
| 用法、用量<br>Les modes d'emploi et la posologie | 催眠：0.1～0.2g；麻醉前给药：手术当日清晨服 0.1g，必要时术前半小时再服 0.1g。极量：1 次 0.2g，1 日 0.6g。<br>Pour l'hypnose : 0,1 à 0,2g ; pour l'administrationavant l'anesthésie : le petit matin du jour de la chirurgie, prendre 0,1g, s'il est nécesaire, reprendre 0,1g 30 minutes avant la chirurgie. La dose maximale : 0,2g par fois, 0,6g par jour. |
| 剂型、规格<br>Les formes pharmaceutiques et les spécifications | 片剂：0.05g；0.1g。<br>注射剂：0.1g；0.5g。<br>Comprimés : 0.05g ou 0,1g.<br>Injection : 0,1g ou 0,5g. |

8.7　抗震颤麻痹药 Antiparkinsoniens

| 药品名称 Drug Names | 左旋多巴 Lévodopa |
|---|---|
| 适应证<br>Les indications | 改善肌强直和运动迟缓效果明显，持续用药对震颤、流涎、姿势不稳及吞咽困难亦有效。①帕金森病（原发性震颤麻痹）；脑炎后或合并有脑动脉硬化及中枢神经系统的一氧化碳与锰中毒后的症状性帕金森综合征（非药源性震颤麻痹综合征）。可减轻没震颤麻痹的症状，改善肌张力，使肢体活动更趋正常。对轻、中度病情者效果较好，重度或老年患者较差。②肝性脑病：可使患者清醒，症状改善。肝性脑病可能与中枢介质多巴胺异常有关，服用后，可改善中枢功能而奏效。亦有学者认为左旋多巴可提高大脑对氨的耐受性，但不能改善肝脏损伤和肝功能。③神经痛：早期服用可缓解神经痛。④高泌乳素血症：可抑制下丘脑的促甲状腺激素释放激素，兴奋泌乳素释放抑制因子，因而减少泌乳素的分泌，用于治疗高泌乳 |

血症，对乳溢症有一定疗效。⑤脱毛症：其机制可能是增加血液到组织的儿茶酚胺浓度，促进毛发生长。⑥促进小儿生长发育：可通过促进生长激素的分泌，加速小儿骨骼的生长发育。治疗垂体功能低下症。

Il est efficace dans l'amélioration de la rigidité musculaire et de la bradykinésie. Avec une administration soutenue, il sert aussi à traiter le tremblement, la salivation, l'instabilité posturale et la dysphagie. ① Le parkinson ; le parkinsonisme symptomatique après l'encéphalite ou après l'artériosclérose cérébral accompagnée de l'empoisonnement au monoxyde de carbone dans le système nerveux central (le parkinsonisme non drogue induit). Il sert à réduire les symptômes du parkinsonisme, à améliorer le tonus musculaire, et à normaliser l'activité physique. Il est plus efficace chez des patients bénins et modérés, moins efficace chez des patients gravement malades et des personnes âgées. ② L'encéphalopathie hépatique : il sert à réveiller les patients et à améliorer les symptômes. L'encéphalopathie hépatique est peut-être liée à l'anormalité de la dopamine neurotransmetteuse centrale. Ce produit peut prendre effet en améliorant les fonctions centrales. Certains pensent que le lévodopa peut améliorer la tolérance du cerveau vis-à-vis de l'ammoniac, mais qu'il ne peut pas améliorer les lésions hépatiques et la fonction hépatique. ③ La névralgie : il peut soulager la névralgie au stade précoce. ④ L'hyperprolactinémie : il peut inhiberla libération de l'hormone par la thyrotropine hypothalamique et peut inciter la prolactine à libérer les facteurs inhibants. Il peut donc réduire la sécrétion de prolactine et sert à traiter ainsi l'hyperprolactinémie. Il est aussi efficace dans le traitement du galactorrhea. ⑤ L'alopécie : il peut augmenter la concentration de la catécholamine dans le sang vers des tissus, et peut ainsi promouvoir la croissance des cheveux. ⑥ La promotion de l'épanouissement des enfants : il sert à favoriser la sécrétion de l'hormone de croissance et peut ainsi favoriser la croissance et le développement des os chez des enfants. Il sert aussi à traiter l'hypopituitarisme.

| | |
|---|---|
| 用法、用量<br>Les modes d'emploi et la posologie | ①治疗震颤麻痹：口服，开始时一日 0.25 ～ 0.5g，分 2 ～ 3 次服用。每服 2 ～ 4 日后，每日量增加 0.125 ～ 0.5g。维持量一日 3 ～ 6g，分 4 ～ 6 次服，连续用药 2 ～ 3 周见效。在剂量递增过程中，如出现恶心等，应停止增量，待症状消失后再增量。②治疗肝性脑病：一日 0.3 ～ 0.4g，加入 5% 葡萄糖溶液 500ml 中静脉滴注，待完全清醒后，减量至一日 0.2g，继续 1 ～ 2 日后停药。或用本品 5g 加入生理盐水 100ml 中，鼻饲或灌肠。<br><br>① Pour traiter le parkinsonisme : par voie orale, au début, 0,25 à 0,5g par jour, à travers 2 à 3 fois. Augmenter tous les 2 à 4 jours de 0,125 à 0,5 g par jour. Pour la dose d'entretien, 3 à 6g par jour, à travers 4 à 6 fois, il commence à prendre effet 2 à 3 semaines après l'administration continue. Au cours de l'augmentation de la dose, en cas de nausée, il faut recommercer à augmenter la dose après la disparition des symptômes. ② Pour traiter l'encéphalopathie hépatique : 0,3 à 0,4g par jour, dissoudre le produit dans 500ml de solution de glucose à 5 %, en perfusion, après le réveil complet, diminuer la dose jusqu'à 0,2g par jour, arrêter l'administration 1 à 2 jours après. Ou dissoudre 5g de ce produit dans 100ml de solution saline, par le sondage naso-gastrique ou par le lavement. |
| 剂型、规格<br>Les formes pharmaceutiques et les spécifications | 片剂：每片 50mg；100mg；250mg。<br>胶囊剂：每粒 100mg；125mg；250mg。<br>Comprimés : 50mg, 100mg ou 250mg par comprimé.<br>Capsules : 100mg, 125mg ou 250mg par capsule. |
| 药品名称 Drug Names | 卡比多巴 Carbidopa |
| 适应证<br>Les indications | ①主要与左旋多巴合用治疗各种原因引起的帕金森症，可获较好临床效果，但晚期重型患者的治疗较差。②本品与左旋多巴联合应用，治疗单眼弱视疗效好，尤其是对屈光参差性单眼弱视、弱视性质为中心注视的弱视。<br><br>① Utilisé en association avec le lévodopa, ce produit sert à traiter le parkinson de toutes sortes, avec un effet clinique satisfaisant, mais il est peu efficace dans le traitement des patients gravement malades au stade avancé. ② Utilisé en association avec le lévodopa, ce produit sert à traiter l'amblyopie monoculaire, surtout efficace dans le traitement de l'amblyopie monoculaire anisométropique et de l'amblyopie à fixation centrale. |

续　表

| 用法、用量<br>Les modes d'emploi et la posologie | 首次剂量，卡比多巴 10mg，左旋多巴 100mg，一日 4 次；以后每隔 3～7 日每日增加卡比多巴 40mg，左旋多巴 400mg，直至每日量卡比多巴 200mg，左旋多巴 2g 为限。多采用其复方制剂如患者先用左旋多巴，需停药 8 小时以上才能再合用二药。<br><br>Pour la première fois, 10mg de carbidopa et 100mg de lévodopa, 4 fois par jour ; ensuite, augmenter tous les 3 à 7 jours de 40mg de carbidopa et de 400mg de lévodopa par jour pour atteindre 200mg de carbidopa et 2g de lévodopa par jour. On utilise souvent la préparation de composés. Si le patient commence par utiliser seulement le lévodopa, il faut arrêter l'administration pendant 8h au moins avant d'utiliser les deux médicaments. |
|---|---|
| 剂型、规格<br>Les formes pharmaceutiques et les spécifications | 片剂：每片 25mg。<br><br>Comprimés : 25mg par comprimé. |
| 药品名称 Drug Names | 苄丝肼 Bensérazide |
| 适应证<br>Les indications | 一般苄丝肼与左旋多巴按 1：4 配伍应用，用于帕金森病和帕金森综合征，可减少左旋多巴的用量，增强其疗效并减其外周不良反应。对药物引起的帕金森症无效。<br><br>Utilisé en association avec le lévodopa à un taux de 1 : 4, il sert à traiter le parkinson et le parkinsonisme. Il aide à réduire la dose du lévodopa, à renforcer son efficacité et à réduire les effets indésirables périphériques. Il est inutile dans le traitement du parkinson induit par les drogues. |
| 用法、用量<br>Les modes d'emploi et la posologie | 多与左旋多巴合用，开始时 1 次，苄丝肼 25mg 以及左旋多巴 100ng，一日 2 次；然后每隔一周将苄丝肼增加 25mg/d 及左旋多巴 100mg/d，至每日剂量苄丝肼达 250mg 及左旋多巴达 100mg 为止。分 3～4 次服用。<br><br>Utilisé souvent association avec le lévodopa, au début, 25mg de bensérazide et 100mg de dévodopa par fois, 2 fois par jour ; ensuite, augmenter toutes les 2 semaines de 25mg de bensérazide et de 100mg de lévodopa par jour pour atteindre 250mg de bensérazide et 100mg de lévodopa par jour. Administration à travers 3 à 4 fois. |
| 剂型、规格<br>Les formes pharmaceutiques et les spécifications | 多巴丝肼：每胶囊 125mg（含苄丝肼 25mg 及左旋多巴 100mg）；250mg（含苄丝肼 50mg 及左旋多巴 200mg）。<br><br>Le lévodopa et la bensérazide : 125mg (25mg de bensérazide et 100mg de lévodopa) ou 250mg (50mg de bensérazide et 200mg de lévodopa) par capsule. |
| 药品名称 Drug Names | 多巴丝肼 Lévodopa et bensérazide |
| 适应证<br>Les indications | 适用于原发性震颤麻痹（帕金森病）、脑炎后或合并有脑动脉硬化的症状性帕金森综合征。<br><br>Ce produit sert à traiter le parkinson et le parkinsonisme symptomatique après l'encéphalite ou après l'artériosclérose cérébrale. |
| 用法、用量<br>Les modes d'emploi et la posologie | 口服，成人，第一周 1 次 125mg，一日 2 次。以后每隔 1 周每日增加 125mg。一般日剂量不得超过 1g，分 3～4 次服用。<br><br>Par voie orale, chez des adultes, pour la première semaine, 125mg par fois, 2 fois par jour. Ensuite, augmenter 125mg par jour toutes les 2 semaines. Pour la dose usuelle, ne pas dépasser 1g par jour, à travers 3 à 4 fois. |
| 剂型、规格<br>Les formes pharmaceutiques et les spécifications | 胶囊剂、片剂：① 125mg：左旋多巴 100mg 和苄丝肼 25mg；② 250mg：左旋多巴 200mg 和苄丝肼 50mg。控释片：125mg。分散片：125mg。<br><br>Capsules, comprimés ： ① 125mg : 100mg de lévodopa et 25mg de bensérazide; ② 250mg : 200mg de lévodopa et 50mg de bensérazide. Comprimés à libération contrôlée : 125mg. Comprimés dispersibles : 125mg. |
| 药品名称 Drug Names | 溴隐亭 Bromocriptine |
| 适应证<br>Les indications | ①抗震颤麻痹，疗效优于金刚烷胺及苯海索，对僵直、少动亦效果好，对重症患者亦效果好，常用于左旋多巴疗效不好或不能耐受患者，症状波动者，对左旋多巴复方制剂无效者。特点是显效快，持续时间长。②治疗慢性精神分裂症和躁狂症，尤其是以阴性症状为主的精神病理基础，是多巴胺功能降低所致。治疗抑郁症，通过增强多巴胺能神经元的活性而对抑郁症 |

**续 表**

有效。治疗抗精神病药恶性综合征。③闭经或乳溢，用于各种原因所致催乳激素过高引起的闭经或乳溢，对垂体瘤诱发者，可作为手术或放射治疗的辅助治疗。④抑制生理性泌乳。⑤用于催乳激素过高的引起的经前期综合征，对周期性乳房痛和乳房结节，可使症状改善，但对非周期性乳房痛和月经正常几乎无效。⑥用于肢端肥大症，无功能性垂体肿瘤，垂体性甲状腺功能亢进。治疗库欣病：大多数库欣病由皮质素瘤引起，少数为下丘脑分泌促甲状腺激素释放激素异常。溴隐亭可以降低皮质素，故可以治疗库欣病。⑦治疗女性不育症。⑧治疗男性性功能减退，对男性乳腺发育、阳痿、精液不足等有一定疗效。⑨治疗可卡因戒断综合征，可有效减轻可卡因的瘾欲和戒断的焦虑症状。⑩可用于 huntington 舞蹈症。

① L'antiparkinsonien. Ce produit est plus efficace que l'amantadine et le trihexyphénidyle. Il est également efficace dans le traitement de la rigidité. Aussi applicable dans le traitement des patients gravement malades, des patients résistants au lévodopa, des patients résistants au composé de lévodopa, avec un effet rapide et soutenu. ② Ce produit sert aussi à traiter la schizophrénie et la manie chronique. Applicable également dans le traitement de la dépression, car il aide à améliorer l'activité des neurones dopaminergiques. Il sert aussi à traiter le syndrome malin des neuroleptiques. ③ L'aménorrhée ou la galactorrhée. Il sert à traiter 3) L'aménorrhée ou la galactorrhée causée par la prolactine excessive. Il sert de traitement adjuvant de la thérapie chirurgicale ou radioactive des inducteurs des tumeurs hypophysaires. ④ L'inhibition de la lactation physiologique. ⑤ Il sert à traiter le syndrome prémenstruel causé par la prolactine excessive. Il permet aussi d'améliorer les symptômes des douleurs mammaires et des nodules mammaires cycliques. Mais il est presque inutile en cas de douleurs mammaires non cycliques et de menstruation normale. ⑥ Il sert à traiter l'acromégalie, les tumeurs hypophysaires non fonctionnelles et l'hyperthyroïdiehypophysaire. La maladie de Cushing : dans la plupart des cas, la maladie de Cushing est causée par la tumeur de cortisol, dans certains cas, elle est provoquée par l'anomalité de la sécrétion hypothalamiqued'hormone de libération de la thyrotropine. La bromocriptine peut diminuer le corticotropin, elle peut donc traiter la maladie de Cushing. ⑦ Il sert à traiter l'infertilité féminine. ⑧ Applicable dans le traitement de la dysfonction sexuelle masculine. Il sert à traiter la gynécomastie, l'impuissance et le manque de sperme. ⑨ Il sert à traiter le syndrome de sevrage de la cocaïne. Il peut atténuer la dépendance de cocaïne et les symptômes de l'anxiété. ⑩ Il est également applicable dans le traitement de la chorée de Huntington.

| | |
|---|---|
| 用法、用量<br>Les modes d'emploi et la posologie | ①震颤麻痹：开始每次 1.25mg，一日 2 次，2 周内逐渐加量，必要时每 2～4 周每日增加 2.5mg，以找到最佳治疗的最小剂量，每日剂量 20mg 为宜。②用于闭经或溢乳、抑制泌乳、不育症、肢端肥大等。<br><br>① Pour traiter le parkinsonisme : au début, 1,25mg par fois, 2 fois par jour, augmenter la dose en 2 semaines, en cas de besoin, augmenter 2,5mg par jour toutes les 2 à 4 semaines, pour trouver la dose minimale efficace. Il vaut mieux prendre 20mg par jour. ② Il est utilisé pour traiter l'aménorrhée, la galactorrhée, l'inhibition de la lactation, l'infertilité féminine et l'acromégalie,etc. |
| 剂型、规格<br>Les formes pharmaceutiques et les spécifications | 片剂：每片 2.5mg。<br>Comprimés : 2,5mg par comprimé. |
| 药品名称 Drug Names | 普拉克索 Pramipexole |
| 适应证<br>Les indications | 单独或与左旋多巴合用于治疗帕金森病，可明显减少静息时的震颤。晚期帕金森病用该药与左旋多巴共同治疗时，可使患者对左旋多巴的治疗量减少 27%～30%，并可延长症状最佳控制时间平均每天 2 小时。<br><br>Utilisé seul ou en association avec le lévodopa, il sert à traiter le parkinson et à réduire efficacement le tremblement de repos. Utilisé en combinaison avec le lévodopa dans le traitement du parkinson au stade avancé, il peut permettre de réduire l'administration du lévodopa de 27 % à 30 %, et prolonger le meilleur moment pour contrôler la maladie de 2 h par jour en moyenne. |

**续　表**

| 用法、用量<br>Les modes d'emploi et la posologie | 按病情程度每次 1.5～4.5mg，一日 3 次。<br>1,5 à 4,5 mg par fois en fonction des maladies, 3 fois par jour. |
|---|---|
| 剂型、规格<br>Les formes pharmaceutiques et les spécifications | 片剂：片剂 0.125mg；0.25mg；0.5mg；1mg；1.5mg。<br>Comprimés : 0,125mg, 0.25mg, 0,5mg, 1mg ou 1,5mg par compirmé. |

| 药品名称 Drug Names | 司来吉兰 Sélégiline |
|---|---|
| 适应证<br>Les indications | 适用于帕金森病，常作为左旋多巴、美多巴或信尼麦的辅助用药。<br>Ce produit sert à traiter le parkinson. Il sert souvent de traitement adjuvant du lévodopa, du madopar et du sinemet. |
| 用法、用量<br>Les modes d'emploi et la posologie | 口服，每日 10mg，早晨 1 次顿服；或每次 5mg，早、晚 2 次服用。<br>Par voir orale, 10mg par jour, une fois par jour, le petit matin ; ou 5mg par fois, 2 fois par jour, le petit matin et le soir. |
| 剂型、规格<br>Les formes pharmaceutiques et les spécifications | 片剂：每片 5mg。<br>Comprimés : 5mg par comprimé. |

| 药品名称 Drug Names | 雷沙吉兰 Rasagiline |
|---|---|
| 适应证<br>Les indications | 用于治疗帕金森病，可单用或作为左旋多巴的辅助用药。<br>Ce produit sert à traiter le parkinson. Il peut être utilisé seul ou en tant qu'adjuvant du lévodopa. |
| 用法、用量<br>Les modes d'emploi et la posologie | 单药治疗：每次 1mg，一日 1 次。与左旋多巴联合治疗：起始剂量每次 0.5mg，一日 1 次，维持剂量为 0.5～1mg，一日 1 次。老年患者需调整剂量。<br>Pour une monothérapie : 1mg par fois, 1 fois par jour. Pour le traitement avec la rasagiline et le lévodopa : au début, 0,5mg par fois, 1 fois par jour, la dose d'entretien, 0,5 à 1mg, 1 fois par jour. Chez des personnes âgées, ajuter la dose. |
| 剂型、规格<br>Les formes pharmaceutiques et les spécifications | 片剂：0.5mg；1mg。<br>Comprimés : 0,5mg ou 1mg. |

| 药品名称 Drug Names | 苯海索 Trihéxyphénidyl |
|---|---|
| 适应证<br>Les indications | ①临床用于震颤麻痹，脑炎后或动脉硬化引起的震颤麻痹，对改善流涎有效，对缓解僵直、运动迟缓疗效较差，改善震颤明显，但总的治疗效果不及左旋多巴、金刚烷胺。主要用于轻症及不耐受左旋多巴的患者。常与左旋多巴合用。②药用利血平和吩噻嗪类引起的锥体外系反应。③肝豆状核变性。④畸形性肌张力障碍、癫痫、慢性精神分裂症、抗精神病药所致的静坐不能。<br>① Il est utilisé dans les cliniques comme traitement du parkinsonisme provoqué par l'encéphalite ou l'athérosclérose. Il est efficace dans l'amélioration de la salivation, mais peu efficace dans le soulagement de la rigidité et de la bradykinésie. Il est utile dans le traitement des tremblements, mais moins efficace que le lévodopa et l'amantadine. Il est généralement applicable dans le traitement des patients bénins et résistants au lévodopa. Il est souvent utilisé en association avec le lévodopa. ② Les réactions extrapyramidales causées par la réserpine et les phénothiazines. ③ La dégénérescence hépatolenticulaire. ④ L'akathisie causée par la déformation de la dystonie, l'épilepsie, la schizophrénie chronique, et l'antipsychotique. |

| 用法、用量<br>Les modes d'emploi et la posologie | 常用量：口服，开始时一日 1 ～ 2mg，一日 2 次；逐日递增至一日 5 ～ 10mg，分次服用。对药物引起的锥体外系反应：口服开始第 1 日 1mg，并逐增剂量直至每日 5 ～ 10mg，一日 2 次。口服，一日最多不超过 10mg。<br><br>Dose usuelle : par voie orale, au début, 1 à 2mg par jour, 2 fois par jour ; augmenter progressivement la dose pour atteindre 5 à 10mg par jour, à travers plusieurs fois. Pour traiter les réactions extrapyramidales causées par des médicaments : par voie orale, pour le premier jour, 1mg, augmenter progressivement la dose pour atteindre 5 à 10mg par jour, 2 fois par jour. Par voie orale, ne pas dépasser 10mg par jour. |
|---|---|
| 剂型、规格<br>Les formes pharmaceutiques et les spécifications | 片剂：每片 2mg。<br>胶囊剂：每粒 5mg。<br>Comprimés : 2mg par comprimé.<br>Capsules : 5mg par capsule. |
| 药品名称 Drug Names | 金刚烷胺 Amantadine |
| 适应证<br>Les indications | ①用于不能耐受左旋多巴治疗的震颤麻痹患者；②亚洲 A- Ⅱ 型流感、病毒性感染发热患者；③脑梗死所致的自发性意识低下。<br><br>① Il est applicable dans le traitement des patients atteints de parkinsonisme résistants au lévodopa. ② Les patients atteints de la grippe asiatiquede type A-II et les patients atteints d'infections virales avec de la fièvre. ③ La faible sensibilisation spontanée causée par l'infarctus cérébral. |
| 用法、用量<br>Les modes d'emploi et la posologie | 口服：成人每次 100mg，早、晚各 1 次，最大剂量每日 400mg。小儿用量酌减，可连用 3 ～ 5 日，最多 10 日。1 ～ 9 岁小儿每日 3mg/kg，最大用量不超过 150mg/d。<br><br>Par voie orale : chez des adultes, 100mg par fois, 2 fois par jour (le petit matin et le soir), la dose maximale, 400mg par jour. Chez des enfants, diminuer la dose, pendant 3 à 5 jours, ne pas dépasser 10 jours. Chez des enfants de 1 à 9 ans, 3 mg/kg par jour, ne pas dépasser 150mg par jour. |
| 剂型、规格<br>Les formes pharmaceutiques et les spécifications | 片剂：每片 100mg。<br>胶囊剂：每粒 100mg。<br>糖浆剂：60ml：300mg。<br>颗粒剂：6g：60mg；12g：140mg。<br>Comprimés : 100mg par comprimé.<br>Capsules : 100mg par capsule.<br>Sirops : 60ml : 300mg.<br>Granules : 6g : 60mg ou 12g : 140mg. |
| 药品名称 Drug Names | 美金刚 Mémantine |
| 适应证<br>Les indications | ①用于震颤麻痹综合征。②能改善阿尔茨海默病患者的认知、行为、日常活动和临床症状，可用于重度患者。<br><br>① Il sert à traiter le parkinsonisme. ② Il sert à améliore la cognition, le comportement, les activités de la vie quotidienne et les symptômes cliniques des patients atteints de la maladie d'Alzheimer. Aussi applicable dans le traitement des patients gravement malades. |
| 用法、用量<br>Les modes d'emploi et la posologie | 口服或胃肠道给药，成人和 14 岁以上青年第 1 周，每日 10mg，分 2 ～ 3 次给药；以后每周增加 10mg/d。维持剂量：一次 10mg，一日 2 ～ 3 次。需要时还可增加。剂量因人而异。14 岁以下儿童的维持量为每日 0.5 ～ 1.0mg/kg。<br><br>Par voie orale ou gastro-intestinale, chez des adultes et des jeunes plus de 14 ans, pour la première semaine, 10mg par jour, à travers 2 à 3 fois ; ensuite, augmenter 10 mg par jour chaque semaine. La dose d'entretien : 10mg par fois, 2 à 3 fois par jour. Le cas échéant, possible d'augmenter la dose. La dose varie en fonction des patients. Chez des enfants moins de 14 ans, la dose d'entretien : 0,5 à 1,0 mg/kg par jour |

续　表

| 剂型、规格<br>Les formes pharmaceutiques et les spécifications | 片剂：每片 10mg。<br>滴剂：10mg。<br>注射液：每支 10mg（2ml）。<br>Comprimés : 10mg par comprimé.<br>Gouttes : 10mg.<br>Injection : 10mg (2ml) par solution. |
|---|---|

8.8　抗精神病药 Antipsychotiques

| 药品名称 Drug Names | 氯丙嗪 Chlorpromazine |
|---|---|
| 适应证<br>Les indications | ①治疗精神病：用于控制精神分裂症或其他精神病的兴奋躁动、紧张不安、幻觉、妄想等症状，对忧郁症状及木僵症状的疗效较差。对Ⅱ型精神分裂症患者无效，甚至加重病情。②镇吐：几乎对各种原因引起的呕吐，如尿毒症、胃肠炎、癌症、妊娠及药物引起的呕吐均有效。也可治疗严重呃逆。但对晕动症呕吐无效。③低温麻醉剂人工冬眠：用于低温麻醉时可以防止休克发生。人工冬眠时，与哌替啶、异丙嗪配成冬眠合剂用于创伤性休克、中毒性休克、烧伤、高热及甲状腺危象的辅助治疗。④与镇痛药合用，治疗癌症晚期患者的剧痛。⑤治疗心力衰竭。⑥试用于治疗巨人症。<br><br>① Ce produit sert à traiter la psychose : il est utilisé pour contrôler la schizophrénie, et les symptômes d'autres maladies mentales, tels que l'agitation, la nervosité, les hallucinations et le délire, mais il est peu efficace dans le traitement de la dépression et de la stupeur. Il est inutile dans le traitement des patients atteints de la schizophrénie de type II. ② L'antiémétique : il est presque applicable dans toutes sortes de votissements, tels que les vomissements causés par l'urémie, la gastro-entérite, le cancer, la grossesse et l'administration de médicaments. Il est aussi utilisé comme traitement du hoquet grave. Mais il est inutile dans le traitement du vomissement causé par le mal de transport. ③ L'anesthésie cryogénique et l'hibernation artificielle : applicable dans l'anesthésie cryogénique, il peut éviter le choc. Utilisé dans l'hibernation artificielle, il peut être appliqué en association avec la mépéridineet la prométhazine dans le traitement adjuvant du choc traumatique, du choc toxique, des brûlures, de la fièvre et la crise de la thyroïde. ④ Utilisé en combinaison avec les analgésiques, il sert à traiter les douleurs chez des patients atteints de cancer avancé. ⑤ L'insuffisance cardiaque. ⑥ Le gigantisme. |
| 用法、用量<br>Les modes d'emploi et la posologie | （1）口服：①用于呕吐，1 次 12.5 ～ 25mg，一日 2 ～ 3 次；②用于精神病，一日 50 ～ 600mg。开始每日 25 ～ 50mg，分 2 ～ 3 次服，逐渐增加至每日 300 ～ 450mg，症状减轻后再减至一日 100 ～ 150mg。极量每次 150mg，每日 600mg。<br>（2）肌内或静脉注射：①用于呕吐，1 次 25 ～ 50mg；②用于神经病，1 次 25 ～ 100mg。目前多采用静脉注射。极量每次 100mg，每日 400mg。③治疗心力衰竭：肌内注射小剂量，每次 5 ～ 10mg，一日 1 ～ 2 次，也可静脉滴注，速度每分钟 0.5mg。<br><br>(1) Par voie orale : ① Pour traiter les vomissements, 12,5 à 25mg par fois, 2 à 3 fois par jour. ② Pour traiter la psychose, 50 à 600mg par jour. Au début, 25 à 50mg par jour, à travers 2 à 3 fois, augmenter progressivement la dose pour atteindre 300 à 450 mg par jour, après l'amélioration des symptômes, 100 à 150 mg par jour.La dose maximale est de 150mg par fois, 600mg par jour.<br>(2) Injeciton par voie IM ou IV : ① Pour traiter les vomissements, 25 à 50mg par fois. ② Pour traiter la psychose, 25 à 100mg par fois. À l'heure actuelle, généralement, injection par voie IV. La dose maximale : 100mg par fois, 400mg par jour. ③ Pour traiter l'insuffisance cardiaque, dose mineure injectée par voie IM, 5 à 10mg par fois, 1 à 2 fois par jour. Il est aussi permissible de l'injecter par voie IV en perfusion, 0,5 mg par minute. |
| 剂型、规格<br>Les formes pharmaceutiques et les spécifications | 片剂：每片 5mg；12.5mg；25mg；50mg。<br>注射液：每支 10mg（1ml）；25g（1ml）；50mg（2ml）。<br>Comprimés : 5mg, 12,5mg, 25mg ou 50mg par comprimé.<br>Injection : 10mg (1ml), 25mg (1ml) ou 50mg (2ml) par solution. |

**续 表**

| 药品名称 Drug Names | 奋乃静 Pérphénazine |
|---|---|
| 适应证<br>Les indications | ①用于治疗偏执性精神病、反应性精神病、症状性精神病，单纯性及慢性精神分裂症。②用于治疗恶心、呕吐、呃逆等症，神经症具焦虑紧张症患者，亦可用小剂量配合其他药物治疗。<br><br>① Ce produit sert à traiter la psychose paranoïde, la psychose réactive, la psychose symptomatique ainsi que les schizophrénies simples et chroniques. ② Il est utilisé comme traitement de la nausée, du vomissement et du hoquet. Chez les catatoniques avec la névrose d'angoisse, il est possible de l'utilisé avec une dose mineure en association avec d'autres médicaments. |
| 用法、用量<br>Les modes d'emploi et la posologie | 口服：用于呕吐焦虑，1次2～4mg，一日2～3次；用于精神病，开始时一日6～12mg，逐日增量至一日30～60mg，分3次服。肌内注射：用于精神病，一次5～10mg，隔6小时1次或酌情调整；用于呕吐一次5mg。<br><br>Par voie orale : pour traiter les vomissements et l'anxiété, 2 à 4mg par fois, 2 à 3 fois par jour ; pour traiter la psychose, au début, 6 à 12mg par jour, ensuite, augmenter la dose pour atteindre 30 à 60mg par jour, à travers 3 fois. Injection par voie IM : pour traiter la psychose, 5 à 10mg par fois, toutes les 6 h ou selon les cas ; pour traiter les vomissements, 5mg par fois. |
| 剂型、规格<br>Les formes pharmaceutiques et les spécifications | 片剂：每片2mg；4mg。<br>注射液：每支5mg（2ml）；5mg（1ml）。<br>Comprimsés : 2mg ou 4mg par comprimé.<br>Injection : 5mg (2ml) ou 5mg (1ml) par solution. |
| 药品名称 Drug Names | 氟奋乃静 Fluphénazine |
| 适应证<br>Les indications | 用于妄想、紧张型精神分裂症、痴呆和中毒性精神病。亦可用于控制恶心呕吐。其癸酸酯注射液有长效作用。<br><br>Il sert à traiter le délire, la schizophrénie catatonique, la démence et la psychose toxique. Il est aussi applicable dans le traitement de la nausée et du vomissement. Son injection de décanoate a un effet à long terme. |
| 用法、用量<br>Les modes d'emploi et la posologie | 口服：成人常用剂量1次2mg，一日1～2次；逐渐递增，日服总量可达20mg。老年或体弱者从最小剂量开始，然后每日用量递增在1～2mg。<br><br>Par voie orale : chez des adultes, dose usuelle, 2mg par fois, 1 à 2 fois par jour ; augmenter progressivement la dose pour atteindre 20 mg par jour. Chez des personnes âgées ou des faibles, commencer par une dose mineure, ensuite, augmenter 1 à 2mg par jour. |
| 剂型、规格<br>Les formes pharmaceutiques et les spécifications | 片剂：1片2mg；5mg。<br>注射液：每支2mg（1m）；5mg（1ml）；10mg（2ml）。<br>Comprimés : 2mg ou 5mg par comprimé.<br>Injection : 2mg (1ml), 5mg (1ml) ou 10mg (2ml) par solution. |
| 药品名称 Drug Names | 三氟拉嗪 Trifluopérazine |
| 适应证<br>Les indications | 主要用于治疗精神病，对急、慢性精神分裂症，尤其对妄想型与紧张型较好。用于镇吐。<br><br>Il sert à traiter la psychose. Il est surtout efficace dans le traitement de la schizophrénie chronique, aigue, notamment paranoïaque et catatonique. Applicable dans l'antiémétique. |
| 用法、用量<br>Les modes d'emploi et la posologie | 口服，一次5～10mg，每日15～30mg。必要时可逐渐递增至每日45mg。也用于镇吐，口服，一次1～2mg，每日2～4mg。<br><br>Par voie orale, 5 à 10mg par fois, 15 à 30 mg par jour. S'il est nécessaire, 45mg par jour. Pour l'antiémétique, par voie orale, 1 à 2mg par fois, 2 à 4mg par jour. |
| 剂型、规格<br>Les formes pharmaceutiques et les spécifications | 片剂：每片1mg；5mg。<br>Comprimés : 1mg ou 5mg par comprimé. |

**续　表**

| 药品名称 Drug Names | 硫利达嗪 Thioridazine |
| --- | --- |
| 适应证<br>Les indications | 主要用于治疗精神分裂症，适用于伴有激动、焦虑、紧张的精神分裂症、躁狂症、更年期精神病。亦用于儿童多动症及行为障碍。因锥体外系反应少而广泛应用。<br><br>Il sert principalement à traiter la chizophrénie. Il est applicable dans le traitement de la schizophrénie,de la manie et de la psychose de la ménopause avec l'agitation, l'angoisse et la nervosité. Il est aussi utilisé dans le traitement du TDAH et des troubles de comportements chez les enfants. Il est largement appliqué grâce à ses réactions extrapyramidales peu importantes. |
| 用法、用量<br>Les modes d'emploi et la posologie | 开始时口服每次 25 ～ 100mg，一日 3 次。然后根据病情及耐受情况逐渐递增至充分治疗剂量每次 100 ～ 200mg，一日 3 次。最多可达每日 800mg。老年或体质弱者，从小剂量开始逐渐增加，每日总量低于成年人。<br><br>Au début, par voie orale, 25 à 100mg par fois, 3 fois par jour. Ensuite, augmenter la dose en fonction des maladies pour atteindre 100 à 200 mg par fois, 3 fois par jour. La dose maximale : 800mg par jour. Chez des personnes âgées ou des faibles, il vaut mieux commencer par une dose mineure avant de l'augmenter. Ne pas dépasser la dose chez des adultes. |
| 剂型、规格<br>Les formes pharmaceutiques et les spécifications | 片剂：每片 10mg；25mg；50mg；100mg；200mg。<br>Comprimés : 10mg, 25mg, 50mg, 100mg ou 200mg par comprimé. |
| 药品名称 Drug Names | 氟哌啶醇 Halopéridol |
| 适应证<br>Les indications | 主要用于：各种急、慢性精神分裂症。特别适合于急性青春型和伴有敌对情绪及攻击行为的偏执型精神分裂症，亦可用于对吩噻嗪类治疗无效的其他类型或慢性精神分裂症、焦虑性神经症、儿童抽动 - 秽语综合征，有称 Tourette 综合征（TS），小剂量本品治疗有效，能消除不自主的运动，又能减轻和消除伴存的精神症状、呕吐及顽固性呃逆。<br><br>Applicable dans le traitement : Les chizophrénies aigues et chroniques. Surtout applicable dans le traitement de la chizophrénie paranoïde aigue de la jeunesse avec l'hostilité et les attaques. Ce produit sert aussi à traiter les chizophrénies chroniques ou d'autres types résistant aux phénothiazines. La névrose d'angoisse. Avec une dose peu importante, ce produit sert aussi à traiter le syndrome de la Tourette, à éliminer des mouvements involontaires, à diminuer ou éliminer les symptômes psychiatriques. Le vomissement et le hoquet réfractaire. |
| 用法、用量<br>Les modes d'emploi et la posologie | ① 口服：用于精神病：成人开始剂量每次 2 ～ 4mg，一日 2 ～ 3 次；逐渐增至 8 ～ 12mg，一日 2 ～ 3 次。一般剂量每日 20 ～ 30mg。维持治疗每次 2 ～ 4mg，一日 2 ～ 3 次。儿童及老年人，剂量减半。用于呕吐和焦虑：每日 0.5 ～ 1.5mg。用于抽动 - 秽语综合征：一般剂量每次 1 ～ 2mg，一日 3 次。② 肌内注射：每次 5 ～ 10mg，一日 2 ～ 3 次。③ 静脉注射：10 ～ 30mg 加入 25% 葡萄糖注射液在 1 ～ 2 分钟缓慢注入，每 8 小时 1 次。好转后可改口服。<br><br>① Par voie orale : pour traiter la psychose : chez des adultes, au début, 2 à 4 mg par fois, 2 à 3 fois par jour ; ensuite, petit à petit, 8 à 12mg, 2 à 3 fois par jour. La dose usuelle, 20 à 30 mg par jour. Pour le traitement d'entretien, 2 à 4 mg par fois, 2 à 3 fois par jour. Chez des enfants et des personnes âgées, diminuer de moitié la dose usuelle. ② Pour traiter les vomissements et l'anxiété : 0.5 à 1.5 mg par jour. Pour traiter le syndrome de la Tourette : 1 à 2 mg par fois, 3 fois par jour. ③ Injection par voie IV : dissoudre 10 à 30 mg de produit dans la solution de glucose à 25 %, injection lente pendant 1 à 2 minutes, toutes les 8 h. Après l'amélioration des symptômes, administration par voie orale. |
| 剂型、规格<br>Les formes pharmaceutiques et les spécifications | 片剂：每片 2mg；4mg；5mg。<br>注射液：每支 5mg（1ml）。<br>Comprimés : 2mg, 4mg ou 5mg par comprimé.<br>Injection : 5mg (1ml) par solution. |

**续　表**

| 药品名称 Drug Names | 氟哌利多 Dropéridol |
|---|---|
| 适应证<br>Les indications | ①治疗精神分裂症的急性精神运动性兴奋躁狂状态。②神经安定镇痛术：利用本药的安定作用及增强镇痛作用的特点，将其与镇痛药芬太尼一起静脉注射，使患者产生一种特殊麻醉状态，用于烧伤大面积换药，各种内镜检查及造影等。③麻醉前给药，具有较好的抗精神紧张、镇吐抗休克的作用等。<br><br>① Ce produit sert à traiter l'exitation et la manie psychomotrices aigues de la schizophrénie. ② L'analgésie neuroleptique : utilisé en association avec le fantanyl dans l'injection en voie IV, il peut permettre aux patients une anesthésie apéciale, ce qui facilite le pansement de brûlure à grande surface, l'endoscopie et radiographie. ③ L'administration avant l'anesthésie. Il pert de lutter contre le stress, le vomissement et le choc. |
| 用法、用量<br>Les modes d'emploi et la posologie | ①治疗精神分裂症：每日 10 ～ 30mg，分 1 ～ 2 次肌内注射。②神经安定镇痛术：每 5mg 加芬太尼 0.1mg，在 2 ～ 3 分钟缓慢静脉注射，5 ～ 6 分钟如未达一级麻醉状态，可追加半倍至一倍剂量。③麻醉前给药：手术前 0.5 小时肌内注射 2.5 ～ 5mg。<br><br>① Pour traiter la schizophrénie : injection par voie IM, 10 à 30 mg par jour, à travers 1 à 2 fois. ② Pour l'analgésie neuroleptique : pour 5mg de produit, ajouter 0,1mg de fantanyl, injection lente par voie IV pendant 2 à 3 minutes. Si l'on n'atteint pas le premier degré de l'anesthésie en 5 à 6 minutes, augmenter moitié la dose ou doubler la dose. ③ L'administration avant l'anesthésie : 0,5h avant la chirurgie, 2,5 à 5 mg, injection par voie IM. |
| 剂型、规格<br>Les formes pharmaceutiques et les spécifications | 注射液：每支 5mg（1ml）。<br>Injection : 5mg (1ml) par solution. |

| 药品名称 Drug Names | 氯哌噻吨 Clopenthixol |
|---|---|
| 适应证<br>Les indications | ①长期使用可预防精神分裂症复发，对慢性患者可改善症状；对幻觉、妄想、思维障碍、行为紊乱、兴奋躁动等效果较好。②对智力障碍伴精神运动性兴奋状态、儿童严重攻击性行为障碍、老年动脉硬化性痴呆疗效较好。<br><br>① Utilisé à long terme, il sert à prévenir la récurrence de la chizophrénie. Chez des patients chroniques, il sert à améliorer les symptômes ; il est efficace dans le traitement de l'hallucination, du délire, des troubles de la pensée, des troubles de la conduite et de l'agitation. ② Il est efficace dans le traitemetn des troubles mentaux avec l'excitation psychomotrice, des troubles graves de comportements agressifs chez les enfants ainsi que la démence artérioscléreuse sénile. |
| 用法、用量<br>Les modes d'emploi et la posologie | 口服：开始剂量每日 10mg，一日 1 次，以后可逐渐增至每日 80mg，分 2 ～ 3 次服；维持剂量每日 10 ～ 40mg。速效针剂：深部肌内注射 50 ～ 100mg，一般 72 小时注射 1 次，累计总量不超过 400mg。癸酸酯长效针剂：一般 200mg 肌内注射，每 2 ～ 4 周 1 次，根据情况调整。<br><br>Par voie orale : au début, 10mg par jour, 1 fois par jour, ensuite, 80mg par jour, à travers 2 à 3 fois; la dose d'entretien, 10 à 40mg par jour. Injection à action rapide : injection par voie IM profonde, 50 à 100mg, une injection toutes les 72h, ne pas dépasser 400mg au total. Injection à action prolongée de décanoate : injection par voie IM 200mg, une fois toutes les 2 à 4 semaines, selon les cas. |
| 剂型、规格<br>Les formes pharmaceutiques et les spécifications | 片剂：每片 10mg。<br>注射剂：速效针剂 50mg（1ml），长效针剂 200mg（1ml）。<br>Comprimés : 10mg par comprimé.<br>Injection : injection à action rapide, 50mg (1ml) ; injection à action prolongée, 200mg (1ml). |

| 药品名称 Drug Names | 氟哌噻吨 Flupentixol |
|---|---|
| 适应证<br>Les indications | ①用于急、慢性精神分裂症，对淡漠，意志减退，违拗症状及分裂症后抑郁效果较好；长效制剂用于维持治疗和慢性精神分裂症的治疗。②各种原因引起的抑郁或焦虑症状。③有癫痫、老年痴呆、精神发育迟滞以及酒、药依赖伴发的精神症状。<br><br>① Il sert à traiter les chizophrénies chroniques et aigues. Il est efficace dans le traitement de l'indifférence, du négavtivisme ainsi que de la dépression post schizophrène. ② La dépression ou l'angoisse. ③ symptômes psychiatriques avec l'épilepsie, la démence, le retard mental et la dépendance à l'alcool et aux médicaments. |

| | |
|---|---|
| 用法、用量<br>Les modes d'emploi et la posologie | ①用于精神病：口服，初始每次 5mg，一日 1 次，以后视情况可逐渐加量，必要时可增至每日 40mg；维持剂量每次 5～20mg，一日 1 次。深部肌内注射，起始剂量 10mg 注射一次，一周后可酌情加量；治疗剂量每次 20～40mg，每 2 周注射一次；维持剂量每次 20mg，每 2～4 周注射一次。②用于治疗忧郁性神经症：口服，每次 1mg，一日 2 次。最大剂量为每日 3mg。<br><br>① Pour traiter la psychose : par voie orale, au début, 5mg par fois, 1 fois par jour, ensuite, augmenter la dose selon les cas, s'il est nécessaire, 40mg par jour ; pour la dose d'entretien, 5 à 20mg par fois, 1 fois par jour. Injection par voie IM profonde, au début, 10mg par injection, 1 semaine après, augmenter la dose selon les cas ; la dose de traitement, 20 à 40mg par fois, une injection toutes les deux semaines ; la dose d'entretien, 20mg par fois, une injection toutes les 2 à 4 semines.  ② Pour traiter la névrose dépressive : par voie orale, 1mg par fois, 2 fois par jour. Ne pas dépasser 3mg par jour. |
| 剂型、规格<br>Les formes pharmaceutiques et les spécifications | 片剂：每片 0.5mg；3mg；5mg。<br>癸酸酯注射剂：每支 20mg（1ml）。<br>Comprimés : 0,5mg, 3mg ou 5mg par comprimé.<br>Injection de décanoate : 20mg (1ml) par solution. |
| 药品名称 Drug Names | 氟哌噻吨美利曲辛 Flupéntixol et Mélitracén |
| 适应证<br>Les indications | ①用于治疗神经症。治疗多种焦虑抑郁状态。②用于治疗神经性头痛、偏头痛、紧张性头痛，某些顽固性疼痛及慢性疼痛等。<br><br>① il sert à traiter la névrose, la dépresssion et l'angoisse.  ② Il sert à traiter la céphalée par tension nerveuse, la céphalée de tension, la migraine, et la céphalée réfractaire ainsi que les douleurs chroniques. |
| 用法、用量<br>Les modes d'emploi et la posologie | 口服：一日 2 片，早晨单次顿服，或早晨中午各服 1 片。严重者一日 3 片，早晨 2 片，中午 1 片。维持剂量为一日 1 片，早晨服。<br><br>Par voie orale : 2 comprimés par jour, le petit matin, une fois par jour, ou à travers 2 fois (le petit matin et le midi). Chez des patients gravement malades, 3 comprimés par jour (2 comprimés le petit matin et 1 comprimé le midi). Pour la dose d'entretien, 1 comprimé par jour, le petit matin. |
| 剂型、规格<br>Les formes pharmaceutiques et les spécifications | 片剂：每片含哌噻吨 0.5mg 和美利曲辛 10mg。<br>Comprimés : chaque comprimé contient 0,5mg de flupentixol et 10mg de melitracen. |
| 药品名称 Drug Names | 舒必利 Sulpiride |
| 适应证<br>Les indications | ①对淡漠、退缩、木僵、抑郁、幻觉和妄想症状的效果较好，适用于精神分裂症单纯型、偏执型、紧张型及慢性精神分裂症的孤僻、退缩、淡漠症状；对抑郁症状有一定疗效。②用于治疗呕吐、酒精中毒性精神病、智力发育不全伴有人格障碍、胃及十二指肠溃疡等。<br><br>① Il est efficace dans le traitement de l'apathie, du retrait, de la stupeur, de la dépression, des hallucinations et des délires. Applicable dans le traitement des chizophrénies simples, paranoïdes et catatoniques, ainsi que dans le traitement du retrait et de l'apathie des chizophrénies chroniques, et un peu efficace pour la dépresssion.  ② Il sert aussi à traiter les vomissements, la psychose alcoolique, le retard mental avec les troubles de la personnalité, l'ulcère gastrique et ulcère duodénal. |
| 用法、用量<br>Les modes d'emploi et la posologie | ①治疗精神病：口服，开始每日 300～600mg，可缓慢增至一日 600～1200mg；肌内注射，每日 200～600mg，分 2 次注射；静脉滴注，每日 300～600mg，稀释后缓慢滴注，滴注时间不少于 4 小时。一般以口服为主，对拒药者或治疗开始 1～2 周可用注射给药，以后改为口服。②治疗呕吐：口服，每次 100～200mg，一日 2～3 次。<br><br>① Pour traiter la psychose : par voie orale, au début, 300 à 600mg par jour, ensuite, petit à petit, 600 à 1 200 mg par jour ; injection par voie IM, 200 à 600 mg par jour, à travers 2 fois ; en perfusion, 300 à 600 mg par jour, perfusion lente après la dilution, pendant 4 h au moins. En général, administration par voie orale. Chez des patients résistants ou pendant les premières 1 à 2 semaines, injection, et puis, par voie orale. ② Pour traiter le vomissement : par voie orale, 100 à 200mg par fois, 2 à 3 fois par jour. |

续 表

| 剂型、规格<br>Les formes pharmaceutiques et les spécifications | 片剂：每片 10mg；50mg；100mg；200mg。<br>注射液：每支 50mg（2ml）；100mg（2ml）。<br>Comprimés : 10mg, 50mg, 100mg ou 200mg par comprimé.<br>Injection : 50mg (2ml) ou 100mg (2ml) par solution. |
|---|---|
| **药品名称 Drug Names** | 氯氮平 Clozapine |
| 适应证<br>Les indications | 对精神分裂症的阳性或阴性症状有较好的疗效，适用于急性和慢性精神分裂的各种亚型，对偏执型、青春型效果好。也可减轻与精神分裂症有关的感情症状（如抑郁、负罪感、焦虑）。本品也用于治疗躁狂症或其他精神障碍的兴奋躁动和幻觉、妄想，适用于难治性精神分裂症。因导致粒细胞减少症，一般不宜作为首选药，而用于患者经历了其他两种抗精神病药充分治疗无效或不耐受其他药物治疗时。<br><br>Ce produit est efficace dans le traitement des symptômes positifs ou négatifs de la schizophrénie. Applicable dans le traitement des sous-types des schizophrénies aigues et chroniques, de la schizophrénie paranoïde et de la schizophrénie de jeunesse. Il permet également de réduire les symptômes émotionnels liés à la schizophrénie (tels que la dépression, la culpabilité et l'anxiété). Il sert aussi à traiter la manie ou l'agitation, les hallucinations et les délires liés à d'autres troubles mentaux, ainsi que la schizophrénie réfractaire. Comme il peut provoquer la granulocytopénie, il ne s'utilise pas comme médicament de choix. Il est utilisé chez des patients résistant à deux autres médicaments antipsychotiques. |
| 用法、用量<br>Les modes d'emploi et la posologie | 口服：开始一次 25mg，一日 1～2 次；然后每日增加 25～50mg，耐受性好，在开始治疗的 2 周末将一日总量增至 300～450mg，均为一日分 1～2 次服用。肌内注射：每次 50～100mg，一日 2 次。<br><br>Par voie orale : au début, 25mg par fois, 1 à 2 fois par jour ; ensuite, augmenter 25 à 50mg par jour, s'il les patients sont résistants, à la fin de deux premières semaines, prendre 300 à 450 mg par jour, à travers 1 à 2 fois par jour. Injection par voie IM : 50 à 100mg par fois, 2 fois par jour. |
| 剂型、规格<br>Les formes pharmaceutiques et les spécifications | 片剂：每片 25mg；50mg。<br>Comprimés : 25mg ou 50mg par comprimé. |
| **药品名称 Drug Names** | 奥氮平 Olanzapine |
| 适应证<br>Les indications | 用于治疗严重阳性症状或阴性症状的精神分裂症和其他精神病的急性期及维持期。亦可用于缓解精神分裂症及相关疾病常见的继发性感情症状。<br><br>Ce produit sert à traiter les symptômes positifs ou négatifs de la schizophrénie, ainsi que la psychose dans la phase aigue ou d'entretien. Il est aussi applicable dans la réduction des symptômes émotionnels secondaires liés à la schizophrénie et aux autres maladies concernées. |
| 用法、用量<br>Les modes d'emploi et la posologie | 口服，每日 10～15mg。可根据病情调整剂量每天 5～20mg。老年人、女性、非吸烟者、有低血压倾向者、严重肾功能损害者或中度肝功能损伤者，起始剂量为每日 5mg，如需加量，剂递增为每次 5mg，递增一次间隔至少 1 周。<br><br>Par voie orale, 10 à 15mg par jour. Il est possible d'ajuster la dose en fonction des maladies, 5 à 20 mg par jour. Chez des personnes âgées, des femmes, des non-fumeurs, ceux qui ont tendance à l'hypotension, les patients insuffisants rénaux graves ou les hépatiques modérés, au début, 5mg par jour, s'il est nécessire d'augmenter la dose, augmenter 5mg par fois, l'intervalle entre deux augmentations de dose doit être une semaine au moins. |
| 剂型、规格<br>Les formes pharmaceutiques et les spécifications | 片剂：每片 2.5mg；5mg；7.5mg；10mg。<br>Comprimés : 2,5mg, 5mg, 7,5mg ou 10mg par comprimé. |

**续　表**

| 药品名称 Drug Names | 喹硫平 Quétiapine |
|---|---|
| 适应证<br>Les indications | ①用于各种精神分裂症，不仅对精神分裂症阳性症状有效，对阴性症状也有一定疗效。②也可以减轻与精神分裂症有关的感情症状如抑郁、焦虑及认知缺陷症状。<br><br>① Ce produit sert à traiter toutes sortes de schizophrénie, non seulement les symptômes positifs de celle-ci, mais aussi un peu efficace dans le traitement de ses symptômes négatifs. ② Il sert aussi à réduire les symptômes émotionnels liés à la schizophrénie, tels que la dépression, l'anxiété et les déficits cognitifs. |
| 用法、用量<br>Les modes d'emploi et la posologie | 口服，成人：起始剂量为 1 次 25mg，一日 2 次。每隔 1～3 日增加 25mg，逐渐加量至一日 300～600mg，分 2～3 次服用。老年人：用本品应慎重，推荐起始剂量为每日 25mg。每日增加剂量幅度为 25～50mg，直至有效剂量，有效剂量可以较一般成人低。<br><br>Par voie orale, chez des adultes : au début, 25mg par fois, 2 fois par jour. Augmenter 25mg tous les 1à 3 jours, pour atteindre 300 à 600mg par jour, à travers 2 à 3 fois. Chez des personnes âgées : il faut être prudent, il est recommandé de prendre 25mg par jour au début. Augmenter 25 à 50mg par jour jusqu'à la dose efficace qui peut être moins importante que chez des adultes ordinaires. |
| 剂型、规格<br>Les formes pharmaceutiques et les spécifications | 片剂：每片 25mg；100mg；200mg。<br>Comprimés : 25mg, 100mg ou 200mg par comprimé. |
| 药品名称 Drug Names | 利培酮 Rispéridone |
| 适应证<br>Les indications | 用于治疗急性和慢性精神分裂症状。特别是对阳性及阴性症状及其伴发的情感症状（如焦虑、抑郁等）有较好的疗效。也可减轻与精神分裂症有关的情感症状。对于急性期治疗有效患者，维持期治疗中，本品可继续发挥临床效果。<br><br>Ce produit sert à traiter les schizophrénies chroniques et aigues. Il est surtout efficace dans le traitement des symptômes positifs, négatifs et émotionnels associés (tels que l'anxiété, la dépression). Il peut également réduire les symptômes émotionnels liés à la schizophrénie. Chez des patients dont le traitement au stade aigu est efficace, il est toujours efficace dans la phase d'entretien. |
| 用法、用量<br>Les modes d'emploi et la posologie | 口服，宜从小剂量开始。初始剂量为每次 1mg，一日 2 次，剂量逐渐增至第 3 日为 3mg，以后每周调整一次剂量，最大疗效剂量为每日 4～6mg。老年患者起始剂量为每次 0.5mg，一日 2 次。<br><br>Par voie orale, il vaut mieux commencer par une dose mineure. Au début, 1mg par fois, 2 fois par jour, pour le troisième jour, 3mg, ensuite, ajuster la dose toutes les semaines, la dose efficace maximale, 4 à 6 mg par jour. Chez des personnes âgées, au début, 0,5mg par fois, 2 fois par jour. |
| 剂型、规格<br>Les formes pharmaceutiques et les spécifications | 片剂：每片 1mg；2mg。<br>Comprimés : 1mg ou 2mg par comprimé. |
| 药品名称 Drug Names | 帕潘立酮 Palipéridone |
| 适应证<br>Les indications | ①用于精神分裂症急性期治疗。②用于精神分裂症、双相情感障碍的躁狂期及孤独症的治疗。<br><br>① Ce produit sert à traiter la schizophrénie aigue. ② Il sert aussi à traiter la schizophrénie et la trouble bipolaire au stade maniaque ainsi que l'autisme. |
| 用法、用量<br>Les modes d'emploi et la posologie | 成人：口服，每次 6mg，一日 1 次，早晨服药。需要进行剂量增加时，推荐增量为每日增加 3mg。一日最大推荐剂量为 12mg。<br><br>Chez des adultes : par voie orale, 6mg par fois, 1 fois par jour, le petit matin. Selon les cas, possible d'augmenter 3mg par jour. Ne pas dépasser 12mg par jour. |
| 剂型、规格<br>Les formes pharmaceutiques et les spécifications | 缓释片：3mg；6mg；9mg。<br>Comprimés à libération prolongée : 3mg, 6mg ou 9mg. |

**续 表**

| 药品名称 Drug Names | 齐拉西酮 Ziprasidone |
|---|---|
| 适应证<br>Les indications | ①主要用于精神分裂症治疗。也能改善分裂症状伴发的抑郁症状。②可用于情感性障碍的狂躁期治疗。<br><br>① Ce produit sert principalement à traiter la schizophrénie. Il est aussi applicable dans la réduction de la dépression liée à la schizophrénie. ② Il sert aussi à traiter les troubles émotionnels au stade maniaque. |
| 用法、用量<br>Les modes d'emploi et la posologie | 口服：初始治疗一日 2 次，每次 20mg，餐时口服。视病情可逐渐增加到一日 2 次，每次 80mg。调整剂量时间间隔一般应不少于 2 日。维持治疗一日 2 次，每次 20mg。肌内注射：用于精神分裂症患者的急性激越期治疗。每次 10 ～ 20mg，最大剂量为每日 40mg。如需长期使用，应改为口服。<br><br>Par voie orale : au début, 2 fois par jour, 20mg par fois, durant le repas, par voie orale. En fonction des maladies, 80mg par fois, 2 fois par jour. L'intervalle pour l'ajustement de la dose doit être 2 jours au moins. Pour le traitement d'entretien, 20 mg par fois, 2 fois par jour. Injection par voir IM : applicable dans le traitement de l'agitation aiguë chez les patients atteints de schizophrénie. 10 à 20 mg par fois, ne pas dépasser 40mg par jour. S'il faut l'administrer à long terme, prendre le médicament par voie orale. |
| 剂型、规格<br>Les formes pharmaceutiques et les spécifications | 片剂：20mg；60mg。<br>胶囊剂：20mg；40mg；60mg；80mg。<br>注射液：10mg（1ml）；20mg（1ml）。<br>Comprimés : 20mg ou 60mg.<br>Capsules : 20mg, 40mg, 60mg ou 80mg.<br>Injection : 10mg (1ml) ou 20mg (1ml). |
| 药品名称 Drug Names | 五氟利多 Penfluridol |
| 适应证<br>Les indications | 对精神分裂症各型和各病程均有疗效，控制幻觉、妄想及淡漠、退缩等症状疗效好。主要用于慢性精神分裂症患者的维持治疗，对急性患者也有效。<br><br>Il est efficace dans le traitement des schizophrénies de toutes sortes et aux différents stades, ainsi que dans le contrôle des symptômes tels que les hallucinations, les délires, l'indifférence et le retrait. Il est aussi applicable dans le traitement d'entretien chez des patients atteints de schizophrénie chronique et également aigue. |
| 用法、用量<br>Les modes d'emploi et la posologie | 口服，每次 20 ～ 60mg，每周 1 次，重症或耐药患者可加至每周 120mg，1 次服或 2 次分服（一半在前半周，一半在后半周服）。<br><br>Par voie orale, 20 à 60 mg par fois, 1 fois par semaine, chez des patients gravement malades ou des patients résistants, 120mg par semaine, à travers 1 ou 2 fois (une fois début semaine, une fois fin de la semaine). |
| 剂型、规格<br>Les formes pharmaceutiques et les spécifications | 片剂：每片 5mg；20mg。<br>Comprimés : 5mg ou 20mg par comprimé. |
| 药品名称 Drug Names | 阿立哌唑 Aripiprazole |
| 适应证<br>Les indications | 用于治疗各类型的精神分裂症。国外临床试验表明，本品对精神分裂症的阳性和阴性症状均有明显疗效，也能改善伴发的情感症状，降低精神分裂症的复发率。<br><br>Ce produit sert à traiter les schizophrénies de toutes sortes. Les essais cliniques étrangers montrent que ce produit est efficace dans le traitement des symptômes positifs et négatifs de la schizophrénie, ainsi que dans la réduction des symptômes émotionnels associés, et la réduction du taux de récurrence de la schizophrénie. |
| 用法、用量<br>Les modes d'emploi et la posologie | 口服，一日 1 次。推荐用法为第 1 周起始剂量每日 5mg，第 2 周为每日 10mg，第 3 周为每日 15mg，之后可根据个体的疗效个耐受情况调整剂量。有效剂量范围每日 10 ～ 30mg，最大剂量不应超过每日 30mg。<br><br>Par voie orale, 1 fois par jour. Dose recommandée : pour la première semaine, 5mg par jour, pour la deuxième semaine, 10mg par jour, pour la troisième semaine, 15mg par jour, ensuite, ajuster la dose en fonction des patients. La dose efficace : 10 à 30 mg par jour, la dose maximale : 30mg par jour. |

**续 表**

| | |
|---|---|
| 剂型、规格<br>Les formes pharmaceutiques et les spécifications | 片剂：每片 5mg；10mg。<br>Comprimés : 5mg ou 10mg par comprimé. |
| **药品名称 Drug Names** | 曲美托嗪 Trimétozine |
| 适应证<br>Les indications | 用于伴有恐惧、紧张和情绪激动的神经精神症状及儿童行为障碍；对于带有神经质综合征的患者，本品可有效地消除兴奋；在精神病的治疗上可作为一种维持治疗用药。<br>Ce produit sert à traiter les symptômes neuropsychiatriques accompagnés de peur, de nervosité et d'agitation, ainsi que les troubles de comportements chez des enfants ; chez les patients atteints de syndrome névrotique, ce produit peut éliminer efficacement l'excitation ; il est aussi applicable dans le traitement d'entretien de la psychose. |
| 用法、用量<br>Les modes d'emploi et la posologie | 每次口服 300mg，一日 3 ～ 6 次。<br>Par voie orale, 300mg par fois, 3 à 6 fois par jour. |
| 剂型、规格<br>Les formes pharmaceutiques et les spécifications | 片剂：每片 300mg。<br>Comprimés : 300mg par comprimé. |
| **药品名称 Drug Names** | 癸氟奋乃静 Fluphénazine décanoate |
| 适应证<br>Les indications | 应用同氟奋乃静。对幻觉、妄想、木僵、淡漠、孤独和紧张性兴奋有较好疗效。对兴奋躁动和焦虑紧张也有效。对慢性精神分裂症可使淡漠和退缩减轻，改善与环境接触的反应。也可用于精神分裂症缓解期的维持治疗。<br>Cf. à la fluphénazine. Il est efficace dans le traitement des hallucinations, des délires, de la stupeur, de l'apathie, de la solitude et de l'excitation nerveuse. Il est aussi applicable dans le traitement de l'agitation et de l'anxiété nerveuse. En cas de schizophrénie chronique, il peut réduire les symptômes tels que l'apathie et le retrait, à améliorer les réactions au contact avec l'environnement. Il est aussi applicable dans le traitement d'entretien de la schizophrénie au stade de la rémission. |
| 用法、用量<br>Les modes d'emploi et la posologie | 深部肌内注射，开始剂量 12.5mg，以后每 2 周肌内注射 25mg。剂量宜从小剂量开始，以后酌情增加或减少。<br>Injection par voie IM profonde, au début, 12,5mg, ensuite, 25mg par voie IM toutes les 2 semaines. Il vaut mieux commencer par une dose mineure, augmenter ou diminuer la dose selon les cas. |
| 剂型、规格<br>Les formes pharmaceutiques et les spécifications | 注射液：每支 25mg（1ml）；25mg（2ml）。<br>Injection : 25mg (1ml) ou 25mg (2ml) par solution. |

8.9 抗焦虑药 Anti-anxietiqués

| | |
|---|---|
| **药品名称 Drug Names** | 地西泮 Diazépam |
| 适应证<br>Les indications | ①焦虑症及各种功能性神经病。②失眠，尤其对焦虑性失眠疗效极佳。③癫痫：可与其他癫痫药合用，治疗癫痫大发作或小发作，控制癫痫持续状态时应静脉注射。④各种原因引起的惊厥，如癫痫、破伤风、小儿高热惊厥等。⑤脑血管意外或脊髓损伤性中枢性僵直或腰肌劳损、内镜检查等所致肌肉痉挛。⑥其他：偏头痛、肌紧张性头痛、呃逆、炎症引起的反射性肌肉痉挛、惊恐症、酒精戒断综合征，还可以治疗家族性、老年性和特发性震颤，可用于麻醉前给药。<br>① Les troubles anxieux et la neuropathie fonctionnelle de toutes sortes. ② L'insomnie, surtout efficace dans le traitement de l'insomnie due à l'anxiété. ③ L'épilepsie : ce produit peut être utilisé en combinaison avec d'autres médicaments antiépileptiques pour traiter les crises tonico-cloniques généralisées et les crises ordinaires de l'épilepsie. En cas de contrôle de l'état de mal épileptique, il faut l'administrer par voie IV. ④ Les convulsions causées par l'épilepsie, le tétanos ou la fièvre chez |

| | |
|---|---|
| | des enfants. ⑤ Les spasmes musculaires causés par l'AVC, la raideur centrale liée aux lésions de la moelle épinière, le claquage musculaire lombaire ou l'endoscopie. ⑥ D'autres : la migraine, la céphalée de tension musculaire, le hoquet,des spasmes musculaires réflexes causés par l'inflammation, le trouble panique, le syndrome de sevrage alcoolique. Il est aussi applicable dans le traitement des tremblements familiaux, séniles et idiopathiques, ainsi que dans l'administration avant l'anesthésie. |
| 用法、用量<br>Les modes d'emploi et la posologie | （1）口服：①抗焦虑：每次 2.5 ～ 10mg，一日 3 次。②催眠：每次 5 ～ 10mg，睡前服用。③麻醉前给药：1 次 10mg。④抗惊厥：成人每次 2.5 ～ 10mg，一日 2 ～ 4 次。6 个月以上儿童，每次 0.1mg/kg，一日 3 次。⑤缓解肌肉阵挛：每次 2.5 ～ 5mg，一日 3 ～ 4 次。<br>（2）静脉注射：①成人基础麻醉：10 ～ 30mg。②癫痫持续状态：开始 5 ～ 10mg，每 5 ～ 10 分钟按需要重复，达 30mg 后必要时每 2 ～ 4 小时重复治疗。静脉注射要缓慢。<br>(1) Par voie orale :　① Pour la lutte contre l'anxiété : 2,5 à 10mg par fois, 3 fois par jour. ② L'hypnose : 5 à 10mg par fois, avant le sommeil. ③ L'administration avant l'anesthésie : 10mg par fois. ④ Pour la lutte contre les convulsions : chez des adultes, 2,5 à 10mg par fois, 2 à 4 fois par jour. Chez des enfants plus de 6 mois, 0,1 mg/kg par fois, 3 fois par jour. ⑤ Pour réduire les spasmes musculaires : 2,5 à 5mg par fois, 3 à 4 fois par jour.<br>(2) Par voie IV ① Pour l'anesthésie de base chez des adultes : 10 à 30mg. ② Pour l'état de mal épileptique : au début, 5 à 10mg, répéter toutes les 5 à 10 minutes en cas de besoin. Après l'administration de 30mg, reprendre la thérapie s'il est nécessaire toutes les 2 à 4h. Injection par voie IV lente. |
| 剂型、规格<br>Les formes pharmaceutiques et les spécifications | 片剂：每片 2.5mg；5mg。<br>胶囊剂：每粒 10mg。<br>注射液：每支 10mg（2ml）。<br>Comprimés : 2,5mg ou 5mg par comprimé.<br>Capsules : 10mg par capsule.<br>Injection : 10mg (2ml) par solution. |
| **药品名称 Drug Names** | 奥沙西泮 Oxazépam |
| 适应证<br>Les indications | 用于焦虑障碍，伴有焦虑的失眠，并能缓解急性酒精戒断症状。<br>Ce produit sert à traiter les troubles anxieux, l'insomnie accompagnée d'anxiété, et à réduire les symptômes de sevrage alcoolique aigus. |
| 用法、用量<br>Les modes d'emploi et la posologie | 口服。焦虑和戒酒症状：每次 15 ～ 30mg，一日 3 ～ 4 次；老年人应当适当减量。失眠：1 次 15mg，睡前服用。<br>Par voie orale. Pour l'anxiété et les symtômes de sevrage alcoolique : 15 à 30 mg par fois, 3 à 4 fois par jour ; chez des personnes âgées, abaisser la dose. Pour l'insomnie, 15mg par fois, avant le sommeil. |
| 剂型、规格<br>Les formes pharmaceutiques et les spécifications | 片剂：每片 10mg；15mg；30mg。<br>Comprimés : 10mg, 15mg ou 30mg par comprimé. |
| **药品名称 Drug Names** | 硝西泮 Nitrazépam |
| 适应证<br>Les indications | ①用于各种失眠的短期治疗，口服后 30 分钟左右起作用，维持睡眠 6 小时。②可用于治疗多种癫痫，尤其对阵挛性发作效果较好。<br>① Il sert de traitement à court terme des insomnies de toutes sortes. Il commence à prendre effet 30 minutes après l'administration par voie orale. Il peut maintenir le sommeil pendant 6h. ② Il sert à traiter l'épilepsie de toutes sortes, il est surtout efficace dans le traitement de la crise clonique. |

续　表

| | |
|---|---|
| 用法、用量<br>Les modes d'emploi et la posologie | 口服。催眠：成人 5 ～ 10mg，儿童 2.5 ～ 5mg，睡前 1 次服用；抗焦虑：每次 5mg，一日 2 ～ 3 次；抗癫痫：每次 5 ～ 30mg，一日 3 次，可酌情增加。老年、体弱者减半。<br><br>Par voie orale. Pour l'hypnose : chez des adultes, 5 à 10mg, chez des enfants, 2,5 à 5mg, une fois avant le sommeil ; pour la lutte contre l'anxiété : 5mg par fois, 2 à 3 fois par jour ; pour la lutte contre l'épilepsie : 5 à 30mg par fois, 3 fois par jour, augmenter la dose selon les cas. Chez des personnes âgées et des faibles, prendre la moitié de la dose usuelle. |
| 剂型、规格<br>Les formes pharmaceutiques et les spécifications | 片剂：每片 5mg；10mg。<br><br>Comprimés : 5mg ou 10mg par comprimé. |
| **药品名称 Drug Names** | 氟西泮 Flurazépam |
| 适应证<br>Les indications | 用于难以入睡、夜间屡醒及早醒的各种失眠。<br><br>Ce produit sert à traiter l'insomnie de toutes sortes, telle que l'endormissement difficile, trop de réveils et réveils trop tôt. |
| 用法、用量<br>Les modes d'emploi et la posologie | 口服：15 ～ 30mg，睡前 1 次服，年老体弱者开始时每次服用 15mg，根据反应适当加量。<br><br>Par voie orale : 15 à 30 mg, une fois avant le sommeil. Chez des personnes âgées, au début, 15mg par fois, ensuite, augmenter la dose en fonction de leur réaction. |
| 剂型、规格<br>Les formes pharmaceutiques et les spécifications | 片剂：每片 15mg。<br>胶囊剂：每粒 5mg；15mg；30mg。<br><br>Comprimés : 15mg par comprimé.<br>Capsules : 5mg, 15mg ou 30mg par capsule. |
| **药品名称 Drug Names** | 氯硝西泮 Clonazépam |
| 适应证<br>Les indications | ①主要用于治疗癫痫和惊厥，对各型癫痫均有效，尤以对小发作和肌阵挛发作疗效最佳。静脉注射治疗癫痫持续状态。②可用于治疗焦虑状态和失眠。③对舞蹈症亦有效。对药物引起的多动症、慢性多发性抽搐、僵人综合征、各类神经痛也有一定疗效。<br><br>① Il sert principalement à traiter l'épilepsie et les convulsions. Il est efficace dans le traitement des épilepsies de toutes sortes, surtout efficace dans le traitement de la crise ordinaire de l'épilepsie et de sa crise myoclonique. Il est administré par voie IV pour traiter l'état de mal épileptique. ② Il est utilisé pour traiter l'anxiété et l'insomnie. ③ Il est aussi efficace dans le traitement de la chorée. Il est un peu efficace dans le traitement des TDAH d'origine médicamenteuse, les tics multiples chroniques, le syndrome de l'homme raide et la névralgie de toutes sortes. |
| 用法、用量<br>Les modes d'emploi et la posologie | ①口服：成人，初始剂量每日 1mg，2 ～ 4 周逐渐增加到每日 4 ～ 8mg，分 3 ～ 4 次服用；儿童，5 岁以下初始剂量每天 0.25mg，5 ～ 12 岁每日 0.5mg，分 3 ～ 4 次服用，逐渐增加剂量到每日 1 ～ 3mg（5 岁以下）和 3 ～ 6mg（5 ～ 12 岁）。②肌内注射：1 次 1 ～ 2mg，一日 2 ～ 4mg。③静脉注射：癫痫持续状态，成人，1 次 1 ～ 4mg；儿童，一次 0.01 ～ 0.1mg/kg，注射速度要缓慢。或将 4mg 溶于 500ml 生理盐水中，以能够控制惊厥发作的速度而缓慢滴注。<br><br>① Par voie orale : chez des adultes, au début, 1mg par jour, 2 à 4 semaines après, 4 à 8 mg par jour, à travers 3 à 4 fois ; chez des enfant, moins de 5ans, au début, 0,25mg par jour, chez des enfants de 5 à 12 ans, 0,5mg par jour, à travers 3 à 4 fois, ensuite, 1 à 3mg (moins de 5 ans) et 3 à 6 mg (5 à 12 ans). ② Injection par voie IM : 1 à 2mg par fois, 2 à 4mg par jour. ③ Injection par voie IV : pour l'état de mal épileptique, chez des adultes, 1 à 4mg par fois ; chez des enfants, 0,01 à 0,1 mg/kg par fois, injection lente. Ou dissoudre 4mg de produit dans 500ml de solution saline, perfusion lente à la vitesse capable de contrôler la crise des convulsions. |
| 剂型、规格<br>Les formes pharmaceutiques et les spécifications | 片剂：每片 0.5mg；1mg；2mg。<br>注射液：每支 1mg（1ml）；2mg（2ml）。<br><br>Comprimés : 0,5mg, 1mg ou 2mg par comprimé.<br>Injection : 1mg (1ml) ou 2mg (2ml) par solution. |

| 药品名称 Drug Names | 劳拉西泮 Lorazépam |
|---|---|
| 适应证<br>Les indications | ①主要用于严重焦虑症、焦虑状态及惊恐焦虑的急性期控制，适宜短期使用。可用于伴有精神抑郁的焦虑，但不推荐用于原发性抑郁症的患者。②失眠。③癫痫。④还可用于癌症化疗时止吐（限注射剂），治疗紧张性头痛，麻醉前及内镜检查前的辅助用药。<br><br>① Ce produit sert principalement à contrôler les troubles d'anxiété et d'angoisse ainsi que l'anxiété panique au stade aigu. Il vaut mieux l'utiliser à court terme. Il est également applicable dans le traitement de l'anxiété accompagnée de dépression, mais il n'est pas recommandé de l'utiliser chez les patients atteints de dépression primaire. ② L'insomnie. ③ L'épilepsie. ④ Aussi applicable dans l'antiémétique au moment de chimiothérapie du cancer (seulement l'administration par injection), dans le traitement de la céphalée de tension. Il sert de médicament adjuvant avant l'anesthésie et avant l'endoscopie. |
| 用法、用量<br>Les modes d'emploi et la posologie | ①焦虑症：口服，每次 1～2mg，一日 2～3 次。②失眠：睡前 1 小时一次服用 1～4mg。③麻醉前给药：术前 1～2 小时，口服 4mg 或肌内注射 2～4mg。④癫痫持续状态：肌内或静脉注射，1 次 1～4mg。⑤化疗止吐：在化疗前 30 分钟注射 1～2mg，预防呕吐发生。<br><br>① Pour les troubles d'anxiété：par voie orale， 1 à 2 mg par fois， 2 à 3 fois par jour. ② Pour l'insomnie：1 à 4 mg par fois， 1h avant le sommeil. ③ L'administration avant l'anesthésie：1 à 2h avant la chirurgie， 4 mg par voie orale， ou 2 à 4mg par voie IM. ④ Pour l'état de mal épileptique：injection par voie IM ou IV， 1 à 4 mg par fois. ⑤ Pour l'antiémétique pendant la chimiothérapie : 1 à 2 mg 30 minutes avant la chimiothérapie pour éviter le vomissement. |
| 剂型、规格<br>Les formes pharmaceutiques et les spécifications | 片剂：每片 0.5mg；1mg；2mg。<br>注射液：每支 2mg（2ml）；4mg（2ml）。<br>Comprimés：0,5mg, 1mg ou 2mg par comprimé.<br>Injection：2mg (2ml) ou 4mg (2ml) par solution. |
| 药品名称 Drug Names | 氟硝西泮 Flunitrazépam |
| 适应证<br>Les indications | 用于催眠（主要用于严重失眠的短期治疗），麻醉前给药和诱导麻醉。<br><br>Ce produit sert à hyphotiser (principalement utilisé dans le traitement à court terme de l'insomnie grave). Il est aussi applicable dans l'administration avant l'anesthésie et l'induction de l'anesthésie. |
| 用法、用量<br>Les modes d'emploi et la posologie | 催眠：口服，1～2mg，睡前一次服。术前给药：肌内注射，1～2mg。诱导麻醉：缓慢静脉注射，1～2mg。<br><br>Pour hyphotiser : par voie orale, 1 à 2mg, une fois avant le sommeil. Pour l'administration avant la chirurgie : injection par voie IM, 1 à 2 mg. Pour l'induction de l'anesthésie : injection lente par voie IV, 1 à 2 mg. |
| 剂型、规格<br>Les formes pharmaceutiques et les spécifications | 片剂：每片 1mg；2mg。<br>注射液：每支 2mg（2ml）。<br>Comprimés : 1mg ou 2mg par comprimé.<br>Injection : 2mg (2ml) par solution. |
| 药品名称 Drug Names | 艾司唑仑 Estazolam |
| 适应证<br>Les indications | ①用于各种类型的失眠。催眠作用强，口服后 20～60 分钟可入睡，维持 5 小时。②用于焦虑、紧张、恐惧及癫痫大、小发作，亦可用于术前镇静。<br><br>① Il est applicable dans l'insomnie de toutes sortes. Il est très efficace dans l'hypnose. On peut s'endormir 20 à 60 minutes après l'administration par voie orle, et dormir pendant 5 h. ② Ce produit sert à traiter l'anxiété, la nervosité, la peur, les crises tonico-cloniques généralisées et les crises ordinaires de l'épilepsie. Il est aussi applicable dans Sédation préopératoire. |

续　表

| 用法、用量<br>Les modes d'emploi et la posologie | 口服。镇静、抗焦虑：1 次 1～2mg，一日 3 次；催眠：1 次 1～2mg，睡前服；抗癫痫：1 次 2～4mg，一日 3 次；麻醉前给药：1 次 2～4mg，术前 1 小时服。<br><br>Par voie orale. Pour la sédation et la lutte contre l'anxiété : 1 à 2mg par fois, 3 fois par jour ; pour l'hypnose : 1 à 2mg par fois, avant le sommeil ; pour la lutte contre l'épilepsie : 2 à 4mg par fois, 3 fois par jour ; pour l'administration avant l'anesthésie : 2 à 4mg par fois, 1h avant la chirurgie. |
|---|---|
| 剂型、规格<br>Les formes pharmaceutiques et les spécifications | 片剂：每片 1mg；2mg。<br>Comprimés : 1mg ou 2mg par comprimé. |
| 药品名称 Drug Names | 阿普唑仑 Alprazolam |
| 适应证<br>Les indications | ①用于治疗焦虑症、抑郁症、失眠。可作为抗惊恐药。②能缓解急性酒精戒断症状。③对药源性顽固性呃逆有较好的治疗作用。<br><br>① Il sert à traiter l'anxiété, la dépresssion et l'insomnie. Il sert aussi de médicament antipanique. ② Il permet de réduire les symptômes de sévrage alcoolique aigus. ③ Il est efficace dans le traitement du hoquet réfractaire d'orgine médicamenteuse. |
| 用法、用量<br>Les modes d'emploi et la posologie | 口服。抗焦虑：一次 0.4mg，一日 3 次，以后酌情增减，量大剂量每日 4mg。抗抑郁：一般为一次 0.8mg，一日 3 次，个别患者可增至每日 10mg。镇静、催眠：0.4～0.8mg，睡前顿服。抗惊恐：每次 0.4mg，一日 3 次，必要时可酌情增量。老年人：初始剂量每次 0.2mg，一日 3 次，根据病情和对药物反应酌情增量。<br><br>Par voie orale. Pour la lutte contre l'anxiété : 0,4mg par fois, 3 fois par jour, ensuite, ajuster la dose en fonction des maladies, ne pas dépasser 4mg par jour. Pour la lutte contre la dépression : 0,8mg par fois, 3 fois par jour, chez certains patients, 10mg par jour. Pour la sédation et l'hypnose : 0,4 à 0,8mg, avant le sommeil, une fois par jour. Pour la lutte contre la panique : 0,4mg par fois, 3 fois par jour, augmenter la dose s'il est nécessaire. Chez des personnes âgées : au début, 0,2mg par fois, 3 fois par jour, augmenter la dose en fonction des maladies et de la réaction des patients au médicament. |
| 剂型、规格<br>Les formes pharmaceutiques et les spécifications | 片剂：每片 0.25mg；0.4mg；0.5mg；1mg。<br>Comprimés : 0,25mg, 0,4mg, 0,5mg ou 1mg par comprimé. |
| 药品名称 Drug Names | 奥沙唑仑 Oxazolam |
| 适应证<br>Les indications | 用于焦虑症、神经症的治疗。亦可用于麻醉前给药。<br>Il sert à traiter l'anxiété et la névrose. Il est aussi applicable dans l'administration avant l'anesthésie. |
| 用法、用量<br>Les modes d'emploi et la posologie | 口服。抗焦虑：每次 10～20mg，一日 3 次。镇静催眠：每次 15～30mg，睡前顿服。麻醉前给药：术前 1 小时给予 1～2mg/kg。<br><br>Par voie orale. Pour la lutte contre l'anxiété : 10 à 20mg par fois, 3 fois par jour. pour la sédation et l'hypnose : 15 à 30 mg par fois, avant le sommeil, une fois par jour. Pour l'administration avant l'anesthésie : 1 à 2mg/kg 1h avant la chirurgie. |
| 剂型、规格<br>Les formes pharmaceutiques et les spécifications | 片剂：每片 5mg；10mg；20mg。<br>胶囊剂：每粒 10mg。<br>Comprimés : 5mg, 10mg ou 20mg par comprimé.<br>Capsules : 10mg par capsule. |
| 药品名称 Drug Names | 美沙唑仑 Méxazolam |
| 适应证<br>Les indications | 可用于神经症、身心疾病，自主神经失调等疾病时的紧张、焦虑、抑郁、易疲劳、睡眠障碍等的治疗。<br><br>Il sert à traiter les symptômes liés à la névrose, aux troubles physiques et mentaux, aux affections du système nerveux autonome, tels que la nervosité, l'anxiété, la dépression, la fatigue et l'insomnie. |

续　表

| 用法、用量<br>Les modes d'emploi et la posologie | 口服，每日 1.5 ～ 3mg，分 3 次服，必要时根据年龄、症状适当调整剂量。老年人每日剂量为 1.5mg。<br>Par voie orale, 1,5 à 3mg, à travers 3 fois, le cas échéant, ajuster la dose en fonction de l'âge et des symptômes. Chez des personnes âgées, 1,5mg par jour. |
|---|---|
| 剂型、规格<br>Les formes pharmaceutiques et les spécifications | 片剂：每片 0.5mg；1mg。<br>Comprimés : 0,5mg ou 1mg par comprimé. |

| 药品名称 Drug Names | 谷维素 Oryzanol |
|---|---|
| 适应证<br>Les indications | 用于自主神经失调（包括胃肠、心血管神经症）、周期性精神病、脑震荡后遗症、精神分裂症和周期型、更年期综合征、月经前期紧张症等，但疗效不够明显。<br>Ce produit sert à traiter les affections du système nerveux autonome (y compris la névrose gastro-intestinale et la névrose cardiovasculaire), la psychose périodique, les séquelles d'une commotion cérébrale, la schizophrénie, le syndrome périodique et de ménopause, ainsi que les troubles de stress prémenstruels. Mais son effet n'est pas assez évident. |
| 用法、用量<br>Les modes d'emploi et la posologie | 口服：每次 10mg，一日 3 次。有时可用至每日 60mg。疗程一般 3 个月左右。<br>Par voie orale : 10mg par fois, 3 fois par jour. Parfois, 60mg par jour. Un traitement médical dure généralement trois mois environ. |
| 剂型、规格<br>Les formes pharmaceutiques et les spécifications | 片剂：每片 5mg；10mg。<br>Comprimés : 5mg ou 10mg par comprimé. |

8.10　抗躁狂药 Anti-maniaques

| 药品名称 Drug Names | 碳酸锂 Carbonate de lithium |
|---|---|
| 适应证<br>Les indications | ①主要用于治疗躁狂症，对躁狂和抑郁交替发作的双相情感性精神障碍有很好的治疗和预防复发作用，对反复发作的抑郁症也有预防发作作用。一般于用药后 6 ～ 7 日症状开始好转。因锂盐无镇静作用，一般主张对严重急性躁狂患者先与氯丙嗪或氟哌啶醇合用，急性症状控制后再单用碳酸锂维持。②还可用于治疗分裂 - 情感性精神病，粒细胞减少，再生障碍性贫血，月经过多症，急性菌痢。<br>① Ce produit sert à traiter et prévenir la récurrence des épisodes maniaques et dépressifs du trouble bipolaire. Il sert aussi à prévenir la crise de la dépression récurrente. Les symptômes commencent à s'améliorer généralement 6 à 7 jours depuis l'administration. Comme le sel de lithium ne sert pas de sédation, il est recommandé d'utiliser d'abord le carbonate de lithium en association avec la chlorpromazine ou l'halopéridol chez des patients souffrant de graves manies aigues, et d'utiliser le carbonate de lithium seul pour maintenir le traitement dès que les symptômes aigus sont sous le contrôle.<br>② Il est aussi utilisé comme traitement de la psychose affective, de la neutropénie, de l'anémie aplasique, de la ménorragie et de la dysenterie aigue. |
| 用法、用量<br>Les modes d'emploi et la posologie | ①躁狂症：口服，一般以小剂量开始，每次 0.125 ～ 0.25g，一日 3 次。可逐渐加到每次 0.25 ～ 0.5g，一般不超过每日 1.5 ～ 2.0g。症状控制后维持一般不超过每日 1g，分 3 ～ 4 次服。预防复发时，需持续用药 2 ～ 3 年。②粒细胞减少、再生障碍性贫血：口服 10 日，每次 0.3g。一日 3 次。③月经过多症：月经第 1 日服 0.6g，以后每日服 0.3g，均分为 3 次服，共服 3 日，总量 1.2g 为 1 个疗程。每一月经周期服 1 个疗程。④急性菌痢：每次 0.1g，一日 3 次，首剂加倍。少数症状较重者，头 1 ～ 3 日每次剂量均可加倍，至症状及粪便明显好转后，以原剂量维持 2 ～ 3 日，再递减剂量，3 ～ 4 日停药。 |

续 表

① Pour traiter la manie : par voie orale, commencer par une dose mineure, 0,125 à 0,25g par fois, 3 fois par jour. Augmenter progressivement la dose pour atteindre 0,25 à 0,5g par fois, ne pas dépasser 1,5 à 2,0g par jour. La dose d'entretien après le contrôle des symptômes, ne pas dépasser 1g par jour, à travers 3 à 4 fois. Pour prévenir la récurrence, il faut prendre le médicament pendant 2 à 3 années consécutives. ② Pour traiter la neutropénie et l'anémie aplasique：par voie orale，0，3g par fois， 3 fois par jour， pendant 10 jours. ③ Pour traiter la ménorragie：prendre 0，6g le premier jour de la menstruation， ensuite， 0，3g par jour， à travers 3 fois， pendant 3 jours au total， la dose totale， 1，2g comme un traitement médical. Prendre un traitement médical par menstruation. ④ Pour traiter la dysenterie aiguë : 0,1g par fois, 3 fois par jour, doubler la dose pour la première fois. Chez certains patients gravement malades, doubler la dose les 1 à 3 premiers jours, jusqu'à 2 à 3 jours après l'amélioration des symptômes, ensuite, diminuer progressivement la dose, 3 à 4 jours après, arrêter l'administration.

| 剂型、规格<br>Les formes pharmaceutiques et les spécifications | 片剂：每片 0.125g；0.25g；0.5g。<br>缓释片剂：每片 0.3g。<br>胶囊剂：每粒 0.25g；0.5g。<br>Comprimés : 0,125g, 0,25g ou 0,5g par comprimé.<br>Comprimés à libération prolongée : 0,3g par comprimé.<br>Capsules : 0,25g ou 0,5g par capsule. |
|---|---|
| 药品名称 Drug Names | 卡马西平 Carbamazépine |
| 适应证<br>Les indications | 可用于急性躁狂发作，抑郁发作及双相情感性精神障碍的维持治疗。锂盐治疗无效或不能耐受时可考虑选用卡马西平代替。<br>Ce produit est utilisé dans le traitement d'entretien de la crise de la manie aigue, de la crise de la dépression et du trouble bipolaire. En cas de l'inefficacité ou de la résistance au traitement avec le sel de lithium, la carbamazépine peut être considérée comme une option. |
| 用法、用量<br>Les modes d'emploi et la posologie | 抗躁狂症：口服，成人开始每日 400mg，分 2 次服。以后隔 1～2 周每日量增加 200mg，分 3～4 次服。治疗量每日 600～1200mg，分 3～4 次服，与其他肝药酶诱导剂合用可达每日 1600mg。急性躁狂症，每日 600～1200mg，分 2 次服。<br>Pour lutter contre la manie : par voie orale, chez des adultes, au début, 400mg par jour, à travers 2 fois. Ensuite, augmenter 200mg par jour toutes les 1 à 2 semaines, à travers 3 à 4 fois. La dose de traitement, 600 à 1 200mg par jour, à travers 3 à 4 fois. S'il est utilisé en combinaison avec d'autres inducteurs d'enzymes métabolisant la drogue du foie, il est possible de prendre 1 600mg par jour. Pour lutter contre la manie aigue, 600 à 1 2000 mg par jour, à travers 2 fois. |
| 剂型、规格<br>Les formes pharmaceutiques et les spécifications | 片剂：每片 100mg；200mg；400mg。<br>胶囊剂：每粒 200mg；300mg。<br>Comprimés : 100mg, 200mg ou 400mg par comprimé.<br>Capsules : 200mg ou 300mg par capsule. |
| 药品名称 Drug Names | 丙戊酸钠 Valproate de sodium |
| 适应证<br>Les indications | 可用于急性躁狂发作的治疗，长期服用对双相情感性神经障碍的反复发作具有预防作用。<br>Ce produit est à traiter la crise de la manie aigue. L'administration à long terme de ce produit peut aider à prévenir la récurrence du trouble bipolaire. |
| 用法、用量<br>Les modes d'emploi et la posologie | 治疗躁狂症：口服，小剂量开始，每次 200mg，一日 2～3 次，逐渐增加至每次 300～400mg，一日 2～3 次。最高剂量不超过每日 1600mg。6 岁以上儿童每日 20～30mg/kg，分 3～4 次服用。<br>Pour traiter la manie : par voie orale, commencer par une dose mineure, 200mg par fois, 2 à 3 fois par jour, augmenter pour atteindre 300 à 400 mg par fois, 2 à 3 fois par jour. Ne pas dépasser 1 600mg par jour. Chez des enfants plus de 6 ans, 20 à 30 mg/kg par jour, à travers 3 à 4 fois. |

| 剂型、规格<br>Les formes pharmaceutiques et les spécifications | 片剂：每片 200mg。<br>Comprimés : 200mg par comprimé. |

## 8.11　抗抑郁药 Anti-dépresseurs

| 药品名称 Drug Names | 丙米嗪 Imipramine |

| 适应证<br>Les indications | ①用于各种类型的抑郁症治疗。对内源性抑郁症、反应性抑郁症及更年期抑郁症均有效，但疗效出现慢（多在 1 周后才出现效果）。对精神分裂症伴发的抑郁状态则几乎无效或疗效差。②可用于惊恐发作的治疗，其疗效与 MAOIs 相当。③可用于小儿遗尿症。<br><br>① Ce produit est utilisé comme traitement de la dépression de toutes sortes. Il est efficace dans le traitement de la dépression endogène, de la dépression réactionnelle et de la dépression de ménopause, mais il prend effet un peu lentement (généralement, une semaine depuis l'administration). Il est inefficace ou peu efficace dans le traitement de l'état dépressif résultant de la schizophrénie. ② Il sert aussi à traiter la crise de la panique, son effet est similaire à MAOIs. ③ Il est aussi applicable dans le traitement de l'énurésie chez des enfants. |
| 用法、用量<br>Les modes d'emploi et la posologie | 口服。①治疗抑郁症、惊恐发作：成人每次 12.5 ～ 25mg，一日 3 次，老年体弱者一次量从 12.5mg 开始，逐渐增加剂量，极量 1 日 200 ～ 300mg。需根据耐受情况调整用量。②小儿遗尿：6 岁以上，每次 12.5 ～ 25mg，每晚 1 次。如在 1 周内未获满意效果，12 岁以下每日可增至 50mg，12 岁以上每日可增至 75mg。<br><br>Par voie orale. ① Pour traiter la crise de la dépression et de la panique : chez des adultes, 12,5 à 25mg par fois, 3 fois par jour, chez des personnes âgées, commencer par 12,5mg par fois, augmenter progressivement la dose pour atteindre 200 à 300mg par jour au maximum. Ajuster la dose selon la tolérance. ② Pour traiter l'énurésie chez des enfants : chez plus de 6 ans, 12,5 à 25mg par fois, une fois par soir. Si on n'a pas d'effets satisfaisants en une semaine, chez des enfants moins de 12 ans, augmenter pour atteindre 50mg par jour, chez plus de 12 ans, 75mg par jour. |
| 剂型、规格<br>Les formes pharmaceutiques et les spécifications | 片剂：每片 10mg；25mg；50mg；75mg。<br>胶囊剂：每粒 75mg；100mg；125mg。<br>缓释胶囊：每粒 50mg。<br>注射剂：每支 25mg（2ml）。<br>Comprimés : 10mg, 25mg, 50mg ou 75mg par comprimé.<br>Capsules : 75mg, 100mg ou 125mg par capsule.<br>Capsules à libération prolongée : 50mg par capsule.<br>Injection : 25mg (2ml) par solution. |

| 药品名称 Drug Names | 氯米帕明 Clomipramine |

| 适应证<br>Les indications | ①用于治疗内源性、反应性、神经性、隐匿性抑郁症及各种抑郁状态；伴有抑郁症的精神分裂症。②对强迫性神经症具有较好的疗效。③对恐怖症、惊恐发作、继发性焦虑、慢性疼痛综合征、神经性厌食及发作性睡病均有一定疗效。<br><br>① Ce produit sert à traiter les dépressions endogène, réactionnelle, neurologique et masquée ainsi que l'état dépressif. Il est aussi applicable dans le traitement de la schizophrénie accompagnée de la dépression. ② Il est efficace dans le traitement du trouble obsessionnel-compulsif. ③ Il est aussi applicable dans le traitement des maladies suivantes : les phobies, les attaques de panique, l'anxiété secondaire, le syndrome de la douleur chronique, l'anorexie mentale et la narcolepsie. |
| 用法、用量<br>Les modes d'emploi et la posologie | （1）治疗抑郁症、强迫症：①口服，成人初始每次 25mg，一日 3 次（或服缓释片，75mg，每晚 1 次），1 周内可渐增至最适宜的治疗量。一日最大剂量为 250mg。症状好转后，改为维持量，每日 50 ～ 100mg（缓释片剂每日 75mg）。老年患者，开始每日 10mg，逐渐增加至 30 ～ 50mg（约 10 日），然后改维持量以每日不超过 75mg 为宜。②静脉滴注：开始每日剂量每日 25 ～ 50mg，用 250ml 葡萄糖注射液稀释，输入时间不低于 2 小时。通常剂量为每日 100mg。 |

**续　表**

（2）治疗慢性痛性疾病：每日 10 ～ 150mg，最好同时服用镇痛药。

(1) Pour traiter la dépression et le trouble obsessionnel-compulsif : ① Par voie orale, chez des adultes, au début, 25mg par fois, 3 fois par jour (ou prendre les comprimés à libération prolongée, 75mg, une fois par soir), augmenter en une semaine pour atteindre la dose la plus efficace. La dose maximale : 250mg par jour. Après l'amélioration des symptômes, prendre la dose d'entretien, soit 50 à 100mg par jour (s'il s'agit des comprimés à libération prolongée, 75mg par jour). Chez des personnes âgées, au début, 10mg par jour, augmenter pour atteindre 30 à 50mg par jour (en 10 jours environ), ensuite, prendre la dose d'entretien, soit 75mg par jour au maximum. ② En perfusion : commencer par 25 à 50mg par jour, utiliser 250ml de solution de glucose pour la dilution, perfusion pendant 2h au moins. La dose usuelle, 100mg par jour.

(2) Traiter les troubles de la douleur chroniques : 10 à 150 mg par jour, il vaut mieux prendre en même temps les analgésiques.

| 剂型、规格<br>Les formes pharmaceutiques et les spécifications | 片剂：每片 10mg；25mg；50mg。<br>缓释片：每片 75mg。<br>胶囊剂：每粒 25mg；50mg；75mg。<br>注射剂：每支 25mg（2ml）。<br><br>Comprimés : 10mg, 25mg ou 50mg par comprimé.<br>Comprimés à libération prolongée : 75mg par comprimé.<br>Capsules : 25mg, 50mg ou 75mg par capsule.<br>Injection : 25mg (2ml) par solution. |
| --- | --- |
| **药品名称 Drug Names** | 阿米替林 Amitriptyline |
| 适应证<br>Les indications | ①用于治疗各型抑郁症或抑郁状态。对内因性抑郁症和更年期抑郁症疗效较好，对反应性抑郁症及神经官能症的抑郁状态亦有效。对兼有焦虑和抑郁症状患者，疗效优于丙米嗪。与电休克联合使用于重症抑郁症，可减少电休克次数。②用于缓解慢性疼痛。③亦用于治疗小儿遗尿症、儿童多动症。<br><br>① Il est à traiter les dépressions de toutes sortes et l'état dépressif. Il est efficace dans le traitement de la dépression endogène et de la dépression de ménopause. Il est aussi applicable dans le traitement de la dépression réactionnelle et de l'état dépressif de la névrose. Chez des patients souffrant de l'anxiété et de la dépression, ce produit est plus efficace que l'imipramine. Utilisé en association avec le choc électrique dans le traitement de la dépression grave, il permet de réduire le nombre du choc électrique. ② Il sert également à atténuer les douleurs chroniques. ③ Il est aussi utilisé comme traitement de l'énurésie et des TDAH chez des enfants. |
| 用法、用量<br>Les modes d'emploi et la posologie | ① 治疗抑郁症、慢性疼痛：口服，每次 25mg，一日 2 ～ 4 次，以后递增至每日 150 ～ 300mg，分次服。维持量每日 50 ～ 200mg。老年患者和青少年，每日 50mg，分次或夜间 1 次服。静脉注射或肌内注射，成人每次 20 ～ 30mg，一日 3 ～ 4 次。②治疗遗尿症：睡前 1 次口服，10 ～ 25mg。③治疗儿童多动症：7 岁以上儿童每次 10 ～ 25mg，一日 2 ～ 3 次。<br><br>① Pour traiter la dépression et les douleurs chroniques : par voie orale, 25mg par fois, 2 à 4 fois par jour, ensuite, augmenter progressivement pour atteindre 150 à 300mg par jour, à travers plusieurs fois. Chez des personnes âgées et des adolescents, 50mg par jour, à travers plusieurs fois ou une fois par nuit. Injection par voie IV ou IM, chez des adultes, 20 à 30mg par fois, 3 à 4 fois par jour. ② Pour traiter l'énurésie : 10 à 25mg, une fois avant le sommeil, par voie orale. ③ Pour traiter les TDAH chez des enfants : chez des enfants plus de 7 ans, 10 à 25 mg par fois, 2 à 3 fois par jour. |
| 剂型、规格<br>Les formes pharmaceutiques et les spécifications | 片剂：每片 10mg；25mg；50mg；75mg；100mg；150mg。<br>缓释胶囊剂：每粒 25mg；50mg；75mg。<br>注射剂：每支 20mg（2ml）；50mg（2ml）；100mg（10ml）。<br><br>Comprimés : 10mg, 25mg, 50mg, 75mg, 100mg ou 150mg par comprimé.<br>Capsules à libération prolongée : 25mg, 50mg ou 75mg par capsule.<br>Injection : 20 mg (2ml), 50mg (2ml) ou 100mg (10ml) par solution. |

续　表

| 药品名称 Drug Names | 多塞平 Doxépine |
|---|---|
| 适应证<br>Les indications | ①用于治疗抑郁症和各种焦虑抑郁为主的神经症，亦可用于更年期精神病，对抑郁和焦虑的躯体性疾病和慢性酒精性精神病也有效。也可用于镇静及催眠。②本品外用膏剂用于治疗慢性单纯性苔藓、湿疹、过敏性皮炎、特应性皮炎等。<br><br>① Ce produit sert à traiter la dépression et la névrose anxieuse et dépressive. Il est également utilisé dans le traitement de la psychose de ménopause, de la dépression et des troubles anxieux somatiques, ainsi que de la psychose alcoolique chronique. Il est aussi applicable dans la sédation et l'hypnose. ② Le produit en pommade est aussi appliqué dans le traitement des maladies, telles que le lichen simplex chronique, l'eczéma, la dermatite atopique, et la dermatite atopique. |
| 用法、用量<br>Les modes d'emploi et la posologie | ①口服，初始剂量每次25mg，一日3次，然后逐渐增至每日150～300mg。宜在餐后服用，以减少胃部刺激。严重的焦虑性抑郁症可肌内注射，每次25～50mg，一日2次。②局部外用：于患处涂布一薄层，一日3次，每次涂布面积不超过总面积的5%，两次使用应间隔4小时。建议短期敷用，不超过7～8日。<br><br>① Par voie orale, commencer par 25mg pa fois, 3 fois par jour, ensuite, augmenter la dose pour atteindre 150 à 300mg par jour. Administration après le repas pour réduire la stimulation gastrique. En cas de dépression d'anxiété grave, injection par voie IM, 25 à 50mg par fois, 2 fois par jour. ② L'usage externe topique : étaler une couche mince sur la zone touchée, 3 fois par jour, avec moins de 5 % de la surface totale, et un intervalle de 4 h entre deux usages. Il est recommandé de l'appliquer pour un court terme, ne pas dépasser 7 à 8 jours. |
| 剂型、规格<br>Les formes pharmaceutiques et les spécifications | 片剂：每片5mg；10mg；25mg；50mg；100mg。<br>胶囊剂：每粒10mg；25mg；50mg；75mg；100mg；150mg。<br>注射剂：每支25mg（1ml）；50mg（2ml）。<br>盐酸多塞平乳膏：每支10g。<br><br>Comprimés :5mg, 10mg, 25mg, 50mg ou 100mg par comprimé.<br>Capsules : 10mg, 25mg, 50mg, 75mg, 100mg ou 150mg par capsule.<br>Injection : 25mg (1ml) ou 50mg (2ml) par solution.<br>Pommade de chlorhydrate de doxépine : 10g par pièce. |
| 药品名称 Drug Names | 吗氯贝胺 Moclobémide |
| 适应证<br>Les indications | ①对双相、单相、激动型、阻滞型及各种亚型抑郁症均有效。对精神运动性阻滞和情绪抑郁症状的改善显著。用于对TCAs不适用或已不再有效的患者。②对睡眠障碍也有一定效果。<br><br>① Ce produit est efficace dans le traitement de la dépression bipolaire, unipolaire, agitée et mélancolique et toutes sortes de sous-types de dépression. Il est efficace dans l'amélioration des troubles psychomoteurs et de la mélancolie. Il est applicable chez des patients résistants à TCAs. ② Il est aussi applicable dans le traitement des troubles du sommeil. |
| 用法、用量<br>Les modes d'emploi et la posologie | 口服：每日100～400mg，分次饭后服，可根据病情增减至每日150～600mg。<br><br>Par voie orale : 100 à 400mg par jour, à travers plusieurs fois, après le repas. Augmenter ou diminuer la dose selon les cas pour atteindre 150 à 600 mg par jour. |
| 剂型、规格<br>Les formes pharmaceutiques et les spécifications | 片剂：每片75mg；100mg；150mg；300mg。<br>胶囊剂：每粒100mg。<br><br>Comprimés : 75mg, 100mg, 150mg ou 300mg par comprimé.<br>Capsules : 100mg par capsule. |
| 药品名称 Drug Names | 氟西汀 Fluoxétine |
| 适应证<br>Les indications | ①用于治疗伴有焦虑的各种抑郁症，尤宜用于老年抑郁症。②用于治疗惊恐状态，对广泛性焦虑障碍也有一定疗效。③用于治疗强迫障碍，但药物剂量应相应加大。④适用于社交恐惧症、进食障碍。<br><br>① Ce produit sert à traiter les dépressions accompagnées de l'anxiété de toutes sortes, surtout la dépression sénile. ② Il sert à traiter l'état panique, et a certain effet sur le trouble d'anxiété généralisée. ③ Il est aussi applicable dans le traitement du trouble obsessionnel-compulsif, il faut augmenter la dose. ④ Il permet de traiter les phobies sociales et les troubles de l'alimentation. |

**续　表**

| | |
|---|---|
| 用法、用量<br>Les modes d'emploi et la posologie | 口服。①治疗抑郁症：最初治疗建议每日 20mg，一般 4 周后才能显效。若未能控制症状，可考虑增加剂量，每日可增加 20mg。最大推荐剂量每日 80mg。维持治疗可以每日使用 20mg。②强迫症：建议初始剂量为每日晨 20mg，维持治疗可以每日 20～60mg。③暴食症：建议每日 60mg。④惊恐障碍：初始剂量每日 10mg，一周后可逐渐增加至每日 20mg，如果症状没有有效控制，可适当增加剂量至每日 60mg。<br><br>Par voie orale. ① Pour traiter la dépression : il est recommandé de commencer par prendre 20mg par jour. Il prendre effet 4 semaines après. Si on ne peut pas contrôler les symptômes, augmenter 20mg par jour. La dose maximale recommandée, 80mg par jour. La dose d'entretien, 20mg par jour. ② Le trouble obsessionnel-compulsif : il est recommandé de commencer par prendre 20mg par jour. La dose d'entretien, 20 à 60mg par jour. ③ Pour traiter la boulimie : 60mg par jour. ④ Pour traiter les troubles de la panique : commencer par 10mg par jour, 1 semaine après, augmenter pour atteindre 20mg par jour, si les symptômes ne se contrôlent pas, augmenter progressivement pour atteindre 60mg par jour. |
| 剂型、规格<br>Les formes pharmaceutiques et les spécifications | 片剂：每片 10mg；20mg。肠溶片：90mg。胶囊剂：每粒 5mg；10mg；20mg；40mg；60mg。<br><br>Comprimés : 10mg ou 20mg par comprimé. Compriméa à enrobage entérique : 90mg. Capsules : 5mg, 10mg, 20mg, 40mg ou 60mg par capsule. |
| **药品名称 Drug Names** | 氟伏沙明 Fluvoxamine |
| 适应证<br>Les indications | ①用于治疗各类抑郁症，特别是持久性抑郁症状及自杀风险大的患者。②还可治疗强迫症和心身性疾病。<br><br>① Ce produit sert à traiter toutes sortes de dépressions, surtout chez des patients présentant des symptômes dépressifs persistants et un gros risque de suicide. ② Il est aussi applicable dans le traitement du trouble obsessionnel-compulsif et des troublespsychosomatiques. |
| 用法、用量<br>Les modes d'emploi et la posologie | 口服。①抗抑郁：初始剂量每日 50～100mg，睡前服。每 4～7 日增加 50mg，剂量可视病情调整，剂量超过每日 150mg 时应分次服用，饭时或饭后服。维持期用药，以 1 日 50～100mg 为宜。②强迫症：初始剂量每日 100～300mg。最大剂量为每日 300mg。<br><br>Par voie orale. ① Pour lutter contre la dépression : commencer par 50 à 100mg par jour, avant le sommeil. Augmenter 50mg tous des 4 à 7 jours, ajuster la dose selon les cas. Si on prendre plus de 150mg par jour, il faut le faire à plusieurs fois, durant ou après le repas. La dose d'entretien, 50 à 100mg par jour. ② Pour traiter le trouble obsessionnel-compulsif : commencer par 100 à 300 mg par jour. La dose maximale, 300mg par jour. |
| 剂型、规格<br>Les formes pharmaceutiques et les spécifications | 片剂：每片 50mg；100mg；200mg。胶囊剂：每粒 20mg。肠溶片：90mg。<br><br>Comprimés : 50mg, 100mg ou 200mg par comprimé. Capsules : 20mg par capsule. Comprimés à enrobage entérique : 90mg. |
| **药品名称 Drug Names** | 帕罗西汀 Paroxétine |
| 适应证<br>Les indications | ①用于治疗抑郁症。适合治疗伴有焦虑症和抑郁症患者，作用比 TCAs 快，而且远期疗效比丙米嗪好。②亦可用于惊恐障碍、社交恐怖症及强迫症的治疗。<br><br>① Il sert à traiter la dépression. Il est applicable dans le traitement des patients présentant de l'anxiété et de la dépression, avec un effet plus rapide que TCAs, un effet à long terme meilleur que l'imipramine. ② Il est aussi utilisé comme traitement des troubles paniques, des phobies sociales et du trouble obsessionnel-compulsif. |
| 用法、用量<br>Les modes d'emploi et la posologie | 口服。通常一日剂量范围在 20～50mg，一般从 20mg 开始，一日 1 次，早餐时顿服。连续用药 3 周。以后根据临床反应增减剂量，每次增减 10mg，间隔不得少于 1 周。最大推荐剂量为每日 50mg（治疗强迫症可用 60mg）。老年人或肝、肾功能不全者可从每日 10mg 开始，每日最高剂量不超过 40mg。对于肌酐清除率 < 30ml/min 的患者，推荐剂量每日 20mg。<br><br>Par voie orale. En général, 20 à 50 mg par jour, commencer par 20mg, 1 fois par jour, une fois par jour, après le petit-déjeuner. Pendant 3 semaines consécutives. Ensuite, augmenter ou diminuer de 10mg par fois selon les réactions cliniques, avec un intervalle de 1 semaine au moins. La dose maximale, 50mg par jour (pour traiter le trouble obsessionnel-compulsif, 60mg par jour). Chez des personnes âgées ou des patients insuffisants rénaux ou hépatiques, commencer par 10mg par jour, ne pas dépasser 40mg par jour. Chez des patients dont la clairance de la créatinine est moins de 30 ml/min, la dose recommandée, 20mg par jour. |

**续 表**

| 剂型、规格 Les formes pharmaceutiques et les spécifications | 片剂：每片 20mg；30mg。<br>Comprimés : 20mg ou 30mg par comprimé. |
|---|---|
| **药品名称 Drug Names** | 舍曲林 Sertraline |
| 适应证 Les indications | 用于治疗抑郁症、强迫症、心境恶劣、性欲倒错等。预防抑郁症复发。<br>Ce produit sert à traite la dépression, le trouble obsessionnel-compulsif, la dysthymie et la paraphilie. Il permet aussi de prévenir la récurrence de la dépression. |
| 用法、用量 Les modes d'emploi et la posologie | 口服。开始每日 50mg，一日 1 次，与食物同服，早晚均可。数周后增加 50mg。调整剂量时间间隔不能短于 1 周。常用剂量为每日 50～100mg，最大剂量为每日 200mg（此剂量不得连续服用超过 8 周以上）。需长期服用者，需用最低有效剂量。<br>Par voie orale. Au début, 50mg par jour, 1 fois par jour, durant le repas, le petit matin ou le soir. Plusieurs semaines après, augmenter 50 mg, avec un intervalle de 1 semaine au moins. La dose usuelle, 50 à 100mg par jour, la dose maximale, 200mg par jour (avec cette dose, ne pas dépasser 8 semaines consécutives). Chez des patients qui ont besoin de prendre ce médicament pour une longue durée, il faut prendre la dose efficace minimale. |
| 剂型、规格 Les formes pharmaceutiques et les spécifications | 片剂：每片 50mg；100mg。胶囊剂：每粒 50mg；100mg。<br>Comprimés : 50mg ou 100mg par comprimé.<br>Capsules : 50mg ou 100mg par capsule. |
| **药品名称 Drug Names** | 西酞普兰 Citalopram |
| 适应证 Les indications | ①用于内源性或非内源性抑郁症。②焦虑性神经症、广场恐惧症、强迫症、经前期心境障碍神经症。③酒精依赖性行为障碍、痴呆的行为问题。④卒中后病理性哭泣。<br>① Ce produit sert à traiter la dépression endogène et non endogène. ② Il sert aussi à traiter la névrose anxieuse, l'agoraphobie, le trouble obsessionnel-compulsif et les troubles de l'humeur prémenstruels. ③ Les troubles du comportement de la dépendance à l'alcool aini que les problèmes comportementaux de la démence. ④ Pleur pathologique après un AVC. |
| 用法、用量 Les modes d'emploi et la posologie | 口服。每日 20～60mg，一日 1 次，晨起或晚间顿服。推荐初始量为每日 20mg，再根据患者症状控制情况酌情增减，逐渐达到稳定控制病情的最小有效剂量。剂量调整间隔时间不能少于 1 周，一般为 2～3 周。通常需要经过 2～3 周的治疗方可判定疗效。为防止复发，治疗至少持续 6 个月。肝功能不全及年龄超过 65 岁的老年人：推荐剂量较常量减半。<br>Par voie orale. 20 à 60mg par jour, 1 fois par jour, le petit matin ou le soir. Il est recommandé de commencer par 20 mg par jour, ajuster la dose selon les cas pour atteindre la dose efficace minimale. Un intervalle de 1 semaine au moins (2 à 3 semaines en général) pour un ajustement de doses. Il faut généralement 2 à 3 semaines pour juger l'efficacité du traitement. Pour prévenir la récurrence, il faut maintenir le traitement pendant 6 mois consécutifs au moins. Chez des patients insuffisants hépatiques et des personnes âgées plus de 65 ans : diminuer de moitié la dose usuelle. |
| 剂型、规格 Les formes pharmaceutiques et les spécifications | 片剂：每片 10mg；20mg；30mg；40mg。口服液：每支 20mg（10ml）。<br>Comprimés : 10mg, 20mg, 30mg ou 40mg par comprimé.<br>La solution buccale : 20mg (10ml) par solution. |
| **药品名称 Drug Names** | 艾司西酞普兰 Escitalopram |
| 适应证 Les indications | ①用于内源性或非内源性抑郁症。②焦虑性神经症、广场恐惧症、强迫症、经前期心境障碍神经症。③酒精依赖性行为障碍、痴呆的行为问题。④卒中后病理性哭泣。<br>① Ce produit sert à traiter la dépression endogène et non endogène. ② Il sert aussi à traiter la névrose anxieuse, l'agoraphobie, le trouble obsessionnel-compulsif et les troubles de l'humeur prémenstruels. ③ Les troubles du comportement de la dépendance à l'alcool aini que les problèmes comportementaux de la démence. ④ Pleur pathologique après un AVC. |

**续　表**

| | |
|---|---|
| 用法、用量<br>Les modes d'emploi et la posologie | 口服。治疗抑郁症：每日 10mg，一日 1 次。根据患者的临床情况最大剂量可增至每日 20mg。通常 2 ～ 4 周可控制抑郁症状，症状缓解后需巩固维持治疗至少 6 个月。伴或不伴恐怖症的患者：初始剂量为每日 5mg，持续 1 周后可考虑增加至每日 10mg。根据患者的个体反应，剂量可增至每日 20mg。老年患者：推荐半量使用本品，最大剂量也不应超过每日 20mg。肝功能不全者或 CYP2C19 慢代谢者：建议起始剂量每日 5mg，持续 2 周后，可根据患者的个体反应，剂量增加至每日 10mg。<br><br>Par voie orale. Pour traiter la dépression : 10mg par jour, 1 fois par jour. Selon les réactions cliniques, la dose maximale peut être de 20mg par jour. Il faut 2 à 4 semaines pour contrôler les symptômes de la dépression, après l'amélioration des symptômes, il est nécessaire de maintenir le traitement pendant 6 moins au moins. Chez des patients avec ou sans phobie : commencer par 5mg par jour, une semaine après, augmenter pour atteindre 10mg par jour. Selon les réactions des patients, il est possible de prendre 20 mg par jour. Chez des personnes âgées : il est recommandé de prendre la moitié de la dose usuelle, et de ne pas dépasser 20 mg par jour. Chez des patients insuffisants hépatiques ou chez des métaboliseurs lents des médicaments métabolisés par le CYP2C19 : il est recommandé de commencer par 5mg par jour, pendant 2 semaines consécutives, ensuite, selon les réactions des patients, il est possible d'augmenter la dose pour atteindre 10mg par jour. |
| 剂型、规格<br>Les formes pharmaceutiques et les spécifications | 片剂：每片 5mg；10mg。<br>Comprimés : 5mg ou 10mg par comprimé. |

8.12　抗脑血管病药 Médicaments contre les maladies cérébrovasculaires

| 药品名称 Drug Names | 尼莫地平 Nimodipine |
|---|---|
| 适应证<br>Les indications | ①用于急性脑血管病恢复期的血液循环改善。各种原因的蛛网膜下腔出血后的脑血管痉挛，以及其所致的缺血性神经障碍高血压、偏头痛等。②也被用作缺血性神经元保护和血管性痴呆的治疗。③对突发性耳聋也有一定疗效。<br><br>① Ce produit est utilisé dans l'amélioration de la circulation sanguine pendant la récupération de maladie cérébrovasculaire aiguë. Il sert à traiter le vasospasme cérébral causé par une hémorragie sous-arachnoïdienne, ainsi que l'hypertention et la migraine résultant des troubles neurologiques ischémiques. ② Il est utilisé dans la protection neuronale ischémique et le traitement de la démence vasculaire. ③ Il est aussi applicable dans le traitement de la surdité subite. |
| 用法、用量<br>Les modes d'emploi et la posologie | 口服：①治疗缺血性脑血管病：片剂，每次 30 ～ 40mg，一日 3 次；缓释剂，每次 60mg，一日 2 次。连用 1 个月。②治疗突发性耳聋：片剂，每次 10 ～ 20mg，一日 3 次；缓释剂，每次 60mg，一日 1 次。5 日为 1 个疗程，可用 3 ～ 4 个疗程。③治疗轻、中度高血压：每次 40mg，一日 3 次。④治疗偏头痛：片剂，每次 40mg，一日 3 次；缓释剂，每次 60mg，一日 2 次，12 周为 1 个疗程。⑤老年性认知功能减退或血管性痴呆：每次 30 ～ 40mg，一日 3 次，连服 2 个月。⑥蛛网膜下腔出血所致脑血管痉挛：片剂，每次 40 ～ 60mg，一日 2 ～ 3 次，发病当日即可服用；缓释剂每次 60mg，一日 2 次。连用 3 ～ 4 周为 1 个疗程。如需手术，术前停药，术后可继续服用。静脉滴注：治疗蛛网膜下腔出血，滴速 0.5μg/（kg·min），随时检测血压，病情稳定后改口服，成人每次 20 ～ 30mg，一日 2 次。<br><br>Par voie orale : ① Pour traiter la maladie cérébrovasculaire ischémique : comprimés, 30 à 40mg par fois, 3 fois par jour ; comprimés à libération prolongée, 60mg par fois, 2 fois par jour, pendant 1 mois consécutif. ② Pour traiter la surdité subite : comprimés, 10 à 20mg par fois, 3 fois par jour ; comprimés à libération prolongée, 60mg par fois, 1 fois par jour. Pendant 5 jours comme un traitement médical, prendre 3 à 4 médicaments. ③ Pour traiter l'hypertension bénigne ou modérée : 40mg par fois, 3 fois par jour. ④ Pour traiter la migraine : comprimés, 40mg par fois, 3 fois par jour ; comprimés à libération prolongée, 60mg par fois, 2 fois par jour, pendant 12 semaines comme un traitement médical. ⑤ Pour traiter le déclin cognitif sénile ou la démence vasculaire : 30 à 40mg par fois, 3 fois par jour, pendant 2 mois consécutifs. ⑥ Pour traiter le vasospasme cérébral causé par une hémorragie sous-arachnoïdienne : comprimés, 40 à 60mg par fois, 2 à 3 fois par jour, administration le jour de la crise de la maladie ; les comprimés à libération prolongée, 60mg par fois, 2 fois par jour. Pendant 3 à 4 semaines consécutives comme un traitement médical. S'il est nécessaire de conduire la chirurgie, arrêter l'administration avant la chirurgie, et la reprendre après la chirurgie. En perfusion : pour traiter l'hémorragie sous-arachnoïdienne, la vitesse de la perfusion, 0.5μg/(kg•min), prendre la tension sanguine tout le temps, après le contrôle des symptômes, par voie orale, chez des adultes, 20 à 30 mg par fois, 2 fois par jour. |

**续 表**

| 剂型、规格<br>Les formes pharmaceutiques et les spécifications | 片剂：每片 10mg；20mg；30mg。胶囊剂：20mg；30mg。控释片：每片 60mg。缓释片：每片 60mg。缓释胶囊：每粒 60mg。注射剂：每支 2mg（10ml）；4mg（20ml）；8mg（40ml）；10mg（50ml）；25mg（50ml）；20mg（100ml）。<br>Comprimés : 10mg, 20mg ou 30mg par comprimé. Capsules : 20mg ou 30mg. Comprimés à libération contrôlée : 60mg par comprimé. Comprimés à libération prolongée : 60mg par comprimé. Capsules à libération prolongée : 60mg par capsule. Injection : 2mg (10ml), 4mg (20ml), 8mg (40ml), 10mg (50ml), 25mg (50ml) ou 20mg (100ml) |
|---|---|

| 药品名称 Drug Names | 桂利嗪 Cinnarizine |
|---|---|
| 适应证<br>Les indications | ①用于脑血栓形成、脑梗死、短暂性缺血发作、脑动脉硬化、脑出血恢复期、蛛网膜下腔出血恢复期、脑外伤后遗症、前庭性眩晕与平衡障碍（包括晕动病等）、冠状动脉硬化及供血障碍，以及由于末梢循环不良引起的疾病（如间歇性跛行及 Raynaud 病等）。②有文献报道，本品还可用于治疗慢性荨麻疹、老年性皮肤瘙痒等过敏性皮肤病。开可以治疗顽固性呃逆。<br>① Ce produit sert à traiter la thrombose cérébrale, l'infarctus cérébral, l'accident ischémique transitoire, l'artériosclérose cérébrale, la récupération de l'hémorragie cérébrale, la récupération de l'hémorragie méningée, les séquelles e lésion cérébrale traumatique, le vertige vestibulaire, les troubles de l'équilibre (y compris le mal des transports, etc), le durcissementde l'artère coronaire, des troubles sanguins ainsi que des maladies dues à la circulation périphérique pauvre (tel que la claudication intermittente et la maladie de Raynaud, etc.). ② Selon certains rapports, ce produit est aussi applicable dans le traitement des dermatoses allergiques, telles que l'urticaire chronique et le prurit sénile. Il sert aussi à traiter le hoquet réfractaire. |
| 用法、用量<br>Les modes d'emploi et la posologie | 口服：一般每次 25 ～ 50mg，一日 3 次，饭后服。晕动病患者于乘车船前 1 ～ 2 小时，1 次服用 30mg；乘车船期间每 6 ～ 8 小时服用 1 次（根据头晕等症状情况）。静脉注射：1 次 20 ～ 40mg，缓慢注入。<br>Par voie orale : 25 à 50mg par fois, 3 fois par jour, après le repas. Chez des patients atteints du mal des transports, 30mg, 1 à 2 h avant de prendre le bateau ou la voiture ; durant le trajet en voiture ou en bateau, prendre une fois toutes les 6 à 8h, selon les cas. Injection par voie IV : 20 à 40 mg par fois, injection lente. |
| 剂型、规格<br>Les formes pharmaceutiques et les spécifications | 片剂：每片 15mg；25mg。<br>胶囊剂：每粒 25mg；75mg。<br>注射剂：每支 20mg（20ml）。<br>Comprimés : 15mg ou 25mg par comprimé.<br>Capsules : 25mg ou 75mg par capsule.<br>Injection : 20mg (20ml) par solution. |

| 药品名称 Drug Names | 氟桂利嗪 Flunarizine |
|---|---|
| 适应证<br>Les indications | ①脑动脉缺血性疾病，如脑动脉硬化、短暂性脑缺血发作、脑血栓形成、脑栓塞和脑血管痉挛。②由前庭刺激或脑缺血引起的头晕、耳鸣、眩晕。③血管性偏头痛的防治。④癫痫辅助治疗。⑤周围血管病：间歇性跛行、下肢静脉曲张及微循环障碍、足踝水肿等。<br>① Les maladies ischémiques de l'artère cérébrale, telles que l'artériosclérose cérébrale, l'accident ischémique transitoire, la thrombose cérébrale, l'embolie cérébrale et le vasospasme cérébral. ② Les vertiges et les acouphènes causés par la stimulation vestibulaire ou l'ischémie cérébrale. ③ Ce produit sert à traiter et à prévenir la migraine vasculaire. ④ Le traitement adjuvant de l'épilepsie. ⑤ Les maladies vasculaires périphériques : la claudication intermittente, les varices, les troubles microcirculatoires, l'œdème de la cheville, etc. |
| 用法、用量<br>Les modes d'emploi et la posologie | 口服。脑动脉硬化、脑梗死恢复期：每日 5 ～ 10mg，一日 1 次，睡前服用。中枢性和外周性眩晕者、椎动脉供血不足者：每日 10 ～ 30mg，2 ～ 8 周为 1 个疗程。特发性耳鸣者：每次 10mg，每晚 1 次，10 日为 1 个疗程。偏头痛预防：每次 5 ～ 10mg，一日 2 次。间歇性跛行：每日 10 ～ 20mg。<br>Par voie orale. Pendant la récupération de l'artériosclérose cérébrale ou de l'infarctus cérébral : 5 à 10 mg par jour, 1 fois par jour, avant le sommeil. Chez des patients atteints de vertige central ou périphérique, ainsi que des patients souffrant del'insuffisance de l'artère vertébrale : 10 à 30mg par jour, pendant 2 à 8 semaines comme un traitement médical. Pour traiter l'acouphène idiopathique : 10mg par fois, une fois par soir, pendant 10 jours comme un traitement médical. Pour prévenir la migraine : 5 à 10mg par fois, 2 fois par jour. Pour traiter la claudication intermittente : 10 à 20mg par jour. |

**续　表**

| | |
|---|---|
| 剂型、规格<br>Les formes pharmaceutiques et les spécifications | 片剂：每片 5mg。胶囊剂：每粒 5mg。滴丸：每丸 1.25mg。<br>Comprimés : 5mg par comprimé. Capsules : 5mg par capsule. Pilules : 1,25mg par pilule. |
| **药品名称 Drug Names** | 降纤酶 Défibrase |
| 适应证<br>Les indications | ①急性脑梗死，短暂性脑缺血发作（TIA），以及脑梗死再复发的预防。②心肌梗死，不稳定型心绞痛以及心肌梗死再复发的预防。③四肢血管病，包括股动脉栓塞，血栓闭塞性脉管炎，雷诺病。④血液呈高黏状态、高凝状态、血栓前状态。⑤突发性耳聋。⑥肺栓塞。<br>① Ce produit sert à traiter l'infarctus aigu cérébral, et l'accident ischémique transitoire (AIT), et à prévenir la récurrence de l'infarctus cérébral. ② L'infarctus du myocarde, l'angine de poitrine instable et la prévention de la récurrence de l'infarctus du myocarde. ③ Maladie vasculaire des membres, y compris l'embolie de l'artère fémorale, l'angéite causée par l'occlusion thrombotique et la maladie de Raynaud. ④ L'hyperviscosité, l'hypercoagulation et l'état prothrombotique sanguins. ⑤ La surdité subite. ⑥ L'embolie pulmonaire. |
| 用法、用量<br>Les modes d'emploi et la posologie | 静脉滴注：急性发作期，1 次 10U，一日 1 次，连用 3～4 日。非急性发作期，首次 10U，维持量 5～10U，每日或隔日 1 次，2 周为 1 个疗程。<br>En perfusion : pendant la crise aigue, 10 U par fois, 1 fois par jour, pendant 3 à 4 jours consécutifs. Durant d'autres périodes, pour la première fois, 10U, la dose d'entretien, 5 à 10U, 1 fois tous les 1 à 2 jours, pendant 2 semaines comme un traitement médical. |
| 剂型、规格<br>Les formes pharmaceutiques et les spécifications | 注射剂（冻干制剂）：每支 5U；10U。<br>Injection (préparation lyophilisée) : 5U ou 10U par solution. |
| **药品名称 Drug Names** | 巴曲酶 Batroxobine |
| 适应证<br>Les indications | 用于急、慢性缺血性脑血管病（以急性效果明显），突发性耳聋，慢性动脉闭塞症，振动病，末梢循环障碍。也用于中、轻度高血压病。<br>Ce produit sert à traiter les maladies cérébrovasculaires ischémiques chroniques et aigues (surtout efficace pour les maladies aigues), la surdité subite, l'artériopathie oblitérante chronique, la maladie des vibrations et le trouble de la circulation périphérique. Il est également applicable dans le traitement de l'hypertension modérée et bénigne. |
| 用法、用量<br>Les modes d'emploi et la posologie | 静脉滴注：首次剂量 10BU，以后维持剂量为 5BU，隔日 1 次。用 100～250ml 生理盐水稀释，1～1.5 小时滴完。给药前血纤溶酶原超过 400mg/dl 或重度突发性耳聋患者剂量应加倍。通常治疗急性缺血性脑血管病一疗程 3 次，治疗突发性耳聋必要时可延长至 3 周，治疗慢性动脉闭塞症可延长至 6 周，但在延长期每次剂量改为 5BU，隔日 1 次。<br>En perfusion : pour la première fois, 10 BU, la dose d'entretien, 5 BU, une fois tous les 2 jours. Dissoudre le produit dans 100 à 250ml de solution saline, perfusion pendant 1 à 1,5h. Chez des patients dont la plasminogène avant l'administration est supérieure à 400mg/dl ou des patients souffrant de la surdité subite grave, il faut doubler la dose. Pour traiter la maladie cérébro-vasculaire ischémique aigue, un traitement médical comporte trois fois d'administration ; pour traiter la surdité subite, s'il est nécessaire, prolonger le traitement jusqu'à 3 semaines ; pour traiter l'artériopathie oblitérante chronique, prolonger le traitement jusqu'à 6 semaines, mais durant la période prolongée, 5BU par fois, une fois tous les 2 jours. |
| 剂型、规格<br>Les formes pharmaceutiques et les spécifications | 注射剂：每支 5BU（0.5ml）；10BU（1ml）。<br>Injection : 5BU (0,5ml) ou 10BU (1ml) par solution. |

| 药品名称 Drug Names | 倍他司汀 Bétahistine |
| --- | --- |
| 适应证<br>Les indications | 　　主要用于梅尼埃综合征、血管性头痛及脑动脉硬化，并可用于治疗急性缺血性脑血管疾病，如脑血栓、脑栓塞、一过性脑供血不足等；对高血压所致直立性眩晕、耳鸣等亦有效。<br>　　Il est principalement utilisé comme traitement du syndrome de Ménière, de la céphalée vasculaire et de l'artériosclérose cérébrale. Il est également applicable dans le traitement des maladies cérébrovasculaires ischémiques, telles que la thrombose cérébrale, l'embolie cérébrale, l'insuffisace cérébrale transitoire, etc. Il sert aussi à traiter les vertiges orthostatiques et la surdité. |
| 用法、用量<br>Les modes d'emploi et la posologie | 　　盐酸倍他司汀片：口服，成人每次 4～8mg，一日 2～4 次，最大日量不得超过 48mg。甲磺酸倍他司汀片：口服，成人每次 2～6mg，一日 3 次，餐后服用。盐酸倍他司汀注射液：肌内注射，每次 2～4mg，一日 2 次；静脉滴注，每次 20mg，一日 1 次。将本品溶于 2ml 5% 葡萄糖溶液或 0.9% 氯化钠溶液中，再溶于静脉滴注液 500ml 中缓慢静脉滴注。<br>　　Comprimés de chlorhydrate de bétahistine : par voie orale, chez des adultes, 4 à 8 mg, 2 à 4 fois par jour, ne pas dépasser 48mg par jour. Comprimés de mésylate de bétahistine : par voie orale, chez des adultes, 2 à 6mg, 3 fois par jour, après le repas. L'injection de chlorhydrate de bétahistine : administrée par voie IM, 2 à 4mg par fois, 2 fois par jour ; en perfusion, 20mg par fois, 1 fois par jour. Dissoudre ce produit dans 20ml de solution de glucose à 5 % ou de solution de chlorure de sodium à 0,9 %, ensuite, dissoudre dans 500ml de liquides par voie intraveineuse, perfusion lente. |
| 剂型、规格<br>Les formes pharmaceutiques et les spécifications | 　　片剂（盐酸盐）：每片 4mg。<br>　　片剂（甲磺酸盐）：每片 6mg。<br>　　注射液：每支 2mg（2ml）；4mg（4ml）。<br>　　Comprimés (chlorhydrate) : 4mg par comprimé.<br>　　Comprimés (mésylate) : 6mg par comprimé.<br>　　Injection : 2mg (2ml) ou 4mg (4ml) par solution. |
| 药品名称 Drug Names | 罂粟碱 Papavérine |
| 适应证<br>Les indications | 　　用于脑血栓形成、脑栓塞、肺栓塞、肢端动脉痉挛及动脉栓塞性疼痛。还可用于调节冠状动脉血流，缓解胃肠道痉挛和咳嗽治疗。海绵体注射用于勃起障碍治疗。<br>　　Ce produit sert à traiter la thrombose cérébrale, l'embolie cérébrale, l'embolie pulmonaire, l'acral spasme de l'artère et les douleurs liées à l'embolie artérielle. Il permet aussi de réguler le débit sanguin coronaire, de soulager les spasmes gastro-intestinaux et de traiter la toux. L'injection intracaverneuse de ce produit sert à traiter la dysfonction érectile. |
| 用法、用量<br>Les modes d'emploi et la posologie | 　　成人常用量：口服，每次 30～60mg，一日 3 次。肌内注射，每次 30mg，一日 90～120mg。静脉注射，每次 30～120mg，3 小时 1 次，应缓慢注射，不少于 1～2 分钟，以免发生心律失常及足以致命的窒息等。用于心脏停搏时，2 次给药要相隔 10 分钟。海绵体注射：推荐 1 次 30mg，每周连续 2 次或不超过 3 次。儿童：肌内或静脉注射，一次按体重 1.5mg/kg，一日 4 次。<br>　　La dose usuelle chez des adultes : par voie orale, 30 à 60 mg par fois, 3 fois par jour. Injection par voie IM, 30 mg par fois, 90 à 120 mg par jour. injection par voie IV, 30 à 120mg par fois, une fois toutes les 3h, injection lente, pendant 1 à 2 minutes au moins, pour éviter l'arythmie et l'asphyxie létale. Lors de l'application dans l'arrêt cardiaque, il faut un intervalle de 10 minutes entre 2 administrations. L'injection intracaverneuse : il est recommandé de prendre 30 mg par fois, 2 fois consécutives par semaine ou 3 fois au maximum. Chez des enfants : injection par voie IM ou IV, 1,5 mg/kg par fois, 4 fois par jour. |
| 剂型、规格<br>Les formes pharmaceutiques et les spécifications | 　　片剂：每片 30mg。注射剂：每支 30mg（1ml）。<br>　　Comprimés : 30mg par comprimé.<br>　　Injection : 30mg (1ml) par solution. |
| 药品名称 Drug Names | 己酮可可碱 Pentoxifylline |
| 适应证<br>Les indications | 　　用于脑血管障碍或脑卒中后引起的后遗症，伴有间歇性跛行的慢性闭塞性脉管炎，血管性头痛；也可用于血管性痴呆的预防和治疗（但目前国际上临床研究结论尚不肯定）。<br>　　Ce produit est utilisé dans le traitement des séquelles causées par les troubles ou accidents cérébro-vasculaires, l'angéite causée par l'occlusion thrombotique chronique accompagnée de la claudication intermittente et de la céphalée vasculaire. Il sert également à prévenir et à traiter la démence vasculaire (mais il n'y a pas encore de conclusions cliniques internationales.) |

**续　表**

| | |
|---|---|
| 用法、用量<br>Les modes d'emploi et la posologie | ①口服：每次 100～400mg，一日 3 次，建议餐后即时服用。控释片，每次 400mg，一日 1 次。口服用药治疗缺血性脑血管病后遗症或血管性痴呆等，需连续 2～8 周可产生治疗效果。②静脉滴注：每次 200～400mg，溶于 250～500ml 静脉滴注液中缓慢滴注，90～180 分钟滴完，每次 1～2 次。配制好的药物需在 24 小时内使用。<br><br>① Par voie orale : 100 à 400mg par fois, 3 fois par jour, immédiatement après le repas. Les comprimés à libération contrôlée, 400mg par fois, 1 fois par jour. Pour traiter les séquelles des maladies cérébrovasculaires ischémiques ou la démence vasculaire, si on administre le médicament par voie orale, il faut prendre pendant 2 à 8 semaines avant de voir l'effet thérapeutique.　② En perfusion : 200 à 400 mg par fois, dissoudre le produit dans 250 à 500ml d'infusion, la perfusion lente, pendant 90 à 180 minutes, 1 à 2 fois par jour.Il faut utiliser le médicament préparé en 24h. |
| 剂型、规格<br>Les formes pharmaceutiques et les spécifications | 片剂（肠溶片）：每片 100mg。控释片：每片 400mg。注射液：每支 100mg（5ml）；300mg（15ml）。<br>Comprimés (comprimés à enrobage entérique) : 100mg par comprimé.<br>Comprimés à libération contrôlée : 400mg par comprimé.<br>Injection : 100mg (5ml) ou 300mg (15ml) par solution. |
| **药品名称 Drug Names** | 丁咯地尔 Buflomédil |
| 适应证<br>Les indications | ①适用于慢性脑血管供血不足引起的症状：眩晕、耳鸣、智力减退、记忆力或注意力减退、定向障碍等。②外周性血管疾病：间歇性跛行、雷诺综合征、血栓闭塞性脉管炎等。<br><br>① Il sert à traiter les symptômes causés par l'insuffisance cérébrovasculaire chronique : les vertiges, la surdité, la détérioration mentale, la perte de mémoire ou de l'attention, ainsi que la désorientation. ② Les maladies vasculaires périphériques : la claudication intermittente, le syndrome de Raynaud, l'angéite causée par l'occlusion thrombotique, etc. |
| 用法、用量<br>Les modes d'emploi et la posologie | 口服：片剂，每次 150～300mg，一日 2～3 次。每日最大剂量为 600mg；缓释片，每次 600mg，一日 1 次。肌内注射或静脉注射：每日 200～400mg。静脉滴注：每日 200～400mg，分 2 次，加于静脉滴注液 250～500ml 中缓慢滴注。轻中度肾功能不全者，用量减半，片剂，每次 150mg，一日 2 次，每日最大推荐剂量为 300mg；不推荐使用缓释片。肝功能不全者考虑减量使用。<br><br>Par voie orale : les comprimés, 150 à 300mg par fois, 2 à 3 fois par jour. La dose maximale est de 600mg par jour ; les comprimés à libération prolongée, 600mg par fois, 1 fois par jour. Injection par voie IM ou IV : 200 à 400mg par jour. En perfusion : 200 à 400 mg par jour, à travers 2 fois, dissoudre le produit dans 250 à 500ml de liquides par voie intraveineuse, perfusion lente. Chez des patients insuffisants rénaux bénins et modérés, diminuer de moitié la dose, les comprimés, 150mg par fois, 2 fois par jour, la dose maximale, 300mg par jour ; il n'est pas recommandé de prendre les comprimés à libération prolongée. Chez des patients insuffisants hépatiques, diminuer la dose. |
| 剂型、规格<br>Les formes pharmaceutiques et les spécifications | 片剂：每片 150mg；300mg。<br>缓释片：600mg。<br>注射液：每支 50mg（5ml）；100mg（10ml）。<br>粉针剂：每支 50mg；100mg；200mg。<br>Comprimés : 150mg ou 300mg par comprimé.<br>Comprimés à libération prolongée : 600mg.<br>Injection : 50mg (5ml) ou 100mg (10ml) par solution.<br>Poudres : 50mg, 100mg ou 200mg par solution. |
| **药品名称 Drug Names** | 尼麦角林 Nicergoline |
| 适应证<br>Les indications | 用于急、慢性脑血管疾病和代谢性脑供血不足，急、慢性外周血管障碍，老年性耳聋和视网膜疾病等。也用于血管性痴呆，尤其在早期治疗时对认知、记忆等有改善，并能减轻疾病严重程度。<br><br>Ce produit sert à traiter les maladies cérébrovasculaires aigues et chroniques, l'insuffisance cérébrale métabolique, les troubles vasculaires périphériques aigus et chroniques, la surdité sénile, les maladies liées à la rétine, etc. Il permet aussi de traiter la démence vasculaire, d'améliorer la cognition et la mémoire dans le traitement précoce et de réduire la gravité des maladies. |

**续 表**

| 用法、用量<br>Les modes d'emploi et la posologie | 口服：每次 10 ～ 20mg，一日 3 次。片剂勿嚼服，可与食物同服。肌内注射：每次 2 ～ 4mg，一日 1 ～ 2 次。静脉注射：每次 2 ～ 4mg，溶于 100ml 的静脉滴注液中缓慢滴注，一日 1 ～ 2 次。<br>Par voie orale : 10 à 20mg par fois, 3 fois par jour. Ne pas mâcher les comprimés, c'est permissible de les prendre durant le repas. Injection par voie IM : 2 à 4 mg par fois, 1 à 2 fois par jour. Injection par voie IV : 2 à 4 mg par fois, dissoudre dans 100mg de liquides par voie intraveineuse, perfusion lente, 1 à 2 fois par jour. |
|---|---|
| 剂型、规格<br>Les formes pharmaceutiques et les spécifications | 片剂：每片 10mg。<br>胶囊剂：每粒 15mg。<br>注射剂：2mg（1ml）；2.5mg（1ml）；4mg（2ml）；8mg（2ml）；8mg（5ml）。<br>Comprimés : 10mg par comprimé.<br>Capsules : 15mg par capsule.<br>Injection : 2mg (1ml), 2,5mg (1ml), 4mg (2ml), 8mg (2ml) ou 8mg (5ml). |

| 药品名称 Drug Names | 川芎嗪 Ligustrazine |
|---|---|
| 适应证<br>Les indications | 适用于脑供血不足、脑栓塞、脉管炎、冠心病、心绞痛、突发性耳聋等。<br>Ce produit sert à traiter l'ischémie cérébrale, la thrombose cérébrale, la vascularite, la maladie coronarienne, l'angine de poitrine, la surdité subite, etc. |
| 用法、用量<br>Les modes d'emploi et la posologie | 口服：每次 100mg，一日 3 次，30 日为 1 个疗程。肌内注射：每次 40 ～ 50mg，一天 1 ～ 2 次，缓慢推注，15 日为 1 个疗程。静脉滴注：每日 50 ～ 100mg，稀释于 250 ～ 500ml 静脉滴注液中缓慢滴注，15 日为 1 个疗程。<br>Par voie orale : 100mg par fois, 3 fois par jour, pendant 30 jours comme un traitement médical. Injection par voie IM : 40 à 50 mg par fois, 1 à 2 fois par jour, injection lente, pendant 15 jours comme un traitement médical. En perfusion : 50 à 100mg par jour, dissoudre dans 250 à 500ml de liquides par voie intraveineuse, pendant 15 jours comme un traitement médical. |
| 剂型、规格<br>Les formes pharmaceutiques et les spécifications | 片剂：每片 50mg。<br>注射用川芎嗪（盐酸盐）：每支 40mg。<br>注射用川芎嗪（磷酸盐）：每支 50mg。<br>Comprimés : 50mg par comprimé.<br>La ligustrazine pour injection (le chlorhydrate) : 40mg par solution.<br>La ligustrazine pour injection (le phosphate) : 50mg par solution. |

| 药品名称 Drug Names | 丁苯酞 Butylphtalide |
|---|---|
| 适应证<br>Les indications | 适用于治疗轻、中度急性缺血性脑卒中及急性缺血性脑卒中患者神经功能缺损的改善。<br>Il sert à traiter l'accident cérébrovasculaire ischémique aigu bénin et modéré et à améliorer le déficit neurologique chez des patients atteints d'accident cérébrobasculaire ischémique aigu. |
| 用法、用量<br>Les modes d'emploi et la posologie | （1）可与复方丹参注射液联合使用。空腹口服。一次两粒（0.2g），一日 3 次，10 日为 1 个疗程。本品应在患者病发后 48 小时内开始服用。<br>（2）静脉滴注，一日 2 次，每次 25mg，每次滴注时间不少于 50 分钟；两次用要间隔不少于 6 小时，疗程 14 日。<br>(1)Ce produit peut être utilisé en association avec les composés Danshen (salvia miltiorrhiza). L'estomac vide. 2 capsules (0,2g) par fois, 3 fois par jour, pendant 10 jours comme un traitement médical. Il faut prendre ce médicament dans les 48 h suivant la crise de la maladie.<br>(2)En perfusion, 2 fois par jour, 25mg par fois, chaque perfusion dure au moins 50 minutes ; avec un intervalle d'au moins 6h entre deux administrations, pendant 14 jours comme un traitement médical. |
| 剂型、规格<br>Les formes pharmaceutiques et les spécifications | 胶囊：每粒 0.1g。丁苯肽氯化钠注射：丁苯肽 25mg 与氯化钠 0.9g（100ml）。<br>Capsules : 0,1g par capsule.<br>Injection de chlorure de sodium de butyl phtalide : 25mg de butyl phtalide et 0,9g (100ml) de chlorure de sodium. |

| 药品名称 Drug Names | 奥扎格雷 Ozagrel |
|---|---|
| 适应证<br>Les indications | 用于缺血性脑卒中急性期，蛛网膜下腔出血术后的脑血管痉挛收缩和伴随的脑缺血症状。<br>Il est utilisé dans la phase aigue de l'accident cérébrovasculaire ischémique, ainsi que dans le traitement de la contraction de vasospasme cérébral et de l'ischémie cérébrale après la chirurgie liée à l'hémorragie méningée. |

续　表

| | |
|---|---|
| 用法、用量<br>Les modes d'emploi et la posologie | ①缺血性脑卒中急性期：每次 40～80mg，溶于 500ml 静脉滴注液中连续静脉滴注，一日 1～2 次，1～2 周为 1 个疗程。②蛛网膜下腔出血术后并发的脑血管痉挛及伴随而产生的脑缺血症状：每次 80mg，一日 1 次，溶于适量滴注液中，24 小时持续静脉滴注，可连续用药 2 周。<br><br>① la phase aigue de l'accident cérébrovasculaire ischémique : 40 à 80mg par fois, dissoudre dans 500ml de liquides par voie intraveineuse, perfusion continue, 1 à 2 fois par jour, pendant 1 à 2 semaines comme un traitement médical. ② Pour traiter la contraction de vasospasme cérébral et de l'ischémie cérébrale après la chirurgie liée à l'hémorragie méningée : 80 mg par fois, 1 fois par jour, dissoudre dans la liquide par voie IV, perfusion pendant 24 h consécutives, pendant 2 semaines consécutives. |
| 剂型、规格<br>Les formes pharmaceutiques et les spécifications | 注射用奥扎格雷：20mg（2ml）；40mg（2ml）。<br>奥扎格雷钠氯化钠（或葡萄糖）注射液：250ml（奥扎格雷钠 80mg）。<br>L'ozagrel pour injection : 20mg (2ml) ou 40mg (2ml).<br>Injection de chlorure de sodium (ou de glucose) de l'ozagrel sodique : 250 ml (80mg d'ozagrel sodique). |
| 药品名称 Drug Names | 曲克芦丁 Troxérutine |
| 适应证<br>Les indications | 用于闭塞性脑血管病引起的偏瘫、失语、冠心病梗死前综合征、中心视网膜炎、血栓性静脉炎、静脉曲张、雷诺综合征、血管通透性升高引起的水肿、淋巴水肿、烧伤及创伤水肿、动脉硬化。<br><br>Ce produit sert à traiter les maladies suivantes causées par les maladies cérébro-vasculaires occlusives : l'hémiplégie, l'aphasie, le syndrome prodromique de la thrombose coronarienne, la rétinite centrale, la thrombophlébite, les varices, le syndrome de Raynaud, l'oedème, le lymphoedème, les brûlures et l'œdème traumatique causés par une perméabilité vasculaire accrue, ainsi que l'athérosclérose. |
| 用法、用量<br>Les modes d'emploi et la posologie | 口服：每次 200～300mg，一日 3 次。肌内注射：每次 100～200mg，一日 2 次。静脉滴注：每次 400mg，一日 1 次，20 日为 1 个疗程，可用 1～3 个疗程，每疗程间隔 3～7 日。<br><br>Par voie orale : 200 à 300mg par fois, 3 fois par jour. Injection par voie IM : 100 à 200mg par fois, 2 fois par jour. En perfusion : 400mg par fois, 1 fois par jour, pendant 20 jours comme un traitement médical. Il est possible de suivre 1 à 3 traitements médicaux, avec un intervalle de 3 à 7 jours entre deux traitements médicaux. |
| 剂型、规格<br>Les formes pharmaceutiques et les spécifications | 片剂：每片 100mg。<br>注射液：每支 100mg（2ml）；200mg（2ml）。<br>Comprimés : 100mg par comprimé.<br>Injection : 100mg (2ml) ou 200mg (2ml) par solution. |
| 药品名称 Drug Names | 维生素 E 烟酸酯 Vitamine E Nicotinate |
| 适应证<br>Les indications | 用于动脉硬化、脑震荡及轻微脑挫伤和脑外伤后遗症、头痛头晕，中心性视网膜炎等血管障碍性疾病，也可用于脂质代谢异常<br><br>Ce produit sert à traiter les maladies liées au trouble vasculaire, telles que l'artériosclérose, les séquelles de la contusion cérébrale, de la légère commotion cérébrale et du traumatisme crânien, la céphalée, les étourdissements, la rétinite centrale, etc. Il est aussi applicable dans le traitement du métabolisme des lipides. |
| 用法、用量<br>Les modes d'emploi et la posologie | 口服，每次 0.1～0.2g，一日 3 次，餐后服。老年人可做适当调整。<br><br>Par voie orale, 0,1 à 0,2 g par fois, 3 fois par jour, après le repas. Chez des personnes âgées, ajuster la dose. |
| 剂型、规格<br>Les formes pharmaceutiques et les spécifications | 片剂：每片 0.1g。<br>胶囊：每粒 0.1g。<br>胶丸：每粒 0.1g。<br>Comprimés : 0,1g par comprimé.<br>Capsules : 0,1g par capsule.<br>Pilules : 0,1g par pilule. |

| 药品名称 Drug Names | 灯盏花素 Bréviscapine |
|---|---|
| 适应证<br>Les indications | ①用于缺血性脑血管病，如脑供血不足、椎基底动脉供血不足、脑出血后遗症。②亦用于冠心病、心绞痛、高血压、高黏滞血症等心血管疾病。<br><br>① Ce produit sert à traiter les maladies cérébrovasculaires ischémiques, telles que l'ischémie cérébrale, l'insuffisance vertébro-basilaire et les séquelles de l'hémorragie cérébrale. ② Il sert aussi à traiter les maladies cérébrovasculaires, telles que la maladie coronarienne, l'angine de poitrine, l'hypertension, l'hyperviscosité, etc. |
| 用法、用量<br>Les modes d'emploi et la posologie | 口服：每次 40mg，一日 3 次。肌内注射：每次 2ml，一日 2 次，15 日为 1 个疗程。静脉滴注：每次 4 ~ 8ml，一日 1 次，加入 500ml 静脉滴注液中稀释应用，10 日为 1 个疗程。<br><br>Par voie orale : 40mg par fois, 3 fois par jour. L'injection par voie IM : 2ml par fois, 2 fois par jour, pendant 15 jours comme un traitement médical. En perfusion : 4 à 8ml par fois, 1 fois par jour, dissoudre dans 500ml de liquides par voie IV avant de l'appliquer, pendant 10 jours comme un traitement médical. |
| 剂型、规格<br>Les formes pharmaceutiques et les spécifications | 片剂：每片 20mg。<br>注射剂：每支 5mg（2ml）；20mg（5ml）。<br><br>Comprimés : 20mg par comprimé.<br>Injection : 5mg (2ml) ou 20mg (5ml) par solution. |
| 药品名称 Drug Names | 地芬尼多 Difénidol |
| 适应证<br>Les indications | 用于治疗各种原因引起的眩晕症（如椎基底动脉供血不足、梅尼埃病等）、恶心呕吐、自主神经功能紊乱、晕车晕船、运动病及外科麻醉手术后的呕吐等。<br><br>Ce produit sert à traiter les vertiges de toutes sortes (tels que l'insuffisance vertébro-basilaire et la maladie de Ménière), les nausées, les vomissements, le dysfonctionnement du système nerveux automatique, le mal des transports, et les vomissements après la chirurgie anesthésique. |
| 用法、用量<br>Les modes d'emploi et la posologie | 口服：成人每次 25 ~ 50mg，一日 3 次；6 个月以上儿童，每次 0.9mg/kg，一日 3 次。肌内注射：每次 10 ~ 20mg，眩晕发作剧烈者可每次 20 ~ 40mg。<br><br>Par voie orale : chez des adultes, 25 à 50 mg par fois, 3 fois par jour ; chez des enfants plus de 6 mois, 0,9 mg/kg par fois, 3 fois par jour. Injection par voie IM : 10 à 20mg par fois. En cas de vertiges intenses, 20 à 40mg par fois. |
| 剂型、规格<br>Les formes pharmaceutiques et les spécifications | 片剂：每片 25mg。<br>注射液：每支 10mg（1ml）。<br><br>Comprimés : 25mg par comprimé.<br>Injection : 10mg (1ml) par solution. |
| 药品名称 Drug Names | 长春西汀 Vinpocétine |
| 适应证<br>Les indications | ①用于改善脑梗死、脑出血后遗症及脑动脉硬化引起的各种症状，如记忆障碍、眩晕、头痛、失语、抑郁症等。②还可用于各种眼底血液循环不良所致的视力障碍；听力损伤、耳鸣前庭功能障碍。③各种颅脑手术后脑功能的康复治疗。<br><br>① Ce produit sert à améliorer les séquelles de l'infarctus cérébral et de l'hémorragie cérébrale, ainsi que les symptômes causés par l'artériosclérose cérébrale, tels que les troubles de la mémoire, les vertiges, la céphalée, l'aphasie, la dépression, etc. ② Il sert aussi traiter la déficience visuelle causée par la mauvaise circulation sanguine au fond d'œil, la perte d'audition, les acouphènes, ainsi que les troubles vestibulaires. ③ La thérapie de réadaptation des fonctions cérébrales après la chirurgie du cerveau. |
| 用法、用量<br>Les modes d'emploi et la posologie | 口服：每次 5 ~ 10mg，一日 3 次，餐时口服。<br>静脉滴注：起始剂量每日 20mg，一日 1 次；以后根据病情可增至每日 30mg，一日 1 次。<br><br>Par voie orale : 5 à 10mg par fois, 3 fois par jour, durant le repas.<br>En perfusion : la dose initiale, 20 mg par jour, 1 fois par jour ; ensuite, augmenter selon les cas pour atteindre 30 mg par jour, 1 fois par jour. |

| 续　表 | |
|---|---|
| 剂型、规格<br>Les formes pharmaceutiques et les spécifications | 片剂：每片 5mg。<br>注射液：20mg（2ml）。<br>长春西汀葡萄糖注射液：100ml（长春西汀 10mg）；200ml（长春西汀 10mg）；250ml（长春西汀 10mg）。<br><br>Comprimés : 5mg par comprimé.<br>Injection : 20mg (2ml).<br>Injection de glucose de vinpocétine : 100ml (10mg de vinpocétine), 200ml (10mg de vinpocétine) ou 250ml (10mg de vinpocétine). |
| **药品名称 Drug Names** | **依达拉奉 Edaravone** |
| 适应证<br>Les indications | 用于改善急性脑梗死所致的神经症状、日常生活活动能力和功能障碍。<br>Ce produit sert à améliorer les symptômes neurologiques et le dysfonctionnement des activités de la vie quotidienne causés pas l'infarctus cérébral aigu. |
| 用法、用量<br>Les modes d'emploi et la posologie | 静脉滴注：一次 30mg，加入适量生理盐水中稀释后静脉滴注，30 分钟内滴完，一日 2 次，14 日为 1 个疗程。尽可能在发病 24 小时内开始给药。<br>En perfusion : 30 mg par fois, dissoudre dans la solution saline pour la dilution, perfusion pendant 30 minutes, 2 fois par jour, pendant 14 jours comme un traitement médical. Essayer de commencer à prendre le médicament dans les 24 h après la crise de la maladie. |
| 剂型、规格<br>Les formes pharmaceutiques et les spécifications | 注射液：每支 10mg（5ml）；30mg（20ml）。<br>Injection : 10mg (5ml) ou 30mg (20ml) par solution. |
| **药品名称 Drug Names** | **血塞通 Xuesaitong** |
| 适应证<br>Les indications | ①用于缺血性脑血管病、冠心病心绞痛，中医证见脑络瘀阻、中风偏瘫、心脉瘀阻、胸痹心痛。②还可用于治疗视网膜血管阻塞、眼前房出血、青光眼；急性黄疸型肝炎、病毒性肝炎；外伤、软组织损伤及骨折恢复期。<br><br>① Ce produit sert à traiter les maladies cérébrovasculaires ischémiques，l'angine de poitrine liée à la maladie coronarienne，et selon la médecine traditionnelle chinoise，il sert à traiter la stase des réseaux cérébraux，l'accident vasculaire cérébral，la paralysie，la stase du sang systolique et la douleur de poitrine. ② Il est aussi utilisé comme traitement de l'occlusion vasculaire rétinienne, de l'hyphéma et du glaucome ; de l'hépatite aiguë avec ictère, de l'hépatite virale, ainsi que de la récupération du traumatisme, des fractures et des lésions des tissus mous. |
| 用法、用量<br>Les modes d'emploi et la posologie | 口服：一次 50～100mg，一日 3 次。肌内注射：一次 100mg。一日 1～2 次。静脉滴注：一次 200～400mg，以 5%～10% 葡萄糖注射液 250～500ml 稀释后缓缓滴注，一日 1 次。静脉注射：每次 200mg，以 25%～50% 葡萄糖注射液 40～60ml 稀释后缓缓注射，一日 1 次。15 日为 1 个疗程。停药 1～3 日后可进行第 2 个疗程。<br><br>Par voie orale : 50 à 100mg par fois, 3 fois par jour. Injection par voie IM : 100mg par fois, 1 à 2 fois par jour. En perfusion : 200 à 400mg par fois, dissoudre dans 250 à 500ml de solution de glucose, perfusion lente, 1 fois par jour. Injection par voie IV : 200mg par fois, dissoudre dans 40 à 60ml de solution de glucose à 25 % à 50 %, injection lente, 1 fois par jour. pendant 15 jours comme un traitement médical. 1 à 3 jours après l'arrêt de l'administration, c'est possible de suivre le deuxième traitement médical. |
| 剂型、规格<br>Les formes pharmaceutiques et les spécifications | 片剂：每片 50mg。<br>胶囊剂：每粒 60mg。<br>注射液：每支 100mg（2ml）。<br><br>Comprimés : 50mg par comprimé.<br>Capsules : 60mg par capsule.<br>Injection : 100mg (2ml) par solution. |
| **药品名称 Drug Names** | **七叶皂苷钠 Aéscinate sodique** |
| 适应证<br>Les indications | ①用于各种病因引起的脑水肿、创伤或手术所致肿胀。②也可用于静脉回流障碍、下肢静脉曲张、血栓性静脉炎、慢性静脉功能不全，下肢动脉阻塞性疾病，运动系统创伤造成的软组织血肿、水肿。③用于周围神经炎性疾病，如吉兰 - 巴雷综合征、多发性神经炎等。 |

**续 表**

| | |
|---|---|
| | ① Il sert à traiter l'œdème cérébral et l'œdème causé par le traumatisme et la chirurgie. ② Il permet aussi de traiter les troubles veineux, les varices, la thrombophlébite, l'insuffisance veineuse chronique, l'artériopathie oblitérante des membres inférieurs, ainsi que l'hématome etl'oedème des tissus mous causées par le traumatisme du système locomoteur. ③ Il est aussi applicable dans le traitement des maladies inflammatoires du système nerveux périphérique, telles que le syndrome de Guillain-Barré et la polynévrite. |
| 用法、用量<br>Les modes d'emploi et la posologie | ① 静脉给药：一日5～10mg溶于250ml滴注液中静脉滴注；或5～10ml溶于10～20ml10%葡萄糖溶液或0.9%氯化钠溶液中，静脉注射。儿童3岁以下一日0.05～0.1mg/kg体重；3～10岁一日0.1～0.2mg/kg体重。重症患者可多次给药，但一日总量不得超过20mg。疗程7～10日。②口服：每次30～60mg，一日2次，餐时或餐后口服，20日为1个疗程。<br><br>① Par voie IV : dissoudre 5 à 10mg par jour dans 250 ml de liquides, en perfusion ; ou dissoudre 5 à 10mg dans 10 à 20 ml de solution de glucose à 10 % ou de solutionde chlorure de sodium à 0,9 %, injection par voie IV. Chez des enfants moins de 3 ans, 0,05 à 0,1 mg/kg par jour ; de 3 à 10 ans, 0,1 à 0,2 mg/kg par jour. Chez des patients gravement malades, administration pendant plusieurs fois, ne pas dépasser 20mg par jour. Pendant 7 à 10 jours comme un traitement médical. ② Par voie orale : 30 à 60 mg par fois, 2 fois par jour, durant ou après le repas, pendant 20 jours comme un traitement médical. |
| 剂型、规格<br>Les formes pharmaceutiques et les spécifications | 片剂：每片30mg。<br>注射剂：每支5mg；10mg；25mg。<br>Comprimés : 30mg par comprimé.<br>Injection : 5mg, 10mg ou 25mg par solution. |
| **药品名称 Drug Names** | 葛根素 Puerarin |
| 适应证<br>Les indications | 可用于辅助治疗冠心病、心绞痛、心肌梗死，缺血性脑血管病，视网膜动、静脉阻塞，青光眼，突发性耳聋，小儿病毒性心肌炎、糖尿病。<br><br>Il sert de traitement adjuvant des maladies suivantes : la maladie coronarienne, l'angine de poitrine, l'infarctus du myocarde, la maladie cérébrovasculaire ischémique, l'occlusion veineuse et artérielle rétinienne, le glaucome, la surdité subite, la myocardite virale chez des enfants ainsi que le diabète. |
| 用法、用量<br>Les modes d'emploi et la posologie | ①静脉滴注：每次0.4～0.6g，一日1次，10～20日为1个疗程，可连续使用2～3个疗程。最大用药剂量为1.0g。②滴眼：一次1～2滴，闭目3～5分钟。首日3次，以后为一日2次。<br><br>① En perfusion : 0,4 à 0,6g par fois, 1 fois par jour, pendant 10 à 20 jours comme un traitement médical, il est possible de suivre 2 à 3 traitements. Ne pas dépasser 1,0 g. ② Les gouttes pour les yeux : 1 à 2 gouttes par fois, fermer les yeux pendant 3 à 5 minutes. Pour le premier jour, 3 fois, ensuite, 2 fois par jour. |
| 剂型、规格<br>Les formes pharmaceutiques et les spécifications | 注射液：每支100mg（2ml）；400mg（8ml）。粉针剂：每支200mg。葛根素氯化钠注射液：100ml（葛根素200mg）。葛根素滴眼液：50mg（5ml）。<br>Injection : 100mg (2ml) ou 400mg (8ml) par solution.<br>Poudre : 200mg par solution.<br>Le chlorure de sodium de puerarin pour injection : 100ml (200mg de puerarin).<br>Les gouttes pour les yeux de puerarin : 50mg (5ml). |

8.13 抗老年痴呆药和改善脑代谢药 Médicaments anti-démence senile et médicaments améliorationdu métabolisme cérébral

| **药品名称 Drug Names** | 加兰他敏 Galantamine |
|---|---|
| 适应证<br>Les indications | ①适用于治疗轻、中度阿尔茨海默病（AD），有效率50%～60%，疗效与他克林相当，但没有肝毒性。用药后6～8周治疗效果开始明显。②用于重症肌无力、脊髓灰质炎后遗症、儿童脑性麻痹、多发性神经炎、脊神经根炎及拮抗氯筒箭毒碱。<br><br>① Ce produit sert à traiter la maladie d'Alzheimer bénigne et modérée, avec un taux de réussite de 50 % à 60 %. Son effet est similaire à celui de la tacrine mais sans hépatotoxémie. L'efficacité de la galantamine commence à être évidenteaprès 6 à 8 semaines d'administration. ② Il est utilisé comme traitement des maladies suivantes : la myasthénie grave, les séquelles de la poliomyélite, la paralysie cérébrale chez dess enfants, la névrite multiple, la radiculite et le chlorure de tubocurarine |

续　表

| 用法、用量<br>Les modes d'emploi et la posologie | 口服：每次 10 ～ 20mg，一日 3 次。小儿每日 0.5 ～ 1mg/kg，分 3 次服。皮下或肌内注射：每次 2.5 ～ 10mg，一日 1 次。小儿每次 0.05 ～ 0.1mg/kg，一日 1 次。每个疗程 8 ～ 10 周。用于抗氯筒箭毒碱时肌内注射起始剂量 5 ～ 10mg，5 分钟或 10 分钟后按需要可逐渐增加至每次 10 ～ 20mg。<br><br>Par voie orale : 10 à 20mg par fois, 3 fois par jour. Chez des enfants, 0,5 à 1 mg/kg par jour, à travers 3 fois. Injection par voie cutanée ou IM : 2,5 à 10 mg par fois, 1 fois par jour. Chez des enfants, 0,05 à 0,1 mg/kg par fois, 1 fois par jour. Chaque traitement médical dure 8 à 10 semaines. Pour contrarier le chlorure de tubocurarine, injection par voie IM, la dose initiale, 5 à 10mg, 5 ou 10 minutes après, augmenter progressivement la dose pour atteindre 10 à 20 mg par fois. |
|---|---|
| 剂型、规格<br>Les formes pharmaceutiques et les spécifications | 口崩片：每片 5mg。<br>分散片：每片 2.5mg。<br>注射剂：每支 1mg（1ml）；2.5mg（1ml）；5mg（1ml）。<br>Comprimés à dissolution orale : 5mg par comprimé.<br>Comprimés dispersibles : 2,5 mg par comprimé.<br>Injection : 1mg (1ml), 2,5mg (1ml) ou 5mg (1ml) par solution. |

| 药品名称 Drug Names | 美金刚 Mémantine |
|---|---|
| 适应证<br>Les indications | 用于治疗中至重度的阿尔茨海默病（AD），以及震颤麻痹综合征的治疗。<br>Ce produit sert à traiter la maladie d'Alzheimer modérée et grave, ainsi que le parkinsonisme. |
| 用法、用量<br>Les modes d'emploi et la posologie | 口服。成人或 14 岁以上青少年：在治疗的前 3 周按每周递增 5mg 的方法逐渐达到维持剂量，即治疗第 1 周每日 5mg（晨服），第 2 周每日 10mg，分 2 次服用；第 3 周每日 15mg（早上 10mg，下午 5mg）；第 4 周开始维持剂量每日 20mg，分 2 次服。片剂可空腹服用，也可随食物同服。14 岁以下小儿：维持量每日 0.55 ～ 1.0mg/kg。中度肾功能损害者，应将剂量减至每日 10mg；不推荐严重肾衰竭患者使用。<br><br>Par voie orale : chez des adultes et des adolescents plus de 14 ans : pendant les 3 premières semaines, augmenter 5mg par semaine pour atteindre progressivement la dose d'entretien, soit 5mg par jour (pris le petit matin) pour la première semaine, 10mg par jour pour la 2ème semaine, à travers 2 fois ; 15mg par jour pour la 3ème semaine (10mg pris le petit matin, 5mg pris l'après-midi) ; à partir de la 4ème semaine, maintenir 20mg par jour, à travers 2 fois. Les comprimés peuvent être pris l'estomac vide ou pendant le repas. Chez des enfants moins de 14 ans : maintenir 0,55 à 1,0 mg/kg par jour. Chez des patients insuffisants rénaux modérés, diminuer la dose pour atteindre 10mg par jour; il n'est pas recommandé de l'utiliser chez des patients atteints d'insuffisance rénale sévère. |
| 剂型、规格<br>Les formes pharmaceutiques et les spécifications | 片剂：每片 5mg；10mg。<br>胶囊：每粒 10mg。<br>Comprimés : 5mg ou 10mg par comprimé.<br>Capsules : 10mg par capsule. |

| 药品名称 Drug Names | 吡拉西坦 Piracétam |
|---|---|
| 适应证<br>Les indications | 由衰老、脑血管病、脑外伤、CO 中毒等引起的记忆和轻中度脑功能障碍。亦可用于儿童发育迟缓。<br>Il sert à traiter le dysfonctionnement de la mémoire et du cerveau bénin et modéré causé par le vieillissement, la maladie cérébrovasculaire, une lésion cérébrale traumatique, une intoxication au CO, etc. Il est également utilisé comme traitement du retard de croissance statural chez l'enfant. |
| 用法、用量<br>Les modes d'emploi et la posologie | ①口服：成人，每次 0.8 ～ 1.2g，一日 2 ～ 3 次，4 ～ 8 周为 1 个疗程。儿童、老年人，剂量酌减。②肌内注射：每次 1g，一日 2 ～ 3 次。③静脉注射：每次 4 ～ 6g，一日 2 次。④静脉滴注：用于改善脑代谢，每次 4 ～ 8g，用 250ml 滴注射液稀释后静脉滴注，一日 1 次。<br><br>① Par voie orale : chez des adultes, 0,8 à 1,2 g par fois, 2 à 3 fois par jour, pendant 4 à 8 semaines comme un traitement médical. Chez des enfants et des personnes âgées, diminuer la dose. ② Injection par voie IM : 1g par fois, 2 à 3 fois par jour. ③ Injection par voie IV : 4 à 6g par fois, 2 fois par jour. ④ En perfusion : pour le métabolisme cérébral, 4 à 8g par fois, dissoudre dans 250 ml de liquides par voie IV, perfusion, 1 fois par jour. |

**续 表**

| | |
|---|---|
| 剂型、规格<br>Les formes pharmaceutiques et les spécifications | 片剂：每片 0.4g。<br>分散片：每片 0.8g。<br>胶囊：每粒 0.2g；0.4g。<br>注射剂：每支 1g（5ml）；2g（10ml）；4g（20ml）。<br>氯化钠注射液：250ml（吡拉西坦 8g，氯化钠 2.25g）。<br>Comprimés : 0,4 g par comprimé.<br>Comprimés dispersibles : 0,8g par comprimé.<br>Capsules : 0,2g ou 0,4g par capsule.<br>Injection : 1g (5ml), 2g (10ml) ou 4g (20ml) par solution.<br>Solution de chlorure de sodium : 250 ml (8g de piracétam et 2,25g de chlorure de sodium). |
| 药品名称 Drug Names | 茴拉西坦 Aniracétam |
| 适应证<br>Les indications | 用于治疗脑血管疾病后的记忆功能减退和血管性痴呆，中、老年记忆减退（健忘症），对帕金森病症状有改善作用，用于脑梗死后遗症的情绪不稳定和抑郁状态。<br><br>Ce produit sert à traiter le dysfonctionnement de la mémoire et la démence vasculaire consécutif de la maladie cérébrovasculaire, le déficit de mémoire chez des personnes d'âge moyen et des personnes âgées (l'amnésie). Il permet aussi d'améliorer les symptômes de la maladie de Parkinson. Il est aussi applicable dans le traitement de l'instabilité émotionnelle et de la dépression comme les séquelles de l'infarctus cérébral. |
| 用法、用量<br>Les modes d'emploi et la posologie | 口服：每次 0.2g，一日 3 次。70 岁以上老年人，每次 0.1g，一日 3 次。1～2 个月为 1 个疗程。可根据病情调整用量和疗程。<br><br>Par voie orale : 0,2g par fois, 3 fois par jour. Chez des personnes âgées plus de 70 ans, 0,1g par fois, 3 fois par jour. Pendant 1 à 2 mois comme un traitement médical. Ajuster la dose et la durée du traitement selon les cas. |
| 剂型、规格<br>Les formes pharmaceutiques et les spécifications | 胶囊：每粒 0.1g。<br>片剂：每片 0.05g。<br>Capsules : 0,1g par capsule.<br>Comprimés : 0,05g par comprimé. |
| 药品名称 Drug Names | 奥拉西坦 Oxiracétam |
| 适应证<br>Les indications | 用于轻中度血管性痴呆、老年性痴呆以及脑外伤等症引起的记忆与智能障碍、大脑功能不全。<br>Ce produit sert à traite le déficit de mémoire, la déficience intellectuelle et le dysfonctionnement cérébral causés par la démence vasculaire bénigne et modérée, la démence sénile ainsi que la lésion cérébrale traumatique. |
| 用法、用量<br>Les modes d'emploi et la posologie | 口服：每次 0.8g，一日 2 次；重症每日 2～8g。静脉滴注：每次 4g，一日 1 次，可酌情减量，用前加入到 100～250ml 静脉滴注液中，摇匀。对功能缺失的治疗通常疗程为 2 周，对记忆与智能障碍的治疗通常疗程为 3 周。<br><br>Par voie orale : 0,8g par fois, 2 fois par jour ; chez des patients gravement malades, 2 à 8g par jour. En perfusion : 4g par fois, 1 fois par jour, diminuer la dose selon les cas, dissoudre d'abord dans 100 à 250 ml de liquides par voie IV, agiter avant de l'utiliser. Pour traiter la dysfonction, le traitement dure 2 semaines, alors que pour le déficit de mémoire et la déficience intellectuelle, le traitement dure 3 semaines. |
| 剂型、规格<br>Les formes pharmaceutiques et les spécifications | 片剂：每片 0.4g。<br>注射液：每支 1g（5ml）。<br>Comprimés : 0,4 g par comprimé.<br>Injection : 1g (5ml) par solution. |
| 药品名称 Drug Names | 银杏叶提取物 Sextrait de Ginkgo biloba Feuille |
| 适应证<br>Les indications | 主要用于脑部、外周血管及冠状动脉血管障碍的患者，包括脑卒中、痴呆症、急慢性脑功能不全及其后遗症。对于阿尔茨海默病、血管性痴呆及缓和性痴呆等患者应用本品后，智力可有所提高，但对明显痴呆者作用仍不佳。<br><br>Ce produit sert principalement à traiter les patients souffrant du trouble vasculaire cérébral, périphérique et coronaire, y compris l'accident cérébrovasculaire, la démence, la dysfonction cérébrale aigue et chronique ainsi que leurs séquelles. Chez des patients atteints de la maladie d'Alzheimer, de la démence vasculaire et de la démence modérée, le traitement avec ce produit peut permettre d'augmenter un peu leur intelligence. Mais il est peu efficace dans le traitement de la démence évidente. |

**续　表**

| 用法、用量<br>Les modes d'emploi et la posologie | 口服：每次 1～2 片，一日 3 次。静脉滴注：1～2 支，加入 250ml 或 500ml 输液剂中静脉滴注，一日 1～2 次。本品不同厂家说明书所列剂量并不一致，主要成分的配比也不同，所以需要根据具体说明书使用药物。<br><br>Par voie orale : 1 à 2 comprimés par fois, 3 fois par jour. En perfusion : 1 à 2 solutions, dissoudre dans 250 à 500ml d'infusion, perfusion, 1 à 2 fois par jour. La dose et le rapport de la composante listés dans les modes d'emploi de diverses usines pharmaceutiques ne sont pas compatibles, il faut donc prendre le médicament selon le mode d'emploi donné. |
|---|---|
| 剂型、规格<br>Les formes pharmaceutiques et les spécifications | 片剂：每片 40mg。<br>注射剂：①金纳多：每支 5ml（含银杏叶提取物 17.5mg）。②舒血宁：2ml（含总黄酮醇苷 1.68mg；银杏内酯 A0.12mg）；5ml（含总黄酮醇苷 4.2mg；银杏内酯 A0.30mg）。<br><br>Comprimés : 40mg par comprimé.<br>Injection : ① le ginaton : 5ml par solution (contient 17,5mg d'extrait de Ginkgo biloba). ② Shuxuening : 2ml (1,68mg de glycosides de flavonol et 17,5mg de ginkgolide A) ou 5ml (4,2mg de glycoside de flavonol et 0,30mg de ginkgolide A). |
| 药品名称 Drug Names | 阿米三嗪 / 萝巴新 Almitrine / Raubasine |
| 适应证<br>Les indications | 用于治疗亚急性或慢性脑功能不全，如记忆力下降；缺血性听觉、前庭、视觉障碍；脑血管意外后的功能恢复。<br><br>Ce produit sert à traiter la dysfonction cérébrale subaiguë et chronique, telle que la perte de mémoire ;les troubles auditifs, vestibulaires et visuels ischémiques ; la récupération fonctionnelle après un accident vasculaire cérébral. |
| 用法、用量<br>Les modes d'emploi et la posologie | 口服，每次 1 片，一日 2 次（早、晚服）。维持量一日 1 次，每次 1 片，餐后服。<br><br>Par voie orale, 1 comprimé par fois, 2 fois par jour (le petit matin et le soir). La dose d'entretien, 1 fois par jour, 1 comprimé par fois, après le repas. |
| 剂型、规格<br>Les formes pharmaceutiques et les spécifications | 片剂：每片含二甲磺酸阿米三嗪 30mg，萝巴新 10mg。<br><br>Comprimés : chaque comprimé contient 30mg de diméthanesulfonate d'almitrine et 10mg de raubasine. |
| 药品名称 Drug Names | 吡硫醇 Pyritinol |
| 适应证<br>Les indications | 用于脑震荡综合征、脑外伤后遗症、脑炎及脑膜炎后遗症等引起的头痛、头晕、失眠、记忆力减退、注意力不集中、情绪变化等症状的改善,也可用于脑动脉硬化、老年痴呆等精神症状。<br><br>Il sert à améliorer la céphalée, les vertiges, l'insomnie, la perte de mémoire, le déficit d'attention, les sautes d'humeur causés par le syndrome de commotion cérébrale, les séquelles d'une lésion cérébrale traumatique ainsi queles séquelles de l'encéphalite et de la méningite. Il permet aussi de traiter l'artériosclérose cérébrale et la démence. |
| 用法、用量<br>Les modes d'emploi et la posologie | 口服：成人每次 100～200mg，一日 3 次。小儿每次 50～100mg，一日 3 次。静脉滴注：每次 200～400mg，一日 1 次，用 250ml 静脉滴注液稀释后使用。<br><br>Par voie orale : chez des adultes, 100 à 200mg par fois, 3 fois par jour. Chez des enfants, 50 à 100mg par fois, 3 fois par jour. En perfusion : 200 à 400mg par fois, 1 fois par jour, dissoudre d'abord dans 250 ml de liquides par voie IV avant de l'utiliser. |
| 剂型、规格<br>Les formes pharmaceutiques et les spécifications | 片剂：每片 100mg；200mg。<br>胶囊剂：每粒 100mg。<br>注射剂：每支 100mg（1ml）；200mg（2ml）。<br>盐酸吡硫醇葡萄糖注射液：250ml（盐酸吡硫醇 200mg，葡萄糖 5g）。<br><br>Comprimés : 100mg ou 200mg par comprimé.<br>Capsules : 100 mg par capsule.<br>Injection : 100mg (1ml) ou 200mg (2ml) par solution.<br>La solution de glucose de chlorhydrate de pyritinol : 250ml (200mg de chlorhydrate de pyritinol et 5g de glucose). |

**续　表**

| 药品名称 Drug Names | 小牛血去蛋白提取物 Extrait déprotéinisé du sang de veau |
|---|---|
| 适应证<br>Les indications | ①用于脑卒中、脑外伤、周围血管病及腿部溃疡。②亦可用于皮移植术、烧伤、烫伤、糜烂、创伤、压疮的伤口愈合；放射所引起的皮肤、黏膜损伤。③各种病因引起的角膜溃疡，角膜损伤，酸或碱引起的角膜灼伤，大疱性角膜炎，神经麻痹性角膜炎，角膜和结膜变性等。<br><br>① Ce produit sert à traiter l'accident vasculaire cérébral (AVC), la lésion cérébrale traumatique, la maladie vasculaire périphérique et les ulcères de jambe.<br>② La cicatrisation des plaies de la greffe de peau, des brûlures, de l'érosion, des traumatismes et des décubitus ; lésions de la peau et de la muqueuse causées par la radiation.<br>③ Les ulcères de la cornée, la lésion de la cornée, lesbrûlures de la cornéeprovoquées par l'acide ou alcalin,la kératite bulleuse,la kératite neuro-paralytique, ainsi que la dégénérescence cornée et conjonctive. |
| 用法、用量<br>Les modes d'emploi et la posologie | 口服：每次 1 ～ 2 片，一日 3 次。整片吞服，一疗程 4 ～ 6 周。静脉注射或缓慢肌内注射：初期每日 10 ～ 20ml，进一步治疗剂量每日 5ml。静脉注射：10 ～ 50ml 加入静脉注射液 250ml 中滴注。皮肤外用：在保证创口或创面清洁的情况下外用。轻者可一日 1 次，涂于创面处；重者可一日 2 ～ 6 次，或酌情增加次数。眼科外用：滴于眼部患处，每次 1 滴，一日 3 ～ 4 次，或视病情而定。口腔外用：涂抹于患处一日 3 ～ 5 次，其中 1 次在睡前使用。<br><br>Par voie orale : 1 à 2 comprimés par fois, 3 fois par jour. Avaler un comprimé en entier, et un traitement médical dure 4 à 6 semaines. Injection par voie IV ou IM lente : la dose initiale, 10 à 20ml par jour, ensuite, 5ml par jour. En perfusion : dissoudre 10 à 50ml de produit dans 250 ml de liquides par voie IV, perfusion. L'usage externe pour la peau : veiller à nettoyer la plaie ou les blessures avant de l'utiliser. Chez des patients légèrement malades, 1 fois par jour, l'appliquer sur la zone touchée ; chez des patients gravement malades, 2 à 6 fois par jour, possible d'augmenter les fois selon les cas. L'usage externe ophtalmique : appliquer sur la zone touchée, 1 goutte par fois, 3 à 4 fois par jour, ou selon les cas. L'usage externe orale : appliquer sur la zone touchée, 3 à 5 fois par jours, dont une fois avant le sommeil. |
| 剂型、规格<br>Les formes pharmaceutiques et les spécifications | 片剂：每片 200mg。<br>注射剂：每支 80mg（2ml）；200mg（5ml）；400mg（10ml）。<br>软膏：10%（20g：2.0g）。<br>眼凝胶制剂：20%（5g：1g）。<br>口腔膏：5%（5g：0.25g）。<br><br>Comprimés : 200mg par comprimé.<br>Injection : 80mg (2ml), 200mg (5ml) ou 400mg (10ml) par solution.<br>La pommade : 10 % (20g : 2,0g).<br>Les gels pour les yeux : 20% (5g : 1g).<br>Pâte orale : 5% (5g : 0,25g). |
| 药品名称 Drug Names | 胞磷胆碱 Citicoline |
| 适应证<br>Les indications | 主要用于急性颅脑外伤和脑手术所引起的意识障碍，以及脑卒中而致偏瘫的患者，也可用于耳鸣及神经性耳聋。对颅内出血引起意识障碍效果较差。<br><br>Ce produit sert à traiter la perturbation de la conscience causée par la chirurgie de lésion cérébrale traumatique aiguë et la chirurgie cérébrale, ainsi que les patients victimes d'AVC qui a causé une hémiplégie. Il est aussi applicable dans le traitement des acouphènes et de la surdité nerveuse. Mais il est peu efficace dans le traitement de la perturbation de la conscience causée par l'hémorragie intracrânienne. |
| 用法、用量<br>Les modes d'emploi et la posologie | 静脉滴注：一日 0.25 ～ 0.5g，用 5% 或 10% 葡萄糖注射液稀释后缓缓滴注，每 5 ～ 10 日为 1 个疗程。单纯静脉注射：每次 0.1 ～ 0.2g。肌内注射：一日 0.1 ～ 0.3g，分 1 ～ 2 次注射，脑出血急性期不宜大剂量应用。一般不采用肌内注射，若用时应经常更换注射部位。口服：每次 0.2g，一日 3 次。用于维持期治疗可为一次 0.1g，一日 3 次口服。<br><br>En perfusion : 0,25 à 0,5g par jour, dissoudre dans la solutionde glucose à 5 % ou à 10 %, la perfusion lente, pendant 5 à 10 jours comme un traitement médical. L'injection par voie IV simple : 0,1 à 0,2g par fois. L'injection par voie IM : 0,1 à 0,3g par jour, à travers 1 à 2 fois. Pendant la phase aigue de l'hémorragie cérébrale, ne pas utiliser une dose importante. En général, ne pas administrer par voie IM. En cas d'administration par voie IM, changer régulièrement le site d'injection. Par voie orale : 0,2g par fois, 3 fois par jour. Pour le traitement d'entretien, 0,1g par fois, 3 fois par jour, par voie orale. |

**续　表**

| | |
|---|---|
| 剂型、规格<br>Les formes pharmaceutiques et les spécifications | 注射剂：每支 0.2g（2ml）；0.25g（2ml）。<br>片剂：每片 0.2g。<br>胶囊剂：每粒 0.1g。<br>Injection : 0,2g (2ml) ou 0,25g (2ml) par solution.<br>Comprimés : 0,2g par comprimé.<br>Capsules : 0,1g par capsule. |
| **药品名称 Drug Names** | 单唾液酸四己糖神经节苷脂 Monosialate de tétrahéxosyle Ganglioside |
| 适应证<br>Les indications | 用于脑脊髓创伤、脑血管意外，可用于帕金森病。<br>Ce produit sert à traiter le traumatisme céphalo rachidien et l'AVC, ainsi que la maladie de Parkinson. |
| 用法、用量<br>Les modes d'emploi et la posologie | 每日 20～40mg，一次或分次肌内注射或缓慢静脉注射。急性期：每日100mg，静脉滴注；2～3周后改为维持量，每日 20～40mg，一般 6 周。对帕金森病，首剂量 500～1000mg，静脉滴注；第 2 日起每日 200mg，皮下、肌内注射或静脉滴注，一般用至 18 周。<br>20 à 40mg par jour, à travers 1 à plusieurs fois, injection par voie IM ou injection par voie IV lente. La phase aigue : 100mg par jour, en perfusion ; 2 à 3 semaines après, la dose d'entretien, 20 à 40 mg par jour, pendant 6 semaines. Pour la maladie de Parkinson, la dose initiale, 500 à 1 000 mg, en perfusion ; à partir du deuxième jour, 200 mg par jour, l'injection sous-cutanée ou par voie IM ou en perfusion, pendant 18 semaines en général. |
| 剂型、规格<br>Les formes pharmaceutiques et les spécifications | 注射液：每支 20mg（2ml）；100mg（5ml）。<br>粉针剂：每支 40mg；100mg。<br>Injection : 20mg (2ml) ou 100mg (5ml) par solution.<br>Poudre : 40mg ou 100mg par solution. |
| **药品名称 Drug Names** | 脑蛋白水解物 Hydrolysats de protéines du cerveau |
| 适应证<br>Les indications | 适用于尤以注意及记忆障碍的器质性脑病性综合征，原发性痴呆（如老年性痴呆），血管性痴呆（如多发梗死性痴呆），混合性痴呆，卒中、颅脑手术后的脑功能障碍，神经衰弱及衰竭症状。<br>Ce produit est utilisé dans le traitement du syndrome cérébral organique lié au déficit d'attention et de mémoire, de la démence primaire (telle que la démence sénile), de la démence vasculaire (telle que la démence multi-infarctus), de la démence mixte, de la dysfonction cérébrale après l'AVC ou une chirurgie cérébrale, ainsi que de la neurasthénie et de l'épuisement nerveux. |
| 用法、用量<br>Les modes d'emploi et la posologie | 成人常用 10～30ml 稀释于 5% 葡萄糖或生理盐水 250ml 中缓慢滴注，60～120 分钟滴完，一日 1 次，每疗程注射 10～20 次，依病情而定。轻微病例或经大剂量用药后为保持疗效者，可用肌注、皮下或静脉注射，每次 1～5ml：皮下注射不超过每次 2ml，肌内注射不超过每次 5ml；静脉注射不超过每次 10ml。应用 10～20 次，以后每周 2～3 次，可重复几个疗程，直至临床表现不再改善为止。<br>Chez des adultes, dissoudre généralement 10 à 30 ml de produit dans 250ml de solution de glucose à 5 % ou de solution saline, perfusion lente, pendant 60 à 120 minutes, 1 fois par jour. Un traitement médical comporte 10 à 20 injections, selon les cas. Chez des cas bénins ou des patients qui veulent maintenir le traitement après avoir pris une dose importante, appliquer les injections sous-cutanées, par voie IM ou IV, 1 à 5ml par fois : pour l'injection sous-cutanée, 2ml au maximum par fois ; pour l'injection par voie IM, ne pas dépasser 5ml par fois ; pour l'injection par voie IV, ne pas dépasser 10ml par fois. Appliquer 10 à 20 fois, avant de prendre 2 à 3 fois par semaine, pendant quelques traitements médicaux, jusqu'à ce que les performances cliniques ne s'améliorent plus. |
| 剂型、规格<br>Les formes pharmaceutiques et les spécifications | 注射液：每支 2ml；5ml；10ml。<br>Injection : 2ml. 5ml ou 10ml par solution. |

**续　表**

| 药品名称 Drug Names | 赖氨酸 Lysine |
|---|---|
| 适应证<br>Les indications | ①用于颅脑损伤综合征、脑血管病、记忆力减退等。②赖氨酸缺乏引起的小儿食欲缺乏、营养不良及脑发育不全等。<br><br>① Applicable dans le traitement du syndrome de lésion cérébrale traumatique, des maladies crérébrovasculaires, et de la perte de mémoire. ② Ce produit sert à traiter la perte d'appétit pédiatrique, la malnutrition et l'hypoplasie cérébrale chez des enfants causées par le manque de lysine. |
| 用法、用量<br>Les modes d'emploi et la posologie | 口服：每次 3g，一日 1 次，10～15 日为 1 个疗程。静脉滴注：一日 1 次，每次 3g，稀释于 250ml 静脉滴注液中缓慢滴注，20 次为 1 个疗程。<br><br>Par voie orale : 3g par fois, 1 fois par jour, pendant 10 à 15 jours comme un traitement médical. En perfusion : 1 fois par jour, 3g par fois, dissoudre dans 250 ml de liquides par voie IV, perfusion lente. Un traitement médical comprend 20 fois. |
| 剂型、规格<br>Les formes pharmaceutiques et les spécifications | 散剂：每袋 3g。<br>注射液：每支 3g（10ml）。<br>Poudre : 3g par sachet.<br>Injection : 3g (10ml) par solution. |

8.14　麻醉药及其辅助用药 Anesthésiques et médicaments auxiliaires

| 药品名称 Drug Names | 恩氟烷 Enflurane |
|---|---|
| 适应证<br>Les indications | 应用于符合全身麻醉（此时浓度 0.5% 即足够，3% 为极限），可与多种静脉全身麻醉药和全身麻醉辅助用药联用或合用。<br><br>Ce produit est utilisé dans l'anesthésie générale (la concentration de 0,5 % suffit, la concentration maximale est de 3 %). Il peut être utilisé en association avec des anesthésiques généraux intraveineux et des anesthésiques généraux adjuvants. |
| 用法、用量<br>Les modes d'emploi et la posologie | 使用量应根据患者的具体情况而定。<br>L'administration du medicament doit etre adaptée aux conditions particulières du patient. |
| 剂型、规格<br>Les formes pharmaceutiques et les spécifications | 液体剂：每瓶 100ml；150ml；250ml。<br>Un agent liquide: 100ml, 150ml ou 250ml, par bouteille. |

| 药品名称 Drug Names | 异氟烷 Isoflurane |
|---|---|
| 适应证<br>Les indications | 可用于各种手术的麻醉。<br>Ce produit est utilisé dans l'anesthésie de diverses chirurgies. |
| 用法、用量<br>Les modes d'emploi et la posologie | 成人诱导麻醉时吸入气体内浓度一般为 1.5%～3%；维持麻醉时气体内浓度为 1%～1.5%。麻醉较深时对循环及呼吸系统均有抑制作用。骨骼肌松弛作用亦较好。<br><br>Lors de l'induction de l'anesethésie chez des adultes, la concentration du gaz inhalé est de 1,5 % à 3 % ; lors de l'entretien de l'anesthésie, la contration du gaz est de 1 % à 1,5 %. Lors d'une anesthésie profonde, les systèmes circulatoires et respiratoires sont aussi inhibés. Ce produit a un effet myorelaxant. |
| 剂型、规格<br>Les formes pharmaceutiques et les spécifications | 液体剂：每瓶 100ml，250ml。<br>Un agent liquide: 100ml, 250ml par bouteille. |

| 药品名称 Drug Names | 七氟烷 Sévoflurane |
|---|---|
| 适应证<br>Les indications | 作为全身麻醉药应用。<br>Il sert d'anesthésique général. |

续　表

| | |
|---|---|
| 用法、用量<br>Les modes d'emploi et la posologie | 麻醉诱导时，以 50% ～ 70% 氧化亚氮与本品 2.5% ～ 4% 吸入。使用睡眠量的静脉麻醉时，本品的诱导量通常为 0.5% ～ 5%。麻醉维持，应以最低有效浓度维持外科麻醉状态，常为 4% 以下。<br><br>Lors de l'induction de l'anesthésie, inhaler le protoxyde d'azote à 50 % à 70 % et le sévoflurane à 2,5 % à 4 %. Lors de l'anesthésie intraveineuse utilisant la quantité de sommeil, la concentration de ce produit pour l'induction est de 0,5 % à 5 %. Pour l'entretien de l'anesthésie, il faut utiliser la concentration efficace la moins importante pour maintenir l'anesthésie, soit moins de 4 % en général. |
| 剂型、规格<br>Les formes pharmaceutiques et les spécifications | 吸入用七氟烷：120ml；250ml。<br>Le sévoflurane pour inhalation : 120ml ; 250 ml. |
| **药品名称 Drug Names** | 硫喷妥钠 Thiopental sodique |
| 适应证<br>Les indications | 常用于静脉麻醉、诱导麻醉、基础麻醉、抗惊厥以及复合麻醉等。<br>Il est souvent utilisé dans l'anesthésie intraveineuse, l'induction de l'anesthésie, l'anesthésie de base, l'anticonvulsivant et l'anesthésie composite. |
| 用法、用量<br>Les modes d'emploi et la posologie | ①静脉麻醉：一般多用 5% 或 2.5% 溶液，缓慢注入。成人，一次 4 ～ 8mg/kg，经 30 秒左右即进入麻醉，神志完全消失，但肌肉松弛不完全，也不能随意调节，麻醉深度，故多用于小手术。如患者有呼吸快、发声、移动等现象，即为苏醒的表现，可再注射少量以持续麻醉。极量：一次 1g（即 5% 溶液 20ml）。②基础麻醉：用于小儿、甲状腺功能亢进症及精神紧张患者。成人，肌内注射，每次 0.5g，以 2.5% 溶液，做深部肌内注射。③诱导麻醉：一般用 2.5% 溶液缓慢静脉注射，1 次 0.3g（1 次不超过 0.5g），继以乙醚吸入。④抗惊厥：每次静脉注射 0.05 ～ 0.1g。<br><br>① L'anesthésie intraveineuse : utiliser souvent la solution à 5 % ou à 2,5 %, injection lente. Chez des adultes, 4 à 8 mg/kg par fois. Dans à peu près 30 secondes, les patients sont en anesthésie, avec la conscience complètement perdue. Mais la relaxation musculaire n'est pas complète. On ne peut pas ajuster la profondeur de l'anesthésie. Ce produit est donc applicable dans la chirurgie mineure. La respiration rapide, le son et le déplacement sont tous des signes de l'éveille, il faut alors injecter une dose mineure du produit pour maintenir l'anesthésie. La dose maximale : 1g par fois (à savoir 20ml de solution à 5 %). ② L'anesthésie de base : appliquée chez des enfants, des patients souffrant de l'hyperthyroïdie et les patients nerveux. Chez des adultes, injection par voie IM, 0,5g par fois, utiliser la solution à 2,5 %, injection par voie IM profonde. ③ L'induction de l'anesthésie : utiliser la solution à 2,5 % pour injection par voie IV profonde, 0,3g par fois (ne pas dépasser 0,5g par fois), ensuite inhaler l'éther. ④ L'anticonvulsivant : 0,05 à 0,1g par fois, par voie IV. |
| 剂型、规格<br>Les formes pharmaceutiques et les spécifications | 注射用硫喷妥钠：每支 0.5g；1g（含无水碳酸钠 6%）。<br>Le thiopental sodique pour injection : 0,5g ou 1g par solution (contient 6 % decarbonate de sodium anhydre). |
| **药品名称 Drug Names** | 氯胺酮 Kétamine |
| 适应证<br>Les indications | 用于：①各种小手术或诊断操作时，可单独使用本品进行麻醉。对于需要肌肉松弛的手术，应加用肌肉松弛剂；对于内脏牵引较重的手术，应配合其他药物以减少牵引反应。②作为其他全身麻醉的诱导剂使用。③辅助麻醉性能较弱的麻醉剂进行麻醉，或与其他全身或局部麻醉复合使用。<br><br>Ce produit est utilisé dans les cas suivants : ① Lors de chirurgies mineures ou d'opérations de diagnostic, le produit peut être utilisé seul dans l'anesthésie ; lors de la chirurgie exigeant la relaxation musculaire, il faut y ajouter les myorelaxants ; lors de la chirurgie dont la traction viscérale est trop lourde, il faut l'utiliser en association avec d'autres médicaments pour réduire la traction viscérale. ② Il sert d'inducteur à d'autres anesthésiques généraux. ③ Il sert d'anesthésique adjuvant à des anesthésiques moins performants ou il est utilisé en association avec d'autres anesthésiques généraux et locaux. |

**续　表**

| | |
|---|---|
| 用法、用量<br>Les modes d'emploi et la posologie | ①成人常用量：全麻诱导，静脉注射 1～2mg/kg，注射应较慢（60 秒以上）。全麻维持，一次静脉注射 0.5～1mg/kg。②极量：静脉注射每分钟 4mg/kg；肌内注射，一次 13mg/kg。<br>① La dose usuelle chez des adultes : l'induction de l'anesthésie générale, 1 à 2 mg/kg, par voie IV, injection lente (pendant 60 secondes au moins). Le maintien de l'anesthésie générale, 0,5 à 1 mg/kg par fois, par voie IV. ② La dose maximale : 4 mg/kg par minute, injection par voie IV ; 13 mg/kg par fois, injection par voie IM. |
| 剂型、规格<br>Les formes pharmaceutiques et les spécifications | 注射液：100mg（2ml）；100mg（1ml）；200mg（20ml）。<br>Injection : 100mg (2ml) ; 100mg (1ml) ou 200mg (20ml). |
| 药品名称 Drug Names | 依托咪酯 Etomidate |
| 适应证<br>Les indications | 可用于诱导麻醉。<br>Il est utilisé dans l'induction de l'anesthésie. |
| 用法、用量<br>Les modes d'emploi et la posologie | 成人：0.3mg/kg，于 15～60 秒静脉注射完毕。<br>Chez des adultes : 0,3 mg/kg, injection par voie IV en 15 à 60 secondes. |
| 剂型、规格<br>Les formes pharmaceutiques et les spécifications | 注射液：每支 20mg（10ml）。<br>Injection : 20mg (10ml) par solution. |
| 药品名称 Drug Names | 羟丁酸钠 Hydroxybutyrate sodique |
| 适应证<br>Les indications | 常用于全身麻醉或诱导麻醉，以及局麻、腰麻的辅助用药，适用于老年人、儿童及脑、神经外科手术，外伤、烧伤患者的麻醉。<br>Ce produit est souvent appliqué dans l'anesthésie générale ou l'induction de l'anesthésie. Il sert aussi d'anesthésique adjuvant à l'anesthésie locale et à la rachianesthésie. Il est applicable dans l'anesthésie chez des personnes âgées, des enfants, des patients recevant la chirurgie cérébrale et la neurochirurgie, ainsi que des patients atteints de traumatisme et de brûlures. |
| 用法、用量<br>Les modes d'emploi et la posologie | ①诱导麻醉：一次静脉注射，成人 60mg/kg；注射速度 1g/min。②维持麻醉：静脉注射，一次 12～80mg/kg。③极量：一次总量 300mg/kg。<br>① L'induction de l'anesthésie : injection par voie IV, une fois, chez des adultes, 60 mg/kg ; la vitesse de l'injection, 1g par minute. ② Le maintien de l'anesthésie：injection par voie IV, 12 à 80 mg/kg, une fois. ③ La dose maximale : 300 mg/kg, une fois. |
| 剂型、规格<br>Les formes pharmaceutiques et les spécifications | 注射液：每支 2.5g（10ml）。<br>Injection : 2,5g (10ml) par solution. |
| 药品名称 Drug Names | 丙泊酚 Propofol |
| 适应证<br>Les indications | 用于全身麻醉的诱导和维持。常与硬膜外或脊髓麻醉同时应用，也常与镇痛药、肌松药及吸入性麻醉药同用。适用于门诊患者。<br>Il est utilisé dans l'induction et l'entretien de l'anesthésie générale. Il souvent utilisé en association avec l'anesthésie péridurale ou rachianesthésie, ainsi que des analgésiques, des relaxants musculaires et des anesthésiques inhalés. Il est applicable dans le traitement des malades ambulatoires. |
| 用法、用量<br>Les modes d'emploi et la posologie | 静脉注射。诱导麻醉：每 10 秒钟注射 40mg，直至产生麻醉。大多数成人用量 2～2.5mg/kg。维持麻醉：常用量为每分钟 0.1～0.2mg/kg。<br>L'injection par voie IV. L'induction de l'anesthésie : injecter 40 mg toutes les 10 secondes, jusqu'à l'anesthésie. Chez la plupart des adultes, 2 à 2,5 mg/kg. L'anesthésie d'entretien : la dose usuelle, 0,1 à 0,2 mg/kg par minute. |

**续　表**

| | |
|---|---|
| 剂型、规格<br>Les formes pharmaceutiques et les spécifications | 注射液：每支 200mg（20ml）；500mg（50ml）；1g（100ml）。<br>丙泊酚中 / 长链脂肪乳注射液：200mg（20ml）。<br>Injection : 200mg (20ml), 500mg (50ml) ou 1g (100ml) par solution.<br>L'émulsion de graisse de propofol à chaîne moyenne ou longue. |
| **药品名称 Drug Names** | 普鲁卡因 Procaïne |
| 适应证<br>Les indications | 主要用于浸润麻醉、蛛网膜下腔阻滞麻醉、神经传导阻滞麻醉和用于治疗某些损伤和炎症，可使发炎损伤部位的症状得到一定的缓解（封闭疗法）。还可用于纠正四肢血管舒缩功能障碍。<br><br>Ce produit est utilisé dans l'anesthésie locale par infiltration, la rachianesthésie, l'anesthésie tronculaire, ainsi que le traitement des lésions et de l'inflammation. Il permet de soulager les symptômes des lésions inflammatoires (le traitement par blocage). Il sert aussi à corriger la dysfonction vasomotrice des membres. |
| 用法、用量<br>Les modes d'emploi et la posologie | ①浸润麻醉，溶液浓度多为 0.25%～0.5%（口腔科有时用其4%的溶液），每次用量0.05～0.25g，每小时不可超过 1.5g。其麻醉时间短，可加入少量肾上腺素 [1 :（100 000～200 000）] 以延长作用的时间。②蛛网膜下腔阻滞麻醉，一次量不宜超过 0.15g，用 5% 溶液，约可麻醉 1 小时，主要用于腹部以下需时不长的手术。③ "封闭疗法"，将 0.25%～0.5% 溶液注射于与病变有关的神经周围或病变部位。<br><br>① Pour l'anesthésie locale par infiltration, la concentration de la solution est de 0,25 % à 0,5 % (en dentisterie, parfois, 4 %), 0,05 à 0,25g par fois, ne pas dépasser 1,5g par h. Son effet est court, c'est possible d'ajouter l'épinéphrine (1 : 100000~200000) pour prolonger la durée de l'anesthésie. ② Pour la rachianesthésie, ne pas dépasser 0,15g par fois, utiliser la solution à 5 %, pour avoir une anesthésie pendant 1 h. Il est principalement appliqué à la chirurgie liée à la partie inférieure à l'abdomen qui ne dure pas longtemps. ③ Le traitement par blocage, injecter la solution à 0,25% à 0,5% autour des nerfs liés aux lésions ou sur des lésions. |
| 剂型、规格<br>Les formes pharmaceutiques et les spécifications | 注射液：每支 100mg（20ml）；50mg（20ml）；100mg（10ml）；40mg（2ml）。<br>注射用盐酸普鲁卡因：每支 150mg；1g。<br>Injection : 100mg (20ml), 50mg (20ml), 100mg (10ml) ou 40mg (2ml).<br>Chlorhydrate de procaïne pour injection : 150mg ou 1g par solution. |
| **药品名称 Drug Names** | 丁卡因 Tétracaïne |
| 适应证<br>Les indications | 用于黏膜表面麻醉、神经阻滞麻醉、硬膜外麻醉和蛛网膜下隙麻醉。<br><br>Ce produit est utilisé dans l'anesthésie sur la moqueuse, l'anesthésie de bloc, l'anesthésie péridurale et la rachianesthésie. |
| 用法、用量<br>Les modes d'emploi et la posologie | ①黏膜麻醉：眼科用 0.5%～1% 溶液，鼻喉科用 1%～2% 溶液，总量不得超过 20ml。应用时应于每 3ml 中加入 0.1% 盐酸肾上腺素溶液 1 滴。浸润麻醉 0.025%～0.03% 溶液。②神经阻滞用 0.1%～0.3% 溶液。③蛛网膜下隙麻醉时用 10～15ml 与脑脊液混合后注入。④硬膜外麻醉用 0.15%～0.3% 溶液，与利多卡因合用时最高浓度为 0.3%。极量：浸润麻醉、神经传导阻滞，一次 0.1g。<br><br>① Pour l'anesthésie sur la moqueuse : en ophtalmologie, utiliser la solution à 0,5 % à 1 %, en rhino-laryngologie, utiliser la solution à 1 % à 2 %, ne pas dépasser 20ml au total. Il faut ajouter une goutte de solution de chlorhydrate de l'épinéphrine à 0,1 % dans 3ml de produit. Pour l'anesthésie d'infiltration, utiliser la solution à 0,025% à 0,03%. ② Pour l'anesthésie de bloc, utiliser la solution à 0,1 % à 0,3 %. ③ Pour la rachianesthésie, mélanger 10 à 15ml de produit et le liquide céphalo-rachidien avant l'injection. ④ Pour l'anesthésie péridurale, utiliser la solution à 0,15 % à 0,3 %, lors de l'utilisation en association avec la lidocaïne, la concentration de la solution ne dépasse par 0,3 %. La dose maximale: pour l'anesthésie par infiltration et le blocage nerveux, 0,1g par fois. |
| 剂型、规格<br>Les formes pharmaceutiques et les spécifications | 注射液：每支 50mg（5ml）。<br>注射用盐酸丁卡因：10mg；15mg；20mg；50mg。<br>盐酸丁卡因凝胶：1.5g；70mg。<br>Injection : 50mg (5ml) par solution.<br>Le chlorhydrate de tétracaïne pour injection : 10mg, 15mg, 20mg ou 50mg.<br>Le gel de chlorhydrate de tétracaine : 1,5g : 70mg. |

**续　表**

| 药品名称 Drug Names | 利多卡因 Lidocaïne |
| --- | --- |
| 适应证<br>Les indications | 主要用于阻滞麻醉及硬膜外麻醉。也用于室性心律失常，如室性心动过速及频发室性早搏。<br>Ce produit est principalement utilisé dans l'anesthésie de bloc et l'anesthésie péridurale. Il est aussi applicable dans le traitement des arythmies ventriculaires, telles que la tachycardie ventriculaire et les fréquentes contractions ventriculaires prématurées. |
| 用法、用量<br>Les modes d'emploi et la posologie | ①局部麻醉：阻滞麻醉用 1% ～ 2% 溶液，每次用量不宜超过 0.4g。表面麻醉用 2% ～ 4% 溶液，喷雾或蘸药贴敷，一次不超过 100mg，也可以 2% 胶浆剂抹于食管、咽喉气管或导尿管的外壁；妇女做阴道检查时可用棉花签蘸 5 ～ 7ml 于局部。尿道扩张术或膀胱镜检查时用量 200 ～ 400mg。气雾剂或喷雾剂 2% ～ 4%，供作内镜检查用，每次 2%10 ～ 30ml，4%5 ～ 15ml。浸润麻醉用 0.25% ～ 0.5% 溶液，每小时用量不超过 0.4g。硬膜外麻醉用 1% ～ 2% 溶液，每次用量不超过 0.5g。②心律失常。<br>① L'anesthésie locale : pour l'anesthésie de bloc, la solution à 1 % à 2 %, ne pas dépasser 0,4g par fois. Pour l'anesthésie superficielle, utiliser la solution à 2 % à 4 %, en vaporisation ou en collage, ne pas dépasser 100mg par fois, ou appliquer les mucilages à 2 % à la paroi externe de l'œsophage, de la trachée ou du cathéter ; lors de l'examen vaginal, appliquer 5 à 7 ml de produit avec un coton-tige sur la zone touchée. Lors de la dilatation de l'urètre ou de la cystoscopie, appliquer 200 à 400mg. L'aérosol à 2 % à 4 % est appliqué pour l'endoscopie, 10 à 30 ml à 2 % par fois, 5 à 15ml à 4 % par fois. Pour l'anesthésie locale par infiltration, utiliser la solution à 0,25 % à 0,5 %, ne pas dépasser 0,4g par h. Pour l'anesthésie péridurale, utiliser la solution à 1 % à 2 %, ne pas dépasser 0,5g par fois. ② L'arythmie. |
| 剂型、规格<br>Les formes pharmaceutiques et les spécifications | 注射液：每支 0.1g（5ml）；0.4g（20ml）。<br>胶浆剂：2%。<br>盐酸利多卡因气雾剂：2%；4%。<br>Injection : 0,1g (5ml) ou 0,4g (20ml) par solution.<br>Mucilages : 2 %.<br>L'aérosol de chlorhydrate de lidocaïne : 2 % ou 4 %. |
| 药品名称 Drug Names | 布比卡因 Bupivacaïne |
| 适应证<br>Les indications | 浸润麻醉用；神经传导阻滞麻醉。<br>Ce produit est utilisé dans l'anesthésie locale par infiltration et l'anesthésie tronculaire. |
| 用法、用量<br>Les modes d'emploi et la posologie | 浸润麻醉用 0.1% ～ 0.25% 溶液；神经传导阻滞用 0.5% ～ 0.75% 溶液。一次极量 200mg，一日极量 400mg。<br>l'anesthésie locale par infiltration utilise la solution à 0,1 % à 0,25 % ; pour l'anesthésie tronculaire, la solution à 0,5 % à 0,75 %. La dose maximale, 200mg par fois, 400mg par jour. |
| 剂型、规格<br>Les formes pharmaceutiques et les spécifications | 注射液：每支 12.5mg（5ml）；25mg（5ml）；37.5mg（5ml）。<br>Injection : 12,5 mg (5ml), 25mg (5ml), 37,5mg (5ml) par solution. |
| 药品名称 Drug Names | 罗哌卡因 Ropivacaïne |
| 适应证<br>Les indications | 用于区域组织麻醉和硬膜外麻醉；也可用于区域组织镇痛，如硬膜外术后或分娩镇痛。<br>Ce produit est appliqué dans l'anesthésie régionale, et l'anesthésie péridurale ; il est aussi applicable dans l'analgésie régionale, telle que l'analgésie après la chirurgie péridurale ou l'analgésie utilisée pour un accouchement. |
| 用法、用量<br>Les modes d'emploi et la posologie | 区域组织麻醉和硬膜外麻醉：0.5% ～ 1% 溶液。一次最大剂量为 200mg。区域组织镇痛：0.2% 溶液。<br>Pour l'anesthésie régionale, et l'anesthésie péridurale : la solution à 0,5 % à 1 %. La dose maximale est de 200mg par fois. Pour l'analgésie régionale : la solution à 0,2 %. |
| 剂型、规格<br>Les formes pharmaceutiques et les spécifications | 注射液：20mg（10ml）；40mg（20ml）；75mg（10ml）；150mg（20ml）；100mg（10ml）；200mg（200ml）。<br>La solution : 20mg (10ml), 40mg (20ml), 75mg (10ml), 150mg (20ml), 100mg (10ml) ou 200mg (200ml). |

**续　表**

| 药品名称 Drug Names | 达克罗宁 Dyclonine |
| --- | --- |
| 适应证<br>Les indications | 对黏膜穿透力强，作用迅速，可做表面麻醉。对皮肤有止痛、止痒及杀菌作用，可用于烧伤、擦伤、痒疹、虫咬伤、痔瘘、溃疡、压疮以及镜检前的准备。<br><br>Comme ce produit est efficace dans la pénétration des muqueuses avec une action rapide, il est applicable dans l'anesthésie superficielle. Il permet l'analgésie, l'antiprurigineux et la stérilisation de la peau. Il est aussi applicable dans le traitement des brûlures, du prurigo, des piqûres d'insectes, des hémorroides, des ulcères, des escarres ainsi que dans la préparation avant un examenmicroscopique. |
| 用法、用量<br>Les modes d'emploi et la posologie | 多制成 1% 的软膏、乳膏或 0.5% 的溶液供用。<br><br>Il est souvent fabriqué en pommade à 1 %, en crème ou en injection à 0,5 %. |
| 剂型、规格<br>Les formes pharmaceutiques et les spécifications | 软膏：1%；乳膏：1%；溶液：0.5%。<br><br>Ouguent: 1%; Crèmes: 1%; La solution: 0.5%. |
| 药品名称 Drug Names | 泮库溴铵 Bromure de Pancuronium |
| 适应证<br>Les indications | 主要用作外科手术麻醉的辅助用药（气管插管和肌松）。<br><br>Il sert de médicament adjuvant à l'anesthésie de la chirurgie (l'intubation trachéale et les myorelaxants). |
| 用法、用量<br>Les modes d'emploi et la posologie | 静脉注射。成人常用量 40～100μg/kg。与乙醚、氟烷合用时应酌减剂量。<br><br>Injection par voie IV. Chez des adultes, la dose usuelle, 40 à 100μg/kg. En cas d'utilisation en association avec l'éther et l'halothane, il faut diminuer la dose du bromure de pancuronium. |
| 剂型、规格<br>Les formes pharmaceutiques et les spécifications | 注射液：每支 4mg（2ml）。<br><br>Injection : 4mg (2ml) par solution. |
| 药品名称 Drug Names | 罗库溴铵 Bromure de Rocuronium |
| 适应证<br>Les indications | 用于气管插管，也可用于各种手术中肌松的维持。<br><br>Il est utilisé dans l'intubation trachéale et aussi dans le maintien des myorelaxants des chirurgies de toutes sortes. |
| 用法、用量<br>Les modes d'emploi et la posologie | 插管：0.6mg/kg 单次静脉注射。维持量：0.15mg/kg，单次静脉注射；每分钟 5～10μg/kg 连续静脉滴注。吸入麻醉下应适当减量。<br><br>L'intubation : 0,6 mg/kg, une fois, injection par voie IV. La dose d'entretien : 0,15 mg/kg, une fois, par voie IV ; 5 à 10 μg/kg, en perfusion continue. Diminuer la dose en cas d'anesthésie par inhalation. |
| 剂型、规格<br>Les formes pharmaceutiques et les spécifications | 注射液：每支 50mg（5ml）；100mg（10ml）。<br><br>Injection : 50mg (5ml) ou 100mg (10ml) par solution. |
| 药品名称 Drug Names | 维库溴铵 Bromure de Vécuronium |
| 适应证<br>Les indications | 为中效非去极化型肌松药。肌松效应及用途等均似于泮库溴铵，但稍强，持续时间为泮库溴铵的 1/3～1/2。<br><br>Ce produit sert de myorelaxants non dépolarisantsà moyen terme. Son effet et utilisation en matière de relaxant musculaire est similaire au bromure de pancuronium, mais plus fort, avec 1/3 à 1/2 de la durée du bromure de celui-ci. |
| 用法、用量<br>Les modes d'emploi et la posologie | 静脉注射，常用量为 70～100μg/kg。<br><br>Injection par voie IV, la dose usuelle, 70 à 100μg/kg. |

**续　表**

| 剂型、规格 Les formes pharmaceutiques et les spécifications | 注射用维库溴铵：每支 4mg，以所附溶剂溶解后应用。<br><br>Le bromure de vécuronium pour injection : 4mg par solution, administré après la dilution avec le solvant proposé. |
| --- | --- |
| 药品名称 Drug Names | 阿库氯铵 Chlorure d'Alcuronium |
| 适应证 Les indications | 为去极化型肌松药，其特点与泮库溴铵相似，其效应比筒箭毒碱强 1.5 ～ 2 倍。静脉注射后肌松起效快（30 秒），2 ～ 3 分钟达高峰，维持 20 ～ 30 分钟。停药后恢复亦快。<br><br>En tant que myorelaxant dépolarisant, sa caratéristique est similaire au bromure de pancuronium, son effet est 1,5 à 2 fois plus fort que la tubocurarine. Administré par voie IV, ce produit peut prendre effet rapidement (en 30 secondes), et peut atteindre le pic en 2 à 3 minutes, maintenir son effet pendant 20 à 30 minutes. On reprend aussi rapidemen après l'arrêt de l'administration. |
| 用法、用量 Les modes d'emploi et la posologie | 静脉注射：首次剂量为 150μg/kg，随后为 300μg/kg，间隔 15 ～ 25 分钟注射一次。<br><br>Injection par voie IV : la dose initiale, 150μg/kg, ensuite, 300μg/kg, avec un intervalle de 15 à 25 minutes entre deux injections. |
| 剂型、规格 Les formes pharmaceutiques et les spécifications | 注射液：每支 10mg（2ml）。<br><br>Injection : 10mg (2ml) par solution. |
| 药品名称 Drug Names | 哌库溴铵 Bromure de Pipecuronium |
| 适应证 Les indications | 为长效非去极化型肌松药，是泮库溴铵的衍生物，作用类似泮库溴铵，肌松持续时间为 20 分钟。也可用作外科手术麻醉的辅助用药。<br><br>Ce produit sert de myorelaxants non dépolarisants à long terme. Il est le dérivé du bromure de pancuronium et a un effet similaire à celui-ci. La durée de relaxation musculaire est de 20 minutes. Il sert aussi de médicamen adjuvant à l'anesthésie chirurgicale. |
| 用法、用量 Les modes d'emploi et la posologie | 气管插管在静脉注射后 3 分钟，用药量为静脉注射 0.08 ～ 0.1mg/kg；肾功能不全者用药量不超过 0.04mg/kg。<br><br>L'intubation est appliquée 3 minutes après l'injection par voie IV. La dose pour l'injection par voie IV est de 0,08 à 0,1 mg/kg ; chez des patients insuffisants rénaux, ne pas dépasser 0,04 mg/kg. |
| 剂型、规格 Les formes pharmaceutiques et les spécifications | 注射剂：每支 4mg（附有溶剂）。<br><br>Injection : 4mg par solution (y compris le solvant). |
| 药品名称 Drug Names | 阿曲库铵 Atracurium |
| 适应证 Les indications | 为非去极化型肌松药。作用与筒箭毒碱同，起效快（1 分钟）、持续时间短（15 分钟）。大剂量可促使组胺释放。用于各种手术时需肌松或控制呼吸情况。<br><br>Ce produit sert de myorelaxants non dépolarisants, avec un effet identique à la tubocurarine. Il prend rapidement effet (en 1 minute), maintien son effet pendant 15 minutes. Avec une dose importante, il permet d'induire la libération d'histamine. Il est appliqué en cas de relaxation musculaire et de contrôle de la respiration lors des chirurgies de toutes sortes. |
| 用法、用量 Les modes d'emploi et la posologie | 静脉注射起始剂量 0.3 ～ 0.6mg/kg，然后可以静脉滴注每分钟 5 ～ 10μg/kg 维持。<br><br>La dose initiale pour l'injection par voie IV, 0,3 à 0,6 mg/kg, ensuite, en perfusion, 5~10μg/kg par minute pour le maintien. |
| 剂型、规格 Les formes pharmaceutiques et les spécifications | 注射液：每支 25mg（2.5ml）；50mg（5ml）。<br><br>Injection : 25mg (2,5ml) ou 50mg (5ml) par solution. |

**续　表**

| 药品名称 Drug Names | 顺阿曲库铵 Cisatracurium |
| --- | --- |
| 适应证<br>Les indications | ①其效能为阿曲库铵的 4 ～ 5 倍；②消除半衰期约为 24 分钟；③作用持续时间 45 ～ 75 分钟；④无组胺释放作用，无心血管不良反应。<br>① Il est 4 à 5 fois plus efficace que l'atracurium. ② L'élimination de la demi-vie pourrait prendre 24 minutes. ③ Il maintient son effet pendant 45 à 75 minutes. ④ Sans libération d'histamine, sans effets indésirables cardiovasculaires. |
| 用法、用量<br>Les modes d'emploi et la posologie | 成人用量为 0.05mg/kg，常用气管插管用量为 0.15 ～ 0.20mg/kg，插管时间在静注后 150 秒左右。<br>Chez des adultes, 0,05 mg/kg. La dose usuelle pour l'intubation est de 0,15 à 0,20 mg/kg. L'introduction d'un tube 150 secondes après la perfusion. |
| 剂型、规格<br>Les formes pharmaceutiques et les spécifications | 注射液：每支 10mg（5ml）；20mg（10ml）；40mg（20ml）。<br>Injection : 10mg (5ml), 20mg (10ml) ou 40mg (20ml) par solution. |
| 药品名称 Drug Names | 琥珀胆碱 Succinylcholine |
| 适应证<br>Les indications | 为速效肌肉松弛药；也用于需快速气管内插管。<br>Il sert de myorelaxant à action rapide et est aussi applicable dans l'intubation endotrachéale rapide. |
| 用法、用量<br>Les modes d'emploi et la posologie | 成人静脉注射一次 1 ～ 2mg/kg。多用其 2% ～ 5% 溶液。注射后 1 分钟即出现肌肉松弛，持续 2 分钟。如需继续维持其作用，可用其 0.1% ～ 0.2% 溶液，以每分钟 2.5mg 的速度静脉注射；亦可静脉滴注，静脉滴注液可用生理盐水或 5% 葡萄糖液稀释至 0.1% 浓度。极量，静脉注射一次 250mg。<br>Chez des adultes, injection par voie IV, 1 à 2 mg/kg par fois. On utilise souvent sa solution à 2 % à 5 %. 1 minute après l'injection, on peut découvrir la relaxation musculaire, qui dure 2 minutes. Si l'on a besoin de maintenir la relaxation musculaire, utiliser la solution de suxaméthonium à 0,1 % à 0,2 %, injection par voie IV, 2,5mg par minute ; ou en perfusion, dissoudre le produit dans la solution saline ou la solution de glucose à 5 % pour que la concentration soit de 0,1 %. La dose maximale, 250mg par voie IV par fois. |
| 剂型、规格<br>Les formes pharmaceutiques et les spécifications | 注射液：每支 50mg（1ml）；100mg（2ml）。<br>Injection : 50mg (1ml), 100mg (2ml). |

9. 作用于自主神经系统的药物 Médicaments agissant sur le système nerveux autonome

9.1　拟胆碱药和抗胆碱药 Médicaments cholinergiques et anticholinergiques

| 药品名称 Drug Names | 卡巴胆碱 Carbachol |
| --- | --- |
| 适应证<br>Les indications | 主要用于治疗青光眼。<br>Ce produit sert à traiter le glaucome. |
| 用法、用量<br>Les modes d'emploi et la posologie | 局部用药。0.75% ～ 3% 溶液滴眼，用于对毛果芸香碱无反应或不能耐受者。成人两眼分别滴入 1 ～ 2 滴，4 ～ 8 小时 1 次。给药后需用手指压迫内眦 1 ～ 2 分钟，以减少吸收，减少全身不良反应。在白内障手术时起缩瞳作用并减少后眼压上升，可用 0.01%0.5ml 滴眼。<br>Un topique. Les gouttes pour les yeux de carbachol à 0,75 % à 3 % sont applicables chez les patients résistants à la pilocarpine. Chez des adultes, 1 à 2 gouttes respectivement pour les deux yeux, toutes les 4 à 8h. Après l'administration, il faut presser avec le doigt sur le canthus intérieur pendant 1 à 2 minutes, pour atténuer l'absorption et réduire les effets indésirables systématiques. Lors de la chirurgie de la cataracte, il peut avoir un effet miotique et réduire la PIO. C'est possible d'utiliser 0,5ml de gouttes pour les yeux à 0,01 %. |

**续　表**

| | |
|---|---|
| 剂型、规格<br>Les formes pharmaceutiques et les spécifications | 滴眼液：0.25%；1.5%；2.25%；3%。<br>注射液：每支 0.1mg（1ml）。<br>Les gouttes pour les yeux : 0,25 %, 1,5 %, 2,25 % ou 3 %.<br>Injection : 0,1mg (1ml) par solution. |
| **药品名称 Drug Names** | **毛果芸香碱 Pilocarpine** |
| 适应证<br>Les indications | 治疗原发性青光眼，包括开角型与闭角型青光眼。滴眼后，缩瞳作用于 10～30 分钟出现，维持 4～8 小时；最大降眼压作用约75分钟内出现，维持 4～14 小时；可缓解或消除青光眼症状。也可用于唾液腺功能。<br>Ce produit sert à traiter le glaucome primaire, ya compris le glaucome à angle ouvert et à angle fermé. Après la goutte, l'effet miotique peut se faire sentir 10 à 30 minutes après, et peut durer pendant 4 à 8 h ; dans les 75 minutes, on peut découvrir la réduction maxiale de la PIO, qui pourrait durer pendant 4 à 14 h. Il permet aussi d'atténuer ou d'éliminuer les symptômes du glaucome. |
| 用法、用量<br>Les modes d'emploi et la posologie | 滴眼液配成 0.5%～4% 毛果芸香碱（常用 1% 及 2%，增加浓度可增加药效，但超过 4% 时，药效无明显增加）。滴眼后 10～15 分钟开始缩瞳，30～50 分钟作用最强，约持续 24 小时，睫状肌痉挛作用约持续 2 小时。滴药后 10～15 分钟开始降眼压，持续 4～8 小时，故应每日滴眼 3～4 次。<br>Les gouttes pour les yeux de pilocarpine à 0,5 % à 4 % (généralement, 1 % ou 2 %, augmenter la concentration pourrait augmenter l'efficacité, mais quand il s'agit de plus de 4 %, l'efficacité n'augmente pas pour autant). Après la goutte, l'effet miotique peut se faire sentir 10 à 15 minutes après, être plus fort 30 à 50 minutes après, et peut durer pendant 24h. Le spasme du muscle ciliaire dure 2 h. Dans les 10 à 15 minutes après la goutte, on peut découvrir la réduction de la PIO, qui pourrait durer 4 à 8h. Il faut donc appliquer les gouttes 3 à 4 fois par jour. |
| 剂型、规格<br>Les formes pharmaceutiques et les spécifications | 滴眼液：1%；2%。片剂（SALAGEN）：每片 5mg。<br>注射液：每支 10mg（1ml）。<br>Les gouttes pour les yeux : 1 % ou 2 %.<br>Comprimés (SALAGEN) : 5mg par comprimé.<br>Injection : 10mg (1ml) par solution. |
| **药品名称 Drug Names** | **毒扁豆碱 Physostigmine** |
| 适应证<br>Les indications | 主要用其 0.2%～0.5% 溶液点眼，用于治疗原发性闭角型青光眼，药效比毛果芸香碱强而持久。它对中枢神经系统的作用是小剂量时兴奋，大剂量时抑制，故已较少做全身给药，只用于眼科。<br>La solution à 0,2 % à 0,5 % de ce produit est souvent appliquée aux yeux pour traiter le glaucome à angle fermé, avec un effet plus fort et plus persistant que la pilocarpine. Il peut exiter le système nerveux central avec une dose mineure et inhiber celui-ci avec une dose importante. Il est donc peu appliqué dans l'administration systématique, mais seulement pour les yeux. |
| 用法、用量<br>Les modes d'emploi et la posologie | 注射液，皮下或肌注，一次 0.5mg 或遵医嘱。眼膏，晚上临睡前点眼，涂于眼睑内，一般白天用毛果芸香碱，晚上用本品。或遵医嘱。<br>Injection par voie sous-cutanée ou IM, 0,5 mg par fois ou selon les ordonnances. Appliquer la pommade pour les yeux à la paupière le soir avant le sommeil. En général, le jour, on applique la pilocarpine, le soir, on utilise la physostigmine. Ou suivre les ordonnances. |
| 剂型、规格<br>Les formes pharmaceutiques et les spécifications | 水杨酸毒扁豆碱滴眼剂：有水杨酸毒扁豆碱 0.25g，硼酸 1.8g，亚硫酸氢钠 0.1g，蒸馏水加至 100ml 配成；或由水杨酸毒扁豆碱 0.46g。氯化钠 0.8g，依地酸二钠 0.1g，尼泊金乙酯 0.03g（加热溶解），蒸馏水加至 100ml 配成。<br>Les gouttes pour les yeux de salicylate de physostigmine : composées de 0,25g de salicylate de physostigmine, de 1,8g d'acide borique, de 0,1g de bisulfite de sodium et de l'eau distillée pour former 100ml de solution. Ou 0,46g de salicylate de physostigmine, 0,8g de chlorure de sodium, 0,1g d'édétate disodique, 0,03g d'ethylparaben (la dissolution chauffée) et de l'eau distillée pour former 100ml de solution. |

**续　表**

| 药品名称 Drug Names | 新斯的明 Néostigmine |
|---|---|
| 适应证<br>Les indications | 多用于重症肌无力及腹部手术后的肠麻痹。<br><br>Il est utilisé comme traitement de la myasthénie grave et la paralysie de l'intestin après la chirurgie abdominale. |
| 用法、用量<br>Les modes d'emploi et la posologie | 口服其溴化物，一次 15mg，一日 45mg；极量：一次 30mg，一日 100mg。皮下注射、肌内注射其甲硫酸盐，一日 1～3 次，每次 0.25～1.0mg；极量：一次 1mg，一日 5mg。以 0.05% 眼药水用于青少年假性近视眼，一日 2 次，每次 1～2 滴，3 个月为 1 个疗程。<br><br>Administrer le bromure de néostigmine par voie orale, 15mg par fois, 45mg par jour ; la dose maximale : 30mg par fois, 100mg par jour. Administrer le sulfate de méthyle de néostigmine par voie sous-cutanée ou IM, 1 à 3 fois par jour, 0,25 à 1,0mg par fois ; la dose maximale : 1mg par fois, 5mg par jour. Appliquer les gouttes pour les yeux à 0,05 % pour traiter la pseudo myopie chez des adolescents, 2 fois par jour, 1 à 2 gouttes par fois, pendant 3 mois comme un traitement médical. |
| 剂型、规格<br>Les formes pharmaceutiques et les spécifications | 片剂：每片 15mg。<br>注射液：每支 0.5mg（1ml）；1mg（2ml）。<br>Comprimés : 15mg par comprimé.<br>Injection : 0,5mg (1ml) ou 1mg (2ml) par solution. |
| 药品名称 Drug Names | 溴吡斯的明 Bromure de pyridostigmine |
| 适应证<br>Les indications | 用于：①重症肌无力；②术后腹气胀或尿潴留；③对抗非去极化型肌松药的肌松作用。<br><br>Il est utilisé dans : ① La myasthénie grave. ② Le ballonnement postopératoire ou la rétention urinaire. ③ Lutter contre la relaxation musculaire des myorelaxants non dépolarisants. |
| 用法、用量<br>Les modes d'emploi et la posologie | ①重症肌无力：口服，一次 60mg，一日 3 次；皮下或肌内注射，每日 1～5mg，或根据病情而定。②术后腹气胀或尿潴留：肌内注射，一次 1～2mg。③对抗非去极化型肌松药的肌松：静脉注射，一次 2～5mg。<br><br>① Pour traiter la myasthésie grave : par voie orale, 60mg par fois, 3 fois par jour ; injection par voie sous-cutanée ou IM, 1 à 5mg par jour, ou selon les cas. ② Pour traiter le ballonnement postopératoire ou la rétention urinaire : injection par voie IM, 1 à 2 mg par fois. ③ Pour lutter contre la relaxation musculaire des myorelaxants non dépolarisant : injection par voie IV, 2 à 5mg par fois. |
| 剂型、规格<br>Les formes pharmaceutiques et les spécifications | 片剂：每片 60mg。<br>缓释片：180mg。<br>注射剂：每支 5mg（1ml）；10mg（2ml）。<br>Comprimés : 60mg par comprimé.<br>Comprimés à libération prolongée : 180mg.<br>Injection : 5mg (1ml) ou 10mg (2ml) par solution. |
| 药品名称 Drug Names | 石杉碱甲 Hupérzine -A |
| 适应证<br>Les indications | 可用于重症肌无力及良性记忆障碍。对阿尔茨海默病和脑器质性病变引起的记忆障碍也有所改善。<br><br>Ce produit sert à traiter la myasthésie grave et les troubles de la mémoire bénins. Il est aussi applicable dans l'amélioration des troubles de la mémoire causés par la maladie d'Alzheimer et l'encéphalopathie organique. |
| 用法、用量<br>Les modes d'emploi et la posologie | ①重症肌无力：肌内注射，每次 0.2～0.4mg，一日 1～2 次。②记忆功能减退：口服，一次 0.1～0.2mg，一日 2 次。因个体差异，一般应从小剂量开始。每日最多不超过 0.45mg。<br><br>① Pour traiter la myasthésie grave : injection par voie IM, 0,2 à 0,4 mg par fois, 1 à 2 fois par jour. ② Pour traiter la perte de la mémoire : par voie orale, 0,1 à 0,2mg par fois, 2 fois par jour. Il vaut mieux commencer par une dose mineure. Ne pas dépasser 0,45mg par jour. |
| 剂型、规格<br>Les formes pharmaceutiques et les spécifications | 片剂：每片 0.05mg。<br>Comprimés : 0.05g par comprimé. |

**续 表**

| 药品名称 Drug Names | 多奈哌齐 Donépézil |
|---|---|
| 适应证<br>Les indications | 可用轻、中度阿尔茨海默病的治疗。<br>Ce produit sert à traiter la maladie d'Alzheimer bénigne et modérée. |
| 用法、用量<br>Les modes d'emploi et la posologie | 口服，一日 1 次，每次 5 ～ 10mg。<br>Par voie orale, 1 fois par jour, 5 à 10mg par fois. |
| 剂型、规格<br>Les formes pharmaceutiques et les spécifications | 片剂：每片 5mg；10mg。<br>Comprimés : 5mg ou 10mg par comprimé. |
| 药品名称 Drug Names | 加兰他敏 Galantamine |
| 适应证<br>Les indications | 本品可用于重症肌无力，进行性肌营养不良，脊髓灰质炎后遗症，儿童脑型麻痹，因神经系统疾患所致感觉或运动障碍，多发性神经炎等。<br>Ce produit sert à traiter la myasthésie grave, la dystrophie musculaire, les séquelles de poliomyélite, la paralysie cérébrale chez des enfants, les troubles sensoriels ou moteurs causés par des maladies du système nerveux, la polynévrite, etc. |
| 用法、用量<br>Les modes d'emploi et la posologie | ①肌内注射或皮下注射：每次 2.5 ～ 10mg，小儿每次 0.05 ～ 0.1mg/kg，一日 1 次，1 疗程 2 ～ 6 周。②口服：每次 10mg，一日 3 次。小儿每日 0.5 ～ 1mg/kg，分 3 次服。<br>① Injection par voie IM ou sous-cutanée : 2,5 à 10mg par fois, chez des enfants, 0,05 à 0,1 mg/kg par fois, 1 fois par jour, pendant 2 à 6 semaines comme un traitement médical. ② Par voie orale : 10mg par fois, 3 fois par jour. Chez des enfants, 0,5 à 1 mg/kg par jour, à travers 3 fois. |
| 剂型、规格<br>Les formes pharmaceutiques et les spécifications | 注射液：1mg（1ml）；2.5mg（1ml）；5mg（1ml）。<br>片剂：5mg。<br>Injection : 1mg (1ml), 2,5 mg (1ml) ou 5mg (1ml).<br>Comprimés : 5mg. |
| 药品名称 Drug Names | 阿托品 Atropine |
| 适应证<br>Les indications | 临床上的用途主要是：①抢救感染中毒性休克。②治疗锑剂引起的阿 - 斯综合征。③治疗有机磷农药中毒。④缓解内脏绞痛，包括胃肠痉挛引起的疼痛、肾绞痛、胆绞痛、胃及十二指肠溃疡。⑤用于麻醉前给药，可减少麻醉过程中支气管黏液分泌，预防术后引起肺炎，并可消除吗啡对呼吸的抑制。⑥眼科用药，用于角膜炎、虹膜睫状体炎。<br>Il est principalement utilisé dans les cliniques comme traitement : ① Sauver le choc septique et toxique. ② Traiter le syndrome d'Adams dû à l'antimoine. ③ Intoxication par les pesticides organophosphorés. ④ Atténuer les coliques viscérales, y compris les douleurs dues aux spasmes gastro-intestinaux, la colique néphrétique, la colique biliaire, ainsi que les ulcères gastriques et duodénaux. ⑤ Appliqué dans l'administration avant l'anesthésie, pour éviterla sécrétion de mucus bronchique durant l'anesthésie, prévenir la pneumonie postopératoire, et éliminier l'inhibition de la respiration par la morphine. ⑥ En tant que médicament ophtalmique, il sert à traiter la kératite et l'iridocyclite. |
| 用法、用量<br>Les modes d'emploi et la posologie | ①感染中毒性休克：成人每次 1 ～ 2mg，小儿每次 0.03 ～ 0.05mg/kg，静脉注射，每 15 ～ 30 分钟 1 次，2 ～ 3 次后加情况不见好转可逐渐增加用量，至情况好转后即减量或停药。②锑剂引起的阿 - 斯综合征：发现严重心律失常时，立即静脉注射 1 ～ 2mg（用 5% ～ 25% 葡萄糖液 10 ～ 20ml 稀释），同时肌内注射或皮下注射 1mg，15 ～ 30 分钟后再静脉注射 1mg。如患者无发作，可根据心律及心率情况改为每 3 ～ 4 小时 1 次皮下注射或肌内注射 1mg，48 小时后如不再发作，可逐渐减量，最后停药。③有机磷农药中毒：a. 与碘解磷定等合用时：对中度中毒，每次皮下注射 0.5 ～ 1mg，隔 30 ～ 60 分钟 1 次；对严重中毒，每次静 |

续　表

脉注射 1 ～ 2mg，隔 15 ～ 30 分钟 1 次，病情稳定后，逐渐减量并改用皮下注射。b. 单用时：对轻度中毒，每次皮下注射 0.5 ～ 1mg，隔 30 ～ 120 分钟 1 次；对中度中毒，每次皮下注射 1 ～ 2mg，隔 15 ～ 30 分钟 1 次；对重度中毒，即刻静脉注射 2 ～ 5mg，以后每次 1 ～ 2mg，隔 15 ～ 30 分钟 1 次，根据病情逐渐减量和延长间隔时间。④缓解内脏绞痛：每次皮下注射 0.5mg。⑤用于麻醉前给药：皮下注射：0.5mg。⑥用于眼科：用 1% ～ 3% 眼药水滴眼或眼膏涂眼。滴时按住内眦部，以免流入鼻腔吸收中毒。

① Pour traiter le choc septique et toxique : chez des adultes, 1 à 2mg par fois, chez des enfants, 0,03 à 0,05 mg/kg par fois, injection par voie IV, toutes les 15 à 30 minutes. Si les symptômes ne s'améliorent pas 2 à 3 administrations, augmenter la dose. Dès les symptômes s'améliorent, diminuer la dose ou arrêter l'administration. ② Pour traiter le syndrome d'Adams dû à l'antimoine : lors de l'arythmie grave, injecter immédiatement 1 à 2 mg par voie IV (utiliser 10 à 20ml de solution de glucose à 5 % à 25 %), injecter en même temps 1mg par voie IM ou sous-cutanée, 15 à 30 minutes après, injecter encore 1mg par voie IV. S'il on ne constate pas la crise de la maladie chez des patients, on peut suivre la dose suivante : injecter 1mg par voie sous-cutanée ou IM toutes les 3 à 4h en fonction du rythme cardiaque, 48h après, s'il n'a toujours pas la crise, diminuer progressivement la dose avant d'arrêter l'administration. ③ Intoxication par les pesticides organophosphorés : a.Utilisé en association avec l'iodure de pralidoxime : pour traiter l'intoxication modérée, injecter 0,5 à 1mg par voie sous-cutanée, toutes les 30 à 60 minutes ; pour traiter l'intoxication grave, injecter 1 à 2mg par voie IV, toutes les 15 à 30 minutes, avec la stabilisation de l'état, diminuer la dose, et injecter par voie sous-cutanée. b. Utilisé seul : pour traiter l'intoxication bénigne, injecter 0,5 à 1mg par voie sous-cutanée, toutes les 30 à 120 minutes ; pour traiter l'intoxication modérée, injecter 1 à 2mg par par voie sous-cutanée, toutes les 15 à 30 minutes ; pour traiter l'intoxication grave, injecter immédiatement 2 à 5mg par voie IV, ensuite, 1 à 2 mg par fois, toutes les 15 à 30 minutes, diminuer progressivement la dose selon les cas et prolonger l'intervalle entre deux administrations. ④ Atténuer les coliques viscérales : injecter 0,5mg par fois par voie sous-cutanée. ⑤ L'administration avant l'anesthésie : injecter 0,5mg par voie sous-cutanée. ⑥ En ophtalmologie : appliquer les gouttes ou les pommades pour les yeux à 1 % à 3 % aux yeux. Lors de la goutte, presser le canthus pour éviter l'empoisonnement si la goutte tombe dans la cavité nasale.

| | |
|---|---|
| 剂型、规格<br>Les formes pharmaceutiques et les spécifications | 片剂：每片 0.3g。<br>注射液：每支 0.5mg（1ml）；1mg（2ml）；5mg（1ml）。<br>滴眼剂：取硫酸阿托品 1g，氯化钠 0.29g，无水磷酸二氢钠 0.4g，无水磷酸氢二钠 0.47g，羟胺乙酯 0.03g，蒸馏水加至 100ml 配成。<br>Comprimés：0，3g par comprimé.<br>Injection：0，5mg（1ml），1mg（2ml）ou 5mg（1ml）par solution.<br>Les gouttes pour les yeux : utiliser 1g de sulfate d'atropine, 0,29g de chlorure de sodium, 0,4g de dihydrogène phosphate de sodium anhydre, 0,47g de Phosphate disodique anhydre, 0,03g d'ethyl hydroxylamine et l'eau distillée pour former 100ml de solutions. |
| 药品名称 Drug Names | 东莨菪碱 Scopolamine |
| 适应证<br>Les indications | 临床用作镇静药，用于全身麻醉前给药、晕动病、震颤麻痹、狂躁性精神病、有机磷农药中毒等。由于本品既兴奋呼吸又对大脑皮质呈镇静作用，故用于抢救极重型流行性乙型脑炎呼吸衰竭（常伴有剧烈频繁的抽搐）亦有效。<br>Il sert d'analgésique clinique. Il est utilisé dans l'administration avant l'anesthésie et dans le traitement du mal de transports, du parkinsonisme, de la psychose maniaque et de l'intoxication par les pesticides organophosphorés. Comme il peut non seulement stimuler la respiration mais aussi servir de sédation au cortex cérébral, il est efficace dans le sauvetage de l'arrêt respiratoire lié à l'encéphalite japonaise de type B extrêmement grave (accompagnée de violentes convulsions fréquentes). |
| 用法、用量<br>Les modes d'emploi et la posologie | 口服：一次 0.3 ～ 0.6mg，一日 0.6 ～ 1.2mg；极量一次 0.6mg，一日 1.8mg。皮下注射：一次 0.2 ～ 0.5mg；极量一次 0.5mg，一日 1.5mg。抢救乙型脑炎呼吸衰竭：以 1ml 含药 0.3mg 的注射液直接静脉注射或稀释于 10% 葡萄糖溶液 30ml 内作静脉注射，常用量为 0.02 ～ 0.04mg/kg，用药间歇时间一般为 20 ～ 30 分钟，用药总量最高达 6.3mg。 |

**续　表**

| | |
|---|---|
| | Par voie orale : 0,3 à 0,6mg par fois, 0,6 à 1,2mg par jour ; la dose maximale, 0,6mg par fois, 1,8 mg par jour. Injection par voie sous-cutanée : 0,2 à 0,5mg par fois ; la dose maximale, 0,5mg par fois, 1,5mg par jour. Pour sauver l'arrêt respiratoire lié à l'encéphalite japonaise de type B : injecter directement 1ml de solution comprenant 0,3mg de produit par voie IV ou le dissoudre dans 30 ml de solution de glucose à 10 % pour injection par voie IV, la dose usuelle, 0,02 à 0,04 mg/kg, toutes les 20 à 30 minutes, la dose totale maximale, 6,3g. |
| 剂型、规格<br>Les formes pharmaceutiques et les spécifications | 片剂：每片 0.3mg。<br>注射液：每支 0.3mg（1ml）；0.5mg（1ml）。<br>晕动片：每片含东莨菪碱 0.2mg、苯巴比妥钠 30mg、阿托品 0.15mg。<br>Comprimés : 0,3mg.<br>Injection : 0,3mg (1ml) ou 0,5mg (1ml) par solution.<br>Comprimés contre le mal : Chaque comprimé contient 0,2 mg de scopolamine, 30mg de sodium phénobarbital, et 0,15mg d'atropine. |
| 药品名称 Drug Names | 山莨菪碱 Anisodamine |
| 适应证<br>Les indications | 适用于下列疾病：①感染中毒性休克：如暴发型流行性脑脊髓膜炎、中毒性痢疾等。②血管性疾病：脑血栓、脑栓塞、瘫痪、脑血管痉挛、血管神经性头痛、血栓闭塞性脉管炎等。③各种神经痛：如三叉神经痛、坐骨神经痛等。④平滑肌痉挛：胃、十二指肠溃疡，胆道痉挛等。⑤眩晕病。⑥眼底疾病：中心性视网膜炎、视网膜色素变性、视网膜动脉血栓等。⑦突发性耳聋：配合新针疗法可治疗其他耳聋。<br><br>Appliquée dans les cas suivants : ① Le choc septique et toxique : tel que la méningite à méningocoque fulminante et la dysenterie fulminante. ② Les maladies vasculaires : la thrombose cérébrale, l'embolie cérébrale, la paralysie, le vasospasme cérébral, la céphalée angioneurotique, oblitérante thrombose, la thromboangéite oblitérante, etc. ③ La névralgie de toutes sortes : la névralgie du trijumeau et la sciatique. ④ Les spasmes des muscles lisses : les ulcères gastriques et duodénaux, ainsi que les spasmes des voies biliaires. ⑤ Les vertiges. ⑥ Les maladies de la rétine : la rétinite centrale, la rétinite pigmentaire, la thrombose de l'artère rétinienne, etc. ⑦ La surdité subite : en association avec le nouveau traitement à l'aiguille, il peut traiter d'autres sortes de surdité. |
| 用法、用量<br>Les modes d'emploi et la posologie | （1）肌内注射或静脉注射：成人一般一次 5～10mg，一日 1～2 次；也可经稀释后静脉注射。用于：①抢救感染中毒性休克：根据病情决定剂量。成人静脉注射每次 10～40mg；小儿 0.3～2mg/kg，需要时每隔 10～30 分钟可重复给药，情况不见好转可加量。病情好转可逐渐延长间隔时间，直至停药。②治疗脑血栓：加入 5% 葡萄糖液中静脉注射，每日 30～40mg。③一般慢性疾病：每次肌内注射 5～10mg，一日 1～2 次，可连用 1 个月以上。④治疗严重三叉神经痛：有时需加大剂量至每次 5～20mg，肌内注射。⑤治疗血栓闭塞性脉管炎：每次静脉注射 10～15mg，一日 1 次。<br>（2）口服：一日 3 次，一次 5～10mg。皮肤或黏膜局部使用，无刺激性。<br><br>(1) Injection par voie IM ou IV : chez des adultes, 5 à 10mg par fois, 1 à 2 fois par jour ; ou injection par voie IV après la dilution.<br>Utilisé pour : ① Sauver le choc septique et toxique : ajuster la dose selon les cas. Chez des adultes, injection par voie IV, 10 à 40 mg par fois ; chez des enfants, 0,3 à 2 mg/kg, s'il est nécessaire, toutes les 10 à 30 minutes, s'il l'état ne s'améliore pas, augmenter la dose. Après l'amélioration de l'état, prolonger progressivement l'intervalle jusqu'à l'arrêt de l'administration. ② Traiter thrombose cérébrale : dissoudre dans la solution de glucose à 5 %, injection par voie IV, 30 à 40mg par jour. ③ Traiter des maladies chroniques : injecter 5 à 10mg par fois par voie IM, 1 à 2 fois par jour, pendant plus d'un mois. ④ Traiter la névralgie du trijumeau grave : parfois, nécessaire d'augmenter la dose pour atteindre 5 à 20mg, injection par voie IM. ⑤ Traiter la thromboangéite oblitérante : injecter 10 à 15mg par fois par voie IV, 1 fois par jour.<br>(2) Par voie orale : 3 fois par jour, 5 à 10mg par fois. Topique cutané ou moqueux, sans irritant. |

续　表

| | |
|---|---|
| 剂型、规格<br>Les formes pharmaceutiques et les spécifications | 氢溴酸山莨菪碱片剂：每片 5mg。<br>注射液：每支 1ml（10mg）；1ml（20mg）。<br>Comprimés alcalins de bromhydrate d'anisodamine : 5mg par comprimé.<br>Injection : 1ml (10mg) ou 1ml (20mg) par solution. |
| 药品名称 Drug Names | 托吡卡胺 Tropicamide |
| 适应证<br>Les indications | 散瞳药，主要用于散瞳检查眼底和散瞳验光。<br>En tant que mydriatique, il est principalement utilisé dans la mydriase lors du fond d'œil et de l'optométrie. |
| 用法、用量<br>Les modes d'emploi et la posologie | 本品 0.5% 溶液滴眼 1～2 次，滴入结膜囊，一次一滴，间隔 5 分钟滴第二次，即可满足三通检查的需要。<br>Instiller la solution à 0,5 % 1 à 2 fois dans le cul-de-sac conjonctival, une goutte par fois, un intervalle de 5 minutes entre ces deux gouttes. |
| 剂型、规格<br>Les formes pharmaceutiques et les spécifications | 滴眼液：每支 12.5mg（5ml）；25mg（5ml）；15mg（6ml）；30mg（6ml）。<br>Les gouttes pour les yeux : 12,5mg (5ml), 25mg (5ml), 15mg (6ml) ou 30mg (6ml) par solution. |
| 药品名称 Drug Names | 颠茄 Belladone |
| 适应证<br>Les indications | 用于胃及十二指肠溃疡、轻度胃肠、肾和胆绞痛等。<br>Ce produit sert à traiter les ulcères gastriques et duodénaux ainsi queles coliques gastro-intestinales, rénales et biliaires bénignes. |
| 用法、用量<br>Les modes d'emploi et la posologie | ① 酊剂：每次服 0.3～1ml。极量：一次 1.5ml，一日 4.5ml。② 片剂：每次服 10～30mg，一日 30～90mg。极量：一次 50mg，一日 150mg。<br>① Teintures : 0,3 à 1ml par fois. La dose maximale : 1,5ml par fois, 4,5ml par jour. ② Comprimés : 10 à 30mg par fois, 30 à 90 mg par jour. La dose maximale : 50mg par fois, 150 mg par jour. |
| 剂型、规格<br>Les formes pharmaceutiques et les spécifications | 酊剂：含生物碱 0.03%；浸膏：含生物碱 1%。<br>片剂：每片含颠茄浸膏 10mg。<br>Teinture: contenant des alcaloïdes 0,03 % ; extrait : contient des alcaloïdes 1 %.<br>Comprimés: Chaque comprimé contient 10 mg d'extrait de belladone |
| 药品名称 Drug Names | 后马托品 Homatropine |
| 适应证<br>Les indications | 用于散瞳检查眼底和散瞳验光。也可用于弱视和斜视的压抑疗法。<br>Ce produit est utilisé dans la mydriase lors du fond d'œil et de l'optométrie. Il est aussi applicable dans le traitement de pénalisation de l'amblyopie et du strabisme. |
| 用法、用量<br>Les modes d'emploi et la posologie | 滴眼液滴入结膜囊，一次一滴。眼膏涂在结膜囊，一次少许。用药次数根据患者的年龄和使用目的以及瞳孔变化而决定。<br>Instiller des gouttes dans le cul-de-sac conjonctival, une goutte par fois. Appliquer la pommade dans le cul-de-sac conjonctival, un peu par fois. Ajuster le nombre d'administrations en fonction de l'âge, de l'objectif et des changements pupillaires. |
| 剂型、规格<br>Les formes pharmaceutiques et les spécifications | 氢溴酸后马托品滴眼剂：1%～5%。<br>眼膏：2%。<br>gouttes oculaires de bromhydrate d'homatropine : 1% à 5 %.<br>Pommade: 2 %. |

**续 表**

9.2 拟肾上腺素药和抗肾上腺素药 Médicaments adrénergiques et médicaments anti-adrénergiques

| 药品名称 Drug Names | 萘甲唑啉 Naphazoline |
|---|---|
| 适应证<br>Les indications | 用于过敏性及炎症性鼻充血、急慢性鼻炎、眼充血等，对细菌性，过敏性结膜炎也有效，并能减轻眼睑痉挛。对麻黄碱有耐受性者，可选用本品。<br><br>Ce produit sert à traiter les congestions nasales allergiques et inflammatoires, la rhinite aiguë et chronique et la congestion ophtalmique. Il est aussi efficace dans le traitement de la conjonctivite bactérienne et allergique, ainsi que dans l'atténuation du blépharospasme. Chez des patients résistants à l'éphédrine, c'est possible de choisir ce produit. |
| 用法、用量<br>Les modes d'emploi et la posologie | 治鼻充血，用其0.05%～0.1%溶液，每侧鼻孔滴2～3滴；治疗充血用其滴眼液，每次1～2滴。<br><br>Pour traiter la congestion nasale, utiliser la solution à 0,05 à 0,1 %, instiller 2 à 3 gouttes dans chaque narine ; pour traiter la congestion ophtalmique, utiliser les gouttes pour les yeux, appliquer 1 à 2 gouttes par fois. |
| 剂型、规格<br>Les formes pharmaceutiques et les spécifications | 滴鼻剂：每瓶0.05%（10ml）；0.1%（10ml）。<br>盐酸萘甲唑啉滴眼液：1.2mg（10ml）。<br>Gouttes nasales : 0,05 % (10ml) ou 0,1 % (10ml) par flacon.<br>Les gouttes pour les yeux de chlorhydrate de naphazoline : 1,2mg (10ml). |
| 药品名称 Drug Names | 米多君 Midodrine |
| 适应证<br>Les indications | 主要用于各种原因引起的低血压、压力性尿失禁、射精功能障碍。<br>Ce produit sert principalement à traiter l'hypotension, l'incontinence urinaire et les troubles de l'éjaculation. |
| 用法、用量<br>Les modes d'emploi et la posologie | 口服：初剂量为1次2.5mg，一日2～3次。必要时可逐渐增加到一次10mg，一日3次的维持剂量。<br><br>Par voie orale : la dose initiale, 2,5mg par fois, 2 à 3 fois par jour. S'il est nécessaire, augmenter la dose pour atteindre 10mg par fois, 3 fois par jour comme dose d'entretien. |
| 剂型、规格<br>Les formes pharmaceutiques et les spécifications | 盐酸米多君片：2.5mg。<br>Comprimés de chlorhydrate de midodrine : 2,5mg. |
| 药品名称 Drug Names | 拉贝洛尔 Labétalol |
| 适应证<br>Les indications | 用于治疗轻度和重度高血压和心绞痛。采用静脉注射能治疗高血压危象。<br>Ce produit sert à traiter l'hypertention artérielle bénigne et grave et l'angine. Administré par voie IV, il permet de traiter la crise hypertensive. |
| 用法、用量<br>Les modes d'emploi et la posologie | 口服：初剂量为1次100mg，一日2～3次。必要时可逐渐增加到一次200mg，一日3～4次。通常对轻、中、重度高血压患者的每日剂量相应为300～800mg、600～1200mg、1200～2400mg，加用利尿剂时可适当减量。静脉注射：一次100～200mg。<br><br>Par voie orale : la dose initiale, 100mg par fois, 2 à 3 fois par jour. S'il est nécessaire, augmenter la dose pour atteindre 200mg par fois, 3 à 4 fois par jour. Chez des patients atteints de l'hypertention bénigne, modérée et grave, prendre respectivement 300 à 800mg, 600 à 1 200mg et 1 200 à 2 400mg par jour. Diminuer la dose s'il on utilise en même temps les diurétiques. Injection par voie IV : 100 à 200mg par fois. |
| 剂型、规格<br>Les formes pharmaceutiques et les spécifications | 片剂：每片100mg；200mg。<br>注射液：每支50mg（5ml）。<br>Comprimés : 100mg ou 200mg par comprimé.<br>Injection : 50mg (5ml) par solution. |
| 药品名称 Drug Names | 卡维地洛 Carvédilol |
| 适应证<br>Les indications | 可用于原发性高血压及心绞痛。<br>Ce produit sert à traiter l'hypertension artérielle essentielle et l'angine. |

**续　表**

| | |
|---|---|
| 用法、用量<br>Les modes d'emploi et la posologie | 口服：初剂量为 25mg/d，一次服用；可根据需要逐渐增剂量至 50mg/d，分 1～2 次服下；最大日剂量不超过 100mg。<br><br>Par voie orale : la dose initiale, 25 mg par jour, une fois par jour ; augmenter la dose selon les cas pour atteindre 50mg par jour, à travers 1 à 2 fois ; la dose maximale, 100mg par jour. |
| 剂型、规格<br>Les formes pharmaceutiques et les spécifications | 片剂：每片 6.25mg；10mg；12.5mg；20mg。<br>胶囊：10mg。<br>Comprimés : 6,25mg, 10mg, 12,5mg ou 20mg par comprimé.<br>Capsules : 10mg. |
| 药品名称 Drug Names | 酚妥拉明 Phentolamine |
| 适应证<br>Les indications | 用于血管痉挛性疾病，如肢端动脉痉挛症（即雷诺病）、手足发绀症等、感染中毒性休克以及嗜铬细胞瘤的诊断试验等。用于室性早搏亦有效。<br><br>Ce produit sert à traiter des maladies angiospastiques, telles que les spasmes artériels des membres (à savoir, la maladie de Raynaud), la cyanose des mains et des pieds, le choc septique et toxique. Il est aussi applicable dans les tests de diagnostic pour le phéochromocytome. Il est également utilisé comme traitement de l'extrasystole ventriculaire. |
| 用法、用量<br>Les modes d'emploi et la posologie | ①治疗血管痉挛性疾病：肌内注射或静脉注射。每次 5～10mg，20～30 分钟后按需要可重复给药。②抗休克：以 0.3mg 每分钟的剂量进行静脉滴注。③室性早搏：开始 2 日，每次口服 50mg，一日 4 次；如无效，则以后 2 日将剂量增加至每次 75mg，一日 4 次；如仍无效，可增至一日 400mg；如再无效，即应停用。无论何种剂量，一旦有效，就按该剂量继续服用 7 日。④诊断嗜铬细胞瘤：静脉注射 5mg。注射后 30 分钟测血压一次，可连续测 10 分钟，如在 2～4 分钟血压降低 4.67/3.3kPa（35/25mmHg）以上为阳性结果。⑤做阴茎海绵体注射，可使阴茎海绵窦平滑肌松弛、扩张而勃起，可用于治疗勃起障碍，一次注射 1mg。<br><br>① Pour traiter les maladies angiospastiques : injection par voie IM ou IV. 5 à 10mg par fois, toutes les 20 à 30 minutes selon les cas. ② Pour lutter contre le choc : injecter 0,3mg par minute par voie IV. ③ Pour traiter l'extrasystole ventriculaire : les deux premiers jour, 50 mg par fois, par voie orale, 4 fois par jour ; s'il est inutile, pendant les deux jours suivants, 75mg par fois, 4 fois par jour; il est encore inutile, 400mg par fois, 4 fois par jour ; il est toujours inutile, arrêter l'administration. Quelle soit la dose, une fois il est utile, continuer de prendre cette dose pendant 7 jours consécutifs. ④ les tests de diagnostic pour le phéochromocytome : injecter 5mg par voie IV. 30 minutes après l'injection, prendre la pression sauguine pendant 10 minutes consécutives. La réduction de 4.67/3.3kPa(35/25mmHg)en 2 à 4 minutes est considérée comme résultat positif. ⑤ L'injection intracaverneuse peut permettre aux muscles lisses des pénis caverneuxla relaxation, la dilatation et l'érection, ce qui permett de traiter la dysfonction érectile. Injecter 1mg par fois. |
| 剂型、规格<br>Les formes pharmaceutiques et les spécifications | 片剂：每片 25mg。<br>甲磺酸酚妥拉明注射液：每支 5mg（1ml）；10mg（1ml）。<br>Comprimés : 25mg par comprimé.<br>Injection de mésylate de phentolamine : 5mg (1ml) ou 10mg (1ml) par solution. |
| 药品名称 Drug Names | 妥拉唑林 Tolazoline |
| 适应证<br>Les indications | 用于血管痉挛性疾病如肢端动脉痉挛症、手足发绀、闭塞性血栓静脉炎等。<br><br>Ce produit sert à traiter des maladies angiospastiques, telles que les spasmes artériels des membres, la cyanose des mains et des pieds ainsi que la thrombophlébite occlusive, etc. |
| 用法、用量<br>Les modes d'emploi et la posologie | 口服，一次 15mg，一日 45～60mg；肌内注射或皮下注射，一次 25mg。<br><br>Par voie orale : 15mg par fois, 45 à 60mg par jour ; injection par voie IM ou sous-cutanée, 25mg par fois. |
| 剂型、规格<br>Les formes pharmaceutiques et les spécifications | 片剂：每片 25mg。<br>注射液：25mg（1ml）。<br>Comprimés : 25mg par comprimé.<br>Injection : 25mg (1ml). |

**续　表**

| 药品名称 Drug Names | 酚苄明 Phénoxybenzamine |
|---|---|
| 适应证<br>Les indications | 用于周围血管疾病，也可用于休克及嗜铬细胞瘤引起的高血压。早泄治疗。<br><br>Ce produit est utilisé pour traiter les maladies vasculaires périphériques, le choc ainsi que l'hypertension artérielle causée par le phéochromocytome. Il sert également à traiter l'éjaculation précoce. |
| 用法、用量<br>Les modes d'emploi et la posologie | 口服：用于血管痉挛性疾患，开始一日1次，10mg，一日2次，隔日增10mg；维持量一次20mg，一日2次。用于早泄，一次10mg，一日3次。静脉注射：每日0.5～1mg/kg。静脉滴注（抗休克）：0.5～1mg/kg，加入5%葡萄糖液250～500ml中静脉滴注（2小时滴完），一日总量不超过2mg/kg。<br><br>Par voie orale : pour traiter des maladies angiospastiques, commencer par 10mg par fois, 2 fois par jour, ensuite, augmenter 10mg tous les deux jours ; la dose d'entretien, 20mg par fois, 2 fois par jour. Pour traiter l'éjaculation précoce, 10mg par fois, 3 fois par jour. Injection par voie IV : 0,5 à 1 mg/kg par jour. En perfusion (antichoc) : 0,5 à 1 mg/kg, dissoudre dans 250 à 500ml de solution de glucose à 5 %, perfusion en 2h, ne pas dépasser 2 mg/kg par jour. |
| 剂型、规格<br>Les formes pharmaceutiques et les spécifications | 片剂：每片5mg；10mg。<br>注射液：每支10mg（1ml）。<br><br>Comprimés : 5mg ou 10mg par comprimé.<br>Injection : 10mg (1ml) par solution. |
| 药品名称 Drug Names | 普萘洛尔 Propranolol |
| 适应证<br>Les indications | 用于治疗多种原因所致的心律失常，如房性及室性早搏(效果较好)、窦性及室上性心动过速、心房颤动等，但室性心动过速应慎用。锑剂中毒引起的心律失常，当其他药物无效时可使用本品。此外也可用于心绞痛、高血压、嗜铬细胞瘤（术前准备）等。治疗心绞痛时，常与硝酸酯类合用，可提高疗效，互相抵消不良反应。对高血压有一定疗效，不易引起直立性低血压的影响的特点。<br><br>Ce produit sert à traiter l'arythmie de toutes sortes, telle que l'extrasystole auriculaire et ventriculaire (efficace), latachycardie sinusale et supraventriculaire, la fibrillation auriculaire, etc. Mais il faut être prudent quant à l'application de ce produit au traitement de la tachycardie ventriculaire. Pour traiter l'arythmie causée par l'intoxication par l'antimoine, quand d'autres médicaments sont inutiles, c'est possible d'appliquer ce produit. Il est également applicable dans le traitement de l'angine de poitrine, l'hypertension artérielle et le phéochromocytome (préparation avant la chirurgie). Lors du traitement de l'angine de poitrine, il est souvent utilisé en association avec les esters de l'acide nitrique, pour améliorer son efficacité ou diminuer les effets indésirables. Il a un certain effet sur l'hypertension artérielle et a la caractéristique de ne pas entraîner facilement l'hypotension orthostatique. |
| 用法、用量<br>Les modes d'emploi et la posologie | （1）口服：①心律失常：每日10～30mg，分3次服，根据心律、心率及血压变化及时调整。②嗜铬细胞瘤：术前3日服，一日60mg，分3次服。③心绞痛：每日40～80mg，分3～4次服，从小剂量开始逐渐加至80mg以上。剂量过小常无效。④高血压：每次5mg，一日4次，1～2周后加1/4量，严密监控下可加至1日100mg。<br>（2）静脉滴注：宜慎用。对麻醉中的心律失常以1mg/min的速度静脉滴注，一次2.5～5mg，稀释于5%～10%葡萄糖液100ml内滴注。严密监控血压、心律和心率变化，随时调整速度。如心率转慢，立即停药。<br><br>(1) Par voie orale : ① L'arythmie : 10 à 30 mg par jour, à travers 3 fois, ajuster la dose en fonction du rythme cardiaque et de la pression sanguine. ② le phéochromocytome : 3 jours avant la chirurgie, 60mg par jour, à travers 3 fois. ③ Pour traiter l'angine de poitrine : 40 à 80mg par jour, à travers 3 à 4 fois, commencer par une dose mineure pour atteindre 80mg et plus. La dose mineure est souvent inefficace. ④ Pour lutter contre l'hypertension : 5mg par fois, 4 fois par jour, 1 à 2 semaines après, augmenter1/4 de la dose précédente, possible de prendre 100mg par jour sous contrôle.<br>(2) En perfusion : soyez prudent. Lors de l'arythmie pendant l'anesthésie, 1mg par minute, 2,5 à 5mg par fois, dissoudre dans 100ml de solution de glucose à 5 % à 10 %. Suivre de près la pression sanguine, le rythme cardiaque et ajuster la vitesse de la perfusion. Lors du ralentissement du rythme cardiaque, arrêter immédiatement l'administration. |

**续　表**

| | |
|---|---|
| 剂型、规格<br>Les formes pharmaceutiques et les spécifications | 片剂：每片 10mg。<br>注射液：每支 5mg（5ml）。<br>Comprimés : 10mg par comprimé.<br>Injection : 5mg (5ml) par solution. |
| 药品名称 Drug Names | 噻吗洛尔 Timolol |
| 适应证<br>Les indications | 治疗高血压病、心绞痛、心动过速及青光眼。①对轻中度高血压疗效较好，无明显不良反应，可与利尿剂合用。②心肌梗死患者长期服用本品可降低发病率和死亡率。对青光眼起效快，不良反应小、耐受性好。滴后 20 分钟，眼压下降，经 1 ～ 2 小时达最大效应，作用持续 24 小时。对瞳孔大小、对光反应及视力无影响。<br><br>Ce produit sert à traiter l'hypertension artérielle, l'angine de poitrine, la tachycardie et le glaucome. ① Il est efficace dans le traitement de l'hypertension bénigne et modérée, sans effets indésirables évidents, possible d'être utilisé en combinaison avec les diurétiques. ② Chez des patients atteints d'infarctus du myocarde, l'utilisation de ce produit à long terme pourrait permettre de réduire la morbidité et la mortalité. Il est efficace dans le traitement du glaucome, avec une action rapide, des effets indésirables mineurs et une bonne torélance.20 minutes après des gouttes, la pression intraoculaire diminue, avant d'atteindre le niveau le plus bas 1 à 2 h après, et de maintenir le niveau pendant 24 h. Il n'affecte pas le diamètre de la pupille, la réaction à la lumière, ni la vision. |
| 用法、用量<br>Les modes d'emploi et la posologie | 口服：每次 5 ～ 10mg，一日 2 ～ 3 次。滴眼：0.25% 滴眼剂，每次 1 滴，一日 2 次。如效果不佳，可改用 5% 滴眼剂，每次 1 滴，一日 2 次。<br><br>Par voie orale : 5 à 10mg par fois, 2 à 3 fois par jour. Les gouttes pour les yeux : les gouttes à 0,25 %, 1 goutte par fois, 2 fois par jour. s'il n'est pas efficace, utiliser les gouttes à 5 %, 1 goutte par fois, 2 fois par jour. |
| 剂型、规格<br>Les formes pharmaceutiques et les spécifications | 片剂：每片 2.5mg；5mg。<br>滴眼剂：12.5mg（5ml）；25mg（5ml）。<br>Comprimés : 2,5mg ou 5mg par comprimé.<br>Gouttes pour les yeux : 12,5mg (5ml) ou 25mg (5ml). |
| 药品名称 Drug Names | 索他洛尔 Sotalol |
| 适应证<br>Les indications | 用于高血压，也可用于心绞痛、心律失常。<br>Ce produit sert à traiter l'hypertention artérielle, l'angine de poitrine et l'arythmie. |
| 用法、用量<br>Les modes d'emploi et la posologie | 高血压：初始 1 日 80mg，分 2 次服，需要时可加至一日 160 ～ 600mg。心绞痛和心律失常：口服，一日 160mg，一日 1 次（清晨）服用。<br><br>Pour traiter l'hypertension : commencer par 80mg par jour, à travers 2 fois, s'il est nécessaire, augmenter la dose pour atteindre 160 à 600mg par jour. Pour traiter l'angine de poitrine et l'arythmie : par voie orale, 160 mg par jour, 1 fois par jour (le petit matin). |
| 剂型、规格<br>Les formes pharmaceutiques et les spécifications | 片剂：每片 20mg；40mg；80mg；160mg；200mg。<br>Comprimés : 20mg, 40mg, 80mg, 160mg ou 200mg par comprimé. |
| 药品名称 Drug Names | 阿替洛尔 Aténolol |
| 适应证<br>Les indications | 用于高血压、心绞痛及心律失常。对青光眼有效。<br>Ce produit sert à traiter l'hypertention artérielle, l'angine de poitrine et l'arythmie. Il est aussi efficace dans le traitement du glaucome. |
| 用法、用量<br>Les modes d'emploi et la posologie | 口服：每日 1 次 100mg 用于心绞痛，每日 1 次 100mg，或每次 25 ～ 50mg，一日 2 次。用于高血压每次 50 ～ 100mg，一日 1 ～ 2 次。青光眼用 4% 溶液滴剂。<br><br>Par voie orale : 100mg par fois par jour, pour traiter l'angine de poitrine, 100mg par fois par jour, ou 25 à 50mg par fois, 2 fois par jour. Pour traiter l'hypertension, 50 à 100mg par fois, 1 à 2 fois par jour. Pour traiter le glaucome, utiliser les gouttes à 4 %. |

**续 表**

| | |
|---|---|
| 剂型、规格<br>Les formes pharmaceutiques et les spécifications | 片剂：每片 12.5mg；25mg；50mg；100mg。<br>Comprimés : 12,5mg, 25mg, 50mg ou 100mg par comprimé. |
| **药品名称 Drug Names** | 美托洛尔 Métoprolol |
| 适应证<br>Les indications | 用于各型高血压及心绞痛。静脉注射对心律失常、特别是室上性心律失常也有效。<br>Ce produit sert à traiter l'hypertension artérielle et l'angine de poitrine. Administré par voie IV, ce produit permet aussi de traiter l'arythmie, surtout l'arythmie supraventriculaire. |
| 用法、用量<br>Les modes d'emploi et la posologie | ①口服：剂量需个体化。一般用于高血压，一日 1 次 100mg，维持量为一日 1 次，100 ~ 200mg，必要时加至每日 400mg，早晚分服。用于心绞痛，每日 100 ~ 150mg，分 2 ~ 3 次服，必要时加至每日 150 ~ 300mg。②静脉注射：用于心律失常。开始为 5mg（每分钟 1 ~ 2mg）每隔 5 分钟重复注射，直至有效，一般总量为 10 ~ 15mg。<br>① Par voie orale : ajuster la dose selon les cas. Pour traiter l'hypertension, 100mg par fois par jour, la dose d'entretien, 100 à 200mg par fois par jour, s'il est nécessaire, 400mg par jour, pris le petit matin et le soir. Pour traiter l'angine de poitrine, 100 à 150 mg par jour, à travers 2 à 3 fois, s'il est nécessaire, 150 à 300mg par jour. ② Injection par voie IV : pour traiter l'arythmie. Commencer par 5mg, (1 à 2mg par minute), toutes les 5 minutes, jusqu'à ce qu'il soit efficace, la dose totale, 10 à 15mg. |
| 剂型、规格<br>Les formes pharmaceutiques et les spécifications | 片剂：25mg；50mg；100mg。胶囊剂：每粒 50mg。缓释片：每片 100mg；200mg。<br>Comprimés : 25mg, 50mg ou 100mg. Capsules : 50mg par capsule. Comprimés à libération prolongée : 100mg ou 200mg par comprimé. |
| **药品名称 Drug Names** | 比索洛尔 Bisoprolol |
| 适应证<br>Les indications | 用于高血压及心绞痛。<br>Ce produit sert à traiter l'hypertension artérielle et l'angine de poitrine. |
| 用法、用量<br>Les modes d'emploi et la posologie | 一日 5 ~ 20mg，一次口服。大多数一日口服 10mg 即可。<br>5 à 20mg par jour, à travers 1 fois, par voie orale. Dans la plupart des cas, l'administration de 10mg par jour par voie orale suffit. |
| 剂型、规格<br>Les formes pharmaceutiques et les spécifications | 片剂：每片 2。5mg；5mg。<br>胶囊：2.5mg；5mg；10mg。<br>Comprimés : 2,5mg ou 5mg par comprimé.<br>Capsules : 2,5mg, 5mg ou 10mg par capsule. |
| **药品名称 Drug Names** | 倍他洛尔 Bétaxolol |
| 适应证<br>Les indications | 用于高血压、开角型青光眼的治疗。<br>Ce produit sert à traiter l'hypertention artérielle et le glaucome à angle ouvert. |
| 用法、用量<br>Les modes d'emploi et la posologie | 高血压：口服，一日 1 次 20mg，在 7 ~ 14 日达良效，如需要可加至一日 1 次 40mg。老年患者酌减。用于开角型青光眼：0.5% 滴眼剂一日 2 次。<br>Pour traiter l'hypertension : par voie orale, 20mg par fois par jour, il est efficace en 7 à 14 jours, s'il est nécessaire, 40mg par fois par jour. Diminuer la dose chez des personnes âgées. Pour traiter le glaucome à angle ouvert : les gouttes à 0,5 %, 2 fois par jour. |
| 剂型、规格<br>Les formes pharmaceutiques et les spécifications | 片剂：每片 20mg。<br>滴眼剂：0.25%；0.5%；1%。<br>Comprimés : 20mg par comprimé.<br>Les gouttes pour les yeux : 0,25 %, 0,5 % ou 1 %. |

续　表

| 药品名称 Drug Names | 艾司洛尔 Esmolol |
| --- | --- |
| 适应证<br>Les indications | 用于轻度高血压和心绞痛。<br>Ce produit sert à traiter l'hypertension artérielle bénigne et l'angine de poitrine. |
| 用法、用量<br>Les modes d'emploi et la posologie | 口服，一日 1 次，100 ～ 200mg。<br>Par voie orale, 100 à 200mg par fois par jour. |
| 剂型、规格<br>Les formes pharmaceutiques et les spécifications | 片剂：每片 200mg；注射剂：每支 200mg（2ml）。<br>Comprimés : 200mg par comprime; Injection : 200mg (2ml) par solution. |

10. 主要作用于心血管系统的药物 Mdicaments agissant sur le système cardiovasculaire

10.1　钙通道阻滞药 Bloqueurs de canaux calciques

| 药品名称 Drug Names | 维拉帕米 Vérapamil |
| --- | --- |
| 适应证<br>Les indications | 用于抗心律失常和抗心绞痛。对于阵发性室上性心动过速最有效；对房室交界区心动过速疗效也很好；也可用于心房颤动、心房扑动、房性早搏。<br>Ce produit sert à lutter contre l'arythmie et l'angine de poitrine. Il est le plus éminent dans le traitement de la tachycardie paroxystique supraventriculaire; il est également efficace dans le traitement des tachycardies de la jonction auriculoventriculaire ; il est aussi applicable dans le traitment dela fibrillation auriculaire, du flutter auriculaire et de l'extrasystole auriculaire. |
| 用法、用量<br>Les modes d'emploi et la posologie | 口服：一次 40 ～ 120mg，一日 3 ～ 4 次。维持剂量每一次 40mg，一日 3 次。稀释后缓慢静脉注射或静脉滴注，0.075 ～ 0.15mg/kg，症状控制后改用片剂口服维持。<br>Par voie orale : 40 à 120mg par fois, 3 à 4 fois par jour. La dose d'entretien, 40mg par fois, 3 fois par jour. Injection par voie IV ou en perfusion lente après la dilution, 0,075 à 0,15 mg/kg, après le contrôle des symptômes, administrer les comprimés par voie orale pour l'entretien. |
| 剂型、规格<br>Les formes pharmaceutiques et les spécifications | 片剂：每片 40mg。<br>注射液：每支 5mg（2ml）。<br>Comprimés : 40mg par comprimé.<br>Injection : 5mg (2ml) par solution. |
| 药品名称 Drug Names | 硝苯地平 Nifédipine |
| 适应证<br>Les indications | 用于预防和治疗冠心病和心绞痛，特别是变异型心绞痛和冠状动脉痉挛所致的心绞痛，对呼吸功能没有不良影响，故适用于患有呼吸道阻塞性疾病的心绞痛患者，其疗效优于 β 受体拮抗剂。还适用于各种类型的高血压，对顽固性、重度高血压也有较好疗效。由于能降低后负荷，对顽固性充血性心力衰竭亦有良好疗效，宜于长期服用。<br>Ce produit sert à prévenir et à traiter la maladie coronarienne et l'angine de poitrine, surtout l'angine de poitrine variante, et l'angine de poitrine causée par le spasme des artères coronaires. Comme il n'a pas d'effet négatif sur la fonction respiratoire, il est applicable chez des patients atteints d'angine de poitrine accompagnée desmaladies respiratoires obstructives, avec un effet meilleur que les antagonistes du récepteurβ. Il est aussi appliqué dans le traitement de l'hypertension artérielle, y compris l'hypertension réfractaire et grave. Étant donné qu'il peut diminuer la post-charge, il est efficace dans le traitement de l'insuffisance cardiaque congestive réfractaire. Il vaut mieux l'appliquer pour une longue durée. |
| 用法、用量<br>Les modes d'emploi et la posologie | 口服：一次 5 ～ 10mg，一日 15 ～ 30mg。急用时可舌下含服。对慢性心力衰竭，每 6 小时 20mg，咽部喷药，每次 1.5 ～ 2mg（喷 3 ～ 4 次）。<br>Par voie orale : 5 à 10mg par fois, 15 à 30mg par jour. En cas d'urgence, prendre le comprimé sublingual. Pour traiter l'insuffisance cardiaque chronique, 20mg toutes les 6h, pulvériser dans la gorge, 1,5 à 2mg par fois, 3 à 4 fois à peu près. |

**续 表**

| 剂型、规格<br>Les formes pharmaceutiques et les spécifications | 片剂：普通片每片 5mg；10mg。<br>控释片：每片 20mg。<br>胶丸剂：每丸 5mg。<br>胶囊剂：每粒 5mg；10mg。<br>喷雾剂：每瓶 100mg。<br>Comprimés : 5mg ou 10mg par comprimé.<br>Comprimés à libération prolongée : 20mg par comprimé.<br>Pilules : 5mg par pilule.<br>Capsules：5mg ou 10mg par capsule.<br>Aérosol : 100mg par flacon. |
|---|---|
| **药品名称 Drug Names** | **尼卡地平 Nicardipine** |
| 适应证<br>Les indications | 用于治疗高血压、脑血管疾病、脑血栓形成或脑出血后遗症及脑动脉硬化症等。<br>Ce produit sert à traiter, l'hypertension artérielle, les maladies cérébrovasculaires, la thrombose cérébrale ou les séquelles d'une hémorragie cérébrale, ainsi que l'artériosclérose cérébrale. |
| 用法、用量<br>Les modes d'emploi et la posologie | 口服：每次 20mg，一日 60mg。静脉滴注：高血压急症时以每分钟 0.5μg/kg 速度开始，根据血压监测调节滴速。<br>Par voie orale : 20mg par fois, 60mg par jour. en perfusion : lors de l'hypertension aigue, commencer par 0,5 µg/kg par minute, ajuster la vitesse en fonction de la pression sanguine. |
| 剂型、规格<br>Les formes pharmaceutiques et les spécifications | 片剂：普通片每片 10mg；20mg；40mg。<br>缓释片：每片 10mg。<br>盐酸尼卡地平注射液：5ml：5mg（以尼卡地平计算）。<br>Comprimés : 10mg, 20mg ou 40mg par comprimé.<br>Comprimés à libération prolongée : 10mg par comprimé.<br>Injection de chlorhydrate de nicardipine : 5ml : 5mg (quantité mesurée par nicardipine). |
| **药品名称 Drug Names** | **尼群地平 Nitrendipine** |
| 适应证<br>Les indications | 用于冠心病及高血压，尤其是患有这两种疾病的患者，也可用于充血性心力衰竭。<br>Ce produit sert àtraiter la maladie coronarienne et l'hypertension artérielle, surtout chez des patients souffrant de ces deux maladies. Il est aussi applicable dans le traitement de l'insuffisance cardiaque congestive. |
| 用法、用量<br>Les modes d'emploi et la posologie | 口服，1 次 10mg，一日 30mg。<br>Par voie orale, 10mg par fois, 30 mg par jour. |
| 剂型、规格<br>Les formes pharmaceutiques et les spécifications | 片剂：每片 10mg。<br>Comprimés : 10mg par comprimé. |
| **药品名称 Drug Names** | **尼莫地平 Nimodipine** |
| 适应证<br>Les indications | 用于脑血管疾病，如脑血管灌注不足、脑血管痉挛、蛛网膜下腔出血、脑卒中和偏头痛等。对突发性耳聋也有一定疗效。<br>Ce produit sert à traiter les maladies cérébrovasculaires, telles que l'hypoperfusion cérébrale, le vasospasme cérébral, l'hémorragie méningée, l'AVC et la migraine. Il a aussi un certain effet sur la surdité subite. |
| 用法、用量<br>Les modes d'emploi et la posologie | 口服：一日剂量 40～60mg，分 2～3 次服。<br>Par voie orale : 40 à 60mg par jour, à travers 2 à 3 fois. |

**续　表**

| 剂型、规格<br>Les formes pharmaceutiques et les spécifications | 片剂：20mg。<br>Comprimés : 20mg. |
| --- | --- |
| 药品名称 Drug Names | 非洛地平 Félodipine |
| 适应证<br>Les indications | 用于高血压病、缺血性心脏病和心力衰竭患者。<br>Ce produit sert à traite l'hypertension artérielle, la cardiopathie ischémique et l'insuffisance cardiaque. |
| 用法、用量<br>Les modes d'emploi et la posologie | 一日剂量 20mg，分次服。<br>20 mg par jour, à travers plusieurs fois. |
| 剂型、规格<br>Les formes pharmaceutiques et les spécifications | 片剂：每片 5mg；10mg。<br>Comprimés : 5mg ou 10mg par comprimé. |
| 药品名称 Drug Names | 氨氯地平 Amlodipine |
| 适应证<br>Les indications | 用于治疗高血压，单独应用或与其他抗高血压药合用均可；也可用于稳定型心绞痛患者，尤其是对硝酸盐和 β 受体拮抗剂无效者。<br>Ce produit sert à traiter l'hypertension artérielle. Il peut être utilisé seul ou en association avec d'autres sntihypertenseurs. Il est aussi applicable chez les patients atteints d'angine de poitrine stable, surtout chez ceux qui sont résistants aux nitrates et auxantagonistes du récepteur β. |
| 用法、用量<br>Les modes d'emploi et la posologie | 口服，开始时 1 次 5mg，一日 1 次，以后可根据患者的临床反应，可将剂量增加，最大可增至每日 10mg。<br>Par voie orale, commencer par 5mg par fois, 1 fois par jour, augmenter ensuite la dose en fonction des réactions cliniques des patients pour atteindre 10mg par jour au maximum. |
| 剂型、规格<br>Les formes pharmaceutiques et les spécifications | 片剂：每片 2.5mg；5mg；10mg。<br>Comprimés : 2,5mg, 5mg ou 10mg par comprimé. |
| 药品名称 Drug Names | 左氨氯地平 Levoamlodipine |
| 适应证<br>Les indications | 用于治疗高血压，单独应用或与其他抗高血压药合用均可；也可用于稳定型心绞痛患者，尤其是对硝酸盐和 β 受体拮抗剂无效者。<br>Ce produit sert à traiter l'hypertension artérielle. Il peut être utilisé seul ou en association avec d'autres sntihypertenseurs. Il est aussi applicable chez les patients atteints d'angine de poitrine stable, surtout chez ceux qui sont résistants aux nitrates et auxantagonistes du récepteur β. |
| 用法、用量<br>Les modes d'emploi et la posologie | 口服，开始时 1 次 2.5mg，一日 1 次；根据患者的临床反应，可将剂量增加，最大可增至每日 5mg，一日 1 次。<br>Par voie orale, commencer par 2,5mg par fois, 1 fois par jour ; augmenter ensuite la dose en fonction des réactions cliniques des patients pour atteindre 5mg par jour, 1 fois par jour au maximum. |
| 剂型、规格<br>Les formes pharmaceutiques et les spécifications | 片剂：每片 2.5mg。<br>Comprimés : 2,5mg par comprimé. |
| 药品名称 Drug Names | 西尼地平 Cilnidipine |
| 适应证<br>Les indications | 用于治疗高血压，可单独应用，或与其他降压药合用。<br>Ce produit sert à traiter l'hypertension artérielle. Il peut être utilisé seul ou en association avec d'autres sntihypertenseurs. |

**续　表**

| 用法、用量 Les modes d'emploi et la posologie | 口服：1 次 5 ～ 10mg，一日 1 次，必要时可增至 20mg，一日 1 次。早餐后服用。根据患者的临床反应，可将剂量增加，最大可增至每次 10mg。<br><br>Par voie orale : 5 à 10mg par fois, 1 fois par jour, s'il est nécessaire, 20mg, 1 fois par jour, après le petit-déjeuner. Augmenter la dose en fonction des réactions cliniques des patients pour atteindre 10mg par fois au maximum. |
|---|---|
| 剂型、规格 Les formes pharmaceutiques et les spécifications | 片剂：每片 5mg。<br><br>Comprimés : 5mg par comprimé. |

| 药品名称 Drug Names | 拉西地平 Lacidipine |
|---|---|
| 适应证 Les indications | 用于治疗高血压。<br><br>Ce produit sert à traiter l'hypertension artérielle. |
| 用法、用量 Les modes d'emploi et la posologie | 开始时每日 1 次，每次 4mg，如效果不佳可增至一日 1 次，每次 6mg。肝功能不全患者，开始时需减半量。<br><br>Commencer par 4mg par fois, 1 fois par jour. s'il n'est pas très efficace, prendre 6mg par fois, 1 fois par jour. Chez des patients insuffisants hépatiques, commencer par prendre la moitié de la dose usuelle. |
| 剂型、规格 Les formes pharmaceutiques et les spécifications | 片剂：每片 2mg；4mg。<br><br>Comprimés : 2mg ou 4mg par comprimé. |

| 药品名称 Drug Names | 地尔硫䓬 Diltiazem |
|---|---|
| 适应证 Les indications | 用于室上性心律失常、典型心绞痛、变异型心绞痛、老年人高血压等。<br><br>Ce produit sert à traiter l'arythmie supraventriculaire, l'angine de poitrine typique, l'angine de poitrine variante et l'hypertension artérielle sénile. |
| 用法、用量 Les modes d'emploi et la posologie | 口服，常用量，1 次 30 ～ 60mg，一日 90 ～ 180mg。用于心律失常：口服，1 次 30 ～ 60mg，一日 4 次；起始剂量为 250μg/kg，于 2 分钟静脉注射；必要时 15 分钟后再给 350μg/kg。以后的剂量应根据患者的情况个体化制定。在房颤或房扑患者，最初输注速率 5 ～ 10mg/h，必要时可增至最大 15mg/h（增幅 5mg/h）。静脉输注最多可维持 24 小时。用于心绞痛：每 6 ～ 8 小时 30 ～ 60mg。用于高血压：一日剂量 120 ～ 240mg，分 3 ～ 4 次服。<br><br>Par voie orale, la dose usuelle, 30 à 60mg par fois, 90 à 180mg par jour. Pour traiter l'arythmie : par voie orale, 30 à 60mg par fois, 4 fois par jour ; la dose initiale, 250μg/kg, injection par voie IV en 2 h ; s'il est nécessaire, encore 350μg/kg 15 minutes après. Ensuite, ajuster la dose selon les cas. Chez des patients souffrant de la fibrillation auriculaire ou du flutter auriculaire, au début, 5 à 10 mg par heure, s'il est nécessaire, 15 mg par h au maximum (augmenter 5mg par heure). La perfusion ne dure que 24h au maximum. Pour traiter l'angine de poitrine : 30 à 60mg toutes les 6 à 8h. Pour traiter l'hypertension : 120 à 240mg par jour, à travers 3 à 4 fois. |
| 剂型、规格 Les formes pharmaceutiques et les spécifications | 片剂：普通片每片 30mg；60mg；90mg；缓释片：每片 30mg；60mg；90mg。<br>缓释胶囊：90mg。<br>注射用盐酸地尔硫䓬：10mg；50mg。<br>Comprimés : 30mg, 60mg ou 90mg par comprimé.<br>Comprimés à libération prolongée : 30mg, 60mg ou 90mg par comprimé.<br>Capsules à liération prolongée : 90mg.<br>Le chlorhydrate de diltiazem pour injection : 10mg ou 50mg. |

| 药品名称 Drug Names | 桂利嗪 Cinnarizine |
|---|---|
| 适应证 Les indications | 用于脑血栓形成、脑栓塞、脑动脉硬化、脑出血恢复期、蛛网膜下腔出血恢复期、脑外伤后遗症、内耳眩晕症、冠状动脉粥样硬化、由于末梢循环不良引起的疾病等。<br><br>Ce produit sert à traiter la thrombose cérébrale, l'embolie cérébrale, l'artériosclérose cérébrale, la récupération de l'hémorragie cérébrale, la récupération de l'hémorragie méningée, les séquelles d'une lésion cérébrale traumatique, le vertige de l'oreille interne, l'athérosclérose coronarienne, ainsi que les maladies liées à la circulation périphérique pauvre. |

**续 表**

| | |
|---|---|
| 用法、用量<br>Les modes d'emploi et la posologie | 口服：每次 25 ～ 50mg，一日 3 次，餐后服。静脉注射：1 次 20 ～ 40mg，缓慢注入。<br>Par voie orale : 25 à 50mg par fois, 3 fois par jour, après le repas. Injection par voie IV : 20 à 40mg par fois, injection lente. |
| 剂型、规格<br>Les formes pharmaceutiques et les spécifications | 片剂及胶囊剂：每片（粒）25mg。<br>注射液：每支 20mg（20ml）。<br>Comprimés et capsules : 25mg par comprimé ou par capsule.<br>Injection : 20mg (20ml) par solution. |
| 药品名称 Drug Names | 氟桂利嗪 Flunarizine |
| 适应证<br>Les indications | 药理及应用同桂利嗪相似，有扩血管作用。此外，对注意力减弱、记忆力障碍、易激动以及平衡功能障碍、眩晕等均有一定疗效。用于老年患者。<br>La pharmacologie et son mode d'emploi sont similaires à la cinnarizine. Il a un effet vasodilatateur. En outre, il permet aussi de traiter le déficit d'attention, les troubles de la mémoire, l'irritabilité, les troubles de l'équilibre, ainsi que le vertige. Il est appliqué chez des personnes âgées. |
| 用法、用量<br>Les modes d'emploi et la posologie | 1 次 5 ～ 10mg，一日 10mg（以氟桂利嗪计），在一般情况下，可于晚上顿服。<br>5 à 10mg par fois, 10 mg par jour (mesuré en flunarizine), en général, pris le soir, une fois par jour. |
| 剂型、规格<br>Les formes pharmaceutiques et les spécifications | 胶囊剂：每粒 5mg（以氟桂利嗪计）。<br>Capsules : 5mg par capsule (mesuré en flunarizine). |
| 药品名称 Drug Names | 利多氟嗪 Lidoflazine |
| 适应证<br>Les indications | 用于心绞痛。<br>Ce produit est utilisé comme traitement de l'angine de poitrine. |
| 用法、用量<br>Les modes d'emploi et la posologie | 口服，1 次 60mg，一日 3 次。<br>Par voie orale, 60mg par fois, 3 fois par jour. |
| 剂型、规格<br>Les formes pharmaceutiques et les spécifications | 片剂：每片 60mg。<br>Comprimés : 60mg par comprimé. |

10.2　治疗慢性心功能不全的药物 Médicaments pour le traitement de l'inefficacité cardiaque chronique

| | |
|---|---|
| 药品名称 Drug Names | 洋地黄毒苷 Digitoxine |
| 适应证<br>Les indications | 用于维持治疗慢性心功能不全。<br>Ce produit permet de traiter l'insuffisance cardiaque chronique. |
| 用法、用量<br>Les modes d'emploi et la posologie | 主要采用口服，不宜口服者可以肌内注射，必要时静脉注射。全效量：成人 0.7 ～ 1.2mg；于 48 ～ 72 小时分次服用。小儿 2 岁以下 0.03 ～ 0.04mg/kg，2 岁以上 0.02 ～ 0.03mg/kg。维持量：成人每日 0.05 ～ 0.1mg，小儿为全效量的 1/10，一日 1 次。<br>Principalement pris par voie orale, s'il est nécessaire, aussi possible d'être pris par voie IM et même IV. La dose pour un effet complet : chez des adultes, 0,7 à 1,2 mg ; à travers plusieurs fois en 48 à 72 h. Chez moins de 2 ans, 0,03 à 0,04 mg/kg, chez plus de 2 ans, 0,02 à 0,03 mg/kg. La dose d'entretien : chez des adultes, 0,05 à 0,1mg par jour, chez des enfants, 1/10 de la dose pour un effet complet, 1 fois par jour. |
| 剂型、规格<br>Les formes pharmaceutiques et les spécifications | 片剂：每片 0.1mg。<br>注射液：每支 0.2mg（1ml）。<br>Comprimés : 0,1mg par comprimé.<br>Injection : 0,2mg (1ml) par solution. |

| 药品名称 Drug Names | 地高辛 Digoxine |
|---|---|
| 适应证<br>Les indications | 用于各种急性和慢性心功能不全和室上性心动过速、心房颤动和扑动等。<br>Ce produit sert à traiter l'insuffisance cardiaque chronique et aigue ainsi que la tachycardie supraventriculaire, la fibrillation auriculaire et le flutter auriculaire. |
| 用法、用量<br>Les modes d'emploi et la posologie | 全效量：成人口服 1～1.5mg；于 24 小时内分次服用。小儿 2 岁以下 0.06～0.08mg/kg，2 岁以上 0.04～0.06mg/kg。不宜口服者也可静脉注射，临用前以 10% 或 25% 葡萄糖注射液稀释后应用,常用量静脉注射 1 次 0.25～0.5mg；极量，1 次 1mg。维持量：成人每日 0.125～0.5mg，分 1～2 次服用；小儿为全效量的 1/4。<br>La dose complète : chez des adultes, 1 à 1,5mg par voie orale ; à plusieurs fois en 24h. Chez moins de 2 ans, 0,06 à 0,08 mg/kg, chez plus de 2 ans, 0,04 à 0,06 mg/kg. Aussi possible de prendre par voie IV, dissoudre dans la solution de glucose à 10 % ou à 25 % avant de l'utiliser, la dose usuelle, injecter 0,25 à 0,5mg par voie IV par fois ; la dose limite, 1mg par fois. La dose d'entretien : chez des adultes, 0,125 à 0,5mg par jour, à travers 1 à 2 fois ; chez des enfants, 1/4 de la dose complète. |
| 剂型、规格<br>Les formes pharmaceutiques et les spécifications | 片剂：每片 0.25mg。<br>注射液：0.5mg（2ml）。<br>Comprimés : 0,25mg par comprimé.<br>Injection : 0,5mg (2ml). |
| 药品名称 Drug Names | 毛花苷 C Lanatoside C |
| 适应证<br>Les indications | 用于急性和慢性心力衰竭。<br>Ce produit sert à traiter l'insuffisance cardiaque chronique et aigue. |
| 用法、用量<br>Les modes d'emploi et la posologie | 缓慢全效量：口服，1 次 0.5mg，一日 4 次。维持量：一般为一日 1mg，分 2 次服用。静脉注射：成人常用量，全效量 1～1.2mg，首次剂量 0.4～0.6mg；2～4 小时后可再给予 0.2～0.4mg，用葡萄糖注射液稀释后缓慢注射。<br>La dose complète ralentie : par voie orale, 0,5mg par fois, 4 fois par jour. La dose d'entretien : 1mg par jour, à travers 2 fois. Injection par voie IV : la dose usuelle chez des adultes, la dose complète, 1 à 1,2mg, la dose initiale, 0,4 à 0,6mg ; 2 à 4 h après, prendre encore 0,2 à 0,4mg, dissoudre dans la solution de glucose avant de l'injecter par voie IV lentement. |
| 剂型、规格<br>Les formes pharmaceutiques et les spécifications | 片剂：每片 0.5mg。<br>注射液：0.4mg（2ml）。<br>Comprimés : 0,5mg par comprimé.<br>Injection : 0,4mg (2ml). |
| 药品名称 Drug Names | 去乙酰毛花苷 Deslanoside |
| 适应证<br>Les indications | 用于急性心力衰竭以及心房颤动及心房扑动等。<br>Ce produit sert à traiter l'insuffisance cardiaque aigue, la fibrillation auriculaire et le flutter auriculaire. |
| 用法、用量<br>Les modes d'emploi et la posologie | 静脉注射 成人常用量：用葡萄糖注射液稀释后缓慢注射，1 次 0.4～0.8mg。全效量 1～1.6mg，于 24 小时内分次注射。儿童每日 20～40μg/kg，分 1～2 次给药。然后改用口服毛花苷 C 维持治疗。<br>La dose usuelle prise par voie IV chez des adultes : dissoudre dans la solution de glucose avant d'injecter lentement 0,4 à 0,8mg par fois. La dose complète, 1 à 1,6mg, à travers plusieurs fois en 24h. Chez des enfants, 20 à 40μg/kg par jour, à travers 1 à 2 fois. Ensuite, prendre la lanatoside par voie orale comme le traitement d'entretien. |
| 剂型、规格<br>Les formes pharmaceutiques et les spécifications | 注射液：每支 0.2mg（1ml）；0.4mg（2ml）。<br>Injection : 0,2mg (1ml) ou 0,4mg (2ml) par solution. |

**续　表**

| 药品名称 Drug Names | 毒毛花苷 K　Strophantine-K |
|---|---|
| 适应证<br>Les indications | 用于急性心力衰竭。动脉硬化性心脏病患者发生心力衰竭时，如心率不快可选用本品。<br><br>Ce produit sert à traiter l'insuffisance cardiaque aigue. Chez les patients atteints de cardiopathie athéroscléreuse, lors de la crise de l'insuffisance cardiaque, si le rythme cardiaque n'est pas rapide, c'est possible d'appliquer ce produit. |
| 用法、用量<br>Les modes d'emploi et la posologie | 静脉注射：首剂 0.125 ～ 0.25mg，加入等渗葡萄糖注射液 20 ～ 40ml 内缓慢注入（时间不少于 5 分钟），1 ～ 2 小时后重复 1 次，总量每日 0.25 ～ 0.5mg。病情转好后，可改用洋地黄苷口服制剂，给予适当的全效量。<br><br>Injection par voie IV : la dose initiale, 0,125 à 0,25mg, dissoudre dans 20 à 40ml de solution de glucose isotonique avant l'injection lente (en 5 minutes au moins), toutes les 1 à 2 h, ne pas dépasser 0,25 à 0,5mg par jour. Dès l'état tourne bien, possible de prendre les formulations orales de glucosides digitaliques, avec une dose complète. |
| 剂型、规格<br>Les formes pharmaceutiques et les spécifications | 注射液：每支 0.25mg（1ml）。<br>Injection : 0,25mg (1ml) par solution. |

| 药品名称 Drug Names | 氨力农 Amrinone |
|---|---|
| 适应证<br>Les indications | 用于对洋地黄、利尿药、血管舒张药治疗无效或效果欠佳的各种原因引起的急性、慢性顽固性充血性心力衰竭的短期治疗。<br><br>Ce produit est utilisé dans le traitement à court terme de l'insuffisance cardiaque congestive réfractaire aigue et chronique, qui est résistante aux digitaliques, aux diurétiques et aux vasodilatateurs. |
| 用法、用量<br>Les modes d'emploi et la posologie | 静脉注射负荷量：0.75mg/kg，2 ～ 3 分钟缓慢静脉注射，继之以每千克 5 ～ 10μg/min 维持静脉滴注，单次剂量最大不超过 2.5mg/kg。每日最大量＜ 10mg/kg。疗程不超过 2 周。<br><br>Dose de charge par voie IV : 0,75 mg/kg, injection lente en 2 à 3 minutes, ensuite, 5 à 10μg par kg par minute en perfusion, ne pas dépasser 2,5 mg/kg par fois. La dose limite est moins de 10 mg/kg par jour. Le traitement médical ne dépasse pas 2 semaines. |
| 剂型、规格<br>Les formes pharmaceutiques et les spécifications | 注射液：每支 50mg（2ml）；100mg（2ml）。<br>Injection : 50mg (2ml) ou 100mg (2ml) par solution. |

| 药品名称 Drug Names | 米力农 Milrinone |
|---|---|
| 适应证<br>Les indications | 用于对洋地黄、利尿药、血管舒张药治疗无效或效果欠佳的各种原因引起的急性、慢性顽固性充血性心力衰竭的短期治疗。<br><br>Ce produit est utilisé dans le traitement à court terme de l'insuffisance cardiaque congestive réfractaire aigue et chronique, qui est résistante aux digitaliques, aux diurétiques et aux vasodilatateurs. |
| 用法、用量<br>Les modes d'emploi et la posologie | 静脉滴注：每分钟 12.5 ～ 75μg/kg。一般开始 10 分钟以 50μg/kg，然后以每分钟 0.375 ～ 0.75μg/kg 维持。每日最大剂量不超过 1.13mg/kg。<br><br>En perfusion : 12,5 à 75μg/kg par minute. En général, 50μg/kg pendant les 10 premières minutes, ensuite, 0,375 à 0,75μg/kg par minute pour l'entretien. Ne pas dépasser 1,13 mg/kg par jour. |
| 剂型、规格<br>Les formes pharmaceutiques et les spécifications | 注射液：每支 10mg（10ml）。<br>Injection : 10mg (10ml) par solution. |

**10.3　抗心律失常药 Antiarrhythmiques**

| 药品名称 Drug Names | 奎尼丁 Quinidine |
|---|---|
| 适应证<br>Les indications | 主要用于阵发性心动过速、心房颤动和早搏等。<br><br>Ce produit sert à traiter la tachycardie paroxystique, la fibrillation auriculaire et l'extrasystole auriculaire. |

**续 表**

| | |
|---|---|
| 用法、用量<br>Les modes d'emploi et la posologie | （1）口服：第 1 天，每次 0.2g，每 2 小时 1 次，连续 5 次；如无效而又无明显毒性反应，第 2 天增至每次 0.3g、第 3 天每次 0.4g，每 2 小时 1 次，连续 5 次。每日总量一般不宜超过 2g。恢复正常心律后，改维持量，每日 0.2 ～ 0.4g。若连服 3 ～ 4 日无效或有毒性反应者，应停药。<br>（2）静脉注射：在十分必要时采用静脉注射并须在心电图观察下进行。每次 0.25g，以 5% 葡萄糖液稀释至 50ml 缓慢静脉注射。<br><br>(1) Par voie orale : le premier jour, 0,2g par fois, toutes les 2 h, pendant 5 fois consécutives ; s'il est inefficace et qu'il n'y a pas d'effets indésirables toxiques évidents, 0,3g pour le deuxième jour, 0,4g pour le troisième jour, toutes les 2 h, pendant 5 fois consécutives. Ne pas dépasser 2g par jour. Dès le rythme cardiaque retourne à la normale, prendre la dose d'entretien, soit 0,2 à 0,4g par jour. S'il est inutile après 3 à 4 jours consécutifs ou s'il y des réactions toxiques, arrêter l'administration.<br>(2) Injection par voie IV : s'il est vraiment nécessaire, injecter par voie IV sous l'observation par l'électrocardiogramme. 0,25g par fois, dissoudre dans la solution de glucose à 5 % pour former 50ml, injection par voie IV lente. |
| 剂型、规格<br>Les formes pharmaceutiques et les spécifications | 片剂：每片 0.2g。<br>葡萄糖酸奎尼丁注射液：每支 0.5g（10ml）。<br><br>Comprimés : 0,2g par comprimé.<br>Injection de gluconate de quinidine : 0,5g (10ml) par solution. |
| 药品名称 Drug Names | 普鲁卡因胺 Procaïnamide |
| 适应证<br>Les indications | 用于阵发性心动过速、频发早搏（对室性早搏疗效较好）、心房颤动和心房扑动，常与奎尼丁交替使用。<br><br>Ce produit sert à traiter la tachycardie paroxystique, l'extrasystole fréquente (surtout efficace pour l'extrasystole ventriculaire), la fibrillation auriculaire et le flutter auriculaire. Il est souvent utilisé en alternance avec la quinidine. |
| 用法、用量<br>Les modes d'emploi et la posologie | ①口服：一日 3 ～ 4 次，每次 0.5 ～ 0.75g，心律正常后逐渐减至一日 2 ～ 6 次，每次 0.25g。②静脉滴注：每次 0.5 ～ 1g，溶于 5% ～ 10% 葡萄糖溶液 100ml 内，开始 10 ～ 30 分钟，点滴速度可适当加快，于 1 小时内滴完。无效者，1 小时后再给一次，24 小时内总量不超过 2g。③静脉注射：每次 0.1 ～ 0.2g。④肌内注射：每次 0.25 ～ 0.5g。<br><br>① Par voie orale : 3 à 4 fois par jour, 0,5 à 0,75g par fois, après la normalisation du rythme cardiaque, diminuer progressivement la dose pour atteindre 0,25 g par fois, 2 à 6 fois par jour. ② En perfusion : 0,5 à 1g par fois, dissoudre dans 100ml de solution de glucose à 5 % à 10 %, pendant les premières 10 à 30 minutes, la vitesse de la perfusion peut être augmentée pour finir la perfusion en 1 h. S'il est inefficace, encore une fois 1 h après, ne pas dépasser 2g par jour. ③ Injection par voie IV : 0,1 à 0,2g par fois. ④ Injection par voie IM : 0,25 à 0,5g par fois. |
| 剂型、规格<br>Les formes pharmaceutiques et les spécifications | 片剂：每片 0.125g；0.25g。<br>注射液：每支 0.1g（1ml）；0.2g（2ml）；0.5g（5ml）；1g（10ml）。<br><br>Comprimés : 0,125g ou 0,25g par comprimé.<br>Injection : 0,1g (1ml), 0,2g (2ml), 0,5g (5ml) ou 1g (10ml) par solution. |
| 药品名称 Drug Names | 丙吡胺 Disopyramide |
| 适应证<br>Les indications | 用于房性早搏、阵发性房性心动过速、房颤、室性早搏等，对室上性心律失常的疗效似较好。<br><br>Il sert à traiter l'extrasystole auriculaire, la tachycardie auriculaire paroxystique, la fibrillation auriculaire, l'extrasystole ventriculaire. Il est surtout efficace dans le traitement de l'arythmie supraventriculaire. |
| 用法、用量<br>Les modes d'emploi et la posologie | 口服，每次 0.1 ～ 0.15g，一日 0.4 ～ 0.8g。最大剂量不超过 800mg/d。静脉注射，每次 1 ～ 2mg/kg，最大剂量每次不超过 150mg，用葡萄糖注射液 20ml 稀释后在 5 ～ 10 分钟注完。必要时，可在 20 分钟后重复一次。静脉滴注，每次 100 ～ 200mg，以 5% 葡萄糖注射液 500ml 稀释，一般滴注量为每小时 20 ～ 30mg。<br><br>Par voie orale, 0,1 à 0,15g par fois, 0,4 à 0,8g par jour. Ne pas dépasser 800mg par jour. Injection par voie IV, 1 à 2 mg/kg par fois, ne pas dépasser 150mg par fois, dissoudre dans 20ml de solution de glucose avant de finir l'injection en 5 à 10 minutes. S'il est nécessaire, encore une fois 20 minutes après. En perfusion, 100 à 200mg par fois, dissoudre dans 500ml de solution de glucose à 5 %, perfusion, 20 à 30 mg par h. |

**续　表**

| | |
|---|---|
| 剂型、规格<br>Les formes pharmaceutiques et les spécifications | 片剂：每片 100mg。<br>注射液：每支 50mg（2ml）；100mg（2ml）。<br>Comprimés : 100mg par comprimé.<br>Injection : 50mg (2ml) ou 100mg (2ml) par solution. |
| **药品名称 Drug Names** | **利多卡因 Lidocaïne** |
| 适应证<br>Les indications | 本品适用于心肌梗死、洋地黄中毒、锑剂中毒、外科手术等所致的室性早搏、室性心动过速和心室颤动。<br>Ce produit est utilisé comme traitement de l'infarctus du myocarde, l'intoxication par les digitaliques, l'intoxication par l'antimoine, ainsi que l'extrasystole ventriculaire, la tachycardie ventriculaire et la fibrillation ventriculaire causées par la chirurgie. |
| 用法、用量<br>Les modes d'emploi et la posologie | 静脉注射，1～2mg/kg，继以 0.1% 溶液静脉滴注，每小时不超过 100mg。也可肌内注射，4～5mg/kg，60～90 分钟重复一次。<br>Injection par voie IV, 1 à 2 mg/kg, ensuite, en perfusion, la solution à 0,1 %, ne pas dépasser 100mg par h. C'est aussi possible d'injecter par voie IM, 4 à 5 mg/kg, toutes les 60 à 90 minutes. |
| 剂型、规格<br>Les formes pharmaceutiques et les spécifications | 注射液：每支 0.1g（5ml）；0.4g（20ml）。<br>Injection : 0,1g (5ml) ou 0,4g (20ml) par solution. |
| **药品名称 Drug Names** | **苯妥英钠 Phénytoïne sodique** |
| 适应证<br>Les indications | 用于洋地黄中毒苷所引起的室上性和室性心律失常及对利多卡因无效的心律失常。<br>Ce produit sert à traiter les arythmies supraventriculaires et ventriculaires causées par les intoxications par les glycosides digitaliques, ainsi que l'arythmie résistante à la lidocaine. |
| 用法、用量<br>Les modes d'emploi et la posologie | 口服：每次 0.1～0.2g，一日 2～3 次。口服极量：每次 0.3g，一日 0.5g。静脉注射：每次 0.125～0.25g，缓慢注入，一日总量不超过 0.5g。<br>Par voie orale : 0,1 à 0,2g par fois, 2 à 3 fois par jour. La dose limite par voie orale : 0,3g par fois, 0,5g par jour. Injection par voie IV : 0,125 à 0,25g par fois, injection lente, ne pas dépasser 0,5g par jour. |
| 剂型、规格<br>Les formes pharmaceutiques et les spécifications | 片剂：每片 0.05g；0.1g。<br>注射用苯妥英钠：每支 0.125g；0.25g。<br>Comprimés : 0,05g ou 0,1g par comprimé.<br>La phénytoïne sodique pour injection : 0,125g ou 0,25g par solution. |
| **药品名称 Drug Names** | **美西律 Mexilétine** |
| 适应证<br>Les indications | 用于急、慢性室性心律失常，如室性早搏、室性心动过速、心室颤动及洋地黄苷中毒引起的心律失常。<br>Ce produit sert à traiter l'arythmie ventriculaire aigue et chronique, telle que l'extrasystole ventriculaire, la tachycardie ventriculaire, la fibrillation ventriculaire ainsi que l'arythmie causée par les intoxications par les glycosides digitaliques. |
| 用法、用量<br>Les modes d'emploi et la posologie | ①口服：每次 50～200mg，一日 150～600mg，或每 6～8 小时 1 次。以后可酌情减量维持。②静脉注射、静脉滴注：开始量 100mg，加入 5% 葡萄糖注射液 20ml 中，缓慢静脉注射（3～5 分钟）。如无效，可在 5～10 分钟后再给 50～100mg1 次。然后以 1.5～2mg/min 的速度静脉滴注，3～4 小时后滴速减至 0.75～1mg/min，并维持 24～48 小时。<br>① Par voie orale : 50 à 200mg par fois, 150 à 600mg par jour, ou toutes les 6 à 8 h. Ensuite, diminuer la dose pour l'entretien. ② Injection par voie IV ou en perfusion : la dose initiale, 100mg, dissoudre dans 20ml de solution de glucose à 5 %, injection par voie IV lente (en 3 à 5 minutes). S'il est inefficace, encore 50 à 100mg 5 à 10 minutes après. Ensuite, en perfusion, 1,5 à 2 mg par minute, pendant 3 à 4 h, puis, 0,75 à 1 mg par minute, pendant 24 à 48h. |

**续 表**

| 剂型、规格<br>Les formes pharmaceutiques et les spécifications | 片剂：每片 50mg；100mg；250mg。<br>胶囊剂：每粒 50mg；100mg；400mg。<br>注射液：100mg（2ml）。<br>Comprimés : 50mg, 100mg ou 250mg par comprimé.<br>Capsules : 50mg, 100mg ou 400mg par capsule.<br>Injection : 100mg (2ml). |
|---|---|
| **药品名称 Drug Names** | **普罗帕酮 Propafénone** |
| 适应证<br>Les indications | 用于预防或治疗室性或室上性异位搏动，室性或室上性心动过速，预激综合征，电转复律后室颤发作等。经临床试用，疗效确切，起效迅速，作用时间持久，对冠心病、高血压所引起的心律失常有较好的疗效。<br>Ce produit sert à traiter les extrasystoles ventriculaire ou supraventriculaire, la tachycardie ventriculaire ou supraventriculaire, le syndrome de WPWet la fibrillation ventriculaire après une cardioversion électrique. L'essai clinique a montré que ce produit avait un effet certain, une action rapide, une efficacité de longue durée, et qu'il était efficace dans le traitement de l'arythmie causée par l'hypertension artérielle. |
| 用法、用量<br>Les modes d'emploi et la posologie | 口服：1 次 100～200mg，一日 3～4 次。治疗量，一日 300～900mg，分 4～6 次服用。维持量，一日 300～600mg，分 2～4 次服用。由于其局部麻醉作用，宜在饭后与饮料或食物同时吞服，不得嚼碎。必要时可在严密监护下缓慢静脉注射或滴注，1 次 70mg，每 8 小时 1 次。一日总量不超过 350mg。<br>Par voie orale : 100 à 200mg par fois, 3 à 4 fois par jour. La dose curative, 300 à 900mg par jour, à travers 4 à 6 fois. La dose d'entretien, 300 à 600mg par jour, à travers 2 à 4 fois. Il vaut mieux le prendre après le repas, avec la boisson ou l'aliment, ne pas le mâcher. S'il est nécessaire, injection par voie IV lente ou en perfusion sous l'observation, 70mg par fois, toutes les 8h. Ne pas dépasser 350mg par jour. |
| 剂型、规格<br>Les formes pharmaceutiques et les spécifications | 片剂：每片 50mg；100mg；150mg。<br>注射液：每支 17.5mg（5ml）；35mg（10ml）。<br>Comprimés : 50mg, 100mg ou 150mg par comprimé.<br>Injection : 17,5mg (5ml) ou 35mg (10ml) par solution. |
| **药品名称 Drug Names** | **恩卡尼 Encaïnide** |
| 适应证<br>Les indications | 用于室性早搏、室性心动过速及心室颤动。也可用于室上性心动过速，对折返性心动过速，尤其是预激综合征有效。<br>Ce produit sert à traiter l'extrasystole ventriculaire, la tachycardie ventriculaire et la fibrillation ventriculaire. Il est également applicable dans le traitement de la tachycardie supraventriculaire. Il est aussi efficace dans le traitement de la tachycardie réentrante, surtout du syndrome de WPW. |
| 用法、用量<br>Les modes d'emploi et la posologie | 口服，每次 25～75mg，一日 3～4 次。静脉注射，以 0.5～1mg/kg，于 15～20 分钟注完。小儿口服一日剂量 60～120mg/m$^2$ 或 2～7.5mg/kg，分 3～4 次服。通常从小剂量开始，在严密观察下逐渐增量。<br>Par voie orale, 25 à 75mg par fois, 3 à 4 fois par jour. Injection par voie IV, 0,5 à 1 mg/kg, en 15 à 20 minutes. Chez des enfants, par voie orale, 60 à 120 mg/m$^2$ ou 2 à 7,5 mg/kg par jour, à travers 3 à 4 fois. Commencer par une faible dose, augmenter progressivement la dose sous l'observation. |
| 剂型、规格<br>Les formes pharmaceutiques et les spécifications | 胶囊剂：每粒 25mg；35mg；50mg。<br>注射液：25mg（1ml）；50mg（2ml）。<br>Capsules : 25mg, 35mg ou 50mg par capsule.<br>Injection : 25mg (1ml) ou 50mg (2ml). |
| **药品名称 Drug Names** | **氟卡尼 Flécaïnide** |
| 适应证<br>Les indications | 用于室上性心动过速、房室结或房室折返心动过速、心房颤动、儿童顽固性交界性心动过速及伴有预激综合征者。对其他抗心律失常药物无效的病例，氟卡尼常有效。<br>Ce produit sert à traiter la tachycardie supraventriculaire, les tachycardies réentrantes nodales ou auriculo-ventriculaires, la fibrillation auriculaire, les tachycardies jonctionnelles réfractaires accompagnées du syndrome de WPW chez des enfants. Chez des cas résistants à d'autres antiarythmiques, laflécaïnide est souvent efficacement utilisée. |

**续　表**

| | |
|---|---|
| 用法、用量<br>Les modes d'emploi et la posologie | 口服：成人开始时每次 100mg，一日 2 次，然后每隔 4 日，每次增加 50mg，最大剂量每次 200mg，一日 2 次；儿童每次 50～100mg，一日 2 次。静脉滴注：成人 2mg/kg，于 15 分钟滴完；儿童 2mg/kg，于 10 分钟内滴完。<br>Par voie orale : chez des adultes, la dose initiale, 100mg par fois, 2 fois par jour, ensuite, augmenter 50mg par fois tous les 4 jours, ne pas dépasser 200mg par fois, 2 fois par jour ; chez des enfants, 50 à 100mg par fois, 2 fois par jour. En perfusion : chez des adultes, 2 mg/kg, en 15 minutes ; chez des enfants, 2 mg/kg, en 10 minutes. |
| 剂型、规格<br>Les formes pharmaceutiques et les spécifications | 片剂：每片 100mg。<br>注射液：50mg（5ml）；100mg（10ml）。<br>Comprimés : 100mg par comprimé.<br>Injection : 50mg (5ml) ou 100mg (10ml). |
| 药品名称 Drug Names | 胺碘酮 Amiodarone |
| 适应证<br>Les indications | 用于室性和室上性心动过速和早搏、阵发性心房扑动和颤动，预激综合征等。也可用于伴有充血性心力衰竭和急性心肌梗死的心律失常患者。对其他抗心律失常药物如丙吡胺、维拉帕米、奎尼丁、β 受体拮抗剂无效的顽固性阵发性心动过速常能奏效。此外，还用于慢性冠脉功能不全和心绞痛。<br>Ce produit sert à traiter la tachycardie et l'extrasystole ventriculaires et supraventriculaires, le flutter et la fibrillation auriculaires paroxystiques, ainsi que le syndrome de WPW. Il est aussi applicable dans le traitement des patients atteints d'arythmie accompagnée de l'insuffisance cardiaque congestive et de l'infarctus du myocarde aigu. Il est souvent efficace dans le traitement de la tachycardie paroxystiqueréfractaire résistante à d'autres antiarythmique, tels que le disopyramide, le vérapamil, la quinidine et l'antagoniste du récepteur β. En outre, il est également utilisé dans le traitement de l'insuffisance coronarienne chronique et de l'angine de poitrine. |
| 用法、用量<br>Les modes d'emploi et la posologie | 口服：每次 0.1～0.2g，一日 1～4 次；或开始每次 0.2g，一日 3 次。餐后服。3 日后改用维持量，每次 0.2g，一日 1～2 次。<br>Par voie orale : 0,1 à 0,2g par fois, 1 à 4 fois par jour, ou commencer par 0,2g par fois, 3 fois par jour, après le repas. 3 jours après, prendre la dose d'entretien, 0,2g par fois, 1 à 2 fois par jour. |
| 剂型、规格<br>Les formes pharmaceutiques et les spécifications | 片剂：每片 0.2g。<br>胶囊剂：每粒 0.1g；0.2g。<br>注射液：150mg（3ml）。<br>Comprimés : 0,2g par comprimé.<br>Capsules : 0,1g ou 0,2g par capsule.<br>Injection : 150mg (3ml). |
| 药品名称 Drug Names | 依地酸二钠 Edétate disodique |
| 适应证<br>Les indications | 常用于洋地黄苷中度所致的心律失常。<br>Ce produit est souvent appliqué dans le traitement des arythmies causées par les intoxications par les glycosides digitaliques. |
| 用法、用量<br>Les modes d'emploi et la posologie | 静脉注射：每次 1～3g，以 50% 的葡萄糖注射液 20～40ml 稀释后注入。静脉滴注：每次 4～6g，用 5%～10% 葡萄糖注射液 500ml 稀释后在 1～3 小时滴完。<br>Injection par voie IV : 1 à 3g par fois, dissoudre dans 20 à 40ml de solution de glucose à 50 %. En perfusion : 4 à 6g par fois, dissoudre dans 500ml de solution de glucose à 5 % à 10 %, finir en 1 à 3 h. |
| 剂型、规格<br>Les formes pharmaceutiques et les spécifications | 注射液：每支 1g（5ml）。<br>Injection : 1g (5ml) par solution. |

| 药品名称 Drug Names | 门冬氨酸钾镁 Aspartate de magnésium et aspartate de potassium |
| --- | --- |
| 适应证<br>Les indications | 　　用于早搏、阵发性心动过速、心绞痛、心力衰竭等。此外还可用于急性黄疸型肝炎、肝细胞功能不全、其他急慢性肝病、低钾血症等。<br><br>　　Ce produit sert à traiter l'extrasystole, la tachycardie paroxystique, l'angine de poitrine, l'insuffisance cardiaque, etc. En outre, il permet aussi de traiter l'hépatite aiguë de la jaunisse, le dysfonctionnement hépatocellulaire, d'autres maladies hépatiques aiguës et chroniques, l'hypokaliémie, etc. |
| 用法、用量<br>Les modes d'emploi et la posologie | 　　静脉滴注：一日量 10～20ml，用时以 10 倍量的输液稀释后缓慢滴注。<br><br>　　En perfusion : 10 à 20 ml par jour, utiliser l'infusion 10 fois plus importante pour le dissoudre, perfusion lente. |
| 剂型、规格<br>Les formes pharmaceutiques et les spécifications | 　　注射液：每支 10ml，含钾盐及镁盐各 500mg。<br><br>　　Injection : 10ml par solution, qui contient 500mg de potassium et 500mg de magnésium. |

10.4 防治心绞痛药 Médicaments pour la prévention et le traitement de l'angine

| 药品名称 Drug Names | 硝酸甘油 Nitroglycérine |
| --- | --- |
| 适应证<br>Les indications | 　　用于防治心绞痛。<br>　　Ce produit sert à prévenir et à traiter l'angine de poitrine. |
| 用法、用量<br>Les modes d'emploi et la posologie | 　　根据不同的临床需求，硝酸甘油可以通过舌下含服给药、黏膜给药、口服给药、透皮给药或静脉途径给药。①用于治疗急性心绞痛：可给予硝酸甘油片舌下含服、舌下喷雾给药或黏膜给药。片剂（每片 0.3～0.6mg）置于舌下，必要时可重复含服。喷雾给药则可每次将 0.4～0.8mg（1～2 揿）喷至舌下，然后闭嘴，必要时可喷 3 次。硝酸甘油黏膜片置于上唇和牙龈之间，1 次 1～2mg。②用于稳定型心绞痛的长期治疗：通常以透皮剂的形式给予。将膜敷贴于皮肤上，药物以恒速进入皮肤。作用时间长，几乎可达 24 小时。③用于控制性降压或治疗心力衰竭：静脉滴注，开始剂量按每分钟 5μg，可每 3～5 分钟增加 5μg/min 以达到满意效果。如在 20μg/min 时无效可以 10μg/min 递增，以后可 20μg/min，一俟有效则剂量渐减小和给药间期延长。<br><br>　　En fonction des besoins cliniques, la nitroglycérine peut être prise par voie sublinguale, mucosale, orale, transdermique, ou intraveineuse. ① Pour traiter l'angine de poitrine aigue : administration par voie sublinguale, par pulvérisation sublinguale ou par voie muqueuse. Le médicament sublingual (0,3 à 0,6mg par comprimé), s'il est nécessaire, encore une fois. En cas de pulvérisation, 0,4 à 0,8 mg (appuyer1 à 2 fois) pour la pulvérisation sublinguale, fermer ensuite la bouche, s'il est nécessaire, 3 fois. Les comprimés de la nitroglycérine absorbés par la muqueuse doivent être palcés entre la lèvre supérieure et la gencive, 1 à 2 mg par fois. ② Pour le traitement à long terme de l'angine de poitrine stable : souvent administré par voie mucosale. Appliquer le film sur la peau pour que le produit s'absorbe à une vitesse constante par la peau. Il a un effet long, pendant 24 h. ③ Pour l'hypotension induite ou pour traiter l'insuffisance cardiaque : en perfusion, commencer par 5μg par minute, augmenter 5μg par minute toutes les 3 à 5 minutes pour atteindre le résultat satisfaisant. S'il est inuitile pour 20μg par minute, augmenter 10μg par minute avant de maintenir 20μg par minute. Une fois qu'il est efficace, diminuer progressivement la dose et prolonger l'intervalle entre deux administrations. |
| 剂型、规格<br>Les formes pharmaceutiques et les spécifications | 　　片剂：每片 0.3mg；0.5mg；0.6mg。<br>　　缓释硝酸甘油片：每片含 2.5mg。<br>　　注射液：1mg（1ml）；2mg（1ml）；5mg（1ml）；10mg（1ml）。<br>　　硝酸甘油膜：每格含硝酸甘油 0.5mg。<br><br>　　Comprimés : 0,3 mg, 0,5mg ou 0,6mg par comprimé.<br>　　Les comprimés à libération prolongée : 2,5mg par comprimé.<br>　　Injection : 1mg (1ml), 2mg (1ml), 5mg (1ml) ou 10mg (1ml).<br>　　Film de nitroglycérine : chaque cellule contient 0,5mg de nitroglycérine. |

**续　表**

| 药品名称 Drug Names | 戊四硝酯 Tétranitrate de Pentaérythritol |
|---|---|
| 适应证<br>Les indications | 用于预防心绞痛的发作。<br>Il sert à prévenir la crise de l'angine de poitrine. |
| 用法、用量<br>Les modes d'emploi et la posologie | 口服：一日 3～4 次，每次 10～30mg。<br>Par voie orale : 3 à 4 fois par jour, 10 à 30 mg par fois. |
| 剂型、规格<br>Les formes pharmaceutiques et les spécifications | 片剂：每片 10mg；20mg。<br>复方制剂：每片含戊四硝醇 20mg、硝酸甘油 0.5mg。<br>Comprimés : 10mg ou 20mg par comprimé.<br>La préparation de composés : chaque comprimé contient 20mg de tétranitrate de pentaérythritol et 0,5mg de nitroglycérine |
| 药品名称 Drug Names | 硝酸异山梨酯 Dinitrate d'isosorbide |
| 适应证<br>Les indications | 急性心绞痛发作的防治。<br>Ce produit sert à prévenir et à traiter l'angine de poitrine aigue. |
| 用法、用量<br>Les modes d'emploi et la posologie | 片剂：急性心绞痛发作时缓解心绞痛，舌下给药，1 次 5mg；预防心绞痛发作，口服，一日 2～3 次，1 次 5～10mg，一日 10～30mg；治疗心力衰竭，口服 1 次 5～20mg，6～8 小时 1 次。外用乳膏：1 次 0.6g，均匀涂抹在心前区约 5cm×5cm，一日 1 次。缓释片：一日 2 次，1 次 1 片。静脉滴注：每小时 2mg，剂量须根据患者反应而调节，且必须密切监测患者脉搏、心率及血压。喷雾吸入：每次 1.25～3.75mg。<br><br>Comprimés : pour le soulagement lors de la crise de l'angine de poitrine aigue, administration par voie sublinguale, 5mg par fois ; pour prévenir la crise de l'angine de poitrine, par voie orale, 2 à 3 fois, 5 à 10mg par fois, 10 à 30mg par jour ; pour traiter l'insuffisance cardiaque, par voie orale, 5 à 20mg par fois, toutes les 6 à 8h. La crème pour un usage externe : 0,6g par fois, appliquer sur la région précordiale 5cm×5cm, 1 fois par jour. Les comprimés à libération prolongée : 2 fois par jour, 1 comprimé par fois. En perfusion : 2mg par h, ajuster la dose selon les réactions des patients, suivre de près l'impulsion, le rythme cardiaque et la pression sanguine. Inhalation d'aérosol : 1,25 à 3,75mg par fois. |
| 剂型、规格<br>Les formes pharmaceutiques et les spécifications | 普通片：每片 2.5mg；5mg；10mg。<br>缓释片：每片 20mg；40mg。<br>注射液：10mg（10ml）。<br>喷雾剂：250mg/200 次。<br>乳膏：1.5g（10g）。<br>Les comprimés ordinaires : 2,5mg, 5mg ou 10mg par comprimé.<br>Les comprimés à libération prolongée : 20mg, 40mg par comprimé.<br>Injection : 10mg (10ml).<br>L'aérosol : 250 mg toutes les 200 fois.<br>La crème : 1,5g (10g). |
| 药品名称 Drug Names | 单硝酸异山梨酯 Mononitrate d'isosorbide |
| 适应证<br>Les indications | 用于冠心病的长期治疗和预防心绞痛发作，也用于心肌梗死后的治疗。<br>Ce produit est utilisé dans le traitement à long terme de la maladie coronarienne et dans la prévention de l'angine de poitrine. Il est aussi appliqué dans le traitement après un infarctus du myocarde. |
| 用法、用量<br>Les modes d'emploi et la posologie | 口服，一日 20mg，一日 2 次，必要时可增至一日 3 次，饭后服。缓释片：1 次 1 片，一日 2 次，不宜嚼碎。<br>Par voie orale, 20mg par jour, 2 fois par jour, s'il est nécessaire, 3 fois par jour, après le repas. Les comprimés à libération prolongée : 1 comprimé par fois, 2 fois par jour, ne pas mâcher. |
| 剂型、规格<br>Les formes pharmaceutiques et les spécifications | 普通片：每片 20mg；40mg；60mg。<br>缓释片：每片 40mg。<br>Les comprimés ordinaires : 20mg, 40mg ou 60mg par comprimé.<br>Les comprimés à libération prolongée : 40mg par comprimé. |

**续　表**

| 药品名称 Drug Names | 曲美他嗪 Trimétazidine |
|---|---|
| 适应证<br>Les indications | 用于冠状动脉功能不全、心绞痛、陈旧性心肌梗死等。对伴有严重心功能不全者，可与洋地黄苷并用。<br><br>Ce produit sert à traiter l'insuffisance coronarienne, l'angine de poitrine et l'ancien infarctus du myocarde. Chez des patients accompagnés de l'insuffisance cardiaque grave, ce produit peut être utilisé en association avec la digitaline. |
| 用法、用量<br>Les modes d'emploi et la posologie | 口服：1 次 2 ～ 6mg，一日 3 次，饭后服；总剂量每日不超过 18mg。常用维持量为 1 次 1mg，一日 3 次。静脉注射：1 次 8 ～ 20mg，加入 25% 葡萄糖注射液 20ml 中。静脉滴注：8 ～ 20mg，加入 5% 葡萄糖注射液 500ml 中。<br><br>Par voie orale : 2 à 6mg par fois, 3 fois par jour, après le repas ; ne pas dépasser 18mg par jour. La dose d'entretien usuelle : 1mg par fois, 3 fois par jour. Injection par voie IV : 8 à 20 mg par fois, dissoudre dans 20ml de solution de glucose à 25 %. En perfusion : 8 à 20mg, dissoudre dans 500ml de solution de glucose à 5 %. |
| 剂型、规格<br>Les formes pharmaceutiques et les spécifications | 片剂：每片 2mg；3mg。<br>注射液：每支 4mg（2ml）。<br>Comprimés : 2mg ou 3mg par comprimé.<br>Injection : 4mg (2ml) par solution. |
| 药品名称 Drug Names | 双嘧达莫 Dipyridamole |
| 适应证<br>Les indications | 弥散性血管内凝血，血栓栓塞性疾病。防止冠心病发展。<br><br>Ce produit sert à traiter les troubles de la coagulation intravasculaire disséminée et la maladie thrombo-embolique. Il permet aussi de prévenir le développement des maladies coronariennes. |
| 用法、用量<br>Les modes d'emploi et la posologie | 口服：每次 25 ～ 100mg，一日 3 次，饭前 1 小时服。在症状改善后，可改为每日 50 ～ 100mg，两次分服。<br><br>Par voie orale : 25 à 100mg par fois, 3 fois par jour, 1 h avant le repas. Après l'amélioration des symptômes, 50 à 100mg par jour, à travers 2 fois. |
| 剂型、规格<br>Les formes pharmaceutiques et les spécifications | 片剂：每片 25mg。<br>Comprimés : 25mg par comprimé. |
| 药品名称 Drug Names | 丹参酮 II A 磺酸钠 Sulfonate de sodium de tanshinone IIA |
| 适应证<br>Les indications | 用于冠心病心绞痛、胸闷及心肌梗死，对室性早搏也可使用。对冠心病患者的疗效与复方丹参注射液相似。<br><br>Ce produit sert à traiter l'angine de poitrine accompagnée des maladies coronariennes, Oppression thoracique et l'infarctus du myocarde. Il est aussi applicable dans le traitement de l'extrasystole ventriculaire. Son effet chez des patients souffrant des maladies coronariennes est similaire à l'injection du composé Danshen. |
| 用法、用量<br>Les modes d'emploi et la posologie | 肌内注射、静脉注射或静脉滴注：一日 1 次 40 ～ 80mg。注射用 25% 葡萄糖注射液 20ml 稀释，静脉滴注用 5% 葡萄糖注射液 250 ～ 500ml 稀释。<br><br>Injection par voie IM, IV ou en perfusion : 40 à 80mg par fois par jour. Pour l'injection, dissoudre dans 20ml de solution de glucose à 25 %, pour la perfusion, dissoudre dans 250 à 500ml de solution de glucose à 5 %. |
| 剂型、规格<br>Les formes pharmaceutiques et les spécifications | 注射液：每支 10mg（2ml）。<br>Injection : 10mg (2ml) par solution. |

续 表

| 药品名称 Drug Names | 川芎嗪 Ligustrazine |
| --- | --- |
| 适应证<br>Les indications | 适用于闭塞性血管疾病、脑血栓形成、脉管炎、冠心病、心绞痛等。对缺血性脑血管病的急性期、恢复期及其后遗症，如脑供血不足、脑血栓形成、脑栓塞、脑动脉硬化等均有较好疗效，能改善这些疾病引起的偏瘫、失语、吞咽困难、肢体麻木、无力、头痛、头晕、失眠、耳鸣、步态不稳、记忆力减退等症状。<br><br>Ce produit sert à traiter des maladies vasculaires occlusives, la thrombose cérébrale, la vasculite, la maladie coronarienne, l'angine de poitrine, etc. Il est aussi efficace dans le traitement de la maladie cérébro-vasculaire ischémique aigue, de sa récupération et de ses séquelles, telles que l'insuffisance cérébrale, la thrombose cérébrale, l'embolie cérébrale, l'artériosclérose cérébrale, etc. Il permet d'améliorer les symptômes de ces maladies précédentes, tels que l'hémiplégie, l'aphasie, la difficulté à avaler, la sensation d'engourdissement, de la faiblesse, la céphalée, les étourdissements, l'insomnie, les acouphènes, l'ataxie, la perte de mémoire, etc. |
| 用法、用量<br>Les modes d'emploi et la posologie | 口服：磷酸盐片剂每次 2 片，一日 3 次，1 个月为 1 个疗程。肌内注射：盐酸盐注射液，每次 2ml，一日 1～2 次。磷酸盐注射液，每次 2～4ml，一日 1～2 次，15 日为 1 个疗程，宜缓慢注射。静脉滴注：盐酸盐注射液，一日 1 次 2～4ml，或磷酸盐注射液一日 1 次 4～6ml，均稀释于 5%～10% 葡萄糖注射液（或氯化钠注射液、低分子右旋糖酐注射液）250～500ml 中缓慢滴注，宜在 3～4 小时滴完，10～15 日为 1 个疗程。<br><br>Par voie orale : 2 comprimés de phosphate par fois, 3 fois par jour, pendant 1 mois comme un traitement médical. Injection par voie IM : 2ml d'injection de chlorhydrate par fois, 1 à 2 fois par jour. 2 à 4ml d'injection de phosphate par fois, 1 à 2 fois par jour, pendant 15 jours comme un traitement médical, injection lente. En perfusion : 2 à 4 ml d'injection de chlorhydrate par fois par jour, ou 4 à 6ml d'injection de phosphate par fois par jour, dissoudre dans 250 à 500ml de solution de glucose à 5 % à 10 % (ou la solution de chlorure de sodium, la solution de dextran à faible poids moléculaire), perfusion lente, en 3 à 4 h, pendant 10 à 15 jours comme une traitement médical. |
| 剂型、规格<br>Les formes pharmaceutiques et les spécifications | 片剂：每片含川芎嗪磷酸盐 50mg。<br>注射液：盐酸盐注射液，每支 40mg（2ml）；磷酸盐注射液，每支 50mg（2ml）。<br>Comprimés : chaque comprimé contient 50mg de phosphate de ligustrazine.<br>Injection : injection de chlorhydrate, 40mg (2ml) par solution; injection de phosphate, 50mg (2ml) par solution. |
| 药品名称 Drug Names | 葛根素 Puerarin |
| 适应证<br>Les indications | 用于辅助治疗冠心病、心绞痛、心肌梗死，视网膜动静脉阻塞、突发性耳聋、血性脑血管病、小儿病毒性心肌炎、糖尿病等。眼科用于原发性开角型青光眼、高眼压症、原发性闭角型青光眼、继发性青光眼。<br><br>Il sert de traitement adjuvant des maladies suivantes : la maladie coronarienne, l'angine de poitrine, l'infarctus du myocarde, l'occlusion veineuse et artérielle rétinienne, la surdité subite, la maladie cérébrovasculaire ischémique, la myocardite virale chez des enfants ainsi que le diabète. Il est aussi utilisé dans le traitement du glaucome primaire à angle ouvert, de l'hypertension oculaire, du glaucome primaire à angle fermé, et du glaucome secondaire. |
| 用法、用量<br>Les modes d'emploi et la posologie | 静脉滴注：每次 200～600mg，加入 5% 葡萄糖注射液 250～500ml 中静脉滴注，一日 1 次，10～20 日为 1 个疗程，可连续使用 2～3 个疗程。超过 65 岁的老年人连续使用总剂量不超过 5g。葛根素葡萄糖注射液：静脉滴注，每次 0.4～0.6g，一日 1 次，15 日为 1 个疗程。滴眼液：1%，一次 1～2 滴，滴入眼睑内，闭目 3～5 分钟。首日 3 次，以后一日 2 次，早晚各一次。偶有一过性异物感或刺激感。<br><br>En perfusion : 200 à 600mg par fois, dissoudre dans 250 à 500ml de solution de glucose à 5 %, une fois par jour, pendant 10 à 20 jours comme un traitement médical, possible de suivre 2 à 3 traitements médicaux consécutifs. Chez des personnes âgées de plus de 65ans, la dose totale pour une administration continue ne dépasse pas 5g. Injection de glucose de puerarin : en perfusion, 0,4 à 0,6g par fois, 1 fois par jour, pendant 15 jours comme un traitement médical. Les gouttes pour les yeux : 1 %, 1 à 2 gouttes par fois, instiller dans la paupière, fermer les yeux pendant 3 à 5 minutes. Le premier jour, 3 fois, ensuite, 2 fois par jour, pris le petit matin et le soir. Parfois, on a une sensation de corsp étranger ou d'irritation dans l'œil. |

**续　表**

| | |
|---|---|
| 剂型、规格<br>Les formes pharmaceutiques et les spécifications | 注射液：每支 100mg（2ml）；250mg（5ml）。<br>注射用葛根素：每支 0.1g。<br>葛根素葡萄糖注射液：每瓶 0.2g（100ml）；0.25g（100ml）；0.3g（150ml）；0.3g（250ml）；0.5g（250ml）。各种规格均含葡萄糖 5%。<br><br>Injection : 100mg (2ml) ou 250 mg (5ml) par solution.<br>Le puerarin pour injection : 0,1g par solution.<br>Injection de glucose de puerarin : 0,2g (100ml), 0,25g (100ml), 0,3g (150ml), 0,3g (250ml) ou 0,5g (250ml) par flacon. Tout contient 5 % de glucose. |
| **药品名称 Drug Names** | **愈风宁心片 Yufengningxin comprimés** |
| 适应证<br>Les indications | 具有增加脑血流量及冠状动脉血流量的作用。可用于缓解高血压症状（颈项强痛）、治疗心绞痛及突发性耳聋，有一定疗效。<br><br>Ce produit sert à augmenter le débit sanguin cérébral et le débit sanguin coronaire. Il permet aussi de soulager les symptômes de l'hypertension artérielle (la douleur cervicale grave), et de traiter l'angine de poitrine ainsi que la surdité subite. |
| 用法、用量<br>Les modes d'emploi et la posologie | 每次 5 片，一日 3 次。<br>5 comprimés par fois, 3 fois par jour. |
| 剂型、规格<br>Les formes pharmaceutiques et les spécifications | 片剂：每片含总黄酮 60mg。<br>Comprimés : chaque comprimé contient 60mg de flavonoïde. |
| **药品名称 Drug Names** | **银杏叶提取物 Extrait de féuilles de Ginkgo biloba** |
| 适应证<br>Les indications | 用于治疗冠心病心绞痛、脑血管痉挛、脑供血不足、记忆力衰退等。也适用于支气管哮喘、老年性痴呆等病。<br><br>Ce produit sert à traiter l'angine de poitrine liée à la maladie coronarienne, le vasospasme cérébral, l'insuffisance cérébrale, la perte de mémoire, etc. Il est aussi applicable dans le traitement de l'asthme bronchique et de la maladie d'Alzheimer. |
| 用法、用量<br>Les modes d'emploi et la posologie | 口服：每次 20 ～ 40mg，一日 3 次。肌内注射：每次 7 ～ 15mg，一日 1 ～ 2 次。静脉滴注：每日 87.5 ～ 175mg。<br><br>Par voie orale : 20 à 40 mg par fois, 3 fois par jour. Injection par voie IM : 7 à 15mg par fois, 1 à 2 fois par jour. En perfusion : 87,5 à 175mg par jour. |
| 剂型、规格<br>Les formes pharmaceutiques et les spécifications | 常用的制剂有片剂、缓释糖衣片、口服液、强化滴剂、酊剂、注射液及静脉滴注剂等。<br>Les comprimés ordinaires, les comprimés dragéifiésà libération lente, la solution buvable, les gouttes renforcées, les teintures, les injections et les injections pour la perfusion, etc. |
| **药品名称 Drug Names** | **地奥心血康 DiAoXinXueKang** |
| 适应证<br>Les indications | 用于冠心病、心绞痛，能改善症状。<br>Ce produit est utilisé dans l'amélioration des symptômes de la maladie coronarienne et de l'angine de poitrine. |
| 用法、用量<br>Les modes d'emploi et la posologie | 口服，一次 0.2g，一日 3 次，有效后可改为 1 次 0.1g，一日 3 次。<br>Par voie orale, 0,2g par fois, 3 fois parjour. Dès qu'il prend effet, 0,1g par fois, 3 fois par jour. |
| 剂型、规格<br>Les formes pharmaceutiques et les spécifications | 常用其胶囊、片剂、颗粒和软胶囊（均为 0.1g）。<br>口服液每支 0.1g（10ml）。<br>Les capsules, les comprimés, les granules et les capsules molles (0,1g pour tous). La solution buvable, 0,1g (10ml) par pièce. |

**续　表**

| 药品名称 Drug Names | 辅酶Ⅰ Coenzyme I |
|---|---|
| 适应证<br>Les indications | 用于冠心病，可改善冠心病的胸闷、心绞痛等症状。<br>Ce produit sert à améliorer les symptômes de la maladie coronarienne, tels que l'oppression thoracique, l'angine de poitrine, etc. |
| 用法、用量<br>Les modes d'emploi et la posologie | 肌内注射：一日1次5mg，溶于0.9%氯化钠注射液2ml，14日为1个疗程。大多应用2个疗程。<br>Injection par voie IM : 5mg par fois par jour, dissoudre dans 2ml de solution de clorure de sodium à 0,9 %, pendant 14 jours comme un traitement médical. En général, on suit 2 traitements médicaux. |
| 剂型、规格<br>Les formes pharmaceutiques et les spécifications | 注射用辅酶Ⅰ：每支5mg。<br>Coenzyme A pour injection : 5mg par solution. |

10.5　周围血管舒张药 Vasodilatateurs périphériques

| 药品名称 Drug Names | 二氢麦角碱 Dihydroergotoxine |
|---|---|
| 适应证<br>Les indications | 主要与异丙嗪、哌替啶等配成冬眠合剂应用。也可用于动脉内膜炎、肢端动脉痉挛症、血管痉挛性偏头痛等。<br>Ce produit est principalement utilisé en association avec la prométhazine et la péthidine pour former le cocktail lytique. Il est aussi applicable dans le traitement de l'endartérite, des spasmes artériels périphériques et de la migraineliée au spasme vasculaire. |
| 用法、用量<br>Les modes d'emploi et la posologie | 肌内注射或皮下注射，每日或隔日1次，每次0.3～0.6mg；亦可舌下给药（含片），每4～6小时1次，每次0.5～2mg。不宜口服。<br>Injection par voie IM ou sous-cutanée, tous les jours ou tous les deux jours, 0,3 à 0,6mg par fois ; ou prendre le médicament sublingual, toutes les 4 à 6h, 0,5 à 2mg par fois. Ne pas administrer par fois orale. |
| 剂型、规格<br>Les formes pharmaceutiques et les spécifications | 含片：每片0.25mg；0.5mg。<br>注射液：每支0.3mg（1ml）。<br>Comprimés sublinguaux : 0,25mg ou 0,5mg par comprimé.<br>Injection : 0,3mg (1ml) par solution. |
| 药品名称 Drug Names | 烟酸 Acide nicotinique |
| 适应证<br>Les indications | 烟酸可用于治疗糙皮病，但因易于产生面部潮红等不良反应，而烟酰胺则无，故一般选用后者。此外，烟酸还有较强的周围血管扩张作用，口服后数分钟即见效，可维持数分钟至1小时，用于治疗血管性偏头痛、头痛、脑动脉血栓形成、肺栓塞、内耳眩晕症、冻伤、中心性视网膜脉络膜炎等。大剂量（一日2～6g）可降低血脂（主要是三酰甘油），适用于Ⅳ、Ⅲ、Ⅴ型高脂血症，亦可用于Ⅱ型患者。烟酰胺无扩张血管及降血脂作用。<br>Ce produit sert à traiter la pellagre, mais il a des effets indésirables tels que la rougeur du visage, alors quele nicotinamiden'en a pas. En conséquence, celui-ci est souvent appliqué dans le traitement de la pellagre. En outre, la niacine est efficace dans la vasodilatation périphérique, avec une action rapide (elle prendre effet quelques minutes après l'administration et l'effet dure entre quelques minutes et 1h). Ce produit est donc applicable dans le traitement des cas suivants : La migraine vasculaire, la céphalée, la thrombose cérébrale artérielle, l'embolie pulmonaire, le vertige de l'oreille interne, les engelures, lachoroïdite centrale de la rétine, etc. Avec une dose importante (2 – 6g par jour), il a un effet hypolipidémiant (principalement les triglycérides), et est applicable dans le traitement des hyperlipidémies de type IV, III et V, mais aussi de type II. Le nicotinamide ne permet ni la vasodilation ni l'hypolipidémiant. |
| 用法、用量<br>Les modes d'emploi et la posologie | ①口服：一次50～200mg，一日3～4次，餐后服。用于降血脂，一日3～6g，分3～4次于餐后服用。②静脉注射或肌内注射：一次10～50mg，一日1～3次。用于脑血管疾病：一次50～200mg，加于5%～10%葡萄糖注射液100～200ml中静脉滴注，一日1次。<br>① Par voie orale : 50 à 200mg par fois, 3 à 4 fois par jour, après le repas. Pour l'hypolipidémiant, 3 à 6g par jour, à travers 3 à 4 fois, après le repas. ② Injection par voie IV ou IM : 10 à 50mg par fois, 1 à 3 fois par jour. pour traiter les maladies cérébrovasculaires : 50 à 200mg par fois, dissoudre dans 100 à 200ml de solution de glucose à 5% à 10 %, en perfusion, 1 fois par jour. |

| | |
|---|---|
| 剂型、规格<br>Les formes pharmaceutiques et les spécifications | 片剂：每片 50mg；100mg。<br>注射液：每支 20mg（2ml）；50mg（1ml）；100mg（2ml）；50mg（5ml）。<br>Comprimés : 50mg ou 100mg par comprimé.<br>Injection : 20mg (2ml), 50mg (1ml), 100mg (2ml) ou 50mg (5ml) par solution. |
| **药品名称 Drug Names** | 烟酸肌醇酯 Nicotinate d'inositol |
| 适应证<br>Les indications | 用于高脂血症、冠心病、各种末梢血管障碍性疾病（如闭塞性动脉硬化症、肢端动脉痉挛症、冻伤、血管性偏头痛等）的辅助治疗。<br>Ce produit est utilisé dans le traitement adjuvant de l'hyperlipidémie, de la maladie coronarienne, d'une variété de troubles vasculaires périphériques (tels que l'artériosclérose oblitérante, les spasmes artériels périphériques, les engelures, la migraine vasculaire, etc.). |
| 用法、用量<br>Les modes d'emploi et la posologie | 口服：一日 3 次，一次 0.2 ～ 0.6g。连续服用 1 ～ 3 个月。<br>Par voie orale : 3 fois par jour, 0,2 à 0,6g par fois, pendant 1 à 3 mois consécutifs. |
| 剂型、规格<br>Les formes pharmaceutiques et les spécifications | 片剂：每片 0.2g。<br>Comprimés : 0,2g par comprimé. |
| **药品名称 Drug Names** | 维生素 E 烟酸酯 Nicotinate de vitamine E |
| 适应证<br>Les indications | 用于治疗脑动脉硬化、脑卒中、脑外伤后遗症、脂质代谢异常、高血压、冠心病及循环障碍引起的各种疾病。其不良反应小，无烟酸样面部潮红等不良反应。<br>Ce produit sert à traiter l'artériosclérose cérébrale, l'accident vasculaire cérébral, les séquelles du traumatisme crânien, le métabolisme lipidique anormal, l'hypertension artérielle, la maladie coronarienne et les maladies causées par les troubles circulatoires. Ses effets indésirables sont mineurs, sans provoquer la rougeur du visage. |
| 用法、用量<br>Les modes d'emploi et la posologie | 口服：每次 100 ～ 200mg，一日 3 次，餐后服用。<br>Par voie orale : 100 à 200mg par fois, 3 fois par jour, après le repas. |
| 剂型、规格<br>Les formes pharmaceutiques et les spécifications | 胶囊剂：每粒 100mg。<br>Capsules : 100mg par capsule. |
| **药品名称 Drug Names** | 罂粟碱 Papavérine |
| 适应证<br>Les indications | 主要用于脑血栓形成、肺栓塞、肢端动脉痉挛症及动脉栓塞性疼痛等。对高血压、心绞痛、幽门痉挛、胆绞痛、肠绞痛、支气管哮喘等在一般剂量下疗效不显著。<br>Ce produit sert à traiter la thrombose cérébrale, l'embolie pulmonaire, lesspasmes artériels des membreset les douleurs liées à l'embolisation artérielle. Avec une dose générale, son effet n'est pas évident dans le traitement de l'hypertension artérielle, de l'angine de poitrine, du spasme du pylore,de la coliquebiliaire, de la colique intestinale, et del'asthme bronchique. |
| 用法、用量<br>Les modes d'emploi et la posologie | 口服：常用量，每次 30 ～ 60mg，一日 3 次；极量，一次 200mg，一日 600mg。肌内注射或静脉滴注：每次 30mg，一日 90 ～ 120mg，一日量不宜超过 300mg。<br>Par voie orale : la dose usuelle, 30 à 60 mg par fois, 3 fois par jour ; la dose limite, 200mg par fois, 600mg par jour. L'injection par voie IM ou en perfusion : 30mg par fois, 90 à 120mg par jour, ne pas dépasser 300mg par jour. |
| 剂型、规格<br>Les formes pharmaceutiques et les spécifications | 片剂：每片 30mg。<br>注射液：每支 30mg（1ml）。<br>Comprimés : 30mg par comprimé.<br>Injection : 30mg (1ml) par solution. |

**续　表**

| 药品名称 Drug Names | 西地那非 Sildénafil |
| --- | --- |
| 适应证<br>Les indications | 用于治疗勃起功能障碍（ED）。<br>Ce produit sert à traiter la dysfonction érectile. |
| 用法、用量<br>Les modes d'emploi et la posologie | 一般剂量为 50mg，在性活动前约 1 小时（或 0.5～4 小时）服用。基于药效和耐药性，剂量可增至 100mg（最大推荐剂量）或降至 25mg。每日最多服用 1 次。<br>La dose usuelle, 50mg, pris 1 h (ou 0,5 à 4h) avant l'activité sexuelle. En fonction de l'efficacité et de la résistance aux médicaments, augmenter jusqu'à 100mg (la dose recommandée maximale) ou diminuer jusqu'à 25mg. Une fois par jour au plus. |
| 剂型、规格<br>Les formes pharmaceutiques et les spécifications | 片剂：25mg；50mg；100mg。<br>Comprimés : 25mg, 50mg ou 100mg. |
| 药品名称 Drug Names | 环扁桃酯 Cyclandelate |
| 适应证<br>Les indications | 用于脑血管意外及其后遗症、脑动脉硬化症、脑外伤后遗症、肢端动脉痉挛症、手足发绀、闭塞性动脉内膜炎、内耳眩晕症等。<br>Ce produit est utilisé comme traitement des cas suivants : l'accident vasculaire cérébral et ses conséquences, l'artériosclérose cérébrale, les séquelles d'un traumatisme cérébral, des spasmes artériels des membres, la cyanose des mains et des pieds, la méningite occlusive artérielle, le vertige de l'oreille interne, etc. |
| 用法、用量<br>Les modes d'emploi et la posologie | 一次服 100～200mg，一日 3～4 次。症状改善后，可减量至一日 300～400mg。对脑血管疾病一般每次服 200～400mg，一日 3 次。<br>100～200mg par fois, 3 à 4 fois par jour. après l'amélioration des symptômes, diminuer pour atteindre 300 à 400mg par jour. Pour traiter les maladies cérébrovasculaires, en général, 200 à 400mg par fois, 3 fois par jour. |
| 剂型、规格<br>Les formes pharmaceutiques et les spécifications | 胶囊剂：每粒 100mg。<br>Capsules : 100mg par capsule. |
| 药品名称 Drug Names | 长春西汀 Vinpocétine |
| 适应证<br>Les indications | 用于治疗由于大脑血液循环障碍引起的精神性或神经性症状如记忆力障碍、失语症、行动障碍、头晕、头痛等，高血压性脑病、大脑血管痉挛、大脑动脉内膜炎、进行性脑血管硬化。眼科用于因视网膜和脉络膜血管硬化及血管痉挛引起的斑点退化。耳科用于治疗老年性耳聋、眩晕等。<br>Ce produit sert à traiter les symptômes psychiatriques ou neurologiques causés par les troubles de la circulation sanguine cérébrale, tels queles troubles de la mémoire, l'aphasie, lestroubles de la mobilité, des étourdissements, la céphalée, l'encéphalopathie hypertensive, le vasospasme cérébral, la méningite de l'artère cérébrale, ainsi que la sclérose cérébrovasculaire progressive. En ophtalmologie, ce produit est utilisé comme traitement de la dégénérescence maculaire causée par la sclérose vasculaire de la rétine et de la choroïde ainsi que par le spasme vasculaire.En otologie, il sert à traiter la surdité sénile et le vertige. |
| 用法、用量<br>Les modes d'emploi et la posologie | 急性病例可用注射剂，每次 10mg，一日 3 次，静脉滴注或静脉注射，用时以 0.9% 氯化钠注射液稀释到 5 倍体积。然后口服片剂，一日 3 次，每次 1～2 片。对慢性患者，一日 3 次，每次 1～2 片。维持剂量时一次 1 片，一日 3 次。<br>Pour traiter les cas aigus, possible d'utiliser l'injection, 10mg par fois, 3 fois par jour, en perfusion ou par voie IV, dissoudre dans la solution de chlorure de sodium à 0,9 % pour obtenir une solution 5 fois plus importante. Ensuite, prendre les comprimés par voie orale, 3 fois par jour, 1 à 2 comprimés par fois. Chez des patients chroniques, 3 fois par jour, 1 à 2 comprimés par fois. La dose d'entretien, 1 comprimé par fois, 3 fois par jour. |

**续 表**

| 剂型、规格<br>Les formes pharmaceutiques et les spécifications | 片剂：每片 5mg。<br>注射液：每支 10mg（2ml）。<br>Comprimés : 5mg par comprimé.<br>Injection : 10mg (2ml) par solution. |
|---|---|
| 药品名称 Drug Names | 倍他司汀 Bétahistine |
| 适应证<br>Les indications | 用于内耳眩晕症，对脑动脉硬化、缺血性脑血管病、头部外伤或高血压所致的体位性眩晕、耳鸣等亦可用。<br>Ce produit sert à traiter le vertige de l'oreille interne. Il est aussi applicable dans le traitement du vertige et des acouphènes posturauxcausés par l'artériosclérose cérébrale, la maladie cérébrovasculaire ischémique, le traumatisme crânien ou l'hypertensionartérielle. |
| 用法、用量<br>Les modes d'emploi et la posologie | 口服每次 4～8mg，一日 2～4 次。肌内注射一次 2～4mg，一日 2 次。<br>Par voie orale, 4 à 8mg par fois, 2 à 4 fois par jour. Injection par voie IM, 2 à 4 mg pa fois, 2 fois par jour. |
| 剂型、规格<br>Les formes pharmaceutiques et les spécifications | 片剂：每片 4mg；5mg。<br>注射液：每支 2mg（2ml）；4mg（2ml）。<br>Comprimés : 4mg ou 5mg par comprimé.<br>Injection : 2mg (2ml) ou 4mg (2ml) par solution. |
| 药品名称 Drug Names | 地芬尼多 Difénidol |
| 适应证<br>Les indications | 用于各种原因引起的眩晕症如椎基底动脉供血不全、梅尼埃病、自主神经功能紊乱、晕车晕船等。<br>Ce produit sert à traiter les vertiges causés par l'insuffisance vertébro, la maladie de Ménière, ladysautonomie, le mal des transports, etc. |
| 用法、用量<br>Les modes d'emploi et la posologie | 口服：一日 3 次，每次 25～50mg。<br>Par voie orale : 3 fois par jour, 25 à 50mg par fois. |
| 剂型、规格<br>Les formes pharmaceutiques et les spécifications | 片剂：每片 25mg。<br>Comprimés : 25mg par comprimé. |
| 药品名称 Drug Names | 血管舒缓素 Kallidinogénase |
| 适应证<br>Les indications | 用于脑动脉硬化症、闭塞性动脉内膜炎、闭塞性血管炎、四肢慢性溃疡、肢端动脉痉挛症、手足发绀、老年性四肢冷感、中央视网膜炎、眼底出血等。由于易被消化酶破坏，口服作用时间短，效力不及注射。<br>Ce produit sert à traiter l'artériosclérose cérébrale, la méningite occlusive artérielle, la vascularite occlusive, les ulcères chroniques des membres, les spasmes artériels périphériques, la cyanose des mains et des pieds, les extrémités froides séniles, la rétinite centrale, l'hémorragie rétinienne, etc. Comme il peut être endommagé par les enzymes digestives, son administration par voie orale a un effet court et moins fort que son administration par l'injection. |
| 用法、用量<br>Les modes d'emploi et la posologie | ①口服，每次 1 片（含 10U），空腹时服。②注射临用时溶解（10U/1.5ml）后进行肌内注射或皮下注射，一次量 10～20U，一日 1～2 次。轻症每日 10U，以 3 周为 1 个疗程。眼科亦可做眼结膜下注射，每次 5U。<br>① Par voie orale, 1 comprimé par fois (contenant 10 unités), l'estomac vide. ② Dissoudre juste avant l'injection par voie IM ou sous-cutanée (10 unités par 1,5ml), 10 à 20 unités par ofis, 1 à 2 fois par jour. Pour les cas bénins, 10 unités par jour, pendant 3 semaines comme un traitement médical. En ophtalmologie, possible d'administrer par injection conjonctivale, 5 unités par fois. |

**续　表**

| | |
|---|---|
| 剂型、规格<br>Les formes pharmaceutiques et les spécifications | 片剂：每片 10U。<br>注射用血管舒缓素：每支 10U。<br>Comprimés : 10 unités par comprimé.<br>Le kallikrein pour injection : 10 unités par pièce. |
| **药品名称 Drug Names** | 二氢麦角胺 Dihydroergotamine |
| 适应证<br>Les indications | 用于偏头痛急性发作及血管性头痛等。<br>Ce produit sert à traiter la crise aigue de la migraine et la céphalée vasculaire. |
| 用法、用量<br>Les modes d'emploi et la posologie | 因口服吸收不好，治偏头痛多采用注射，肌内注射一次 1～2mg，一日 1～2 次。口服一次 1～3mg，一日 2～3 次。<br>Comme le produit ne s'absorbe par très bien par voie orale, pour traiter la migraine, il est souvent administré par injection. Injection par voie IM, 1 à 2 mg par fois, 1 à 2 fois par jour. Par voie orale, 1 à 3 mg par fois, 2 à 3 fois par jour. |
| 剂型、规格<br>Les formes pharmaceutiques et les spécifications | 片剂：1mg。<br>注射液：1mg（1ml）。<br>Comprimés : 1mg.<br>Injection : 1mg (1ml). |
| **药品名称 Drug Names** | 尼麦角林 Nicergoline |
| 适应证<br>Les indications | 用于脑血管疾病及下肢闭塞性动脉内膜炎等。<br>Ce produit sert à traiter les maladies cérébrovasculaires, et la méningiteartérielle occlusive des extrémités inférieures. |
| 用法、用量<br>Les modes d'emploi et la posologie | 口服：一次 5mg，一日 3 次；肌内注射或静脉注射：一次 2.5～5mg。<br>Par voie orale : 5mg par fois, 3 fois par jour. Injection par voie IM ou IV : 2,5 à 5mg par fois. |
| 剂型、规格<br>Les formes pharmaceutiques et les spécifications | 片剂：5mg。<br>注射液：2.5mg（1ml）。<br>Comprimés : 5mg.<br>Injection : 2,5mg (1ml). |
| **药品名称 Drug Names** | 长春胺 Vincamine |
| 适应证<br>Les indications | 用于脑血管障碍、脑栓塞、脑血栓形成及出血后遗症等。对脑动脉硬化症的疗效比二氢麦角碱和罂粟碱强，需长期应用方见效。<br>Ce produit sert à traiter les troubles cérébro-vasculaires, l'embolie cérébrale, la thrombose cérébrale et les séquellesd'une hémorragie, etc. Il est plus efficace dans le traitement de l'artériosclérose cérébraleque la dihydroergotoxine et la papavérine. Il faut l'utiliser pour une longue durée avant de découvrir son effet. |
| 用法、用量<br>Les modes d'emploi et la posologie | 口服：一次 5～20mg，一日 2～3 次；肌内注射：一次 5～15mg，一日 2～3 次。<br>Par voie orale : 5 à 20mg par fois, 2 à 3 fois par jour ; injection par voie IM : 5 à 15mg par fois, 2 à 3 fois par jour. |
| 剂型、规格<br>Les formes pharmaceutiques et les spécifications | 片剂：5mg。<br>注射液：5mg（2ml）。<br>Comprimés : 5mg.<br>Injection : 5mg (2ml). |

10.6　抗高血压药 Médicaments antihypertensifs

| | |
|---|---|
| **药品名称 Drug Names** | 可乐定 Clonidine |
| 适应证<br>Les indications | 本品预防偏头痛亦有效。亦能降低眼压，可用于治疗开角型青光眼。<br>Ce produit est efficace dans la prévention de la migraine. Il sert aussi à réduire la pression intraoculaire et à traiter le glaucome à angle ouvert. |

**续　表**

| | |
|---|---|
| 用法、用量<br>Les modes d'emploi et la posologie | ①治疗高血压：口服，常用量，每次服 0.075～0.15mg，一日 3 次。可逐渐增加剂量，通常维持剂量为每日 0.2～0.8mg。极量，一次 0.6mg。缓慢静脉注射：每次 0.15～0.3mg，加入 50% 葡萄糖注射液 20～40ml 中（多用于三期高血压及其他危重高血压病）注射。②预防偏头痛：一日 0.1mg，分 2 次服，8 周为 1 个疗程（第 4 周以后，一日量可增至 0.15mg）。③治青光眼：用 0.25% 液滴眼。低血压患者慎用。<br><br>① Pour traiter l'hypertension : par voie orale, la dose usuelle, 0,075 à 0,15mg par fois, 3 fois par jour. Possible d'augmenter la dose. La dose d'entretien, 0,2 à 0,8mg par jour. La dose limite, 0,6mg par fois. Injection par voie IV lente : 0,15 à 0,3mg par fois, dissoudre dans 20 à 40ml de solution de glucose à 50 % (souvent utilisé pour traiter l'hypertension artérielle stade III et l'hypertension artérielle extrêmement grave). ② Pour prévenir la migraine : 0,1mg par jour, à travers 2 fois, pendant 8 semaines comme un traitement médical (4 semaines après, 0,15mg par jour). ③ Pour traiter le glaucome : appliquer les gouttes pour les yeux à 0,25 %. Soyez prudent chez des patients souffrant de l'hypotension. |
| 剂型、规格<br>Les formes pharmaceutiques et les spécifications | 片剂：每片 0.075mg；0.15mg。<br>贴片：每片 2mg。<br>注射液：每支 0.15mg（1ml）。<br>滴眼液：12.5mg（5ml）。<br><br>Comprimés : 0,075mg ou 0,15mg par comprimé.<br>Patch : 2mg par patch.<br>Injection : 0,15mg (1ml) par solution.<br>Les gouttes pour les yeux : 12,5mg (5ml). |
| **药品名称 Drug Names** | 哌唑嗪 Prazosine |
| 适应证<br>Les indications | 用于治疗轻、中度高血压，常与 β 受体拮抗剂或利尿剂合用，降压效果更好。由于本品既能扩张容量血管，降低前负荷，又能扩张阻力血管，降低后负荷，可用于治疗中、重度慢性充血性心力衰竭及心肌梗死后心力衰竭。对常规疗法（洋地黄类、利尿剂）无效或效果不显著的心力衰竭患者也有效。<br><br>Ce produit sert à traiter l'hypertension artérelle bénigne et modérée. Il est souvent utilisé en association avec les antagonistes du récepteur β ou des diurétiques, pour renforcer leur efficacité. Comme il peut permettre non seulement l'extension de la capacité des vaisseaux sanguins, réduisant la précharge, mais aussi l'expansion des vaisseaux de résistance, réduisant la postcharge, il peut être appliqué dans le traitement de l'insuffisance cardiaque congestive chronique modérée ou grave ainsi que le traitement de l'insuffisance consécutive à l'infarctus du myocarde. Il est aussi applicable dans le traitement des patients souffrant de l'insuffisance et résistant au traitement conventionnel (les digitaliques ou les diurétiques). |
| 用法、用量<br>Les modes d'emploi et la posologie | 口服：开始每次 0.5～1mg，一日 1.5～3mg，以后逐渐增至一日 6～15mg。对充血性心力衰竭，维持量通常为每日 4～20mg，分次服用。<br><br>Par voie orale : commencer par 0,5 à 1mg par fois, 1,5 à 3mg par jour, ensuite, augmenter pour atteindre 6 à 15mg par jour. Pour traiter l'insuffisance cardiaque congestive, la dose d'entretien, 4 à 20mg par jour, à travers plusieurs fois. |
| 剂型、规格<br>Les formes pharmaceutiques et les spécifications | 片剂：每片 0.5mg；1mg；2mg；5mg。<br>Comprimés : 0,5mg, 1mg, 2mg ou 5mg par comprimé. |
| **药品名称 Drug Names** | 特拉唑嗪 Térazosine |
| 适应证<br>Les indications | 用于高血压，也可用于良性前列腺增生。<br>Ce produit sert à traiter l'hypertension artérielle et aussi l'hyperplasie bénigne de la prostate. |
| 用法、用量<br>Les modes d'emploi et la posologie | 口服：开始时，一次不超过 1mg，睡前服用，以后可根据情况逐渐增量，一般为一日 8～10mg；一日最大剂量 20mg。用于前列腺肥大，一日剂量为 5～10mg。<br><br>Par voie orale : au début, ne pas dépasser 1mg par fois, avant le sommeil, ensuite, augmenter la dose selon les cas, en général, 8 à 10mg par jour ; la dose maximale est de 20mg par jour. Pour traiter l'hypertrophie prostatique, 5 à 10mg par jour. |

**续　表**

| 剂型、规格<br>Les formes pharmaceutiques et les spécifications | 片剂：每片 0.5mg；1mg；2mg；5mg；10mg。<br>Comprimés : 0,5mg, 1mg, 2mg, 5mg ou 10mg par comprimé. |
|---|---|
| **药品名称 Drug Names** | 多沙唑嗪 Doxazosine |
| 适应证<br>Les indications | 用于高血压。<br>Applicable dans le traitement de l'hypertension artérielle. |
| 用法、用量<br>Les modes d'emploi et la posologie | 开始时，口服一日 1 次 0.5mg，根据情况可每 1 ～ 2 周逐渐增加剂量至一日 2mg，然后再增量至一日 4 ～ 8mg。<br>Au début, 0,5mg par fois par jour, par voie orale, ensuite, augmenter la dose toutes les 1 à 2 semaines pour atteindre 2mg par jour, ensuite, augmenter jusqu'à 4 à 8mg par jour. |
| 剂型、规格<br>Les formes pharmaceutiques et les spécifications | 常用甲磺酸盐的片剂：每片 0.5mg；1mg；2mg；4mg；8mg。<br>Les comprimés de mésylate de doxazosine : 0,5mg, 1mg, 2mg, 4mg ou 8mg par comprimé. |
| **药品名称 Drug Names** | 乌拉地尔 Urapidil |
| 适应证<br>Les indications | 用于各类型的高血压（口服）。可与利尿降压药、β 受体拮抗药合用；也用于高血压危象及手术前、中、后对高血压升高的控制性降压（静脉注射）。<br>Ce produit sert à traiter l'hypertension artérielle de toutes sortes (par voie orale). Il peut être utilisé en association avec des diurétiques ou des antagoniste de récepteur β ; il est aussi applicable dans le traitement de la crise hypertensive ainsi que le contrôle de la pression artérielle élevée de l'hypertension avant, durant et après la chirurgie (injection par voie IV). |
| 用法、用量<br>Les modes d'emploi et la posologie | 口服：开始时一次 60mg，早晚各服 1 次，如血压逐渐下降，可减量为每次 30mg。维持量一日 30 ～ 180mg。静脉注射：一般剂量为 25 ～ 50mg，如用 50mg，应分 2 次给药，其间隔为 5 分钟。静脉滴注：将 250mg 溶于输液 500ml 中，开始滴速为 6mg/min，维持剂量滴速平均为 120mg/h。<br>Par voie orale : commencer par 60mg par fois, pris le petit matin et le soir, en cas de diminution progressive de la pression sanguine, possible de diminuer la dose pour prendre 30mg par fois. La dose d'entretien, 30 à 180mg par jour. Injection par voie IV : 25 à 50mg en général, si on prend 50mg, il faut le faire à travers 2 fois, avec un intervalle de 5 minutes. En perfusion : dissoudre 250mg de produit dans 500ml d'infusion, 6mg par minute au début. La vitesse de la perfusion pour l'entretien est de 120mg par h. |
| 剂型、规格<br>Les formes pharmaceutiques et les spécifications | 缓释胶囊剂：每胶囊 30mg；60mg。<br>注射液：每支 25mg（5ml）；50mg（10ml）。<br>Capsules à libération prolongée : 30mg ou 60mg par capsule.<br>Injection : 25mg (5ml) ou 50mg (10ml) par solution. |
| **药品名称 Drug Names** | 利血平 Réserpine |
| 适应证<br>Les indications | 对于轻度至中等度的早期高血压，疗效显著（精神紧张病例疗效尤好），长期应用小量，可将多数患者的血压稳定于正常范围内，但对严重和晚期病例，单用本品疗效较差，常与肼屈嗪、氢氯噻嗪等合用，以增加疗效。<br>Ce produit sert à traiter l'hypertension bénigne et modérée au stade précoce, avec un effet évident (surtout dans le cas de stress mental). S'il est utilisé pour une longue durée, il faut prendre une dose mineure. Il permet de maintenir la pression sanguine chez la plupart des patients à un niveau normal, mais pour des cas graves ou avancés, l'utilisation unique de ce produit est peu efficace, il faut utiliser en même temps l'hydralazine ou l'hydrochlorothiazide pour renforcer l'efficacité. |
| 用法、用量<br>Les modes d'emploi et la posologie | 作为降压药，每日服 0.25 ～ 0.5mg，一次顿服或 3 次分服。如长期应用，须酌减剂量只求维持药效即可。作为安定药，每日量 0.5 ～ 5mg。亦可肌内注射或静脉注射。<br>Pris comme antihypertenseur, 0,25 à 0.5 mg par jour, une fois par jour ou à travers 3 fois. S'il est pris pour une longue durée, diminuer la dose à seule condition de maintenir l'effet. Pris comme antipsychotiques, 0,5 à 5mg par jour. C'est aussi possible d'injecter par voie IM ou IV. |

| 剂型、规格<br>Les formes pharmaceutiques et les spécifications | 片剂：每片 0.25mg。<br>注射液：每支 1mg（1ml）。<br>Comprimés : 0,25mg par comprimé.<br>Injection : 1mg (1ml) par solution. |
|---|---|
| 药品名称 Drug Names | 肼屈嗪 Hydralazine |
| 适应证<br>Les indications | 现多用于肾性高血压及舒张压较高的患者。单独使用效果不甚好，且易引起不良反应，故多与利血平、氢氯噻嗪、胍乙啶或普萘洛尔合用以增加疗效。<br>À l'heure actuelle, ce produit est souvent appliqué chez des patients souffrant de l'hypertension rénovasculaire ou la pression artérielle diastolique élevée. Utilisé seul, il n'est pas très efficace et peut entraîner des effets indésirables. Il est donc souvent appliqué en combinaison avec la réserpine, l'hydrochlorothiazide, la guanéthidine ou le propranolol pour renforcer l'efficacité. |
| 用法、用量<br>Les modes d'emploi et la posologie | 口服或静脉注射、肌内注射。一般开始时用小量，每次 10mg，一日 3～4 次，用药 2～4 日。以后用量逐渐增加。维持量，一日 30～200mg，分次服用。<br>Par voie orale, injection par voie IV ou IM. Commencer par une dose faible, 10mg par fois, 3 à 4 fois par jour, pendant 2 à 4 jours. Ensuite, augmenter progressivement la dose. La dose d'entretien, 30 à 200mg par jour, à travers plusieurs fois. |
| 剂型、规格<br>Les formes pharmaceutiques et les spécifications | 片剂：每片 10mg；25mg；50mg。<br>缓释片：每片 50mg。<br>注射液：每支 20mg（1ml）。<br>Comprimés : 10mg, 25mg ou 50mg par comprimé.<br>Comprimés à libération prolongée : 50mg par comprimé.<br>Injection : 20mg (1ml) par solution. |
| 药品名称 Drug Names | 双肼屈嗪 Dihydralazine |
| 适应证<br>Les indications | 现多用于肾性高血压及舒张压较高的患者。单独使用效果不甚好，且易引起不良反应，故多与利血平、氢氯噻嗪、胍乙啶或普萘洛尔合用以增加疗效。<br>À l'heure actuelle, ce produit est souvent appliqué chez des patients souffrant de l'hypertension rénovasculaire ou la pression artérielle diastolique élevée. Utilisé seul, il n'est pas très efficace et peut entraîner des effets indésirables. Il est donc souvent appliqué en combinaison avec la réserpine, l'hydrochlorothiazide, la guanéthidine ou le propranolol pour renforcer l'efficacité. |
| 用法、用量<br>Les modes d'emploi et la posologie | 口服：一次 12.5～25mg，一日 25～50mg。发生耐受性后，可加大到每次 50mg，一日 3 次。<br>Par voie orale : 12,5 à 25mg par fois, 25 à 50 mg par jour. Après la résistance au médicament, augmenter la dose pour atteindre 50mg par fois, 3 fois par jour. |
| 剂型、规格<br>Les formes pharmaceutiques et les spécifications | 片剂：每片 12.5mg；25mg。<br>注射用双肼屈嗪：25mg。<br>Comprimés : 12.5mg ou 25mg par comprimé.<br>La dihydralazine pour injection : 25mg. |
| 药品名称 Drug Names | 硝普钠 Nitroprusside de sodium |
| 适应证<br>Les indications | 用于其他降压药无效的高血压危象，疗效可靠，且由于其作用持续时间较短，易于掌握。用于心力衰竭，能使衰竭的左心室排血量增加，心力衰竭症状得以缓解。<br>Ce produit est utilisé comme traitement de la crise hypertensive résistante à d'autres antihypertenseurs, avec un effet sûr. Et son effet ne dure pas longtemps et il est donc facile à contrôler. Appliqué dans le traitement de l'insuffisance cardiaque, il peut permettre l'augmentation du débit cardiaque du ventricule gauche défaillant, et l'amélioration des symptômes de l'insuffisance cardiaque. |
| 用法、用量<br>Les modes d'emploi et la posologie | 临用前，先用 5% 葡萄糖注射液溶解，再用 5% 葡萄糖注射液 250～1000ml 稀释。静脉滴注，每分钟 1～3μg/kg。开始时速度可略快，血压下降后可减慢。但用于心力衰竭、心源性休克时，开始宜缓慢，以 10 滴 / 分为宜，以后再酌情加快速度。用药不宜超过 72 小时。 |

**续　表**

| | |
|---|---|
| | Dissoudre dans la solution de glucose à 5 % avant d'utiliser 250 à 1 000 ml de solution de glucose à 5 % pour la dilution. En perfusion, 1 à 3µg/kg par minute. Commencer par une vitesse un peu rapide avant de ralentir dès la diminution de la pression sanguine. Lors du traitement de l'insuffisance cardiaque ou du choc cardiogénique, la perfusion doit être effectuée lentement au début, avec une vitesse de 10 gouttes par minute, avant d'accélérer. L'administration ne dépasse pas 72h. |
| 剂型、规格<br>Les formes pharmaceutiques et les spécifications | 注射用硝普钠：每支 50mg。<br>Le nitroprusside de sodium pour injection : 50mg par solution. |
| **药品名称 Drug Names** | 卡托普利 Captopril |
| 适应证<br>Les indications | 用于治疗各种类型高血压，特别是常规疗法无效的高血压。由于本品通过降低血浆血管紧张素Ⅱ和醛固酮水平，而使心脏前、后负荷减轻，故可用于顽固性慢性心力衰竭，对洋地黄、利尿剂和血管扩张剂无效的心力衰竭患者也有效。<br>Ce produit sert à traite rl'hypertension artérielle de toutes sortes, surtout celle résistant au traitement conventionnel. Comme il peut réduire la précharge et la postcharge cardiaques en diminuant l'angiotensine plasmatiq II et le niveau de l'aldostérone, il peut être utilisé pour prévenir l'insuffisance chronique et réfractaire. Il est aussi efficace dans le traitement de l'insuffisance cardiaque résistant aux digitalis, aux diurétiques et aux vasodilatateurs. |
| 用法、用量<br>Les modes d'emploi et la posologie | 口服：一次 25～50mg，一日 75～150mg。开始时每次 25mg，一日 3 次（饭前服用）；渐增至每次 50mg，一日 3 次。每日最大剂量为 450mg。儿童，开始每日 1mg/kg，最大 6mg/kg，分 3 次服。<br>Par voie orale : 25 à 50 mg par fois, 75 à 150 mg par jour. Commencer par 25mg par fois, 3 fois par jour, avant le repas ; augmenter progressivement pour atteindre 50mg par fois, 3 fois par jour. La dose maximale est de 450mg par jour. Chez des enfants, commencer par 1 mg/kg par jour, ne pas dépasser 6 mg/kg, à travers 3 fois. |
| 剂型、规格<br>Les formes pharmaceutiques et les spécifications | 片剂：12.5mg；25mg；50mg；100mg。<br>复方卡托普利片：每片含卡托普利 10mg，氢氯噻嗪 6mg。<br>Comprimés : 12,5 mg, 25mg, 50mg ou 100mg.<br>Les comprimés de composé de captopril : chaque comprimé contient 10mg de captopril et 6mg d'hydrochlorothiazide. |
| **药品名称 Drug Names** | 依那普利 Enalapril |
| 适应证<br>Les indications | 用于高血压及充血性心力衰竭的治疗。<br>Ce produit sert à traiter l'hypertension artérielle et l'insuffisance cardiaque congestive. |
| 用法、用量<br>Les modes d'emploi et la posologie | 口服 10mg，日服 1 次，必要时也可静脉注射以加速起效。可根据患者情况增加至日剂量 40mg。<br>Par voie orale, 10mg, 1 fois par jour, s'il est nécessaire, injection par voie IV pour renforcer son efficacité. Augmenter progressivement la dose pour atteindre 40mg par jour selon les cas. |
| 剂型、规格<br>Les formes pharmaceutiques et les spécifications | 片剂：每片 5mg；10mg；20mg。<br>Comprimés : 5mg, 10mg ou 20mg par comprimé. |
| **药品名称 Drug Names** | 贝那普利 Bénazépril |
| 适应证<br>Les indications | 用于各型高血压和充血性心力衰竭患者。对正在服用地高辛和利尿药的充血性心力衰竭患者可使心排血量增加，全身和肺血管阻力、平均动脉压、肺动脉压及右房压下降。<br>Ce produit sert à traiter l'hypertension artérielle de toutes sortes et l'insuffisance cardiaque congestive. Il permet aux patients souffrant de l'insuffisance cardiaque congestive et prenant la digoxine et auxdiurétiques d'augmenter le débit cardiaque, et de diminuer la résistance vasculaire systémique et pulmonaire, la pression artérielle moyenne, la pression de l'artère pulmonaire ainsi que la pression de l'oreillettedroite. |

**续 表**

| | |
|---|---|
| 用法、用量<br>Les modes d'emploi et la posologie | 　用于降压，口服，开始剂量为一日 1 次 10mg，然后可根据病情渐增剂量至每日 40mg，一次或分 2 次服用。严重肾功能不全者或心力衰竭患者或服用利尿药的患者，初始剂量为每日 5mg，充血性心力衰竭患者，每日剂量为 2.5 ～ 20mg。<br>　Pour la lutte contre l'hypertension, par voie orale, commencer par 10 mg par fois par jour, augmenter ensuite progressivement la dose pour atteindre 40mg par jour, à travers 1 à 2 fois. Chez des patients insuffisants rénaux, des patients souffrant de l'insuffisance cardiaque ou des malades prenant des diurétiques, commencer par 5mg par jour, chez des patients atteints de l'insuffisance cardiaque congestive, 2,5 à 20mg par jour. |
| 剂型、规格<br>Les formes pharmaceutiques et les spécifications | 　片剂：每片 5mg；10mg；20mg。<br>　Comprimés : 5mg, 10mg ou 20mg par comprimé. |
| 药品名称 Drug Names | 培哚普利 Périndopril |
| 适应证<br>Les indications | 　用于治疗高血压。<br>　Il sert à traiter l'hypertension artérielle. |
| 用法、用量<br>Les modes d'emploi et la posologie | 　口服，一日 1 次 4mg，可根据病情增至一日 8mg。老年患者及肾功能低下患者酌情减量。<br>　Par voie orale, 4mg par fois par jour, possible d'augmenter jusqu'à 8 mg par jour. Chez des personnes âgées et des patients insuffisants rénaux, diminuer la dose. |
| 剂型、规格<br>Les formes pharmaceutiques et les spécifications | 　片剂：每片 2mg；4mg。<br>　Comprimés : 2mg ou 4mg par comprimé. |
| 药品名称 Drug Names | 氯沙坦 Losartan |
| 适应证<br>Les indications | 　用于高血压和充血性心力衰竭的治疗。<br>　Il sert à traiter l'hypertension artérielle et l'insuffisance cardiaque congestive. |
| 用法、用量<br>Les modes d'emploi et la posologie | 　口服，一日 1 次，10 ～ 100mg；一般维持量一日 1 次 50mg，剂量增加，抗高血压效果不再增加。<br>　Par voie orale, 1 fois par jour, 10 à 100mg ; la dose d'entretien usuelle, 50mg par fois par jour. L'effet de lutte contre l'hypertension artérielle ne s'améliore pas avec l'augmentation de la dose. |
| 剂型、规格<br>Les formes pharmaceutiques et les spécifications | 　氯沙坦钾，片剂：50mg，100mg；胶囊：50mg。<br>　Le potassium de Losartan, comprimés: 50mg, 100mg; capsule: 50mg. |
| 药品名称 Drug Names | 缬沙坦 Valsartan |
| 适应证<br>Les indications | 　用于治疗高血压。<br>　Il sert à traiter l'hypertension artérielle. |
| 用法、用量<br>Les modes d'emploi et la posologie | 　常口服其胶囊剂，每粒含 80mg 或 160mg，每次 80mg，一日 1 次，亦可根据需要增加至每次 160mg，或加用利尿药。也可与其他降压药合用。<br>　Pris souvent en capsules par voie orale. Chaque capsule contient 80mg ou 160mg, 80mg par fois, 1 fois par jour. C'est aussi possible d'augmenter la dose pour atteindre 160mg par fois, ou de prendre en même temps des diurétiques. Il est souvent pris en association avec d'autres antihypertenseurs. |
| 剂型、规格<br>Les formes pharmaceutiques et les spécifications | 　胶囊：80mg；160mg。<br>　Capsules : 80mg ou 160mg. |

**续　表**

| 药品名称 Drug Names | 厄贝沙坦 Irbésartan |
| --- | --- |
| 适应证<br>Les indications | 用于治疗原发性高血压。<br>Il sert à traiter l'hypertension essentielle. |
| 用法、用量<br>Les modes d'emploi et<br>la posologie | 口服每次 150mg，一日 1 次，对血压控制不佳者可加至 300mg 或合用小剂量噻嗪类利尿药。<br>Par voie orale, 150mg par fois, 1 fois par jour. Quand il est peu efficace, possible d'augmenter la dose pour atteindre 300mg ou de prendre en même temps des diurétiques thiazidiques à faible dose. |
| 剂型、规格<br>Les formes<br>pharmaceutiques et les<br>spécifications | 片剂：每片 150mg。<br>Comprimés : 150mg par comprimé. |
| 药品名称 Drug Names | 坎地沙坦 Candésartan |
| 适应证<br>Les indications | 用于高血压治疗。<br>Il sert à traiter l'hypertension artérielle. |
| 用法、用量<br>Les modes d'emploi et<br>la posologie | 口服，每次 8～16mg，一日 1 次。也可与氨氯地平、氢氯噻嗪合用。中、重度肝、肾功能不全患者应适当调整剂量。<br>Par voie orale, 8 à 16mg par fois, 1 fois par jour. Il peut être utilisé en association avec l'amlodipine et l'hydrochlorothiazide. Chez des patients insuffisants rénaux et hépatiques modérés ou graves, diminuer la dose. |
| 剂型、规格<br>Les formes<br>pharmaceutiques et les<br>spécifications | 片剂：4mg，8mg；胶囊：4mg，8mg；分散片：4mg。<br>Comprimés : 4mg, 8mg; Capsules : 4mg, 8mg; Comprimés de dispersion: 4mg. |
| 药品名称 Drug Names | 替米沙坦 Telmisartan |
| 适应证<br>Les indications | 用于原发性高血压的治疗。<br>Il sert à traiter l'hypertension essentielle. |
| 用法、用量<br>Les modes d'emploi et<br>la posologie | 一日 1 次，每次 1 片，40mg/ 片。<br>1 fois par jour, 1 comprimé par fois, 40mg par comprimé. |
| 剂型、规格<br>Les formes<br>pharmaceutiques et les<br>spécifications | 片剂：每片 40mg。<br>Comprimés : 40mg par comprimé. |
| 药品名称 Drug Names | 吲达帕胺 Indapamide |
| 适应证<br>Les indications | 对轻、中度原发性高血压具有良好效果。单独服用降压效果显著，不必加用其他利尿剂。可与 β 受体拮抗剂合并应用。<br>1 est efficace dans le traitement de l'hypertension essentielle bénigne et modérée. Utilisé seul, il est déjà efficace, sans avoir à être appliqué en association avec des diurétiques. Il peut être utilisé en combinaison avec les antagonistes du récepteur β. |
| 用法、用量<br>Les modes d'emploi et<br>la posologie | 口服：一次 2.5mg，一日 1 次，维持量可 2 日一次 2.5mg。<br>Par voie orale : 2,5mg pas fois, 1 fois par jour, la dose d'entretien, 2,5mg par fois tous les deux jours. |
| 剂型、规格<br>Les formes<br>pharmaceutiques et les<br>spécifications | 片剂：每片 2.5mg。<br>Comprimés : 2,5mg par comprimé. |

续 表

| 药品名称 Drug Names | 甲基多巴 Méthyldopa |
|---|---|
| 适应证<br>Les indications | 用于中、重度、恶性高血压。<br>Ce produit sert à traiter l'hypertension modérée, grave ou maligne. |
| 用法、用量<br>Les modes d'emploi et la posologie | 每次服 250mg，一日 3 次。<br>250mg par fois, 3 fois par jour. |
| 剂型、规格<br>Les formes pharmaceutiques et les spécifications | 片剂：250mg。<br>Comprimés : 250mg. |
| 药品名称 Drug Names | 胍乙啶 Guanethidine |
| 适应证<br>Les indications | 用于中、重度舒张压高的高血压。<br>Ce produit sert à traiter l'hypertension modérée et grave dont la pression artérielle diastolique est élevée. |
| 用法、用量<br>Les modes d'emploi et la posologie | 开始每日 10mg，以后视病情每隔 5～7 日递增 10mg，分次服用。一般一日不超过 100mg。<br>Commencer par 10mg par jour, ensuite, augmenter 10mg tous les 5 à 7 jours selon les cas, pris à travers plusieurs fois. Ne pas dépasser 100mg par jour. |
| 剂型、规格<br>Les formes pharmaceutiques et les spécifications | 片剂：10mg；25mg。<br>Comprimés : 10mg ou 25mg. |
| 药品名称 Drug Names | 倍他尼定 Bétanidine |
| 适应证<br>Les indications | 用于中、重度舒张压高的高血压。<br>Ce produit sert à traiter l'hypertension modérée et grave dont la pression artérielle diastolique est élevée. |
| 用法、用量<br>Les modes d'emploi et la posologie | 开始：一次 10mg，一日 3 次；维持：20～200mg/d。<br>La dose initiale : 10 mg par fois, 3 fois par jour ; la dose d'entretien : 20 à 200mg par jour. |
| 剂型、规格<br>Les formes pharmaceutiques et les spécifications | 片剂：10mg；50mg。<br>Comprimés : 10mg ou 50mg. |
| 药品名称 Drug Names | 异喹胍 Debrisoquine |
| 适应证<br>Les indications | 用于中、重度舒张压高的高血压。<br>Ce produit sert à traiter l'hypertension modérée et grave dont la pression artérielle diastolique est élevée. |
| 用法、用量<br>Les modes d'emploi et la posologie | 开始：一次 10mg，一日 1～2 次；维持：40～120mg/d。<br>La dose initiale : 10mg par fois, 1 à 2 fois par jour ; la dose d'entretien : 40 à 120 mg par jour. |
| 剂型、规格<br>Les formes pharmaceutiques et les spécifications | 片剂：10mg；20mg。<br>Comprimés : 10mg ou 20mg. |

**续 表**

| 药品名称 Drug Names | 西拉普利 Cilazapril |
|---|---|
| 适应证<br>Les indications | 用于治疗各种程度原发性高血压和肾性高血压，也可与洋地黄和（或）利尿剂合用作为治疗慢性心力衰竭的辅助药物。<br><br>Ce produit sert à traiter l'hypertension essentielle et l'hypertension rénovasculaire de tous degrés. Utilisé en association avec lesdigitalis et (ou) les diurétiques, il est aussi applicable dans le traitement adjuvant de l'insuffisance cardiaque chronique. |
| 用法、用量<br>Les modes d'emploi et la posologie | 口服：一日 1 次 2.5 ～ 5mg。<br>Par voie orale : 2,5 à 5mg par fois par jour. |
| 剂型、规格<br>Les formes pharmaceutiques et les spécifications | 片剂：2.5mg；5mg。<br>Comprimés : 2,5 mg ou 5mg. |
| 药品名称 Drug Names | 喹那普利 Quinapril |
| 适应证<br>Les indications | 高血压、充血性心力衰竭。<br>Ce produit sert à traite l'hypertension et l'insuffisance cardiaque. |
| 用法、用量<br>Les modes d'emploi et la posologie | 口服：一日 10 ～ 80mg，1 次或分 2 次服。<br>Par voie orale : 10 à 80mg par jour, à travers 1 à 2 fois. |
| 剂型、规格<br>Les formes pharmaceutiques et les spécifications | 片剂：10mg。<br>Comprimés : 10mg. |
| 药品名称 Drug Names | 雷米普利 Ramipril |
| 适应证<br>Les indications | 用于治疗原发性高血压。<br>Il sert à traiter l'hypertension essentielle. |
| 用法、用量<br>Les modes d'emploi et la posologie | 口服：一日 1 次 2.5 ～ 5mg。<br>Par voie orale : 2,5 à 5mg par fois par jour. |
| 剂型、规格<br>Les formes pharmaceutiques et les spécifications | 片剂：1.25mg，2.5mg，5mg。<br>Comprimés : 1.25mg, 2.5mg, 5mg. |
| 药品名称 Drug Names | 咪达普利 Imidapril |
| 适应证<br>Les indications | （1）原发性高血压；<br>（2）肾实质性病变所致继发性高血压。<br>(1)Il sert à traiter l'hypertension essentielle.<br>(2)Il sert aussi à traiter l'hypertension causée par les lésions du parenchyme rénal. |
| 用法、用量<br>Les modes d'emploi et la posologie | 口服：一日 1 次 5 ～ 10mg。<br>Par voie orale : 5 à 10mg par fois par jour. |
| 剂型、规格<br>Les formes pharmaceutiques et les spécifications | 片剂：5mg；10mg。<br>Comprimés : 5mg ou 10mg. |

**续 表**

| 药品名称 Drug Names | 赖诺普利 Lisinopril |
|---|---|
| 适应证<br>Les indications | 用于高血压和充血性心力衰竭。<br>Ce produit sert à traite l'hypertension et l'insuffisance cardiaque. |
| 用法、用量<br>Les modes d'emploi et la posologie | 口服：一日 1 次 5 ～ 20mg。最多一日不超过 80mg。<br>Par voie orale : 5 à 20mg par fois par jour. Ne pas dépasser 80mg par jour. |
| 剂型、规格<br>Les formes pharmaceutiques et les spécifications | 片剂：5mg；10mg；20mg。<br>Comprimés : 5mg, 10mg ou 20mg. |
| 药品名称 Drug Names | 福辛普利 Fosinopril |
| 适应证<br>Les indications | 适用于治疗高血压和心力衰竭。治疗高血压时，可单独使用作为初始治疗药物，或与其他抗高血压药物联合使用。治疗心力衰竭时，可与利尿剂合用。<br>Ce produit sert à traiter l'hypertension et l'insuffisance cardiaque. Lors du traitement de l'hypertension, il peut être utilisé seul comme médicament du traitement initial ou utilisé en association avec d'autres antihypertenseurs. Lors du traitement de l'insuffisance cardiaque, il peut être appliqué en combinaison avec des diurétiques. |
| 用法、用量<br>Les modes d'emploi et la posologie | 口服：一日 1 次 5 ～ 40mg。最大剂量一日 80mg。<br>Par voie orale : 5 à 40mg par fois par jour. Ne pas dépasser 80 mg par jour. |
| 剂型、规格<br>Les formes pharmaceutiques et les spécifications | 片剂：10mg；20mg。<br>Comprimés : 10mg ou 20mg. |

10.7 抗休克的血管活性药 Médicaments antichoc activité vasculaire

| 药品名称 Drug Names | 去甲肾上腺素 Norépinéphrine (Noradrénaline) |
|---|---|
| 适应证<br>Les indications | 临床上主要用它的升压作用，静脉滴注用于各种休克（但出血性休克禁用），以升高血压，保证对重要器官（如脑）的血液供应。<br>Ce produit est principalement utilisé dans les cliniques pour augmenter la pression sanguine. Administré en perfusion, il est appliqué dans le traitement du choc de toutes sortes (sauf le choc hémorragique) en augmentant la pression sanguine, afin de veiller à l'approvisionnement en sang vers les organes vitaux (comme le cerveau). |
| 用法、用量<br>Les modes d'emploi et la posologie | ①静脉滴注：临用前稀释，每分钟滴入 4 ～ 10μg，根据病情调整剂量。可用 1 ～ 2mg 加入生理盐水或 5% 葡萄糖注射液 100ml 内静脉滴注，根据情况掌握滴注速度，待血压升至所需水平后，减慢滴速，以维持血压正常范围。如效果不好，应换用其他升压药。对危急病例可用 1 ～ 2mg 稀释到 10 ～ 20ml，徐徐注射入静脉，同时根据血压以调节其剂量，待血压回升后，再用滴注法维持。②口服：治上消化道出血，每次服注射液 1 ～ 3ml（1 ～ 3mg），一日 3 次，加入适量冷盐水服下。<br>① En perfusion : la dilution avant l'utilisation, 4 à 10μg par minute, ajuster la dose selon les cas. Dissoudre 1 à 2 mg dans 100ml de solution de glucose à 5 % ou de solution saline, ajuster la vitesse de la perfusion selon les cas, dès la pression sanguine atteint le niveau désiré, ralentir la perfusion pour maintenir la pression sanguine à un niveau normal. S'il n'est pas très efficace, utiliser d'autres médicaments pour augmenter la pression sanguine. Pour traiter les cas extrêment graves, diluer 1 à 2mg pour obtenir 10 à 20ml, injection lente par voie IV, ajuster la dose en fonction de la pression sanguine. Après l'augmentation de la pression sanguine, reprendre la perfusion pour l'entretien. ② Par voie orale : pour traiter le saignement des voies gastro-intestinales suprérieures, prendre 1 à 3ml d'injection (1à 3mg), 3 fois par jour, avec de l'eau salée froide. |

| 剂型、规格<br>Les formes pharmaceutiques et les spécifications | 注射液：每支 2mg（1ml）（以重酒石酸盐计）；10mg（2ml）（以重酒石酸盐计）。<br>Injection : 2mg (1ml) (mesuré en bitartrate) ou 10mg (2ml) (mesuré en bitartrate) par solution. |
|---|---|
| 药品名称 Drug Names | 去氧肾上腺素 Phényléphrine |
| 适应证<br>Les indications | 用于感染中毒性及过敏性休克、室上性心动过速、防治全身麻醉及腰麻时的低血压。眼科用于散瞳检查，特点是作用时间短，不麻痹调节功能，不引起眼压升高。<br>Ce produit sert à traiter l'hypotension liée au choc septique et anaphylactique, à la tachycardie supraventriculaire, àla prévention de l'anesthésie générale et de l'anesthésie lombaire. En ophtalmologie, il est appliqué à l'examen avec pupilles dilatées. Il a un effet court, ne paralyse pas la fonction de réglage, et n'entraîne pas l'augmentation de la pression intraoculaire. |
| 用法、用量<br>Les modes d'emploi et la posologie | （1）肌内注射或静脉滴注：①常用量：肌内注射，一次 2 ~ 5mg；静脉滴注，一次 10 ~ 20mg。稀释后缓慢滴注。②极量：肌内注射，一次 10mg；静脉滴注，每分钟 0.1mg。<br>（2）滴眼：用于散瞳检查，用 2% ~ 5% 溶液滴眼。<br>(1) Injection par voie IM ou en perfusion　① La dose usuelle : injection par voie IM, 2 à 5mg par fois ; en perfusion, 10 à 20 mg par fois. La dilution avant la perfusion lente. ② La dose limite : injection par voie IM, 10mg par fois ; en perfusion, 0,1 mg par minute.<br>(2) Les gouttes pour les yeux : pour l'examen avec pupilles dilatées, utiliser la solution à 2 % à 5 %. |
| 剂型、规格<br>Les formes pharmaceutiques et les spécifications | 注射液：每支 10mg（1ml）。<br>滴眼剂：为 2% ~ 5% 溶液。<br>njection : 10mg (1ml) par solution.<br>Les gouttes pour les yeux : la solution à 2 % à 5 %. |
| 药品名称 Drug Names | 甲氧胺 Méthoxamine |
| 适应证<br>Les indications | 用于外科手术，以维持或恢复动脉压，尤其适用于脊椎麻醉造成的血压降低。又用于大出血、创伤及外科手术所引起的低血压、心肌梗死所致休克及室上性心动过速。<br>Ce produit est appliqué lors de la chirurgie pour maintenir ou rétablir la pression artérielle, surtout applicable dans le traitement de la réduction de la pression artérielle causée par l'achianesthésie. Il est aussi applicable dans le traitement de l'hypotension causée par l'hémorragie massive, le traumatisme et la chirurgie, ainsi que dans le traitement du choc causé par l'infarctus du myocarde, et de la tachycardie supraventriculaire. |
| 用法、用量<br>Les modes d'emploi et la posologie | （1）肌内注射、静脉注射或静脉滴注。①常用量：肌内注射，一次 10 ~ 20mg；静脉注射：一次 5 ~ 10mg；静脉滴注，一次 20 ~ 60mg，稀释后缓慢滴注。②极量：肌内注射，一次 20mg，一日 60mg；静脉注射：一次 10mg。<br>（2）对急症病例或收缩压降至 8kPa（60mmHg）甚至更低的病例，缓慢静脉注射 5 ~ 10mg，注射一次量不超过 10mg，并严密观察血压变动。静脉注射后，继续肌内注射 15mg，以维持较长药效。<br>（3）对室上性心动过速病例，用 10 ~ 20mg，以 5% 葡萄糖注射液 100ml 稀释，做静脉滴注。也可用 10mg 加入 5% ~ 10% 葡萄糖注射液 20ml 中缓缓静脉注射。注射时应观察心率及血压，当心率突然减慢时，应停注。<br>（4）对处理心肌梗死的休克病例，开始肌内注射 15mg，接着静脉滴注，静脉滴注液为 5% ~ 10% 葡萄糖注射液 500ml 内含本品 60mg，滴速应随血压反应而调整，每分钟不宜超过 20 滴。<br>(1) Injection par voie IM, IV ou en perfusion : ① La dose usuelle : par voie IM, 10 à 20mg par fois ; injection par voie IV, 5 à 10mg par fois ; en perfusion, 20 à 60mg par fois, après la dilution, la perfusion lente. ② La dose limite : injection par voie IM, 20mg par fois, 60mg par jour ; injection par voie IV, 10mg par fois.<br>(2) Pour traiter les cas urgents ou des patients dont la pression artérielle systolique atteint 8 kPa(60mmHg)ou moins, injection par voie IV lente, 5 à 10mg, ne pas dépasser 10mg par fois, suivre de près la pression artérielle. Après l'injection par voie IV, injecter 15 mg par voie IM, pour maintenir un effet pour une longue durée. |

**续 表**

(3) Pour traiter la tachycardie supraventriculaire, dissoudre 10 à 20mg dans 100ml de solution de glucose à 5 %, en perfusion. Ou dissoudre 10mg dans 20ml de solution de glucose à 5 % à 10 %, injection par voie IV lente. Suivre de près le rythme cardiaque et la pression artérielle, lors du ralentissement subite du rythme cardiaque, arrêter l'injection.

(4) Pour traiter le choc lié à l'infarctus du myocarde, commencer par injecter 15mg par voie IM, ensuite, dissoudre 60mg dans 500ml de solution de glucose à 5 % à 10 %, en perfusion, la vitesse de la perfusion s'ajuste avec la réaction de la pression artérielle, ne pas dépasser 20 gouttes par minute.

| 剂型、规格<br>Les formes pharmaceutiques et les spécifications | 注射液：每支 10mg（1ml）；20mg（1ml）。<br>Injection : 10mg (1ml) ou 20mg (1ml) par solution. |
|---|---|
| 药品名称 Drug Names | 间羟胺 Métaraminol |
| 适应证<br>Les indications | 用于各种休克及手术时低血压。在一般用量下，不致引起心律失常，因此也可用于心肌梗死性休克。<br>Ce produit sert à traiter le choc et l'hypotension chirurgicale. Avec une dose usuelle, il n'entraîne pas l'arythmie, il est donc aussi applicable dans le traitement du choc lié à l'infarctus du myocarde. |
| 用法、用量<br>Les modes d'emploi et la posologie | （1）肌内注射或静脉滴注：① 常用量：肌内注射一次 10～20mg；静脉滴注，一次 10～40mg，稀释后缓慢滴注，如以 15～100mg 加入 0.9% 氯化钠注射液或 5%～10% 葡萄糖注射液 250～500ml 中静脉滴注，每分钟 20～30 滴，用量及滴速随血压情况而定。② 极量：静脉滴注一次 100mg（每分钟 0.2～0.4mg）。<br>（2）局部鼻充血可用 0.25%～0.5% 的等渗缓冲液（pH=6）每小时喷入或滴入 2～3 滴，每天不超过 4 次，一疗程为 7 日。<br>(1) Injection par voie IM ou en perfusion : ① La dose usuelle : injecter 10 à 20mg par fois par voie IM ; en perfusion, 10 à 40 mg par fois, après la dilution, perfusion lente, par exemple, dissoudre 15 à 100mg dans 250 à 500ml de solution de chlorure de sodium à 0,9 % ou de solution de glucose à 5% à 10 %, 20 à 30 gouttes par minute, ajuster la dose et la vitesse de la perfusion en fonction de la pression artérielle. ② La dose usuelle : en perfusion, 100mg par fois, 0,2 à 0,4mg par minute.<br>(2) Pour traiter la congestion nasale topique, utiliser la solution isotonique à 0,25% à 0,5 % (pH=6), pulvériser ou instiller 2 à 3 gouttes par h, ne pas dépasser 4 fois, pendant 7 jours comme un traitement médical. |
| 剂型、规格<br>Les formes pharmaceutiques et les spécifications | 注射液：每支 10mg（1ml）（以间羟胺计）；50mg（5ml）（以间羟胺计）。<br>Injection : 10mg (1ml) ou 50mg (5ml) (mesuré en métaraminol) par solution. |
| 药品名称 Drug Names | 肾上腺素 Adrénaline(Epinehrine) |
| 适应证<br>Les indications | 用于抢救过敏性休克、心搏骤停、支气管哮喘急性发作。与局麻药合用延长其药效。<br>Ce produit sert à sauver le choc anaphylactique, l'arrêt cardiaque et l'exacerbation aiguë de l'asthme bronchique. L'utilisation en association avec des anesthésiques locaux peut prolonger son efficacité. |
| 用法、用量<br>Les modes d'emploi et la posologie | 常用量：皮下注射，一次 0.25～1mg；心室内注射，一次 0.25～1mg。极量：皮下注射，一次 1mg。<br>La dose usuelle : injection sous-cutanée, 0,25 à 1mg par fois, injection intraventriculaire, 0,25 à 1mg par fois. La dose limite, injection sous-cutanée, 1mg par fois. |
| 剂型、规格<br>Les formes pharmaceutiques et les spécifications | 注射液：1mg（1ml）。<br>Injection : 1mg (1ml). |

**续　表**

| 药品名称 Drug Names | 多巴胺 Dopamine |
|---|---|
| 适应证<br>Les indications | 　　用于各种类型休克，包括中毒性休克、心源性休克、出血性休克、中枢性休克，特别对伴有肾功能不全、心排血量降低、周围血管阻力增高而已补足血容量的患者更有意义。<br>　　Le produit sert à traiter le choc de toutes sortes, y compris le choc toxique, lechoc cardiogénique,le choc hémorragique et le choc central. Il est surtout efficace dans le traitement des patients insuffisants rénaux, accompagnés de la réduction du débit cardiaque, de la croissance de la résistance vasculaire périphérique et ayant le volume sanguin. |
| 用法、用量<br>Les modes d'emploi et la posologie | 　　静脉注射，一次 20mg，稀释后缓慢滴注；极量，每分钟 20μg/kg。将 20mg 加入 5% 葡萄糖注射液 200 ~ 300ml 中静脉滴注，开始每分钟 20 滴左右（即每分钟滴入 75 ~ 100μg），以后根据血压情况，可加快速度或加大浓度。<br>　　Injection par voie IV, 20mg par fois, après la dilution, la perfusion lente ; la dose limite, 20μg/kg par minute. Dissoudre 20mg dans 200 à 300ml de solution de glucose à 5 %, en perfusion, commencer par 20 gouttes par minute (à savoir 75 à 100μg par minute), augmenter la concentration ou la vitesse de la perfusion en fonction de la pression artérielle. |
| 剂型、规格<br>Les formes pharmaceutiques et les spécifications | 　　注射液：每支 20mg（2ml）。<br>　　Injection : 20mg (2ml) par solution. |
| 药品名称 Drug Names | 多巴酚丁胺 Dobutamine |
| 适应证<br>Les indications | 　　用于心排血量低和心率慢的心力衰竭患者，其改善左心室功能的作用优于多巴胺。<br>　　Ce produit sert à traiter les patients accompagnés d'un faible débit cardiaque et et du rythme cardiaque ralenti. Il est plus efficace dans l'amélioration de la fonction du ventricule gauche que la dopamine. |
| 用法、用量<br>Les modes d'emploi et la posologie | 　　静脉滴注：250mg 加入 5% 葡萄糖注射液 250ml 或 500ml 中滴注，每分钟 2.5 ~ 10μg/kg。<br>　　En perfusion : dissoudre 250mg dans 250 ou 500ml de solution de glucose à 5 %, 2,5 à 10μg/kg par minute. |
| 剂型、规格<br>Les formes pharmaceutiques et les spécifications | 　　注射液：每支 20mg（按多巴酚丁胺计）（2ml）；200mg（按多巴酚丁胺计）（2ml）。<br>　　Injection : 20mg (2ml) ou 200mg (2ml) (mesuré en dobutamine) par solution. |
| 药品名称 Drug Names | 血管紧张素胺 Angioténsinamide |
| 适应证<br>Les indications | 　　用于外伤或手术后休克和全身麻醉或腰椎麻醉时所致的低血压症等。<br>　　Ce produit sert à traiter l'hypotention causée par le choc lié au traumatisme ou après la chirurgie, ainsi que par l'anesthésie générale ou la rachianesthésie. |
| 用法、用量<br>Les modes d'emploi et la posologie | 　　静脉滴注：每次 1 ~ 1.25mg，溶解于 5% 葡萄糖或 0.9% 氯化钠注射液 500ml 中，滴速一般每分钟 3 ~ 10μg，应经常测定血压，随时调整滴速。<br>　　En perfusion : 1 à 1,25mg par fois, dissoudre dans 500ml de solution de glucose à 5% ou de solution de chlorure de sodium à 0,9%, 3 à 10μg par minute, ajuster la vitesse de la perfusion en fonction de la pression artérielle. |
| 剂型、规格<br>Les formes pharmaceutiques et les spécifications | 　　注射用血管紧张素胺：每支 1mg。<br>　　L'angiotensine-amine pour injection : 1mg par solution. |

10.8　调节血脂药及抗动脉粥样硬化药 Médicaments régulateurs des lipides et antiathérosclérotiques

| 药品名称 Drug Names | 氯贝丁酯 Clofibrate |
|---|---|
| 适应证<br>Les indications | 　　用于动脉粥样硬化及其继发症，如冠状动脉病、脑血管疾病、周围血管病及糖尿病所致动脉疾病等。<br>　　Ce produit sert à traiter l'athérosclérose et sa maladie secondaire, telle que la maladie de l'artère coronaire, la maladie vasculaire cérébrale, la maladie vasculaire périphérique et la maladie de l'artère causée par le diabète, etc. |

**续　表**

| 用法、用量<br>Les modes d'emploi et la posologie | 口服，一次 0.25～0.5g，一日 3 次，饭后服。<br>Par voie orale, 0,25 à 0,5g par fois, 3 fois par jour, après le repas. |
|---|---|
| 剂型、规格<br>Les formes pharmaceutiques et les spécifications | 胶囊剂：每粒 0.25g；0.5g。<br>Capsules : 0,25g ou 0,5g par capsule. |
| **药品名称 Drug Names** | 非诺贝特 Fénofibrate |
| 适应证<br>Les indications | 用于高胆固醇血症、高三酰甘油血症及混合性高脂血症，疗效确切，且耐受性好。<br>Ce produit sert à traiter l'hypercholestérolémie, l'hypertriglycéridémie et l'hyperlipidémie mixte, avec un effet sûr et une bonne tolérance. |
| 用法、用量<br>Les modes d'emploi et la posologie | 口服：一次 100mg，一日 2～3 次。<br>Par voie orale : 100mg par fois, 2 à 3 fois par jour. |
| 剂型、规格<br>Les formes pharmaceutiques et les spécifications | 胶囊（片）剂；每粒（片）100mg；200mg；300mg。<br>Capsules (comprimés) : 100mg, 200mg ou 300mg par capsule ou par comprimé. |
| **药品名称 Drug Names** | 洛伐他汀 Lovastatine |
| 适应证<br>Les indications | 用于原发性高胆固醇血症（Ⅱa 及Ⅱb 型）。也用于合并有高胆固醇血症和高三酰甘油血症，而以高胆固醇血症为主的患者。<br>Ce produit sert à traiter l'hypercholestérolémie primaire (de type Ⅱa et de type Ⅱb). Il est aussi applicable dans le traitement des patients souffrant à la fois de l'hypercholestérolémie et de l'hypertriglycéridémie, et surtout souffrant de la première. |
| 用法、用量<br>Les modes d'emploi et la posologie | 口服，开始剂量一日 1 次 20mg，晚餐时服用，必要时于 4 周内调整剂量，最大剂量一日 80mg，1 次或分 2 次服。<br>Par voie orale, commencer par 20mg par fois par jour, durant le dîner, s'il est nécessaire, ajuster la dose en 4 semaines, ne pas dépasser 80 mg par jour, à travers 1 à 2 fois. |
| 剂型、规格<br>Les formes pharmaceutiques et les spécifications | 片剂：每片 10mg；20mg；40mg。<br>Comprimés : 10mg, 20mg ou 40mg par comprimé. |
| **药品名称 Drug Names** | 辛伐他汀 Simvastatine |
| 适应证<br>Les indications | 用于原发性高胆固醇血症（Ⅱa 及Ⅱb 型）。也用于合并有高胆固醇血症和高三酰甘油血症，而以高胆固醇血症为主的患者。<br>Ce produit sert à traiter l'hypercholestérolémie primaire (de type Ⅱa et de type Ⅱb). Il est aussi applicable dans le traitement des patients souffrant à la fois de l'hypercholestérolémie et de l'hypertriglycéridémie, et surtout souffrant de la première. |
| 用法、用量<br>Les modes d'emploi et la posologie | 口服，一日 1 次 10mg，晚餐时服，必要时于 4 周内增量至一日 1 次 40mg。<br>Par voie orale, 10 mg par fois par jour, durant le dîner, s'il est nécessaire, augmenter en 4 semaines pour atteindre 40mg par fois par jour. |
| 剂型、规格<br>Les formes pharmaceutiques et les spécifications | 片剂：每片 10mg；20mg。<br>Comprimés : 10mg ou 20mg par comprimé. |

续　表

| 药品名称 Drug Names | 普伐他汀 Pravastatine |
|---|---|
| 适应证<br>Les indications | 用于原发性高胆固醇血症（Ⅱa 及Ⅱb 型）。也用于合并有高胆固醇血症和高三酰甘油血症，而以高胆固醇血症为主的患者。<br><br>Ce produit sert à traiter l'hypercholestérolémie primaire (de type II a et de type II b). Il est aussi applicable dans le traitement des patients souffrant à la fois de l'hypercholestérolémie et de l'hypertriglycéridémie, et surtout souffrant de la première. |
| 用法、用量<br>Les modes d'emploi et la posologie | 口服，一日 10mg，分 2 次服，可根据情况增量至一日 20mg。<br><br>Par voie orale, 10mg par jour, à travers 2 fois, selon les cas, possible d'augmenter jusqu'à 20mg par jour. |
| 剂型、规格<br>Les formes pharmaceutiques et les spécifications | 片剂：每片 5mg；10mg。<br><br>Comprimés : 5mg ou 10mg par comprimé. |
| 药品名称 Drug Names | 氟伐他汀 Fluvastatine |
| 适应证<br>Les indications | 用于饮食控制无效的高胆固醇血症。<br>Ce produit sert à traiter l'hypercholestérolémie pour laquelle le régime alimentaire n'est pas valide. |
| 用法、用量<br>Les modes d'emploi et la posologie | 用量：口服每日 1 次 20mg，晚间服用。<br>La dose : 20mg par fois par jour, pris le soir. |
| 剂型、规格<br>Les formes pharmaceutiques et les spécifications | 胶囊剂：每粒 20mg；40mg。<br>Capsules : 20mg ou 40mg par capsule. |
| 药品名称 Drug Names | 阿托伐他汀 Atorvastatine |
| 适应证<br>Les indications | 用于原发性高胆固醇血症、混合型高脂血症或饮食控制无效杂合子家族型高胆固醇血症患者。<br><br>Ce produit sert à traiter l'hypercholestérolémie primaire, l'hyperlipidémie mixte ou des patients souffrants de l'hypercholestérolémie familiale pour laquelle le régime alimentaire est inutile. |
| 用法、用量<br>Les modes d'emploi et la posologie | 口服：每日 10mg，如需要，4 周后可增至每日 80mg。<br>Par voie orale : 10mg par jour, s'il nécessaire, augmenter en 4 semaines pour atteindre 80 mg par jour. |
| 剂型、规格<br>Les formes pharmaceutiques et les spécifications | 片剂：每片 10mg；20mg；40mg。<br>Comprimés : 10mg, 20mg ou 40mg par comprimé. |
| 药品名称 Drug Names | 瑞舒伐他汀 Rosuvastatine |
| 适应证<br>Les indications | 用于高脂血症和高胆固醇血症。<br>Ce produit sert à traiter l'hyperlipidémie et l'hypercholestérolémie. |
| 用法、用量<br>Les modes d'emploi et la posologie | 口服，一日 5～40mg，开始治疗时应从 10mg 开始，需要时增至 20～40mg，不宜开始时直接用 40mg。<br>Par voie orale, 5 à 40mg par jour, commencer par 10mg, s'il est nécessaire, augmenter jusqu'à 20 à 40mg, ne pas commencer directement par 40mg. |
| 剂型、规格<br>Les formes pharmaceutiques et les spécifications | 片剂：每片 5mg；10mg；20mg。<br>Comprimés : 5mg, 10mg ou 20mg par comprimé. |

**续 表**

| 药品名称 Drug Names | 普罗布考 Probucol |
|---|---|
| 适应证<br>Les indications | 用于Ⅱa型高脂血症，与其他降脂药物可用于Ⅱb和Ⅲ、Ⅳ型高脂血症。<br>Ce produit sert à traiter l'hyperlipidémie de type II a. utilisé en association avec d'autres médicaments hypolipidémiants, il permet aussi de traiter l'hyperlipidémie de type II b, III et IV. |
| 用法、用量<br>Les modes d'emploi et la posologie | 口服，每次500mg，一日2次，早、晚餐时服用。<br>Par voie orale, 500mg par fois, 2 fois par jour, pris le petit déjeuner et le dîner. |
| 剂型、规格<br>Les formes pharmaceutiques et les spécifications | 片剂：每片500mg。<br>Comprimés : 500mg par comprimé. |
| 药品名称 Drug Names | 考来烯胺 Coléstyramine |
| 适应证<br>Les indications | 用于Ⅱ型高脂血症、动脉粥样硬化及肝硬化、胆石病引起的瘙痒。其缺点是用量大，约2%的患者产生胃肠道反应。<br>Ce produit sert à traiter l'hyperlipidémie, l'athérosclérose ainsi que les démangeaisons causées par la cirrhose du foie et la lithiase biliaire. Son inconvénient est sa dose forte, ce qui entraîne des réactions gastro-intestinales chez environ 2 % des patients. |
| 用法、用量<br>Les modes d'emploi et la posologie | ①治疗动脉粥样硬化：一日3次，每次服粉剂4～5g。②止痒：开始时一日量6～10g，维持量每日3g，分3次服。<br>① Pour traiter l'athérosclérose : 3 fois par jour, 4 à 5g par fois en poudre. ② Pour les démangeaisons : commencer par 6 à 10g par jour, la dose d'entretien, 3g par jour, à travers 3 fois. |
| 剂型、规格<br>Les formes pharmaceutiques et les spécifications | 散剂：每包4g。<br>Poudre : 4g par sachet. |
| 药品名称 Drug Names | 依折麦布 Ezetimibe |
| 适应证<br>Les indications | 治疗原发性高胆固醇血症。<br>Ce produit sert à traiter l'hypercholestérolémie primaire. |
| 用法、用量<br>Les modes d'emploi et la posologie | 一日1次，每次10mg，可单独服用或与他汀类联合应用。<br>1 fois par jour, 10mg par fois, utilisé seul ou en association avec des statinesr . |
| 剂型、规格<br>Les formes pharmaceutiques et les spécifications | 片剂：每片10mg。<br>Comprimés : 10mg par comprimé. |
| 药品名称 Drug Names | 血脂康 XueZhiKang |
| 适应证<br>Les indications | 治疗动脉粥样硬化及原发性高脂血症。<br>Ce produit sert à traiter l'athérosclérose et l'hyperlipidémie primaire. |
| 用法、用量<br>Les modes d'emploi et la posologie | 口服2粒/次，一日2次。<br>Par voie orale, 2 capsules par fois, 2 fois par jour. |
| 剂型、规格<br>Les formes pharmaceutiques et les spécifications | 胶囊（丸）：0.3g/粒。<br>Capsules (pilules) : 0,3g par capsule. |

**续　表**

| 药品名称 Drug Names | 心脑康 XinNaoKang |
|---|---|
| 适应证<br>Les indications | 用于治疗动脉粥样硬化、冠心病、心绞痛、高脂血症、高血压、脑动脉硬化、偏瘫（脑出血和脑血栓形成）等。亦可作为动脉粥样硬化症的预防用药。<br><br>Ce produit sert à traiter l'athérosclérose,la maladie coronarienne,l'angine de poitrine,l'hyperlipidémie, l'hypertension artérielle, l'artériosclérose cérébrale,l'hémiplégie (l'hémorragie cérébrale et la thrombose cérébrale), etc. Il sert aussi à prévenir l'athérosclérose. |
| 用法、用量<br>Les modes d'emploi et la posologie | 口服：每次 2 粒，一日 3 次，饭后服用，1 个月为 1 个疗程，一般以连用 2～3 个疗程为宜。偏瘫患者每次 3 粒，一日 3 次，连服至症状好转或基本痊愈。<br><br>Par voie orale : 2 capsule par fois, 3 fois par jour, après le repas, pendant un mois comme un traitement mdécial, en général, il vaut mieux suivre 2 à 3 traitement médicaux consécutifs. Chez des patients atteints de l'hémiplégie, 3 capsules par fois, 3 fois par jour, administration continue jusqu'à l'amélioration des symptômes ou à la guérison générale. |
| 剂型、规格<br>Les formes pharmaceutiques et les spécifications | 软胶囊剂：每粒 415mg。<br>Capsules molles : 415mg par capsule. |

11. 主要作用于呼吸系统的药物 Médicaments agissant princepalement sur le système respiratoire

11.1 祛痰药 Expectorants

| 药品名称 Drug Names | 氯化铵 Chlorure d'ammonium |
|---|---|
| 适应证<br>Les indications | 用于急性呼吸道炎症时痰黏稠不易咳出者。常与其他复方制剂合用。纠正代谢性碱中毒。其酸化尿液作用可使一些需要在酸性尿液中显效的药物产生作用。也可增加汞剂的利尿作用以及四环素和青霉素的抗菌作用；还可促进碱性药物的排泄。<br><br>Ce produit est applicable dans le traitement des patients dont l'expectoration collante est difficile à expectorer en cas d'inflammation respiratoire aiguë. Il est souvent utilisé en association avec la préparation de composés. Il permet aussi de corriger l'alcalose métabolique. Son effet de l'acidification de l'urine peut permettre aux médicaments qui exigent l'urine acide de prendre effet. Il sert également à améliorer la diurèse de l'amalgame et l'effet antibactérien de la tétracycline et de la pénicilline. Il facilite aussi l'excrétion des médicaments de base. |
| 用法、用量<br>Les modes d'emploi et la posologie | ①祛痰：口服，成人一次 0.3～0.6g，一日 3 次。②治疗代谢性碱中毒或酸化尿液：静脉滴注，每日 2～20g，每小时不超过 5g。<br><br>① L'expectorant : par voie orale, chez des adultes, 0,3 à 0,6g par fois, 3 fois par jour. ② Pour traiter l'alcalose métabolique ou pour l'acidification de l'urine : en perfusion, 2 à 20g par jour, ne pas dépasser 5g par h. |
| 剂型、规格<br>Les formes pharmaceutiques et les spécifications | 片剂：每片 0.3mg。<br>注射液：每支 5g（500ml）。<br>Comprimés : 0,3mg par comprimé.<br>Injection : 5g (500ml) par solution. |
| 药品名称 Drug Names | 溴己新 Bromhexine |
| 适应证<br>Les indications | 用于慢性支气管炎、哮喘、支气管扩张、矽肺等有白色痰液不易咳出的患者，脓性痰患者需加用抗生素控制感染。<br><br>Ce produit est applicable dans le traitement des patients souffrant de la bronchite chronique, de l'asthme, de la dilatation des bronches ou de la silicose, et ayantdes expectorations blanches difficiles à expectorer. Chez les patients atteints d'expectoration purulente, il faut appliquer aussi des antibiotiques pour prévenir les infections. |
| 用法、用量<br>Les modes d'emploi et la posologie | 口服：成人一次 8～16mg。肌内注射：一次 4～8mg，一日 2 次。静脉注射：一日 4～8mg，加入 5% 葡萄糖氯化钠溶液 500ml 中。气雾吸入：一次 2ml，一日 2～3 次。<br><br>Par voie orale : chez des adultes, 8 à 16mg par fois. Injection par voie IM : 4 à 8mg par fois, 2 fois par jour. Injection par voie IV : 4 à 8 mg par jour, dissourdre dans 500ml de solution de glucose à 5 % ou de solution de chlorure de sodium. L'inhalation d'aérosol : 2ml par fois, 2 à 3 fois par jour. |

**续　表**

| 剂型、规格<br>Les formes pharmaceutiques et les spécifications | 片剂：每片 4mg；8mg。<br>注射液：每支 0.2%，2mg（1ml）；4mg（2ml）。<br>气雾剂：0.2% 溶液。<br>Comprimés：4mg ou 8mg par comprimé.<br>Injection：0,2 %, 2mg (1ml) ou 4mg (2ml) par solution.<br>Aérosol：la solution à 0,2 %. |
|---|---|
| **药品名称 Drug Names** | 氨溴索 Ambroxol |
| 适应证<br>Les indications | 用于急慢性支气管炎及支气管哮喘、支气管扩张、肺气肿、肺结核、肺尘埃沉着病、术后的咳痰困难等。注射药可用于术后肺部并发症的预防及早产儿、新生儿呼吸窘迫综合征的治疗。本品高剂量有降低血浆尿酸浓度和促进尿酸排泄的作用。可用于治疗痛风。<br>Ce produit sert à traiter la bronchite aiguë et chronique, l'asthme bronchique, la dilatation des bronches, l'emphysème, la tuberculose, la pneumoconiose, l'expectoration difficile postopératoire, etc. Son injection est utilisée dans la prévention des complications pulmonaires postopératoires et dans le traitement du syndrome de détresse respiratoire chez les enfants prématurés et les nouveau-nés. Le produit à forte dose pourrait réduire la concentration plasmatique d'acide urique et favoriser l'excrétion d'acide urique. Il est aussi applicable dans le traitement de la goutte. |
| 用法、用量<br>Les modes d'emploi et la posologie | 口服：成人及 12 岁以上儿童，每次 30mg，一日 3 次。长期使用剂量可减半。静脉注射、肌内注射及皮下注射：成人每次 15mg，一日 2 次。亦可加入生理盐水或葡萄糖溶液中静脉滴注。<br>Par voie orale：chez des adultes et des enfants plus de 12 ans, 30mg par fois, 3 fois par jour. Pour un usage à long terme, prendre la moitié de la dose usuelle. Injection par voie IV, IM et sous-cutanée : chez des adultes, 15mg par fois, 2 fois par jour. Possible de dissoudre dans la solution saline ou la solution de glucose pour la perfusion. |
| 剂型、规格<br>Les formes pharmaceutiques et les spécifications | 片剂：每片 15mg；30mg。<br>胶囊剂：每粒 30mg。<br>缓释胶囊：每粒 75mg。<br>口服溶液剂：每支 15mg（5ml）；180mg（60ml）；300mg（100ml）；600mg（100ml）。<br>气雾剂：每瓶 15mg（2ml）。<br>注射液：每支 15mg（2ml）。<br>Comprimés：15mg ou 30mg par comprimé.<br>Capsules：30mg par capsule.<br>Capsules à libération prolongée：75mg par capsule.<br>La solution orale：15mg (5ml), 180mg (60ml), 300mg (100ml) ou 600mg (100ml) par solution.<br>Aérosol：15mg (2ml) par flacon.<br>Injection：15mg (2ml) par solution. |
| **药品名称 Drug Names** | 乙酰半胱氨酸 Acétylcystéine |
| 适应证<br>Les indications | ①用于术后、急慢性支气管炎、支气管扩张、肺结核、肺炎、肺气肿等引起的黏稠分泌物过多所致的咳痰困难。②用于对乙酰氨基酚中毒的解毒以及环磷酰胺引起的出血性膀胱炎的治疗。<br>① Ce produit sert à traiter l'expectoration difficile en raison des sécrétions collantes excessives causées par la chirurgie, la bronchite aiguë et chronique, la bronchectasie, la tuberculose, la pneumonie, l'emphysème, etc. ② Ce produit est utilisé dans la désintoxication de l'intoxication à l'acétaminophène et dans le traitement de la cystite hémorragique provoquée par la cyclophosphamide. |
| 用法、用量<br>Les modes d'emploi et la posologie | ①喷雾吸入：仅用于非紧急情况下，临用下溶解于氯化钠液中成 10% 溶液，每次 1～3ml，一日 2～3 次。②气管滴入：急救时 5% 溶液经气管插管或气管套管直接滴入，每次 0.5～2ml，一日 2～4 次。③气管注入：急救时 5% 溶液用 1ml 注射器自甲状软骨环骨膜处注入管腔内，每次 0.5～2ml（婴儿每次 0.5ml，儿童每次 1ml，成人每次 2ml）。④口服：成人每次 200mg，一日 2～3 次。<br>① L'inhalation d'aérosol：seulement utilisé dans les cas non urgents, dissoudre dans la solution de chlorure de sodium pour former une solution à 10 %, prendre 1 à 3 ml par fois, 2 à 3 fois par jour. ② L'instillation intratrachéale：en cas d'urgence, instiller la solution à 5 %à travers l'intubation trachéale, 0,5 à 2 ml par fois, 2 à 4 fois par jour. ③ L'injection intratrachéale：en cas d'urgence, injecter la solution à 0,5 % avec la seringue de 1ml dans la cavité trachéale via le périoste du cartilage thyroïde, 0,5 à 2ml par fois (chez des bébés, 0,5ml par fois, chez des enfants, 1ml par fois, chez des adultes, 2ml par fois). ④ Par voie orale：chez des adultes, 200mg par fois, 2 à 3 fois par jour. |

**续　表**

| 剂型、规格<br>Les formes pharmaccutiqucs ct lcs spécifications | 片剂：每片 200mg；500mg。<br>喷雾剂：每瓶 0.5g；1g。<br>颗粒剂：每袋 100mg。<br>泡腾片：每片 600mg。<br>Comprimés : 200mg ou 500mg par comprimé.<br>Aérosol : 0,5g ou 1g par flacon.<br>Granules : 100mg par sachet.<br>Comprimés effervescents : 600mg par comprimé. |
|---|---|
| **药品名称 Drug Names** | 羧甲司坦 Carbocystéine |
| 适应证<br>Les indications | 用于慢性支气管炎、支气管哮喘等引起的痰液黏稠、咳痰困难和痰阻气管等。亦可用于术后咳痰困难和肺炎合并症。用于小儿非化脓性中耳炎，有预防耳聋效果。<br>Ce produit sert à traiter l'expectoration collante, l'expectoration difficile, le flegme accumulé dans la trachée causés par la bronchite chronique, l'asthme bronchique, etc. Il est aussi applicable dans le traitement de l'expectoration difficile postopératoire et des complications de la pneumonie. Il permet aussi de traiter l'otite moyenne non suppurée chez des enfants et de prévenir la surdité. |
| 用法、用量<br>Les modes d'emploi et la posologie | 口服，成人每次 0.25 ~ 0.5g，一日 3 次。儿童 1 日 30mg/kg。<br>Par voie orale, chez des adultes, 0,25 à 0,5g par fois, 3 fois par jour. Chez des enfants, 30 mg/kg par jour. |
| 剂型、规格<br>Les formes pharmaceutiques et les spécifications | 口服液：每支 0.2g（10ml）；0.5g（10ml）。<br>糖浆剂：2%（20mg/ml）。<br>片剂：每片 0.25g。<br>泡腾剂：每包 0.25g。<br>La solution orale : 0,2g (10ml) ou 0,5g (10ml) par solution.<br>Sirops : 2% (20mg/ml).<br>Comprimés : 0,25g par comprimé.<br>Comprimés effervescents : 0,25g par sachet. |
| **药品名称 Drug Names** | 标准桃金娘油 Gelomyrtol |
| 适应证<br>Les indications | 用于急慢性支气管炎、鼻窦炎、支气管扩张、肺结核、矽肺及各种原因引起的慢性阻塞性肺疾病。亦可用于支气管造影术后，可促进造影剂的排除。<br>Ce produit sert à la maladie pulmonaire obstructive chronique causée par la bronchite aiguë et chronique, la sinusite, la dilatation des bronches, la tuberculose, la silicose et d'autres maladies. Il est aussi applicable après l'artériographie bronchique pour promouvoir l'exclusion du contraste. |
| 用法、用量<br>Les modes d'emploi et la posologie | 口服。成人：每次 300mg，一日 2 ~ 3 次；4 ~ 10 岁儿童：每次 120mg，一日 2 次。<br>Par voie orale. Chez des adultes : 300mg par fois, 2 à 3 fois par jour ; chez des enfants de 4 à 10 ans : 120mg par fois, 2 fois par jour. |
| 剂型、规格<br>Les formes pharmaceutiques et les spécifications | 胶囊剂：每粒 120mg；300mg。<br>Capsules : 120mg ou 300mg par capsule. |
| **药品名称 Drug Names** | 碘化钾 Iodure de potassium |
| 适应证<br>Les indications | 为刺激性祛痰剂，可使痰液变稀，易于咳出，并可增加支气管分泌。配成含碘食盐，预防地方性甲状腺肿。<br>En tant qu'expectorant irritant,ce produit permet l'amincissement des expectorations et l'augmentation de la sécrétion bronchique. Appliqué dans le sel iodé, il sert à prévenir le goitre endémique. |
| 用法、用量<br>Les modes d'emploi et la posologie | 口服：每次 6 ~ 10ml，一日 3 次。<br>Par voie orale : 6 à 10ml par fois, 3 fois par jour. |
| 剂型、规格<br>Les formes pharmaceutiques et les spécifications | 合剂：每 100ml 含碘化钾 5g。<br>Composés : chaque 100ml contient 5g d'iodure de potassium. |

续　表

| 药品名称 Drug Names | 美司钠 Mésna |
|---|---|
| 适应证<br>Les indications | 用于慢性支气管炎、肺炎、肺癌患者痰液黏稠、术后肺不张等所致咳痰困难者。<br><br>Ce produit sert à traiter l'expectoration difficile causée par l'expectoration collante et l'atélectasie postopératoire chez des patients atteints de la bronchite chronique, de la pneumonie ou du cancer du poumon. |
| 用法、用量<br>Les modes d'emploi et la posologie | 雾化吸入或气管内滴入，每次20%溶液1～2ml。局部刺激作用，可引起咳嗽及支气管痉挛。不宜与红霉素、四环素、氨茶碱合用。<br><br>L'inhalation d'aérosol ou l'instillation intratrachéale, 1 à 2 ml de solution à 20 % par fois. Il peut avoir une stimulation locale et causer la toux et les spasmes bronchiques. Il vaut mieux éviter de l'utiliser en association avec l'érythromycine, la tétracycline et la théophylline. |
| 剂型、规格<br>Les formes pharmaceutiques et les spécifications | 气雾剂：0.2g/ml。<br>溶液剂：10% 水溶液。<br>Aérosol : 0.2g/ml.<br>Solution : la solution à 10%. |

11.2　镇咳药 Antitoux

| 药品名称 Drug Names | 可待因 Codéine |
|---|---|
| 适应证<br>Les indications | ①各种原因引起的剧烈干咳和刺激性咳嗽，尤适用于伴有胸痛的剧烈咳嗽。由于本品能抑制呼吸道腺体分泌和纤毛运动，故对少量痰液的剧烈咳嗽，应与祛痰药并用。②用于中度疼痛的镇痛。③局部麻醉或全身麻醉时的辅助用药，具有镇静作用。<br><br>① Ce produit sert à traiter une toux sévère et une toux irritante causées par diverses raisons, notamment pour la toux sévère accompagnée des douleurs à la poitrine. Comme ce produit peut inhiberla sécrétion glandulaire et le mouvement de cils des voies respiratoires, il doit être utilisé en association avec des expectorants pour traiter les toux sévères accompagnées des crachats de petite quantité. ② Il sert d'analgésique de la douleur modérée. ③ Il sert de médicament adjuvant lors de l'anesthésie locale ou de l'anesthésie générale, et il a un effet sédatif. |
| 用法、用量<br>Les modes d'emploi et la posologie | （1）成人：①常用量：口服或皮下注射，一次15～30mg，1日30～90mg。缓释片剂一次1片（45mg），一日2次；②极量：一次100mg，一日250mg。<br>（2）儿童：镇痛，口服，每次0.5～1.0mg/kg，一日3次，或一日3mg/kg；镇咳，为镇痛剂量的1/3～1/2。<br><br>(1) Chez des adultes : ① La dose usuelle : par voie orale ou injection sous-cutanée, 15 à 30mg par fois, 30 à 90mg par jour. Les comprimés à liberation prolongée, 1 comprimé (45mg) par fois, 2 fois par jour. ② La dose limite : 100mg par fois, 250 mg par jour.<br>(2) Chez des enfants : l'analgésie, par voie orale, 0,5 à 1,0 mg/kg par fois, 3 fois par jour, ou 3 mg/kg par jour ; pour l'expectorant, 1/3 à 1/2 de la dose pour l'analgésie. |
| 剂型、规格<br>Les formes pharmaceutiques et les spécifications | 片剂：每片15mg；30mg。<br>缓释胶囊：每粒45mg。<br>糖浆剂：0.5%，10ml，100ml。<br>注射液：每支15mg（1ml）；30mg（1ml）。<br><br>Comprimés : 15mg ou 30mg par comprimé.<br>Capsules à libération prolongée : 45mg par capsule.<br>Sirops : 0,5%, 10ml ou 100ml.<br>Injection : 15mg (1ml) ou 30mg (1ml). |
| 药品名称 Drug Names | 福尔可定 Pholcodine |
| 适应证<br>Les indications | 用于剧烈干咳和中等度疼痛。<br>Ce produit sert à traiter les toux sévères et des douleurs modérées. |
| 用法、用量<br>Les modes d'emploi et la posologie | 口服：常量，一次5～10mg，一日3～4次；极量，一日60mg。<br>Par voie orale : la dose usuelle, 5 à 10mg par fois, 3 à 4 fois par jour ; la dose limite, 60mg par jour. |

续　表

| 剂型、规格<br>Les formes pharmaceutiques et les spécifications | 片剂：每片 5mg；10mg；15mg；30mg。<br>Comprimés : 5mg, 10mg, 15mg ou 30mg par comprimé. |
|---|---|
| 药品名称 Drug Names | 喷托维林 Pentoxyvérine |
| 适应证<br>Les indications | 用于上呼吸道感染引起的无痰干咳和百日咳等，对小儿疗效优于成人。<br>Ce produit sert à traiter la toux sans flegme et la coqueluche causées par les infections des voies respiratoires supérieures. Il est plus efficace chez des enfants que chez des adultes. |
| 用法、用量<br>Les modes d'emploi et la posologie | 口服，成人，每次 25mg，一日 3 ～ 4 次。<br>Par voie orale, chez des adultes, 25mg par fois, 3 à 4 fois par jour. |
| 剂型、规格<br>Les formes pharmaceutiques et les spécifications | 片剂：每片 25mg。<br>滴丸：每丸 25mg。<br>冲剂：每袋 10g。<br>糖浆剂：0.145%；0.2%；0.25%。<br>Comprimés : 25mg par comprimé.<br>Pilules : 25mg par pilule.<br>Granules : 10g par sachet.<br>Sirops : 0,145 %, 0,2 % ou 0,25 %. |
| 药品名称 Drug Names | 右美沙芬 Dextrométhorphane |
| 适应证<br>Les indications | 用于干咳，适用于感冒、急慢性支气管炎、支气管哮喘、咽喉炎、肺结核以及其他上呼吸道感染时的咳嗽。<br>Ce produit sert à traiter la doux causée par le rhume, la bronchite aiguë et chronique, l'asthme bronchique, la laryngite, la tuberculose et d'autres infections des voies respiratoires supérieures. |
| 用法、用量<br>Les modes d'emploi et la posologie | 口服，成人，每次 10 ～ 30mg，一日 3 次。一日最大剂量 120mg。<br>Par voie orale, chez des adultes, 10 à 30mg par fois, 3 fois par jour. La dose maximale, 120mg par jour. |
| 剂型、规格<br>Les formes pharmaceutiques et les spécifications | 片剂：每片 10mg；15mg。<br>分散片：每片 15mg；30mg。<br>胶囊剂：每粒 15mg。<br>颗粒剂：每袋 7.5mg；15mg。<br>糖浆剂：每瓶 15mg（20ml）；150mg（100ml）。<br>注射剂：每支 5mg。<br>Comprimés : 10mg ou 15mg par comprimé.<br>Comprimés dispersibles : 15mg ou 30mg par comprimé.<br>Capsules : 15mg par capsule.<br>Granules : 7,5mg ou 15mg par sachet.<br>Sirops : 15mg (20ml) ou 150 mg (100ml) par flacon.<br>Injection : 5mg par solution. |

11.3　平喘药 Anti-Asthmatiques

| 药品名称 Drug Names | 麻黄碱 Ephédrine |
|---|---|
| 适应证<br>Les indications | ①预防支气管哮喘发作和缓解轻度哮喘发作，对急性重度哮喘发作效果不佳。②用于蛛网膜下隙麻醉或硬膜外麻醉引起的低血压及慢性低血压。③治疗各种原因引起的鼻黏膜充血、肿胀引起的鼻塞。<br>① Ce produit sert à prévenir l'asthme bronchique et à soulager la crise d'asthme léger. Il est peu efficace dans le traitement de la crise d'asthme aiguë et grave. ② Il permet de traiter l'hypotension causée par la rachianesthésie ou l'anesthésie péridurale ainsi que l'hypotension chronique. ② Ce produit sert à traiter la congestion nasale et le nez bouché causé par le gonflement. |
| 用法、用量<br>Les modes d'emploi et la posologie | ①支气管哮喘：口服：成人，常用量一次 15 ～ 30mg，一日 45 ～ 90mg；极量，一次 60mg，一日 150mg。皮下或肌内注射：成人，常用量一次 15 ～ 30mg，一日 45 ～ 60mg；极量，一次 60mg，一日 150mg。②蛛网膜下隙麻醉或硬膜外麻醉时维持血压：麻醉前皮下或肌内注射 20 ～ 50mg。慢性低血压症，每次口服 20 ～ 50mg，一日 150mg。③解除鼻黏膜充血、水肿：以 0.5% ～ 1% 溶液滴鼻。 |

续　表

|  | ① Pour traiter l'asthme bronchique : par voie orale : chez des adultes, la dose usuelle, 15 à 30mg par fois, 45 à 90mg par jour ; la dose limite, 60mg par fois, 150 mg par jour. Injection sous-cutanée ou IM : chez des adultes, la dose usuelle, 15 à 30mg par fois, 45 à 60mg par jour ; la dose limite, 60mg par fois, 150mg par jour. ② Pour maintenir la pression artérielle lors de la rachianesthésie ou de l'anesthésie péridurale : injection sous-cutanée ou par voie IM avant l'anesthésie, 20 à 50mg. Pour traiter l'hypotension chronique, 20 à 50mg, par voie orale, 150mg par jour. ③ Pour traiter la congestion nasale et l'œdème : instiller la solution à 0,5% à 1% dans le nez. |
|---|---|
| 剂型、规格<br>Les formes pharmaceutiques et les spécifications | 片剂：每片 15mg；25mg；30mg。<br>注射液：每支 30mg（1ml）；50mg（1ml）。<br>滴鼻剂：0.5%（小儿）；1%（成人）；2%（检查、手术或止血时用）。<br>Comprimés : 15mg, 25mg ou 30mg par comprimé.<br>Injection : 30mg (1ml), 50mg (1ml) par solution.<br>Les gouttes nasales : 0,5% (chez des enfants), 1%(chez des adultes), 2% (lors de l'examen, de la chirurgie ou de l'hémostase). |
| 药品名称 Drug Names | 异丙肾上腺素 Isoprotérénol |
| 适应证<br>Les indications | ①支气管哮喘：适用于控制哮喘发作，常气雾吸入给药，作用快而强，但持续时间短。②心搏骤停：治疗各种原因及溺水、电击、手术意外和药物中毒等引起的心搏骤停。必要时可与肾上腺素和去甲肾上腺素配合使用。③房室传导阻滞。④抗休克：心源性休克和感染性休克。对中心静脉压高、心排血量低者，应在不足血容量的基础上使用本品。<br>① L'asthme bronchique : ce produit sert à contrôler la crise de l'asthme. Il est souvent administré par voie de l'inhalation d'aérosols, avec un effet rapide et fort mais qui dure peu. ② L'arrêt du cœur : il permet de traiter l'arrêt du cœur causé par la noyade, l'électrocution, les accidents chirurgicaux et les intoxications par le médicament. S'il est nécessaire, il peut être utilisé en association avec l'adrénaline et la noradrénaline. ③ Le bloc auriculo-ventriculaire. ④ L'anti-choc : le choc cardiogénique et le choc septique. Chez des patients dont la pression veineuse centrale est élevée et le débit cardiaque est bas, il peut être appliqué à condition de l'hypovolémie. |
| 用法、用量<br>Les modes d'emploi et la posologie | ①支气管哮喘：舌下含服，成人常用量一次 10～15mg，一日 3 次；极量，一次 20mg，一日 60mg。气雾剂吸入，常用量，一次 0.1～0.4mg；极量，一次 0.4mg，一日 2.4mg。重复使用的间隔时间不宜少于 2 小时。②心搏骤停：心腔内注射 0.5～1mg。③房室传导阻滞：二度者采用舌下含服，每次 10mg，每 4 小时一次；三度者如心率低于 40 次/分时，可用 0.5～1mg 溶于 5% 葡萄糖液 200～300ml 中缓慢静脉滴入。④抗休克：以 0.5～1mg 加入 5% 葡萄糖液 200ml 中，静脉滴注，滴速 0.5～2μg/min，根据心率调整滴速，使收缩压维持在 12kPa（90mmHg）脉压维持在 2.7kPa（20mmHg）以上，心率 120 次/分以下。<br>① L'asthme bronchique : administration sublinguale, chez des adultes, la dose usuelle, 10 à 15mg par fois, 3 fois par jour ; la dose limite, 20mg par fois, 60mg par jour. L'inhalation d'aérosol, la dose usuelle, 0,1 à 0,4mg par fois ; la dose limite, 0,4mg par fois, 2,4mg par jour. L'intervalle entre deux administrations est de 2 h au moins. ② Pour traiter l'arrêt cardiaque : l'injection intracardiaque, 0,5 à 1mg. ③ Pour traiter le bloc auriculo-ventriculaire : chez les patients de degré II, administration sublinguale, 10mg par fois, toutes les 4h ; chez les patients de degré III, si le rythme cardiaque est inférieur à 40 fois par minute, dissoudre 0,5 à 1mg dans 200 à 300ml de solution de glucose à 5%, en perfusion lente. ④ Pour l'anti-choc : dissoudre 0,5 à 1mg dans 200ml de solution de glucose à 5%, en perfusion, 0,5 à 2μg par minute, ajuster la vitesse de la perfusion en fonction du rythme cardiaque, pour maintenir la pression artérielle systolique à 12kPa (90mmHg), la pression du pouls supérieure à 2,7 kPa (20mmHg), et le rythme cardique inférieur à 120 fois par minute. |
| 剂型、规格<br>Les formes pharmaceutiques et les spécifications | 片剂：每片 10mg。纸片：每片 5mg。<br>气雾剂：浓度为 0.25%，每瓶可喷吸 200 次左右，每揿约 0.175mg。<br>注射液：每支 1mg（2ml）。<br>Comprimés : 10mg par comprimé.<br>Papier : 5mg par pièce.<br>Aérosol : 0,025%, chaque flacon permet de pulvériser 200 fois, avec chaque pulvérisation de 0,175mg.<br>Injection : 1mg (2ml) par solution. |

**续　表**

| 药品名称 Drug Names | 沙丁胺醇 Salbutamol |
|---|---|
| 适应证<br>Les indications | 用于防治支气管哮喘，哮喘型支气管和肺气肿的支气管痉挛。制止发作多用气雾吸入，预防可用口服。<br><br>Ce produit sert à prévenir et à traiter l'asthme bronchique, l'asthme bronchique et l'emphysème bronchospasme. Pour arrêter la crise, il est souvent administré par voie de l'inhalation d'aérosols ; pour prévenir la maladie, il est souvent administré par voie orale. |
| 用法、用量<br>Les modes d'emploi et la posologie | 口服：成人，每次 2 ~ 4mg，一日 3 次。气雾吸入：每次 0.1 ~ 0.2mg，必要时每 4 小时重复一次，但 24 小时内不宜超过 8 次，粉雾吸入，成人每次吸入 0.4mg，一日 3 ~ 4 次。静脉注射：一次 0.4mg，用 5% 葡萄糖液 20ml 或氯化钠液 20ml 稀释后，缓慢注射。静脉滴注：一次 0.4mg，用 5% 葡萄糖液 100ml 稀释后滴入。肌内注射：一次 0.4mg，必要时可重复注射。<br><br>Par voie orale : chez des adultes, 2 à 4mg par fois, 3 fois par jour. L'inhalation d'aérosol : 0,1 à 0,2mg par fois, s'il est nécessaire, toutes les 4 h, mais ne pas dépasser 8 fois par jour. Inhalation de poudre sèche, chez des adultes, 0,4mg par fois, 3 à 4 fois par jour. Injection par voie IV : 0,4mg par fois, dissoudre dans 20ml de solution de glucose à 5% ou dans 20ml de solution de chlorure de sodium, injection lente. En perfusion : 0,4mg par fois, dissoudre dans 100ml de solution de glucose à 5%, la perfusion. Injection par voie IM : 0,4mg par fois, s'il est nécessaire, injection répétée. |
| 剂型、规格<br>Les formes pharmaceutiques et les spécifications | 片（胶囊）剂：每片（粒）0.5mg；2mg。<br>缓释片（胶囊）剂：每粒 4mg；8mg。<br>气雾剂：溶液型 0.2%（g/g），每瓶 20mg（200 揿）每揿 0.1mg。<br>粉雾剂胶囊：每粒 0.2mg；0.4mg，用粉物吸入器吸入。<br>注射液：每支 0.4mg（2ml）。<br>糖浆剂：4mg（1ml）。<br>Comprimés (capsules) : 0,5mg ou 2mg par comprimé ou par capsule.<br>Comprimé (capsule) à libération prolongée : 4mg ou 8mg par comprimé ou par capsule.<br>Aérosol : la solution à 0,2% (g/g), 20mg par flaocn (200 pulvérisations), 0,1mg par pulvérisation.<br>Capsules de poudre pour inhalation : 0,2mg ou 0,4mg par capsule, inhaler avec un inhalateur de poudre.<br>Injection : 0,4mg (2ml) par solution.<br>Sirops : 4mg (1ml). |
| 药品名称 Drug Names | 福莫特罗 Formotérol |
| 适应证<br>Les indications | 用于慢性哮喘于慢性阻塞性肺疾病的维持治疗与预防发作，因其为长效制剂，特别适用于哮喘夜间发作患者，疗效尤佳。能有效预防运动型哮喘的发作。<br><br>Ce produit est utilisé dans le traitement d'entretien et la prévention de la crise de l'asthme chronique et de la maladie pulmonaire obstructive chronique. Comme il s'agit d'une formulation à action prolongée, il est surtout efficace dans le traitement des patients atteints de la crise nocturne d'asthme. Il est aussi applicable dans la prévention de la crise de l'asthme lié à l'activité sportive. |
| 用法、用量<br>Les modes d'emploi et la posologie | 口服：成人每次 40 ~ 80μg，一日 2 次。气雾吸入：成人每次 4.5 ~ 9μg，一日 2 次。<br><br>Par voie orale : chez des adultes, 40 à 80μg par fois, 2 fois par jour. L'inhalation d'aérosol : chez des adultes, 4,5 à 9μg par fois, 2 fois par jour. |
| 剂型、规格<br>Les formes pharmaceutiques et les spécifications | 片剂：每片 20μg；40μg。<br>干糖浆：20mg（0.5g）。<br>气雾剂：每瓶 60 喷（每喷含本品 9μg）。<br>干粉吸入剂：每瓶 60 喷（每喷含本品 4.5μg）。<br>Comprimés : 20μg, 40μg par comprimé.<br>Agent pour sirop: 20mg (0.5g).<br>Aerosol : 60 pressions（9 μg par pression）.<br>Poudres: 60 pressions (4.5μg, par pression). |
| 药品名称 Drug Names | 丙卡特罗 Procatérol |
| 适应证<br>Les indications | 用于防治支气管哮喘，喘息性支气管炎和慢性阻塞性肺疾病所致喘息症状。<br><br>Ce produit sert à prévenir et à traiter l'asthme bronchique, la bronchite asthmatique et la maladie pulmonaire obstructive chronique. |
| 用法、用量<br>Les modes d'emploi et la posologie | 口服，成人，每晚睡前一次服 50μg，或每次 25 ~ 50μg，早晚（睡前）各服一次。<br><br>Par voie orale, chez des adultes, 50μg pris avant le sommeil du soir, ou 25 à 50μg par fois, deux fois par jour, le petit matien et avant le sommeil du soir. |

**续　表**

| | |
|---|---|
| 剂型、规格<br>Les formes pharmaceutiques et les spécifications | 片剂（胶囊）剂：每片（粒）含本品 25μg；50μg。<br>口服液：0.15mg（30ml）。<br>气雾剂：2mg，每揿含 10μg。<br>Comprimés (capsules) : 25μg ou 50μg par comprimé ou capsule.<br>La solution orale : 0,15mg (30ml).<br>Aerosol : 2mg, chaque pression contient 10μg. |
| **药品名称 Drug Names** | 沙美特罗 Salmétérol |
| 适应证<br>Les indications | 用于哮喘、喘息性支气管炎和可逆性气管阻塞。<br>Ce produit sert à traiter l'asthme, la bronchite asthmatique et l'obstruction réversible des voies respiratoires. |
| 用法、用量<br>Les modes d'emploi et la posologie | 粉物吸入：成人，每次 50μg，一日 2 次；儿童，每次 25μg，一日 2 次。气雾吸入：剂量用法同上。<br>L'inhalation de poudre sèche : chez des adultes, 50μg par fois, 2 fois par jour ; chez des enfants, 25μg par fois, 2 fois par jour. L'inhalation d'aérosol : la même dose. |
| 剂型、规格<br>Les formes pharmaceutiques et les spécifications | 粉雾剂胶囊：每粒含本品 50μg。<br>气雾剂：每喷含本品 25μg。<br>Capsules de poudre pour inhalation : chaque capsule contient 50μgde salmétérol.<br>Aérosol : chaque pulvérisation contient 25μg de salmétérol. |
| **药品名称 Drug Names** | 班布特罗 Bambutérol |
| 适应证<br>Les indications | 用于支气管哮喘、慢性喘息性支气管炎、阻塞性肺气肿及其他伴有支气管痉挛的肺部疾病。<br>Ce produit sert à traiter l'asthme bronchique, la bronchite asthmatique chronique, l'emphysème obstructif et d'autres maladies pulmonaires accompagnées dubronchospasme. |
| 用法、用量<br>Les modes d'emploi et la posologie | 每晚睡前口服一次，成人 10mg，12 岁以下儿童 5mg。<br>Pris par voie orale, une fois avant le sommeil du soir, chez des adultes, 10mg, chez des enfants moins de 12 ans, 5mg. |
| 剂型、规格<br>Les formes pharmaceutiques et les spécifications | 片剂（胶囊）：每片（粒）10mg；20mg。<br>口服液：10mg（10ml）。<br>Comprimés (capsules) : 10mg ou 20mg par comprimé ou par capsule.<br>Solution orale : 10mg (10ml). |
| **药品名称 Drug Names** | 异丙托溴铵 Bromure d'ipratropium |
| 适应证<br>Les indications | ①用于缓解慢性阻塞性肺疾病（COPD）引起的支气管痉挛、喘息症状。②防治哮喘，尤适用于因用 β 受体激动药产生肌肉震颤、激动过速而不能耐受此类药物的患者。<br>① Ce produit sert à soulager le bronchospasme et la respiration sifflante causés par la maladie pulmonaire obstructive chronique. ② Il permet de prévenir et de traiter l'asthme, surtout chez des patients souffrant du tremblement musculaire et de l'agitation trop vite causés par les agonistes du récepteur β et résistant à ceux-ci. |
| 用法、用量<br>Les modes d'emploi et la posologie | 气雾吸入：成人一次 40～80μg，一日 3～4 次。雾化吸入：成人，一次 100～500μg（14 岁以下 50～250μg），用生理盐水稀释到 3～4ml，至雾化器中吸入。<br>L'inhalation d'aérosol : chez des adultes, 40 à 80μg par fois, 3 à 4 fois par jour. L'inhalation de brouillard : chez des adultes, 100 à 500μg (chez moins de 14ans, 50 à 250μg), utiliser la solution saline pour la dilution, pour former 3 à 4ml, inhaler avec le nébuliseur. |
| 剂型、规格<br>Les formes pharmaceutiques et les spécifications | 气雾剂：每喷 20μg，40μg；每瓶 200 喷（10ml）。<br>吸入溶液剂：2ml：异丙托溴铵 500μg。<br>雾化溶液剂：50μg（2ml）；250μg（2ml）；500μg（2ml）；500μg（20ml）<br>Aérosol : 20μg ou 40μg par pulvérisation ; 200 pulvérisations par flacon (10ml).<br>La solution pour inhalation : 2ml : 500 μg de bromue d'ipratropium.<br>La solution pour atomisation : 50μg (2ml), 250 μg (2ml), 500 μg (2ml) ou 500 μg (20ml). |

续　表

| 药品名称 Drug Names | 噻托溴铵 Bromure de tiotropium |
|---|---|
| 适应证<br>Les indications | 用于治疗慢性阻塞性肺疾病及支气管哮喘，对于急性哮喘发作无效。<br>Ce produit sert à traiter la maladie pulmonaire obstructive chronique et l'asthme bronchique. Mais il est inutile dans le traitement de la crise de l'asthme aigu. |
| 用法、用量<br>Les modes d'emploi et la posologie | 噻托溴铵粉吸入剂（胶囊）；每粒 18μg，每次吸入 1 粒，一日 1 次。<br>Capsules de poudre pour inhalation de bromure de tiotropium : 18 μg par capsule, inhaler 1 capsule par fois, 1 fois par jour. |
| 剂型、规格<br>Les formes pharmaceutiques et les spécifications | 粉雾剂：18μg；吸入剂：18μg。<br>Pouders : 18μg; Inhalation : 18μg. |
| 药品名称 Drug Names | 氨茶碱 Aminophylline |
| 适应证<br>Les indications | 用于①支气管哮喘和喘息性支气管炎，与 β 受体激动剂合用可提高疗效。在哮喘持续状态，常选用本品与肾上腺皮质激素配伍进行治疗；②治疗急性心功能不全和心源性哮喘；③胆绞痛。<br>① Ce produit sert à traiter l'asthme bronchique et la bronchite asthmatique. L'utilisation en association avec les agonistes du récepteur β peut permettre d'augmenter l'efficacité. Il est souvent appliqué en combinaison avec l'hormone corticotrope pour traiter l'état de mal asthmatique. ② Il permet de traiter l'insuffisance cardiaque aiguë et l'asthme cardiaque. ③ Il sert aussi à traiter les coliques. |
| 用法、用量<br>Les modes d'emploi et la posologie | 口服：成人，常用量，每次 0.1 ~ 0.2g，一日 0.3 ~ 0.6g；极量，一次 0.5g，一日 1g。肌内注射或静脉注射：成人，常用量，每次 0.25 ~ 0.5g，一日 0.5 ~ 1g；极量，一次 0.5g。以 50% 葡萄糖注射液 20 ~ 40mg 稀释后缓慢静脉注射（不少于 10 分钟）。静脉滴注：以 5% 葡萄糖注射液 500ml 稀释后滴注。直肠给药：栓剂或保留灌肠，每次 0.3 ~ 0.5g，一日 1 ~ 2 次。<br>Par voie orale : chez des adultes, la dose usuelle, 0,1 à 0,2g par fois, 0,3 à 0,6g par jour ; la dose limite, 0,5g par fois, 1g par jour. Injection par voie IM ou IV : chez des adultes, la dose usuelle, 0,25 à 0,5g par fois, 0,5 à 1g par jour ; la dose limite, 0,5g par jour. Dissoudre dans 20 à 40mg de solution de glucose à 50%, injection par voie IV lente (10 minutes au moins). En perfusion : dissoudre dans 500ml de solution de glusoe à 5%, la perfusion. L'administration rectale : suppositoires ou le lavement à garder, 0,3 à 0,5g par fois, 1 à 2 fois par jour. |
| 剂型、规格<br>Les formes pharmaceutiques et les spécifications | 片剂：每片 0.05g；0.1g；0.2g。<br>肠溶片：每片 0.05g；0.1g。<br>注射液：①肌内注射用每支 0.125g（2ml）；0.25g（2ml）；0.5g（2ml）。②静脉注射用每支 0.25g（10ml）。<br>栓剂：每粒 0.25g。缓释片每片 0.15g；0.2g。<br>Comprimés : 0,05g, 0,1g ou 0,2 par comprimé.<br>Comprimés à enrobage entérique : 0,05g, 0,1g par comprimé.<br>Injection : ① injection par voie IM, 0,125g (2ml), 0,25g (2ml) ou 0,5g (2ml) par solution. ② injection par voie IV, 0,25g (10ml).<br>Suppositoires : 0,25g par suppositoire.<br>Comprimé à libération prolongée : 0,15g ou 0,2g par comprimé. |
| 药品名称 Drug Names | 多索茶碱 Doxofylline |
| 适应证<br>Les indications | 适用于支气管哮喘、喘息性支气管炎及其他伴支气管痉挛的肺部疾病。<br>Ce produit sert à traiter l'asthme bronchique, la bronchite asthmatique et d'autres maladies pulmonaires associées à un bronchospasme. |
| 用法、用量<br>Les modes d'emploi et la posologie | 口服：每日 2 片或每 12 小时 1 ~ 2 粒胶囊，或每日 1 ~ 3 包散剂冲服。急症可先注射 100mg，然后每 6 小时静脉注射一次，也可每日静脉滴注 300mg。<br>Par voie orale : 2 comprimés par jour ou 1 à 2 capsules toutes les 12h, ou 1 à 3 sachets en poudre. En cas d'urgence, injecter 100mg d'abord, ensuite, injection par voie IV toutes les 6h, ou 300mg en perfusion par jour. |

**续 表**

| 剂型、规格<br>Les formes pharmaceutiques et les spécifications | 片剂：每片 200mg；300mg；400mg。<br>胶囊剂：每粒 200mg；300mg。<br>散剂：每包 200mg。<br>注射液：每支 100mg（10ml）。<br>葡萄糖注射液：每瓶 0.3g 与葡萄糖 5g（100ml）。<br>Comprimés : 200mg, 300mg ou 400mg par comprimé.<br>Capsules : 200mg ou 300mg par capsule.<br>Poudre : 200mg par sachet.<br>Injection : 100mg (10ml) par solution.<br>Injection de glucose : 0,3g de doxofylline et 5g de glucose par flacon (100ml). |
| --- | --- |
| 药品名称 Drug Names | 二羟丙茶碱 Diprophylline |
| 适应证<br>Les indications | 用于支气管哮喘、喘息性支气管炎，尤适用于伴有心动过速的哮喘患者。亦可用于心源性肺水肿引起的喘息。<br>Ce produit sert à traiter l'asthme bronchique, la bronchite asthmatique, en particulier pour les patients asthmatiques atteints de tachycardie. Il est aussi applicable dans le traitement de la respiration causée par un œdème pulmonaire cardiogénique. |
| 用法、用量<br>Les modes d'emploi et la posologie | 口服：每次 0.1～0.2g，一日 3 次。极量，一次 0.5g，一日 1.5g。肌内注射：每次 0.25～0.5g，静脉滴注：用于严重哮喘发作，每日 0.5～1g，加于 5% 葡萄糖液 1500～2000ml 中滴入。直肠给药：每次 0.25～0.5g。<br>Par voie orale : 0,1 à 0,2g par fois, 3 fois par jour. La dose limite, 0,5g par fois, 1,5g par jour. Injection par voie IM : 0,25 à 0,5g par fois. En perfusion : appliqué pour traiter la crise de l'asthme grave, 0,5 à 1g par jour, dissoudre dans 1 500 à 2 000ml de solution de glocuse à 5%, la perfusion. L'administration rectale : 0,25 à 0,5g par fois. |
| 剂型、规格<br>Les formes pharmaceutiques et les spécifications | 片剂：每片 0.1g；0.2g。<br>注射液：每支 0.25g（2ml）。<br>葡萄糖注射液：每瓶 0.25g 与葡萄糖 5g（100ml）。<br>栓剂：每粒 0.25g。<br>Comprimés : 0,1g ou 0,2g par comprimé.<br>Injection : 0,25g (2ml) par solution.<br>Injection de glucose : 0,25g de diprophylline et 5g de glucose par flacon (100ml).<br>Suppositoires : 0,25g par suppositoire. |
| 药品名称 Drug Names | 色甘酸钠 Cromoglicate de sodium |
| 适应证<br>Les indications | ①支气管哮喘：可用于预防各型哮喘发作。对外源性哮喘疗效显著，特别是对已知抗原的年轻患者疗效更佳，对内源性哮喘和慢性哮喘亦有一定疗效，约半数患者的症状改善或完全控制。对依赖肾上腺皮质激素的哮喘患者，经本品后可减少或完全停用肾上腺皮质激素。运动性哮喘患者预先给药几乎可防止全部病例发作。一般应于接触抗原前一周给药，但运动性哮喘可在运动前 15 分钟给药。β 肾上腺素受体激动剂合用可提高疗效。②过敏性鼻炎，季节性花粉症，春季角膜、结膜炎，过敏性湿疹及某些皮肤瘙痒症。③溃疡性结肠炎和直肠炎：本品灌肠后可改善症状，内镜检查和活检均可见炎症及损伤减轻。<br>① L'asthme bronchique : ce produit sert à prévenir la crise de l'asthme de tous types. Il est surtout efficace dans le traitement de l'asthme extrinsèque, en particulier chezles jeunes patients avec antigène connu. Il a aussi un certain effet sur l'asthme intrinsèque et l'asthme chronique. Chez la moitié des patients, il permet l'amélioration des symptômes ou le contrôle total. Chez des asthmatiques dépendants des hormonescorticotropes, il permet de diminuer ou d'arrêter l'administration de celleci. Le prétraitement chez des patients atteints de l'asthme induit par l'exercice physique pourrait prévenir la crise de tous les cas. Il faut généralement prendre des médicaments une semaine avant de contacter des antigènes, mais il faut l'administration 15 minutes avant l'exercice physique dans le cas de l'asthme lié à l'activité sportive. L'utilisation en association avec des agonistes adrénergiques du récepteur β peut renforcer l'efficacité. ② La rhinite allergique, le pollinose saisonnier, la cornée du printemps, la conjonctivite, l'eczéma atopique et certains prurits. ③ La colite ulcéreuse et la proctite : l'administration par voie de lavement peut permettre de soulager les symptômes. On voit le soulagement de l'inflammation et des blessures à travers l'endoscopie et la biopsie. |

**续　表**

| | |
|---|---|
| 用法、用量<br>Les modes d'emploi et la posologie | ①支气管哮喘：粉物吸入，每次 20mg，一日 4 次；症状减轻后，一日 40 ～ 60mg；维持量，一日 20mg。气雾吸入，每次 2.5 ～ 7mg，一日 3 ～ 4 次，每日最大剂量 32mg。②过敏性鼻炎：干粉吸入或吹入鼻腔，每次 10mg，一日 4 次。③季节性花粉症和春季角膜、结膜炎：滴眼，2% 溶液，每次 2 滴，一日数次。④过敏性湿疹、皮肤瘙痒症：外用 5% ～ 10% 软膏。⑤溃疡性结肠炎、直肠炎：灌肠，每次 200mg。<br><br>① Pour traiter l'asthme bronchique : l'inhalation de poudre, 20mg par fois, 4 fois par jour ; après l'amélioration des symptômes, 40 à 60mg par jour ; la dose d'entretien, 20mg par jour. L'inhalation d'aérosol, 2,5 à 7mg par fois, 3 à 4 fois par jour, ne pas dépasser 32mg par jour. ② Pour traiter la rhinite allergique : l'inhalation de poudre sèche ou l'inhalation nasale, 10mg par fois, 4 fois par jour. ③ Pour traiter le pollinose saisonnier, la cornée du printemps, la conjonctivite : les gouttes pour les yeux, la solution à 2%, 2 gouttes par fois, plusieurs fois par jour. ④ 4) Pour traiter l'eczéma atopique et certains prurits : la pommade à 5% à 10% pour un usage externe. ⑤ Pour traire la colite ulcéreuse et la proctite : le lavement, 200mg par fois. |
| 剂型、规格<br>Les formes pharmaceutiques et les spécifications | 粉雾剂胶囊：每粒 20mg，装于专用喷雾器内吸入。<br>气雾剂：每瓶 700mg（200 揿），每揿 3.5mg。软膏：5% ～ 10%。<br>滴眼剂：0.16g/8ml（2%）。<br><br>Capsule de poudre pour inhalation : 20mg par capsule, inhaler avec le pulvérisateur.<br>Aérosol : 700mg (200 pressions) par flacon, chaque pression contient 3,5mg de produit.<br>Pommade : 5% à 10%.<br>Les gouttes pour les yeux : 0.16g/8ml(2%). |
| **药品名称 Drug Names** | 酮替芬 Kétotifène |
| 适应证<br>Les indications | ①支气管哮喘，对过敏性、感染性和混合性哮喘均有预防发作效果。②哮喘性支气管炎、过敏性咳嗽。③过敏性鼻炎、过敏性结膜炎及过敏性皮炎。<br><br>① Ce produit sert à traiter l'asthme bronchique,et à prévenir l'asthme allergique, infectieuse et mixte. ② La bronchite asthmatique et latoux allergique. ③ La rhinite allergique, la conjonctivite allergique et la dermatite atopique. |
| 用法、用量<br>Les modes d'emploi et la posologie | ①口服：a. 片剂，成人及儿童均为每次 1mg，一日 2 次，早、晚服用；b. 小儿可服其口服溶液，一日 1 ～ 2 次（一次量：4 ～ 6 岁，2ml；6 ～ 9 岁，2.5ml；9 ～ 14 岁，3ml）。②滴鼻：一次 1 ～ 2 滴，一日 1 ～ 3 次。③滴眼：滴入结膜囊，一日 2 次，一次 1 滴，或每 8 ～ 12 小时滴 1 次。<br><br>① Par voie orale : a. Comprimés, chez des enfants et des enfants, 1mg par fois, 2 fois par jour, pris le petit matien et le soir. b. Chez des enfants, possible de prendre la solution orale de kétotifène, 1 à 2 fois par jour (chez de 4 à 6 ans, 2ml par fois ; de 6 à 9 ans, 2,5ml par fois ; de 9 à 14 ans, 3ml par fois). ② Les gouttes nasales : 1 à 2 gouttes par fois, 1 à 3 fois par jour. ③ Les gouttes pour les yeux : instiller dans le cul-sac conjonctival, 2 fois par jour, 1 goutte par fois, ou toutes les 8 à 12h. |
| 剂型、规格<br>Les formes pharmaceutiques et les spécifications | 片剂：每片 0.5mg；1mg。<br>胶囊剂：每粒 0.5mg；1mg。<br>口服溶液：1mg（5ml）。<br>滴鼻液：15mg（10ml）。<br>滴眼液：2.5mg（5ml）。<br><br>Comprimés : 0,5mg ou 1mg par comprimé.<br>Capsules : 0,5mg ou 1mg par capsule.<br>La solution orale : 1mg (5ml).<br>Les gouttes nasales : 15mg (10ml).<br>Les gouttes pour les yeux : 2,5mg (5ml). |
| **药品名称 Drug Names** | 氮䓬司汀 Azelastine |
| 适应证<br>Les indications | 用于治疗支气管哮喘、过敏性鼻炎或过敏性结膜炎。<br>Ce produit sert à traiter l'asthme bronchique, la rhinite allergique ou la conjonctivite allergique. |

**续 表**

| | |
|---|---|
| 用法、用量<br>Les modes d'emploi et la posologie | 支气管哮喘：口服，成人每次 2～4mg，6～12 岁儿童每次 1mg，一日 2 次。过敏性鼻炎：口服，每次 1mg，一日 2 次，在早餐后及睡前各服 1 次；喷鼻，一次 1 喷，一日 2～4 次。过敏性结膜炎：滴眼，一次 1 滴，一日 2～4 次。<br><br>Pour traiter l'asthme bronchique : par voie orale, chez des adultes, 2 à 4mg par fois, chez des enfants de 6 à 12ans, 1mg par fois, 2 fois par jour. pour traiter la rhinite allergique : par voie orale, 1mg par fois, 2 fois par jour, après le petit-déjeuner et avant le sommeil du soir ; la pulvérisation nasale : 1 pulvérisation par fois, 2 à 4 fois par jour. Pour traiter la conjonctivite allergique : les gouttes pour les yeux, une goutte par fois, 2 à 4 fois par jour. |
| 剂型、规格<br>Les formes pharmaceutiques et les spécifications | 片剂：每片 1mg；2mg。<br>颗粒剂：0.2%。<br>喷鼻剂：10mg（10ml）。<br>滴眼液：2.5mg（5ml）。<br><br>Comprimés : 1mg ou 2mg par comprimé.<br>Granules : 0,2%.<br>La pulvérisation nasale : 10mg (10ml).<br>Les gouttes pour les yeux : 2,5mg (5ml). |
| 药品名称 Drug Names | 倍氯米松 Béclométhasone |
| 适应证<br>Les indications | ①本品吸入给药可用于慢性哮喘患者；②鼻喷用于过敏性鼻炎；③外用治疗过敏所致炎症性皮肤病如湿疹、神经性或接触性皮炎、瘙痒症等。<br><br>① L'administration de ce produit par l'inhalation d'aérosol est applicable dans le traitement des patients atteints d'asthme chronique. ② Son administration par la pulvérisation nasale est applicable dans le traitement de la rhinite allergique. ③ Son usage externe sert à traiter les maladies inflammatoires de la peau causées par les allergies telles que l'eczéma, la dermatite de contact ou neurologiques, le prurit, etc. |
| 用法、用量<br>Les modes d'emploi et la posologie | 气雾吸入，成人开始剂量每次 50～200μg，一日 2 次或 3 次，每日最大剂量 1mg。儿童用量依年龄酌减，每日最大剂量 0.8mg。长期吸入的维持量应个体化，以减至最低剂量又能控制症状为准。粉雾吸入，成人每次 200μg，一日 3～4 次。儿童每次 100μg，一日 2 次或遵医嘱。<br><br>L'inhalation d'aérosol, chez des adultes, la dose initiale, 50 à 200μgpar fois, 2 à 3 fois par jour, ne pas dépasser 1mg par jour. Diminuer la dose chez des enfants en fonction de l'âge, ne pas dépasser 0,8mg par jour. La dose d'entretien pour l'inhalation à long terme doit être personnalisée, diminuée pour atteindre la dose efficace la moins importante. L'inhalation de poudre, chez des adultes, 200μg par fois, 3 à 4 fois par jour. chez des enfants, 100 μg par fois, 2 fois par jour ou selon les ordonnances. |
| 剂型、规格<br>Les formes pharmaceutiques et les spécifications | 气雾剂：每瓶 200 喷（每喷 50μg；80μg；100μg；200μg；250μg）；每瓶 80 喷（每喷 250μg）。<br>粉雾剂胶囊：每粒 50μg；100μg；200μg。<br>喷鼻剂：每瓶 10mg（每喷 50μg）。<br>软膏剂：2.5mg/10g。<br>霜剂：2.5mg/10g。<br><br>Aérosol : 200 pulvérisations par flacon (chaque pulvérisation contient 50 μg, 80μg, 100μg, 200μg ou 250 μg de produit) ou 80 pulvérisations par flacon (250μg par pulvérisation).<br>Capsules de poudre pour inhalation : 50 μg, 100μg ou 200μg par capsule.<br>La pulvérisation nasale : 10mg par flacon (50μg par pulvérisation).<br>Pommade : 2.5mg/10g.<br>Crème : 2.5mg/10g. |
| 药品名称 Drug Names | 布地奈德 Budésonide |
| 适应证<br>Les indications | ①用于肾上腺皮质激素依赖性或非依赖性支气管哮喘及喘息性支气管炎患者，可有效地减少口服肾上腺皮质激素的用量，有助于减轻肾上腺皮质激素的不良反应。②用于慢性阻塞性肺病。<br><br>① Ce produit est appliqué chez des patients atteints de bronchite asthmatique et d'asthme bronchique hormono corticotrope -dépendant ou non dépendant. Il peut réduire efficement l'administration par voie orale de l'hormone corticotrope, ce qui permet de diminuer les effets indésirables liés à l'hormone corticotrope. ② Ce produit sert à traiter la maladie pulmonaire obstructive chronique. |

**续　表**

| | |
|---|---|
| 用法、用量<br>Les modes d'emploi et la posologie | 气雾吸入：成人，开始剂量每次 200～800μg，一日 2 次，维持量因人而异，通常为每次 200～400μg，一日 2 次；儿童，开始剂量每次 100～200μg，一日 2 次，维持量也应个体化，以减至最低剂量义能控制症状为准。<br><br>L'inhalation d'aérosol : chez des adultes, la dose initiale, 200 à 800 μg par fois, 2 fois par jour, la dose d'entretien personnalisée, en général, 200 à 400μg par fois, 2 fois par jour ; chez des enfants, la dose initiale, 100 à 200 μg par fois, 2 fois par jour, la dose d'entretien personnalisée, pour atteindre la dose efficace la moins importante. |
| 剂型、规格<br>Les formes pharmaceutiques et les spécifications | 气雾剂：每瓶 10mg（100 喷，200 喷），每喷 100μg，50μg；每瓶 20mg（100 喷），每喷 200μg；每瓶 60mg（300 喷），每喷 200μg。粉雾剂：每瓶 20mg；40mg，每喷 200μg。<br><br>Aérosol : 10mg par flacon (100 pulvérisations ou 200 pulvérisations), 100 μg ou 50 μg par pulvérisation ; 20mg par flacon (100 pulvérisations), 200 μg par pulvérisation ; 60mg par flacon (300 pulvérisations), 200 μg par pulvérisation. Poudre : 20mg ou 40 mg par flacon, 200 μg par pulvérisation. |
| **药品名称 Drug Names** | 氟替卡松 Fluticasone |
| 适应证<br>Les indications | 雾化吸入用于慢性持续性哮喘的长期治疗，亦可治疗过敏性鼻炎。<br><br>Son administration par l'inhalation d'aérosol peut être appliquée dans le traitement à long terme de l'asthme chronique persistant. Il est aussi applicable dans le traitement de la rhinite allergique. |
| 用法、用量<br>Les modes d'emploi et la posologie | （1）支气管哮喘：雾化吸入，成人和 16 岁以上青少年起始剂量：①轻度持续，一日 200～500μg，分 2 次给予；②中度持续，一日 500～1000μg，分 2 次给予；③重度持续，一日 1000～2000μg，分 2 次给予。16 岁以下儿童起始剂量，根据病情及身体发育情况酌情给予，一日 100～400μg；5 岁以下 1 日 100～200μg。维持量亦应个体化，以减至最低剂量又能控制症状为准。<br><br>（2）过敏性鼻炎：鼻喷，一次 50～200μg，一日 2 次。<br><br>(1)Pour traiter l'asthme bronchique : l'inhalation d'aérosol, chez des adultes et des adolescents plus de 16ans, la dose initiale : ① persistant léger, 200 à 500μg par jour, à travers 2 fois ; ② persistant modéré, 500 à 1000μg par jour, à travers 2 fois ; ③ persistant sévère, 1 000 à 2 000μg par jour, à travers 2 fois. Chez des enfants moinsde 16ans, ajuster la dose initiale selon les cas, 100 à 400 μg par jour ; chez moins de 5 ans, 100 à 200 μg par jour. La dose d'entretien doit être personnalisée pour atteindre la dose efficace la moins importante.<br><br>(2)Pour traiter la rhinite allergique : la pulvérisation nasale, 50 à 200 μg par fois, 2 fois par jour. |
| 剂型、规格<br>Les formes pharmaceutiques et les spécifications | 气雾剂：每瓶 60 喷；120 喷（每喷 25μg；50μg；125μg；250μg）。<br>喷鼻剂：每瓶 120 喷（每喷 50μg）。<br><br>Aérosol : 60 pulvérisations ou 120 pulvérisations par flacon (25 μg, 50 μg, 125 μg ou 250 μg par pulvérisation).<br>La pulvérisation nasale : 120 pulvérisations par flacon (50μg par pulvérisation). |
| **药品名称 Drug Names** | 曲安奈德 Triamcinolone Acétonide |
| 适应证<br>Les indications | 用于支气管哮喘。<br>Ce produit sert à traiter l'asthme bronchique. |
| 用法、用量<br>Les modes d'emploi et la posologie | 常用气雾吸入：成人每日 0.8～1.0mg，儿童每日 0.4mg，分 4 次给药。<br><br>L'inhalation d'aérosol : chez des adultes, 0,8 à 1,0 mg par jour, chez des enfants, 0,4mg par jour, à travers 4 fois. |
| 剂型、规格<br>Les formes pharmaceutiques et les spécifications | 鼻喷雾剂：每支 6ml [6.6mg，120 喷（55μg/ 喷）]。<br>L'aérosole nasal :6ml par pièce. [6,6mg, 120 pulvérisations (55μg par pulvérisation)]. |
| **药品名称 Drug Names** | 糠酸莫米松 Furoate de mométasone |
| 适应证<br>Les indications | 用于预防和治疗各种过敏性鼻炎，亦可试用于支气管哮喘。<br><br>Ce produit sert à prévenir et à traiter la rhinite allergique de toutes sortes. Il est aussi applicable dans le traitement de l'asthme bronchique. |

**续　表**

| | |
|---|---|
| 用法、用量<br>Les modes d'emploi et la posologie | 　　成人常用量：每侧鼻孔 2 喷，每喷 50 μg，一日 1 次，一日总量 200 μg。症状控制后，剂量减至一日总量 100 μg 以维持疗效。12 岁以下儿童：每侧鼻孔 1 喷，每喷 50 μg，一日 1 次，一日总量 100 μg。维持量酌减。<br>　　La dose chez des adultes : 2 pulvérisations pour chaque côté du nez, 50μg par pulvérisation, 1 fois par jour, 200μgpar jour. Après le contrôle des symptômes, diminuer la dose pour atteindre 100μg par jour pour le traitement d'entretien. Chez des enfants moins de 12ans : 1 pulvérisation pour chaque côté du nez, 50 μg par pulvérisation, 1 fois par jour, 100μg par jour. Diminuer la dose pour le traitement d'entretien. |
| 剂型、规格<br>Les formes pharmaceutiques et les spécifications | 　　喷鼻剂：每支 60 喷，每喷 50 μg。<br>　　La pulvérisation nasale : 6 pulvérisations par pièce, 50 μg par pulvérisation. |
| 药品名称 Drug Names | 扎鲁司特 Zafirlukast |
| 适应证<br>Les indications | 　　用于①慢性轻至中度支气管哮喘的预防和治疗，尤其适于对阿司匹林敏感或有阿司匹林哮喘的患者或伴有上呼吸道疾病（如鼻息肉、过敏性鼻炎）者，但不宜用于治疗急性哮喘；②激素抵抗型哮喘或拒绝使用激素的哮喘患者；③严重哮喘时加用本品以维持控制哮喘发作或用以减少激素用量。<br>　　Ce produit est applicable dans :<br>　　① La prévention et le traitement de l'asthme bronchique chronique bénin et modéré, surtout chez les patients sensibles à l'aspirineou atteints d'asthme dû à l'aspirine, ou accompagnés des maladies des voies respiratoires supérieures (comme les polypes nasaux et la rhinite allergique). Mais il n'est pas applicable dans le traitement de l'asthme aigu. ② Applicable dans le traitement de l'asthme résistant aux stéroïdes ou des patients atteints d'asthme et rejetant l'utilisation de l'hormone. ③ Lors du traitement de l'asthme grave, l'utilisastion adjuvante de ce produit permet de prévenir la crise de l'asthme et de réduire l'utilisation d'hormone. |
| 用法、用量<br>Les modes d'emploi et la posologie | 　　口服：成人及 12 岁以上儿童，每次 20mg，一日 2 次，餐前 1 小时或餐后 2 小时服，用于预防哮喘时，应持续用药。<br>　　Par voie orale : chez des adultes ou des enfants de plus de 12ans, 20mg par fois, 2 fois par jour, 1h avant le repas ou 2h après le repas, pour la prévention de l'asthme, il faut prendre le médicament pour une longue durée. |
| 剂型、规格<br>Les formes pharmaceutiques et les spécifications | 　　片剂：每片 20mg；40mg。<br>　　Comprimés : 20mg ou 40mg par comprimé. |
| 药品名称 Drug Names | 孟鲁司特钠 Montélukast de sodium |
| 适应证<br>Les indications | 　　用于预防支气管哮喘和支气管哮喘的长期治疗。也用于治疗阿司匹林敏感的哮喘，预防运动性哮喘。对激素已耐药的患者本品亦有效。<br>　　Ce produit est utilisé dans la prévention et le traitement à long terme de l'asthme bronchique. Il est aussi applicable dans le traitement de l'asthme sensible à l'aspirine et dans la prévention de l'asthme lié à l'exercice physique. Il sert également à traiter les patients résistant à l'hormone. |
| 用法、用量<br>Les modes d'emploi et la posologie | 　　口服：成人 10mg，一日 1 次，每晚睡前服。6～14 岁儿童 5mg，一日 1 次。2～6 岁儿童 4mg，一日 1 次。<br>　　Par voie orale : chez des adultes, 10mg, 1 fois par jour, avant le sommeil du soir. Chez des enfants de 6 à 14 ans, 5mg, 1 fois par jour. Chez des enfants de 2 à 6 ans, 4mg, 1 fois par jour. |
| 剂型、规格<br>Les formes pharmaceutiques et les spécifications | 　　片剂：每片 4mg；5mg。<br>　　包衣片：10mg。<br>　　Comprimés : 4mg ou 5mg par comprimé.<br>　　Comprimés enrobés : 10mg. |

**续　表**

| 药品名称 Drug Names | 普仑司特 Pranlukast |
|---|---|
| 适应证<br>Les indications | 用于支气管哮喘的预防和治疗。<br>Ce produit sert à prévenir et à traiter l'asthme bronchique. |
| 用法、用量<br>Les modes d'emploi et la posologie | 口服，成人一次 225mg，一日 2 次（餐后服）。<br>Par voie orale, chez des adultes, 225mg par fois, 2 fois par jour (après le repas). |
| 剂型、规格<br>Les formes pharmaceutiques et les spécifications | 胶囊剂：每粒 112.5mg。<br>Capsules : 112,5mg par capsule. |
| 药品名称 Drug Names | 吡嘧司特 Pémirolast |
| 适应证<br>Les indications | 用于预防或减轻支气管哮喘发作，不能迅速缓解急性哮喘发作。<br>Ce produit sert à prévenir et à réduire la crise de l'asthme bronchique. Il ne peut pas soulager rapidement la crise de l'asthme aigu. |
| 用法、用量<br>Les modes d'emploi et la posologie | 口服：成人常用量每次 10mg，一日 2 次，早、午或临睡前服用。<br>Par voie orale : la dose usuelle chez des adultes, 10mg par fois, 2 fois par jour, pris le petit matin, le midi ou avant le sommeil. |
| 剂型、规格<br>Les formes pharmaceutiques et les spécifications | 片剂：每片 10mg。<br>Comprimés : 10mg par comprimé. |
| 药品名称 Drug Names | 阿桔片 Comprimés opiacées et platycodon grandiflorum composés |
| 适应证<br>Les indications | 镇咳、祛痰。<br>Il a un effet antitussif et expectorant. |
| 用法、用量<br>Les modes d'emploi et la posologie | 每次 3～4 片，一日 3 次。<br>3 à 4 comprimés par fois, 3 fois par jour. |
| 剂型、规格<br>Les formes pharmaceutiques et les spécifications | 片剂：300mg。<br>Comprimés:300mg. |
| 药品名称 Drug Names | 川贝枇杷糖浆 ChuanbeiPipa Sirop |
| 适应证<br>Les indications | 化痰止咳。<br>Il a un effet antitussif et expectorant. |
| 用法、用量<br>Les modes d'emploi et la posologie | 一次 10ml，一日 3 次。<br>10ml par fois, 3 fois par jour. |
| 剂型、规格<br>Les formes pharmaceutiques et les spécifications | 糖浆：100ml，120ml，150ml。<br>Sirop: 100ml, 120ml, 150ml. |
| 药品名称 Drug Names | 复方鲜竹沥液 FufangXianzhuLi Solution |
| 适应证<br>Les indications | 清热化痰，止咳。<br>Il a un effet antitussif et expectorant. |

**续　表**

| 用法、用量 Les modes d'emploi et la posologie | 口服：一次 20ml，一日 2 ～ 3 次。<br>Par voie orale: 20ml par fois, 2 à 3 fois par jour. |
|---|---|
| 剂型、规格 Les formes pharmaceutiques et les spécifications | 口服溶液：10ml，20ml，30ml。<br>Solution orale: 10ml, 20ml, 30ml. |

| 药品名称 Drug Names | 急支糖浆 Jizhi Sirop |
|---|---|
| 适应证 Les indications | 清热化痰。用于外感风热咳嗽。<br>Il a un effet antitussif et expectorant. Il est appliqué dans le traitement de la toux liée à la chaleur et au rhume. |
| 用法、用量 Les modes d'emploi et la posologie | 口服：一次 20 ～ 30ml，一日 3 ～ 4 次。<br>Par voie orale: 20 à 30ml par fois, 3 à 4 fois par jour. |
| 剂型、规格 Les formes pharmaceutiques et les spécifications | 糖浆：100ml，200ml。<br>Sirop: 100ml, 200ml. |

12. 主要作用于消化系统的药物 Médicaments agissant princepalement sur le système digestif

12.1 抗酸药 Antiacides

| 药品名称 Drug Names | 氢氧化铝 Hydroxyde d'aluminium |
|---|---|
| 适应证 Les indications | 主要用于胃酸过多、胃及十二指肠溃疡、反流性食管炎及上消化道出血等。由于铝离子在肠内与磷酸盐结合成不溶解的磷酸铝自粪便排出，故尿毒症患者服用大剂量氢氧化铝后可减少磷酸盐的吸收，减轻酸血症（但同时应注意上述不良反应）。<br>Ce produit sert à traiter principalement l'hyperacidité, les ulcères gastriques et duodénaux, l'oesophagite par reflux et les saignements gastro-intestinaux. Comme les ions d'aluminium et le phosphate se combinent dans les intestins en phosphate d'aluminium insolublele et sont être excrétés, l'administration de ce produit à forte dose peut permettre aux patients urémiques de réduire l'absorption de phosphate, ce qui permet ainsi de réduire l'acidose (mais il faut faire attention aux réactions indésirables précédentes). |
| 用法、用量 Les modes d'emploi et la posologie | 口服，一次 0.6 ～ 0.9g，一日 1.8 ～ 2.7g。<br>现多用氢氧化铝凝胶。治胃酸过多和溃疡病等，每次 4 ～ 8ml，一日 12 ～ 24ml，饭前 1 小时和睡前服；病情严重时剂量可加倍。<br>Par voie orale, 0,6 à 0,9g par foie, 1,8 à 2,7g par jour.<br>On utilise aujourd'hui souvent les gels d'hydroxyde d'aluminium. Pour traiter l'hyperacidité et les ulcères, 4 à 8ml par fois, 12 à 24ml par jour, 1 h avant le repas et avant le sommeil ; en cas grave, il est possible de doubler la dose. |
| 剂型、规格 Les formes pharmaceutiques et les spécifications | 片剂：每片 0.3g。<br>Comprimés : 0,3g par comprimé. |

| 药品名称 Drug Names | 铝碳酸镁 Hydrotalcite |
|---|---|
| 适应证 Les indications | 主要用于胃及十二指肠溃疡、反流性食管炎、急慢性胃炎和十二指肠球炎等。也用于胃酸过多引起的胃部不适，如胃灼痛、胃灼热、反酸及腹胀、恶心、呕吐等的对症治疗。<br>Ce produit sert à traiter les ulcères gastriques et duodénaux, l'oesophagite par reflux, la gastrite aiguë et chronique et l'inflammation du duodénum. Il est aussi applicable dans le traitement de l'inconfort de l'estomac causé par l'hyperacidité, tel que les brûlures d'estomac, les brûlures d'estomac, le reflux acide, des ballonnements, des nausées, des vomissements, etc. |

**续　表**

| | |
|---|---|
| 用法、用量<br>Les modes d'emploi et la posologie | 一般每日 3 次，每次 1.0g，餐后 1 小时服用。十二指肠球部溃疡 6 周为 1 个疗程，胃溃疡 8 周为 1 个疗程。<br><br>En général, 3 fois par jour, 1,0g par fois, 1h après le repas. Pour tratier l'ulcère duodénal, prendre le médicament pendant 6 semaines comme un traitement médical, alors pour l'ulcère gastrique, pendant 8 semaines. |
| 剂型、规格<br>Les formes pharmaceutiques et les spécifications | 片剂（咀嚼片）：每片 0.5g。<br>Comprimés (comprimés à mâcher) : 0,5g par. |
| **药品名称 Drug Names** | 碳酸钙 Carbonate de calcium |
| 适应证<br>Les indications | 用于胃酸过多引起的反酸、胃灼热等症状。适用于胃、十二指肠溃疡及反流性食管炎的治疗。也用于补充机体钙缺乏，如各种机体对钙需求量增加的情况，可作为骨质疏松症的辅助治疗。另外，本品也用于治疗肾衰竭患者的高磷血症，同时纠正轻度代谢性酸中毒。作为磷酸盐结合剂，治疗继发性甲状旁腺功能亢进纤维性骨炎所致的高磷血症。<br><br>Ce produit sert à traiter le reflux acideet les brûlures d'estomaccausés par l'hyperacidité. Il est aussi applicable dans le traitement des ulcères gastriques et duodénaux, de l'oesophagite par reflux. Il permet aussi de compléter une carence en calcium de l'organisme, et servir de traitement adjuvant de l'ostéoporose. En outre, il est également appliqué dans le traitement de l'hyperphosphatémie chez les patients atteints d'insuffisance rénale, et dans la correction de l'acidose métabolique légère. En tant que chélateur de phosphate, il sert à traiter l'hyperphosphatémie causée par l'hyperparathyroïdie secondaire et l'ostéite fibreuse. |
| 用法、用量<br>Les modes d'emploi et la posologie | 用于中和胃酸，每次 0.5 ～ 1g，一日 3 ～ 4 次，餐后 1 ～ 1.5 小时服用可维持缓冲时间长达 3 ～ 4 小时，如餐后即服，因随食物一起排空而失去作用。用于高磷血症，每日 1.5g，最高每日可用至 13g，进餐时服用或与氢氧化铝合用。用于补钙，每日 1 ～ 2g，分 2 ～ 3 次与食物同服，老年人可适当补充维生素 D。<br><br>Pour traiter l'hyperacidité, 0,5 à 1g par fois, 3 à 4 fois par jour, 1 à 1,5h après le repas pour une action prolongée de 3 à 4 h, s'il est pris immédiatement après le repas, il sera vidé avec des aliments sans prendre effet. Pour traiter l'hyperphosphatémie, 1,5g par jour, ne pas dépasser 13g par jour, pris durant le repas ou en association avec l'hydroxyde d'aluminium. Pour compléter une carence en calcium, 1 à 2g par jour, à travers 2 à 3 fois durant le repas, chez des personnes âgées, il est recommandé de prendre aussi la vitamine D. |
| 剂型、规格<br>Les formes pharmaceutiques et les spécifications | 片剂：每片 0.5g（相当于元素钙 200mg）。<br>Comprimés : 0,5g par comprimé (équivalent à 200mg de calcium élémentaire). |

12.2　胃酸分泌抑制剂 Inhibitéurs de la sécrétion d'acide gastrique

| | |
|---|---|
| **药品名称 Drug Names** | 西咪替丁 Cimétidine |
| 适应证<br>Les indications | 用于治疗十二指肠溃疡、胃溃疡、上消化道出血等。治疗十二指肠溃疡愈合率为 74%（对照组为 37%），愈合时间大多在 4 周左右。对胃溃疡疗效不及十二指肠溃疡。另据报道，还可用于治疗带状疱疹和包括生殖器在内的其他疱疹性感染。<br><br>Ce produit sert à traiter l'ulcère duodénal, l'ulcère gastrique, le saignement gastro-intestinal supérieur, etc. Le taux de guérison pour le traitement de l'ulcère duodénal est de 74 % (le groupe de référence est de 37 %) et le temps de guérison est de 4 semaines. Il est moins efficace dans le traitement de l'ulcère gastrique que dans le traitement de l'ulcère duodénal. Selon des sources, il est aussi applicable dans le traitement du zona et d'autres infections herpétiques y compris l'herpès génital. |

**续　表**

| | |
|---|---|
| 用法、用量<br>Les modes d'emploi et la posologie | ①口服，每次 200～400mg，一日 800～1600mg，一般于餐后及睡前各服一次，疗程一般为 4～6 周。亦有主张 1 次 400mg，一日 2 次的疗法。另外，也有报道夜间一次给予双倍剂量（800mg）的疗法。②注射：用葡萄糖注射液或葡萄糖氯化钠注射液稀释后静脉滴注，每次 200～600mg；或用上述溶液 20ml 稀释后缓慢静脉注射，每次 200mg，4～6 小时 1 次。一日剂量不宜超过 2g。也可直接肌内注射。<br><br>① Par voie orale, 200 à 400mg par fois, 800 à 1 600 mg par jour, après le repas et avant le sommeil, pendant 4 à 6 semaines. Ou 400mg par fois, 2 fois par jour. En outre, selons certains rapports, douber la dose (800mg) le soir. ② Injection : 200 à 600mg par fois, dissoudre dans la solution de glucose ou la solution de chlorure de sodium, perfusion lente ; ou dissoudre dans 20ml de solution précédente, injection par voie IV lente, 200mg par fois, toutes les 4 à 6h. Ne pas dépasser 2g par jour. Il est aussi possible d'injecter par voie IM. |
| 剂型、规格<br>Les formes pharmaceutiques et les spécifications | 片剂：每片 0.2g；0.8g。<br>胶囊剂：每粒 0.2g。<br>注射液：每支 0.2g（2ml）。<br><br>Comprimés : 0,2g ou 0,8g par comprimé.<br>Capsules : 0,2g par capsule.<br>Injection : 0,2g (2ml) par solution. |
| 药品名称 Drug Names | 雷尼替丁 Ranitidine |
| 适应证<br>Les indications | 用于治疗十二指肠溃疡、良性胃溃疡、术后溃疡、反流性食管炎及卓 - 艾综合征等。静脉注射可用于上消化道出血。<br><br>Ce produit sert à traiter l'ulcère duodénal, l'ulcère gastrique bénin, l'ulcère post-opératoire, l'oesophagite par reflux, le syndrome Zhuo -Ellison, etc. Son administration par voie IV est aussi applicable dans le traitement du saignement gastro-intestinal supérieur. |
| 用法、用量<br>Les modes d'emploi et la posologie | 口服：一日 2 次，每次 150mg，早晚饭时服。维持剂量每日 150mg，于餐前顿服。用于反流性食管炎的治疗，一日 2 次，每次 150mg，共用 8 周。对卓 - 艾综合征，开始一日 3 次，每次 150mg，必要时剂量可加至每日 900mg。对慢性溃疡病有复发史患者，应在睡前给予维持剂量。治疗上消化道出血，可用本品 50mg 肌内注射或缓慢静脉注射（1 分钟以上），或以每小时 25mg 的速率间歇静脉滴注 2 小时。以上方法一般一日 2 次或每 6～8 小时 1 次。<br><br>Par voie orale : 2 fois par jour, 150mg par fois, le petit-déjeuner et le dîner. La dose d'entretien, 150mg par jour, une fois par jour, avant le repas. Pour traiter l'oesophagite par reflux, 2 fois par jour, 150mg par fois, pendant 8 semaines. Pour traiter le syndrome Zhuo-Ellison, la dose initiale, 3 fois par jour, 150mg par fois. En cas de besoin, augmenter pour atteindre 900mg par jour. Pour les patients atteints d'ulcère gastrique récurrent, prendre la dose d'entretien avant le sommeil. Pour traiter le saignement gastro-intestinal supérieur, injecter 50mg par voie IM ou IV lente (pendant 1 minute au moins), ou en perfusion intermittente, avec une vitesse de 25mg par h, pendant 2 h. Pour tous ces modes d'emploi précédents, en général, 2 fois par jour ou toutes les 6 à 8h. |
| 剂型、规格<br>Les formes pharmaceutiques et les spécifications | 片（胶囊）剂：每片（粒）150mg。<br>泡腾颗粒：0.15g/1.5g。<br>糖浆剂：1.5g/100ml。<br>注射液：每支 50mg（2ml）；50mg（5ml）。<br><br>Comprimés (capsules) : 150mg par comprimé ou par capsule.<br>Les granules effervescents : 0.15g/1.5g.<br>Sirop : 1.5g/100ml<br>Injection : 50mg (2ml) ou 50mg (5ml) par solution. |
| 药品名称 Drug Names | 枸橼酸铋雷尼替丁 Citrate de bismuth et Ranitidine |
| 适应证<br>Les indications | 用于胃及十二指肠溃疡。与抗生素合用可协同根除幽门螺杆菌，预防十二指肠溃疡的复发。<br><br>Ce produit sert à traiter l'ulcère duodénal et l'ulcère gastrique. Utilisé en association avec l'antibiotique, il permet d'éradiquer l'helicobacter pylori et de prévenir la récurrence de l'ulcère duodénal. |

**续表**

| 用法、用量<br>Les modes d'emploi et la posologie | 成人每次 1 粒，一日 2 次，餐前服。治疗胃溃疡 8 周 1 个疗程，治疗十二指肠溃疡 4 周为 1 个疗程。轻至中度肾功能损害及肝功能不全者无须改变剂量。<br>Chez des adultes, 1 capsule par fois, 2 fois par jour, avant le repas. Pour traiter l'ulcère gastrique, pendant 8 semaines comme un traitement médical, alors que pour l'ulcère duodénal, 4 semaines. Chez des patients insuffisants rénaux bénins et modérés, pas nécessaire de changer la dose. |
|---|---|
| 剂型、规格<br>Les formes pharmaceutiques et les spécifications | 胶囊剂：每粒含枸橼酸铋雷尼替丁 350mg。<br>Capsule : 350mg de ranitidine citrate de bismuth par capsule. |

| 药品名称 Drug Names | 法莫替丁 Famotidine |
|---|---|
| 适应证<br>Les indications | 口服用于胃及十二指肠溃疡、吻合口溃疡，反流性食管炎；口服或静脉注射用于上消化道出血（消化性溃疡、急性应激性溃疡，出血性胃炎所致），卓 - 艾综合征。<br>Son administration par voie orale est utilisée dans le traitement de l'ulcère duodénal, de l'ulcère gastrique, de l'ulcère anastomotique, et de l'oesophagite par reflux ; administré par voie orale ou IV, il permet de traiter le saignement gastro-intestinal supérieur (causé par l'ulcère gastro-duodénal, l'ulcère de stress aigu, et la gastrite hémorragique) ainsi que lesyndrome Zhuo-Ellison. |
| 用法、用量<br>Les modes d'emploi et la posologie | 口服，每次 20mg，一日 2 次（早餐后，晚餐后或临睡前），4～6 周为 1 个疗程，溃疡愈合后维持量减半，睡前服。肾功能不全者应调整剂量。缓慢静脉注射或静脉滴注 20mg（溶于生理盐水或葡萄糖注射液 20ml 中），一日 2 次（间隔 12 小时），疗程 5 日，一旦病情许可，应迅速将静脉给药改为口服给药。<br>Par voie orale, 20mg par fois, 2 fois par jour (après le petit-déjeuner, après le dîner ou avant le sommeil), pendant 4 à 6 semaines comme un traitement médical. Après la guérison de l'ulcère, pour le traitement d'entretien, diminuer de moitié la dose, avant le sommeil. Chez des patients insuffisants rénaux, ajuster la dose. Injection par voie IV lente ou en perfusion, dissoudre 20mg dans 20ml de solution saline ou de solution de glucose, 2 fois par jour (toutes les 12h), pendant 5 jours, une fois la condition des malades le permet, prendre lemédicament par voie orale. |
| 剂型、规格<br>Les formes pharmaceutiques et les spécifications | 片剂：每片 10mg；20mg。<br>分散片：每片 20mg。<br>胶囊剂：每粒 20mg。<br>散剂：10%（100mg/g）。<br>注射液：每支 20mg（2ml）；每瓶 20mg/100ml。<br>Comprimés : 10mg ou 20mg par comprimé.<br>Comprimés dispersibles : 20mg par comprimé.<br>Capsules : 20mg par capsule.<br>Dispersants : 10% (100 mg/g).<br>Injection : 20mg (2ml) par solution ou 20mg /100ml par flacon. |

| 药品名称 Drug Names | 奥美拉唑 Oméprazole |
|---|---|
| 适应证<br>Les indications | 主要用于十二指肠溃疡和卓 - 艾综合征，也可用于胃溃疡和反流性食管炎；静脉注射可用于消化性溃疡急性出血的治疗。与阿莫西林和克拉霉素或与甲硝唑与克拉霉素合用，以杀灭幽门螺杆菌。<br>Ce produit est principalement utilisé dans le traitement de l'ulcère duodénal et du syndrome Zhuo-Ellison. Il est aussi applicable dans le traitement de l'ulcère gastrique et de l'oesophagite par reflux ; administré par voie IV, il permet aussi de traiter le saignement de l'ulcère gastroduodénal aigu. Utilisé en association avec l'amoxicilline et la clarithromycine ou avec le métronidazole et la clarithromycine, il sert à éradiquer l'helicobacter pylori. |
| 用法、用量<br>Les modes d'emploi et la posologie | 可口服或静脉给药。治疗十二指肠溃疡，一日 1 次，每次 20mg，疗程 2～4 周。治疗卓 - 艾综合征，初始剂量为一日 1 次，每次 60mg，90% 以上患者用每日 20～120mg 即可控制症状，如剂量大于每日 80mg，则应分 2 次给药，治疗反流性食管炎，剂量为每日 20～60mg，治疗消化性溃疡出血，静脉注射，一次 40mg，每 12 小时 1 次，连用 3 日。 |

**续 表**

| | |
|---|---|
| | Par voie orale ou IV. Pour traiter l'ulcère duodénal, 1 fois par jour, 20mg par fois, pendant 2 à 4 semaines. Pour traiter le syndrome Zhuo-Ellison, la dose initiale, 1 fois par jour, 60mg par fois, dans 90% des cas, l'administration de 20 à 120mg par jour suffit pour contrôler les symptômes. Si on prendre plus de 80mg par jour, il faut le faire à travers 2 fois. Pour traiter l'oesophagite par reflux, 20 à 60mg par jour, pour traiter le saignement de l'ulcère gastrointestinal, injection par voie IV, 40mg par fois, toutes les 12h, pendant 3 jours consécutifs. |
| 剂型、规格<br>Les formes pharmaceutiques et les spécifications | 胶囊剂：每粒 20mg。<br>肠溶片：每片 20mg。<br>注射用奥美拉唑：每支 40mg。<br>Capsules : 20mg par capsule.<br>Comprimés à enrobage entérique : 20mg par comprimé.<br>L'oméprazole pour injection : 40mg par solution. |
| **药品名称 Drug Names** | **兰索拉唑 Lansoprazole** |
| 适应证<br>Les indications | 用于胃溃疡、十二指肠溃疡、吻合口溃疡及反流性食管炎、卓 - 艾综合征等。<br>Ce produit sert à traiter l'ulcère gastrique, l'ulcère duodénal, l'ulcère anastomotique, l'oesophagite par reflux, le syndrome Zhuo-Ellison, etc. |
| 用法、用量<br>Les modes d'emploi et la posologie | 成年人一般每日口服 1 次，每次 1 粒（片）。胃溃疡、吻合口溃疡、反流性食管炎 8 周为 1 个疗程。十二指肠溃疡 6 周为 1 个疗程。<br>Chez des adultes, en général, 1 fois par jour par voie orale, 1 capsule ou comprimé par fois. Pour l'ulcère gastrique, l'ulcère anastomotique, l'oesophagite par reflux, pendant 8 semaines comme un traitement médical, alors que pour l'ulcère duodénal, 6 semaines. |
| 剂型、规格<br>Les formes pharmaceutiques et les spécifications | 片（胶囊）剂：每片（粒）30mg。<br>Comprimés (capsules) : 30mg par comprimé ou par capsule. |
| **药品名称 Drug Names** | **泮托拉唑 Pantoprazole** |
| 适应证<br>Les indications | 主要用于胃及十二指肠溃疡、胃 - 食管反流性疾病、卓 - 艾综合征等。<br>Ce produit sert principalement à traiter l'ulcère gastrique, l'ulcère duodénal, le reflux gastro-oesophagien, le syndrome Zhuo-Ellison, etc. |
| 用法、用量<br>Les modes d'emploi et la posologie | 一般患者每日服用 1 片（40mg），早餐前或早餐间用少量水送服，不可嚼碎。个别对其他药物无反应的病例可每日服用 2 次；老年患者及肝功能受损者，每日剂量不得超过 40mg。十二指肠溃疡疗程 2 周，必要时再服 2 周；胃溃疡及反流性食管炎疗程 4 周，必要时再服 4 周。总疗程不超过 8 周。静脉滴注：一日 1 次 40mg，疗程依需要而定，但一般不超过 8 周。<br>Chez des patients ordinaires, 1 comprimé (40mg) par jour, avant ou durant le petit-déjeuner avec un peu d'eau, ne pas mâcher. Chez certains patients résistants à d'autres médicaments, 2 fois par jour; chez des personnes âgées et des patients insuffisants hépatiques, ne pas dépasser 40mg par jour. Pour l'ulcère duodénal, pendant 2 semaines comme un traitement médical, s'il est nécessaire, encore 2 semaines ; pour l'ulcère gastrique et l'oesophagite par reflux, pendant 4 semaines, en cas de besoins, encore 4 semaines. Ne pas dépasser 8 semaines. Perfusion : 40mg par fois par jour, la durée d'un traitement médical varie selon les cas, mais ne pas dépasser 8 semaines en général. |
| 剂型、规格<br>Les formes pharmaceutiques et les spécifications | 片（肠溶）剂：每片 40mg。<br>注射用泮托拉唑：每支 40mg。<br>Comprimés (comprimés à enrobage entérique) : 40mg par comprimé.<br>Le pantoprazole pour injection : 40mg par solution. |
| **药品名称 Drug Names** | **雷贝拉唑 Rabéprazole** |
| 适应证<br>Les indications | 用于治疗活动性十二指肠溃疡、活动性良性胃溃疡、弥散性或溃疡性胃 - 食管反流症。<br>Ce produit sert à traiter l'ulcère duodénal actif, l'ulcère gastrique bénin actifet le reflux gastro-œsophagiendisséminé ou ulcéreux. |

**续　表**

| | |
|---|---|
| 用法、用量<br>Les modes d'emploi et la posologie | 活动性十二指肠溃疡：每次 10 ～ 20mg，一日 1 次，连服 2 ～ 4 周；活动性良性胃溃疡：每次 20mg，一日 1 次，连服 4 ～ 6 周；胃 - 食管反流症：每次 20mg，一日 1 次，连服 6 ～ 10 周。均早晨服用，片剂必须整片吞服。<br><br>Pour traiter l'ulcère duodénal actif : 10 à 20mg par fois, 1 fois par jour, pendant 2 à 4 semaines consécutives ; pour l'ulcère gastrique actif bénin, 20 mg par fois, 1 fois par jour, pendant 4 à 6 semaines consécutives ; pour le reflux gastro-oesophagien : 20mg par fois, 1 fois par jour, pendant 6 à 10 semaines consécutives. Pris le petit matin, avaler les comprimés en entier. |
| 剂型、规格<br>Les formes pharmaceutiques et les spécifications | 片（肠溶）剂：每片 10mg；20mg。<br>Comprimés (comprimés à enrobage entérique) : 10mg ou 20mg par comprimé. |
| **药品名称 Drug Names** | 艾司奥美拉唑 Esoméprazole |
| 适应证<br>Les indications | 用于食管反流性疾病。①治疗糜烂性反流性食管炎。②已经治愈的食管炎患者长期维持治疗，以防止复发。③为食管反流性疾病的症状控制。本品联合适当的抗菌疗法，用于根除幽门螺杆菌，使幽门螺杆菌感染相关的消化性溃疡愈合，并防止其复发。<br><br>Ce produit sert à traiter le reflux gastro-œsophagien. ① Il permet de traiter l'oesophagite érosive par reflux. ② Il sert de traitement d'entretien à long terme des patients atteints de l'oesophagite guéris, pour éviter la récurrence. ③ Il sert à contrôler les symptômes du reflux gastro-oesophagien. Utilisé en association avec le traitement antimicrobien, il permet d'éradiquer l'helicobacter pylori, de guérir l'ulcère gastroduodénal lié à l'helicobacter pylori, et d'éviter sa récurrence. |
| 用法、用量<br>Les modes d'emploi et la posologie | ①治疗糜烂性反流性食管炎：一次 40mg，一日 1 次，连服 4 周。对于食管炎未治愈或症状持续的患者，建议再治疗 4 周。②已经治愈的食管炎患者长期维持治疗，以防止复发：一次 20mg，一日 1 次。③胃食管反流性疾病的症状控制：无食管炎的患者一次 20mg，一日 1 次，如用药 4 周后症状未得到控制，应对患者做进一步检查，症状消除后，可采用即时疗法（即需要时口服 20mg，一日 1 次）。④联合适当的抗菌疗法，用于根除幽门螺杆菌：采用联合用药方案，本品一次 20mg，阿莫西林一次 1g，克拉霉素一次 500mg，均为一日 2 次，共用 7 日。老年人和轻度肾功能损害者，无须调整剂量；轻中度肝功能损害的患者无须调整剂量。严重肝功能损害的患者，一日用量为 20mg。本品对酸不稳定，口服制剂均为肠溶制剂，服用时应整片（粒）吞服，不应嚼碎或压碎，至少应于餐前 1 小时服用。<br><br>① Pour traiter l'oesophagite érosive par reflux : 40mg par fois, 1 fois par jour, pendant 4 semaines consécutives. Pour les patients atteints d'oesophagite non guérie, il est recommandé de prendre le médicament pendant 4 semaines supplémentaires. ② Pour le traitement d'entretien de l'oesophagite guérie : 20mg par fois, 1 fois par jour. ③ Pour contrôler les symptômes du reflux gastro-oesophagien : chez des patients qui ne souffrent pas de l'oesophagite, 20mg par fois, 1 fois par jour, si les symptômes ne se contrôlent pas 4 semaines après l'administration, conduire un examen en profondeur, après la disparition des symptômes, appliquer la thérapie instante (à savoir, en cas de besoin, 20mg par voir orale, 1 fois par jour). ④ Utilisé en association avec le traitement antimicrobien, il permet d'éradiquer l'helicobacter pylori : 20mg d'ésoméprazole par fois, 1g d'amoxicillinem 500mg de clarithromycine par fois, 2 fois par jour, pendant 7 jours. Chez des personnes âgées et des patients insuffisants rénaux bénins, pas nécessaire d'ajuster la dose ; chez des patients insuffiants hépatiques bénins et modérés, pas nécessaire d'ajuster la dose. Chez des patients insuffisants hépatiques graves, 20mg par jour. Ce produit est labile en milieu acide, sa préparation orale est le comprimé à enrobage entérique. Il faut l'avaler en entier, au lieu de le mâcher ou le casser, au moins 1 h avant le repas. |
| 剂型、规格<br>Les formes pharmaceutiques et les spécifications | 片（肠溶）剂：每片 20mg；40mg（以埃索美拉唑计）。<br>Comprimés (comprimés à enrobage entérique) : 20mg ou 40mg par comprimé (mesuré en ésoméprazole). |

续　表

| 药品名称 Drug Names | 丙谷胺 Proglumide |
|---|---|
| 适应证<br>Les indications | 用于治疗胃溃疡和十二指肠溃疡、胃炎等。由于本品抑制胃酸分泌的作用较弱，临床已不再单独用于治疗溃疡病，但其利胆作用较受重视。也可与非甾体抗炎药合用，预防后者对胃黏膜的损害。<br><br>Ce produit sert à traiter l'ulcère gastrique, l'ulcère duodénal, la gastrite, etc. Comme il est peu efficace dans l'inhibition de la sécrétion d'acide gastrique, il est rarement utilisé seul dans les cliniques pour traiter l'ulcère, mais son effet cholérétique est bien apprécié. Il peut être aussi appliqué en combinaison avec les médicaments anti- inflammatoires non stéroïdiens pour éviter les dommages causés par ceux-ci sur la muqueuse gastrique. |
| 用法、用量<br>Les modes d'emploi et la posologie | 口服，每次 0.4g，一日 3 ～ 4 次，餐前 15 分钟给药，连续服 30 ～ 60 日（可根据胃镜或 X 线检查结果决定用药期限）。<br><br>Par voie orale, 0,4g par fois, 3 à 4 fois par jour, 15 semaines avant le repas, pendant 30 à 60 jours consécutifs (la durée du traitement dépendant du résultat de l'examen par l'endoscopie ou par rayon X). |
| 剂型、规格<br>Les formes pharmaceutiques et les spécifications | 片（胶囊）剂：每片（粒）0.2g。<br><br>Comprimés ou capsules : 0,2g par comprimé ou par capsule. |

12.3　胃黏膜保护剂 Médicaments Protectteur des muqueuses de l'estomac

| 药品名称 Drug Names | 枸橼酸铋钾 Citrate de bismuth potassium |
|---|---|
| 适应证<br>Les indications | 用于胃及十二指肠溃疡的治疗，也用于复合溃疡、多发溃疡、吻合口溃疡和糜烂性胃炎等。本品与抗生素合用，可根除幽门螺杆菌。用于幽门螺杆菌相关的胃、十二指肠溃疡及慢性胃炎、胃 M A L T 淋巴瘤、早期胃癌术后、胃食管反流病及功能性消化不良等。也可与抑制胃酸分泌药（质子泵抑制剂和 H$_2$ 受体拮抗剂）组成四联方案，作为根除幽门螺杆菌失败的补救治疗。<br><br>Ce produit sert à traiter l'ulcère gastrique, l'ulcère duodénal. Il est aussi applicable dans le traitement de l'ulcère composite, de l'ulcèremultiple, de l'ulcère anastomotique et de la gastrite érosive. Utilisé en association avec l'antibiotique, il permet d'éradiquer l'helicobacter pylori. Il est aussi appliqué dans le traitement del'ulcère gastrique et l'ulcère duodénal liés à l'helicobacter pylori, de la gastrite chronique,du lymphome gastrique du MALT,du cancer gastrique précoce postopératoire,de la maladie de reflux gastro-oesophagien ainsi que de la dyspepsie fonctionnelle. Utilisé en association avec des médicaments inhibant la sécrétion d'acide gastrique (les inhibiteurs de la pompe à protons et des antagonistes du récepteur H2), il sert de traitement curatif de l'échec d'un traitement anti-helicobacter pylori. |
| 用法、用量<br>Les modes d'emploi et la posologie | 颗粒剂：一次一袋，一日 3 ～ 4 次，餐前半小时和睡前服用。片剂或胶囊剂：一次 2 片（粒），一日 2 次，早餐前半小时与睡前用温水送服，忌用含碳酸饮料（如啤酒等）；服药前、后半小时，不要喝牛奶或服用抗酸剂和其他碱性药物，疗程 4 ～ 8 周，然后停用含铋药物 4 ～ 8 周，如有必要，可再继续服用 4 ～ 8 周。<br><br>Les granules : 1 cachet par fois, 3 à 4 fois par jour, 0,5h avant le repas et avant le sommeil. Les comprimés ou les capsules : 2 comprimés ou capsules par fois, 2 fois par jour, 0,5h avant le petit-déjeuner et avant le sommeil avec de l'eau chaude, ne pas utiliser les boissons gazeuses comme la bière ; 0,5 h avant et après l'administration, ne pas boire de lait ni antiacides nid'autres médicaments de base, pendant 4 à 8 semaines comme un traitement médical, ensuite, prendre des médicaments contenant du bismuth pendant 4 à 8 semaines, s'il est nécessaire, rependre le médicament encore 4 à 8 semaines. |
| 剂型、规格<br>Les formes pharmaceutiques et les spécifications | 颗粒剂：每袋 1.2g，含本品 300mg。<br>片（胶囊）剂：每片（粒）120mg。<br><br>Granules : 1,2g par cachet, qui contient 300mg de citrate de potassium de bismuth.<br>Comprimés ou capsules : 120mg par comprimé ou capsule. |

**续　表**

| 药品名称 Drug Names | 胶体果胶铋 Colloïdale Bismuth Pectine |
| --- | --- |
| 适应证<br>Les indications | 用于胃及十二指肠溃疡，也可用于慢性浅表性胃炎、慢性萎缩性胃炎和消化道出血的治疗。本品与抗生素合用，可根除幽门螺杆菌。用于幽门螺杆菌相关的胃、十二指肠溃疡及慢性胃炎、胃MALT　淋巴瘤、早期胃癌术后、胃食管反流病及功能性消化不良等。也可与抑制胃酸分泌药（质子泵抑制剂和 $H_2$ 受体拮抗药）组成四联方案，作为根除幽门螺杆菌失败的补救治疗。<br><br>Ce produit sert à traiter l'ulcère gastrique, l'ulcère duodénal.Il est aussi applicable dans le traitement de la gastrite chronique superficielle, de la gastrite atrophique chronique et des saignements gastro-intestinaux.Utilisé en association avec l'antibiotique, il permet d'éradiquer l'helicobacter pylori. Il est aussi appliqué dans le traitement de l'ulcère gastrique et l'ulcère duodénal liés à l'helicobacter pylori, de la gastrite chronique, du lymphome gastrique du MALT, du cancer gastrique précoce postopératoire, de la maladie de reflux gastro-oesophagien ainsi que de la dyspepsie fonctionnelle. Utilisé en association avec des médicaments inhibant la sécrétion d'acide gastrique (les inhibiteurs de la pompe à protons et des antagonistes du récepteur $H_2$), il sert de traitement curatif de l'échec d'un traitement anti-helicobacter pylori. |
| 用法、用量<br>Les modes d'emploi et la posologie | 治疗消化性溃疡和慢性胃炎：每次 3～4 粒，一日 4 次，于三餐前半小时各服一次，睡前加服 1 次。疗程一般为 4 周。治疗消化道出血：将胶囊内药物倒出，用水冲开搅匀服用，日剂量一次服用，儿童用量酌减。<br><br>Pour traiter l'ulcère gastro-duodénal et la gastrite chronique : 3 à 4 capsules par fois, 4 fois par jour, 0,5 h avant les trois repas et une fois avant le sommeil. Pendant 4 semaines comme un traitement médical. Pour les saignements gastro-intestinaux : retirer les médicaments de la capsule, les infuser avec de l'eau, remuer avant de les prendre. Une fois par jour, ajuster la dose chez des enfants. |
| 剂型、规格<br>Les formes pharmaceutiques et les spécifications | 胶囊剂：每粒 50mg。<br>Capsules : 50mg par capsule. |

| 药品名称 Drug Names | 胶体酒石酸铋 Colloïdal de Bismuth Tartrate |
| --- | --- |
| 适应证<br>Les indications | 用于治疗慢性结肠炎、溃疡性结肠炎、肠功能紊乱及与幽门螺杆菌有关的消化性溃疡和慢性胃炎。<br><br>Ce produit sert à traiter la colite chronique, la colite ulcéreuse, les troubles intestinaux, l'ulcère gastro-duodénal associé à Helicobacter pylori et la gastrite chronique. |
| 用法、用量<br>Les modes d'emploi et la posologie | 口服，每次 165mg（3 粒），一日 3～4 次，儿童用量酌减。一般 4 周为 1 个疗程。<br><br>Par voie orale, 165mg par fois (3 capsules), 3 à 4 fois par jour, ajuster la dose chez des enfants. Pendant 4 semaines comme un traitement médical. |
| 剂型、规格<br>Les formes pharmaceutiques et les spécifications | 胶囊剂：每粒 55mg（以铋计）。<br>Capsules : 55mg par capsule (mesuré en bismuth). |

| 药品名称 Drug Names | 米索前列醇 Misoprostol |
| --- | --- |
| 适应证<br>Les indications | 用于为及十二指肠溃疡。对十二指肠溃疡，口服本品 $200\mu g$ 一日 4 次，4 周后愈合率为 54%，对照组口服西咪替丁 300mg 一日 4 次，4 周后愈合率为 61%，疗效略低于西咪替丁，但本品在保护胃黏膜不受损伤方面比西咪替丁更为有效。<br><br>Ce produit sert à traiter l'ulcère gastrique et l'ulcère duodénal.Lors du traitement de l'ulcère duodénal, administrer par voie orale 200μg de ce produit, 4 fois par jour, le taux de guérison est de 54 % 4 semaines après ; alors que pour le groupe de référence, administrer 300mg de cimétidine 4 fois par jour, le taux de guérison est de 61 % 4 semaines après. Le misoprostol est donc moins efficace que la cimétidine. Mais il est plus efficace que celle-ci dans la protection de la muqueuse gastrique contre les blessures. |

**续 表**

| 用法、用量 Les modes d'emploi et la posologie | 每次 200μg，一日 4 次，于餐前和睡前口服。疗程 4～8 周。<br>200μg par fois, 4 fois par jour, avant les repas et le sommeil, pendant 4 à 8 semaines comme un traitement médical. |
|---|---|
| 剂型、规格 Les formes pharmaceutiques et les spécifications | 片剂：每片 200μg。<br>Comprimés : 200μg par comprimé. |

| 药品名称 Drug Names | 硫糖铝 Sucralfate |
|---|---|
| 适应证 Les indications | 用于胃及十二指肠溃疡，也用于胃炎。<br>Ce produit sert à traiter l'ulcère gastrique et l'ulcère duodénal.Il est aussi applicable dans le traitement de la gastrite. |
| 用法、用量 Les modes d'emploi et la posologie | 口服，每次 1g，一日 3～4 次，餐前 1 小时及睡前服用。<br>Par voie orale, 1g par fois, 3 à 4 fois par jour, 1h avant les repas et avant le sommeil. |
| 剂型、规格 Les formes pharmaceutiques et les spécifications | 片剂：每片 0.25g；0.5g。<br>分散片：每片 0.5g。<br>胶囊剂：每粒 0.25g。<br>悬胶剂：每袋 5ml（含硫糖铝 1g）。<br>Comprimés : 0,25g ou 0,5g par comprimé.<br>Comprimés dispersibles : 0,5g par comprimé.<br>Capsules : 0,25g par capsule.<br>Gel suspendu : 5ml (contenant 1g de sucralfate) par sachet. |

| 药品名称 Drug Names | 麦滋林 -S　Marzulene-S |
|---|---|
| 适应证 Les indications | 用于胃炎、胃溃疡和十二指肠溃疡，可明显缓解临床症状，并有较好的预防溃疡复发的作用。<br>Ce produit sert à traiter la gastrite, l'ulcère gastrique et l'ulcère duodénal, permettant une amélioration évidente des symptômes cliniques. Il est aussi efficace dans la prévention de la récurrence de l'ulcère. |
| 用法、用量 Les modes d'emploi et la posologie | 成人一般每日 1.5～2.5g，分 3～4 次口服，剂量可随年龄与症状适当增减。<br>Chez des adultes, en général, 1,5 à 2,5g par jour, à travers 3 à 4 fois par voie orale, ajuster la dose en fonction de l'âge et des maladies. |
| 剂型、规格 Les formes pharmaceutiques et les spécifications | 颗粒剂：1g 内含水溶性薁 3mg 和 L- 谷酰胺 990mg。<br>Granules : 1g de marzulene-S contient 3mg d'azulène soluble dans l'eau et 990mg de L- glutamine. |

| 药品名称 Drug Names | 替普瑞酮 Téprenone |
|---|---|
| 适应证 Les indications | 用于胃溃疡，也用于急性胃炎和慢性胃炎的急性加重期。<br>Ce produit sert à traiter l'ulcère gastrique. Il est aussi applicable dans le traitement de la gastrite aiguë et de l'exacerbation aiguë de la gastrite chronique. |
| 用法、用量 Les modes d'emploi et la posologie | 餐后 30 分钟内口服，一日 3 次，每次 1 粒胶囊（50mg）或颗粒剂 0.5g（含本品 50mg）。<br>Prendre 30 minutes après le repas par voie orale, 3 fois par jour, 1 capsule (50mg) ou 0,5g de granule (contenant 50mg de téprenone) par fois. |
| 剂型、规格 Les formes pharmaceutiques et les spécifications | 胶囊剂：每粒 50mg。<br>颗粒剂：100mg（含本品）/g。<br>Capsules : 50mg par capsule.<br>Granules : 100mg (contenant le téprenone) /g. |

续　表

| 药品名称 Drug Names | 吉法酯 Géfarnate |
| --- | --- |
| 适应证<br>Les indications | 用于治疗胃及十二指肠溃疡、急慢性胃炎、结肠炎、胃痉挛等。<br>Ce produit sert à traiter les ulcères gastriques et duodénaux, la gastrite aiguë et chronique, la colite, les crampes d'estomac, etc. |
| 用法、用量<br>Les modes d'emploi et la posologie | 口服，对一般肠胃不适、胃酸过多、胃胀及消化不良等，可根据病情每次 1～2 片，一日 3 次。治疗消化性溃疡及急慢性胃炎，每次 2 片，一日 3 次，餐后服用；症状较轻者疗程 4～5 周，重症者疗程 2～3 个月。儿童剂量酌减。<br>Par voie orale, pour traiter le malaise gastro-intestinal, l'hyperacidité, les ballonnements et l'indigestion, prendre 1 à 2 compriés par fois, 3 fois par jour selon les cas. Pour traiter l'ulcère gastro-intestinal et la gastrite aigue et chronique, 2 comprimés par fois, 3 fois par jour, après le repas ; chez des cas bénins, 4 à 5 semaines comme un traitement médical, chez des cas graves, pendant 2 à 3 mois. Diminuer la dose chez des enfants. |
| 剂型、规格<br>Les formes pharmaceutiques et les spécifications | 片剂：每片 0.4g。<br>Comprimés : 0,4g par comprimé. |

| 药品名称 Drug Names | 甘草锌 Licorzinc |
| --- | --- |
| 适应证<br>Les indications | 用于口腔、胃、十二指肠及其他部位的溃疡症，还可用于促进刀口、创伤和烧伤的愈合。儿童厌食、异食癖、生长发育不良、肠病性肢端皮炎及其他儿童、成人锌缺乏症也可用本品治疗。本品还可用于青春期痤疮。<br>Ce produit sert à traiter les ulcères buccaux, gastriques et duodénaux. Il permet aussi de favoriser la guérison des plaies, du traumatisme et des brûlures. Il est également applicable dans le traitement de l'anorexie, du pica, du retard de croissance, et de l'entéropathie acrodermatitis chez des enfants, ainsi que dans le traitement de la carence en zinc chez des enfants et des adultes. Il sert aussi à traiter l'acné de l'adolescent. |
| 用法、用量<br>Les modes d'emploi et la posologie | （1）治疗消化性溃疡：片剂 1 次 0.5g，或颗粒剂 1 次 10g，一日 3 次，疗程 4～6 周。必要时可减半再服 1 个疗程巩固疗效。<br>（2）治疗青春期痤疮，口腔溃疡及其他病症：片剂 1 次 0.25g，或颗粒剂 1 次 5g，一日 2～3 次。治疗青春期痤疮疗程 4～6 周。愈后每日服药 1 次，片剂 0.25g，或颗粒剂 5g，服 4～6 周，以减少复发。<br>（3）保健营养性补锌，一日片剂 0.25g 即可，1 次或分 2 次服用；或颗粒剂 1 次 1.5g，一日 2～3 次。<br>（4）儿童用量每日按 0.5～1.5mg（以元素锌计）/kg 计算，分 3 次服用。<br>(1)Pour traiter l'ulcère gastro-intestinal : 0,5g par fois en comprimé ou 10g par fois en granule, 3 fois par jour, pendant 4 à 6 semaines comme un traitement médical. En cas de besoin, prendre encore un traitement médical avec la moitié de la dose usuelle.<br>(2)Pour traiter l'acné de l'adolescent, l'ulcère buccal et d'autres symptômes : 0,25g par fois en comprimé ou 5g par fois en granul, 2 à 3 fois par jour. Pour traiter l'acné de l'adolescent, pendant 4 à 6 semaines comme un traitement médical. Après la guérison, prendre 1 fois par jour, 0,25g en comprimés ou 5g en granul, pendant 4 à 6 semaines pour réduire la récurrence.<br>(3)Pour compléter la carence en zinc, 0,25g par jour en comprimé, à travers 1 ou 2 fois ; ou 1,5g par fois en granul, 2 à 3 fois par jour.<br>(4)Chez des enfants, 0,5 à 1,5 mg/kg par jour (mesuré en zinc), à travers 3 fois. |
| 剂型、规格<br>Les formes pharmaceutiques et les spécifications | 片剂：每片 0.25g（相当于含锌 12.5mg，甘草酸 87.5mg）。<br>颗粒剂：每小袋 1.5g（相当于含元素锌 3.6～4.35mg）。<br>Comprimés : 0,25g par comprimé (équivalent à 12,5mg de zinc et 87,5mg de licorzince).<br>Granules : 1,5g par sachet (équivalent à 3,6 à 4,35mg de zinc). |

| 药品名称 Drug Names | 瑞巴派特 Rébamipide |
| --- | --- |
| 适应证<br>Les indications | 主要用于胃溃疡，但不宜单独用于 Hp 感染。也用于改善急性胃炎及慢性胃炎急性加重期的胃黏膜病变（如糜烂、出血、充血、水肿等）。<br><br>Ce produit sert principalement à traiter l'ulcère gastrique. Il vaut mieux éviter de l'utiliser seul dans le traitement des infections par H. pylori. Il permet également d'améliorer la gastrite aiguë et les lésions de la muqueuse gastrique lors de l'exacerbation aiguë de la gastrite chronique (comme l'érosion, l'hémorragie, la congestion et l'œdème). |
| 用法、用量<br>Les modes d'emploi et la posologie | 口服，一般每次 0.1g，一日 3 次，早、晚及睡前服用。<br><br>Par voie orale, 0,1 g par fois, 3 fois par jour, le petit matin, le soir et avant le sommeil. |
| 剂型、规格<br>Les formes pharmaceutiques et les spécifications | 片剂：每片 0.1g。<br><br>Comprimés : 0,1g par comprimé. |

| 药品名称 Drug Names | 复方铝酸铋 Aluminate de bismuth composé |
| --- | --- |
| 适应证<br>Les indications | 用于胃及十二指肠溃疡、慢性浅表性胃炎、十二指肠球炎、胃酸过多症及功能性消化不良等。<br><br>Ce produit sert à traiter les ulcères gastriques et duodénaux, la gastrite chronique superficielle, l'inflammation duodénale, l'hyperacidité et la dyspepsie fonctionnelle. |
| 用法、用量<br>Les modes d'emploi et la posologie | 成人一日 3 次，每次 1～2 片，餐后嚼碎服。疗程为 1～3 个月；以后可减量维持防止复发。<br><br>Chez des adultes, 3 fois par jour, 1 à 2 comprimés par fois, mâcher après le repas. Pendant 1 à 3 mois comme un traitement médical ; ensuite, possible de prendre la dose diminuée pour l'entretien afin d'éviter la récurrence. |
| 剂型、规格<br>Les formes pharmaceutiques et les spécifications | 复方片剂，每片含铝酸铋 200mg、甘草浸膏粉 300mg、重质碳酸镁 400mg、碳酸氢钠 200mg、弗朗鼠李皮 25mg、茴香 10mg。<br><br>Comprimés composés : chaque comprimé contient 200mg d'aluminate de bismuth, 300mgd'extrait de réglisse en poudre, 400mg de carbonate lourd de magnésium, 200 mg de bicarbonate de sodium, 25mg deCortex Frangulae et 10mg de fenouil. |

12.4　胃肠解痉药 Médicaments levée des spasmes gastro intestinaux

| 药品名称 Drug Names | 丁溴东莨菪碱 Butylbromures de Scopolamine |
| --- | --- |
| 适应证<br>Les indications | ①用于胃、十二指肠、结肠纤维内镜检查的术前准备，内镜逆行胰胆管造影和胃、十二指肠、结肠的气钡低张造影或计算机腹部体层扫描（CT 扫描）的术前准备，可有效减少或抑制胃肠道蠕动。②用于治疗各种病因引起的胃肠道痉挛、胆绞痛、肾绞痛或胃肠道蠕动亢进等。<br><br>① Ce produit est applicable dans la préparation préopératoire de la fibroscopiegastrique, duodénale et de la fibre du côlon. Il est également appliqué dans la préparation préopératoire de la cholangiopancréatographie rétrograde endoscopique et du CT-scan, permettant de réduire ou d'inhiber efficacement la motilité gastro-intestinale. ② Ce produit sert à traiter les spasmes gastro-intestinaux, les coliques, la colique néphrétique ou la motilité gastro-intestinale hyperthyroïde. |
| 用法、用量<br>Les modes d'emploi et la posologie | 口服：1 次 10mg，一日 3 次。肌内注射、静脉注射或静脉滴注（溶于葡萄糖注射液、0.9% 路华纳注射液中滴注）：每次 20～40mg；或 1 次 20mg，间隔 20～30 分钟后再用 20mg。<br><br>Par voie orale : 10mg par fois, 3 fois par jour. Injection par voie IM ou IV ou en perfusion (dissoudre dans la solution de glucose, la solution de chlorure de sodium à 0,9% pour la perfusion) : 20 à 40mg par fois ; ou 20mg par fois, toutes les 20 à 30 minutes. |
| 剂型、规格<br>Les formes pharmaceutiques et les spécifications | 注射液：每支 20mg（1ml）。<br>胶囊剂：每粒 10mg。<br>片剂：每片 10mg。<br><br>Injection : 20mg (1ml) par solution.<br>Capsules : 10mg par capsule.<br>Comprimés : 10mg par comprimé. |

**续　表**

| 药品名称 Drug Names | 曲美布汀 Trimébutine |
|---|---|
| 适应证<br>Les indications | 用于慢性胃炎引起的胃肠道症状，如腹部胀满感、腹痛和嗳气等；也用于肠道易激综合征。<br>Ce produit sert à traiter les symptômes gastro-intestinaux causés par la gastrite chronique, comme la plénitude abdominale,la douleur abdominale, les éructations, etc ; il est également utilisédans le traitement du syndrome du côlon irritable. |
| 用法、用量<br>Les modes d'emploi et la posologie | 治疗慢性胃炎，通常成人每次 100mg，一日 3 次。可根据年龄、症状适当增减剂量。治疗肠易激综合征，一般每次 100 ～ 200mg，一日 3 次。<br>Pour traiter la gastrite chronique, en général, chez des adultes, 100mg par fois, 3 fois par jour. Ajuster la dose en fonction de l'âge ou des maladies. Pour traiter le syndrome du côlon irritable, 100 à 200mg par fois, 3 fois par jour. |
| 剂型、规格<br>Les formes pharmaceutiques et les spécifications | 片剂：每片 100mg；200mg。<br>Comprimés : 100mg ou 200mg par comprimé. |
| 药品名称 Drug Names | 溴丙胺太林 Bromures de Propanthéline |
| 适应证<br>Les indications | 用于胃及十二指肠溃疡的辅助治疗，也用于胃炎、胰腺炎、胆汁排泄障碍、遗尿和多汗症。<br>Il est utilisé dans le traitement adjuvant de l'ulcère gastrique et duodénal. Il sert aussi à traiter la gastrite, la pancréatite, les troubles de l'excrétion biliaire, l'incontinence urinaire et l'hyperhidrose. |
| 用法、用量<br>Les modes d'emploi et la posologie | 每次 15mg，一日 3 ～ 4 次，餐前服，睡前 30mg；治疗遗尿可于睡前口服 15 ～ 45mg。<br>15mg par fois, 3 à 4 fois par jour, avant le repas, 30mg pris avant le sommeil ; pour traiter l'incontinence urinaire, 15 à 45mg pris avant le sommeil. |
| 剂型、规格<br>Les formes pharmaceutiques et les spécifications | 片剂：15mg。<br>Comprimés : 15mg. |

12.5　助消化药 Médicaments pour la digestion

| 药品名称 Drug Names | 多酶 Multienzyme |
|---|---|
| 适应证<br>Les indications | 用于多种消化酶缺乏的消化不良症。<br>Ce produit sert à traiter l'indigestion causée par une carence en diverses enzymes. |
| 用法、用量<br>Les modes d'emploi et la posologie | 口服，一次 1 ～ 2 片，一日 3 次，餐前服。<br>Par voie orale, 1 à 2 comprimés par fois, 3 fois par jour, avant le repas. |
| 剂型、规格<br>Les formes pharmaceutiques et les spécifications | 13mg（胃蛋白酶）-300mg（胰酶）。<br>13 mg (pepsine) -300mg (trypsine). |
| 药品名称 Drug Names | 复方慷彼申 Composés de Combizym |
| 适应证<br>Les indications | 用于各种原因所致的消化不良症。<br>Ce produit sert à traiter l'indigestion de touets sortes. |
| 用法、用量<br>Les modes d'emploi et la posologie | 口服：每次 1 片，一日 3 次，饭时或餐后服用。<br>Par voie orale : 1 comprimé par fois, 3 fois par jour, durant ou après le repas. |
| 剂型、规格<br>Les formes pharmaceutiques et les spécifications | 肠溶片剂：24mg（米曲菌酶提取物）-220mg（胰酶）。<br>Enrobage entérique comprimés: 24 mg (m aspergillose extraits enzymatiques) -220mg (trypsine). |

| 药品名称 Drug Names | 干酵母 Levure sèchèes |
|---|---|
| 适应证<br>Les indications | 用于营养不良、消化不良、食欲缺乏、腹泻及胃肠胀气。<br>Ce produit sert à traiter la malnutrition, l'indigestion, la perte d'appétit, la diarrhée et la flatulence. |
| 用法、用量<br>Les modes d'emploi et la posologie | 口服：每次 0.5 ～ 4g，嚼碎服。剂量过大可引起腹泻。<br>Par voie orale : 0,5 à 4g par fois, mâcher le médicament. La dose trop forte pourrait entraîner la diarrhée. |
| 剂型、规格<br>Les formes pharmaceutiques et les spécifications | 片剂：每片 0.2g；0.3g；0.5g。<br>Comprimés : 0,2g, 0,3g ou 0,5g par comprimé. |

12.6　促胃肠动力药 Médicaments favorisant la motilité gastrointestinale

| 药品名称 Drug Names | 甲氧氯普胺 Métoclopramide |
|---|---|
| 适应证<br>Les indications | ①因脑部肿瘤手术、肿瘤放疗及化疗、脑外伤后遗症、急性颅脑损伤及药物所引起的呕吐。②胃胀气性消化不良、食欲缺乏、嗳气、恶心、呕吐。③海空作业引起的呕吐及晕车。④可增加食管括约肌压力，从而减少全身麻醉时胃肠道反流所致吸入性肺炎的发生率；可减轻钡剂检查时的恶心、呕吐反应，促进钡剂通过；十二指肠插管前服用，有助于顺利插管。⑤对糖尿病性胃轻瘫，胃下垂等。⑥可减轻偏头痛引起的恶心，并可能由于提高胃通过率而促进麦角胺的吸收。⑦其催乳作用可试用于乳量严重不足的产妇。⑧胆道疾病和慢性胰腺炎的辅助治疗。<br><br>① Ce produit sert à traiter les vomissements causés par la chirurgie des tumeurs du cerveau, la radiothérapie et la chimiothérapie, les séquelles du traumatisme crânien, une lésion cérébrale aiguë ou des médicaments. ② Les ballonnements, l'indigestion, la perte d'appétit, des éructations, des nausées et des vomissements. ③ Les vomissements et le mal de transport causés par les opérations aériennes et maritimes. ④ Il permet d'augmenter la pression du sphincter œsophagien, réduisant la pneumonie par aspirationle causée par le reflux gastro-intestinallors de l'anesthésie générale. Il permet aussi de soulager les nausées et les vomissements lors de l'examen de repas de Baryum, favorisant le passage du baryum. Il est aussi administré avant l'intubation duodénale, favorisant l'intubation. ⑤ Ce produit sert à traiter la gastroparésie et le gastroptosis diabétiques. ⑥ Il permet de réduire les nausées causées par la migraine et de favoriser l'absorption gastrique de l'ergotamine. ⑦ Son rôle de la prolactine lui permet de s'utiliser dans le traitement d'une pénurie de lait maternel. ⑧ Il sert de traitement adjuvant des maladies des voies biliaires et de la pancréatite chronique. |
| 用法、用量<br>Les modes d'emploi et la posologie | ① 口服：一次 5 ～ 10mg，一日 10 ～ 30mg。餐前半小时服用。② 肌内注射：1 次 10 ～ 20mg。每日剂量一般不超过 0.5mg/kg，否则易引起锥体外系反应。<br>① Par voie orale : 5 à 10mg par fois, 10 à 30 mg par jour, 0,5h avant le repas. ② Injection par voie IM : 10 à 20mg par fois. Ne pas dépasser 0,5 mg/kg par jour, sinon, la dose trop forte pourrait entraîner les réactions extrapyramidales. |
| 剂型、规格<br>Les formes pharmaceutiques et les spécifications | 片剂：每片 5mg。<br>注射液：每支 10mg（1ml）。<br>Comprimés : 5mg par comprimé.<br>Injection : 10mg (1ml) par solution. |
| 药品名称 Drug Names | 多潘立酮 Dompéridone |
| 适应证<br>Les indications | ①由胃排空延缓、反流性胃炎、慢性胃炎、反流性食管炎引起的消化不良症状；其他消化系统疾病引起的呕吐。②胃轻瘫，尤其是糖尿病性胃轻瘫可缩短胃排空时间，使胃潴留症状消失。③各种原因引起的恶心呕吐；抗帕金森综合征药物引起的胃肠道症状及多巴胺受体激动药所致的恶心呕吐。偏头痛、痛经、颅外伤及颅内病灶、放射治疗以及左旋多巴非甾体抗炎药等引起的恶心呕吐。检查和治疗措施引起的恶心呕吐；儿童因各种原因引起的急性和持续性呕吐等。对细胞毒性药物引起的呕吐只在不太严重时有效。④可作为消化性溃疡的辅助治疗药物，用于消除胃窦部潴留。 |

**续　表**

| | ① Ce produit sert à traiter l'indigestion causée par la vidange gastrique retardée, la gastrite de reflux, la gastrite chronique et l'oesophagite par reflux ; ainis que les vomissements causés par d'autres maladies digestives. ② Il permet de traiter la gastroparésie, de raccourcir le temps de vidange gastrique dans le traitement de la gastroparésie diabétique, et de faire dispaître les symptômes de la rétention gastrique. ③ Ce produit sert à traiter les vomissements et les nausées de toutes sortes: ceux causés par les médicaments anti- parkinsonisme et par les agonistes des récepteurs de la dopamine ; ceux causés par la migraine, la dysménorrhée, les lésions intracrâniennes, les blessures extracrâniennes, la radiothérapie et les médicaments anti- inflammatoires non stéroïdiens comme le lévodopa ; ceux causés par l'examen et le traitement ; les vomissements aigus et persisitants chez des enfants. Pour traiter les vomissements causés par les médicaments cytotoxiques, il n'est efficace que dans les cas pas très graves. ④ Il sert aussi de traitement adjuvent de l'ulcère gastroduodénal pour traiter la rétention de l'antre gastrique. |
|---|---|
| 用法、用量<br>Les modes d'emploi et la posologie | ①肌内注射：每次 10mg，必要时可重复给药。②口服：每次 10～20mg，一日 3 次，餐前服。③直肠给药：每次 60mg，一日 2～3 次。栓剂最好在直肠空时插入。<br><br>① Injection par voie IM : 10mg par fois, en cas de besoin, l'administration répétée. ② Par voie orale : 10 à 20mg par fois, 3 fois par jour, avant le repas. ③ Administration rectale : 60mg par fois, 2 à 3 fois par jour. Il vaut mieux insérer les suppositoires dans le rectum vide. |
| 剂型、规格<br>Les formes pharmaceutiques et les spécifications | 片剂：每片 10mg。<br>栓剂：每粒 60mg。<br>注射液：每支 10mg（2ml）。<br>滴剂：10mg/ml。<br>混悬液：1mg/ml。<br><br>Comprimés : 10mg par comprimé.<br>Suppositoires : 60mg par suppositoire.<br>Injection : 10mg (2ml) par solution.<br>Gouttes : 10 mg/ml.<br>Suspension : 1 mg/ml. |
| 药品名称 Drug Names | 西沙必利 Cisapride |
| 适应证<br>Les indications | ①可增加胃肠动力，用于胃轻瘫综合征，或上消化道不适，X 线、内镜检查阴性的症候群，特征为早饱、餐后饱胀、食量减低、胃胀、过多的嗳气、食欲缺乏、恶心、呕吐或类似溃疡的主诉（上腹部灼痛）。②胃 - 食管反流：包括食管炎的治疗及维持治疗。③与运动功能失调有关的假性肠梗阻导致的推进性蠕动不足和胃肠内容物滞留。④可恢复结肠的推进性运动，作为慢性便秘患者的长期治疗。<br><br>① Ce produit permet d'augmenter la motilité gastro-intestinale, de traiter le syndrome de gastroparésie, ou l'inconfort gastro-intestinal supérieur, ainsi que les symptômes du syndrome de X -ray, endoscopie négative, caractérisés par lasatiété précoce, la plénitude postprandiale, la perte de l'appétit, les ballonnements, l'éructationexcessive,l'anorexie, les nausées, les vomissements, ou les ulcères (la combustion de l'abdomensupérieur). ② Le reflux gastro-oesophagien : y compris la thérapie et le traitement d'entretien de l'oesophagite. ③ La motilité propulsive insuffisante et la rétention gastrique causées par la pseudo-obstruction intestinale liée aux troubles de la motilité. ④ Il permet la récupération du mouvement de propulsion du côlon et sert de traitement à long terme des patients souffrant de constipation chronique. |
| 用法、用量<br>Les modes d'emploi et la posologie | 口服，根据病情，一日总量为 15～40mg，分 2～4 次给药。食管炎的维持治疗：一次 10mg，一日 2 次，早餐前和睡前服用；或一次 20mg，一日 1 次，睡前服用。病情严重者剂量可加倍。<br><br>Par voie orale, selon les cas, 15 à 40mg par jour, à travers 2 à 4 fois. Le traitement d'entretien de l'oesophagite : 10mg par fois, 2 fois par jour, avant le petit-déjeuner et le sommeil ; ou 20mg par fois, 1 fois par jour, pris avant le sommeil. Possible de doubler la dose chez des patients graves. |

**续 表**

| 剂型、规格<br>Les formes pharmaceutiques et les spécifications | 片剂：每片 5mg；10mg。<br>胶囊剂：每粒 5mg。<br>干混悬剂：100mg。<br>Comprimés : 5mg ou 10mg par comprimé.<br>Capsules : 5mg par capsule.<br>Suspension sèche : 100mg. |
|---|---|
| **药品名称 Drug Names** | **莫沙必利 Mosapride** |
| 适应证<br>Les indications | ①慢性胃炎或功能性消化不良引起的消化道症状，如上腹部胀满感、腹胀、上腹部疼痛；嗳气、恶心、呕吐；胃烧灼感等。②胃食管反流病和糖尿病胃轻瘫。③胃大部切除术患者的胃功能障碍。<br>① Ce produit sert à traiter les symptômes gastro-intestinaux causés par la gastrite chronique ou la dyspepsie fonctionnelle, tels que la lourdeur abdominale, des ballonnements, des douleurs abdominales, deséructations, desnausées, des vomissements, ainsi que la sensation de brûlure gastrique. ② Le reflux gastro-oesophagien et la gastroparésie diabétique. ③ Le dysfonctionnement gastrique chez des patients de gastrectomie. |
| 用法、用量<br>Les modes d'emploi et la posologie | 每次 5mg，一日 3 次，餐前服用。<br>5mg par fois, 3 fois par jour, pris avant le repas. |
| 剂型、规格<br>Les formes pharmaceutiques et les spécifications | 片剂：每片 5mg。<br>Comprimés : 5mg par comprimé. |

12.7　止吐药和催吐药 Les antiémétiques et les émétiques

| **药品名称 Drug Names** | **昂丹司琼 Ondansétron** |
|---|---|
| 适应证<br>Les indications | 用于治疗由化疗和放疗引起的恶心、呕吐，也可用于预防和治疗手术后引起的恶心呕吐。<br>Ce produit sert à traiter les nausées et les vomissements causés par la chimiothérapie et la radiothérapie. Il est aussi applicable dans la prévention et le traitement des nausées et des vomissements postopératoires. |
| 用法、用量<br>Les modes d'emploi et la posologie | （1）治疗由化疗和放疗引起的恶心呕吐。①成人：给药途径和剂量应视患者情况因人而异，剂量一般为 8～32mg，为避免治疗 24 小时后出现恶心呕吐，均应让患者持续服药，每次 8mg，一日 2 次，连服 5 日。②儿童：$5mg/m^2$ 静脉注射，12 小时后再口服 4mg，化疗后应持续给患儿口服 4mg，一日 2 次，连服 5 日。③老年人：可依成年人给药法给药，一般无须调整。<br>（2）预防或治疗手术后呕吐：①成人：一般可于麻醉诱导同时静脉滴注 4mg，或于麻醉前 1 小时口服 8mg，之后每隔 8 小时口服 8mg，共 2 次。已出现术后恶心呕吐时，可缓慢静脉滴注 4mg 进行治疗。②肾衰竭患者：无须调整剂量、用药次数或用药途径。③肝衰竭患者：由于主要自肝脏代谢，对中度或严重肝衰竭患者，每日用药剂量不应超过 8mg。<br>(1) Pour traiter les nausées et les vomissements causés par la chimiothérapie et la radiothérapie : ① Chez des adultes : les modes d'emploi et la dose varient selon les cas, en général, 8 à 32mg, pour éviter les nausées et les vomissements 24h après l'administration, il faut prendre les médicaments de manière consécutive, 8mg par fois, 2 fois par jour, pendant 5 jours consécutifs. ② Chez des enfants : $5mg/m^2$, injection par voie IV, 12h après, reprendre 4mg par voie orale, après la chimiothérapie, il faut prendre 4mg par voie orale, 2 fois par jour, pendant 5 jours consécutifs. ③ Chez des personnes âgées : la même dose que chez des adultes, pas besoin d'ajuster la dose.<br>(2) Pour prévenir ou traiter les vomissements postopératoires : ① Chez des adultes : en général, durant l'induction de l'anesthésie, 4mg en perfusion, ou 1h avant l'anesthésie, prendre 8mg par voie orale, 8h après, reprendre 8mg. En cas de nausées ou de vomissements postopératoires, perfusion lente, 4mg. ② Chez des patients insuffisants rénaux : pas nécessaire d'ajuster la dose, le nombre d'administration et les modes d'emploi. ③ Chez des patients insuffisants hépatiques : pour les patients modérés ou graves, ne pas dépasser 8mg par jour. |

**续　表**

| | |
|---|---|
| 剂型、规格<br>Les formes pharmaceutiques et les spécifications | 注射液：每支 4mg（1ml）；8mg（2ml）。<br>片剂：每片 4mg；8mg。<br>Injection : 4mg (1ml) ou 8mg (2ml) par solution.<br>Comprimés : 4mg ou 8mg par comprimé. |
| **药品名称 Drug Names** | 托烷司琼 Tropisétron |
| 适应证<br>Les indications | 主要用于预防和治疗癌症化疗引起的恶心、呕吐。<br>Il est principalement utilisé dans la prévention et le traitement des nausées et des vomissements causés par la chimiothérapie anticancéreuse. |
| 用法、用量<br>Les modes d'emploi et la posologie | 每日 5mg，总疗程 6 日。第 1 日，静脉给药，在化疗前将本品 5mg 溶于 100ml 生理盐水、林格液或 5% 葡萄糖注射液中静脉滴注或缓慢静脉注射，第 2～6 日，口服给药，一日 1 次，每次 1 粒胶囊（5mg），于进食前至少 1 小时服用，或于早上起床后立即用水送服。疗程 2～6 日，轻症者可适当缩短疗程。<br>5mg par jour, pendant 6 jours consécutifs. Le premier jour, injection par voie IV, avant la chimiothérapie, dissoudre 5mg dans 10ml de solution saline, de solution de Linger ou de solution de glucose à 5%, perfusion ou injection par voie IV lente. Du 2ème au 6ème jour, l'administration parv oie orale, 1 fois par jour, 1 capsule (5mg) par fois, au moins 1 h avant le repas, ou immédiatement après le lever du matin avec de l'eau. Pendant 2 à 6 jours consécutifs, possible de raccourcir la durée du traitement médical chez des patients bénins. |
| 剂型、规格<br>Les formes pharmaceutiques et les spécifications | 注射液：每支 5mg（1ml）。<br>胶囊剂：每粒 5mg。<br>Injection : 5mg (1ml) par solution.<br>Capsules : 5mg par capsule. |
| **药品名称 Drug Names** | 格拉司琼 Granisétron |
| 适应证<br>Les indications | 用于预防和治疗化疗、放疗及手术后引起的恶心和呕吐。<br>Ce produit sert à prévenir et à traiter les nausées et les vomissements causés par la chimiothérapie et la radiothérapie et après la chirurgie. |
| 用法、用量<br>Les modes d'emploi et la posologie | 将本品以注射用生理盐水 20～50ml 稀释后，于化疗或放疗前一日 1 次静脉滴注，成人剂量每次 40μg/kg，或给予标准剂量 3mg，如症状未见改善，可再增补一次，对老年患者及肾功能不全患者一般无须调整剂量。每一疗程可连续使用 5 日。<br>Dissoudre dans 20 à 50ml de solution saline pour injection, avant la chimiothérapie ou la radiothérapie, perfusion, 1 fois par jour, chez des adultes, 40μg/kg par fois, ou prendre la dose standard, 3mg, s'il les symptômes ne s'améliorent pas, reprendre une fois encore ; chez des personnes âgées et des patients insuffisants rénaux, pas nécessaire d'ajuster la dose. Pendant 5 jours consécutifs comme un traitement médical. |
| 剂型、规格<br>Les formes pharmaceutiques et les spécifications | 注射液：每支 3mg（3ml）。<br>片（胶囊）剂：每片（粒）1mg。<br>Injection : 3mg (3ml) par solution.<br>Comprimés (capsules) : 1mg par comprimé ou par capsule. |
| **药品名称 Drug Names** | 阿扎司琼 Azasétron |
| 适应证<br>Les indications | 用于化疗及放疗引起的消化系统症状，如恶心、呕吐等。<br>Il sert à traiter les symptômes gastro-intestinaux causés par la chimiothérapie et la radiothérapie, tels que les nausées et les vomissements. |
| 用法、用量<br>Les modes d'emploi et la posologie | 成人一般用量为 10mg，一日 1 次静脉注射。<br>Chez des adultes, 10mg par fois par jour, injection par voie IV. |
| 剂型、规格<br>Les formes pharmaceutiques et les spécifications | 注射剂：每支 10mg（2ml）。<br>Injection : 10mg (2ml) par solution. |

**续　表**

| 药品名称 Drug Names | 地芬尼多 Difénidol |
|---|---|
| 适应证<br>Les indications | 用于各种原因引起的眩晕、恶心、呕吐等症状。<br>Il permet de traiter les vertiges, les nausées, les vomissements, etc. |
| 用法、用量<br>Les modes d'emploi et<br>la posologie | 口服：每次 25～50mg，一日 3 次；肌内注射：每次 20～40mg，一日 4 次。儿童（6 个月以上）：每次 0.9mg/kg，一日 3 次。<br>Par voie orale : 25 à 50mg par fois, 3 fois par jour ; injection par voie IM : 20 à 40 mg par fois, 4 fois par jour. chez des enfants (plus de 6 mois) : 0,9 mg/kg par fois, 3 fois par jour. |
| 剂型、规格<br>Les formes<br>pharmaceutiques et les<br>spécifications | 片剂：25mg。<br>注射液：10mg/1ml。<br>Comprimés : 25mg.<br>Injection : 10mg/1ml. |

12.8　泻药 Laxalifs

| 药品名称 Drug Names | 硫酸镁 Sulfate de magnésium |
|---|---|
| 适应证<br>Les indications | ①导泻，肠内异常发酵，亦可与驱虫剂并用；与药用炭合用，可治疗食物或药物中毒。②阻塞性黄疸及慢性胆囊炎。③惊厥、子痫、尿毒症、破伤风、高血压脑病及急性肾性高血压危象等。④也用于发作频繁而其他治疗效果不佳的心绞痛患者，对伴有高血压的患者效果较好。⑤外用热敷消炎去肿。<br>① Il a un effetcathartique, et peut traiter la fermentation anormale intestinale. Il peut être utilisé en association avec des insectifuges. Utilisé en combinaison avec le charbon médicinal, il sert aussi à traiter l'intoxication médicamenteuse et alimentaire. ② La jaunisse obstructive et cholécystite chronique. ③ Les convulsions, l'éclampsie, l'urémie, le tétanos, l'encéphalopathie hypertensive et la crise d'hypertension rénale aiguë. ④ Il est aussi appliqué chez les patients atteints d'angine de poitrine fréquente et résistant à d'autres traitements. Il est surtout efficace chez des patients souffrant de l'angine de poitrine et accompagnés de l'hypertension artérielle. ⑤ L'usage externe pour l'anti-inflammation et l'anti-oedème. |
| 用法、用量<br>Les modes d'emploi et<br>la posologie | ①导泻：每次口服 5～20g，清晨空腹服，同时饮 100～400ml 水，也可用水溶解后服用。②利胆：每次 2～5g，一日 3 次，餐前或两餐间服。也可服用 33% 溶液，每次 10ml。③抗惊厥、降血压等：肌内注射，一次 1g，10% 溶液，每次 10ml；静脉滴注，一次 1～2.5g，将 25% 溶液 10ml 用 5% 葡萄糖注射液稀释成 1% 浓度缓慢静脉滴注。<br>① Pour l'effet cathartique : 5 à 20g par fois par voie orale, le petit matin, l'estomac vide, prendre en même temps 100 à 400ml d'eau, ou dissoudre dans l'eau avant de le prendre. ② Pour traiter les maladies biliaires : 2 à 5g par fois, 3 fois par jour, avant le repas ou entre les deux repas. Ou prendre la solution à 33%, 10ml par fois. ③ Pour l'anticonvulsivant ou l'anti-hypertenseur : injection par voie IM, 1g par fois, la solution à 10%, 10ml par fois ; la perfusion, 1 à 2,5 g par fois, diluer 10ml de solution à 25% avec la solution de glocuse à 5% pour que la concentration de la solution soit 1%, la perfusion lente. |
| 剂型、规格<br>Les formes<br>pharmaceutiques et les<br>spécifications | 注射液：每支 1g（10ml）；2.5g（10ml）。<br>Injection : 1g (10ml) ou 2,5g (10ml) par solution. |

| 药品名称 Drug Names | 甘油 Glycérol |
|---|---|
| 适应证<br>Les indications | 用于便秘、降眼压和颅内压。<br>Ce produit sert à traiter la constipation, à diminuer la pression intraoculaire et la pression intracrânienne. |

**续　表**

| | |
|---|---|
| 用法、用量<br>Les modes d'emploi et la posologie | ①便秘：使用栓剂，每次 1 粒塞入肛门（成人用大号栓、小儿用小儿栓），对小儿及年老体弱者较为适宜。也可用本品 50% 溶液灌肠。②降眼压和降颅内压：口服 50% 甘油溶液（含 0.9% 氯化钠），每次 200ml，日服 1 次，必要时日服 2 次，但要间隔 6 ～ 8 小时。<br><br>① Pour traiter la constipation : utiliser les suppositoires, insérér 1 suppositoire par fois dans l'anus (grand suppositoire chez des adultes, petit suppositoire chez des enfants), il est applicable chez des petits enfants et des personnes âgées faibles. Ou utiliser la solution à 50% de glycérol pour le lavement. ② Pour diminuer la PIO et la pression intracrânienne : prendre la solution à 50 % de glycérol par voie orale (contenant le chlorure de sodium à 0,9%), 200ml par fois, 1 fois par jour, s'il est nécessaire, 2 fois par jour, toutes les 6 à 8h. |
| 剂型、规格<br>Les formes pharmaceutiques et les spécifications | 栓剂：含甘油约 90%，大号每个约重 3g，小号每个约重 1.5g。<br>甘油溶液：包括 10% 甘油生理盐水溶液、10% 甘油葡萄糖溶液、10% 甘油甘露醇溶液和 50% 甘油盐水溶液。<br><br>Suppositoires : contenant 90% de glycérol, grand suppositoire pesant 3g, petit suppositoire pesant 1,5g.<br>La solution de glycérol : contenant la solution saline de glycérol à 10%, la solution de glucose de glycérol à 10%, la solution de mannitol glycérolà 10% et la solution aqueuse de sel de glycérol à 50%. |
| 药品名称 Drug Names | 开塞露 Enéma Glycérini |
| 适应证<br>Les indications | 本品为治疗便秘的直肠用溶液剂。<br>Il s'agit de solutions rectales traitant la constipation. |
| 用法、用量<br>Les modes d'emploi et la posologie | 用时将容器顶端刺破，外面涂油脂少许，徐徐插入肛门，然后将药液挤入直肠内，引起排便。成人用量每次 20ml（1 支）。<br><br>Percer d'abord la partie supérieure du récipient, mettre un peu de graisse à l'extérieur, insérer lentement dans l'anus avant de pousser le médicament dans le rectum pour faciliter la constipation. Chez des adultes, 20ml (une solution) par fois. |
| 剂型、规格<br>Les formes pharmaceutiques et les spécifications | 每支 20ml。<br>20ml par pièce. |
| 药品名称 Drug Names | 硫酸钠 Sulfate de sodium |
| 适应证<br>Les indications | 为容积性泻药。<br>Il s'agit de laxatifs de volume. |
| 用法、用量<br>Les modes d'emploi et la posologie | 散剂：一次 5 ～ 20g，溶于 250ml 水，清晨空腹服用；肠溶胶囊：一次 5g，一日 1 ～ 3 次。排便后即可停药，如 12 小时后未排便，可追加服药 1 ～ 2 次。<br><br>Poudre : 5 à 20g par fois, dissoudre dans 250ml d'eau, pris le petit matin, l'estomac vide ; les capsules à enrobage entérique, 5g par fois, 1 à 3 fois par jour. Arrêter l'administion après la défécation. S'il on ne défèque pas 12h après l'administration, reprendre le médicament 1 à 2 fois. |
| 剂型、规格<br>Les formes pharmaceutiques et les spécifications | 散剂：500g。<br>肠溶胶囊：1g/ 粒。<br>Poudre : 500g.<br>Les capsules à enrobage entérique : 1g par capsule. |
| 药品名称 Drug Names | 液状石蜡 Paraffine liquide |
| 适应证<br>Les indications | 使粪便稀释变软，同时润滑肠壁，使粪便易于排出。<br>Ce produit permet de ramollir et de diluer des selles tout en lubrifiant la paroi intestinalepour faciliter la défécation. |
| 用法、用量<br>Les modes d'emploi et la posologie | 每次 15 ～ 30ml，睡前服。<br>15 à 30ml par fois, pris avant le sommeil. |

**续　表**

| 剂型、规格<br>Les formes pharmaceutiques et les spécifications | 原液：500ml。<br>stoste : 500ml. |
| --- | --- |

## 12.9　止泻药 Antidiarrhéiques

| 药品名称 Drug Names | 双八面体蒙脱石 Smectite dioctaédrique |
| --- | --- |
| 适应证<br>Les indications | 用于急慢性腹泻，尤以对儿童急性腹泻疗效为佳，但在必要时应同时治疗脱水，也用于食管炎及与胃、十二指肠、结肠疾病有关的疼痛的对症治疗。<br><br>Ce produit sert à traiter la diarrhée aiguë et chronique. Il est surtout efficace dans le traitement de la diarrhée aigue chez des enfants. Mais en cas de besoin, il faut traiter en même temps la déshydration. Il est aussi applicable dans le traitement symptomatique de l'oesophagite et des douleurs liées à l'estomac, au duodénum et à la maladie du côlon. |
| 用法、用量<br>Les modes d'emploi et la posologie | 成人每次 1 袋，一日 3 次，治疗急性腹泻首剂应加倍。食管炎患者宜于餐后服用，其他患者于餐前服用，将本品溶于半杯温水中送服。<br><br>Chez des adultes, 1 sachet par fois, 3 fois par jour, pour traiter la diarrhée aigue, il faut doubler la dose pour la première fois. Chez des patients atteints d'oesophagite, il vaut mieux prendre le médicament après le raps, chez les autres patients, le prendre avant le repas, dissoudre ce produit dans l'eau chaude avant de le prendre. |
| 剂型、规格<br>Les formes pharmaceutiques et les spécifications | 散剂：每小袋内含双八面体蒙脱石 3g、葡萄糖 0.749g、糖精钠 0.007g、香兰素 0.004g。<br><br>Poudre : chaque sachet contient 3g de smectite dioctaédrique, 0,749g de glucose, 0,007g de saccharine sodique et 0,004g de vanilline. |

| 药品名称 Drug Names | 鞣酸蛋白 Tannalbin |
| --- | --- |
| 适应证<br>Les indications | 用于急性胃肠炎非细菌性腹泻。<br>Ce produit sert à traiter la diarrhée non bactérienne liée à la gastro-entérite aiguë. |
| 用法、用量<br>Les modes d'emploi et la posologie | 一日 3 次，每次 1～2g，空腹服。<br>3 fois par jour, 1 à 2 g par fois, l'estomac vide. |
| 剂型、规格<br>Les formes pharmaceutiques et les spécifications | 片剂：0.25g；0.5g。<br>Comprimés : 0,25g ou 0,5g. |

| 药品名称 Drug Names | 碱式碳酸铋 Subcarbonate de bismuth |
| --- | --- |
| 适应证<br>Les indications | 用于腹泻、慢性胃肠炎、胃及十二指肠溃疡。<br>Ce produit sert à traiter la diarrhée, la gastro-entérite chronique, les ulcères gastriques et duodénaux. |
| 用法、用量<br>Les modes d'emploi et la posologie | 一日 3 次，每次 0.3～0.9g，餐前服。<br>3 fois par jour, 0,3 à 0,9g par fois, pris avant le repas. |
| 剂型、规格<br>Les formes pharmaceutiques et les spécifications | 片剂：0.3g。<br>Comprimés : 0,3g. |

**续　表**

12.10　微生态药物 Médicaments microécologie

| 药品名称 Drug Names | 地衣芽孢杆菌活菌 Bacillus licheniformis vivants |
|---|---|
| 适应证<br>Les indications | 用于细菌与真菌引起的急慢性腹泻及各种原因所致的肠道菌群失调的防治。<br>Ce produit sert à traiter la diarrhée aiguë et chronique causée par des bactéries et des champignons. Il est aussi applicable dans la prévention et le traitement des perturbations de la flore intestinale. |
| 用法、用量<br>Les modes d'emploi et la posologie | 口服：每次 0.5g，一日 3 次，小儿减半或遵医嘱。<br>Par voie orale : 0,5g par fois, 3 fois par jour, chez des enfants, diminuer de moitié la dose ou selon les ordonnances. |
| 剂型、规格<br>Les formes pharmaceutiques et les spécifications | 胶囊剂：每粒 0.25g（含 2.5 亿活菌）。<br>Capsules : 0,25g par capsule (contenant 250 millions de bactéries vivantes). |

| 药品名称 Drug Names | 嗜酸乳杆菌 Lactobacillus LB |
|---|---|
| 适应证<br>Les indications | 用于急慢性腹泻的对症治疗。<br>Il sert de traitement symptomatique de la diarrhée aiguë et chronique. |
| 用法、用量<br>Les modes d'emploi et la posologie | 胶囊剂：成人及儿童一日 2 次，每次 2 粒，成人首剂量加倍；婴儿一日 2 次，每次 1～2 粒，首剂量 2 粒。散剂：成人及儿童一日 2 次，每次 1 袋，成人首剂量加倍；婴儿一日 2 次，每次 1 袋。胶囊剂可用水吞服亦可倒出内容物混合于水中饮服。<br>Capsules : chez des adultes et des enfants, 2 fois par jour, 2 capsules par fois, chez des adultes, doubler la dose pour la première fois ; chez des bébés, 2 fois par jour, 1 à 2 capsules par fois, pour la dose initiale, 2 capsule. Poudre : chez des adultes et des enfants, 2 fois par jour, 1 sachet par fois, doubler la dose pour la première fois chez des adultes ; chez des bébés, 2 fois par jour, 1 sachet par fois. Pour les capsules, possible de les avaler avec de l'eau ou de verser les contenants, de les dissoudre dans l'eau avant de les prendre. |
| 剂型、规格<br>Les formes pharmaceutiques et les spécifications | 胶囊剂：每胶囊含灭活冻干的嗜酸乳杆菌 50 亿和中和后冻干的培养基 80mg。<br>散剂：每小袋含灭活冻干的嗜酸乳杆菌 50 亿和中和后冻干的培养基 160mg。<br>Capsules : chaque capsule contient 5 milliards de lactobacillus acidophilus inactivés et lyophilisés ainsi que 80mg de médium neutralisé et lyophilisé.<br>Poudre : chaque sachet contient 5 milliards de lactobacillus acidophilus inactivés et lyophilisés ainsi que 160mg de médium neutralisé et lyophilisé. |

| 药品名称 Drug Names | 复合乳酸菌 Lactobacillus complexe |
|---|---|
| 适应证<br>Les indications | 用于各种原因引起的肠道菌群紊乱、急慢性腹泻、肠易激综合征、抗生素相关性腹泻的治疗。亦可用于预防或减少抗生素及化疗药物所致的肠道菌群紊乱的辅助治疗。<br>Ce produit sert à traiter les perturbations de la flore intestinale, la diarrhée aiguë ou chronique, le syndrome du côlon irritable, et la diarrhée associée aux antibiotiques.Il est aussi applicable dans la prévention ou le traitement adjuvant visant à réduire les perturbations de la flore intestinale causées par les antibiotiques et les médicaments de chimiothérapie. |
| 用法、用量<br>Les modes d'emploi et la posologie | 口服：一次 1～2 粒，一日 1～3 次，根据病情和年龄可适当增减。<br>Par voie orale : 1 à 2 capsule par fois, 1 à 3 fois par jour, ajuster la dose selon les maladies et l'âge. |
| 剂型、规格<br>Les formes pharmaceutiques et les spécifications | 胶囊剂：每粒 0.33g（含活乳酸菌 2 万个以上）。<br>Capsules : 0,33g par capsule (contenant plus de 20 000 lactobacillus actifs). |

**续　表**

| 药品名称 Drug Names | 双歧杆菌嗜酸乳杆菌肠球菌三联活菌 Combinaison Bifidobactérium Lactobacillus et Entérococcus, Viable |
|---|---|
| 适应证<br>Les indications | 　　用于肠道菌群失调引起的腹泻、腹胀等，也用于慢性腹泻和轻中型急性腹泻，以调节肠道功能；对缓解便秘也有较好疗效，还可作为肝硬化、急慢性肝炎及肿瘤化疗等的辅助用药。<br><br>　　Il sert à traiter la diarrhée et la distension abdominalecausées par les perturbations de la flore intestinale. Il est aussi applicable dans le traitement de la diarrhée chronique et de la diarrhée aiguë bénigne et modérée pour réguler la fonction intestinale. Il est également efficace dans le soulagement de la constipation. Il sert aussi de traitement adjuvant de la cirrhose,de l'hépatite aiguë et chronique et de la chimiothérapie du cancer. |
| 用法、用量<br>Les modes d'emploi et la posologie | 　　口服：每次 420～630mg，一日 2～3 次，餐后服用。小于 1 岁儿童每次 105mg；1～6 岁每次 210mg；6～13 岁每次 210～420mg。婴幼儿可取胶囊内药粉用温开水调服。<br><br>　　Par voie orale : 420 à 630mg par fois, 2 à 3 fois par jour, pris après le repas. Chez des enfants moins de 1 an, 105mg par fois ; chez des enfants de 1 à 6 ans, 210mg par fois ; de 6 à 13 ans, 210 à 420mg par fois. Chez des bébés et des petits enfants, possible de retirer les contenus de la capsule, dissoudre avec de l'eau chaude, avant de les prendre. |
| 剂型、规格<br>Les formes pharmaceutiques et les spécifications | 　　胶囊剂：每粒 210mg。<br>　　散剂：每包 1g；2g。<br><br>　　Capsules : 210mg par capsule.<br>　　Poudre : 1g ou 2g par sachet. |
| 药品名称 Drug Names | 枯草杆菌肠球菌二联活菌 Viable combinaison de bacillus subtilis et d'enterococcus |
| 适应证<br>Les indications | 　　治疗和预防抗生素相关性腹泻、旅行者腹泻及其他腹泻；也可用于肠易激综合征（IBS）及炎症性肠病的辅助治疗。<br><br>　　Ce produit sert à traiter et à prévenir la diarrhée associée aux antibiotiques, la diarrhée du voyageur et d'autres sortes de diarrhée. Il est aussi applicable dans le traitement adjuvant du syndrome du côlon irritable (IBS) et des maladies inflammatoires de l'intestin. |
| 用法、用量<br>Les modes d'emploi et la posologie | 　　12 岁以上儿童及成人：口服，每次 1～2 粒，一日 2～3 次。<br><br>　　Chez des enfants plus de 12ans et des adultes : par voie orale, 1 à 2 capsules par fois, 2 à 3 jours par fois. |
| 剂型、规格<br>Les formes pharmaceutiques et les spécifications | 　　胶囊（肠溶）剂：每粒 250mg。<br><br>　　Capsules (à enrobage entérique) : 250mg par capsule. |
| 药品名称 Drug Names | 乳酶生 Lactasine |
| 适应证<br>Les indications | 　　用于消化不良、肠发酵、小儿饮食不当引起的腹泻等。<br><br>　　Ce produitsert à traiter la diarrhée causée par l'indigestion, la fermentation intestinale ou la mauvaise alimentation chez les enfants. |
| 用法、用量<br>Les modes d'emploi et la posologie | 　　每次 0.3～1.0g，一日 3 次，餐前服。<br><br>　　0,3 à 1,0g par fois, 3 fois par jour, pris avant le repas. |
| 剂型、规格<br>Les formes pharmaceutiques et les spécifications | 　　片剂：0.15g；0.3g。<br><br>　　Comprimés : 0,15g ou 0,3g. |

12.11　治疗肝性脑病药 Médicaments destinés au traitement de l'encéphalopathie hépatique

| 药品名称 Drug Names | 乳果糖 Lactulose |
|---|---|
| 适应证<br>Les indications | 　　用于肝性脑病的辅助治疗，也用于内毒素血症和治疗便秘。<br><br>　　Ce produit sert de traitement adjuvant de l'encéphalopathie hépatique. Il permet aussi de traiter l'endotoxémie et la constipation. |

| | |
|---|---|
| 用法、用量<br>Les modes d'emploi et la posologie | 治疗肝性脑病和内毒素血症：开始每次 10～20mg，一日 2 次，后改为每次 3～5g，一日 2～3 次；以每日排软便 2～3 次为宜。治疗肝性脑病时可将本品 200g 加入 700ml 水或生理盐水中，保留灌肠 30～60 分钟，每 4～6 小时 1 次。本品与新霉素合用可提高对肝性脑病的疗效。治疗便秘：每次 5～10mg，一日 1～2 次，应根据个人反应调节，如 48 小时未见效果，可适当增加剂量。<br><br>Pour traiter l'encéphalopathie hépatique et l'endotoxémie : la dose initiale, 10 à 20mg par fois, 2 fois par jour, ensuite, 3 à 5g par fois, 2 à 3 fois par jour ; expulser des selles molles 2 à 3 fois par jour. Pour traiter l'encéphalopathie, possible de dissoudre 200g de lactulose dans 700ml d'eau ou de solution saline, le lavement pendant 30 à 60 minutes, toutes les 4 à 6h. L'utilisation en association avec la néomycine peut renforcer l'efficacité du lactulose dans le traitement de l'encéphalopathie. Pour traiter la constipation : 5 à 10mg par fois, 1 à 2 fois par jour, selon les réactions des patients, s'il est inefficace dans les 48h, augmenter un peu la dose. |
| 剂型、规格<br>Les formes pharmaceutiques et les spécifications | 乳果糖粉：每袋 5g；100g；500g。<br>乳果糖颗粒：每袋 10g。<br>乳果糖口服液：5g（10ml）；50g（100ml）。<br>乳果糖糖浆：60%。<br><br>Le lactulose en poudre : 5g, 100mg ou 500g par sachet.<br>Le lactulose en granule : 10g par sachet.<br>La solution orale de lactulose : 5g (10ml) ou 50g (100ml).<br>Sirop de lactulose : 60%. |
| 药品名称 Drug Names | 谷氨酸钠 Glutamate de sodium |
| 适应证<br>Les indications | 用于肝性脑病及酸血症。<br>Ce produit sert à traiter l'encéphalopathie hépatique et l'acidémie. |
| 用法、用量<br>Les modes d'emploi et la posologie | 肝性脑病：每次静脉滴注 11.5g，用 5% 葡萄糖注射液 750～1000ml 或 10% 葡萄糖注射液 250～500ml 稀释，于 1～4 小时滴完，滴注过快可引起流涎、潮红、呕吐等。必要时可于 8～12 小时后重复给药，一日量不宜超过 23g。酸血症：用量根据病情决定。<br><br>Pour traiter l'encéphalopathie : 11,5g par fois en perfusion, dissoudre dans 750 à 1 000 ml de solution de glucose à 5% ou dans 250 à 500ml de solution de glucose à 10%, finir en 1 à 4 h, la vitesse excessive de la perfusion pourrait entraîner la salivation, la rougeur et des vomissements. S'il est nécessaire, reprendre le médicament 8 à 12h après, ne pas dépasser 23g par jour. Pour traiter l'acidémie: ajuster la dose selon les cas. |
| 剂型、规格<br>Les formes pharmaceutiques et les spécifications | 注射液：每支 5.75g/20ml。<br>Injection : 5.75g/20ml par solution. |
| 药品名称 Drug Names | 支链氨基酸 Acides aminés ramifiés |
| 适应证<br>Les indications | 支链氨基酸 3H 注射液、六合氨基酸注射液主要用于支 / 芳比失调引起的肝性脑病及各种肝病引起的氨基酸代谢紊乱。14 氨基酸 -800 主要用于肝功能不全合并蛋白营养缺乏症和肝性脑病。<br><br>Son injection 3H et l'injection des acides aminés sont utilisées dans le traitement de l'encéphalopathie hépatique et des troubles du métabolisme des acides aminés causés par des maladies hépatiques. Les acides aminés 14-800 sont appliqués dans le traitement du dysfonctionnement hépatique accompagné de la carence nutritionnelleen protéine et dans le traitement de l'encéphalopathie hépatique. |
| 用法、用量<br>Les modes d'emploi et la posologie | 静脉滴注：一日 2 次，每次 250ml，与等量 10% 葡萄糖注射液串联后做缓慢滴注（不宜超过 3ml/min）。如疗效显著者（完全清醒），后阶段剂量可减半。疗程一般为 10～15 日。中心静脉滴注：每日量以 0.68～0.87g/kg 计，成人剂量相当于每日 500～750ml，与 25%～50% 高渗葡萄糖注射液等量混匀后，经中心静脉缓慢滴注，低速不得超过 40 滴 / 分。. |

**续 表**

| | |
|---|---|
| | La perfusion : 2 fois par jour, 250ml par fois, dissoudre dans 250ml de solution de glucose à 10%, la perfusion lente (ne pas dépasser 3ml par minute). Si l'effet est évident, diminuer de moitié la dose pendant la deuxième partie du traitement. Un traitement médical dure entre 10 et 15 jours. La perfusion veineuse centrale : 0,68 à 0,87 g/kg par jour, chez des adultes, à savoir 500 à 750 ml par jour, dissoudre dans la solution de glucose hypertonique à 25% à 50 % de même quantité, la perfusion veineuse centrale lente, ne pas dépasser 40 gouttes par minute |
| 剂型、规格<br>Les formes pharmaceutiques et les spécifications | 注射液：250ml-10.65g（总氨基酸）。<br>Injection: 250ml-10.65g (acides aminés totale). |
| 药品名称 Drug Names | 谷氨酸钾 Glutamate de potassium |
| 适应证<br>Les indications | 用于肝性脑病、酸血症，常与谷氨酸钠合用，以维持电解质平衡。<br>Ce produit sert à traiter l'encéphalopathie hépatique et l'acidemia. Il est souvent utilisé en association avec le glutamate de sodium pour maintenir l'équilibre électrolytique. |
| 用法、用量<br>Les modes d'emploi et la posologie | 静脉滴注：每次 6.3g，其余用法、注意同谷氨酸钠。<br>En perfusion : 6,3g par fois, pour les modes d'emploi et les notes, c.f. au glutamate de sodium. |
| 剂型、规格<br>Les formes pharmaceutiques et les spécifications | 注射液：6.3g（20ml）。<br>Injection : 6,3g (20ml). |
| 药品名称 Drug Names | 精氨酸 Arginine |
| 适应证<br>Les indications | 用于肝性脑病，适用于忌钠患者。也适用于其他原因引起血氨过高所致的精神病状。<br>Ce produit sert à traiter l'encéphalopathie hépatique chez des patients résistant au sodium. Il est aussi applicable dans le traitement de l'état psychotique causé par l'hyperammoniémie. |
| 用法、用量<br>Les modes d'emploi et la posologie | 静脉滴注：一次 15～20g，以5%葡萄糖液 500～1000ml 稀释，滴注宜慢（每次4小时以上）。用其盐酸盐，可引起高氯性酸血症，肾功能不全者禁用。滴注太快可引起流涎、潮红、呕吐等。<br>En perfusion : 15 à 20g par fois, dissoudre dans 500 à 1 000ml de solution de glucose à 5%, perfusion lente (au moins 4h par fois). L'utilisation du chlorhydrate d'arginine pourrait entraîner l'acidémie haut en chlorure. Chez des patients insuffisants rénaux, il est interdit de l'utiliser. La vitesse excessive de la perfusion pourrait entraîner la salivation, la rougeur et des vomissements. |
| 剂型、规格<br>Les formes pharmaceutiques et les spécifications | 注射液：5g（20ml）。<br>Injection : 5g (20ml). |
| 药品名称 Drug Names | 谷氨酸 Acide Glutamique |
| 适应证<br>Les indications | 可预防肝性脑病；减少癫痫小发作发作次数；治疗胃酸不足。<br>Ce produit sert à traiter l'encéphalopathie hépatique, à réduire le nombre d'épisodes de l'épilepsie mineure et à traiterle manque d'acidité gastrique. |
| 用法、用量<br>Les modes d'emploi et la posologie | 预防肝性脑病：每次 2.5～5g，一日4次；用于癫痫小发作：每次 2～3g，一日 3～4次；治疗胃酸不足：一次 0.3g，一日3次。肾功能不全或无尿患者慎用。不宜与碱性药物合用。与抗胆碱药合用有可能减弱后者的药效。<br>Pour prévenir l'encéphalopathie : 2,5 à 5g par fois, 4 fois par jour ; pour traiter la crise mineure de l'épilepsie : 2 à 3g par fois, 3 à 4 fois par jour ; pour traiter le manque d'acidité gastrique : 0,3g par fois, 3 fois par jour. Chez des patients insuffisants rénaux ou des patients avec anurie, il faut faire attention. Il vaut mieux éviter l'utilisation en association avec des médicaments de base. L'utilisation en association avecles anticholinergiques pourrait réduire l'efficacité de ceux-ci. |

**续　表**

| 剂型、规格<br>Les formes pharmaceutiques et les spécifications | 片剂：每片 0.3g；0.5g。<br>Comprimés : 0,3g ou 0,5g par comprimé. |
|---|---|

**12.12　治疗肝炎辅助用药 Médicaments adjuvants pour traiter l'hépatite**

| 药品名称 Drug Names | 联苯双酯 Bifendate |
|---|---|
| 适应证<br>Les indications | 用于迁延性肝炎及长期单项丙氨酸氨基转移酶异常者。对肝炎主要症状如肝区痛、乏力、腹胀等的改善有一定疗效，但对肝脾大的改变无影响。<br><br>Ce produit sert à traiter l'hépatite persistante et les patients dont l'alanine aminotransférase est anormale pour une longue durée. Il est efficace dans l'amélioration de principaux symptômes de l'hépatite, tesl que les douleurs hépatiques, la fatigue et les ballonnements, mais il est peu efficace dans le traitement de l'hépatosplénomégalie. |
| 用法、用量<br>Les modes d'emploi et la posologie | 口服，一日量 75～150mg。多采用一日 3 次，每次服 25mg。<br>Par voie orale, 75 à 150mg par jour. Pour la plupart des cas, 3 fois par jour, 25mg par fois. |
| 剂型、规格<br>Les formes pharmaceutiques et les spécifications | 片剂：每片 25mg。<br>滴丸：每丸 1.5mg，口服，一次 7.5～15mg，一日 22.5～45mg。<br>Comprimés : 25mg par comprimé.<br>Pilules : 1,5mg par pilule, par voie orale, 7,5 à 15mg par fois, 22,5 à 45mg par jour. |

| 药品名称 Drug Names | 门冬氨酸钾镁 Aaspartate de magnésium potassium |
|---|---|
| 适应证<br>Les indications | 用于急性黄疸型肝炎、肝细胞功能不全，也可用于其他急慢性肝病。本品还可用于低钾血症、洋地黄中毒引起的心律失常、心肌炎后遗症、慢性心功能不全、冠心病等。<br><br>Ce produit sert à traiter l'hépatite de jaunisse aiguë, le dysfonctionnement hépatocellulaire ainsi que d'autres maladies aigues et chroniques hépatiques. Il est aussi applicable dans le traitement de l'arythmie, des séquelles de la myocardite, de l'insuffisance cardiaque chronique, ainsi que la maladie coronarienne causées par l'hypokaliémie et l'intoxication digitalique. |
| 用法、用量<br>Les modes d'emploi et la posologie | 注射液：一般为成人 10～20ml，加入 5% 或 10% 葡萄糖注射液 250～500ml 中缓慢静脉滴注，一日 1 次。儿童用量酌减。对重症黄疸患者，每日可用 2 次。对低血钾患者可适当加大剂量。口服：一般为一次 1 片，一日 3 次。由于各制品的含量有所不同，应用前须详阅产品说明书，并按其规定使用。<br><br>Injection : en général, chez des adultes, 10 à 20ml, dissoudre dans 250 à 500ml de solution de glucose à 5% ou à 10%, la perfusion lente, 1 fois par jour. Diminuer un peu la dose chez des enfants. Chez les patients atteints d'une jaunisse grave, possible de prendre 2 fois par jour. Pour les patients présentant une hypokaliémie, augmenter un peu la dose. Par voie orale : en général, 1 comprimé par fois, 3 fois par jour. Il faut lire attentivement les modes d'emploi pour chaque médicament, et suivre les indications, car la dose pour chaque médicament se différencie. |
| 剂型、规格<br>Les formes pharmaceutiques et les spécifications | 片剂：含门冬氨酸 252mg，钾 36.1mg，镁 11.8mg。<br>口服液：含无水 L- 门冬氨酸钾 451mg（钾 103mg），无水门冬氨酸镁 403.6mg（镁 34mg），按门冬氨酸计为 723mg，每支 5ml 或 10ml。<br>门冬氨酸钾镁注射液：每支 10ml（每 1ml 含无水 L- 门冬氨酸 85mg，钾 11.4mg、镁 4.2mg）。<br>注射用门冬氨酸钾镁：每瓶含无水 L- 门冬氨酸 850mg、钾 114mg、镁 42mg。<br>Comprimés : contenant 252mg d'aspartate, 36,1mg de potassium et 11,8mg de magnésium.<br>Solution orale : contenant 451mg de L-aspartate de potassium anhydrate (103mg de potassium), 403,6mg de L-aspartate de magnésium anhydrate (34mg de magnésium), mesuré en aspartate, 723mg, 5ml ou 10ml par solution.<br>Injection de l'aspartate de magnésium potassium : 10ml (1ml de produit contient 85mg de L-aspartate anhydrate, 11,4mg de potassium et 4,2mg de magnésium) par solution.<br>L'aspartate de magnésium potassium pour injection : chaque flacon contient 850mg de L-aspartate anhydrate, 114mg de potassium et 42mg de magnésium. |

**续 表**

| 药品名称 Drug Names | 水飞蓟宾 Silibinine |
|---|---|
| 适应证<br>Les indications | 慢性迁延性肝炎、慢性活动性肝炎、初期肝硬化、中毒性肝损伤等。<br>Ce produit sert à traiter l'hépatite chronique persistante, l'hépatite chronique active, la cirrhose précoce, l'atteinte hépatique toxique, etc. |
| 用法、用量<br>Les modes d'emploi et la posologie | 口服，每次 70～140mg，一日 3 次，餐后服。维持量可减半。<br>Par voie orale, 70 à 140mg par fois, 3 fois par jour, pris après le repas. Diminuer de moitié pour la dose d'entretien. |
| 剂型、规格<br>Les formes pharmaceutiques et les spécifications | 水飞蓟宾片：35mg，38.5mg。<br>水飞蓟宾胶囊剂：每粒 35mg，140mg。<br>水飞蓟宾葡甲胺片：50mg（相当于水飞蓟宾 35.6mg）。<br>Comprimés de silibinin : 35mg, 38,5mg.<br>Capsules de silibinin : 35mg ou 140mg par capsule.<br>Comprimés de méglumine de silibinin : 50mg (équivalent à 35,6mg de silibinin). |
| 药品名称 Drug Names | 牛磺酸 Taurine |
| 适应证<br>Les indications | 可用于急慢性肝炎、脂肪肝、胆囊炎等，也可用于支气管炎、扁桃体炎、眼炎等感染性疾病。感冒、乙醇戒断症状、关节炎、肌强直等可试用本品治疗。<br>Ce produit sert à traiter l'hépatite aiguë et chronique, la stéatose hépatique, la cholécystite. Il est aussi applicable dans le traitement des maladies infectieuses telles que la bronchite, l'amygdalite et l'ophtalmie. Il est aussi appliqué dans le traitement du rhume, des symptômes de sevrage de l'éthanol, de l'arthrite et de la rigidité musculaire. |
| 用法、用量<br>Les modes d'emploi et la posologie | 治疗急慢性肝炎，成人每次服 0.5g，一日 3 次；儿童每次 0.5g，一日 2 次。<br>Pour traiter l'hépatite aigue et chronique, 0,5g par fois chez des adultes, 3 fois par jour ; chez des enfants, 0,5g par fois, 2 fois par jour. |
| 剂型、规格<br>Les formes pharmaceutiques et les spécifications | 片（胶囊）剂：每片（粒）0.5g。<br>冲剂：每袋含牛磺酸 0.5g。<br>Comprimés (capsules) : 0,5g par comprimé ou par capsule.<br>Granules : chaque sachet contient 0,5g de taurine. |
| 药品名称 Drug Names | 促肝细胞生长因子 Facteur de croissance des hépatocytes |
| 适应证<br>Les indications | 用于亚急性重型肝炎（病毒性；肝衰竭早期或中期）的辅助治疗。<br>Ce produit sert de traitement adjuvant de hépatitesévèresubaiguë (virale ; l'insuffisance hépatique au stade précoce ou intermédiaire). |
| 用法、用量<br>Les modes d'emploi et la posologie | 口服，每次 100～150mg，一日 3 次，疗程 3 个月，可连续使用 2～4 个疗程；肌内注射，每次 40mg，一日 2 次；必要时也可将本品 80～120mg 加入 10% 葡萄糖注射液中静脉滴注，一日 1 次。疗程视病情而定，一般为 1 个月。<br>Par voie orale, 100 à 150mg par fois, 3 fois par jour, pendant 3 mois comme un traitement médical, possible de prendre 2 à 4 traitements de manière consécutive ; injection par voie IM, 40mg par fois, 2 fois par jour ; s'il est nécessaire, dissoudre dans 80 à 120mg de solution de glucose à 10%, en perfusion, 1 fois par jour. La durée du traitement varie en fonction des maladies, en général, pendant un moi. |
| 剂型、规格<br>Les formes pharmaceutiques et les spécifications | 颗粒剂：每袋 50mg。<br>注射用促肝细胞生长素：20mg。<br>Granules : 50mg par sachet.<br>Le facteur de croissance des hépatocytes pour injection : 20mg. |
| 药品名称 Drug Names | 甘草酸二铵 Glycyrrhiate de diammonium |
| 适应证<br>Les indications | 用于伴有 ALT 升高的慢性肝炎。<br>Ce produit sert à traiter l'hépatite chronique avec élévation des ALAT. |

**续　表**

| | |
|---|---|
| 用法、用量<br>Les modes d'emploi et la posologie | 口服，每次 150mg，一日 3 次；静脉滴注，30ml 用 10% 葡萄糖注射液 250ml 稀释后缓慢静脉滴注，一日 1 次。<br>Par voie orale, 150mg par fois, 3 fois par jour ; la perfusion, dissoudre 30ml de produit dans 250ml de solution de glucose à 10%, en perfusion lente, 1 fois par jour. |
| 剂型、规格<br>Les formes pharmaceutiques et les spécifications | 胶囊：每粒 50mg。<br>注射液：每支 50mg（10ml）。<br>Capsules : 50mg par capsule.<br>Injection : 50mg (10ml) par solution. |
| 药品名称 Drug Names | 硫普罗宁 Tiopronine |
| 适应证<br>Les indications | 用于：①脂肪肝、早期肝硬化、急慢性肝炎、酒精及药物引起的肝炎。②重金属中毒。③降低化疗及放疗的不良反应，升高白细胞，并可预防化疗、放疗所致二次肿瘤的发生。<br>Il est utilisé dans le traitement des cas suivants :<br>① La stéatose hépatique, lacirrhose précoce, l'hépatite aiguë et chronique etles hépatites causées par l'alcool et les médicaments. ② L'empoisonnement aux métaux lourds. ③ La réduction des effets indésirables de la chimiothérapie et de la radiothérapie, l'élévation du leucocyte ainsi que la prévention des tumeurs secondairescausées par la chimiothérapie et de la radiothérapie. |
| 用法、用量<br>Les modes d'emploi et la posologie | ①肝病治疗：餐后口服，每次 1～2 片，一日 3 次，连服 12 周，停药 3 个月后继续下一疗程；急性病毒性肝炎初期每次 2～4 片，一日 3 次，连服 1～3 周，以后每次 1～2 片，一日 3 次。②重金属中毒：每次 1～2 片，一日 2 次。③化疗及放疗引起的白细胞减少症：餐后口服，化疗及放疗前一周开始服用，每次 2～4 片，一日 2 次，连服 3 周。<br>① Pour traiter les maladies hépatiques : prendre après le repas par voie orale, 1 à 2 comprimés par fois, 3 fois par jour, pendant 12 semaines consécutives, 3 mois après l'arrêt de l'administration, reprendre un nouveau traitement ; pour traiter l'hépatite virale aigue, au début, 2 à 4 comprimés par fois, 3 fois par jour, pendant 1 à 3 semaines consécutives, ensuite, 1 à 2 comprimés par fois, 3 fois par jour. ② Pour traiter l'empoisonnement aux métaux lourds : 1 à 2 comprimés par fois, 2 fois par jour. ③ Pour traiter la leucopénie causée par la chimiothérapie et la radiothérapie : prendre après le repas par voie orale, commencer à prendre le médicament 1 semaine avant la chimiothérapie et la radiothérapie, 2 à 4 comprimés par fois, 2 fois par jour, pendant 3 semaines consécutives. |
| 剂型、规格<br>Les formes pharmaceutiques et les spécifications | 片剂：每片 0.1g。<br>Comprimés : 0,1g par comprimé. |
| 药品名称 Drug Names | 葡醛内酯 Glucurolactone |
| 适应证<br>Les indications | 用于急慢性肝炎、肝硬化；本品又有一定的解毒作用，可用于食物或药物中毒。<br>Il sert à traiter l'hépatite aiguë et chronique et la cirrhose hépatique. Il permet la désintoxication et est aussi applicable dans le traitement de l'intoxication alimentaire ou médicamenteuse. |
| 用法、用量<br>Les modes d'emploi et la posologie | 口服：一日 3 次，每次 0.1～0.2g。肌内或静脉注射：一日 1～2 次，每次 0.1～0.2g。<br>Par voie orale : 3 fois par jour, 0,1 à 0,2 g par fois. Injection par voie IM ou IV : 1 à 2 fois par jour, 0,1 à 0,2g par fois. |
| 剂型、规格<br>Les formes pharmaceutiques et les spécifications | 片剂：0.05g；0.1g。<br>注射液：0.1g（2ml）。<br>Comprimés : 0,05g ou 0,1g.<br>Injection : 0,1g (2ml). |

| 药品名称 Drug Names | 辅酶 A Coenzyme A |
|---|---|
| 适应证<br>Les indications | 用于白细胞减少症、原发性血小板减少性紫癜、功能性低热等，对脂肪肝、肝性脑病、急慢性肝炎、冠脉硬化、慢性动脉炎、心肌梗死、慢性肾功能减退引起的肾病综合征、尿毒症等可作为辅助治疗药。<br><br>Ce produit sert à traiter la leucopénie, le purpura thrombopénique idiopathique, la fièvre fonctionnelle, etc. Il est aussi applicable dans le traitement adjuvant de la stéatose hépatique, de l'encéphalopathie hépatique, l'hépatite aiguë et chronique, de la sclérose coronaire, de l'artérite chronique, de l'infarctus du myocarde, le syndrome néphrotique causé par une insuffisance rénale chronique, l'urémie, etc. |
| 用法、用量<br>Les modes d'emploi et la posologie | 静脉滴注：一日 1～2 次或隔日 1 次，每次 50～100U；肌内注射：一日 1 次，每次 50～100U。一般以 7～14 日为 1 个疗程。<br><br>En perfusion : 1 à 2 fois par jour ou tous les deux jours, 50 à 100 unités par fois ; injection par voie IM : 1 fois par jour, 50 à 100 unités par fois. En général, pendant 7 à 14 jours comme un traitement médical. |
| 剂型、规格<br>Les formes pharmaceutiques et les spécifications | 注射用辅酶 A：50U；100U。<br><br>Le coenzyme A pour injection : 50 unités ou 100 unités. |

## 12.13 利胆药 Cholésiques

| 药品名称 Drug Names | 熊去氧胆酸 Acide ursodésoxycholique |
|---|---|
| 适应证<br>Les indications | 用于不宜手术治疗的胆固醇型胆结石。应用时，仔细选择病例十分重要。对胆囊功能基本正常，结石直径在 5mm 以下，X 线能透过，非钙化型的浮动胆固醇型结石有较高的治愈率。结石的大小与溶石成功率密切相关，直径小于 5mm 者为 70%，5～10mm 者约为 50%。由于表面积/体积的比值较大，故较小的结石对治疗反应较好。本品不能溶解胆色素结石、混合结石及不透过 X 线的结石。对中毒性肝障碍、胆囊炎、胆道炎和胆汁性消化不良等也有一定的治疗效果。<br><br>Ce produit sert à traiter les calculs biliaires de cholestérol qui ne peuvent pas être traités par la chirurgie. Il faut sélectionner attentivement les cas. Il dispose d'un taux de guérison élevé dans le traitement des calculs flottants et non calcifiés de cholestérol, dont le diamètre est inférieur à 5mm, que les rayons X peuvent traverser et dont la fonction de la vésicule biliaire est normale. Son taux de réussite est étroitement lié à la taille des calculs : 70 % chez des calculs dont le diamètre est moins de 5mm et 50 % chez des calculs dont le diamètre est entre 5 et 10 mm. Il est plus efficace dans le traitement des calculs de petite taille. Il ne peut pas dissoudre les calculs de pigment biliaire, les calculs mixtes ni les calculs que les rayons X ne peuvent pas traverser. Il a aussi un certain effet sur les troubles toxiques hépatiques, lacholécystite, la cholangite ainsi que la dyspepsie biliaire. |
| 用法、用量<br>Les modes d'emploi et la posologie | 口服，利胆，1 次 50mg，一日 150mg。早、晚进餐时分次给予。疗程最短为 6 个月，6 个月后超声波检查及胆囊造影无改善者可停药；如结石已有部分溶解，则继续服药直至结石完全溶解。如治疗中有反复胆绞痛发作，症状无改善甚至加重，或出现明显结石钙化时，则宜终止治疗，并进行外科手术。溶胆石，一日 450～600mg，分 2 次服用。<br><br>Par voie orale : pour traite les maladies biliaires, 50mg par fois, 150mg par jour, pris durant le petit-déjeuner et le dîner. Pendant 6 mois au moins comme un traitement médical. S'il les symptômes ne s'améliorent pas à travers l'examen à ultrason et la cholécystographie après 6 mois de traitement, arrêter l'administration ; si les calculs sont partiellement dissous, continuer l'administration jusqu'à la dissolution totale des calculs. S'il y a une crise récurrente de la colique, et que les symptômes ne s'améliorent pas et même s'aggravent ou s'il y a une calcification évidente des calculs, il vaut mieux arrêter le traitement, et mener la chirurgie. Pour dissoudre les calculs biliaires, 450 à 600mg par jour, à travers 2 fois. |
| 剂型、规格<br>Les formes pharmaceutiques et les spécifications | 片剂：每片 50mg。<br><br>Comprimés : 50mg par comprimé. |

**续　表**

| 12.14　治疗炎性肠病药 Médicaments traitant la maladie inflammatoire de l'intestin | |
|---|---|
| 药品名称 Drug Names | 美沙拉秦 Mésalazine |
| 适应证<br>Les indications | 用于治疗溃疡性结肠炎、克罗恩病（Crohn 病）；栓剂用于治疗溃疡性直肠炎。<br>Ce produit sert à traiter la colite ulcéreuse et la maladie de Crohn. Administré en suppositoires, il permet aussi de traiter la proctite ulcéreuse. |
| 用法、用量<br>Les modes d'emploi et la posologie | ①口服：溃疡性结肠炎急性发作，每次 1g，一日 4 次。维持治疗，每次 0.5g，一日 3 次。克罗恩病，每次 1g，一日 4 次。儿童及老年人用量应酌减。②直肠给药：每次 1g，一日 1～2 次。<br>① Par voie orale : pour traiter la crise aigue de la colite ulcéreuse, 1g par fois, 4 fois par jour. Pour le traitement d'entretien, 0,5g par fois, 3 fois par jour. Pour traiter la maladie de Crohn, 1 g par fois, 4 fois par jour. Chez des enfants et des personnes âgées, diminuer un peu la dose. ② L'administration rectale : 1g par fois, 1 à 2 fois par jour. |
| 剂型、规格<br>Les formes pharmaceutiques et les spécifications | 片剂：每片 0.25g；0.4g；0.5g。<br>缓释片：每片 0.5g。<br>缓释颗粒：每袋 0.5g。<br>肠溶片：每片 0.5g。<br>栓剂：每粒 1g。<br>Comprimés : 0,25g, 0,4g ou 0,5g par comprimé.<br>Comprimés à libération prolongée : 0,5g par comprimé.<br>Capsules à libération prolongée : 0,5g par sachet.<br>Comprimé à enrobage entérique : 0,5g par comprimé.<br>Suppositoires : 1g par suppositoire. |
| 药品名称 Drug Names | 柳氮磺吡啶 Sulfasalazine |
| 适应证<br>Les indications | 主要用于炎症性肠炎，即 Crohn 病和溃疡性结肠炎。<br>Ce produit sert principalement à traiter l'entérite inflammatoire, à savoir la maladie de Crohn, et la proctite ulcéreuse. |
| 用法、用量<br>Les modes d'emploi et la posologie | 口服。成人常用量：初始剂量为一日 2～3g，分 3～4 次口服，无明显不适者，可渐增至一日 4～6g。待肠病症状缓解后逐渐减量至维持量，一日 1.5～2g。小儿初始剂量为一日 40～60mg/kg，分 3～6 次口服，病情缓解后改为维持量一日 30mg/kg，分 3～4 次口服。<br>Par voie orale. La dose usuelle chez des adultes : la dose initiale, 2 à 3g par jour, à travers 3 à 4 fois par voie orale, ensuite, possible d'augmenter progressivement pour atteindre 4 à 6g par jour. Après l'amélioration des symptômes, diminuer progressivement pour atteindre la dose d'entretien, soit 1,5 à 2g par jour. La dose initiale pour des enfants, 40 à 60 mg/kg par jour, à travers 3 à 6 fois par voie orale, après l'amélioration des symptômes, prendre la dose d'entretien, 30 mg/kg par jour, à travers 3 à 4 fois par voie orale. |
| 剂型、规格<br>Les formes pharmaceutiques et les spécifications | 片剂（胶囊剂）：每片（粒）0.25g。<br>栓剂：每粒 0.5g。<br>Comprimés (capsules) : 0,25g par comprimé ou par capsule.<br>Suppositoires : 0,5g par suppositoire. |
| 药品名称 Drug Names | 奥沙拉秦 Olsalazine |
| 适应证<br>Les indications | 用于治疗急慢性溃疡性结肠炎与节段性回肠炎，并用于缓解期的长期维持治疗。<br>Ce produit sert à traiter la colite ulcéreuse aiguë et chronique ainsi que l'iléite segmentaire. Il est aussi applicable dans le traitement d'entretien de la rémission à long terme. |
| 用法、用量<br>Les modes d'emploi et la posologie | 口服，治疗开始时每日 1g，分次服用，根据患者反应逐渐提高剂量至每日 3g，分 3～4 次服用。儿童为每日 20～40mg/kg。长期维持治疗，成人每日 1g，分 2 次服用；儿童每日 15～30mg/kg。本品随食物同服。<br>Par voie orale, la dose initiale, 1g par jour, à travers plusieurs fois, augmenter selon les réactions des patients la dose pour atteindre 3g par jour, à travers 3 à 4 fois. Chez des enfants, 20 à 40 mg/kg par jour. Pour le traitement d'entretien à long terme, chez des adultes, 1 g par jour, à travers 2 fois ; chez des enfants, 15 à 30 mg/kg par jour, pris avec des aliments. |

| 剂型、规格<br>Les formes pharmaceutiques et les spécifications | 胶囊剂：每粒 250mg。<br>Capsules : 250mg par capsule. |
|---|---|

### 12.15　其他消化系统用药 Autres médicaments pour l'appareil digestif

| 药品名称 Drug Names | 奥曲肽 Octréotide |
|---|---|
| 适应证<br>Les indications | 用于：①门静脉高压引起的食管静脉曲张破裂出血。②应激性溃疡及消化道出血。③重型胰腺炎及内镜逆行胰胆管造影（ＥＲＣＰ）术后急性胰腺炎并发症。④缓解由胃、肠及胰内分泌系统肿瘤所引起的症状。⑤突眼性甲状腺肿和肢端肥大症。⑥胃肠道瘘管。<br><br>Il sert à traiter : ① Les varices et les saignements oesophagiens causés par l'hypertension portale. ② L'ulcère de stress et les saignements gastro-intestinaux. ③ La pancréatite sévère et les complications de la pancréatite aiguë après la cholangiopancréatographie rétrograde endoscopique. ④ Soulager les symptômes causés par les tumeurs endocrines gastriques, intestinaux, pancréatiques. ⑤ Le goitreexophtalmique et l'acromégalie. ⑥ La fistule gastro-intestinale. |
| 用法、用量<br>Les modes d'emploi et la posologie | ①预防胰腺手术后并发症：手术前 1 小时，0.1mg 皮下注射；以后 0.1mg 皮下注射，一日 3 次，连续 7 日。②治门静脉高压引起的食管静脉曲张破裂出血：静脉注射开始 0.1mg，以后 0.5mg，每 2 小时 1 次静脉滴注。③应激性溃疡及消化道出血：皮下注射 0.1mg，一日 3 次。④重型胰腺炎：皮下注射 0.1mg，一日 4 次，疗程 3 ～ 7 日。⑤胃肠道瘘管和消化道内分泌系统肿瘤的辅助治疗：皮下注射 0.1mg，一日 3 次，疗程 10 ～ 14 日。⑥突眼性甲状腺肿和肢端肥大症：皮下注射 0.1mg，一日 3 次；肢端肥大症疗程和剂量需视疗效而定，有时可长达数月。<br><br>① Pour prévenir les complications après la chirurgie pancréatique : 1h avant la chirurgie, injecter 0,1mg par voie sous-cutanée ; après la chirurgie, injecter 0,1mg par voie sous-cutanée, 3 fois par jour, pendant 7 jours consécutifs. ② Pour traiter Les varices et les saignements oesophagiens causés par l'hypertension portale : injection par voie IV, au début, 0,1mg, ensuite, 0,5mg, toutes les 2h, en perfusion. ③ Pour traiter l'ulcère de stress et les saignements gastro-intestinaux : injecter par voie sous-cutanée 0,1mg, 3 fois par jour. ④ Pour traiter la pancréatite sévère : injection sous-cutanée, 0,1mg, 4 fois par jour, pendant 3 à 7 jours comme un traitement médical. ⑤ Pour le traitement adjuvant des tumeurs endocrines gastriques, intestinaux, pancréatiques : injecter 0,1mg par voie sous-cutanée, 3 fois par jour, pendant 10 à 14 jours comme un traitement médical. ⑥ Pour traiter le goitreexophtalmique et l'acromégalie, injecter par voie sous-cutanée 0,1mg, 3 fois par jour. La durée du traitement médical et sa dose pour le traitement de l'acromégalie dépendent de l'effet réel. Quelquefois, il faut prendre le médicament pendant plusieurs mois. |
| 剂型、规格<br>Les formes pharmaceutiques et les spécifications | 注射液：每支 0.1mg（1ml）。<br>Injection : 0,1mg (1ml) par solution. |

| 药品名称 Drug Names | 生长抑素 Somatostatine |
|---|---|
| 适应证<br>Les indications | 用于严重急性上消化道出血，如胃出血、十二指肠出血、胃和十二指肠溃疡出血、出血性胃炎、食管静脉曲张破裂出血等；预防胰腺术后及 ERCP 术后的并发症，急性胰腺炎，胰腺、胆囊和肠道瘘管的辅助性治疗；治疗类风湿关节炎引起的严重疼痛。<br><br>Ce produit sert à traiter le saignement gastro-intestinal supérieur aigu sévère, tel que le saignement gastrique, le saignement duodénal, le saignement des ulcères gastriques et duodénaux, la gastrite hémorragique, le saignement lié aux varices oesophagiennes. Il permet aussi de prévenir les complications après la chirurgie pancréatique et la CPRE. Il est aussi applicable dans le traitement adjuvant de la pancréatite aiguëet la fistule pancréatique, intestinale et de la vésicule biliaire. Il est également appliqué dans le traitement des douleurs causées par la polyarthrite rhumatoïde. |

**续　表**

| | |
|---|---|
| 用法、用量<br>Les modes d'emploi et la posologie | ①治疗上消化道出血，以 3mg 溶于 500ml0.9% 氯化钠或 5% 葡萄糖注射液中，连续 12 小时静脉滴注。某些病例可在连续滴注前给予 250μg 缓慢（不少于 3 分钟）静脉注射。为避免再出血，在止血后用同一剂量维持治疗 48～72 小时，总疗程不应超过 120 小时，延长静脉滴注时间并不加强效果。②预防胰腺术后并发症，在手术开始时以 250μg/h 速度连续静脉滴注，术后连续静脉滴注 5 日。③预防 ERCP 术后并发症，术前 1 小时以 250μg/h 速度连续静脉滴注，持续 12 小时。④急性胰腺炎：以 250μg/h 速度连续静脉滴注 5～7 日。⑤胰腺、胆囊及肠道瘘管的辅助性治疗，以 250μg/h 速度连续静脉滴注，直到瘘管闭合之后 2 日，在此期间应结合全胃肠外营养治疗，疗程应不超过 20 日。⑥治疗类风湿关节炎引起的严重疼痛，以 750μg 溶于 2ml0.9% 氯化钠注射液中做关节腔内注射，每隔 7 日或 15 日重复一次，连续 4～6 次。<br><br>① Pour traiter le saignement gastro-intestinal, dissoudre 3mg dans 500ml de solution de chlorure de sodium à 0,9% ou de solution de glucose à 5%, perfusion pendant 12 h consécutives. Chez certains patients, possible d'injecter 250 μg lentement (pendant 3 minutes au moins) avant la perfusion consécutive. Pour éviter le resaignement, prendre la même dose pendant 48 à 72h après l'arrêt du saignement comme traitement d'entretien. Mais le traitement médical ne dépasse pas 120 h, le prolongement du traitement n'augmente pas l'efficacité. ② Pour prévenir les complications de la chirurgie pancréatique, au début de la chirurgie, la perfusion continue avec une vitesse de 250 μg par h, après la chirurgie, la perfusion pendant 5 jours consécutifs. ③ Pour prévenir les complications de la CPRE, 1 h avant la chirurgie, la perfusion continue avec une vitesse de 250 μg par h, pendant 12 h consécutives. ④ Pour traiter la pancréatite aigue : la perfusion avec une vitesse de 250 μg par h, pendant 5 à 7 jours. ⑤ Pour le traitement adjuvant de la fistule pancréatique, intestinale et de la vésicule biliaire, la perfusion avec une vitesse de 250 μg par h jusqu'à 2 jours après la fermeture de la fistule. Pendant ce temps-là, il faut prendre en même temps la thérapie de nutrition parentérale totale. Le traitement ne dépasse pas 20 jours. ⑥ Pour traiter les douleurs graves causées par la polyarthrite rhumatoide, dissoudre 750 μg dans 2ml de solution de chlorure de sodium à 0,9% pour l'injection intra-articulaire, tous les 7 ou 15 jours, pendant 4 à 6 fois consécutives. |
| 剂型、规格<br>Les formes pharmaceutiques et les spécifications | 注射用生长抑素：每支 250μg；750μg；3mg。<br>La somatostatine pour injection : 250μg, 750μg ou 3mg par solution. |
| 药品名称 Drug Names | 抑肽酶 Aprotinine |
| 适应证<br>Les indications | 用于预防和治疗急性胰腺炎、纤维蛋白溶解所引起的出血、弥散性血管内凝血。也用于抗休克治疗。腹腔手术后，直接注入腹腔可预防术后肠粘连。<br><br>Ce produit sert à prévenir et à traiter la pancréatite aiguë, le saignement causé par la fibrinolyse et la coagulation intravasculaire disséminée. Il est aussi applicable dans l'anti-choc. Après la chirurgie abdominale, injecter directement ce produit dans la cavité abdominale peut prévenir les adhérences intestinales postopératoires. |
| 用法、用量<br>Les modes d'emploi et la posologie | 第 1～2 日，每日 8 万～12 万 U，首剂用量应大些，缓慢静脉注射（每分钟不超过 2ml）。维持剂量宜采用静脉滴注，每日 2 万～4 万 U。由纤维蛋白溶解引起的出血，应立即静脉注射 8 万～12 万 U，以后每 2 小时 1 万 U，直至出血停止。预防剂量：手术前一日开始，每日 2 万 U，共 3 日。治疗肠瘘及连续渗血也可局部应用。预防术后肠粘连，在手术切口闭合前，腹腔直接注入 2 万～4 万 U，注意勿与伤口接触。<br><br>Pendant les 1 à 2 premiers jours, 80 000 à 120 000 unités par jour, la dose initiale doit être importante, injection lente (ne pas dépasser 2ml par minute). Pour le traitement d'entretien, la perfusion, 20 000 à 40 000 unités par jour. Pour traiter le saignement causé par la fibrinolyse, injecter immédiatement 80 000 à 120 000 unités par voie IV, ensuite, 10 000 unités toutes les 2 h, jusqu'à l'arrêt de saignement. La dose pour la prévention : 1 jour avant la chirurgie, 20 000 unités par jour, pendant 3 jours. Pour traiter la fistule intestinale et l'hémorragie continue, possible d'appliquer l'administration topique. Pour prévenir les adhérences intestinales postopératoires, avant la fermeture de l'incision chirurgicale, injecter directement 20 000 à 40 000 unités dans la cavité abdominale. Éviter le contact avec les plaies. |

| 剂型、规格<br>Les formes pharmaceutiques et les spécifications | 注射抑肽酶：每支1万U；5万U；10万U；50万U。<br>L'aprotinine pour injection : 10 000 unités, 50 000 unités, 100 000 unités ou 500 000 unités par solution. |
|---|---|
| **药品名称 Drug Names** | **加贝酯 Gabexate** |
| 适应证<br>Les indications | 用于急性轻型（水肿型）胰腺炎；也可用于急性出血性坏死型胰腺炎的辅助治疗。<br>Ce produit sert à traiter la pancréatite aiguë bénigne (oedémateuse). Il est aussi applicable dans le traitement adjuvant de lapancréatite aiguë hémorragique nécrosante. |
| 用法、用量<br>Les modes d'emploi et la posologie | 仅供静脉滴注。每次100mg，治疗开始3日，每日用量300mg，症状减轻后改为每日100mg，疗程6～10日。先以5ml注射用水注入冻干粉针瓶内，待溶解后注入5%葡萄糖注射液或林格液500ml中，供静脉滴注用。滴注速度不宜过快，应控制在1mg/（kg·h）以内，不宜超过2.5mg/（kg·h）。<br>Il ne peut être administré qu'en perfusion. 100mg par fois, 3 jours après, 300mg par jour, après l'amélioration des symptômes, 100mg par jour, pendant 6 à 10 jours comme un traitement médical. Injecter d'abord 5ml d'eau pour injection dans la bouteille de poudre lyophilisée, après la dilution, injecter dans 500ml de solution de glucose à 5% ou de solution de Linger, pour la perfusion. La perfusion ne doit pas être trop vite, avec une vitesse de1mg/(kg•h), ne pas dépasser 2,5mg/(kg•h). |
| 剂型、规格<br>Les formes pharmaceutiques et les spécifications | 注射用加贝酯：每支0.1g。<br>Le gabexate pour injection : 0,1g par solution. |
| **药品名称 Drug Names** | **二甲硅油 Diméthicone** |
| 适应证<br>Les indications | 用于胃肠道胀气及急性肺气肿。<br>Ce produit sert à traiter la flatulence gastro-intestinale et l'emphysèmepulmonaire aigu. |
| 用法、用量<br>Les modes d'emploi et la posologie | ①消胀气：一次0.1～0.2g，一日3次，嚼碎服。②抢救急性肺水肿：使用气雾剂，用时将瓶倒置，距患者口鼻约15cm处，揿压瓶帽，在吸气时（或呼气终末时）连续喷入或与给氧同时进行，直至泡沫减少、症状改善为止。必要时可反复适用。<br>① Pour traiter la flatulence : 0,1 à 0,2g par fois, 3 fois par jour, les comprimés à mâcher. ② Pour sauver l'emphysème pulmonaire aigu : utiliser l'aérosol, inverser la bouteille, placer 15cm devant la bouche et le nez du patient, lors de l'inhalation, pulvériser de manière continue ou en association avec la pulvérisation de l'oxygène, jusqu'à la réduction des mousses et à l'amélioration des symplôtmes. S'il est nécessaire, l'administration répétée. |
| 剂型、规格<br>Les formes pharmaceutiques et les spécifications | 片剂：每片含二甲硅油25mg或50mg，另含氢氧化铝40mg或80mg，为分散剂。<br>二甲硅油气雾剂：每瓶总量18g，内含二甲硅油0.15g，此外尚含适量薄荷脑及抛射剂氟利昂（F12）。<br>二甲硅油散：含二甲硅油6%，为抗泡沫药。<br>Comprimés : chaque comprimé contient 25mg ou 50mg de siméthicone, et 40mg ou 80mg de d'hydroxyde d'aluminium, les comprimés dispersibles.<br>L'aérosol de siméthicone : chaque bouteille contient 18g, y compris 0,15g de siméthicone et certain menthol et propuleur fréon (F12).<br>La siméthicone en poudre : contenant la siméthicone à 6%, il s'agit de médicament anti-mousse. |

13. 影响血液及造血系统的药物 Médicaments affectant le système sanguin et hématopoïétique

13.1 促凝血药 Médicaments procoagulants

| **药品名称 Drug Names** | **亚硫酸氢钠甲萘醌 Bisulfite Ménadione de Sodium** |
|---|---|
| 适应证<br>Les indications | ①止血：用于阻塞性黄疸、胆瘘、慢性腹泻、广泛性切除所致肠吸收功能不全者，早产儿、新生儿低凝血酶原血症，香豆素类或水杨酸类过量以及其他原因所致凝血酶原过低等引起的出血。亦可用于预防长期口服广谱抗生素类药物引起的维生素K缺乏症。②镇痛：用于胆石症、胆道蛔虫病引起的胆绞痛。③解救杀鼠药"敌鼠钠"（diphacin）中毒：此时宜用大剂量。 |

|  | ① Il est utilisé dans l'hémostase : traiter les le dysfonctionnement de l'absorption intestinale caué par la jaunisse obstructive, la fistule biliaire, la diarrhée chronique et une large excision. Il permet aussi de traiter l'hypoprothrombinémiechez les enfants prématurés et les nouveau-nés, ainsi que le saignement causé par l'hypoprothrombinémie provoquée par la coumarine ou le surdosage d'acide salicylique.Il est également applicable dans la prévention de la carence en vitamine K causée par l'administration des antibiotiques à large spectre par voie orale à long terme. ② Il sert d'analgésique : utilisé dans el traitement des coliques biliaires causées par la lithiase biliaire,et l'ascaridiose biliaire. ③ Il sert aussi sauver l'empoisonnement par les rodenticides (Diphacinone de sodium) : il faut utiliser une forte dose. |
|---|---|
| 用法、用量<br>Les modes d'emploi et la posologie | ①止血：成人口服，一次 2～4mg，一日 6～20mg；肌内注射，每次 2～4mg，一日 4～8mg。防止新生儿出血，可在产前 1 周给妊娠期妇女肌内注射，每日 2～4mg。②胆绞痛：肌内注射，每次 8～16mg。<br><br>① Pour l'hémostase : chez des adultes, par voie orale, 2 à 4mg par fois, 6 à 20mg par jour ; injection par voie IM, 2 à 4mg par fois, 4 à 8mg par jour.Pour prévenir le saignement des nouveau-nés, injecter par voie IM 1 semaine avant l'accouchement des femmes pendant la grossesse, 2 à 4mg par jour. ② Pour traiter la colique : injection par voie IM, 8 à 16mg par fois. |
| 剂型、规格<br>Les formes pharmaceutiques et les spécifications | 片剂：每片 2mg。<br>注射液：每支 2mg（1ml）；4mg（1ml）。<br>Comprimés : 2mg par comprimé.<br>Injection : 2mg (1ml) ou 4mg (1ml) par solution. |
| 药品名称 Drug Names | 维生素 $K_1$ Phytoménadione (Vitamine $K_1$) |
| 适应证<br>Les indications | ①止血：用于阻塞性黄疸、胆瘘、慢性腹泻、广泛性切除所致肠吸收功能不全者、早产儿、新生儿低凝血酶原血症、香豆素类或水杨酸类过量以及其他原因所致凝血酶原过低等引起的出血。亦可用于预防长期口服广谱抗生素类药物引起的维生素 K 缺乏症。②镇痛：用于胆石症、胆道蛔虫病引起的胆绞痛。③解救杀鼠药"敌鼠钠"（diphacin）中毒：此时宜用大剂量。<br><br>① Il est utilisé dans l'hémostase : traiter les le dysfonctionnement de l'absorption intestinale caué par la jaunisse obstructive, la fistule biliaire, la diarrhée chronique et une large excision. Il permet aussi de traiter l'hypoprothrombinémiechez les enfants prématurés et les nouveau-nés, ainsi que le saignement causé par l'hypoprothrombinémie provoquée par la coumarine ou le surdosage d'acide salicylique.Il est également applicable dans la prévention de la carence en vitamine K causée par l'administration des antibiotiques à large spectre par voie orale à long terme. ② Il sert d'analgésique : utilisé dans el traitement des coliques biliaires causées par la lithiase biliaire,et l'ascaridiose biliaire. ③ Il sert aussi sauver l'empoisonnement par les rodenticides (Diphacinone de sodium) : il faut utiliser une forte dose. |
| 用法、用量<br>Les modes d'emploi et la posologie | 肌内注射或静脉注射：每次 10mg，一日 1～2 次，或根据具体病情而定；口服：每次 10mg，一日 3 次。<br><br>Injection par voie IM ou IV : 10mg par fois, 1 à 2 fois par jour, ou selon les maladies ; par voie orale, 10mg par fois, 3 fois par jour. |
| 剂型、规格<br>Les formes pharmaceutiques et les spécifications | 片剂：10mg。<br>注射液：10mg（1ml）；2mg（1ml）。<br>Comprimés : 10mg.<br>Injection : 10mg (1ml) ou 2mg (1ml). |
| 药品名称 Drug Names | 氨基己酸 Acide aminocaproïque |
| 适应证<br>Les indications | 用于纤溶性出血、如脑、肺、子宫、前列腺、肾上腺、甲状腺等外伤或手术出血。术中早期用药或术前用药，可减少手术中渗血，并减少输血量。亦用于肺出血、肝硬化出血及上消化道出血。 |

**续 表**

| | |
|---|---|
| | Ce produit sert à traiter l'hémorragie fibrinolytique, telle que le saignement lié au traumatisme du cerveau, du poumon, de l'utérus, de la prostate, des glandes surrénales et de la thyroïdeou le saignement chirurgical. Administré avant la chirurgie ou au stade précoce de la chirurgie, il permet de réduire le saignement chirurgical et ainsi la transfusion sanguine. Il est également applicable dans le traitement de l'hémorragie pulmonaire,du saignement lié à la cirrhose et du saignement gastro-intestinal supérieur. |
| 用法、用量<br>Les modes d'emploi et la posologie | 静脉滴注，初用量 4～6g，以 5%～10% 葡萄糖注射液或生理盐水 100ml 稀释，15～30 分钟滴完，维持量为每小时 1g，维持时间依病情而定，一日量不超过 20g，可连用 3～4 日。口服，成人，每次 2g，依病情服用 7～10 日或更久。<br><br>La perfusion, la dose initiale, 4 à 6g, dissoudre dans 100ml de solution de glucose à 5% à 10% ou de solution saline, finir en 15 à 30 minutes. La dose d'entretien, 1g par h, la durée du traitement d'entretien varie en fonction des maladies. Ne pas dépasser 20g par jour, pendant 3 à 4 jours consécutifs. Par voie orale, chez des adultes, 2g par fois, pendant 7 à 10 jours ou plus selon les cas. |
| 剂型、规格<br>Les formes pharmaceutiques et les spécifications | 片剂：每片 0.5g。<br>注射液：每支 1g（10ml）；2g（10ml）。<br>Comprimés : 0,5g par comprimé.<br>Injection : 1g (10ml) ou 2g (10ml) par solution. |
| 药品名称 Drug Names | 氨甲苯酸 Acide aminométhylbenzoïque |
| 适应证<br>Les indications | 用于纤维蛋白溶解过程亢进所致的出血，如肺、肝、胰、前列腺、肾上腺等手术时的异常出血，妇产科和产后出血以及肺结核咳血或痰中带血、血尿、前列腺肥大出血、上消化道出血等，对一般慢性渗血效果较显著，但对癌症出血以及创伤出血无止血作用。此外，尚可用于链激酶或尿激酶过量引起的出血。<br><br>Ce produit sert à traiter le saignement causé par l'hyperthyroïdie au processus de fibrinolytique, tel que lessaignements anormaux lors de la chirurgie liée au poumon, au foie, au pancréa, à la prostate, et aux glandes surrénales, le saignement obstétrique, l'hémorragie du post-partum, l'hémoptysie liée à la tuberculose, des expectorations sanglantes, l'hématurie, le saignement de l'hypertrophie de la prostate, le saignement gastro-intestinal supérieur, etc. Il est surtout efficace dans le traitement du saignement chronique, mais inefficace dans le traitement du saignement cancéreux et du saignement traumatique. En outre, il est aussi appliqué dans le traitement du saignement causé parle surdosage de la streptokinase ou de l'urokinase. |
| 用法、用量<br>Les modes d'emploi et la posologie | 静脉注射，每次 0.1～0.3g，用 5% 葡萄糖注射液或 0.9% 氯化钠注射液 10～20ml 稀释后缓慢注射，一日最大用量 0.6g。<br><br>Injection par voie IV, 0,1 à 0,3g par fois, dissoudre dans 10 à 20ml de solution de glucose à 5% ou de solution de chlorure de sodium à 0,9%, injection lente, ne pas dépasser 0,6g par jour. |
| 剂型、规格<br>Les formes pharmaceutiques et les spécifications | 片剂：每片 0.125g；0.25g。<br>注射液：每支 0.05g（5ml）；0.1g（10ml）。<br>Comprimés : 0,125g ou 0,25g par comprimé.<br>Injection : 0,05g (5ml) ou 0,1g (10ml) par solution. |
| 药品名称 Drug Names | 血凝酶 Hémocoagulase |
| 适应证<br>Les indications | 可用于治疗和防治多种原因引起的出血。<br>Il sert à prévenir et à traiter les saignements d'origine multiple. |
| 用法、用量<br>Les modes d'emploi et la posologie | 静脉注射、肌内注射，也可局部使用。成人：每次 1000～2000U，紧急情况下，立即静脉注射 1000U，同时肌内注射 1000U。各类外科手术：手术前 1 小时，肌内注射 1000U；或手术前 15 分钟，静脉注射 1000U。手术后每日肌内注射 1000U，连用 3 日，或遵医嘱。<br><br>Injection par voie IV ou IM, ou l'administration topique. Chez des adultes : 1000 à 2000U par fois, en cas d'urgence, injecter immédiatement 1000U par voie IV, injecter en même temps 1000U par voie IM. Pour la chirurgie de toutes sortes : 1h avant la chirurgie, injecter 1000U par voie IM ; ou 15 minutes avant la chirurgie, injecter 1000U par voie IV. Après la chirurgie, injecter 1000U par voie IM par jour, pendant 3 jours consécutifs, ou selon les ordonnances. |

**续　表**

| | |
|---|---|
| 剂型、规格<br>Les formes pharmaceutiques et les spécifications | 注射用凝血酶（REPTILASE）每支 0.5kU；1kU；2kU。<br>L'hémocoagulase pour injection : 0.5kU, 1kU ou 2kU par solution. |
| **药品名称 Drug Names** | 酚磺乙胺 Etamsylate |
| 适应证<br>Les indications | 用于预防和治疗外科手术出血过多，血小板减少性紫癜或过敏性紫癜以及其他原因引起的出血，如脑出血、胃肠道出血、泌尿道出血、眼底出血、牙龈出血、鼻出血和皮肤出血等。<br>Ce produit sert à prévenir et à traiter les saignements excessifs chirurgicaux, le purpura hémorragique, le purpura anaphylactique ou d'autres saignements, tels que l'hémorragie cérébrale, l'hémorragie gastro-intestinale, l'hémorragie du tractus urinaire, l'hémorragie rétinienne, des saignements des gencives, desépistaxis et le saignement de la peau. |
| 用法、用量<br>Les modes d'emploi et la posologie | ①预防手术出血：术前 15～30 分钟静脉注射或肌内注射，一次 0.25～0.5g，必要时 2 小时后再注射 0.25g，一日 0.5～1.5g。②治疗出血：成人，口服，每次 0.5～1g，一日 3 次。肌内注射或静脉注射每次 0.25～0.5g，一日 2 次或 3 次。也可与 5% 葡萄糖注射液或生理盐水混合静脉滴注，每次 0.25～0.75g，一日 2 次或 3 次，必要时可根据病情增加剂量。<br>① Pour prévenir les saignements chirurgicaux : 15 à 30 minutes avant la chirurgie, injection par voie IV ou IM, 0,25 à 0,5g par fois, s'il est nécessaire, 2 h après, injecter 0,25g, administrer 0,5 à 1,5g par jour. ② Pour traiter les saignements : chez des adultes, par voie orale, 0,5 à 1g par fois, 3 fois par jour. Injection par voie IM ou IV, 0,25 à 0,5g par fois, 2 à 3 fois par jour. Ou dissoudre dans la solution de glucose à 5% ou de solution saline pour la perfusion, 0,25 à 0,75g par fois, 2 à 3 fois par jour, s'il est nécessaire, augmenter la dose selon les cas. |
| 剂型、规格<br>Les formes pharmaceutiques et les spécifications | 片剂：每片 0.25g；0.5g。<br>注射液：每支 0.25g（2ml）；0.5g（5ml）；1.0g（5ml）。<br>Comprimés : 0,25g ou 0,5g par comprimé.<br>Injection : 0,25g (2ml), 0,5g (5ml) ou 1,0g (5ml) par solution. |
| **药品名称 Drug Names** | 卡巴克络 Carbazochrome |
| 适应证<br>Les indications | 用于毛细血管通透性增加所致的出血，如特发性紫癜、视网膜出血、慢性肺出血、肠胃出血、鼻出血、咯血、血尿、痔出血、子宫出血、脑出血等。<br>Ce produit sert à traiter les saignements causés par l'augmentation de la perméabilité capillaire, tels que le purpura idiopathique, l'hémorragie rétinienne, l'hémorragie pulmonaire chronique, l'hémorragie gastro-intestinale, les épistaxis, l'hémoptysie, l'hématurie, les saignements des hémorroïdes, les saignements utérins, et l'hémorragie cérébrale. |
| 用法、用量<br>Les modes d'emploi et la posologie | ①卡络柳钠片：口服，每次 2.5～5mg，一日 3 次。卡络柳钠注射液：肌内注射，每次 5～10mg，一日 2～3 次。不可静脉注射。②注射用卡络磺钠：肌内注射，每次 20mg，一日 2 次；静脉注射，每次 25～50mg，一日 1 次；静脉滴注，每次 60～80mg，加入输液中滴注。<br>① Carbazochrome salicylate de sodium comprimés: par voie orale, 0,5~1g par fois, 3 fois par jour. Carbazochrome salicylate de sodium injection: par injection IM, 5~10mg par fois, 2~3 fois par jour. Non injectable par voie intraveineuse. ② Carbazochrome sulfonate de sodium pour injection: par injection IM, 20mg par fois, 2 fois par jour; par injection IV, 25~50mg par fois, 1 fois par jour; Goutte intraveineuse: 60~80mg par fois, ajouter à la perfusion. |
| 剂型、规格<br>Les formes pharmaceutiques et les spécifications | 卡络柳钠片：每片 2.5mg；5mg。<br>卡络柳钠注射液：每支 5mg（1ml）；10mg（2ml）。<br>注射用卡络磺钠：20mg。<br>Les comprimés de salicylate de sodium de carbazochrome : 2,5mg ou 5mg par comprimé.<br>L'injection de salicylate de sodium de carbazochrome : 5mg (1ml) ou 10mg (2ml) par solution.<br>Le sulfonate de sodium de carbazochrome pour injection : 20mg. |
| **药品名称 Drug Names** | 重组人凝血因子Ⅷ Facteur Ⅷ de Coagulation Humain Recombinante |
| 适应证<br>Les indications | 用于纠正和预防凝血因子Ⅷ缺乏或因患获得性因子Ⅷ抑制物增多症而引起的出血。主要用于治疗甲型血友病。<br>Ce produit sert à traiter et à prévenir l'hémorragie causée par le manque de facteur VIII de coagulation. Il est principalement utilisé comme traitement de l'hémophilie A. |

**续 表**

| 用法、用量<br>Les modes d'emploi et la posologie | 　静脉滴注：①轻度关节出血：一次 8 ～ 10U/kg，一日 1 ～ 2 次，连用 1 ～ 4 日；使 F Ⅷ c 水平提高到正常水平的 15% ～ 20%。②中度关节，肌肉出血：一次 15U/kg，一日 2 次，需用 3 ～ 7 日，使 F Ⅷ c 水平提高到正常水平的 30%。③大出血或严重外伤而无出血证据：一次 25U/kg，一日 2 次，至少用 7 日；使 F Ⅷ c 水平提高到正常水平的 50%。④外科手术或严重外伤伴出血：40 ～ 50U/kg 于术前 1 小时开始输注，使 F Ⅷ c 水平达到正常水平的 80% ～ 100%，随后使 F Ⅷ c 水平维持在正常水平的 30% ～ 60%，10 ～ 14 日。⑤预防出血：体重大于 50kg，一日 500U；小于 50kg 者，一日 250U。使 F Ⅷ c 水平达到到正常水平的 5% ～ 10%。⑥抗 F Ⅷ c 抗体生成伴出血：首剂 5000 ～ 10 000U/h，维持剂量为 300 ～ 1000U/h，使体内 F Ⅷ c 水平维持在 30 ～ 50U/ml，如联合应用血浆交换术，宜追加本品 40U/kg，以增强疗效。<br><br>　La perfusion : ① Pour traiter le saignement articulaire bénin : 8 à 10 U/kg par fois, 1 à 2 fois par jour, pendant 1 à 4 jours consécutifs ; augmenter le niveau du F VIIIc à 15 à 20 % du niveau normal. ② Pour traiter le saignement articulaire ou musculaire modéré : 15 U par kg par fois, 2 fois par jour pendant 3 à 7 jours, augmenter le niveau du F VIII c à 30% du niveau normal. ③ Pour traiter une hémorragie sévère ou un traumatisme sans preuve de saignement : 25 U par kg par fois, 2 fois par jour, pendant 7 jours au moins, augmenter le niveau du F VIIIc à 50% du niveau normal. ④ Pour la chirurgie ou un traumatisme sévère accompagné de saignement : 1 h avant la chirurgie, 40 à 50 U par kg, augmenter le niveau F VIIIc à 80 à 100 % du niveau normal, ensuite, ensuite maintenir le niveau F VIII c à 30 à 60 % du niveau normal, pendant 10 à 14 jours. ⑤ Pour prévenir le saignement : chez plus de 50kg, 500 U par jour ; chez moins de 50kg, 250 U par jour. Augmenter le niveau du F VIIIc à 5 à 10 % du niveau normal. ⑥ Pour lutter contre la formtion d'anticorps du F VIII accompagnée de l'hémorragie : la dose initiale, 5 000 à 10 000 U par h, la dose d'entretien, 30 à 50 U par ml, s'il est utilisé en association avec l'échange de plasma, il faut prendre encore 40 U par kg pour renforcer l'efficacité. |
| --- | --- |
| 剂型、规格<br>Les formes pharmaceutiques et les spécifications | 　人凝血因子Ⅷ：每瓶 100U；200U；250U；300U；400U；500U；750U；1000U。<br>　Le facteur VIII de coagulation humain : 100U, 200U, 250U, 300U, 400U, 500U, 750U ou 1 000 par flacon. |
| **药品名称 Drug Names** | 重组人血小板生成素 Thrombopoïétine humaine recombinante |
| 适应证<br>Les indications | 　用于治疗实体瘤化疗后所致的血小板减少症，适用对象为血小板低于 $50 \times 10^9$/L 且医师认为有必要升高血小板治疗的患者。<br>　Ce produit sert à traiter la thrombocytopénie causée par la chimiothérapie des tumeurs solides. Il est applicable chez des patients dont la plaquette sanguine est inférieure à $50 \times 10^9$/L et dont le médecin pense qu'il est nécessaire d'augmenter la plaquette sanguine. |
| 用法、用量<br>Les modes d'emploi et la posologie | 　恶性实体肿瘤化疗时，可于给药结束后 6 ～ 24 小时皮下注射本品，剂量为每日 300U/kg，一日 1 次，连用 14 日。<br>　Lors de la chimiothérapie des tumeurs solides, injecter ce produit par voie sous-cutanée 6 à 24 h après l'administration, 300 U par kg, 1 fois par jour, pendant 14 jours. |
| 剂型、规格<br>Les formes pharmaceutiques et les spécifications | 　注射液：7500 U（1ml）；15 000 U（1ml）。<br>　Injection : 7500 U (1ml) ou 15 000 U (1ml). |
| **药品名称 Drug Names** | 重组人白细胞介素 -11 Interleukine-11 humaine recombinante |
| 适应证<br>Les indications | 　用于实体瘤和白血病放、化疗后血小板减少症的预防和治疗及其他原因引起的血小板减少症的治疗。<br>　Ce produit sert à prévenir et à traiter la thrombocytopénie causée par la radiothérapie et la chimiothérapiedes tumeurs solides et de la leucémie. Il est également applicable dans le traitement de la thrombocytopénie causée par d'autres facteurs. |

续　表

| 用法、用量<br>Les modes d'emploi et la posologie | 应用剂量为 25μg/kg，于化疗结束后 24～48 小时起或发生血小板减少症后皮下注射，一日 1 次，疗程一般为 7～14 日。血小板计数恢复后应及时停药。<br>25 μg par kg, 24 à 48 h après la chimiothérapie, ou lors de la thrombocytopénie, injection par voie sous-cutanée, 1 fois par jour, pendant 7 à 14 jours comme un traitement médical. Après la récupération du nombre plaquettaire, il faut arrêter immédiatement l'administration. |
|---|---|
| 剂型、规格<br>Les formes pharmaceutiques et les spécifications | 注射用重组人白介素 -11：每支 1.5mg；3.0mg。<br>L'interleukine-11 recombinante humaine pour injection : 1,5mg ou 3,0 mg par solution. |
| 药品名称 Drug Names | 云南白药 YunNanBaiYao |
| 适应证<br>Les indications | 缩短凝血时间，具有止血作用。<br>Il sert à raccourcir le temps de coagulation et permet l'hémostase. |
| 用法、用量<br>Les modes d'emploi et la posologie | 成人每次服 0.2～0.3g，重症可酌加，但一次不宜超过 0.5g，每隔 4 小时服 1 次。若初服无反应，可连续服用。小儿 2 岁以上者，每次服 0.03g；5 岁以上者，每次服 0.06g。<br>Chez des adultes, 0,2 à 0,3g par fois, augmenter la dose pour traiter les cas sévères. Mais ne pas dépasser 0,5g par fois, toutes les 4 h. S'il n'y pas de réaction pour la première dose, possible de le prendre de manière consécutive. Chez des enfants plus de 2 ans, 0,03g par fois ; chez des enfants de plus de 5 ans, 0,06g par fois. |
| 剂型、规格<br>Les formes pharmaceutiques et les spécifications | 胶囊：250mg；气雾剂：85g。<br>Capsules : 250mg. Aérosol : 85g. |
| 药品名称 Drug Names | 氨甲环酸 Acide tranexamique |
| 适应证<br>Les indications | 用于各种出血性疾病、手术时异常出血等。<br>Ce produit sert à traiter des maladies hémorragiques, des saignements anormaux pendant la chirurgie, etc. |
| 用法、用量<br>Les modes d'emploi et la posologie | 口服，每次 1.0～1.5g，一日 2～6g。静脉注射或静脉滴注：每次 0.25～0.5g，一日 0.75～2g。静脉注射以 25% 葡萄糖注射液稀释，静脉滴注液以 5%～10% 葡萄糖注射液稀释。<br>Par voie orale, 1,0 à 1,5g par fois, 2 à 6g par jour. Injection par voie IV ou en perfusion : 0,25 à 0,5g par fois, 0,75 à 2g par jour. Pour l'injection IV, utiliser la solution de glucose à 25% pour la dilution ; pour la perfusion, utiliser la solution de glucose à 5 % à 10% pour la dilution. |
| 剂型、规格<br>Les formes pharmaceutiques et les spécifications | 片剂：0.125g；0.25g。<br>胶囊：0.25g。<br>注射液：0.1g（2ml）；0.2g（2ml）；0.25g（5ml）；0.5g（5ml）；1.0g（10ml）。<br>注射用氨甲环酸：0.2g；0.4g；0.5g；1.0g。<br>Comprimés : 0,125g ou 0,25g.<br>Capsules : 0,25g.<br>Injection : 0,1g (2ml), 0,2g (2ml), 0,25g (5ml), 0,5g (5ml) ou 1,0g (10ml).<br>L'acide tranexamique pour injection : 0,2g, 0,4g, 0,5g ou 1,0g. |
| 药品名称 Drug Names | 鱼精蛋白 Protamine |
| 适应证<br>Les indications | 用于因注射肝素过量而引起的出血，以及自发性出血如咳血。<br>Ce produit est utilisé comme traitement de l'hémorragie causée par le surdosage d'héparine et des saignements spontanés tels que l'hémoptysie. |
| 用法、用量<br>Les modes d'emploi et la posologie | ①抗肝素过量：静脉注射，用量应与最后一次作用肝素量相当（本品 1mg 中可中和肝素 100U），但一次不超过 50mg。②抗自发性出血：静脉滴注，每日 5～8mg/kg，分 2 次，间隔 6 小时。每次以生理盐水 300～500ml 稀释。连用不宜超过 3 日。注射宜缓慢（10 分钟内注入量以不超过 50mg 为度）。 |

续表

| | ① Pour lutter contre le surdosage d'héparine : injection par voie IV, en fonction de la dose de l'héparine de la dernière fois (1mg de protamine peut neutraliser 100 unités d'héparine), mais ne pas dépasser 50mg par fois. ② Pour lutter contre les saignements spontanés : injection par voie IV, 5 à 8 mg/kg par fois, à travers 2 fois, toutes les 6h. Utiliser 300 à 500ml de solution saline pour la dilution. Ne pas administrer pendant plus de 3 jours consécutifs. Injection doit être lente (ne pas dépasser 50 mg en 10 minutes). |
|---|---|
| 剂型、规格<br>Les formes pharmaceutiques et les spécifications | 硫酸鱼精蛋白注射液：50mg（5ml）；100mg（10ml）。<br>注射用硫酸鱼精蛋白：50mg。<br>L'injection de sulfate de protamine : 50mg (5ml) ou 100mg (10ml).<br>Le sulfate de protamine pour injection : 50mg. |
| 药品名称 Drug Names | 凝血酶 Thrombine |
| 适应证<br>Les indications | 局部止血药。可用于局部出血及消化道出血。<br>Ce produit sert d'hémostatique topique. Il est applicable dans le traitement du saignement local et des saignements gastro-intestinaux. |
| 用法、用量<br>Les modes d'emploi et la posologie | 局部出血：以干燥粉末或溶液（50～250U/ml）喷洒或喷雾于创伤表面。消化道出血：以溶液（10～100U/ml）口服或局部灌注。严禁注射。<br>Pour l'hémostatique topique : pulvériser la poudre sèche ou la solution (50 à 250 U par ml) sur la zone touchée. Pour traiter les saignements gastro-intestinaux : prendre la solution (10 à 100U par ml) par voie orale ou par la perfusion locale. L'injection est interdite. |
| 剂型、规格<br>Les formes pharmaceutiques et les spécifications | 凝血酶冻干粉剂：200U；500U；1000U；2000U；5000U；10 000U。<br>La poudre lyophilisée de thrombine : 200U；500U; 1000U；2 000u；5000U；10 000U. |
| 药品名称 Drug Names | 凝血酶原复合物 Complexe de prothrombine |
| 适应证<br>Les indications | 用于手术、急性肝坏死、肝硬化等所致出血的防治。<br>Ce produit sert à prévenir et à traiter l'hémorragie causée par la chirurgie, la nécrose hépatique aiguë, la cirrhose, etc. |
| 用法、用量<br>Les modes d'emploi et la posologie | 本品仅供静脉滴注，且用前新鲜配制。每瓶加注射用水 25ml 使溶，按输血法过滤，滴速不超过 60 滴 / 分。<br>Ce produit n'est administré qu'en perfusion. Préparer la solution juste avant de l'utiliser. Ajouter 25ml d'eau pour injection pour la dissolution, filtrer par transfusion, ne pas dépasser 60 gouttes par minute. |
| 剂型、规格<br>Les formes pharmaceutiques et les spécifications | 注射剂（冻干粉）：200U；400U。<br>Injection (poudre lyophilisée) : 200U ou 400U. |

13.2 抗凝血药 Anticoagulants

| 药品名称 Drug Names | 枸橼酸钠 Citrate Sodique |
|---|---|
| 适应证<br>Les indications | 仅用于体外抗凝血。<br>Il n'est applicable que dans l'anticoagulantextracorporel. |
| 用法、用量<br>Les modes d'emploi et la posologie | 输血时预防凝血，每 100ml 全血加入 2.5% 输血用枸橼酸钠注射液 10ml。<br>Pour prévenir la coagulation pendant la transfusion, ajouter 10ml d'injection de citrate de sodium pour transfusion à 2,5% dans 100ml de sang total. |
| 剂型、规格<br>Les formes pharmaceutiques et les spécifications | 输血用枸橼酸钠注射液：为枸橼酸钠的灭菌水溶液，含枸橼酸钠 2.35%～2.65%。<br>L'injection de citrate de sodium pour transfusion : la solution aqueuse stérile de citrate de sodium, contenant 2,35 % à 2,65% de citrate de sodium. |

**续　表**

| 药品名称 Drug Names | 肝素钠 Héparine Sodique |
|---|---|
| 适应证<br>Les indications | ①预防血栓形成和栓塞，如深部静脉血栓、心肌梗死、肺栓塞、血栓静脉炎及术后血栓形成等。②治疗各种原因引起的弥散性血管内凝血（DIC），如细菌性脓毒血症、胎盘早期剥离、恶性肿瘤细胞溶解所致的 DIC，但蛇咬伤所致的 DIC 除外。早期应用可防止纤维蛋白原和其他凝血因子的消耗。③其他体外抗凝血，如心导管检查、心脏手术外循环、血液透析等。<br><br>① Ce produit permet de prévenir la thrombose et l'embolie, telles que la thrombose veineuse profonde, l'infarctus du myocarde, l'emboliepulmonaire,la thrombophlébite et la thrombose postopératoire. ② Il sert à traiter la coagulation intravasculaire disséminée (CID) causée par divers facteurs, telle que la septicémie bactérienne, le décollement placentaire, la CID causée par la lyse des cellules cancéreuses, non compris la CID causée par la morsure de serpent. Appliqué au stade précoce, il permet de prévenir la consommation du fibrinogène et d'autres facteurs de la coagulation. ③ Autres anticoagulantsextracorporels, tels que le cathétérisme cardiaque, la chirurgie cardiaque de pontage, l'hémodialyse, etc. |
| 用法、用量<br>Les modes d'emploi et la posologie | ①静脉注射：成人首剂 5000U 加入 100ml0.9% 氯化钠注射液中，在 30～60 分钟滴完。需要时可每隔 4～6 小时重复静脉滴注 1 次，每次 5000U，总量可达 25 000U/d。为维持恒定血药浓度，也可每 24 小时 10 000～20 000U 加入 1000ml0.9% 氯化钠注射液中静脉滴注，速度 20 滴 / 分。用于体外循环时，375U/kg；体外循环超过 1 小时者，每 1kg 体重加 125U。②静脉注射或深部肌内注射（或皮下注射）：每次 5000～10 000U。<br><br>① La perfusion : chez des adultes, la dose initiale, dissoudre 5000 U de produit dans 100ml de solution de chlorure de sodium à 0,9%, la perfusion pendant 30 à 60 minutes. En cas de besoin, reprendre la perfusion toutes les 4 à 6 h, 5000U par fois, ne pas dépasser 25 000 U par jour. Pour maintenir une concentration constante du médicament dans le sang, possible de dissoudre 10 000 à 20 000 U dans 100ml de solution de chlorure de sodium à 0,9% pour la perfusion toutes les 24h, avec une vitesse de 20 gouttes par minute. Pour la circulation extraporelle, 375U par kg ; chez des patients dont la circulation extraporelle dépasse 1 h, utiliser 125U supplémentaire par kg. ② L'injection par voie IV ou IM profonde (ou sous-cutanée) : 5000 à 10 000 unités par fois. |
| 剂型、规格<br>Les formes pharmaceutiques et les spécifications | 注射液：每支 1000U（2ml）；5000U（2ml）；12 500U（2ml）。<br>Injection : 1000U (2ml), 5000U (2ml) ou 12 500U (2ml) par solution. |

| 药品名称 Drug Names | 肝素钙 Héparine Calcique |
|---|---|
| 适应证<br>Les indications | 用于预防和治疗血栓 - 栓塞性疾病及血栓形成。本品具有较明显的抗醛固酮活性，故亦适于人工肾、人工肝和体外循环使用。<br><br>Ce produit sert à prévenir et à traiter la thrombose et des maladies thrombus-emboliques. Comme il a une activité anti-aldostérone évidente, il est applicable dans le rein artificiel, lefoie artificiel et la circulation extracorporelle. |
| 用法、用量<br>Les modes d'emploi et la posologie | ①用于血栓 - 栓塞意外：皮下注射，首次 0.01ml/kg，5～7 小时后以 APTT 检测剂量是否合适，12 小时 1 次，每次注射后 5～7 小时进行新的检查，连续 3～4 日。②用于内科预防：皮下注射，首剂 0.005ml/kg，注射后 5～7 小时以 APTT 检测调整合适剂量，一次 0.2ml，一日 2～3 次，或一次 0.3ml，一日 2 次。③用于外科预防：皮下注射，术前 0.2ml，术后每 12 小时 0.2ml，至少持续 10 日。<br><br>① Pour traiter des accidents thrombus-emboliques : injection sous-cutanée, au début, 0,01ml par kg, 5 à 7h après, conduire la TCA pour juger si la dose est pertinente, toutes les 12h. 5 à 7 h après l'injection, conduire la TCA, pendant 3 à 4 jours. ② Pour la prévention de la médecine générale : injection sous-cutanée, la dose initiale, 0,005ml par kg, 5 à 7h après, conduire la TCA pour juger si la dose est pertinente, 0,2ml par fois, 2 à 3 fois par jour, ou 0,3ml par fois, 2 fois par jour. ③ Pour la prévention chirurgicale : injection sous-cutanée, 0,2ml avant la chirurgie, après la chirurgie, 0,2ml toutes les 12h, pendant 10 jours consécutifs au moins. |

**续 表**

| 剂型、规格<br>Les formes pharmaceutiques et les spécifications | 注射液：2500U（0.3ml）。<br>Injection : 2500U (0,3ml). |
|---|---|
| **药品名称 Drug Names** | 低分子量肝素 Héparine de faible poids moléculaire |
| 适应证<br>Les indications | ①预防深部静脉血栓形成和肺栓塞。②治疗已形成的急性深部静脉血栓。③在血液透析或血液滤过时，防止体外循环系统中发生血栓或血液凝固。④治疗不稳定型心绞痛及非 ST 段抬高心肌梗死。<br>① Ce produit sert à prévenir la thrombose veineuse profonde et l'embolie pulmonaire. ② Il sert à traiter la thrombose veineuse profonde aiguë formée. ③ Lors de l'hémodialyse ou de l'hémofiltration, il permet de prévenir la thrombose ou la coagulation sanguine dans le système de circulation extracorporelle. ④ Il permet aussi de traiter l'angine de poitrine instable et l'infarctus du myocarde sans élévation du segment ST. |
| 用法、用量<br>Les modes d'emploi et la posologie | ①本品给药途径为腹壁皮下注射或静脉注射或遵医嘱。②血透时预防血凝块形成。<br>① Administré par voie sous-cutanée abdominale ou IV ou selon les ordonnances. ② Lors de l'hémodialyse, prévenir la coagulation sanguine. |
| 剂型、规格<br>Les formes pharmaceutiques et les spécifications | 针剂：5000U。<br>Injection : 5000U. |
| **药品名称 Drug Names** | 华法林 Warfarine |
| 适应证<br>Les indications | ①防治血栓栓塞性疾病，可防止血栓形成与发展，如治疗血栓栓塞性静脉炎，降低肺栓塞的发病率和死亡率，减少外科大手术、风湿性心脏病、髋关节固定术、人工置换心脏瓣膜手术等的静脉血栓发生率。②心肌梗死的治疗辅助用药。<br>① Ce produit sert à prévenir et à traiter la maladie thromboembolique, à prévenir la thrombose et son développement, à traiter la phlébite thromboembolique, àréduire l'incidence et la mortalité de l'embolie pulmonaire, et à réduire l'incidence de la thrombose veineuse lors de l'intervention chirurgicale majeure, des cardiopathies rhumatismales, dela fixation de la hanche,et de la chirurgie de prothèse de valve cardiaque. ② Il sert aussi de traitement adjuvant de l'infarctus du myocarde. |
| 用法、用量<br>Les modes d'emploi et la posologie | 口服，第 1 日 5 ～ 20mg，次日起用维持量，一日 2.5 ～ 7.5mg。<br>Par voie orale, le premeir jour, 5 à 20mg, à partir du 2ème jour, prendre la dose d'entretien, 2,5 à 7,5 mg par jour. |
| 剂型、规格<br>Les formes pharmaceutiques et les spécifications | 片剂：每片 2.5mg；5mg。<br>Comprimés : 2,5mg ou 5mg par comprimé. |
| **药品名称 Drug Names** | 利伐沙班 Rivaroxaban |
| 适应证<br>Les indications | 用于髋关节或膝关节置换手术成年患者，以预防静脉血栓形成（VTE）。<br>Il est applicable chez des patients faisant l'objet de l'arthroplastie de la hanche ou du genou pour prévenir la thrombose veineuse. |
| 用法、用量<br>Les modes d'emploi et la posologie | 口服，10mg，一日 1 次。如伤口已止血，首次用药时间应于手术后 6 ～ 10 小时进行。<br>Par voie orale, 10mg, 1 fois par jour. S'il le saignement s'arrête sur la zone touchée, la première administration doit être conduite 6 à 10 h après la chirurgie. |

| 续　表 | |
|---|---|
| 剂型、规格<br>Les formes pharmaceutiques et les spécifications | 片剂：每片 10mg。<br>Comprimés : 10mg par comprimé. |
| **药品名称 Drug Names** | 重组链激酶 Streptokinase Recombinante |
| 适应证<br>Les indications | 用于治疗血栓栓塞性疾病，如深静脉血栓、周围动脉栓塞、急性肺栓塞、血管外科手术后的血栓形成、导管给药所致血栓形成、新鲜心肌梗死、中央视网膜动静脉栓塞等。<br>Ce produit sert à traiter les maladies thromboemboliques, telles que la thrombose veineuse profonde, la thrombose artérielle périphérique, l'embolie pulmonaire, la formation de thrombose après la chirurgie vasculaire, la thrombosedue au cathétérisme,l'infarctus du myocarde frais, la thrombose de la veine rétinienne centrale, etc. |
| 用法、用量<br>Les modes d'emploi et la posologie | 一般推荐本品 150 万 U 溶解于 5% 葡萄糖 100ml，静脉滴注 1 小时。<br>Il est généralement recommandé de dissoudre 1,5 million d'unités de streptokinase dans 100ml de solution de glucose à 5%, la perfusion pendant 1h. |
| 剂型、规格<br>Les formes pharmaceutiques et les spécifications | 注射用冻干链激酶：每支 10 万 U；15 万 U；20 万 U；25 万 U；30 万 U；50 万 U；75 万 U；150 万 U。<br>La streptokinase lyophilisée pour injection : 100 000 U, 150 000 U, 200 000 U, 250 000U, 300 000U, 500 000U, 750 000U ou 1,5 million d'u par solution. |
| **药品名称 Drug Names** | 尿激酶 Urokinase |
| 适应证<br>Les indications | 用于急性心肌梗死、肺栓塞、脑血管栓塞、周围动脉或静脉栓塞、视网膜动脉或静脉栓塞等。也可用于眼部炎症、外伤性组织水肿、血肿等。<br>Ce produit sert à traiter l'infarctus aigu du myocarde, l'embolie pulmonaire, l'embolie cérébrale, la thrombose artérielle ou veineuse périphérique, la thrombose de l'artère ou la veine rétinienne, etc. Il est aussi applicable dans le traitement de l'inflammation oculaire, de l'œdème et de l'hématome traumatiques. |
| 用法、用量<br>Les modes d'emploi et la posologie | ①肺栓塞：初次剂量 3 万～4 万 U，间隔 24 小时重复给药一次，最多使用 3 次。②心肌梗死：建议 0.9% 氯化钠注射液配制后，按 6000U/min 的给药速度冠状动脉内连续滴注 2 小时，滴注前应先行静脉给予肝素 2500～10 000U。<br>① Pour traiter l'embolie pulmonaire : la dose initiale, 30 000 à 40 000U, toutes les 24h, ne pas dépasser 3 fois. ② Pour traiter l'infarctus du myocarde : il est recommandé de dissoudre dans la solution de chlorure de sodium à 0,9%, la perfusion continue intracoronaire pendant 2h avec une vitesse de 6 000unités par minute. Avant la perfusion, il faut d'abord injecter par voie iV 2 500 à 10 000 unités d'héparine. |
| 剂型、规格<br>Les formes pharmaceutiques et les spécifications | 注射用尿激酶：每瓶 1 万 U；5 万 U；10 万 U；20 万 U；25 万 U；50 万 U；150 万 U；250 万 U。<br>L'urokinase pour injection : 10 000U, 50 000U, 100 000U, 200 000U, 250 000 U, 500 000 U, 1,5 million d'u ou 2,5 million d'u par flacon. |
| **药品名称 Drug Names** | 阿替普酶 Alteplase |
| 适应证<br>Les indications | 用于急性心肌梗死和肺栓塞的溶栓治疗。<br>Ce produit sert de traitement thrombolytique de l'infarctus aigu du myocarde et de l'embolie pulmonaire. |
| 用法、用量<br>Les modes d'emploi et la posologie | ①静脉注射：将本品 50mg 溶于灭菌注射用水中，使溶液浓度为 1mg/ml，给予静脉注射。②静脉滴注：将本品 100mg 溶于 0.9% 氯化钠注射液 500ml 中，在 3 小时内按以下方式滴完，即：前 2 分钟先注入 10mg，以后 60 分钟内滴入 50mg，最后剩余时间内滴完所余 40mg。<br>① Injection par voie IV : dissoudre 50mg d'alteplase dans l'eau stérile pour injection, pour que la concentration de la solutoin soit de 1mg par ml, injection par voie iV. ② La perfusion : dissoudre 100mg d'alteplase dans 500ml de solution de chlorure de sodium à 0,9%, la perfusion en 3h en suivant les démarches suivantes : administrer 10mg en 2 minutes, pendant les 60 minutes suivantes, administrer 50mg en perfusion, pour le reste du temps, administrer les autres 40mg en perfusion. |

**续 表**

| 剂型、规格<br>Les formes pharmaceutiques et les spécifications | 注射用：每瓶 20mg；50mg。<br>L'alteplase pour injection : 20mg ou 50mg par flacon. |
|---|---|
| **药品名称 Drug Names** | **瑞替普酶 Retéplase** |
| 适应证<br>Les indications | 用于成人由冠状动脉梗死引起的急性心肌梗死的溶栓疗法，能改善心功能。<br>Appliqué chez des adultes, ce produit sert de traitement thrombolytique de l'infarctus aigu du myocarde causé par l'infarctus artériel coronarien. Il permet d'améliorer la fonction cardiaque. |
| 用法、用量<br>Les modes d'emploi et la posologie | 10MU 缓慢静脉注射 2～3 分钟以上，间隔 30 分钟后可重复给药（10MU）1 次，目前尚无 2 次以上重复给药的经验。<br>10MU, injecter lentement par voie IV pendant 2 à 3 minutes au moins, 30 minutes après, possible d'administrer 10MU encore une fois. Pour le moment, l'administration se limite à 2 fois. |
| 剂型、规格<br>Les formes pharmaceutiques et les spécifications | 注射用：每支 5.0MU。<br>La retéplase pour injection : 5,0 MU pour injection. |
| **药品名称 Drug Names** | **巴曲酶 Defibrine** |
| 适应证<br>Les indications | 用于急性缺血性脑血管病，突发性耳聋，慢性动脉闭塞症如闭塞性血栓脉管炎、闭塞性动脉硬化症和末梢循环障碍等。<br>Ce produit sert à traiter les maladies cérébro-vasculaires ischémiques aigues, la surdité brusque, l'artériopathie oblitérante chronique, telle que la vascularite thrombus occlusive, l'artériosclérose oblitérante et les troubles circulatoires périphériques. |
| 用法、用量<br>Les modes d'emploi et la posologie | 静脉滴注：成人首次 10 巴曲酶单位（BU），以后隔日 1 次，5BU。使用前用 100～200ml 的 0.9% 氯化钠注射液静脉滴注 1 小时以上。通常疗程为 1 周，必要时可增至 3～6 周。<br>La perfusion : chez des adultes, la dose initiale, 10BU, ensuite, 5 BU tous les deux jours. Dissoudre dans 100 à 200ml de solution de chlorure de sodium à 0,9% pour la perfusion pendant 1h au moins. Pendant 1 semaine comme un traitement médical, s'il est nécessaire, pendant 3 à 6 semaines. |
| 剂型、规格<br>Les formes pharmaceutiques et les spécifications | 注射液：每支 10BU（1ml）；5BU（0.5ml）。<br>Injection : 10 BU (1ml) ou 5BU (0,5ml) par solution. |
| **药品名称 Drug Names** | **蚓激酶 Lumbrokinase** |
| 适应证<br>Les indications | 用于缺血性脑血管病中纤维蛋白原增高及血小板聚集率增高的患者。<br>Ce produit sert à traiter des patients atteints de maladies cérébro-vasculaires ischémiques et accompagnés d'une augmentation du fibrinogène et de l'agrégation des plaquettes taux accrue. |
| 用法、用量<br>Les modes d'emploi et la posologie | 口服：一次 2 粒，一日 3 次，餐前半小时服用。3～4 周为 1 个疗程，也可连续服用。<br>Par voie orale : 2 capsule par fois, 3 fois par jour, pris 0,5h avant le repas. Pendant 3 à 4 semaines comme un traitement médical, possible de le prendre de manière consécutive. |
| 剂型、规格<br>Les formes pharmaceutiques et les spécifications | 肠溶胶囊：每粒 30 万 U。<br>Capsules à enrobage entérique : 300 000 unités par capsule. |

**续　表**

### 13.3　血浆代用品 Substituts plasmatiques

| 药品名称 Drug Names | 右旋糖酐 40 Dextrane 40 |
|---|---|
| 适应证<br>Les indications | ①各种休克：用于失血、创伤、烧伤及中毒性休克，还可早期预防因休克引起的弥散性血管内凝血。②体外循环时，还可代替部分血液预充心肺机。③血栓性疾病如脑血栓形成、心绞痛和心肌梗死、血栓闭塞性脉管炎、视网膜动静脉血栓、皮肤缺血性溃疡等。④肢体再植和血管外科手术，可预防术后血栓形成，并可改善血液循环，提高再植成功率。<br><br>① Ce produit sert à lutter contre toutes sortes de choc : le choc hémorragique, traumatique, le choc lié aux brûlures et le choc toxique, il permet aussi de prévenir au stade précoce la coagulation intravasculaire disséminée causée par le choc. ② Lors de la circulation extracorporelle, il sert à préremplir la machine cœur-poumon en remplaçant du sang. ③ Il sert à traiter les maladies thrombotiques telles que la thrombose cérébrale, l'angine de poitrine, l'infarctus du myocarde, la thromboangéite oblitérante, la thrombose de la veine et de l'artère rétiniennes, les ulcères ischémiques de la peau, etc. ④ Il est utilisé dans la réimplantation des membres et la chirurgie vasculaire pour prévenir la thrombose postopératoire, améliorer la circulation sanguine et améliorer le taux de succès de la réimplantation. |
| 用法、用量<br>Les modes d'emploi et la posologie | 静脉滴注（10% 溶液），每次 250～500ml，成人和儿童每日不超过 20ml/kg。抗休克时滴注速度为 20～40ml/min，在 15～30 分钟注入 500ml。对冠心病和脑血栓患者应缓慢静脉滴注。疗程视病情而定，通常每日或隔日 1 次，7～14 次为 1 个疗程。<br><br>La perfusion (la solution à 10%), 250 à 500ml par fois, chez des adultes et des enfants, ne pas dépasser 20ml par kg. Pour l'anti-choc, 20 à 40 ml par minute pour la perfusion, administrer 500ml en 15 à 30 minutes. Chez des patients atteints de maladie coronarienne et la thrombose cérébrale, la perfusion doit être lente. Ajuster la durée du traitement en fonction des maladies, en général, 1 fois par jour ou tous les 2 jours, pendant 7 à 14 fois comme un traitement médical. |
| 剂型、规格<br>Les formes pharmaceutiques et les spécifications | 右旋糖酐 40（低分子右旋糖酐）葡萄糖注射液：每瓶 10g（100ml）；25g（250ml）；50g（500ml）；6g（100ml）；15g（250ml）；30g（500ml）。均含葡萄糖 5%。<br>右旋糖酐 40（低分子右旋糖酐）氯化钠注射液：每瓶 10g（100ml）；25g（250ml）；50g（500ml）；6g（100ml）；15g（250ml）；30g（500ml）。均含氯化钠 0.9%。<br><br>L'injection de glucose de dextran 40 (dextran à faible poids moléculaire): 10g (100ml), 25g (250ml), 50g (500ml), 6g (100ml), 15g (250ml), 30mg (500ml) par flacon. Tout cela contient le glucose à 5%.<br>L'injection de chlorure de sodium de dextran 40 (dextran à faible poids moléculaire) : 10g (100ml), 25g (250ml), 50g (500ml), 6g (100ml), 15g (250ml), 30mg (500ml) par flacon. Tout cela contient le chlorure de sodium à 0,9%. |
| 药品名称 Drug Names | 右旋糖酐 70 Dextrane 70 |
| 适应证<br>Les indications | 用于防治低血容量休克如出血性休克、手术中休克、烧伤性休克。也可用于预防手术后血栓形成和血栓性静脉炎。<br><br>Ce produit sert à prévenir et à traiter le choc hypovolémique, tel que le choc hémorragique, le choc opératoire et le choc lié aux brûlures. Il est aussi applicable dans la prévention de la thrombose postopératoire et de la thrombophlébite. |
| 用法、用量<br>Les modes d'emploi et la posologie | 静脉滴注，每次 500ml，每分钟注入 20～40ml。每日最大量不超过 1000～1500ml。<br><br>En perfusion, 500ml par fois, 20 à 40ml par minute. Ne pas dépasser 1 000 à 1 500 ml par jour. |
| 剂型、规格<br>Les formes pharmaceutiques et les spécifications | 右旋糖酐 70（中分子右旋糖酐）葡萄糖注射液：每瓶 30g（500ml），含葡萄糖 5%。右旋糖酐 70（中分子右旋糖酐）氯化钠注射液：每瓶 30g（500ml），含氯化钠 0.9%。<br><br>L'injection de glucose de dextran 70 (le dextran àpoids moléculaire moyen) : 30g (500ml) par flacon, qui contient le glucose à 5%. L'injection de chlorure de sodium de dextran 70 (le dextran àpoids moléculaire moyen) : 30g (500ml) par flacon, qui contient le chlorure de sodium à 0,9%. |

**续　表**

| 药品名称 Drug Names | 右旋糖酐 10　Dextrane 10 |
|---|---|
| 适应证<br>Les indications | 　　用于急性失血性休克、创伤及烧伤性休克、急性心肌梗死、心绞痛、脑血栓形成、脑供血不足、血栓闭塞性脉管炎、雷诺病等。此外，术前有低血容量以及硬膜外麻醉后所致的低血压者均可使用本品升压。<br><br>　　Ce produit sert à traiter le choc hémorragique aigu, le choc traumatique, le choc lié aux brûlures, l'infarctus aigu du myocarde, l'angine de poitrine, la thrombose cérébrale, l'insuffisance cérébrale, la thrombose oblitérante, la maladie de Raynaud, etc. En plus, il est aussi applicable chez des patients accompagnés de l'hypovolémique préopératoire ou atteints d'hypotension causée par l'anesthésie péridurale, pour permettre l'augmentation de la pression artérielle. |
| 用法、用量<br>Les modes d'emploi et la posologic | 　　静脉滴注：速度为 5～15ml/min，血压上升后，可酌情减慢。每次 500～1000ml（参见药品说明书）。<br><br>　　En perfusion : 5 à 15 ml par minute, après l'augmentation de la pression artérielle, ralendir un peu. 500 à 1 00ml par fois (consulter les modes d'emploi). |
| 剂型、规格<br>Les formes pharmaceutiques et les spécifications | 　　右旋糖酐 10（低分子右旋糖酐）葡萄糖注射液：每瓶 30g（500ml）；50g（500ml），均含葡萄糖 5%。<br>　　右旋糖酐 10（低分子右旋糖酐）氯化钠注射液：每瓶 30g（500ml）；50g（500ml），均含氯化钠 0.9%。<br><br>　　L'injection de glucose de dextran 10 (le dextran à petit poids moléculaire) : 30g (500ml) ou 50g (500ml) par flacon, qui contient le glucose à 5%.<br>　　L'injection de chlorure de sodium de dextran 10 (le dextran à petit poids moléculaire) : 30g (500ml) par flacon ou 50g (500ml) par flacon, qui contient le chlorure de sodium à 0,9%. |
| 药品名称 Drug Names | 琥珀酰明胶 Gélatine succinylée |
| 适应证<br>Les indications | 　　用于各种原因引起的低血容量休克的早期治疗，如失血、创伤或手术、烧伤、败血症、腹膜炎、胰腺炎或挤压伤等引起的休克。也可用于体外循环或预防麻醉时出现的低血压。<br><br>　　Ce produit est utilisé dans le traitement précoce du choc hypovolémique, tel que le choc causé par la perte de sang, un traumatisme ou une intervention chirurgicale, les brûlures, la septicémie, la péritonite, la pancréatite, ou les blessures d'écrasement. Il est aussi applicable dans le traitement de l'hypotention lors de la circulation extracorporelle ou de la prévention de l'anesthésie. |
| 用法、用量<br>Les modes d'emploi et la posologie | 　　静脉输入的剂量和速度取决于患者的实际情况。严重急性失血时可在 5～10 分钟输入 500ml，直至低血容量症状缓解。快速输入时应加温液体但不超过 37℃。大量输入时应确保维持血细胞比容不低于 25%。大出血者，本品可于血液同时使用。可经同一输液器输入本品和血液。成人少量出血，可在 1～3 小时输入 500～1000ml。<br><br>　　La dose et la vitesse de la perfusion intraveineuse dépendent de la situation des patients. Lors de l'hémorragie aigue et sévère, possible d'administrer 500ml en perfusion en 5 à 10 minutes, jusqu'à l'amélioration des symptômes de l'hypovolémie. Lors de la perfusion rapide, il faut chauffer le liquide jusqu'à 37 degré au maximum. Lors de la perfusion massive, il faut maintenir l'hématocritesupérieur à 25%. Chez des patients souffrant d'hémorragie massive, ce produit peut être administré en perfusion avec le sang en même temps. Chez des adultes souffrant d'hémorragie peu importante, possible d'administrer en perfusion 500 à 1000ml en 1 à 3h. |
| 剂型、规格<br>Les formes pharmaceutiques et les spécifications | 　　注射液：每瓶 500ml。<br>　　Injection : 500ml par flacon. |
| 药品名称 Drug Names | 羟乙基淀粉 200/0.5 Hydroxyéthy lamidon 200/0.5 |
| 适应证<br>Les indications | 　　用于预防和治疗各种原因引起的血容量不足和休克，如手术、创伤、感染、烧伤等；急性等容血液稀释，减少手术中对供血的需要，节约用血；治疗性血液稀释，改善血液流变学指标，使红细胞聚集减少，血细胞和血液黏稠度下降，改善微循环。据报道，本品还有防止和堵塞毛细血管漏的作用，在毛细血管通透性增加的情况下使用本品，可减少白蛋白渗漏，减轻组织水肿，减少炎症介质产生，对危重患者更有利。 |

| 续　表 |
|---|

| | Ce produit sert à prévenir et à traiter l'hypovolémie et le choc causés par divers facteurs, tels que la chirurgie, le traumatisme, l'infection, labrûlure, etc. Il est appliqué dans l'hémodilution normovolémique aiguë, réduisant la demande de sang lors de la chrurgie ; il est aussi utilisé dans l'hémodilution thérapeutique,ce qui améliore la rhéologie du sang, réduit l'agrégation des globules rouges,diminue la viscositédes globules et du sang, et améliore la microcirculation. Selon des rapports, il est aussi applicable dans la prévention du colmatage de la fuite de capillaires. En cas d'augmentation de la perméabilité capillaire, l'utilisation de ce produit permet de réduire les fuites d'albumine, l'œdème des tissus et le nombre des médiateurs de l'inflammation, favorisant ainsi les patients gravement malades. |
|---|---|
| 用法、用量<br>Les modes d'emploi et la posologie | 静脉滴注。由于会有过敏反应发生，开始的 10～20ml 应缓慢滴注，每日用量和滴注速度取决于失血量、血液浓缩程度，每日总量不应大于 33ml/kg（6% 浓度），在心肺功能正常的患者，其血细胞比容应不低于 30%。①治疗和预防容量不足或休克（容量替代治疗）：使用不同浓度中分子羟乙基淀粉溶液最大剂量 6% 的为 33ml/kg，10% 的为 20ml/kg。②急性等容血液稀释（ANH）：手术前即刻开展 ANH，按 1∶1 比例，每日剂量（2～3）×500ml（6%），采血量：（2～3）×500ml（自体血），输注速度 1000ml/（15～30min），采血速度 1000ml/（15～30min）。③治疗性血液稀释：治疗可分为等容血液稀释（放血）和高容血液稀释（不放血），按药物不同浓度，给药剂量每日可分为低（250ml）、中（500ml）、高（1000ml）三种，滴注速度：0.5～2 小时 250ml，4～6 小时 500ml，8～24 小时 1000ml，建议治疗 10 日。<br><br>En perfusion. Comme il y a des réactions allergiques, pour les premiers 10 à 20ml, la perfusion doit être lente. La dose par jour et la vitesse de la perfusion dépendent de la perte de sang et du degré d'enrichissement de sang. La dose totale ne doit pas dépasser 33ml par kg (à 6%) par jour. Chez des patients dont la fonction cardiaque et pulmonaire est normale, l'hématocrite ne doit pas être inférieure à 30 %.<br>① Pour prévenir et traiter l'hypovolémie et le choc : la dose maximale pour l'injection d'hydroxyéthylamidon de poids moléculaire à 6 % est de 33 ml par kg, alors que pour l'injection d'hydroxyéthylamidon de poids moléculaire à 10%, la dose maximale est de 20ml par kg. ② Pour l'hémodilution normovolémique aiguë (HNA) : appliquer l'HNA immédiatement avant la chirurgie, à un ratio de 1 : 1, la dose par jour : (2 à 3) ×500ml (6%), le volume de l'échantillonage du sang : (2 à 3)×500ml(le sang autologue), la vitesse de la transfusion : 1 000ml /(15 ～ 30min), la même vitesse pour l'échantillonage du sang. ③ Pour l'hémodilution thérapeutique : il y a l'hémodilution normovolémique (avec saignée) et l'hémodilution hypervolémique (sans saignée), selon la concentration du médicament, la dose par jour se divise en 3 catégories : 250 ml, 500ml et 1 000ml. La vitesse de la perfusion : 250ml en 0,5 à 2h, 500ml en 4 à 6h, 1 000ml en 8 à 24h. Il est recommandé de suivre le traitement pendant 10 jours. |
| 剂型、规格<br>Les formes pharmaceutiques et les spécifications | 6% 中分子羟乙基淀粉 200/0.5 氯化钠注射液：每瓶 500ml。<br>10% 中分子羟乙基淀粉 200/0.5 氯化钠注射液：每瓶 500ml。<br>L'injection de chlorure de sodium d'hydroxyéthylamidon de poids moléculaire200/0.5 à 6 % : 500ml par flacon.<br>L'injection de chlorure de sodium d'hydroxyéthylamidon de poids moléculaire200/0.5 à 10 % : 500ml par flacon. |
| 药品名称 Drug Names | 羟乙基淀粉 130/0.4 Hydroxyéthyl Amidon130/0.4 |
| 适应证<br>Les indications | 用于治疗和预防血容量不足、急性等容血液稀释（ＡＮＨ）。<br>Ce produit sert à traiter et à prévenir l'hypovolémie et est utilisé dans l'hémodilution normovolémique aiguë. |
| 用法、用量<br>Les modes d'emploi et la posologie | 同中分子羟乙基淀粉 200/0.5，每日最大剂量按体重 33ml/kg，据患者需要可持续使用数日，治疗持续时间取决于低血容量程度及血流动力学参数和稀释效果。在欧洲已批准用于 0～2 岁儿童，每日最大剂量 50ml/kg。国内儿童用药正在研究中。<br>c.f. à l'hydroxyéthylamidon de poids moléculaire 200/0.5. La dose maximale est mesurée comme la dose de 33ml par kg. En fonction du besoin des patients, possible de prendre le médicament pendant plusieurs jours consécutifs. La durée du traitement dépend de l'hypovolémie, des paramètres hémodynamiques et de l'effet de dilution. En Europe, il est autorisé de l'appliquer chez des enfants de 0 à 2 ans, avec la dose maximale de 50 mg/kg par jour. En Chine, l'administration de ce médicament chez des enfants est en cours de recherche. |

**续 表**

| 剂型、规格<br>Les formes pharmaceutiques et les spécifications | 6% 中分子羟乙基淀粉 130/0.4 氯化钠注射液：每瓶 250ml；500ml。<br>L'injection d'hydroxyéthylamidon de poids moléculaire130/0.4 à 6 % : 250 ml ou 500ml par flacon. |
|---|---|
| **药品名称 Drug Names** | 包醛氧淀粉 Aldéhyde oxygène amidon |
| 适应证<br>Les indications | 用于各种原因造成的氮质血症。<br>Ce produit sert à traiter l'azotémie causée par divers facteurs. |
| 用法、用量<br>Les modes d'emploi et la posologie | 口服：餐后用温开水送服。一日 2～3 次，一次 5～10g，或遵医嘱。<br>Par voie orale : pris après le repas avec de l'eau chaude. 2 à 3 fois par jour, 5 à 10g par fois, ou selon les ordonnances. |
| 剂型、规格<br>Les formes pharmaceutiques et les spécifications | 胶囊：每粒 0.625g。<br>粉剂：每袋 5g。<br>Capsules : 0,625g par capsule.<br>Poudre : 5g par sachet. |
| **药品名称 Drug Names** | 聚维酮 Polyvidone |
| 适应证<br>Les indications | 用于外伤性出血及其他原因引起的血容量减少。<br>Ce produit sert à traiter l'hypovolémie causée par l'hémorragie traumatique et d'autres facteurs. |
| 用法、用量<br>Les modes d'emploi et la posologie | 视病情而定，一般为 500～1000ml 静脉滴注。<br>Selon les cas, en général, 500 à 1 000ml, en perfusion. |
| 剂型、规格<br>Les formes pharmaceutiques et les spécifications | 注射液：3.5%（250ml）。<br>Injection : 3,5 % (250ml). |
| **药品名称 Drug Names** | 羟乙基淀粉 40 Hydroxyéthyl amidon 40 |
| 适应证<br>Les indications | 为血容量扩充剂。用于各种手术、外伤的失血，中毒性休克等的补液。<br>ce produit sert d'expanseur du volume sanguin. Il est utilisé comme perfusion sanguine lors de la perte de sang chirurgicale et traumatique ou comme hydratation lors du choc toxique. |
| 用法、用量<br>Les modes d'emploi et la posologie | 视病情而定，一般为 500～1000ml 静脉滴注。<br>Selon les cas, en général, 500 à 1 000ml, en perfusion. |
| 剂型、规格<br>Les formes pharmaceutiques et les spécifications | 注射液：6%（500ml）。<br>Injection : 6% (500ml). |
| **药品名称 Drug Names** | 人血白蛋白 Albumine humaine |
| 适应证<br>Les indications | 用于失血性休克、脑水肿、流产等引起的白蛋白缺乏、肾病等。<br>Ce produit sert à traiter la carence en albumine et les maladies rénales causées par le choc hémorragique, l'œdème cérébral, l'avortement, etc. |
| 用法、用量<br>Les modes d'emploi et la posologie | 静脉注射或静脉滴注：用量视病情而定。<br>Injection par voie IV ou en perfusion : selon les cas. |

**续　表**

| 剂型、规格<br>Les formes pharmaceutiques et les spécifications | 注射液：5%；10%；20%；25%。<br>冻干粉：5g；10g。<br>Injection：5%；10%；20%；25%.<br>Poudre lyophilisée：5g ou 10g. |
|---|---|

**13.4　抗贫血药 Médicaments contre l'anémie**

| 药品名称 Drug Names | 硫酸亚铁 Sulfate ferreux |
|---|---|
| 适应证<br>Les indications | 用于慢性失血（月经过多、慢性消化道出血、子宫肌瘤出血、钩虫病失血等）、营养不良、妊娠、儿童发育期等引起的缺铁性贫血。用药后贫血症状迅速改善，用药 1 周左右即可见网织红细胞增多，血红蛋白每日可增加 0.1% ～ 0.3%，4 ～ 8 周可恢复至正常。<br>Ce produit sert à traiter l'anémie ferriprive causée par le saignement chronique (la ménorragie, les saignements gastro-intestinaux chroniques, les hémorragies dufibrome utérin, perte de sang liée à l'ankylostome, etc), la malnutrition, la grossesse, la période de développement de l'enfant. On assiste à l'amélioration rapide de l'anémie après l'administration, à l'augmentation des réticulocytesen 1 semaine, et à l'augmentation de l'hémoglobine de 0,1% à 0,3% par jour qui retourne à la normale en 4 à 8 semaines. |
| 用法、用量<br>Les modes d'emploi et la posologie | 口服，成人，每次 0.3g，一日 3 次，餐后服用。<br>Par voie orale, chez des adultes, 0,3g par fois, 3 fois par jour, pris après le repas. |
| 剂型、规格<br>Les formes pharmaceutiques et les spécifications | 硫酸亚铁片：每片 0.3g。<br>硫酸亚铁缓释片：每片 0.25g；0.45g。<br>Les comprimés de sulfate ferreux：0,3g par comprimé.<br>Les comprimés à libération prolongée：0,25g ou 0,45g par comprimé. |

| 药品名称 Drug Names | 葡萄糖酸亚铁 Gluconate ferreux |
|---|---|
| 适应证<br>Les indications | 用于各种原因引起的缺铁性贫血，如营养不良、慢性失血、月经过多、妊娠、儿童生长期等所致的缺铁性贫血。<br>Ce produit sert à traiter l'anémie ferriprive causée par la malnutrition, les saignements chroniques, la ménorragie, la grossesse, la période de développement de l'enfant, etc. |
| 用法、用量<br>Les modes d'emploi et la posologie | 口服：预防，成人，每次 0.3g，一日 1 次；儿童：每次 0.1g，一日 2 次。治疗，成人，每次 0.3 ～ 0.6g，一日 3 次；儿童：每次 0.1 ～ 0.2g，一日 3 次。<br>Par voie orale：pour la prévention, chez des adultes, 0,3g par fois, 1 fois par jour；chez des enfants：0,1g par fois, 2 fois par jour. Pour le traitement, chez des adultes, 0,3 à 0,6g par fois, 3 fois par jour；chez des enfants：0,1 à 0,2g par fois, 3 fois par jour. |
| 剂型、规格<br>Les formes pharmaceutiques et les spécifications | 片剂（糖衣片）：每片 0.1g；0.3g。<br>胶囊剂：每粒 0.25g；0.3g；0.4g。<br>糖浆：每瓶 0.25g（10ml）；0.3g（10ml）。<br>Comprimés (comprimés dragéifiés)：0,1g ou 0,3g par comprimé.<br>Capsules：0,25g, 0,3g ou 0,4g par capsule.<br>Sirop：0,25g (10ml) ou 0,3g (10ml) par flacon. |

| 药品名称 Drug Names | 蔗糖铁 Saccharose Fer |
|---|---|
| 适应证<br>Les indications | 主要用于治疗口服铁不能有效缓解的缺铁性贫血。<br>Ce produit sert à traiter l'anémie ferriprive qui ne peut pas être traitée par l'administration par voie orale du fer. |
| 用法、用量<br>Les modes d'emploi et la posologie | 本品只能与 0.9%w/v 生理盐水混合使用。应以滴注或缓慢注射的方式给药，或直接注射到透析器的静脉端给药。<br>Ce médicament ne peut être utilisé en association avec la solution saline à0.9%w/v. Il faut l'administrer par voie IV lente ou en perfusion, ou l'injecter directement dans le dialyseur veineux. |

**续　表**

| 剂型、规格<br>Les formes pharmaceutiques et les spécifications | 蔗糖铁注射液：5ml：100mg（铁元素）。<br>L'injection de fer-saccharose : 5ml : 100mg (fer). |
|---|---|
| **药品名称 Drug Names** | **叶酸 Acide folique** |
| 适应证<br>Les indications | 巨幼红细胞性贫血，尤适用于营养不良或婴儿期、妊娠期叶酸需要增加所致的巨幼红细胞贫血。用于治疗恶性贫血时，虽可纠正异常血象，但不能改善神经损害症状，故应以维生素 $B_{12}$ 为主，叶酸为辅。也用于妊娠期和哺乳期妇女的预防用药。<br><br>Ce produit sert à traiter l'anémie mégaloblastique, surtout celle causée par la malnutrition ou le besoin croissant en acide folique pendant le petit enfance et la grossesse. Lors du traitement de l'anémie pernicieuse, il ne peut pas améliorer les lésions nerveuses, donc il faut prendre la vitamine $B_{12}$ comme le médicament principal et l'acide folique comme le traitement adjuvant. Il est aussi applicable dans la prévention chez des femmes pendant la grossesse et la lactation. |
| 用法、用量<br>Les modes d'emploi et la posologie | 口服：成人，每次 5～10mg，一日 5～30mg。肌内注射：每次 10～20mg。妊娠期和哺乳期妇女的预防用药：口服一次 0.4mg，一日 1 次。<br><br>Par voie orale : chez des adultes, 5 à 10mg par fois, 5 à 30mg par jour. Injection par voie IM : 10 à 20mg par fois. Pour la prophylaxie chez des femmes pendant la grossesse et la lactation : par voie orale, 0,4mg par fois, 1 fois par jour. |
| 剂型、规格<br>Les formes pharmaceutiques et les spécifications | 叶酸片：每片 0.4mg；5mg。<br>注射液：每支 15mg（1ml）。<br>复方叶酸注射液：每支 1ml，含叶酸 5mg、维生素 $B_{12}$ 30μg。<br>Comprimés d'acide folique : 0,4mg ou 5mg par comprimé.<br>Injection : 15mg (1ml) par solution.<br>L'injection composée d'acide folique : 1ml par solution, qui contient 5mg d'acide folique et 30 μgde vitamine $B_{12}$. |
| **药品名称 Drug Names** | **氰钴胺（维生素 $B_{12}$)Cyanocobalamine(Vitamine $B_{12}$)** |
| 适应证<br>Les indications | 用于治疗恶性贫血，亦与叶酸合用于治疗各种巨幼红细胞性贫血、抗叶酸药引起的贫血及脂肪泻、全胃切除或胃大部切除。尚用于神经系统疾病（如神经炎、神经萎缩等）、肝脏疾病（肝炎、肝硬化等）等。<br><br>Ce produit sert à traiter l'anémie pernicieuse. Utilisé en association avec l'acide folique, il sert à traiter l'anémie mégaloblastique, l'anémie causée par des antifoliques, la stéatorrhée, la gastrectomie totale ou la gastrectomie subtotale. Il est également utilisé dans le traitement desmaladies du système nerveux (telles que la névrite, l'atrophie du nerf, etc.), des maladieshépatiques (l'hépatite, la cirrhose, etc.). |
| 用法、用量<br>Les modes d'emploi et la posologie | 肌内注射，成人，一日内 0.025～0.1mg 或隔日 0.05～0.2mg。用于神经系统疾病时，用量可酌增。<br><br>Injection par voie IM, chez des adultes, 0,025 à 0,1mg par jour ou 0,05 à 0,2mg tous les deux jours. Pour traiter des maladies du système nerveux, possible d'augmenter un peu la dose. |
| 剂型、规格<br>Les formes pharmaceutiques et les spécifications | 注射液：每支 0.05mg（1ml）；0.1ng（1ml）；0.25mg（1ml）；0.5mg（1ml）；1mg（1ml）.<br>Injection : 0.05mg (1ml), 0.1mg (1ml), 0.25mg (1ml), 0.5mg (1ml), 1mg (1ml) par solution. |
| **药品名称 Drug Names** | **腺苷钴胺 Cobamamide** |
| 适应证<br>Les indications | 主要用于巨幼红细胞型贫血、营养不良性贫血、妊娠期贫血，亦用于神经性疾病如多发性神经炎、神经根炎、三叉神经痛、坐骨神经痛、神经麻痹、营养性神经疾病，以及放射线和药物引起的白细胞减少症。<br><br>Ce produit sert à traiter l'anémie mégaloblastique, l'anémie causée par la malnutrition, l'anémie pendant la grossesse. Il est aussi applicable dans le traitement des troubles neurologiques, tels que la polynévrite, la radiculite, la névralgie, la sciatique, la paralysie, lestroubles neurologiques nutritionnels ainsi que la leucopénie induite par le rayonnement et le médicament. |

**续　表**

| | |
|---|---|
| 用法、用量<br>Les modes d'emploi et la posologie | 口服，成人，每次 0.5～1.5mg，一日 1.5～4.5mg。肌内注射，每日 0.5～1mg。<br>Par voie orale, chez des adultes, 0,5 à 1,5mg par fois, 1,5 à 4,5mg par jour. Injection par voie IM, 0,5 à 1mg par jour. |
| 剂型、规格<br>Les formes pharmaceutiques et les spécifications | 片剂：每片 0.25mg。<br>注射液：每支 0.5mg（1ml）。<br>冻干粉针：0.5mg；1.0mg；1.5mg。<br>Comprimés : 0,25mg par comprimé.<br>Injection : 0,5mg (1ml) par solution.<br>Poudre lyophilisée : 0,5mg, 1,0mg ou 1,5mg. |
| 药品名称 Drug Names | 甲钴胺 Mécobalamine |
| 适应证<br>Les indications | 用于治疗缺乏维生素 $B_{12}$ 引起的巨幼细胞性贫血，也用于周围神经病。<br>Ce produit sert à traiter l'anémie mégaloblastique induite par le manque de la vitamine $B_{12}$, ainsi que la neuropathie périphérique. |
| 用法、用量<br>Les modes d'emploi et la posologie | 肌内注射或静脉注射。①成人巨红细胞性贫血：通常一次 500μg，一日 1 次，隔日 1 次。给药约 2 个月后，可维持治疗，一次 500μg，每 1～3 个月 1 次。②周围神经病：通常，成人一次 500μg，一日 1 次，一周 3 次，可按年龄、症状酌情增减。<br>Injection par voie IM ou IV.<br>① Pour traiter l'anémie mégaloblastique : en général, 500μg par fois, 1 fois par jour, une fois tous les deux jours. 2 mois après l'administration, possible de suivre le traitement d'entretien, soit 500μg par fois, tous les 1 à 3 mois. ② Pour traiter la neuropathie périphérique : en général, chez des adultes, 500μg par fois, 1 fois par jour, 3 fois par semaine, ajuster la dose selon l'âge et des symptômes. |
| 剂型、规格<br>Les formes pharmaceutiques et les spécifications | 注射液：1ml：500μg。<br>Injection : 1ml : 500μg. |
| 药品名称 Drug Names | 重组人促红细胞生成素 Recombinant Humaine Erythropoïétine |
| 适应证<br>Les indications | 用于慢性肾衰竭和晚期肾病所致的贫血，也用于多发性骨髓瘤相关的贫血和骨髓增生异常综合征（MDS）及骨癌引起的贫血。对结缔组织病（类风湿关节炎和系统性红斑狼疮）所致的贫血也有效。<br>Ce produit sert à traiter l'anémie causée par l'insuffisance rénale chronique et les maladies rénales avancées. Il est aussi applicable dans le traitement de l'anémie liée au myélome multiple, de l'anémie causée par le syndrome myélodysplasique et le cancer osseux. Il a aussi un certain effet sur l'anémie causée par la maladie du tissu conjonctif (la polyarthrite rhumatoïde et le lupus érythémateux disséminé). |
| 用法、用量<br>Les modes d'emploi et la posologie | 可静脉注射或皮下注射，剂量应个体化，一般开始剂量为 50～150U/kg，每周 3 次。治疗过程中需视血细胞比容或血红蛋白水平调整剂量或调节维持量。建议以血细胞比容 30%～33% 或血红蛋白 100～120g/L 为指标，调节维持剂量。<br>Injection IV ou sous-cutanée, la dose doit être personnalisée, en général, la dose initiale, 50 à 150 unités par kg, 3 fois par semaine. Au cours du traitement, il faut ajuster la dose en fonction de l'hématocrite et du taux d'hémoglobine. Il est recommandé de consider l'hématocrite à 30 % à 33% et l'hémoglobine à 100 à 120 g par L comme un critère pour ajuster la dose. |
| 剂型、规格<br>Les formes pharmaceutiques et les spécifications | 重组人促红细胞生成素注射液（CHO 细胞）：每支 2000U（1ml）；4000U（1ml）；10 000U（1ml）。<br>注射用重组人促红细胞生成素（CHO 细胞）：每支 2000U；4000U；10 000U。<br>L'injection d'érythropoïétine humaine recombinant : 2000U (1ml), 4000U (1ml), 10 000U (1ml) par solution.<br>L'érythropoïétine humaine recombinant pour injection : 2 000U, 4 000U ou 10 000U. |

**续 表**

| 药品名称 Drug Names | 琥珀酸亚铁 Succinate ferreux |
|---|---|
| 适应证<br>Les indications | 用于缺铁性贫血的预防和治疗。<br>Ce produit sert à prévenir et à traiter l'anémie ferriprive. |
| 用法、用量<br>Les modes d'emploi et la posologie | 预防：普通成人每日 0.1g；妊娠期妇女每日 0.2g；儿童每日 0.03 ～ 0.06g。治疗：成人一次 0.1 ～ 0.2g，一日 3 次；儿童一次 0.05 ～ 0.1g，一日 1 ～ 2 次餐后服。<br>Pour la prévention : la dose ordinaire, chez des adultes, 0,1g par jour ; chez des femmes pendant la grossesse, 0,2g par jour ; chez des enfants, 0,03 à 0,06g par jour. Pour le traitement : chez des adultes, 0,1 à 0,2g par fois, 3 fois par jour ; chez des enfants, 0,05 à 0,1g par fois, 1 à 2 fois par jour, pris après le repas. |
| 剂型、规格<br>Les formes pharmaceutiques et les spécifications | 片剂：0.1g。<br>胶囊剂：0.1g。<br>Comprimés : 0,1g.<br>Capsules : 0,1g. |
| 药品名称 Drug Names | 富马酸亚铁 Fumarate ferreux |
| 适应证<br>Les indications | 用于治疗缺铁性贫血。<br>Ce produit sert à traiter l'anémie ferriprive. |
| 用法、用量<br>Les modes d'emploi et la posologie | 口服，一次 0.2 ～ 0.4g，一日 3 次，疗程：轻症 2 ～ 3 周，重症 3 ～ 4 周。<br>Par voie orale, 0,2 à 0,4g par fois, 3 fois par jour, la durée du traitement médical : pour des cas bénins, 2 à 3 semaines, pour des cas sévères, 3 à 4 semaines. |
| 剂型、规格<br>Les formes pharmaceutiques et les spécifications | 片剂：0.2g；0.05g。<br>胶囊剂：0.2g。<br>Comprimés : 0,2g ou 0,05g.<br>Capsules : 0,2g. |
| 药品名称 Drug Names | 枸橼酸铁铵 Citrate d'ammonium ferrique |
| 适应证<br>Les indications | 适用于儿童及不能吞服药片的患者。由于含铁量低，不适于重症贫血病例。<br>Ce produit est applicable chez des enfants et des patients résistants aux préparations orales de fer. Comme il contient une faible dose de fer, il n'est pas applicable chez des cas graves d'anémie. |
| 用法、用量<br>Les modes d'emploi et la posologie | 口服，一次 0.5 ～ 2g，一日 3 次，餐后服。<br>Par voie orale, 0,5 à 2g par fois, 3 fois par jour, pris après le repas. |
| 剂型、规格<br>Les formes pharmaceutiques et les spécifications | 溶液：10%。<br>Solution : 10%. |
| 药品名称 Drug Names | 右旋糖酐铁 Fer dextran |
| 适应证<br>Les indications | 适用于不能耐受口服铁制剂的缺铁性贫血患者或者需要迅速纠正缺铁者。<br>Ce produit est applicable dans le traitement des patients atteints de l'anémie ferriprive et résistant aux préparations orales de fer ou chez des patients qui nécessitent la correction rapide du déficit en fer. |
| 用法、用量<br>Les modes d'emploi et la posologie | 深部肌内注射：每日 1ml。<br>Injection par voie IM profonde : 1ml par jour. |
| 剂型、规格<br>Les formes pharmaceutiques et les spécifications | 注射液：每毫升含元素铁 25mg。<br>Injection : chaque ml contient 25mg de fer. |

**续　表**

| 药品名称 Drug Names | 山梨醇铁 Fer sorbitol |
| --- | --- |
| 适应证<br>Les indications | 适用于不能耐受口服铁制剂的缺铁性贫血患者或者需要迅速纠正缺铁者。<br>Ce produit est applicable dans le traitement des patients atteints de l'anémie ferriprive et résistant aux préparations orales de fer ou chez des patients qui nécessitent la correction rapide du déficit en fer. |
| 用法、用量<br>Les modes d'emploi et la posologie | 深部肌内注射，一次 1.5 ～ 2ml（相当于铁 75 ～ 100mg）。<br>Injection IM profonde, 1,5 à 2ml par fois (équivalent à 75 à 100mg de fer). |
| 剂型、规格<br>Les formes pharmaceutiques et les spécifications | 注射剂。<br>injection. |
| 药品名称 Drug Names | 亚叶酸钙 Folinate de calcium |
| 适应证<br>Les indications | 常用作氨蝶呤及甲氨蝶呤过量时的解毒剂。此外尚可用于巨幼红细胞性贫血及白细胞减少症。<br>Ce produit sert d'antidotelors du surdosage du méthotrexate. Il permet aussi de traiter l'anémie mégaloblastique et la leucopénie. |
| 用法、用量<br>Les modes d'emploi et la posologie | 肌内注射：①抗叶酸代谢药中度中毒，一次 6 ～ 12mg，每 6 小时 1 次，共 4 次。②巨幼红细胞性贫血：一日 1mg，一日 1 次。③白细胞减少症：每次 3 ～ 6mg，一日 1 次。静脉滴注：抗叶酸代谢药重度中毒：75mg 于 12 小时内滴注完毕，随后改为肌内注射。<br>Injection IM : ① Pour lutter contre l'empoisonnement modéré au métabolisme du folate, 6 à 12mg par fois ,toutes les 6h, 4 fois au total. ② Pour traiter l'anémie mégaloblastique : 1mg par jour, 1 fois par jour. ③ Pour traiter la leucopénie : 3 à 6mg par fois, 1 fois par jour. En perfusion : pour lutter contre l'empoisonnement modéré au métabolisme du folate : administrer 75mg en perfusion en 12h, ensuite, administrer par voie IM. |
| 剂型、规格<br>Les formes pharmaceutiques et les spécifications | 注射用冻干粉：3mg；5mg。<br>Poudre lyophilisée pour injection : 3mg ou 5mg. |

13.5　促进白细胞增生药 Médicament destiné à promouvoir la prolifération des leucocytes

| 药品名称 Drug Names | 腺嘌呤（维生素 $B_4$）　　Adénine(Vitamine $B_4$) |
| --- | --- |
| 适应证<br>Les indications | 用于各种原因如放射治疗、苯中毒、抗肿瘤药和抗甲状腺药物等引起的白细胞减少症，也用于急性粒细胞减少症。<br>Ce produit sert à traiter la leucopénie causée par la radiothérapie, l'empoisonnement de benzène, des anticancéreux et des anti-thyroïdiens, etc. il est aussi applicable dans le traitement de la neutropénie aiguë. |
| 用法、用量<br>Les modes d'emploi et la posologie | 口服，成人，每次 10 ～ 20mg，一日 3 次。肌内注射或静脉注射，每日 20 ～ 30mg。<br>Par voie orale, chez des adultes, 10 à 20mg par fois, 3 fois par jour. Injection par voie IM ou IV, 20 à 30mg par jour. |
| 剂型、规格<br>Les formes pharmaceutiques et les spécifications | 片剂：每片 10mg；25mg。<br>注射用维生素 $B_4$：每支 20mg。<br>Comprimés : 10mg ou 25mg par comprimé.<br>La vitamine $B_4$ pour injection : 20mg par solution. |

**续 表**

| 药品名称 Drug Names | 苦参总碱 Alcaloïdes du Sophora |
|---|---|
| 适应证<br>Les indications | 用于肿瘤放疗、化疗及其他原因引起的白细胞减少症（包括再生障碍性贫血、慢性放射病、慢性肝炎等）。<br><br>Ce produit sert à traiter la leucopénie causée parla radiothérapie et la chimiothérapie (y compris l'anémie aplasique, la maladie des rayons chronique, l'hépatite chronique, etc.). |
| 用法、用量<br>Les modes d'emploi et la posologie | 肌内注射，每次 0.2g，一日 2 次。<br>Injection par voie IM, 0,2g par fois, 2 fois par jour. |
| 剂型、规格<br>Les formes pharmaceutiques et les spécifications | 注射液：0.2g（1ml）。<br>Injection : 0,2g (1ml). |
| 药品名称 Drug Names | 鲨肝醇 Batilol |
| 适应证<br>Les indications | 用于各种原因引起的粒细胞减少。<br>Ce produit sert à traiter la neutropénie induite par divers facteurs. |
| 用法、用量<br>Les modes d'emploi et la posologie | 一日 50 ～ 150mg，分 3 次口服。<br>50 à 150mg par jour, à travers 3 fois. |
| 剂型、规格<br>Les formes pharmaceutiques et les spécifications | 片剂：25mg；50mg。<br>Comprimés : 25mg ou 50mg. |
| 药品名称 Drug Names | 利可君 Léucogen |
| 适应证<br>Les indications | 用于防治各种原因引起的白细胞较少、再生障碍性贫血。<br>Ce produit sert à prévenir et à traiter la leucopénie induite par divers facteurs, et l'anémie aplasique. |
| 用法、用量<br>Les modes d'emploi et la posologie | 口服，一次 20mg，一日 3 次。<br>Par voie orale, 20mg par fois, 3 fois par jour. |
| 剂型、规格<br>Les formes pharmaceutiques et les spécifications | 片剂：10mg；20mg。<br>Comprimés : 10mg ou 20mg. |
| 药品名称 Drug Names | 肌苷 Inosine |
| 适应证<br>Les indications | 用于治疗各种原因所致的白细胞较少、血小板减少等。<br>Ce produit sert à traiter la leucopénie et la thrombocytopénie causées par divers facteurs. |
| 用法、用量<br>Les modes d'emploi et la posologie | 口服：一次 200 ～ 600mg，一日 3 次。静脉注射或静脉滴注：一次 200 ～ 600mg，一日 1 ～ 2 次。<br>Par voie orale : 200 à 600mg par fois, 3 fois par jour. injection par voie IV ou en perfusion : 200 à 600mg par fois, 1 à 2 fois par jour. |
| 剂型、规格<br>Les formes pharmaceutiques et les spécifications | 片剂：200mg。<br>注射液：100mg（2ml）；200mg（5ml）。<br>Comprimés : 200mg.<br>Injection : 100mg (2ml) ou 200mg (5ml). |

**续　表**

| 药品名称 Drug Names | 氨肽素 Aminopolypeptide |
|---|---|
| 适应证<br>Les indications | 用于原发性血小板减少性紫癜、过敏性紫癜、白细胞减少症和再生障碍性贫血。<br>Ce produit sert à traiter le purpura thrombopénique idiopathique, le purpura allergique, la leucopénie et l'anémie aplasique. |
| 用法、用量<br>Les modes d'emploi et la posologie | 口服：成人一次 1g，一日 3 次；小儿酌减。用药至少 4 周，有效者可连续服用。<br>Par voie orale : chez des adultes, 1g par fois, 3 fois par jour ; chez des enfants, diminuer un peu la dose. Pendant au moins 4 semaines. S'il est efficace, possible de le prendre de manière continue. |
| 剂型、规格<br>Les formes pharmaceutiques et les spécifications | 片剂：0.2g。<br>Comprimés : 0,2g. |

### 13.6　抗血小板药物 Antiplaquettes

| 药品名称 Drug Names | 阿司匹林 Aspirine |
|---|---|
| 适应证<br>Les indications | 可用于预防心、脑血管疾病的发作及人工心脏瓣膜或其他手术后的血栓形成。临床研究发现在男性患者预防脑卒中的效果似乎较女性患者为好，这可能与女性的血小板环氧酶对阿司匹林的耐受性较高有关。<br>Ce produit sert à prévenir les maladiescérébrovasculaires et la thrombose après la chirurgie valvulaire cardiaque artificielle et d'autres chirurgies. Les recherches cliniques montrent qu'il est plus efficace dans le traitement de l'accident vasculaire cérébral chez des hommes et chez des femmes, cela est peut-être lié à la bonne résistance de la cyclooxygénase plaquettaire à l'aspirine chez des femmes. |
| 用法、用量<br>Les modes d'emploi et la posologie | 用于防治短暂性脑缺血和卒中：成人常用量，每次 75～300mg，一日 1 次。预防用，一般一日 75～150mg；治疗用，一般一日 300mg。用于缺血性心脏病，可预防心肌梗死，减少心律失常的发生率和死亡率。<br>Ce produit est utilisé dans la prévention et le traitement de l'ischémie cérébrale et de l'AVC provisoires : la dose usuelle chez des adultes, 75 à 300mg par fois, 1 fois par jour. Pour la prévention, en général, 75 à 150 mg par jour ; pour le traitement, en général, 300mg par jour. Il est appliqué pour traiter la cardiopathie ischémique, prévenir l'infarctus du myocarde et réduire le taux d'incidence et la mortalité de l'arythmie. |
| 剂型、规格<br>Les formes pharmaceutiques et les spécifications | 肠溶片：每片 25mg；40mg；100mg。<br>Comprimés à enrobage entérique : 25mg, 40mg ou 100mg par comprimé. |
| 药品名称 Drug Names | 双嘧达莫 Dipyridamole |
| 适应证<br>Les indications | 用于血栓栓塞性疾病及缺血性心脏病。<br>Ce produit sert à traiter la maladie thrombo-embolique et la maladie cardiaque ischémique. |
| 用法、用量<br>Les modes d'emploi et la posologie | 单独应用疗效不及与阿司匹林合用者。单独应用时，每日口服 3 次，每次 25～100mg；与阿司匹林合用时其剂量可减少至每日 100～200mg。<br>Utilisé seul, il est moins efficace que l'utilisation en association avec l'aspirine. Lors de l'utilisation seule du dipyridamole, prendre 25 à 100mg par fois, 3 fois par jour par voie orale ; lors de l'utilisation en association avec l'aspirine, prendre 100 à 200mg par jour. |
| 剂型、规格<br>Les formes pharmaceutiques et les spécifications | 片剂：每片 25mg。<br>Comprimés : 25mg par comprimé. |

**续 表**

| 药品名称 Drug Names | 氯吡格雷 Clopidogrél |
|---|---|
| 适应证<br>Les indications | 用于预防和治疗因血小板高聚集引起的心、脑及其他动脉循环障碍疾病，如近期发作的脑卒中、心肌梗死和确诊的外周动脉疾病。<br><br>Ce produit sert à prévenir et à traiter la maladie cérébrovasculaire et d'autres troubles de la circulation artérielle induits par l'agrégation plaquettaire élevée, tels que l'accident vasculaire cérébral, l'infarctus du myocarde et la maladie artérielle périphérique. |
| 用法、用量<br>Les modes d'emploi et la posologie | 一日一次，每次 75mg。<br>1 fois par jour, 75mg par fois. |
| 剂型、规格<br>Les formes pharmaceutiques et les spécifications | 片剂：每片 25mg。<br>Comprimés : 25mg par comprimé. |
| 药品名称 Drug Names | 替罗非班 Tirofiban |
| 适应证<br>Les indications | 用于急性冠脉综合征、不稳定型心绞痛和非 Q 波心肌梗死、急性心肌梗死和急性缺血性心脏猝死等，包括可用药控制的患者和需做 PTCA、血管成形术或动脉粥样硬化血管切除术的患者。替罗非班可减少急性冠脉综合征和冠状动脉内介入治疗后冠心病事件发生率，改善患者症状和预后。<br><br>Ce produit sert à traiter le syndrome coronarien aigu, l'angine de poitrine instable, l'infarctus du myocarde sans onde Q, l'infarctus aigu du myocarde etla mort cardiaque ischémique aigue, y compris chez des patients qui peuvent être traités par les médicaments et des patients qui ont besoin de PTCA, d'uneangioplastie ou d'une chirurgie vasculaire athéroscléreuse. Le tirofiban permet aussi de réduire le taux d'incidence du syndrome coronarien aigu et de la maladie coronarienne après l'intervention coronarienne et d'améliorer les symptômes. |
| 用法、用量<br>Les modes d'emploi et la posologie | 与肝素合用，静脉给药。开始30分钟给药速度为 0.4 μg/（kg·min），然后减为维持量 0.1 μg/（kg·min）。2～5 日为 1 个疗程。患者至少给药 48 小时，此期间不进行手术治疗（除非患者发病为顽固性心肌缺血或新的心肌梗死）。<br><br>Utilisé en association avec l'héparine, il est administré par voie IV. Durant les 30 premières minutes, 0,4μg/(kg•min), ensuite, prendre la dose d'entretien, soit 0,1μg/(kg•min). Un traitement médical dure 2 à 5 jours. L'administration doit être appliquée pendant 48h, pendant ce temps-là, on ne conduit pas la chirurgie, sauf chez des patients atteints d'ischémie myocardique réfractaire ou de nouveau infarctus du myocarde. |
| 剂型、规格<br>Les formes pharmaceutiques et les spécifications | 注射液：每瓶 5mg（100ml）。<br>Injection : 5mg (100ml) par flacon. |
| 药品名称 Drug Names | 奥扎格雷 Ozagrél |
| 适应证<br>Les indications | 用于治疗急性血栓性脑梗死及伴发的运动障碍，改善蛛网膜下腔出血手术后血管痉挛及其并发的脑缺血症状。<br><br>Ce produit sert à traiter l'infarctus thrombotique aigu et les troubles de mouvements accompagnés, et à améliorer les vasospasme et les symptômes ischémiques cérébraux après la chirurgie de l'hémorragie méningée. |
| 用法、用量<br>Les modes d'emploi et la posologie | 常用制剂为奥扎格雷钠注射液，每支 20mg。以生理盐水或葡萄糖注射液稀释后静脉滴注，一日 80mg。如与其他抗血小板药合用时，本品剂量宜酌减。<br><br>Il est souvent utilisé en injection, 20mg par solution. Dissoudre dans la solution saline ou de glucose pour la perfusion, 80mg par jour. Lors de l'utilisation avec d'autres médicaments antiplaquettaires, il faut diminuer un peu la dose de l'ozagrel. |

**续　表**

| | |
|---|---|
| 剂型、规格<br>Les formes pharmaceutiques et les spécifications | 注射用奥扎格雷：20mg；40mg。<br>奥扎格雷注射液：每支 20mg（1ml）；40mg（2ml）。<br>L'ozagrel pour injection : 20mg ou 40mg.<br>L'injection d'ozagrel : 20mg (1ml) ou 40mg (2ml). |

| 药品名称 Drug Names | 曲克芦丁 Troxérutine |
|---|---|
| 适应证<br>Les indications | 用于脑血栓形成和脑栓塞所致的偏瘫、失语以及心肌梗死前综合征、动脉硬化、中心性视网膜炎、血栓性静脉炎、静脉曲张、血管通透性高引起的水肿等。<br>Ce produit sert à traiter les cas suivants causés par la thrombose cérébrale et l'embolie cérébrale: l'hémiplégie, l'aphasie, le syndrome avant l'infarctus du myocarde, l'artériosclérose, la rétinite centrale, la thrombophlébite, les varices et l'œdème provoqué par une forte perméabilité vasculaire, etc. |
| 用法、用量<br>Les modes d'emploi et la posologie | 口服：每次 300mg，一日 2～3 次。肌内注射：每次 100～200mg，一日 2 次，20 日为 1 个疗程，可用 1～3 个疗程，每疗程间隔 3～7 日。静脉滴注：每次 400mg，一日 1 次，用 5%～10% 葡萄糖注射液稀释。<br>Par voie orale : 300mg par fois, 2 à 3 fois par jour. Injection par voie IM : 100 à 200mg par fois, 2 fois par jour, pendant 20 jours comme un traitement médical, possible de suivre 1 à 3 traitements, avec un intervalle de 3 à 7 jours entre deux traitements. En perfusion : 400mg par fois, 1 fois par jour, utiliser la solution de glucose à 5% à 10% pour la dilution. |
| 剂型、规格<br>Les formes pharmaceutiques et les spécifications | 片剂：每片 100mg。<br>注射液：每支 100mg（2ml）。<br>Comprimés : 100mg par comprimé.<br>Injection : 100mg (2ml) par solution. |

| 药品名称 Drug Names | 氯贝丁酯 Clofibrate |
|---|---|
| 适应证<br>Les indications | 能降低血小板的黏附作用，它能降低血小板对 ADP 和肾上腺素导致聚集的敏感性，并可抑制 ADP 诱导的血小板聚集。它还可延长血小板寿期。可单独应用或与抗凝剂合用于缺血性心脏病的患者。<br>Il permet de réduire l'adhésion des plaquettes, de réduire la sensibilité des plaquettes àl'agrégation causée par l'ADP et l'épinéphrine et d'inhiber l'agrégation plaquettaire induite par l'ADP. Il sert aussi à prolonger la vie de plaquettes. Utilisé suel ou en association avec les anticoagulants, il permet de traiter la cardiopathie ischémique. |
| 用法、用量<br>Les modes d'emploi et la posologie | 口服。每日 3 次，每次 0.25～0.5g。<br>Par voie orale. 3 fois par jour, 0,25 à 0,5g par fois. |
| 剂型、规格<br>Les formes pharmaceutiques et les spécifications | 胶囊：0.25g；0.5g。<br>Capsules : 0,25g ou 0,5g. |

**14. 主要作用于泌尿系统的药物 Médicaments agissant sur le système urinaire**

**14.1　利尿药 Diurétiques**

| 药品名称 Drug Names | 呋塞米 Furosémide |
|---|---|
| 适应证<br>Les indications | ①水肿性疾病：包括心脏性水肿、肾性水肿（肾炎、肾病及各种原因所致的急、慢性肾衰竭）、肝硬化腹水、功能障碍或血管障碍所引起的周围性水肿，尤其是应用其他利尿药效果不佳时，应用本品仍可能有效。静脉给药或与其他药物合用，可治疗急性肺水肿和急性脑水肿等。②高血压：不作为原发性高血压的首选药，但当噻嗪类药物疗效不佳，尤其当伴有肾功能不全或出现高血压危象时，尤为适用。③预防急性肾衰竭：用于各种原因导致的肾脏血流灌注不足，例如失水、休克、中毒、麻醉意外以及循环功能不全等，及时应用可减少急性肾小管坏死的机会。④高钾血症及高钙血症。⑤抗利尿激素分泌过多症（SIADH）。⑥稀释性低钠血症，尤其时当血钠浓度低于 120mmol/L 时。⑦急性药物中毒：用本品可加速毒物排泄。 |

**续　表**

| | |
|---|---|
| | ① Les maladies liées à l'oedème : l'oedème cardiaque, l'œdème rénal (la néphrite, la néphrotique et l'insuffisance rénale aiguë et chronique), la cirrhose du foie, l'œdème périphérique causé par le dysfonctionnement ou des troubles vasculaires. Surtout quand les autres diurétiques ne sont pas efficaces, ce produit est encore efficace. Administré par voie IV ou en association avec d'autres médicaments, il sert à traiter l'oedème pulmonaire aigu et l'œdème cérébral aigu. ② L'hypertension artérielle : il est pas considéré comme le médicament de choix chans le traitement de l'hypertension essentielle. Mais lorsque les diurétiques thiazidiques ne sont pas efficaces, et surtout quand l'hypertension s'accompagne de l'insuffisance rénale ou de la crise hypertensive, il est applicable. ③ La prévention de l'insuffisance rénale aigue : il permet de traiter l'hypoperfusion rénale causée par la déshydratation, le choc, l'intoxication, les accidents d'anesthésie et l'insuffisance circulatoire. Sonapplication en temps opportun peut réduire le risque de nécrose tubulaire aiguë. ④ L'hyperkaliémie et l'hypercalcémie. ⑤ Le syndrome de sécrétion inappropriée d'hormone antidiurétique. ⑥ L'hyponatrémie de dilution, surtout quand la concentration de sodium dans le sang est inférieuré à120mmol/L. ⑦ L'intoxications médicamenteuse aigue : ce produit permet d'accélérer l'excrétion de substances toxiques. |
| 用法、用量<br>Les modes d'emploi et la posologie | 成人：水肿：① 口服，开始每日 20 ～ 40mg，一日 1 ～ 2 次，必要时 6 ～ 8 小时后追加 20 ～ 40mg，直至出现满意的利尿效果。最大剂量虽可达一日 600mg，但一般应控制在 100mg 以下，分 2 ～ 3 次服用。以防过度利尿和发生不良反应。部分患者剂量可减至 20 ～ 40mg，隔日 1 次，或一周中连续服药 2 ～ 4 日，一日 20 ～ 40mg。②肌内注射或静脉注射，一次 20 ～ 40mg，隔日一次，根据需要亦可一日 1 ～ 2 次，必要时可每 2 小时追加剂量。一日量视需要可增至 120mg。静脉注射宜用氯化钠注射液稀释后缓慢注射，不宜与其他药物混合。<br><br>Chez des adultes : l'œdème ① Par voie orale, commencer par 20 à 40mg par jour, 1 à 2 fois par jour, en cas de besoin, 6 à 8 h après, reprendre 20 à 40mg, jusqu'à l'apparition de l'effet diurétique satisfaisant. La dose maximale est de 600mg par jour, mais il faut maintenir à 100mg au maximum en général, pris à travers 2 à 3 fois, pour éviter l'effet diurétique excessif et d'autres réactions indésirables. Chez certains patients, possible de diminuer la dose jusqu'à 20 à 40 mg, tous les 2 jours, ou 2 à 4 jours consécutifs par semaine, 20 à 40mg par jour. ② Injection IM ou IV, 20 à 40mg par fois, tous les deux jours, ou selon les cas, 1 à 2 fois par jour, en cas de besoin, augmenter la dose toutes les 2h. Il est aussi permissible de prendre 120mg par jour en fonction des maladies. Il vaut mieux utiliser la solution de chlorure de sodium pour la dilution avant d'injecter par voie IV. Il vaut mieux éviter l'utilisation avec d'autres médicaments. |
| 剂型、规格<br>Les formes pharmaceutiques et les spécifications | 片剂：每片 20mg。<br>注射液：每支 20mg（2ml）。<br><br>Comprimés : 20mg par comprimé.<br>Injection : 20mg (2ml) par solution. |
| 药品名称 Drug Names | 布美他尼 Bumétanide |
| 适应证<br>Les indications | ①水肿性疾病：包括心脏性水肿、肾性水肿（肾炎、肾病及各种原因所致的急、慢性肾衰竭）、肝硬化腹水、功能障碍或血管障碍所引起的周围性水肿，尤其是应用其他利尿药效果不佳时，应用本品仍可能有效。静脉给药或与其他药物合用，可治疗急性肺水肿和急性脑水肿等。②高血压：不作为原发性高血压的首选药，但当噻嗪类药物疗效不佳，尤其当伴有肾功能不全或出现高血压危象时，尤为适用。③预防急性肾衰竭：用于各种原因导致的肾脏血流灌注不足，例如失水、休克、中毒、麻醉意外以及循环功能不全等，及时应用可减少急性肾小管坏死的机会。④高钾血症及高钙血症。⑤抗利尿激素分泌过多症（SIADH）。⑥稀释性低钠血症，尤其时当血钠浓度低于 120mmol/L 时。⑦急性药物中毒：用本品可加速毒物排泄。<br><br>① Les maladies liées à l'oedème : l'oedème cardiaque, l'œdème rénal (la néphrite, la néphrotique et l'insuffisance rénale aiguë et chronique), la cirrhose du foie, l'œdème périphérique causé par le dysfonctionnement ou des troubles vasculaires. Surtout quand les autres diurétiques ne sont pas efficaces, ce produit est encore efficace. Administré par voie IV ou en association avec d'autres médicaments, il sert à traiter l'oedème pulmonaire aigu et l'œdème cérébral aigu. ② L'hypertension |

**续　表**

<table>
<tr>
<td></td>
<td>artérielle : il est pas considéré comme le médicament de choix chans le traitement de l'hypertension essentielle. Mais lorsque les diurétiques thiazidiques ne sont pas efficaces, et surtout quand l'hypertension s'accompagne de l'insuffisance rénale ou de la crise hypertensive, il est applicable. ③ La prévention de l'insuffisance rénale aigue : il permet de traiter l'hypoperfusion rénale causée par la déshydratation, le choc, l'intoxication, les accidents d'anesthésie et l'insuffisance circulatoire. Sonapplication en temps opportun peut réduire le risque de nécrose tubulaire aiguë. ④ L'hyperkaliémie et l'hypercalcémie. ⑤ Le syndrome de sécrétion inappropriée d'hormone antidiurétique. ⑥ L'hyponatrémie de dilution, surtout quand la concentration de sodium dans le sang est inférieuré à120mmol/L. ⑦ L'intoxications médicamenteuse aigue : ce produit permet d'accélérer l'excrétion de substances toxiques.</td>
</tr>
<tr>
<td>用法、用量<br>Les modes d'emploi et la posologie</td>
<td>　　（1）成人：①水肿：口服，一次 0.5 ～ 2mg，一日 1 次，必要时可一日 2 ～ 3 次，总量有时可高达一日 10mg；肌内或静脉注射，起始 0.5 ～ 1mg，必要时每隔 2 ～ 3 小时重复，最大剂量为一日 10mg。②急性肺水肿及左心衰竭：将本品 2 ～ 5mg 加入 500ml 氯化钠注射液中静脉滴注，30 ～ 60 分钟滴完。也可肌内注射或静脉注射，一次 1 ～ 2mg，必要时间隔 20 分钟再给药 1 次。<br>　　（2）儿童：口服，一次 0.01 ～ 0.02mg/kg，必要时 4 ～ 6 小时 1 次；肌内或静脉注射：剂量同口服。<br><br>　　(1) Chez des adultes : ① Pour traite l'œdème : par voie orale, 0,5 à 2mg par fois, 1 fois par jour, s'il est nécessaire, 2 à 3 fois par jour, la dose totale pourrait atteindre 10mg par jour ; l'injection IM ou IV, commencer par 0,5 à 1mg, s'il est nécessaire, reprendre toutes les 2 à 3h, la dose maximale est de 10mg par jour. ② Pour traiter l'œdème pulmonaire aigu et l'insuffisance cardiaque gauche : dissoudre 2 à 5mg de bumétanide dans 500ml de solution de chlorure de sodium pour la perfusion, finir en 30 à 60 minutes. Aussi possible d'administrer par voie IM ou IV, 1 à 2mg par fois, s'il est nécessaire, reprendre toutes les 20 minutes.<br>　　(2) Chez des enfants : par voie orale, 0,01 à 0,02 mg/kg par fois, s'il est nécessaire, toutes les 4 à 6h ; injection IM ou IV : la même dose que celle prise par voie orale.</td>
</tr>
<tr>
<td>剂型、规格<br>Les formes pharmaceutiques et les spécifications</td>
<td>片剂：每片 1mg。<br>注射液：每支 0.5mg（2ml）。<br>Comprimés : 1mg par comprimé.<br>Injection : 0,5mg (2ml) par solution.</td>
</tr>
<tr>
<td>药品名称 Drug Names</td>
<td>托拉塞米 Torasémide</td>
</tr>
<tr>
<td>适应证<br>Les indications</td>
<td>　　①各种原因所致水肿：如，由于原发或继发性肾脏疾病及何种原因所致急、慢性肾衰竭、充血性心力衰竭，以及肝硬化等所致的水肿；与其他药合用治疗急性脑水肿等。②急、慢性心力衰竭。③原发或继发性高血压。④急、慢性肾衰竭，本品可增加尿量，促进尿钠排出。⑤肝硬化腹水。⑥急性毒物或药物中毒。本品通过强效、迅速的利尿作用，配合充分的液体补充，不仅可以加速毒性物质和药物的排泄，而且由于其肾脏保护作用，还可减轻有毒物质对近曲小管上皮细胞的损害。<br><br>　　① L'œdème induite par divers facteurs : tel que l'œdème causé par les maladies rénales primaires ou secondaire, l'insuffisance rénale aigue ou chronique, l'insuffisance cardiaque congestive ainsi que la cirrhose. Utilisé en association avec d'autres médicaments, il peut traiter l'œdème cérébral aigu. ② L'insuffisance cardiaque aigue ou chronique. ③ L'hypertension artérielle primaire ou secondaire. ④ L'insuffisance rénale aigue ou chronique. il permet d'augmenter la production d'urine et de favoriser l'excrétion urinaire de sodium. ⑤ Les ascites en raison de la cirrhose. ⑥ L'intoxication aigue par des substances toxiques ou des médicaments. Ce produit a une diurèse forte et rapide, permettant l'accélération de l'excrétion des substances toxiques et des médicaments. Avec son effet protecteur réna, il permet de réduire l'atteinte des substances toxiques sur les cellules épithéliales du tubule proximal.</td>
</tr>
</table>

**续　表**

| | |
|---|---|
| 用法、用量<br>Les modes d'emploi et la posologie | ①心力衰竭：口服或静脉注射（用5%葡萄糖注射液或氯化钠注射液稀释），初始剂量一般为一次5～10mg，一日1次，递增至一次10～20mg，一日1次。②急性或慢性肾衰竭：口服，开始5mg，可增加至20mg，均为一日1次。需要时可静脉注射，一次10～20mg，一日1次。必要时可由初始剂量逐渐增加为每日100～200mg。③肝硬化腹水：口服，开始5～10mg，一日1次；以后可增加至一次20mg，一日1次，但最多不超过40mg。静脉注射同口服，一日剂量不超过40mg。④高血压：口服，开始每日2.5mg或5mg，需要时可增至每日10mg，单用或与其他降压药合用。<br><br>① Pour traite l'insuffisance cardiaque : par voie orale ou IV (utiliser la solution de glucose ou de chlorure de sodium pour la dilution), commencer par 5 à 10mg par fois, 1 fois par jour, augmenter progressivement pour atteindre 10 à 20mg par fois, 1 fois par jour. ② Pour traiter l'insuffisance rénale aigue ou chronique : par voie orale, commencer par 5mg, augmenter jusqu'à 20mg, 1 fois par jour. S'il est nécessaire, injecter par voie IV, 10 à 20mg par fois, 1 fois par jour. En cas de besoin, augmenter à partir de la dose initiale pour atteindre 100 à 200mg par jour. ③ Pour traiter les ascites en raison de la cirrhose : par voie orale, commencer par 5 à 10mg, 1 fois par jour ; ensuite, augmenter pour atteindre 20mg par fois, 1 fois par jour, ne pas dépasser 40mg. La dose maximale pour l'injection IV est aussi de 49mg par jour. ④ Pour traiter l'hypertension artérielle : par voie orale, commencer par 2,5mg ou 5mg par jour, s'il est nécessaire, augmenter pour atteindre 10mg par jour, utilisé seul ou en association avec d'autres antihypertenseurs. |
| 剂型、规格<br>Les formes pharmaceutiques et les spécifications | 片剂：每片2.5mg；5mg；10mg；20mg。<br>注射液：每支10mg（1ml）；20mg（2ml）。<br>Comprimés : 2,5mg, 5mg, 10mg ou 20mg par comprimé.<br>Injection : 10mg (1ml) ou 20mg (2ml) par solution. |
| 药品名称 Drug Names | 氢氯噻嗪 Hydrochlorothiazide |
| 适应证<br>Les indications | ①各种水肿性疾病：排泄体内过多的钠和水，减少细胞外液容量，消除水肿。常见的适应证包括充血性心力衰竭、肝硬化腹水、肾病综合征、急慢性肾炎水肿、慢性肾衰竭早期、肾上腺皮质激素和雌激素治疗所致的钠、水潴留。②高血压：可单独或与其他降压药联合应用，主要用于治疗原发性高血压。③肾性尿崩症、中枢性尿崩症：单独用于肾性尿崩症，与其他抗利尿剂联合亦可用于中枢性尿崩症。④肾结石：主要用于预防含钙成分形成的结石。<br><br>① Les maladies liées à l'œdème : excréter l'excès de sodium et de l'eau du corps, réduire le volume de fluide extracellulaire, éliminer oedèmes. Il est applicable dans le traitement des cas suivants : l'insuffisance cardiaque congestive, les ascites en raison de la cirrhose, le syndrome néphrotique, l'œdème lié à la néphrite aiguë et chronique, l'insuffisance rénale chronique précoce ainsi que la rétention de sodium et de l'eau induite par la thérapie d'hormone corticotrope et d'œstrogène. ② L'hypertension artérielle : utilisé seul ou en association avec d'autres antihypertenseurs, il sert à traiter l'hypertension essentielle. ③ Le diabète insipide néphrogénique et le diabète insipide centraldiurétique : utilisé seul, il sert à traiter la diabète insipide néphrogénique et utilisé en association avec d'autres diurétiques, il permet de traiter le diabète insipide central. ④ les calculs rénaux : il est principalement utilisé comme prévention des calculs formés dans des ingrédients contenant du calcium. |
| 用法、用量<br>Les modes d'emploi et la posologie | 成人口服：①治疗水肿性疾病：一次25～50mg，一日1～2次，或隔日治疗，或每周连服3～5日。为预防电解质紊乱及血容量骤降，宜从小剂量（12.5～25mg/d）用起，以后根据利尿情况逐渐加重。②心源性水肿：开始用小剂量，一日12.5～25mg，以免因盐及水分排泄过快而引起循环障碍或其他症状；同时注意调整洋地黄用量，以免由于钾的丢失而导致洋地黄中毒。③肝性腹水：最好与螺内酯合用，以防血钾过低诱发肝性脑病。④高血压：常与其他药合用，可减少后者剂量，减少不良反应。开始一日50～100mg，分1～2次服用，并按降压效果调整剂量，一周后为每日25～50mg的维持量。⑤尿崩症：成人口服：一次25mg，一日3次；或一次50mg，一日2次。儿童口服：一日按体重1～2mg/kg，或按体表面积30～60mg/m²，分1～2次服用，并按疗效调整剂量。小于6个月的婴儿，剂量可达一日3mg/kg。 |

**续　表**

| | |
|---|---|
| | Chez des adultes, par voie orale : ① pour traiter les maladies liées à l'œdème : 25 à 50mg par fois, 1 à 2 fois par jour, ou tous les 2 jours, ou pendant 3 à 5 jours consécutifs par semaine. Pour prévenir le déséquilibre électrolytique ou l'hypovolémie soudaine, il vaut mieux commencer par une dose mineure (12,5 à 25mg par jour), augmenter progressivement la dose en fonction de l'effet diurétique. ② Pour traiter l'œdème cardiogénique : commencer par une faible dose, 12,5 à 25mg par jour, pour éviter les troubles ciruculatoires causés par l'excrétion de sel et d'eau excessive ; il faut penser à ajuster la dose de la digitale pour éviter une intoxication digitalique à cause de la perte de potassium. ③ Pour traite l'ascite hépatique : il vau mieux utiliser ce médicament en association avec la spironolactone pour éviter la crise des maladies hépatiques induites par l'hypokaliémie. ④ Pour traite l'hypertension artérielle : utilisé souvent en association avec d'autre médicaments, permettant de réduire la dose de ceux-ci et de réduire les réactions indésirables. Commencer par 50 à 100mg par jour, à travers 1 à 2 fois, ajuster la dose en fonction de l'effet antihypertenseur, 1 semaine après, prendre la dose d'entretien, soit 25 à 50mg par jour. ⑤ Pour traiter le diabète insipide : chez des adultes, par voie orale : 25mg par fois, 3 fois par jour; ou 50mg par fois, 2 fois par jour. chez des enfants, par voie orale : 1 à 2 mg/kg par jour, ou 30 à 60 mg/m$^2$, à travers 1 à 2 fois, ajuster la dose en fonction de l'effet du traitement. Chez des bébés moins de 6 mois, possible de prendre 3 mg/kg par jour. |
| 剂型、规格<br>Les formes pharmaceutiques et les spécifications | 片剂：每片 10mg；25mg；50mg。<br>Comprimés : 10mg, 25mg ou 50mg par comprimé. |
| **药品名称 Drug Names** | 吲达帕胺 Indapamide |
| 适应证<br>Les indications | 作用与氢氯噻嗪相似，但比后者利尿作用强 10 倍。可用于慢性肾衰竭。<br>Il a un effet similaire à l'hydrochlorothiazide, mais sa diurèse est 10 fois plus forte que celle-ci. Il est applicable dans le traitement de l'insuffisance rénale chronique. |
| 用法、用量<br>Les modes d'emploi et la posologie | 水肿，口服，一次 2.5mg，必要时 5mg，一日 1 次；降压，一次 2.5mg，一日 1 次，维持量可每 2 日 2.5 ～ 5mg。<br>Pour traiter l'œdème, par voie orale, 2,5mg par fois, s'il est nécessaire, 5mg, 1 fois par jour ; pour traiter l'hypertension artérielle, 2,5mg par fois, 1 fois par jour, la dose d'entretien, 2,5 à 5mg tous les 2 jours. |
| 剂型、规格<br>Les formes pharmaceutiques et les spécifications | 片剂：2.5mg。<br>Comprimés : 2,5mg. |
| **药品名称 Drug Names** | 螺内酯 Spironolactone |
| 适应证<br>Les indications | ①治疗与醛固酮升高有关的顽固性水肿，故对肝硬化和肾病综合征的患者较有效，而对充血性心力衰竭效果较差（除非因缺钠而引起的继发性醛固酮增多者外）。也可用于特发性水肿的治疗。单用本品时利尿效果往往较差，故常与噻嗪类、髓袢利尿药合用，既能增强利尿效果，又可防止低血钾。②治疗高血压，可作为原发性或继发性高血压的辅助用药，尤其是应用于有排钾离子作用的利尿药时。③原发性醛固酮增多症的诊断与治疗。④低钾血症的预防，与噻嗪类利尿药合用，增强利尿效果并预防低钾血症。<br>① Il sert à traiter l'oedème réfractaire lié à l'élévation de l'aldostérone, il est donc efficace dans le traitement des patients souffrant de la cirrhose et du syndrome néphrotique. Mais il est peu efficace dans le traitement de l'insuffisance cardiaque congestive (sauf l'hyperaldostéronisme secondaire causé par l'absence de sodium). Il est aussi applicable dans le traitement de l'oedème idiopathique. Utilisé seul, il a un effet diurétique faible. Il est donc souvent utilisé en association avec des thiazidiques et des diurétiques de l'anseanse de henlépour renforcer sa diurèse tout en évitant l'hypokaliémie. ② Il sert à traiter l'hypertension artérielle. Il sert de traitement adjuvant de l'hypertension essentielle ou secondaire, surtout quand il est utilisé en association avec des diurétiques facilitant l'excrétion des ions de potassium. ③ L'examen et le traitement de l'hyperaldostéronisme primaire. ④ La prévention de l'hypokaliémie. Utilisé en combinaison avec les diurétiques thiazidiques, il peut renforcer sa diurèse tout en évitant l'hypokaliémie. |

| | |
|---|---|
| 用法、用量<br>Les modes d'emploi et la posologie | 　　成人口服。①治疗水肿：一次 20 ～ 40mg，一日 3 次。用药 5 日后，如疗效满意，继续用原量。②治疗高血压：开始每日 40 ～ 80mg，分 2 ～ 4 次服用，至少 2 周，以后酌情调整剂量。本品不宜与血管紧张素转化酶抑制剂合用，以免增加发生高钾血症的机会。③治疗原发性醛固酮增多症：手术前患者一日用量 100 ～ 400mg，分 2 ～ 4 次服用。不宜手术的患者，则选用较小剂量维持。④诊断原发性醛固酮增多症：长期试验，一日 400mg，分 2 ～ 4 次服用，连续 3 ～ 4 周。短期试验，一日 400mg，分 2 ～ 4 次服用，连续 4 日。老年人对本药较敏感，开始用量宜偏小。<br>　　儿童口服，治疗水肿性疾病，开始一日按体重 1 ～ 3mg/kg 或按体表面积 30 ～ 90mg/m²，单次或分 2 ～ 4 次服用，连用 5 日后酌情调整剂量。最大剂量一日 3 ～ 9mg/kg 或 90 ～ 270mg/m²。<br><br>　　Chez des adultes, par voie orale. ① Pour traiter l'œdème : 20 à 40mg par fois, 3 fois par jour. 5 jours après, si l'effet est satisfaisant, continuer la dose initiale. ② Pour traiter l'hypertension artérielle : commencer par 40 à 80 mg par jour, à travers 2 à 4 fois, pendant au moins 2 semaines, ensuite, ajuster la dose selon les cas. Ce médicament ne doit pas être utilisé en association avec les inhibiteurs de l'enzyme de conversion de l'angiotensine, pour éviter l'incidence de l'hyperkaliémie. ③ Pour traiter l'hyperaldostéronisme primaire : avant la chirurgie, 100 à 400mg par jour, à travers 2 à 4 fois. Chez des patients qui ne peuvent pas être traités par la chirurgie, il faut prendre une faible dose pour le traitement d'entretien. ④ Pour le diagnostic de l'hyperaldostéronisme primaire : pour le test à long terme, 400 mg par jour, à travers 2 à 4 fois, pendant 3 à 4 semaines consécutives. Pour l'examen à court terme, 400mg par jour, à travers 2 à 4 fois, pendant 4 jours consécutifs. Comme les personnes âgées sont sensibles à ce médicament, il faut commencer par une dose mineure.<br>　　Chez des enfants, par voie orale, pour traiter les maladies liées à l'œdème, commencer par 1 à 3 mg/kg par jour ou 30 à 90 mg/m², une fois par jour ou à travers 2 à 4 fois, pendant 5 jours consécutifs avant d'ajuster la dose selon les cas. La dose maximale est de 3 à 9 mg/kg par jour ou de 90 à 270 mg/m² par jour. |
| 剂型、规格<br>Les formes pharmaceutiques et les spécifications | 　　片剂：每片 20mg。<br>　　胶囊剂：每粒 20mg（微粒制剂 20mg 与普通制剂 100mg 的疗效相仿）。<br>　　Comprimés : 20mg par comprimé.<br>　　Capsules : 20mg par capsule (l'effet de 20mg de préparations à base de particules est similaire à celui de 100mg de préparations ordinaires.) |
| 药品名称 Drug Names | 氨苯蝶啶 Triamtérène |
| 适应证<br>Les indications | 　　用于治疗各类水肿，如心力衰竭、肝硬化及慢性肾炎引起的水肿或腹水，以及糖皮质激素治疗过程中发生的水钠潴留。常与排钾利尿药合用。亦用于对氢氯噻嗪或螺内酯无效的病例。<br><br>　　Il sert à traiter l'œdème de toutes sortes, tel que l'oedème ou l'ascite provoqués par l'insuffisance cardiaque, la cirrhose et la néphrite chronique, ainsi que la rétention de l'eau et de sodium lors de la corticothérapie. Il est souvent utilisé en association avec des diurétiques facilitant l'excrétion des ions de potassium. Il est aussi appliqué dans le traitement des cas résistant àl'hydrochlorothiazideou à la spironolactone. |
| 用法、用量<br>Les modes d'emploi et la posologie | 　　口服，成人，开始一次 25 ～ 50mg，一日 2 次，餐后服，最大剂量每日不宜超过 300mg。维持阶段可改为隔日疗法。与其他利尿剂合用时，两者均应减量。儿童，开始一日按体重 2 ～ 4mg/kg 或按体表面积 120mg/m²，分 2 次服，每日或隔日疗法。以后酌情调整剂量。最大剂量不超过每日 6mg/kg 或 300mg/m²。<br><br>　　Par voie orale, chez des adultes, commencer par 25 à 50mg par fois, 2 fois par jour, pris après le repas, ne pas dépasser 300mg par jour. Pour le traitement d'entretien, possible de prendre le médicament tous les deux jours. Lors de l'utilisation avec d'autres médicaments diurétiques, il faut diminuer la dose pour les deux. Chez des enfants, commencer par 2 à 4 mg/kg par jour ou 120 mg/m² par jour, à travers 2 fois, tous les 1 à 2 jours. Ensuite, ajuster la dose selon les cas. La dose maximale est de 6 de 6 mg/kg par jour ou de 300 mg/m² par jour. |
| 剂型、规格<br>Les formes pharmaceutiques et les spécifications | 　　片剂：每片 50mg。<br>　　Comprimés : 50mg par comprimé. |

**续　表**

| 药品名称 Drug Names | 阿米洛利 Amiloride |
|---|---|
| 适应证<br>Les indications | 本品同氨苯蝶啶，主要用于治疗水肿性疾病，亦可用于难治性低钾血症的辅助治疗。氨苯蝶啶和螺内酯均大部分经肝脏代谢，当肝功能严重损害时，剂量不易控制，此时则可应用不经肝脏代谢的本品。另外，本品可增加氢氯噻嗪和利尿酸等利尿药的作用，并减少钾的丢失，故一般不单独应用。<br><br>Comme le triamtérène, il sert à traiter les maladies liées à l'œdème. Il est aussi applicable dans le traitement adjuvant de l'hypokaliémie réfractaire. Le triamtérène et la spironolactone sont principalement métabolisés par le foie. Quand il s'agit de l'insuffisance hépatique et qu'il est difficile de contrôler la dose, il faut utiliser l'amiloride qui n'est pas métabolisé à travers le foie. En outre, ce produit peut renforcer l'efficacité des diutériques comme l'hydrochlorothiazideet l'acide étacrynique, tout en réduisant la perte de potassium. Il n'est donc pas souvent utilisé seul. |
| 用法、用量<br>Les modes d'emploi et la posologie | 口服：开始一次 2.5 ~ 5mg，一日 1 次；必要时可增加剂量，但每日不宜超过 20mg。<br>Par voie orale : commencer par 2,5 à 5mg par fois, 1 fois par jour ; s'il est nécessaire, augmenter la dose, ne pas dépasser 20mg par jour. |
| 剂型、规格<br>Les formes pharmaceutiques et les spécifications | 片剂：每片含 2.5mg；5mg。<br>Comprimés : 2,5mg ou 5mg par comprimé. |
| 药品名称 Drug Names | 乙酰唑胺 Acétazolamide |
| 适应证<br>Les indications | 用于治疗青光眼、心脏性水肿、脑水肿，亦用于癫痫小发作。<br>Ce produit sert à traiter le glaucome, l'œdème cardiaque, l'œdème cérébral ainsi que la crise mineure de l'épilepsie. |
| 用法、用量<br>Les modes d'emploi et la posologie | （1）青光眼：一般口服给药，①开角型青光眼，首量 0.25g，一日 1 ~ 3 次。维持剂量根据患者对药物的反应而定，尽量使用较小剂量使眼压得到控制，一般 1 次 0.25g，一日 2 次就可使眼压控制在正常范围。②继发性青光眼和手术前降眼压，一次 0.25g，一般一日 2 ~ 3 次。③闭角型青光眼急性发作，首次 0.5g，以后一次 0.125 ~ 0.25g，一日 2 ~ 3 次维持。④青光眼急性发作时的抢救或某些恶心、呕吐不能口服的患者，可静脉或肌内注射本品。将本品 2.5g 溶于 5 ~ 10ml 灭菌注射用水静脉注射，或溶于 2.5ml 灭菌注射用水肌内注射；也可静脉注射 0.25g 或肌内注射 0.25g 交替使用。对于一些急性发作的青光眼患者，可在 2 ~ 4 小时重复上述剂量，但继续治疗应根据患者情况改为口服给药。<br>（2）脑水肿：口服，一次 0.25g，一日 2 ~ 3 次。<br>（3）心源性水肿：口服，一次 0.25 ~ 0.5g，一日 1 次，早餐后服用药效最佳。<br>（4）癫痫小发作：其作用可能与抑制脑组织中的碳酸酐酶有关。口服，一次 0.5 ~ 1g，一日 1 次。与其他药物合用时则不超过 0.25g。儿童：①青光眼：口服，一日 5 ~ 10mg/kg，分 2 ~ 3 次服用；②青光眼急性发作：静脉或肌内注射，一次 5 ~ 10mg/kg，每 6 小时 1 次。<br><br>(1) Pour traiter le glaucome : en général, par voie orale<br>① Pour traiter le glaucome à angle ouvert : la dose initiale, 0,25g, 1 à 3 fois par jour. La dose d'entretien est dépendante des réactions des patients. Essayer de prendre une faible dose pour contrôler la PIO, en général, 0,25g par fois, 2 fois par jour, cela suffit pour maintenir la PIO à un niveau normal. ② Pour traiter le glaucome secondaire et diminuer la PIO avant la chirurgie, 0,25g par fois, en général, 2 à 3 fois par jour. ③ Pour traiter la crise aigue du glaucome à angle fermé, la dose initiale, 0,5g, ensuite, 0,125 à 0,25g par fois, 2 à 3 fois par jour.<br>④ Utilisé lors dc la crise aigue du glaucome ou chez des patients atteints de glaucome mais qui ne peuvent pas prendre le médicament à cause des nausées et des vomissements, possible d'injecter ce médicament par voie IV ou IM. Dissoudre 0,5g d'acétazolamide dans 5 à 10ml d'eau stérile pour injection pour l'injection IV, ou dissoudre dans 2,5ml d'eau stérile pour injection pour l'injection IM ; ou injection IV de 0,25g et l'injection IM de 0,25g en alternative. Pour la crise aigue du glaucome, possible de reprendre la dose précédente dans les 2 à 4h, mais pour continuer le traitement, il faut commencer à prendre par voie orale.<br>(2) Pour traiter l'odème cérébral : par voie orale, 0,25g par fois, 2 à 3 fois par jour.<br>(3) Pour traiter l'œdème cardiogénique : par voie orale, 0,25 à 0,5g par fois, 1 fois par jour, pris après le petit-déjeuner au mieux. |

|  |  |
|---|---|
|  | (4) Pour traiter la crise mineure de l'épilepsie : son action est peut-être liée à l'inhibition de l'anhydrase carbonique de l'organiseme cérébral. Par voie orale, 0,5 à 1 g par fois, 1 fois par jour. Lors de l'utilisation en association avec d'autres médicaments, ne pas dépasser 0,25g.Chez des enfants: ① Pour traiter le glaucome : par voie orale, 5 à 10 mg/kg par jour, à travers 2 à 3 fois. ② Pour traiter la crise aigue du glaucome : injection IV ou IM, 5 à 10 mg/kg par fois, toutes les 6h. |
| 剂型、规格<br>Les formes pharmaceutiques et les spécifications | 片剂：每片 0.25g。<br>注射用乙酰唑胺：每支 500mg。<br>Comprimés : 0,25g par comprimé.<br>L'acétazolamide pour injection : 500mg par solution. |

14.2　脱水药 Médicaments de déshydratation

| 药品名称 Drug Names | 甘露醇 Mannitol |
|---|---|
| 适应证<br>Les indications | ①治疗各种原因引起的脑水肿，降低颅内压，防止脑疝；②降低眼压：当在应用其他降眼压药无效或青光眼的术前准备时应用；③预防急性肾小管坏死：在大面积烧伤、严重创伤、广泛外科手术时，常因肾小球滤过率降低及血容量减少而出现少尿、无尿，极易发生肾衰竭，应及时用本品预防；④作为其他利尿药的辅助药，治疗某些伴有低钠血症的顽固性水肿（因本品排水多于排钠，故不适用于全身性水肿的治疗）；⑤鉴别肾前性因素或急性肾衰竭引起的少尿；⑥对于某些药物过量或毒物引起的重度，可促进上述物质的排泄，防止肾毒性；⑦术前肠道准备；⑧作清洗剂，应用于经尿道内做前列腺切除术。<br><br>① Ce produit sert à traiter l'œdème cérébral causé par divers facteurs, à réduire la pression intracrânienne et à prévenir l'hernie cérébrale. ② Réduire la pression intraoculaire : utilisé lorsque d'autres médicaments capables de réduire la PIO sont inefficaces ou avant la chirurgie liée au glaucome. ③ Prévenir la nécrose tubulaire rénale aiguë : lors des brûlures étendues, du traumatisme sévère et d'une importante intervention chirurgicale, la diminution du taux de filtration glomérulaire et une hypovolémie peuvent souvent entraîner l'oligurie, l'anurie et l'insuffisance rénale. Il faut donc utiliser ce produit en temps opportun pour la prévention. ④ En tant que médicament adjuvant des autres diurétiques, il sert à traiter l'œdème réfractaire accompagné de l'hypokaliémie (comme son drainage est plus important que sa natriurèse, il n'est pas applicable dans le traitement de l'œdème systématique). ⑤ Distinguer l'oligurie causée par le facteurs prérénales ou par l'insuffisance rénale. ⑥ Lors de l'intoxication par le surdosage ou des substances toxiques, il permet l'excrétion de ces objects et d'éviter la néphrotoxicité. ⑦ La préparation de l'intestin préopératoire. ⑧ Commme nettoyeur, il est utilisé dans la résection transurétrale de la prostate. |
| 用法、用量<br>Les modes d'emploi et la posologie | ①利尿：静脉滴注，按体重 1～2g/kg，一般为 20% 溶液 250～500ml，并调整剂量使尿量维持在每小时 30～50ml。②脑水肿、颅内高压和青光眼：静脉滴注，按体重 1.5～2g/kg，配成 15%～20% 浓度于 30～60 分钟滴完（当患者衰弱时，剂量可减为 0.5g/kg）。③预防急性肾小管坏死：先给予 12.5～25g，10 分钟内静脉滴注，若无特殊情况，再给 50g，1 小时内静脉滴注，若尿量能维持在每小时 50ml 以上，则可继续应用 5% 溶液静滴；若无效则立即停药。同时需注意补足血容量。④鉴别肾前性少尿和肾性少尿：按体重 0.2g/kg，以 20% 浓度于 3～5 分钟静脉滴注。如用药 2～3 小时以后尿量仍低于 30～50ml/h，最多再试用一次，若仍无反应则应停药。心功能减退或心力衰竭者，慎用或不宜使用。⑤药物或毒物中毒：50g 以 20% 溶液静脉滴注，调整剂量使尿量维持在每小时 100～500ml。⑥术前肠道准备：口服，于术前 4～8 小时以 10% 溶液 1000ml 于 30 分钟内口服完毕。<br><br>① Pour l'effet diurétique : la perfusion, 1 à 2 g/kg, 250 à 500ml de solution à 20%, ajuster la dose pour maintenir 30 à 50ml d'urine par h. ② Pour traiter l'œdème cérébra, la pression intracrânienne élevée et le glaucome : en perfusion, 1,5 à 2 g/kg, la solution à 15% à 20% pour la perfusion, finir en 30 à 60 minutes (chez des patients faibles, 0,5 g/kg). ③ Pour prévenir la nécrose tubulaire rénale |

续　表

<table>
<tr>
<td></td>
<td>aigue : commencer par 12,5 à 25g, la perfusion en 10 minutes, si tout est normal, reprendre 50g en perfusion, finir en 1h, s'il on peut maintenir 50ml ou plus d'urine par h, possible d'administrer la solution à 5% en perfusion ; s'il est inefficace, il faut arrêter immédiatement l'administration. Il faut compléter le volume sanguin. ④ Pour distinguer l'oligurie prérénale et l'oligurie rénale : 0,2 g par kg, administrer la solution à 20% en perfusion en 3 à 5 minutes. Si 2 à 3 h après l'administration, la quantité de l'urine est encore inférieure à 30 à 50ml par h, il faut essayer encore une fois au plus, s'il est toujours inefficace, il faut arrêter l'administration. Chez des patients insuffisants cardiaques, soyez prudent ou ne pas l'appliquer. ⑤ Pour traiter l'intoxication par le surdosage ou des substances toxiques : administrer la solution de 50g à 20% en perfusion, ajuster la dose pour maintenir 100 à 500ml d'urine par h. ⑥ Pour la préparation de l'intestin préopératoire : par voie orale, 4 à 8 h avant la chirurgie, administrer par voie orale 1 000ml de solution à 10% en 30 minutes.</td>
</tr>
<tr>
<td>剂型、规格<br>Les formes pharmaceutiques et les spécifications</td>
<td>注射液：每瓶 10g（50ml）；20g（100ml）；50g（250ml）；100g（500ml）；150g（3000ml）。<br>Injection : 10g (50ml), 20g (100ml), 50g (250ml), 100g (500ml) ou 150g (3 000ml).</td>
</tr>
<tr>
<td>药品名称 Drug Names</td>
<td>甘油果糖氯化钠 Glycérine-Fructoseet Chlorure de Sodium</td>
</tr>
<tr>
<td>适应证<br>Les indications</td>
<td>①由脑血管疾病、脑外伤、脑肿瘤、颅内炎症及其他原因引起的急、慢性颅内压增高，脑水肿症；②改善下列疾病的意识障碍、神经障碍和自觉症状，如脑梗死（脑栓死、脑血栓）、脑内出血、蛛网膜下腔出血、头部外伤、脑脊髓膜炎等；③脑外科手术术前缩小脑容积；④脑外科手术后降颅内压；⑤青光眼患者降低眼压或眼科手术缩小眼容积。<br><br>① L'élévation de la pression intracrânienne aiguë et chronique, ainsi que l'oedème cérébral causés par les maladies vasculaires cérébrales, un traumatisme cérébral, les tumeurs cérébrales, une inflammation intracrânienne et d'autres facteurs. ② Améliorer les troubles de conscience, les troubles neurologiques liés aux maladies suivantes: l'infarctus cérébral (la mort du thrombus cérébral, la thrombose cérébrale), une hémorragie intracérébrale, l'hémorragie méningée, le traumatisme crânien, la méningite cérébrale, etc. ③ Réduire le volume du cerveau avant la chirurgie cérébrale. ④ Réduction de la pression intracrânienne après la chirurgie cérébrale. ⑤ Chez des patients souffrant du glaucome, il permet de réduire la pression intraoculaire ou de réduire le volume oculaire lors de la chirurgie ophtalmique.</td>
</tr>
<tr>
<td>用法、用量<br>Les modes d'emploi et la posologie</td>
<td>静脉滴注。①治疗颅内压增高、脑水肿：成人一次 250 ～ 500ml，一日 1 ～ 2 次；儿童用量为 5 ～ 10ml/kg。每 500ml 需滴注 2 ～ 3 小时，连续给药 1 ～ 2 周。②脑外科手术时缩小脑容积：每次 500ml，静脉滴注时间为 30 分钟。③降低眼压或眼科手术时缩小眼容积：每次 250 ～ 500ml，静脉滴注时间为 45 ～ 90 分钟。<br><br>En perfusion. ① Pour traiter l'élévation de la pression intracrânienne, l'œdème cérébral : chez des adultes, 250 à 500ml par fois, 1 à 2 fois par jour ; chez des enfants, 5 à 10 ml/kg. La perfusion de 500ml en 2 à 3 h. L'administration continue pendant 1 à 2 semaines. ② Pour réduire le volume du cerveau avant la chirurgie cérébrale : 500ml par fois, la perfusion pendant 30 minutes. ③ Pour réduire la PIO ou réduire le volume oculaire lors de la chirurgie ophtalmique : 250 à 500ml par fois, la perfusion pendant 45 à 90 minutes.</td>
</tr>
<tr>
<td>剂型、规格<br>Les formes pharmaceutiques et les spécifications</td>
<td>注射液：每瓶 250ml；500ml（每 1ml 中含甘油 100mg、果糖 50mg、氯化钠 9mg）。<br>Injection : 250 ml ou 500ml par flacon (chaque 1ml contient 100mg de glycérine, 50mg de fructose et 9mg de chlorure de sodium).</td>
</tr>
</table>

14.3　治疗尿崩症用药 Médicaments traitant le diabète insipide

<table>
<tr>
<td>药品名称 Drug Names</td>
<td>鞣酸加压素 Vasopréssine Tannique</td>
</tr>
<tr>
<td>适应证<br>Les indications</td>
<td>①中枢性尿崩症、头部手术或外伤所致的暂时性尿崩症的治疗。②用于中枢性尿崩症、肾性尿崩症的鉴别诊断试验。③食管静脉曲张破裂出血及咯血。</td>
</tr>
</table>

| | |
|---|---|
| | ① Traiter le diabète insipide temporaire causé par le diabète insipide central, la chirurgie ou un traumatismecraniens. ② Utilisé dans le test de diagnostic pour distinguer le diabète insipide central etle diabète insipide néphrogénique. ③ L'hémoptysie et le saignement liés aux varices oesophagiennes. |
| 用法、用量<br>Les modes d'emploi et la posologie | ①中枢性尿崩症：a. 成人，加压素注射液 3mg 皮下或肌内注射，一日 2～3 次。b. 儿童，加压素注射液 1～1.5mg 皮下或肌内注射，一日 2～3 次。②中枢性尿崩症的诊断：禁水 - 加压素试验时，皮下注射加压素注射液 3mg，继续禁水 2 小时测血和尿渗透压、尿量、尿比重、血压、脉率等。儿童酌情减量。③食管静脉曲张破裂出血及咯血：加压素注射液 3mg 稀释后缓慢静脉注射，或 6～12mg 加入 200～500ml 的 5% 葡萄糖注射液中缓慢静脉滴注。<br><br>① Pour traiter le diabète insipide central : a. Chez des adultes, injecter par voie sous-cutanée ou IM 3mg d'injection de vasopressine, 2 à 3 fois par jour.b.Chez des enfants, 1 à 1,5 mg d'injection de vasopressine administré par voie sous-cutanée ou IM, 2 à 3 fois par jour. ② Pour diagnostiquer le diabète insipide central : lors du test de privation d'eau –vasopressine, injection sous-cutanée de 3mg d'injection de vasopressine, continuer la privation d'eau pour tester l'osmolalité anguine et urinaire, la quantité d'urine, la tensité urinaire, la pression artérielle, le pouls, etc. Chez des enfants, diminuer un peu la dose. ③ Pour traiter l'hémoptysie et le saignement liés aux varices oesophagiennes : diluer 3mg d'injection de vasopressine avant de l'injecter par voie IV lentement, ou dissoudre 6 à 12mg dans 200 à 500ml de solution de glucose à 5% pour la perfusion lente. |
| 剂型、规格<br>Les formes pharmaceutiques et les spécifications | 注射液：每支 6mg（1ml）；12mg（1ml）。<br>Injection : 6mg (1ml) ou 12mg (1ml) par solution. |
| 药品名称 Drug Names | 垂体后叶粉 Poudre hypophyse postérieure |
| 适应证<br>Les indications | 治疗尿崩症。<br>Traiter le diabète insipide. |
| 用法、用量<br>Les modes d'emploi et la posologie | 用特制小匙（每匙装量为 30～40mg）取出本品 1 小匙，以小指头抹在鼻黏膜上；亦可将取出的粉剂倒在纸上，卷成卷纸，用左手压住左鼻孔，用右手将纸卷插入右鼻孔内，抬头轻轻将粉剂吸进鼻腔内。一日 3～4 次。<br><br>Retirer une cuillère de ce médicament (30 à 40mg par cuillère), essuyer sur la muqueuse nasale avec le petit doigt ; ou verser la poudre sur un papier, rouler, presser la narine gauche avec la main gauche, insérer le rouleau dans la narine droite avec la main droite, hausser la tête avant d'inhaler la poudre dans la cavité nasale. 3 à 4 fois par jour. |
| 剂型、规格<br>Les formes pharmaceutiques et les spécifications | 鼻吸入粉剂：每瓶 1g（附小匙）。<br>Poudre pour inhalation nasale : 1g par flacon (y compris une cuillère). |
| 药品名称 Drug Names | 去氨加压素 Desmopressine |
| 适应证<br>Les indications | ①中枢性尿崩症及颅外伤或手术所致的暂时性尿崩症：用后可减少尿排出，增加尿渗透压，减低血浆渗透压，减少尿频和夜尿（一般对肾源性尿崩症无效）。②治疗 5 岁以上患有夜间遗尿症的患者。③肾尿液浓缩功能试验：有助于对肾功能的鉴别，对于诊断不同部位的尿道感染尤其有效。④对于轻度血友病及 I 型血管性血友病患者，在进行小型外科手术时可控制出血或预防出血。⑤因尿毒症、肝硬化以及先天的或用药诱发的血小板功能障碍而引起的出血时间过长和不明原因的出血，用本品可使出血时间缩短或恢复正常。<br><br>① Traiter le diabète insipide temporaire causé par le diabète insipide central, la chirurgie ou un traumatisme crâniens :il permet de réduire l'urine, d'augmenter l'osmolalité urinaire, de réduire l'osmolalité plasmatique et de réduire la fréquence urinaire et nycturie (en général, il est inutile pour le diabète insipide néphrogénique). ② Traiter les patients âgés de plus de 5 ans atteints de l'énurésie |

**续　表**

<table>
<tr>
<td></td>
<td>nocturne. ③ Le test sur la fonction rénale de la concentration de l'urine : il faciliter l'identification de la fonction rénale. Il est surtout efficace dans le diagnostic des infections des voies urinaires dans les différentes parties. ④ Chez des patients atteints de l'hémophilie légère et de l'hémophilie vasculaire de type I, il permet de contrôler ou de prévenir les saignements lors de la chirurgie mineure. ⑤ Pour les saignements prolongés causés par l'urémie, la cirrhose et la dysfonction plaquettaire congénitale ou induite par les médicaments, ainsi que des saignements de cause inconnue, le produit permet de raccourcir le temps de saignements ou de faire retourner à la normale.</td>
</tr>
<tr>
<td>用法、用量<br>Les modes d'emploi et la posologie</td>
<td>（1）中枢性尿崩症①鼻腔给药：a. 鼻喷剂：成人开始 10μg，睡前喷鼻，以后根据尿量每晚递增 2.5μg，直至获得良好睡眠。b. 成人开始一次 10μg，逐渐调整到最适剂量，一日 3～4 次，儿童用量酌减。②口服：因人而异，区分调整。③静脉注射。<br>　　（2）夜间遗尿症：鼻腔给药或口服。<br>　　（3）肾尿液浓缩功能试验：鼻腔给药或肌内、皮下注射。<br>　　（4）治疗性控制出血或手术前预防出血：静脉滴注。<br>　　(1) Pour traiter le diabète insipide central : ① L'administration nasale : a. l'aérosol nasal : chez des adultes, commencer par 10 μg, la pulvérisation nasale avant le sommeil, augmenter ensuite de 2,5 μg par soit, jusqu'à un bon sommeil. b. Chez des adultes, commencer par 10 μg, ajuster la dose pour atteindre la dose la plus pertinente, 3 à 4 fois par jour. chez des enfants, diminuer un peu la dose. ② Par voie orale : la dose est personnalisée. ③ Injection par voie IV.<br>　　(2) Pour traiter l'énurésie nocturne : administration nasale ou orale.<br>　　(3) Pour le test sur la fonction rénale de la concentration de l'urine : administration nasale, IM ou sous-cutanée.<br>　　(4) Pour le contrôle thérapeutique de saignement ou pour prévenir les saignements avant la chirurgie: en perfusion.</td>
</tr>
<tr>
<td>剂型、规格<br>Les formes pharmaceutiques et les spécifications</td>
<td>片剂：每片 100μg；200μg。<br>鼻喷雾剂：每支 250μg（2.5ml，每喷 0.1ml，含 10μg）。<br>滴鼻液：每支 250μg（2.5ml）。<br>注射液：每支 4μg（1ml）。<br>Comprimés : 100μg ou 200μg par comprimé.<br>L'aérosol nasal : 250 μg (2,5ml, chaque pulvérisation de 0,1ml contient 10 μg de desmopressine).<br>Les gouttes nasales : 250μg (2,5ml) par solution.<br>Injection : 4 μg (1ml) par solution.</td>
</tr>
</table>

15. 主要作用于生殖系统的药物 Médicaments agissant principalement sur le système reproducteur

15.1　子宫收缩药及引产药 Médicaments contractions utérines et de l'avortement

<table>
<tr>
<td>药品名称 Drug Names</td>
<td>垂体后叶素 Pituitrine</td>
</tr>
<tr>
<td>适应证<br>Les indications</td>
<td>产后出血、产后子宫复原不全、促进宫缩引产（由于有升高血压作用，现产科已少用）、肺出血、食管及胃底静脉曲张破裂出血和尿崩症等。<br>　　L'hémorragie du post-partum, la récupération incomplèteutérine du post-partum, la promotion des contractions utérines (comme il peut entraîner l'élévation de la pression artérielle, il est peu utilisé en obstétrique), l'hémorragie pulmonaire, les saignements liés aux varices œsophagiennes et gastriques ainsi que le diabète insipide.</td>
</tr>
<tr>
<td>用法、用量<br>Les modes d'emploi et la posologie</td>
<td>①一般应用：肌内注射，每次 5～10U。②肺出血：可静脉注射或静脉滴注。③产后出血：必须在胎儿和胎盘均已分娩出之后方可肌内注射 10U，如作预防性应用，可在胎儿前肩娩出后立即静脉注射 10U。④临产阵缩弛缓不正常者（偶亦用于催生，但须谨慎）：将 5～10U 本品以 5% 葡萄糖注射液 500ml 稀释后缓慢静脉滴注，并严密观察宫缩情况，适时调整滴速。⑤尿崩症：肌内注射，常用量为每次 5U，一日 2 次。⑥消化道出血：可用本品静脉滴注，其用量和溶媒同肺出血，每分钟 0.1～0.5U。</td>
</tr>
</table>

**续 表**

| | |
|---|---|
| | ① L'application générale : injection IM, 5 à 10u par fois. ② Pour traiter l'hémorragie pulmonaire : injection IV ou en perfusion. ③ Pour traiter l'hémorragie du post-partum : après l'accouchement du fœtus et du placenta, injecter 10U par voie IM. Pour la prévention, injecter 10 U par voie IV immédiatement après l'accouchement de l'épaule du fœtus. ④ Lors de la contraction utérine avant l'accouchement flasque et anormal : dissoudre 5 à 10 U de pituitrine dans 500ml de solution de glucose à 5% pour la perfusion lente, ajuster la vitesse de la perfusion en fonction de la contraction utérine. ⑤ Pour traiter le diabète insipide : injection IM, la dose usuelle, 5U par fois, 2 fois par jour. ⑥ Pour traiter les saignements gastro-intestinaux : en perfusion, 0,1 à 0,5U par minute. Sa dose et ses solvants sont les mêmes que ceux pour traiter l'hémorragie pulmonaire. |
| 剂型、规格<br>Les formes pharmaceutiques et les spécifications | 注射液：每支 5U（1ml）；10U（1ml）。<br>Injection : 5U (1ml) ou 10U (1ml) par solution. |
| 药品名称 Drug Names | 缩宫素 Ocytocine |
| 适应证<br>Les indications | 用于引产、催产、产后出血和子宫复原不全；滴鼻用于促排乳；催产素激惹试验。<br>Ce produit est utilisé dans le déclenchement du travail, la provocation de la contraction utérine, le traitement de l'hémorragie du post-partum et de la récupération incomplètede l'utérus. Ses gouttes nasales sont utilisées dansla promotion de l'allaitement maternel. Il est aussi applicable dans letest de provocation à l'ocytocine. |
| 用法、用量<br>Les modes d'emploi et la posologie | ①引产或催产：静脉滴注。②防治产后出血或促进子宫复原：将本品 5 ～ 10U 加于 5% 葡萄糖注射液中静脉滴注，每分钟滴注 0.02 ～ 0.04U，胎盘排出后可肌内注射 5 ～ 10U。③子宫出血：肌内注射，1 次 5 ～ 10U。肌内注射极量，1 次 20U。④催乳：在哺乳前 2 ～ 3 分钟，用滴鼻液，每次 3 滴或少量喷于一侧或双侧鼻孔内。⑤催产素激惹试验：试验剂量同引产，用稀释后的缩宫素作静脉滴注，直到 10 分钟出现 3 次有效宫缩。<br><br>① Pour le déclenchement du travail et la provocation de la contraction utérine : en perfusion. ② Pour prévenir l'hémorragie du post-partum ou promouvoir la récupération de l'utérus : dissoudre 5 à 10U d'ocytocine dans la solution de glucose à 5% pour la perfusion, 0,02 à 0,04U par minute, après l'accouchement du placenta, injecter 5 à 10U par voie IM. ③ Pour traiter l'hémorragie utérine : injection IM, 5 à 10U par fois. La dose limite pour injection IM, 20U par fois. ④ Pour la prolactine : 2 à 3 minutes avant l'allaitement maternel, utiliser les gouttes nasales, instiller 3 gouttes ou moins dans une ou deux narines. ⑤ Pour le test de provocation à l'ocytocine : la dose pour le test est la même que celle pour le déclenchement du travail, administrer l'ocytocine en perfusion après la dilution, jusqu'à l'apparition de 3 contractions utérines en 10 minutes. |
| 剂型、规格<br>Les formes pharmaceutiques et les spécifications | 注射液：每支 2.5U（0.5ml）；5U（1ml）；10U（1ml）。<br>滴鼻液：每支 40U（1ml）。<br>鼻喷雾剂：每瓶 200U（5ml）（每喷 0.1ml，相当于 4U）。<br>Injection : 2,5U (0,5ml), 5U (1ml) ou 10U (1ml) par solution.<br>Les gouttes nasales : 4U (1ml) par solution.<br>L'aérosol nasal : 200U (5ml) par flacon (une pulvérisation de 0,1ml contient 4U d'ocytocine). |
| 药品名称 Drug Names | 米非司酮 Mifépristone |
| 适应证<br>Les indications | 本品除用于抗早孕、催经止孕外，尚可用于中期妊娠引产（与前列腺素合用）、死胎引产、扩宫颈。<br>Ce produit est utilisé dans l'interruption de grossesse précoce. Il est aussi applicable dans l'avortement du deuxième trimestre (en association avec les prostaglandines), le déclenchement du travail lors d'une mort fœtale et la dilatation instrumentale du col de l'utérus. |
| 用法、用量<br>Les modes d'emploi et la posologie | ①中期妊娠引产（在妊娠 13 ～ 24 周用人工方法终止妊娠）a. 与米索前列醇配伍；b. 与卡前列甲酯配伍。②宫内死胎引产：口服，一次 200mg，一日 2 次或一日 1 次 400 ～ 600mg，连服 2 日，一般在 72 小时后排出死胎。③扩宫颈：口服，1 次 100 ～ 200mg。宫内手术前软化和扩张宫颈：于术前 48 小时口服 600mg。 |

| 续　表 | |
|---|---|
| | ① Pour l'avortement du deuxième trimestre (l'interruption artificielle de grossesse de la 13ème à 24ème semaine de grossesse) a. Utilisé en association avec le misoprostol. b. Utilisé en association avec. ② Pour le déclenchement du travail lors d'une mort fœtale : par voie orale, 200mg par fois, 2 fois par jour ou 400 à 600mg par fois par jour, pendant 2 jours consécutifs, en général, l'expulsion du fœtus mort 72 h après. ③ Pour la dilatation instrumentale du col de l'utérus : par voie orale, 100 à 200mg par fois. Pour le ramollissement et la dilatation du col de l'utérus avant la chirurgie intra-utérine : administrer 600mg par voie orale 48 h avant la chirurgie. |
| 剂型、规格<br>Les formes pharmaceutiques et les spécifications | 片剂：每片 25mg；200mg。<br>Comprimés : 25mg ou 200mg par comprimé. |
| 药品名称 Drug Names | 地诺前列酮 Dinoprostone |
| 适应证<br>Les indications | 可用于中期妊娠引产、足月妊娠引产和治疗性流产，对妊娠毒血症（先兆子痫、高血压）、妊娠合并肾病患者、过期妊娠、死胎不下、水泡状胎块、羊膜早破、高龄初产妇等均可应用。<br>Ce produit est utilisé dans l'avortement du deuxième trimestre, le déclenchement artificiel du travail en cas de grossesse à terme et l'avortement thérapeutique. Il est aussi applicable dans le traitement dela toxémie gravidique (la pré-éclampsie, l'hypertension),des patients atteints de maladie rénale pendant la grossesse, de la grossesse prolongée, des taupes hydatiformes, de la rupture prématurée de la membrane amniotique, ainsi que des primipares âgées. |
| 用法、用量<br>Les modes d'emploi et la posologie | ①催产：普通阴道栓，一次 3mg，置于阴道后穹窿深处，6～8 小时后若产程无进展，可再放置一次。②引产：a. 静脉滴注法；b. 宫腔内羊膜腔外注射法（中期妊娠引产）；c. 阴道内给药法；d. 宫颈内给药法。③产后出血：将本品注射液 5mg 用所吸附的稀释液稀释后溶于氯化钠注射液中，缓慢静脉滴注（开始宜慢，以后可酌情加快）。<br>① Pour la provocation de la contraction utérine au cours de l'accouchement : le pressaire ordinaire: 3mg par fois, introduire dans le fornix postérieur profond du vagin, s'il n'est pas efficace 6 à 8 après, introduire un autre pressaire dans le vagin. ② Pour le déclenchement artificiel du travail a. En perfusion. b. Injection intra-utérine en dehors de la cavité amniotique (pour l'avortement du deuxième trimestre). c. Administration intravaginale. d. Administration dans le col de l'utérus. ③ Pour traiter l'hémorragie du post-partum : diluer 5mg d'injection de dinoprostone avant de le dissoudre dans la solution de chlorure de sodium, perfusion lente (commencer lentement, ensuite, accélérer un peu selon les cas). |
| 剂型、规格<br>Les formes pharmaceutiques et les spécifications | 注射液：每支 2mg（1ml）。<br>阴道栓：每粒 3mg；20mg。<br>控释阴道栓（普贝生）：每粒 10mg。<br>凝胶剂：普比迪，每支 0.5mg/3g；普洛舒定，每支 1mg/3g；2mg/3g。<br>Injection : 2mg (1ml) par solution.<br>Le pressaire : 3mg ou 20mg par pièce.<br>Le suppositoire vagin à libération contrôlée (Puluosheng) : 10mg par pièce.<br>Les gels : Pubidi, 0,5 mg/3g par pièce ; Puluoshuding, 1 mg/3g ou 2 mg/3g par pièce. |
| 药品名称 Drug Names | 米索前列醇 Misoprostol |
| 适应证<br>Les indications | 本品单用于中期引产，效果不好，一般均与米非司酮联合应用，不良反应比卡前列甲酯栓轻。<br>Utilisé seul dans l'avortement du deuxième trimestre, il est peu efficace. Il est donc généralementappliqué en association avecla mifépristone. Ses réations indésirables sont moins importantes que l'ester decarboprost. |

**续 表**

| 用法、用量<br>Les modes d'emploi et la posologie | 中期妊娠引产：①先顿服米非司酮 200mg，36 小时后在阴道后穹窿放置米索前列醇 3 片（600μg）。②在服用米非司酮 36～48 小时后，一次口服米索前列醇 500μg。<br>Pour l'avortement du deuxième trimestre :<br>① Prendre d'abord 200mg de mifépristone une fois par jour, 36h après, introduire 3 comprimés de misoprostol (600μg) dans le fornix postérieur profond du vagin. ② 36 à 48 h après l'administration de la mifépristone, prendre 500μg de misoprostol par voie orale pour une fois. |
| --- | --- |
| 剂型、规格<br>Les formes pharmaceutiques et les spécifications | 片剂：每片 200μg。<br>Comprimés : 200μg par comprimé. |

| 药品名称 Drug Names | 依沙吖啶 Ethacridine |
| --- | --- |

| 适应证<br>Les indications | ①中期妊娠引产，终止 12～26 周妊娠。②用于外科创伤、黏膜感染等消毒。<br>① L'avortement du deuxième trimestre, de la 12ème à 26ème semaine de grossesse. ② La désinfection appliquée dans le traumatisme chirurgical etles infections des muqueuses. |
| --- | --- |
| 用法、用量<br>Les modes d'emploi et la posologie | ①羊膜腔内注射：由下腹壁向羊膜腔内注射本品 1% 溶液 5～10ml（含药 50～100mg）。每周用量不超过 100mg。妊娠 20 在 20 周以内者用 50mg，在 20 周以上者用 100mg。②羊膜腔外注射：先冲洗阴道，一日 1 次，冲洗 3 日。在消毒的情况下，将橡皮导尿管送入羊膜腔外，经导尿管注入药液 50ml（取本品 1% 的注射液 10ml，加注射用水 40ml，含药 100mg）。注药后将导尿管折叠结扎放入阴道，保留 24 小时后取出。③外用灭菌：用 0.1%～0.2%（用片剂溶解配制而成）溶液，局部洗涤、湿敷。<br>① Injection intra-amniotique : injecter 5 à 10 solution d'étracridine à 1% dans la cavité amniotique (contenant 50 à 100mg d'éthacridine). Ne pas dépasser 100mg par semaine. Pour moins de 20 semaines de grossesse, utiliser 50mg, pour plus de 20 semaines de grossesse, utiliser 100mg. ② Injection extra-amniotique : laver d'abord le vagin, 1 fois par jour, pendant 3 jours. Dans des conditions stériles, introduire le cathéter de caoutchouc à l'extérieur de la cavité amniotique, injecter 50ml de médicament à travers le cathéter (utiliser 10ml d'injection d'éthacridine à 1%, ajouter 40ml d,eau pour injection, contenant 100mg d'éthacridine). Après l'injection du médicament, plier le cathéter et faire une ligature avant de la mettre dans le vagin et de la tirer 24 h après. ③ Pour la désinfection pour un usage externe: utiliser la solution à 0,1% à 0,2% (diluer les comprimés), le lavage topique et l'application humide. |
| 剂型、规格<br>Les formes pharmaceutiques et les spécifications | 片剂：每片 100mg。<br>注射用依沙吖啶：每支 100mg。<br>Comprimés : 100mg par comprimé.<br>L'éthacridine pour injection : 100mg par solution. |

15.2 退乳药物 Médicaments de retrait de laitmaternel

| 药品名称 Drug Names | 溴隐亭 Bromocriptine |
| --- | --- |

| 适应证<br>Les indications | ①分娩后、自发性、肿瘤性、药物等引起的闭经；②高泌乳素血症引起的月经紊乱、不孕、继发性闭经、排卵减少；③抑制泌乳，预防分娩后和早产后的泌乳；④产后的乳房充血、高泌乳素血症引起的特殊的乳房触痛、乳房胀痛和烦躁不安；⑤高泌乳素血症引起男性性功能低下（如阳痿和精子减少引起的不育）；⑥肢端肥大症的辅助治疗。<br>① L'aménorrhée induite après l'accouchement, ou l'aménorrhée spontanée, néoplasique ou médicamenteuse. ② Les troubles menstruels, la stérilité, l'aménorrhée secondaire etla réduction de l'ovulation induites par l'hyperprolactinémie. ③ Inhiber la lactation et prévenir la lactation après l'accouchement et la prématurité. ④ La congestion mammaire du post-partum, la sensibilité des seins, les douleurs mammaires et l'irritabilitécausées par l'hyperprolactinémie. ⑤ La dysfonction sexuelle masculine causée par l'hyperprolactinémie (comme l'impuissance et l'infertilité due à la réduction du sperme). ⑥ Le traitement adjuvant de l'acromégalie. |
| --- | --- |

**续　表**

| | |
|---|---|
| 用法、用量<br>Les modes d'emploi et la posologie | ①产后回乳：口服，如为预防性用药，分娩后 4 小时开始服用 2.5mg，以后改为一日 2 次，1 次 2.5mg，连用 14 日；如已有乳汁分泌，则每日用 2.5mg，2～3 日后改为一日 2 次，一次 2.5mg，连用 14 日。②高泌乳素血症引起的闭经溢乳、不孕症：口服，常用起始量为一次 1.25mg，一日 2～3 次；若症状未得到控制，可逐渐增量至一次 2.5mg，一日 2～3 次，餐后服用，直至月经恢复正常，再继续用药几周，完全停止则需 12～13 周，以防复发。③产后乳房充血：轻者可口服，一次 2.5mg，如需要又没停止泌乳，则 6～12 小时后可重复一次。短时间用药不会抑制泌乳。④男性高泌乳素血症引起的性功能低下：口服，1 次 1.25mg，一日 2～3 次，逐渐增加至一日 5～10mg，分 3 次服用。⑤肢端肥大症：开始一日 2.5mg，经 7～14 日后根据临床反应可逐渐增至一日 10～20mg，分 4 次与食物同服。⑥垂体泌乳素瘤：口服，起始量为每日 1.25mg，维持量为每日 5～7.5mg，最大量为每日 15mg。<br><br>① Pour le retrait du lait maternel après l'accouchement : Par voie orale, pour la prévention, 4 h après l'accouchement, prendre 2,5mg, ensuite, 2 fois par jour, 2,5 mg par fois, pendant 14 jours consécutifs ; s'il y a déjà la lactation, prendre 2,5mg par jour, 2 à 3 jours après, 2 fois par jour, 2,5mg par fois, pendant 14 jours consécutifs. ② Pour traiter l'aménorrhée, la galactorrhée, l'infertilité causées par l'hyperprolactinémie : par voie orale, la dose initiale usuelle, 1,25mg par fois, 2 à 3 fois par jour ; si les symptômes ne se contrôlent pas, augmenter progressivement pour atteindre 2,5mg par fois, 2 à 3 fois par jour, pris après le repas, jusqu'à la normalisation de la règle, continuer l'administration pendant plusieurs semaines, et arrêter complètement l'administration 12 à 13 semaines après pour éviter la récurrence. ③ Pour traiter la congestion mammaire du post-partum : pour des cas bénins, par voie orale, 2,5 mg par fois, s'il est nécessaire et que la lactation ne s'arrête pas, reprendre l'administration 6 à 12h après. L'administration à court terme n'inhibe pas la lactation. ④ Pour traiter la dysfonction sexuelle masculine causée par l'hyperprolactinémie : par voie orale, 1,25mg par fois, 2 à 3 fois par jour, augmenter pour atteindre 5 à 10mg par jour, à travers 3 fois. ⑤ Pour traiter l'acromégalie : commencer par prendre 2,5mg par jour, 7 à 14 jours après, augmenter pour atteindre 10 à 20 mg par jour selon les réactions cliniques, à travers 4 fois, pris avec des aliments. ⑥ Pour traiter la prolactinome hypophysaire : par voie orale, commencer par prendre 1,25mg par jour, la dose d'entretien, 5 à 7,5mg par jour, la dose maximale, 15mg par jour. |
| 剂型、规格<br>Les formes pharmaceutiques et les spécifications | 片剂：每片 4mg。<br>Comprimés : 4mg par comprimé. |

16. 主要作用于内分泌系统药物 Médicaments agissant principalement sur le système endocrinien

16.1　肾上腺皮质激素和促肾上腺皮质激素 Corticoïdes surrénaux et corticotrophine

| 药品名称 Drug Names | 氢化可的松 Hydrocortisone |
|---|---|
| 适应证<br>Les indications | 用于结缔组织病、系统性红斑狼疮、严重的支气管哮喘、皮肌炎、血管炎等过敏性疾病、急性白血病、恶性淋巴瘤等病症。<br>Ce produit sert à traiter la maladie du tissu conjonctif, le lupus érythémateux systématique, l'asthme bronchique grave, la dermatomyosite, la vascularite et d'autres maladies allergiques, ainsi que la leucémie aiguë et le lymphome malin. |
| 用法、用量<br>Les modes d'emploi et la posologie | 氢化可的松注射液：每次 100～200mg，与 0.9% 氯化钠注射液或 5% 葡萄糖注射液 500ml 混合均匀后做静脉滴注。注射用氢化可的松琥珀酸钠：50mg 或 100mg。临用时，以生理盐水或 5% 葡萄糖注射液稀释后静脉滴注或肌内注射。醋酸氢化可的松片：一日 1～2 次，每次 1 片。醋酸氢化可的松眼膏：一日 2～3 次。醋酸氢化可的松滴眼液：用前摇匀。<br><br>Injection d'hydrocortisone : 100 à 200mg par fois, dissoudre dans 500ml de solution de chlorure de sodium ou de solution de glucose à 5%, en perfusion. Le succinate de sodium d'hydrocortisone pour injection : 50mg ou 100mg. Dissoudre dans la solution saline ou la solution de glucose, en perfusion ou injection IM. Comprimés d'acétate d'hydrocortisone : 1 à 2 fois par jour, 1 comprimé par fois. La pommade ophtalmique d'acétate d'hydrocortisone : 2 à 3 fois par jour. Les gouttes pour les yeux d'acétate d'hydrocortisone : agiter avant de l'utiliser. |

**续　表**

| | |
|---|---|
| 剂型、规格<br>Les formes pharmaceutiques et les spécifications | 氢化可的松注射液：10mg（2ml）；25mg（5ml）；50mg（10ml）；100mg（20ml）（为氢化可的松的稀乙醇溶液）。<br>醋酸氢化可的松注射液：125mg（5ml）（为醋酸氢化可的松的无菌混悬液）。<br>注射用氢化可的松琥珀酸钠：50mg 或 100mg（按氢化可的松算）。<br>醋酸氢化可的松片：每片 20mg。<br>醋酸氢化可的松软膏：1%。<br>醋酸氢化可的松眼膏：0.5%。<br>醋酸氢化可的松滴眼液：3ml：15mg。<br>Injection d'hydrocortisone : 10mg(2ml)；25mg(5ml)；50mg(10ml)；100mg(20ml).<br>Injection d'acétate d'hycrocortisone : 125mg (5ml).<br>Le succinate de sodium d'hydrocortisone pour injection : 50mg ou 100mg (mesuré en hydrocortisone).<br>Comprimés d'acétate d'hydrocortisone : 20mg par comprimé.<br>La pommade d'acétate d'hydrocortisone : 1%.<br>La pommade ophtalmique d'acétate d'hydrocortisone : 0.5%.<br>Les gouttes pour les yeux d'acétate d'hydrocortisone : 3ml : 15mg. |
| **药品名称 Drug Names** | 泼尼松 Prednisone |
| 适应证<br>Les indications | 用于结缔组织病、系统性红斑狼疮、严重的支气管哮喘、皮肌炎、血管炎等过敏性疾病，急性白血病、恶性淋巴瘤等病症。<br>Ce produit sert à traiter la maladie du tissu conjonctif, le lupus érythémateux systématique, l'asthme bronchique grave, la dermatomyosite, la vascularite et d'autres maladies allergiques, ainsi que la leucémie aiguë et le lymphome malin. |
| 用法、用量<br>Les modes d'emploi et la posologie | ①补充替代疗法口服，1 次 5 ～ 10mg，一日 10 ～ 60mg，早晨起床后服用 2/3，下午服用 1/3。②抗炎口服，一日 5 ～ 60mg。③自身免疫性疾病口服，每日 40 ～ 60mg，病情稳定后可逐渐减量。④过敏性疾病，口服每日 20 ～ 40mg，病情症状减轻后减量，每隔 1 ～ 2 日减少 5mg。⑤防止器官移植排异反应，一般在术前 1 ～ 2 日开始每日口服 100mg，术后 1 周改为每日 60mg，以后逐渐减量。⑥治疗急性白血病、恶性肿瘤等，每日口服 60 ～ 80mg，症状缓解后减量。<br>① Les thérapies complémentaires et alternatives, par voie orale, 5 à 10mg par fois, 10 à 60mg par jour, 2/3 de la dose prise après le lever du matin, 1/3 de la dose prise après-midi. ② Pour lutter contre l'inflammation, par voie orale, 5 à 60mg par jour. ③ Pour traiter des maladies auto-immunes, par voie orale, 40 à 60mg par jour, augmenter la dose avec la stabilisation des cas. ④ Pour traiter les maladies allergiques, par voie orale, 20 à 40mg par jour, diminuer la dose après le soulagement des symptômes, diminuer de 5mg tous les 1 à 2 jours. ⑤ Pour l'anti-rejet de la transplantation d'organes, commencer de prendre 100mg par voie orale par jour 1 à 2 jours avant la chirurgie, 1 semaine après la chirurgie, prendre 60mg par jour, diminuer ensuite la dose. ⑥ Pour traiter la leucémie et le cancer, par voie orale 60 à 80mg par jour, diminuer la dose après l'amélioration des symptômes. |
| 剂型、规格<br>Les formes pharmaceutiques et les spécifications | 醋酸泼尼松片：每片 5mg。<br>醋酸泼尼松眼膏：0.5%。<br>Les comprimés d'acétate de prednisone : 5mg par comprimé.<br>La pommade ophtalmique d'acétate de prednisone : 0,5%. |
| **药品名称 Drug Names** | 泼尼松龙 Prednisolone |
| 适应证<br>Les indications | 用于过敏性和自身免疫性疾病。<br>Les maladies allergiques et les maladies autoimmunes. |

**续 表**

| | |
|---|---|
| 用法、用量<br>Les modes d'emploi et la posologie | 口服：成人开始一日 15 ～ 40mg，需用时可用到 60mg 或每日 0.5 ～ 1mg/kg，发热患者分 3 次服用，体温正常者每日晨起一次顿服。病情稳定后应逐渐减量，维持量 5 ～ 10mg，视病情而定。小儿开始用量 1mg/kg。肌内注射：一日 10 ～ 30mg。静脉滴注：1 次 10 ～ 25mg，溶于 5% ～ 10% 葡萄糖溶液 500ml 中应用。关节腔或软组织内注射（混悬液）：1 次 5 ～ 50mg，用量依关节大小而定，应在无菌条件下操作，以防引起感染。滴眼：一次 1 ～ 2 滴，一日 2 ～ 4 次，治疗开始的 24 ～ 48 小时，剂量可酌情加大至每小时 2 滴，注意不宜过早停药。<br><br>Par voie orale : chez des adultes, commencer par 15 à 40mg par jour, s'il est nécessaire, 60mg par jour ou 0,5 à 1 mg/kg par jour, chez des patients atteints de fièvre, pris à travers 3 fois, chez des patients dont la température corporelle est normale, pris une fois par jour, le lever du matin. Après l'amélioration des symptômes, diminuer la dose, la dose d'entretien est de 5 à 10mg, selon les cas. Chez des enfants, commencer par 1 mg/kg. Injection IM : 10 à 30 mg par jour. En perfusion : 10 à 25mg par fois, dissoudre dans 500ml de solution de glucose à 5% à 10%. Injection intra-articulaire ou dans les tissus mous : 5 à 50mg par fois, ajuster la dose en fonction de la taille articulaire. Il faut conduire dans des conditions stériles pour éviter l'infection. Les gouttes pour les yeux : 1 à 2 gouttes par fois, 2 à 4 fois par jour, les 24 à 48 premières heures, augmenter la dose pour atteindre 2 gouttes toutes les 2 h, ne pas arrêter l'administration trop tôt. |
| 剂型、规格<br>Les formes pharmaceutiques et les spécifications | 醋酸泼尼松龙片：每片 5mg。<br>醋酸泼尼松龙注射液（混悬液）：125mg（5ml）。<br>泼尼松龙磷酸钠注射液：20mg（1ml）。<br>泼尼松龙软膏：0.25% ～ 0.5%。<br>泼尼松龙眼膏：0.25%。<br>泼尼松龙滴眼液：1%。<br><br>Les comprimés d'acétate de prednisolone : 5mg par comprimé.<br>Injection d'acétate de prednisolone : 125mg (5ml).<br>Injection de phosphate sodique de prednisolone : 20mg (1ml).<br>La pommade de prednisolone : 0,25% à 0,5%.<br>La pommade ophtalmique de prednisolone : 0.25%.<br>Prednisolone gouttes pour les yeux : 1%. |
| 药品名称 Drug Names | 甲泼尼龙 Méthylprednisolone |
| 适应证<br>Les indications | 用于抗炎治疗风湿性疾病、肌原疾病、皮肤疾病、过敏状态、眼部疾病、胃肠道疾病、呼吸道疾病、水肿状态；免疫抑制治疗、休克、内分泌失调等。<br><br>Ce produit sert à traiter les maladies rhumatismales, les maladies myogéniques, les maladies de la peau, l'état allergique, les troubles oculaires, les maladies gastro-intestinales, les maladies respiratoires, l'état de l'œdème ; le traitement immunosuppresseur, le choc, des troubles endocriniens, etc. |
| 用法、用量<br>Les modes d'emploi et la posologie | 口服：开始一日 16 ～ 24mg，分 2 次，维持量一日 4 ～ 8mg。关节腔内及肌内注射：一次 10 ～ 40mg。用于危重病情作为辅助疗法时，推荐剂量是 30mg/kg 体重，将已溶解的药物与 5% 葡萄糖注射液、生理盐水注射液或者二者混合后至少静脉输注 30 分钟。此剂量可于 48 小时内，每 4 ～ 6 小时重复一次。冲击疗法：每日 1g，静脉注射，使用 1 ～ 4 日；或每月 1g，静脉注射，使用 6 个月。系统性红斑狼疮：每日 1g，静脉注射，使用 3 日。多发性硬化症：每日 1g，静脉注射，使用 3 日或 5 日。肾小球肾炎、狼疮性肾炎：每日 1g，静脉注射，使用 3、5 或 7 日。<br><br>Par voie orale : commencer par 16 à 24mg par jour, 2 fois par jour, la dose d'entretien, 4 à 8 mg par jour. Injection intra-articulaire ou IM : 10 à 40mg par fois. Utilisé comme traitement adjuvant des cas sévères, la dose recommandée est de 30 mg/kg, dissoudre dans la solutionde glucose à 5% ou la solution saline, en perfusion pendant 30 minutes au moins. Il est permissible de reprendre cette dose toutes les 4 à 6h en 48h. La thérapie de choc : 1g par jour, injection par voie IV, pendant 1 à 4 jours ; ou 1g par mois, injection par voie IV, pendant 6 mois. Pour traiter le lupus érythémateux disséminé : 1g par jour, injection IV, pendant 3 jours. La sclérose en plaques : 1g par jour, injection IV, pendant 3 ou 5 jours. La glomérulonéphrite et la néphrite lupique : 1g par jour, injection IV, pendant 3, 5 ou 7 jours. |

| | |
|---|---|
| 剂型、规格<br>Les formes pharmaceutiques et les spécifications | 片剂：每片 2mg；4mg。<br>甲泼尼龙醋酸酯混悬注射液（局部注射）：每支 20mg（1ml）；40mg（1ml）。<br>甲泼尼龙琥珀酸钠注射液：每支相当于甲泼尼龙 40mg；125mg；500mg。<br>Comprimés : 2mg, 4mg par comprimé.<br>L'injection d'une suspension d'acétate de méthylprednisolone (injection topique) : 20mg (1ml), 40 mg(1ml) par solution.<br>L'injection desuccinate de sodium de méthylprednisolone : chaque solution contient 40mg, 125mg ou 500mg de méthylprednisolone. |
| **药品名称 Drug Names** | 曲安西龙 Triamcinolone |
| 适应证<br>Les indications | 用于类风湿关节炎、其他结缔组织炎症、支气管哮喘、过敏性皮炎、神经性皮炎、湿疹等，尤其适用于对皮质激素禁忌的伴有高血压或水肿的关节炎患者。<br>Ce produit sert à traiter la polyarthrite rhumatoïde, d'autres inflammations du tissu conjonctif, l'asthme bronchique, la dermatite allergique, la neurodermite, l'eczéma, etc. Il est surtout efficace dans le traitement des patients souffrant d'arthrite accompagnée de l'hypertension artérielle ou de l'œdème et ayant des contre-indications de corticostéroïdes. |
| 用法、用量<br>Les modes d'emploi et la posologie | ①口服：开始时 1 次 4mg，一日 2～4 次。维持量为 1 次 1～4mg，一日 1～2 次，通常维持量不超过 8mg。②肌内注射：每 1～4 周一次 40～80mg。③皮下注射：一次 5～20mg。④关节腔内注射：每 1～7 周一次 5～40mg。<br>① Par voie orale : commencer par prendre 4mg par fois, 2 à 4 fois par jour. La dose d'entretien, 1 à 4mg par fois, 1 à 2 fois par jour, ne pas dépasser 8mg pour l'entretien. ② Injection IM : 40 à 80mg par fois toutes les 1 à 4 semaines. ③ Injection sous-cutanée : 5 à 20mg par fois. ④ Injection intra-articulaire : 5 à 40mg par fois, toutes les 1 à 7 semaines. |
| 剂型、规格<br>Les formes pharmaceutiques et les spécifications | 片剂：每片 1mg；2mg；4mg。<br>曲安西龙双醋酸酯混悬注射液：每支 125mg（5ml）；200mg（5ml）。<br>Comprimés : 1mg, 2mg ou 4mg par comprimé.<br>L'injection d'une suspension de diacétate de triamcinolone : 125mg (5ml) ou 200mg (5ml) par solution. |
| **药品名称 Drug Names** | 曲安奈德 Acétonide de triamcinolone |
| 适应证<br>Les indications | 用于各种皮肤病（如神经性皮炎、湿疹、牛皮癣等）、支气管哮喘、过敏性鼻炎、关节痛、肩周围炎、腱鞘炎、急性扭伤、慢性腰腿痛及眼科炎症等。鼻喷雾剂用于治疗常年性过敏性鼻炎或季节性过敏性鼻炎。<br>Ce produit sert à traiter diverses maladies de la peau (comme le neurodermatitis, l'eczéma, le psoriasis, etc.), l'asthme bronchique, la rhinite allergique, les douleurs articulaires, la périarthrite de l'épaule, la ténosynovite, l'entorse aiguë, la lombalgie chronique, l'inflammation des yeux, etc. Son aérosol nasal est appliqué dans le traitement de la rhinite allergiqueperannuelle et de la rhinite allergique saisonnière. |
| 用法、用量<br>Les modes d'emploi et la posologie | ①支气管哮喘：肌内注射，成人每次 1ml（40mg），每 3 周 1 次，5 次为 1 个疗程，患者症状较重者可用 80mg；6～12 岁儿童减半，在必要时 3～6 岁幼儿可用成人剂量的 1/3。穴位或局部注射，成人每次 1ml（40mg），在扁桃体穴或颈前甲状软骨旁注射，每周 1 次，5 次为 1 个疗程，注射前先用少量普鲁卡因局麻。②过敏性鼻炎：肌内注射，每次 1ml（40mg），每 3 周 1 次，5 次为 1 个疗程；下鼻甲注射，鼻腔先喷 1% 利多卡因表面麻醉后，在双下鼻甲前端各注入本品 0.5ml，每周 1 次，4～5 次为 1 个疗程。③各种关节病：每次 10～20mg，加 0.25% 利多卡因液 10～20ml，用 5 号针头，一次进针直至病灶，每周 2～3 次或隔日一次，症状好转后每周 1～2 次，4～5 次为 1 个疗程。④皮肤病：直接注入皮损部分，通常每一部位用 0.2～0.3mg，视患部大小而定，每处每次不超过 0.5mg，必要时每隔 1～2 周重复使用。局部外用：一日 2～3 次，一般早晚各一次。治疗皮炎、湿疹时，疗程 2～4 周。⑤鼻腔内用药：用前须振摇 5 次以上；12 岁以上的儿童、成人及老年人，推荐剂量为每鼻孔 2 喷（共 220μg），一日 1 次。症状得到控制时，可降低剂量至每鼻孔 1 喷（共 110μg），一日 1 次。如 3 周后症状无改善应就医。 |

① L'asthme bronchique : injection IM, chez des adultes, 1ml (40mg) par fois, toutes les 3 semaines, 5 fois au total comme un traitement médical. Chez des patients gravement maladies, 80mg; chez des enfants de 6 à 12ans, diminuer de moitié la dose, s'il est nécessaire, chez des enfants de 3 à 6ans, prendre 1/3 de la dose chez des adultes. Injection topique ou sur le point d'acupuncture, chez des adultes, 1 ml (40mg) par fois, l'injection latérale antérieure du cartilage thyroïde, 1 fois par semaine, 5 fois au total comme un traitement médical, utiliser la procaine pour l'anesthésie locale avant l'injection. ② Pour traiter la rhinite allergique : injection IM, 1ml (40mg) par fois, toutes les 3 semaines, 5 fois au total comme un traitment médical ; injection de cornet inférieur, pulvériser d'abord la lidocaine à 1% dans la cavité nasale pour l'anesthésie superficielle, avant d'injecter 0,5ml de ce médicament dans les deux cornets, une fois par semaine, 4 à 5 fois au total comme un traitement mécial. ③ Diverses arthropathies:10 à 20mg chaque fois, avec 10 à 20ml de la solution de La lidocaine 0.25%, avec l'aiguille no.5, une fois dans la lésion, 2 à 3 fois par semaine ou un jour alterné. Après l'améliration des symptômes, 1 à 2 fois par semaine. 4 à 5 fois pour 1 traitement. ④ Injection directe sur le site de la blessure cutanée. La dose habituelle est de 0.2 à 0.3 mg. Chaque site ne doit pas être administré plus de 0,5 mg par dose. Si nécessaire, répéter ladministration à intervalles de 1 à 2 semaines. Application locale et externe: 2 à 3 fois par jour, une fois le matin et une fois le soir. Pour le traitement de la dermatite et de l'eczéma, le cours est de 2 à 4 semaines. ⑤ Pour administration intra-nasale: Secouez le médicament plus de 5 fois avant utilisation. La dose recommandée pour les enfants de plus de 12 ans, les adultes et les personnes âgées est de 2 vaporisations par narine (la dose totale est de 220µg) une fois par jour. Lorsque les symptômes sont maîtrisés, la dose administrée peut être réduite à 1 spray par narine (la dose est de 110µg) une fois par jour. Si les symptômes ne s'améliorent pas après 3 semaines d'administration, vous devriez aller à l'hôpitaux.

| 剂型、规格<br>Les formes pharmaceutiques et les spécifications | 注射液（混悬剂）：每支 40mg（1ml）。<br>复方曲安奈德霜：每支 5g；10g；15g；20g。<br>鼻喷雾剂：每支 6ml [6.6mg，120 喷（55μg/喷）]。<br>Injection : 40mg (1ml) par soluton.<br>La crème composée d'acétonide de triamcinolone : 5g, 10g, 15g ou 20g par pièce.<br>L'aérosole nasal : 6ml [6,6mg, 120 pulvérisations (55µg par pulvérisation)]. |
|---|---|
| **药品名称 Drug Names** | 布地奈德 Budésonide |
| 适应证<br>Les indications | 用于支气管哮喘的症状和体征的长期控制。粉吸入剂用于需使用糖皮质激素维持治疗以控制基础炎症的支气管哮喘、慢性阻塞性肺疾病患者。鼻喷雾剂用于季节性和常年性过敏性鼻炎、血管运动性鼻炎；预防鼻息肉切除术后鼻息肉的再生，对症治疗鼻息肉。<br><br>Ce produit est appliqué dans le contrôle à long terme des symptômes et des signesde l'asthme. Sa poudre pour inhalation est applicable chez des patients atteints de l'asthme bronchique et de la maladie pulmonaire obstructive et ayant besoin des glucocorticoïdes pour le traitement d'entretien de l'inflammation de base. Son aérosol nasal est applicable dans le traitement de la rhinite allergiqueperannuelle, saisonnière et dela rhinite vasomotrice, dans la prévention de la régénération des polypes nasaux après l'excision de ces derniers ainsi que dans le traitement symptomatique des polypes nasaux. |
| 用法、用量<br>Les modes d'emploi et la posologie | 剂量应个体化，成人初始剂量为 200～1600μg/d，分 2～4 次给药（较轻微的病例 200～800μg/d，较严重的 800～1600μg/d）。一般一次 200μg，早晚各一次，病情严重时一日 4 次。7 岁以上儿童：200～800μg/d，分 2～4 次使用。2～7 岁儿童：200～400μg/d，分成 2～4 次使用。维持剂量成人一日 100～600μg，儿童 100～800μg；当哮喘控制后可减量至最低有效维持剂量。鼻喷，成人及 6 岁以上儿童，起始剂量为一日 256μg，次剂量可早晨一次喷入和早晚 2 次喷入（即早晨每个鼻孔内喷入 2 喷；或早晚 2 次，每个鼻孔内喷 1 喷）。<br><br>La dose doit être personnalisée, chez des adultes, la dose initiale est de 200 à 1 600µgpar jour, à travers 2 à 4 fois (pour des cas bénins, 200 à 800 µg par jour, pour des cas graves, 800 à 1 600µg par jour). En général, 200 µg par fois, pris le petit matin et le soir, pour des cas sévères, 4 fois par jour. Chez des enfants de plus de 7 ans : 200 à 800 µg par jour, à tavers 2 à 4 fois. Chez des enfants de 2 à 7 ans : 200 à 400 µg par jour, à travers 2 à 4 fois. La dose d'entretien, chez des adultes, 100 à 600 µg par jour, chez des enfants, 100 à 800 µg ; après le contrôle de l'asthme, possible de diminuer jusqu'à la dose efficace minimale. Pour la pulvérisation nasale, chez des adultes et des enfants plus de 6 ans, la dose initiale, 256µgpar jour, ensuite, 2 pulvérisations pour chaque narine prises le petit matin ou 1 pulvérisation pour chaque narine, prise le petit matin et le soir. |

**续 表**

| | |
|---|---|
| 剂型、规格<br>Les formes pharmaceutiques et les spécifications | 气雾剂：10ml：10mg（50μg/喷，200喷/瓶）；10ml：20mg（100μg/喷，200喷/瓶）；5ml：20mg（200μg/喷，100喷/瓶）。<br>雷诺考特鼻喷雾剂（白色或类白色黏稠混悬液）：64μg/喷（120喷/支，药液浓度1.28mg/ml）。<br>粉吸入剂：0.1mg/吸（200吸/支）。<br>细微颗粒混悬液：0.5mg/2ml；1mg/2ml。<br>L'aérosol : 10ml : 10mg (50 µg par pulvérisation, 200 pulvérisations par bouteille), 10ml : 20mg (100µgpar pulvérisation, 200 pulvérisations par bouteille), 5ml : 20mg (200µg par pulvérisation, 100 pulvérisations par bouteille).<br>L'aérosol nasal : 64 µg par pulvérisation (120 pulvérisations par pièce, la concentration est de 1,28mg par ml).<br>Poudre pour inhalation : 0,1mg par inhalation (200 inhalations par pièce).<br>La solution de suspension de particules fines : 0,5mg par 2ml ; 1mg par 2ml. |
| 药品名称 Drug Names | 氟替卡松 Fluticasone |
| 适应证<br>Les indications | 用作持续性哮喘的长期治疗，季节性过敏性鼻炎（包括枯草热）和常年性过敏性鼻炎的预防和治疗。外用可缓解炎症性和瘙痒性皮肤病。吸入剂适用于12岁及以上患者预防用药维持治疗哮喘。<br>Ce produit est utilisé dans le traitement à long terme de l'asthme persistant, dans la prévention et le traitement de la rhinite allergique saisonnière (y compris le rhume des foins) et de la rhinite allergique perannuelle. Son usage externe est aussi applicable dans le soulagement des maladies de la peau inflammatoires et accompagnées des démangeaisons. Son inhalation est appliquée dans le traitement d'entretien de l'asthme chez des patients de plus de 12 ans. |
| 用法、用量<br>Les modes d'emploi et la posologie | 成人，老年患者和12岁以上儿童：一日1次，每个鼻孔各2喷，以早晨用药为好，某些患者需一日2次，每个鼻孔各2喷。当症状得到控制时，维持剂量为一日1次，每个鼻孔各1喷。若症状复发，可相应增加剂量，每日最大剂量为每个鼻孔不超过4喷。4～11岁儿童：一日1次，每个鼻孔各1喷。某些患者需一日2次，每个鼻孔各1喷，最大剂量为每个鼻孔不超过2喷。湿疹/皮炎：成人及1岁以上儿童，一日1次涂于患处。其他适应证，一日2次。吸入剂：轻度哮喘：100～250μg，一日2次；中度哮喘：250～500μg，一日2次；重度哮喘：500～1000μg，一日2次。<br>Chez des personnes âgées, des adultes, chez des enfants de plus de 12 ans : 1 fois par jour, 2 pulvérisations par narine, le petit matin au mieux, chez certains patients, 2 fois par jour, 2 pulvérisations par narine. Après le contrôle des symptômes, la dose d'entretien, 1 fois par jour, 1 pulvérisation par narine. Lors de la récurrence des symptômes, augmenter la dose, la dose maximale est de 4 pulvérisations par narine. Chez des enfants de 4 à 11 ans : 1 fois par jour, 1 pulvérisation par narine. Chez certains patients, 2 fois par jour, 1 pulvérisation par narine. La dose maxiale est de 2 pulvérisations par narine. Pour traier l'eczéma et la dermatite : chez des adultes et des enfants plus de 1 ans, essuyer sur la zone touchée, une fois par jour. Pour les autres indications : 2 fois par jour. L'inhalation : pour l'asthme bénin, 100 à 250 µg, 2 fois par jour ; pour l'asthme modéré, 250 à 500 µg, 2 fois par jour ; pour l'asthme grave, 500 à 1 000 µg, 2 fois par jour. |
| 剂型、规格<br>Les formes pharmaceutiques et les spécifications | 鼻喷剂：50μg×120喷。<br>吸入气雾剂：125μg×60喷/支，250μg×60泡/盒。<br>乳膏：15g：7.5mg（0.05%）；30g：15mg（0.05%）。<br>L'aérosol nasal : 50 µg×120 pulvérisations.<br>L'aérosol pour inhalation : 125µg×60 pulvérisations par pièce, 250 µg×60 ampoules par boite.<br>La crème : 15g : 7,5mg (0,05%) ; 30g : 15mg (0,05%). |
| 药品名称 Drug Names | 莫米松 Mométasone |
| 适应证<br>Les indications | 用于治疗成人及12岁以上儿童的季节性或常年性鼻炎。对于中至重度季节性过敏性鼻炎的患者，建议在花粉季节开始前2～4周使用本品作预防治疗。也用于对皮脂类固醇有效的皮肤病如异位性皮炎。<br>Il sert à traiter la rhinite saisonnière ou perannuelle chez des adultes et des enfants de plus de 12 ans. Chez des patients atteints de la rhinite allergique saisonnière modérée ou grave, il est recommandé de prendre ce médicament 2 à 4 semaines avant le début de la saison de pollen. Il est aussi applicable dans le traitement de la maladie de la peau qui n'est pas résistante aux corticostéroïdes, telle que la dermatite atopique. |

续　表

| | |
|---|---|
| 用法、用量<br>Les modes d'emploi et la posologie | 鼻喷剂：成人（包括老年患者）和 12 岁以上儿童，常用推荐剂量为每侧鼻孔 2 喷（每喷为 50μg），一日 1 次（总量为 200μg）。当症状被控制时，可减至每侧鼻孔 1 喷（总量为 100μg），如果症状未被有效控制，则可增至每侧鼻孔 4 喷（400μg），在症状控制后减少剂量。乳膏：一日 1 次，涂于患处。<br><br>L'aérosol nasal : chez des adultes (y compris les personnes âgées) et des enfants de plus de 12 ans, la dose usuelle recommandée est de 2 pulvérisations par narine (50 μg par pulvérisation), 1 fois par jour (200μg au total). Quand les symtômes se contrôlent, diminuer jusqu'à 1 pulvérisation par narine (100μg au total). Si les symptômes ne se contrôlent pas, augmenter jusqu'à 4 pulvérisations par narine (400μg), diminuer la dose après le contrôle des symptômes. La crème : 1 fois par jour, essuyer sur la zone touchée. |
| 剂型、规格<br>Les formes pharmaceutiques et les spécifications | 鼻喷剂：50μg×60 揿 / 支；50μg×120 揿 / 支。<br>乳膏：5g：5mg。<br><br>L'aérosol nasal : 50 μg×60 compresses par pièce, 50 μg×120 compresses par pièce.<br>L'cream : 5g : 5mg. |
| 药品名称 Drug Names | 地塞米松 Dexaméthasone |
| 适应证<br>Les indications | 用于过敏性与自身免疫性炎症性疾病。多用于结缔组织病、活动性风湿病、类风湿关节炎、红斑狼疮、严重支气管哮喘、严重皮炎、溃疡性结肠炎、急性白血病等，也用于某些严重感染及中毒、恶性淋巴瘤的综合治疗。片剂还用于某些肾上腺皮质疾病的诊断。<br><br>Il est applicable dans le traitement des maladies inflammatoires auto-immunes et allergiques. Il sert souvent à traiter la maladie du tissu conjonctif, des rhumatismes actifs, la polyarthrite rhumatoïde, le lupus, l'asthme sévère, la dermatite sévère, la colite ulcéreuse, la leucémie aiguë, etc. Il est également appliqué dans le traitement complet de certaines infections, des intoxications graves et du lymphome malin. Ses comprimés sont utilisés dans le diagnostic de maladie des glandes surrénales. |
| 用法、用量<br>Les modes d'emploi et la posologie | 口服，每日 0.75～3mg，一日 2～4 次；维持剂量每日 0.75mg。一般剂量静脉注射每次 2～20mg；静脉滴注时，应以 5% 葡萄糖注射液稀释，可 2～6 小时重复给药至病情稳定，但大剂量连续给药一般不超过 72 小时。还可用于缓解恶性肿瘤所致的脑水肿，首剂静脉推注 10mg，随后每 6 小时肌内注射 4mg，一般 12～24 小时患者可有所好转，2～4 日后逐渐减量，5～7 日停药。对不宜手术的脑肿瘤，首剂可静脉推注 50mg，以后每 2 小时重复给予 8mg，数天后再减至每天 2mg，分 2～3 次静脉给予。用于鞘内注射每次 5mg，间隔 1～3 周注射一次；关节腔内注射一般每次 0.8～4mg，按关节腔大小而定。<br><br>Par voie orale, 0,75 à 3mg par jour, 2 à 4 fois par jour ; la dose d'entretien, 0,75mg par jour. La dose usuelle pour injection IV, 2 à 20mg par fois, en perfusion, dissoudre dans la solution de glucose à 5%, toutes les 2 à 6h jusqu'à la stabilisation des maladies. Mais l'administration consécutive à forte dose ne dépasse pas 72h. Il est aussi appliqué dans le soulagement de l'œdème cérébral causé par le cancer, la dose initiale, 10mg en injection IV, ensuite, 4mg injecté par voie IM toutes les 6h, en général, les symptômes s'améliorent 12 à 24 h après, diminuer la dose 2 à 4 jours après, arrêter l'administration 5 à 7 jours après. Pour traiter le cancer cérébral qui ne peut pas être traité par la chirurgie, la dose initiale, 50mg injecté par voie IV, ensuite, 8mg toutes les 2h, quelques jours après, diminuer jusqu'à 2mg par jour, à travers 2 à 3 fois, injecté par voie IV. 5mg par fois, injection intrathécale, toutes les 1 à 3 semaines ; injection intra-articulaire, 0,8 à 4mg par fois, en fonction de la taille articulaire. |
| 剂型、规格<br>Les formes pharmaceutiques et les spécifications | 醋酸地塞米松片：每片 0.75mg。<br>地塞米松磷酸钠注射液：2mg（1ml）；5mg（1ml）。<br><br>Les comprimés d'acétate de dexaméthasone : 0,75mg par comprimé.<br>L'injection de phosphate de sodium de dexaméthasone : 2mg (1ml) ou 5mg (1ml). |
| 药品名称 Drug Names | 倍他米松 Bétaméthasone |
| 适应证<br>Les indications | 用于治疗活动性风湿病、类风湿关节炎、红斑性狼疮、严重支气管哮喘、严重皮炎、急性白血病等，也可用于某些感染的综合治疗。<br><br>Il sert à traiter les rhumatismes actifs, l'arthrite rhumatoïde, le lupus érythémateux, l'asthme bronchique grave, la dermatite sévère, la leucémie aiguë, etc. Il est aussi applicable dans le traitement complet de certaines infections. |

**续　表**

| | |
|---|---|
| 用法、用量<br>Les modes d'emploi et la posologie | 口服：成人开始每日 0.5 ～ 2mg，分次服用。维持量为每日 0.5 ～ 1mg。肌内注射、静脉注射或静脉滴注用倍他米松磷酸钠；用于危急患者的抢救。<br><br>Par voie orale : chez des adultes, commencer par 0,5 à 2mg par jour, à travers plusieurs fois. La dose d'entretien, 0,5 à 1mg par jour. Injecter IM, IV ou en perfusion le phosphate sodique de bétaméthasone : pour le sauvetage des patients extrêmement malades. |
| 剂型、规格<br>Les formes pharmaceutiques et les spécifications | 片剂：每片 0.5mg。<br>倍他米松醋酸酯注射液：每支 1.5mg（1ml）。<br>Comprimés : 0,5mg par comprimé.<br>L'injection d'acétate de bétaméthasone : 1,5mg (1ml) par solution. |
| 药品名称 Drug Names | 氟氢可的松 Fludrocortisone |
| 适应证<br>Les indications | 可与糖皮质类固醇一起用于原发性肾上腺皮质功能减退症的替代治疗。也适用于低肾素低醛固酮综合征和自主神经病变所致直立性低血压等。因本品内服易致水肿，多供外用局部涂敷治疗皮脂溢性湿疹、接触性皮炎、肛门、阴部瘙痒等症。<br><br>Utilisé en association avec des glucocorticoïdes, il sert de traitement de substitution de l'hypofonctionnement des glandes surrénales primiare.Il est également applicable dans le traitement de l'hypotension orthostatique causée par le syndrome de faible rénine et aldostérone, et par la neuropathie autonome. Comme son utilisation interne peut entraîner facilement l'œdème, il est souvent appliqué dans le traitement pour un usage externe de l'eczéma séborrhéique, de la dermatite de contact etdes démangeaisons vaginales et anales. |
| 用法、用量<br>Les modes d'emploi et la posologie | 替代治疗：成人口服，每日 0.1 ～ 0.2mg，分 2 次。局部皮肤涂敷一日 2 ～ 4 次。<br>Le traitement de substitution : chez des adultes, par voie orale, 0,1 à 0,2mg par jour, à travers 2 fois. Essuyer sur la peau pour un usage topique, 2 à 4 fois par jour. |
| 剂型、规格<br>Les formes pharmaceutiques et les spécifications | 片剂：每片 0.1mg。<br>醋酸氟氢可的松软膏：0.025%。<br>Comprimés : 0,1mg par comprimé.<br>La pommade d'acétate de fludrocortisone : 0,025%. |
| 药品名称 Drug Names | 氯倍他索 Clobétasol |
| 适应证<br>Les indications | 治疗皮肤炎症和瘙痒症，如神经性皮炎、接触性皮炎、脂溢性皮炎、湿疹、局限性瘙痒症、盘状红斑狼疮等。<br><br>Ce produit sert à traiter l'inflammation et le prurit de la peau, comme la névrodermite, la dermatite de contact, la dermatite séborrhéique, l'eczéma, le prurit localisé, le lupus érythémateux discoïde, etc. |
| 用法、用量<br>Les modes d'emploi et la posologie | 外用：涂于患处，一日 2 ～ 3 次，待病情控制后，改为一日 1 次。<br>Pour un usage externe : essuyer sur la zone touchée, 2 à 3 fois par jour, après le contrôle des symptômes, 1 fois par jour. |
| 剂型、规格<br>Les formes pharmaceutiques et les spécifications | 软膏：0.05%。<br>霜剂：0.025%。<br>La pommade : 0,05%.<br>La crème : 0,025%. |
| 药品名称 Drug Names | 氟轻松 Fluocinolone |
| 适应证<br>Les indications | 湿疹（特别是婴儿湿疹）、神经性皮炎、皮肤瘙痒症、接触性皮炎、牛皮癣、盘状红斑狼疮、扁平苔藓、外耳炎、日光性皮炎等。<br><br>L'eczéma (en particulier l'eczéma chez des bébés), le neurodermatitis, le prurit de la peau, la dermatite de contact, le psoriasis, le lupus érythémateux discoïde, le lichen plan, l'otite externe, la dermatite solaire, etc. |
| 用法、用量<br>Les modes d'emploi et la posologie | 皮肤洗净后局部外用，薄薄涂于患处，可轻揉促其渗入皮肤，一日 3 ～ 4 次。<br>Application topique sur la zone touchée après le lavage, essuyer doucement, 3 à 4 fois par jour. |

**续　表**

| | |
|---|---|
| 剂型、规格<br>Les formes pharmaceutiques et les spécifications | 醋酸氟轻松软膏、乳膏：0.025%。<br>La pommade et la crème de fluocinolone acétonide : 0,025%. |
| 药品名称 Drug Names | 倍氯米松 Béclométhasone |
| 适应证<br>Les indications | 外用可治疗各种炎症皮肤病如湿疹、过敏性皮炎、神经性皮炎、接触性皮炎、牛皮癣、瘙痒等。气雾剂可用于预防和治疗常年性及季节性的过敏性鼻炎和血管舒缩性鼻炎。<br>Il est appliqué pour un usage externe pour traiter les maladies inflammatoires de la peau, comme l'eczéma, la dermatite allergique, la neurodermatite, la dermatite de contact, le psoriasis, le prurit, etc. Son aérosol nasal est aussi applicable dans la prévention et le traitement de la rhinite allergiqueperannuelle, saisonnière et de la rhinite vasomotrice. |
| 用法、用量<br>Les modes d'emploi et la posologie | 乳膏或软膏用于皮肤病：一日 2～3 次，涂于患处，必要时包扎。气雾剂用于治疗哮喘：成人，一日 3～4 次，每次 2 揿，严重者每日 12～16 揿，根据病情好转逐渐减量；儿童，一日 2～4 次，每次 1～2 揿。鼻气雾剂，用于防止过敏性鼻炎，鼻腔喷雾给药，成人，一次每鼻孔 2 揿，一日 2 次，也可一次每鼻孔 1 揿（50μg），一日 3～4 次。一日总量不可超过 8 揿（400μg）。<br>Sa pommade ou sa crème sont utilisées dans le traitement des maladies de la peau : 2 à 3 fois par jour, essuyer sur la zone touchée, s'il est nécessaire, appliquer le pansement. Son aérosol est appliqué dans le traitement de l'asthme : chez des adultes, 3 à 4 fois par jour, 2 pulvérisations par fois, chez des patients gravement malades, 12 à 16 pulvérisations par jour, diminuer la dose avec l'amélioration des symptômes ; chez des enfants, 2 à 4 fois par jour, 1 à 2 pulvérisations par fois. L'aérosol nasal, pour prévenir la rhinite allergique, chez des adultes, 2 pulvérisations dans chaque narine, 2 fois par jour, ou 1 pulvérisation par narine par fois (50 μg), 3 à 4 fois par jour. Ne pas dépasser 8 pulvérisations par jour (400 μg). |
| 剂型、规格<br>Les formes pharmaceutiques et les spécifications | 软膏：0.025%。<br>鼻气雾剂、喷雾剂：50μg/揿（200 揿/支），250μg/揿（80 揿/支），50μg/揿（200 揿、支）。<br>L'aérosol nasal, l'aérosol : 50μg par pulvérisation (200 pulvérisations par pièce), 250 μg par pulvérisation (80 pulvérisations par pièce), 50 μg par pulvérisation (200 pulvérisations par pièce). |
| 药品名称 Drug Names | 哈西奈德 Halcinonide |
| 适应证<br>Les indications | 用于银屑病和湿疹性皮炎。用于银屑病，具有疗程短、不良反应少的特点。<br>Ce produit sert à traiter le psoriasis et la dermatite eczémateuse. Lors de son application dans le traitement du psoriasis, il a un traitement médical court et des effets indésirables peu importants. |
| 用法、用量<br>Les modes d'emploi et la posologie | 一日 2～3 次，涂于患处。<br>2 à 3 fois par jour, essuyer sur la zone touchée. |
| 剂型、规格<br>Les formes pharmaceutiques et les spécifications | 乳膏、软膏：0.1%。<br>La crème ou la pommade : 0,1 %. |
| 药品名称 Drug Names | 可的松 Cortisone |
| 适应证<br>Les indications | 主要用于肾上腺皮质功能减退症的替代治疗。<br>Ce produit est principalement utilisé dans le traitement de substitution de l'hypofonctionnement des glandes surrénales. |
| 用法、用量<br>Les modes d'emploi et la posologie | 口服：成人，每日剂量 25～37.5mg，清晨服 2/3，午后服 1/3。当患者有应激状况时（如发热、感染）可适当加量，增到每日 100mg。肌内注射：每日 25mg，有应激状况适当加量，有严重应激时，应改用氢化可的松静脉滴注。<br>Par voie orale : chez des adultes, 25 à 37,5mg par jour, prendre 2/3 le petit matin, 1/3 après-midi. En condition de stress chez des patients (telle que la fièvre ou l'infection), augmenter un peu la dose pour atteindre 100mg par jour. Injection IM : 25 mg par jour, augmenter un peu la dose en condition de stress. En condition de stress grave, il faut administrer l'hydrocortisone par voie IV en perfusion. |

**续 表**

| 剂型、规格<br>Les formes pharmaceutiques et les spécifications | 醋酸可的松注射液（混悬液）：每瓶 125mg（5ml）。<br>醋酸可的松片：每片 5mg；25mg。<br>Injection de l'acétate de cortisone (suspension) : 125mg (5ml) par flacon.<br>Comprimés d'acétate de cortisone : 5mg ou 25mg par comprimé. |
|---|---|

16.2　雄激素及蛋白同化激素 Androgènes et hormones d' assimilation des protéines

| 药品名称 Drug Names | 丙酸睾酮 Propionate de Téstostérone |
|---|---|
| 适应证<br>Les indications | 原发性或继发性男性性功能低减，男性青春期发育迟缓；绝经期后女性晚期乳腺癌的姑息治疗等。<br>La réduction de la fonction sexuelle masculine primaire ou secondaire, le retard de croissance chez les adolescents masculins ; lessoins palliatifs chez les femmes ménopausées atteintes d'un cancer du sein avancé. |
| 用法、用量<br>Les modes d'emploi et la posologie | ①成人常用量深部肌内注射，每次 25～50mg，每周 2～3 次。儿童常用量，每次 12.5～25mg，每周 2～3 次，疗程不超过 4～6 个月。②功能性子宫出血，配合黄体酮使用肌内注射，每次 25～50mg，一日 1 次，共 3～4 次。③绝经妇女晚期乳腺癌姑息性治疗，每次 50～100mg，每周 3 次，共 2～3 个月。<br>① La dose usuelle chez des adultes, injection IM profonde, 25 à 50mg par fois, 2 à 3 fois par semaine. La dose usuelle chez des enfants, 12,5 à 25mg par fois, 2 à 3 fois par semaine, ne pas dépasser 4 à 6 mois comme un traitement médical. ② Pour traiter les saignements utérins fonctionnels, utilisé en association avec la progestérone, injection IM, 25 à 50mg par fois, 1 fois par jour, 3 à 4 fois au total. ③ Pour les lessoins palliatifs chez les femmes ménopausées atteintes d'un cancer du sein avancé, 50 à 100mg par fois, 3 fois par semaine, pendant 2 à 3 mois. |
| 剂型、规格<br>Les formes pharmaceutiques et les spécifications | 注射剂（油溶液）：每支 10mg（1ml）；25mg（1ml）；50mg（1ml）。<br>Injection (la solution d'huile) : 10mg (1ml), 25mg (1ml) ou 50mg (1ml) par solution. |

| 药品名称 Drug Names | 苯丙酸诺龙 Phénylpropionate de nandrolone |
|---|---|
| 适应证<br>Les indications | 慢性消耗性疾病、严重灼伤、手术前后骨折不易愈合和骨质疏松症、早产儿、儿童发育不良等。尚可用于不可手术的乳腺癌、功能性子宫出血、子宫肌瘤等。<br>La maladie du dépérissement chronique, de graves brûlures, fractures difficiles à guérir avant et après la chirurgie et l'ostéoporose, ainsi que la dysplasie des enfants prématurés et des enfants. Il est aussi applicable dans le traitement du cancer du sein qui ne peut pas être traité par la chirurgie, des saignements utérins anormaux, et des fibromes utérins, etc. |
| 用法、用量<br>Les modes d'emploi et la posologie | 深部肌内注射：成人每次 25mg，每 1～2 周 1 次，儿童每次 10mg，婴儿每次 5mg。女性转移性乳腺癌姑息性治疗，每周 25～100mg，疗程的长短视疗效及不良反应而定。<br>Injection IM profonde : chez des adultes, 25mg par fois, toutes les 1 à 2 semaines, chez des enfants, 10 mg par fois, chez des bébés, 5mg par fois. Pour le traitement palliatif des femmes avec cancer du sein métastatique, 25 à 100mg par semaine, la durée du traitement dépend de l'efficacité et des réactions indésirables. |
| 剂型、规格<br>Les formes pharmaceutiques et les spécifications | 注射液（油溶液）：每支 10mg（1ml）；25mg（1ml）。<br>Injection (la solution d'huile) : 10mg (1ml) ou 25mg (1ml) par solution. |

| 药品名称 Drug Names | 司坦唑醇 Stanozolol |
|---|---|
| 适应证<br>Les indications | 预防和治疗遗传性血管神经性水肿、慢性消耗性疾病、重病及手术后体弱消瘦，年老体弱、骨质疏松症、小儿发育不良、再生障碍性贫血、白细胞减少症、血小板减少症、高脂血症等。还用于防治长期使用皮脂激素引起的肾上腺皮质功能减退。 |

**续　表**

|  | Il sert à prévenir et à traiter l'angio-œdème héréditaire, la maladie générale ou grave du dépérissement chronique,la fragilité après la chirurgie, l'ostéoporose chez des personnes âgées, la dysplasie chez des enfants, l'anémie aplasique, la leucopénie, la thrombocytopénie, l'hyperlipidémie, etc. Il est aussi applicable dans la prévention de l'insuffisance surrénale causée par l'utilisation à long terme de l'hormone de sébum. |
|---|---|
| 用法、用量<br>Les modes d'emploi et la posologie | 口服：成人，开始时每次 2mg，一日 2～3 次（女性酌减）。如治疗效果明显，可每隔 1～3 个月减量，直至每日 2mg 维持量。儿童，每日 1～2mg，仅在发作时应用。<br><br>Par voie orale : chez des adultes, commencer par prendre 2mg par fois, 2 à 3 fois par jour (diminuer un peu la dose chez des femmes). Si l'effet est évident, diminuer la dose tous les 1 à 3 mois, jusqu'à la dose d'entretien, soit 2mg par jour. Chez des enfants, 1 à 2mg par jour, appliquer seulement lors de la crise de la maladie. |
| 剂型、规格<br>Les formes pharmaceutiques et les spécifications | 片剂：每片 2mg。<br>Comprimés : 2mg par comprimé. |

| 药品名称 Drug Names | 达那唑 Danazol |
|---|---|
| 适应证<br>Les indications | 治疗子宫内膜异位症，尚用于纤维性乳腺炎、男性乳房发育、乳腺痛、痛经、腹痛等，可使肿块消失、软化或缩小，使疼痛消失或减轻。还用于性早熟、自发性血小板减少性紫癜、血友病和 Christmas 病（凝血因子IX缺乏）、遗传性血管性水肿、系统性红斑狼疮等。<br><br>Il sert à traiter l'endométriose. Il est aussi applicable dans le traitement de la mammite fibreuse, la gynécomastie,les douleurs mammaires, la dysménorrhée, des douleurs abdominales, etc. Il peut faire disparaître, ramollir ou réduire les grumeaux, et faire disparaître ou diminuer les douleurs. Il est également appliqué dans le traitement de la puberté précoce, du purpura thrombopénique idiopathique, de l'hémophilie, de la maladie de Christmas (le déficit dufacteur IX de coagulation),de l'angio-œdème héréditaire, du lupus érythémateux disséminé, etc. |
| 用法、用量<br>Les modes d'emploi et la posologie | ① 子宫内膜异位症：口服，从月经周期第 1～3 日开始服用，一日 2 次，每次 200～400mg，总量一天不超过 800mg，连续 3～6 个月为 1 个疗程，必要时可继续到第 9 个月。②纤维性乳腺炎：口服，每次 50～200mg，一日 2 次，连用 3～6 个月。③男性乳房发育：口服，每日 200～600mg。④性早熟：口服，每日 200～400mg。⑤血小板减少性紫癜：口服，每次 200mg，一日 2～4 次。⑥血友病：口服，每日 600mg，连用 14 日。⑦遗传性血管性水肿：口服，开始每次 200mg，一日 2～3 次。急性发作时，剂量可提高到 200mg。⑧红斑狼疮：每日 400～600mg。<br><br>① Pour traiter l'endométriose : par voie orale, commencer à prendre à partir des 1 à 3 premiers jours du cycle mensuel, 2 fois par jour, 200 à 400mg par fois, ne pas dépasser 800mg par jour, pendant 3 à 6 mois comme un traitement médical, s'il est nécessaire, jusqu'à 9ème mois. ② Pour traiter la mammite fibreuse : par voie orale, 50 à 200mg par fois, 2 fois par jour, pendant 3 à 6 mois consécutifs. ③ Pour traiter la gynécomastie : par voie orale, 200 à 600mg par jour. ④ Pour traiter la puberté précoce : par voie orale, 200 à 400 mg par jour. ⑤ Pour traiter purpura thrombopénique idiopathique : par voie orale, 200mg par fois, 2 à 4 fois par jour. ⑥ Pour traiter l'hémophilie : par voie orale, 600mg par jour, pendant 14 jours consécutifs. ⑦ Pour traiter l'angio-œdème héréditaire : par voie orale, commencer par 200mg par fois, 2 à 3 fois par jour. Lors de la crise aigue, augmenter la dose pour atteindre 200mg. ⑧ Pour traiter le lupus érythémateux disséminé : 400 à 600 mg par jour. |
| 剂型、规格<br>Les formes pharmaceutiques et les spécifications | 胶囊剂：每粒 100mg；200mg。<br>Capsules : 100mg ou 200mg par capsule. |

**续　表**

16.3　雌激素及其类似合成药物 Oestrogènes et leurs analogues synthétiques

| 药品名称 Drug Names | 雌二醇 Estradiol |
|---|---|
| 适应证<br>Les indications | 卵巢功能不全或卵巢激素不足引起的各种症状，主要是功能性子宫出血、原发性闭经、绝经期综合征及前列腺癌等。<br><br>Il sert à traiter les symptômes causés pas le dysfonctionnement ovarien ou le manque d'hormones ovariennes, y compris le saignement utérin fonctionnel, l'aménorrhée primaire, le syndrome de la ménopause, lecancer de la prostate, etc. |
| 用法、用量<br>Les modes d'emploi et la posologie | 肌内注射：每次 0.5 ～ 1.5mg，每周 2 ～ 3 次。口服，一日 1 片。<br><br>Injection IM : 0,5 à 1,5mg par fois, 2 à 3 fois par semaine. Par voie orale, 1 comprimé par jour. |
| 剂型、规格<br>Les formes pharmaceutiques et les spécifications | 注射液：每支 2mg（1ml）。<br>凝胶：每支 80g；0.06%。<br>片剂：每片 1mg。<br>微粒化 17β 雌二醇片：每片 1mg；2mg。<br>控释贴片：周效片，每片 2.5mg；3 ～ 4 日效片：每片 4mg。<br><br>Injection : 2mg (1ml) par solution.<br>Les gels : 80g ; 0,06% par pièce.<br>Comprimés : 1mg par comprimé.<br>Comprimés de 17β estradiol micronisés : 1mg ou 2mg par comprimé.<br>Les patchs à libération contrôlée : les patchs à action en une semaine, 2,5mg par patch ; les patchs à action en 3 à 4 jours : 4mg par patch. |
| 药品名称 Drug Names | 苯甲酸雌二醇 Benzoate d'estradiol |
| 适应证<br>Les indications | 卵巢功能不全、闭经、绝经期综合征、退奶及前列腺癌等。<br><br>Il sert à traiter le dysfonctionnement ovarien, l'aménorrhée, lesyndrome de la ménopause, le retrait de lait et le cancer de la prostate. |
| 用法、用量<br>Les modes d'emploi et la posologie | ①绝经期综合征：肌内注射，每次 1 ～ 2mg，每 3 日 1 次。②子宫发育不良：肌内注射，每次 1 ～ 2mg，每 2 ～ 3 日 1 次。③子宫出血：肌内注射，每次 1mg，一日 1 次，1 周后继续用黄体酮。<br><br>① Pour traiter le syndrome de la ménopause : injection IM, 1 à 2mg par fois, tous les 3 jours. ② Pour traiter l'hypoplaisie utérine : injection IM, 1 à 2mg par fois, tous les 2 à 3 jours. ③ L'hémorragie utérine : injection IM, 1mg par fois, 1 fois par jour, une semaine apèrs, continuer de prendre la progestérone. |
| 剂型、规格<br>Les formes pharmaceutiques et les spécifications | 注射液：每支 1mg（1ml）；2mg（1ml）。<br><br>Injection : 1mg (1ml) ou 2mg (1ml) par solution. |
| 药品名称 Drug Names | 戊酸雌二醇 Valérate d'estradiol |
| 适应证<br>Les indications | 口服缓解绝经后更年期症状、卵巢切除后及非癌性疾病、放疗性去势的雌激素缺乏引起的症状，外用于治疗扁平疣。<br><br>Son administration par voie orale permet de soulager les symptômes de la ménopause, les maladies non cancéreuses aprèsl'ablation des ovaires,les symptômes causés par la carence en oestrogènesaprès la radiothérapie. Son usage externe permet de traiterla verrue plate. |
| 用法、用量<br>Les modes d'emploi et la posologie | 肌内注射：每次 5 ～ 10mg，每 1 ～ 2 周 1 次，平均替代治疗剂量为每 2 周 5 ～ 20mg，用于卵巢功能不全，每次 5 ～ 20mg，每月 1 次。口服，每天 1 ～ 2mg，连续 21 日，停服 1 周后开始下一疗程。<br><br>Injection IM : 5 à 10mg par fois, toutes les 1 à 2 semaines, la dose pour le traitement de substitution en moyenne, 5 à 20mg toutes les 2 semaines. Pour traiter le dysfonctionnement ovarien, 5 à 20mg par fois, une fois par mois. Par voie orale, 1 à 2mg par jour, pendant 21 jours consécutifs, un intervalle de 1 semaine entre deux traitements. |

**续　表**

| | |
|---|---|
| 剂型、规格<br>Les formes pharmaceutiques et les spécifications | 注射液：每支 5mg（1ml）；10mg（1ml）。<br>片剂：每片 0.5mg；1mg；2mg。<br>Injection : 5mg (1ml) ou 10mg (1ml) par solution.<br>Comprimés : 0,5mg, 1mg ou 2mg par comprimé. |
| 药品名称 Drug Names | 炔雌醇 Ethinyléstradiol |
| 适应证<br>Les indications | 月经紊乱，如闭经、月经过少、功能性子宫出血、绝经期综合征、子宫发育不全、前列腺癌等。也做口服避孕药中常用的雌激素成分。<br><br>Il sert à traiter les troubles menstruels, tels que l'aménorrhée, le saignement utérin fonctionnel, le syndrome de la ménopause, l'hypoplasie utérine, le cancer de la prostate, etc. Il sert aussi d'oestrogènedes contraceptifs oraux. |
| 用法、用量<br>Les modes d'emploi et la posologie | 口服：每次 0.0125～0.05mg，每晚服用 1 次，用于前列腺癌每次 0.05～0.5mg，一日 3 次。<br><br>Par voie orale : 0,0125 à 0,05mg par fois, une fois par voir. Pour traiter le cancer de la prostate, 0,05 à 0,5mg par fois, 3 fois par jour. |
| 剂型、规格<br>Les formes pharmaceutiques et les spécifications | 片剂：每片 5μg；12.5μg；50μg；500μg。<br>Comprimés : 5 μg, 12,5μg, 50μg ou 500μg. |
| 药品名称 Drug Names | 雌三醇 Estriol |
| 适应证<br>Les indications | 绝经后妇女因雌激素缺乏而引起的泌尿生殖道萎缩和萎缩性阴道炎（及老年性阴道炎），表现为外阴或阴道干燥、瘙痒、灼热、阴道分泌物异常及性交疼痛或尿频、尿急、尿失禁等症状。<br><br>Ce produit sert à traiter l'atrophie urogénitale et la vaginite atrophique (et la vaginite sénile), causées par la carence en œstrogènes chez des femmes ménopausées, y compris la sécheresse vaginale ou de la vulve, les démangeaisons, des brûlures, des pertes vaginales anormales, des douleurs pendant les rapports sexuels, la miction, l'urgence urinaire, l'incontinence urinaire, etc. |
| 用法、用量<br>Les modes d'emploi et la posologie | 阴道给药，常用剂量为一日 2mg，连续治疗 1 周，以后每周放置 1 粒维持或遵医嘱。绝经后妇女阴道手术前后，在手术前 2 周，每天使用 1 次 0.5g 软膏，术后 2 周内每周用药 2 次。可疑宫颈涂片辅助诊断检查前 1 周内，每 2 天用药 1 次，每次用 0.5g 乳膏。<br><br>Administration par voie vaginale, la dose usuelle, 2mg par jour, pendant une semaine consécutive. Ensuite, mettre 1 suppositoire par semaine pour le traitement d'entretien ou selon les ordonnances. Avant et après la chirurgie vaginale chez desfemmes ménopausées, 2 semaines avant la chirurgie, appliquer 0,5g de pommade par fois par jour, 2 semaines après la chirurgie, appliquer 2 fois par semaine. Possible d'utiliser les frottis cervicaux comme diagnostic adjuvant, 1 semaine avant la chirurgie, 1 fois tous les 2 jours, 0,5g de crème par fois. |
| 剂型、规格<br>Les formes pharmaceutiques et les spécifications | 栓剂：每枚 0.5mg；1mg；2mg。<br>乳膏：15g；15mg。<br>Suppositoires : 0,5mg, 1mg ou 2mg par suppositoire.<br>Crème : 15g : 15mg. |
| 药品名称 Drug Names | 尼尔雌醇 Nilestriol |
| 适应证<br>Les indications | 用于雌激素缺乏引起的绝经期或更年期综合征，如潮热、出汗、头痛、目眩、疲劳、烦躁易怒、神经过敏、外阴干燥、老年性阴道炎等。<br><br>Il sert à traiter le syndrome de ménopause causé par la carence en œstrogènes, tel que les bouffées de chaleur, la transpiration, les maux de tête, des étourdissements, la fatigue, l'irritabilité, la nervosité, la vulve sèche, la vaginite sénile, etc. |
| 用法、用量<br>Les modes d'emploi et la posologie | 口服：一次 5mg，每月 1 次。症状改善后维持量为每次 1～2mg，每月 2 次，3 个月为 1 个疗程。<br><br>Par voie orale : 5mg par fois, 1 fois par mois. La dose d'entretien après l'amélioration des symptômes, 1 à 2 mg par fois, 2 fois par mois, pendant 3 mois comme un traitement médical. |

| 剂型、规格<br>Les formes pharmaceutiques et les spécifications | 片剂：每片 1mg；2mg；5mg。<br>Comprimés : 1mg, 2mg ou 5mg par comprimé. |
|---|---|
| **药品名称 Drug Names** | 己烯雌酚 Diéthylstilbestrol |
| 适应证<br>Les indications | 卵巢功能不全或垂体功能异常引起的各种疾病、闭经、子宫发育不全、功能性子宫出血、绝经期综合征、老年性阴道炎等。也用于不能进行手术的晚期前列腺癌。<br><br>Il sert à traiter les maladies cauées par le dysfonctionnement ovarien ou le dysfonctionnement de l'hypophyse, l'aménorrhée, l'hypoplasie utérine, les saignements utérins anormaux, le syndrome de la ménopause, la vaginite sénile. Il es aussi application dans le traitement du cancer de la prostate avancé qui ne peut pas être traité par la chirurgie. |
| 用法、用量<br>Les modes d'emploi et la posologie | ①闭经：口服小剂量刺激垂体前叶分泌促性腺激素，每日不超过 0.25mg。②用于人工月经周期：每日服 0.25mg，连用 20 日，待来月经后再用同法治疗，共 3 个周期。③用于月经周期延长及子宫发育不全：每日服 0.1～0.2mg，持续半年，经期停服。④治疗功能性子宫出血：每晚服 0.5～1mg，连服 20 日。⑤用于绝经期综合征：每日服 0.25mg，症状控制后改为每日 0.1mg。⑥老年性阴道炎：阴道塞药，每晚塞入 0.2～0.4mg，共用 7 日。⑦配合手术用于前列腺癌：每日 3mg，分 3 次服，连用 2～3 个月，维持量每日 1mg。⑧用于因子宫发育不良及子宫颈分泌物黏稠所致不育症：以小剂量促使宫颈黏液稀薄，精子宜透入，于月经后每日服 0.1mg，共 15 日，疗程 3～6 个月。⑨用于稽留流产（妊娠 7 个月内死胎经 2 个月或以上仍未娩出）：每次服 5mg，每日 3 次，5～7 日为 1 个疗程，停药 5 日，如无效，可重复一疗程。<br><br>① Pour traiter l'aménorrhée : prendre une faible dose par voie orale pour stimuler la sécrétion de gonadotrophine de l'hypophyse antérieure, ne pas dépasser 0,25mg par jour. ② Pour le cycle mensuel artificiel : 0,25mg par jour, pendant 20 jours consécutifs, après la rège, poursuivre le même traitement pendant 3 cycles au total. ③ Pour traiter le cycle mensuel prolongé et l'hypoplasie utérine : 0,1 à 0,2mg par jour, pendant 6 mois, arrêter l'administration pendant la règle. ④ Pour traiter les saignement utérins anormaux :0,5 à 1mg par soir, pendant 20 jours consécutifs. ⑤ Pour traiter le syndrome de la ménopause : 0,25mg par jour, après le contrôle des symptômes, 0,1mg par jour. ⑥ Pour traiter la vaginite sénile : introduire le médicament dans le vagin, 0,2 à 0,4mg par soir, pendant 7 jours consécutifs. ⑦ Pour traiter le cancer de la prostate comme traitement adjuvant : 3mg par jour, à travers 3 fois, pendant 2 à 3 mois consécutifs, la dose d'entretien, 1mg par jour. ⑧ Pour traiter l'infertilité causée par l'hypoplasie utérine et les sécrécations cervicales collantes: utiliser une faible dose pour fluidifier les sécrécations cervicales, facilitant la pénétration des spermatozoïdes. 0,1mg par jour après la règle, pendant 15 jous, le traitement dure 3 à 6 mois. ⑨ Pour l'avortement manqué (l'accouchement manqué du fœtus pendant 2 mois ou plus en 7 mois de la grossesse) : 5mg par fois, 3 fois par jour, pendant 5 à 7 jours comme un traitement médical, arrêter l'administration pendant 5 jours, s'il est inefficace, possible reprendre un traitement. |
| 剂型、规格<br>Les formes pharmaceutiques et les spécifications | 片剂：每片 0.5mg；1mg；2mg。<br>注射液：每支 0.5mg（1ml）；1mg（1ml）；2mg（1ml）。<br>Comprimés : 0,5mg, 1mg ou 2mg par comprimé.<br>Injection : 0,5mg (1ml), 1mg (1ml) ou 2mg (1ml). |

16.4 孕激素类 Progestérines

| **药品名称 Drug Names** | 黄体酮 Progestérone |
|---|---|
| 适应证<br>Les indications | 用于习惯性流产、痛经、经血过多或血崩症、闭经等。口服大剂量也用于黄体酮不足所致疾病，如经前综合征、排卵停止所致月经紊乱、良性乳腺病、围绝经期激素替代疗法。<br><br>Il sert à traiter l'avortement habituel, la dysménorrhée, la ménorragie, les troubles de saignement vaginal, l'aménorrhée, etc. L'administration par voie orale d'une forte dose est aussi appliquée dans le traitement des maladies causées par le manque de progestéron, telles que le syndrome prémenstruel, les troubles menstruels provoqués par l'arrêt de l'ovulation, la maladie bénigne du sein, et la thérapie de remplacement d'hormone périménopause. |

**续 表**

| | |
|---|---|
| 用法、用量<br>Les modes d'emploi et la posologie | ①习惯性流产：肌内注射，一次 10～20mg，一日 1 次，或每周 2～3 次，一直用到妊娠第 4 个月。②先兆流产：肌内注射，一般每日 20～50mg，待疼痛及出血停止后减为每日 10～20mg。③痛经：在月经之前 6～8 日每天肌内注射 5～10mg，共 4～6 日，疗程可重复若干次，对子宫发育不全所致的痛经，可与雌激素配合使用。④经血过多和血崩症：肌内注射，每日 10～20mg，5～7 日为 1 个疗程，可重复 3～4 个疗程，每疗程间隔 15～20 日。⑤闭经：先肌内注射雌激素 2～3 周后，立即给予本品，每日肌内注射 3～5mg，6～8 日为 1 个疗程，总剂量不宜超过 300～350mg，疗程可重复 2～3 次。⑥功能性出血：肌内注射，每日 5～10mg，连用 5～10 日，如在用药期间月经来潮，应立即停药。<br><br>① Pour traiter l'avortement habituel : injection IM, 10 à 20mg par fois, 1 fois par jour, ou 2 à 3 fois par semaine, jusqu'au 4ème mois de la grossesse. ② Pour traiter la manace d'avortement : injection IM, 20 à 50mg par jour, après l'arrêt des douleurs et des saignements, 10 à 20mg par jour. ③ Pour traiter la dysménorrhée : 6 à 8 jours avant la règle, injecter 5 à 10mg par voie IM par jour, pendant 4 à 6 jours, possible de reprendre plusieurs traitements. Pour traiter la ménorragie causée par l'hypoplasie utérine, possible d'être utilisé en association avec l'œstrogène. ④ Pour traiter la ménorragie et les troubles de saignement vaginal : injection IM, 10 à 20mg par jour, pendant 5 à 7 jours comme un traitement médical, possible de reprendre 3 à 4 traitements, avec un intervalle de 15 à 20 jours entre deux traitements. ⑤ Pour traiter l'aménorrhée : injecter l'œstrogène par voie IM, 2 à 3 semaines après, injecter immédiatement la progestérone, 3 à 5 mg par voie IM par jour, pendant 6 à 8 jours comme un traitement médical, ne pas dépasser 300 à 350mg au total, possible de reprendre 2 à 3 traitements. ⑥ Pour traiter les saignements fonctionnels : injection IM, 5 à 10mg par jour, pendant 5 à 10 jours consécutifs. Lors de la règle, arrêter immédiatement l'administration. |
| 剂型、规格<br>Les formes pharmaceutiques et les spécifications | 注射液：每支 10mg（1ml）；20mg（1ml）。<br>胶囊：每粒 100mg。<br>Injection : 10mg (1ml) ou 20mg (1ml) par solution.<br>Capsules : 100mg par capsule. |

| 药品名称 Drug Names | 甲羟孕酮 Médroxyprogestérone |
|---|---|
| 适应证<br>Les indications | 痛经、功能性闭经、功能性子宫出血、先兆流产或习惯性流产、子宫内膜异位症等。大剂量可用作长效避孕针，肌内注射 1 次 150mg，可避孕 3 个月。<br><br>Il sert à traiter la dysménorrhée, l'aménorrhée fonctionnelle, les saignements utérins anormaux, la menace d'avortement ou l'avortement habituel, l'endométriose, etc. Utilisé à forte dose, il est utilisé pour la contraception pour une longue durée. Une injection de 150mg par voie IM peut permettre la contraception de 3 mois. |
| 用法、用量<br>Les modes d'emploi et la posologie | ①功能性闭经：每日口服 4～8mg，连用 5～10 日。②子宫内膜癌或肾癌：口服，一次 100mg，一日 3 次，肌内注射，起始 0.4～1g，1 周后可重复一次，待病情改善或稳定后，剂量改为 400mg，每月 1 次。③避孕：肌内注射，每 3 个月一次 150mg，于月经来潮第 2～7 日内注射。<br><br>① Pour traiter l'aménorrhée fonctionnelle : par voie orale, 4 à 8mg par jour, pendant 5 à 10 jours consécutifs. ② Pour traiter le cancer de l'endomètre ou le cancer du rein : par voie orale, 100mg par fois, 3 fois par jour. Injection IM, commencer par 0,4 à 1g, possible de reprendre une fois 1 semaine après, après l'amélioration des symptômes, 400mg, 1 fois par mois. ③ Pour la contraception : injection IM, 150mg par fois tous les 3 mois, injecter du 2ème au 7ème jour de la règle. |
| 剂型、规格<br>Les formes pharmaceutiques et les spécifications | 片剂：每片 2mg，4mg；10mg。<br>注射液：100mg；150mg。<br>Comprimés : 2mg, 4mg ou 10mg par comprimé.<br>Injection : 100mg ou 150mg. |

**续　表**

| 药品名称 Drug Names | 炔孕酮 Ethistérone |
| --- | --- |
| 适应证<br>Les indications | 功能性子宫出血、月经异常、闭经、痛经等。也用于防止先兆性流产和习惯性流产，但由于维持妊娠作用较弱，效果并不好。如与雌激素炔雌醇合用，则疗效较好。<br><br>Il sert à traiter les saignements utérins anormaux, des troubles menstruels, l'aménorrhée, la dysménorrhée, etc. Il est aussi appliqué dans la prévention de la menace d'avortement et de l'avortement habituel, mais à cause de son faible effet de l'entretien de la grossesse, il n'est pas très efficace. S'il est utilisé en association l'avecéthinylestradiol (un œstrogène), il sera plus efficace. |
| 用法、用量<br>Les modes d'emploi et la posologie | 口服：一次 10mg，一日 3 次。<br>舌下含服：一次 10 ～ 20mg，一日 2 ～ 3 次。<br>Par voie orale : 10mg par fois, 3 fois par jour.<br>Administration par voie sublinguale : 10 à 20mg par fois, 2 à 3 fois par jour. |
| 剂型、规格<br>Les formes pharmaceutiques et les spécifications | 片剂：每片 5mg；10mg；25mg。<br>Comprimés : 5mg, 10mg ou 25mg par comprimé. |

| 药品名称 Drug Names | 屈螺酮 Drospirénone |
| --- | --- |
| 适应证<br>Les indications | 女性避孕。<br>La contraception féminine. |
| 用法、用量<br>Les modes d'emploi et la posologie | 必须按照包装所表明的顺序，每天约在同一时间用少量液体送服。每日 1 片，连服 21 日。停药 7 日后开始服用下一盒药，其间通常会出现撤退性出血。<br><br>suivre l'ordre indiqué sur le baquet, administrer la drospirénone avec un peu de liquide au même moment du jour. 1 comprimé par jour, pendant 21 jours consécutifs. Avec un intervalle de 7 jours entre deux traitements. Pendant cet intervalle, il y a souvent un saignement de retrait. |
| 剂型、规格<br>Les formes pharmaceutiques et les spécifications | 复方制剂（优思明）：每片含屈螺酮 3mg 和炔雌醇 0.03mg。<br>La préparation de composés : chaque comprimé contient 3mg de drospirénone et 0,03mg d'éthinylestradiol. |

16.5　促性腺激素 Gonadotrophine

| 药品名称 Drug Names | 绒毛膜促性腺激素 Gonadotropine Corionique |
| --- | --- |
| 适应证<br>Les indications | ①青春期隐睾症的诊断和治疗。②垂体功能低下所致的男性不育。③垂体促性腺激素不足所致的女性无排卵性不孕症。④用于体外受精以获取多个卵母细胞。⑤女性黄体功能不足、功能性子宫出血、妊娠早期先兆流产、习惯性流产。<br><br>① Ce produit est utilisé dans le diagnostic et le traitement de la cryptorchidie chez les adolescents. ② L'infertilité masculine due à hypopituitarisme. ③ L'infertilité anovulatoire féminine due àla carence en hypophyse gonadotrophine. ④ Applicable dans la FIV pour obtenir des vocytes multiples. ⑤ L'insuffisance lutéale chez des femmes, des saignements utérins anormaux, l'avortement menacé pendant la grossesse précoce et l'avortement habituel. |
| 用法、用量<br>Les modes d'emploi et la posologie | ①促排卵：于绝经后促性腺激素末次给药后一天或氯米芬末次给药后 5 ～ 7 日肌内注射一次 5000 ～ 10 000U，连续治疗 3 ～ 6 周期，如无效，应停药。②黄体功能不足：于经期第 15 ～ 17 天排卵之日起，隔日注射一次 1500U，连用 5 次，剂量可根据患者的反应作调整，妊娠后需维持原剂量直至 7 ～ 10 孕周。③功能性子宫出血：肌内注射一次 1000 ～ 3000U。④青春期前隐睾症，肌内注射一次，1000 ～ 5000U，每周 2 ～ 3 次。⑤男性性功能减退症：肌内注射一次 1000 ～ 4000U，每周 2 ～ 3 次，持续数周至数月。⑥先兆流产或习惯性流产：肌内注射一次 1000 ～ 5000U。 |

**续　表**

| | |
|---|---|
| | ① Pour la promotion de l'ovulation :après la ménopause, 1 jour après la dernière administration de lagonadotrophine ou 5 à 7 jours après la dernière administration de laclomifène, injecter par voie IM 5000 à 10 000 U, pendant 3 à 6 semines consécutives, s'il est inefficace, arrêter l'administration. ② Pour traiter l'insuffisance lutéale : à partir du 15 à 17ème jour du cycle mensuel, le jour de l'ovulation, injecter 1 500U tous les 2 jours, pour 5 fois consécutives, ajuster la dose en fonction des réactions des patients, après la grossesse, il faut maintenir l'ancienne dose jusqu'à 7 à 10ème semaine de la grossesse. ③ Pour traiter les saignements utérins fonctionnels : injecter par voie IM 1000 à 3000 U. ④ Pour traiter la cryptorchidie chez les adolescents : injecter 1000 à 5000 U par voie IM, 2 à 3 fois par semaine. ⑤ Pour traiter la dysfonction sexuelle masculine : injecter 1000 à 4000U par voie IM, 2 à 3 fois par semaine, pendant quelques semaines ou des mois. ⑥ Pour traiter la menace d'avortement ou l'avortement habitul, injecter 1000 à 5000 U par voie IM. |
| 剂型、规格 Les formes pharmaceutiques et les spécifications | 注射用绒促性素：每支 500U；1000U；2000U；5000U。 L'hormone chorionique gonadotrope pour injection : 500U, 1 000U, 2 000U ou 5 000U par solution. |

| 药品名称 Drug Names | 尿促性素 Ménotrophine |
|---|---|
| 适应证 Les indications | ①与绒促性素或氯米芬配合使用以治疗无排卵性不孕症。②用于原发性或继发性闭经，男性精子缺乏症及卵巢功能试验等。 ① Utilisé en associaiton avec l'HCG ou le clomifènepour traiter l'infertilité anovulatoire. ② Utilisé dans le traitement de l'aménorrhée primaire ou secondaire, de la carence de sperme et les tests de la fonction de l'ovaire. |
| 用法、用量 Les modes d'emploi et la posologie | 肌内注射：用于诱导排卵，开始每天 75～150U，连用 7～12 日，至雌激素水平增高后，再肌内注射绒促性素，经 12 小时即排卵。用于男性性功能低下，开始一周给予 HCG 每次 2000U，共 2～3 次，以产生适当的男性特征。然后肌内注射本品，每次 75～150U，每周 3 次，同时给予 HCG 每次 2000U，每周 2 次。至少治疗 4 个月。 Injection IM : pour la promotion de l'ovulation, commencer par 75 à 150U par jour, pendant 7 à 12 jours consécutifs, jusqu'à l'augmentation du niveau de l'œstrogène, injecter par voie IM l'hormone chorionique gonadotrope (HCG), 12 h après, l'ovulation aura lieu. Pour traiter la dysfonction sexuelle masculine, pendant la première semaine, prendre 2000U d'HCG par fois, 2 à 3 fois au total. Ensuite, injecter par voie IM ce médicament, 75 à 150 U par fois, 3 fois par semaine, en même temps, prendre 2000 U d'HCG par fois, 2 fois par semaine. Pendant 4 mois au moins. |
| 剂型、规格 Les formes pharmaceutiques et les spécifications | 注射用尿促性素：每支 75U；150U。 La gonadtrophine urinaire pour injection : 75U ou 150U par solution. |

| 药品名称 Drug Names | 普罗瑞林 Protiréline |
|---|---|
| 适应证 Les indications | 用于诊断 Graves 病、甲状腺功能减退症及促甲状腺素性突眼等。 Utilisé dans le diagnostic de la maladie de Graves, de l'hypothyroïdieet de l'exophtalmie thyrotrophique. |
| 用法、用量 Les modes d'emploi et la posologie | 静脉注射本品 200～500μg，观察血中促甲状腺激素水平的变化，正常人于注射后 15～30 分钟达峰值，为基础值的 2～3 倍以上。 Injecter par voie IV 200 à 500μg de protiréline, observer le changement du niveau de la thyrotrophine dans le sang, en général, le pic arrive 15 à 30 minutes après l'injection, soit 2 à 3 fois plus important que le niveau de base. |

续　表

| 剂型、规格 Les formes pharmaceutiques et les spécifications | 注射用普罗瑞林：0.5mg。<br>La protiréline pour injection : 0,5mg. |
|---|---|

| 药品名称 Drug Names | 亮丙瑞林 Leuproreline |
|---|---|
| 适应证 Les indications | 子宫内膜异位症，对伴有月经过多、下腹痛、腰痛及贫血等的子宫肌瘤，可使肌瘤缩小和（或）症状改善，绝经前乳腺癌且雌激素受体阳性患者；前列腺癌、中枢性性早熟症。<br><br>Il sert à traiter l'endométriose. Pour les fibromes utérinsaccompagnés de la ménorragie, des douleurs abdominales basses, de l'anémie et des douleurs lombaires, il permet de réduire les fibromes et (ou) d'améliorer les symptômes. Il est aussi applicable dans le traitement des patients atteints de cancer du sein avant la ménopauseet dontle récepteur de l'hormone oestrogène est positif. Il permet aussi de traiter le cancer de la prostateet la puberté précoce centrale. |
| 用法、用量 Les modes d'emploi et la posologie | 前列腺癌、绝经前乳腺癌，皮下注射，每次 3.75mg，每 4 周 1 次。子宫内膜异位症：通常成人皮下注射，每次 3.75mg，每 4 周 1 次，对体重低于 50kg 时，可以使用 1.88mg 的制剂。初次给药于经期开始后的第 1～5 日。子宫肌瘤：通常成人皮下注射每次 1.88mg，每 4 周 1 次，对体重过重或子宫明显增大的患者，应注射 3.75mg。初次给药于经期开始后的 1～5 日。中枢性性早熟症：通常皮下注射 30μg/kg，每 4 周 1 次，根据患者症状可增量至 90μg/kg。<br><br>Pour traiter le cancer de prostate et le cancer du sein avant la ménopause, injection sous-cutanée, 3,75mg par fois, toutes les 4 semaines. Pour traiter l'endométriose : chez des adultes, en général, injection sous-cutanée, 3,75mg par fois, toutes les 4 semaines, chez des patients de moins de 50kg, possible de prendre la préparation de 1,88mg. La première administration est appliquée le 1 à 5ème jours de la menstruation. Pour traiter les fibromes utérins : en général, chez des adultes, injecter 1,88mg par fois par voie sous-cutanée, toutes les 4 semaines. Chez des patients en surpoids ou dont l'utérus augmente de manière évidente, injecter 3,75mg. La première administration doit être appliquée le 1 au 5ème jours de la menstruation. Pour traiter la puberté précoce centrale : en général, injecter par voie sous-cutanée 30 µg par kg, toutes les 4 semaines, selon les cas, possbile d'augmenter jusqu'à 90 µgµg par kg. |
| 剂型、规格 Les formes pharmaceutiques et les spécifications | 注射用亮丙瑞林微球：3.75mg/ 瓶。<br>Microsphères de leuprolide pour injection : 3,75 mg par flacon. |

| 药品名称 Drug Names | 戈舍瑞林 Goséréline |
|---|---|
| 适应证 Les indications | 前列腺癌：本品适用于可用激素治疗的前列腺癌。<br>乳腺癌：适用于可用激素治疗的绝经前期及围绝经期妇女的乳腺癌。<br>子宫内膜异位症：缓解症状包括减轻疼痛并减少子宫内膜损伤的大小和数目。<br><br>Le cancer de la prostate : ce produit est applicable dans le traitement du cancer de la prostate qui ne peut pas être traité par l'hormone.<br>Le cancer du sein : applicable chez les femmes préménopausées et de périménopause avec le cancer du sein qui peut être traité par l'hormone.<br>L'endométriose : il permet de réduire les symptômes, y compris l'atténuation des douleurs et la réduction deslésions de l'endomètre en taille et en nombre. |
| 用法、用量 Les modes d'emploi et la posologie | 腹部皮下注射植入剂：每 28 日 1 次，每次 3.6mg，如果必要可使用局部麻醉。子宫内膜异位症者治疗不应超过 6 个月。<br><br>Implant sous-cutané abdominal : 3,6 mg par fois, tous les 28 jours. S'il est nécessaire, appliquer l'anesthésie locale. Le traitement de l'endométriose ne doit pas dépasser 6 mois. |
| 剂型、规格 Les formes pharmaceutiques et les spécifications | 缓释植入剂：每支 3.6mg。<br>Implant à libération prolongée : 3,6mg par pièce. |

**续　表**

| 药品名称 Drug Names | 丙氨瑞林 Alareline |
|---|---|
| 适应证<br>Les indications | 子宫内膜异位症。<br>Il sert à traiter l'endométriose. |
| 用法、用量<br>Les modes d'emploi et<br>la posologie | 皮下或肌内注射，从月经来潮的第 1～2 日开始治疗，每次 150μg，一日 1 次，或遵医嘱。制剂在临用前用 2ml 灭菌生理盐水溶解。对子宫内膜异位症，3～6 个月为 1 个疗程。<br>Injection sous-cutanée ou IM. Commencer à partir du 1 à 2ème jour de la menstruation, 150 μg par fois, 1 fois par jour, ou selon les ordonnances. Dissoudre dans 2ml de solution saline stérile avant l'injection. Pour l'endométriose, le traitement dure 3 à 6 mois. |
| 剂型、规格<br>Les formes<br>pharmaceutiques et les<br>spécifications | 注射用阿拉瑞林：每支 25μg；150μg。<br>L'alarelin pour injection : 25μg ou 150μg par solution. |
| 药品名称 Drug Names | 曲普瑞林 Triptoréline |
| 适应证<br>Les indications | 临床主要用于前列腺癌，还用于促排卵，治疗妇女不孕症。<br>Il est est utilisé dans les cliniques dans le traitement du cancer du sein. Il est aussi applicale dans la promotion de l'ovulation et le traitement de l'infertilité chez les femmes. |
| 用法、用量<br>Les modes d'emploi et<br>la posologie | 缓释剂型仅可肌内注射，一次一支，每 4 周 1 次。皮下注射：每日 1 次 0.1mg。用于促排卵：于月经周期第 2 日开始，一日 1 次，0.1mg，连续 10～12 日。<br>La préparation à libération prolongée est seulement injectée par voie IM, une pièce par fois, toutes les 4 semaines. injection sous-cutanée : 0,1mg par fois par jour. Pour la promotion de l'ovulation : à partir du 2ème de la menstruation, 1 fois par jour, 0,1mg, pendant 10 à 12 jours. |
| 剂型、规格<br>Les formes<br>pharmaceutiques et les<br>spécifications | 粉针剂：每支 0.1mg。<br>Poudre : 0,1mg par pièce. |

16.6　短效口服避孕药 Contraceptifs oraux à action courte

| 药品名称 Drug Names | 炔诺酮 Noréthindrone |
|---|---|
| 适应证<br>Les indications | 除作为口服避孕药外，还可用于功能性子宫出血、妇女不孕症、痛经、闭经、子宫内膜异位症、子宫内膜增生等。<br>Il sert de contraceptifs oraux. Ce produit sert aussi à traiter les saignements utérins anormaux, l'infertilité chez les femmes, la dysménorrhée, l'aménorrhée, l'endométriose, l'hyperplasie de l'endomètre, etc. |
| 用法、用量<br>Les modes d'emploi et<br>la posologie | 口服，一次 1.25～5mg，一日 1～2 次。<br>Par voie orale, 1,25 à 5mg par fois, 1 à 2 fois par jour. |
| 剂型、规格<br>Les formes<br>pharmaceutiques et les<br>spécifications | 复方炔诺酮片（避孕片一号）：每片含炔诺酮 0.6mg 和炔雌醇 0.035mg。<br>Les comprimés composés de noréthindrone：chaque comprimé contient 0，6mg de noréthindrone et 0，035mg d'éthinylestradiol. |
| 药品名称 Drug Names | 甲地孕酮 Mégestrol |
| 适应证<br>Les indications | 主要用作短效口服避孕药，也可作肌内注射长效避孕药，还可用于治疗痛经、闭经、功能性子宫出血、子宫内膜异位症及子宫内膜腺癌等。由于其抗雌激素活性，近年亦用于乳腺癌的姑息治疗。<br>Il sert de contraceptifs oraux à action brève. Il est aussi utilisé comme contraceptifs à action prolongée administrés par voie IM. Il sert aussi à traiter la dysménorrhée, l'aménorrhée, les saignements utérins anormaux, l'endométriose et l'adénocarcinome de l'endomètre. En raison de son activité anti- oestrogénique, il est récemment utilisé dans les soins palliatifs du cancer du sein. |

| 续 表 | |
|---|---|
| 用法、用量<br>Les modes d'emploi et la posologie | ①用作短效口服避孕药：从月经周期第 5 日起，每天口服一片甲地孕酮片、膜或纸片，连服 22 日为一周期，停药后 2～4 日来月经，然后于第 5 日继续服下一个月的药。②治疗功能性子宫出血：口服甲地孕酮片、膜或纸片，每 8 小时 1 次，每次 2mg，然后将剂量每 3 日递减一次，直至维持量每天 4mg，连服 20 日，出血停止后，每天加服炔雌醇 0.05mg 或己烯雌酚 1mg，共 20 日。③闭经：口服，每次一片甲地孕酮片和炔雌醇 0.05mg，共 20 日，连服 3 个月。④痛经和子宫内膜增生过长：于月经第 5～7 日开始，一天口服一片，共 20 日。⑤子宫内膜异位症：每次一片，一日 2 次，共 7 日，然后一日 3 次，每次 1 片，共 7 日，再后，一日 2 次，每次 2 片，共 7 日，最后每天 20mg，共 6 周。⑥子宫内膜癌：口服，一日 4 次，每次 10～80mg，连续 2 个月。⑦乳腺癌：口服，一日 4 次，每次 40mg，连续 2 个月为 1 个疗程。<br><br>① Utilisé comme contraceptif oral à action brève : à partir du 5ème jour du cycle menstruel, prendre un comprié (film ou papier) de mégestrol par voie orale, pendant 22 jours comme un traitement médical. 2 à 4 jours après l'arrêt de l'administration viendra la menstruation, reprendre un nouveau traitement au 5ème jour da la menstruation. ② Pour traiter les saignements utérins fonctionnels : prendre le mégestrol en comprimé, film ou papier par voie orale, toutes les 8 h, 2mg par fois, ensuite, diminuer la dose tous les 3 jours, jusqu'à 4mg par jour, pendant 20 jours consécutifs. Après l'arrêt des saingments, prendre en supplément 0,05mg de mégestrol ou 1mg de diéthylstilbestrol, pendant 20 jours au total. ③ Pour traiter l'aménorrhée : par voie orale, 1 comprimé de mégestrol et 0,05mg d'éthinylestradiol par fois, 20 jours au total, pendant 3 mois consécutifs. ④ Pour traiter la dysménorrhée et l'hyperplasie de l'endomètre : commencer du 5ème au 7ème jour du cycle menstruel, 1 comprimé par jour, 20 jours au total. ⑤ Pour traiter l'endométriose : 1 comprimé par fois, 2 fois par jour, pendant 7 jours, ensuite, 3 fois par jour, 1 comprimé par fois, pedant 7 jours, ensuite, 2 fois par jour, 2 comprimés par fois, pendant 7 jours, enfin, 20mg par jour, pendant 6 semaines. ⑥ Pour traiter l'adénocarcinome de l'endomètre :par voie orale, 4 fois par jour, 10 à 80mg par fois, pendant 2 mois consécutifs. ⑦ Pour traiter le cancer du sein : par voie orale, 4 fois par jour, 40mg par fois, pendant 2 mois comme un traitement médical. |
| 剂型、规格<br>Les formes pharmaceutiques et les spécifications | 片剂：每片 1mg；4mg。<br>膜剂：每片 1mg；4mg。<br>纸片：每片 1mg；4mg。<br>Comprimés : 1mg ou 4mg par comprimé.<br>Film : 1mg ou 4mg par pièce.<br>Papier : 1mg ou 4mg par pièce. |
| 药品名称 Drug Names | 炔诺孕酮 Norgestrel |
| 适应证<br>Les indications | 主要以炔雌醇组成复方作为短效口服避孕药，也可通过剂型改变用作长效避孕药，还可用于治疗痛经、月经不调。<br><br>Utilisé en combinaison avec l'éthinylestradiol, il sert de contraceptifs oraux à action brève. À travers le changement des formes posologiques, il sert aussi de contraceptifs oraux à action prolongée. Il permet aussi de traiter la dysménorrhée et les règles irrégulières. |
| 用法、用量<br>Les modes d'emploi et la posologie | ①用作短效口服避孕药：口服复方炔诺孕酮一号片或滴丸，从月经第 5 日开始，每天服 1 片（丸），连服 22 日，不能间断，服完后 3～4 日即来月经，并于月经的第 5 日再服下一个月的药。②用作探亲避孕药：于探亲当晚开始服炔诺孕酮探亲避孕药，每日 1 片，服法同炔诺酮。③用作房事后避孕药：房事后 72 小时内口服 2 片事后避孕药，12 小时后再服 2 片。<br><br>① Comme contraceptif oral à action brève : prendre par voie orale les comprimés ou granules composés de norgestrel de numéro 1, à partir du 5ème jour du cycle menstruel, 1 comprimé ou granule par jour, pendant 22 jours consécutifs, 3 à 4 jours après l'administration viendra la règle, reprendre le médicament le 5ème jour du cycle menstrul du mois prochain. ② Comme contraceptif pour la visite familiale : commencer à prendre le norgestrel le soir de la visite, 1 comprimé par jour, suivre les modes d'emploi que la noréthindrone. ③ Comme contraceptif après l'activité sexuelle : dans les 72h après l'activité sexuelle, 2 comprimés, 12h après, reprendre 2 comprimés. |

**续　表**

| 剂型、规格<br>Les formes pharmaceutiques et les spécifications | 复方炔诺酮一号片（复甲一号）：每片含炔诺孕酮 0.3mg 和炔雌醇 0.03mg。<br>Comprimés composés de norgestrel numéro 1 : chaque comprimé contient 0,3mg de norgestrel et 0,03mg d'éthinylestradiol. |
|---|---|

### 16.7　抗早孕药 Médicaments contre la grossesse précoce

| 药品名称 Drug Names | 米非司酮 Mifépristone |
|---|---|
| 适应证<br>Les indications | 除用于抗早孕、催经止孕、胎死宫内引产外，还用于妇科手术操作，如宫内节育器的放置和取出、取内膜标本、宫颈管发育异常的激光分离以及宫颈扩张和刮宫术。<br>Ce produit est utilisé dans l'interruption de grossesse précoce, l'induction de la mort fœtale. Il est aussi applicable dans les interventions chirurgicales gynécologiques, telles que le placement et le retrait du DIU, le prélevement des échantillons de l'endomètre, la séparationde laser de la dysplasie cervicale, la dilatation du col et le curetage. |
| 用法、用量<br>Les modes d'emploi et la posologie | 停经 ≤ 49 日的健康早妊娠期妇女，于空腹或进食后 1 小时口服，①顿服 200mg；②每次 25mg，一日 2 次，连续 3 日，服药后禁食 1 小时。<br>Les femmes saines pendant la grossesse précoce qui arrêtent les règles pendant moins de 49 jours, administrer par voie orale à jeun ou 1h après la nourriture, 1)200mg, une fois par jour; 2)25mg par fois, 2 fois par jour, pendant 3 jours consécutifs, l'alimentation interdite pendant 1 h suivant l'administration. |
| 剂型、规格<br>Les formes pharmaceutiques et les spécifications | 片剂：每片 25mg；200mg。<br>Comprimés : 25mg ou 200mg par comprimé. |

### 16.8　高血糖素 Glucagon

| 药品名称 Drug Names | 高血糖素 Glucagon |
|---|---|
| 适应证<br>Les indications | 用于低血糖症，在一时不能口服或静脉注射葡萄糖时特别有用。用于心源性休克有效。<br>Applicable dans le traitement de l'hypoglycémie. Il est surtout efficace quant on ne peut pas administrer le glucose par voie orale ou IV. Il sert aussi à traiter le choc cardiogénique. |
| 用法、用量<br>Les modes d'emploi et la posologie | 肌内注射、皮下注射或静脉注射，用于低血糖症，每次 0.5 ～ 1.0mg，5 分钟左右即可见效。用于心源性休克，连续静脉滴注，每小时 1 ～ 12mg。<br>Injection IM, sous-cutanée ou IV, pour traiter l'hypoglycémie, 0,5 à 1,0mg par fois, efficace en 5minutes. Pour traiter le choc cardiogénique, la perfusion continue, 1 à 12mg par h. |
| 剂型、规格<br>Les formes pharmaceutiques et les spécifications | 注射用高血糖素：每支 1mg；10mg。<br>Le glucagon pour injection : 1mg ou 10mg par solution. |

### 16.9　胰岛素 Insulines

| 药品名称 Drug Names | 胰岛素 Insuline |
|---|---|
| 适应证<br>Les indications | 用于糖尿病患者，控制血糖，特别是餐后血糖。<br>Il est applicable chez des patients atteints dediabète en permettant le contrôle de la glycémie, en particulier la glycémie postprandiale. |
| 用法、用量<br>Les modes d'emploi et la posologie | 餐前 30 分钟皮下注射，用药后 30 分钟内须进食含碳水化合物的食物，一日 3 ～ 4 次。<br>30 minutes avant le repas, injection sous-cutanée, durant les 30 minutes suivant l'administration, il faut prendre des aliments contenant le glucide, 3 à 4 fois par jour. |

**续　表**

| | |
|---|---|
| 剂型、规格<br>Les formes pharmaceutiques et les spécifications | 注射液：重组人胰岛素注射液：每瓶 400U（10ml）。笔芯：300U（3ml）。<br>生物合成人胰岛素注射液：每瓶 400U（10ml）。笔芯：300uU（3ml）。<br>胰岛素（猪）注射液：每瓶 400U（10ml）。<br>Injection : injection de l'insuline recomposante : 400U (10ml) par flacon. Le penfill : 300U (3ml).<br>Injection de l'insuline humaine biosynthétique : 400U (10ml) par flacon. Le penfill : 300U (3ml).<br>Injection de l'insuline : 400U (10ml) par flacon. |
| **药品名称 Drug Names** | 门冬胰岛素 Insuline aspartate |
| 适应证<br>Les indications | 用于控制餐后血糖，也可与中效胰岛素合用控制晚间或晨起高血糖。<br>Il sert à contrôler la glycémie postprandiale. Il peut être aussi utilisé en association avec l'insuline à action moyenne pour contrôler une glycémie élevée le soir ou le petit matien. |
| 用法、用量<br>Les modes d'emploi et la posologie | 于 3 餐前 15 分钟至进餐开始时皮下注射一次，根据血糖情况调整剂量。<br>Injecter une fois par voie sous-cutanée 15 minutes avant les trois repas, ajuster la dose en fonction de la glycémie. |
| 剂型、规格<br>Les formes pharmaceutiques et les spécifications | 注射液：300U（3ml）。<br>Injection : 300U (3ml). |
| **药品名称 Drug Names** | 赖脯胰岛素 Insuline lispro |
| 适应证<br>Les indications | 用于控制餐后血糖，也可与中效胰岛素合用控制晚间或晨起高血糖。<br>Il sert à contrôler la glycémie postprandiale. Il peut être aussi utilisé en association avec l'insuline à action moyenne pour contrôler une glycémie élevée le soir ou le petit matien. |
| 用法、用量<br>Les modes d'emploi et la posologie | 于 3 餐前 15 分钟至进餐开始时皮下注射一次，根据血糖情况调整剂量。<br>Injecter une fois par voie sous-cutanée 15 minutes avant les trois repas, ajuster la dose en fonction de la glycémie. |
| 剂型、规格<br>Les formes pharmaceutiques et les spécifications | 注射液：300U（3ml）。<br>Injection : 300U (3ml). |
| **药品名称 Drug Names** | 低精蛋白锌胰岛素 Insuline isophane |
| 适应证<br>Les indications | 用于糖尿病控制血糖，一般与短效胰岛素配合使用，提供胰岛素的日基础用量。<br>Il permet le contrôle de la glycémie chez les patients atteints de diabète. Utilisé souvent en association avec l'insuline à action brève, il sert à fournir la quantitéquotidienne d'insuline. |
| 用法、用量<br>Les modes d'emploi et la posologie | 于睡前或早餐前每天一次给药或者早晚每日 2 次给药，以控制空腹血糖。<br>Une fois par jour, avant le sommeil ou le petit matin ; ou deux fois par jour, le petit matin et le soir, pour contrôler la glycémie à jeun. |
| 剂型、规格<br>Les formes pharmaceutiques et les spécifications | 注射液：每瓶 400U（10ml）。<br>笔芯：300U（3ml）。<br>Injection : 400U (1ml) par flacon.<br>Le penfill : 300U (3ml). |
| **药品名称 Drug Names** | 精蛋白锌胰岛素 Insuline Protamine Zinc |
| 适应证<br>Les indications | 用于糖尿病控制血糖，一般与短效胰岛素配合使用，提供胰岛素的日基础用量。<br>Il permet le contrôle de la glycémie chez les patients atteints de diabète. Utilisé souvent en association avec l'insuline à action brève, il sert à fournir la quantitéquotidienne d'insuline. |
| 用法、用量<br>Les modes d'emploi et la posologie | 于早餐前 0.5 小时皮下注射一次，剂量根据病情而定，每日用量一般为 10 ～ 20U。<br>0,5h avant le repas, injection par voie sous-cutanée, ajuster la dose en fonction des maladies, la dose usuelle est de 10 à 20U par jour. |

**续　表**

| | |
|---|---|
| 剂型、规格<br>Les formes pharmaceutiques et les spécifications | 注射液：每瓶 400U（10ml）。<br>Injection : 400U (10ml) par flacon. |
| 药品名称 Drug Names | 甘精胰岛素 Insuline glargine |
| 适应证<br>Les indications | 用于基础胰岛素替代治疗，一般也和短效胰岛素或口服降糖药配合使用。<br>Il est applicable dans la thérapie de remplacement de l'insuline basale. Il est aussi utilisé en association avec l'insuline à action brève et des hypoglycémiants oraux. |
| 用法、用量<br>Les modes d'emploi et la posologie | 每日傍晚注射一次，满足糖尿病患者的基础胰岛素需要量。<br>Injecter une fois le coucher du soleil pour fournir la quantité quotidienne d'insuline. |
| 剂型、规格<br>Les formes pharmaceutiques et les spécifications | 注射液：300U（3ml）。<br>Injection : 300U (3ml). |
| 药品名称 Drug Names | 地特胰岛素 Insuline détémir |
| 适应证<br>Les indications | 用于治疗糖尿病。<br>Il permet de traiter le diabète. |
| 用法、用量<br>Les modes d'emploi et la posologie | 与口服降糖药联合治疗：起始剂量为 10U 或 0.1～0.2U/kg，一日 1 次，皮下注射，以后根据早餐前平均自测血糖浓度进行个体化的调整。<br>Utilisé en association avec des antidiabétiques oraux : la dose initiale, 10U ou 0,1 à 0,2U par kg, 1 fois par jour, injection sous-cutanée, ensuite, personnaliser la dose en fonction de la glycémie testée avant le petit-déjeuner. |
| 剂型、规格<br>Les formes pharmaceutiques et les spécifications | 注射液：300U（3ml）。<br>Injection : 300U (3ml). |
| 药品名称 Drug Names | 胰岛素预混制剂 Insuline Prémix |
| 适应证<br>Les indications | 用于糖尿病控制血糖。<br>Il permet le contrôle de la glycémie chez des patients atteints de diabète. |
| 用法、用量<br>Les modes d'emploi et la posologie | 于早餐前 0.5 小时皮下注射一次，剂量根据病情而定，每日用量一般为 10～20U。有时需要于晚餐前再注射一次。<br>0,5h avant le petit-déjeuner, injection sous-cutanée, ajuster la dose en fonction des maladies, la dose usuelle est de 10 à 20 U par jour. Quelquefois, il est nécessaire de reprendre une injection avant le dîner. |
| 剂型、规格<br>Les formes pharmaceutiques et les spécifications | 注射液：每瓶 400U（10ml）。<br>笔芯：300U（3ml）。<br>Injection : 400U (10ml) par flacon.<br>Le penfill : 300U (3ml). |
| 16.10　口服降糖药 Médicaments hypoglycériques par voie orale | |
| 药品名称 Drug Names | 甲苯磺丁脲 Tolbutamide |
| 适应证<br>Les indications | 一般用于成年后发病，单用饮食控制无效而胰岛功能尚存的轻、中度糖尿病患者，对胰岛素抵抗患者，可加用本品。对胰岛素依赖型患者及酸中毒昏迷者无效，不能完全代替胰岛素。<br>Ce produit est généralement utilisé dans le traitement des patients adultes atteints de diabète bénin ou modéré dont l'îlot fonctionne encore mais qui ne peut pas être traité par le régime alimentaire seul. Il est aussi applicable chez les patients résistants à l'insuline. Mais il est inefficace chez les patients insulinodépendants et les patients souffrant de l'acidose coma. Il ne peut pas remplacer complètement l'insuline. |

**续　表**

| 用法、用量<br>Les modes d'emploi et la posologie | 餐前服药效果较好，如有胃肠反应，进餐时服药可减少反应。口服，每日剂量 1～2g，分次服用，一日 2～3 次，从小剂量开始，每 1～2 周加量一次。<br>L'administration avant le repas a un meilleur effet. S'il y a des réactions gastro-intestinales, l'administration durant le repas peut permettre de réduire ces réactions. Par voie orale, 1 à 2g par jour, à travers plusieurs fois, 2 à 3 fois par jour, commencer par une dose mineure, augmenter la dose toutes les 1 à 2 semaines. |
|---|---|
| 剂型、规格<br>Les formes pharmaceutiques et les spécifications | 片剂：每片 0.5g。<br>Comprimés : 0,5g par comprimé. |

| 药品名称 Drug Names | 格列本脲 Glibénclamide |
|---|---|
| 适应证<br>Les indications | 用于饮食不能控制的轻、中度 2 型糖尿病。<br>Ce produit sert à traiter le diabète bénin et modéré de type II qui ne peut pas être contrôlé par le régime alimentaire. |
| 用法、用量<br>Les modes d'emploi et la posologie | 开始时每日剂量 2.5～5mg，早餐前 1 次服，或一日 2 次，早晚餐前各一次，然后根据情况每周增加 2.5mg，一般每日量为 5～10mg，最大不超过 15mg。<br>Commencer par 2,5 à 5mg par jour, une fois pris avant le petit-déjeuner, ou 2 fois par jour, pris avant le petit-déjeuner et le dîner, ensuite, augmenter 2,5mg par semaine, la dose usuelle est de 5 à 10mg par jour, ne pas dépasser 15mg par jour. |
| 剂型、规格<br>Les formes pharmaceutiques et les spécifications | 片剂：每片 2.5mg。<br>Comprimés : 2,5mg par comprimé. |

| 药品名称 Drug Names | 格列吡嗪 Glipizide |
|---|---|
| 适应证<br>Les indications | 本品主要用于单用饮食控制治疗未能达到良好控制的轻、中度非胰岛素依赖型患者；对胰岛素抵抗患者可加用本品，但用量应在 30～40U 以下者。<br>Ce produit est principalement utilisé chez lespatients atteints de diabète bénin ou modéré non insulino- dépendant qui ne peut pas être contrôlé par le régime alimentaire seul. Chez des patients résistant à l'insuline, il est applicable, mais avec une dose inférieure à 30 – 40U. |
| 用法、用量<br>Les modes d'emploi et la posologie | 一般一日 2.5～20mg，先从小量 2.5～5mg 开始，餐前 30 分钟服用，一日剂量超过 15mg 时，应分成 2～3 次餐前服用。<br>En général, 2,5 à 20mg par jour, commencer par une dose mineure de 2,5 à 5mg, pris 30 minutes avant le repas, ne pas dépasser 15mg par jour, à travers 2 à 3 fois avant le repas. |
| 剂型、规格<br>Les formes pharmaceutiques et les spécifications | 片剂：每片 2.5mg；5mg。<br>控释片：每片 5mg。<br>Comprimés : 2,5mg ou 5mg par comprimé.<br>Comprimés à libération contrôlée : 5mg par comprimé. |

| 药品名称 Drug Names | 格列齐特 Gliclazide |
|---|---|
| 适应证<br>Les indications | 成人 2 型糖尿病。<br>Ce produit sert à traiter le diabète de type II chez des adultes. |
| 用法、用量<br>Les modes d'emploi et la posologie | 开始时一日 2 次，一日 40～80mg，早晚 2 餐前服用；连服 2～3 周，然后根据血糖调整用量，一般剂量一日 80～240mg，最大日剂量不超过 240mg。<br>Commencer par 40 à 80mg par jour, 2 fois par jour, pris avant le petit-déjeuner et le dîner ; pendant 2 à 3 semaines consécutives, ensuite, ajuster la dose en fonction de la glycémie, la dose usuelle, 80 à 240mg par jour, ne pas dépasser 240mg par jour. |

**续　表**

| | |
|---|---|
| 剂型、规格<br>Les formes pharmaceutiques et les spécifications | 片剂：每片 80mg。<br>缓释片：每片 30mg。<br>Comprimés : 80mg par comprimé.<br>Comprimés à libération prolongée : 30mg par comprimé. |
| 药品名称 Drug Names | 格列喹酮 Gliquidone |
| 适应证<br>Les indications | 2 型糖尿病合并轻至中度肾病者，但严重肾功能不全时应改用胰岛素治疗。<br>Il est applicable dans le traitement des patients atteints de diabète de type II et de néphropathie bénigne ou modérée. Mais chez des patients insuffisants rénaux sévères, il faut utiliser l'insuline. |
| 用法、用量<br>Les modes d'emploi et la posologie | 口服，开始时 15mg，应在餐前 30 分钟服用。1 周后按需调整，必要时逐步加量，一般日剂量为 15 ～ 20mg，日剂量为 30mg 以内者，可于早餐前一次服用，更大剂量应分 3 次，分别与 3 餐前服用，最大日剂量不超过 180mg。<br>Par voie orale, commencer par 15mg, pris 30 minutes avant le repas. Une semaine après, ajuster la dose en fonction du besoin, s'il est nécessaire, augmenter progressivement la dose, la dose usuelle est de 15 à 20mg par jour. Pour la dose de 30mg par jour, pris une seule fois avant le petit-déjeuner, pour une dose plus forte, pris à travers 3 fois, avant les 3 repas. Ne pas dépasser 180mg par jour. |
| 剂型、规格<br>Les formes pharmaceutiques et les spécifications | 片剂：每片 30mg。<br>Comprimés : 30mg par comprimé. |
| 药品名称 Drug Names | 格列美脲 Glimépiride |
| 适应证<br>Les indications | 成人 2 型糖尿病。<br>Ce produit sert à traiter le diabète de type II chez des adultes. |
| 用法、用量<br>Les modes d'emploi et la posologie | 开始用量一日 1mg，一次顿服，如不能满意控制血糖，每隔 1 ～ 2 周逐步增加剂量至每日 2mg、3mg、4mg，最大推荐剂量为每日 6mg。<br>Commencer par 1mg par jour, une fois par jour. S'il la glycémie ne se contrôle pas, augmenter la dose toutes les 1 à 2 semaines pour atteindre 2mg, 3mg ou 4mg par jour. La dose recommandée maximale est de 6mg par jour. |
| 剂型、规格<br>Les formes pharmaceutiques et les spécifications | 片剂：每片 1mg；2mg。<br>Comprimés : 1mg ou 2mg par comprimé. |
| 药品名称 Drug Names | 二甲双胍 Metformine |
| 适应证<br>Les indications | ①首选用于单纯饮食控制及体育锻炼治疗无效的 2 型糖尿病，特别是肥胖的 2 型糖尿病。②与胰岛素合用可减少胰岛素用量，防止低血糖发生。③与磺酰脲类降血糖药合用具协同作用。<br>① Il est principalement utilisé chez des patients atteints de diabète de type II et qui ne peut pas être contrôlé par le régime alimentaire et des exercices physiques, surtout le diabète de type II lié à l'obésité. ② Utilisé en association avec l'insuline, il permet de réduire l'utilisation de celle-ci, et de prévenir l'hypoglycémie. ③ Il peut travailler en synergie avec des hypoglycémiants de sulfonylurée. |
| 用法、用量<br>Les modes d'emploi et la posologie | ①普通片：开始时一次 0.25g，一日 2 ～ 3 次，以后可根据病情调整剂量。口服，一次 0.5g，一日 1 ～ 1.5g，最大剂量不超过 2g。餐中服药可减轻胃肠反应。②缓释片：开始时一日 1 次，每次 0.5g，晚餐时服用。后根据血糖调整剂量。日最大剂量不超过 2g。<br>① Les comprimés ordinaires : commencer par 0,25g par fois, 2 à 3 fois par jour, ensuite, ajuster la dose en fonction des maladies. Par voie orale, 0,5g par fois, 1 à 1,5g par jour. Ne pas dépasser 2g. L'administration pendant le repas permet de réduire les réactions indésirables. ② Les comprimés à libération prolongée : commencer par 0,5g par fois, 1 fois par jour, pris durant le dîner. Ensuite, ajuster la dose en fonction de la glycémie. Ne pas dépasser 2g par jour. |

**续　表**

| 剂型、规格<br>Les formes pharmaceutiques et les spécifications | 片剂：每片 0.25g；0.5g；0.85g。<br>缓释片：0.5g。<br>Comprimés : 0,25g, 0,5g ou 0,85g par comprimé.<br>Comprimés à libération prolongée : 0,5g. |
| --- | --- |
| **药品名称 Drug Names** | **苯乙双胍 Phenformin** |
| 适应证<br>Les indications | 用于单纯饮食控制不满意的 2 型糖尿病患者，尤其是肥胖者和伴高胰岛素血症者。与磺酰脲类降血糖药合用具协同作用。<br>Il est principalement utilisé chez des patients atteints de diabète de type II et qui ne peut pas être contrôlé par le régime alimentaire, surtout chez des patients obèses et accompagnés de l'hyperinsulinémie. Il peut travailler en synergie avec des hypoglycémiants de sulfonylurée. |
| 用法、用量<br>Les modes d'emploi et la posologie | 口服：成人开始时一次 25mg，一日 2 次，餐前服，数日后可再增加 25mg，但最多每日不超过 75mg。<br>Par voie orale : chez des adultes, commence par 25mg par fois, 2 fois par jour, pris avant le repas, quelques jours après, possible d'augmenter 25mg. Ne pas dépasser 75mg par jour. |
| 剂型、规格<br>Les formes pharmaceutiques et les spécifications | 片剂：每片 25mg。<br>Comprimés : 25mg par comprimé. |
| **药品名称 Drug Names** | **瑞格列奈 Répaglinide** |
| 适应证<br>Les indications | 用于饮食控制、降低体重与运动不能有效控制高血糖的 2 型糖尿病。与二甲双胍合用对控制血糖有协同作用。<br>Il est utilisé chez des patients atteints de diabète de type II et qui ne peut pas être contrôlé par le régime alimentaire, la perte du poids et des exercices physiques. Il peut travailler en synergie avec la metformine. |
| 用法、用量<br>Les modes d'emploi et la posologie | 服药时间应在餐前 30 分钟内服用，剂量依个人血糖而定。推荐起始剂量为 0.5mg，最大的推荐单次剂量为 4mg，但最大日剂量不应超过 16mg。<br>Il faut prendre le médicament 30 minutes avant le repas, ajuster la dose en fonction de la glycémie. La dose initiale recommandée est de 0,5mg. Ne pas dépasser 4mg par fois, et 16mg par jour. |
| 剂型、规格<br>Les formes pharmaceutiques et les spécifications | 片剂：每片 0.5mg；1mg；2mg。<br>Comprimés : 0,5mg, 1mg ou 2mg par comprimé. |
| **药品名称 Drug Names** | **那格列奈 Natéglinide** |
| 适应证<br>Les indications | 用于饮食控制、降低体重与运动不能有效控制高血糖的 2 型糖尿病。与二甲双胍合用对控制血糖有协同作用。<br>Il est utilisé chez des patients atteints de diabète de type II et qui ne peut pas être contrôlé par le régime alimentaire, la perte du poids et des exercices physiques. Il peut travailler en synergie avec la metformine. |
| 用法、用量<br>Les modes d'emploi et la posologie | 本品可单独应用，也可与二甲双胍合用，起始剂量一日 3 次，一次 60mg，餐前 15 分钟服药。常用剂量为餐前 60 ～ 120mg，并根据 HbAlc 检测结果调整剂量。<br>Ce médicament peut être utilisé seul ou en association avec la metformine. La dose initiale est de 60mg par fois, 3 fois par jour, pris 15 minutes avant le repas. La dose usuelle est de 60 à 120 mg pris avant le repas, ajuster la dose en fonction du résultat de l'HbAlc. |
| 剂型、规格<br>Les formes pharmaceutiques et les spécifications | 片剂：每片 30mg；60mg；120mg。<br>Comprimés : 30mg, 60mg ou 120mg par comprimé. |

**续　表**

| 药品名称 Drug Names | 罗格列酮 Rosiglitazone |
| --- | --- |
| 适应证<br>Les indications | 本品仅适用于其他降糖药无法达到血糖控制目标的 2 型糖尿病患者。<br>Ce produit n'est applicable que dans le traitement des patients atteints de diabète de type II qui ne peut pas êtré traité par d'autres hypoglycémiants. |
| 用法、用量<br>Les modes d'emploi et la posologie | 单独用药：初始剂量为每日 4mg，单次或分 2 次口服，12 周后如空腹血糖下降不满意，剂量可加至每日 8mg，单次或分 2 次口服。<br>Utilisé seul : la dose initiale est de 4mg par jour, à travers une fois ou 2 fois, par voie orale, 12 semaines après, si la glycémie à jeun n'est pas satisfaisante, augmenter la dose pour atteindre 8mg par jour, à travers 1 à 2 fois, pris par voie orale. |
| 剂型、规格<br>Les formes pharmaceutiques et les spécifications | 片剂：每片 2mg；4mg；8mg。<br>Comprimés : 2mg, 4mg ou 8mg par comprimé. |
| 药品名称 Drug Names | 吡格列酮 Pioglitazone |
| 适应证<br>Les indications | 用于 2 型糖尿病，可于饮食控制和体育锻炼联合以改善血糖控制，可单独使用。当饮食控制、体育锻炼和单药治疗不能满意控制血糖时，也可与磺脲、二甲双胍或胰岛素合用。<br>Ce produit sert à traiter le diabète de type II et peut être utilisé en association avec le régime alimentaire et des exercices physiques. Il peut être aussi appliqué seul. Quand le régime alimentaire, des exercices physiques ou l'utilisation seule de la pioglitazone, celle-ci peut être appliquée en association avec la sulfonylurée, la metformine ou l'insuline. |
| 用法、用量<br>Les modes d'emploi et la posologie | 口服，单药治疗初始剂量可为 15mg 或 30mg，一日 1 次；反应不佳时，可加量直至 45mg，一日 1 次。<br>Par voie orale, utilisé seul, la dose initiale, 15mg ou 30mg, 1 fois par jour ; si l'effet n'est pas très satisfaisant, possible de prendre 45mg, 1 fois par jour. |
| 剂型、规格<br>Les formes pharmaceutiques et les spécifications | 片剂：每片 15mg。<br>Comprimés : 15mg par comprimé. |
| 药品名称 Drug Names | 阿卡波糖 Acarbose |
| 适应证<br>Les indications | 可与其他口服降血糖药或胰岛素联合应用于胰岛素依赖型或非胰岛素依赖型的糖尿病。<br>Ce prosuit peut être appliqué en association avec d'autres hypoglycémiants oraux ou l'insuline pour traiter le diabète insulino-dépendant ou non insulino-dépendant. |
| 用法、用量<br>Les modes d'emploi et la posologie | 口服剂量需个体化。一般维持量为一次 50～100mg，一日 3 次，餐前即刻吞服，或与第一口主食一起咀嚼服用。开始时从小剂量 25mg，一日 3 次，6～8 周后加量至 50mg，必要时可加至 100mg，一日 3 次，一日量不宜超过 300mg。<br>La dose orale doit être personnalisée. La dose d'entretien usuelle est de 50 à 100mg par fois, 3 fois par jour, avaler avant le repas, ou mâcher avec la première bouchée du repas. Commencer par une dose mineure de 25mg, 3 fois par jour, 6 à 8 semaines après, augmenter pour atteindre 50mg, s'il est nécessaire, 100mg, 3 fois par jour, ne pas dépasser 300mg par jour. |
| 剂型、规格<br>Les formes pharmaceutiques et les spécifications | 片剂：每片 50mg；100mg。<br>Comprimés : 50mg ou 100mg par comprimé. |
| 药品名称 Drug Names | 伏格列波糖 Voglibose |
| 适应证<br>Les indications | 改善糖尿病餐后高血糖。<br>Ce produit permet d'améliorer l'hyperglycémie postprandiale du diabète. |

| 用法、用量<br>Les modes d'emploi et la posologie | 口服，成人一次 200μg，一日 3 次，餐前服，疗效不明显时根据临床观察可将一次量增至 300μg。<br>Par voie orale, chez des adultes, 200μg par fois, 3 fois par jour, pris avant le repas. Si l'effet n'est pas évident, possible de prendre 300μg par fois. |
|---|---|
| 剂型、规格<br>Les formes pharmaceutiques et les spécifications | 片剂：每片 200μg。<br>Comprimés : 200 μg par comprimé. |
| **药品名称 Drug Names** | **西格列汀 Sitagliptine** |
| 适应证<br>Les indications | 用于经生活方式干预无法达标的 2 型糖尿病患者。可采用单药治疗或与其他口服降糖药联合治疗。<br>Ce produit sert à traiter le diabète qui ne peut pas être contrôlé par l'amélioration du mode de vie. Il peut être utlisé seul ou en association avec d'autres hypoglycémiants oraux. |
| 用法、用量<br>Les modes d'emploi et la posologie | 本品单药治疗的推荐剂量为 100mg，一日 1 次。本品可与或不与食物同服。<br>La dose recommdée pour l'utilisation seule de ce médicament est de 100mg, 1 fois par jour. Il peut être administré avec ou sans aliments. |
| 剂型、规格<br>Les formes pharmaceutiques et les spécifications | 每片 100mg。<br>100mg par comprimé. |

16.11　甲状腺激素类药物 Médicaments à base de thyroides

| **药品名称 Drug Names** | **左甲状腺素 Lévothyroxine** |
|---|---|
| 适应证<br>Les indications | 适用于甲状腺激素缺乏的替代治疗。<br>Ce produit est applicable dans la thérapie de remplacement d'une déficience en hormone de la thyroïde. |
| 用法、用量<br>Les modes d'emploi et la posologie | 口服一般开始剂量每日 25～50μg，每 2 周增加 25μg，直到 100～150μg，成人维持量为每日 75～125μg，高龄患者、心功能不全者及严重黏液性水肿患者开始剂量应减为每日 12.5～25μg，以后每 2～4 周递增 25μg，不必要求达到完全替代剂量，一般每日 75～100μg 即可。婴儿及儿童甲状腺功能减退症，每日完全替代剂量为：6 个月以内 6～8μg/kg；6～12 个月，6μg/kg；1～5 岁 5μg/kg，6～12 岁，4μg/kg。静脉注射适用于黏液性水肿昏迷，首次剂量宜较大，200～400μg，以后每日 50～100μg，直到患者清醒改为口服。<br>Par voie orale, commencer par 25 à 50 μg par jour, augmenter 25 μg toutes les 2 semaines, jusqu'à 100 à 150 μg, la dose d'entretien chez des adultes est de 75 à 125μg par jour. Chez des personnes âgées, des patients insuffisants cardiaques, des patients atteints d'œdème muqueux sévère, la dose initiale est de 12,5 à 25μg par jour, ensuite, augmenter 25 μg toutes les 2 à 4 semaines, pas nécessaire d'atteindre la dose de substitution, 75 à 100 μg par jour suffit. Chez des bébés et des enfants atteints d'hypothyroïdie, la dose de substitution par jour : moins de 6 mois, 6 à 8 μg par kg ; de 6 à 12 mois, 6 μg par kg ; de 1 à 5 ans, 5 μg par kg ; de 6 à 12 ans, 4 μg par kg. L'injection IV est applicable dans le traitement du coma lié à l'œdème muqueux, la dose initiale doit être forte, 200 à 400 μg, ensuite, 50 à 100 μg par jour, jusqu'au réveil des patients, prendre par voie orale. |
| 剂型、规格<br>Les formes pharmaceutiques et les spécifications | 片剂：每片 25μg；50μg；100μg。<br>注射液：每支 100μg（1ml）；200μg（2ml）；500μg（5ml）。<br>Comprimés : 25μg, 50μg ou 100μg par comprimé.<br>Injection : 100 μg (1ml), 200 μg (2ml) ou 500 μg (5ml) par solution. |
| **药品名称 Drug Names** | **甲状腺片 Thyroxine en Comprimés** |
| 适应证<br>Les indications | 主要用甲状腺功能减退症的治疗。包括甲减引起的呆小病及黏液性水肿等。<br>Ce produit est principalement appliqué dans le traitement de l'hypothyroïdie, y compris le crétinisme et le myxedema causés par l'hypothyroïdie. |

**续 表**

| | |
|---|---|
| 用法、用量<br>Les modes d'emploi et la posologie | 常用量开始时一日 10～20mg，逐渐加量，维持量一般为一日 40～80mg。<br>La dose usuelle, commencer par 10 à 20mg par jour, augmenter progressivement la dose, la dose d'entretien est de 40 à 80mg par jour. |
| 剂型、规格<br>Les formes pharmaceutiques et les spécifications | 片剂：每片 10mg；40mg；60mg。<br>Comprimés : 10mg, 40mg ou 60mg par comprimé. |
| **药品名称 Drug Names** | 促甲状腺素 Thyrotropine(Hormones stimulantes de la thyroïde) |
| 适应证<br>Les indications | 用于 TSH 试验及甲状腺癌诊断。<br>Ce produit est appliqué dans le test TSH et le diagnostic du cancer de la thyroïde. |
| 用法、用量<br>Les modes d'emploi et la posologie | ① TSH 试验：每日肌内注射 2 次，每次 10μg，共 3 日。②提高甲状腺癌转移病灶吸 [131]I：甲状腺全切除后。每日肌内注射 10μg，共 7 日。使转移病灶吸 [131]I 率提高后再给予治疗量碘。<br>① Le test TSH : injection sous-cutanée, 2 fois par jour, 10μg par fois, 3 jours au total. ② Après la thyroïdectomie totale, injection IM, 10μg par jour, pendant 7 jours au total. Après l'augmentation du taux de métastases d'absorption [131]I, administrer une quantité thérapeutique d'iode. |
| 剂型、规格<br>Les formes pharmaceutiques et les spécifications | 注射液：每支 10μg（6ml）。<br>Injection : 10μg (6ml) par solution. |

16.12　抗甲状腺药 Médicaments anti- thyroïdiens

| | |
|---|---|
| **药品名称 Drug Names** | 丙硫氧嘧啶 Propylthiouracil |
| 适应证<br>Les indications | ①甲亢的内科治疗。②甲状腺危象的治疗。③术前准备。<br>① Le traitement médical de l'hyperthyroïdie. ② Le traitement de la crise de la thyroïde. ③ La préparation préopératoire. |
| 用法、用量<br>Les modes d'emploi et la posologie | ①成人甲亢：口服常用量 300～450mg/d，分 3 次口服，极量一次 0.2g，一日 0.6g。小儿开始剂量每日按 4mg/kg 分次口服，维持量酌减。②甲状腺危象：一日 0.4～0.8g，分 3～4 次服用，疗程不超过 1 周。③甲亢的术前准备：术前服用本品一次 100mg，一日 3～4 次，使甲状腺功能恢复到正常或接近正常，然后加服 2 周碘剂再进行手术。<br>① Traiter l'hyperthyroïdie chez des adultes : par voie orale, la dose usuelle, 300 à 450 mg par jour, à travers 3 fois, la dose limite, 0,2g par fois, 0,6g par jour. Chez des enfants, commencer par 4mg/kg par jour, à travers plusieurs fois, par voie orale, diminuer un peu la dose pour l'entretien. ② Pour la crise de la thyroide : 0,4 à 0,8 g par jour, à travers 3 à 4 fois. Le traitement médical ne dépasse pas une semaine. ③ Pour la préparation préopératoire de l'hyperthyroide : prendre 100mg par fois avant la chirurgie, 3 à 4 fois par jour, normaliser la fonction thyroïdienne, ensuite, prendre l'iode pendant 2 semaines avant de suivre la chrurgie. |
| 剂型、规格<br>Les formes pharmaceutiques et les spécifications | 片剂：每片 50mg；100mg。<br>Comprimés : 50mg ou 100mg par comprimé. |
| **药品名称 Drug Names** | 甲巯咪唑 Méthimazole |
| 适应证<br>Les indications | ①甲亢的内科治疗。②甲状腺危象的治疗。③术前准备。<br>① Le traitement médical de l'hyperthyroïdie. ② Le traitement de la crise de la thyroïde. ③ La prépartion préopératoire. |

| | |
|---|---|
| 用法、用量<br>Les modes d'emploi et la posologie | 成人：开始时每天30mg，可按病情轻重调节为每日15～40mg，每日最大量60mg，分次口服，病情控制后逐渐减量，维持量：一日5～15mg，疗程一般12～18个月。小儿：开始剂量为每日0.4mg/kg，分3次口服。维持量约减半或按病情轻重调节。<br><br>Chez des adultes : commencer par prendre 30mg par jour, ensuite, 15 à 40 mg par jour selon les cas, ne pas dépasser 60mg par jour, pris à travers plusieurs fois, par voie orale, diminuer la dose après le contrôle des symptômes. La dose d'entretien : 5 à 15mg par jour, pendant 12 à 18 mois comme un traitement médical. Chez des enfants : commencer par prendre 0,4 mg/kg par jour, pris à travers 3 fois, par voie orale. La dose d'entretien est la moitié de la dose initiale ou selon les cas. |
| 剂型、规格<br>Les formes pharmaceutiques et les spécifications | 片剂：每片5mg。<br>Comprimés : 5mg par comprimé. |

### 17. 主要影响变态反应和免疫功能的药物 Médicaments qui affectent principalement allergiques et les fonctions immunitaires

### 17.1 抗变态反应药物 Médicaments antiallergie

| 药品名称 Drug Names | 苯海拉明 Diphénhydramine |
|---|---|
| 适应证<br>Les indications | ①主要用于Ⅰ型和Ⅳ型变态反应，对毛细血管通透性增加所致渗出、水肿、分泌物增多的疾病疗效较好，尤其适用于皮肤黏膜的过敏性疾病，如过敏性药疹、过敏性湿疹、血管性神经水肿和荨麻疹等。对平滑肌痉挛所致支气管哮喘的效果较差，需与氨茶碱、麻黄碱等合用。②镇静催眠和手术前给药。③抗帕金森和药物所致锥体外系症状。④防晕止吐：可用于乘船乘车所致晕动病，以及放射病术后及药物引起的恶心呕吐。⑤乳膏外用，治虫咬、神经性皮炎、瘙痒症等。<br><br>① Ce produit est principalement utilisé dans le traitement de l'hypersensibilité de type I et II. Il est efficace dans l'exsudation, l'œdème et l'augmentation des sécrétions cauées par l'augmentation de la perméabilité capillaire. Il est surtout efficace dans le traitement des maladies allergiques cutanéo-muqueuses, telles que l'éruption médicamenteuse allergique, l'eczéma atopique, l'œdème du nerf vasculaire et l'urticaire. Il est peu efficace dans le traitement de l'asthme bronchiquespasmes causé par des muscles lisses, il doit être utilisé en combinaison avec la théophylline et l'éphédrine. ② L'hypnotique, le sédatif et l'administration avant la chirurgie. ③ Les symptômes extrapyramidaux causés par l'anti-parkinson et des médicaments. ④ L'antiémétique : le mal de transport ou les nausées et les vomissements causés par l'irradiation, la radiation et des médicaments. ⑤ Utilisé en crème pour un usage externe, pour traiter les piqûres d'insectes, le neurodermatitis, le prurit, etc. |
| 用法、用量<br>Les modes d'emploi et la posologie | 可口服、肌内注射及局部应用。不能皮下注射，因有刺激性。成人：口服，一次25～50mg，一日2～3次。饭后服。肌内注射，一次12.5～25mg，一日3～4次；或一日5mg/kg，分次给药，或一日150mg/m²，分次给药。<br><br>Administration orale, IM ou topique. Interdit d'administrer par voie sous-cutanée. Chez des adultes: par voie orale, 25 à 50mg par fois, 2 à 3 fois par jour, pris après le repas. Injection IM, 12,5 à 25mg par fois, 3 à 4 fois par jour ; ou 5 mg/kg par jour, à travers plusieurs fois ; ou 150 mg/ m² par jour, à travers plusieurs fois. |
| 剂型、规格<br>Les formes pharmaceutiques et les spécifications | 片剂：每片25mg；50mg。<br>注射液：每支20mg（1ml）。<br>乳膏：每支20g。<br>Comprimés : 25mg ou 50mg par comprimé.<br>Injection : 20mg (1ml) par solution.<br>La crème : 20g par pièce. |
| 药品名称 Drug Names | 异丙嗪 Prométhazine |
| 适应证<br>Les indications | ①抗过敏：适用于各种过敏症（如哮喘、荨麻疹等）。②镇吐抗眩晕：可用于一些麻醉和手术后的恶心呕吐，乘车、船等引起的眩晕症等。③镇静催眠：可在外科手术和分娩时与哌替啶合用，缓解患者紧张情绪，或用于晚间催眠药。亦可与氯丙嗪等配成冬眠注射液用于人工冬眠。 |

**续　表**

| | |
|---|---|
| | ① L'anti-allergie : applicable dans le traitement de l'allergie de toutes sortes, telle que l'asthme, l'urticaire, etc. ② L'anti-vertige et l'antiémétique : applicable dans le traitement des nausées et des vomissements après l'anesthésie et la chirurgie, et du vertige causé par le transport en voiture ou en bateau. ③ Le sédatif et l'hypnotique : applicable en association avec la péthidine lors de la chirurgie ou de l'accouchement, pour apaiser le stress des paitents ou applicable en tant qu'hypnotiquesdu soir. Il est aussi appliqué en association avec lachlorpromazine pour former l'injectiond'hibernation comme l'hibernation artificielle. |
| 用法、用量<br>Les modes d'emploi et la posologie | ①抗过敏：成人，口服，一次 6.25～12.5mg，一日 3 次，饭后及睡前服用，必要时睡前 25mg；儿童，口服，每次按体重 0.125mg/kg 或按体表面积 7.5～15mg/m²，每 4～6 小时 1 次，或睡前按体重 0.25～0.5mg/kg 或按体表面积 7.5～15mg/m²；按年龄计算，每日量 5 岁 5～15mg，6 岁以上 10～15mg，可一日 1 次或分次服用。肌内注射，每次按体重 0.125mg/kg 或按体表面积 3.75mg/m²，每 4～6 小时肌内注射 1 次。②止吐：成人，口服，开始时一次 12.5～25mg，必要时可每 4～6 小时服 12.5～25mg，通常 24 小时不超过 100mg。③抗眩晕：成人，旅行前口服，一次 12.5～25mg，必要时一日 2 次；儿童，口服，剂量减半。④镇静催眠：成人，口服，一次 12.5～25mg，睡前服用。儿童，口服，5 岁 6.25mg，6～12 岁 6.25～12.5mg。<br><br>① L'anti-allergie : chez des adultes, par voie orale, 6,25 à 12,5 mg par fois, 3 fois par jour, pris après le repas et avant le sommeil, s'il est nécessaire, prendre 25mg avant le sommeil ; chez des enfants, par voie orlae, 0,125 mg/kg par fois, ou 7,5 à 15 mg/ ㎡ par fois, toutes les 4 à 6h, ou prendre 0,25 à 0,5mg/kg avant le sommeil, ou prendre 7,5 à 15 mg/ ㎡ avant le sommeil ; chez des patients de 5 ans, 5 à 15mg par jour, chez des patients de plus de 6 ans, 10 à 15mg par jour, à travers 1 ou plusieurs fois. Injection IM, prendre 0,125 mg/kg par fois ou 3,75 mg/ ㎡ , toute les 4 à 6 h. ② Pour l'antiémétique : chez des adultes, par voie orale, commencer par 12,5 à 25mg par fois, s'il est nécessaire, 12,5 à 25mg toutes les 4 à 6h, ne pas dépasser 100mg en 24h. ③ Pour l'anti-vertige : chez des adultes, avant le voyage, par voie orale, 12,5 à 25mg par fois, s'il est nécessaire, 2 fois par jour ; chez des enfants, par voie orale, diminuer de moitié la dose. ④ Pour le sédatif et l'hypnotique : chez des adultes, par voie orale, 12,5 à 25mg par fois, pris avant le sommeil. Chez des enfants, par voie orale, chez les enfants de 5 ans, 6,25mg, chez de 6 à 12ans, 6,25 à 12,5mg. |
| 剂型、规格<br>Les formes pharmaceutiques et les spécifications | 片剂：每片 12.5mg；25mg。<br>注射液：每支 25mg（1ml）；50mg（2ml）。<br>Comprimés : 12,5mg ou 25mg par comprimé.<br>Injection : 25mg (1ml) ou 50mg (2ml) par solution. |
| **药品名称 Drug Names** | 去氯羟嗪 Décloxizine |
| 适应证<br>Les indications | 用于支气管哮喘、急慢性荨麻疹、皮肤划痕症、血管神经性水肿、接触性皮炎、光敏性皮炎、季节性花粉症、过敏性鼻炎及结膜炎等。<br>Ce produit sert à traiter l'asthme bronchique, l'urticaire aiguë et chronique, la maladie des griffes de la peau, l'œdème angioneurotique, la dermatite de contact, la dermatite de photosensibilité, la fièvre des foins saisonnière, la rhinite allergique et la conjonctivite, etc. |
| 用法、用量<br>Les modes d'emploi et la posologie | 口服：一日 3 次，一次 25～50mg。<br>Par voie orale : 3 fois par jour, 25 à 50 mg par fois. |
| 剂型、规格<br>Les formes pharmaceutiques et les spécifications | 片剂：每片 25mg；50mg。<br>Comprimés : 25mg ou 50mg par comprimé. |
| **药品名称 Drug Names** | 阿伐斯汀 Acrivastine |
| 适应证<br>Les indications | 用于过敏性鼻炎及荨麻疹等。<br>Ce produit sert à traiter la rhinite allergique et l'urticaire. |
| 用法、用量<br>Les modes d'emploi et la posologie | 成人及 12 岁以上儿童口服：1 次 8mg，一日不超过 3 次。<br>Chez des adultes ou des enfants de plus de 12 ans : par voie orale, 8mg par fois, ne pas dépasser 3 fois par jour. |

**续　表**

| 剂型、规格<br>Les formes pharmaceutiques et les spécifications | 胶囊剂：每粒 8mg。<br>Capsules : 8mg par capsule. |
|---|---|
| **药品名称 Drug Names** | 左卡巴斯汀 Lévocabastine |
| 适应证<br>Les indications | 用于局部治疗的滴眼剂和喷鼻剂，缓解过敏性鼻炎，预防包括鼻炎及结膜炎在内的过敏反应。<br>Ce produit est utilisé comme des gouttes pour les yeux et le spray nasalpour un traitement topique. Il est appliqué pour soulager la rhinite allergique,et prévenir la rhinite allergique et la conjonctivite. |
| 用法、用量<br>Les modes d'emploi et la posologie | ①喷鼻：成人及12岁以上儿童常用量为每个鼻孔喷2下，一日2次。必要时可增至每次喷2下，一日3～4次。连续用药直至症状消除。②滴眼：每次1滴，一日2～4次。<br>① La pulvérisation nasale : chez des adultes et des enfants de plus de 12 ans, la dose usuelle est de 2 pulvérisations dans chaque narine, 2 fois par jour. s'il est nécessaire, possible de prendre 2 pulvérisations par fois, 3 à 4 fois par jour. L'adminstration continue jusqu'à la disparition des symptômes. ② Les gouttes pour les yeux : 1 goutte par fois, 2 à 4 fois par jour. |
| 剂型、规格<br>Les formes pharmaceutiques et les spécifications | 喷鼻剂（微悬浮液）：每支 10ml（0.5g/ml）。<br>滴眼剂：0.5mg/kg。<br>L'aérosol nasal (suspension) : 10ml (0,5g par ml).<br>Les gouttes pour les yuex : 0,5mg/kg. |
| **药品名称 Drug Names** | 咪唑斯汀 Mizolastine |
| 适应证<br>Les indications | 本品用于长效 $H_1$ 受体拮抗药，适用于季节性过敏性鼻炎、花粉症、常年性过敏性鼻炎及荨麻疹等皮肤过敏症状。<br>Ce produit sert d'antagoniste du récepteur $H_1$ à action prolongé pour traiterla rhinite allergique saisonnière, le rhume des foins, la rhinite allergique apériodique, l'urticaire et d'autres allergies cutanées. |
| 用法、用量<br>Les modes d'emploi et la posologie | 口服，成人（包括老年人）和12岁以上儿童，推荐剂量为一次 10mg，一日 1 次。<br>Par voie orale, chez des adultes (y compris des personnes âgées) et des enfants de plus de 12ans, la dose recommandée est de 10mg par fois, 1 fois par jour. |
| 剂型、规格<br>Les formes pharmaceutiques et les spécifications | 片剂：每片 10mg。<br>Comprimés : 10mg par comprimé. |
| **药品名称 Drug Names** | 赛庚啶 Cyproheptadine |
| 适应证<br>Les indications | 用于荨麻疹、湿疹、过敏性和接触性皮炎、皮肤瘙痒、鼻炎、偏头痛、支气管哮喘等。皮肤瘙痒通常在服药后2～3日消失。对库欣病、肢端肥大症也有一定疗效。<br>Ce produit sert à traiter l'urticaire,l'eczéma, la dermatite atopique et de contact,le prurit,la rhinite, la migraine, l'asthme bronchique, etc. Il a aussi un certain effet sur la maladie de Cushing et l'acromégalie. |
| 用法、用量<br>Les modes d'emploi et la posologie | ①口服，成人，一次2～4mg，一日3次。儿童，口服，2～6岁，一次2mg，一日2～3次，7～14岁，一次4mg，一日2～3次，极量：一次 0.2mg/kg。作为食欲增进剂应用时，用药时间不超过6个月。②乳膏外用。<br>① Par voie orale, chez des adultes, 2 à 4mg par fois, 3 fois par jour. chez des enfants, par voie orale, de 2 à 6 ans, 2 mg par fois, 2 à 3 fois par jour ; de 7 à 14 ans, 4mg par fois, 2 à 3 fois par jour. La dose limite : 0,2 mg/kg par fois. Utilisé comme activateur d'appétit, le traitement ne dépasse pas 6 mois. ② La crème pour un usage externe. |
| 剂型、规格<br>Les formes pharmaceutiques et les spécifications | 片剂：每片 2mg。<br>糖浆剂：4mg/kg。<br>霜剂：每支 10g（0.5%），20g（0.5%）。<br>乳膏剂：0.5%。<br>Comprimés : 2mg par comprimé.<br>Sirop : 4mg/kg.<br>La crème : 10g (0,5%) ou 20g (0,5%) par solution.<br>La crème : 0,5%. |

**续　表**

| 药品名称 Drug Names | 氯雷他定 Loratadine |
|---|---|
| 适应证<br>Les indications | 用于过敏性鼻炎、急性或慢性荨麻疹、过敏性结膜炎、花粉症及其他过敏性皮肤病。<br><br>Ce produit sert à traiter la rhinite allergique, l'urticaire aiguë ou chronique, la conjonctivite allergique, le rhume des foins et d'autres affections allergiques cutanées. |
| 用法、用量<br>Les modes d'emploi et la posologie | 口服，成人及 12 岁以上儿童，1 次 10mg，一日 1 次，空腹服用。日夜均有发作者，可一次 5mg，每日晨、晚各一次。儿童，口服，2～12 岁，体重大于 30kg 者，一次 5mg，一次 5mg，一日 1 次。复方氯雷他定片：成人及 12 岁以上儿童，一次 1 片，一日 2 次。<br><br>Par voie orale, chez des adultes et des enfants de plus de 12ans, 10mg par fois, 1 fois par jour, l'estomac vide. Chez des patients souffrant des maladies le jour comme le soir, 5mg par fois, pris le petit matin et le soir. Chez des enfants, par voie orale, de 2 à 12 ans, plus de 30kg, 5mg par fois, 1 fois par jour. Les comprimés composés de loratadine : chez des adultes et des enfants de plus de 12ans, 1 comprimé par fois, 2 fois par jour. |
| 剂型、规格<br>Les formes pharmaceutiques et les spécifications | 片剂：每片 10mg。<br>胶囊剂：每粒 10mg。<br>颗粒剂：5mg。<br>糖浆剂：60mg/60ml。<br><br>Comprimés : 10mg par comprimé.<br>Capsules : 10mg par capsule.<br>Granules : 5mg.<br>Sirop : 60 mg par 60ml. |
| 药品名称 Drug Names | 西替利嗪 Cétirizine |
| 适应证<br>Les indications | 用于季节性和常年性过敏性鼻炎、结膜炎及过敏反应所致的瘙痒和荨麻疹。<br><br>Ce produit sert à traiter la rhinite saisonnière et perannuelle allergique, la conjonctivite ainsi quedes démangeaisons et l'urticaire causées par des réactions allergiques. |
| 用法、用量<br>Les modes d'emploi et la posologie | 口服，成人及 12 岁以上儿童，1 次 10～20mg，一日 1 次，或早晚各服 5mg。肾功能损害者需减量。儿童，2～6 岁者，每日 5mg；7～11 岁者，每日 10mg。<br><br>Par voie orale, chez des adultes et des enfants de plus de 12ans, 10 à 20mg par fois, 1 fois par jour, ou prendre 5mg le petit matin et le soir. Chez des patients insuffisants rénaux, diminuer la dose. Chez des enfants, de 2 à 6 ans, 5mg par jour ; de 7 à 11 ans, 10 mg par jour. |
| 剂型、规格<br>Les formes pharmaceutiques et les spécifications | 片剂：每片 10mg。<br>胶囊剂：每粒 10mg。<br>分散片：每片 10mg。<br>口服液：10mg/10ml。<br><br>Comprimés : 10mg par comprimé.<br>Capsules : 10mg par capsule.<br>Comprimés dispersibles : 10mg par comprimé.<br>La solution buccale : 10mg par 10ml. |
| 药品名称 Drug Names | 依巴斯汀 Ebastine |
| 适应证<br>Les indications | 用于季节性和常年性过敏性鼻炎和慢性荨麻疹、湿疹、皮炎、痒疹、皮肤瘙痒等。<br><br>Ce produit sert à traiter la rhinite allergique et l'urticaire chronique saisonnière et perannuelles, l'eczéma, la dermatite, les éruptions cutanées, lesdémangeaisons de la peau, etc. |
| 用法、用量<br>Les modes d'emploi et la posologie | ①常年性过敏性鼻炎：成人，一日 1 次，每次 10mg；儿童（12～17），一日 1 次，每次 5mg。②季节性过敏性鼻炎：成人，一日 1 次，每次 10mg，早上服用效果更好。如严重过敏患者可日服 20mg，但应从小剂量开始。儿童（2～15 岁），一日 1 次，每次 2.5～5mg。<br><br>① Pour traiter la rhinite allergique perannuelle : chez des adultes, 1 fois par jour, 10mg par fois; chez des enfants (12 à 17 ans), 1 fois par jour, 5mg par fois. ② Pour traiter la rhinite allergique saisonnière : chez des adultes, 1 fois par jour, 10mg par fois, pris le petit matin au mieux. Pour l'allergie grave, 20mg par jour, commencer par une dose faible. Chez des enfants (2 à15 ans), 1 fois par jour, 2,5 à 5mg par fois. |

| 续　表 | |
|---|---|
| 剂型、规格<br>Les formes<br>pharmaceutiques et les<br>spécifications | 片剂：每片 10mg。<br>Comprimés : 10mg par comprimé. |
| 药品名称 Drug Names | 地氯雷他定 Desloratadine |
| 适应证<br>Les indications | 用于治疗慢性特发性荨麻疹、常年过敏性鼻炎及季节过敏性鼻炎。<br>Ce produit sert à traiter l'urticaire chronique idiopathique, la rhinite allergique perannuelle et la rhinite allergique saisonnière. |
| 用法、用量<br>Les modes d'emploi et<br>la posologie | ①慢性特发性荨麻疹、常年过敏性鼻炎及季节过敏性鼻炎：成人口服，一日 1 次，每次 5mg。②慢性特发性荨麻疹、常年过敏性鼻炎：儿童，口服，12 岁以上，每次 5mg，一日 1 次；6～11 岁者，每次 2.5mg，一日 1 次；12 个月～5 岁者，每次 1.25mg，一日 1 次；6 个月～11 个月者，每次 1mg，一日 1 次。③季节性过敏性鼻炎：儿童口服，12 岁以上者，每次 5mg，一日 1 次；6～11 岁者，每次 2.5mg，一日 1 次；2～5 岁者，每次 1.25mg，一日 1 次。④肝、肾功能不全患者，在开始治疗时可隔日服用 5mg。<br><br>① Pour traiter l'urticaire chronique idiopathique, la rhinite allergique perannuelle et saisonnière : chez des adultes, par voie orale, 1 fois par jour, 5mg par fois. ② Pour traiter l'urticaire chronique idiopathique, la rhinite allergique perannuelle : chez des enfants, par voie orale, plus de 12 ans, 5mg par fois, 1 fois par jour ; de 6 à 11 ans, 2,5mg par fois, 1 fois par jour ; de 12 mois à 5 ans, 1,25mg par fois, 1 fois par jour ; de 6 mois à 11 mois, 1mg par fois, 1 fois par jour. ③ Pour traiter la rhinite allergique saisonnière : chez des enfants, par voie orale, plus de 12ans, 5mg par fois, 1 fois par jour ; de 6 à 11 ans, 2,5mg par fois, 1 fois par jour ; de 2 à 5 ans, 1,25mg par fois, 1 fois par jour. ④ Chez des patients insuffisants rénaux et hépatiques, au début du traitement, prendre 5mg tous les 2 jours. |
| 剂型、规格<br>Les formes<br>pharmaceutiques et les<br>spécifications | 片剂：每片 5mg。<br>Comprimés : 5mg par comprimé. |
| 药品名称 Drug Names | 氮䓬斯汀 Azélastine |
| 适应证<br>Les indications | 口服或喷鼻可控制季节性或非季节性鼻炎以及非过敏性血管收缩性鼻炎症状。滴眼剂可用于治疗过敏性结膜炎。<br>Administré par voie orale ou enpulvérisation nasale, ce produit permet de contrôler la rhinite saisonnière et non saisonnière ainsi que les symptômes vasomoteurs de la rhinite non allergique. Ses gouttes pour les yeux peuvent traiter la conjonctivite allergique. |
| 用法、用量<br>Les modes d'emploi et<br>la posologie | ①过敏性鼻炎（季节性或非季节性）：a. 成人及 12 岁以上儿童，经鼻给药：每次每鼻孔 1 喷（每喷 0.137mg），一日 2 次，作用持续时间 12 小时。在花粉季节连续用药对控制鼻部症状优于临时用药。对于非季节性过敏性鼻炎，可长期用药 6 个月，安全性和疗效良好。口服：每次 1～2mg，一日 2 次。或遵医嘱。b. 5～11 岁儿童，经鼻给药：每次每鼻孔 1 喷，一日 2 次。口服：6 岁以上儿童，每次 1～2mg，一日 2 次。或遵医嘱。②血管收缩性鼻炎：成人及 12 岁以上患者，每次每鼻孔 1 喷（每喷 0.137mg），一日 2 次，或遵医嘱。③过敏性结膜炎：成人滴患眼，每次 1 滴（0.05%），一日 2 次。有报道 1 个疗程可用 8 个月。儿童滴眼剂只能用于 3 岁以上儿童。每次 1 滴（0.05%），一日 2 次。有报道 1 个疗程可用至 8 个月。或遵医嘱。④治疗和预防哮喘：成人或 6 岁以上儿童，口服，每次 1～4mg，一日 2 次；或每次 8mg，一日 1 次，睡前服。睡前服可用于控制哮喘夜间和晨起发作。遵医嘱。⑤）肝功能不全和老年患者无须调整剂量。 |

**续　表**

| | |
|---|---|
| | ① Pour traiter la rhinite allergique saisonnière ou non saisonnière :a. Chez des adultes et des enfants de plus de 12 ans, par voie nasale : 1 pulvérisation dans chaque narine par fois (0,137mg par pulvérisation), 2 fois par jour, avec une action de 12h. Pendant la saison de pollen, l'administration continue est plus efficace que l'administration provisoire. Pour traiter la rhinite allergique non saisonnière, possible de prendre le médicament pendant 6 mois, avec une meilleure sûreté et un meilleur effet. Par voie orale : 1 à 2mg par fois, 2 fois par jour. ou selon les ordonnances. b. Chez des enfants de 5 à 11 ans, par voie nasale : 1 pulvérisation dans chaque narine par fois, 2 fois par jour. par voie orale : chez des enfants plus de 6 ans, 1 à 2mg par fois, 2 fois par jour. Ou selon les ordonnance. ② Pour traiter la rhinite vasomotrice : chez des adultes et des enfants de plus de 12ans, 1 pulvérisation dans chaque narine (0,137mg par pulvérisation) par fois, 2 fois par jour, ou selon les ordonnances. ③ Pour traiter la conjonctivite allergique : chez des adultes, instiller des gouttes sur les yeux touchés, 1 goutte par fois (0,05%), 2 fois par jour. Selon des rapports, 1 traitement est appliqué pendant 8 mois. Les gouttes pour les yeux des enfants ne peuvent être appliquées que chez des enfants plus de 3 ans. 1 goutte par fois (0,05%), 2 fois par jour. selon des rapports, un traitement peut dure 8 mois. Ou selon des ordonnances. ④ Pour traiter et prévenir l'asthme : chez des adultes et des enfants de plus de 6 ans, par voie orale, 1 à 4mg par fois, 2 fois par jour ; ou 8mg par fois, 1 fois par jour, pris avant le sommeil. L'administration avant le sommeil permet de contrôler la crise de l'asthme la nuit et le petit matin. Ou selon les ordonnances. ⑤ Chez des patients insuffisants hépatiques ou des personnes âgées, pas nécessaire d'ajuster la dose. |
| 剂型、规格<br>Les formes pharmaceutiques et les spécifications | 片剂：每片 0.5mg；1mg。<br>颗粒剂：2mg/g。<br>喷鼻剂：10mg/10ml。<br>滴眼剂：2.5mg/5ml。<br>Comprimés : 0,5mg ou 1mg par comprimé.<br>Granules : 2mg par g.<br>L'aérosol nasal : 10mg par 10ml.<br>Les gouttes pour les yeux : 2,5 mg par 5ml. |
| 药品名称 Drug Names | 溴苯那敏 Bromphéniramine |
| 适应证<br>Les indications | 可用于慢性荨麻疹。<br>Ce produit sert à traiter l'urticaire chronique. |
| 用法、用量<br>Les modes d'emploi et la posologie | 口服：一日 3～4 次，一次 4～8mg。<br>Par voie orale : 3 à 4 fois par jour, 4 à 8mg par fois. |
| 剂型、规格<br>Les formes pharmaceutiques et les spécifications | 片剂：4mg。<br>缓释片：12mg。<br>Comprimés : 4mg.<br>Comprimés à libération prolongée : 12mg. |
| 药品名称 Drug Names | 氯苯那敏 Chlorphéniramine |
| 适应证<br>Les indications | 用于过敏性鼻炎、感冒和鼻窦炎及过敏性皮肤疾病如荨麻疹、过敏性药疹或湿疹、血管神经性水肿、虫咬所致皮肤瘙痒。<br>Ce produit sert à traiter la rhinite allergique, le rhume, la sinusite aisni que les troubles allergiques cutanés tels que l'urticaire,l'éruption allergique ou l'eczéma,l'œdème angioneurotique et le prurit causé par les piqûres d'insectes. |
| 用法、用量<br>Les modes d'emploi et la posologie | 口服，成人一次量 4mg，一日 3 次。肌内注射，一次 5～20mg。<br>Par voie orale, chez des adultes, 4mg par fois, 3 fois par jour. Injection IM, 5 à 20mg par fois. |
| 剂型、规格<br>Les formes pharmaceutiques et les spécifications | 片剂：每片 4mg。<br>胶囊剂：每粒 8mg。<br>注射液：每支 10mg（1ml）；20mg（2ml）。<br>Comprimés : 4mg par comprimé.<br>Capsules : 8mg par capsule.<br>Injection : 10mg (1ml) ou 20mg (2ml) par solution. |

**续　表**

| 药品名称 Drug Names | 茶苯海明 Dimenhydrinate |
|---|---|
| 适应证<br>Les indications | 有镇吐、防晕作用、可用于妊娠、晕动症、放射线治疗及术后引起的恶心、呕吐。<br><br>Il sert d'antiémétique et d'anti-verge. Il peut être utilisé pour la grossesse, le mal des transports,des nauséeset des vomissements postopératoires ou provoqués par la radiothérapie. |
| 用法、用量<br>Les modes d'emploi et la posologie | 一次 25 ～ 50mg，一日 3 次。<br>25 à 50mg par fois, 3 fois par jour. |
| 剂型、规格<br>Les formes pharmaceutiques et les spécifications | 片剂：25mg；50mg。<br>Comprimés : 25mg ou 50mg. |

| 药品名称 Drug Names | 色甘酸钠 Cromoglycate de sodium |
|---|---|
| 适应证<br>Les indications | 　用于预防过敏性哮喘的发作，改善主观症状，增加患者对运动的耐受能力，对于依赖皮质激素的患者，服用本品后可使之减量或完全缓解。患有慢性难治性哮喘的儿童应用本品大部分或完全缓解。与异丙肾上腺素合用，较单用时的效率显著增高。但本品起效较慢，需连续用药数天后才能见效。如已发病，用药多无效。对变态反应作用不明显的慢性哮喘也有疗效。用于过敏性鼻炎和季节性花粉症，能迅速控制症状。软膏外用于慢性过敏性湿疹及某些皮肤瘙痒症也有显著疗效。2% ～ 4% 滴眼液适用于花粉症、结膜炎和春季角膜炎结膜炎。<br><br>Il sert à prévenir la crise de l'asthme allergique, à améliorer les symptômes, à renforcer la tolérance des patients vis-à-vis du sport. Chez des patients cortico- dépendants, l'administration de ce produit permet de réduire les corticostéroïdes ou de soulager les symptômes. Chez des enfants atteints d'asthme réfractaire chronique, l'utilisation de ce produit peut permettre de réduire partiellement ou complètement les symptômes. Utilisé en association avec l'isoprotérénol, il sera plus efficace que l'utilisation seule. Mais il prend effet lentement, il faut donc attendre quelques jours après l'administration avant de percevoir l'effet. Mais il est peu efficace, quand la crise de l'asthme a eu lieu. Il a aussi un certain effet sur l'asthme chronique peu sentible à l'effet allergique. Appliqué pour le traitement dela rhinite allergique et du rhume des foins saisonnier, il permet de contrôler rapidement les symptômes. Sa pommade est aussi utilisée dans le traitement de l'eczéma atopique chronique et de certains prurits. Ses gouttes pour les yeux à 2% à 4% sont aussi applicables dans le traitementdu rhume des foins, de la conjonctivite, de laconjonctivite vernale et de la kératite. |
| 用法、用量<br>Les modes d'emploi et la posologie | ①支气管哮喘：干粉喷雾吸入：成人，一次 20mg，一日 4 次。症状减轻后，一日 2 ～ 3 次；维持量一日 20mg。5 岁以上儿童用量同成人。②过敏性鼻炎：干粉鼻吸入：一次 10mg，一日 4 次；2% 或 4% 溶液滴鼻或喷雾，每次用药量约含色甘酸钠 5mg，一日 6 次。③食物过敏：成人，一次 200mg，一日 4 次，饭前服。2 岁以上儿童，一次 100mg，一日 4 次。如 2 ～ 3 周效果不佳，剂量可增加，每日不超过 40mg/kg，症状控制后可减量。④滴眼：2% 或 4% 滴眼剂滴眼，一日数次。⑤外用：5% ～ 10% 软膏，涂于患处，一日 2 次。<br><br>① Pour traiter l'asthme bronchique : la poudre pour inhalation : chez des adultes, 20mg par fois, 4 fois par jour. Après l'amélioration des symptômes, 2 à 3 fois par jour ; la dose d'entetien, 20mg par jour. Chez des enfants de plus de 5 ans, la même dose que chez des adultes. ② Pour traiter la rhinite allergique : la poudre pour inhalation : 10mg par fois, 4 fois par jour ; utiliser la solution à 2% ou 4% pour les gouttes nasales ou la pulvérisation, chaque administration contient 5mg de cromoglycate de sodium, 6 fois par jour. ③ Pour traiter les allergies alimentaires : chez des adultes, 200mg par fois, 4 fois par jour, pris avant le repas. Chez des enfants de plus de 2 ans, 100mg par fois, 4 fois par jour. s'il est toujours peu efficace après 2 à 3 semaines, augmenter la dose, mais ne pas dépasser 40 mg/kg par jour, possible de diminuer la dose après le contrôle des symptômes. ④ Les gouttes pour les yeux : les gouttes pour les yeux à 2% ou 4%, plusieurs fois par jour. ⑤ Pour un usage externe : appliquer la pommade à 5% à 10% sur la zone touchée, 2 fois par jour. |
| 剂型、规格<br>Les formes pharmaceutiques et les spécifications | 气雾剂：每瓶总量约 14g，内含色甘酸钠 0.7g，每揿含药量 3.5mg。<br>胶囊剂：每粒 20mg。<br>软膏：5% ～ 10%。<br>滴眼剂：2%（8ml）；4%（8ml）。<br>L'aérosol : 14g par flacon, contenant 0,7g de cromoglycate de sodium, chaque pulvérisation contient 3,5mg de médicament.<br>Capsule : 20mg par capsule.<br>La pommade : 5% à 10%.<br>Les gouttes pour les yeux : 2% (8ml) ou 4% (8ml). |

| 药品名称 Drug Names | 酮替芬 Kétotifène |
|---|---|
| 适应证<br>Les indications | ①用于多种类型支气管哮喘，均有明显疗效，对过敏性哮喘疗效尤为明显，混合性次之，感染型约半数以上有效。对过敏性哮喘效果优于色甘酸钠。②也可用于过敏性鼻炎、过敏性结膜炎、花粉症、急慢性荨麻疹、药物、食物或昆虫所致变态反应的预防和治疗。<br><br>① Ce produit sert à traiter l'asthme bronchique de toutes sortes, avec un effet évident. Il est surtout efficace pour l'asthme allergique, assez efficace pour l'asthme mixte. Chez plus de 50% d'asthme infectieux, il est efficace. Il est plus efficace que le cromoglycate de sodium dans le traitement de l'asthme allergique. ② Il est aussi applicable dans la prévention et le traitement de la rhinite allergique, de la conjonctivite allergique,du rhume des foins,de l'urticaire aiguë et chronique ainsi que l'effet allergique causé par des médicaments, des aliments ou des insectes. |
| 用法、用量<br>Les modes d'emploi et la posologie | 口服：成人，一次 1mg，早、晚各服一次；若困意明显，可只在睡前服 1 次。<br><br>Par voie orale : chez des adultes, 1mg par fois, pris le petit matin et le soir ; si le sommeil est évident, possible de prendre seulement avant le sommeil. |
| 剂型、规格<br>Les formes pharmaceutiques et les spécifications | 片剂：每片 1mg。<br>胶囊剂：每粒 1mg。<br>口服液：每支 1mg/5ml。<br>滴眼液：2.5mg/5ml。<br>滴鼻液：15mg/10ml。<br>分散片：每片 1mg。<br>鼻吸入粉雾剂：15.5mg/14g。<br>Comprimés : 1mg par comprimé.<br>Capsules : 1mg par capsule.<br>La solution buccale : 1mg par 5ml par solution.<br>Les gouttes pour les yeux : 2,5mg par 5ml.<br>Les gouttes nasales : 15mg par 10ml.<br>Les compriés dispersibles : 1mg par comprimé.<br>La poudre pour inhalation nasale : 15,5mg par 14g. |

17.2　免疫抑制药 Immunosuppresseurs

| 药品名称 Drug Names | 环孢素 Cyclosporine |
|---|---|
| 适应证<br>Les indications | 主要用于肾、肝、心、肺、骨髓移植的抗排异反应，可与肾上腺皮质激素或其他免疫抑制剂合用，也可用于治疗类风湿关节炎、系统性红斑狼疮、肾病型慢性肾炎、自身免疫性溶血性贫血、银屑病、葡萄膜炎等自身免疫性疾病。<br><br>Ce produit est utilisé dans l'anti-rejet de la transplantation rénale, hépatique, cardique, pulmonaire ou de moelle osseuse. Il peut être utilisé en association avec des corticostéroïdes ou d'autres agents immunosuppresseurs. Il sert aussi à traiter des maladies auto-immunes, telles que la polyarthrite rhumatoïde, le lupus érythémateux disséminé, la néphropathie, la maladie rénale chronique, l'anémie hémolytique auto-immune, le psoriasis et l'uvéite. |
| 用法、用量<br>Les modes d'emploi et la posologie | ①器官移植：a. 口服：于移植前 12 小时起每日服 8～10mg/kg，维持术后 1～2 周，根据血药浓度减至每日 2～6mg/kg，分 2 次服。b.静脉注射：仅用于不能口服的患者，于移植前 4～12 小时每日给予 3～5mg/kg，以 5% 葡萄糖或生理盐水稀释至 1：20 至 1：100 的浓度于 2～6 小时缓慢滴注。②自身免疫性疾病：口服，初始剂量为每日 2.5～5mg/kg，分 2 次服；症状缓解后改为最小剂量维持，但成人不应超过每日 5mg/kg，儿童不应超过 6mg/kg。<br><br>① Pour la transplantation d'organes : a. Par voie orale : 12 h avant la transplantation, 8 à 10 mg/kg par jour, jusqu'à 1 à 2 semaines après la chirurgie, diminuer la dose pour atteindre 2 à 6mg/kg par jour, à travers 2 fois. b. Injection IV : seulement applicable chez des patients ne peuvent pas administrer par voie orale. Prendre 3 à 5 mg/kg par jour 4 à 12 h avant la transplantation, dissoudre dans la solution de glucose à 5% ou la solution saline pour obtenir une concentration de 1：20 à 1：100, la perfusion en 2 à 6h. ② Pour traiter des maladies auto-immunes : par voie orale, la dose initiale, 2,5 à 5 mg/kg par jour, à travers 2 fois ; après l'amélioration des symptômes, prendre la dose minimale pour l'entretien, mais pas dépasser 5mg/kg par jour chez des adultes, et 6 mg/kg par jour chez des enfants. |

续 表

| | |
|---|---|
| 剂型、规格<br>Les formes pharmaceutiques et les spécifications | 胶囊剂：每粒 25mg；100mg。<br>微乳化软胶囊：每粒 10mg；25mg；50mg；100mg。<br>口服液：100mg/ml（50ml）。<br>微乳化口服液：100mg/ml（50ml）。<br>静脉滴注浓缩液：250mg/5ml；500mg/10ml。<br><br>Capsules : 25mg ou 100mg par capsule.<br>Capsules molles microémulsionnables : 10mg, 25mg, 50mg ou 100mg par capsule.<br>La solution buccale : 100mg par ml (50ml).<br>La solution buccale microémulsionnable : 100mg par ml (50ml).<br>Concentré pour la perfusion intraveineuse : 250mg par 5ml ou 500mg par 10ml. |
| **药品名称 Drug Names** | 他克莫司 Tacrolimus |
| 适应证<br>Les indications | 主要用于器官移植的抗排异反应，尤其适用于肝移植，还可用于肾、心、肺、胰、骨髓及角膜移植等。<br><br>Il est principalement utilisé dans l'anti-rejet de la transplantation d'organes, surtout la transplantation hépatique. Il est aussi applicable dans la transplantation rénale, cardiaque, pulmonaire, de pancréas, de moelle osseuse et de la cornée. |
| 用法、用量<br>Les modes d'emploi et la posologie | 开始采用每日 0.05～0.1mg/kg（肾移植），或 0.01～0.05mg/kg（肝移植）持续静脉滴注。能进行口服时，改为口服胶囊，开始剂量为每日 0.15～0.3mg/kg，分 2 次服；在逐渐减至维持剂量，每日 0.1mg/kg，分 2 次服，亦可根据病情调整剂量，通常低于首次免疫抑制剂量。本品外用皮肤涂布可用于其他免疫抑制药疗效不佳或无法耐受的中重度特应性皮炎。<br><br>Commencer par prendre 0,05 à 0,1 mg/kg par jour (la transplantation rénale), ou 0,01 à 0,05 mg/kg par jour (la transplantation hépatique), en perfusion continue. Quand le patient peut administrer par voie orale, prendre les capsules par voie orale, la dose initiale, 0,15 à 0,3 mg/kg par jour, à travers 2 fois ; diminuer ensuite pour atteindre la dose d'entretien, soit 0,1 mg/kg par jour, à travers 2 fois, ou ajuster la dose selon les cas, mais en général la dose d'entretien est inférieure à la dose initiale. Son usage externe est applicable dans le traitement de la dermatite atopique résistant à d'autres immunosuppresseurs. |
| 剂型、规格<br>Les formes pharmaceutiques et les spécifications | 胶囊剂：每粒 0.5mg；1mg；5mg。<br>注射液：每支 5mg（1ml），用时稀释在 5% 葡萄糖或生理盐水中缓慢静脉滴注。<br>外用软膏剂：3mg/10g；10mg/10g。<br><br>Capsules : 0,5mg, 1mg ou 5mg par capsule.<br>Injection : 5mg (1ml) par solution, dissoudre dans la solution de glucose à 5% ou la solution saline pour la perfusion lente.<br>La pommade pour un usage externe : 3mg par 10g ou 10mg par 1g. |
| **药品名称 Drug Names** | 吗替麦考酚酯 Mycophénolate mofétil |
| 适应证<br>Les indications | 主要用于预防和治疗肾、肝、心脏及骨髓移植的排斥反应。也可用于不能耐受其他免疫抑制剂或疗效不佳的类风湿关节炎、全身性红斑狼疮、原发性肾小球肾炎、牛皮癣等自身免疫性疾病。<br><br>Ce produit est utilisé dans l'anti-rejet de la transplantation rénale, hépatique, cardique ou de moelle osseuse.Il est aussi applicable dans le traitement des maladies auto-immunes résistant à d'autres immunosuppresseurs, y compris la polyarthrite rhumatoïde, le lupus érythémateux disséminé, la glomérulonéphrite primaire et le psoriasis. |
| 用法、用量<br>Les modes d'emploi et la posologie | 用于器官移植：空腹口服，成人每日 1.5～2.0g，小儿 30mg/kg，分 2 次服，首剂量应在器官移植后 72 小时内服用；静脉注射，主要用于口服不能耐受者，每次注射时间多于 2 小时。用于自身免疫病：成人每日 1.5～2.0g，维持量 0.25～0.5g，一日 2 次，空腹服用。<br><br>Pour la transplantation d'organes : par voie orale, l'estomac vide, chez des adultes, 1,5 à 2,0g par jour, chez des enfants, 30 mg/kg par jour, à travers 2 fois, la dose initiale doit être administrée en 72h suivant la transplantation d'organes ; injection IV, principalement applicable chez des patients qui ne peuvent pas tolérer l'administration orale, une injection de plus de 2h par fois. Pour le traitement des maladies auto-immunes : chez des adultes, 1,5 à 2,0g par jour, la dose d'entretien, 0,25 à 0,5g par jour, 2 fois par jour, à jeun. |

**续　表**

| 剂型、规格 Les formes pharmaceutiques et les spécifications | 胶囊剂：每粒 250mg。<br>片剂：每片 500mg。<br>注射剂：每支 500mg。<br>Capsules : 250mg par capsule.<br>Comprimés : 500mg par comprimé.<br>Injection : 500mg par solution. |
|---|---|
| 药品名称 Drug Names | 来氟米特 Léflunomide |
| 适应证 Les indications | 用于治疗风湿性关节炎、系统性红斑狼疮等自身免疫性疾病，亦可用于器官移植抗排异反应。<br>Ce produit sert à traiter les maladies auto-immunes telles que la polyarthrite rhumatoïde et le lupus érythémateux disséminé. Il est aussi utilisé dans l'anti-rejet de la transplantation d'organes. |
| 用法、用量 Les modes d'emploi et la posologie | 口服，成人常用量：①类风湿关节炎、系统性红斑狼疮及银屑病关节炎，一次 20mg，一日 1 次；病情控制后可以一日 10 ～ 20mg 维持。②韦格纳肉芽肿病，一日 20 ～ 40mg 维持。③器官移植，负荷剂量一日 200mg，维持剂量一日 40 ～ 60mg。<br>Par voie orale, chez des adultes la dose usuelle :<br>① pour traiter la polyarthrite rhumatoïde et le lupus érythémateux disséminé et l'arthrite psoriasique, 20mg par fois, 1 fois par jour ; après le contrôle des symptômes, 10 à 20mg par jour pour l'entretien. ② pour traiter la granulomatose de Wegener, 20 à 40mg par jour pour l'entretien. ③ pour la transplantation d'organes : 200mg par jour pour la dose de charge, 40 à 60mg par jour pour la dose d'entretien. |
| 剂型、规格 Les formes pharmaceutiques et les spécifications | 片剂：每片 10mg；20mg；100mg。<br>Comprimés : 10mg, 20mg ou 100mg par comprimé. |
| 药品名称 Drug Names | 泼尼松 Prednisone |
| 适应证 Les indications | 糖皮质激素对 Ⅰ、Ⅱ、Ⅲ、Ⅳ型变态反性疾病具有程度不同的治疗效果。①在 Ⅰ 型变态反应疾病中，糖皮质激素应用广泛，可全身给药或局部给药，如用于过敏性鼻炎、异位性皮炎、过敏性哮喘等。②糖皮质激素用于治疗 Ⅱ 型的自身免疫性疾病往往有效，是寻常性天疱疮、自身免疫性溶血性贫血的首选药物，如泼尼松可使 60% ～ 80% 的自身免疫性溶血性贫血缓解。③糖皮质激素广泛应用于治疗免疫复合物疾病（Ⅲ 型变态反应性疾病），主要是依靠其抗炎作用，但仅仅可缓解症状，无消除病因作用。对系统性红斑狼疮，糖皮质激素往往可降低抗核抗体的浓度以及减少狼疮红细胞的出现，而且某些证据表明，对肾损伤的患者应用大剂量的糖皮质激素能改善肾功能并延长患者生命。④糖皮质激素是 Ⅳ 型变态反应性疾病的强力抑制剂，临床上用于移植器官或组织的排异反应、接触性皮炎等。<br>Les effets de traitement des glucocorticoïdes sont différents chez des maladies allergiques de typs I, II, III et IV.<br>① Les glucocorticoïdes sont largement appliqués dans le traitement des maladies allergiques de type I. Administrés systémiquement ou localement, ils permettent de traiter la rhinite allergique, la dermatite atopique, l'asthme allergique, etc. ② Les glucocorticoïdessont aussi efficaces dans le traitement des maladies auto-immunes de type II. Ils sont des médicaments de choix pour traiter le pemphigus vulgaire et l'anémie hémolytique auto-immune. La prednisone peut permettre de soulager l'anémie hémolytique auto-immune dans 60% à 80% des cas. ③ Les glucocorticoïdes sont largement appliqués dans le traitement de maladies complexes immunes (maladies allergiques de typs III), grâce à leurs effets anti – inflammatoires. Mais ils ne peuvent que soulager les symptômes, au lieu d'éradiquer les maladies. Pour le lupus érythémateux disséminé, les glucocorticoïdes permettent de réduire la concentration d'anticorps anti- nucléaires et de réduire l'apparence des globules rouges dans le lupus. Certains rapports montrent que l'utilisation des glucocorticoides à forte dose chez des patients insuffisants rénaux peut permettre d'améliorer la fonction rénale et de prolongée la vie des patients. ④ Les glucocorticoides sont des inhibiteurs puissants des maladies allergiques de type IV. Ils sont utilisés dans les cliniques pour l'anti-rejet de la transplantation d'organes ou de tissus et le traitement de la dermatite de contact. |
| 用法、用量 Les modes d'emploi et la posologie | 口服：一般每日 20 ～ 60mg，如疗效不明显可逐渐增至每日 100mg，维持量为每日 10mg。用于肾、肝、心脏等器官移植：一般术后每日 4mg/kg，加硫唑嘌呤每日 5mg/kg；维持剂量每日 10 ～ 20mg，加硫唑嘌呤每日 1 ～ 2mg/kg。<br>Par voie orale : en général, 20 à 60mg par jour, s'il n'est pas très efficace, augmenter la dose pour atteindre 100mg par jour, la dose d'entretien, 10mg par jour. Pour la transplantation rénale, hépatique et cardiaque : en général après la chirurgie, 4mg/kg par jour, ajouter l'azathioprine, 5 mg/kg par jour ; la dose initiale, 10 à 20mg par jour, ajouter l'azathioprine, 1 à 2mg/kg par jour. |

**续 表**

| | |
|---|---|
| 剂型、规格<br>Les formes pharmaceutiques et les spécifications | 片剂：每片 5mg。<br>Comprimés : 5mg par comprimé. |
| 药品名称 Drug Names | 硫唑嘌呤 Azathioprine |
| 适应证<br>Les indications | 主要用于器官移植时的排异反应，多与糖皮质激素并用，或加用淋巴细胞球蛋白（ALG），疗效好。也广泛用于类风湿关节炎、系统性红斑狼疮，自身免疫性溶血性贫血、特发性血小板减少性紫癜、活动性慢性肝炎、溃疡性结肠炎、重症肌无力、硬皮病等自身免疫性疾病。对慢性肾炎及肾病综合征，其疗效似不及环磷酰胺。由于其不良反应较多且严重，对上述疾病治疗不作为首选，通常是在单用糖皮质激素不能控制时才使用。<br>Ce produit est utilisé pour l'anti-rejet de la transplantation d'organes. Il est souvent utilisé en association avec les corticostéroïdeset les lymphocytes globulines, avec un effet évident. Il est aussi largement appliqué dans le traitement des maladies auto-immunes, telles que la polyarthrite rhumatoïde, le lupus érythémateux disséminé, l'anémie hémolytique auto-immune, le purpura thrombopénique idiopathique, l'hépatite chronique active, la colite ulcéreuse, la myasthénie grave ainsi que la sclérodermie. Pour le traiment de la néphrite chronique et du syndrome néphrotique, il est moins efficace que lacyclophosphamide. Comme ses effets secondaires sont nombreux et graves, il n'est pas le médicament de choix pour traiter les maladies précédentes. Il n'est appliqué que quand l'utilisation seule des glucocorticoides n'est pas efficace. |
| 用法、用量<br>Les modes d'emploi et la posologie | 口服：每日 1～3mg/kg，一般每日 100mg，一次服用，可连服数月。用于器官移植：每日 2～5mg/kg，维持量每日 0.5～3mg/kg。<br>Par voie orale : 1 à 3 mg/kg par jour, en général, 100mg par jour, une fois par jour, pendant quelques mois consécutifs. Pour la transplantation d'organes : 2 à 5 mg/kg par jour, la dose initiale est de 0,5 à 3 mg/kg par jour. |
| 剂型、规格<br>Les formes pharmaceutiques et les spécifications | 片剂：每片 25mg；50mg；100mg。<br>注射液：50mg（以硫唑嘌呤计量）。<br>Comprimés : 25mg, 50mg ou 100mg par comprimé.<br>Injection : 50mg (mesuré en azathioprine). |
| 药品名称 Drug Names | 羟基脲 Hydroxyurée |
| 适应证<br>Les indications | 用于顽固性银屑病和脓疱性银屑病均有效，能减轻全身性脓疱性银屑病的脓疱、发热和中毒症状。短期用药，其毒性作用较甲氨蝶呤小，对有肝脏损伤不宜用甲氨蝶呤或用甲氨蝶呤无效的严重银屑病患者，可选用本品治疗。<br>Ce produit est efficace dans le traitement du psoriasis réfractaire et du psoriasis pustuleux. Il permet d'atténuer les pustules, la fièvre et l'empoissonement du psoriasis pustuleux généralisé. Utilisé pour une courte durée, il a effet toxique mois important que le méthotrexate. Chez des patients atteints de psoriasis grave insuffisants hépatiques et résistants au méthotrexate, ce produit peut être appliqué. |
| 用法、用量<br>Les modes d'emploi et la posologie | 口服：每日 0.5～1.5g，4～8 周为 1 个疗程。<br>Par voie orale : 0,5 à 1,5g par jour, pendant 4 à 8 semaines comme un traitement médical. |
| 剂型、规格<br>Les formes pharmaceutiques et les spécifications | 片剂：每片 400mg；500mg。<br>胶囊剂：每粒 250mg；400mg；500mg。<br>Comprimés : 400mg ou 500mg par comprimé.<br>Capsules : 250mg, 400mg ou 500mg par capsule. |
| 药品名称 Drug Names | 甲氨蝶呤 Méthotrexate |
| 适应证<br>Les indications | 本品原为抗肿瘤药，经剂量、用法调整后用作免疫抑制药。主要用于类风湿关节炎、银屑病关节炎、红斑狼疮、脊柱关节病的周围关节炎、多肌炎、多发性肉芽肿等自身免疫性疾病。甲氨蝶呤间歇疗法治疗多发性肉芽肿起效较糖皮质激素、烷化剂或硫唑嘌呤迅速，故急性患者应首选本品。用于糖皮质激素无效的多肌炎、皮肌炎均见肌力改善、皮疹消退。根据报道甲氨蝶呤特别适用于顽固的进行性多发性肌炎和顽固的进行性眼色素层炎，治疗 1～2 周后可使麻 |

|  | 痹或失明的患者恢复一定功能。其作用机制不明，可能与其抗炎作用有关。应用免疫抑制量的甲氨蝶呤后 24 小时内再给适量的甲酰四氢叶酸，可对抗甲氨蝶呤的毒性，但几乎不影响其免疫抑制作用。<br><br>Ancien antinéoplasique, il est utilisé comme immunosuppresseur après la modification de la posologie et du mode l'emploi. il sert principalement à traiter la polyarthrite rhumatoïde, l'arthrite psoriasique, le lupus érythémateux, l'arthrite périphérique des spondylarthropathies, la polymyosite, de multiples granulomes, etc. Son traitement intermittent permet de traiter les granulomes multiples, avec un effet plus rapide que les corticostéroïdes, les agents alkylants ou l'azathioprine. Il s'agit de médicament de choix chez des patients aigus. Utilisé dans le traitement de la polymyosite et de la dermatomyositerésistant aux corticostéroïdes, il permet d'améliorer la force musculaire et de réduire l'éruption cutanée. Selon certains rapports, il est surtout applicable dans le traitement de la polymyosite progressive réfractaire et de l'uvéite progressive réfractaire. 1 à 2 semaines après son traitement, les patients atteints de paralysie ou de cécité peuvent reprendre certaines fonctions. Son mécanisme est inconnu, il est peut-être lié aux effets anti –inflammatoires. Il faut prendre une dose d'immunosuppression du métrotrexate avant de prendre la leucovorine 24 h après. Celle- ci aide à lutter contre la toxicité du méthotrexate sans affecter son effet d'immunosuppression. |
|---|---|
| 用法、用量<br>Les modes d'emploi et la posologie | 口服：初始剂量一次 7.5mg，一周 1 次；可酌情增加至 20mg，一周 1 次，分 2 次服。肌内注射：每次 10mg，一周 1 次。静脉注射：每次 10～15mg，一周 1 次。银屑病，口服，一次 0.25～5mg，一日 1 次，6～7 日为 1 个疗程。<br><br>Par voie orale : la dose initiale, 7,5 mg par fois, 1 fois par semaine ; possible d'augmenter jusqu'à 20mg par semaine, à travers 2 fois. Injection IM : 10mg par fois, une fois par semaine. Injection IV : 10 à 15mg par fois, 1 fois par semaine. Pour traiter le psoriasis, par voie orale, 0,25 à 5mg par fois, 1 fois par jour, pendant 6 à 7 jours comme un traitement médical. |
| 剂型、规格<br>Les formes pharmaceutiques et les spécifications | 片剂：每片 2.5mg；5mg；10mg。<br>注射液：每支 5mg；10mg；20mg；25mg；50mg；100mg。<br>Comprimés : 2,5mg, 5mg ou 10mg par comprimé.<br>Injection : 5mg, 10mg 20mg, 25mg, 50mg ou 100mg par solution. |
| 药品名称 Drug Names | 环磷酰胺 Cyclophosphamide |
| 适应证<br>Les indications | 用于各种自身免疫性疾病，对严重类风湿关节炎及全身系统性红斑狼疮，大部分病例有效；对儿童肾病综合征，其疗效较硫唑嘌呤好，可长期缓解。可单独用药，但与糖皮质激素并用则疗效较佳，且不良反应较少。对多发性肉芽肿亦常用。与皮质激素并用则疗效较佳，且不良反应较少。与糖皮质激素并用于治疗天疱疮疗效也较好。此外，也用于治疗溃疡性结肠炎、特发性血小板减少性紫癜等自身免疫性疾病。<br><br>也用于器官移植时抗排异反应，通常是与泼尼松、抗淋巴细胞球蛋白并用，其效果与硫唑嘌呤、泼尼松、抗淋巴细胞球蛋白的效果相似，且可避免硫唑嘌呤对肝脏可能产生的不良影响。<br><br>Ce produit sert à traiter des maladies auto-immunes de toutes sortes. Il est efficace dans le traitement de la polyarthrite rhumatoïde sévère et du lupus érythémateux disséminépour la plupart des cas. Il est plus efficace dans le traitement dusyndrome néphrotiqueque l'azathioprine, avec une action prolongée. Il peut être utilisé seul mais il est plus efficace quand il est appliqué en association avec les corticostéroïdes, avec des effets secondaires moins nombreux. Il est aussi souvent applicable dans le traitement des granulomes multiples. Appliqué en association avec les corticostéroïdes, il est aussi applicable dans le traitement du pemphigus, avec un effet satisfaisant.<br><br>En outre, il sert aussi à traiter la colite ulcéreuse etle purpura thrombopénique idiopathique. Il est aussi applicable dans l'anti-rejet de la transplantation d'organes, souvent en association avec la prednisone et la globuline anti- lymphocyte, avec un effet similaire à l'azathioprine, à la prednisone et à la globuline anti- lymphocyte. Il peut aussi permettre d'éviter les effets secondaires hépatiques de la prednisone. |
| 用法、用量<br>Les modes d'emploi et la posologie | 自身免疫性疾病：口服，一日 2～3mg/kg，一日 1 次或隔日 1 次，连用 4～6 周。器官移植：口服，一日 50～150mg；静脉注射，一次 0.2g，一日或隔日 1 次，总量 8～10g 为 1 个疗程。<br><br>Pour traiter les maladies auto-immunes : par voie orale, 2 à 3 mg/kg par jour, une fois par jour ou tous les 2 jours, pendant 4 à 6 semaines consécutives. Pour la transplantation d'organes : par voie orale, 50 à 150mg par jour ; injection IV, 0,2g par fois, une fois par jour ou tous les 2 jours, la dose totale est de 8 à 10g comme un traitement médical. |

**续 表**

| 剂型、规格<br>Les formes<br>pharmaceutiques et les<br>spécifications | 片剂：50mg。<br>注射剂：100mg；200mg。<br>滴眼液：1%。<br>Comprimés : 50mg.<br>Injection : 100mg ou 200mg.<br>Les gouttes pour les yeux : 1%. |
|---|---|

| 药品名称 Drug Names | 苯丁酸氮芥 Chlorambucil |
|---|---|
| 适应证<br>Les indications | 对于切特综合征、红斑狼疮病有较好疗效。尚用于治疗类风湿关节炎并发的脉管炎、伴有寒冷凝集素的自身免疫性溶血性贫血以及依赖糖皮质激素的肾病综合征，与泼尼松龙并用于频发的肾病综合征。用于硬皮病可迅速阻止其发展，使皮肤溃疡痊愈，肺功能改善。<br><br>Il est efficace dans le traitement du syndrome Chet et du lupus érythémateux. Il est aussi applicable dans le traitement de la vascularite compliquée par la polyarthrite rhumatoïde, de l'anémie hémolytique auto-immune accompagnée d'agglutinines froides ainsi du syndrome néphrotique cortico- dépendant. Utilisé en association avec laprednisolone, il permet aussi de traiter le syndrome néphrotique fréquent. Appliqué dans le traitement de la sclérodermie, il permet la guérison de l'ulcèrecutanée et l'amélioration de la fonction pulmonaire. |
| 用法、用量<br>Les modes d'emploi et<br>la posologie | 口服：每日 3 ～ 6mg，早饭前 1 小时或晚饭后 2 小时服用，连服数周，待疗效或骨髓抑制出现后减量，总量一般为 300 ～ 500mg。<br><br>Par voie orale : 3 à 6 mg par jour, pris 1 h avant le petit-déjeuner ou 2h après le dîner, pendant plusieurs semaines consécutives, après l'améolioration des symptômes, diminuer la dose, la dose totale est de 300 à 500mg en général. |
| 剂型、规格<br>Les formes<br>pharmaceutiques et les<br>spécifications | 片剂：每片 1mg；2mg。<br>纸型片：每格 2mg。<br>Comprimés : 1mg ou 2mg par comprimé.<br>Papier : 2mg par grille. |

### 17.3 免疫增强药 Immunostimulants

| 药品名称 Drug Names | 香菇多糖 Lentinan |
|---|---|
| 适应证<br>Les indications | 用于急慢性白血病、胃癌、肺癌、乳腺癌等肿瘤的辅助治疗，提高患者免疫功能，减轻放射治疗和化学治疗的副作用。亦可用于治疗乙型病毒性肝炎。<br><br>Il est utilisé dans le traitement adjuvant de la leucémie aiguë et chronique, du cancer de l'estomac, du cancer du poumon et du cancer du sein. Il permet d'améliorer la fonction immunitaire chez des patients et de réduire les effets secondaires de la radiothérapie et de la chimiothérapie. Il est aussi applicable dans le traitement de l'hépatite virale B. |
| 用法、用量<br>Les modes d'emploi et<br>la posologie | 口服：成人每次 12.5mg，一日 2 次；儿童每次 5 ～ 7.5mg，一日 2 次。静脉注射或静脉滴注：一次 2mg，每周 1 次。一般 3 个月为 1 个疗程。<br><br>Par voie orale : chez des adultes, 12,5mg par fois, 2 fois par jour ; chez des enfants, 5 à 7,5 mg par fois, 2 fois par jour. Injection IV ou en perfusion : 2mg par fois, 1 fois par semaine. Pendant 3 mois comme un traitement médical. |
| 剂型、规格<br>Les formes<br>pharmaceutiques et les<br>spécifications | 片剂：每片 2.5mg。<br>注射剂：每支 1mg。<br>Comprimés : 2,5mg par comprimé.<br>Injection : 1mg par solution. |

| 药品名称 Drug Names | 重组人白细胞介素 -2 　Interleukine 2 humaine recombinante |
|---|---|
| 适应证<br>Les indications | 用于肾细胞癌、黑色素瘤，控制癌性胸、腹水及其他晚期肿瘤；先天或后天免疫缺陷症，如艾滋病等；细菌、真菌及病毒感染，如慢性活动性乙型肝炎、慢性活动性 EB 病毒感染、麻风病、肺结核、白念珠菌感染等。<br><br>Il permet de traiter le carcinome rénal, lemélanome, le cancer du sein, l'ascite et d'autres tumeurs avancées. Il est aussi applicable dans le traitement du syndrome d'immunodéficience congénitale ou acquise, comme le sida ; les infections bactériennes, fongiques et virales, telles que l'hépatite chronique active B, l'infection par le virus EB chronique active, la lèpre, la tuberculose, l'infection par Candida albicans, etc. |

续　表

| | |
|---|---|
| 用法、用量<br>Les modes d'emploi et la posologie | 　皮下注射：每日 20 万～ 40 万 U/m²，加入无菌注射用水 2ml，一日 1 次，每周连用 4 日，4 周为 1 个疗程。肌内注射：慢性乙型肝炎每次 20 万 U，隔日 1 次。静脉滴注：20 万～ 40 万 U/m²，加入生理盐水 500ml，一日 1 次，每周连用 4 日，4 周为 1 个疗程。腔内注射：癌性胸、腹水时先抽取胸腔内积液，在将本品 40 万～ 50 万 /m² 加入生理盐水 20ml 注入，每周 1 ～ 2 次，3 ～ 4 周为 1 个疗程。瘤内或瘤周注射：10 万～ 30 万 U/m²，加至 3 ～ 5ml 注射用生理盐水中，分多点注射到瘤内或瘤周。每周 2 次，连用 2 周为 1 个疗程。<br>　Injection sous-cutanée : 200 000U à 400 000U par m² par jour, ajouter 2ml d'eau stérile pour injection, 1 fois par jour, pendant 4 jours consécutifs par semaine, 4 semaines comme un traitement médical. Injection IM : pour traiter l'hépatite chronique B, 200 000U par fois, tous les 2 jours. En perfusion : 200 000U à 400 000U par m², ajouter 500ml de solution saline, une fois par jour, pendant 4 jours consécutifs par semaine, 4 semaines comme un traitement médical. Injectionintra-thoracique: sortir l'épanchement intra-thoracique lors du traitement du cancer du sein et de l'ascite, injecter ensuite 400 000U à 500 000U par m² plus 20ml de solution saline, 1 à 2 fois par semaine, pendant 3 à 4 semaines comme un traitement médical. Injection péri-tumorale ou intratumorale : 100 000U à 300 000U par m², ajouter 3 à 5ml de solution saline, injection de multi-point dans la tumeur ou autour de la tumeur, 2 fois par semaine, pendant 2 semaine comme un traitement médical. |
| 剂型、规格<br>Les formes pharmaceutiques et les spécifications | 　注射剂：每支 2.5 万 U；5 万 U；10 万 U；20 万 U；50 万 U；100 万 U；200 万 U。<br>　Injection : 25 000U, 50 000U, 100 000U, 200 000U, 500 000U, 1 million d'U ou 2 million d'U par solution. |
| 药品名称 Drug Names | 重组人白细胞介素 -11Interleukine-11 humaine recombinante |
| 适应证<br>Les indications | 　用于实体瘤、非髓性白细胞病化疗后Ⅲ、Ⅳ度血小板减少症的治疗。<br>　Il est applicable dans le traitement de la thrombopénie de degré III et IV après la chimiothérapie des tumeurs solides etde la maladie de leucocytes non myéloïde. |
| 用法、用量<br>Les modes d'emploi et la posologie | 　皮下注射，一次 25 ～ 50μg/kg（以 1ml 注射用水稀释），一日 1 次，7 ～ 14 日为 1 个疗程。于化疗结束后 24 ～ 48 小时开始或发生血小板减少症后给药，血小板计数恢复后应及时停药。<br>　Injection sous-cutanée, 25 à 50 μg par kg par fois (utiliser 1ml d'eau pour injection pour la dilution), 1 fois par jour, pendant 7 à 14 jours comme un traitement médical. Commener à partir de 24 à 48h après la chimiothérapie ou à partir de la crise de la thrombopénie, arrêter immédiatement l'administration après la reprise du nombre plaquettaire. |
| 剂型、规格<br>Les formes pharmaceutiques et les spécifications | 　注射用粉针剂：每支 0.75mg（600 万 U）；1.5mg（1200 万 U）；3mg（2400 万 U）。<br>　Poudre pour injection : 0,75mg (6 millions d'u) ou 1,5mg (12 millions d'u) ou 3mg (24 millions d'u) par solution. |
| 药品名称 Drug Names | 重组人干扰素 Interféron humaine recombinante |
| 适应证<br>Les indications | 　干扰素可用于肿瘤、病毒感染及慢性活动性乙型肝炎等。<br>　L'interféron est applicable dans le traitement du cancer, des infections virales, del'hépatite active chronique, etc. |
| 用法、用量<br>Les modes d'emploi et la posologie | 　各种不同干扰素制剂的用法不同，简介于下，详见说明书。<br>　Les modes d'emplois pour les interférons se différnecient, consulter les modes d'emploi de chaque médicament. |
| 剂型、规格<br>Les formes pharmaceutiques et les spécifications | 　详见下述干扰素 α、β、γ 各亚型内容。<br>　c.f. aux indications suivantes sur les interférons de type α, β ou γ. |

| 药品名称 Drug Names | 重组人干扰素 α -2a Interféron α -2a humaine recombinante |
|---|---|
| 适应证<br>Les indications | 用于治疗：①某些病毒性疾病：乙型肝炎、丙型肝炎、尖锐湿疣、带状疱疹、小儿病毒性肺炎和上呼吸道感染、慢性宫颈炎等。②某些恶性肿瘤：毛细胞白血病、慢性粒细胞白血病、多发性骨髓瘤、非霍奇金淋巴瘤、卡波济氏肉瘤、肾癌、喉乳头状瘤、黑色素瘤、蕈样肉芽肿、膀胱癌、基底细胞癌等。<br><br>Il permet de traiter : ① Certaines maladies virales : l'hépatite B, l'hépatite C, les verrues génitales, l'herpès zoster, la pneumonie virale chez des enfants, l'infection des voies respiratoires supérieures, la cervicite chronique, etc. ② Certains cancers : la leucémie de cellule poilue, la leucémie myéloïde chronique, le myélome multiple, le lymphome non - Hodgkin, le sarcome de Kaposi, le cancer du rein, le papillome laryngé, le mélanome, le mycosis fongoïde, le carcinome de la vessie, le basal Carcinome, etc. |
| 用法、用量<br>Les modes d'emploi et la posologie | 皮下或肌内注射给药，剂量和疗程如下：①慢性活动性乙型肝炎：每次 500 万 U，一周 3 次，共用 6 个月。一个月后病毒复制标志物如未见下降，剂量可增加至患者能耐受水平；如疗程 3 ～ 4 个月后症状未获改善，则应停止治疗。②急、慢性丙型肝炎：起始剂量为一次 300 万 ～ 500 万 U，一周 3 次，持续 3 个月。对血清谷丙转氨酶（ALT）正常的患者给予维持治疗：一次 300 万 U，一周 3 次，持续 3 个月。ALT 异常者停止使用。③多发性骨髓瘤：起始剂量为一次 300 万 U，一周 3 次，可根据患者的耐受性，逐周增加至最大耐受量（900 万 ～ 1800 万 U）。④毛细胞白血病：起始剂量为一次 300 万 U，一日 1 次，持续 16 ～ 24 周。如患者难以忍受，则剂量减为一次 150 万 U，一周 3 次。⑤慢性粒细胞白血病：采用逐渐增加剂量给药方案，即第 1 ～ 3 日，每日 300 万 U；第 4 ～ 6 日，每日 600 万 U；第 7 ～ 84 日，每日 900 万 U。治疗 8 ～ 12 周后，时视其疗效决定是否继续治疗。⑥非霍奇金淋巴瘤：作为肿瘤化疗的辅助用药，推荐剂量为：一次 300 万 U，一周 3 次，至少持续 12 周。⑦尖锐湿疣：皮下或肌内注射，一次 100 万 ～ 300 万 U，一周 3 次，使用 1 ～ 2 个月。⑧宫颈糜烂：非月经期睡前用手指将一枚栓剂放入阴道贴近子宫颈处，隔日 1 次，9 次为 1 个疗程。<br><br>Injection sous-cutanée ou IM :<br>① Pour traiter l'hépatite B chronique active : 5 millions d'u par fois, 3 fois par semaine, pendant 6 mois au total. Un mois après, si les marqueurs de la réplication virale ne diminuent pas, augmenter la dose jusqu'au niveau tolérable ; s'il est toujours inefficace pendant 3 à 4 mois de traitement, arrêter le traitement.Alanine aminotransférase sérique. ② Pour traiter l'hépatite C aigue et chronique : la dose initiale, 3 millions d'u à 5 millions d'u par fois, 3 fois par semaine, pendant 3 mois consécutifs. Chez les patients dont l'alanine aminotransférase (ALT) est normale, prendre la dose d'entretien : 3 millions d'u par fois, 3 fois par semaine, pendant 3 mois consécutifs. Chez les patients dont l'ALT est anormale, arrêter l'administration. ③ Pour traiter le myélome multiple : la dose initiale, 3 millions d'u par fois, 3 fois par semaine, selon la tolérance des patients, augmenter la dose jusqu'à la dose tolérée maximale (9 millions d'u à 18 millions d'u). ④ Pour traiter la leucémie de cellule poilue : la dose initiale est de 3 millions d'u par fois, 1 fois par jour, pendant 16 à 24 semaines consécutives. S'il est mal toléré, diminuer la dose pour atteindre 1,5 million d'u par fois, 3 fois par semaine. ⑤ Pour traiter la leucémie myéloïde chronique : augmenter progressivement la dose, à savoir, du 1er au 3ème jour, 3 millions d'u par jour ; du 4ème au 6ème jour, 6 millions d'u par jour ; du 7ème au 84ème jour, 9 millions d'u par jour. 8 à 12 semaines après, continuer ou arrêter le traitement selon les cas. ⑥ Pour traiter le lymphome non – Hodgkin : comme traitement adjuvant de la chimiothérapie, la dose recommandée est de 3 millions d'u par fois, 3 fois par semaine, pendant 12 semaines au moins. ⑦ Pour traiter les verrues génitales : injection sous-cutanée ou IM, 1 million à 3 millions d'u par fois, 3 fois par semaine, pendant 1 à 2mois. ⑧ Pour traiter l'érosion du col utérin : introduire un suppositoire dans le vagin près du col utérin avant le sommeil en dehors de la menstruation, une fois tous les 2 jours, 9 fois comme un traitement médical. |
| 剂型、规格<br>Les formes pharmaceutiques et les spécifications | 注射剂：每支 100 万 U；300 万 U；450 万 U；500 万 U；600 万 U；900 万 U；1800 万 U。栓剂：每支 6 万 U；50 万 U。<br><br>Injection : 1 million d'U, 3 millions d'U, 4,5 millions d'U, 5 millions d'U, 6 millions d'U, 9 millions d'U, 18 millions d'U par solution.<br>Suppositoires : 60 000 U ou 500 000U par pièce. |

**续　表**

| 药品名称 Drug Names | 聚乙二醇干扰素 α-2a Péginterféron alfa-2a |
| --- | --- |
| 适应证<br>Les indications | 用于治疗慢性丙型肝炎，适用于无肝硬化和非肝硬化代偿期的患者。<br>Il sert à traiter l'hépatite C chronique. Il est applicable chez les patients sans cirrhose et non cirrhotiques décompensée. |
| 用法、用量<br>Les modes d'emploi et la posologie | 皮下注射，一次 180μg（1ml），每周 1 次，共 48 周。可根据发生的不良反应调整剂量，可减至 45～90μg 乃至 135μg，不良反应减轻后可增加或恢复规定剂量。<br>Injection sous-cutanée, 180μg (1ml) par fois, 1 fois par semaine, pendant 48 semaines au total. Ajuster la dose en fonction des réactions indésirables, possible de diminuer jusqu'à 45 à 90μg ou 135μg, après le soulagement des réactions indésirables, augmenter la dose ou reprendre la dose usuelle. |
| 剂型、规格<br>Les formes pharmaceutiques et les spécifications | 注射剂：每支 45μg/1ml；90μg/ml；135μg/1ml；180μg/1ml。<br>注射剂（预充式注射器）：每支 135μg/0.5ml；180μg/0.5ml。<br>Injection : 45μg/1ml；90μg/ml；135μg/1ml；180μg/1ml par solution.<br>Injection (Seringues pré-remplies) :135μg/0.5ml；180μg/0.5ml par solution. |
| 药品名称 Drug Names | 重组人干扰素 α-1b Interféron α-1b humaine recombinante |
| 适应证<br>Les indications | 用于病毒性疾病和某些恶性肿瘤。①已批准用于临床治疗慢性乙型肝炎、丙型肝炎和毛细胞白血病。②已有临床试验结果和文献的有：带状疱疹、尖锐湿疣、流行性出血热和小儿呼吸道合胞病毒性肺炎等病毒性疾病，以及慢性粒细胞白血病、黑色素瘤、淋巴瘤、肝细胞瘤、肺癌、直肠癌、膀胱癌、多发性骨髓瘤等恶性肿瘤。③滴眼液可用于眼部病毒性疾病。<br>Il sert à traiter des maladies virales et certains cancers. ① Il est déjà autorisé de l'utiliser dans le traitement des maladies suivantes : l'hépatite chronique B, l'hépatite C et la leucémie à tricholeucocytes. ② Selon les résultats cliniques et des documents de référence, il peut être appliqué dans le traitement des maladies suivantes : le zona, les verrues génitales, l'épidémie de fièvre hémorragique, la pneumonie du virus respiratoire syncytial chez des enfants et d'autres maladies virales ; la leucémie myéloïde chronique, le mélanome, le lymphome, l'hépatome, le cancer du poumon, le cancer colorectal, le cancer de la vessie, le myélome multiple et d'autres tumeurs malignes. ③ Ses gouttes pour les yeux sont applicables dans le traitement des maladies virales oculaires. |
| 用法、用量<br>Les modes d'emploi et la posologie | 皮下或肌内注射给药，一次 30～50μg，隔日或一日 1 次，疗程不超过 6 个月或视病情而定。<br>Injection sous-cutanée ou IM, 30 à 50μg par fois, tous les 2 jours ou une fois par jour, ne pas dépasser 6 mois ou selon les cas. |
| 剂型、规格<br>Les formes pharmaceutiques et les spécifications | 注射剂：每支 10μg（100 万 U）；20μg（200 万 U）；30μg（300 万 U）；50μg（500 万 U）。<br>滴眼液：20 万 U/2ml。<br>Injection : 10μg (1 million d'U), 20μg (2 millions d'U), 30μg (2 millions d'U) ou 50μg (5 millions d'U) par solution.<br>Les gouttes pour les yeux : 200 000 U par 2ml. |
| 药品名称 Drug Names | 重组人干扰素 α-2b Interféron α-2b humaine recombinante |
| 适应证<br>Les indications | 用于：①慢性活动性乙型、丙型、丁型病毒性肝炎、带状疱疹、尖锐湿疣等病毒性疾病；②毛细血管性白血病、慢性粒细胞性白血病、多发性骨髓瘤、非霍奇金淋巴瘤、艾滋病相关的喉乳头状瘤或卡波西肉瘤、肾细胞癌、卵巢癌、恶性黑色素瘤等恶性肿瘤。<br>Ce produit sert à traiter :<br>① L'hépatite B chronique active, l'hépatite C, l'hépatite D hépatite virale , l'herpès zoster , les verrues génitales et d'autres maladies virales. ② La leucémie capillaire, la leucémie myéloïde chronique, le myélome multiple, le lymphome non - Hodgkin, le papillome laryngé ou le sarcome de Kaposi lié au sida, le carcinome des cellules rénales, le cancer des ovaires, le mélanome malin et d'autres tumeurs malignes. |

**续　表**

| 用法、用量<br>Les modes d'emploi et la posologie | 推荐的给药途径、剂量及疗程如下：①慢性乙型、丙型肝炎：皮下注射，一次 300 万 U ～ 500 万 U，每日或隔日 1 次，3 ～ 6 个月为 1 个疗程。②慢性丁型肝炎：皮下注射，一次 300 万 U，一周 3 次，至少使用 3 ～ 4 个月。③毛细胞性白血病或喉乳头状瘤：皮下注射，一次 300 万 U，一周 3 次（隔日 1 次）。④慢性粒细胞白血病：单药治疗：皮下注射，一次 400 万 ～ 500 万 U，一日 1 次，至白细胞计数得到控制后，给予最大耐受量维持治疗；与阿糖胞苷合用：先用本药一次 500 万 U，一日 1 次，2 周后加用阿糖胞苷。若以上方案 8 ～ 12 周未见效应停止治疗。⑤多发性骨髓瘤：皮下注射，一次 300 万 ～ 500 万 U，一周 3 次（隔日 1 次）。⑥非霍奇金淋巴瘤：皮下注射，一次 500 万 U，一周 3 次（隔日 1 次），与化疗药合用。⑦艾滋病相关的卡波西肉瘤：皮下注射，一次 300 万 U，一周 3 ～ 5 次，也可每天 100 万 ～ 1200 万 U。⑧肾细胞癌：皮下注射或静脉给药，单药治疗，一次 300 万 ～ 400 万 U，可以一周 3 次、5 次或一日 1 次。⑨转移性类癌瘤：皮下注射，一次 300 万 U，一周 3 次，每日或隔日 1 次。⑩恶性黑色素瘤：诱导治疗，可先静脉给药，剂量为一次 2000 万 U，一周 5 次，共 4 周，然后皮下注射，一次 1000 万 U，一周 3 次，共 48 周。⑪尖锐湿疣：皮下注射，一次 100 万 ～ 300 万 U，一周隔日注射 3 次，1 ～ 2 个月为 1 个疗程。<br><br>① Pour traiter l'hépatite B et C chronique : injection sous-cutanée, 3 millions d'U à 5 millions d'U par fois, une fois par jour ou tous les 2 jours, pendant 3 à 6 mois comme un traitement médical. ② Pour traiter l'hépatite D chronique : injection sous-cutanée, 3 millions d'u par fois, 3 fois par semaine, pendant 3 à 4 mois au moins. ③ Pour traiter la leucémie capillaire ou le papillome laryngé : injection sous-cutanée, 3 millions d'U par fois, 3 fois par semaine (tous les 2 jours). ④ Pour traiter la leucémie myéloide chronique : l'utilisation seule de ce médicament : injection sous-cutanée, 4 millions à 5 millions d'u par fois, 1 fois par jour, après le contrôle du nombre des leucocytes, prendre la dose tolérée maximale comme le traitement d'entretien ; utilisation en association avec ARA : appliquer ce médicament seul, 5 millions d'u par fois, 1 fois par jour, 2 semaines après, ajouter l'ARA. S'il est toujours inefficace pendant 8 à 12 semaines, arrêter le traitement. ⑤ Pour traiter le myélome multiple : injection sous-cutanée, 3 millions d'u à 5 millions d'U par fois, 3 fois par semaine (tous les 2 jours). ⑥ Pour traiter le lymphome non – Hodgkin : injection sous-cutanée, 5 millions d'U par fois, 3 fois par semaine (tous les 2 jours), en association avec la chimiothérapie. ⑦ Pour traiter le sarcome de Kaposi lié au sida : injection sous-cutanée, 3 millions d'U par fois, 3 à 5 fois par semaine, ou 1 millions d'U à 12 millions d' U par jour. ⑧ Pour traiter le carcinome des cellules rénales : injection sous-cutanée ou IM, la monothérapie, 3 millions d'u à 4 millions d'U par fois, 3 fois ou 5 fois par semaine, ou une fois par jour. ⑨ Pour traiter la carcinoïde métastatique : injection sous-cutanée, 3 millions d'U par fois, 3 fois par semaine, ou une fois par jour ou tous les 2 jours. ⑩ Pour traiter le mélanome malin : le traitement d'induction, injection IV, 20 millions d'U par fois, 5 fois par semaine, pendant 4 semaines au total, ensuite, injection sous-cutanée, 10 millions d'U, 3 fois par semaine, pendant 48 semaines. ⑪ Pour traiter les verrues génitales : injection sous-cutanée, 1 million à 3 millions d'U par fois, 3 fois par semaine (tous les 2 jours), pendant 1 à 2 mois comme un traitement médical. |
|---|---|
| 剂型、规格<br>Les formes pharmaceutiques et les spécifications | 注射用粉针剂：每支 100 万 U；300 万 U；500 万 U；1000 万 U；1800 万 U；3000 万 U。<br>注射液（多剂量笔）：180 万 U/1（2）ml。<br>栓剂：每支 50 万 U。<br>Poudre pour injection : 1 million d'U, 3 millions d'U, 5 millions d'U, 10 millions d'U, 18 millions d'U, 30 millions d'U par solution.<br>Injection : 1,8 million d'U par 1 (2) ml.<br>Suppositoires : 500 000U par pièce. |
| **药品名称 Drug Names** | **重组人干扰素 β Interféron β humaine recombinante** |
| 适应证<br>Les indications | ①用于病毒性疾病的治疗，对 RNA、DNA 病毒均敏感，皮下或静脉注射给药用于治疗慢性活动性肝炎、新生儿巨细胞病毒性脑炎。外涂、滴鼻、病灶局部给药用于防治流感 A2 和 B 病毒、鼻病毒所致的感冒、带状疱疹、甚至起疱疹等。②用于多发性硬化疾病。③用于肿瘤性胸腔积液、毛细胞白血病、宫颈上皮肿瘤、或乳腺及子宫内膜肿瘤的甾体激素受体诱导治疗。 |

**续　表**

|  |  |
|---|---|
|  | ① Ce produit sert à traiter des maladies virales. Il est sensible aux virus ARN et ADN. Son administration sous-cutanée ou par voie IV est applicable dans le traitement de l'hépatite chronique active et de l'encéphalite néonatale liée au cytomégalovirus. Son administration à un usage externe, intranasale ou topique est appliquée dans le traitement du rhume, du zona, de l'herpès causés par les virus de la grippe A2 et B ainsi que les rhinovirus. ② Applicable dans le traitement des maladies de la sclérose en plaques. ③ Ce produit est utilisé dans le traitement d'induction des récepteurs d'hormones stéroïdes liés à l'épanchement pleural, àla leucémie à tricholeucocytes, à la néoplasie intra-épithéliale cervicale,au cancer du sein ou au cancer de l'endomètre. |
| 用法、用量<br>Les modes d'emploi et la posologie | ①多发性硬化疾病：皮下注射，每次 44μg，每周 3 次。②生殖器疱疹、带状疱疹：肌内注射，一次 200 万 U，一日 1 次，连续 10 日。③扁平或尖锐湿疣：皮下或病灶局部注射，每日 100 万～300 万 U，连用 5 日为 1 个疗程，每次 1～3 个疗程。或肌内注射，每日 200 万 U，连续 10 日。④慢性乙型肝炎：肌内注射，一次 500 万 U，每周 3 次，连续 6 个月。慢性丙型或丁型肝炎：前 2 个月每次 600 万 U，每周 3 次；后改为每次 300 万 U，每周 3 次，连续 3～6 个月。⑤宫颈上皮肿瘤：病灶内注射，300 万 U，一日 1 次，连续 5 日。后改为隔日 1 次，连续 2 周。⑥肿瘤性胸腔积液：胸穿后将 500 万 U 的本品注入胸膜腔。若 7～15 日后又出现胸腔积液，再次胸穿，注入本品 1000 万 U。若 15 日后再复发，用 50ml 生理盐水稀释 2000 万 U 药物注入胸腔。⑦毛细胞白血病：静脉内缓慢注入，诱导剂量每天 600 万 U，连续 7 日为 1 个疗程，共 3 周（隔周）。维持剂量 600 万 U，每周 2 次，连续 24 周。⑧乳腺肿瘤和子宫内膜肿瘤：肌内注射，每次 200 万～600 万 U，每周 3 次（隔天），共 2 周。此方案在激素治疗期每间隔 4 周可重复使用。<br><br>① Pour traiter les maladies de la sclérose en plaques : injection sous-cutanée, 44μg par fois, 3 fois par semine. ② Pour traiter l'herpès génital, le zona : injection IM, 2 millions d'u par fois, 1 fois par jour, pendant 10 jours consécutifs. ③ Pour traiter les verrues planes ou génitales : injection sous-cutanée ou injection topique sur la zone touchée, 1 million à 3 millions d'u par jour, pendant 5 jours consécutifs comme un traitement, 1 à 3 traitements. Ou Injection IM, 2 millions d'u par jour, pendant 10 jours. ④ Pour traiter l'hépatite B chronique : injection IM, 5 millions d'u par fois, 3 fois par semaine, pendant 6 mois consécutifs. Pour traiter l'hépatite C ou D chronique : les deux premiers mois, 6 millions d'u par fois, 3 fois par semaine ; ensuite, 3 millions d'u par fois, 3 fois par semaine, pendant 3 à 6 mois. ⑤ Pour traiter la néoplasie intra-épithéliale cervicale : injection topique sur la zone touchée, 3 millions d'u, 1 fois par jour, pendant 5 jours consécutifs. Ensuite, tous les 2 jours, pendant 2 semaines consécutives. ⑥ Pour traiter l'épanchement pleural : injecter 5 millions d'u dans la cavité pleurale. S'il y a un autre épanchement pleural dans les 7 à 15 jours, injecter 10 millions d'u dans la cavité pleurale. S'il y a une récurrence 15 jours après, utiliser 50ml de solution saline pour diluer 20 millions d'u, injecter ensuite dans la cavité pleurale. ⑦ Pour traiter Leucémie à tricholeucocytes : injection lente IV, la dose d'induction est de 6 millions d'u par jour, pendant 7 jours comme un traitement, 3 semaines au total (avec un intervalle d'une semaine). La dose d'entretien est de 6 millions d'u, 2 fois par semaine, pendant 24 semaines consécutives. ⑧ Pour traiter cancer du sein ou au cancer de l'endomètre : injection IM, 2 millions à 6 millions d'u par fois, 3 fois par semaine (tous les 2 jours), pendant 2 semaines au total. Ce médicament peut être repris pendant la période de traitement hormonal avec un intervalle de 4 semaines. |
| 剂型、规格<br>Les formes pharmaceutiques et les spécifications | 注射用冻干粉：每安瓿 11μg/2ml（300 万 U）。<br>注射液（预装式注射器）：22μg/0.5ml（600 万 U）；44μg/0.5ml（1200 万 U）。<br>Poudre lyophilisée pour injection : 11μg/2ml (3 millions d'U) par ampoule.<br>Injection (Seringues préchargées) : 22μg/0.5ml(6millions d'U)；44μg/0.5ml(12 millions d'U). |
| **药品名称 Drug Names** | 重组人干扰素 γ Interféron γ humaine recombinante |
| 适应证<br>Les indications | 用于类风湿关节炎、迁延性肝病及肝纤维化的治疗。<br>Ce produit est utilisé dans le traitement de la polyarthrite rhumatoïde, de la maladie du foie persistante et de la fibrose hépatique. |

**续　表**

| | |
|---|---|
| 用法、用量<br>Les modes d'emploi et la posologie | ①类风湿关节炎：皮下注射，初始剂量为一次 50 万 U，一日 1 次，连续 3～4 日，如无不良反应，将剂量加至每日 100 万 U；第二个月改为一次 150 万～200 万 U，隔日 1 次，总疗程为 3 个月。<br>②肝纤维化：皮下注射，前 3 个月，一次 50 万 U，一日 1 次，后 6 个月，一次 100 万 U，隔日 1 次。<br><br>① Pour traiter la polyarthrite rhumatoide : injection sous-cutanée, la dose initiale, 500 000 U par fois, 1 fois par jour, pendant 3 à 4 jours consécutifs, s'il n'y pas de réactions indésirables, augmenter jusqu'à 1 million d'u par jour ; le deuxième mois, 1,5 million à 2 millions d'u par fois, tous les 2 jours, pendant 3 mois au total. ② Pour traiter la fibrose hépatique : injection sous-cutanée, les 3 premiers mois, 500 000u par fois, 1 fois par jour, les 6 derniers mois, 1million d'u par fois, tous les 2 jours. |
| 剂型、规格<br>Les formes pharmaceutiques et les spécifications | 注射剂：每支 50 万 U；100 万 U；200 万 U。<br><br>Injection : 500 000 U, 1 million d'U, 2 millions d'U par solution. |
| **药品名称 Drug Names** | 人免疫球蛋白 Immunoglobuline humaine |
| 适应证<br>Les indications | 用于免疫缺陷疾病和传染性肝炎、麻疹、水痘、腮腺炎、带状疱疹等病毒感染和细菌感染的防治，也用于哮喘、过敏性鼻炎、湿疹等内源性过敏性疾病。<br><br>Ce produit sert à prévenir et à traiter les infections virales ou bactériennes, telles que les maladies d'immunodéficience, l'hépatite infectieuse, la rougeole, la varicelle, les oreillons et l'herpès zoster. Il est aussi applicable dans le traitement de l'asthme, dela rhinite allergique, del'eczéma et d'autres maladies allergiques endogènes. |
| 用法、用量<br>Les modes d'emploi et la posologie | 肌内注射：①预防麻疹：0.05～0.15ml/kg 或儿童 5 岁以下 1.5～3ml，成人不超过 6ml，预防效果 1 个月。②预防甲型肝炎：0.05～0.15ml/kg 或儿童 1.5～3ml，成人每次 3ml，预防效果 1 个月。③预防乙型肝炎：成人一次 200U，儿童 100U，必要时隔 3～4 周再注射一次。母为乙肝表面抗原或核心抗原双阳者，婴儿出生 24 小时内注射 100U，阻断预防。<br><br>Injection IM :<br>① Pour prévenir la rougeole : 0,05 à 0,15 ml par kg ou chez des enfants moins de 5 ans, 1,5 à 3ml, ne pas dépasser 6ml chez des adultes, l'effet préventif dure 1 mois. ② Pour prévenir l'hépatite A : 0,05 à 0,15 ml par kg ou chez des enfants, 1,5 à 3ml, chez des adultes, 3ml par fois, l'effet préventif dure 1 mois. ③ Pour prévenir l'hépatitie B : chez des adultes, 200U par fois, chez des enfants, 100 U, s'il est nécessaire, encore une injection toutes les 3 à 4 semaines. Si les antigènes de surface et de base du virus de l'hépatite B de la mère sont tous positifs, il faut injecter chez son bébé 100U en 24 h suivant sa naissance pour la prévention de blocage. |
| 剂型、规格<br>Les formes pharmaceutiques et les spécifications | 注射液（10%）：每支 150mg/1.5ml，300mg/3ml，500mg/5ml。<br>注射冻干粉：每支 150mg；300mg；500mg。<br>注射液：每支 100U；200U；400U。<br><br>Injection (10%) : 150mg/1.5ml,300mg/3ml,500mg/5ml par solution.<br>Poudre lyophilisée pour injection : 150mg, 300mg ou 500mg par solution.<br>Injection : 100U, 200U ou 400U par solution. |
| **药品名称 Drug Names** | 静脉注射用人免疫球蛋白 Immunoglobuline pour injection |
| 适应证<br>Les indications | 用于原发性和继发性免疫球蛋白缺乏症如 X 连锁低免疫球蛋白血症、重症感染、艾滋病；自身免疫性疾病如原发性血小板减少性紫癜、川崎病、重症系统性红斑狼疮等。<br><br>Ce produit sert à traiter la déficience en immunoglobuline primaire et secondaire, tel que l'immunoglobuline faible liée à l'X, l'infection sévère, le SIDA ; et les maladies auto-immunes telles que le purpura thrombocytopénique idiopathique, la maladie de Kawasaki, le lupus érythémateux systémique sévère, etc. |
| 用法、用量<br>Les modes d'emploi et la posologie | ①免疫球蛋白缺乏或低下症：按体重一日 400mg/kg，维持量为 200～400mg/kg，用药间隔视血清 IgG 水平定。②特发性血小板减少性紫癜：开始一日 400mg/kg，连续 5 日，维持量一次 400mg/kg，每周一次或视血小板计数而定。③川崎病：发病 10 日内使用。儿童一次 2.0g/kg，一次静脉滴注。④严重感染：一日 200～400mg/kg，连续 3～5 日。 |

续　表

| | |
|---|---|
| | ① Pour traiter la déficience en immunoglobuline : 400 mg/kg par jour, la dose d'entretien, 200 à 400 mg/kg par jour, l'intervalle dépend du taux des IgG sériques. ② Pour traiter le purpura thrombocytopénique idiopathique : commencer par 400mg/kg par jour, pendant 5 jours consécutifs, la dose d'entretien, 400mg/kg par fois, une fois par semaine ou en fonction du nombre plaquettaire. ③ Pour traiter la maladie de Kawasaki : utilisée en 10 jours suivant la crise de la maladie. Chez des enfants, 2,0 g par kg par fois, une perfusion. ④ Pour des infections sévères : 200 à 400 mg/kg par jour, pendant 3 à 5 jours consécutifs. |
| 剂型、规格<br>Les formes pharmaceutiques et les spécifications | 注射液 pH4 每瓶 1g；1.25g；2.5g；4g。<br>Injection pH4 : 1g, 1,25g, 2,5g ou 4g par flacon. |
| 药品名称 Drug Names | 乌苯美司 Ubénimex |
| 适应证<br>Les indications | 竞争性抑制氨肽酶 B 及亮氨酸肽酶。可刺激骨髓细胞再生及分化。<br>Il sert d'inhibition compétitive de l'aminopeptidase B et de la leucine peptidase. Il est capable de stimuler la régénération et la différenciation des cellules de la moelle osseuse. |
| 用法、用量<br>Les modes d'emploi et la posologie | 口服，每日 30 ～ 100mg，1 次或分 2 次服。也可每周服 2 ～ 3 日，10 个月为 1 个疗程。<br>Par voie orale, 30 à 100mg par jour, à travers 1 ou 2 fois. Aussi possible de prendre 2 à 3 jours par semaine, pendant 10 mois comme un traitement médical. |
| 剂型、规格<br>Les formes pharmaceutiques et les spécifications | 片剂：每片 10mg。<br>胶囊剂：每粒 10mg；30mg。<br>Comprimés : 10mg par comprimé.<br>Capsules : 10mg ou 30mg par capsule. |
| 药品名称 Drug Names | 白芍总苷 Glucoside total de paeonia alba |
| 适应证<br>Les indications | 免疫调节药，改善类风湿关节炎患者症状。<br>En tant qu'agent immunomodulateur, ce produit permet d'améliorer les symptômes des patients atteints de polyarthrite rhumatoïde. |
| 用法、用量<br>Les modes d'emploi et la posologie | 口服，一次 300mg，一日 2 ～ 3 次。<br>Par voie orale, 300mg par fois, 2 à 3 fois par jour. |
| 剂型、规格<br>Les formes pharmaceutiques et les spécifications | 胶囊剂：每粒 300mg。<br>Capsules : 300mg par capsule. |

18. 维生素类、酶及生化制剂，调节水、电解质及酸碱平衡和营养类药物 Vitamines, enzymes et agents biochimiques, médicament régulateur de l'équilibre eau, électrolyte et acide-base,et médicaments nutritionnels

18.1　维生素类 Les vitamines

| 药品名称 Drug Names | 维生素 A Vitamine A(Retinol) |
|---|---|
| 适应证<br>Les indications | 用于：①维生素 A 缺乏症：如夜盲症、眼干燥症、角膜软化症和皮肤粗糙等。②用于补充需要，如妊娠、哺乳期妇女和婴儿等。③有学者认为对预防上皮癌、食管癌的发生有一定意义。<br>Ce produit sert à traiter : ① La carence en vitamine A : comme la cécité nocturne, le syndrome de l'oeil sec, le keratomalacia et la peau rugueuse. ② Pour des besoins supplémentaires, tels que la grossesse, les femmes allaitant et les bébés. ③ Certains croient qu'il a un certain effet sur la prévention du cancer épithélial et du cancer de l'œsophage. |

**续 表**

| | |
|---|---|
| 用法、用量<br>Les modes d'emploi et la posologie | ①严重维生素A缺乏症：口服，成人每日10万U，3日后改为每日5万U，给药2周，然后每日1万～2万U，再用药2个月。吸收功能障碍或口服困难者可用肌内注射，成人每日5万～10万U，3日后改为每日5万U，给药2周；1～8岁儿童，每日0.5万～1.5万U，给药10日；婴儿，每日0.5万～1万U，给药10日。②轻度维生素A缺乏症：每日1万～2.5万U，分2～3次口服。③补充需要：成人每日5000U，哺乳期妇女每日5000U，婴儿每日600～1500U，儿童每日2000～3000U。<br><br>① Pour traiter la carence grave en vitamine A : par voie orale, chez des adutles, 100 000 U par jour, 3 jours après, 50 000 U par jour, pendant 2 semaines, ensuite, 10 000 U à 20 000 U par jour, pendant 2 mois. En cas d'absorption ou d'administration orale difficiles, possible d'injecter par IM, chez des adultes, 50 000 à 100 000 U par jour, 3 jours après, 50 000 U par jour, pendant 2 semaines ; 1 à 8 ans, 5 000 à 15 000 U par jour, pendant 10 jours ; chez des bébés, 5 000 U à 10 000 U par jour, pendant 10 jours. ② Pour traiter la carence bénigne en vitamine A : 10 000 à 25 000 U par jour, à travers 2 à 3 fois, par voie orale. ③ Pour le besoin supplémentaire : chez des adultes, 5 000U par jour, chez des femmes pendant l'allaitement, 5 000 U par jour, chez des bébés, 600 à 1 500 U par jour, chez des enfants, 2 000 à 3 000 U par jour. |
| 剂型、规格<br>Les formes pharmaceutiques et les spécifications | 胶丸剂：每丸5000U；2.5万U。<br>Granules : 5 000 U ou 25 000 U par granule. |
| 药品名称 Drug Names | 维生素D　Vitamine D |
| 适应证<br>Les indications | 维生素D缺乏，防治佝偻病、骨软化症和婴儿手足搐搦症。<br><br>Ce produit est utilisé pour traiter la carence en vitamine D. Il permet aussi de prévenir et de traiter le rachitisme, l'ostéomalacie et la tétanie chez des bébés. |
| 用法、用量<br>Les modes d'emploi et la posologie | ①治疗佝偻病：口服一日2500～5000U，1～2个月后待症状开始消失时即改用预防量。若不能口服者、重症的患者，肌内注射一次30万～60万U，如需要，1个月后再肌内注射1次，两次总量不超过90万U。用大剂量维生素D时如缺钙，应口服10%氯化钙，一次5～10ml，一日3次，用2～3日。②婴儿手足搐搦症：口服一日2000～5000U，1个月后改为每日400U。③预防维生素D缺乏症：用母乳喂养的婴儿一日400U，妊娠期必要时1日400U。<br><br>① Pour traiter le rachitisme : par voie orale, 2 500 à 5 000 U par jour, 1 à 2 mois après quand il y a une disparition des symptômes, prendre la dose d'entretien. Chez des patiens gravement malades incapables d'administrer par voie orale, injection IM, 300 000 à 600 000 U par fois, s'il est nécessaire, 1 mois après, injection IM encore une fois, ne pas dépasser 900 000 U par ces deux fois. Lors d'une forte dose de la vitamine D pour traiter la carence en calcium par exemple, il faut prendre par voie orale le chlorure de calcium à 10%, 5 à 10ml par fois, 3 fois par jour, pendant 2 à 3 jours. ② Pour traiter la tétanie chez des bébés : par voie orale, 2 000 à 5 000 U par jour, un mois après, 400U par jour. ③ Pour prévenir la carence en vitamine D : chez des bébés allaités, 400U par jour, pendant la grossesse, s'il est nécessaire, 400U par jour. |
| 剂型、规格<br>Les formes pharmaceutiques et les spécifications | 维生素$D_2$胶丸：每粒含1万U。维生素$D_2$片：每片5000U；10 000U。维生素$D_2$胶性钙注射液：每支1ml；10ml。每1ml含D25万U，胶性钙0.5mg。维生素$D_3$注射液：每支15万U（0.5ml）；30万U（1ml）；60万U（1ml）。用前及用时需服钙剂。维生素AD胶丸：每粒含维生素A 3000U，维生素D 300U。浓维生素AD胶丸：每粒含维生素A 1万U，维生素D 1000U。维生素AD滴剂：每1g含维生素A 5000U，维生素D 500U；每1g含维生素A 5万U，维生素D 5000U；每1g含维生素A 9000U，维生素D 3000U。<br><br>Granules de vitamine $D_2$ : 10 000U par granule. Comprimés de vitamine $D_2$ : 5000U ou 10 000U par comprimé. Injection plastique de calcium de vitamine $D_2$ : 1ml ou a0ml par solution. Chaque 1ml de solution contient 250 000 U de vitamine D et 0,5 mg de calcium plastique. Injection de vitamine $D_3$ : 150 000 U (0,5ml), 300 000 U (1ml), 600 000U (1ml) par oslution. Avant et durant l'injection, il faut prendre le calcium. Granules de vitamine AD : 3000 U de vitamine A et 300U de vitamine D par granule. Granules concentrés de vitamine AD : 5000U de vitamine A et 500U de vitamine D par 1g ; 50 000U de vitamine A et 5 000 U de vitamine D par 1g ; 9 000 U de vitamine A et 3000 U de vitamine D par 1g. |

**续　表**

| 药品名称 Drug Names | 骨化三醇 Calcitriol |
|---|---|
| 适应证<br>Les indications | 　　应用于甲状腺功能低下症及血液透析患者的肾性营养不良，骨质疏松症，维生素 D 依赖性佝偻病（肾小管缺乏 1-α 羟化酶）。<br><br>　　Ce produit sert à traiter l'hypothyroïdie, la malnutrition rénale chez des patients hémodialysés, l'ostéoporose, le rachitisme de vitamine D dépendant (lacarence en hydroxylase 1 – α de tubules rénaux). |
| 用法、用量<br>Les modes d'emploi et la posologie | 　　口服剂量应根据患者的血钙浓度来决定。①血液透析患者的肾性营养不良：如患者血钙浓度正常或略低，口服，一日 0.25μg。如 2～4 周生化指标及病情无明显改变，则一日剂量可达到 0.5μg。每周应测两次血钙浓度，随时调整剂量。大多数血透患者用量在一日 0.5～1μg。②甲状腺功能低下：儿童 1～5 岁，一日 0.25～0.75μg；6 岁以上和成人，一日 0.5～2μg（用量须个体化）。<br><br>　　La dose orale dépend de la concentration du calcium dans le sang.<br>　　① Pour traiter la malnutrition réanle chez des patients hémodialysés : si la concentration du calcium dans le sang est normale ou un peu basse, par voie orale, 0,25μg par jour. S'il n'y pas d'amélioration évidente des symptômes, 0,5 μg par jour. il faut examiner la concentration du calcium dans le sang 2 fois par semaine pour ajuster la dose. Chez la plupart des patients hémodialysés, 0,5 à 1μg par jour.<br>　　② Pour traiter l'hypothyroide : chez des enfants de 1 à 5 ans, 0,25 à 0,75 μg par jour ; chez plus de 6 ans et des adultes, 0,5 à 2 μg par jour (il faut personnaliser la dose). |
| 剂型、规格<br>Les formes pharmaceutiques et les spécifications | 　　胶囊剂：每粒 0.25μg；0.5μg。<br>　　Capsules : 0,25μg ou 0,5 μg par capsule. |
| 药品名称 Drug Names | 阿法骨化醇 Alfacalcidol |
| 适应证<br>Les indications | 　　用于慢性肾衰竭合并骨质疏松症、甲状腺功能低下及抗维生素 D 的佝偻病患者。<br>　　Ce produit sert à traiter l'insuffisance rénale chronique combinée de l'ostéoporose, l'hypothyroïdie et des patients atteints de rachitisme résistant à la vitaine D. |
| 用法、用量<br>Les modes d'emploi et la posologie | 　　①慢性肾衰竭合并骨质疏松：成人，口服，一次 0.5～1.0μg，一日 1 次。②甲状腺功能低下和抗维生素 D 的佝偻病：成人，口服，一日 1.0～4.0μg，一日 2～3 次。<br><br>　　① Pour traiter l'insuffisance rénale chronique combinée de l'ostéoporose : chez des adultes, par voie orale, 0,5 à 1,0 μg par fois, 1 fois par jour. ② Pour traiter l'hypothyroïdie et le rachitisme résistant à la vitaine D : chez des adultes, par voie orale, 1,0 à 4,0 μg par jour, 2 à 3 fois par jour. |
| 剂型、规格<br>Les formes pharmaceutiques et les spécifications | 　　胶囊剂：每粒 0.25μg；0.5μg；1.0μg。<br>　　Capsules : 0,25 μg, 0,5 μg ou 1,0 μg par capsule. |
| 药品名称 Drug Names | 维生素 B$_1$　Vitamine B$_1$(Thiamine) |
| 适应证<br>Les indications | 　　用于脚气病防治及各种疾病的辅助治疗（如全身感染、高热、糖尿病、多发性神经炎、小儿麻痹后遗症以及小儿遗尿症、心肌炎、食欲缺乏、消化不良、甲状腺功能亢进和妊娠期等）。对解除某些药物如链霉素、庆大霉素等引起的听觉障碍有帮助。<br><br>　　Ce produit est utilisé dans la prévention du béribéri etle traitement adjuvant de diverses maladies ( telles que les infections systémiques, la fièvre, le diabète, la névrite multiple, les séquelles de poliomyélite et l'énurésie chez des enfants, la myocardite, une perte d'appétit, l'indigestion, l'hyperthyroïdie et la grossesse , etc ). Il permet aussi de soulager les malentendants causés par certains médicaments tels que la streptomycine et la gentamicine. |
| 用法、用量<br>Les modes d'emploi et la posologie | 　　成人每日的最小必需量为 1mg，孕妇及小儿因发育原因需要较多。在治疗脚气病及消化不良时可根据病情调整。成人 1 次 10～20mg，一日 3 次，口服；或 1 次 50～100mg，一日 1 次，肌内注射。儿童 1 次 5～10mg，一日 3 次，口服；或 1 次 10～20mg，一日 1 次，肌内注射。不宜静脉注射。 |

**续 表**

|  | Chez des adultes, la dose minimale nécessaire est de 1mg par jour, chez des femmes enceintes et des enfants, la dose est plus importante. Ajuster la dose selon les cas pour traiter le béribéri et l'indigestion. Chez des adultes, 10 à 20mg par fois, 3 fois par jour, par voie orale ; ou 50 à 100mg par fois, 1 fois par jour, injection IM. Chez des enfants, 5 à 10mg par fois, 3 fois par jour, par voie orale ; ou 10 à 20mg par fois, 1 fois par jour, injection IM. Il faut éviter l'injection IM. |
|---|---|
| 剂型、规格<br>Les formes pharmaceutiques et les spécifications | 片剂：每片 5mg；10mg。<br>注射液：每支 10mg（1ml）；25mg（1ml）；50mg（2ml）；100mg（2ml）。<br>Comprimés : 5mg ou 10mg par comprimé.<br>Injection : 10mg (1ml), 25mg (1ml), 50mg (2ml) ou 100mg (2ml) par solution. |
| 药品名称 Drug Names | 维生素 B$_2$　Vitamine B$_2$(Riboflavine) |
| 适应证<br>Les indications | 用于口角炎、唇炎、舌炎、眼结膜炎和阴囊炎等的防治。<br>Ce produit sert à prévenir et à traiter la perlèche,la chéilite,la glossite, la conjonctivite et le scrotum. |
| 用法、用量<br>Les modes d'emploi et la posologie | 成人每日的需要量为 2～3mg。治疗口角炎、舌炎、阴囊炎等时，一次可服 5～10mg，一日 3 次，或皮下注射或肌内注射 5～10mg，一日 1 次，连用数周，至病势减退为止。<br>Chez des adultes, la dose nécessaire est de 2 à 3mg par jour. pour traiter la perlèche, la glossite, le scrotum, 5 à 10mg par fois, 3 fois par jour, ou injecter par voie sous-cutanée ou IM 5 à 10mg, 1 fois par jour, pendant plusieurs semaines consécutives, jusqu'à la réduction des symptômes. |
| 剂型、规格<br>Les formes pharmaceutiques et les spécifications | 片剂：每片 5mg；10mg。<br>注射液：每支 1mg（2ml）；5mg（2ml）；10mg（2ml）。<br>Comprimés : 5mg ou 10mg par comprimé.<br>Injection : 1mg (2ml), 5mg (2ml) ou 10mg (2ml) par solution. |
| 药品名称 Drug Names | 烟酸 Acide nicotinique |
| 适应证<br>Les indications | 用于预防和治疗因烟酸缺乏引起的糙皮病等。也用作血管扩张药及治疗高脂血症。对于严格控制或选择饮食或接受肠道外营养的患者，因营养不良体重骤减，妊娠期、哺乳期妇女，以及服用异烟肼者，严重烟瘾、酗酒、吸毒者，烟酸的需要量均需增加。<br>Ce produit sert à prévenir et à traiter la pellagre causée par la carence en acide nicotinique. Il sert aussi de vasodilatateur et permet le traitement de l'hyperlipidémie. Chez des patients choisissant la nutrition parentérale, chez des personnes dont lePoid chute en raison de la malnutrition, chez des femmes pendant la grossesse et l'allaitement, chez des patients prenant l'isoniazide et chez des patients dépendant gravement de la cigarette, de l'alcool et de drogue, l'utilisation de l'acide nicotimique doit être augmentée. |
| 用法、用量<br>Les modes d'emploi et la posologie | ①推荐膳食每日摄入量：出生至 3 岁 5～9mg，4～6 岁 12mg，7～10 岁 12mg，男性青少年及成人 15～20mg，女性青少年及成人 13～15mg，孕妇 17mg，哺乳期妇女 20mg。②糙皮病：成人口服：1 次 50～100mg，一日 5 次；静注：1 次 25～100mg，一日 2 次或多次。儿童口服：1 次 25～50mg，一日 2～3 次；静脉缓慢注射：一日 300mg。③抗高血脂：成人口服，缓释片或缓释胶囊，推荐 1～4 周一次 0.5g，一日 1 次；5～8 周为一次 1g，一日 1 次；8 周后，根据患者的疗效和耐受性逐渐增加，如有必要，最大剂量可加至 2g。应在少量低脂肪饮食就睡前服用。须整片（粒）吞服。维持剂量：每日 1～2g。女性患者的剂量低于男性患者。<br>① Apport quotidien recommandé en diététique : chez 3 ans ou moins, 5 à 9mg, de 4 à 6 ans, 12mg, de 7 à 10 ans, 12mg, chez des adolescents et des adultes masculins, 15 à 20mg, chez des adolescents et des adultes féminins, 13 à 15mg, chez des femmes enceintes, 17mg, chez des femmes pendant l'allaitement, 20mg. ② Pour traiter la pellagre : chez des adultes, par voie orale : 50 à 100mg par fois, 5 fois par jour ; injection IM : 25 à 100mg par fois, 2 fois ou plusieurs fois par jour. Chez des enfants par voie orale : 25 à 50mg par fois, 2 à 3 fois par jour ; injection IM lente : 300mg par jour. ③ Pour traiter l'hyperlipidémie : chez des adultes, par voie orale, comprimés à libération prolongée ou capsules à libération prolongée, il est recommandé de prendre 0,5g par fois, 1 fois par jour pendant 1 à 4 semaines ; de 5ème à la 8ème semaine, 1g par fois, 1 fois par jour ; 8 semaines après, augmenter progressivement la dose en fonction de l'efficacité et de la tolérance des patients, s'il est nécessaire, 2g au maximum. Il faut le prendre avant le sommeil avec des aliments de petite quantité et faibles en gras. Il faut l'avaler en entier. La dose d'entretien : 1 à 2g par jour. La dose chez des femmes est moins importante que chez des hommes. |

续　表

| | |
|---|---|
| 剂型、规格<br>Les formes pharmaceutiques et les spécifications | 片剂、胶囊剂：每片 50mg；100mg。<br>注射液：50mg/ml；100mg/ml。<br>Comprimés ou capsules : 50mg ou 100mg par comprimé.<br>Injection : 50 mg par ml ou 100mg par ml. |
| 药品名称 Drug Names | 维生素 B₆　Vitamine B₆(Pyridoxine) |
| 适应证<br>Les indications | 用于：①防治因大量或长期服用异烟肼、肼屈嗪等引起的周围神经炎、失眠、不安；减轻抗癌药和放射治疗引起恶心、呕吐或妊娠呕吐等。②治疗因而惊厥或给孕妇服用以预防婴儿惊厥。③白细胞减少症。④局部涂搽治疗痤疮、酒糟鼻、脂溢性湿疹等。<br>Ce produit sert à : ① Prévenir et traiter la névrite périphérique, l'insomnie, l'anxiété causées par l'administration à long terme de l'isoniazide et de l'hydralazine. Il sert aussi à atténuer les nausées, les vomissements ou les vomissements de la grossesse induits par les médicaments anticancéreux et la radiothérapie. ② Traiter les convulsions infantiles ou faire adminitrer aux femmes enceintes pour prévenir les convulsions infantiles. ③ Traiter la leucopénie. ④ L'application topique permet de traiterl'acné, la rosacée, l'eczéma séborrhéique, etc. |
| 用法、用量<br>Les modes d'emploi et la posologie | 口服：一次 10～20mg，一日 3 次（缓释片一次 50mg，一日 1～2 次）。皮下注射、肌内注射、静脉注射：一次 50mg，一日 1～2 次。皮下注射、肌内注射、静脉注射：一次 50～100mg，一日 1 次。治疗白细胞减少症时，以 50～100mg，加入 5% 葡萄糖注射液 20ml 中做静脉注射，一日 1 次。<br>Par voie orale : 10 à 20mg par fois, 3 fois par jour (pour les comprimés à libération prolongée, 50mg par fois, 1 à 2 fois par jour). Injection sous-cutanée, IM ou IV : 50mg par fois, 1 à 2 fois par jour. Injection sous-cutanée, IM ou IV : 50 à 100mg par fois, 1 fois par jour. Pour traiter la leucopénie, 50 à 100mg, dissoudre dans 20ml de solution de glucose à 5%, injection IM, 1 fois par jour. |
| 剂型、规格<br>Les formes pharmaceutiques et les spécifications | 片剂：每片 10mg。<br>维生素 B₆ 缓释片：每片 50mg。<br>注射液：每支 25mg（1ml）；50mg（1ml）；100mg（22ml）。霜剂：每支含 12mg。<br>Comprimés : 10mg par comprimé.<br>Comprimés à libération prolongée de vitamine B₆ : 50mg par comprimé.<br>Injection : 25mg (1ml), 50mg (1ml) ou 100mg (22ml).<br>Crème : 12mg par pièce. |
| 药品名称 Drug Names | 干酵母 Levure sèche |
| 适应证<br>Les indications | 用于防止脚气病、多发性神经炎、糙皮病等。<br>Ce produit sert à traiter le béribéri,la polynévrite, la pellagre, etc. |
| 用法、用量<br>Les modes d'emploi et la posologie | 每次服 0.5～4g，一日 3 次，服时嚼碎。<br>0,5 à 4g par fois, 3 fois par jour, comprimés à mâcher. |
| 剂型、规格<br>Les formes pharmaceutiques et les spécifications | 片剂：0.3g；0.5g。<br>Comprimés : 0,3g ou 0,5g. |
| 药品名称 Drug Names | 维生素 C　Vitamine C(Acide ascorbique) |
| 适应证<br>Les indications | 用于：①坏血病的预防及治疗。②急慢性传染病时，消耗量增加，宜适当补充。病后恢复期，创伤愈合不良者，也应适当补充。③克山病患者在发生心源性休克时，可用大剂量治疗。④用于肝硬化、急性肝炎和砷、汞、铅、苯等慢性中毒时的肝脏损害。⑤其他：用于各种贫血、过敏性皮肤病、口疮、促进伤口愈合等。<br>Ce produit sert à :<br>① La prévention et le traitement du scorbut. ② Pour traiter les infections aigues ou chroniques, il faut administrer la vitamine C pour compenser une consommation plus importante. Lors de la convalescence, il faut prendre un peu la vitamine C chez des patiens dont la cicatrisation des plaies n'est pas très satisfaisante. ③ Chez des patients atteints de la maladie de Keshan en état de choc |

| | |
|---|---|
| | cardiogénique, il faut administrer une forte dose de la vitamine C. ④ Ce produit permet de traiter des dommages au foie liés à la cirrhose, àl'hépatite aiguë et à l'intoxication chronique de l'arsenic, du mercure, du plomb, et du benzène. ⑤ Il permet aussi de traiter l'anémie, les maladies allergiques de la peau,l'aphte et de promouvoir la cicatrisation des plaies, etc. |
| 用法、用量<br>Les modes d'emploi et la posologie | ①一般应用：口服（饭后）一次 0.05～0.1g，一日 2～3 次；亦可静脉注射或肌内注射，或以 5%～10% 葡萄糖液稀释进行静脉滴注，每日 0.25～0.5g（小儿 0.05～0.3g），必要时可酌增剂量。②克山病：首剂 5～10g，加入 25% 葡萄糖注射液中，缓慢静脉注射。③口疮：将本品 1 片（0.1g）压碎，撒于溃疡面上，令患者闭口片刻，一日 2 次，一般 3～4 次即可治愈。<br><br>① Application générale : par voie orale, après le repas, 0,05 à 0,1g par fois, 2 à 3 fois par jour ; ou injection IV ou IM, ou dissoudre dans la solution à 5% à 10% pour la perfusion, 0,25 à 0,5g par jour (chez des enfants, 0,05 à 0,3g), s'il est nécessaire, augmenter un peu la dose. ② Pour la maladie de Keshan : la dose initiale, 5 à 10g, dissoudre dans la solution de glucose à 25%, injection IV lente. ③ Pour traiter l'aphte : casser 1 comprimé (0,1g), appliquer sur la zone touchée, fermer la bouche pour un instant, 2 fois par jour. L'aphte sera guéri après 3 à 4 fois. |
| 剂型、规格<br>Les formes pharmaceutiques et les spécifications | 片剂：每片 20mg；25mg；50mg；100mg；250mg。<br>咀嚼片剂：每片 100mg。<br>泡腾片：每片 500mg。<br>注射液：每支 100mg（2ml）；250mg（2ml）；500mg（2ml）；2.5g（20ml）。<br><br>Comprimés : 20mg, 25mg, 50mg, 100mg ou 250mg par comprimé.<br>Comprimés à mâcher : 100mg par comprimé.<br>Comprimés effervescents : 500mg par comprimé.<br>Injection : 100mg (2ml), 250 mg (2ml), 500mg (2ml) ou 2,5g (20ml) par solution. |
| 药品名称 Drug Names | 维生素 E　Vitamine E(Tocopherol) |
| 适应证<br>Les indications | 用于：①未进食强化奶或有严重脂肪吸收不良母亲所生的新生儿、早产儿、低出生体重儿。②未成熟儿、低出生体重儿常规应用于预防维生素 E 缺乏。③进行性肌营养不良的辅助治疗。④维生素 E 需要量增加的情况，如甲状腺功能亢进、吸收功能不良综合征、肝胆系统疾病等。<br><br>① Applicable chez les nouveau-nés, les enfants prématurés ou les enfants ayant un faible poids à la naissance nés de mères n'ayant pas pris de lait enrichiou atteintes de grave malabsorption des graisses. ② Applicable dans la prévention de la carence en vitamine E chez des enfants immatures et les enfants ayant un faible poids à la naissance. ③ Applicable dans le traitement adjuvant de la dystrophie musculaire progressive. ④ Applicable dans l'augmentation du besoin en vitamine E, telle que l'hyperthyroïdie, le syndrome de dysfonction d'absorption, des affections hépatobiliaires, etc. |
| 用法、用量<br>Les modes d'emploi et la posologie | 口服或肌内注射：一次 10～100mg，一日 1～3 次。<br><br>Par voie orale ou injection IM : 10 à 100mg par fois, 1 à 3 fois par jour. |
| 剂型、规格<br>Les formes pharmaceutiques et les spécifications | 片剂：每片 5mg；10mg；100mg。<br>胶丸：每丸 5mg；10mg；50mg；100mg；200mg。<br>粉剂：每克粉剂中含维生素 E0.5mg。<br>注射液：每支 5mg（1ml）；50mg（1ml）。<br><br>Comprimés : 5mg, 10mg ou 100mg par comprimé.<br>Granules : 5mg, 10mg, 50mg, 100mg ou 200mg par granule.<br>Poudre : 0,5mg de vitamine E par g.<br>Injection : 5mg (1ml) ou 50mg (1ml) par solution. |
| 18.2　酶类和生化制剂 Enzyme et Agents Biochimiques | |
| 药品名称 Drug Names | 胰蛋白酶 Trypsine |
| 适应证<br>Les indications | 临床上主要用于脓胸、血胸、外科炎症、溃疡、创伤性损伤、瘘管等所产生的局部水肿、血肿、脓肿等，虹膜睫状体炎、急性泪囊炎、视网膜周围炎、眼外伤等。喷雾吸入，用于呼吸道疾病。因对蛇毒蛋白（蛇毒的主要毒成分）有水解作用，故有将本品用于治疗毒蛇咬伤，曾试用于竹叶青、银环蛇、眼镜蛇、蝮蛇等毒蛇咬伤的各型病例。 |

续　表

| | |
|---|---|
| | Ce produit est utilisé dans les cliniques comme traitement de l'oedème local, de l'hématome, de l'abcès causés par l'empyème, l'hémothorax, l'inflammation chirurgicale, les ulcères, les lésions traumatiques et la fistule, ainsi de l'iridocyclite, de la dacryocystite aiguë, de l'inflammation autour de la rétine, et du traumatisme de l'œil, etc. Son aérosol pour inhalation est applicable dans le traitement des maladies respiratoires. Comme il permet l'hydrolysedes protéines de venin, il est apppliqué dans le traitement desmorsures de serpent. Il est appliqué dans le traitement des morsures de serpent de plusieurs types, comme le trimeresurus, le serpent corail, le cobra, la vipère, etc. |
| 用法、用量<br>Les modes d'emploi et la posologie | ①一般应用：每次 5000U，一日 1 次，肌内注射，用量斟酌情况决定。为防止疼痛，可加适量普鲁卡因。局部用药视情况而定，可配成溶液剂（pH7.4 ～ 8.2，微碱性时活性最强）、喷雾剂、粉剂、软膏等，用于体腔内注射、患部注射、喷涂、湿敷、涂搽等。②滴眼：0.25%溶液，一日 4 ～ 6 次。冲洗泪道：0.25% ～ 0.5% 溶液（内加 2% 普鲁卡因少量），一日 1 次。眼浴 1：5000 ～ 1：10 000 溶液 10 ～ 20ml，1 次 10 ～ 20ml，一次 10 ～ 15 分钟，一日 1 次，或隔日 1 次。球后注射 1 次 1 ～ 2.5mg，隔日 1 次。肌内注射 1 次 2.5 ～ 5mg。一日 1 ～ 2 次。③治蛇毒：取注射用结晶胰蛋白酶 2000 ～ 6000U，加 0.25% ～ 0.5% 盐酸普鲁卡因（或注射用水）4 ～ 20ml 稀释，以牙痕为中心，在伤口周围做浸润注射，或在肿胀部位上方做环状封闭 1 ～ 2 次。如病情需要，可重复使用。若伤肢肿胀明显，可于注射 30 分钟后，切开伤口排毒减压（严重出血者例外），也可在肿胀部位针刺排毒。如伤口已坏死、溃疡，可用其 0.1% 溶液湿敷患处。<br><br>① Application générale : 5000U par fois, 1 fois par jour, injection IM, ajuster la dose selon les cas. Pour éviter la douleur, ajouter un peu de procaine. Pour l'administration topique, possible d'utiliser la solution (pH7,4 à 8,2, plus actif quand il est légèrement alcalin), l'aérosol, la poudre ou la pommade, pour l'injection intra-cavité, l'injection topique sur la zone touchée, la pulvérisation, etc. ② Les gouttes pour les yeux : la solution à 0,25%, 4 à 6 fois par jour. Pour l'irrigation lacrymale : la solution à 0,25% à 0,5% (y compris un peu de procaine à 2%), 1 fois par jour. Pour le bain oculaire : 10 à 20ml de solution à 1:5000 à 1:10000, 10 à 20ml par fois, 10 à 15 minutes par fois, 1 fois par jour, ou tous les 2 jours. Pour l'injection Rétrooculaire, 1 à 2,5mg par fois, tous les 2 jours. Injection IM, 2,5 à 5mg par fois, 1 à 2 fois par jour. ③ Pour traiter l'intoxiation par la morsure de serpent : prendre 2000 à 6000 U de trypsine cristalline pour injection, dissoudre dans 4 à 20ml de chlorydrate de procaine à 0,25 à 0,5% (ou la solution saline), les injections d'infiltration autour de la plaie 1 à 2 fois. s'il est nécessaire, possible de répéter. Possible d'inciser les plaies pour la décompression (non compris les saignements graves). Aussi possible de faire l'acupuncture sur le site de gonflement pour la désinfection. Sion constate la nécrose et l'ulcération des plaies, possible d'utiliser la solution de trypsine à 0,1% pour l'usage externe sur la zone touchée. |
| 剂型、规格<br>Les formes pharmaceutiques et les spécifications | 注射用胰蛋白酶：每支 1.25 万 U；2.5 万 U；5 万 U；10 万 U（附灭菌缓冲液 1 瓶）。<br><br>La trypsine pour injection : 12 500 U, 25 000 U, 50 000 U ou 100 000U par solution (y compris 1 flacon de tampon stérile). |
| 药品名称 Drug Names | 糜蛋白酶 Chymotrypsine |
| 适应证<br>Les indications | 主要用于创伤或手术后创口愈合、抗炎及防止局部水肿、积血、扭伤血肿、乳房手术后水肿、中耳炎、鼻炎、角膜溃疡、泪道疾病、眼外伤、眼睑水肿、出血和玻璃体积血、慢性支气管炎、支气管扩张、肺脓肿以及毒蛇咬伤等。<br><br>Ce produit est principalement utilisé dans la cicatrisation des plaies après un traumatisme ou une intervention chirurgicale, dans l'anti –inflammation. Il permet de prévenir et de traiter un œdème local, l'hématocèle, l'hématome de l'entorse, l'œdème après une chirurgie mammaire, l'otite moyenne, la rhinite, des ulcères cornéens, la maladie lacrymale, les traumatismes de l'oeil, l'œdème et l'hémorragie de la paupière, l'hémotocèle intravitréenne, la bronchite chronique, la dilatation des bronches, l'abcès du poumon et les morsures de serpent, etc. |
| 用法、用量<br>Les modes d'emploi et la posologie | ①肌内注射：以 0.9% 氯化钠注射液 5ml 溶解 4000U 后注射。②经眼用药：本品对眼球睫状韧带有选择性松弛作用，故可用于白内障摘除，使晶状体比较容易移去。眼科注入后房，一次 800U，以 0.9% 氯化钠注射液配成 1：5000 溶液，由瞳孔注入后房，经 2 ～ 3 分钟，在晶状体浮动后以生理盐水冲洗前后方中遗留的本品。③喷雾吸入：每次 5mg，以 0.9%% 氯化钠注射液配成 0.5mg/ml 浓度溶液使用。④用于处理软组织炎症或创伤，800U 糜蛋白酶溶于 |

续表

<table>
<tr>
<td></td>
<td>1ml0.9% 氯化钠注射液注于创面。⑤毒蛇咬伤：糜蛋白酶 10 ～ 20mg 用注射用水 4ml 稀释后，以蛇牙痕迹为中心区域向后浸润注射，并在伤口中心区域注射 2 针，再在肿胀上方 3cm 做环状封闭 1 ～ 2 层，根据不同部位 0.3 ～ 0.7ml，至少 10 针，最多 26 针。

① Injection IM : dissoudre 4 000U dans 5ml de solution de glucose à 0,9%, injecter par voie IM. ② Pour l'administration oculaire : il a un effet relaxant sélectif sur le ligament ciliaire du globe oculaire, il est ainsi applicable dans l'extraction de la cataracte. En ophtalmologie, dissoudre 800U de ce produit dans la solution de chlorure de sodium à 0,9% pour former la solution à 1 ： 5000, injecter ensuite dans la chambre postérieure au travers de la pupille, 2 à 3 minutes après, laver avec la solution saline les résidus de ce produit. ③ La pulvérisation pour inhalation : 5mg par fois, dissoudre dans la solution de chlorure de sodium à 0.9% pour former la solution à 0,5mg par ml. ④ Pour traiter l'inflammation du tissu mous ou le traumatisme, dissoudre 800U de chymotrypsine dans 1ml de solution de chlorure de sodium à 0,9%, injecter sur la zone touchée. ⑤ La morsure de serpent : dissoudre 10 à 20mg de chymotrypsine dans 4ml d'eau pour injection, à partir des marques de dents de serpent, injection d'infiltration, en même temps, 2 injections au centre de plaies, appliquer 1-2 couches de fermeture annulaire 3 cm au-dessus du gonflement. Pour différentes zones, 0,3 à 0,7ml, au moins 10 injections, au plus 26 injections.</td>
</tr>
<tr>
<td>剂型、规格<br>Les formes pharmaceutiques et les spécifications</td>
<td>注射用糜蛋白酶：每支 800U；4000U。<br>La chymotrypsine pour injection : 800U ou 4 000U par solution.</td>
</tr>
<tr>
<td>药品名称 Drug Names</td>
<td>抑肽酶 Aprotinine</td>
</tr>
<tr>
<td>适应证<br>Les indications</td>
<td>用于各型胰腺炎的治疗与预防；能抑制纤维蛋白溶酶，阻止胰腺中其他活性蛋白酶原的激活及胰蛋白酶原的活化，用于治疗和预防各种纤维蛋白溶解所引起的急性出血；能抑制血管舒张素，从而抑制其舒张血管、增加毛细血管通透性、降低血压的作用，用于各种严重休克状态。此外，在腹腔手术后直接注入腹腔，能预防肠粘连。

Ce médicament est applicable dans le traitement et la prévention de la pancréatite de toutes sortes. En permettant l'inhibition de la plasmine et l'inhibition del'activation du trypsinogène, il est appliqué dans le traitement et la prévention de l'hémorragie aiguë causée par la fibrinolyse. Il permet d'inhiber le vasorelaxant, empêchant sa vasodilatation, sonaugmentation de la perméabilité capillaire et son abaissement de la pression artérielle. Il est donc appliqué dans le traitement de l'état de choc sévère. En outre, injecté directement dans la cavité abdominale lors de la chirurgie abdominale, il peut empêcher l'adhérence intestinale.</td>
</tr>
<tr>
<td>用法、用量<br>Les modes d'emploi et la posologie</td>
<td>①第 1、2 日每日注射 5 万～ 12 万 U，首剂用量应大一些，缓慢静脉注射（每分钟不超过 2ml）。维持剂量采用静脉滴注，一般一日 4 次，每日总量 2 万～ 4 万 U。②对由纤维蛋白溶解引起的急性出血，立即静脉注射 5 万～ 10 万 U，以后每 2 小时 1 万 U，直至出血停止。③预防剂量：手术前 1 日开始，每日注射 2 万 U，共 3 日。治疗肠瘘及连续渗血也可局部使用。④预防术后肠粘连：在手术切后闭合前，腹腔内直接注入 2 万～ 4 万 U，注意勿与伤口接触。⑤用于体外循环心脏直视手术。

① Les deux premiers jours, injecter 50 000 à 120 000U par jour, la dose initiale doit être importante, injection IV lente (ne pas dépasser 2ml par minute). La dose d'entretien doit être administrée en perfusion, 4 fois par jour, 20 000U à 40 000U par jour. ② Pour traiter l'hémorragie aigue causée par la fibrinolyse, injecter immédiatement 50 000U à 100 000U par voie IV, ensuite, 10 000U toutes les 2 h, jusqu'à l'arrêt de l'hémorragie. ③ La dose pour la prévention : 1 jour avant la chirurgie, injecter 20 000U par jour, pendant 3 jours au total. Pour traiter la fistule intestinale et l'hémorragie continue, possible de l'appliquer de manière topique. ④ Pour prévenir l'adhérence intestinale : avant la fermeture de l'incision chirurgicale, injecter directement 20 000uU à 40 000U dans la cavité abdominale, éviter le contact avec les plaies. ⑤ Applicable dans la chirurgie de pontage cardiopulmonaire.</td>
</tr>
<tr>
<td>剂型、规格<br>Les formes pharmaceutiques et les spécifications</td>
<td>注射液：每支 5 万 U（5ml）；10 万 U（5ml）；50 万 U（5ml）。<br>Injection : 50 000U (5ml), 100 000U (5ml), 500 000 U (5ml) par solution.</td>
</tr>
</table>

**续　表**

| 药品名称 Drug Names | 玻璃酸酶 Hyaluronidase |
|---|---|
| 适应证<br>Les indications | 　　一些以缓慢速度进行静脉滴注的药物如各种氨基酸、水解蛋白等，在与本品合用的情况下可改为皮下注射或肌内注射，使吸收加快。<br><br>L'utilisation en assoication avec l'hyaluronidase permet à certains médicaments qui doivent administrés en perfusion à une vitesse lente, tels que les acides aminés et les protéines hydrolysées, d'être administrés par voie sous-cutanée ou IM, ce qui accélère l'absorption. |
| 用法、用量<br>Les modes d'emploi et la posologie | 　　①临用时将本品粉末溶于生理盐水中，常用量 50U 或 150U，配成每毫升含 0.7U、1.5U 或 2.0U 的注射液，事先注射于灌注部位。②皮下注射大量的某些抗生素（如链霉素）或其他化疗药物（如异烟肼等）以及麦角制剂时，合用本品，可使扩散加速，减轻痛感。③以 150U 溶解在 25～50ml 局部麻醉药中，如加入肾上腺素，可加速麻醉，并减少麻醉药的用量。④与胰岛素合用，可防止注射局部浓度过高而出现的脂肪组织萎缩。胰岛素休克疗法中用本品 100～150U，促使胰岛素吸收量增加，注射较小量即可达血中有效浓度，因而减少其危险性。⑤球后注射促进玻璃体浑浊或出血的吸收，1 次 100～300U/ml，一日 1 次。⑥结膜下注射促使球后血肿的吸收，1 次 50～100U/0.5ml，1 日或隔日 1 次。⑦滴眼预防结膜化学烧伤后睑球粘连，治疗外伤性眼眶出血、外伤性视网膜水肿，150U/ml，每 2 小时滴眼一次。⑧关节腔内注射，一次 2ml，一周 1 次，连续 3～5 周。<br><br>① Dissoudre la poudre d'hyaluronidase dans la solution saline, la dose usuelle est de 50 ou 150U, pour former l'injection de 0,7U, de 1,5U ou de 2,0U par ml, injecter au site de perfusion. ② Lors de l'injection sous-cutanée d'une forte dose de certains antibiotiques (tels que la streptomycine) ou d'autres médicaments chimiothérapeutiques (tels que l'isoniazide), et des préparations de l'ergot, l'utilisation de l'hyaluronidase permet d'accélérer la prolifération et de réduire la douleur. ③ Dissoudre 150U dans 25 à 50ml d'anesthésiques locaux. Si on ajoute aussi l'épinéphrine, cela peut accélérer l'anesthésie et réduire la consommation des anesthésiques. ④ Utilisé en association avec l'insuline, il permet de prévenir l'atrophie du tissu adipeux causée par la concentration trop élevée au site d'injection. Dans la thérapie de choc à l'insuline, prendre 100 à 150g d'hyaluronidase, permettant de promouvoir l'absorption de l'insuline et d'atteindre la concentration désirée dans le sang avec une faible dose, réduisant ainsi le risque. ⑤ L'injection rétrooculaire peut favoriser l'absorption de l'opacitéou des saignements du vitré, 100 à 300U par ml par fois, 1 fois par jour. ⑥ L'injection sous-conjonctivale contribue à l'absorption de l'hématome rétrooculaire, 50 à 100U par 0,5ml par fois, tous les 1 à 2 jours. ⑦ Les gouttes pour les yeux permettent de prévenir les adhérences des paupières après les brûlures chimiques de la conjonctive. Elles permettent également de traiter l'hémorragie traumatique orbitaire et l'oedème de la rétine traumatique. 150 U par ml, toutes les 2 h. ⑧ Injection intra-articulaire, 2ml par fois, 1 fois par semaine, pendant 3 à 5 semaines. |
| 剂型、规格<br>Les formes pharmaceutiques et les spécifications | 　　注射用玻璃酸酶：每支 150U；1500U。<br>L'hyaluronidase pour injection : 150U ou 1 500U par solution. |
| 药品名称 Drug Names | 三磷酸腺苷 Adénosine Triphosphate |
| 适应证<br>Les indications | 　　用于心力衰竭、心肌炎、心肌梗死、脑动脉硬化、冠状动脉硬化、心绞痛、阵发性心动过速、急性脊髓灰质炎、进行性肌萎缩性疾病、肝炎、肾炎、视疲劳、眼肌麻痹、视网膜出血、中心性视网膜炎、视神经炎、视神经萎缩等。本品不易透过细胞膜，能否发挥其生理效应，值得怀疑。其能量注射液为本品与辅酶 A 等配制的复方注射液，用于肝炎、肾炎、心力衰竭等。<br><br>Ce médicament sert à traiter l'insuffisance cardiaque, la myocardite, l'infarctus du myocarde, l'artériosclérose cérébrale, la maladie coronarienne, l'angine de poitrine, la tachycardie paroxystique, la poliomyélite aiguë, la maladie de l'atrophie musculaire progressive, l'hépatite, lanéphrite, la fatigue visuelle, laparalysie musculaire, l'hémorragierétinienne, la rétinite centrale, lanévrite optique, l'atrophie optique, etc. À cause de sa difficulté à pénétrer la membrane cellulaire, son efficacité est mise en doute.Son injection d'énergieest l'injection composée avec le coenzyme A. Elle est appliquée pour traiterl'hépatite, la néphrite, l'insuffisance cardiaque, etc. |

**续 表**

| 用法、用量<br>Les modes d'emploi et la posologie | 肌内注射或静脉注射，每次 20mg，一日 1～3 次。肌内注射多用注射液，静脉注射多用注射用三磷腺苷，另附有缓冲液溶解，再以 5%～10% 葡萄糖注射液 10～20ml 稀释后缓慢静脉注射，也可用 5%～10% 葡萄糖注射液稀释后静脉滴注。1% 生理盐水溶液滴眼，治疗弥漫性表层角膜炎和角膜外伤。<br><br>Injection IM ou IV, 20mg par fois, 1 à 3 fois par jour. Pour l'injection IM, on applique souvent l'injection d'adénosine diphosphate. Pour l'injection IV, on utilise souvent l'adénosine diphosphate pour injection, avec le tampon. Dissoudre dans 10 à 20ml de solution de glucose à 5% à 10%, injection IV lente, ou dissoudre dans la solution de glucose à 5% à 10% pour la perfusion. Utiliser les gouttes pour les yeux de solution saline à 1% pourtraiter la kératite superficielle et le traumatisme de la cornée. |
|---|---|
| 剂型、规格<br>Les formes pharmaceutiques et les spécifications | 注射液：每支 20mg（2ml）。<br>注射用三磷腺苷：每支 20mg；另附磷酸缓冲液 2ml。<br>Injection : 20mg (2ml) par solution.<br>L'adénosine diphosphate pour injection : 20mg par solution, y compris 2ml de tampon de phosphate. |

**18.3　调节水、电解质和酸碱平衡药 Médicaments régulateur de l'équilibre eau, électrolyte et acide-base**

| 药品名称 Drug Names | 氯化钠 Chlorure de sodium |
|---|---|
| 适应证<br>Les indications | 氯化钠注射液可补充血容量和钠离子，用于各种缺盐性失水症（如大面积烧伤、严重吐泻、大量发汗、强利尿药、出血等引起）。在大量出血而又无法进行输血时，可输入氯化钠注射液以维持血容量进行急救。还用于慢性肾上腺皮质功能不全（艾迪生病）治疗过程中补充氯化钠，每日约 10g。此外，生理盐水可用于洗伤口、洗眼、洗鼻以及产科水囊引产等。<br><br>L'injection de chlorure de sodium permet de compléter le volume sanguin et l'ion sodium. Il est applicable dans le traitement des symptômes de déshydratationliés à la carence en sel (souvent causés par des brûlures étendues, des vomissements et des diarrhées sévères,la transpiration excessive, les diurétiques forts, des saignements, etc.) Lors de l'hémorragie massive qui ne peut pas être complétée par la transfusion sanguine, l'injection de chlorure de sodium permet de maintenir le volume sanguin. il est aussi applicable dans le supplément de chlorure de sodium au cours du traitement de l'insuffisance surrénale chronique, 10g par jour. En outre, la solution saline est également appliquée dans le lavage des plaies, le lavage des yeux, le lavage nasal et l'avortement par les vessies obstétricales. |
| 用法、用量<br>Les modes d'emploi et la posologie | ①口服：用于轻度急性胃肠患者恶心、呕吐不严重者。②高渗性失水：高渗性失水时，患者脑细胞和脊髓液渗透浓度升高，若对其治疗则会使血浆和细胞外液钠浓度和渗透浓度下降过快，可致脑水肿。一般认为，在治疗开始的 48 小时内，血浆钠浓度每小时下降应不超过 0.5mmol/L。③等渗性失水：原则给予等渗溶液，如 0.9% 氯化钠注射液或复方氯化钠注射液，但上述溶液氯浓度明显高于血浆，单独大量使用可致高氯血症，故可将 0.9% 氯化钠注射液和 1.25% 碳酸氢钠或 1.86%（1/6M）乳酸钠以 7：3 的比例配制后补给。后者氯浓度为 107mmol/L，并可纠正代谢性酸中毒。④低渗性失水：严重低渗性失水时，脑细胞内溶质减少以维持细胞容积。若治疗使血浆和细胞外液钠浓度和渗透浓度迅速回升，可致脑细胞损伤。一般认为，当血钠低于 120mmol/L 时，治疗使血钠上升速度在每小时 0.5mmol/L，不超过每小时 1.5mmol/L（稀释性低钠血症不需要补钠）。当急性血钠低于 120mmol/L 或出现中枢神经系统症状时，可给予 3% 氯化钠注射液静脉滴注。一般要求在 6 小时内将血钠浓度提高至 120mmol/L 以上。参考补钠量为 3% 氯化钠 1ml/kg，可提高血钠 1mmol/L。待血钠回升至 120～125mmol/L 以上，可改用等渗溶液。慢性缺钠补钠速度要慢，剂量要少，使血钠浓度逐日回升至 130mmol/L。⑤低氯性碱中毒：给予 0.9% 氯化钠注射液或复方氯化钠注射液（林格液）500～1000ml，以后根据碱中毒情况决定用量。⑥外用：用生理氯化钠溶液洗涤伤口、冲洗眼部。<br><br>① Par voie orale : pour traiter les patients atteints de maladies aigues bénignes gastro-intestinales dont les vomissements et les nausées ne sont pas très graves. ② Pour traiter la déshydratation hypertonique : lors de la déshydration hypertonique, l'osmolalité des cellules cérébrales et du liquide céphalo-rachidien va augmenter. Le traitement pourrait conduire à la chute trop rapide de l'osmolalité et de la concentration de sodium dans le plasma et dans le liquide extracellulaire, provoquant ainsi l'œdème cérébral. il est gnénéralement reconnu qu'en 48 h après le traitement, la diminution de la concentration de sodium dans le plasma ne doit pas dépasser 0,5 mmol/L par h. ③ Pour traiter la |

déshydratation isotonique : en principe, il faut prendre la solution isotonique, telle que la solution de chlorure de sodium à 0.9% ou la solution composée de chlorure de sodium, mais la concentration de chlorure dans ces solutions est évidement supérieure à celle dans le plasma, son utilisatio seule peut donc entraîner l'hyperchlorémie. On peut alors utiliser la solution de chlorure de sodium à 0,9% en association avec le bicarbonate de sodium à 1,25% ou le lactate de sodium à 1,86% (1/6M) avec une proportion de 7 ： 3. La concentration de chlorure de cette solution composée est de 107 mmol par L, il peut donc permettre de corriger l'acidose métabolique.　④ Pour traiter la déshydratation hypotonique: lors de la déshydratation hypotonique sévère, le soluté dans les cellules cérébrales va diminuer pour maintenir le volume cellulaire. Le traitement pourrait conduire à l'augmentation trop rapide de l'osmolalité et de la concentration de sodium dans le plasma et dans le liquide extracellulaire, provoquant ainsi les lésions cérébrales. Il est généralement reconnu que lorsque la concentration de sodium dans le sang est inférieure à 120 mmol/L, le traitement pourrait conduire à l'augmentation de la concentration de sodium dans le sang à un débit de 0,5mmol/L (1,5mmol/L au maximum) (pas nécessaire de compléter le sodium pour l'hyponatrémie de dilution). Lorsque la cencentration de sodium dans le sang aigue est inférieure à 120 mmol/L ou que les symptômes du système nerveux central, possible d'administrer la solution de chlorure de sodium à 3% en perfusion. En général, il est demandé d'augmenter la concentration de sodium dans le sang jusqu'à 120 mmol/L ou plus en 6h. La dose de référence pour compléter le sodium est de 1ml par kg de solution de chlorure de sodium à 3mg/kg par fois pour augmenter 1 mmol/L de concentration. Quand la concentration revient à 120 à 125 mmol/L ou plus, prendre la solution isotonique. Pour la carence en sodium chronique, le complément doit être lent, avec une faible dose, pour permettre à la concentration de revenir progressivement à 130 mmol/L. ⑤ Pour traiter l'alcalose à faible chlore : injecter 500 à 1000ml de solution de chlorure de sodium ou de solution composée de chlorrue de sodium (solution de Linger), ensuite ajuster la dose en fonction de l'alcalose. ⑥ Pour un usage externe : utiliser une solution physiologique de chlorure de sodium pour laver des plaies et les yeux.

| 剂型、规格<br>Les formes pharmaceutiques et les spécifications | 注射液：为含 0.9% 氯化钠的灭菌水溶液。每支（瓶）2ml；10ml；250ml；500ml；1000ml。浓氯化钠注射液：每支 1g（1ml），0.3g（10ml）。临用前稀释。复方氯化钠注射液（林格液）：灭菌溶液，每 100ml 中含氯化钠 0.85g，氯化钾 0.03g，氯化钙 0.033g，比生理盐水成分完全，可替代生理盐水用。葡萄糖氯化钠注射液：每 1000ml 中含葡萄糖 5% 及氯化钠 0.9%。每瓶 250ml；500ml；1000ml。口服补液盐：①每包 14.75g（大包中含氯化钠 1.75g，葡萄糖 11g；小包中含氯化钾 0.75g，碳酸氢钠 1.25g）。②每包 13.95g（氯化钠 1.75g，葡萄糖 10g，枸橼酸钠 1.45g，氯化钾 0.75g）。治疗和预防轻度急性腹泻。<br><br>Injection : la solution stérile de chlorure de sodium à 0,9%, 2ml, 10ml, 250ml, 500ml ou 1 000ml par flacon. Injection concentrée de chlorure de sodium : 1g (1ml), 0,3g (10ml). Diluer avant d'utiliser. La solution composée de chlorure de sodium (la solution de Linger) : la solution stérile, 100ml de solution contient 0,85g de chlorure de sodium 0,03g de chlorure de potassium, 0,033g de chlorure de calcium. Sa composition est plus complète que la solution saline, et elle peut remplacer la solution saline. Injection de glucose de chlorure de sodium : 1000ml contient la glucose à 5% et le chlorure de sodium à 0,9%. 250ml, 500ml ou 1000ml par flacon. Sels de réhydratation orale : 1) 14,75g par sachet (grand sachet contient 1,75g de chlorure de sodium, 11g de glucose ; petit sachet contient 0,75g de chlorure de potassium, 1,25g de bicarbonate de sodium). 2) 13,95g par sachet (1,75g de chlorure de sodium, 10g de glucose, 1,45g de citrate de sodium, 0,75g de chlorure de potassium). Prévenir et traiter la diarrhée aigue bénigne. |
|---|---|
| **药品名称 Drug Names** | 氯化钾 Chlorure de potassium |
| 适应证<br>Les indications | 用于低钾血症（多由严重吐泻不能进食、长期应用排钾利尿剂或肾上腺皮质激素所引起）的防治，亦可用于强心苷中毒引起的阵发性心动过速或频发室性期外收缩。<br><br>Il est utilisé comme prévention et traitement de l'hypokaliémie (souvent causée par des vomissements et des diarrhées graves, l'utilisation à long terme de diurétiques épargneurs de potassium ou de l'hormone corticotrope). Il est aussi applicable dans le traitment de la tachycardie paroxystique et de la contraction ventriculaire externe fréquente causées par l'intoxication du glycoside cardiaque. |
| 用法、用量<br>Les modes d'emploi et la posologie | 补充钾盐大多采用口服，一次 1g，一日 3 次。血钾过低，病情危急或吐泻严重口服不易吸收时，可用静脉滴注，每次用 10% ～ 15% 液 10ml，用 5% ～ 10% 葡萄糖注射液 500ml 稀释或根据病情酌定用量。<br><br>Pour compléter le potassium, prendre généralement par voie, 1g par fois, 3 fois par jour. Lors del'hypokaliémie, des vomissements et des diarrhées sévères dans un état critique ou difficile d'absorber par voie orale, possible d'administrer en perfusion, utiliser 10ml de solution à 10% à 15%, dissoudre dans 500ml de solution de glucose à 5% à 10%, ou ajuster la dose selon les cas. |

**续　表**

| | |
|---|---|
| 剂型、规格<br>Les formes pharmaceutiques et les spécifications | 片剂：每片 0.25g；0.5g。<br>控释片（SLOW-K）：每片 0.6g。<br>微囊片（PEL-K）：每片 0.75g。<br>氯化钾口服液：100ml：10g。<br>注射液：每支 1g（10ml）。<br>复方氯化钾注射液：内含氯化钾 0.28%、氯化钠 0.42% 及乳酸钠 0.63%，可用于代谢性酸血症及低血钾。用量视病情而定，一般每日量 500 ～ 1000ml，静脉滴注。<br><br>Comprimés : 0,25g ou 0,5g par comprimé.<br>Comprimés à libération contrôlée (SLOW-K) : 0,6g par comprimé.<br>Les comprimés de microcapsule (PEL-K) : 0,75g par comprimé.<br>La solution buccale de chlorure de potassium : 100ml : 10g.<br>Injection : 1g (10ml) par solution.<br>Injection composée de chlorure de potassium : chaque injection contient le chlorure de potassium à 0,28%, le chlorure de sodium à 0,42% et le lactate de sodium à 0,63%, applicable dans le traitement de l'acidose métabolique et de l'hypokaliémie. Ajuster la dose selon les cas, 500 à 1 000ml par jour en général, en perfusion. |
| 药品名称 Drug Names | 门冬氨酸钾镁 Aspartates de magnésium et de potassium |
| 适应证<br>Les indications | 用于低钾血症、低钾及洋地黄中毒引起的心律失常、病毒性肝炎、肝硬化和肝性脑病的治疗。<br><br>Ce produit sert à traiter l'hypokaliémie, l'arythmie causée par l'hypokaliémie et l'empoisonnement digitalique, l'hépatite virale, la cirrhose et l'encéphalopathie hépatique. |
| 用法、用量<br>Les modes d'emploi et la posologie | 口服：每次 1 ～ 2 片，一日 3 次。静滴：心律失常、心肌梗死，每次 10 ～ 20ml，加入 5% ～ 10% 葡萄糖液 50 ～ 100ml 中缓慢滴注，4 ～ 6 小时后有必要可重复。<br><br>Par voie orale : 1 à 2 comprimés par fois, 3 fois par jour. En perfusion : pour traiter l'rythmie, l'infarctus du myocarde, 10 à 20ml par fois, dissoudre dans 50 à 100ml de solution de glucose à 5% à 10%, s'il est nécessaire, reprendre une fois 4 à 6 h après. |
| 剂型、规格<br>Les formes pharmaceutiques et les spécifications | 片剂：（钾 0.9mmol+ 镁 0.4mmol）。<br>注射剂：（钾 2.7 ～ 3.1mmol+ 镁 1.5 ～ 1.9mmol）/10ml。<br>Comprimés : (0,9 mmol de potassium + 0,4 mmol de magnésium).<br>Injection : (2,7 à 3,1 mmol de potassium + 1,5 à 1,9 mmol de magnésium) par 10ml. |
| 药品名称 Drug Names | 枸橼酸钾 Citrate de potassium |
| 适应证<br>Les indications | 用于低钾血症。<br>Ce produit sert à traiter l'hypokaliémie. |
| 用法、用量<br>Les modes d'emploi et la posologie | 口服：每次 10 ～ 20ml<br>Par voio orale: 10 à 20ml par fois. |
| 剂型、规格<br>Les formes pharmaceutiques et les spécifications | 10% 溶液剂。<br>10% Solution. |
| 药品名称 Drug Names | 氯化钙 Chlorure de calcium |
| 适应证<br>Les indications | 本品可用于血钙降低引起的手足搐搦症以及肠绞痛、输尿管绞痛，荨麻疹、渗出性水肿、瘙痒性皮肤病，镁盐中毒、佝偻病、软骨病、孕妇及哺乳期妇女钙盐补充，高血钾等。<br><br>Ce produit sert à traiter la tétanie causée par la baisse de la calcémie. Il permet aussi de traiter les coliques intestinales, les coliques urétérales, l'urticaire, l'œdème exsudatif, des démangeaisons de la peau, l'empoisonnement de magnésium, le rachitisme, l'ostéomalacie. Il est aussi applicable dans le supplément de calcium chez les femmes pendant la grossesse et l'allaitement. Il permet également de traiter l'hyperkaliémie. |

续　表

| 用法、用量<br>Les modes d'emploi et la posologie | ①成人：a.治疗低钙血症，500～1000mg（含 Ca 离子 136～272mg）缓慢静脉注射，速度不超过每分钟 50mg，根据反应和血钙浓度，必要时 1～3 日后重复。b.心脏复苏：静脉或心室腔内注射，每次 200～400mg。应避免注入心肌内。c.治疗高钾血症：先静脉注射 500mg，每分钟速度不超过 100mg，以后酌情用药。②小儿：a.治疗低钙血症，按体重 25mg/kg（含 Ca 离子 6.8mg）缓慢静脉注射。但一般情况下本品不用于小儿，因刺激性较大。b.心脏复苏心室内注射，一次 10mg/kg，间隔 10 分钟可重复注射。<br><br>① Chez des adultes : a. Pour traiter l'hypocalcémie, 500 à 1 000mg (conteant 136 à 272mg de calcium), injection IV lente, ne pas dépasser 50mg par minute, selon les réactions et la concentration du calcium dans le sang, s'il est nécessaire, reprendre encore une fois 1 à 3 jours après. b. Pour la réanimation du cœur : injection IV ou intra-ventriculaire, 200 à 400mg par fois. Éviter d'injecter dans le myocarde. c. Pour traiter l'hyperkaliémie : injecter d'abord 500mg par voie IV, ne pas dépasser 100mg par minute, ensuite, ajuster la dose selon les cas. ② Chez des enfants :a. Pour traiter l'hypocalcémie, 25 mg/kg (contenant 6,8mg de calcium), injection IV lente. Mais en général, ce produit n'est pas appliqué chez des enfants, parce qu'il est irritant. b. Pour la réanimation du cœur, 10 mg/kg par fois, possible de reprendre 10 minutes après. |
|---|---|
| 剂型、规格<br>Les formes pharmaceutiques et les spécifications | 注射液：每支 0.3g（10ml）；0.5g（10ml）；0.6g（20ml）；1g（20ml）。<br>氯化钙葡萄糖注射液：为含氯化钙 5% 及葡萄糖 25% 的灭菌溶液，用于因血钙降低而致的手足搐搦、荨麻疹、血清反应等，1 次量 10～20ml，静脉注射，每日或隔日 1 次。禁用于肌内注射，以免引起组织坏死。<br>氯化钙溴化钠注射液：每支 5ml，含氯化钙 0.1g，溴化钠 0.25g。<br>每次静脉注射 5ml（重症可用 10ml），一日 1～2 次。静脉注射时宜缓慢，以免引起全身发热反应。禁用于肌内注射。<br><br>Injection : 0,3g (10ml), 0,5g (10ml), 0,6g (20ml) ou 1g (20ml) par solution.<br>Injection de glucose de chlorure de calcium : la solution stérile contenant le chlorure de calcium à 5% et la glucose à 25%, pour traiter la ténanie, l'urticaire et la réaction de sérum causées par la baisse de la calcémie, 10 à 20ml par fois, injection IV, tous les jours ou tous les 2 jours. Interdit d'injecter par voie IM, pour éviter la nécrose tissulaire.<br>Injection de bromure de sodium de chlorure de calcium : injecter 5ml par voie IV (chez des cas graves, 10ml) par fois, 1 à 2 fois par jour. L'injection IV doit être lente pour éviter la fièvre du corps. Interdit d'utiliser l'injection IM. |
| **药品名称 Drug Names** | 碳酸钙 Carbonate de calcium |
| 适应证<br>Les indications | 用于低钙血症和高磷血症。<br>Ce produit sert à traiter l'hypocalcémie et l'hyperphosphatémie. |
| 用法、用量<br>Les modes d'emploi et la posologie | ①低钙血症：成人口服，每次 1.25～1.5g，一日 1～3 次，进食时或进食后服用。尤其慢性肾衰竭患者伴高磷血症。②制酸：成人口服：1 次 0.5～2g，一日 3～4 次。③高磷血症：成人口服：每日 3～12g，分次在进食时服用。每日 2g 以上钙时即可发生高钙血症，故应密切监测血清钙浓度。<br><br>① Pour l'hypocalcémie : chez des adultes, par voie orale, 1,25 à 1,5g par fois, 1 à 3 fois par jour, durant ou après le repas. Surtant chez des patients insuffisants rénaux chroniques accompagnés de l'hyperprhosphatémie. ② Pour l'antacide : chez des adultes, par voie orale : 0,5 à 2g par fois, 3 à 4 fois par jour. ③ Pour traiter l'hyperphosphatémie : chez des adultes, par voie orale : 3 à 12g par jour, pris à travers plusieurs fois durant le repas. Comme l'administration de 2g de calcium par jour pourrait conduire à l'hypercalcémie, il faut suivre de près la concentration de calcium sérique. |
| 剂型、规格<br>Les formes pharmaceutiques et les spécifications | 片剂：每片 0.5g( 相当于元素钙 200mg)。<br>Comprimés : 0.5g par comprimé (eguivalent à calcium 200mg). |

**续 表**

| 药品名称 Drug Names | 葡萄糖酸钙 Gluconate de calcium |
|---|---|
| 适应证<br>Les indications | 本品可用于血钙降低引起的手足搐搦症以及肠绞痛、输尿管绞痛，荨麻疹、渗出性水肿、瘙痒性皮肤病，镁盐中毒，佝偻病、软骨病、孕妇及哺乳期妇女钙盐补充，高血钾等。<br><br>Ce produit sert à traiter la tétanie causée par la baisse de la calcémie. Il permet aussi de traiter les coliques intestinales, les coliques urétérales, l'urticaire, l'œdème exsudatif, des démangeaisons de la peau, l'empoisonnement de magnésium, le rachitisme, l'ostéomalacie. Il est aussi applicable dans lesupplément de calcium chez les femmes pendant la grossesse et l'allaitement. Il permet également de traiter l'hyperkaliémie. |
| 用法、用量<br>Les modes d'emploi et la posologie | ①口服：成人一次 0.5～2g，一日 3 次；儿童一次 0.5～1g，一日 3 次。②静脉注射：每次 10% 注射液 10～20ml（对小儿手足搐搦症，每次 5～10ml）。加等量 5%～25% 葡萄糖注射液稀释后缓慢静脉注射（每分钟不超过 2ml）。<br><br>① Par voie orale : chez des adultes, 0,5 à 2g par fois, 3 fois par jour ; chez des enfants, 0,5 à 1g par fois, 3 fois par jour. ② Injection IV : 10 à 20ml d'injection à 10% par fois (pour traiter la tétanie chez des enfants, 5 à 10ml par fois). Ajouter la même quantité de solution de glucose à 5% à 25% pour la dilution avant l'injection IV lente (ne pas dépasser 2ml par minute). |
| 剂型、规格<br>Les formes pharmaceutiques et les spécifications | 片剂：每片 0.1g；0.5g。<br>含片：每片 0.1g；0.15g；0.2g。<br>口服液：每支 1g（10ml）。<br>注射液：每支 1g（10ml）。<br><br>Comprimés : 0,1g ou 0,5g par comprimé.<br>Comprimés sublinguaux : 0,1g, 0,15g ou 0,2g par comprimé.<br>La solution buccale : 1g (10ml) par solution.<br>Injection : 1g (10ml) par solution. |
| 药品名称 Drug Names | 乳酸钙 Lactate de calcium |
| 适应证<br>Les indications | 用于防治钙缺乏症如手足搐搦症、骨发育不全、佝偻病，以及结核病、妊娠和哺乳期妇女的钙盐补充。<br><br>Ce produit permet de prévenir et de traiter la carence en calcium comme la tétanie, l'hypoplasie de la moelle, et le rachitisme, ainsi que la tuberculose. Il est aussi applicable dans le supplément de calcium chez les femmes pendant la grossesse et l'allaitement. |
| 用法、用量<br>Les modes d'emploi et la posologie | 每 1g 乳酸钙含钙为 130mg。成人：口服，一日 1～2g，分 2～3 次口服。小儿：按体重一日 45～65mg/kg，分 2～3 次口服。<br><br>1g de lactate de calcium contient 130mg de calcium. Chez des adultes : par voie orale, 1 à 2g par jour, à travers 2 à 3 fois. Chez des enfants : 45 à 65 mg/kg par jour, à travers 2 à 3 fois par voie orale. |
| 剂型、规格<br>Les formes pharmaceutiques et les spécifications | 片剂：每片 0.25g；0.5g。<br>Comprimés : 0,25g ou 0,5g par comprimé. |
| 药品名称 Drug Names | 硫酸镁 Sulfate de magnésium |
| 适应证<br>Les indications | ①可预防和治疗低镁血症，特别是急性低镁血症伴有肌肉痉挛、手足搐搦。②先兆子痫和子痫、早产子宫肌肉痉挛等。③导泻、利胆。<br><br>① Ce produit permet de prévenir et de traiter l'hypomagnésémie, surtout l'hypomagnésémie associée à des spasmes musculaires et à la tétanie. ② La pré-éclampsie et l'éclampsie, ainsi que les spasmes musculaires utérins prématurés. ③ Le laxatif et le cholagogue. |
| 用法、用量<br>Les modes d'emploi et la posologie | ①防止低镁血症：成人轻度镁缺乏，1g 硫酸镁，肌内注射或溶于 500ml5% 葡萄糖注射液内缓慢滴注，每日总量 2g。重度镁缺乏，一次按体重 0.25mmol/kg 硫酸镁，也可静脉滴注，将 2.5g 硫酸镁溶于 5% 葡萄糖注射液或氯化钠注射液 500ml 中，缓慢滴注 3 小时。严密观察呼吸等生命体征。②全静脉内营养，按体重每日 0.125～0.25mmol 镁 /kg 添加。儿童全静脉内营养，按体重每日 0.125mmol 镁 /kg 添加。③治疗先兆子痫和子痫，肌内注射：每次 1～2.5g 硫酸镁，根据病情决定剂量，最多每日肌内注射 6 次，并监测心电图、肌腱反射、呼吸和血压。静脉注射： |

续　表

将 1 ~ 2g 硫酸镁，以 5% 葡萄糖液稀释，推注速度每分钟不超过 150mg，静注硫酸镁可使血镁浓度突增至接近中毒浓度，必须严格掌握剂量，并严密观察呼吸、肌腱反射和心电图。静脉滴注：4g 硫酸镁加入 5% 葡萄糖注射液或氯化钠注射液 250ml 内，滴注速度每分钟不超过 4ml。④抗惊厥：儿童按体重 20 ~ 40mg/kg，配成 20% 注射液肌内注射。慎用，不作为首选药物。⑤导泻：成人口服：1 次 5 ~ 20g，用水 200 ~ 400ml 溶解后顿服。⑥利胆：成人口服：1 次 2 ~ 5g，一日 3 次，用水配成 33% 溶液服用。

① Pour prévenir et traiter l'hypomagnésémie : pour la carence en magnésium bénigne, 1g de sulfate de magnésium, injecter par voie IM ou dissoudre dans 500ml de solution de glucose à 5% pour la perfusion lente, 2g par jour. Pour la carence grave en magnésium, 0,25 mmol par kg de sulfate de magnésium pa fois, ou en perfusion, dissoudre 2,5g de sulfate de magnésium dans 500ml de solution de glucose à 5% ou dans la solution de chlorure de sodium, perfusion lente en 3h. Suivre de près des signes vitaux tels que la respiration. ② Pour la nutrition intraveineuse complète, 0,125 à 0,25 mmol de magnésium par kg par jour. Chez des enfants, 0,125 mmol de magnésium par kg par jour. ③ Pour traiter la pré-éclampsie et l'éclampsie, injection IM : 1 à 2,5g de sulfate de magnésium, ajuster la dose selon les cas, 6 fois d'injections IM par jour au plus, observer ECG , réflexes tendineux, la respiration et la pression artérielle en même temps. Injection IV : diluer 1 à 2g de sulfate de magnésium dans la solution de glucose à 5%, avec un débit de 150mg par minute au maximum. L'injection IV de sulfate de magnésoum pourrait entraîner l'augmentation de la concentration de magnésium dans le sang jusqu'à la concentration toxique, il faut donc contrôler strictement la dose et observer la respiration, les réflexes tendineux et ECG. En perfusion : dissoudre 4g de sulfate de magnésium dans 250ml de solution de glucose à 5% ou de solution de chlorure, avec un débit de 4ml par minute au maximum. ④ Pour l'anti-convulsion : chez des enfants, 20 à 40 mg/kg, former la solution à 20%, injection IM. Soyez prudent, ne pas utiliser comme un médicament de choix. ⑤ Le laxatif : chez des adultes, par voie orale : 5 à 20g par fois, utiliser 200 à 400ml d'eau pour la dissolution, une fois par jour. ⑥ Le cholagogue : chez des adultes, par voie orale : 2 à 5g par fois, 3 fois par jour, prendre la solution à 33% préparée avec l'eau.

| 剂型、规格<br>Les formes pharmaceutiques et les spécifications | 注射剂：1g/10ml；2.5g/10ml。<br>口服粉剂，按需要取用，配成溶液服用。<br>Injection : 1g/10ml；2.5g/10ml.<br>La poudre orale, en function des besoins, prendre la solution preparée. |
| --- | --- |
| 药品名称 Drug Names | 乳酸钠 Lactate de sodium |
| 适应证<br>Les indications | 可用于纠正代谢性酸血症。由于作用不及碳酸氢钠迅速，现已渐少用。但在高钾血症或普鲁卡因等引起的心律失常伴有酸血症者，仍以应用本品为宜。<br>Ce produit permet de corriger l'acidose métabolique. Il est peu appliqué aujourd'hui, car son effet est mois rapide que le bicarbonate de sodium. Mais chez des patients atteints d'arythmie associée à une acidose causée par l'hyperkaliémie ou la procaine, il vaut mieux appliquer ce produit. |
| 用法、用量<br>Les modes d'emploi et la posologie | 静脉滴注：每次 11.2% 液 5 ~ 8ml/kg，先用半量，以后根据病情再给其余量。用时须以 5% ~ 10% 葡萄糖液 5 倍量稀释（成为 1.87%，即 1/6 克分子溶液）后静脉滴注。成人每次量一般为 1.87% 液 500 ~ 2000ml。<br>En perfusion : 5 à 8 ml par kg de solution à 11,2% par fois, commencer par la moitié de la dose, ensuite, prendre le reste de la dose selon les cas. Il faut utiliser la solution de glucose à 5% à 10% 5 fois plus importante pour la dilution, en perfusion. Chez des adultes, 500 à 2 000ml de solution à 1,87% par fois en général. |
| 剂型、规格<br>Les formes pharmaceutiques et les spécifications | 注射液：每支 1.12g（10ml）；2.24g（20ml）；5.6g（50ml）.<br>Injection : 1,12g (10ml), 2,24g (20ml) ou 5,6g (50ml) par solution. |

**续　表**

| 药品名称 Drug Names | 葡萄糖 Glucose |
|---|---|
| 适应证<br>Les indications | 　　用于：①腹泻、呕吐、重伤大失血等，体内损失大量水分时，可静脉滴注含本品 5%～10% 的溶液 200～1000ml，同时静脉滴注适宜生理盐水，以补充体液的损失及钠的不足。②不能摄取食物的重病患者，可注射本品或灌肠，以补助营养。③血糖过低症或胰岛素过量，静脉注射 50% 溶液 40～100ml，以保护肝脏。对糖尿病的酮中毒须与胰岛素同用。④降低眼压及因颅压增加引起的各种病症如脑出血、颅骨骨折、尿毒症等，25%～50% 溶液静脉注射，因其高渗压作用，将组织（特别是脑组织）内液体进入循环系统内由肾排出。注射时切勿注于血管之外，以免刺激组织。⑤高钾血症。<br><br>　　Il est appliqué dans le traitement des cas suivants : ① La diarrhée, des vomissements, des blessures graves de perte de sang, etc. Lors de la perte d'une grande quantité d'eau dans le corp, injecter 200 à 1 000ml de solution de glucose à 5% à 10% en perfusion. Il est aussi applicable dans la perfusion de la solution saline pour la réhydratation et améliorer le déficit de sodium. ② Chez des patients gravement malades incapables de prendre des aliments, l'injection ou le lavement du glucose permet d'absorber la nutrition. ③ Pour traiter le syndrome de l'hypoglycémie ou le surdosage d'insuline, injecter 40 à 100ml de solution à 50%, pour protéger le foie. Pour traiter l'acidocétose du diabète, il faut appliquer en même temps l'insuline. ④ Il permet d'atténuer les symptômes causés par la PIO et l'augmentation de la pression intracrânienne, tels que l'hémorragie cérébrale, des fractures du crâne, l'urémie, etc. Injecter par voie IV la solution à 25% à 50%. Grâce à soneffet de la pression hypertonique, il permet l'excrétion rénale du fluide tissulaire dans le système circulatoire. Ne pas injecter le glucose à l'extérieur des vaisseaux sanguins pour éviter l'irritation tissulaire. ⑤ L'hyperkaliémie. |
| 用法、用量<br>Les modes d'emploi et la posologie | 　　①补充热量：患者因为某些原因进食减少或不能进食，一般可予 10%～25% 葡萄糖注射液静脉滴注，并同时补充体液。②全静脉营养疗法：葡萄糖是此疗法中最重要的能量供给物质。在非蛋白质热能中，葡萄糖与脂肪供给热量之比为 2∶1。③低糖血症：轻者口服，重者可先给予 50% 葡萄糖注射液 20～40ml 静脉滴注。④饥饿性酮症：轻者口服，重者可先给予 5%～25% 葡萄糖注射液静脉滴注，每日 100g 葡萄糖可基本控制病情。⑤失水：等渗性失水给予 5% 葡萄糖注射液静脉滴注。⑥高钾血症：应用 10%～25% 注射液，每 2～4g 葡萄糖加正规胰岛素 1U，可降低血清钾浓度。但此疗法仅使细胞外钾离子进入细胞内，体内总钾含量不变。如不采取排钾措施，仍有再次出现高钾血症的可能。⑦组织脱水：高渗溶液（一般采用 50% 注射液）快速静脉注射 20～50ml，但作用短暂。应注意防止高血糖，目前少用。用于调节腹膜透析液渗透压时，50% 葡萄糖注射液 20ml 即 10g 葡萄糖可使 1L 透析渗透压提高 55mOsm/（kg·H$_2$O）。⑧葡萄糖耐量试验：空腹口服葡萄糖 1.75g/kg，于服后 0.5、1、2、3 小时抽血测血糖。血糖浓度正常上限分别为 6.9mmol/L、11.1mmol/L、10.5mmol/L、8.3mmol/L。<br><br>　　① Compléter les calories : chez des patients incapables de prendre d'aliments pour certaines raisons, administrer la solution de glucose à 10% à 25% en perfusion, et faire en même temps la déhydratation. ② Thérapie de nutrition parentérale totale : le glucose est la substance la plus importante contributrice aux calories dans cette thérapie. Dans l'énergie non protéique, le taux pour la fourniture des calories du glucose et de la graisse est de 2 ∶ 1. ③ Pour traiter l'hypoglycémie : pour des cas bénins, prendre par voie orale, pour des cas graves, administrer 20 à 40ml de solution de glucose à 50% en perfusion. ④ Pour traiter la cétose liée à la faim : pour des cas bénins, prendre par voie orale, pour des cas graves, administrer la solution de glucose à 5% à 25% en perfusion. 100g de glucose par jour suffit pour contrôler les symptômes. ⑤ Pour traiter la déshydration : pour la déshydration isotonique, administrer la solution de glucose à 5% en perfusion. ⑥ Pour traiter l'hyperkaliémie : utiliser la solution à 10% à 25%, ajouter 1 unité de l'insuline Actrapid pour 2 à 4 g de glucose, pour diminuer la concentration en potassium sérique. Mais cette thérapie peut permettre seulement au potassium extra-cellulaire d'entrer dans les cellules, sans changer la quantité totale du potassium du corps. S'il on ne prend pas des mesures pour évacuer le potassium, il y a encore le risque de récurrence de l'hyperkaliémie. ⑦ La déshydration du tissu : injecter 20 à 50 ml de solution hypertonique par voie IV rapidement, avec une action brève. Il faut faire attention à l'hyperglycémie, il est donc peu appliqué. Lors de la réglementation de l'osmolalitédu liquide de la dialyse péritonéale, 20ml de solution de glucose à 50% (à savoir 10g de glucose) peut permettre d'augmenter l'osmolalité de 1L de dialyse de 55mOsm/(kg•H$_2$O) ⑧ Test de tolérance au glucose : prendre 1,75g par kg de glucose par voie orale à jeun, ensuite, examiner la glycémie 0,5, 1, 2, 3 h après. Le limite supérieur norml de la glycémie est respectivement 6.9mmol/L, 11.1mmol/L, 10.5mmol/L, 8.3mmol/L. |

**续 表**

| 剂型、规格<br>Les formes pharmaceutiques et les spécifications | 粉剂：每袋 250g；500g。<br>注射液：每支（瓶）50g（1000ml）；100g（1000ml）；50g（500ml）；25g（500ml）；12.5g（250ml）；25g（250ml）；1g（20ml）；5g（20ml）；10g（20ml）；2g（10ml）；0.5g（10ml）。<br>Poudre : 250g ou 500g par sachet.<br>Injection : 50g(1000ml)；100g(1000ml)；50g(500ml)；25g(500ml)；12.5g(250ml)；25g(250ml)；1g(20ml)；5g(20ml)；10g(20ml)；2g(10ml)；0.5g(10ml)par solution. |
|---|---|
| **药品名称 Drug Names** | 果糖 Fructose |
| 适应证<br>Les indications | 对糖尿病、肝病患者供给能力、补充体液。此外，能加速乙醇代谢，用于急性中毒的辅助治疗。<br>Ce médicament permet l'approvisionnement en énergie et la réhydratation chez des patients atteints de diabète et des malades hépatiques. En outre, il peutaccélérer le métabolisme de l'alcool, servant ainsi de traitement adjuvant de l'intoxication aigue. |
| 用法、用量<br>Les modes d'emploi et la posologie | 用以静脉注射或静脉滴注，用量视病情而定。常用量为每次 500 ~ 1000ml。<br>Injection IV ou en perfusion. Ajuster la dose selon les cas. La dose usuelle est de 500 à 1 000ml par fois. |
| 剂型、规格<br>Les formes pharmaceutiques et les spécifications | 注射液：每瓶 12.5g（250ml）；25g（250ml；500ml）；50g（500ml）。<br>Injection : 12,5g (250ml), 25g (250ml ; 500ml) ou 50g (500ml) par flacon. |
| **药品名称 Drug Names** | 口服补液盐 Sels de réhydratation orale |
| 适应证<br>Les indications | 用于补充水、钠和钾丢失的失水。治疗急性腹泻。<br>Il permet de traiter la déshydratation causée par la perte d'eau, de sodium et de potassium. Il sert à traiter la diarrhée aiguë. |
| 用法、用量<br>Les modes d'emploi et la posologie | 每份必须加水 500ml 溶解混匀后服用。①预防和治疗因腹泻、呕吐、经皮肤和呼吸道等液体丢失引起的轻、中度失水，可补充水、钾和钠，重度失水需静脉补液。a.轻度失水：成人口服：开始时 50ml/kg，4 ~ 6 小时饮完，以后酌情调整剂量。儿童口服：开始时 50ml/kg，4 小时内饮完，直至腹泻停止。b. 中度失水：成人口服：开始时 50ml/kg，6 小时内饮完，其余应以静脉补液。儿童应以静脉补液为主。②急性腹泻：a.轻度腹泻，口服：成人每日 50ml/kg。b. 重度腹泻，应以静脉滴注为主，直至腹泻停止。<br>Il est nécessaire d'ajouter 500ml d'eau pour la dissolution avant d'utiliser le produit. ① Pour prévenir et traiter la déshydratation bénigne ou modérée causée par la perte de liquide liée aux vomissements ou à la diarrhée, possible de compléter de l'eau, du potassium et du sodium, pour la déshydratation grave, il faut la réhydratation par voie intraveineuse.a. La déshydratation bénigne : chez des adultes par voie orale : commencer par 50 ml par kg, finir en 4 à 6 h, ensuite, ajuster la dose selon les cas. Chez des enfants par voie orale : commencer par 50ml par kg, finir en 4h, jusqu'à l'arrêt de la diarrhée. b. La déshydratation modérée : chez des adultes par voie orale : commencer par 50 ml par kg, finir en 6 h, pour le reste, il faut la réhydratation par voie intraveineuse. Chez des enfants, la réhydratation doit être principalement conduite par voie intraveineuse. ② Pour traiter la diarrhée aigue: a. La diarrhée bénigne, par voie orale : chez des adultes, 50ml par kg par jour.b. La diarrhée grave, en perfusion, jusqu'à l'arrêt de la diarrhée. |

| | |
|---|---|
| 剂型、规格<br>Les formes pharmaceutiques et les spécifications | 　　口服补液盐Ⅰ：口服补液盐：每包总重 14.75g（大包中含氯化钠 1.75g，葡萄糖 11g；小包中含氯化钾 0.75g，碳酸氢钠 1.25g）（为 500ml 用量）。<br>　　口服补液盐Ⅱ，每包总重 13.95g（氯化钠 1.75g，葡萄糖 10g，枸橼酸钠 1.45g，氯化钾 0.75g）（为 500ml 用量）。<br><br>　　Les sels de réhydratation orale de type I : les sels de réhydratation : 14,75g par sachet (grand sachet contient 1,75g de chlorure de sodium et 11g de glucose ; le petit sachet contient 0,75g de chlorure de potassium et 1,25g de bicarbonate de sodium) (500ml).<br>　　Les sels de réhydratation orale de type I : chaque sachet pèse 13,95g (1,75g de chlorure de sodium, 10g de glucose, 1,45g de citrate de sodium et 0,75g de chlorure de potassium) (500ml). |
| **药品名称 Drug Names** | 腹膜透析液 Solution de dialyse péritonéale |
| 适应证<br>Les indications | 　　腹膜透析液可用于：①急性或慢性肾衰竭；②药物中毒；③顽固性心力衰竭；④电解质紊乱和酸碱平衡失调；⑤急性出血性胰腺炎和广泛化脓性腹膜炎等。<br><br>　　La solution pour dialyse péritonéale sert à traiter : ① L'insuffisance aigue ou chronique rénale. ② L'intoxication médicamenteuse. ③ L'insuffisance cardiaque réfractaire. ④ La déséquilibre électrolytique et la perte d'équilibre acide-base. ⑤ La pancréatite aiguë hémorragique et la péritonite purulente généralisée. |
| 用法、用量<br>Les modes d'emploi et la posologie | 　　①治疗急、慢性肾衰竭伴水潴留者，用间歇性腹膜透析每次 2L，留置 1～2 小时，每日交换 4～6 次。无水潴留者，用连续不卧床腹膜透析（CAPD），一般一日 4 次，每次 2L，日间每次间隔 4～5 小时，夜间一次留置 9～12 小时，以增加中分子尿症毒素清除。一般每日透析液量为 8L。②治疗急性左心衰竭，酌情用 2.5% 或 4.25% 葡萄糖透析液 2L；后者留置 30 分钟，可脱水 300～500ml；前者留置 1 小时，可脱水 100～300ml。③儿童：每次交换量一般为 50mg/kg 体重。<br><br>　　① Pour traiter l'insuffisance rénale chronique et aigue accompagnée de la rétention d'eau, utiliser la dialyse péritonéale intermittente, 2L par fois, pendant 1 à 2 h, échanger 4 à 6 fois par jour. Chez des patients sans rétention d'eau, utiliser la dialyse péritonéale continue ambulatoire, 4 fois par jour, 2L par fois, pendant la journée, toutes les 4 à 5 h, pendant la nuit, demeurer pendan 9 à 12h, pour aider à effacer les toxines urémiques moléculaires de poids moyen. La quantité de la solution pour dialyse est de 8L par jour en général. ② Pour traiter l'insuffisance ventriculaire gauche aigue : utiliser 2L de solution de glucose pour dialyse à 2,5% ou à 4,25% ; pour la solution à 4,25%, demeurer pendant 30 minutes, permettant la désydratation de 300 à 500ml ; pour la solution à 2,5%, demeurer pendant 1h, permettant la désydration de 100 à 300ml. ③ Chez des enfants : la dose d'échange est de 50 mg/kg par fois. |
| 剂型、规格<br>Les formes pharmaceutiques et les spécifications | 　　（1）腹膜透析液（乳酸盐）：①含 1.5% 葡萄糖（1L，1.5L，2L，2.5L，5L，6L）；②含 2.5% 葡萄糖（1L，1.5L，2L，2.5L，5L，6L）；③含 4.25% 葡萄糖（1L，1.5L，2L，2.5L，5L，6L）；④含葡萄糖 4.0%（1000ml）。（2）腹膜透析液（乳酸盐）（低钙）：①含葡萄糖 4.0%（2000ml）；②含葡萄糖 2.5%（1000ml）；③含葡萄糖 2.5%（2000ml）；④含葡萄糖 1.5%（2000ml）。<br><br>　　(1) La solution pour dialyse péritonéale (lactate) : ① Contenant la glucose à 1,5% (1L, 1,5L, 2L, 2,5L, 5L et 6L). ② Contenant la glucose à 2.5% (1L, 1,5L, 2L, 2,5L, 5L et 6L). ③ Contenant la glucose à 4,25% (1L, 1,5L, 2L, 2,5L, 5L et 6L). ④ Contenant la glucose à 4,0% (1 000ml).<br>　　(2) La solution pour dialyse péritonéale (lactate) (pauvre en calcium) : ① Contenant la glucose à 4,0% (2 000ml). ② Contenant la glucose à 2,5% (1 000ml). ③ Contenant la glucose à 2,5% (2 000ml). ④ Contenant la glucose à 1,5% (2 000ml). |

### 18.4　营养药 Médicaments de nutrition

| | |
|---|---|
| **药品名称 Drug Names** | 安素 Ensure |
| 适应证<br>Les indications | 　　用于乳糖不耐受患者，无法进固体饮食的外伤、慢性病、年老体弱、产妇、术前后及某些必须限制饮食的患者等。<br><br>　　Pour les personnes intolérantes au lactose, les traumatismes, les maladies chroniques, les personnes âgées et affaiblies qui ne peuvent pas entrer dans un régime solide, après l'accouchement et les patients qui doivent limiter leur alimentation. |

**续　表**

| 用法、用量<br>Les modes d'emploi et la posologie | 口服或鼻饲：取 5 量匙（约 55g）本品，加入开水溶解稀释至 250ml，按 1ml 标准稀释液提供 1 cal 热量计算患者每日用量。<br>Par voie orale ou nasogastrique : prendre 5 cuillères d'ensure (environ 55g), ajouter l'eau chaude pour diluer jusqu'à 250ml, décider la dose du jour pour les patients en fonction du critère : 1ml de dilution standard propose 1 calorie. |
|---|---|
| 剂型、规格<br>Les formes pharmaceutiques et les spécifications | 粉剂：每罐 400g。<br>Poudre : 400g par pot. |
| 药品名称 Drug Names | 肠内营养乳剂 (TP)Emulsion Nutritive Entérale |
| 适应证<br>Les indications | 用于有胃肠功能的营养不良或摄入障碍、重症或手术后需要补充营养的患者。<br>Ce produit est applicable chez des patients nécessitant le complément de la nutrition à cause de la malnutrition ou destroubles de l'apport nutritionnel liés à la fonction gastro-intestinale, ou à cause des maladies graves ou de la chirurgie. |
| 用法、用量<br>Les modes d'emploi et la posologie | 通过管饲或口服使用，应按照患者的体重和营养状况计算每日用量。①对作为唯一营养来源的患者：推荐剂量为一日 30ml/kg（30kcal/kg）。②作为补充营养的患者：根据患者需要推荐剂量为一日 500 ～ 1000ml。③管饲给药时，应逐渐增加给药速度，第一天的速度约为 20ml/h，以后每日逐增至最大滴速 150ml/h。通过重力或泵调整输注速度。<br>L'administration par sonde ou par voie orale, décider la dose en fonction du poids et de l'état nutritionnel des patients. ① Chez des patients qui considèrent ce médicament comme la seule source de nutrition : la dose recommandée est de 30 ml par kg par jour (30 kcal par kg). ② Chez des patients qui utilisent ce médicament pour le supplément nutritionnel : la dose recommandée est de 500 à 1 000ml par jour. ③ L'administration par sonde, augmenter progressivement la vistesse de l'administration, 20ml par h pour le premier jour, ensuite, augmenter jusqu'à 150ml par h au maximum. Ajuster la vitesse de la perfusion par gravité ou par pompage. |
| 剂型、规格<br>Les formes pharmaceutiques et les spécifications | 乳剂：500ml。<br>Émulsion : 500ml. |
| 药品名称 Drug Names | 水解蛋白 Protéines hydrolysées |
| 适应证<br>Les indications | 用于各种原因的蛋白质缺乏和衰弱患者以及对一般蛋白质消化吸收障碍的病例。用量视病情酌定。<br>Ce produit est appliqué chez des patients qui souffrent de la carence en protéine et des patients qui souffrent des troubles de digestion et d'absorption de la protéine. Ajuster la dose selon les cas. |
| 用法、用量<br>Les modes d'emploi et la posologie | 口服：一次 1 ～ 5g/kg。<br>静脉滴注：一般每次用 5% 溶液 500ml。<br>Par voie orale : 1 à 5g par kg par fois. En perfusion : 500ml de solution à 5% par fois. |
| 剂型、规格<br>Les formes pharmaceutiques et les spécifications | 注射用水解蛋白：每瓶 500g。注射液：每瓶 25g（500ml）。<br>Les protéines hydrolysées pour injection : 500mg par flacon.<br>Injection : 25g (500ml) par flacon. |
| 药品名称 Drug Names | 复方氨基酸 (18AA) Composée d'acide aminé (18AA) |
| 适应证<br>Les indications | 用于营养不良或有发生营养不良危险的患者，分解代谢旺盛疾病的营养支持和蛋白质消耗或丢失过多或合成障碍引起的低蛋白血症。<br>Ce produit sert à traiter les maladies souffrant de la malnutrition ou de la malnutrition potentielle. Il permet aussi de traiter l'hypoprotéinémie induite par la consommation excessive de la protéine ou par les troubles de synthèse de la protéine. |

续　表

| 用法、用量<br>Les modes d'emploi et la posologie | 静脉滴注，每次 250～500ml，一日 1～4 次，滴速 40～50 滴/分。<br>En perfusion, 250 à 500ml par fois, 1 à 4 fois par jour, 40 à 50 gouttes par minute. |
| --- | --- |
| 剂型、规格<br>Les formes pharmaceutiques et les spécifications | 注射液：250ml：12.5g（总氨基酸）；500ml：25g（总氨基酸）；500ml：60g（总氨基酸）。<br>Injection: 250ml : 12,5g (acide aminé total), 500ml : 25g (acide aminé total); 500ml : 60g (acide aminé total). |
| **药品名称 Drug Names** | 复方氨基酸 (9AA) Composée d'acide aminé (9AA) |
| 适应证<br>Les indications | 用于急性和慢性肾功能不全患者的肠道外支持；大手术、外伤或脓毒血症引起的严重肾衰竭。<br>Ce produit sert d'apport parentéral chez des patients insuffisants rénaux chroniques et aigus. Il permet aussi de traiter l'insuffisance rénale grave induite par l'intervention chirurgicale majeure, le traumatisme ou la septicémie. |
| 用法、用量<br>Les modes d'emploi et la posologie | 静脉滴注：成人一日 250～500ml，缓慢滴注。小儿用量遵医嘱。进行透析的急、慢性肾衰竭患者一日 1000ml，最大剂量不超过 1500ml。滴速不超过每分钟 15 滴。<br>En perfusion : chez des adultes, 250 à 500ml par jour, perfusion lente. Chez des enfants, selon les ordonnances. Chez des patients dialysés insuffisants rénaux chroniques et aigus, 1 000ml par jour, la dose maximale est de 1 500ml. Ne pas dépasser 15 gouttes par minute. |
| 剂型、规格<br>Les formes pharmaceutiques et les spécifications | 注射液：每瓶 250ml。<br>Injection : 250ml par flacon. |
| **药品名称 Drug Names** | 复方 α - 酮酸 Composés α-Acid Cetone |
| 适应证<br>Les indications | 配合低蛋白质和高热量饮食，预防和治疗因慢性肾功能不全而造成蛋白质代谢失调引起的损害，延缓肾脏病进展。<br>Doté d'un régime alimentaire hypercalorique et faible en protéine, il permet de prévenir et de traiter les dommages causés par les troubles du métabolisme des protéines induits par l'insuffisance rénale chronique et aigue, et de ralentir le développement des maladies rénales. |
| 用法、用量<br>Les modes d'emploi et la posologie | 口服：慢性肾功能不全，一般每次 4～8 片，一日 3 次，饭时服用；代偿期：每次 4～6 片，一日 3 次，服药期间配合低蛋白、高热量饮食。蛋白质摄入量为一日 0.5～0.6g/kg，高热量饮食为一日 146.44～167.36kJ/kg；失代偿期：每次 4～8 片，一日 3 次，配合低蛋白、高热量饮食。蛋白质摄入量为一日 0.3～0.4g/kg，高热量饮食为 146.44～167.36kJ/kg。<br>Par voie orale : pour traiter l'insuffisance rénale chronique, 4 à 8 comprimés par fois, 3 fois par jour, durant le repas ; pendant la phase compensée : 4 à 6 comprimés par fois, 3 fois par jour, prendre avec un régime alimentaire hypercalorique et faible en protéine. L'apport en protéine est de 0,5 à 0,6g par kg par jour, l'apport calorique est de 146,44 à 167,36 kj par kg par jour ; pendant la phase décompensée : 4 à 8 comprimés par fois, 3 fois par jour, avec un régime alimentaire hypercalorique et faible en protéine. L'apport en protéine est de 0,3 à 0,4g par kg par jour, l'apport calorique est de 146,44 à 167,36 kj par kg par jour. |
| 剂型、规格<br>Les formes pharmaceutiques et les spécifications | 片剂：0.63g。<br>Comprimés : 0.63g. |
| **药品名称 Drug Names** | 复方氨基酸 (3AA) Composée d'acide aminé (3AA) |
| 适应证<br>Les indications | 用于：①急性、亚急性、慢性重症肝炎以及肝硬化、慢性活动肝炎等；②促进胰岛素的分泌；③胆固醇合成的前体；④供给合成蛋白质的必需氨基酸原料；⑤促进蛋白质的合成；⑥抑制蛋白质的分解。<br>Ce produit est appliqué dans les cas suivants : ① Le traitement de l'hépatite sévère aiguë, subaiguë et chronique ainsi que de la cirrhose et de l'hépatite chronique active. ② La promotion de la sécrétion |

| | |
|---|---|
| 续　表 | |
| | d'insuline. ③ Les précurseurs de la synthèse du cholestérol. ④ L'approvisionnement en matières premières d'acides aminés essentiels pour la synthèse des protéines. ⑤ La promotion de la synthèse des protéines. ⑥ L'inhibition de la dégradation des protéines. |
| 用法、用量<br>Les modes d'emploi et la posologie | 静脉滴注：一日 250～500ml，或用 5%～10% 葡萄糖注射液适量混合后，缓慢静脉滴注，每分钟不超过 40 滴。一般昏迷期可酌情加量，疗程根据病情遵医嘱。<br>En perfusion : 250 à 500ml par jour, ou dissoudre dans la solution de glucose à 5% à 10%, perfusion lente, ne pas dépasser 40 gouttes par minute. Pendant le coma, augmenter un peu la dose, la durée du traitement dépend des ordonnances. |
| 剂型、规格<br>Les formes pharmaceutiques et les spécifications | 注射液：每瓶 250ml。<br>Injection : 250ml par flacon. |
| 药品名称 Drug Names | 复方氨基酸 (15AA) Composée d'acide aminé (15AA) |
| 适应证<br>Les indications | 用于大面积烧伤、创伤及严重感染等应激状态下肌肉分解代谢亢进、消化系统功能障碍、营养恶化及免疫功能下降的患者的营养支持，亦用于手术后患者，改善其营养状态。<br>Ce produit sert d'apport nutritionnel chez des patients souffrant du catabolisme musculaire hyperactif, du dysfonctionnement digestif, de la diminution de la fonction immunitaire et de la détérioration nutritionnelle sous l'état de stress à cause des brûlures étendues, du traumatisme et des infestions graves. Il est aussi applicable chez des patients postopératoires pour améliorer leur état de nutrition. |
| 用法、用量<br>Les modes d'emploi et la posologie | 静脉滴注一日 250～500ml，用适量 5%～10% 葡萄糖注射液混合后缓慢滴注。滴速不宜超过每 1 分钟 20 滴。<br>En perfusion : 250 à 500ml par jour, dissoudre dans la solution de glucose à 5% à 10%, perfusion lente, ne pas dépasser 20 gouttes par minute. |
| 剂型、规格<br>Les formes pharmaceutiques et les spécifications | 每瓶 250ml（总氨基酸 20g）。<br>250ml par flacon (20g d'acide aminé total). |
| 药品名称 Drug Names | 脂肪乳 Emulsion de graisse |
| 适应证<br>Les indications | 适用于需要高热量的患者（如肿瘤及其他恶性病）、肾损害、禁用蛋白质的患者和由于某种原因不能经胃肠道摄取营养的患者，以补充适当热量和必需脂肪酸。<br>Il permet de compléter les calories appropriées et des acides gras essentiels, chez des patients qui nécessitent l'alimentation d'une grande quantité de calories (tels que les patients atteints de tumeurs ou de maladies malignes), chez des paitents qui ne peuvent pas prendre des protéines à cause des lésions rénales, et des patients qui ne peuvent pas absorber les nutriments par voie gastro-intestinale pour certaines raisons. |
| 用法、用量<br>Les modes d'emploi et la posologie | 静脉滴注：第一日脂肪量不应超过 1g/kg，以后剂量可酌增，但脂肪量不得超过 2.5g/kg，静脉滴注速度最初 10 分钟为 20 滴 / 分，如无不良反应出现，以后可逐渐增加，30 分钟后维持 40～60 滴 / 分。<br>En perfusion : pour le premier jour, la quantité de la grasse ne doit pas dépasser 1g par kg, augmenter progressivement la dsoe, mais ne pas dépasser 2,5g par kg. La vitesse de la perfusion est de 20 gouttes par minute pour les 10 premières minutes, s'il n'y a pas de réactions indésirables, augmenter progressivement la vitesse pour maintenir à 40 à 60 gouttes par minute 30 minutes après. |
| 剂型、规格<br>Les formes pharmaceutiques et les spécifications | 注射乳剂：每瓶 100ml（10g）；100ml（20g）；100ml（30g）；250ml（25g）；250ml（50g）。<br>Émulsion injectable : 100ml (10g), 100ml (20g), 100ml (30g), 250ml (25g ) ou 250ml (50g) par flacon. |

| 药品名称 Drug Names | ω-3 鱼油脂肪乳注射液 Injéction d'émulsion Emulsion d'Huile de Poisson ω-3 |
|---|---|
| 适应证<br>Les indications | 用于全身炎症反应综合征较严重但又需要肠外营养的患者。<br><br>Ce produit est applicable chez des patients atteints d'un sévère syndrome de réponse inflammatoire systémique, mais qui nécessitent une nutrition parentérale. |
| 用法、用量<br>Les modes d'emploi et la posologie | 按体重一日 1～2ml/kg，即按体重一日 0.1g～0.2g 鱼油 /kg，70kg 患者每日用量不超过 140ml。最大输注速率按体重不超过每小时 0.5ml/kg。必须与其他类型脂肪乳剂同时输注时，推荐鱼油剂量应占其中的 10%～20%。<br><br>1 à 2ml par kg, soit 0,1 à 0,2g d'huile de poisson par kg, chez des patients de 70kg, ne pas dépasser 140ml par jour. Le débit de perfusion maximal est de 0,5ml par kg par h. Lors de l'utilisation avec d'autres émulsions de grasse, l'huile de graisse recommandée doit représenter 10% à 20%. |
| 剂型、规格<br>Les formes pharmaceutiques et les spécifications | 注射剂：50ml；100ml。<br>Injection : 50ml ou 100ml. |
| 药品名称 Drug Names | 多种微量元素（Ⅰ）Multi-Oligo-éléments (I) |
| 适应证<br>Les indications | 本品用于新生儿和婴儿全肠外营养时补充电解质和微量元素日常需求。<br><br>Ce produit permet de satisfaire aux besoins quotidiens en électrolytes et en oligo-éléments lors de la nutrition parentérale totale pour les nouveau-nés et les bébés. |
| 用法、用量<br>Les modes d'emploi et la posologie | 新生儿和婴儿：一般每日用本品 4ml/kg，可根据患儿对电解质和微量元素需要的不同而调节用量。<br><br>Chez des nouveau-nés et des bébés : en général, 4ml par kg par jour, ajuster la dose en fonction du besoin des patients en électrolytes et en oligo-éléments. |
| 剂型、规格<br>Les formes pharmaceutiques et les spécifications | 注射液：每支 10ml。<br>Injection : 10ml par solution. |
| 药品名称 Drug Names | 多种微量元素（Ⅱ）Multi-oligo-éléments (II) |
| 适应证<br>Les indications | 一般饮食摄入不会引起微量元素的缺乏和过量，但长期肠外营养，可造成微量元素摄入不足，本品可满足成人每日对所含微量元素的生理需要。仅用于 15kg 以儿童及成人长期肠外全营养时补充电解质和微量元素。妊娠期妇女对微量元素的需要量轻度增高，本品也适用于妊娠期妇女。<br><br>L'apport alimentaire général ne provoque pasle manque ni l'excèsd'oligo-éléments, mais la nutrition parentérale à long terme peut entraîner un apport insuffisant en oligo-éléments. Ce produit permet de satisfaire aubesoin physiologique quotidien d'un adulte pour les oligo-éléments. Il n'est applicable que chez des enfants plus de 15kg et des adultes pour permettre de compléter les électrolytes et les oligo-éléments lors de la nutrition parentérale totale. Comme le besoin en oligo-éléments des femmes pendant la grossesse connaît une légère augmentation, ce produit est aussi applicable chez les femmes pendant la grossesse. |
| 用法、用量<br>Les modes d'emploi et la posologie | 成人推荐剂量为每日 10ml。加于复方氨基酸注射液或葡萄糖注射液 500ml 内滴注，滴注时间为 6～8 小时。配制好的输液必须在 24 小时内输注完毕，以免被污染。<br><br>La dose recommandée chez des adultes est de 10ml par jour. Dissoudre dans 500ml d'injection composée d'acide animé ou de solution de glucose pour la perfusion, en 6 à 8h. La perfusion préparée doit être administrée en 24h pour éviter la contamination. |
| 剂型、规格<br>Les formes pharmaceutiques et les spécifications | 注射液：每支 10ml。<br>Injection : 10ml par solution. |

**续　表**

| 药品名称 Drug Names | 脂溶性维生素（Ⅰ）Vitamine liposoluble (I) |
| --- | --- |
| 适应证<br>Les indications | 为长期肠外全营养患者补充需要的脂溶性维生素 A、D、E、K。<br>Ce produit permet de compléter les besoins en vitamine liposoluble A, D, E et K des patients nécessitant une nutrition parentérale à long terme. |
| 用法、用量<br>Les modes d'emploi et la posologie | 用于 11 岁以下儿童及婴儿，每日 1ml/kg 体重，每日最大剂量 10ml。使用前在无菌条件下，将本品加入到脂肪乳注射液内（100ml 或以上量），轻轻摇匀后输注，并在 24 小时内用完。<br>Applicable chez des enfants moins de 11ans et des bébés, 1ml par kg par jour, ne pas dépasser 10ml par jour. sous des conditions stériles, ajouter ce produit dans l'injection d'émulsion de graisse (100ml ou plus), agiter doucement avant la perfusion, en 24h. |
| 剂型、规格<br>Les formes pharmaceutiques et les spécifications | 注射液：每支 10ml。<br>Injection : 10ml par solution. |
| 药品名称 Drug Names | 脂溶性维生素（Ⅱ）Vitamine liposoluble (II) |
| 适应证<br>Les indications | 为长期肠外全营养患者补充需要量的脂溶性维生素 A、D、E、K。<br>Ce produit permet de compléter les besoins en vitamine liposoluble A, D, E et K des patients nécessitant une nutrition parentérale à long terme. |
| 用法、用量<br>Les modes d'emploi et la posologie | 静脉滴注：将本品 1 支（10ml）加到脂肪乳注射剂内，轻摇混合后输注。11 岁以上儿童及成人用成人注射液，每日 10ml。<br>En perfusion : ajouter 1 solution de ce produit (10ml) dans l'injection d'émulsion de graisse, agiter doucement pour la perfusion. Chez des enfants plus de 11 ans et des adultes, 10ml par jour. |
| 剂型、规格<br>Les formes pharmaceutiques et les spécifications | 注射液：每支 10ml。<br>Injection : 10ml par solution. |
| 药品名称 Drug Names | 水溶性维生素 Vitamine solubles dans l'eau |
| 适应证<br>Les indications | 用于长期肠外全营养患者补充水溶性维生素。<br>Ce produit permet de compléter les besoins en vitamine soluble dans l'eau des patients nécessitant une nutrition parentérale à long terme. |
| 用法、用量<br>Les modes d'emploi et la posologie | 10kg 以上儿童及成人，每日 1 瓶，10kg 以下儿童每日按每千克体重给予 1/10 瓶。本品用注射用水或葡萄糖注射液 10ml 溶解后再稀释于同一类型药液中静脉滴注。<br>Chez des enfant plus de 10kg ou des adultes, 1 flacon par jour, chez des enfants moins de 10kg, 1/10 de flacon par kg par jour. Dissoudre dans 10ml d'eau pour injection ou de solution de glucose, diluer ensuite dans les liquides de même sorte pour la perfusion. |
| 剂型、规格<br>Les formes pharmaceutiques et les spécifications | 冻干粉剂：每瓶含有硝酸硫胺 3.1mg，核黄素磷酸钠 4.9mg，烟酸胺 40mg，盐酸吡多辛 4.9mg，泛酸钠 16.5mg，维生素 C 钠 113mg，生物素 60μg，叶酸 0.4mg，维生素 $B_{12}$ 5.0μg。<br>Poudre lyophilisée: Chaque flacon contient 3.1mg de nitrate de thiamine, 4.9mg de riboflavine phosphate de sodium, 40mg de niacinamide, 4.9mg de chlorhydrate de pyridoxine, 16.5mg de pantothénate de sodium, 113mg de vitamine de sodium, 60μg de biotine, 0.4mg de acide folique et 5.0μg vitamine $B_{12}$. |

### 19. 专科用药 Médicaments spécialisés

### 19.1　老年病用药 Médicaments pour la vieillesse

| 药品名称 Drug Names | 帕米膦酸二钠 Pamidronate disodique |
| --- | --- |
| 适应证<br>Les indications | ①用于治疗恶性肿瘤患者骨转移疼痛和高钙血症。②治疗骨质疏松症和骨质愈合不良。③也用于甲状旁腺功能亢进症。<br>① Ce produit sert à traiter la douleur liée aux métastases osseuses et l'hypercalcémie chez les patients cancéreux. ② Il permet de traiter l'ostéoporose et la guérison osseuse pauvre. ③ Il sert aussi à traiter l'hyperparathyroïdie. |

**续 表**

| 用法、用量<br>Les modes d'emploi et la posologie | ①用于治疗骨质疏松症：每月 1 次 30mg 静脉滴注，连续 6 个月，改为预防量；每 3 个月 1 次 30mg 静脉滴注，连续 2 年。②治疗癌症骨转移性疼痛：一次用药 30～60mg，静脉缓慢滴注 4 小时以上，浓度不得超过 15mg/125ml，滴速不得大于 15～30mg/2h。③治疗高钙血症：当血钙浓度＜ 3.0、3.0～3.5、3.5～4.0、＞ 4.0mmol/L，或＜ 12.0、12.0～14.0、14.0～16.0、＞ 16.0mg，用本品剂量为 15～30mg、30～60mg、60～90mg、90mg。④治疗变形性骨炎及骨愈合不良：每日 30～60mg，连续 1～3 日；或每日 30mg，连续 6 周。⑤预防癌症骨转移，每 4 周静脉滴注 30～60mg。<br><br>① Pour traiter l'ostéoporose : 30mg par fois par mois, en perfusion, pendant 6 mois consécutifs, ensuite, la dose pour la prévention ; 30mg par fois, tous les 3 mois, pendant 2 ans consécutifs. ② Pour traiter la douleur liée aux métastases osseuses chez des patients cancéreux : 30 à 60mg par fois, perfusion lente, pendant plus de 4 h, la concentration ne dépasse pas 15mg par 125ml, le débit de la perfusion ne dépasse pas 15 à 30mg par 2h. ③ Pour traiter l'hypercalcémie : quand la concentration de calcium dans le sang est inférieure à 3,0 mmol par L (inférieure à 12,0 mg), prendre 15 à 30mg de ce produit ; quand la concentration est de3,0 à 3,5 mmol par L (12,0 à 14,0mg), prendre 30 à 60mg; quand la concentration est de 3,5 à 4,0 mmol par L (14,0 à 16,0mg), prendre 60 à 90mg ; quand la concentration est supérieure à 4,0 mmol par L (supérieure à 16,0mg), prendre 90mg. ④ Pour traiter la maladie de Paget et la guérison osseuse pauvre : 30 à 60mg par jour, penant 1 à 3 jours ; ou 30mg par jour, pendant 6 semaines consécutives. ⑤ Pour prévenir les métastases osseuses du cancer, 30 à 60mg, en perfusion, toutes les 4 semaines. |
| --- | --- |
| 剂型、规格<br>Les formes pharmaceutiques et les spécifications | 片剂：每片 150mg。<br>注射液：每支 15mg（5ml）。<br>Comprimés : 150mg par comprimé.<br>Injection : 15mg (5ml) par solution. |

| 药品名称 Drug Names | 阿仑膦酸钠 Alendronate sodique |
| --- | --- |
| 适应证<br>Les indications | 用于治疗绝经后妇女骨质疏松症，预防髋部和脊柱骨折，也适用于男性骨质疏松症及增加骨质。<br><br>Il permet de traiter l'ostéoporose chez les femmes ménopausées, de prévenir fracturesvertébrales et de la hanche. Il est aussi applicable dans le traitement de l'ostéoporose et l'augmentation osseuse chez des hommes. |
| 用法、用量<br>Les modes d'emploi et la posologie | 口服，一日 1 次 10mg，或每周一次 70mg，早餐前 30 分钟用至少 200ml 白开水送服，不要咀嚼或吮吸药片。<br><br>Par voie orale, 10mg par fois par jour, ou 70mg par fois par semaine, pris 30 minutes avant le petit-déjeuner avec 200ml d'eau chaude au moins, ne pas mâcher ni sucer les comprimés. |
| 剂型、规格<br>Les formes pharmaceutiques et les spécifications | 片剂：每片 10mg；70mg。<br>Comprimés : 10mg ou 70mg par comprimé. |

| 药品名称 Drug Names | 伊班膦酸钠 Ibandronate Sodique |
| --- | --- |
| 适应证<br>Les indications | 用于伴有或不伴有骨转移的恶性肿瘤引起的高钙血症。<br>Ce produit permet de traiter l'hypercalcémie induite par les tumeurs malignes avec ou sans métastases osseuses. |
| 用法、用量<br>Les modes d'emploi et la posologie | 缓慢静脉滴注，滴注时间不得少于 2 小时。严格按照血钙浓度，治疗前适当给予 0.9% 氯化钠注射液进行水化治疗。中、重度单剂量给 2～4mg。<br><br>Perfusion lente, pendant 2 h au moins. Suivre de près la concentration de calcium dans le sang. Avant le traitement, suivre la thérapie d'hydratation avec l'injection de chlorure de sodium à 0,9%. La dose unique chez des cas modéré et grave est de 2 à 4mg. |
| 剂型、规格<br>Les formes pharmaceutiques et les spécifications | 注射液：每支 1mg（1ml）。<br>Injection : 1mg (1ml) par solution. |

**续　表**

| 药品名称 Drug Names | 利塞膦酸钠 Risédronate sodique |
|---|---|
| 适应证<br>Les indications | ①用于治疗绝经后妇女骨质疏松症，预防髋部和脊柱骨折，也适用于男性骨质疏松症，糖皮质激素诱导的骨质疏松症。②治疗 Paget 病。<br><br>① Il permet de traiter l'ostéoporose chez les femmes ménopausées, et de prévenir fractures vertébrales et de la hanche. Il est aussi applicable dans le traitement de l'ostéoporose masculine et de l'ostéoporose induite par les glucocorticoïdes. ② Il permet de traiter la maladie de Paget. |
| 用法、用量<br>Les modes d'emploi et la posologie | 口服，餐前 30 分钟直立服用，200ml 左右清水送服，服后 30 分钟内不应躺下。一日 1 次，一次 5mg。绝经后骨质疏松症：15mg/ 片，一日 1 次；35mg/ 片，一周 1 次；75mg/ 片，1 个月连服 2 片；150mg/ 片，1 个月一次。治疗男性骨质疏松症：15mg/ 片，一日 1 次。治疗 Paget 病：30mg/ 片，一日 1 次，连服 2 个月。<br><br>Par voie orale, prendre de manière verticale (debout) 30 minutes avant le repas, avec 200ml d'eau, durant les 30 minutes suivantes, ne pas n'allonger. 1 fois par jour, 5mg par fois. Pour traiter l'ostéoporose chez les femmes ménopausées : 15mg par comprimé, 1 fois par jour ; 35mg par comprimé, une fois par semaine ; 75mg par comprimé, 2 comprimés par mois, pris de manière consécutif ; 150 mg par comprimé, une fois par mois. Pour traiter l'ostéoporose masculine : 15mg par comprimé, une fois par jour. Pour traiter la maladie de Paget : 30mg par comprimé, une fois par jour, pendant 2 mois consécutifs. |
| 剂型、规格<br>Les formes pharmaceutiques et les spécifications | 片剂：每片 5mg；15mg；30mg；35mg；75mg；150mg。<br>Comprimés : 5mg, 15mg, 30mg, 35mg, 75mg ou 150mg par comprimé. |
| 药品名称 Drug Names | 降钙素 Calcitonine |
| 适应证<br>Les indications | ①用于治疗绝经后妇女骨质疏松症，老年骨质疏松症。②用于治疗恶性肿瘤患者骨转移疼痛和高钙血症。③各种骨代谢疾病所致的骨痛。④也用于甲状旁腺功能亢进症，缺乏动力或维生素 D 中毒导致的应变性骨炎。⑤ Paget 病。⑥高钙血症和高钙血症危象。<br><br>① Il permet de traiter l'ostéoporose chez les femmes ménopausées et l'ostéoporose sénile. ② Ce produit sert à traiter la douleur liée aux métastases osseuses et l'hypercalcémie chez les patients cancéreux. ③ Il permet de traiter la douleur osseuse causée par des maladies métaboliques osseuses. ④ Il est aussi applicable dans le traitement de l'hyperparathyroïdie et de l'ostéite causée par le manque de motivation ou l'intoxicationà la vitamine D. ⑤ Il permet de traiter la maladie de Paget. ⑥ L'hypercalcémie et la crise de l'hypercalcémie. |
| 用法、用量<br>Les modes d'emploi et la posologie | ①绝经后或老年骨质疏松症：a. 皮下或肌内注射，每日 50 ～ 100U；或隔日 100U。b. 鼻内用药，每次 100U，一日 1 ～ 2 次；或每次 50U，一日 2 ～ 4 次；或隔日 200U。12 周为 1 个疗程。治疗期间，应日服钙元素 0.5 ～ 1.0g，维生素 D 400U。② Paget 病：a. 皮下或肌内注射，每日 100U，改善后，隔日或每日注射 50U，必要时日剂量增至 200U。b. 鼻内用药：每次 100U，一日 2 次；或每次 50U，一日 4 次，少数病例可能需要每次 200U，一日 2 次。③高钙血症：危象紧急处理每日 5 ～ 10U ／ kg，溶于 500ml 生理盐水中，静脉滴注至少 6 小时或日剂量分 2 ～ 4 次缓慢静脉注射，同时补液。慢性症状每日 5 ～ 10U/kg，1 次或 2 次皮下或肌内注射。也可每日 200 ～ 400U，分数次鼻内给药。④痛性神经营养不良症：a. 皮下或肌内注射，每日 100U，持续 2 ～ 4 周，然后每次 100U，每周 3 次，维持 6 周以上。b. 鼻内给药，每日 200U，分 2 ～ 4 次给药，持续 2 ～ 4 周，然后每次 200U，每周 3 次，持续 6 周以上。<br><br>① Pour traiter l'ostéoporose chez les femmes ménopausées et l'ostéoporose sénile : a. Injection sous-cutanée ou IM, 50 à 100U par jour ; ou 100 U tous les 2 jours. b. Administration par voie nasale, 100 U par fois, 1 à 2 fois par jour ; ou 50 U par fois, 2 à 4 fois par jour ; ou 200 U tous les 2 jours. Pendant 12 semaines comme un traitement médical. Durant le traitement, il faut prendre 0,5 à 1,0g de calcium, 400 U de vitamine D. ② Pour traiter la maladie de Paget : a. Injection sous-cutanée ou IM, 100U par jour, après l'amélioration des symptômes, 50 U tous les 1 à 2 jours, en cas de besoin, 200U |

续　表

<table>
<tr>
<td colspan="2">par jour. b. Administration par voie nasale : 100 U par fois, 2 fois par jour; ou 50 U par fois, 4 fois par jour, pour certains cas, 200 U par fois, 2 fois par jour. ③ Pour traiter l'hypercalcémie : lors de la crise, 5 à 10 U par kg par jour, dissoudre dans 500ml de solution saline, en perfusion pendant 6 h au mois ou injecter par voie IV la dose du jour à travers 2 à 4 fois, faire l'hydratation en même temps. Pour des cas chroniques, 5 à 10 U par kg par jour, injection sous-cutanée ou IM, 1 à 2 fois. Ou 200 à 400 U par jour, administration nasale à plusieurs fois. ④ Pour traiter la maladie de Sudeck : a. Injection sous-cutanée ou IM, 100 U par jour, pendant 2 à 4 semaines, ensuite, 100 U par fois, 3 fois par semaine, pendant 6 semaines au moins.b. Administration nasale, 200 U par jour, à travers 2 à 4 fois, pendant 2 à 4 semaines, ensuite, 200 U par fois, 3 fois par semaine, pendant 6 semaines au moins.</td>
</tr>
<tr>
<td>剂型、规格<br>Les formes pharmaceutiques et les spécifications</td>
<td>注射液：每支 1ml；2ml。<br>喷鼻剂：每瓶 2ml。<br><br>Injection : 1ml ou 2ml par solution.<br>L'aérosol nasal : 2ml par flacon.</td>
</tr>
<tr>
<td>药品名称 Drug Names</td>
<td>骨化三醇 Calcitriol</td>
</tr>
<tr>
<td>适应证<br>Les indications</td>
<td>①绝经后或老年骨质疏松症。②肾性骨营养不良。③特发性、假性或术后甲状旁腺功能低下。④维生素 D 依赖型佝偻病，低血磷性抗维生素 D 型佝偻病。<br><br>① Il permet de traiter l'ostéoporose chez les femmes ménopausées et l'ostéoporose sénile. ② L'ostéodystrophie rénale. ③ L'hypoparathyroïdie idiopathique, pseudo ou postopératoire. ④ Le rachitisme vitamine D-dépendant et le rachitisme hypophosphatémique résistant à la vitamine D.</td>
</tr>
<tr>
<td>用法、用量<br>Les modes d'emploi et la posologie</td>
<td>①绝经后或老年骨质疏松症：推荐剂量为每次 0.25μg，一日 2 次，最大剂量可至每次 0.5μg，一日 2 次。用药后第 1、3、6 个月应监测血钙及血肌酐，正常以后，可每 6 个月检测一次。调整剂量期间，需每周检测血钙。②肾性骨营养不良症：最初剂量为 0.25μg，每日口服一次，连服 2～4 周。对血清钙正常或偏低者，口服 0.25μg，每 2 日一次即可。注射剂的剂量为开始每次 0.5μg（0.01μg/kg），每周 3 次。如用药后 2～4 周，患者生化指标和临床症状无明显改善，可每隔 2～4 周将用量增高 0.25μg/d。在此期间，应每周监测血钙至少 2 次。③甲状旁腺功能低或佝偻病患者：初始剂量 0.25μg，每晨服用。如生化指标和临床症状无明显改善，可每隔 2～4 周提高药物剂量。<br><br>① Pour traiter l'ostéoporose chez les femmes ménopausées et l'ostéoporose sénile : la dose recommandée est de 0,25μg par fois, 2 fois par jour, la dose maximale est de 0,5μg par fois, 2 fois par jour. 1, 3, 6 mois après l'administration, il faut examiner la concentration de calcium dans le sang et la créatinine sérique, après la normalisation, examiner tous les 6 mois. Lors de l'ajustement de la dose, il faut examiner la concentration de calcium dans le sang toutes les semaines. ② Pour traiter l'ostéodystrophie rénale : commencer par 0,25μg, une fois par jour, pendant 2 à 4 semaines. Chez des patients dont la cencentration en calcium sérique est normale ou légèrement basse, prendre 0,25μg par voie orale, une fois tous les 2 jours. Pour l'injection, commencer par 0.5μg(0.01μg/kg) par fois, 3 fois par semaine. S'il n'y a pas l'amélioration évidente des symptômes cliniques 2 à 4 semaines après l'administration, il faut augmenter 0,25μg par jour toutes les 2 à 4 semaiens. Pendant ce temps-là, examinier la concentration en calcium sérique 2 fois par semaine au moins. ③ Pour traiter l'hypoparathyroïdie ou le rachitisme : la dose initiale est de 0,25μg, prendre chaque petit matin. S'il n'y a pas l'amélioration des symptômes cliniques, augmenter la dose toutes les 2 à 4 semaines.</td>
</tr>
<tr>
<td>剂型、规格<br>Les formes pharmaceutiques et les spécifications</td>
<td>胶囊剂：每粒 0.25μg。<br>注射剂：每支 1μg（1ml）；2μg（1ml）。<br>Capsules : 0,25ug par capsule.<br>Injection : 1μg (1ml) ou 2μg (1ml) par solution.</td>
</tr>
<tr>
<td>药品名称 Drug Names</td>
<td>阿法骨化醇 Alfacalcidol</td>
</tr>
<tr>
<td>适应证<br>Les indications</td>
<td>用于：预防骨质疏松症、佝偻病和软骨病、肾源性骨病、甲状旁腺功能减退症。<br>Il permet de prévenir l'ostéoporose, le rachitisme et l'ostéomalacie, source de l'ostéodystrophie rénale, et l'hypoparathyroïdie.</td>
</tr>
</table>

**续　表**

| | |
|---|---|
| 用法、用量<br>Les modes d'emploi et la posologie | 口服。骨质疏松症：成人，初始剂量每日 0.5μg，维持量为每日 0.25～0.5μg。其他指征患者：成人或体重 20kg 以上儿童初始剂量每日 1μg，老年人每日 0.5μg，维持剂量为每日 0.25～1μg。<br>Par voie orale. Pour traiter l'ostéoporose : chez des adultes, la dose initiale, 0,5μg par jour, la dose d'entretien, 0,25 à 0,5μg par jour. Pour les autres cas : chez des adultes ou des enfants plus de 20kg, la dose initiale, 1ug par jour, chez des personnes âgées, 0,5μg par jour, la dose d'entretien est de 0,25 à 1μg par jour. |
| 剂型、规格<br>Les formes pharmaceutiques et les spécifications | 胶囊剂：每粒 0.25μg。<br>片剂：每片 0.25μg；0.5μg。<br>Capsules : 0,25μg par capsule.<br>Comprimés : 0,25μg ou 0,5μg par comprimé. |
| 药品名称 Drug Names | 碳酸钙 Carbonate de calcium |
| 适应证<br>Les indications | 用于预防和治疗钙缺乏症，以及妊娠和哺乳期妇女、绝经期妇女钙的补充。<br>Ce produit permet de prévenir et de traiter la carence en calcium. Il est également applicable dans le supplément de calcium chez les femmes enceintes et les mères allaitantes, les femmes ménopausées. |
| 用法、用量<br>Les modes d'emploi et la posologie | 口服，一日 1～3 次，分次服。可根据个人情况酌情进行补充。<br>Par voie orale, 1 à 3 fois par jour, à travers plusieurs fois. Possible de compléter selon les cas personnels. |
| 剂型、规格<br>Les formes pharmaceutiques et les spécifications | 片剂：0.75g。<br>咀嚼片：每片 1.25g。<br>Comprimés : 0,75g.<br>Comprimés à mâcher : 1,25g par comprimé. |
| 药品名称 Drug Names | 替勃龙 Tibolone |
| 适应证<br>Les indications | 用于绝经后引起的多种症状。<br>Il sert à traiter des symptômes post-ménopausiques. |
| 用法、用量<br>Les modes d'emploi et la posologie | 口服，每日一次 2.5mg，最好固定时间服用，症状消除后可每日服半量，连续服用 3 个月或更长时间。<br>Par voie orale, 2,5mg par fois par jour, il vaut mieux fixer le moment pour l'administration. Après la disparition des symptômes, prendre la moitié de la dose, pendant 3 mois ou plus de manière consécutive. |
| 剂型、规格<br>Les formes pharmaceutiques et les spécifications | 片剂：每片 2.5mg。<br>Comprimés : 2,5mg par comprimé. |
| 药品名称 Drug Names | 雌二醇 Estradiol |
| 适应证<br>Les indications | 卵巢功能不全或卵巢激素不足引起的各种症状，主要是功能性子宫出血、原发性闭经、绝经期综合征以及前列腺癌等。<br>Il sert à traiter les symptômes causés pas le dysfonctionnement ovarien ou le manque d'hormones ovariennes, y compris le saignement utérin fonctionnel, l'aménorrhée primaire, le syndrome de la ménopause, lecancer de la prostate, etc. |
| 用法、用量<br>Les modes d'emploi et la posologie | 肌内注射：每次 0.5～1.5mg，每周 2～3 次。口服，一日 1 片。<br>Injection IM : 0,5 à 1,5mg par fois, 2 à 3 fois par semaine. Par voie orale, 1 comprimé par jour. |
| 剂型、规格<br>Les formes pharmaceutiques et les spécifications | 注射液：每支 2mg（1ml）。<br>凝胶：每支 80g；0.06%。<br>片剂：每片 1mg。<br>微粒化 17β 雌二醇片：每片 1mg；2mg。<br>控释贴片：周效片，每片 2.5mg；3～4 日效片：每片 4mg。 |

续 表

|  | Injection : 2mg (1ml) par solution.<br>Les gels : 80g ; 0,06% par pièce.<br>Comprimés : 1mg par comprimé.<br>Comprimés de 17β estradiol micronisés : 1mg ou 2mg par comprimé.<br>Les patchs à libération contrôlée : les patchs à action en une semaine, 2,5mg par patch ; les patchs à action en 3 à 4 jours : 4mg par patch. |
|---|---|
| 药品名称 Drug Names | 雷洛昔芬 Raloxifène |
| 适应证<br>Les indications | 主要用于预防绝经后妇女的骨质疏松症。<br>Ce médicament est principalement utilisé dans le traitement de l'ostéoporose chez les femmes ménopausées. |
| 用法、用量<br>Les modes d'emploi et la posologie | 口服，每日 60mg，不受进食限制。老年人无须调整剂量。由于疾病的必然过程，本品需要长期使用。<br>Par voie orale, 60mg par jour. Pas nécessaire d'ajuster la dose. Il faut prendre ce médicament pour une longue durée. |
| 剂型、规格<br>Les formes pharmaceutiques et les spécifications | 片剂：每日 60mg。<br>Comprimés : 60mg par comprimé. |
| 药品名称 Drug Names | 氨基葡萄糖 Glucosamine |
| 适应证<br>Les indications | 用于治疗和预防全身部位的骨关节炎。可缓解和消除骨关节炎的疼痛、肿胀等症状，改善关节活动功能。<br>Ce produit permet de traiter et de prévenir l'arthrose de toutes les parties du corps. Il permet aussi d'atténuer ou de supprimer la douleur et le gonflement liés à l'arthrose et d'améliorer les fonctions articulaires. |
| 用法、用量<br>Les modes d'emploi et la posologie | 口服，每次 1～2 粒，一日 3 次，一般疗程 4～12 周，如有必要可延长服药时间。每年重复治疗 2～3 次。<br>Par voie orale, 1 à 2 capsules par fois, 3 fois par jour, pendant 4 à 12 semaines, s'il est nécessaire, prolonger la durée du traitement. Répéter le traitement 2 à 3 fois par an. |
| 剂型、规格<br>Les formes pharmaceutiques et les spécifications | 胶囊剂：每粒 0.24mg。<br>Capsules : 0,24mg par capsule. |
| 药品名称 Drug Names | 酚苄明 Phénoxybenzamine |
| 适应证<br>Les indications | ①用于前列腺增生引起的尿潴留。②嗜铬细胞瘤的治疗和术前准备。③周围血管痉挛性疾病。<br>① La rétention urinaire due à l'hyperplasie bénigne de la prostate. ② Le traitement et la préparation préopératoire du phéochromocytome. ③ Les maladies liées au spasme vasculaire périphérique. |
| 用法、用量<br>Les modes d'emploi et la posologie | 开始每次 10mg，一日 2 次，以后隔日加量 10mg，直至获得临床效果或出现轻微不良反应。以每次 20～40mg，每日 2～3 次维持。<br>Commencer par 10mg par fois, 2 fois par jour, ensuite, augmenter 10mg tous les jours, jusqu'à l'obtention des résultats cliniques ou à l'apparition des réactions indésirables mineures. Pour l'entretien, 20 à 40mg par fois, 2 à 3 fois par jour. |
| 剂型、规格<br>Les formes pharmaceutiques et les spécifications | 片剂：每片 10mg。<br>Comprimés : 10mg par comprimé. |

**续 表**

| 药品名称 Drug Names | 特拉唑嗪 Térazosine |
|---|---|
| 适应证<br>Les indications | ①用于改善良性前列腺增生患者的排尿症状。②还用于治疗慢性、非细菌性前列腺炎和前列腺痛，女性膀胱颈梗阻，结肠手术拔出导尿管前服用，预防急性尿潴留的发生。③用于治疗高血压，可单独使用或与其他药合用。<br><br>① Il permet d'améliorer la miction chez les patients présentant des symptômes de l'hyperplasie bénigne de la prostate. ② Il permet de traiter la prostatite et la prostatodynie chroniques non bactériennes, l'obstruction du col de la vessie féminine. Il faut le prendre avant de tirer le cathéter lors de la chirurgie du côlon. Il permet aussi de prévenir la rétention urinaire aiguë. ③ Utilisé seul ou en association avec d'autres médicaments, il permet de traiter l'hypertension artérielle. |
| 用法、用量<br>Les modes d'emploi et la posologie | ①良性前列腺增生：口服，每次 2mg，一日 1 次，每晚睡前服用。②高血压：初始剂量为睡前服用 1mg，且不应超过，以尽量减少首次低血压事件的发生。一周后，每日单剂量可加倍以达到预期效果。常用维持剂量为一日 2～10mg。<br><br>① Pour traiter l'hyperplasie bénigne de la prostate : par voie orale, 2mg par fois, 1 fois par jour, avant le sommeil du soir. ② Pour traiter l'hypertension artérielle : la dose initiale est de 1mg avant le sommeil du soir, ne pas dépasser 1mg pour éviter l'hypotension. Une semaine après, possible de doubler la dose pour atteindre le résultat désiré. La dose d'entretien usuelle est de 2 à 10mg par jour. |
| 剂型、规格<br>Les formes pharmaceutiques et les spécifications | 片剂：每片 1mg；2mg；5mg。<br>胶囊剂：每粒 2mg。<br>Comprimés : 1mg, 2mg ou 5mg par comprimé.<br>Capsules : 2mg par capsule. |
| 药品名称 Drug Names | 坦洛新 Tamsulosine |
| 适应证<br>Les indications | 主要用于治疗前列腺增生而导致的异常排尿症状，适用于轻、中度患者及未导致排尿障碍者，如已发生严重尿潴留患者不宜单独服用此药。<br><br>Il permet d'améliorer la miction chez les patients présentant des symptômes de l'hyperplasie de la prostate. Il est applicable chez des patients bénins et modérés qui n'a pas encore ledysfonctionnement mictionnel. Chez les patients souffrant de rétention urinaire sévère, il ne faut pas appliquer ce médicament tout seul. |
| 用法、用量<br>Les modes d'emploi et la posologie | 口服，每次 0.2mg，一日 1 次，餐后服。<br>Par voie orale, 0,2mg par fois, 1 fois par jour, après le repas. |
| 剂型、规格<br>Les formes pharmaceutiques et les spécifications | 缓释胶囊剂：每粒 0.2mg。<br>Capsules à libération prolongée : 0,2mg par capsule. |
| 药品名称 Drug Names | 非那雄胺 Finastéride |
| 适应证<br>Les indications | ①用于治疗良性前列腺增生，使增大的前列腺缩小，其逆转过程需要 3 个月以上；可以改善排尿症状，使最大尿流率增加；减少发生尿潴留和手术概率。②可以治疗男性秃发，能促进头发增长并防止继续脱发。<br><br>① Il permet de traiter l'hyperplasie bénigne de la prostate, permettant deréduire la prostate. Ce processus d'inversiondure plus de trois mois. Il peut améliorer la miction et augmenter ledébit maximum urinaire. Il sert aussi à réduire le risque de rétention urinaire. ② Il sert à traiter la calvitie masculine, en promouvant la croissance des cheveux et prévenant la chute des cheveux. |

**续　表**

| 用法、用量<br>Les modes d'emploi et la posologie | 口服。①治疗良性前列腺增生：每次 5mg，一日 1 次，6 个月为 1 个疗程。空腹或与食物同时服用均可。肾功能程度不全者、老年人不需要调整剂量。②治疗脱发：每次 1mg，一日 1 次，睡前服用。一般连续服用 3 个月或更长时间才达到效果。<br><br>Par voie orale. ① Pour traiter l'hyperplasie bénigne de la prostate : 5mg par fois, 1 fois par jour, pendant 6 mois comme un traitement médical. À jeun ou avec des aliments. Chez des patients insuffisants rénaux ou des personnes âgées, pas nécessaire d'ajuster la dose. ② Pour traiter la calvitie: 1mg par fois, 1 fois par jour, avant le sommeil du soir. Prendre pendant 3 mois consécutifs ou plus pour atteindre le résultat désiré. |
|---|---|
| 剂型、规格<br>Les formes pharmaceutiques et les spécifications | 片剂：每片 1mg；5mg。<br><br>Comprimés : 1mg ou 5mg par comprimé. |
| **药品名称 Drug Names** | **舍尼通 Cernilton** |
| 适应证<br>Les indications | 用于良性前列腺增生，慢性、非细菌性前列腺炎及前列腺疼痛等。<br><br>Il permet de traiter l'hyperplasie bénigne de la prostate, la prostatite et la prostatodynie chroniques non bactériennes. |
| 用法、用量<br>Les modes d'emploi et la posologie | 口服，一次 1 片，一日 2 次，早晚各 1 片，疗程 3～6 个月。衰老或肾功能不全者无须改变剂量。<br><br>Par voie orale, 1 comprimé par fois, 2 fois par jour, le petit matin et le soir, pendant 3 à 6 mois comme un traitement médical. Chez des personnes âgées ou des patients insuffisants rénaux, pas nécessaire d'ajuster la dose. |
| 剂型、规格<br>Les formes pharmaceutiques et les spécifications | 片剂：每片含 p5 70mg，E A10 4mg。<br><br>Comprimés : 70mg de p5 et 4mg de E A10 par comprimé. |
| **药品名称 Drug Names** | **前列通 QianLieTong** |
| 适应证<br>Les indications | 用于急性前列腺炎、前列腺增生引起的尿潴留、尿血、尿频等症。<br><br>Il permet de traiter la rétention urinaire, l'hématurie et la pollakiurie causée par la prostatite aiguë et l'hyperplasie bénigne de la prostate. |
| 用法、用量<br>Les modes d'emploi et la posologie | 口服：大片每次服 4 片，或小片每次 6 片，一日 3 次。30～45 日为 1 个疗程。<br><br>Par voie orale : prendre 4 grands comprimés par fois, ou 6 petits comprimés par fois, 3 fois par jour. Pendant 30 à 45 jours comme un traitement médical. |
| 剂型、规格<br>Les formes pharmaceutiques et les spécifications | 片剂：340mg。<br>胶囊：250mg，380mg，400mg。<br>Tablette: 340mg.<br>gélule: 250mg, 380mg, 400mg. |
| **药品名称 Drug Names** | **谷丙甘氨酸 Acide glutamique, Alanine et Glycine** |
| 适应证<br>Les indications | 用于治疗前列腺增生引起的尿频、排尿困难及尿潴留。尤适用于心肺功能不全和不易手术的高龄患者。本品为氨基酸制剂，适合老年患者使用。<br><br>Ce produit sert à traiter la pollakiurie, la dysurie et la rétention urinaire causées par l'hyperplasie de la prostate. Il est surtout applicable chez des patients âgés insuffisants cardiaques et incapables de suivre la chirurgie. Il s'agit de la préparation d'acides aminés et il est applicable donc chez des personnes âgées. |
| 用法、用量<br>Les modes d'emploi et la posologie | 口服，一次 2 片，一日 3 次，或根据病情适当增减。<br>Par voie orale, 2 comprimés par fois, 3 fois par jour, ou ajuster la dose selon les cas. |

| 剂型、规格<br>Les formes pharmaceutiques et les spécifications | 片剂：每片 0.41g。<br>Comprimés : 0,41g par comprimé. |
|---|---|
| 药品名称 Drug Names | 吡诺克辛 Pirénoxine |
| 适应证<br>Les indications | 用于治疗初期老年性白内障、轻度糖尿病性白内障或并发性白内障等。<br>Ce produit sert à traiter la cataracte sénile précoce, la cataracte diabétique ou la cataracte compliquée légère. |
| 用法、用量<br>Les modes d'emploi et la posologie | 滴眼，用前充分摇匀，每次 1～2 滴，一日 3～5 次。<br>Les gouttes pour les yeux, agiter avant de l'utiliser, 1 à 2 gouttes par fois, 3 à 5 fois par jour. |
| 剂型、规格<br>Les formes pharmaceutiques et les spécifications | 滴眼剂：每瓶装有密封的药片 1 片；每瓶内装溶剂 15ml。<br>Les gouttes pour les yeux : chaque flacon contient 1 comprimé scellé et 15ml de solvant. |

19.2　消毒防腐收敛药 Médicaments utilisés pour la désinfection, l'antiseptique et l'astringent

| 药品名称 Drug Names | 过氧乙酸 Acide peracétique |
|---|---|
| 适应证<br>Les indications | 用于空气、环境消毒和预防消毒。<br>Ce produit est utilisé dans la désinfection de l'air, de l'environnement et dans la désinfection préventive. |
| 用法、用量<br>Les modes d'emploi et la posologie | 用前按比例稀释。最常用为稀释 500 倍，即用 20% 的本品 2ml 加水 998ml 制得，含过氧乙酸 0.04%。①空气消毒：1∶200 液对空气喷雾，每立方米空间含药 30ml。②预防性消毒：食具、毛巾、水果、蔬菜等用 1∶500 液洗刷浸泡，禽蛋用 1∶1000 液浸泡，时间为 5 分钟，密封 50～60 分钟。<br>　　Diluer avant de l'utiliser. La proportion la plus usuelle pour la dilution est de 1∶500, à savoir dissoudre 2ml d'acide peracétique à 20% dans 998ml d'eau. La solution préparée contient 0,04 %d'acide peracétique.<br>　　① Pour la désinfection de l'air : utiliser la solution à 1∶200 pour la pulvérisation d'air, 30ml d'acide peracétique par $m^3$. ② Pour la désinfection préventive : laver et faire tremper des ustensiles, des serviettes, des fruits, et des légumes avec la solution à 1∶500, et faire tremper des œufs dans la solution à 1∶1 000, pendant 5 minutes, sceller pendant 50 à 60 minutes. |
| 剂型、规格<br>Les formes pharmaceutiques et les spécifications | 溶液：16%～20%。<br>La solution : 16% à 20%. |
| 药品名称 Drug Names | 聚维酮碘 Povidone iodée |
| 适应证<br>Les indications | 用于皮肤、黏膜的窗口消毒，也用于化脓性皮炎、皮肤真菌感染、小面积烧烫伤及念珠菌阴道炎、细菌性阴道炎、混合感染性阴道炎、老年性阴道炎等。<br>　　Ce produit est utilisé dans la désinfection de la peau et de la muqueuse. Il sert aussi à traiter la dermatite purulente, les infections fongiques de la peau, des brûlures mineures,la vaginite à Candida, la vaginose bactérienne,la vaginite infectieuse mixte, la vaginite sénile, etc. |
| 用法、用量<br>Les modes d'emploi et la posologie | ①外科手术消毒，0.5% 溶液刷洗 5 分钟。注射部位消毒，30 分钟以上。②术野皮肤消毒，0.5% 溶液均匀涂抹 2 次。③黏膜创伤或感染，用 0.1%～0.025% 溶液冲洗或软膏涂抹病患部位。④皮肤感染 0.5% 溶液局部涂擦或软膏涂抹患处。⑤阴道或直肠给药，每晚睡前 1 次，一次 1 支软膏或 1 个栓剂，7～10 日为 1 个疗程。 |

**续 表**

| | |
|---|---|
| | ① Pour la désinfection chirurgicale, laver avec la solution à 0.5% pendant 5 minutes. Pour la désinfection du site d'injection à, pendant 30 minutes au moins. ② La désinfection de la peau au champ opératoire : appliquer la solution à 0.5% sur la peau, 2 fois. ③ Lors du traumatisme ou des infections de la muqueuse, laver la zone touchée avec la solution de 0,1% à 0.025% ou essuyer la zone touchée avec la pommade. ④ Pour traiter des infections cutanées, appliquer la solution à 0,5% ou la pommade sur la zone touchée. ⑤ L'administration par voie vaginale ou rectale, une fois par soir, avant le sommeil, une pommade ou un suppositoire par fois, pendant 7 à 10 jours comme un traitement médical. |
| 剂型、规格<br>Les formes pharmaceutiques et les spécifications | 溶液：0.5%；1%；5%。<br>软膏、乳膏或凝胶：10%。<br>栓剂：每个 0.29g。<br>La solution : 0,5%, 1% ou 5%.<br>Pommade, crème ou gel : 10%.<br>Suppositoire : 0,29g par pièce. |
| **药品名称 Drug Names** | 氯己定 Chlorhexidine |
| 适应证<br>Les indications | 用于皮肤、创面、妇产科、泌尿外科的消毒及卫生用品的消毒，也用于急性坏死性溃疡性牙龈炎、牙科术后口腔感染，预防和治疗癌肿和白血病患者的口腔感染、义齿引起的创伤性磨损继发细菌和真菌感染、滤泡性口炎等。<br><br>Ce produit est utilisé dans la désinfection de la peau et des plaies, dans la désinfection obstétrique, gynécologique, urologique et dans la désinfection de l'hygiène. Il est aussi applicable dans le traitement de la gingivite ulcéro-nécrotique aiguë, et des infections buccales après la chirurgie dentaire. Il est aussi applicable dans la prévention et le traitement des infections buccales chez les patients atteints de cancer et de leucémie. Il permet aussi de traiter les infections bactériennes et fongiques secondaires traumatiques cauées par les dentiers, ainsi que la stomatite folliculaire. |
| 用法、用量<br>Les modes d'emploi et la posologie | ①手术消毒：以 1∶5000 水溶液泡手 3 分钟。②术野消毒：用 0.5% 乙醇（70%）溶液，其功效约与碘酊相当，但无皮肤刺激、亦不染色，因而特别适于面部、会阴部及儿童的术野消毒。③创伤伤口消毒：用 1∶2000 水溶液冲洗。④含漱：以 1∶5000 溶液漱口，对咽峡炎及口腔溃疡有效。⑤烧伤、烫伤：用 0.5% 乳膏或气雾剂。⑥分娩时产妇外阴及周围皮肤消毒，会阴镜检的润滑：用 1% 乳膏涂抹。⑦器械消毒：消毒用 1∶1000 水溶液，贮存用 1∶5000 水溶液，加入 0.1% 亚硝酸钠浸泡，隔两周换一次。⑧房间、家具等消毒：用 0.02% 溶液膀胱冲洗。⑨滴眼液防腐：用 0.01% 溶液。⑩伤口护理：用贴剂，清洁患处后，将中间护创贴在创伤处，两端用胶带固定。<br><br>① Pour la désinfection chirurgicale : faire tremper les mains avec la solution à 1∶5000 pendant 3 minutes. ② La désinfection au champ opératoire : utiliser la solution d'éthanol à 0,5% (70%). Son effet est similaire à la teinture d'iode mais sans irriter la peau ni faire la teinture, il est donc surtout applicable dans la désinfection du visage et du périnée au champ opératoire ainsi que la désinfection au champ opératoire chez des enfants. ③ Pour la désinfection des plaies traumatiques : laver avec la solution à 1∶2000. ④ Pour le gargarisme : utiliser la solution à 1∶5000 pour le gargrisme. Il est efficace dans le traitement de l'angine et l'aphte. ⑤ Pour traiter des brûlures : utilise la pommade à 0.5% ou l'aérosol. ⑥ Pour la désinfection de la vulve et de la peau périphérique chez des femmes lors de son accouchement, et pour la lubrification lors de la microscorpie du périnée : utiliser la pommade à 1%. ⑦ Pour la désinfecton des équipements : pour la désinfection, utiliser la solution à 1∶1000, pour la conservation, utiliser la solution à 1∶5000, ajouter le nitrite de sodium à 0,1%, changer toutes les 2 semaines. ⑧ Pour la désinfection des chambres et des meubles : utiliser la solution à 0,02% pour l'irrigation de la vessie. ⑨ Les gouttes pour les yeux pour l'anticorrosion : utiliser la solution à 0.01%. ⑩ Pour le soin des plaies : utiliser le pensement, après le nettoyage de la zone touchée, appliquer le pensement sur la zone touchée et fixer les deux extrémités avec les bandes. |

**续　表**

| 剂型、规格<br>Les formes<br>pharmaceutiques et les<br>spécifications | 葡萄糖酸氯己定含漱剂：0.016g（200ml）；0.04g（500ml）。<br>葡萄糖酸氯己定溶液：50g（250ml）。<br>稀葡萄糖酸氯己定溶液：12.5g（250ml）。<br>醋酸氯己定片：每片 5mg。<br>醋酸氯己定霜：1%。<br>醋酸氯己定软膏：1%。<br>Le gargarisme de gluconate de chlorhexidine : 0,016g (200ml), 0,04g (500ml).<br>La solution de gluconate de chlorhexidine : 50g (250ml).<br>La solution diluée de gluconate de chlorhexidine : 12,5g (250ml).<br>Les comprimés d'acétate de chlorhexidine : 5mg par comprimé.<br>La rème d'acétate de chlorhexidine : 1%.<br>La pommade d'acétate de chlorhexidine : 1%. |
|---|---|
| **药品名称 Drug Names** | 戊二醛 Glutaraldéhyde |
| 适应证<br>Les indications | 用于器械消毒，也可用于治疗寻常疣、甲癣和多汗症。<br>Il est applicable dans la désinfection des instruments. Il est aussi appliqué dans le traitement des verrues vulgaires, de l'onychomycose et de l'hyperhidrose. |
| 用法、用量<br>Les modes d'emploi et<br>la posologie | ①碱性戊二醛水溶液或异丙醇溶液（浓度为 2%，pH 为 7.5 ～ 8.5）：对细菌繁殖体的作用时间为 10 ～ 20 分钟，对细菌芽孢为 4 ～ 12 小时。10% 溶液用于治疗寻常疣、甲癣和多汗症，局部涂擦，一日 1 ～ 2 次。配制好的 2% 碱性水溶液在室温下经 14 日后，杀菌作用即明显减退。②酸性强化戊二醛液：是在 2% 戊二醛溶液中加入某些非离子型化合物作为强化剂配制而成。所加强化剂有稳定作用，又有协同增效作用。国外商品名为 Sonacide。国内曾用 0.25% 聚氧乙烯脂肪醇醚作为强化剂配制。此溶液因仍保持酸性（pH3.4），故稳定，室温下放置 18 个月，杀菌效能不减。同时加强药物表面活性，协同增效。杀菌力与碱性戊二醛相似，用法也相同。唯一缺点易导致金属生锈。③人造心脏瓣膜消毒液：为其 0.65% 溶液，pH（7.4）与血液相似，系磷酸盐缓冲液。④戊二醛气体：用于密封空间内表面的熏蒸消毒，因其不易在物体表面聚合，故优于甲醛。<br><br>① La solution de glutaraldéhyde alcaline ou la solution de l'isopropanol (la concentration est de 2%, pH : 7,5 à 8,5) : l'effet sur la multiplication des bactéries dure 10 à 20 minutes, sur les spores bactériennes 4 à 12h. La solution à 10% est appliquée dans le traitement des verrues vulgaires, de l'onychomycose et de l'hyperhidrose, application topique, 1 à 2 foispa rjour. La solution alcaline préparée à 2% diminue son effet de désinfection de manière évidente 14 jours après l'exposition à température ambiante. ② La solution acide de glutaraldéhyde : elle est préparée par l'introduction des composés non ioniques dans la solution de glutaraldéhyde à 2%. L'introduction de ces composés peut permettre de renforcer et de stabiliser l'efficcité. Elle est connue sous le nom Sonacide à l'étranger. En Chine, on a utilisé l'éther d'alcool gras de polyoxyéthylène à 0,25 % comme ces composés. Cette solution peut être conservée pendant 18 mois à température ambiante sans avoir l'effet diminué, car elle peut maintenir acide (pH3,4) et est stable. Elle peut renforcer l'activité de surface des médicaments et renforcer ainsi l'efficacité. Son effet bactéricide est similaire à celui du glutaraldéhyde alcaline, avec un même mode d'emploi. Mias elle peut entraîner la rouille des métaux. ③ Le désinfectant des valvules cardiaques artificielles : la solution de glutaraldéhyde à 0,65%, avec pH (7,4) similaire au sang. Il s'agit de tampon de phosphate. ④ Le gaz de glutaraldéhyde : appliqué dans la fumigation superficielle d'une zone fermée. Il est meilleur que le formaldéhyde, car il entraîne peu la polymérisation en surface. |
| 剂型、规格<br>Les formes<br>pharmaceutiques et les<br>spécifications | 溶液：20%；25%，稀释后使用。<br>La solution : 20% ou 25%, utilisée après la dilution. |
| **药品名称 Drug Names** | 洗消净 Hypochlorite de sodium et dodécylsulfonate de sodium |
| 适应证<br>Les indications | 适用范围广泛，可供器械、用具、衣物及排泄物消毒。<br>Il est appliqué dans plusieurs domaines. Il permet la déinfection des équipements, des appareils, des vêtements et des excréments. |
| 用法、用量<br>Les modes d'emploi et<br>la posologie | 取本品 50ml，用 10kg 水稀释，将被洗涤物品放在其中刷洗，即可达到消毒洗净的目的。也可浸泡 3 ～ 5 分钟，然后再刷洗，配制本品可用自来水，最适水温为 40℃左右。<br>Prendre 50ml de ce produit, diluer avec 10kg d'eau, laver des objets pour la désinfection. Ou faire tremper ces objects avant de les laver. Possible d'utiliser l'eau courante, à une température de 40 degrés. |

**续 表**

| | |
|---|---|
| 剂型、规格<br>Les formes pharmaceutiques et les spécifications | 溶液<br>La solution à |
| **药品名称 Drug Names** | 苯酚 Phénol |
| 适应证<br>Les indications | 常用于消毒痰、脓、粪便和医疗器械。液化苯酚用于涂拭阑尾残端。<br>Il est souvent appliqué dans la désinfection des crachats, des pus, des matières fécales et des dispositifs médicaux. Le phénol liquéfié permet aussi d'essuyer le moignon appendiculaire. |
| 用法、用量<br>Les modes d'emploi et la posologie | 外用消毒防腐剂。本品对人有腐蚀性、毒性，可引起新生儿黄疸，不宜长期使用。<br>Il s'agit d'un désinfectant antiseptique topique. Il est corrosif et toxique et peut entraîner l'ictère néonatal. Éviter l'utilisation à long terme. |
| 剂型、规格<br>Les formes pharmaceutiques et les spécifications | 1% ～ 5% 溶液。<br>La solution à 1% à 5%. |
| **药品名称 Drug Names** | 鱼石脂 Ichthammol |
| 适应证<br>Les indications | 有抑菌、消炎、抑制分泌和消肿等作用，可用于疖肿及外耳道炎等。<br>Il permet l'antibactérien, l'anti- inflammation, l'inhibition de la sécrétion et l'amélioration du gonflement. Il sert aussi à traiter lefuroncleet l'otite externe. |
| 用法、用量<br>Les modes d'emploi et la posologie | 外用涂擦，一日 2 次。滴耳，一日 3 次，一次 2 滴。<br>Essuyer ce produit 2 fois par jour. Pour les gouttes auriculaires, 3 fois par jour, 2 gouttes par fois. |
| 剂型、规格<br>Les formes pharmaceutiques et les spécifications | 10% 软膏。<br>鱼石脂甘油滴耳剂。<br>La pommade à 10%.<br>Les gouttes auriculaires de glycérol d'ichtyol. |
| **药品名称 Drug Names** | 乙醇 Ethanol |
| 适应证<br>Les indications | 75% 用于杀菌消毒。50% 用于防压疮。25% ～ 50% 擦浴用于高热患者物理退热。还可用于小面积烫伤的湿敷浸泡。在配制剂时用作溶剂。<br>L'éthanol à 75% permet la désinfection. L'éthanol à 50% permet la prévention de l'escarre de décubitus. L'éthanol à 25% à 50% est utilisé dans le bain à l'éponge pour faire tomber la fièvre. Il est appliqué dans le trempage pour les brûlures mineures. Il sert aussi de solvant dans les formulations. |
| 用法、用量<br>Les modes d'emploi et la posologie | 用作消毒剂时注意浓度，过高或过低均影响杀菌效果。不宜用于伤口或破损的皮肤面。<br>Lors de la désinfection, faire attention à la concentration, un taux trop bas ou élevé peut affecter l'effet de désinfection. Il n'est pas applicable sur les plaies ou sur la peau endommagée. |
| 剂型、规格<br>Les formes pharmaceutiques et les spécifications | 各种不同浓度的乙醇溶液。<br>La solution d'éthanol à différente concentration. |
| **药品名称 Drug Names** | 甲紫 Méthylrosanilinium |
| 适应证<br>Les indications | 有较好的杀菌作用，且无刺激性。用于皮肤革兰阳性菌和皮肤黏膜念珠菌病。<br>Il a un bon effet bactéricide, non irritant. Il sert à traiter les bactéries cutanées à Gram positif les candidoses cutanéo-muqueuses. |
| 用法、用量<br>Les modes d'emploi et la posologie | 外用涂擦。据报道，有一定致癌作用，故在伤口处禁用。<br>Appliquer ce produit pour un usage externe. Selon des rapports, il a un certain effet cancérogène. Il faut éviter de l'appliquer sur les plaies. |

**续　表**

| 剂型、规格<br>Les formes pharmaceutiques et les spécifications | 1% 溶液。<br>1% 糊。<br>La solution à 1%.<br>Le collage à 1%. |
|---|---|
| **药品名称 Drug Names** | 依沙吖啶 Ethacridine |
| 适应证<br>Les indications | 有消毒防腐作用，用于有感染及糜烂渗液的皮肤或创面。<br>Il permet la désinfection antiseptique. Il est appliqué dans le traitement de la peau ou de la plaie souffrant des infections ou de l'exsudat érosif. |
| 用法、用量<br>Les modes d'emploi et la posologie | 外用冲洗、湿敷。<br>Pour le lavage et l'application humide. |
| 剂型、规格<br>Les formes pharmaceutiques et les spécifications | 0.1% 溶液。<br>La solution à 0.1%. |
| **药品名称 Drug Names** | 高锰酸钾 Permanganate de potassium |
| 适应证<br>Les indications | 有强氧化作用，可除臭消毒，但作用短暂表浅。冲洗感染创面及膀胱炎用 0.1%～0.5% 溶液，清除皮损表面的脓性分泌物和恶臭、湿敷治疗湿疹 0.025%～0.01% 溶液，眼科用 0.01%～0.02% 溶液，洗胃 1：1000～1：5000，坐浴 0.02%，水果、食具消毒 0.1%。<br>Il a une oxydation forte et peut servir dedésodorisant et de désinfectant, mais avec une action brève. Sa solutuion à 0,1 % à 0.5% est appliquée dans le lavage des plaies infectées et le traitemen t de la cystite. Sa solution à 0,025 % à 0,01% permet de chasser les sécrétions purulentes et la puanteurdes lésions de surface, et de traiter l'eczéma. Sa solution à 0,01% à 0,02% est appliquée en ophtalmologie, sa solution à 1：1000 à 1：5000 est appliquée dans le lavage gastrique. Sa solution à 0,02% est utilisée dans le bain de siège. Sa solution à 0,1% est utilisée dans la désinfection des fruits et desustensiles. |
| 用法、用量<br>Les modes d'emploi et la posologie | 溶液应新配，久置或加热可迅速失效。其褐色斑可以用过氧化氢溶液或草酸溶液拭去。<br>Il faut préparer la solution juste avant l'utilisation. La solution devient perd son effet avec le temps et le chauffage. On peut utiliser la solution de peroxyde d'hydrogène ou la solution d'acide oxalique pour effacer ses taches brunes. |
| 剂型、规格<br>Les formes pharmaceutiques et les spécifications | 外用片：100mg。<br>Comprimés pour un usage externe : 100mg. |
| **药品名称 Drug Names** | 过氧化氢溶液 Solution de peroxyde d'hydrogène |
| 适应证<br>Les indications | 为强氧化剂，具有消毒、防腐、除臭及清洁作用，用于清洗创面、溃疡、脓窦、耳内脓液；涂擦治疗面部褐斑；在换药时可以去痂皮和黏附在伤口的敷料；稀释至 1% 浓度用于扁桃体炎、口腔炎、白喉等含漱。<br>Il s'agit d'un oxydant fort. Il peut avoir un effet désinfectant, antiseptique, désodorisant et un effet de nettoyage. Il est appliqué dans le lavage des blessures, des ulcères, du sinus purulent, et du pus de l'oreille. Il permet aussi de traiter les taches brunes du visage. Il sert à enlever la gale et le pansement adhésif lors du pansement. Dilué à 1%, il est utilisé dans le gargarismedu traitement de l'amygdalite, de la stomatite et de la diphtérie. |
| 用法、用量<br>Les modes d'emploi et la posologie | 除用于恶臭不洁的创面外，尤适用于厌氧菌感染以及破损伤口、气性坏疽的创面，用 3% 溶液冲洗或湿敷，根据情况每日多次使用。<br>Non seulement sur des plaies sales et malodorantes, ce produit est surtout applicable sur des plaies de la gangrène gazeuse, sur des plaies endomangées et sur des plaies infectées par des anaérobies. Utiliser la solution à 3% pour le lavage ou l'application humide, plusieurs fois par jour selon les cas. |

**续　表**

| 剂型、规格<br>Les formes pharmaceutiques et les spécifications | 本品为过氧化氢的 3% 水溶液。<br>La solution de peroxyde d'hydrogène à 3%. |
|---|---|

| 药品名称 Drug Names | 呋喃西林 Furacilline |
|---|---|
| 适应证<br>Les indications | 有广谱抗菌活性，但对假单胞菌属疗效甚微，对真菌和病毒无效。表面消毒用 0.001%～0.01% 水溶液，冲洗、湿敷患处，冲洗腔道或用于滴耳、滴鼻。<br>Ce produit a une activité antimicrobienne à large spectre, mais il est peu efficace dans le traitement du pseudomonas et inutile dans la lutte contre les champignons et le virus. Sa solution à 0,001% à 0,01% est appliquée dans la désinfection de surface, dans le lavage de la zone touchée, le lavage de la cavité ou dans la goutte nasale et la goutte auriculaire. |
| 用法、用量<br>Les modes d'emploi et la posologie | ①对本品过敏者禁用。<br>②口服毒性较大，目前仅供外用。<br>① Interdit de l'appliquer chez des patients allergiques à ce produit.<br>② Son administration par voie orale est toxique, il est aujourd'hui administré seulement pour un usage externe. |
| 剂型、规格<br>Les formes pharmaceutiques et les spécifications | 0.02% 溶液；0.2% 溶液。<br>La solution à 0,02% ou à 0.2%. |

| 药品名称 Drug Names | 苯扎溴铵 Bromure de benzalkonium |
|---|---|
| 适应证<br>Les indications | 阳离子活性的广谱杀菌剂，杀菌力强，对皮肤和局部组织无刺激性，对金属、橡胶制品无腐蚀作用。1：1000～1：2000 溶液广泛用于手、皮肤、黏膜、器械等的消毒。可长期保存效力不减。<br>Il sert de fongicide cationique à large spectre actif, avec uneforte bactéricide, non irritant pour la peau et des tissus locaux, et non corrosif pour les objets enmétal,et en caoutchouc. Sa solution à 1：1000 à 1：2000 est largement appliquée dans la désinfection des mains, de la peau, de la muqueuse et des équipements. On peut le conserver pour une longue durée et son efficacité ne diminue pas avec le temps. |
| 用法、用量<br>Les modes d'emploi et la posologie | ①不可与普通肥皂配伍。②泡器械加 0.5% 亚硝酸钠。③不适用于膀胱镜、眼科器械、橡胶、铝制品及排泄物消毒。<br>① Interdit de l'utiliser en association avec des savons ordinaires. ② Pour faire tremper des équipements, ajouter le nitrite de sodium à 0,5%. ③ Il n'est pas applicable dans la désinfection de la cystoscopie, des équipements d'ophtalmologie, du caoutchouc, des produits en aluminium et des excréments. |
| 剂型、规格<br>Les formes pharmaceutiques et les spécifications | 1：1000～1：2000 溶液。<br>La solution à 1：1 000 à 1：2 000. |

19.3　皮肤科用药 Medicamentos para dermatología

| 药品名称 Drug Names | 莫匹罗星 Mupirocine |
|---|---|
| 适应证<br>Les indications | 用于多种病菌引起的皮肤感染和湿疹、皮炎、糜烂、溃疡等继发性感染。有报道称，本品预防或治疗给药，对降低皮肤外科手术后伤口化脓十分有效。<br>Ce produit permet de traiter des infections secondaires causées par diverses bactéries, telles que les infections de la peau, l'eczéma, la dermatite, des érosions, des ulcères, etc. Selon des rapports, il est efficace dans la prévention et le traitement de la maturation des plaies après la chirurgie de la peau. |
| 用法、用量<br>Les modes d'emploi et la posologie | 涂于患处，也可用敷料包扎或覆盖，一日 3 次，5 日为 1 个疗程。必要时可重复一疗程。<br>Appliquer sur la zone touchée. Aussi applicable dans le pansement ou la couverture, 3 fois par jour, pendant 5 jours comme un traitement médical. S'il est nécessaire, reprendre un traitement. |
| 剂型、规格<br>Les formes pharmaceutiques et les spécifications | 软膏：2%。<br>La pommade : 2%. |

**续　表**

| 药品名称 Drug Names | 夫西地酸 Acide fusidique |
|---|---|
| 适应证<br>Les indications | 对与皮肤感染有关的革兰阳性球菌，尤其对葡萄球菌高度敏感，对耐药金葡菌也有效，对革兰阴性菌有一定作用。与其他抗生素无交叉耐药性。<br><br>Il est allergique à la cocci à Gram positif lié aux infections cutanées, surtout le staphylococcus aureus résistant. Il a un certain effet sur la cocci à Gram négatif. Il n'a aucune résistance croisée avec d'autres antibiotiques. |
| 用法、用量<br>Les modes d'emploi et la posologie | 涂于患处，并缓和摩擦。也可用敷料包扎，一日 2～3 次，7 日为 1 个疗程，必要时可重复一疗程。<br><br>Appliquer sur la zone touchée et frotter doucement. 2 à 3 fois par jour, pendant 7 jours comme un traitement médical. S'il est nécessaire, reprendre un traitement. |
| 剂型、规格<br>Les formes pharmaceutiques et les spécifications | 乳膏：2%。<br>La crème : 2%. |
| 药品名称 Drug Names | 环吡酮胺 Ciclopirox olamine |
| 适应证<br>Les indications | 外用于治疗各种皮肤浅表或黏膜的癣菌病。<br><br>Son usage externe est applicable dans le traitement des teignes cutanéo-superficielles et cutanéo-muqueuses. |
| 用法、用量<br>Les modes d'emploi et la posologie | 涂于患处，一日 2 次，甲癣，先用温水泡软灰指甲，再削薄病甲，涂药包扎。疗程一般 1～4 周（甲癣 13 周）。阴道栓用于治疗阴道念珠菌感染。<br><br>Appliquer sur la zone touchée, 2 fois par jour, pour traiter l'onychomycose, faire tremper d'abord l'onychomycose dans l'eau chaude, ensuite, l'amincir avant d'appliquer ce produit et le pansement, pendant 1 à 4 semaines comme un traitement (13 semines pour l'onychomycose). Le suppositoire vaginal est utilisé pour traiter la candidose vaginale. |
| 剂型、规格<br>Les formes pharmaceutiques et les spécifications | 溶液或乳膏：均为 1%。<br>阴道栓：每个含药 50mg 或 100mg。<br>栓剂：1%。洗剂：1%。<br>La solution ou la crème : 1%.<br>Le suppositoire vaginal : chaque pièce contient 5mg ou 100mg de ciclopirox olamine.<br>Suppositoire : 1%.<br>Lotion : 1% |
| 药品名称 Drug Names | 联苯苄唑 Bifonazole |
| 适应证<br>Les indications | 用于体癣、股癣、手足癣、花斑癣、红癣及皮肤念球菌病等表浅皮肤真菌感染及短小杆状菌引起的皮肤念球菌性外阴道炎。<br><br>Il permet de traiter le tinea corporal, la démangeaison de Jock, le tinea pedis, le pityriasis versicolor, l'érythrasmaet,la maladie cutanée liée à la candidose, et d'autres infections fongiques de la peau superficielle, ainsi que la vaginite externe liée à candiodose cutanée. |
| 用法、用量<br>Les modes d'emploi et la posologie | 涂于患处，一日 1 次，2～4 周为 1 个疗程。阴道给药，于睡前将阴道片放入阴道深处，一日 1 次，一次 1 片。<br><br>Appliquer sur la zone touchée, 1 fois par jour, pendant 2 à 4 semaines comme un traitement médical. L'administration vaginale, introduire le comprimé vaginal au fond du vagin avant le sommeil, 1 fois par jour, 1 comprimé par fois. |
| 剂型、规格<br>Les formes pharmaceutiques et les spécifications | 溶液：1%。<br>乳膏：1%。<br>凝胶：1%。<br>阴道片：每片 100mg。<br>La crème : 1%. crèmes : 1%.<br>Gel : 1%.<br>Le comprimé vaginal : 100mg par comprimé. |

**续　表**

| 药品名称 Drug Names | 酞丁安 Ftibamzone |
|---|---|
| 适应证<br>Les indications | 用于带状疱疹、单纯疱疹、尖锐湿疣、浅部真菌感染及各型沙眼等。<br>Il permet de traiter le zona, l'herpès simplex, les verrues génitales, des infections fongiques superficielles et le trachome de toutes sortes. |
| 用法、用量<br>Les modes d'emploi et la posologie | 涂于患处，一日 2～3 次，体癣、股癣连用 3 周，手足癣连用 4 周；滴眼，一次 1～2 滴，一日 3～4 次，连用 4 周。<br>Appliquer sur la zone touchée, 2 à 3 fois par jour, pour traiter le tinea corporal et la démangeaison de Jock, pendant 3 semaines consécutives, pour traiter le tinea pedis, pendant 4 semaines consécutives ; les gouttes pour les yeux, 1 à 2 gouttes par fois, 3 à 4 fois par jour, pendant 4 semaines consécutives. |
| 剂型、规格<br>Les formes pharmaceutiques et les spécifications | 软膏或乳膏：1%。<br>搽剂：0.5%（5ml）。<br>滴眼液：0.1%。<br>La pommade ou la crème : 1%.<br>Le liniment : 0,5% (5ml).<br>Les gouttes pour les yeux : 0,1%. |
| 药品名称 Drug Names | 克罗米通 Crotamiton |
| 适应证<br>Les indications | 用于治疗疥疮、皮肤瘙痒及继发性皮肤感染。<br>Il permet de traiter la gale, des démangeaisons de la peau et des infections secondaires de la peau. |
| 用法、用量<br>Les modes d'emploi et la posologie | ①疥疮：治疗前应洗澡并擦干，将本品从颈部以下涂搽全身皮肤，特别应涂搽在手足、指趾间、腋下和腹股沟；24 小时后涂第 2 次，再隔 48 小时洗澡将药洗去，更换干净衣服和床单。必要时，1 周后重复 1 次；也可一日涂搽 1 次，连续 5～10 日。②瘙痒症：局部涂于患处，一日 3 次。③脓性皮肤病：将患处用浸渍本品的敷料覆盖。<br>① Pour traiter la gale : avant le traitement, il faut se laver et s'essuyer, appliquer ce produit du cou jusqu'au reste du corps, surtout sur la main, sur le pied, entre des orteils de doigts, sous l'aine et sur les aisselles ; appliquer pour la deuxième fois 24 après, 48 h après, se laver, se changer de vêtements et changer le drap propre. S'il est nécessaire, répéter le traitement 1 semaine après ; ou appliquer 1 fois par jour, pendant 5 à 10 jours consécutifs. ② Pour traiter les démangeaisons : une application topique sur la zone touchée, 3 fois par jour. ③ Pour traiter les maladies de la peau purulente : couvrir la zone touchée du pensement trempé de crotamiton. |
| 剂型、规格<br>Les formes pharmaceutiques et les spécifications | 片剂：每片 10mg；20mg。<br>乳膏或软膏：0.025%；0.05%；0.1%。<br>凝胶剂：0.05%。<br>乙醇溶液：0.05～0.1%。<br>Comprimés : 10mg ou 20mg par comprimé.<br>La pommade ou la crème : 0,025%, 0,05% ou 0,1%.<br>Gel : 0,05%.<br>La solution d'éthanol : 0,05 % à 0,1%. |
| 药品名称 Drug Names | 维 A 酸 Trétinoine |
| 适应证<br>Les indications | 适用于寻常痤疮、扁平苔藓、白斑、毛发红糠疹和面部单纯糠疹。还用作银屑病的辅助治疗，亦用于治疗多发性寻常疣以及角化异常类的各种皮肤病如鱼鳞病、毛囊角化异常。<br>Ce produit permet de traiter l'acné vulgaire, le lichen plan, la leucoplasie, le pityriasis rubra pilaireet le pityriasis simplex facial. Il sert aussi de traitement adjuvant du psoriasis. Il est aussi applicable dans le traitement de diverses verrues de la peau et le traitement de la kératose anormale de plusieurs classes telles que l'ichtyose et la kératose folliculaire anormale. |
| 用法、用量<br>Les modes d'emploi et la posologie | 口服：一日 2～3 次，一次 10mg。外用 0.025% 乳膏或软膏治疗痤疮、单纯面部糠疹；0.1% 乳膏或软膏治疗扁平苔藓、毛发红糠疹、白斑等皮肤病，一日涂药 2 次，或遵医嘱。<br>Par voie orale : 2 à 3 fois par jour, 10mg par fois. Pour un usage externe, utiliser la pommade ou la crème à 0,025% pour traiter l'acné et le pityriasis simplex facial ; appliquer la pommade ou la crème à 0,1% pour traiter le lichen plan, le pityriasis rubra pilaire, la leucoplasie, 2 fois par jour, ou selon des ordonnances. |

**续　表**

| | |
|---|---|
| 剂型、规格<br>Les formes pharmaceutiques et les spécifications | 片剂：每片 10mg；20mg。<br>软膏或乳膏：0.025%；0.05%；0.1%。<br>凝胶：0.05%。<br>乙醇溶液：0.05% ～ 0.1%。<br><br>Comprimés : 10mg ou 20mg par comprimé.<br>La pommade ou la crème : 0,025%, 0,05% ou 0,1%.<br>Gel : 0,05%.<br>La solution d'éthanol : 0,05% à 0,1%. |
| 药品名称 Drug Names | 异维 A 酸 Isotrétinoïne |
| 适应证<br>Les indications | 用于其他药物治疗无效的严重痤疮，尤其是囊肿性痤疮及聚合性痤疮。<br>Il sert à traiter l'acné sévère qui ne peut pas être traitée par d'autres médicaments, surtout l'acné kystique et l'acné conglobata. |
| 用法、用量<br>Les modes d'emploi et la posologie | 口服：开始量为每日 0.5mg/kg，4 周后改用维持量，按每日 0.1 ～ 1mg/kg 计，视患者耐受性决定，但最高每日不超过 1mg/kg。饭间或饭后服用，用量大时分次服用，一般 16 周为 1 个疗程。如需要，停药 8 周后再进行下一疗程。局部外用：取适量涂于患处，每晚睡前涂一次。<br>Par voie orale : commencer par 0,5 mg par kg, 4 semaines après, prendre la dose d'entretien, 0,1 à 1 mg par kg, en fonction de la tolérance des patients, mais ne pas dépasser 1mg par kg par jour. Prendre le médicament durant ou après le repas, et à plusieurs fois pour une dose forte. Un traitement médical dure généralement 16 semaines. S'il est nécessaire, arrêter pendant 8 seamines pour continuer un nouveau traitement. L'usage externe topique : appliquer sur la zone touchée, une fois par soir avant le sommeil. |
| 剂型、规格<br>Les formes pharmaceutiques et les spécifications | 胶丸：每粒 5mg；10mg。<br>凝胶：0.05%。<br>Granules : 5mg ou 10mg par granule.<br>Gel : 0,05%. |
| 药品名称 Drug Names | 糠酸莫米松 Furoate de mométasone |
| 适应证<br>Les indications | 用于缓解对皮质激素有效的湿疹、接触性皮炎、特应性皮炎。神经性皮炎及皮肤瘙痒症等。<br>Il permet d'atténuer l'eczéma, la dermatite de contact et la dermatite atopique pour lesquels les corticostéroïdes sont efficaces. Il sert aussi à traiter le neurodermatitis et le prurit. |
| 用法、用量<br>Les modes d'emploi et la posologie | 涂于患处，一日 1 次，不应封闭敷裹。<br>Appliquer sur la zone touchée, 1 fois par our, ne pas faire le pensement fermé. |
| 剂型、规格<br>Les formes pharmaceutiques et les spécifications | 乳膏或软膏：0.1%。<br>La crème ou la pommade : 0,1%. |

19.4　眼科用药 Médicaments en ophtalmologie

| | |
|---|---|
| 药品名称 Drug Names | 吡诺克辛 Pirénoxine |
| 适应证<br>Les indications | 用于老年性白内障、外伤性白内障、轻度糖尿病性白内障、并发性白内障和先天性白内障。<br>Ce produit sert à traiter la cataracte sénile, la cataracte traumatique, la cataracte diabétique bénigne,la cataracte compliquée et les cataractes congénitales. |
| 用法、用量<br>Les modes d'emploi et la posologie | 滴眼，用前摇匀，一日 3 ～ 5 次，一次 1 ～ 2 滴。<br>Les gouttes pour les yeux, agiter avant d'utiliser, 3 à 5 fois par jour, 1 à 2 gouttes par fois. |
| 剂型、规格<br>Les formes pharmaceutiques et les spécifications | 滴眼液：含药片 7.5mg，溶剂 15ml 溶解药片后，浓度为 0.005%。<br>Les gouttes pour les yeux : contenant 7,5mg de comprimé, 15ml de solvant, après la dissolution, la concentration est de 0,005%. |

**续 表**

| 药品名称 Drug Names | 布林佐胺 Brinzolamide |
|---|---|
| 适应证<br>Les indications | 用于治疗原发性及继发性开角型青光眼和高眼压症。也可用于防止激光手术后的眼压升高。<br>Ce produit permet de traiter le glaucome à angle ouvert et l'hypertension oculaire primaireset secondaires. Il sert aussi à prévenir l'augmentation de la pression intra-oculaire après une intervention chirurgicale au laser. |
| 用法、用量<br>Les modes d'emploi et la posologie | 用前摇匀，滴眼，一日 2～3 次，一次 1 滴，滴于结膜囊内，滴后用手指压迫眦泪囊部 3～5 分钟。<br>Agiter fortement avant d'utiliser, les gouttes pour les yeux, 2 à 3 fois par jour, 1 goutte par fois, instiller dans la conjonctive, après la goutte, presser le sac lacrymal du canthus avec les doigts pendant 3 à 5 minutes. |
| 剂型、规格<br>Les formes pharmaceutiques et les spécifications | 滴眼液：每支 1%（5ml）。<br>Les gouttes pour les yeux : 1% (5ml) par pièce. |
| 药品名称 Drug Names | 拉坦前列腺素 Latanoprost |
| 适应证<br>Les indications | 用于治疗青光眼、高眼压症和其他各种眼压升高。<br>Il permet de traiter le glaucome, l'hypertension oculaire et l'augmentation de la pression intraoculaire de d'autres types. |
| 用法、用量<br>Les modes d'emploi et la posologie | 滴眼，一日 1 次，一次 1 滴，最好在睡前用。<br>Les gouttes pour les yeux, 1 fois par jour, 1 goutte par fois, avant le sommeil au mieux. |
| 剂型、规格<br>Les formes pharmaceutiques et les spécifications | 滴眼液：每支 125μg（2.5ml）。<br>Les gouttes pour les yeux : 125μg (2,5ml) par pièce. |
| 药品名称 Drug Names | 托吡卡胺 Tropicamide |
| 适应证<br>Les indications | 用于散瞳检查眼底和散瞳验光。<br>Ce produit est applicable dans la mydriase lors du fond d'œil et de l'optométrie. |
| 用法、用量<br>Les modes d'emploi et la posologie | 滴眼，一次 1 滴，间隔 5 分钟滴第二次，即可满足散瞳检查之需。<br>Les gouttes pour les yeux, 1 goutte par fois, 5 minutes après, instiller la deuxième fois, cela suffit pour l'examen avec pupilles dilatées. |
| 剂型、规格<br>Les formes pharmaceutiques et les spécifications | 滴眼液：每支 0.25%（6ml）；0.5%（6ml）；1%（8ml）。<br>Les gouttes pour les yeux : 0,25% (6ml), 0,5% (6ml) ou 1% (8ml) par pièce. |
| 药品名称 Drug Names | 玻璃酸钠 Hyaluronate de sodium |
| 适应证<br>Les indications | 滴眼用于防治干眼症、眼疲劳、斯 - 约综合征等内因性疾病和术后药物性、外伤、光线对眼造成的刺激及戴软性接触镜引起的外因性疾病。眼科手术用其注射液。<br>Ses gouttes pour les yeux servent à traiter les maladies endogènes telles que la sécheresse oculaire, la fatigue oculaire, etc. ainsi que des maladies exogènes causées par l'irritation oculaire liée au médicament postopératoire, au traumatisme età la lumière, etpar le port de lentilles de contact souples. Son injection est appliquée dans la chirurgie ophtalmologique. |
| 用法、用量<br>Les modes d'emploi et la posologie | 前房内注射，一次 0.5～0.75ml。滴眼，一日 4～6 次，一次 1～2 滴。<br>Injection dans la chambre antérieure de l'œil, 0,5 à 0,75ml par fois. Les gouttes pour les yeux, 4 à 6 fois par jour, 1 à 2 gouttes par fois. |

**续　表**

| 剂型、规格<br>Les formes pharmaceutiques et les spécifications | 注射液：每支 5mg（0.5ml）。<br>滴眼液：每支 0.1%（5ml）。<br>L'injection : 5mg (0,5ml).<br>Les gouttes pour les yeux : 0,1% (5ml) par pièce. |
|---|---|

**19.5　耳鼻喉科和口腔科用药 Médicaments en otolaryngologie et en stomatologie**

| 药品名称 Drug Names | 羟甲唑啉 Oxymétazoline |
|---|---|
| 适应证<br>Les indications | 用于急性鼻炎、慢性单纯性鼻炎、慢性肥厚性鼻炎、变态反应性鼻炎（过敏性鼻炎）、鼻息肉、航空性鼻炎、航空性中耳炎、鼻出血、鼻阻塞性打喷嚏或其他鼻阻塞性疾病。<br>Ce produit sert à traiter la rhinite aiguë, larhinite chronique simple, la rhinite hypertrophique chronique,la rhinite allergique (la rhinite allergique), les polypes nasaux, la rhinite d'aviation, l'otite moyenne, les saignements de nez, des éternuements, des troubles obstructifs nasaux ou d'autres obstructions nasales. |
| 用法、用量<br>Les modes d'emploi et la posologie | 每揿定量为 0.065ml。将 1/4 喷头伸入鼻孔内，揿压喷鼻。成人和 6 岁以上儿童，一次一侧 1 ～ 3 喷，早晨和睡前各一次；或滴鼻，一日 2 ～ 3 次，一次 1 ～ 2 滴。若需长期用药，可采用连续用于 7 日停药一段时间在用药的间歇用药方式。<br>0,065ml par pulvérisation. Insérer 1/4 de la buse dans la narine, appuyer pour la pulvérisation nasale. Chez des adultes et des enfants plus de 6 ans, 1 à 3 pulvérisations dans chaque narine par fois, le petit matin et avant le sommeil ; ou les gouttes nasales, 2 à 3 fois par jour, 1 à 2 gouttes par fois. S'il nécessite une administration à long terme, possible d'appliquer pendant 7 jours consécutifs avant d'arrêter l'administration pendant certains temps. |
| 剂型、规格<br>Les formes pharmaceutiques et les spécifications | 滴鼻剂：每支 1.5mg（3ml）；2.5mg（5ml）；5mg（10ml）。<br>喷雾剂：每支 2.5mg（5ml）；5mg（10ml）。<br>Les gouttes nasales : 1,5mg (3ml), 2,5mg (5ml) ou 5mg (10ml) par pièce.<br>L'aérosol : 2,5mg (5ml) ou 5mg (10ml) par pièce. |

| 药品名称 Drug Names | 西地碘 Cydiodine |
|---|---|
| 适应证<br>Les indications | 用于治疗慢性咽喉炎、白念珠菌性口炎、口腔溃疡、慢性牙龈炎及糜烂扁平苔藓等。<br>Ce produit est applicable dans le traitement de la pharyngite chronique, de la stomatite à Candida albicans,de l'aphte, du lichen plan érosif et de la gingivite chronique. |
| 用法、用量<br>Les modes d'emploi et la posologie | 含化，一次 1.5mg，一日 3 ～ 5 次。<br>Pour les comprimés sublinguaux, 1,5mg par fois, 3 à 5 fois par jour. |
| 剂型、规格<br>Les formes pharmaceutiques et les spécifications | 含片：每片 1.5mg。<br>Comprimés sublinguaux : 1,5mg par comprimé. |

| 药品名称 Drug Names | 氯霉素滴耳液 Chloramphénicol gouttes pour oreilles |
|---|---|
| 适应证<br>Les indications | 用于外耳炎、中耳炎。<br>Ce produit sert à traiter l'otite externe et l'otite moyenne |
| 用法、用量<br>Les modes d'emploi et la posologie | 滴耳，一日 3 次。宜遮光保存。<br>Les gouttes auriculaires, 3 fois par jour. Il faut conserver le produit à l'abri de la lumière. |
| 剂型、规格<br>Les formes pharmaceutiques et les spécifications | 氯霉素 2g，乙醇 16ml，甘油加至 100ml。<br>2g de chloramphénicol, 16ml d'éthanol, la glycérine jusqu'à 100ml. |

**续 表**

| 药品名称 Drug Names | 氧氟沙星滴耳液 Ofloxacine gouttes pour oreilles |
|---|---|
| 适应证<br>Les indications | 用于化脓性中耳炎。<br>Il est utilisé comme traitement de l'otite moyenne suppurée. |
| 用法、用量<br>Les modes d'emploi et<br>la posologie | 耳浴，一日 1 ～ 2 次。<br>Bain d'oreille, 1 ~ 2 fois par jour. |
| 剂型、规格<br>Les formes<br>pharmaceutiques et les<br>spécifications | 氧氟沙星 0.3g，醋酸适量，甘油 20ml，乙醇（70%）加至 100ml。<br>Ajouter 0,3g d'ofloxacine, l'acide acétique, 20ml de glycérine et l'éthanol (70%) pour atteindre 100ml. |
| 药品名称 Drug Names | 酚甘油滴耳液 Phénoglycérol gouttes pour oreilles |
| 适应证<br>Les indications | 有消炎杀菌及镇痛作用，用于急性及慢性中耳炎及外耳道炎。<br>Il a un effet anti -inflammatoire et analgésique. Il sert à traiter l'otite moyenne aiguë et chronique et l'otite externe. |
| 用法、用量<br>Les modes d'emploi et<br>la posologie | 滴耳，一日 3 次。<br>Les gouttes auriculaires, 3 fois par jour. |
| 剂型、规格<br>Les formes<br>pharmaceutiques et les<br>spécifications | 酚 2g，甘油加至 100ml。<br>2g de phénol et le glycérol pour atteindre 100 ml. |
| 药品名称 Drug Names | 硼酸滴耳液 Acide Borique gouttes pour oreilles |
| 适应证<br>Les indications | 用于慢性化脓性中耳炎。<br>Il sert à traiter l'otite moyenne chronique suppurée. |
| 用法、用量<br>Les modes d'emploi et<br>la posologie | 滴耳，一日 3 次。<br>Les gouttes auriculaires, 3 fois par jour. |
| 剂型、规格<br>Les formes<br>pharmaceutiques et les<br>spécifications | 硼酸 2 ～ 3g，乙醇（70%）加至 100ml。<br>2 à 3g d'acide borique, l'éthanol (70%), pour atteindre 100ml. |
| 药品名称 Drug Names | 碳酸氢钠滴耳液（耵聍液）Bicarbonate de Sodium gouttes pour oreilles |
| 适应证<br>Les indications | 软化耵聍（耳垢）及冲洗耳道。<br>l permet le ramollissement du cérumen (cérumen) et de rincer le canal de l'oreille. |
| 用法、用量<br>Les modes d'emploi et<br>la posologie | 滴耳，一日 3 次。每次用量要大，应将药液充满耳内。<br>Les gouttes auriculaires, 3 fois par jour. Utiliser une dose forte par fois, remplir l'oreille du produit. |
| 剂型、规格<br>Les formes<br>pharmaceutiques et les<br>spécifications | 碳酸氢钠 5g，甘油 30ml，蒸馏水加至 100ml。<br>5g de bicarbonate de sodium, 30ml de glycérol, l'eau distillée pour atteindre 100ml. |

## 续　表

| 药品名称 Drug Names | 碘甘油 Iodo Glyérine |
|---|---|
| 适应证<br>Les indications | 有防腐消毒作用，用于咽部慢性炎症及角化症，也可用于慢性萎缩性鼻炎。<br>Ce produit a un effet désinfectant et antiseptique. Il permet de traiter l'inflammation chronique du pharynx et de la kératose. Il est applicable dans le traitement de la rhinite atrophique chronique. |
| 用法、用量<br>Les modes d'emploi et la posologie | 涂于患处，一日 2 ~ 3 次。<br>Appliquer sur la zone touchée, 2 à 3 fois par jour. |
| 剂型、规格<br>Les formes pharmaceutiques et les spécifications | 碘 2g，碘化钾 1g，甘油加至 100ml。<br>2g d'iode, 1g d'iodure de potassium, la glycérine pour atteindre 100ml. |
| 药品名称 Drug Names | 呋喃西林/麻黄碱滴鼻液 Furacilline/Ephédrine gouttes nasales |
| 适应证<br>Les indications | 用于鼻炎或鼻黏膜肿胀。<br>Il sert à traiter la rhinite ou le gonflement nasal. |
| 用法、用量<br>Les modes d'emploi et la posologie | 滴鼻，一日 3 次，遮光保存。<br>Les gouttes nasales, 3 fois par jour, conserver le produit à l'abri de la lumière. |
| 剂型、规格<br>Les formes pharmaceutiques et les spécifications | 盐酸麻黄碱 10g，羟苯乙酯 0.3g，0.01% 呋喃西林溶液加至 1000ml。<br>10g de chlorhydrate d'éphédrine, 0,3g d'hydroxyle d'éthylbenzène, la solution de nitrofurazone à 0,01% pour atteindre 1 000ml. |
| 药品名称 Drug Names | 复方薄荷滴鼻液 Composés Menthe gouttes nasales |
| 适应证<br>Les indications | 用于干燥性鼻炎、萎缩性鼻炎、鼻出血，有除臭及滋养黏膜的作用。<br>Il sert à traiter la rhinite sèche,la rhinite atrophique,et l'épistaxis. Il sert de déodorant et permet de nourrir la muqueuse. |
| 用法、用量<br>Les modes d'emploi et la posologie | 滴鼻或涂鼻。<br>Les gouttes nasales ou application nasale. |
| 剂型、规格<br>Les formes pharmaceutiques et les spécifications | 薄荷脑 1g，樟脑 1g，液状石蜡加至 100ml。<br>1g de menthe, 1g de camphre, la paraffine liquide pour atteindre 100ml. |
| 药品名称 Drug Names | 盐酸麻黄碱滴鼻液 Chlorhydrate d'éphédrine Gouttes nasales |
| 适应证<br>Les indications | 有收缩血管作用，用于急性鼻炎、鼻窦炎、慢性肥大性鼻炎。<br>Il a un effet vasoconstricteur. Il sert à traiter la rhinite aiguë,la sinusite,la rhinite chronique hypertrophique. |
| 用法、用量<br>Les modes d'emploi et la posologie | 滴鼻，一日 3 次。<br>Les gouttes nasales, 3 fois par jour. |
| 剂型、规格<br>Les formes pharmaceutiques et les spécifications | 盐酸麻黄碱 10g，氯化钠 0.6g，羟苯乙酯 0.03g，蒸馏水加至 1000ml。<br>10g de chlorhydrate d'éphédrine, 0,6g de chlorure de sodium, 0,03g d'hydroxyle d'éthylbenzène, l'eau distillée pour atteindre 1000ml. |

续 表

| 药品名称 Drug Names | 复方硼砂片（漱口）Comprimés de borax composé(pour Bouche) |
| --- | --- |
| 适应证<br>Les indications | 用于口腔炎、咽喉炎及扁桃体炎等。<br>Ce produit sert à traiter la stomatite,la pharyngite et l'amygdalite. |
| 用法、用量<br>Les modes d'emploi et<br>la posologie | 一片加温开水一杯（60～90ml）溶后含漱，一日数次。<br>Dissoudre un comprimé dans un verre d'eau chaude (60 à 90ml) pour le gargarisme, plusieurs fois par jour. |
| 剂型、规格<br>Les formes<br>pharmaceutiques et les<br>spécifications | 每片含：硼砂 0.324g，碳酸氢钠 0.162g，氯化钠 0.162g，麝香草酚 0.0032g。<br>Chaque comprimé contient : 0,324g de boraz, 0,162g de bicarbonate de sodium, 0,162g de chlorure de sodium, 0,0032g de thymol. |

19.6 妇科外用药 Médicaments gynécologiques (topique)

| 药品名称 Drug Names | 硝呋太尔/制霉素（阴道用）Nifuratel/Nysfungin(Pour vagin) |
| --- | --- |
| 适应证<br>Les indications | 硝呋太尔制霉素在体外具有抗真菌、抗滴虫、抗细菌的广谱活性。用于细菌性阴道病、滴虫性阴道炎、念珠菌性外阴阴道炎、阴道混合感染。<br>Le Nifuratel nystatine a un large spectre d'activité permettant l'anti-fongique, l'anti- trichomonas, l'anti –bactérien, etc. Il sert à traiter la vaginose bactérienne, latrichomonase vaginite,la candidose vulvo-vaginale,les infections vaginales mixtes, etc. |
| 用法、用量<br>Les modes d'emploi et<br>la posologie | 阴道给药，每晚一粒，连用 6 日。亦可遵医嘱调整。<br>L'administration vaginale, l'capsule par soir, pendant 6 jours consécutifs. Ou ajuster la dose selon les ordonnances. |
| 剂型、规格<br>Les formes<br>pharmaceutiques et les<br>spécifications | 每粒含硝呋太尔 0.5g，制霉素 20 万 U。<br>Chaque capsule contient 0,5g de nifuratel et 200 000 U de nystatine. |

20. 其他药物 Autres médicaments

20.1 解毒药 Médicaments pour soigner l'intoxication

| 药品名称 Drug Names | 谷胱甘肽 Glutathion |
| --- | --- |
| 适应证<br>Les indications | 临床上用于：①解毒：对丙烯腈、氟化物、一氧化碳、重金属及有机溶剂等的中毒均有解毒作用。对红细胞膜有保护作用，故防止溶血，从而减少高铁血红蛋白。②对某些损伤的保护作用：由于放射线治疗、放射性药物或由于使用肿瘤药物所引起白细胞减少症以及由于放射线引起的骨髓组织炎症，本品均可改善其症状。③保护肝脏：能抑制脂肪肝的形成，也能改善中毒性肝炎和感染性肝炎的症状。④抗过敏：能纠正乙酰胆碱、胆碱酯酶的不平衡，从而消除由于这种不平衡所引起的过敏症状。⑤改善某些疾病的症状：对缺氧血症的不适、恶心、呕吐、瘙痒等症状以及由于肝脏疾病引起的其他症状，均有改善作用。⑥防止皮肤色素沉着：可防止新的黑色素形成并减少其氧化。⑦眼科疾病：可抑制晶体蛋白质巯基的不稳定，因而可以抑制进行性白内障及控制角膜及视网膜疾病的发展等。<br><br>Il est appliqué dans les cliniques : ① La désintoxication : il permet la désintoxication de l'intoxication à l'acrylonitrile, au fluorure, au monoxyde de carbone, aux métaux lourds et aux solvants organique. Comme il peut protéger lamembrane érythrocytaire, il permet d'empêcher l'hémolyse, réduisant ainsi la méthémoglobine. ② La protection de certaines lésions : il permet de traiter la leucopénie cauée par la radiothérapie, des médicaments radioactifs ou l'utilisation de médicaments contre le cancer. Il sert aussi à traiter l'inflammation des tissus de la moelle osseuse causée par la radiation. ③ La protection du foie : il peut inhiber la formation dea stéatose hépatique, et améliorer les symptômes de l'hépatite toxique et de l'hépatite infectieuse. ④ L'anti-allergie : il peut corriger le déséquilibre de l'acétylcholine et du cholinestérase, permettant ainsi de supprimer les symptômes allergiques causés par ce déséquilibre. ⑤ L'amélioration des symptômes de certaines maladies : |

| | |
|---|---|
| | les malaises, les nausées, les vomissements, le pruritcausés par l'anoxémie, ainsi que des symptômes liés aux maladies hépatiques. ⑥ La prévention de la pigmentation de la peau : il permet de prévenir et de réduire la formation de la nouvelle mélanineet son oxydation. ⑦ Les maladies ophtalmologiques: il peut supprimer l'instabilité des groupes sulfhydryle de la protéine cristalline, permettant ainsi d'inhiber la cataracte progressive et de contrôler le développement de la maladie de la cornée et de la rétine. |
| 用法、用量<br>Les modes d'emploi et la posologie | 肌内或静脉注射，将本品注射剂用所附的 2ml 维生素 C 注射液溶解后使用。肝脏患者一般 30 日为 1 个疗程，其他情况根据病情决定。滴眼，一次 1～2 滴，一日 4～8 次。<br><br>Injection IM ou IV, dissoudre dans 2ml d'injection de vitamine C jointe pour l'injection. Chez des patients atteints de maladies hépatiques, un traitement médical dure 30 jours. Les gouttes pour les yeux, 1 à 2 gouttes par fois, 4 à 8 fois par jour. |
| 剂型、规格<br>Les formes pharmaceutiques et les spécifications | 注射剂：每支 300mg；600mg。<br>Injection : 300mg ou 600mg par solution. |
| 药品名称 Drug Names | 二巯丙醇 Dimercaprol |
| 适应证<br>Les indications | 对砷、汞及金的中毒有解救作用，但治疗慢性汞中毒效果差。对锑中毒的作用因锑化合物的不同而异，它能够减轻酒石酸锑钾的毒性而能增加锑波芬与新斯锑波散等的毒性。能减轻镉对肺的损害，故使用时要注意掌握。它还能减轻发泡性砷化合物战争毒气所引起的损害。<br><br>Ce produit permet de sauver l'intoxication à l'arsenic, au mercure et à l'or, mais il est peu efficace dans le sauvetage de l'intoxication au mercure chronique. Son effet dans le traitement de l'intoxication à l'antimoineest différent pour les composés d'antimoine différents : il permet de réduire la toxicité de l'antimoine tartrate de potassium mais aussi d'augmenter la toxicité de l'antimoine Bofen. Il peut réduire les dommages caués par le cadmiumsur le poumon, il faut donc faire attention. Il permet aussi de réduire les dommages causés par les composés moussantsde l'arsenic. |
| 用法、用量<br>Les modes d'emploi et la posologie | 成人，肌内注射，按体重 2～3mg/kg，最初 2 日，每 4 小时注射 1 次。第 3 日，每 6 小时注射 1 次，以后每 12 小时注射 1 次，一个疗程为 10 日。小儿用量同成人。治疗小儿铅脑病，与依地酸钙钠同用。<br><br>Chez des adultes, injection IM, 2 à 3mg par kg, pendant les 2 premiers jours, injection toutes les 4h. Pour le 3ème jour, injection toutes les 6h, ensuite, toutes les 12h, pendant 10 jours comme un traitement. La dose est la même chez des enfants que chez des adultes. Pour traiter l'encéphalopathie liée à l'intoxication au plomb, il faut utiliser le dimercaprol en association avec EDTA. |
| 剂型、规格<br>Les formes pharmaceutiques et les spécifications | 注射液：每支 0.1g/1ml，0.2g/ml。<br>Injection : 0,1g par 1ml ou 0,2g par ml par solution. |
| 药品名称 Drug Names | 二巯丁二钠 Dimercaptosuccinate de sodium |
| 适应证<br>Les indications | 用于治疗锑、铅、汞、砷、铜的中毒（治疗汞中毒的效果不如二巯丙磺钠）及预防镉、钴、镍中毒，对肝豆状核变性病有驱铜及减轻症状的作用。<br><br>Ce produit sert à traiter l'intoxication à l'antimoine, auplomb, aumercure, àl'arsenic et au cuivre (il est moins efficace que la dimercaptopropane sulfonate de sodium dans le traitement de l'intoxication au mercure). Il sert aussi à prévenir l'intoxication au cadmium, au cobalt et au nickel. Il permet aussi de réduire les symptômes de la dégénérescence hépato-lenticulaire. |
| 用法、用量<br>Les modes d'emploi et la posologie | ①成人解毒：1g，临用时配成 10% 溶液，立即缓慢静脉注射，10～15 分钟注射完毕。②急性锑中毒引起的心律失常：本品首次剂量为 2g，用 5% 葡萄糖液 20ml 溶解后，静脉缓慢注射。以后每小时 1g，共 4～5 次。用于亚急性金属中毒：每次 1g，一日 2～3 次，共用 3～5 日。用于慢性中毒，每日 1g，共 5～7 日，或每日 1g，连续 3 日，停药 4 日为 1 个疗程，按病情可用 2～4 疗程。③小儿常用量：按体重 20mg/kg。 |

**续　表**

| | |
|---|---|
| | ① Pour la désintoxication chez des adultes : 1g, former la solution à 10% avant l'administration, injecter par voie IV lentement, en 10 à 15 minutes. ② Pour traiter l'arythmie causée par l'intoxication à l'antimoine : la dose initiale est de 2g, dissoudre dans 20ml de solution de glucose à 5%, injection IV lente. Ensuite, 1g par h, 4 à 5 fois au total. Pour traiter l'intoxication subaiguë aux métaux : 2g par fois, 2 à 3 fois par jour, pendant 3 à 5 jours au total. Pour traiter l'intoxication chronique, 1g par jour, 5 à 7 jours au total, ou 1g par jour, pendant 3 jours consécutifs, arrêter l'administration pendant 4 jours comme un traitement. Selon les cas, prendre 2 à 4 traitements. ③ La dose usuelle chez des enfants : 20 mg/kg par jour. |
| 剂型、规格<br>Les formes pharmaceutiques et les spécifications | 注射剂：每支：0.5g；1g。<br>Injection : 0,5g ou 1g par pièce. |
| 药品名称 Drug Names | 去铁胺 Déféroxamine |
| 适应证<br>Les indications | 本品主要用于急性铁中毒和海洋性贫血、铁粒幼细胞贫血、溶血性贫血、再生障碍性贫血或其他慢性贫血，因反复输血引起的继发性含铁血黄素沉着症；亦用于特发性血色病有放血禁忌证者。对慢性肾衰竭伴有铝过量负荷引起的脑病、骨病和贫血，在进行透析过程中亦可应用。本品还可用作铁负荷试验。<br><br>Ce produit est princiaplement appliqué dans le traitement de l'empoisonnement de fer aigu, de lathalassémie,de l'anémie sidéroblastique,de l'anémie hémolytique,de l'anémie aplasique ou d'autres anémies chroniques. Il sert aussi à traiter l'hémosidérose secondairecausée par les transfusions sanguines répétées et l'hémochromatose idiopathique. Chez des patients atteints d'insuffisance rénale chronique accompagnée des maladies cérébrale, osseuses et de l'anémie causées par l'aluminium excessif, il est applicable dans la dislyse. Il est également appliqué dans le test de charge en fer. |
| 用法、用量<br>Les modes d'emploi et la posologie | ①成人：a. 急性铁中毒：肌内注射，首次 0.5～1g，隔 4 小时 0.5g，共 2 次，以后根据病情 4～12 小时 1 次，24 小时总量不超过 6g。静脉滴注，一次 0.5g，加入 5%～10% 葡萄糖注射液 50～500ml 中滴注，滴注速度，按体重 1 小时不超过 15mg/kg，24 小时总量不超过 90mg/kg。b. 慢性铁负荷过量，肌内注射，一日 0.5～1g。腹壁皮下注射，按体重 20～40mg/kg，8～24 小时，以微型泵作动力。②小儿：a. 急性铁中毒：按体重一次 20mg/kg。b. 慢性铁负荷过量，按体重一日 10mg/kg，腹壁皮下注射，8～12 小时或 24 小时，用微型泵作动力。c. 慢性肾衰竭伴铁负荷过量：按体重 20mg/kg，一周 1～2 次，在透析初 2 小时通过动脉导管滴注，一周总量一般不超过 6g。铁负荷试验：成人肌内注射本品 0.5g。注射前，排空膀胱内剩余尿，注射后留 6 小时尿。尿铁超过 1mg，提示有过量铁负荷；超过 1.5mg，对机体可引起病理性损害。<br><br>① Chez des adultes : a. Pour traiter l'intoxication au fer aigue : injection IV, la dose initiale, 0,5 à 1g, 4 h après, 0,5g, 2 fois au total, ensuite, selon les cas, une fois toutes les 4 à 12h, ne pas dépasser 6g par jour. En perfusion, 0,5g par fois, dissoudre dans 50 à 500ml de solution de glucose à 5% à 10% pour la perfusion, la vitesse est de 15 mg/kg par h au maximum, ne pas dépasser 90mg/kg pendant 24h.b. Pour traiter la charge de fer excessive, injection IM, 0,5 à 1g par jour. Injection sous-cutanée abdominale, 20 à 40 mg/kg, 8 à 24h, utiliser la micro-pompe comme moteur. ② Chez des enfants : a. Pour traiter l'intoxication aigue au fer : 20 mg/kg par fois. b. Pour traiter la charge de fer excessive chronique : 10 mg/kg par jour, injection sous-cutanée abdominale, 8 à 12h ou 24h, utiliser la micro-pompe comme moteur. c. Pour traiter l'insuffisance rénale chronique accompagnée de la charge de fer excessive : 20 mg/kg, 1 à 2 fois par semaine, pendant les 2 premières heures de la dislyse, en perfusion à travers le cathéter artériel, ne pas dépasser 6g par semaine. Pour le test de charge de fer : chez des adultes, injection IM, 0,5g. Avant l'injection, vider l'urine résiduelle dans la vessie, après l'injection, conserver l'urine pendant 6h. Le fer urinaire supérieur à 1mg montre la charge de fer excessif, le fer urinaire supérieur à 1,5mg peut entraîner les dommages pathologiques au corps. |
| 剂型、规格<br>Les formes pharmaceutiques et les spécifications | 注射剂：0.5g。<br>Injection : 0,5g. |

**续　表**

| 药品名称 Drug Names | 碘解磷定 Iodure de pralidoxime |
|---|---|
| 适应证<br>Les indications | 该药物用于治疗有机磷中毒。<br>Ce médicament sert à traiter l'intoxication aux composés organophosphorés. |
| 用法、用量<br>Les modes d'emploi et la posologie | ①治疗轻度中毒：成人 0.4 ～ 0.8g/ 次，以葡萄糖液或生理盐水稀释后静脉滴注或缓慢静脉注射，必要时 2 ～ 4 小时重复一次。小儿 1 次 15mg/kg。②治疗中度中毒：成人首次 0.8 ～ 1.6g，缓慢静注，以后每 1 小时重复 0.4 ～ 0.8g，肌颤缓解和血液胆碱酯酶活性恢复至正常的 60% 以上后酌情减量或停药。或以静脉滴注给药维持，每小时给 0.4g，共 4 ～ 6 次。小儿 1 次 20 ～ 30mg/kg。③治疗重度中毒：成人首次用 1.6 ～ 2.4g，缓慢静脉注射，以后每小时重复 0.8 ～ 1.6g，肌颤缓解和血液胆碱酯酶活性恢复至正常以后的 60% 以上后酌情减量或停药。小儿 1 次 30mg/kg。<br><br>① Pour traiter l'intoxication bénigne : chez des adultes, 0,4 à 0,8g par fois, dissoudre dans la solution de glucose ou la solution saline pour la perfusion ou l'injection IV lente, s'il est nécessaire, répéter une fois toutes les 2 à 4 h. chez des enfants, 15mg/kg par fois. ② Pour traiter l'intoxication modérée : chez des adultes, la dose initiale, 0,8 à 1,6g, injection IV, ensuite 0,4 à 0,8g par h, après l'atténuation de la fibrillation masculaire et le retour de l'activité du cholinestérase dans le sang à 60% du niveau normal, diminuer la dose ou arrêter l'administration. Ou la perfusion pour l'entretien, 0,4g par h, 4 à 6 fois au total. Chez des enfants, 20 à 30 mg/kg par fois. ③ Pour traiter l'intoxication sévère : chez des adultes, la dose initiale est de 1,6 à 2,4g, injection IV lente, ensuite, 0,8 à 1,6g par h. Après l'atténuation de la fibrillation masculaire et le retour de l'activité du cholinestérase dans le sang à 60% du niveau normal, diminuer la dose ou arrêter l'administration. Chez des enfants, 30 mg/kg par fois. |
| 剂型、规格<br>Les formes pharmaceutiques et les spécifications | 注射剂：0.5g(20ml), 0.4g(10ml)。<br>Injection : 0.5g(20ml), 0.4g(10ml). |
| 药品名称 Drug Names | 氯解磷定 Chlorure de pralidoxime |
| 适应证<br>Les indications | 该药物用于治疗有机磷中毒。<br>Ce médicament sert à traiter l'intoxication aux composés organophosphorés. |
| 用法、用量<br>Les modes d'emploi et la posologie | ①成人：a. 轻度中毒：0.5 ～ 0.75g 肌内注射，必要时一小时后重复一次。b. 中度中毒：首次 0.75 ～ 1.5g，肌注或稀释后缓慢静注，以后每小时重复以后每小时重复 0.5 ～ 1.0g，肌颤消失或胆碱酯酶活性恢复至正常的 60% 以上后酌情减量或停药。c. 重度中毒：成人首次用 1.5 ～ 2.5g 分两处肌注或稀释后缓慢静脉注射，以后每 0.5 ～ 1 小时重复 1.0 ～ 1.5g，肌颤消失或血液胆碱酯酶活性恢复至正常以后的 60% 以上后酌情减量或停药。②小儿：用法与成人同，a. 轻度中毒：按体重 15 ～ 20mg/kg；b. 中度中毒：按体重 20 ～ 30mg/kg；c. 重度中毒：按体重 30mg/kg。<br><br>① Chez des adultes : a. Pour traiter l'intoxication bénigne : 0,5 à 0,75g, injection IM, s'il est nécessaire, répéter encore une fois une heure après. b. Pour traiter l'intoxication modérée : la dose initiale, 0,75 à 1,5g, injection IM ou l'injection IV lente après la dilution, ensuite, 0,5 à 1,0g par h, après la disparition de la fibrillation masculaire et le retour de l'activité du cholinestérase dans le sang à 60% du niveau normal, diminuer la dose ou arrêter l'administration. c. Pour traiter l'intoxication sévère : chez des adultes, la dose initiale est de 1,5 à 2,5g, à deux sites d'injection, injection IM ou injection IV lente après la dilution, ensuite 1,0 à 1,5g toutes les 0,5 à 1h, après la disparition de la fibrillation masculaire et le retour de l'activité du cholinestérase dans le sang à 60% du niveau normal, diminuer la dose ou arrêter l'administration. ② Chez des enfants : les modes d'emploi sont les mêmes que chez des adultes a. Pour traiter l'intoxication bénigne : 15 à 20 mg/kg. b. Pour traiter l'intoxication modérée : 20 à 30 mg/kg. c. Pour traiter l'intoxication sévère : 30 mg/kg. |

**续 表**

| 剂型、规格<br>Les formes pharmaceutiques et les spécifications | 注射液：0.5g/2ml。<br>La solution : 0,5g par 2ml. |
|---|---|
| 药品名称 Drug Names | 阿托品 Atropine |
| 适应证<br>Les indications | 做解毒药使用时：①治疗有机磷类（包括有机磷农药及军用神经性毒剂）与氨基甲酸酯类农药中毒。应与胆碱酯酶复活剂合用，单独使用效果差（除西维因中毒外）。②治疗胃肠型毒蕈（如捕蝇蕈）中毒。③治疗中药乌头中毒。④治疗锑剂中毒引起的心律失常与钙通道阻滞剂引起的心动过缓。<br><br>Quand ce produit sert d'antidote, il permet de traiter les maladies suivantes : ① L'intoxication par les pesticides organophosphorés (y compris les agents neurotoxiques à usage militaire) et l'intoxication par les pesticides de carbamate. Il doit être utilisé en association avec lecholinestérase, car il est inefficace quand il est utilisé seul (sauf pour l'empoisonnement de carbaryl). ② L'intoxication gastro-intestinale aux champignons vénéneux (par exemple l'amanitaceae). ③ L'intoxication par l'aconitum. ④ L'arythmie causée par l'empoisonnement de l'agent antimoine et la bradycardie causée par les bloqueurs des canaux calciques. |
| 用法、用量<br>Les modes d'emploi et la posologie | 静脉注射或静脉滴注。①成人：a.治疗有机磷中毒：首次，轻度中毒，2.0～4.0mg；中度中毒，4.0～10mg；重度中毒，10～20mg。重复用药剂量为其半数，重复的次数依病情而异，达到阿托品化后减量或改用维持量。b.治疗氨基甲酸酯类农药中毒，根据病情给药，首次应给足量，用量范围为0.5～3.0mg，经口严重中毒可用5mg；如毒蕈碱症状未消失，可重新给0.5～1mg，除经口严重中毒外，一般不需达到阿托品化。c.治疗锑剂中毒引起的阿-斯综合征，立即静脉注射1.0～2.0mg，15～30分钟后再注射1mg。d.治疗乌头中毒及钙拮抗剂过量，按消化系统用药的用量给药，一次0.5～1mg，肌内注射，1～4小时一次，至中毒症状缓解为止。②小儿：用量可根据体重折算，用法与成人同。<br><br>Injection IV ou en perfusion. ① Chez des adultes : a. Pour traiter l'intoxication aux composés organophosphorés : la dose initiale, pour l'intoxication bénigne, 2,0 à 4,0mg ; pour l'intoxication modérée, 4,0 à 10mg ; pour l'intoxication grave, 10 à 20mg. La dose répétée est la moitié de la dose initiale, le nombre d'administration dépend des cas. b. Pour traiter l'intoxication par les pesticides de carbamate, ajuster la dose selon les cas, la première dose doit être suffisante, 0,5 à 3,0mg, en cas d'intoxication grave, 5mg ; si le syndrome muscarinique ne disparaît pas, reprendre 0,5 à 1mg. c. Pour traiter le syndrome d'Adams causé par l'intoxication à l'antimoine, injecter immédiatement par voie IV 1,0 à 2,0mg, 15 à 30mg, injecter encore 1mg. d. Pour traiter l'intoxication par l'aconitum, le surdosage des antagonistes de calsium, 0,5 à 1mg par fois, injection IM, toutes les 1 à 4 h, jusqu'à l'atténuation des symptômes. ② chez des enfants : la dose peut être mesuée en fonction du poids et les modes d'emploi sont les mêmes que chez des adultes. |
| 剂型、规格<br>Les formes pharmaceutiques et les spécifications | 注射液：每支 0.5mg/1ml；1mg/2ml；5mg/1ml。<br>Injection : 0.5mg/1ml；1mg/2ml；5mg/1ml par solution. |
| 药品名称 Drug Names | 东莨菪碱 Scopolamine |
| 适应证<br>Les indications | 有机磷农药类中毒的治疗。<br>Il permet de traiter l'intoxication par les pesticides organophosphorés. |
| 用法、用量<br>Les modes d'emploi et la posologie | 成人首次为：轻度中毒：0.3～0.5mg；中度中毒：0.5～1.0mg；重度中毒：2.0～4.0mg。重复用药量0.3～0.6mg。<br><br>La dose initiale chez des adultes : l'intoxication bénigne : 0,3 à 0,5mg ; l'intoxication modérée, 0,5 à 1,0mg ; l'intoxication sévère : 2,0 à 4,0mg. La dose répétée est de 0,3 à 0,6mg. |

续 表

| 剂型、规格<br>Les formes pharmaceutiques et les spécifications | 注射液：1ml：0.3mg；1mg：0.5mg。<br>Injection : 1ml : 0,3mg ; 1mg : 0,5mg. |
|---|---|
| **药品名称 Drug Names** | 亚甲蓝 Chlorures de Méthylthionine |
| 适应证<br>Les indications | ①治疗亚硝酸盐及苯胺类引起的中毒。②治疗氰化物中毒。<br>① Il sert à traiter l'empoisonnement de nitrite et de l'aniline. ② Il permet de traiter l'intoxication au cyanure. |
| 用法、用量<br>Les modes d'emploi et la posologie | ①治疗亚硝酸盐中毒：用1%溶液5～10ml（1～2mg/kg），稀释于25%葡萄糖溶液20～40ml中，缓慢静脉注射（10分钟注完）。若注射后30～60分钟发绀不消退，可重复注射首次剂量。3～4小时后，根据病情还可注射半量。若口服本品，可用150～250mg，每4小时1次。②治疗氰化物中毒用1%溶液50～100ml（5～10mg/kg），以25%葡萄糖溶液稀释后缓慢注射，尔后，再注入25%硫代硫酸钠20～40ml。严重者二者交替使用。<br>① Pour traiter l'impoisonnement de nitrite : dissoudre 5 à 10ml de solution à 1% (1 à 2 mg/kg) dans 20 à 40ml de solution de glucose à 25%, injection IV lente, finir en 10 minutes. Si le cyanose ne disparaît pas 30 à 60 minutes après l'injection, répéter la dose initiale. 3 à 4 h après, possible de prendre la moitié de la dose initiale. Par voie orale, 150 à 250 mg, toutes les 4 h. ② Pour traiter l'intoxication au cyanure, dissoudre 50 à 100ml de solution à 1% (5 à 10 mg/kg) dans la solution de glucose à 25% pour l'injection IV lente, ensuite, injecter 20 à 40ml dethiosulfate de sodium. Pour des cas graves, possible d'utiliser les deux en alternative. |
| 剂型、规格<br>Les formes pharmaceutiques et les spécifications | 注射液：20mg/2ml。<br>Injection : 20mg/2ml |
| **药品名称 Drug Names** | 硫代硫酸钠 Thiosulfate de sodium |
| 适应证<br>Les indications | ①抢救氰化物中毒。②抗过敏。③治疗降压药硝普钠过量中毒。④治疗可溶性钡盐（如硝酸钡）中毒。⑤治疗砷、汞、铋、铅等金属中毒。<br>① Le sauvetage de l'intoxication au cyanure. ② L'anti-allergie. ③ Le traitement de l'intoxication par le surdosage de médicament antihypertenseur de nitroprussiate de sodium. ④ Le traitement de l'intoxication par le sel de baryum soluble (par exemple le nitrate de baryum). ⑤ Le traitement des intoxications à l'arsenic, au mercure, aubismuth, au plomb et à d'autres métaux. |
| 用法、用量<br>Les modes d'emploi et la posologie | ①成人：a.抢救氰化物中毒：由于本品解毒作用较慢，须先用作用迅速的亚硝酸钠、亚硝酸异戊酯或亚甲蓝，然后缓慢静脉注射10～30g（25%～50%溶液40～60ml），每分钟5ml以下。必要时，1小时后再与高铁血红蛋白形成剂合用半量至全量。口服中毒者，还须用5%溶液洗胃，洗后留本品溶液适量于胃内。b.硝普钠过量中毒：单独使用25%溶液20～40ml，缓慢静脉注射。c.可溶性钡盐中毒：缓慢静脉注射25%溶液20～40ml。d.治疗砷、汞、铋、铅等金属中毒：静脉注射，0.5～1.0g/次。e.抗过敏：0.5～1.0g（5%10～20ml）静脉注射，一日1次，10～14日为1个疗程。②小儿：按体重计算，25%溶液1.0～1.5ml/kg（250～375mg/kg）。<br>① Chez des adultes :a. Pour sauver l'intoxication au cyanure : comme son effet de désintoxication est lent, il faut utiliser le nitrite de sodium, le nitrite d'amyle ou le bleu de méthylène à action rapide, ensuite injecter lentement par voie IV 10 à 30g (40 à 60ml de solution à 25% à 50%), à un débit de 5ml au maximum par minute. S'il est nécessaire, 1 h après, utiliser la moitié ou la totalité de la dose initiale en association avec des agents de formtion de méthémoglobine. En cas d'intoxication par voie orale, il est encore nécessaire d'utiliser la solution à 5% pour le lavage gastrique, avant de mettre la |

续 表

solution de ce produit dans l'estomac. b. Pour traiter l'intoxication par le surdosage de nitroprussiate de sodium : utiliser 20 à 40ml de solution à 25%, injection IV lente.c. pour traiter l'intoxication par le sel de baryum soluble : injecter lentement par voie IV 20 à 40ml de solution à 25%.d. Pour traiter l'intoxication à l'arsenic, aur mercure, au bismuth, au plomb et à d'autres métaux : injection IV, 0,5 à 1,0g par fois.e. pour l'anti-allergie : 0,5 à 1,0g (5% 10 à 20ml), injection IV, une fois par jour, pendant 10 à 14 jours comme un traitement. ② chez des enfants : 1,0 à 1,5 ml par kg (250 à 375mg/kg) de solution à 25%.

| | |
|---|---|
| 剂型、规格<br>Les formes pharmaceutiques et les spécifications | 注射用硫代硫酸钠：有无水物 0.32g （相当于含结晶水者 0.5g），无水物 0.64g （相当于含结晶水者 1.0g）。<br>注射液：每支 0.5g/10ml，1.0g/20ml。<br>Le thiosulfate de sodium pour injection : 0,32g anhydre (équivalent à 0,5g de produit aqueux) ou 0,64g anhydre (équivalent à 1,0g de produit aqueux).<br>Injection : 0,5 g par 10ml, ou 1,0g par 20ml par solution. |
| 药品名称 Drug Names | 亚硝酸钠 Nitrite de sodium |
| 适应证<br>Les indications | 治疗氰化物中毒及硫化氢中毒。<br>Il permet de traiter l'intoxication au cyanure et l'empoisonnement de sulfure d'hydrogène. |
| 用法、用量<br>Les modes d'emploi et la posologie | ①成人，静脉注射：每次 3% 溶液 10～15ml （或 6～12mg/kg），注射速度宜慢（按 2ml/mim）。合用氯化钠注射液稀释至 100ml 后静脉注射（5～20 分钟），随后静脉注射 25% 硫代硫酸钠 40ml （硫化氢中毒不需要注射硫代硫酸钠）。必要时，0.5～1 小时后可重复给半量或全量。②小儿：按体重 3% 溶液 0.15～0.3mg/kg。本品 3% 溶液，仅供静脉注射用，每次 10～20ml，每分钟注射 2～3ml；需要时在 1 小时后重复半量或全量。<br>① Chez des adultes, injection IV : 10 à 15ml de solution à 3% (6 à 12 mg/kg), injection IV lente (2ml par minute). Dissoudre la solution de chlorure pour former 10ml de solution, injection IV pendant 5 à 20 minutes, ensuite, injecter par voie IV 40ml de thiosulfate de sodium à 25%(en cas d'empoisonnement de sulfure d'hydrogène, pas nécessaire d'injecter le thiosulfate de sodium). En cas de besoin, 0,5 à 1 h après, reprendre la moitié ou la totalité de la dose initiale. ② Chez des enfants : 0,15 à 0,3mg/kg de solutiton à 3mg/kg par fois. La solution de nitrite de sodium à 3mg/kg par fois n'est applicable que dans l'injection IV, 10 à 20ml par fois, injecter 2 à 3ml par minute ; en cas de besoin, 1 h après, reprendre la moitié ou la totalité de la dose initiale. |
| 剂型、规格<br>Les formes pharmaceutiques et les spécifications | 注射液：0.3g/10ml。<br>Injection : 0.3g/10ml. |
| 药品名称 Drug Names | 氟马西尼 Flumazénil |
| 适应证<br>Les indications | 苯二氮䓬类药物的中毒解救。也可用于乙醇中毒的解救。<br>Il permet de sauver l'intoxication aux benzodiazépines. Il sert aussi à sauver l'intoxication à l'éthanol. |
| 用法、用量<br>Les modes d'emploi et la posologie | 成人常用量 0.5～2mg，静脉注射。小儿常用量：0.01mg/kg，静脉注射。最大剂量 1mg。<br>①麻醉后：因苯二氮䓬类常用于术前的麻醉诱导和术中的麻醉维持。本药则于术后使用，以终止 BZD 类的镇静作用。开始用量是 15 秒内缓慢静脉注射 0.2mg，如 30 秒内尚未清醒，可再注射 0.1～0.3mg，必要时，60 秒重复一次，直至总量达 3mg 为止。通常使用 0.3～0.6mg 即可。②急救：对原因不明的神志丧失患者，可用本品来鉴别是否为苯二氮䓬类所致，如反复给药也不能使意识或呼吸功能改善，则可判定为非苯二氮䓬所致。开始用量是 0.2mg，以氯化钠注射液或 5% 葡萄糖注射液稀释后静脉注射；重复给药每次增加 0.1mg，或每小时 0.1～0.4mg/h，滴速个体化，直至清醒为止。 |

续　表

|  | La dose usuelle chez des adultes est de 0,5 à 2mg, injection IV. La dose usuelle chez des enfants est de 0,01mg/kg, injection IV. La dose maximale est de 1mg. ① Après l'anesthésie : comme les benzodiazépines sont souvent utilisés dans l'induction préopératoire de l'anesthésie et l'entretien de l'anesthésie durant la chirurgie, le flumazénil est appliqué après la chirurgie pour terminer l'anesthésie introduite par les benzodiazépines. La dose initiale est de 0,2mg injecté par voie IV en 15 secondes. S'il le patient ne se réveille pas en 30 secondes, injecter 0,1 à 0,3mg, s'il est nécessaire, reprendre toutes les 60 secondes jusqu'à 3mg au total. En général, 0,3 à 0,6mg suffit. ② Pour le sauvetage urgent : chez des patients inconscients pour des raisons inconnues, l'administration du flumazénil permet de distinguer si cela est induit par les benzodiazépines. Si l'administration répétée ne peut toujours pas améliorer la conscience ni la fonction respiratoire, cela veut dire que ce cas n'est pas lié aux benzodiazépines. La dose initiale est de 0,2mg, dissoudre dans la solution de chlorure de sodium ou la solution de glucose à 5%, injection IV ; augmenter 0,1mg par fois lors de l'administration répétée, ou 0,1 à 0,4 mg par h en perfusion, avec un débit personnalisé, jusqu'à la reprise de conscience. |
|---|---|
| 剂型、规格<br>Les formes pharmaceutiques et les spécifications | 注射液：每支 0.5mg/5ml，1mg/10ml。<br>Injection : 0.5mg/5ml，1mg/10ml. |
| 药品名称 Drug Names | 纳洛酮 Naloxone |
| 适应证<br>Les indications | ①治疗阿片类药物及其他麻醉性镇痛药（如哌替啶、阿法罗定、美沙酮、芬太尼、二氢埃托啡、依托尼嗪等）中毒。②治疗镇静催眠药与急性酒精中毒。③阿片类及其他麻醉性镇痛药依赖性的诊断。<br>① 1) Il sert à traiter l'empoisonnement d'opiacés et d'autres analgésiques narcotiques (par exemple, la mépéridine, le fentanyl, la méthadone, DHE, etc.). ② Il sert à traiter l'intoxication alcoolique aiguë et l'intoxication par le sédatif et l'hypnotique. ③ Il permet le diagnostic de la dépendance à des analgésiques narcotiques. |
| 用法、用量<br>Les modes d'emploi et la posologie | 成人：静脉注射 0.4 ～ 0.8mg（小儿用量与成人同）。治疗阿片类。镇静催眠药类与急性酒精中毒，首剂 0.4 ～ 0.8mg，无效时可重复一次。因纳洛酮的作用只能持续 45 ～ 90 分钟，以后必须根据病情重复用药，以巩固疗效。<br>Chez des adultes : injecter par voie IV 0,4 à 0,8mg (chez des enfants comme chez des adultes). Pour traiter l'empoisonnement d'opiacés, l'intoxication alcoolique aigue et l'intoxication par le sédatif et l'hyphotique, la dose initiale est de 0,4 à 0,8mg, s'il est inefficace, répéter une fois. Comme l'action de la naloxone ne peut durer que 45 à 90 minutes, il faut reprendre l'administration selon les cas pour renforcer son efficacité. |
| 剂型、规格<br>Les formes pharmaceutiques et les spécifications | 注射液：0.4mg/1ml。<br>Injection : 0.4mg/1ml |
| 药品名称 Drug Names | 乙酰半胱氨酸 Acétylcystéine |
| 适应证<br>Les indications | 对乙酰氨基酚中毒。<br>Il sert à traiter l'empoisonnement de l'acétaminophène. |
| 用法、用量<br>Les modes d'emploi et la posologie | 5% 乙酰半胱氨酸（痰易净）水溶液加果汁内服，如服后 1 小时呕吐，可再补服一次，如连续呕吐可下胃管将药液直接导入十二指肠内。用量：140mg/kg 为起始量，70mg/kg 为后续量，每 4 小时一次，17 次可达解救的负荷量。静脉滴注：成人，第一阶段，140mg/kg 加入葡萄糖液 200ml 中，静脉滴注 15 ～ 20 分钟。第二阶段，70mg/kg 加入 5% 葡萄糖液 500ml 中静脉滴注。每 4 小时 1 次，共给 17 次。儿童，根据患儿的年龄和体重调整用量，解毒剂量同成人，但需按体重折算（将成人剂量按 50 ～ 69kg 折算成每千克的剂量）。 |

**续　表**

| | |
|---|---|
| | Administrater par voie orale la solution d'acétylcystéine à 5% et des jus de fruit, s'il y a des vomissements 1 h après, répéter une fois, s'il y a des vomissements continus, introduire la solution directement dans le duodénum de l'estomac à travers le cathéter gastrique. La dose : au début, 140 mg/kg, ensuite, 70 mg/kg, toutes les 4 h, 17 fois pourrait permettre la désintoxicatin. En perfusion : chez des adultes, au début, dissoudre 140 mg/kg dans 200ml de solution de glucose, en perfusion pendant 15 à 20 minutes. Ensuite, dissoudre 70 mg/kg dans 500ml de solution de glucose à 5%. Toutes les 4 h, 17 fois au total. Chez des enfants, ajuster la dose en fonction de l'âge et du poids, la dose pour la désinfection est la même que chez des adultes, mais il faut mesurer en fonction du poids (convertir la dose chez des adultes (50 à 69kg en dose par kg). |
| 剂型、规格<br>Les formes pharmaceutiques et les spécifications | 颗粒剂：100mg。<br>泡腾片：600mg。<br>Granules : 100mg.<br>Comprimés effervescents : 600mg. |

| 药品名称 Drug Names | 亚叶酸钙 Folinate de calcium |
|---|---|
| 适应证<br>Les indications | 用于抗叶酸代谢药过量中毒和甲醇中毒。<br>Il sert à traiter l'empoisonnement de surdosage du médicament métabolique anti- folate ainsi que l'empoisonnement du méthanol. |
| 用法、用量<br>Les modes d'emploi et la posologie | ①抗叶酸代谢药过量中毒：用量相当于抗叶酸代谢药的剂量（15～100mg），静脉注射。以后，如为甲氨蝶呤过量中毒，每3～6小时再注射或口服15mg，共8次；如为甲氧苄啶过量中毒，口服15mg，一日1次，共5～7日。②甲醇中毒：亚叶酸钙50mg，静脉注射，每4小时1次，共2日。<br>① Pour traiter l'empoisonnement de surdosage du médicament métabolique anti-folate : la dose équivaut à celle du médicament métabolique anti-folate (15 à 100mg), injection IV. Ensuite, s'il s'agit de l'empoisonnement de surdosage duméthotrexate, répéter toutes les 3 à 6 h ou prendre 15mg par voie orale, 8 fois au total ; s'il s'agit de l'empoisonnement de surdosage du triméthoprime, prendre 15mg par voie orale, 1 fois par jour, pendant 5 à 7 jours. ② Pour traiter l'empoisonnement du méthanol : 50mg de folinate de calcium, injection IV, toutes les 4h, 2 jours au total. |
| 剂型、规格<br>Les formes pharmaceutiques et les spécifications | 片剂：5mg，15mg，25mg。<br>注射液：50mg，100mg，300mg。<br>胶囊：25mg。<br>Comprimés: 5mg, 15mg, 25mg.<br>injection: 50mg, 100mg.<br>300mg; capsule: 25mg. |

20.2　诊断用药 Médicaments diagnostiques

| 药品名称 Drug Names | 碘海醇 Iohexol |
|---|---|
| 适应证<br>Les indications | 心血管造影、冠状动脉造影、尿路造影、CT增强扫描及脊髓造影等。<br>Ce produit est utilisé dans l'angiographie cardiovasculaire, la coronarographie, l'urographie, la TDM avec injection et la myélographie. |
| 用法、用量<br>Les modes d'emploi et la posologie | ①脊髓造影：腰穿注入造影剂7～10ml。②泌尿系造影（300mgI/ml）：成人，静脉注射40～80ml；儿童，＜7kg，3ml/kg；＞7kg，2ml/kg（最高40ml）。③主动脉血管造影：注射30～40ml/次。④CT增强扫描（300mgI/ml）：成人，100～180ml静脉注射；儿童，按1.5～2mg/kg体重计。<br>① Pour la myélographie : injecter 7 à 10ml de contraste par la ponction lombaire. ② Pour l'urographie (300mgI/ml) : chez des adultes, injecter par voie IV 40 à 80ml ; chez des enfants, ＜ 7kg, 3ml/kg ; ＞ 7kg, 2ml/kg, (40ml au maximum). ③ Pour l'angiographie aortique : injecter 30 à 40ml par fois. ④ Pour la TDM avec injection (300mgI/ml) : chez des adultes, injecter par voie IV 100 à 180ml ; chez des enfants, 1,5 à 2 mg/kg. |
| 剂型、规格<br>Les formes pharmaceutiques et les spécifications | 注射液：每支20ml。<br>Injection : 20ml par solution. |

**续　表**

| 药品名称 Drug Names | 碘佛醇 Ioversol |
| --- | --- |
| 适应证<br>Les indications | 心血管造影、冠状动脉造影、尿路造影、CT 增强扫描及脊髓造影等。<br>Ce produit est utilisé dans l'angiographie cardiovasculaire, la coronarographie, l'urographie, la TDM avec injection et la myélographie. |
| 用法、用量<br>Les modes d'emploi et la posologie | ①脊髓造影：腰穿注入造影剂 7 ～ 10ml。②泌尿系造影（300mgI/ml）：成人，静脉注射 40 ～ 80ml；儿童，＜ 7kg，3ml/kg；＞ 7kg，2ml/kg（最高 40ml）。③主动脉血管造影：注射 30 ～ 40ml/ 次。④ CT 增强扫描（300mgI/ml）：成人，100 ～ 180ml 静脉注射；儿童，按 1.5 ～ 2mg/kg 体重计。<br>① Pour la myélographie : injecter 7 à 10ml de contraste par la ponction lombaire. ② Pour l'urographie (300mgI/ml) : chez des adultes, injecter par voie IV 40 à 80ml ; chez des enfants, ＜ 7kg, 3ml/kg ; ＞ 7kg, 2ml/kg, (40ml au maximum). ③ Pour l'angiographie aortique : injecter 30 à 40ml par fois. ④ Pour la TDM avec injection (300mgI/ml) : chez des adultes, injecter par voie IV 100 à 180ml ; chez des enfants, 1,5 à 2 mg/kg. |
| 剂型、规格<br>Les formes pharmaceutiques et les spécifications | 注射液：20ml，50ml，100ml。<br>Injection : 20ml, 50ml ou 100ml. |
| 药品名称 Drug Names | 碘帕醇 Iopamidol |
| 适应证<br>Les indications | 主要适用于腰、胸及颈段脊髓造影，脑血管造影，周围动、静脉造影，心血管造影，冠状动脉造影，尿路、关节造影及 CT 增强扫描等。<br>Il est principalement appliqué dans la radiographie du thorax, la myélographie, l'angiographie cérébrale, l'artériographie et la phlébographie périphériques, la phlébographie, l'angiographie cardiovasculaire, lacoronarographie, l'urographie, l'arthrographie et la TDM avec injection. |
| 用法、用量<br>Les modes d'emploi et la posologie | 脊髓造影，成人用浓度为 200 ～ 300mgI/ml 溶液 5 ～ 15ml。大脑血管造影用 300mgI/ml 溶液 5 ～ 10ml（成人）。3 ～ 7ml（儿童）。周围动静脉造影用 300mgI/ml 溶液 20 ～ 50ml（成人）。冠状动脉造影用 370mgI/ml 溶液 4 ～ 8ml（成人）。主动脉造影（逆行）用 370mgI/ml 溶液 50 ～ 80ml（成人）。尿路造影用 300 ～ 370mgI/ml 溶液 20 ～ 50ml（成人），1 ～ 2.5ml（儿童）。CT 扫描用 300 ～ 370mgI/ml 溶液 50 ～ 100ml（成人）等。<br>Pour la myélographie, chez des adultes, utiliser 5 à 15ml de solution à 200~300mgI/ml. Pour l'angiographie cérébrale, utiliser 5 à 10ml de solution à 300mgI/ml chez des adultes, et 3 à 7 ml de solution chez des enfants. Pour l'artériographie et la phlébographie périphériques, utiliser 20 à 50ml de solution à 300mgI/ml chez des adultes. Pour la coronarographie (rétrograde), utiliser 50 à 80ml de solution à 370mgI/ml chez des adultes. Pour l'urographie, utiliser 20 à 50ml de solution à 300 à 370 mgI/ml chez des adultes, et 1 à 2,5ml de solution chez des enfants. Pour la TDM avec injection, utiliser 50 à 100ml de solution à 300 à 370 mgI/ml chez des adultes. |
| 剂型、规格<br>Les formes pharmaceutiques et les spécifications | 注射液：每支 20ml，50ml，100ml。<br>Injection : 20ml, 50ml ou 100ml par solution. |
| 药品名称 Drug Names | 碘克沙醇 Iodixanol |
| 适应证<br>Les indications | 成人的心、脑血管造影（常规的与 i.a.DSA）、外周动脉造影（常规的与 i.a.DSA）腹部血管造影（i.a.DSA）尿路造影、静脉造影以及 CT 增强检查。<br>Il est applicable dans l'angiographie cardiovasculaire, l'artériographie périphérique, l'angiographie abdominale, l'urographie, la phlébographie et la TDM avec injection chez des adultes. |
| 用法、用量<br>Les modes d'emploi et la posologie | 用药剂量取决于检查类型、年龄、体重、心排血量和患者全身情况及所使用的技术。<br>La dose dépend du type d'examen, de l'âge, du poids, du débit cardiaque, de l'état général du patient et de la technologie employée. |

**续 表**

| 剂型、规格<br>Les formes pharmaceutiques et les spécifications | 注射液：150mg/ml（50ml；200ml）；270mg/ml（20ml；50ml；100ml）；320mg/ml（20ml；50ml；100ml）。<br>Injection：150mg/ml(50ml；200ml)；270mg/ml(20ml；50ml；100ml)；320mg/ml(20ml；50ml；100ml). |
|---|---|
| **药品名称 Drug Names** | 硫酸钡 Sulfate de Baryum |
| 适应证<br>Les indications | 适用于上、下消化道造影。<br>Il est applicable dans la radiographie gastro-intestinale supérieure et inférieure. |
| 用法、用量<br>Les modes d'emploi et la posologie | ①上消化道造影，根据检查部位和检查方法不同，加适量水调成不同浓度的混悬液，通常成人使用量食管：检查方法：经口，浓度为100%～180%（W/V），用量为50～150ml；胃、十二指肠：检查方法：经口，浓度为100%～180%（W/V），用量为50～150ml。②下消化道造影：经肛门灌入肠内。灌前准备：按常规肠清洗（控制饮食、大量饮水、加用泻剂），肌注解痉灵（可根据医院临床经验及习惯选择）。使用前，加适量水调成180%（W/V）浓度混悬液，按照自动灌肠机操作程序进行，250～300ml/次。<br><br>1) Pour la radiographie gastro-intestinale supérieure, en fonction de la partie examinée et des modes d'examen, préparer la solution en suspension avec l'eau, en général, chez des adultes, pour la radiographie de l'œsophage, par voie orale, 50 à 150ml de solution à 100% à 180% (W/V) ; pour la radiographie gastrique et duodénale, par voie orale, 50 à 150ml de solution à100% à 180% (W/V).<br>2) Pour la radiographie gastro-intestinale inférieure : le lavement par l'anus. La préparation pou le lavement : le nettoyage du côlon régulier (régime alimentaire, boire beaucoup d'eau et prendre des laxatifs), injecter le remède antispasmodique (en fonction de l'expérience clinique d'hôpitaux). Avant l'utilisation, préparer la solution en suspension à 180% (W/V) avec l'eau. Suivre les procédures de fonctionnement de la machine de lavement automatique, 250 à 300ml par fois. |
| 剂型、规格<br>Les formes pharmaceutiques et les spécifications | 混悬液：（W/V）100%，120%，130%，140%。<br>Suspension: (W/V) 100%, 120%, 130%, 140%. |
| **药品名称 Drug Names** | 碘化油 Huile iodée |
| 适应证<br>Les indications | 主要用于支气管及子宫、输卵管、瘘管、腔道等的造影检查，亦用于肝癌的栓塞治疗及地方性甲状腺肿。<br>Il est princiaplament appliquée dans la bronchographie, la radiographie utérine, l'hysterosalpingographie, la radiographie de la fistule et la radiographie de la cavité. Il est aussi applicable dans le traitement del'embolisation du cancer hépatique et du goitre endémique. |
| 用法、用量<br>Les modes d'emploi et la posologie | ①支气管造影：经气管导管直接注入气管或支气管腔内。成人单侧15～20ml（40%），双侧30～40ml；小儿酌减。注入应缓慢，采用体位使各叶支气管充盈。②子宫输卵管造影：经宫颈管直接注入子宫腔内，5～12ml（40%）。③各种腔室（如鼻旁窦、腮腺管、泪腺管等）和窦道、瘘管造影：依据病灶大小酌量直接注入。④肝癌栓塞治疗：先作选择性或超选择性肝动脉插管造影，将与抗癌药混合的碘化油5～10ml注入肿瘤供血动脉内。⑤预防地方甲状腺肿：多用肌内注射，亦可口服（应用其胶丸剂）。肌内注射：学龄前儿童1次剂量0.5ml，学龄期儿童或成人1次量1ml，每2～3年注射1次；口服，学龄前儿童每次服0.2～0.3g，学龄期至成人服0.4～0.6g，每1～2年服1次。<br><br>① Pour la bronchographie : injecter directement dans la cavité cachérale ou bronchique à travers le cathéter trachéal. Chez des adultes, le seul côté, 15 à 20ml (40%), les deux côtés, 30 à 40ml ; chez des enfants, diminuer un peu la dose. Injection lente afin de remplir chaque bronche lobaire. ② Pour la radiographie utérine et l'hysterosalpingographie : injecter directement dans la cavité utérine par le cathérer cervical, 5 à 12ml (40%). ③ Pour la radiographie de la cavité (sinus paranasals, la glande parotide, la glande lacrymale), du sinus et de la fistule de toutes sortes : injecter directement dans la |

续　表

| | zone touchée, ajuster la dose en fonction de la taille de la zone touchée. ④ Pour le traitement de l'embolisation du cancer hépatique : conduire d'abord l'angiographie de l'artère hépatique sélective ou super- sélective, injecter 5 à 10ml d'huile iodée associés aux anticancéreux dans l'artère de la tumeur. ⑤ Pour traiter le goitre endémique : injection IM dans la plupart des cas, aussi possible d'administrer par voie orale (utiliser les pilules). Injection IM : chez des enfants préscolaires, 0,5ml par fois, chez des enfants scolaires ou chez des adultes, 1ml par fois, une fois tous les 2 à 3 ans ; par voie orale, chez des enfants préscolaires, 0,2 à 0,3g par fois, chez des enfants scolaires ou chez des adultes, 0,4 à 0,6g, tous les 1 à 2 ans. |
|---|---|
| 剂型、规格<br>Les formes pharmaceutiques et les spécifications | 油注射液：每支 10ml（含碘 40%）。<br>胶丸剂：每丸 0.1g，0.2g。<br>Injection d'huile : 10ml (contenant 40% d'iode) par solution.<br>Pilules : 0,1g ou 0,2g par pilule. |
| 药品名称 Drug Names | 复方泛影葡胺 Composé diatrizoate de méglumine |
| 适应证<br>Les indications | 常用于尿路造影，也可用于肾上腺肾盂、心、脑血管等的造影。<br>Il est souvent utilisé dans l'urographie. Il est aussi applicable dans l'urographie surrénale, l'angiographie cérébrale et l'angiographie cardiaque. |
| 用法、用量<br>Les modes d'emploi et la posologie | ①逆行肾盂造影：20%，6～10ml。②尿路造影 50%，20～30ml。③脑血管造影：45% 以下溶液，10ml。④心脏大血管造影：50%，40ml。<br>① Pour l'urographie surrénale retrograde : 20%, 6 à 10ml. ② Pour l'urographie : 50%, 20 à 30ml. ③ Pour l'angiographie cérébrale : la solution inférieure à 45%, 10ml. ④ Pour l'angiographie cardiaque : 50%, 40ml. |
| 剂型、规格<br>Les formes pharmaceutiques et les spécifications | 注射液：60%20ml；76%20ml。<br>Injection : 60% 20ml ou 76% 20ml. |
| 药品名称 Drug Names | 钆喷酸葡胺 Gadopentétate diméthylglumine |
| 适应证<br>Les indications | 本品适用于中枢神经（脑脊髓）、腹、盆腔、四肢等人体脏器和组织的磁共振成像。还可替代 X 线含碘造影剂，用于不能使用者。<br>Ce produit est utilisé dans l'imagerie par la résonance magnétique des organes et tissus du corps, y comprisle système nerveux central (cerveau et moelle épinière), l'abdomen, le bassin, des membres, etc. Il sert aussi à remplacer le contrasteaux rayons X contenant l'iode et est appliqué chez des patients qui ne peuvent pas utiliser le dernier. |
| 用法、用量<br>Les modes d'emploi et la posologie | ①静脉注射：成人及 2 岁以上儿童，按体重一次 0.2ml/kg（或 0.1mmol/kg），最大用量为按体重一次 0.4ml/kg。颅脑及脊髓磁共振成像：为获得充分的强化，可按体重一次 0.4ml/kg 给药。最佳强化时间，一般在注射后数分钟之内（不超过 45 分钟）。②将 1ml 钆喷酸葡胺（相当于 2mmol/L GD-DTPA）加 2449ml 氯化钠注射液或用 1mlGD-DTPA 加 49ml 氯化钠注射液稀释后，可直接用于体腔的造影，如关节造影或腹腔造影等。③将 1ml 钆喷酸葡胺 +15g/L 甘露醇和 25mmol/L 缓冲剂枸橼酸钠配合，有较佳效果，胃肠涂布穿透力强，不易产生腔内浓缩的胃肠道阳性磁共振造影剂。尽管钆喷酸葡胺在大鼠脑池内注射的神经毒性，低于泛影葡胺及优维显等含碘造影剂，但目前仍不主张将它用于直接鞘内注射造影。④利用钆喷酸葡胺中 Gd 元素原子序数高（157.3）有吸收 X 线的特点，可用于碘过敏患者的肾动脉 X 线造影或肾排泄性造影（即代替 X 线含碘造影剂）。<br>① Injection IV : chez des adultes et des enfants de plus de 2 ans, 0.2ml/kg(ou 0.1mmol/kg) par fois, la dose maximale est de 0,4 ml/kg par fois. L'imagerie par la résonance magnétique du cerveau et de la moelle épinière : pour renforcer l'efficacité, prendre 0,4 ml/kg. Le meilleur moment pour le renforcement, c'est dans les quelques minutes après l'injection (moins de 45 minutes). ② Dissoudre |

1ml de gadopentétate de diméglumine (équivalent à 2mmol/L GD-DTPA) dans 2449ml de solution de chlorure de sodium ou dissoudre 1ml de GD-DTPA dans 49ml de chlorure de sodium, pour la radiographie de la cavité, telle que la radiographie articulaire ou abdominale. ③ Utiliser 1ml de gadopentétate de diméglumine, 15g/L de mannitol et 25 mmol/L de tampon de citrate de sodium, avec une action renforcée. Cela a l'avantage d'avoir une pénétration gastro-intestinale forte, et de ne pas former le contraste d'IRM positif gastro-intestinal concentré. Bien que sa neurotoxicité dans l'injection intracisternale chez le rat soit moins importante que les contrastes iodés tels que le diatrizoate et ULTRAVIST, il n'est pas recommandé de l'appliquer comme contraste injecté par voie intrathécale. ④ Comme le gadopentétate de diméglumine se caractérise par le nombre atomique élevé de l'élément Gd (157,3) et par son absorption des rayons X, il est applicable dans la radiographie de l'artère rénal aux rayons X ou la radiographie de l'excrétion rénale chez des patients allergiques à l'iode (à savoir remplacer le contraste iodé aux rayons X).

| 剂型、规格<br>Les formes pharmaceutiques et les spécifications | 注射液：每支 7.42g（20ml）；5.57g（15ml）；3.71g（10ml）。<br>Injection : 7,42g (20ml), 5,57g (15ml) ou 3,71g (10ml) par solution. |
|---|---|
| **药品名称 Drug Names** | 吲哚菁绿 Indocyanine vert |
| 适应证<br>Les indications | 本品用于诊断肝硬化、肝纤维化、韧性肝炎，对职业和药物中毒性肝病的诊断极有价值。也可用于循环系统功能（心排血量、平均循环时间或异常血流量）的检查测定。<br><br>Ce produit est utilisé dans le diagnostic de la cirrhose, dela fibrose hépatique et de l'hépatite réfractaire. Il est surtout efficace dans le diagnostic de la maladie hépatique professionnele ou liée à l'empoisonnement médicamenteux. Il est aussi applicable dans le diagnostic du fonctionnement du système circulatoire (le débitcardiaque, le temps de cycle moyen ou un flux sanguin anormal). |
| 用法、用量<br>Les modes d'emploi et la posologie | 静脉注射：①血浆消失率及血中停滞率的测定：0.5mg/kg，用蒸馏水稀释为5mg/ml 浓度，在 30 秒从肘静脉慢慢注入。②肝血流量的测定：将本品 25mg 用少量蒸馏水溶解后，稀释成 2.5 ～ 5.90mg/ml 浓度，开始时，注射相当于 3mg 的此浓度溶液，以后再 50 分钟内慢慢静滴至采血完毕。③用于循环功能检查：通常从前臂静脉注入，成人 1 次量 5 ～ 10mg，小儿按体重酌减。<br><br>Injection IV ① L'examen du taux de disparition de plasma sanguin et du taux de stagnation de sang : 0,5mg/kg, dilluer avec l'eau distillée pour former la solution à 5mg par ml, injecter par la veine cubitale lentement en 30 secondes. ② L'examen du débit sanguin hépatique : diluer 25mg de ce produit avec l'eau distillée pour former la solution à 2,5 à 5,90 mg par ml, au début, injecter 3mg de ce solution, ensuite, administrer cette solution en perfusion en 50 minutes jusqu'à la collection du sang. ③ L'examen de la fonction circulatoire : injecter dans la veine d'avant-bras, chez des adultes, 5 à 10mg par fois, diminuer un peu la dose chez des enfants. |
| 剂型、规格<br>Les formes pharmaceutiques et les spécifications | 注射剂：每支 25mg（附注射用水 10ml）。<br>Injection : 25mg par solution (y compris 10ml d'eau pour injection). |
| **药品名称 Drug Names** | 荧光素钠 Fluorescéine de sodium |
| 适应证<br>Les indications | ①滴眼液用于眼科诊断，正常角膜不显色，异常角膜显色。②针剂用于测血液循环时间，静脉注射后，在紫外线灯下观察，以 10 ～ 15 秒唇部黏膜能见到黄绿色荧光为正常。<br><br>① Ses gouttes pour les yeux sont appliquées dans le diagnostic ophtalmologique. La couleur est invisible s'il la cornée est normale, visible si elle est anormale. ② Son injection est utilisée comme mesure du temps de circulation sanguine. Après l'injection IV, observer sous la lampe UV, si on remarque la fluorescence jaune et verte dans la muqueuse labialeune en 10 à 15 secondes, cela est considéré comme normal. |

**续 表**

| 用法、用量<br>Les modes d'emploi et la posologie | ①滴眼后于角膜显微镜下观察颜色。②测血循环时间，于臂静脉注 2ml，每次用量 0.4 ~ 0.8g（2 ~ 4ml）。<br><br>① Après les gouttes pour les yeux, observer la couleur sous le microscope de la cornée. ② Pour mesurer le temps de circulation sanguine, injecter 2ml dans la veine du bras, 0,4 à 0,8g par fois (2 à 4ml). |
|---|---|
| 剂型、规格<br>Les formes pharmaceutiques et les spécifications | 滴眼液：2%。<br>注射液：0.4g（2ml）。<br>Les gouttes pour les yeux : 2%.<br>Injection : 0,4g (2ml). |

## 20.3 生物制品 Agents biologiques

| 药品名称 Drug Names | 人用狂犬病疫苗 (vero 细胞) Vaccins antirabiquesà usage humain (Cellules vero) |
|---|---|
| 适应证<br>Les indications | 用于预防狂犬病。凡被狂犬或其他疯动物咬伤、抓伤时，不分年龄、性别均应立即处理局部伤口（用清水或肥皂水反复冲洗后，再用碘酊或酒精消毒数次），并及时按暴露后免疫程序注射本疫苗；凡有接触狂犬病病毒危险的人员（如兽医、动物饲养员、林业从业人员、屠宰厂工人、狂犬病实验人员等），按暴露前免疫程序预防接种。<br><br>Ce médicament est applicable dans la prévention de la rage.Une fois mordusou rayés par la rage ou d'autres animaux fous, les patients doivent mener le traitement local des plaies (le lavage répété avec de l'eau ou de l'eau savonneuse, ensuite, la désinfection avec l'iode ou l'alcool), et être vacciné en suivant des démarches de vaccination post-exposition ; chez le personnel qui court le risque d'être en contact avec le virus de la rage (tel que les vétérinaires, les éleveurs des animaux, les forestiers, les travailleurs de l'abattoir, le personnel de laboratoire de la rage, etc.), il faut conduire al vaccination suivant des démarches de vaccination pré-exposition. |
| 用法、用量<br>Les modes d'emploi et la posologie | ①于上臂三角肌处肌内注射，幼儿可在大腿前外侧区肌内注射。②暴露后免疫程序：一般咬伤者于 0 日（第 1 天，当天）、3 日（第 4 天，以下类推）7 日、14 日和 28 日各注射本疫苗 1 剂，全程免疫共注射 5 剂，儿童用量相同。对有下列情况之一的，建议首剂狂犬疫苗剂量加倍给予：a. 注射疫苗前一天或更早一些时间内，注射过狂犬病人免疫球蛋白或狂犬病血清的慢性患者。b. 先天性或获得性免疫缺陷患者。c. 接受免疫抑制剂（包括抗疟疾药物）治疗的患者。d. 老年人。e. 于暴露后 48 小时或更长时间后才注射狂犬病疫苗的人员。f. 暴露后免疫程序按下述伤及程度分级处理：Ⅰ级暴露：触摸动物，被动物舔及无破损皮肤，一般不需要处理，不必注射狂犬疫苗。Ⅱ级暴露：未出血的皮肤咬伤、抓伤，应按暴露后免疫程序接种狂犬病疫苗。Ⅲ级暴露：一处或多处皮肤出血性咬伤或被抓伤出血，可疑或确诊的疯动物唾液污染黏膜，破损的皮肤被舔，应按暴露后程序立即接种狂犬病疫苗和抗狂犬病血清或抗狂犬病人免疫球蛋白按 20U/kg 给予。将尽可能多的抗狂犬病血清或抗狂犬病人免疫球蛋白做咬伤局部浸润注射，剩余部分做肌内注射，抗狂犬病血清或抗狂犬病人免疫球蛋白仅为单次应用。③暴露前免疫程序：按 0 日、7 日、21 日或 28 日各注射 1 剂，全程免疫共注射 3 剂。④对曾经接种过狂犬病疫苗的一般患者，再需接种疫苗的建议：a. 1 年内进行过全程免疫，被可疑疯动物咬伤者，应于 0 日或 3 日各注射 1 剂疫苗。b. 1 年前进行过全程免疫，被可疑疯动物咬伤者，则应全程接种疫苗。c. 3 年内进行过全程免疫，并且进行过加强免疫，被可疑疯动物咬伤者，应于 0 日或 3 日各注射 1 剂疫苗。d. 3 年前进行过全程免疫，并且进行过加强免疫，被可疑疯动物咬伤者，应全程接种疫苗。<br><br>① Injection IM dans le deltoide du haut-bras, chez des petits enfants, injection IM sur la zone antérolatérale de la cuisse. ② Les démarches de vaccination post-exposition : en général, injecter chez des personnes mordues 1 vaccin le premier jour (le jour de la morsure), le 4ème jour, le 8ème jour, le 15ème jour et le 29ème jour, 5 injections au total. La même dose chez des enfants que chez des adultes. Dans les cas suivants, il est recommandé de doubler la dose initiale du vaccin contre la rage : a. Le jour ou quelques temps précédant la vaccination, les patients chroniques ont administré l'immunoglobuline antirabique ou sérum antirabique. b. Patients atteints de déficit immunitaire congénital ou acquis. c. Les paitents qui administrent les immunosuppresseurs (y compris les antipaludismes). d. Les personnes âgées. e. Les personnes qui sont vaccinées 48 h ou plus après la |

**续　表**

morsure. f. Dans des démarches de vaccination post-exposition, il faut traiter les malades selon les niveaux.L'exposition de premier degré : toucher des animaux, être léché par des animaux et ne pas avoir la peau endommagée, dans les cas précédents, en général, pas nécessaire d'injecter le vaccin contre la rage. L'expoxition de deuxième degré : pour les morsures et les griffures sans saignement, il faut être vacciné suivant les démarches de vaccination post-exposition. L'exposition de troisième degré : une ou plusieurs morsures ou griffures avec saignement, la muqueuse condaminée par la salive des animaux enragés suspects ou confirmés, la peau avec lésions léchée, dans des cas précédents, il faut injecter le vaccin contre la rage et administer 20U par kg d'immunoglobuline antirabique ou de sérum antirabique princiaplement à travers l'injection d'infiltration sur la zone touchée en grande partie et aussi à travers l'injection IM. L'administration de l'immunoglobuline antirabique et du sérum antirabique n'est applicable que pour une fois. ③ Les démarches de vaccination pré-exposition : injecter un vaccin le 1er jour, le 8ème jour, le 22ème ou le 29ème jour, 3 injections au total pour toutes les démarches. ④ Chez des patients vaccinés contre la rage, il est recommandé de reprendre la vaccination dans ces cas suivants : a. Chez des personnes mordues par des animaux enragés suspects et qui sont vaccinés il y a moins d'un an, il faut injecter 1 vaccin le premier jour ou le 4ème jour. b. Chez des personnes mordues par des animaux enragés suspects et qui sont vaccinés il y a plus d'un an, il faut suivre toutes les démarches de la vaccination. c. Chez des personnes mordues par des animaux enragés suspects et qui sont vaccinés il y a moins de trois ans et qui a reçu la vaccination renforcée, il faut injecter un vaccin 1er jour ou le 4ème jour. d. Chez des personnes mordues par des animaux enragés suspects et qui sont vaccinés il y a plus de trois ans et qui ont reçu la vaccination renforcée, il faut suivre toutes les démarches de la vaccination.

| | |
|---|---|
| 剂型、规格<br>Les formes pharmaceutiques et les spécifications | 注射液：每瓶 1ml，每人 1 次用量为 1ml。<br>狂犬病疫苗效价应不低于 2.5U。<br><br>Injection : 1ml par flacon, 1ml par fois par personne.<br>Le titre de vaccin antirabique ne doit pas être inférieur à 2,5 U. |
| **药品名称 Drug Names** | 破伤风抗毒素 Antitoxine tétanique |
| 适应证<br>Les indications | 本品用于预防和治疗破伤风。已出现破伤风或可疑症状时，应在进行外科处理及其他疗法的同时，及时使用抗毒素治疗。开放性外伤（特别是伤口深、污染严重者）有感染破伤风的危险时，应注射抗毒素进行紧急预防。凡已接受过破伤风的危险时，应在再受伤后，再注射 1 剂疫苗，以加强免疫，不必注射抗毒素；如受伤者未接受过破伤风疫苗免疫或免疫史不清者，须注射抗毒素预防，但也应同时开始疫苗预防注射，以获得持久免疫。<br><br>Ce produit sert à prévenir et à traiter le tétanos. Lorsque le tétanos ou des symptômes suspects apparaissent, il faut conduire le traitement chirurgical ou d'autres traitements tout en prenant l'antitoxine. Lorsque le traumatisme ouvert risque d'être infecté par le le tétanos, il faut injecter en temps opportun l'antitoxine pour une prévention urgente. Chez des patients qui ont résisté au risque d'infection par le tétanos, il faut injecter encore une fois un vaccin lorsqu'ils se blessent, pour renforcer l'immunisation, pas nécessaire d'injecter l'antitoxine ; si les blessés ne sont pas vaccinés contre le tétanos, il faut injecter l'antitoxine pour la prévention, mais il faut injecter en même temps le vaccin pour obtenir une immunisation persistante. |
| 用法、用量<br>Les modes d'emploi et la posologie | ①预防用：皮下或肌内注射，一次 1500～3000U，儿童与成人用量相同；伤势严重者可增加用量 1～2 倍。经 5～6 日，如破伤风感染危险还未消除，应重复注射。②治疗用：肌内注射或静脉注射，第 1 次肌内或静脉注射 50 000～200 000U，儿童与成人用量相同；以后视病情决定注射剂量和间隔时间，同时还可将适量的抗毒素注射于伤口周围的组织中。初生儿破伤风，24 小时内分次或 1 次肌内或静脉注射 20 000～100 000U。皮下注射应在上臂三角肌处，同时注射疫苗时，注射部位应分开。肌内注射应在上臂三角肌处或臀部。只有经过皮下或肌内注射未发生异常反应者，方可作静脉注射。静脉注射应缓慢，开始每分钟不超过 1ml，以后每分钟亦不宜超过 4ml。一次静脉注射总量不应超过 40ml。儿童每千克体重不宜超过 0.8ml。亦可将抗毒素加入葡萄糖注射液或氯化钠注射液等溶液中静脉滴注。静脉注射前应将安瓿置温水浴中加温至接近体温，注射中如发现异常反应，应立即停止。 |

续　表

| | |
|---|---|
| | ① Pour la prévention : injection sous-cutanée ou IM, 1500 à 3000 U, la même dose chez des enfants que chez des adultes ; pour les cas sévères, doubler ou tripler la dose. S'il le risque des infections par le tétanos ne se dissipe pas 5 à 6 jour après l'injection, répéter l'injection. ② Pour le traitement : injection IM ou IV, pour la première fois, 50 000 à 200 000U, la même dose chez des enfants que chez des adultes ; ensuite, ajuster la dose et l'intervalle selon les cas, injecter en même temps l'antitoxine dans les tissus au tour des plaies. Chez des nouveau-nés, injecter 20 000 à 100 000U par voie sous-cutanée ou IM en 24h à travers plusieurs fois. L'injection sous-cutanée doit être conduite dans le deltoïde du haut-bras, le site de vaccination doit être différent. L'injection IM doit être menée dans le deltoide du haut –bras ou sur la fesse.L'injection IV n'est applicable que chez des patients qui ne présentent pas de réaction anormale après l'injection sous-cutanée ou IM. L'injection IV doit être lente, commencer par 1ml par minute au plus, ensuite 4ml par minute au plus. Ne pas dépasser 40ml par fois pour une injection IV. Chez des enfants, ne pas dépasser 0,8ml par kg. Aussi possible d'administrer en perfusion après avoir ajouté l'antitoxine dans la solution de glucose ou la solution de chlorure de sodium. Avant l'injection IV, réchauffer l'ampoule dans le bain chaud pour qu'elle s'approche de la température du corps. S'il y a des réactions anormales, arrêter l'injection. |
| 剂型、规格 Les formes pharmaceutiques et les spécifications | 注射液：预防用：每瓶 1500IU；治疗用：每瓶 10000IU。<br>Injection: Pour la prévention:1500IU par flacon; pour le traitement:10000IU par flacon. |
| **药品名称 Drug Names** | 抗蛇毒血清 Antivenin |
| 适应证 Les indications | 用于毒蛇咬伤中毒。<br>Il est applicable dans le traitement de l'intoxication liée à la morsure de serpent. |
| 用法、用量 Les modes d'emploi et la posologie | 稀释后静脉注射或静脉滴注，也可肌内或皮下注射。用量根据被咬伤者的受毒量及血清效价而定。以下为中和一条毒蛇的剂量：①抗蝮蛇毒血清：主要用于蝮蛇咬伤的治疗，对竹叶青和烙铁头毒蛇也有交叉中和作用。一次用 6000 ～ 16 000U，以氯化钠或 25% 葡萄糖注射液稀释 1 倍，缓慢静脉注射。②抗五步蛇毒血清：主要用于五步蛇咬伤的治疗，对蝮蛇蛇毒也有交叉中和作用。每次用 8000U，以氯化钠注射液稀释 1 倍，缓慢静脉注射。③抗银环蛇毒血清：主要用于银环蛇咬伤的治疗，一次用 10 000U，缓慢静脉注射。④抗眼镜蛇毒血清：主要用于眼镜蛇咬伤的治疗，对其他科的毒蛇蛇毒也有交叉中和作用。一次用 2500 ～ 10 000U，缓慢静脉注射。<br><br>Après l'injection IV ou la perfusion, aussi possible l'injection IM ou sous-cutanée. La dose dépend de la quantité de poisson et le titre de sérum chez des personnes mordues. La dose suivante est celle pour neutraliser un serpent : ① Le sérum d'anti-vipère : applicable dans le traitement de la morsure par une vipère. Il peut neutraliser dans certaines mesures le venin de la vipère couleur de bambou. 6000 à 16 0000 U par fois, diluer de moitié avec la solution de glucose à 25% ou la solution de chlorure de sodium, injection IV lente. ② Le sérum d'anti- Deinagkistrodon acutus : applicable dans le traitement de la morsure par un Deinagkistrodon acutus. Il peut exercer une neutralisation coisée sur le venin de la vipère. 8 000U par fois, diluer de moitié avec la solution de chlorure de sodium, injection IV lente. ③ Le sérum d'anti-serpent corail : il est principalement appliqué dans le traitement de la morsure par le serpent corail, 10 000 U par fois, injection IV lente. ④ Le sérum d'anti-cobra : il est principalement appliqué dans le traitement de la morsure par le cobra, il exerce aussi une neutralisation croisée sur le venin d'autres serpents. 2 500 à 10 000U, injection IV lente. |
| 剂型、规格 Les formes pharmaceutiques et les spécifications | 注射液：①抗蝮蛇蛇毒血清：每瓶含抗蝮蛇毒血清 6000U。②抗五步蛇蛇毒血清：每瓶含抗眼镜蛇毒血清：2000U。③抗银环蛇毒血清：每瓶含抗银环蛇毒血清：10 000U。④抗眼镜蛇毒血清：每瓶含抗眼镜蛇毒血清：1000U。<br>Injection : ① Le sérum d'anti-vipère : 6000 U de sérum d'anti-vipère par flacon. ② Le sérum d'anti-Deinagkistrodon acutus : 2000U de sérum d'anti-Deinagkistrodon acutus par flacon. ③ Le sérum d'anti-serpent corail : 10 000U de sérum d'anti-serpent corail par flacon. ④ Le sérum d'anti-cobra : 1000U de sérum d'anti-cobra par flacon. |

**续　表**

| 药品名称 Drug Names | 人血白蛋白 Albumine humaine |
| --- | --- |
| 适应证<br>Les indications | 用于治疗因失血、创伤及烧伤等引起的休克，脑水肿及大脑损伤所致的脑压增高，防治低蛋白血症以及肝硬化或肾病引起的水肿和腹水，有较好的疗效。<br>Ce produit permet de traiter le choc causé par le saignement, les brûlures et le traumatisme, l'hypertension intracrânienne induite par l'oedème cérébral et le traumatisme crânien. Il sert aussi à prévenir l'œdème et l'ascite caués par l'hypoalbuminémie, la cirrhose du foie ou des maladies rénales, avec un effet satisfaisant. |
| 用法、用量<br>Les modes d'emploi et la posologie | 静脉滴注，用量由医师酌定。一般因严重烧伤或失血等所致的休克可直接注射本品 5～10g，隔 4～6 小时重复注射一次。在治疗肾病及肝硬化等慢性白蛋白缺乏症时，可每日注射本品 5～10g，直至水肿消失、血清白蛋白恢复正常为止。<br>En perfusion, la dose est décidée par le médecin. Pour le choc causé par des brûlures ou des saignements, injecter directement 5 à 10g de ce produit, répéter une fois 4 à 6 h après. Pour traiter l'hypoalbuminémie liée aux maladies rénales et la cirrhose, injecter 5 à 10g par jour, jusqu'à la disparition de l'œdème et à la normalisation de l'albumine sérique. |
| 剂型、规格<br>Les formes pharmaceutiques et les spécifications | 注射液：1g (10ml)；2g (10ml)；2.5g (10ml)；5g (10ml)；10g (50ml)；12.5g (50ml)；25g (125ml)。<br>冻干品：10g；20g。<br>Injection : 1g(10ml)；2g(10ml)；2.5g(10ml)；5g(10ml)；10g(50ml)；12.5g(50ml)；25g(125ml).<br>Agent lyophilisé : 10g ou 20g. |
| 药品名称 Drug Names | 人免疫球蛋白 Immunoglobuline humaine |
| 适应证<br>Les indications | 主要用于预防麻疹和甲型肝炎等病毒性感染。<br>Ce médicament est principalement appliqué dans la prévention de la rougeole, de l'hépatite A et d'autres infections virales. |
| 用法、用量<br>Les modes d'emploi et la posologie | ①预防麻疹：0.05～0.15ml/kg 或 5 岁以内儿童注射 1.5～3ml，成人不得超过 6ml，预防效果为 1 个月。②预防甲型肝炎：按每千克体重注射 0.05～0.1ml/kg 或儿童每次注射 1.5～3ml，成人每次注射 3ml。1 次注射，预防效果为 1 个月。<br>① Pour prévenir la rougeole : 0,05 à 0,15ml par kg ou injecter 1,5 à 3ml chez des enfants moins de 5 ans, ne pas dépasser 6ml chez des adultes, l'action de prévention dure 1 mois. ② Pour prévenir l'hépatite A : 0,05 à 0,1 ml par kg ou chez des enfants, injecter 1,5 à 3ml, chez des adultes, injecter 3ml par fois. Une injection peut avoir une action de prévention pendant 1 mois. |
| 剂型、规格<br>Les formes pharmaceutiques et les spécifications | 注射液：10%/1.5ml (150mg)；10%/3ml (300mg)。<br>Injection : 10%/1.5ml(150mg)；10%/3ml(300mg) |
| 药品名称 Drug Names | 乙型肝炎人免疫球蛋白 Immunoglobuline humaine hépatite B |
| 适应证<br>Les indications | 用于乙型肝炎的预防。主要适用于：①乙型肝炎表面抗原阳性母亲的新生儿。②预防意外感染人群，如血友病患者、肾透析患者、医务人员或皮肤破损被乙型肝炎表面抗原阳性的血液或分泌物污染的人员等。③与乙型肝炎患者或携带者密切接触的易感人群。<br>Ce produit permet de prévenir l'hépatite B. Il est applicable dans des cas suivants : ① Les nouveau-nés dont la mère est atteinte de l'hépatite B dont l'antigène de surface est positif. ② Les personnes infectées accidentellement, telles que les patients atteints d'hémophilie, les patients de dialyse rénale, le personnel médical, le personnel avec les lésions cutanées et qui est contaminé par les sécrétions ou par le sang de l'antigène positif de surface de l'hépatite B. ③ Les populations sensibles en contact étroit avec les patients ou des porteurs de l'hépatite B. |
| 用法、用量<br>Les modes d'emploi et la posologie | ①母婴阻断：乙型肝炎表面抗原阳性母亲的婴儿出生 24 小时内，肌内注射 100～200U，同时联合乙型肝炎疫苗，按乙型肝炎疫苗注射程序全程注射（按照 0、1、6、个月或医师推荐的适宜方案）；亦可在婴儿出生 24 小时内肌内注射 100～200U，1 个月时在注射一次，同时按乙型肝炎疫苗注射程序全程注射。单独使用乙型肝炎免疫球蛋白很少获得满意结果，如果单独使用应多次注射，每 3～4 周 1 次，每次肌内注射 100～200U。②乙型肝炎预防：用于预防意外暴露时，注射越早越好，一般应在 24 小时内进行肌内注射，最迟不超过 7 日。一次注射量，儿童为 100U，成人为 200U，必要时剂量可加倍，每 3～4 周再注射 1 次，必要时按注射程序全程注射乙型肝炎疫苗。 |

续　表

① La prévention de la transmission mère-enfant (PTME) : en 24h après la naissance du bébé de la mère atteinte de l'hépatite B dont l'antigène de surface est positif, injecter 100 à 200U par voie IM, en même temps, suivre toutes les démarches de la vaccination contre l'hépatite B (injecter le vaccin le premier mois, le 2ème, le 7ème mois ou selon des ordonnances) ; aussi possible d'injecter 100 à 200U par voie IM en 24h après la naissance du bébé, répéter une fois en un mois, en même temps, suivre toutes les démarches de la vaccination contre l'hépatite B. L'utilisation seule de l'immunoglobuline de l'hépatite B peut rarement avoir des effets satisfaisants. S'il est utilisé seul, il faut injecter plusieurs fois, une fois toutes les 3 à 4 semaines, 100 à 200 U par fois par voie IM. ② Pour prévenir l'hépatite B : pour prévenir l'exposition accidentelle, il faut injecter le plus tôt possible, en général, injection IM en 24h, en 7 jours au plus. 100U par fois chez des enfants, 200 U par fois chez des adultes, s'il est nécessaire, doubler la dose, injection toutes les 3 à 4 semaines, en cas de besoin, suivre toutes les démarches de la vaccination contre l'hépatite B.

| 剂型、规格<br>Les formes pharmaceutiques et les spécifications | 注射液（冻干）：乙型肝炎免疫球蛋白　100U；200U；400U。<br>Injection (lyophilisée) : 100 U, 200 U ou 400 U d'immunoglobuline de l'hépatite B. |

| 药品名称 Drug Names | 破伤风人免疫球蛋白 Humaine Tetanos Immunoglobuline |
| --- | --- |
| 适应证<br>Les indications | 用于预防和治疗破伤风，尤其适用于对破伤风抗毒素（TAT）有过敏反应的患者。<br>Ce médicament sert à prévenir et à traiter le tétanos. Il est surtout applicable chez des patients allergiques à l'antitoxine. |
| 用法、用量<br>Les modes d'emploi et la posologie | 肌内注射。①预防用：儿童、成人一次用量均为250U。创面严重或创面严重和感染严重者可加倍注射。②治疗用：3000～6000U。可多点注射。<br>Injection IM : ① Pour la prévention : chez des enfants et chez des adultes, 250 U par fois. En cas de blessures graves ou d'infections graves, doubler la dose. ② Pour le traitement : 3 000 à 6 000 U, possible d'injecter à plusieurs sites. |
| 剂型、规格<br>Les formes pharmaceutiques et les spécifications | 注射液：100U；200U；250U。<br>注射剂（冻干品）：100U；200U；250U。<br>Injection : 100 U, 200 U ou 250 U.<br>Injection (lyophilisée) : 100 U, 200 U ou 250 U. |
| 药品名称 Drug Names | 狂犬病人免疫球蛋白 Humaine Rabique Immunoglobuline |
| 适应证<br>Les indications | 本品主要配合狂犬病疫苗使用，当被狂犬或其他疯动物严重咬伤者，进行狂犬病疫苗预防注射的同时，配合使用本品，对狂犬病做紧急的被动免疫，以提高预防性治疗效果。<br>Il est principalement utilisé en association avec le vaccin contre la rage. Lorsque le patient a été gravement mordu par la rage ou d'autres animaux déjantés, il faut injecter le vaccin contre la rage ainsi que ce médicament pour une immunisation passive urgente afin de renforcer l'efficacité du traitement prophylactique. |
| 用法、用量<br>Les modes d'emploi et la posologie | 肌内注射：动物咬伤部位及时清创后，于受伤部位用本品总剂量的1/2 做皮下浸润注射，余下制剂进行肌内注射（头部咬伤者可于背部肌内注射），按体重每千克20U（或遵医嘱），一次注射，如所需总剂量大于10ml，可于1～2日分次注射。同时或随后即可进行狂犬病疫苗注射，但两种制品的注射部位和器具应严格分开。<br>Injection IM : après le nettoyage des zones mordues par des animaux, suivre l'injection d'infiltration sous-cutanée avec la moitié de la dose totale sur la zone touchée, injecter le reste de la dose par voie IM (pour les morsures sur la tête, possible d'injecter au dos par voie IM), 20 U par kg (ou selon des ordonnances), une fois, si la dose nécessaire totale est supérieure à 10ml, injecter à plusieurs fois en 1 à 2 jours. Il est possible de mener la vaccination contre la rage en même temps ou après l'injection. Mais il faut distinguer strictement les sites d'injection et les outils utilisés. |
| 剂型、规格<br>Les formes pharmaceutiques et les spécifications | 注射液：100U；200U；500U。<br>注射剂（冻干品）：100U；200U；500U。<br>Injection : 100U, 200 U ou 500 U.<br>Injection (lyophilisée) : 100 U, 200U ou 500 U. |

续 表

| 药品名称 Drug Names | 人纤维蛋白原 Fibrinogène humaine |
|---|---|
| 适应证<br>Les indications | ①遗传性纤维蛋白原减少症，包括遗传性异常纤维蛋白原血症或遗传性纤维蛋白原缺乏症。②获得性纤维蛋白原减少症，主要见于严重肝脏损害所致的纤维蛋白原合成不足及局部或弥散性血管内凝血导致纤维蛋白原消耗量增加。<br><br>① Le fibrinogène héréditaire, y compris la dysfibrinogénémie héréditaire et le déficit en fibrinogène héréditaire. ② Le déficit en fibrinogène acquis, comme le déficit de synthèse de fibrinogène causé par les lésions hépatiques sévères, ou l'augmentation de la consommation du fibrinogène induite par la coagulation intravasculaire disséminée. |
| 用法、用量<br>Les modes d'emploi et la posologie | 静脉注射：其用量视血浆纤维蛋白原水平及要达到止血所需的纤维蛋白原水平（1g/L）而定。由于纤维蛋白原的生物半衰期长达 96 ～ 144 小时，故开始每 1 ～ 2 日，以后每 3 ～ 4 日，滴注 1 次即可。能够按每 2g 纤维蛋白原可使血浆纤维蛋白原水平升至 0.5g/L 的原则推算所需剂量，一般首次用量 1 ～ 2g，必要时可加量。大出血时应立即给予 4 ～ 8g。<br><br>Injection IV : fixer la dose en fonction du fibrinogène du plasma et du niveau de fibrinogène nécessaire pour arrêter le saignement. Comme la demi-vie biologique du fibrinogène est de 96 à 144h, commencer par la perfusion une fois tous les 1 à 2 jours, ensuite tous les 3 à 4 jours. En fonction du principe selon lequel 2g de fibrinogène peut permettre au fibrinogène plasmatique d'atteindre 0,5 g par L, la dose initiale en général est de 1 à 2g, s'il est nécessaire, augmenter la dose. Lors de l'hémorragie massive, injecter immédiatement 4 à 8g. |
| 剂型、规格<br>Les formes pharmaceutiques et les spécifications | 注射剂（冻干品）：每支 0.5g。<br>Injection (lyophilisée) : 0,5g par solution. |
| 药品名称 Drug Names | 重组人干扰素 α - 1b Interféron α -1b humaine recombinante |
| 适应证<br>Les indications | 用于病毒性疾病和某些恶性肿瘤。①已批准用于治疗慢性乙型肝炎、丙型肝炎和毛细胞血友病。②已有临床试验结果或文献报道，用于病毒性疾病，如带状疱疹、尖锐湿疣、流行性出血热和小儿呼吸道合胞病毒肺炎等。③用于治疗恶性肿瘤，如慢性粒细胞白血病、黑色素瘤、淋巴瘤等。④滴眼液，可用于眼部病毒性疾病。<br><br>Il est applicable dans le traitement des maladies virales et de certaines tumeurs malignes.<br>① Il est autorisé de l'appliquer dans le traitement de l'hépatite chronique B, del'hépatite C et de l'hémophilie des cellules ciliées. ② Selon des tests cliniques ou des documents de référence, il peut être appliqué dans les maladies virales, telles que l'herpès, les verrues génitales,la fièvre hémorragique épidémiqueet la pneumonie liée au virus syncytialrespiratoire chez les enfants. ③ Il permet de traiter les tumeurs malignes, telles que la leucémie myéloïde chronique, le mélanome, le lymphome, etc. ④ Ses gouttes pour les yeux sont applicables dans le traitement des maladies virales oculaires. |
| 用法、用量<br>Les modes d'emploi et la posologie | ①慢性乙型肝炎：一次 30 ～ 50μg，隔日一次，疗程 4 ～ 6 个月，可根据病情延长疗程至一年，也可进行诱导治疗，即在治疗开始时，每天用药 1 次，0.5 ～ 1 个月后改为每周 3 次，直到疗程结束。②慢性丙型肝炎：一次 30 ～ 50μgμ，隔日一次，疗程 4 ～ 6 个月，无效者停用。有效者可继续治疗至 12 个月。根据病情需要，可延长至 18 个月。在治疗的第 1 个月，一日 1 次。疗程结束后随访 6 ～ 12 个月。急性丙型肝炎，应及早使用本品治疗，可减少慢性化。③慢性粒细胞白血病：一次 30 ～ 50μg，一日 1 次，连续用药 6 个月以上。可根据病情适当调整，缓解后可改为隔日注射。④肿瘤：视病情可延长疗程。如患者未出现病情恶化或严重不良反应，应当在适当剂量下继续用药。<br><br>① Pour traiter l'hépatite B : 20 à 50 µg par fois, tous les 2 jours, pendant 4 à 6 mois comme un traitement médical, possible de prolonger jusqu'à un an selon les cas. Aussi possible de suivre le traitement d'induction, au début, 1 fois par jour, 0,5 à 1 mois après, 3 fois par semaine, jusqu'à la fin du traitement. ② Pour traiter l'hépatite C chronique : 30 à 50 µg par fois, tous les 2 jours, pendant 4 à 6 |

| | |
|---|---|
| | mois. S'il est inutile, arrêter l'administration. S'il est efficace, continuer jusqu'à 12 mois. Selon les cas, possible de prolonger jusqu'à 18 mois. Durant le premier mois du traitement, 1 fois par jour. Après la fin du traitement, suivre de près pendant 6 à 12 mois. Pour traiter l'hépatite C aigue, il faut prendre ce produit le plus tôt possible pour réduire le risque d'être chronique. ③ Pour traiter la leucémie myéloïde chronique : 30 à 50 μg par fois, 1 fois par jour, pendant 6 mois consécutifs. Ajuster la dose selon les cas, après l'amélioration des symptômes, injecter tous les 2 jours. ④ Pour traiter les tumeurs: possible de prolonger le traitement selon les cas. S'il n'y a pas la détérioration des symptômes ou l'apparition des réactions indésirables, il faut continuer l'administration avec une dose pertinente. |
| 剂型、规格<br>Les formes pharmaceutiques et les spécifications | 注射剂（冻干品）：10μg（10万U）；20μg（20万U）；30μg（30万U）；50μg（50万U）。<br>Injection (lyophilisée) : 10 μg (100 000 U), 20 μg (200 000 U), 30μg (300 000 U) ou 50 μg (500 000 U). |
| 药品名称 Drug Names | 重组人白细胞介素 -2 Interleukine-2 Humaine Recombinante |
| 适应证<br>Les indications | ①用于肾细胞癌、黑色素瘤，用于控制晚期腹水及其他晚期肿瘤。②用于先天或后天免疫缺陷症，如艾滋病等。③对某些病毒性、细菌性疾病、胞内寄生感染性疾病，如乙型肝炎、麻风病、肺结核、白念珠菌感染等，有一定作用。<br>① Ce médicament est appliqué dans le traitement du carcinome rénal, du mélanome, et dans le contrôle de l'ascite avancée et de la tumeur avancée. ② Il sert à traiter le syndrome d'immunodéficience congénitale ou acquise, comme le sida. ③ Il a un certain effet sur certaines maladies infectieuses, bactériennes et parasitaires intracellulaires, telles que l'hépatite B, la lèpre, la tuberculose, l'infection de Candida albicans, etc. |
| 用法、用量<br>Les modes d'emploi et la posologie | 皮下注射：20万～40万 U/m² 加入灭菌注射用水 2ml，一日 1 次，每周注射 4 日，4 周为 1 个疗程。肌内注射：慢性乙型肝炎，一次 20 万 U，隔日 1 次。静脉滴注：20万～40万 U/m²，加入注射用生理盐水 500ml，一日 1 次，每周连用 4 日，4 周为 1 个疗程。腔内注射：先抽去腔内积液，再将本品 40 万～50 万 U/m² 加入注射用生理盐水 20ml 注入，一周 1～2 次，3～4 周为 1 个疗程。瘤内、瘤周注射：10 万～30 万 U 加入注射用生理盐水 3～5ml，分多点注射到瘤内或瘤周，一周 2 次，连用 2 周为 1 个疗程。<br>Injection sous-cutanée : dissoudre 200 000 U ou 400 000 U par m² dans 2ml d'eau stérile pour injection, 1 fois par jour, 4 fois par semaine, pendant 4 semaines comme un traitement. Injection IM : pour traiter l'hépatite B chronique, 200 000 U par fois, tous les 2 jours. La perfusion : dissoudre 200 000 U à 400 000 U par m² dans 500ml de solution saline, 1 fois par jour, 4 jours consécutifs par semaine, pendant 4 semaines comme un traitement médical. Injection articulaire : retirer l'épanchement articulaire, ensuite, dissoudre 400 000 U à 500 000 U par m² dans 20ml de solution saline, 1 à 2 fois par semaine, pendant 3 à 4 semaines comme un traitement médical. Injection intratumorale ou péri-tumorale : dissoudre 100 000 U à 300 000 U dans 3 à 5ml de solution saline, mener l'injection intratumorale ou péri-tumorale à plusieurs sites, 2 fois par semaine, pendant 2 semaines consécutives comme un traitement médical. |
| 剂型、规格<br>Les formes pharmaceutiques et les spécifications | 注射剂（冻干品）：每支 50 万 U；100 万 U；200 万 U；1800 万 U。<br>Injection (lyophilisée) : 500 000U, 1 million d'U, 2 millions d'U ou 18 millions d'U par solution. |
| 药品名称 Drug Names | 结核菌素纯蛋白衍生物 Dérivés Protéiques purs de la Tuberculine(TB-PPD) |
| 适应证<br>Les indications | 本品 5U 用于结核病的临床诊断，卡介苗接种对象的选择及卡介苗接种后机体免疫反应的监测。2U 制品用于临床诊断及流行病学监测。<br>5U de ce médicament est appliqué dans le disgnostic clinique de la tuberculose, le choix des objets de la vaccination duBCG et le suivi de la réponse immunitaire après l'injection d'un BCG. 2U de ce médicament est appliqué dans le diagnostic clinique et les enquêtes épidémiologiques. |

**续 表**

| 用法、用量<br>Les modes d'emploi et la posologie | ①婴儿、儿童及成人均可用。②皮内注射，吸取本品 0.1ml（5U），皮内注射于前臂掌侧，于注射后 48～72 小时检查注射部位反应。测量应以硬的横径及其垂直径的 mm 数记录之。5U 制品反应平均直径应不低于 5mm 为阳性反应。凡有水疱、坏死、淋巴管炎者均属阳性反应，应详细注明。<br><br>① Il est applicable chez des bébés, des enfants et des adultes. ② Injection intradermique, prendre 0,1ml (5U) de ce produit, injecter par voie intradermique dans l'avant-bras, examiner les réactions du site d'injection 48 à 72 h. Noter le diamète transversal et le diamète vertical de l'induration en mm. Le diamète moyen supérieur à 5mm à la réation de 5 U de produit est considéré comme réaction positive. Les cloques, la nécrose, la lymphangite sont toutes des réactions positives, il faut les noter précisément. |
|---|---|
| 剂型、规格<br>Les formes pharmaceutiques et les spécifications | 注射剂：每瓶 1ml；2ml。<br>①每 1 次人用剂量为 0.1ml 含 5UTB-PPD。<br>②每 1 次人用剂量为 0.1ml 含 2U TB-PPD。<br><br>njection : 1ml ou 2ml par flacon.<br>① La dose par fois par personne est de 0,1ml contenant 5U de dérivé protéinique purifié de tuberculine.<br>② La dose par fois par personne est de 0,1ml contenant 2U de dérivé protéinique purifié de tuberculine. |
| 药品名称 Drug Names | 布氏菌纯蛋白衍生物 Dérivés Protéiques purs de la Brucella(BR-PPD) |
| 适应证<br>Les indications | 可用于布氏疫苗接种对象的选择及布氏疫苗接种后机体免疫反应的监测和布氏菌的临床诊断与流行病学调查。<br><br>Ce médicament est utilisé dans le choix des objets de la vaccination du vaccin de Brucella et le suivi de la réponse immunitaire après l'injection d'un vaccin de Brucella ainsi que le diagnostic et les enquêtes épidémiologiques de la brucellose. |
| 用法、用量<br>Les modes d'emploi et la posologie | 用药途径：吸取本品 0.1ml（1U）皮内注射于前臂掌侧。于注射后 48～72 小时的检查注射部位反应，测量时应以硬节的横径及其垂直径的毫米数记录之。反应平均直径应不低于 5mm 为阳性。凡有水疱、坏死、淋巴管炎者均属阳性反应，应详细注明。<br><br>Injecter 0,1ml (1U) de ce produit par voie intradermique dans l'avant-bras, examiner les réactions du site d'injection 48 à 72 h. Noter le diamète transversal et le diamète vertical de l'induration en mm. Le diamète moyen supérieur à 5mm est considéré comme réaction positive. Les cloques, la nécrose, la lymphangite sont toutes des réactions positives, il faut les noter précisément. |
| 剂型、规格<br>Les formes pharmaceutiques et les spécifications | 注射液：每支 1ml；2ml。<br>每人用量为 0.1ml 含 1U UBR-PPD。<br><br>Injection : 1ml ou 2ml par solution.<br>La dose par personne est de 0,1ml contenant 1U de dérivé protéique purifié de Brucella. |

# 第4章

# 中文—西班牙文对照药品临床使用说明

Instrucciones para la aplicación clínica del medicamento(Chino – Español)

| 1. 抗生素 Antibióticos |
| --- |

| 1.1　青霉素类 Penicillina |
| --- |

| 药品名称 Drug Names | 青霉素 Penicilina |
| --- | --- |
| 适应证<br>Indicaciones | 　　青霉素用于敏感菌所致的急性感染，如：菌血症、败血症、猩红热、丹毒、肺炎、脓胸、扁桃体炎、中耳炎、蜂窝织炎、疖、痈、急性乳腺炎、心内膜炎、骨髓炎、流行性脑膜炎（流脑）、钩端螺旋体病（对本病早期疗效较好），奋森咽峡炎、创伤感染、回归热、气性坏疽、炭疽、淋病、放线菌病等。治疗破伤风、白喉宜与相应的抗毒素联用。<br>　　普鲁卡因青霉素吸收缓慢，肌内注射30万U，血药浓度峰值约2U/ml，24小时仍可测得。适用于梅毒和一些敏感菌所致的慢性感染。<br>　　苄星青霉素吸收极缓慢，血药浓度低，适用于需长期使用青霉素预防的患者，如慢性风湿性心脏病患者。<br>　　Se usa para infecciones agudas producidas por gérmenes sensibles, tales como: septicemia, bacteriemia, escarlatina, erisipela, neumonía, empireuma, amigdalitis, otitis media, celulitis, forúnculos, despreciable, mastitis aguda, endocarditis, osteomielitis, la epidemia de meningitis (EEM), leptospirosis (la eficacia es mejor en la etapa temprana), vincent angina de pecho, infección de la herida, fiebre recurrente, gangrena gaseosa, el ántrax, gonorrea y la actinomicosis.Para tratar el tétanos y la difteria se debe usar en combinación con la correspondiente antitoxina.<br>　　La penicilina procaína se absorbe lentamente en la circulación. Tras la administración de una inyección intramuscular de 300 mil unidades, la concentración plasmática máxima se mantiene en aproximadamente 2 unidades/ml y al cabo de 24 horas puede ser medido.Se usa para el tratamiento de la sífilis e infecciones crónicas causadas por cepas sensibles.<br>　　La absorción de benzatina penicilina es muy lenta, con una baja concentración plasmática, aplicable a los pacientes con la necesidad de la penicilina como uso de prevención a largo plazo, por ejemplo,pacientes con Cardiopatía Reumática Crónica. |
| 用法、用量<br>Administración y dosis | 　　青霉素钠常用于肌内注射或静脉滴注。肌内注射成人一日量为80万～320万U，儿童一日量为3万～5万U/kg，分为2～4次给予。静脉滴注适用于重病，如感染性心内膜炎、化脓性脑膜炎患者。成人一日量为240万～2000万U，儿童一日量为20万～40万U/kg，分4～6次加至少量输液中做间歇快速滴注。输液的青霉素（钠盐）浓度一般为1万～4万U/ml。本品溶液[20万～40万U/（2～4ml）]可用于气雾吸入，一日2次。青霉素钾通常用于肌内注射，由于注射局部较痛，可以用0.25%利多卡因注射液作为溶剂（2%苯甲醇注射液已不用）。钾盐也可静脉滴注，但必须注意患者体内血钾浓度和输液的钾含量（每100万U青霉素G钾中含钾量为65mg，与氯化钾125mg中的含钾量相近），并注意滴注速度不可太快。普鲁卡因青霉素仅供肌内注射，1次量40万～80万U，一日1次。苄星青霉素仅供肌内注射，1次60万U，10～14日1次；1次120万U，10～21日1次。 |

**续　表**

La Penicilina sódica se usa frecuentemente en la inyección intramuscular o infusión intravenosa. Para inyección intramuscular, el volumen de día para adultos es de 800,000 a 3,200,000 unidades, para niños es de 30,000 a 50,000 unidades/kg, divididas en 2 a 4 veces. La infusión intravenosa se aplica a enfermedades graves, como la endocarditis infecciosa y meningitis purulenta y el volumen de día para adultos es de 2,400,000 a 20,000,000 unidades, para niños es de 200,000 a 40,000 unidades/kg, divididas en 4 a 6 veces, agregándose a una pequeña cantidad de la infusión como infusión rápida intermitente. La concentración de la infusión penicilina (sal de sodio) es de 10,000 a 40,000 unidades/ml. La solución (200 000 ~ 400 000 unidades / 2 ~ 4 ml) se puede utilizar para la inhalación, 2 veces al día. El potasio de enicilina generalmente se utiliza para la inyección intramuscular, y como la. inyección local duele mucho, se puede utilizar el 0.25% de la inyección de lidocaína como solvente (2% de la inyección de alcohol bencílico no se usa ya). La silvita puede ser infusión intravenosa, pero se debe prestar atención a la concentración de potasio corporal y el contenido de potasio infundido (por 1 millón de unidades de penicilina G potasio el contenido de potasio es de 65 mg, similar al contenido de potasio en 125 mg de cloruro de potasio), y velocidad de perfusión no puede ser demasiado rápida. Penicilina procaína se inyecta por vía intramuscular, un volumen de 400,000 a 800,000 unidades al día. Benzatina sólo para inyección intramuscular, un volumen de 600,000 unidades por cada 10 a 14 días; un volumen de 1,200,000 unidades por cada 10 a 21 días

| | |
|---|---|
| 剂型、规格<br>Formulaciones y especificaciones | 注射用青霉素钠：每支（瓶）0.24g（40万U）、0.48g（80万U）或0.6g（100万U）。注射用青霉素钾：每支0.25g（40万U）。注射用普鲁卡因青霉素：每瓶40万U者，含普鲁卡因青霉素30万U及青霉素钾盐或钠盐10万U；每瓶80万U者其含量加倍。既有长效，又有速效作用。每次肌内注射40万～80万U，一日1次。注射用苄星青霉素（长效青霉素，长效西林）：每瓶120万U，肌内注射。<br><br>Penicilina sódica para inyección: 0.24g(400000 unidades) cada dosis(botella), 0.48g(800000 unidades) o 0.6g(1000000 unidades). Penicilina de potasio para inyección: 0.25g(400000 unidades) cada dosis(botella). Penicilina G procaína para inyección: la botella de 400000 unidades contiene 300000 unidades de penicilina G procaína y 100000 unidades de penicilina sódica o de potasio; la botella de 800000 unidades contiene la dosis duplicada. No sólo tiene efecto duraderos sino también efecto inmediatos. Cada vez se inyectan por vía intramuscular 400000 ～ 800000 unidades, 1 vez al día. Benzatina para inyección (penicilina o amoxicilina de efecto duradero): cada botella contiene 1200000 unidades, por vía intramuscular. |
| 药品名称 Drug Names | 青霉素 V　Fenoximetilpenicilina |
| 适应证<br>Indicaciones | 青霉素用于敏感菌所致的急性感染，如：菌血症、败血症、猩红热、丹毒、肺炎、脓胸、扁桃体炎、中耳炎、蜂窝织炎、疖、痈、急性乳腺炎、心内膜炎、骨髓炎、流行性脑膜炎（流脑）、钩端螺旋体病（对本病早期疗效较好），奋森咽峡炎、创伤感染、回归热、气性坏疽、炭疽、淋病、放线菌病等。治疗破伤风、白喉宜与相应的抗毒素联用。<br><br>普鲁卡因青霉素吸收缓慢，肌内注射30万U，血药浓度峰值约2U/ml，24小时仍可测得。适用于梅毒和一些敏感菌所致的慢性感染。<br><br>苄星青霉素吸收极缓慢，血药浓度低，适用于需长期使用青霉素预防的患者，如慢性风湿性心脏病患者。<br><br>Se usa para infecciones agudas producidas por gérmenes sensibles, tales como: septicemia, bacteriemia, escarlatina, erisipela, neumonía, empireuma, amigdalitis, otitis media, celulitis, forúnculos, despreciable, mastitis aguda, endocarditis, osteomielitis, la epidemia de meningitis (EEM), leptospirosis (la eficacia es mejor en la etapa temprana), vincent angina de pecho, infección de la herida, fiebre recurrente, gangrena gaseosa, el ántrax, gonorrea y la actinomicosis.Para tratar el tétanos y la difteria se debe usar en combinación con la correspondiente antitoxina.<br><br>La penicilina procaína se absorbe lentamente en la circulación. Tras la administración de una inyección intramuscular de 300 mil unidades, la concentración plasmática máxima se mantiene en aproximadamente 2 unidades/ml y al cabo de 24 horas puede ser medido.Se usa para el tratamiento de la sífilis e infecciones crónicas causadas por cepas sensibles.<br><br>La absorción de benzatina penicilina es muy lenta, con una baja concentración plasmática, aplicable a los pacientes con la necesidad de la penicilina como uso de prevención a largo plazo, por ejemplo,pacientes con Cardiopatía Reumática Crónica. |

**续　表**

| 用法、用量<br>Administración y dosis | 口服。成人：125～500mg（20万～80万U）/次，每6～8小时1次。儿童：每日15～50mg/kg，分3～6次服用。<br><br>Se toma por vía oral. Adulto: 125～500 mg (200,000-800,000 unidades)/vez, cada 6 a 8 horas. Niños: todos los días 15～50mg/kg, divididos en 3～6 dosis. |
|---|---|
| 剂型、规格<br>Formulaciones y especificaciones | 片剂、胶囊剂：每片或颗粒125mg（20万U）；250mg（40万U）；500mg（80万U）。颗粒剂或口服干糖浆。<br><br>Una tableta o cápsula: 125mg (200000 unidades); 250mg(400000 unidades); 500mg(800000 unidades).<br>También hay gránulos o jarabe seco oral. |

| 药品名称 Drug Names | 苯唑西林钠 Oxacilina sódica |
|---|---|
| 适应证<br>Indicaciones | 本品主要用于产酶的金黄色葡萄球菌和表皮葡萄球菌的周围感染，包括内脏、皮肤和软组织等部位的感染，但对耐甲氧西林金黄色葡萄球菌（MSRA）感染无效。对中枢感染不适用。<br><br>Se usa principalmente para infecciones periféricas por los estafilococos dorados que producen enzimas y staphylococcus epidermidis, incluyendo infecciones viscerales, de la piel y de tejidos blandos entre otras partes.Para staphylococcus aureus resistente a la meticilina（infección MRSA）no es válida. A las infecciones del sistema nervioso central, no se aplica. |
| 用法、用量<br>Administración y dosis | 静脉滴注：1次1～2g，必要时可用到3g，溶于100ml输液内滴注0.5～1小时，一日3～4次。小儿每日用量50～100mg/kg，分次给予。肌内注射：一次1g，一日3～4次。口服、肌内注射均较少用。肾功能轻中度不足者可按正常用量，重度不足者应适当减量。<br><br>Infusión intravenosa：1～2 g/vez, si es necesario, se puede utilizar 3g, disuelto en 100 ml de la infusión dentro de 0, 5～1h, 3 a 4 veces al día. La dosis diaria para niños es de 50～100mg/kg, dada en varias veces. Inyección intramuscular：1g cada vez, 3～4 veces al día. Se usa menos por vía oral o inyección intramuscular. A los pacientes con leve a moderada insuficiencia renal se los puede aolicar dosis normal, a los con deficiencias graves se debe reducir la dosis oportunamente. |
| 剂型、规格<br>Formulaciones y especificaciones | 注射用苯唑西林钠：每瓶0.5g；1g（效价）。<br>Oxacilina sódica para inyección：0.5g/botella；1g（potencia）. |

| 药品名称 Drug Names | 氯唑西林钠 Cloxacilina sódica |
|---|---|
| 适应证<br>Indicaciones | 主要用于产酶金黄色葡萄球菌或不产酶葡萄球菌所致的败血症、肺炎、心内膜炎、骨髓炎或皮肤软组织感染等。但对耐甲氧西林金黄色葡萄球菌（MSRA）感染无效。<br><br>Se usa principalmente para septicemia, neumonía, endocarditis, osteomielitis e infecciones de tejidos blandos en la piel causados por los estafilococos dorados que producen enzimas y staphylococcus que no producen enzimas.Para staphylococcus aureus resistente a la meticilina (infección MRSA) no es válida. |
| 用法、用量<br>Administración y dosis | 肌内注射：1次0.5～1g，一日3～4次。静脉滴注：一次1～2g，溶于100ml输液中，滴注0.5～1小时，一日3～4次。小儿每日用量30～50mg/kg，分次给予。口服剂量：每次0.25～0.5g，一日4次，空腹服用。<br><br>Inyección intramuscular: 0.5～1g cada vez, 3～4 veces al día. Infusión intravenosa: 1～2 g/vez, disuelto en 100 ml de la infusión dentro de 0.5～1h, 3 a 4 veces al día. La dosis diaria para niños es de 30～50mg/kg, dada en varias veces. Dosis por vía oral: 0.25～0.5g cada vez, 4 veces al día, en un estomago vacío. |
| 剂型、规格<br>Formulaciones y especificaciones | 注射用氯唑西林钠：每瓶0.5g（效价）。<br>胶囊剂：每胶囊0.125g；0.25g；0.5g。颗粒剂：50mg。<br>Cloxacilina sódica para inyección: 0.5g/botella(potencia).<br>Una cápsula: 0.125g;0.25g;0.5g. Un gránulo: 50mg. |

**续 表**

| 药品名称 Drug Names | 氟氯西林 Flucloxacilina |
|---|---|
| 适应证<br>Indicaciones | 主要应用于葡萄球菌所致的各种周围感染，但对耐甲氧西林金黄色葡萄球菌（MSRA）感染无效。<br><br>Se usa principalmente para todo tipo de infecciones periféricas debido a staphylococcus. Para staphylococcus aureus resistente a la meticilina (infección MRSA) no es válida. |
| 用法、用量<br>Administración y dosis | 口服（用游离酸）：常用量为每次 250mg，每日 3 次；重症用量为每次 500mg，一日 4 次，于食前 0.5 ～ 1 小时空腹服用。肌内注射：常用量为每次 250mg，一日 3 次；重症用量为每次 500mg，一日 4 次。静脉注射：每次 500mg，一日 4 次，将药物溶于 10 ～ 20ml 注射用水或葡萄糖溶液中使用，每 4 ～ 6 小时 1 次。一日量不超过 8g。<br>儿童：2 岁以下按成人量的 1/4；2 ～ 10 岁按成人量的 1/2，根据体重适当调整。也可按照每日 25 ～ 50mg/kg，分次给予。<br><br>Por vía oral(con el ácido libre): dosis normal es de 250 mg cada vez, 3 veces al día; dosis para síntomas severos es de 500 mg cada vez, 4 veces al día, se toma 0,5 a 1 hora antes de comer con el estómago vacío. Inyección intramuscular: dosis normal es de 250 mg cada vez, 3 veces al día; dosis para síntomas severos es de 500 mg cada vez, 4 veces al día. Infusión intravenosa: 500 mg cada vez, 4 veces al día, disuelto en 10 ～ 20 ml de agua para inyección o infusión de glucosa, 4 ～ 6h cada vez, la dosis diaria no debe sobrepasar 8g.<br>Niños: menos de 2 años, 1/4 la dosis de adultos; 2 a 10 años, 1/2 la dosis de adultos, ajustada oportunamente de acuerdo con el peso. También se puede adoptar la dosis diaria de 25 ～ 50mg/kg, dada en varias veces. |
| 剂型、规格<br>Formulaciones y especificaciones | 片剂（游离酸）：每片 125mg。<br>注射用氟氯西林钠：每瓶 500mg；1000mg。<br>Una tableta(ácidos libres): 125mg.<br>Flucloxacilina para inyección: 500mg/botella; 1000mg. |
| 药品名称 Drug Names | 氨苄西林 Ampicilina |
| 适应证<br>Indicaciones | 本品主要用于敏感菌所致的泌尿系统、呼吸系统、胆道、肠道感染以及脑膜炎、心内膜炎等。<br>Se usa principalmente para infecciones en el sistema urinario, en el sistema respiratorio, en el tracto biliar, en el intestino producidas debido a gérmenes sensibles así como en el tratamiento de la meningitis y la endocarditis. |
| 用法、用量<br>Administración y dosis | 口服：一日 50 ～ 100mg/kg，分成 4 次空腹服用；儿童一日 50 ～ 100mg/kg，分成 4 次。肌内注射：一次 0.5 ～ 1g，一日 4 次；儿童一日 50 ～ 100mg/kg，分成 4 次。静脉滴注：一次 1 ～ 2g，必要时可用到 3g，溶于 100ml 溶液中，滴注 0.5 ～ 1 小时，一日 2 ～ 4 次，必要时每 4 小时 1 次；儿童一日 100 ～ 150mg/kg，分 4 次给予。<br><br>Por vía oral: 50 ～ 100mg/kg al día, 4 veces al día con el estómago vacío; niños: 50 ～ 100mg/kg al día, en 4 veces. Inyección intramuscular: 0.5 ～ 1g cada vez, 4 veces al día; niños: 50 ～ 100mg/kg al día, en 4 veces. Infusión intravenosa: 1 ～ 2g cada vez, si es necesario se puede usar 3g, disuelto en 100 ml de agua para inyección, 0.5 ～ 1h cada vez, 2 ～ 4 veces al día, si es necesario se puede usar una vez cada 4 horas; niños: 100 ～ 150mg/kg al día, dada en 4 veces. |
| 剂型、规格<br>Formulaciones y especificaciones | 胶囊剂：每粒 0.25g。注射用氨苄西林钠：每瓶 0.5g；1.0g。<br>Una cápsula：0.25g. Ampicilina para inyección：0.5g/botella；1.0g. |
| 药品名称 Drug Names | 阿莫西林 Amoxicilina |
| 适应证<br>Indicaciones | 常用于敏感菌所致的呼吸道、尿路和胆道感染及伤寒等。<br>Se usa normalmente para infecciones respiratorias, urinarias y del tracto biliar causadas por gérmenes sensibles así como en el tratamiento de la tifoidea entre otros. |
| 用法、用量<br>Administración y dosis | 口服：成人每日 1 ～ 4g，分 3 ～ 4 次服。儿童每日 50 ～ 100mg/kg，分 3 ～ 4 次服。肾功能严重不足者，应延长用药间隔时间；肾小球率过滤（GFR）为 10 ～ 15ml/min 者，8 ～ 12 小时给药 1 次；< 10ml/min 者，12 ～ 16 小时给药 1 次。<br><br>Por vía oral: adultos 1 ～ 4 g al día, en 3 a 4 veces. Niños 50 ～ 100mg/kg al día en 3 a 4 veces. Los con deficiencia renal grave deben ampliarse el intervalo de dosificación; a los con tasa de filtración glomerular (TFG) de 10 ～ 15ml/min, administran cada 8 a 12 horas; < a los de 10ml/min administran cada 12 a 16 horas. |

续　表

| 剂型、规格<br>Formulaciones y especificaciones | 片剂（胶囊）：每片（粒）0.125g；0.25g（效价）。<br>Una tableta(cápsula): 0.125g; 0.25g (potencia). |
|---|---|
| 药品名称 Drug Names | 哌拉西林钠 Piperacilina sódica |
| 适应证<br>Indicaciones | 临床上用于上述敏感菌中所引起的感染（对中枢感染疗效不确切）。<br>En la clínica se usa para infecciones arriba-mencionadas debido a gérmenes sensibles(eficacia para infección en el sistema nervioso central inexacta). |
| 用法、用量<br>Administración y dosis | 尿路感染，一次 1g，一日 4 次，肌内注射或静脉注射。其他部位（呼吸道、腹腔、胆道等）感染：一日 4～12g，分 3～4 次静脉注射或静脉滴注。严重感染一日可用 10～24g。<br>Infección urinaria, 1g cada vez, 4 veces al día por inyección intramuscular o por vía intravenosa. Infecciones de otras partes(tracto respiratorio, abdomen, tracto biliar, etc.) 4 ～ 12g al día, en 3 a 4 veces por vía intravenosa o infusión intravenosa. Para infecciones graves se puede usar hasta 10 ～ 24g al día. |
| 剂型、规格<br>Formulaciones y especificaciones | 注射用哌拉西林钠：每瓶 0.5g；1.0g（效价）。<br>Piperacilina sódica para inyección: 0.5g/botella; 1.0g(potencia). |
| 药品名称 Drug Names | 替卡西林 Ticarcilina |
| 适应证<br>Indicaciones | 主要用于革兰阴性菌感染，包括变形杆菌、大肠埃希菌、肠杆菌属、淋球菌、流感杆菌等所致全身感染，对尿路感染的效果好。对于铜绿假单胞菌感染，常需与氨基糖苷类抗生素联合应用。本品不耐酶，对 MRSA 也无效。<br>Se usa principalmente para infecciones causadas por bacterias Gram - negativas,tales como infecciones sistémicas debido a proteus, E. coli, enterobacter, neisseria gonorrhoeae y haemophilus influenzae. Cura bien a la infección del tracto urinario. Para la infección por pseudomonas aeruginosa, se suele usar en combinación con antibióticos aminoglucósidos. No es resistente a la enzima, tampoco eficaz contra MRSA. |
| 用法、用量<br>Administración y dosis | 成人一日 200～300mg/kg，分次给予或一次 3g，根据病情，每 3、4 或 6 小时 1 次。按每 1g 药物用 4ml 溶剂溶解后缓缓静脉注射或加入适量溶剂中静脉滴注 0.5～1 小时。泌尿系统感染可肌内注射给药，一次 1g，一日 4 次，用 0.25%～0.5% 利多卡因注射液 2～3ml 溶解后深部肌内注射。儿童一日为 200～300mg/kg。婴儿一日为 225mg/kg，7 日龄以下婴儿则一日 150mg/kg，均分 3 次给予。<br>Adultos 200 ～ 300mg/kg al día, dado en varias veces o 3g cada vez, dado cada 3, 4 o 6 horas una vez de acuerdo la enfermedad. Disuelve 1 g por 4 ml de disolvente para inyectar lentamente por vía intravenosa o agrega disolvente para tener infusión intravenosa de 0,5 a 1 hora. Para infección urinaria se puede administrar por vía intramuscular 1g cada vez, 4 veces al día, disuelto con 2 ~ 3 ml de solución de lidocaína 0.25% ～ 0.5% para inyección intramuscular profunda.Para niños 200 ～ 300mg/kg al día. Para bebés 225mg/kg al día, y los bebés menores de 7 días de edad, 150mg/kg al día, dado en tres veces. |
| 剂型、规格<br>Formulaciones y especificaciones | 注射用替卡西林钠：每瓶 1g；3g；6g（效价）。<br>Ticarcilina para inyección: 1g;3g;6g(potencia) cada botella. |
| 药品名称 Drug Names | 美洛西林钠 Mezlocilina sódica |
| 适应证<br>Indicaciones | 本品主要用于一些革兰阴性病原菌，如假单胞菌、克雷伯菌、肠杆菌属、沙雷菌、变形杆菌、大肠埃希菌、嗜血杆菌、以及拟杆菌和其他一些厌氧菌（包括革兰阳性的粪链球菌）所致的下呼吸道、腹腔、胆道、尿路、妇科、皮肤及软组织部位感染以及败血症。<br>Se usa principalmente para infecciones causadas por bacterias Gram - negativas, tales como infecciones del tracto inferior respiratorio, abdominal, vías biliares, vías urinarias, ginecológicas, la piel y tejidos blandos así como septicemia entre otros debido a pseudomonas, klebsiella, enterobacter, serratia, proteus, E. coli, haemophilus, bacteroides y otras bacterias anaerobias (incluyendo estreptococos fecales Gram-positivas). |

**续　表**

| | |
|---|---|
| 用法、用量<br>Administración y dosis | 用氯化钠液、葡萄糖液或乳酸钠林格液溶解后静脉注射或静脉滴注，也可肌内注射给药。成人一般感染每日 150 ～ 200mg/kg，或每次 2 ～ 3g，每 6 小时 1 次；重症感染每日 200 ～ 300mg/kg，或每次 3g，每 4 小时 1 次；极重感染可用到每日 24g 分 6 次用；淋球菌尿道炎，1 ～ 2g，只用 1 次，用前 0.5 小时服用丙磺舒 1g。新生儿用量：≤ 7 日龄者，每日 150mg/kg 或 75mg/kg，每 12 小时 1 次。> 7 日龄者，根据体重不同可按每日 225 ～ 300mg/kg，或每次 75mg/kg，一日 3 ～ 4 次。肾功能受损者：肌酐清除率 > 30ml/min 者，可按正常用量；10 ～ 30ml/min 者，按疾病轻重用每次 1.5 ～ 3g，每 8 小时一次；< 10ml/min 者，用 1.5g，每 8 小时 1 次，重症可用到 2g，每 8 小时 1 次。手术预防感染给药：每次 4g，与术前 1 小时及术后 6 ～ 12 小时各给药 1 次。<br><br>Se disuelve en la solución de cloruro sódico, solución de glucosa o solución de lactato de Ringer para inyectar por vía intravenosa o por infusión intravenosa, y también puede administrarse por vía intramuscular. Infecciones generales de adultos 150 ～ 200mg/kg al día o 2 ～ 3g una vez, cada 6 horas; infecciones graves 200 ～ 300mg/kg al día o 3g cada vez, cada 4 horas;infecciones pesadas, hasta 24g al día en 6 veces; uretritis gonocócica, 1 ～ 2g, sólo una vez, y se debe tomar 1g de probenecid media hora antes de usarlo. Dosis para recién nacidos: para los de o menos de 7 días de edad, 150mg/kg o 75mg/kg al día, cada 12 horas. Para los mayores de 7 días de edad, 225 ～ 300mg/kg al día, 3 o 4 veces al día. Los con insuficiencia renal: aclaramiento de creatinina > 30ml/min, la dosis normal; 10 ～ 30ml/min, 1.5 ～ 3g cada vez, cada 8 horas, según la gravedad; < 10ml/min, 1.5g, cada 8 horas, si se trata de síntomas graves, se usa hasta 2g, cada 8 horas. Administración para prevenir infección quirúrgica: 4g cada vez, una hora antes y 6 ～ 12 horas después de la operación una vez respectivamente. |
| 剂型、规格<br>Formulaciones y especificaciones | 粉针剂：每瓶 1g。<br>Inyección de polvo: 1g/botella. |

| 药品名称 Drug Names | 阿洛西林钠 Azlocilina sódica |
|---|---|
| 适应证<br>Indicaciones | 主要用于铜绿假单胞菌与其他革兰阴性菌所致的系统感染，如败血症、脑膜炎、肺炎及尿路和软组织感染。必要时可与氨基糖苷类联合以加强抗铜绿假单胞菌的作用。<br><br>Se usa principalmente para infecciones sistemáticas causadas por pseudomonas aeruginosa y bacterias Gram - negativas tales como septicemia, meningitis, neumonía, infección del tracto urinario y tejidos blandos. Si es necesario, se puede usar en combinación con el aminoglucósido para fortalecer el efecto de anti-pseudomonas aeruginosa. |
| 用法、用量<br>Administración y dosis | 尿路感染：每日 50 ～ 100mg/kg；重症感染，成人每日 200 ～ 250mg/kg，儿童每日 50 ～ 150mg/kg。以上量分 4 次，静脉注射或静脉滴注，也可肌内注射给予。可用氯化钠注射液、葡萄糖液或乳酸钠林格液溶解后给予，也可加入墨菲管中，随输液进入（但要掌握速度，不宜过快）。<br><br>Infección urinaria, 50 ～ 100mg/kg al día; infecciones graves, 200 ～ 250mg/kg al día para adultos y 50 ～ 150mg/kg al día para niños. Se administra en 4 veces, por vía intravenosa o infusión intravenosa, también por vía intramuscular. Puede disolverse en inyección de cloruro sódico, solución de glucosa o lactato de Ringer para dar, o se puede añadir al tubo Murphy con la infusión (pero se debe controlar la velocidad, no demasiado rápida). |
| 剂型、规格<br>Formulaciones y especificaciones | 粉针剂：每支 2g；3g；4g。<br>Una inyección de polvo: 2g;3g;4g. |

| 药品名称 Drug Names | 磺苄西林钠 Sulbenicilina sódica |
|---|---|
| 适应证<br>Indicaciones | 临床上用于敏感的铜绿假单胞菌、某些变形杆菌属及其他敏感革兰阴性菌所致肺炎、尿路感染、复杂性皮肤软组织感染和败血症等。对本品敏感菌所致腹腔感染、盆腔感染宜与抗厌氧菌药物联合应用。<br><br>En clínica se usa principalmente para neumonía, infecciones urinarias, infecciones complicadas de la piel y tejidos blandos así como septicemia entre otros causados por pseudomonas aeruginosa sensibles, determinados proteus y otras bacterias gram-negativas sensibles. En cuanto a las infecciones abdominales y pélvicas causadas por cepas sensibles se debe usar drogas anti-anaerobias en combinación. |

**续　表**

| 用法、用量<br>Administración y dosis | 中度感染，成人一日 8g，重症感染或铜绿假单胞菌感染时剂量需增至一日 20g，分 4 次静脉滴注或可静脉注射；儿童根据病情每日剂量按体重 80 ～ 300mg/kg，分 4 次给药。<br><br>Infecciones moderadas, para adultos 8g al día, infecciones graves o infecciones por pseudomonas aeruginosa, la dosis diaria puede ser hasta 20g, en 4 veces, por infusión intravenosa o por vía intravenosa; para niños la dosis diaria puede ser entre 80 y 300mg/kg variándose según la gravedad y el peso, administrada en 4 veces. |
|---|---|
| 剂型、规格<br>Formulaciones y especificaciones | 注射用磺苄西林钠：每瓶 1.0g；2g；4g。<br>Sulbenicilina sódica para inyección: 1.0g；2g；4g cada botella. |
| 药品名称 Drug Names | 阿帕西林钠 Apalcilina sódica |
| 适应证<br>Indicaciones | 临床可用于敏感革兰阳性或阴性菌感染，如呼吸道、尿路、胆道、妇科感染，也可用于术后感染和五官科感染的治疗。<br><br>En clínica se puede usar para infecciones bacterianas gram-positivos o negativos sensibles, tales como infecciones respiratorias, del tracto urinario, tracto biliar y ginecológicas.También se usa para el tratamiento de infección postoperatoria y infecciones de los cinco órganos sensoriales. |
| 用法、用量<br>Administración y dosis | 成人 1 次 2 ～ 3g，一日 3 次，肌内或静脉给药。10 岁以下儿童，一日 60 ～ 220mg/kg，分 3 ～ 4 次静脉滴注。10 岁以上儿童剂量同成人。<br><br>Adultos 2 ～ 3g una vez, 3 veces al día, por vía intramuscular o intravenosa. Para niños menores de 10 años de edad, 60 ～ 220mg/kg al día, 3 ～ 4 veces de infusión intravenosa. Para niños mayores de 10 años de edad la dosis es igual que adultos. |
| 剂型、规格<br>Formulaciones y especificaciones | 注射用阿帕西林钠：每瓶 1g；3g。<br>Apalcilina sódica para inyección: 1g；3g cada botella. |

1.2　头孢菌素类 Cefalosporinas

| 药品名称 Drug Names | 头孢氨苄 Cefalexina |
|---|---|
| 适应证<br>Indicaciones | 用于敏感菌所致的呼吸道、泌尿道、皮肤和软组织、生殖器官（包括前列腺）等部位的感染，也常用于中耳炎。<br><br>Se usa para infecciones de vías respiratorias, de tracto urinario, la piel y tejidos blandos, órganos reproductivos (incluyendo la próstata) entre otras partes causadas por cepas susceptibles. También se utiliza comúnmente en la otitis media. |
| 用法、用量<br>Administración y dosis | 成人：一日 1 ～ 2g，分 3 ～ 4 次服用，空腹服用。小儿：一日 25 ～ 50mg/kg，分 3 ～ 4 次服用。<br>Adultos: 1 ～ 2g al día en 3 a 4 veces con estómago vacío. Niños: 25 ～ 50mg/kg al día en 3 a 4 veces. |
| 剂型、规格<br>Formulaciones y especificaciones | 片（胶囊）剂：每片（粒）0.125g；0.25g。<br>颗粒剂：1g 含药 50mg。<br>Una tableta(cápsula): 0.125g; 0.25g.<br>Un gránulo: cada 1g contiene 50mg del medicamento. |
| 药品名称 Drug Names | 头孢唑林钠 Cefazolina sódica |
| 适应证<br>Indicaciones | 用于敏感菌所致的呼吸道、泌尿生殖系统、皮肤软组织、骨和关节、胆道等感染，也可用于心内膜炎、败血症、咽和耳部感染。<br><br>Se usa para infecciones respiratoria, genitourinaria, de la piel y tejidos blandos, de huesos y articulaciones, de tracto biliar causadas por cepas sensibles, también se puede utilizar para endocarditis, septicemia, infecciones de garganta y oído. |
| 用法、用量<br>Administración y dosis | 肌内或静脉注射，1 次 0.5 ～ 1g，一日 3 ～ 4 次。革兰阳性菌所致轻度感染一日 0.5g，一日 2 ～ 3 次；中度或重症感染：1 次 0.5 ～ 1g，一日 3 ～ 4 次；极重感染：1 次 1 ～ 1.5g，一日 4 次。泌尿系感染：1 次 1g，一日 2 次。儿童一日量为：20 ～ 40mg/kg，分 3 ～ 4 次给药；重症可用到一日 100mg/kg。新生儿 1 次不超过 20mg/kg，一日 2 次。 |

| | |
|---|---|
| | Inyección intramuscular o intravenosa, 0.5～1g una vez, entre 3 y 4 veces al día. Para infecciones bacterianas gram-positivos 0.5g al día, entre 2 y 3 veces; infecciones moderadas o graves: cada toma de 0.5～1g, 3～4 tomas al día; infecciones pesadas: cada toma de 1～1.5g, 4 tomas al día. Infección urinaria: cada toma de 1g, 2 tomas al día. La dosis diaria para niños: 20～40mg/kg, entre 3 y 4 dosis divididas; en caso de síntomas grave se puede utilizar dosis diaria de 100mg/kg. Recién nacidos: cada toma no sobrepasa 20mg/kg, 2 tomas al día. |
| 剂型、规格 Formulaciones y especificaciones | 注射用头孢唑林钠：每瓶 0.5g；1g；2g。<br>Cefazolina sódica para inyección: 0.5g; 1g; 2g cada botella. |
| 药品名称 Drug Names | 头孢羟氨苄 Cefadroxilo |
| 适应证 Indicaciones | 用于呼吸道、泌尿道、咽部、皮肤等部位敏感菌感染。<br>Se usa para infecciones del tracto respiratorio, tracto urinario, garganta, la piel y otras partes causadas por cepas susceptibles. |
| 用法、用量 Administración y dosis | 成人平均用量：一日 1～2g，分 2～3 次口服，泌尿道感染时，也可 1 次服下。小儿一日量 50mg/kg，分 2 次服用。肾功能不全者，首次服 1g，以后按肌酐清除率制订给药方案：肌酐清除率为 25～50ml/min 者，每 12 小时服 0.5g；10～25ml/min 者，每 24 小时服 0.5g；< 10ml/min 者，每 36 小时服 0.5g。<br>Dosis de promedio de los adultos: 1～2g al día, en 2～3 tomas, en caso de infección urinaria, se toma por una vez. Dosis diaria de niños es 50mg/kg, dividida en dos tomas. Los con insuficiencia renal: toman 1g la primera dosis, y luego administran según el aclaramiento de creatinina: los de 25～50ml/min, 0.5g cada 12 horas; los de 10～25ml/min, 0.5g cada 24 horas; los < 10ml/min, 0.5g cada 36 horas. |
| 剂型、规格 Formulaciones y especificaciones | 片剂（胶囊剂）：每片（粒）0.125g；0.25g。<br>Una tableta(cápsula): 0.125g；0.25g. |
| 药品名称 Drug Names | 头孢拉定 Cefradina |
| 适应证 Indicaciones | 用于呼吸道、泌尿道、咽部、皮肤等部位的敏感菌感染，注射剂也可用于败血症和骨感染。<br>Se usa para infecciones del tracto respiratorio, tracto urinario, garganta, la piel y otras partes causadas por cepas susceptibles.La inyección también se puede usar en el tratamiento de septicemia e infecciones óseas. |
| 用法、用量 Administración y dosis | 口服：成人一日 1～2g，分 3～4 次服用。小儿每日 25～50mg/kg，分 3～4 次服用。肌内注射、静脉注射或静脉滴注：成人一日 2～4g，分 4 次注射。小儿每日 50～100mg/kg，分 4 次注射。肾功能不全者按患者肌酐清除率制订给药方案：肌酐清除率为 > 20ml/min 者，每 6 小时服 500mg；15～20ml/min 者，每 6 小时服 250mg；< 15ml/min 者，每 12 小时服 250mg。<br>Dosis por vía oral: adultos: 1～2g al día, en 3～4 tomas. Dosis diaria de niños es 25～50mg/kg, dividida en 3～4 tomas. Administración por vía intramuscular, intravenosa o por infusión intravenosa, adultos: 2～4g al día, en 4 inyecciones. Niños: 50～100mg/kg al día, en 4 inyecciones. Los con insuficiencia renal: administran según el aclaramiento de creatinina: los > 20ml/min, 500mg cada 6 horas; los de 15～20ml/min, 250mg cada 6 horas; los < 15ml/min, 250mg cada 12 horas. |
| 剂型、规格 Formulaciones y especificaciones | 胶囊剂：每粒 0.25g；0.5g。干混悬剂：0.125g；0.25g。注射用头孢拉定（添加碳酸钠）：每瓶 0.5g；1g。注射用头孢拉定 A（添加精氨酸）：每瓶 0.5g；1g。<br>Una cápsula: 0.25g; 0.5g. Una suspensión: 0.125g; 0.25g. Cefradina para inyección(agregado de carbonato de sodio): 0.5g; 1g cada botella. Cefradina A para inyección(agregado de arginina): 0.5g; 1g cada botella. |
| 药品名称 Drug Names | 头孢呋辛钠 Cefuroxima sódica |
| 适应证 Indicaciones | 临床应用于敏感的革兰阴性菌所致的下呼吸道、泌尿系、皮肤和软组织、骨和关节、女性生殖器等部位的感染。对败血症、脑膜炎也有效。<br>En clínica se usa para infecciones del tracto respiratorio inferior, tracto urinario, la piel y tejidos blandos, huesos y articulaciones, genitales femeninas entre otras partes causdas por bacterias negativas Glenn sensible. También es eficaz para septicemia y meningitis. |

**续　表**

| 用法、用量<br>Administración y dosis | 肌内注射或静脉注射，成人：1 次 750 ～ 1500mg，一日 3 次；对严重感染，可按 1 次 1500mg，一日 4 次。应用于脑膜炎，一日剂量在 9g 以下。儿童：平均一日量为 60mg/kg，严重感染可用到 100mg/kg，分 3 ～ 4 次给予。肾功能不全者按患者肌酐清除率制订给药方案：肌酐清除率为 > 20ml/min 者，一日 3 次，每次 0.75 ～ 1.5g；10 ～ 20ml/min 者，每次 0.75g，一日 2 次；< 10ml/min 者，每次 0.75g，一日 1 次。肌内注射：1 次用 0.75g，加注射用水 3ml，振摇使成混悬液，用粗针头做深部肌内注射。静脉给药：每 0.75g 本品，用注射用水约 10ml，使其溶解成澄明溶液，缓慢静脉注射或加到莫菲管中随输液滴入。<br><br>Administración por vía intramuscular o intravenosa, adultos: 3 inyecciones al día, 750 ～ 1500mg cada una; infecciones graves, 4 inyecciones al día, 1500mg cada una. Si se aplica a meningitis, la dosis diaria debe ser inferior a 9g. Niños: la dosis diaria de promedio es 60mg/kg, infecciones graves, puede se hasta 100mg/kg, en 3 ～ 4 inyecciones. Los con insuficiencia renal: administran según el aclaramiento de creatinina: los > 20ml/min, 3 inyecciones al día, 0.75 ～ 1.5g cada una; los de 10 ～ 20ml/min, 250mg cada 6 horas; los < 10ml/min, 1 inyección al día, 0.75g cada una. Inyección intramuscular: 0.75g cada inyección, agregando 3ml de agua para disolverlo en solución transparente, por inyección intravenosa lenta o Murphy con el tubo de goteo de infusión. |
|---|---|
| 剂型、规格<br>Formulaciones y especificaciones | 注射用头孢呋辛钠：每瓶 0.75g；1.5g。<br>Cefuroxima sódica para inyección: 0.75g；1.5g cada botella. |

| 药品名称 Drug Names | 头孢呋辛酯 Cefuroxima axetilo |
|---|---|
| 适应证<br>Indicaciones | 临床用于敏感菌所致的上、下呼吸道及泌尿系统、皮肤和软组织等部位的感染。<br>En clínica se usa para infecciones del tracto respiratorio superior e inferior y tracto urinario, la piel y tejidos blandos entre otras partes causadas por cepas susceptibles. |
| 用法、用量<br>Administración y dosis | 成人每次口服 250mg，一日 2 次，重症可每次 500mg。儿童每次 125mg，一日 2 次。一般疗程为 7 日。<br>Adultos: dos tomas al día, 250mg cada una, infecciones graves, puede ser hasta 500mg cada toma. Niños: dos tomas al día, 125mg cada una. Ciclo general de tratamiento es de 7 días. |
| 剂型、规格<br>Formulaciones y especificaciones | 片剂（薄膜衣片）：每片 125mg；250mg。<br>Una tableta(recubierta con película): 125mg；250mg. |

| 药品名称 Drug Names | 头孢克洛 Cefaclor |
|---|---|
| 适应证<br>Indicaciones | 用于上述敏感菌所致的呼吸道、泌尿道和皮肤、软组织感染，以及中耳炎等。<br>Se usa para infecciones del tracto respiratorio, tracto urinario, la piel, tejidos blandos y la otitis media causadas por cepas susceptibles. |
| 用法、用量<br>Administración y dosis | 成人口服常用量为 250mg，每 8 小时 1 次。重病或微生物敏感性较差时，剂量可加倍，但一日量不可超过 4g。儿童：一日口服剂量为 20mg/kg，分 3 次（每 8 小时 1 次）；重症可按一日 40mg/kg 给予，但一日量不超过 1g。<br>La dosis habitual por vía oral para adultos es de 250mg, cada 8 horas. En caso de enfermedad grave o sensibilidad microbiana pobre, la dosis puede duplicarse, pero la dosis diaria no debe sobrepasar 4g. Niños: la dosis diaria por vía oral es de 20mg/kg, en 3 tomas(cada 8 horas); en caso de enfermedad grave, la administración diaria puede ser hasta 40mg/kg, pero la dosis diaria no sobrepasa 1g. |
| 剂型、规格<br>Formulaciones y especificaciones | 胶囊剂（片剂）：每粒（片）0.125g；0.25g。干混悬剂：0.125g；1.5g。<br>Una cápsula（tableta）：0.125g；0.25g. Una suspensión：0.125g；1.5g. |

| 药品名称 Drug Names | 头孢噻肟钠 Cefotaxima sódica |
|---|---|
| 适应证<br>Indicaciones | 用于敏感菌所致的呼吸道、泌尿道、骨和关节、皮肤和软组织、腹腔、胆道、消化道、五官、生殖器等部位的感染，对烧伤、外伤引起的感染以及败血症、中枢感染也有效。<br>Se usa para infecciones del tracto respiratorio, tracto urinario, huesos y articulaciones, la piel, tejidos blandos, abdominal, tracto biliar, tracto digestivo, los cinco órganos sensoriales, genitales y otras partes causadas por cepas sensibles. También es eficaz para las infecciones causadas por quemaduras y traumatismos, eficaz para septicemia y infecciones del sistema nervioso central. |

**续 表**

| 用法、用量<br>Administración y dosis | 临用前，加灭菌注射用水使溶解，溶解后立即使用。成人：肌内或静脉注射，1 次 0.5 ～ 1g，一日 2 ～ 4 次。一般感染用 2g/d，分成 2 次肌内注射或静脉注射；中等或较重感染 3 ～ 6g/d，分为 3 次肌内注射或静脉注射；败血症等 6 ～ 8g/d，分为 3 ～ 4 次静脉给药，极重感染一日不超过 12g，分为 6 次静脉给药；淋病用 1g 肌内注射（单次给药已足）。静脉滴注，2 ～ 3g/d。小儿：肌内注射或静脉注射一日量为 50 ～ 100mg/kg，分成 2 ～ 3 次给予。婴幼儿不能肌内注射。<br><br>Antes del uso, se debe agregar agua estéril de inyección para disolverlo y luego utilizarlo de inmediato. Adultos: por vía intramuscular o intravenosa, 2 ～ 4 inyecciones al día, 0.5 ～ 1g cada una. Infecciones generales: 2g/d, en dos inyecciones por vía intramuscular o intravenosa; infecciones moderadas o graves: 3 ～ 6g/d, en tres inyecciones por vía intramuscular o intravenosa; septicemia, etc.: 6 ～ 8g/d, en 3 ～ 4 inyecciones por vía intravenosa; infecciones pesadas: la dosis diaria no debe sobrepasar 12g, en 6 inyecciones por vía intravenosa; gonorrea: 1g, por vía intramuscular (una sola administración suficiente). Infusión intravenosa: 2 ～ 3g/d. Niños: por vía intramuscular o intravenosa, dosis diaria de 50 ～ 100mg/kg, en 2 ～ 3 inyecciones. Infantiles: no puede ser por vía intramuscular. |
|---|---|
| 剂型、规格<br>Formulaciones y especificaciones | 注射用头孢噻肟钠：每瓶 0.5g；1g；2g。<br>Cefotaxima sódica para inyección: : 0.5g；1g；2g cada botella. |

| 药品名称 Drug Names | 头孢匹胺钠 Cefpiramida sodica |
|---|---|
| 适应证<br>Indicaciones | 用于敏感菌所致的下呼吸道、胆道、泌尿道、生殖系统、皮肤和软组织等部位的感染及败血症，腹腔炎时与甲硝唑或克林霉素合用。<br><br>Se usa para infecciones del tracto respiratorio inferior, tracto biliar, tracto urinario, sistema reproductivo, la piel, tejidos blandos y otras partes así como septicemia causadas por cepas sensibles. Para la inflamación abdominal se usa en combinación con metronidazol o clindamicina. |
| 用法、用量<br>Administración y dosis | 成人：轻中度感染，口服，一日 1 ～ 2g，分 2 次给予；肌内注射，用 0.5% ～ 1% 利多卡因注射液作溶剂，进行深部肌内注射；静脉注射，溶于 5% 的葡萄糖注射液或 0.9% 氯化钠注射液中，缓慢滴注 30 ～ 60 分钟。重度感染，一日剂量 4g，用法同上。<br>儿童：静脉给药，轻中度感染，一日 20 ～ 80mg/kg，分成 2 ～ 3 次给予；重度感染，一日剂量增至 150mg/kg，分 2 ～ 3 次缓慢静脉注射或静脉滴注。<br><br>Adultos: infecciones leves y moderadas, por vía oral, 1 ～ 2g al día, en 2 tomas; por vía intramuscular, 0.5% ～ 1% Lidocaína como disolvente, inyección en un músculo profundo; por vía intravenosa, disolverse en 5% solución de glucosa o 0.9% solución de cloruro de sodio, perfusión lenta de 30 ～ 60 minutos. Infecciones graves: dosis diaria de 4g, uso igual.<br>Niños: administración por vía intravenosa, infecciones leves y moderadas, 20 ～ 80mg/kg al día, en 2 ～ 3 inyecciones; infecciones graves: la administración diaria puede ser hasta 150mg/kg, en 2 ～ 3 inyecciones, por intravenosa lenta o infusión intravenosa. |
| 剂型、规格<br>Formulaciones y especificaciones | 注射用头孢匹胺钠：每瓶 0.5g；1g。<br>Cefpiramide de sodio para inyección: 0.5g；1g cada botella. |

| 药品名称 Drug Names | 头孢曲松钠 Ceftriaxona sódica |
|---|---|
| 适应证<br>Indicaciones | 对罗氏芬敏感的致病菌引起的感染，如脓毒血症，脑膜炎，播散性莱姆病（早、晚期），腹部感染（腹膜炎、胆道及胃肠道感染），骨、关节、软组织、皮肤及伤口感染，免疫机制低下患者的感染，肾脏及泌尿道感染，呼吸道感染，尤其是肺炎、耳鼻喉感染，生殖系统感染，包括淋病，术前预防感染。<br><br>Se usa para infecciones causadas por gérmenes patógenos sensibles a la ceftriaxona, tales como sepsis, meningitis, enfermedad de Lyme(fase primaria y terciaria), infecciones abdominales(peritonitis, infecciones biliares y gastrointestinales), infecciones de huesos, articulaciones, tejidos blandos, la piel y la herida,infecciones de pacientes con mecanismo inmunológico bajo, infecciones renales y del tracto urinario, infecciones respiratorias, sobre todo neumonía y infecciones ORL, infecciones del sistema reproductor, incluyendo gonorrea y infecciones antes de la cirugía. |

**续　表**

| | |
|---|---|
| 用法、用量<br>Administración y dosis | 一般感染，一日 1g，1 次肌内注射或静注。严重感染，一日 2g，分 2 次给予。脑膜炎，可按一日 100mg/kg（但总量不超过 4g），分 2 次给予。淋病，单次用药 250mg 即足。儿童用量一般按成人量的 1/2 给予。肌内注射：将 1 次药量溶于适量 0.5% 盐酸利多卡因注射液，做深部肌内注射。静脉注射：按 1g 药物用 10ml 灭菌注射用水溶解，缓缓注入，历时 2 ～ 4 分钟。静脉滴注：成人 1 次量 1g 或一日量 2g，溶于等渗氯化钠注射液或 5% ～ 10% 葡萄糖液 50 ～ 100ml 中，于 0.5 ～ 1 小时滴入。<br><br>Infecciones generales: 1g al día, en una inyección intramuscular o intravenosa. Infecciones graves: 2g al día, en 2 inyecciones. Meningitis: 100mg/kg al día( la dosis total no debe sobrepasar 4g), en 2 inyecciones. Gonorrea: una inyección de 250mg suficiente. La dosis para niños comúnmente es la mitad de la de adultos. Inyección intramuscular: disolver una dosis en 0.5% Lidocaína para hacer inyección en un músculo profundo. Inyección intravenosa: disolver 1g en 10ml del agua estéril, inyección lenta, duración de 2 ～ 4 minutos. Infusión intravenosa: adultos: 1g una infusión o 2g dosis diaria, disolverse en inyección isotónica de cloruro de sodio o 50 ～ 100ml de 5% ～ 10% solución de glucosa, dentro de 0.5 ～ 1 hora. |
| 剂型、规格<br>Formulaciones y especificaciones | 注射用头孢曲松钠：每瓶 0.5g；1g；2g。<br>Ceftriaxona sódica para inyección: 0.5g；1g；2g cada botella. |
| 药品名称 Drug Names | 头孢哌酮钠 Cefoperazona sódica |
| 适应证<br>Indicaciones | 用于各种敏感菌所致的呼吸道、泌尿道、腹膜、胸膜、皮肤和软组织、骨和关节、五官等部位的感染，还可用于败血症和脑膜炎等。<br><br>Se usa para infecciones del tracto respiratorio, tracto urinario, peritoneo, la pleura, la piel y los tejidos blandos, los huesos y las articulaciones, los rasgos faciales y otras partes causadas por una variedad de cepas sensibles. También se puede usar para la septicemia y la meningitis. |
| 用法、用量<br>Administración y dosis | 肌内或静脉注射，成人一次 1 ～ 2g，一日 2 ～ 4g。严重感染，一次 2 ～ 4g，一日 6 ～ 8g。小儿每日 50 ～ 100mg/kg，分 2 ～ 4 次注射。<br><br>Por vía intramuscular o intravenosa, adultos, 1 ～ 2g cada inyección, 2 ～ 4g al día. Infecciones graves: 2 ～ 4g cada inyección, 6 ～ 8g al día. Niños: 50 ～ 100mg/kg al día, en 2 ～ 4 inyecciones. |
| 剂型、规格<br>Formulaciones y especificaciones | 注射用头孢哌酮钠：每瓶 0.5g；1g；2g。注射用头孢哌酮钠 / 舒巴坦（1 : 1；2 : 1；4 : 1；8 : 1）。<br><br>Cefoperazona sódica para inyección: 0.5g；1g；2g cada botella. Cefoperazona sódica/ sulbactam para inyección: (1 : 1；2 : 1；4 : 1；8 : 1). |
| 药品名称 Drug Names | 头孢他啶 Ceftazidima |
| 适应证<br>Indicaciones | 用于革兰阴性菌的敏感菌株所致的下呼吸道、皮肤和软组织、骨和关节、胸腔、腹腔、泌尿生殖系及中枢等部位感染，也用于败血症。<br><br>Se usa para infecciones del tracto respiratorio inferior, la piel y tejidos blandos, huesos y articulaciones, el tórax, el abdomen, sistema genitourinario, sistema nervioso central entre otras partes debido a las cepas sensibles de bacterias Gram-negativas. También se puede usar para la septicemia. |
| 用法、用量<br>Administración y dosis | 轻症一日剂量为 1g，分 2 次肌内注射。中度感染一次 1g，一日 2 ～ 3 次肌内注射或静脉注射；重症一次 2g，一日 2 ～ 3 次，肌内注射或静脉注射。本品可加入氯化钠注射液、5% ～ 10% 葡萄糖注射液、含乳酸钠的输液、右旋糖酐输液中。<br><br>Síntomas leves: 1g al día, por vía intramuscular, en 2 inyecciones. Infecciones moderadas: 1g cada inyección, por vía intramuscular o intravenosa, en 2 ～ 3 inyecciones. Infecciones graves: 2g cada inyección, por vía intramuscular o intravenosa, en 2 ～ 3 inyecciones. Este medicamento se puede agregar a la inyección de cloruro de sodio, 5% ～ 10% inyección de glucosa, infusión que contiene lactato de sodio o infusión de dextrano. |
| 剂型、规格<br>Formulaciones y especificaciones | 注射用头孢他啶：每瓶 1g；2g。<br>Ceftazidima para inyección: 1g；2g cada botella. |

**续 表**

| 药品名称 Drug Names | 头孢美唑 Cefmetazol |
| --- | --- |
| 适应证<br>Indicaciones | 用于葡萄球菌、大肠埃希菌、克雷伯杆菌、吲哚阴性和阳性杆菌、拟杆菌等微生物的敏感菌株所致的肺炎、支气管炎、胆道感染、腹膜炎、泌尿系统感染、子宫及附件感染等。<br><br>Se usa para neumonía, bronquitis, infecciones de las vías biliares, peritonitis, infecciones del tracto urinario, infecciones uterinas y accesorios entre otros debido a cepas sensibles de Staphylococcus aureus, Escherichia coli, Klebsiella, bacterias negativas y positivas de indol, y otros microorganismos Bacteroides. |
| 用法、用量<br>Administración y dosis | 成人，一日 1～2g，分 2 次静脉注射或静脉滴注。小儿，一日 25～100mg/kg，分 2～4 次静脉注射或者静脉滴注。重症或顽症时，成人可用到一日 4g，儿童可用到一日 150mg/kg。溶剂可选用等渗氯化钠注射液或 5% 葡萄糖液，静脉注射时还可用灭菌注射用水（但不可用于静脉滴注，因渗透压过低）。<br><br>Adultos: 1～2g al día, en 2 inyecciones o infusiones intravenosas. Niños: 25～100mg/kg al día, en 2～4 inyecciones o infusiones intravenosas. La enfermedad grave o crónica: la administración puede ser 4g diario para adultos y 150mg/kg diario para niños. El disolvente puede ser inyección isotónica de cloruro de sodio o 5% solución de glucosa, y puede usar agua estéril para inyección intravenosa( pero la infusión intravenosa no puede usarlo porque al presión osmótica del agua es demasiado baja). |
| 剂型、规格<br>Formulaciones y especificaciones | 注射用头孢美唑钠：每瓶 0.25g；0.5g；1g；2g（效价）。<br>Cefmetazol para inyección: 0.25g；0.5g；1g；2g(potencia) cada botella. |
| 药品名称 Drug Names | 头孢克肟 Cefixima |
| 适应证<br>Indicaciones | 用于上述敏感菌所引起的肺炎、支气管炎、泌尿道炎、淋病、胆囊炎、胆管炎、猩红热、中耳炎、鼻旁窦炎。<br><br>Se usa para neumonía, bronquitis, uretritis sangrado, gonorrea, colecistitis, colangitis, escarlatina, otitis media, sinusitis debido a cepas susceptibles. |
| 用法、用量<br>Administración y dosis | 成人及体重为 30kg 以上的儿童：每次 50～100mg，一日 2 次；重症每次口服量可增至 200mg。体重为 30kg 以下的儿童：每次 1.5～3mg/kg，一日 2 次；重症每次量可增至 6mg/kg。<br><br>Adultos y niños más de 30kg de pesos: 2 tomas al día, 50～100mg cada una; enfermedad grave: la dosis de una toma puede aumentarse a 200mg. Niños menos de 30kg de pesos: 2 tomas al día, 1.5～3mg/kg cada una; enfermedad grave: la dosis de una toma puede aumentarse a 6mg/kg. |
| 剂型、规格<br>Formulaciones y especificaciones | 胶囊剂：每粒 50mg 或 100mg；颗粒：每 1g 中含本品 50mg（效价）。<br>Una cápsula: 50mg o 100mg; Un gránulo: cada 1g contiene 50mg(potencia) del medicamento. |
| 药品名称 Drug Names | 头孢西丁钠 Cefoxitina sódica |
| 适应证<br>Indicaciones | 临床应用于敏感的革兰阴性菌或厌氧菌所致的下呼吸道、泌尿生殖系、腹腔、骨和关节、皮肤和软组织等部位感染，也可用于败血症。<br><br>En clínica se usa para infecciones del tracto respiratorio inferior, sistema genitourinario, el abdomen, la piel y los tejidos blandos así como los huesos y las articulaciones entre otras partes causadas por las cepas sensibles de bacterias Gram-negativas o anaerobios. También se puede usar para la septicemia. |
| 用法、用量<br>Administración y dosis | 成人：每次 1～2g，一日 3～4 次。肾功能不全者按患者肌酐清除率制订给药方案：肌酐清除率为 30～50mg/min 者，每 8～12 小时用 1～2g；10～29ml/min 者，每 12～24 小时用 1～2g；5～9ml/min 者，每 12～24 小时用 0.5～1g；<5ml/min 者，每 24～48 小时用 0.5～1g。<br><br>Adultos: 3～4 tomas al día, 1～2g cada una. Los con insuficiencia renal: administran según el aclaramiento de creatinina: los de 30～50mg/min, 1～2g cada 8～12 horas; los de 10～29ml/min, 0.5～1g cada 12～24 horas; los <5ml/min, 0.5～1g cada 24～48 horas. |
| 剂型、规格<br>Formulaciones y especificaciones | 注射用头孢西丁钠：每瓶 1g。<br>Cefoxitina sódical para inyección: 1g cada botella. |

续　表

| 药品名称 Drug Names | 头孢米诺钠 Cefminox sódico |
| --- | --- |
| 适应证<br>Indicaciones | 用于上述敏感菌所致的扁桃体、呼吸道、泌尿道、胆道、腹腔、子宫等部位的感染，也可用于败血症。<br><br>Se usa para infecciones de amígdalas, el tracto respiratorio, tracto urinario,tracto biliar, abdominal y útero entre otras partes debido a cepas susceptibles. También se puede usar para la septicemia. |
| 用法、用量<br>Administración y dosis | 静脉注射或静脉滴注。成人每次 1g，一日 2 次；儿童每次 20mg/kg，一日 3 ～ 4 次。败血症时，成人一日可用到 6g，分 3 ～ 4 次给予。本品静脉注射，每 1g 药物用 20ml 注射用水、5% ～ 10% 葡萄糖液或 0.9% 氯化钠液溶解。滴注时，每 1g 药物溶于输液 100 ～ 200ml 中，静脉滴注 1 ～ 2 小时。<br><br>Inyección o infusión intravenosa. Adultos: 2 veces al día, 1g cada una; niños: 3 ～ 4 veces al día, 20mg/kg cada una. Septicemia: la dosis diaria para adultos puede ser hasta 6g, dosis dividida en 3 ～ 4 veces. Inyección intravenosa: 1g del medicamento se disuelve en 20ml de agua de inyección , usando 5% ～ 10% solución de glucosa o 0.9% solución de cloruro de sodio. En infusión, 1g del medicamento se disuelve en 100 ～ 200ml de la infusión, goteando 1 ～ 2 horas. |
| 剂型、规格<br>Formulaciones y especificaciones | 注射用头孢米诺钠：每瓶 0.5g；1g（效价）。<br>Cefminox sódico para inyección: 0.5g；1g(potencia) cada botella. |
| 药品名称 Drug Names | 头孢吡肟 Cefepima |
| 适应证<br>Indicaciones | 用于敏感菌所致的下呼吸道、皮肤和骨组织、泌尿系、妇科和腹腔感染及菌血症等。<br><br>Se usa para infecciones del tracto respiratorio inferior, la piel, el tejido óseo, el sistema urinario, infecciones ginecológicas y de abdominal así como bacteriemia debido a cepas susceptibles. |
| 用法、用量<br>Administración y dosis | 常用剂量每日 2 ～ 4g，分 2 次给予。治疗泌尿系感染每日 1g。极严重感染每日 6g，分 3 次给予。可用 0.9% 氯化钠、5% ～ 10% 葡萄糖、0.16mol/L 乳酸钠、林格液等溶解。溶解液在室温 24 小时内应用。<br><br>La dosis habitual: 2 ～ 4g al día, dividida en dos. Tratamiento la infección urinaria: 1g al día. Infecciones pesadas: 6g al día, dividida en tres. El disolvente puede ser 0.9% solución de cloruro de sodio, 5% ～ 10% solución de glucosa, 0.16mol/L lactato de sodio o solución de Ringer, etc. El disolvente se aplica bajo al temperatura ambiental dentro de 24 horas. |
| 剂型、规格<br>Formulaciones y especificaciones | 粉针剂：每瓶 0.5g；1g；2g。<br>Inyección de polvo: 0.5g；1g；2g cada botella. |
| 药品名称 Drug Names | 头孢布烯 Ceftibuteno |
| 适应证<br>Indicaciones | 主要用于上述敏感菌所致的呼吸道感染，如慢性气管炎急性发作、咽炎、扁桃体炎、泌尿道感染等。<br><br>Se usa para infecciones del tracto respiratorio debido a cepas susceptibles, tales como la exacerbación aguda de la bronquitis crónica, faringitis, amigdalitis e infecciones del tracto urinario entre otras partes. |
| 用法、用量<br>Administración y dosis | 成人和体重 45kg 以上儿童：每日 1 次 400mg。儿童：体重 10kg 服 90mg，20kg 服 180mg，40kg 服 360mg。服用混悬剂必须避开进食（食前 1 小时或食后 2 小时服用）；胶囊剂则无碍。肾功能不全者，肌酐清除率＞ 50ml/min 者，可按正常剂量服用（9mg/kg 或 400mg/QD）；肌酐清除率 30 ～ 49ml/min 者，照上量减半；肌酐清除率为 5 ～ 29ml/min 者，给上量的 1/4。<br><br>Adultos y niños más de 45kg de pesos: 1 toma al día, 400mg cada una. Niños de 10kg de peso: 90mg, 20kg: 180mg, 40kg: 360mg. La toma de suspensión debe evitar alimentarse(se toma 1 hora antes o 2 horas después de la comida); la toma de cápsula no tiene nada que ver con esto. Los con insuficiencia renal: administran según el aclaramiento de creatinina: los ＞ 50ml/min, dosis habitual (9mg/kg o 400mg/QD); los de 30 ～ 49ml/min, la mitad de la dosis habitual; los de 5 ～ 29ml/min, el cuarto de la dosis habitual. |

**续 表**

| 剂型、规格<br>Formulaciones y especificaciones | 胶囊剂：每粒 200mg，400mg。 混悬剂：90mg/5ml、180mg/5ml，每瓶 30ml、60ml、120ml。<br>Una cápsula: 200mg，400mg. Una suspensión: 90mg/5ml、180mg/5ml、30ml、60ml、120ml cada botella. |
|---|---|
| **药品名称 Drug Names** | **头孢丙烯 Cefprozilo** |
| 适应证<br>Indicaciones | 用于敏感菌所致上呼吸道、下呼吸道、中耳、皮肤和皮肤组织、尿路等部位感染。<br>Se usa para infecciones del tracto respiratorio inferior, tracto respiratorio superior, el oído medio, la piel y los tejidos blandos y tracto urinario entre otras partes debido a cepas susceptibles. |
| 用法、用量<br>Administración y dosis | 成人（含 13 岁以上）：上呼吸道感染，每次 500mg，一日 1 次；下呼吸道感染，每次 500mg，一日 2 次；皮肤感染，250mg，一日 1 次（重症一日 2 次）。儿童（2～12 岁）：上呼吸道感染，每次 7.5mg/kg，一日 2 次；皮肤感染，每次 20mg/kg，一日 2 次；中耳炎，每次 15mg/kg，一日 2 次。肾功能不全：肌酐清除率小于 30mg/min 者，用量减半。<br>Adultos(incluyendo los de 13 años): infección del tracto respiratorio superior: una toma al día, 500mg cada una; infección del tracto respiratorio inferior: dos tomas al día, 500mg cada una; infección de la piel: dos tomas al día, 20mg/kg cada una; otitis media: dos tomas al día, 15mg/kg cada una; los con insuficiencia renal: aclaramiento de creatinina menor de 30ml/min: la mitad de la dosis. |
| 剂型、规格<br>Formulaciones y especificaciones | 片剂：每片 250mg；500mg。 干混悬剂：每瓶 2.5g、5g，加水后成为 125mg/5ml 和 250mg/5ml。<br>Una tableta: 250mg；500mg. Una suspensión: 2.5g、5g cada botella, al agregarse auga se convierte en 125mg/5ml y 250mg/5ml. |
| **药品名称 Drug Names** | **头孢泊肟酯 Cefpodoxime proxetilo** |
| 适应证<br>Indicaciones | 用于敏感菌所致支气管炎、肺炎、泌尿系统、皮肤组织、中耳、扁桃体等部位的感染。<br>Se usa para bronquitis, neumonía, infecciones del sistema urinario, el oído medio y amígdalas entre otras partes debido a cepas susceptibles. |
| 用法、用量<br>Administración y dosis | 成人（或大于 12 岁儿童）用量：一般感染，每日 200mg；重度感染，每日 400mg；皮肤及皮肤组织感染，每日 800mg，以上均分为 2 次服用。妇女淋球菌感染，服用单剂量 200mg。儿童：每日 10mg/kg，一般分为 2 次给予（单次剂量不超过 400mg）。<br>肾功能严重不足（肌酐清除率＜ 30ml/min）者给药间隔延长至 24 小时（按以上每日剂量的 1/2），透析患者于透析后一日给药 3 次。<br>Adultos ( o niños más de 12 años): infecciones generales: 200mg al día; infecciones graves: 400mg al día; infecciones de la piel y tejidos blandos: 800mg al día, todos en dos tomas por vía oral. Niños: 10mg/kg al día, comúnmente en dos tomas(cada una no debe sobrepasar 400mg.<br>Los con insuficiencia renal (aclaramiento de creatinina menor de 30ml/min): el intervalo de dosificación se extiende a 24 horas( la mitad de la dosis diaria de arriba) y se administra a pacientes en diálisis 3 veces al día después de la diálisis. |
| 剂型、规格<br>Formulaciones y especificaciones | 片剂：每片 100mg；200mg。<br>干混悬剂：每瓶 1000mg，加水至 100ml，得 50mg/5ml 混悬剂。<br>Una tableta: 100mg；200mg.<br>Una suspensión: 1000mg cada botella, al agregarse auga al 100ml se convierte en 50mg/5ml. |
| **药品名称 Drug Names** | **头孢托仑匹酯 Cefditoren pivoxilo** |
| 适应证<br>Indicaciones | 临床用于敏感菌引起的皮肤感染、乳腺炎、肛周脓肿、泌尿生殖系统感染、胆囊炎、胆管炎、中耳炎、鼻窦炎、牙周炎、睑腺炎、泪囊炎、咽喉炎、扁桃体炎、急慢性支气管炎。<br>En clínica se usa para infecciones de la piel, la mastitis, abscesos, infecciones urogenitales, colecistitis, colangitis, otitis media, sinusitis, periodontitis, orzuelo, dacriocistitis, faringitis, amigdalitis, bronquitis aguda y crónica debido a cepas susceptibles. |
| 用法、用量<br>Administración y dosis | 口服：成人每次 200～400mg，一日 2 次，连续用药 10～14 日。肾功能不全者，肌酐清除率＜ 30ml/min 者，每次用量不应超过 200mg，一日 1 次，肌酐清除率为 30～49ml/min 者，每次用量不应超过 200mg，一日 2 次。 |

续　表

| | Vía oral: adultos: dos tomas al día, 200mg ～ 400mg cada una, administración continua de 10 ～ 14 días. Los con insuficiencia renal, aclaramiento de creatinina menor de 30ml/min: cada dosis no dede sobreapsar 200mg, una dosis al día, los de 30 ～ 49ml/min: cada dosis no dede sobreapsar 200mg, dos dosis al día. |
|---|---|
| 剂型、规格<br>Formulaciones y<br>especificaciones | 片剂：每片 100mg；200mg。<br>Una tableta：100mg；200mg. |
| 药品名称 Drug Names | 头孢地嗪钠 Cefodizima sodica |
| 适应证<br>Indicaciones | 临床用于敏感菌所致的下呼吸道、泌尿系感染。<br>En clínica se usa para infecciones del tracto respiratorio inferior y sistema urinario debido a cepas susceptibles. |
| 用法、用量<br>Administración y dosis | 成人：每次 1g（重症可用到 2g），溶于注射用水 10ml，再加入其他输液中，使成 50 ～ 100ml，静脉滴注，一日 2 次。肌内注射：用注射用水 4ml 溶解，也可用 0.5% ～ 1% 利多卡因注射液溶解，以减轻疼痛。淋病的治疗只注射 1 次，用量 0.5g。<br>Adultos: una dosis de 1g ( enfermedad grave hasta 2g), se disuelve en un total de 50 ～ 100ml, 10ml de agua de inyección más otra infusión, por goteo intravenoso, 2 veces al día. Inyección intramuscular: se disuelve en 4ml de agua de inyección, o también 0.5% ～ 1% inyección de lidocaína para aliviar el dolor. Gonorrea: una inyección, dosis de 0.5g. |
| 剂型、规格<br>Formulaciones y<br>especificaciones | 粉针剂：每瓶 1g；2g。<br>Una inyección de polvo: 1g；2g. |
| 药品名称 Drug Names | 头孢硫脒 Cefatiamidina |
| 适应证<br>Indicaciones | 用于上述敏感菌所引起的呼吸道、泌尿道、胆道、皮肤及软组织感染，对心内膜炎、败血症也有较好疗效。<br>Se usa para infecciones del tracto respiratorio, tracto urinario, tracto biliar, la piel y los tejidos blandos debido a cepas susceptibles. También tiene un buen efecto para la endocarditis y septicemia. |
| 用法、用量<br>Administración y dosis | 成人：一日 2 ～ 4g，分 2 ～ 4 次给药，肌内注射或静脉滴注，严重者可增至一日 8g。儿童：一日 50 ～ 100mg/kg，分 2 ～ 4 次给药，肌内注射或静脉滴注。先用生理盐水或注射用水溶解后，再用生理盐水或 5% 葡萄糖注射液 250ml 稀释。<br>Adultos: 2 ～ 4g al día, se administra en 2 ～ 4 veces por inyección intramuscular o goteo intravenoso, los de síntomas graves, la dosis puede aumentarse hasta 8g al día. Niños: 50 ～ 100mg/kg al día, se administra en 2 ～ 4 veces por inyección intramuscular o goteo intravenoso. Se disuelve primero en solución salina fisiológica o agua de inyección y luego se diluye en 250ml de solución salina fisiológica o 5% inyección de glucosa. |
| 剂型、规格<br>Formulaciones y<br>especificaciones | 注射用头孢硫脒：每瓶 0.5g；1g。<br>Cefathiamidine para inyección: 0.5g/botella；1g/botella. |
| 药品名称 Drug Names | 头孢替安 Cefotiam |
| 适应证<br>Indicaciones | 用于敏感菌所引起的术后感染、烧伤感染、皮肤软组织感染、骨及关节感染、呼吸系统扁桃体炎、肺炎、支气管炎、泌尿道炎、前列腺炎、胆囊炎、胆管炎，以及子宫内膜炎、盆腔炎。<br>Se usa para infecciones postoperatoria, infecciones por quemaduras, infecciones de la piel y los tejidos blandos, infecciones de los huesos y las articulaciones, amigdalitis respiratoria, neumonía, bronquitis, uretritis sangrado, prostatitis, colecistitis, colangitis así como endometritis y enfermedad inflamatoria pélvica debido a cepas susceptibles. |
| 用法、用量<br>Administración y dosis | 成人：静脉给药，一日 1 ～ 2g，2 ～ 4 次缓慢静脉注射或静脉滴注；严重感染增至一日 4g。儿童：一日 40 ～ 80mg/kg，分 3 ～ 4 次静脉给药；重症时剂量可增至一日 160mg/kg。<br>Adultos: se administra por vía intravenosa, 1 ～ 2g al día, 2 ～ 4 veces por inyección intravenosa lenta o goteo intravenoso; los de infecciones graves pueden aumentar la dosis hasta 4g al día. Niños: 40 ～ 80mg/kg al día, dividido en 3 ～ 4 veces por vía intravenosa; los de infecciones graves pueden aumentar la dosis hasta 160mg/kg al día. |

**续 表**

| 剂型、规格<br>Formulaciones y especificaciones | 注射用盐酸头孢替安：每瓶 0.25g；0.5g；1g。<br>Cefotiam para inyección: 0.25g/botella；0.5g/botella；1g/botella. |
|---|---|
| **药品名称 Drug Names** | 头孢替坦 Cefotetán |
| 适应证<br>Indicaciones | 用于敏感菌所引起的呼吸道、肺部感染、腹部感染、尿路感染、妇科感染及皮肤软组织感染。<br>Se usa para infecciones del tracto respiratorio, infecciones pulmonares, abdominales, del tracto urinario, infecciones ginecológicas así como de la piel y los tejidos blandos debido a cepas susceptibles. |
| 用法、用量<br>Administración y dosis | 深部肌内注射、静脉注射或静脉滴注。成人：常用量每次 1～2g，每 12 小时 1 次，每日最大剂量不超过 6g。儿童：每日 40～60mg/kg，病情严重者可增至 100mg/kg，分 2～3 次。<br>Inyección intramuscular profunda, inyección intravenosa o goteo intravenoso. Adultos: una dosis habitual de 1～2g, cada 12 horas, la dosis dairia máxima no puede sobrepasar 6g. Niños: dosis dairia de 40～60mg/kg, los con síntomas graves pueden aumentar la dosis hasta 100mg/kg, dividida en 2～3 veces. |
| 剂型、规格<br>Formulaciones y especificaciones | 注射用头孢替坦二钠：每瓶 1g；2g；10g。<br>Cefotetán para inyección: 1g；2g；10g cada botella. |
| **药品名称 Drug Names** | 头孢唑肟 Ceftizoxima |
| 适应证<br>Indicaciones | 敏感菌所致的下呼吸道感染、尿路感染、腹腔感染、盆腔感染、败血症、皮肤软组织感染、骨和关节感染、肺炎链球菌或流感嗜血杆菌所致脑膜炎和单纯性淋病。<br>Se usa para infecciones del tracto respiratorio inferior, tracto urinario, abdominal, infecciones pélvicas, septicemia, infecciones de la piel y los tejidos blandos, los huesos y las articulaciones debido a cepas susceptibles,el haemophilus influenzae causado por streptococcus pneumoniae o meningitis así como gonorrea no complicada. |
| 用法、用量<br>Administración y dosis | 静脉滴注静脉注射。成人：1 次 1～2g，每 8～12 小时 1 次；严重感染者的剂量可增至 1 次 3～4g，每 8 小时一次；治疗非复杂性尿路感染时，1 次 0.5g，每 12 小时 1 次。6 个月及 6 个月以上的婴儿及儿童常用量：按体重 1 次 50mg/kg，每 6～8 小时 1 次。<br>Inyección intravenosa o goteo intravenoso. Adultos: una dosis de 1～2g, cada 8～12 horas, los con infecciones graves pueden aumentar la dosis hasta 3～4g, cada 8 horas; en tratamiento de infecciones urinarias no complicadas: una dosis de 0.5g, cada 12 horas. Infantes de o más de 6 meses y niños: la dosis habitual de 50mg/kg cada vez según su peso, cada 6～8 horas. |
| 剂型、规格<br>Formulaciones y especificaciones | 注射用头孢唑肟钠：每瓶 0.5g；1g。<br>Ceftizoxima para inyección: 0.5g；1g cada botella. |
| **药品名称 Drug Names** | 头孢孟多 Cefamandol |
| 适应证<br>Indicaciones | 临床应用于敏感的革兰阴性菌所致的呼吸道、泌尿生殖系、皮肤和软组织、骨和关节、咽耳鼻喉等部位感染以及腹膜炎、败血症等。对胆道和肠道感染有较好疗效。<br>En clínica se usa para infecciones del tracto respiratorio, sistema genitourinario, la piel y los tejidos blandos, los huesos y las articulaciones, faringe, oídos, nariz y garganta entre otras partes, así como peritonitis y septicemia entre otros debido a las cepas sensibles de bacterias Gram-negativas. También tiene buen efecto para infecciones del tracto biliar e infecciones intestinales. |
| 用法、用量<br>Administración y dosis | 静脉注射或静脉滴注。成人，一般感染 1 次 0.5～1g，一日 4 次；较重感染 1 次 1g，一日 6 次；极严重感染一日可用到 12g。儿童，一日剂量为 50～100mg/kg；极重感染可用到 150mg/kg，分 3～4 次给予。<br>Inyección intravenosa o goteo intravenoso. Adultos: infecciones generales: 4 veces al diá, 0.5～1g cada una; infecciones graves: 6 veces al diá, 1g cada una; infecciones pesadas: la dosis diaria puede ser 12g. Niños: la dosis diaria debe ser 50～100mg/kg, y puede alcanzar a 150mg/kg, dividida en 3～4 veces. |

**续　表**

| | |
|---|---|
| 剂型、规格<br>Formulaciones y<br>especificaciones | 注射用头孢孟多甲酸酯钠：每瓶 0.5g、1g。每 1g 药物添加碳酸钠 63mg。<br>Cefamandol para inyección: 0.5g、1g cada botella. Cada 1g del medicamento contiene 63mg de sodio. |
| 药品名称 Drug Names | 头孢尼西钠 Cefonicida sodica |
| 适应证<br>Indicaciones | 用于上述敏感菌所致的下呼吸道感染、尿路感染、败血症、皮肤软组织感染、骨和关节感染。也可用于手术预防感染。<br>Se usa para infecciones del tracto respiratorio inferior y tracto urinario, septicemia, infecciones de la piel y los tejidos blandos, los huesos y las articulaciones debido a cepas susceptibles. También se puede usar para prevención de infecciones antes de la cirugía. |
| 用法、用量<br>Administración y dosis | 一般轻度至中度感染成人每日剂量为 1g，一天 1 次；在严重感染或危及生命的感染中，可一日 2g，每 24 小时给药 1 次；无并发症的尿路感染：每日 0.5g，每 24 小时 1 次；手术预防感染：手术前 1 小时单剂量给药 1g，术中和术后没有必要再用。必要时如关节成型手术或开胸手术可重复给药 2 天；剖宫产手术中，应在脐带结扎后才给予本品。<br>Infecciones generales de intensidad leve a moderada: dosis diaria de adultos: 1g, una toma al día; los con infecciones graves o infecciones que amenazan la vida: 2g al día, una administración cada 24 horas; infecciones urinarias sin complicaciones: 0.5g al día, una administración cada 24 horas; prevención para infección quirúrgica: una hora antes de la operación, administración única de 1g, y durante y después de la cirugía no hace falta administrarse. En casos necesarios, como artroplastia o toracotomía, la administración puede duplicarse; en cesárea, deben administrarse después de la ligadura del cordón umbilical. |
| 剂型、规格<br>Formulaciones y<br>especificaciones | 注射用头孢尼西钠：每瓶 0.5g；1g；2g。<br>Cefonicida para inyección: 0.5g；1g；2g cada botella. |
| 药品名称 Drug Names | 拉氧头孢钠 Latamoxef de sodio |
| 适应证<br>Indicaciones | 用于上述敏感菌所致肺炎、气管炎、胸膜炎、腹膜炎，以及皮肤和软组织、骨和关节、五官、创面等部位的感染，还可用于败血症和脑膜炎。<br>Se usa para neumonía, bronquitis, pleuresía, peritonitis así como infecciones de la piel y los tejidos blandos, los huesos y las articulaciones, rasgos faciales y la herida entre otras partes debido a cepas susceptibles. También se puede usar para la septicemia y meningitis. |
| 用法、用量<br>Administración y dosis | 肌内注射：每次 0.5 ～ 1 g，一日 2 次，用 0.5% 利多卡因注射液溶解，做深部肌内注射。静脉注射：每次 1 g，一日 2 次，溶解于 10 ～ 20ml 液体中，缓缓注入。静脉滴注：每次 1g，一日 2 次，溶于液体 100ml 中滴入，重症可加倍量给予。儿童用量：一日 40 ～ 80mg/kg，分 2 ～ 4 次。静脉注射和静脉滴注可用等渗氯化钠溶液或 5% ～ 10% 葡萄糖注射液、灭菌注射用水、低分子右旋糖酐注射液等做溶剂，但不得与甘露醇注射液配伍。<br>Inyección intramuscular: dos veces al día, 0.5 ～ 1 g cada vez, se disuelve en 0.5% inyección de lidocaína, por vía intramuscular profunda. Inyección intravenosa: dos veces al día, 1 g cada vez, se disuelve en 10 ～ 20ml de líquido y se inyecta lentamente. Goteo intravenoso: dos veces al día, 1 g cada vez, se disuelve en 100ml de líquido y en caso de enfermedad grave, la dosis puede duplicarse. Dosis para niños: 40 ～ 80mg/kg al día, dividida en 2 ～ 4 administraciones. El disolvente de inyección o goteo intravenoso puede ser solución isotónica de cloruro de sodio, 5% ～ 10% inyección de glucosa, agua estéril de inyección, inyección de dextrano de bajo peso molecular, etc. pero no se prepara con inyección de manitol. |
| 剂型、规格<br>Formulaciones y<br>especificaciones | 注射用拉氧头孢钠：每瓶 0.25g；0.5g；1g。<br>Latamoxef de sodio para inyección: 0.25g；0.5g；1g cada botella. |
| 药品名称 Drug Names | 氟氧头孢钠 Flomoxef de sodio |
| 适应证<br>Indicaciones | 用于上述敏感菌所致的咽炎、扁桃体炎、支气管炎、肺炎、肾盂肾炎、膀胱炎、前列腺炎、胆道感染、腹膜炎、盆腔炎、子宫及附属组织炎症、中耳炎、创口感染、心内膜炎及败血症等。<br>Se usa para faringitis, amigdalitis, bronquitis, neumonía, pielonefritis, cistitis, prostatitis, infecciones del tracto biliar, peritonitis, enfermedad inflamatoria pélvica, inflamación del útero y de las organizaciones afiliadas, otitis media, infecciones de la herida, endocarditis y septicemia debido a cepas susceptibles. |

**续 表**

| 用法、用量<br>Administración y dosis | 轻症：成人一日量 1～2g，分成 2 次静脉注射；儿童一日 60～80mg/kg，分 2 次静脉注射或静脉滴注。重症：成人一日 4g，分 2～4 次用；儿童一日 150mg/kg，分 3～4 次用。<br>Síntomas leves: adultos: dosis diaria, 1～2g, en dos inyecciones intravenosas; niños: 60～80mg/kg al día, en dos inyecciones o goteos intravenosos. Síntomas graves: adultos: 4g al día, dividida en 2～4 administraciones; niños: 150mg/kg al día, dividida en 3～4 administraciones. |
|---|---|
| 剂型、规格<br>Formulaciones y especificaciones | 注射用氟氧头孢钠：每瓶 0.5g；1g；2g。<br>Flomoxef de sodio para inyección: 0.5g；1g；2g cada botella. |

**1.3** β - 内酰胺酶抑制剂及其与 β - 内酰胺类抗生素配伍的复方制剂 Iinhibidor de la β-lactamasa y compuesto de compatibilidad con antibióticos β-lactámicos

| 药品名称 Drug Names | 克拉维酸钾 Clavulanato de potasio |
|---|---|
| 适应证<br>Indicaciones | 与 β - 内酰胺类抗生素联用于敏感菌所致的下呼吸道感染、耳鼻喉科感染、尿路感染、腹腔感染、盆腔感染、骨和关节感染、皮肤软组织感染、血流感染及败血症等。<br>Y ß-lactámicos en combinación con, para el tratamiento de infecciones del tracto respiratorio inferior causadas por cepas sensibles, infecciones ORL, infecciones del tracto urinario, infecciones abdominales, infecciones pélvicas, infecciones óseas y articulares, piel y tejidos blandos, infecciones del torrente sanguíneo y septicemia. |
| 用法、用量<br>Administración y dosis | 本药单用无效，常与 β - 内酰胺类抗生素组成复方制剂应用。各复方制剂的具体用法与用量参见"阿莫西林克拉维酸钾""替卡西林钠克拉维酸钾"。<br>El fármaco solo ineficaz, a menudo con la composición lactámicos β- aplicaciones de preparación de compuestos. El uso específico y la cantidad de cada preparación compuesto Ver "amoxicilina y clavulanato de potasio", "Ticarcilina clavulanato de potasio y sodio". |
| 剂型、规格<br>Formulaciones y especificaciones | 参见"阿莫西林克拉维酸钾""替卡西林钠克拉维酸钾"的相关项。<br>Consulte "amoxicilina y clavulanato de potasio", "Ticarcilina clavulanato de potasio de sodio" artículos relacionados. |

| 药品名称 Drug Names | 舒巴坦钠 Sulbactam sodica |
|---|---|
| 适应证<br>Indicaciones | 与青霉素类或头孢菌素类药联用于治疗敏感菌所致的败血症、尿路感染、肺部感染、支气管感染、胆道感染、腹腔感染、盆腔感染、皮肤软组织感染及耳、鼻、喉部感染等。<br>Las drogas y las penicilinas o cefalosporinas combinadas con, para el tratamiento de la sepsis causada por cepas sensibles, infecciones del tracto urinario, infecciones pulmonares, infecciones bronquiales, infecciones de las vías biliares, infecciones abdominales, infecciones pélvicas, de la piel y las infecciones de tejidos blandos y del oído, la nariz , infecciones de garganta. |
| 用法、用量<br>Administración y dosis | 静脉滴注 与氨苄西林联用，本药一日 1～2g，氨苄西林一日 2～4g，分 2～3 次给药。<br>La infusión intravenosa, y ampicilina en conjunto con, el día de drogas 1～2g, día ampicilina 2～4g, 2～3 dosis |
| 剂型、规格<br>Formulaciones y especificaciones | 注射用舒巴坦钠：0.5g；1g。<br>Sulbactam para inyección: 0.5g；1g. |

| 药品名称 Drug Names | 他唑巴坦 Tazobactam |
|---|---|
| 适应证<br>Indicaciones | 参见"哌拉西林钠 - 他唑巴坦钠"的相关项。<br>Artículos - "sodio tazobactam piperacilina sódica" relacionados Ver. |
| 用法、用量<br>Administración y dosis | 参见"哌拉西林钠 - 他唑巴坦钠"的相关项。<br>Artículos - "sodio tazobactam piperacilina sódica" relacionados Ver. |
| 剂型、规格<br>Formulaciones y especificaciones | 参见"哌拉西林钠 - 他唑巴坦钠"的相关项。<br>Artículos - "sodio tazobactam piperacilina sódica" relacionados Ver. |

续　表

| 药品名称 Drug Names | 阿莫西林 - 克拉维酸钾 Amoxicilina y clavulanato de potasio |
| --- | --- |
| 适应证<br>Indicaciones | 用于上述敏感菌所致的下呼吸道、中耳、鼻窦、皮肤组织、尿路等部位感染。对肠杆菌属尿路感染也可有效。<br><br>Se usa para infecciones del tracto respiratorio inferior, oído medio, los senos nasales, tejido de la piel y tracto urinario entre otras partes debido a cepas susceptibles. También es eficaz para enterobacter spp infecciones del tracto urinario. |
| 用法、用量<br>Administración y dosis | 一般感染：用 2 ：1 比例片，每次 1 片，每 8 小时 1 次。重症或呼吸道感染，用 4 ：1 比例片，每次 1 片，每 6 ～ 8 小时 1 次。注射应用见阿莫西林。<br><br>Infecciones generales: se usan tabletas con una relación de 2 ：1, una tableta una vez, cada 8 horas. Síntomas graves o infecciones del tracto respiratorio: se usan tabletas con una relación de 4 ：1, una tableta una vez, cada 6 ～ 8 horas. Las aplicaciones de inyección pueden referirse a Amoxicilina. |
| 剂型、规格<br>Formulaciones y especificaciones | 片剂：0.375g（2 ：1）；0.625g（4 ：1）；0.3125g（4 ：1）；0.475g（7 ：1）；1.0g（7 ：1）。<br>注射用阿莫西林钠 - 克拉维酸钾：1.2g/ 瓶（5 ：1）。<br>Una tableta: 0.375g(2 ：1); 0.625g(4 ：1); 0.3125g(4 ：1); 0.475g(7 ：1); 1.0g(7 ：1).<br>Amoxicilina y clavulanato de potasio para inyección: 1.2g/botella(5 ：1). |
| 药品名称 Drug Names | 替卡西林钠 - 克拉维酸钾 Ticarcilina de sodio y clavulanato de potasio |
| 适应证<br>Indicaciones | 本品适用于上述敏感菌引起的呼吸道、骨和关节、皮肤组织、尿路等部位的感染及败血症、骨髓炎和各种手术后感染。<br><br>Se usa para infecciones del tracto respiratorio,los huesos y las articulaciones, tejidos de la piel, tracto urinario así como septicemia, osteomielitis y todo tipo de infecciones postoperatorias entre otras partes debido a cepas susceptibles. |
| 用法、用量<br>Administración y dosis | 每次注射 3g，每 4 ～ 6 小时 1 次，溶于 13ml 等渗盐水或灭菌注射用水中，缓缓静脉推注，或溶于适量溶剂中静脉滴注，30 分钟内滴完。<br><br>De 3g cada vez, con un intervalo de 4 ～ 6 horas, disuelto en 13ml de solución salina isotónica o agua estéril de inyección, se lo inyecta a la vena lentamente o se lo diluye y se lo gotea en la vena dentro de 30 minutos. |
| 剂型、规格<br>Formulaciones y especificaciones | 注射用替卡西林钠 - 克拉维酸钾：3g（3 ：0.1）；3g（3 ：0.2）。<br>Ticarcilina de sodio y clavulanato de potasio para inyección: 3g(3 ：0.1)；3g(3 ：0.2). |
| 药品名称 Drug Names | 氨苄西林钠 - 舒巴坦钠 Ampicilina sódica y sulbactam sódico |
| 适应证<br>Indicaciones | 可用于治疗上述敏感菌所致的下呼吸道、泌尿道、胆道、皮肤和软组织、中耳、鼻窦等部位感染。<br><br>Se usa para infecciones del tracto respiratorio inferior, tracto urinario, tracto biliar, la piel y los tejidos blandos, oído medio, los senos nasales entre otras partes debido a cepas susceptibles. |
| 用法、用量<br>Administración y dosis | 氨苄西林和舒巴坦钠以 2 ：1（效价）的比率联合应用。肌内注射：一次 0.75g（氨苄西林 0.5g 和舒巴坦钠 0.25g），一日 2 ～ 4 次。静脉注射或静脉滴注：每次 1.5g，一日 2 ～ 4 次。静脉滴注时以 100ml 等渗氯化钠液或注射用水溶解，滴注 0.5 ～ 1 小时。<br><br>Se aplican ampicilina sódica y sulbactam sódico con una proporción de 2 ：1(titre). Inyección intramuscular: 0.75g cada vez(0.5g de ampicilina sódica y 0.25g de sulbactam sódico), 2 ～ 4 veces al día. Inyección o goteo intravenoso: 1.5g cada vez, 2 ～ 4 veces al día. Se lo gotea por vía intravenosa, disuelto en 100ml de solución isotónica de cloruro de sodio o auga de inyección. |
| 剂型、规格<br>Formulaciones y especificaciones | 注射用氨苄西林钠 - 舒巴坦钠：0.75g；1.5g [ 含氨苄西林钠和舒巴坦钠（重量效价比）2 ：1]。<br>Ampicilina sódica y sulbactam sódico para inyección: 0.75g；1.5g (que contiene ampicilina sódica y sulbactam (relación en peso potencia 2 ：1). |

**续　表**

| 药品名称 Drug Names | 舒他西林 Sultamicilina |
|---|---|
| 适应证<br>Indicaciones | 用于治疗敏感细菌引起的下列感染：<br>　（1）上呼吸道感染：鼻窦炎、中耳炎、扁桃体炎等。<br>　（2）下呼吸道感染：支气管炎、肺炎等。<br>　（3）泌尿道感染及肾盂肾炎。<br>　（4）皮肤、软组织感染。<br>　（5）淋病。<br>Para el tratamiento de las siguientes infecciones causadas por bacterias sensibles:<br>(1)Infecciones del tracto respiratorio superior: sinusitis, otitis media, amigdalitis<br>(2)Infecciones del tracto respiratorio inferior: bronquitis, neumonía.<br>(3)Infecciones del tracto urinario y pielonefritis.<br>(4)Infecciones de piel y tejidos blandos.<br>(5)gonorrea |
| 用法、用量<br>Administración y dosis | 每次 375mg，一日 2～4 次，在餐前 1 小时或餐后 2 小时服用。<br>375mg cada administración, 2～4 veces al día, se l toma 1 hora antes o 2 horas después de la comida. |
| 剂型、规格<br>Formulaciones y especificaciones | 片剂：375mg（效价）。<br>Una tableta: 375mg(potencia). |
| 药品名称 Drug Names | 哌拉西林钠 - 他唑巴坦钠 Piperacilina de sodio y tazobactam sódico |
| 适应证<br>Indicaciones | 临床主要用于敏感菌所致下呼吸道、腹腔、妇科、泌尿、骨及关节、皮肤组织等部位感染和败血症。也可用于多种细菌的混合感染和患中性粒细胞缺乏者的感染。<br>En clínica se usa para infecciones del tracto respiratorio, abdominal, infecciones ginecológicas, de tracto urinario, los huesos y las articulaciones, la piel y los tejidos blandos entre otras partes así como septicemia debido a cepas susceptibles. También se puede usar para infecciones mixtas de una variedad de bacterias e infecciones de los pacientes neutropénicos. |
| 用法、用量<br>Administración y dosis | 成人和 12 岁以上儿童的常用量为：每次 4.5g，一日 3 次静脉滴注（静脉滴注 30 分钟），也可静脉注射。<br>Dosis habitual para adultos y niños de más de 12 años: 4.5g cada vez, tres veces por infusión intravenosa al día(goteo de 30 minutos) o por inyección intravenosa. |
| 剂型、规格<br>Formulaciones y especificaciones | 注射用哌拉西林钠 - 他唑巴坦：2.25g（8∶1）；4.5g（8∶1）。<br>Piperacilina de sodio y tazobactam sódico para inyección: 2.25g(8∶1); 4.5g(8∶1). |

1.4 碳青霉烯类和其他 β - 内酰胺类 Carbapenems y otros β -lactámicos

| 药品名称 Drug Names | 亚胺培南 - 西司他汀钠 Imipenem / cilastatina sódica |
|---|---|
| 适应证<br>Indicaciones | 用于敏感菌所致的腹膜炎、肝胆感染、腹腔内脓肿、阑尾炎、妇科感染、下呼吸道感染、皮肤和软组织感染、尿路感染、骨和关节感染以及败血症等。<br>Se usa para peritonitis, infecciones hepatobiliares, absceso intraabdominal, apendicitis, infecciones ginecológicas, infecciones del tracto respiratorio inferior, la piel y los tejidos blandos, tracto urinario, los huesos y las articulaciones así como septicemia debido a cepas susceptibles. |
| 用法、用量<br>Administración y dosis | 静脉滴注或肌内注射。用量以亚胺培南计量，根据病情，一次 0.25～1g，一日 2～4 次，对中度感染一般可按 1 次 1g，一日 2 次给予。静脉滴注可选用等渗氯化钠注射液、5%～10% 葡萄糖液作溶剂。每 0.5g 药物用 100ml 溶剂，制成 5mg/ml 液体，缓缓滴入。肌内注射用 1% 利多卡因注射液为溶剂，以减轻疼痛。<br>对肾功能不全者应按肌酐清除率调整剂量：肌酐清除率为 31～70ml/min 的患者，每 6～8 小时用 0.5g，每日最高剂量为 1.5～2g；肌酐清除率为 21～30ml/min 的患者，每 8～12 小时用 0.5g，每日最高剂量为 1～1.5g；肌酐清除率为 < 20ml/min 的患者，每 12 小时用 0.25～0.5g，每日最高剂量为 0.5～1g。 |

**续　表**

Infusión intravenosa o inyección intramuscular. La dosis se calcula por imipenem, de acuerdo con la gravedad, 0.25 ～ 1g cada vez, 2 ～ 4 veces al día, y para infecciones moderadas, se administra 1g una vez, dos veces al día. Para infusión intravenosa se usa inyección isotónica de cloruro de sodio o 5% ～ 10% infusión de glucosa como disolvente. Se hace la solución con 0.5g del medicamento disuelto en 100ml del disolvente para gotearla lentamente. En caso de inyección intramuscular se usa inyección de lidocaína como disolvente para aliviar el dolor.

Los con insuficiencia renal: se administra la dosis según el aclaramiento de creatinina: los de 31 ～ 70ml/min, 0.5g cada 6 ～ 8 horas, la dosis diaria máxima 1.5 ～ 2g; los de 21 ～ 30ml/min, 0.5g cada 8 ～ 12 horas, la dosis diaria máxima 1 ～ 1.5g; los menor de < 20ml/min, 0.25 ～ 0.5g cada 12 horas, la dosis diaria máxima 0.5 ～ 1g.

| 剂型、规格 Formulaciones y especificaciones | 注射用亚胺培南 - 西司他汀：每支 0.25g；0.5g；1g（以亚胺培南计量）。其中含有等量的西司他汀钠。<br><br>Imipenem / cilastatina sódica para inyección: 0.25g；0.5g；1g(calculado en imipenem) cada una. Contiene igual dosis de cilastatina sódica. |
|---|---|

**药品名称 Drug Names**　美罗培南 Meropenem

| 适应证 Indicaciones | 用于敏感菌所致的呼吸道、尿路、肝胆、外科、骨科、妇科、五官科感染及腹膜炎、皮肤化脓性疾病等。本品可适用于敏感菌所致脑膜炎。<br><br>Se usa para infecciones del tracto respiratorio, tracto urinario, hígado y vesícula biliar, así como infecciones quirúrgicas, ortopédicas,ORL y ginecológicas,peritonitis, enfermedades de la piel purulenta entre otros debido a cepas susceptibles. También se aplica a meningitis debido a cepas susceptibles. |
|---|---|
| 用法、用量 Administración y dosis | 成人每日 0.5 ～ 1g，分为 2 ～ 3 次，稀释后静脉滴注每次 30 分钟。重症每日计量可增至 2g。连续应用不超过 2 周。本品每 0.5g 用生理盐水约 100ml 溶解，不可用注射用水。儿童（3 月龄以上）推荐用量：周围感染 20mg/kg，每 8 小时 1 次；脑膜炎 40mg/kg，每 8 小时一次。肾功能减退者应按肌酐清除率调整剂量：肌酐清除率为 26 ～ 50ml/min 的患者，每 12 小时用 1g；肌酐清除率为 10 ～ 25ml/min 的患者，每 12 小时用 0.5g；肌酐清除率为< 10/min 的患者，每 24 小时用 0.5g。<br><br>Adultos: 0.5 ～ 1g al día, en 2 ～ 3 veces, tras la dilusión se gotea por vía intravenosa durante 30 minutos cada vez. Para síntomas graves la dosis diaria puede alcanzar 2g. La aplicación contínua no debe sobrepasar 2 semanas. Cada 0.5g del medicamento se disuelve en 100ml de solución salina fisiológica en vez de agua de inyección. Dosis recomendada para niños(mayores de 3 meses): 20mg/kg de infección periférica, cada 8 horas; 40mg/kg de meningitis, cada 8 horas. Los con insuficiencia renal: se administra la dosis según el aclaramiento de creatinina: los de 26 ～ 50ml/min, 1g cada 12 horas; los de 10 ～ 25ml/min, 0.5g cada 12 horas; los menor de < 10ml/min, 0.5g cada 24 horas. |
| 剂型、规格 Formulaciones y especificaciones | 粉针剂：每瓶 0.5g；1g。<br>Una inyección de polvo: 0.5g；1g cada botella. |

**药品名称 Drug Names**　帕尼培南 - 倍他米隆 Panipenem y betamiprón

| 适应证 Indicaciones | 用于治疗敏感菌引起的呼吸系统、泌尿生殖系统、腹内、眼科、皮肤及软组织、骨及关节的感染。如急慢性支气管炎、肺炎、肺脓肿、胆囊炎、腹膜炎、肝脓肿，肾盂肾炎、前列腺炎、子宫内感染，角膜溃疡、眼球炎、丹毒、蜂窝织炎，骨髓炎、关节炎等。还可用于败血症、感染性心内膜炎等严重感染。<br><br>Se usa para infecciones del tracto respiratorio, sistema genitourinario, abdominal, los ojos, la piel y los tejidos blandos, los huesos y las articulaciones debido a cepas susceptibles tales como bronquitis aguda y crónica, neumonía, absceso pulmonar, colecistitis, peritonitis, abscesos hepáticos, pielonefritis, prostatitis, infecciones intrauterinas, úlceras corneales, inflamación de los ojos, la erisipela, celulitis, osteomielitis, artritis entre otros. También se puede usar para infecciones graves como la septicemia y endocarditis infecciosa. |
|---|---|

| | |
|---|---|
| 用法、用量<br>Administración y dosis | 静脉滴注：成人，一般感染，每次 0.5g，一日 2 次，用不少于 100ml 的生理盐水或 5% 葡萄糖注射液溶解后，于 30 ～ 60 分钟滴注；重症或顽固性感染，剂量为每次 1g，一日 2 次，静脉滴注时间不少于 1 小时。儿童，每日 30 ～ 60mg/kg，分 2 ～ 3 次，每次 30 分钟静脉滴注；严重感染可增加至每日 100mg/kg，分 3 ～ 4 次。 |
| | Infusión intravenosa: adultos: para infecciones generales, dos veces al día, 0.5g cada vez, disuelto en la solución salina fisiológica o 5% inyección de glucosa, se gotea durante 30 ～ 60 minutos; para síntomas graves o crónicos, dos veces al día, 1g cada vez, la duración del goteo intravenoso no debe ser menos de 1 hora. Niños: 30 ～ 60mg/kg al día, en 2 ～ 3 infusiones intravenosas, 30min cada vez; para infección grave: la administración puede ser 100mg/kg diario en 3 ～ 4 infusiones. |
| 剂型、规格<br>Formulaciones y especificaciones | 注射用帕尼培南 - 倍他米隆：250mg/ 瓶；500mg/ 瓶。帕尼培南与等量倍他米隆配伍，以帕尼培南含量计。 |
| | Panipenem y betamiprón para inyección: 250mg/botella; 500mg/botella. Se prepara igual dosis de panipenem y betamiprón, calculado en la dosis de panipenem. |

| 药品名称 Drug Names | 厄他培南 Ertapenem |
|---|---|
| 适应证<br>Indicaciones | 用于治疗敏感菌引起的呼吸系统、泌尿生殖系统、腹腔、皮肤及软组织、盆腔等部位的感染。 |
| | Se usa para infecciones de sistema respiratorio, sistema genitourinario, abdominal, la piel y los tejidos blandos y pélvis entre otras partes debido a cepas susceptibles. |
| 用法、用量<br>Administración y dosis | 静脉滴注：成人，每日 1g，用不少于 100ml 的生理盐水稀释。肾功能不全者，肌酐清除率＜ 30ml/min，每天剂量 0.5g。3 个月及以上的儿童一天 2 次按 15mg/kg 给予肌内注射或静脉滴注，日剂量不超过 1g。 |
| | Infusión intravenosa: adultos: 1g al día, se disuelve en la solución salina fisiológica no menos de 100ml. Los con insuficiencia renal: aclaramiento de creatinina ＜ 30ml/min, 0.5g al día. Niños de 3 meses o más: 15mg/kg, 2 veces al día, por vía intramuscular o infusión intravenosa, la dosis diaria no debe sobrepasar 1g. |
| 剂型、规格<br>Formulaciones y especificaciones | 注射用厄他培南：每支 1g。 |
| | Etapenem para inyección: 1g cada una. |

| 药品名称 Drug Names | 比阿培南 Biapenem |
|---|---|
| 适应证<br>Indicaciones | 用于肠杆菌属、假单胞属、不动杆菌、枸橼酸杆菌、脆弱拟杆菌所致慢性呼吸道感染急性发作、肺炎、肺脓肿、腹膜炎、复杂性膀胱炎、女性生殖器感染。对某些革兰阳性菌也有效。 |
| | Se usa para exacerbación aguda de infecciones respiratorias crónicas, neumonía, absceso pulmonar, peritonitis, complicada cistitis e infecciones genitales femeninos debido a enterobacter, especies de pseudomonas, acinetobacter, citrobacter y bacteroides fragilis. También tiene efecto para bacterias Gram-positivas. |
| 用法、用量<br>Administración y dosis | 静脉滴注：成人一般感染，每次 0.3g，一日 2 次。可根据病情增加剂量，但每日不可超过 1.2g。用 0.9% 的生理盐水或 5% 葡萄糖注射液稀释。 |
| | Infusión intravenosa: infecciones generales de adultos: dos veces al día, 0.3g cada vez. Se puede incrementar la dosis según la gravedad, pero la dosis diaria no debe sobrepasar 1.2g. Se disuelve en la 0.9% solución salina fisiológica o se diluye en 5% inyección de glucosa. |
| 剂型、规格<br>Formulaciones y especificaciones | 注射用比阿培南：每支 300mg。 |
| | Biapenem para inyección: 300mg cada una. |

| 药品名称 Drug Names | 法罗培南钠 Faropenem de sodio |
|---|---|
| 适应证<br>Indicaciones | 用于皮肤及软组织、呼吸系统、泌尿生殖系统及眼、耳、鼻、喉、口腔等部位的敏感菌感染。 |
| | Se usa para infecciones la piel y los tejidos blandos, sistema respiratorio, sistema genitourinario, ojos, oídos, nariz, garganta, boca y entre otras partes debido a cepas susceptibles. |
| 用法、用量<br>Administración y dosis | 口服：成人常用量每次 150 ～ 200mg，一日 3 次。重症每次 200 ～ 300mg，一日 3 次。 |
| | Se toma por vía oral: la dosis habitual de adultos es de 150 ～ 200mg cada vez, 3 veces al día. Para síntomas graves: 200 ～ 300mg cada vez, 3 veces al día. |

**续　表**

| 剂型、规格<br>Formulaciones y<br>especificaciones | 片剂：每片 150mg；300mg。<br>Una tableta: 150mg；300mg. |
|---|---|

| 药品名称 Drug Names | 氨曲南 Aztreonam |
|---|---|

| 适应证<br>Indicaciones | 用于敏感的革兰阴性菌所致的感染，包括肺炎、胸膜炎、腹腔感染、胆道感染、骨和关节感染、皮肤和软组织炎症，尤适用于尿路感染，也用于败血症。由于本品有较好的耐酶性能，因此，当细菌对青霉素类、头孢菌素类、氨基糖苷类等药物不敏感时，可试用本品。<br><br>Se usa para infecciones debido a las cepas sensibles de bacterias Gram-negativas tales como neumonía, pleuresía, infecciones abdominales, infecciones de las vías biliares, los huesos y articulaciones, inflamación de la piel y los tejidos blandos, sobre todo para infecciones del tracto urinario así como la septicemia. Por lo tanto, cuando las bacterias no son sensibles a las penicilinas, cefalosporinas, aminoglucósidos y otros fármacos se puede usar este medicamento. |
|---|---|
| 用法、用量<br>Administración y dosis | 肌内注射、静脉注射、静脉滴注。成人，一般感染，3～4g/d，分2～3次给予；严重感染，每次2g，一日3～4次，一日最大剂量为8g；无其他并发症的尿路感染，只需用1g，分1～2次给予。儿童，每次30mg/kg，一日3次，重症感染可增加至一日4次给药，一日最大剂量为120mg/kg。肌内注射：每1g药物，加液体3～4ml溶解。静脉注射：每1g药物，加液体10ml溶解，缓慢注射。静脉滴注：每1g药物，加液体50ml以上溶解（浓度不超过2%），滴注时间20～60分钟。<br><br>注射时，下列药液可用做本品的溶解-稀释液：灭菌注射用水、等渗氯化钠注射液、林格液、乳酸钠林格液、5%～10%葡萄糖液、葡萄糖氯化钠注射液等。用于肌内注射时，还可用含苯甲醇的氯化钠注射液作溶剂。<br><br>Inyección intramuscular, inyección intravenosa o infusión intravenosa. Adultos: infecciones generales: 3～4g al día, administrado en 2～3 veces; infecciones graves: 3～4 veces al día, la dosis diaria máxima de 8g; infecciones urinarias sin complicaciones: sólo se necesita 1g, dividido en 1～2 veces. Niños: 30mg/kg cada vez, tres veces al día, para infecciones graves, se puede administrase hasta 4 veces, la dosis máxima es de 120mg/kg. Inyección intramuscular: disolver 1g del medicamento en líquido de 3～4ml. Inyección intravenosa: disolver 1g en 10ml del líquido, inyección lenta. Infusión intravenosa: 1g en más de 50ml del líquido(la concentración no debe sobrepasar 2%), duración de 20～60 minutos.<br><br>Los siguientes líquidos médicos pueden usarse como disolución - diluyente durante la inyección: agua estéril, inyección isotónica de cloruro de sodio, ringer-locke licor, ringer lactato, 5%～10% solución de glucosa y saline glucosa, etc. En la inyección intramuscular, también se puede usar inyección de cloruro de sodio con alcohol bencílico como disolvente. |
| 剂型、规格<br>Formulaciones y<br>especificaciones | 注射用氨曲南：每天1g（效价）。内含精氨酸0.78g（稳定、助溶用）。<br>Aztreonam para inyección: 1g al día(potencia). Contiene 0.78g de arginina(estable y solubilizable). |

## 1.5　氨基糖苷类 Aminoglucósidos

| 药品名称 Drug Names | 卡那霉素 Kanamicina |
|---|---|

| 适应证<br>Indicaciones | 口服用于治疗敏感菌所致的肠道感染及用作肠道手术前准备，并有减少肠道细菌产生氨的作用，对肝硬化消化道出血患者的肝性脑病有一定防治作用。<br><br>肌内注射用于敏感菌所致的系统感染，如肺炎、败血症、尿路感染等，常与其他抗菌药物联合应用。<br><br>Se toma por vía oral para el tratamiento de infecciones intestinales, puede servir de preparación de una operación intestinal, tiene el efecto de reducir amoniacos producidos por las bacterias intestinales y el efecto de prevenir encefalopatía hepática sufrido por pacientes con el sangrado gastrointestinal de cirrosis.<br><br>Inyección intramuscular se usa para infecciones del sistema debido a cepas susceptibles tales como neumonía, septicemia, infecciones del tracto urinario etc.Suele aplicarse en combinación con otros antimicrobianos. |
|---|---|

**续 表**

| | |
|---|---|
| 用法、用量<br>Administración y dosis | 肌内注射或静脉滴注：每次 0.5g，一日 1～1.2g；小儿每日 15～25mg/kg，分 2 次给予。静脉滴注时应将一次用量以输液约 100ml 稀释，滴入时间为 30～60 分钟，切勿过速。口服：用于防治肝性脑病，一日 4g，分次给予。腹部手术前准备：每小时 1g，连续 4 次（常与甲硝唑联合应用）后，改为每 6 小时 1 次，连服 36～72 小时。<br><br>Inyección intramuscular o goteo intravenoso: 0.5g cada vez, 1～1.2g al día; niños: 15～25mg/kg al día, en dos veces. En goteo intravenoso, la dosis de una vez se debe diluir en 100ml de infusión, durante 30～60 minutos, cuidando por no exceder la velocidad. Se toma por vía oral: para prevenir encefalopatía hepática, 4g al día, dividido en varias veces. Preparación antes de la cirugía abdominal: 1g cada hora, tras 4 veces consecutivas(habitualmente con metronidazol), se convierte en 6 horas una vez durante 36～72 horas. |
| 剂型、规格<br>Formulaciones y especificaciones | 注射用硫酸卡那霉素：每瓶 0.5g；1g。<br>注射液（含单硫酸卡那霉素）：每支 500mg（2ml）。<br>滴眼液：8ml（40mg）。<br>Kanamicina para inyección: 0.5g; 1g cada botella.<br>Inyección(que contiene kanamicina monosulfato): 500mg(2ml)cada una.<br>Gotas para los ojos: 8ml(40mg). |
| 药品名称 Drug Names | 阿米卡星 Amikacina |
| 适应证<br>Indicaciones | 临床主要用于对卡那霉素或庆大霉素耐药的革兰阴性杆菌所致的尿路、下呼吸道、腹腔、软组织、骨和关节、生殖系统等部位的感染，以及败血症等。<br><br>En clínica se usa para infecciones del tracto urinario, tracto respiratorio inferior, abdominal, los tejidos blandos, los huesos y las articulaciones y sistema reproductivo entre otras partes así como septicemia etc. debido a kanamicina o bacilos gramnegativos resistentes a la gentamicina. |
| 用法、用量<br>Administración y dosis | 肌内注射或静脉滴注：成人 7.5mg/kg，每 12 小时一次，每日总量不超过 1.5g，可用 7～10 日；无并发症的尿路感染，每次 0.2g，每 12 小时一次；小儿，开始用 10mg/kg，以后 7.5mg/kg，每 12 小时一次；较大儿童可按成人用量。<br>给药途径以肌内注射为主，也可用 100～200ml 输液稀释后静脉滴注，30～60 分钟进入体内，儿童则为 1～2 小时。疗程一般不超过 10 日。<br>肾功能不全者首次剂量 7.5mg/kg，以后则调整使血药峰浓度为 25μg/ml，谷浓度 5～8μg/ml.<br><br>Inyección intramuscular o goteo intravenoso: adultos: 7.5mg/kg, cada 12 horas, dosis diaria máxima no debe sobrepasar 1.5g, durante 7～10 días; infecciones urinarias sin complicaciones: 0.2g cada vez, cada 12 horas; niños: 10mg/kg al principio, 7.5mg/kg luego, cada 12 horas; los niños mayores: se puede administrar la dosis de adultos.<br>La forma principal de administración es inyección intramuscular. También se lo puede diluir en 100～200ml de infusión y gotear en la vena durante 30～60 minutos, 1～2 horas para niños. El ciclo de tratamiento generalmente no sobrepasa 10 días.<br>Los con insuficiencia renal: la primera dosis es de 7.5mg/kg, y ajustan la concentración plasmática máxima al 25μg/ml, mínima al 5～8μg/ml. |
| 剂型、规格<br>Formulaciones y especificaciones | 注射液：每支 0.1g（1ml）；0.2g（2ml）。注射用硫酸阿米卡星：每瓶：0.2g。<br>Inyección: 0.1g(1ml)cada una; 0.2g(2ml). Amikacina para inyección: 0.2g cada botella. |
| 药品名称 Drug Names | 妥布霉素 Tobramicina |
| 适应证<br>Indicaciones | 临床主要用于铜绿假单胞菌感染。如烧伤、败血症等。对其他敏感革兰阴性杆菌所致的感染也可应用。与庆大霉素间存在较密切的交叉耐药性。<br><br>En clínica se usa para infecciones causadas por pseudomonas aeruginosa, tales como quemadura y septicemia etc. También se aplica a infecciones debido a las cepas sensibles de bacterias Gram-negativas. Tiene una mayor resistencia cruzada con gentamicina. |
| 用法、用量<br>Administración y dosis | 肌内注射或静脉滴注，一日 4.5mg/kg，分为 2 次给予，一日剂量不可超过 5mg/kg。静脉滴注时 1 次量用输液 100ml 稀释，于 30 分钟左右滴入。新生儿一日量 4mg/kg，分为 2 次给予。一般用药不超过 7～10 日。<br><br>Inyección intramuscular o goteo intravenoso: 4.5mg/kg al día, en dos veces, la dosis diaria máxima no debe sobrepasar 5mg/kg. En goteo intravenoso: se diluye una dosis en 100ml de infusión y gotear en la vena durante apróximamente 30 minutos. La dosis diaria de recién nacidos es de 4mg/kg, dividido en dos veces. En general, la dosis administrada no debe sobrepasar 7～10 días. |

**续　表**

| 剂型、规格<br>Formulaciones y especificaciones | 注射液：每支 80mg（2ml）。<br>Inyección: 80mg(2ml)cada una. |
|---|---|
| **药品名称 Drug Names** | **庆大霉素 Gentamicina** |
| 适应证<br>Indicaciones | 临床主要用于大肠埃希菌、痢疾杆菌、克雷伯肺炎杆菌、变形杆菌、铜绿假单胞菌等革兰阴性菌引起的系统或局部感染（对中枢感染无效）。<br><br>En clínica se usa para infecciones sistémicas o locales debido a E. coli, shigella, klebsiella pneumoniae, proteus y pseudomonas aeruginosa entre otras bacterias Gram-negativas(sin efecto para infección del sistema nervioso central). |
| 用法、用量<br>Administración y dosis | 肌内注射或静脉滴注，一次 80mg，一日 2 ～ 3 次（间隔 8 小时）。对于革兰阴性杆菌所致重症感染或铜绿假单胞菌全身感染，一日量可用到 5mg/kg。静脉滴注给药可将 1 次量（80mg），用输液 100ml 稀释，于 30 分钟左右滴入。小儿一日 3 ～ 5mg/kg，分 2 ～ 3 次给予。<br>口服：一次 80 ～ 160mg，一日 3 ～ 4 次。小儿每日 5 ～ 10mg/kg，分 3 ～ 4 次服用，用于肠道感染或术前准备。<br><br>Inyección intramuscular o goteo intravenoso: 80mg cada vez, 2 ～ 3 veces al día(con intervalo de 8 horas). Para infecciones graves causadas por bacterias Gram-negativas o infecciones sistémicas debido a pseudomonas aeruginosa, la dosis diaria puede alcanzar a 5mg/kg. En goteo intravenoso: se diluye una dosis(80mg) en 100ml de infusión y gotear en la vena durante apróximamente 30 minutos. La dosis diaria de niños es de 3 ～ 5mg/kg, dividida en 2 ～ 3 veces.<br>Se toma por vía oral: 80 ～ 160mg cada vez, 3 ～ 4 veces al día. La dosis diaria de niños es de 5 ～ 10mg/kg, dividida en 3 ～ 4 veces, para el tratamiento de las infecciones intestinales o como preparación preoperatoria. |
| 剂型、规格<br>Formulaciones y especificaciones | 注射液：每支 20mg（1ml）；40mg（1ml）；80mg（2ml）。<br>片剂：每片 40mg。<br>滴眼液：8ml（40mg）。<br><br>Inyección: 20mg(1ml)cada una; 40mg(1ml)；80mg(2ml).<br>Una tableta: 40mg.<br>Gotas para los ojos: 8ml(40mg). |
| **药品名称 Drug Names** | **西索米星 Sisomicina** |
| 适应证<br>Indicaciones | 临床主要用于大肠埃希菌、痢疾杆菌、克雷伯杆菌、变形杆菌等革兰阴性菌引起的局部或系统感染（对中枢感染无效），对尿路感染作用尤佳。<br><br>En clínica se usa para infecciones sistémicas o locales debido a E. coli, shigella, klebsiella pneumoniae y proteus entre otras bacterias Gram-negativas, (sin efecto para infección del sistema nervioso central). Tiene efecto extraordinario para infección del tracto urinario. |
| 用法、用量<br>Administración y dosis | 成人一日量 3mg/kg，分为 3 次，肌内注射。疗程不超过 7 ～ 10 日。<br><br>La dosis diaria de adultos es de 3mg/kg, en tres veces, por inyección intramuscular. El ciclo de tratamiento no debe sobrepasar a 7 ～ 10 días. |
| 剂型、规格<br>Formulaciones y especificaciones | 注射液：每支 75mg（1.5ml）；100mg（2ml）。<br>Inyección: 75mg(1.5ml)cada una; 100mg(2ml). |
| **药品名称 Drug Names** | **奈替米星 Netilmicina** |
| 适应证<br>Indicaciones | 临床主要用于大肠埃希菌、克雷伯杆菌、变形杆菌、肠杆菌属、枸橼酸杆菌、沙雷杆菌、流感嗜血杆菌、沙门杆菌、志贺杆菌、奈瑟球菌等革兰阴性菌所致呼吸道、消化道、泌尿生殖系、皮肤和软组织、骨和关节、腹腔、创伤等部位的感染，也适用于败血症。<br><br>Se usa para infecciones del tracto respiratorio, tracto gastrointestinal, sistema genitourinario, la piel y los tejidos blandos, los huesos y las articulaciones, abdominal y la herida entre otras partes así como la septicemia debido a E. coli, klebsiella, proteus,enterobacter, citrobacter, bacterias Serratia, haemophilus influenzae, salmonella, shigella, neisseria entre otras bacterias Gram-negativas. |

续　表

| 用法、用量<br>Administración y dosis | 单纯泌尿系感染：成人一日量为 3 ～ 4mg/kg，分为 2 次。较严重的系统感染：成人一日量为 4 ～ 6.5mg/kg，分为 2 ～ 3 次给予；新生儿（6 周龄以内）：一日 4 ～ 6.5mg/kg；婴儿和儿童：一日 5 ～ 8mg/kg，分为 2 ～ 3 次给予，肌内注射给药。如必须静脉滴注，则将 1 次药量加入 50 ～ 200ml 输液中，缓慢滴入。有报道，本品一日按 4.5 ～ 6mg/kg 量，1 次肌内注射，效果好，且不良反应少。<br><br>Infección del tracto urinario simple: la dosis diaria de adultos es de 3 ～ 4mg/kg, dividida en dos veces. Infección sistémica grave: la dosis diaria de adultos es de 4 ～ 6.5mg/kg, dividida en 2 ～ 3 veces; recién nacidos(menores a 6 semanas de edad): 4 ～ 6.5mg/kg al día; bebés y niños: 5 ～ 8mg/kg al día, dividido en 2 ～ 3 veces, administrado por inyección intramuscular. Si se debe efectuar el goteo intravenoso, se agrega una dosis lentamente a 50 ～ 200ml de infusión. Se ha informado que si se administra una dosis de 4.5 ～ 6mg/kg al día, por una inyección intramuscular, tendrá buenos efectos y menos reacciones adversas. |
| --- | --- |
| 剂型、规格<br>Formulaciones y especificaciones | 注射液：每支 150mg（1.5ml）。<br>Inyección: 150mg(1.5ml)cada una. |
| 药品名称 Drug Names | 小诺米星 Micronomicina |
| 适应证<br>Indicaciones | 临床主要用于大肠埃希菌、克雷伯杆菌、变形杆菌、肠杆菌属、沙雷杆菌、铜绿假单胞菌等革兰阴性杆菌引起的呼吸道、泌尿道、腹腔及外伤感染，也适用于败血症。<br><br>En clínica se usa para infecciones del tracto respiratorio, tracto urinario, abdominal, debido a E. coli, klebsiella, proteus,enterobacter, bacterias Gram-negativas. También se puede usar para la septicemia. |
| 用法、用量<br>Administración y dosis | 泌尿道感染：每次 120mg，肌内注射，一日 2 次。其他感染：每次 60mg，一日 2 ～ 3 次，肌内注射。用药疗程一般不超过 2 周。<br><br>Infección del tracto urinario: 120mg cada vez, por inyección intramuscular, dos veces al día. Otras infecciones: 60mg cada vez, por inyección intramuscular, 2 ～ 3 veces al día. Habitualmente, el ciclo de tratamiento no sobrepasa dos semanas. |
| 剂型、规格<br>Formulaciones y especificaciones | 注射液：每支 60mg（2ml）。<br>Inyección: 60mg(2ml)cada una. |
| 药品名称 Drug Names | 异帕米星 Isepamicina |
| 适应证<br>Indicaciones | 临床适用于上述敏感菌所致外伤或烧伤创口感染、肺炎、支气管炎、肾盂肾炎、膀胱炎、腹膜炎及败血症。<br><br>En clínica se usa para infecciones de la herida de trauma o quemadura, neumonía, bronquitis, pielonefritis, cistitis, peritonitis y septicemia debido a cepas susceptibles. |
| 用法、用量<br>Administración y dosis | 成人一日量 400mg，通常分为 2 次（或一日 1 次）肌内注射或静脉滴注。静脉滴注速度控制 0.5 ～ 1 小时滴毕，按年龄、体重和症状适当调整。<br><br>La dosis diaria para adultos: 400mg, normalmente dividida en dos veces(o una vez al día) por inyección intramuscular o goteo intravenoso. Se controla el tiempo para efectuar el goteo intravenoso entre media y una hora, ajustado oportunamente según la edad, el físico y los síntomas. |
| 剂型、规格<br>Formulaciones y especificaciones | 注射液：每支 200mg（2ml）。<br>Inyección: 200mg(2ml)cada una. |
| 药品名称 Drug Names | 依替米星 Etimicina |
| 适应证<br>Indicaciones | 临床主要用于革兰阴性杆菌、大肠埃希菌、肺炎克雷伯菌、沙雷菌属、奇异变形杆菌、沙门菌属、流感嗜血杆菌等敏感菌株所引起的呼吸道、泌尿生殖系统、腹腔、皮肤和软组织等部位的感染以及败血症。<br><br>En clínica se usa para infecciones del tracto respiratorio, sistema genitourinario, abdominal, la piel y los tejidos blandos entre otras partes así como septicemia debido a bacterias Gram-negativas, escherichia coli, klebsiella pneumoniae, serratia, proteus mirabilis, salmonella y haemophilus influenzae entre otras cepas susceptibles. |

**续　表**

| | |
|---|---|
| 用法、用量<br>Administración y dosis | 成人量每日 200mg，一次加入输液（0.9% 氯化钠液或 5% 葡萄糖液）100ml 中，静脉滴注 1 小时，每日只用 1 次，连用 3 ～ 7 日。<br><br>La dosis diaria de adultos: 200mg, de una vez se agrega a 100ml de infusión(0.9% solución de cloruro de sodio o 5% solución de glucosa), geteando por una hora, una vez al día, durante 3 ～ 7 días consecutivos. |
| 剂型、规格<br>Formulaciones y especificaciones | 注射用粉针：每支 50mg；100mg。<br>注射液：50mg（1ml）；100mg（2ml）。<br>Una inyección de polvo: 50mg；100mg.<br>Inyección: 50mg(1ml)；100mg(2ml). |
| 药品名称 Drug Names | 大观霉素 Espectinomicina |
| 适应证<br>Indicaciones | 临床主要应用于淋球菌所引起的泌尿系感染，适用于对青霉素、四环素等耐药的病例。<br><br>En clínica se usa principalmente para infecciones del tracto urinario debido a neisseria gonorrhoeae. Se aplica a los casos resistentes a la penicilina, la tetraciclina, etc. |
| 用法、用量<br>Administración y dosis | 1 次肌内注射 2g。将特殊稀释液（0.9% 苯甲醇溶液）3.2ml 注入安瓿中，猛力振摇，使成混悬液（约 5ml），用粗针头注入臀上部外侧深部肌内。一般只用 1 次即可。对于使用其他抗生素治疗而迁延未愈的患者，可按 4g 剂量给药，即 1 次用药 4g，分注于两侧臀上外侧肌内，或 1 次肌内注射 2g，一日内用药 2 次。<br><br>Una inyección intramuscular de 2g. Se inyecta 3,2 ml del diluyente especial(0.9% solución de alcohol bencílico) a la botella, se lo agita vigorosamente para hacer una suspensión (aproximadamente 5 ml), con una aguja gruesa se inyecta en la parte lateral de los profundos músculos de los glúteos superiores. Generalmente se usa sólo una vez. A los pacientes con el uso persistente de otros antibióticos sin haberse curado, se los puede aplicar una dosis de 4g, es decir, 4g cada administración, en los lados exteriores de la inyección intramuscular glútea superior o 2g de cada inyección intramuscular, dos veces al día. |
| 剂型、规格<br>Formulaciones y especificaciones | 注射用盐酸大观霉素：每支 2g；4g（附 0.9% 苯甲醇注射液 1 支）。<br>Clorhidrato de espectinomicina para inyección: 2g；4g cada una (se agrega una 0.9% inyección de alcohol bencílico). |

1.6　四环素类 Tetraciclina

| | |
|---|---|
| 药品名称 Drug Names | 四环素 Tetraciclina |
| 适应证<br>Indicaciones | 现主要用于立克次体病、布氏杆菌病、淋巴肉芽肿、支原体肺炎、螺旋体病、衣原体病，也可用于敏感的革兰阳性球菌或革兰阴性杆菌所引起的轻症感染。<br><br>Se usa para enfermedades por rickettsias, brucelosis, linfogranuloma venéreo, neumonía por micoplasma, leptospirosis y clamidiosis.También se puede usar para infección leve debido a cepas susceptibles de bacterias Gram-negativas o bacterias Gram-positivas. |
| 用法、用量<br>Administración y dosis | 口服：成人一日 3 ～ 4 次，每次 0.5g；8 岁以上小儿一日 30 ～ 40mg/kg，分 3 ～ 4 次用。<br><br>Se toma por vía oral: adultos 3 ～ 4 veces al día, 0.5g cada vez; niños mayores a 8 años de edad, 30 ～ 40mg/kg al día, en 3 ～ 4 veces. |
| 剂型、规格<br>Formulaciones y especificaciones | 片剂：每片 0.125g；0.25g。胶囊剂：每粒 0.25g。<br>Una tableta: 0.125g；0.25g. Una cápsula: 0.25g. |
| 药品名称 Drug Names | 土霉素 Oxitetraciclina |
| 适应证<br>Indicaciones | 现主要用于立克次体病、布氏杆菌病、淋巴肉芽肿、支原体肺炎、螺旋体病、衣原体病，也可用于敏感的革兰阳性球菌或革兰阴性杆菌所引起的轻症感染。<br><br>Se usa para enfermedades por rickettsias, brucelosis, linfogranuloma venéreo, neumonía por micoplasma, leptospirosis y clamidiosis.También se puede usar para infección leve debido a cepas susceptibles de bacterias Gram-negativas o bacterias Gram-positivas. |
| 用法、用量<br>Administración y dosis | 口服：每次 0.5g，一日 3 ～ 4 次。8 岁以上小儿每日 30 ～ 40mg/kg，分 3 ～ 4 次服用。<br><br>Se toma por vía oral: 0.5g cada vez, 3 ～ 4 veces al día. Niños mayores a 8 años de edad, 30 ～ 40mg/kg al día, en 3 ～ 4 veces. |

**续 表**

| 剂型、规格<br>Formulaciones y especificaciones | 片剂：每片 0.125g；0.25g（1mg= 盐酸土霉素 1000U）。<br>Una tableta: 0.125g；0.25g (1mg=1000 unidades de clorhidrato de oxitetraciclina). |
| --- | --- |
| 药品名称 Drug Names | 多西环素 Doxiciclina |
| 适应证<br>Indicaciones | 临床主要用于敏感的革兰阳性球菌和革兰阴性杆菌所致的上呼吸道感染、扁桃体炎、胆道感染、淋巴结炎、蜂窝织炎、老年慢性支气管炎等，也用于斑疹伤寒、恙虫病、支原体肺炎等。尚可用于治疗霍乱，也可用于预防恶性疟疾和钩端螺旋体感染。<br>En clínica se usa para infecciones del tracto respiratorio superior, amigdalitis, infección del tracto biliar, linfadenitis, celulitis y bronquitis crónica etc., así como tifus, tifus de los matorrales, la neumonía por micoplasma etc. debido a cepas susceptibles de bacterias Gram-positivas y bacterias Gram-negativas. También se puede usar para tratar cólera y prevenir falciparum malaria e infección por Leptospira. |
| 用法、用量<br>Administración y dosis | 口服，首次 0.2g，以后每次 0.1g，一日 1～2 次。8 岁以上儿童，首次 4mg/kg，以后每次 2～4mg/kg，一日 1～2 次。一般疗程为 3～7 日。预防恶性疟：每周 0.1g；预防钩端螺旋体病：每周 2 次，每次 0.1g。<br>Se toma por vía oral: 0.2g la primera vez, 0.1g cada vez en adelante, 1～2 veces al día. Niños mayores a 8 años, 4mg/kg la primera vez, 2～4mg/kg cada vez en adelante, 1～2 veces al día. El ciclo general es de 3～7 días. Prevención de falciparum malaria: 0.1g a la semana; prevención de leptospirosis: 0.1g cada vez, dos veces a la semana. |
| 剂型、规格<br>Formulaciones y especificaciones | 片剂：每片 0.05g；0.1g。胶囊剂：每粒 0.1g（1mg= 盐酸多西环素 1000U）。<br>Una tableta: 0.05g；0.1g. Una cápsula: 0.1g(1mg=1000 unidades de clorhidrato de doxiciclina). |
| 药品名称 Drug Names | 米诺环素 Minociclina |
| 适应证<br>Indicaciones | 临床主要用于立克次体病、支原体肺炎、淋巴肉芽肿、下疳、鼠疫、霍乱、布氏杆菌病（与链霉素联合应用）等引起的泌尿系、呼吸道、胆道、乳腺及皮肤软组织感染。<br>En clínica se usa para infecciones del tracto urinario, tracto respiratorio, tracto biliar, pecho, la piel y los tejidos blandos debido a rickettsiosis, neumonía por micoplasma, linfogranuloma venéreo, chancro, la peste, el cólera, la brucelosis (en combinación con estreptomicina). |
| 用法、用量<br>Administración y dosis | 成人一般首次量 200mg，以后每 12 小时服 100mg。或在首次量后，每 6 小时服用 50mg。<br>Generalmente, la primera dosis de adultos es de 200mg, y se toma 100mg cada 12 horas en adelante. O tras la primera dosis, se toma 50mg cada 6 horas. |
| 剂型、规格<br>Formulaciones y especificaciones | 片剂：每片 0.1g（效价）。<br>Una tableta: 0.1g(potencia). |

## 1.7 林可霉素类 Lincomicina

| 药品名称 Drug Names | 氯霉素 Cloramfenicol |
| --- | --- |
| 适应证<br>Indicaciones | 临床主要用于伤寒、副伤寒和其他沙门菌、脆弱拟杆菌感染。与氨苄西林合用于流感嗜血杆菌性脑膜炎。由脑膜炎球菌或肺炎链球菌引起的脑膜炎，在患者不宜用青霉素时，也可用本品。外用治疗沙眼或化脓菌感染。<br>En clínica se usa para tifoidea, paratifoidea e otras infecciones cuasadas por salmonella y bacteroides fragilis. Se usa en combinación con ampicilina para meningitis causada por haemophilus influenzae. En caso de pacientes con meningitis causada por bacteria meningocócica o neumocócica no deben utilizar la penicilina, también se puede optar este medicamento. En uso externo puede tratar clamidia o infección por bacterias piógenas. |
| 用法、用量<br>Administración y dosis | 口服：成人每次 0.25～0.5g，一日 1～2g；小儿每日 25～50mg/kg，分 3～4 次服用；新生儿每日不超过 25mg/kg。<br>静脉滴注：一日量为 1～2g，分 2 次注射。以输液稀释，1 支氯霉素（250mg）至少用稀释液 100ml。氯霉素注射液（含乙醇、甘油或丙二醇等溶媒），宜用干燥注射器抽取，边稀释边振荡，防止析出结晶。症状消退后应酌情减量或停药。 |

**续　表**

| | |
|---|---|
| | Se toma por vía oral: adultos: 0.25 ～ 0.5g cada vez, 1 ～ 2g al día; niños: 25 ～ 50mg/kg al día, en 3 ～ 4 veces; recién nacidos: la dosis diaria no sobrepasa 25mg/kg.<br><br>Goteo intravenoso: dosis diaria de 1 ～ 2g, dividida en dos inyecciones. Se diluye por la infusión: un cloranfenicol(250mg) con al menos 100ml del dilución. La inyección de cloranfenicol (incluyendo etanol, glicerol o propilenglicol disolvente) conviene extraerse por la jeringa secada y agitarse durante la dilución para evitar la precipitación de cristales. Después de que los síntomas desaparezcan, se debe reducir la dosis correspondientemente o dejar de administrarse por completo. |
| 剂型、规格<br>Formulaciones y especificaciones | 片剂（胶囊剂）：每片（粒）0.25g。注射液：每支 0.25g（2ml）。滴眼液：8ml（20mg）。滴耳液：10ml（0.25g）。眼膏：1%；3%。<br><br>Una tableta(cápsula): 0.25g. Una inyección: 0.25g(2ml). Gotas para los ojos: 8ml(20mg). Gotas para el oído:10ml(0.25g). Ungüento para los ojos: 1%；3%. |
| 药品名称 Drug Names | 林可霉素 Lincomicina |
| 适应证<br>Indicaciones | 用于葡萄球菌、链球菌、肺炎链球菌引起的呼吸道感染、骨髓炎、关节和软组织感染及胆道感染。对一些厌氧菌感染也可应用。外用治疗革兰阳性菌化脓性感染。<br><br>Se usa para infección del tracto repiratorio, osteomielitis, infecciones de articulaciones, tejidos blandos y tracto biliar debido a staphylococcus aureus, streptococcus pneumoniae y streptococcus. También se aplica a infecciones por anaerobios. En uso externo se puede tratar infecciones piógenas por bacterias Gram-positivas. |
| 用法、用量<br>Administración y dosis | 口服（空腹）：成人，每次 0.25 ～ 0.5g（活性），一日 3 ～ 4 次；小儿一日 30 ～ 50mg（活性）/kg，分 3 ～ 4 次服用。肌内注射：成人 1 次 0.6g（活性），一日 2 ～ 3 次；小儿一日 10 ～ 20mg（活性）/kg，分 2 ～ 3 次给药。静脉滴注：成人 1 次 0.6g（活性），溶于 100 ～ 200ml 输液内，滴注 1 ～ 2 小时，每 8 ～ 12 小时 1 次。<br><br>Se toma por vía oral(con estómago vacío): adultos, 0.25 ～ 0.5g a la vez(activo), 3 ～ 4 veces al día; niños, 30 ～ 50mg al día(activo), administrado en 3 ～ 4 veces. Inyección intramuscular: adultos, 0.6g a la vez(activo), 2 ～ 3 veces al día; niños, 10 ～ 20mg al día(activo), administrado en 2 ～ 3 veces. Infusión intravenosa: adultos, 0.6g a la vez(activo), disuelto en 100 ～ 200ml de infusión, por un período de 1 ～ 2 horas, cada 8 ～ 12 horas una vez. |
| 剂型、规格<br>Formulaciones y especificaciones | 片（胶囊）剂：每片（粒）0.25g（活性）；0.5g（活性）。注射液：每支 0.2g（活性）(1ml）；0.6g（活性）(2ml）。滴眼液：每支 3%（8ml）。<br><br>Una tableta（cápsula）：0.25g（activo）；0.5g（activo）. Una inyección：0.2g（activo）(1ml）；0.6g（activo）(2ml）. Gotas para los ojos: 3%（8ml）. |
| 药品名称 Drug Names | 克林霉素 Clindamicina |
| 适应证<br>Indicaciones | 主要用于厌氧菌（包括脆弱拟杆菌、产气荚膜杆菌、放线菌等）引起的腹腔和妇科感染（常需与氨基糖苷类联合以消除需氧病原菌）。还用于敏感的革兰阳性菌引起的呼吸道、关节和软组织、骨组织、胆道等感染及败血症、心内膜炎等。本品是金黄色葡萄球菌骨髓炎的首选治疗药物。<br><br>Se usa principalmente para infecciones abdominales y ginecológicas debido a anaerobios(incluyendo bacteroides fragilis, clostridium perfringens, actinomicetos, etc.). También se usa para blandos,tejido óseo, tracto biliar así como septicemia,endocarditis, etc. debido a bacterias Gram-positivas. Es la primera opción para tratar la osteomielitis causada por staphylococcus aureus.)infecciones del tracto repiratorio, articulaciones y tejidos . |
| 用法、用量<br>Administración y dosis | 盐酸盐口服：成人，每次 0.15 ～ 0.3g（活性），一日 3 ～ 4 次；小儿，每日 10 ～ 20mg（活性）/kg，分 3 ～ 4 次给予。棕榈酸酯盐酸盐（供儿童应用）：一日 8 ～ 12mg/kg，极严重时可增至 20 ～ 25mg/kg，分为 3 ～ 4 次给予；10kg 以下体重的婴儿可按一日 8 ～ 12mg/kg 用药，分为 3 次给予；磷酸酯（注射剂）：成人革兰阳性需氧菌感染，一日 600 ～ 1200mg，分为 2 ～ 4 次肌内注射或静脉滴注；厌氧菌感染，一般用一日 1200 ～ 2700mg，极严重感染可用到 4800mg/d。儿童（1 月龄以上），重症感染一日量 15 ～ 25mg/kg，极严重可按 25 ～ 40mg/kg，均分为 3 ～ 4 次应用。肌内注射量一次不超过 600mg，超过此量应静脉给予。静脉滴注前应先将药物用输液稀释，600mg 药物应加入不少于 100ml 输液中，至少输注 20 分钟。1 小时输注的药量不应超过 1200mg。 |

**续 表**

| | |
|---|---|
| | Clorhidrato orales: adultos, 0.15 ～ 0.3 a la vez(activo), 3 ～ 4 veces al día; niños, 10 ～ 20mg al día(activo), administrado en 3 ～ 4 veces. Hidrocloruro de palmitato(para niños): 8 ～ 12mg/kg al día, en casos graves se aumenta hasta 20 ～ 25mg/kg, administrado en 3 ～ 4 veces; bebés de peso corporal menos de 10kg, se administra 8 ～ 12mg/kg al día, en 3 veces; fosfato(inyección): adultos, infección por bacterias aeróbicas gram-positivas, 600 ～ 1200mg al día, en 2 ～ 4 veces por inyección intramuscular o infusión intravenosa; infecciones por anaerobios, 1200 ～ 2700mg al día, en casos pesados, puede alcanzar a 4800mg/d. Niños(mayores a un mes de edad), en casos de infecciones graves, dosis diaria de 15 ～ 25mg/kg, en casos pesados, 25 ～ 40mg/kg, en 3 ～ 4 veces. La dosis de una inyección intramuscular no sobrepasa 600mg, en dosis excesiva, se debe administra por vía intravenosa. Antes del goteo intravenoso, se debe diluir el medicamento en la infusión, 600mg del medicamento en no menos de 100ml de infusión por al menos 20 minutos. La dosis goteada en una hora no debe ser más de 1200mg. |
| 剂型、规格<br>Formulaciones y especificaciones | 盐酸克林霉素胶囊剂：每胶囊75mg（活性）；150mg（活性）。盐酸克林霉素注射液：每支 150mg（2ml）；300mg（2ml）；600mg（4ml）。<br><br>Una cápsula de clorhidrato de clindamicina: 75mg (activo); 150mg (activo). Una inyección de clorhidrato de clindamicina: 150mg(2ml)；300mg(2ml)；600mg(4ml). |
| **药品名称 Drug Names** | 甲砜霉素 Tiamfenicol |
| 适应证<br>Indicaciones | 临床主要用于伤寒、副伤寒和其他沙门菌感染，也用于敏感菌所致的呼吸道、胆道、尿路感染。<br><br>En clínica se usa para tifoidea, paratifoidea e otras infecciones causadas por salmonela. También se usa para infecciones del tracto respiratorio, tracto respiratorio y tracto urinario. |
| 用法、用量<br>Administración y dosis | 每次 0.25 ～ 0.5g，一日 3 ～ 4 次。<br>0.25 ～ 0.5g una vez, 3 ～ 4 veces al día. |
| 剂型、规格<br>Formulaciones y especificaciones | 片剂／胶囊剂：0.125g；0.25g。<br>Una tableta/cápsula: 0.125g；0.25g. |

1.8 大环内酯类 Macrolidos

| | |
|---|---|
| **药品名称 Drug Names** | 红霉素 Eritromicina |
| 适应证<br>Indicaciones | 临床主要应用于链球菌引起的扁桃体炎、猩红热、白喉及带菌者、淋病、李斯特菌病、肺炎链球菌下呼吸道感染（以上适用于不耐受青霉素的患者）。对于军团菌肺炎和支原体肺炎，本品可作为首选药应用。尚可应用于流感杆菌引起的上呼吸道感染、金黄色葡萄球菌皮肤及软组织感染、梅毒、肠道阿米巴病等。<br><br>En clínica se usa para amigdalitis, fiebre escarlatina, la difteria y portadores, gonorrea y listeriosis a causa del estreptococo, así como infecciones del tracto respiratorio inferior causadas por streptococcus pneumoniae( lo anterior se aplica a los pacientes que no toleran la penicilina). También se aplica a infecciones del tracto respiratorio superior causadas por haemophilus influenzae, infecciones de la piel y los tejidos blandos, sífilis, amebiasis intestinal etc. causadas por staphylococcus aureus. |
| 用法、用量<br>Administración y dosis | 口服：成人一日 1 ～ 2g，分 3 ～ 4 次服用，整片吞服；小儿，每日 30 ～ 50mg/kg，分 3 ～ 4 次服用。静脉滴注：成人一日 1 ～ 2g，分 3 ～ 4 次滴注；小儿每日 30 ～ 50mg/kg，分 3 ～ 4 次滴注。用时，将乳糖酸红霉素溶于 10ml 灭菌注射用水中，再添加到输液 500ml 中，缓慢滴入（最后稀释浓度一般小于 0.1%）。不能直接用含盐输液溶解。<br><br>Se toma por vía oral: adultos, 1 ～ 2g al día, en 3 ～ 4 veces, toda la pieza; niños, 30 ～ 50mg/kg al día, en 3 ～ 4 veces. Goteo intravenoso: 1 ～ 2g al día, en 3 ～ 4 veces; niños, 30 ～ 50mg/kg al día, en 3 ～ 4 veces. Al usarlo, se lo diluye en 10ml de agua eséril de inyección, se lo agrega a 500ml de infusión y se lo gotea lentamente(la concentración final de dilución es generalmente menor a 0.1%). No se lo puede diluir en la infusión de solución salina. |
| 剂型、规格<br>Formulaciones y especificaciones | 片剂（肠溶）：每片 0.1g（10 万 U）；0.125g（12.5 万 U）；0.25g（25 万 U）。注射用乳糖酸红霉素：每瓶 0.25g（25 万 U）；0.3g（30 万 U）。红霉素软膏：1%。红霉素眼膏：0.5%。<br><br>Una tableta (entérica): 0.1g(100000 unidades); 0.125g(125000 unidades); 0.25g(250000 unidades). Lactobionato de eritromicina para inyección: 0.25g(250000 unidades); 0.3g(300000 unidades) cada botella. Pomada de eritromicina: 1%. Ungüento para los ojos de eritromicina: 0.5%. |

续　表

| 药品名称 Drug Names | 琥乙红霉素 Eritromicina Etilsuccinato |
|---|---|
| 适应证<br>Indicaciones | 　　临床主要应用于链球菌引起的扁桃体炎、猩红热、白喉及带菌者、淋病、李斯特菌病、肺炎链球菌下呼吸道感染（以上适用于不耐青霉素的患者）。对于军团菌肺炎和支原体肺炎，本品可作为首选药应用。尚可应用于流感杆菌引起的上呼吸道感染、金黄色葡萄球菌皮肤及软组织感染、梅毒、肠道阿米巴病等。<br><br>　　En clínica se usa para amigdalitis, fiebre escarlatina, la difteria y portadores, gonorrea y listeriosis a causa del estreptococo, así como infecciones del tracto respiratorio inferior causadas por streptococcus pneumoniae( lo anterior se aplica a los pacientes que no toleran la penicilina). También se aplica a infecciones del tracto respiratorio superior causadas por haemophilus influenzae, infecciones de la piel y los tejidos blandos, sífilis, amebiasis intestinal etc. causadas por staphylococcus aureus. |
| 用法、用量<br>Administración y dosis | 　　口服：成人一次 0.25 ～ 0.5g，一日 3 ～ 4 次；小儿一日量 30 ～ 50mg/kg，分 3 ～ 4 次用。或按下列方案应用：体重＜ 5kg 者，1 次 40mg/kg，一日 4 次；5 ～ 7kg 者，1 次 50mg，一日 4 次；7 ～ 11kg 者，1 次 100mg，一日 4 次；11 ～ 23kg 者，1 次 200mg，一日 4 次；23 ～ 45kg 者，1 次 300mg，一日 4 次；＞ 45kg 者，按成人量给予。<br><br>　　Se toma por vía oral: para adultos 0.25 ～ 0.5g cada vez, 3 ～ 4 veces al día; para niños la dosis diaria de 30 ～ 50mg/kg, en 3 ～ 4 veces. O se lo aplica según el programa siguiente: los pacientes con peso corporal ＜ 5kg, 40mg/kg cada vez, 4 veces al día; de 5 ～ 7kg, 50mg cada vez, 4 veces al día; de 7 ～ 11kg, 100mg cada vez, 4 veces al día; de 11 ～ 23kg, 200mg cada vez, 4 veces al día; de 23 ～ 45kg, 300mg cada vez, 4 veces al día; ＞ 45kg, se los administra según la dosis de adultos. |
| 剂型、规格<br>Formulaciones y especificaciones | 　　片剂：每片 0.1g；0.125g（按红霉素计量）。<br>　　颗粒剂：每袋 0.05g；0.1g；0.125g；0.25g（按红霉素计量）。<br>　　Una tableta: 0.1g；0.125g(calculado en la dosis de eritromicina).<br>　　Gránulos: 0.05g；0.1g；0.125g；0.25g cada saco(calculado en la dosis de eritromicina). |
| 药品名称 Drug Names | 罗红霉素 Roxitromicina |
| 适应证<br>Indicaciones | 　　临床应用于上述敏感菌所致的呼吸道、泌尿道、皮肤和软组织、五官科感染。<br>　　En clínica se usa para infecciones del tracto respiratorio, tracto urinario, la piel y los tejidos blandos e infecciones ORL debido a cepas susceptibles. |
| 用法、用量<br>Administración y dosis | 　　成人 一次 150mg，一日 2 次，餐前服。幼儿：每次 2.5 ～ 5mg/kg，一日 2 次。老年人与肾功能一般减退者不需调整剂量。严重肝硬化者，每日 150mg。<br><br>　　Adultos: 150mg una vez, dos veces al día, antes de la comida. Niños: 2.5 ～ 5mg/kg una vez, dos veces al día. Para los ancianos y pacientes con insuficiencia renal la dosis no hace falta ajustar. Los pacientes con cirrosis severa, 150mg al día. |
| 剂型、规格<br>Formulaciones y especificaciones | 　　片剂：每片 150mg；250mg；300mg。<br>　　Una tableta: 150mg；250mg；300mg. |
| 药品名称 Drug Names | 克拉霉素 Claritromicina |
| 适应证<br>Indicaciones | 　　临床用于化脓性链球菌所致的咽炎和扁桃体炎，肺炎链球菌所致的急性中耳炎、肺炎和支气管炎，流感嗜血杆菌、卡他球菌所致支气管炎，支原体肺炎及葡萄球菌、链球菌所致皮肤及软组织感染。<br><br>　　En clínica se usa para infecciones de faringitis y amigdalitis debido a streptococcus pyogenes, otitis media aguda, neumonía y bronquitis debido a streptococcus pneumoniae, bronquitis y neumonía por micoplasma debido a haemophilus influenzae y bacterias catarral así como infecciones de la piel y los. tejidos blandos debido a staphylococcus aureus y streptococcus. |
| 用法、用量<br>Administración y dosis | 　　轻症：每次 250mg，重症每次 500mg，均为 12 小时 1 次口服，疗程 7 ～ 14 日。12 岁以上儿童按成人量。6 个月以上小儿至 12 岁以下儿童用量每日 15mg/kg，分为 2 次；或按以下方法口服给药：8 ～ 11kg 体重每次 62.5mg，12 ～ 19kg 体重每次 125mg，20 ～ 29kg 体重每次 187.5mg，30 ～ 40kg 体重每次 250mg，按上量一日用药 2 次。 |

|  | Síntomas leves: 250mg cada vez, síntomas graves: 500mg cada vez, por vía oral, cada 12 horas, ciclo de tratamiento 7 ~ 14 días. Para niños mayores de 12 años de edad se administra por la dosis de adultos. De infantes mayores a 6 meses de edad a niños menores a 12 años de edad: 15mg/kg añ día, en dos veces; o se administra por vía oral de la forma siguiente: peso corporal entre 8 ~ 11 kg, 62.5mg cada vez; 12 ~ 19kg, 125mg; 20 ~ 29kg, 187.5mg; 30 ~ 40kg, 250mg; la dosis de arriba, dos veces al día. |
|---|---|
| 剂型、规格<br>Formulaciones y especificaciones | 片剂：每片 250mg 或 500mg。<br>Una tableta: 250mg o 500mg. |
| **药品名称 Drug Names** | **阿奇霉素 Azitromicina** |
| 适应证<br>Indicaciones | 临床应用于敏感微生物所致的呼吸道、皮肤和软组织感染。<br>En clínica se usa para infecciones del tracto respiratorio, la piel y los tejidos blandos debido a microorganismos sensibles. |
| 用法、用量<br>Administración y dosis | 每日只需服 1 次，成人 500mg；儿童 10mg/kg，连用 3 日。<br>重症可注射给药，每日 1 次，每次 500mg，以注射用水 5ml 溶解后，加入 0.9% 氯化钠液或 5% 葡萄糖液中使成 1 ~ 2mg/ml 浓度，静脉滴注 1 ~ 2 小时，约 2 日症状控制后改成口服巩固疗效。<br>Sólo se toma una dosis al día, adultos 500mg; niños 10mg/kg, por tres días consecutivos. Síntomas graves: se administra por inyección, una vez al día, 500mg cada vez, disuelto en 5ml de agua de inyección, se agrega a la 0.9% solución de cloruro de sodio o 5% solución de glucosa para tener la concentración de 1 ~ 2mg/ml, se gotea por vena durante 1 ~ 2 horas y se controlan los síntomas tras dos días de inyección, se toma por vía oral para fortalecer los efectos. |
| 剂型、规格<br>Formulaciones y especificaciones | 片剂（胶囊）：每粒 250mg 或 500mg。乳糖酸阿奇霉素（冻干粉针）：每支 500mg。<br>Una tableta (cápsula): 250mg o 500mg. Lactobionato azitromicina(polvo liofilizado): 500mg cada uno. |
| **药品名称 Drug Names** | **泰利霉素 Telitromicina** |
| 适应证<br>Indicaciones | 临床主要用于敏感菌所致的呼吸道感染，包括社区获得性肺炎、慢性支气管炎、急性上颌窦咽炎及扁桃体炎。<br>En clínica se usa para infecciones del tracto respiratorio, tales como neumonía adquirida en la comunidad, la bronquitis crónica, faringitis maxilar aguda y amigdalitis debido a cepas susceptibles. |
| 用法、用量<br>Administración y dosis | 口服，一日 1 次 800mg，疗程 5 ~ 10 日。<br>Se toma por vía oral, 800mg una vez al día, con un ciclo de tratamiento de 5 ~ 10 días. |
| 剂型、规格<br>Formulaciones y especificaciones | 片剂：400mg；800mg。<br>Una tableta: 400mg；800mg. |
| **药品名称 Drug Names** | **地红霉素 Diritromicina** |
| 适应证<br>Indicaciones | 本品适用于敏感菌所致的轻、中度感染，慢性支气管炎（包括急性发作）、社区获得性肺炎、咽炎、扁桃体炎等。<br>Se usa para infecciones leves a moderadas, bronquitis crónica (incluyendo episodios agudos), neumonía adquirida en la comunidad, faringitis y amigdalitis debido a cepas susceptibles. |
| 用法、用量<br>Administración y dosis | 每次 500mg，每日 1 次，餐时服用，疗程根据病情为 7 ~ 14 日。<br>500mg cada vez, una vez al día, se toma durante la comida, con el ciclo de tratamiento de 7 ~ 14 días según la gravedad. |
| 剂型、规格<br>Formulaciones y especificaciones | 片剂（肠溶衣片）：每片 250mg。<br>Una tableta (con recubrimiento entérico): 250mg. |

**续　表**

| 药品名称 Drug Names | 吉他霉素 Kitasamicina |
| --- | --- |
| 适应证<br>Indicaciones | 可作为红霉素的替代品，用于上述敏感菌所致的口咽部、呼吸道、皮肤和软组织、胆道等感染。<br>Se usa como una alternativa a la eritromicina para infecciones del orofaríngeo, tracto respiratorio, la piel y los tejidos blandos así como el tracto biliar entre otros debido a cepas susceptibles. |
| 用法、用量<br>Administración y dosis | 口服：每次 0.3 ～ 0.4g，一日 3 ～ 4 次。静脉注射：1 次 0.2 ～ 0.4g，一日 2 ～ 3 次，将 1 次用量溶于 20ml 氯化钠注射液或葡萄糖液中，缓慢注射。<br>Se toma por vía oral: 0.3 ～ 0.4g cada vez, 3 ～ 4 veces al día. Inyección intravenosa: 0.2 ～ 0.4g cada vez, 2 ～ 3 veces al día, con una dosis disuelta en 20ml de inyección de cloruro de sodio o solución de glucosa, inyección lenta. |
| 剂型、规格<br>Formulaciones y especificaciones | 片剂：每片 0.1g。<br>注射用酒石酸吉他霉素：每瓶 0.2g。<br>Una tableta：0.1g.<br>Tartrato kitasamycin para inyección：0.1g cada botella. |
| 药品名称 Drug Names | 麦迪霉素 Midecamicina |
| 适应证<br>Indicaciones | 可作为红霉素的替代品，用于上述敏感菌所致的口咽部、呼吸道、皮肤和软组织、胆道等感染。<br>Se usa como una alternativa a la eritromicina para infecciones del orofaríngeo, tracto respiratorio, la piel y los tejidos blandos así como el tracto biliar entre otros debido a cepas susceptibles. |
| 用法、用量<br>Administración y dosis | 口服，成人一日量 0.8 ～ 1.2g，分 3 ～ 4 次服用。儿童一日量 30mg/kg，分 3 ～ 4 次给予。<br>Se toma por vía oral, la dosis diaria de adultos 0.8 ～ 1.2g, en 3 ～ 4 veces. La dosis diaria de niños 30mg/kg, en 3 ～ 4 veces. |
| 剂型、规格<br>Formulaciones y especificaciones | 麦迪霉素片：每片 0.1g。<br>Una tableta de midecamicina: 0.1g. |
| 药品名称 Drug Names | 乙酰麦迪霉素 Acetilmi-decamicina |
| 适应证<br>Indicaciones | 主要适用于金黄色葡萄球菌、溶血性链球菌、肺炎球菌等所致的呼吸道感染及皮肤、软组织感染，也可用于支原体肺炎。<br>Principalmente aplicable a infecciones de las vías respiratorias y la piel e infecciones de tejidos blandos por Staphylococcus aureus, bacteria streptococcus pneumoniae hemolíticas causadas, también se puede utilizar para la neumonía por micoplasma. |
| 用法、用量<br>Administración y dosis | 成人：一日 300 ～ 900mg，分 3 ～ 4 次服用。儿童：一日 15 ～ 30mg/kg，分 3 ～ 4 次给予。<br>Adultos: 300 ～ 900mg al día, en 3 ～ 4 veces. Niños: 15 ～ 30mg/kg al día, en 3 ～ 4 veces. |
| 剂型、规格<br>Formulaciones y especificaciones | 醋酸乙酰麦迪霉素颗粒剂：1.0g；0.2g；干混悬剂：0.1g。<br>Acetil acetato midecamicina gránulos: 1.0 g: 0.2 g; suspensión seca: 0.1g. |
| 药品名称 Drug Names | 交沙霉素 Josamicina |
| 适应证<br>Indicaciones | 临床应用于敏感菌所致的口咽部、呼吸道、肺、鼻窦、中耳、皮肤及软组织、胆道等部位的感染。<br>En clínica se usa para infecciones del orofaríngeo, tracto respiratorio, pulmones, senos, oído medio, la piel y los tejidos blandos, tracto biliar entre otras partes debido a cepas susceptibles. |
| 用法、用量<br>Administración y dosis | 成人：一日量 0.8 ～ 1.2g，分 3 ～ 4 次服用。儿童：一日量为 30mg/kg，分 3 ～ 4 次给予。空腹服用吸收好。<br>Adultos: 0.8 ～ 1.2g al día, en 3 ～ 4 veces. Niños: 30mg/kg al día, en 3 ～ 4 veces. Se absorbe bien con el estómago vacío. |
| 剂型、规格<br>Formulaciones y especificaciones | 交沙霉素片剂：每片 0.1g。丙酸交沙霉素散剂：每包含药 0.1g（效价）。<br>Una tableta de Josamicina: 0.1g. Josamicina polvo propionato: cada saco contiene 0.1g(potencia). |

**续 表**

| 药品名称 Drug Names | 麦白霉素 Meleumicina |
|---|---|
| 适应证<br>Indicaciones | 用于敏感菌所致的呼吸道感染、皮肤感染、软组织感染、胆道感染、支原体性肺炎等。<br><br>Infecciones del tracto respiratorio, infecciones de la piel, infecciones de tejidos blandos, infecciones del tracto biliar, neumonía por micoplasma, causadas por las cepas sensibles. |
| 用法、用量<br>Administración y dosis | 成人一日量 0.8 ～ 1.2g，分 3 ～ 4 次服用。儿童一日量 30mg/kg，分 3 ～ 4 次服用。<br><br>Adultos: 0.8 ～ 1.2g al día, en 3 ～ 4 veces. Niños: 30mg/kg al día, en 3 ～ 4 veces. |
| 剂型、规格<br>Formulaciones y especificaciones | 片剂：每片 0.1g。<br>Una tableta：0.1g. |

| 药品名称 Drug Names | 罗他霉素 Rokitamicina |
|---|---|
| 适应证<br>Indicaciones | 临床应用于上述敏感菌所致的咽、扁桃体、支气管、肺、中耳、鼻旁窦、牙周、皮肤及软组织等部位的感染。<br><br>En clínica se usa para infecciones del faringe, amígdalas, bronquio, pulmones, senos, oído medio, la piel y los tejidos blandos y periodontal entre otras partes debido a cepas susceptibles. |
| 用法、用量<br>Administración y dosis | 口服，成人每次 200mg，一日 3 次。儿童：一日量 20 ～ 30mg/kg，分 3 次服用。<br><br>Se toma por vía oral: adultos: 200mg una vez, 3 veces al día. Niños: 20 ～ 30mg/kg al día, en 3 veces. |
| 剂型、规格<br>Formulaciones y especificaciones | 片剂：每片 100mg。<br>Una tableta: 100mg. |

| 药品名称 Drug Names | 乙酰螺旋霉素 Acetilspiramicina |
|---|---|
| 适应证<br>Indicaciones | 适用于上述敏感菌所致的扁桃体炎、支气管炎、肺炎、咽炎、中耳炎、皮肤和软组织感染、乳腺炎、胆囊炎、猩红热、牙科和眼科感染等。<br><br>Se usa para amigdalitis, bronquitis, neumonía, faringitis, otitis media, infecciones de la piel y los tejidos blandos, mastitis, colecistitis, escarlatina, infecciones dentales y oculares entre otras debido a cepas susceptibles. |
| 用法、用量<br>Administración y dosis | 成人一次 0.2g，一日 4 ～ 6 次。重症一日可用至 1.6 ～ 2g。儿童一日量 30mg/kg，分 4 次给予。<br><br>Adultos 0.2g una vez, 4 ～ 6 veces al día. Síntomas graves: la dosis diaria puede alcanzar a 1.6 ～ 2g. La dosis diaria de niños es de 30mg/kg, en 4 veces. |
| 剂型、规格<br>Formulaciones y especificaciones | 乙酰螺旋霉素片（肠溶）剂：每片 0.1g（效价）。<br>Una tableta de acetylspiramycin(entérica): 0.1g(potencia). |

1.9 糖肽类 Glucopéptidos

| 药品名称 Drug Names | 去甲万古霉素 Norvancomicina |
|---|---|
| 适应证<br>Indicaciones | 主要用于葡萄球菌（包括产酶株和耐甲氧西林株）、肠球菌（耐氨苄西林株）、难辨梭状芽孢杆菌等所致的系统感染和肠道感染，如心内膜炎、败血症，以及假膜性肠炎等。<br><br>Se usa para infecciones sistemáticas e intestinales tales como endocarditis, septicemia así como colitis seudomembranosa etc. debido a estafilococo(incluyendo cepas productoras y cepas resistentes a la meticilina), enterococcus(resistente a la ampicilina) y clostridium difficile entre otros. |
| 用法、用量<br>Administración y dosis | 口服（治疗假膜性肠炎）：成人一次 0.4g，每 6 小时 1 次，每日量不可超过 4g；儿童酌减。静脉滴注：成人一日量 0.8 ～ 1.6g，1 次或分次给予；小儿一日量 16 ～ 24mg/kg，1 次或分次给予。一般将 1 次量的药物先用 10ml 灭菌注射用水溶解，再加入到适量等渗氯化钠注射液或葡萄糖输液中，缓慢滴注。如采取连续滴注给药，则可将一日量药物加到 24 小时内所用的输液中给予。 |

| | Se toma por vía oral( para tratar colitis seudomembranosa): adultos 0.4g cada vez, con intervalo de 6 horas, la dosis diaria no sobrepasa 4g; la dosis para niños con reducciones apropiadas. Goteo intravenoso: dosis diaria de adultos 0.8 ～ 1.6g, dividida en una o varias veces; dosis diaria de niños 16 ～ 24mg/kg, dividida en una o varias veces. Generalmente se diluye una dosis en 10ml de agua estéril para inyección y se agrega cierta cantidad de inyección isotónica de cloruro de sodio o infusión de glucosa para efectuar el goteo lentamente. Si se adopta la administración de infusión continua, se puede agregar la dosis diaria a la infusión dada por 24 horas. |
|---|---|
| 剂型、规格<br>Formulaciones y especificaciones | 注射用盐酸去甲万古霉素：每瓶 0.4g（40 万 U）［相当万古霉素约 0.5g（50 万 U）］。<br>Clorhidrato Norvancomycin para inyección: 0.4g cada botella(400000 unidades)[equivalente a 0.5g de vancomicina(500000 unidades)]. |
| 药品名称 Drug Names | 万古霉素 Vancomicina |
| 适应证<br>Indicaciones | 临床用于革兰阳性菌严重感染，尤其是对其他抗菌药耐药的耐甲氧西林菌株。血液透析患者发生葡萄球菌属所致的动静脉分流感染。口服用于对甲硝唑无效的假膜性结肠炎或多重耐药葡萄球菌小肠结肠炎。<br>En clínica se usa para infecciones graves debido a bacterias Gram-positivas, sobre todo cepas resistentes a la meticilina resistente a otros antimicrobianos. Se usa para infección de la derivación arteriovenosa causada por el estafilococo en pacientes sometidos a hemodiálisis. Se toma por vía oral para tratar colitis pseudomembranosa inválido de metronidazol o multirresistente staphylococcus enterocolitis. |
| 用法、用量<br>Administración y dosis | 口服：每次 125 ～ 500mg，每 6 小时 1 次，每日剂量不宜超过 4g，疗程 5 ～ 10 日；小儿 1 次 10mg/kg，每 6 小时 1 次，疗程 5 ～ 10 日。<br>静脉滴注：全身感染，成人每 6 小时 7.5mg/kg，或每 12 小时 15mg/kg。严重感染，可一日 3 ～ 4g 短期应用；新生儿（0 ～ 7 日）首次 15mg/kg，以后 10mg/kg，每 12 小时给药 1 次；婴儿（7 日～ 1 个月）首次 15mg/kg，以后 10mg/kg，每 8 小时给药 1 次；儿童每次 10mg/kg，每 6 小时给药 1 次，或每次 20mg/kg，每 12 小时 1 次。<br>Se toma por vía oral: 125 ～ 500mg cada vez, con intervalo de 6 horas, la dosis diaria no debe sobrepasar 4g, con ciclo de tratamiento de 5 ～ 10 días; niños 10mg/kg cada vez, con intervalo de 6 horas, con ciclo de tratamiento de 5 ～ 10 días.<br>Infusiión intravenosa: infección sistémica, adultos 7.5mg/kg, con intervalo de 6 horas, o 15mg/kg, con intervalo de 12 horas. Infecciones graves, 3 ～ 4g al día a corto plazo; recién nacidos(de 0 ～ 7 días) 15mg/kg la primera dosis, 10mg/kg en adelante, una administración cada 12 horas; bebés(de 7 días a un mes) 15mg/kg la primera dosis, 10mg/kg en adelante, una administración cada 8 horas; niños 10mg/kg cada vez, cada 6 horas o 20mg/kg cada vez, cada 12 horas. |
| 剂型、规格<br>Formulaciones y especificaciones | 胶囊：每粒 20mg；250mg。注射用盐酸万古霉素：每支 0.5g；1.0g。<br>Una cápsula: 20mg；250mg. Clorhidrato de vancomicina para inyección: 0.5g；1.0g cada una. |
| 药品名称 Drug Names | 替考拉宁 Teicoplanina |
| 适应证<br>Indicaciones | 临床用于耐甲氧西林金黄色葡萄球菌和耐氨苄西林肠球菌所致的系统感染（对中枢感染无效）。本类药物（万古霉素与本品）现用于上述适应证，其目的是防止过度应用（即用于其他抗生素能控制的一些病原菌感染而造成耐药菌滋长）。<br>En clínica se usa para infección sistemática debido a staphylococcus aureus resistente a la meticilina y enterococos resistentes a la ampicilina(inválida para infección del sistema nervioso central). Este tipo de medicamentos(vancomicina y éste) ahora se aplican a los casos anteriores con el fin de prevenir la aplicación excesiva( Es decir si se usa para infecciones de cepas que se pueden controlar otros antibióticos, ayudará a crecer cepas resistentes). |
| 用法、用量<br>Administración y dosis | 首剂（第一日）400mg，次日开始每日 200mg，静脉注射或肌内注射；严重感染，每次 400mg，一日 2 次，3 日后减为一日 200 ～ 400mg。用前以注射用水溶解，静脉注射应不少于 1 分钟。若采取静脉滴注，则将药物加入 0.9% 氯化钠溶液中，静脉滴注不少于 30 分钟。也可采用肌内注射。<br>La primera dosis(el primer día) 400mg, en adelante 200mg al día, por inyección intravenosa o intramuscular; infecciones graves 400mg cada vez, dos veces al día, reducido al 200 ～ 400mg al día dentro de 3 días. Antes del uso, se disuelve en agua para inyección y la inyección no debe ser menos de un minuto. Si se adopta la infusión intravenosa, se agega el medicamento a 0.9% solución de cloruro de sodio con un período no menos a 30 minutos. También se puede adoptar inyección intramuscular. |

**续　表**

| 剂型、规格<br>Formulaciones y especificaciones | 粉针：每支 200mg；400mg。<br>Una inyección de polvo: 200mg；400mg。 |
|---|---|

### 1.10　其他抗菌抗生素 Otros antibióticos antibacterianos

| 药品名称 Drug Names | 磷霉素 Fosfomicina |
|---|---|
| 适应证<br>Indicaciones | 临床主要用于敏感菌引起的尿路、皮肤及软组织、肠道等部位感染。对肺部、脑膜感染和败血症也可考虑应用。可与其他抗生素联合治疗由敏感菌所致重症感染。也可与万古霉素合用治疗 MRSA 感染。<br><br>En clínica se usa para infecciones del tracto urinario, la piel y tejidos blandos y tracto intestinal entre otras partes debido a cepas susceptibles. Considere la posibilidad de la aplicación para infección de pulmones, infección meníngea y septicemia. También se puede usar en combinación con otros antibiótocos para tratar infecciones graves debido a cepas susceptibles. También se puede usar en combinación con vancomicina para tratar infección MRSA. |
| 用法、用量<br>Administración y dosis | 口服磷霉素钙，适用于尿路感染及轻症感染，成人 2～4g/d，儿童一日量为 50～100mg/kg，分 3～4 次服用。静脉注射或静脉滴注磷霉素钠，用于中度或重度系统感染，成人 4～12g/d，重症可用到 16g/d；儿童一日量为 100～300mg/kg，均分为 2～4 次给予。1g 药物至少应用 10ml 溶剂，如一次用数克，则应按每 1g 药物用 25ml 溶剂的比率进行溶解，予以静脉滴注或缓慢静脉注射。适用的溶剂有：灭菌注射用水、5%～10% 葡萄糖液、0.9% 氯化钠注射液、含乳酸钠的输液等。<br><br>Administración oral de calcio fosfomicina: aplicada a infección urinaria e infecciones leves, adultos, 2～4g/d, niños, dosis diaria de 50～100mg/kg, administrada en 3～4 veces. Inyección intravenosa o infusión intravenosa de fosfomicina, para infecciones sistémicas moderadas o graves, adultos, 4～12g/d, en síntomas graves, se puede alcanzar a 16g/d; niños: dosis diaria de 100～300mg/kg, administrada en 2～4 veces. Se disuelve 1g del medicamento en al menos 10ml de solución, si se administra varios gramos en una vez, se disuelve 1g del medicamento en 25ml de solución como proporción por infusión intravenosa o inyección lenta intravenosa. Solución apropiada: agua estéril para inyección, 5%～10% solución de glucosa, 0.9% inyección de cloruro de sodio, infusión de lactato de sodio, etc. |
| 剂型、规格<br>Formulaciones y especificaciones | 磷霉素钙胶囊：每粒 0.1g；0.2g；0.5g。<br>注射用磷霉素钠：每瓶 1g；4g。<br>Una cápsula de calcio fosfomicina：0.1g；0.2g；0.5g.<br>Inyección de fosfomicina：1g；4g cada botella. |

| 药品名称 Drug Names | 达托霉素 Daptomicina |
|---|---|
| 适应证<br>Indicaciones | 临床用于复杂性皮肤及皮肤软组织感染。<br>En clínica se usa para infecciones complicadas de la piel e infecciones de la piel y tejidos blandos. |
| 用法、用量<br>Administración y dosis | 静脉注射：每次 4mg/kg，一日 1 次，连续用药 7～14 日。肌酐清除率低于 30ml/min 者，每次 4mg/kg，每 2 日 1 次。<br><br>Inyección intravenosa: 4mg/kg cada vez, una vez al día, por 7～14 días consecutivos. Los pacientes con aclaramiento de creatinina menor a 30ml/min, 4mg/kg cada vez, una vez cada dos días. |
| 剂型、规格<br>Formulaciones y especificaciones | 注射用达托霉素：每支 250mg；500mg。<br>Una inyección de daptomicina: 250mg；500mg。 |

| 药品名称 Drug Names | 利福昔明 Rifaximina |
|---|---|
| 适应证<br>Indicaciones | 临床用于敏感菌所致的肠道感染，预防胃肠道围术期感染性并发症，也可用于高氨血症的辅助治疗。<br><br>En clínica se usa para infecciones intestinales debido a cepas susceptibles, prevención de complicaciones infecciosas de la operación gastrointestinal perioperatoria así como tratamiento adyuvante del hiperamonemia. |

**续　表**

| | |
|---|---|
| 用法、用量<br>Administración y dosis | 口服，肠道感染：成人每次 200mg，一日 4 次，连续使用 5～7 日。6～12 岁儿童，每次 100～200mg，一日 4 次。手术前后预防感染：成人每次 400mg，6～12 岁儿童每次 200～400mg，一日 2 次，在手术前 3 日给药。高氨血症的辅助治疗：成人每次 400mg，疗程 7～21 日。6～12 岁儿童每次 200～300mg，一日 3 次。<br><br>Se toma por vía oral, infecciones intestinales: adultos, 200mg cada vez, cuatro veces al día, por 5～7 días consecutivos. Niños de 6～12 años de edad, 100～200mg cada vez, cuatro veces al día. Prevención de infecciones postoperarias y preoperarias: adultos, 400mg cada vez, niños de 6～12 años de edad, 200～400mg cada vez, dos veces al día, se administra tres días antes de la operación. Tratamiento adyuvante del hiperamonemia: adultos, 400mg cada vez, ciclo de tratamiento 7～21 días. Niños de 6～12 años de edad, 200～300mg cada vez, tres veces al día. |
| 剂型、规格<br>Formulaciones y especificaciones | 片剂（胶囊剂）：每片（粒）200mg。<br>Una tabletaz(cápsula): 200mg. |
| 药品名称 Drug Names | 多黏菌素 B　Polimixina B |
| 适应证<br>Indicaciones | 临床主要应用于铜绿假单胞菌及其他假单胞菌引起的创面、尿路及眼、耳、气管等部位感染，也可用于败血症。鞘内注射用于铜绿假单胞菌脑膜炎。<br><br>En clínica se usa para infecciones de la herida, el tracto urinario, los ojos, oídos, la tráquea entre otras partes debido a pseudomonas aeruginosa y otras pseudomonas. También se puede usar para la septicemia. Con la inyección intratecal puede tratar meningitis por pseudomonas aeruginosa. |
| 用法、用量<br>Administración y dosis | 静脉滴注：成人及儿童肾功能正常者一日 1.5～2.5mg/kg（一般不超过 2.5mg/kg），分 2 次给予，每 12 小时静脉滴注 1 次。每 50mg 本品，以 5% 葡萄糖液 500ml 稀释后滴入。婴儿肾功能正常者可耐受一日 4mg/kg 的用量。肌内注射：成人及儿童一日 2.5～3mg/kg，分次给予，每 4～6 小时用药 1 次。婴儿一日量可用到 4mg/kg，新生儿可用到 4.5mg/kg，滴眼液浓度 1～2.5mg/ml。<br><br>Infusión intravenosa: adultos y niños con función renal normal, 1.5～2.5mg/kg al día(generalmente no sobrepasa 2.5mg/kg), administrado en dos veces, cada 12 horas. Se disuelve 50mg del medicamento en 500ml de 5% solución de glucosa disolvente. Bebés con función renal normal pueden tolerar la dosis diaria de 4mg/kg. Inyección intramuscular: adultos y niños, 2.5～3mg/kg al día, dividido en varias veces, se administra cada 4～6 horas una vez. La dosis diaria de bebés puede alcanzar a 4mg/kg y la dosis diaria de recén nacidos puede alcanzar a 4.5mg/kg. La concentración de gotas es de 1～2.5mg/ml. |
| 剂型、规格<br>Formulaciones y especificaciones | 注射用硫酸多黏菌素 B：每瓶 50mg（1mg=10 000U）。<br>Polimixina B Sulfato para inyección: 50mg cada botella(1mg=10 000 unidades). |
| 药品名称 Drug Names | 黏菌素 Colistina |
| 适应证<br>Indicaciones | 用于治疗大肠埃希菌性肠炎和对其他药物耐药的菌痢。外用于烧伤和外伤引起的铜绿假单胞菌局部感染和耳、咽等部位敏感菌感染。<br><br>Se usa para tratar enteritis por E. coli y disentería resistente a otros fármacos. Con uso externo, se usa para quemadura, trauma causado por infección local Pseudomonas aeruginosa e infecciones de los oídos y faringe entre otras partes debido a cepas susceptibles. |
| 用法、用量<br>Administración y dosis | 口服：成人一日 150 万～300 万 U，分 3 次服。儿童 1 次量 25 万～50 万 U，一日 3～4 次。重症时上述剂量可加倍。外用：溶液剂 1 万～5 万 U/ml，氯化钠注射液溶解。<br><br>Se toma por vía oral: adultos entre 1.5 y 3 millones de unidades al día, dividida en tres veces. Niños: entre 0.25 y 0.5 millones de unidades una vez, 3～4 veces al día. En casos graves, la dosis puede duplicarse. Uso exterior: solución de 10000～50000 unidades/ml, disuelta en la inyección de de cloruro de sodio. |
| 剂型、规格<br>Formulaciones y especificaciones | 片剂：每片 50 万 U；100 万 U；300 万 U。灭菌粉剂：每瓶 100 万 U，供制备溶液用（1mg=6500U）。<br>Una tableta: 500 000 unidades; 1 000 000 unidades; 3 000 000 unidades. Inyección de polvo estéril: 1 000 000 unidades cada botella, para preparar la solución (1mg=6500 unidades). |

**续 表**

| 药品名称 Drug Names | 夫西地酸钠 Fusidato de sodio |
|---|---|
| 适应证<br>Indicaciones | 　　主治由各种敏感细菌，尤其是葡萄球菌引起的各种感染，如骨髓炎、败血症、心内膜炎，反复感染的囊型纤维化、肺炎、皮肤及软组织感染，外科及创伤性感染等。<br><br>　　Se usa principalmente todo tipo de infecciones tales como osteomielitis, septicemia, endocarditis, infecciones recurrentes de fibrosis quística, neumonía, infecciones de piel y tejidos blandos, infecciones quirúrgicas y traumáticas,etc. debido a cepas susceptibles, sobre todo estafilococo. |
| 用法、用量<br>Administración y dosis | 　　口服：每8小时500mg，重症感染可加倍服用；儿童1岁以下，每日50mg/kg，分次给予；1～5岁，每次250mg，一日3次；5～12岁，可按成人量给予。静脉滴注：成人每次500mg，一日3次；儿童及婴儿每日20mg/kg，分3次给药。将本品500mg溶于10ml所附的无菌缓冲溶液中，然后用氯化钠注射液或5%葡萄糖注射液稀释至250～500ml静脉输注。若葡萄糖注射液过酸，溶液会呈乳状，如出现此情况即不能使用。输注时间不应少于2～4小时。<br><br>　　Se toma por vía oral: 500mg cada 8 horas, en casos graves, la dosis puede duplicarse; niños menores a un años de edad, 50mg/kg al día, dividida en varias veces; 1～5 años de edad, se administra con la cantidad dada a adultos. Infusión intravenosa: adultos, 500mg cada vez, tres veces al día; niños y bebés: 20mg/kg al día, administrado en tres veces. Se disuelve 500mg del medicamento en 10ml de solución tampón estéril, y se diluye en 250～500ml de inyección de cloruro de sodio o 5% inyección de glucosa para efectuar infusión intravenosa. Si la inyección de glucosa es demasiado ácida, la solución será lechosa, en este caso, no se puede utilizarlo. El período de infusión no debe ser inferior a 2～4 horas. |
| 剂型、规格<br>Formulaciones y especificaciones | 　　片剂：每片250mg。注射用夫西地酸：每瓶500mg（钠盐）；580mg（二乙醇胺盐）。<br><br>　　Una tableta: 250mg. Fusidato de sodio para inyección: 500mg cada botella (sodio); 580mg(dietanolamina). |

2. 化学合成的抗菌药 Medicamentos antibacterianos sintéticos

2.1　磺胺类 Sulfamidas

| 药品名称 Drug Names | 磺胺嘧啶 Sulfadiazina |
|---|---|
| 适应证<br>Indicaciones | 　　防治敏感脑膜炎球菌所致的流行性脑膜炎。<br>　　Se usa para prevenir y tratar epidemia de meningitis debido a meningococo sensible. |
| 用法、用量<br>Administración y dosis | 　　口服：成人：预防脑膜炎，1次1g，一日2g；治疗脑膜炎：1次1g，一日4g。儿童：一般感染，可按一日50～75mg/kg，分为2次服用；流脑：则按一日100～150mg/kg应用。缓慢静脉注射或静脉滴注：治疗严重感染，成人1次1～1.5g，一日3～4.5g。本品注射液为钠盐，需用灭菌注射用水或等渗氯化钠注射液稀释，静脉注射时浓度应低于5%；静脉滴注时浓度约为1%（稀释20倍），混匀后应用。<br><br>　　Se toma por vía oral: adultos: para prevenir meningitis, 1g cada vez, 2g al día; para tratar meningitis: 1g cada vez, 4g al día. Niños: infecciones comunes, se administra 50～75mg/kg al día, en dos veces; epidemia de meningitis: se aplica 100～150mg/kg al día. Inyección lenta o infusión intravenosa: para tratar infecciones graves, adultos 1～1.5g cada vez, 3～4.5g al día. La inyección del medicamento es sal sódica, y se debe diluirlo en agua estéril para inyección o inyección isotónica de cloruro de sodio. Se aplica tras la mezcla homogénea con una concentración inferior a 5% en la inyección intravenosa y cerca de 1% en la infusión intravenosa(diluido 20 veces). |
| 剂型、规格<br>Formulaciones y especificaciones | 　　片剂：每片0.5g。磺胺嘧啶混悬液：10%（g/ml）。磺胺嘧啶钠注射液：每支0.4g（2ml）；1g（5ml）。注射用磺胺嘧啶钠：每瓶0.4g；1g。复方磺胺嘧啶（双嘧啶，SD-TMP）片：每片含磺胺嘧啶（SD）400mg和甲氧苄啶（TMP）50mg。本品的治疗效果约与复方磺胺甲噁唑（SMZ-TMP）片相近。<br><br>　　Una tableta: 0.5g. Una suspensión de sulfadiazina: 10%(g/ml).Una inyección de sodio sulfadiazina: 0.4g(2ml);1g(5ml). Sodio sulfadiazina para inyección: 0.4g;1g cada botella. Sulfadiazina Compuesto (doble pirimidina, SD-TMP) pieza: 400mg de sulfadiazina(SD) y 50mg de trimetoprima(TMP). El efecto del tratamiento es similar al sulfametoxazol(SMZ-TMP). |
| 药品名称 Drug Names | 磺胺甲噁唑 Sulfametoxazol |
| 适应证<br>Indicaciones | 　　用于急性支气管炎、肺部感染、尿路感染、伤寒、布氏杆菌病、菌痢等，疗效与氨苄西林、氯霉素、四环素等相近。<br><br>　　Se usa para bronquitis aguda, infección pulmonar, infecciones del tracto urinario, fiebre tifoidea, brucelosis, disentería etc. La eficacia es similar a ampicilina, cloranfenicol, tetraciclina, etc. |

**续　表**

| 用法、用量<br>Administración y dosis | 一日 2 次，每次服 1g。<br>Dos veces al día, 1g cada vez. |
|---|---|
| 剂型、规格<br>Formulaciones y especificaciones | 片剂：每片 0.5g。复方磺胺甲噁唑（复方新诺明，SMZ-TMP）片：每片含 SMZ0.4g、TMP0.08g。联磺甲氧苄啶片（增效联磺片）：每片含 SMZ0.2g、SD0.2g、TMP0.08g。复方磺胺甲噁唑（复方新诺明；SMZ-TMP）注射液：每支 2ml，含 SMZ0.4g、TMP0.08g。<br><br>Una tableta: 0.5g. Sulfametoxazol (Bactrim, SMZ-TMP) pieza: 0.4g de SMZ, 0.08g de TMP. Tableta trimetoprim sulfametoxazol (tableta plug-sulfametoxazol): 0.2g de SMZ, 0.2g de SD, 0.08g de TMP. El sulfametoxazol (Bactrim, SMZ-TMP) inyección: 2ml, 0.4g de SMZ, 0.08g de TMP. |
| **药品名称 Drug Names** | 柳氮磺吡啶 Sulfasalazina |
| 适应证<br>Indicaciones | 用于治疗轻中度溃疡性结肠炎，活动期的克罗恩病，类风湿关节炎。<br><br>Se usa para tratar la colitis ulcerosa leve a moderada, el período de actividad de la enfermedad de Crohn y artritis reumatoide. |
| 用法、用量<br>Administración y dosis | 口服：治疗溃疡性结肠炎，1 次 0.5 ~ 1g，一日 2 ~ 4g。如需要可逐渐增量至一日 4 ~ 6g，好转后减量为一日 1.5g，直至症状消失。也可用于灌肠，一日 2g，混悬于生理盐水 20 ~ 50ml 中，作保留灌肠，也可添加白及粉以增大药液黏滞度。治疗类风湿关节炎：用肠溶片，每次 1g（4 片），一日 2 次。直肠给药：重症患者，1 次 0.5g，早、中、晚各 1 次。轻、中度患者，早、晚各 0.5g。症状明显改善后，每晚或隔日睡前 0.5g。用药后需侧卧半小时。<br><br>Se toma por vía oral: para tratar colitis ulcerosa, 0.5 ~ 1g cada vez, 2 ~ 4g al día. En casos necesarios, se puede aumentar la dosis gradualmente hasta 4 ~ 6g al día y cuando se mejore, se podrá reducir la dosis a 1.5g al día, hasta que los síntomas desaparezcan. También se puede aplicar al enema, 2g al día, suspendido en 20 ~ 50ml de solución salina. En un enema de retención, también se pueden agregar polvo rhizoma bletillae para aumentar la viscosidad del líquido. Para tratar artritis reumatoide: se usan tabletas con recubrimiento entérico, 1g cada vez(4 tabletas), dos veces al día. Se administra por vía rectal: pacientes con síntomas graves, 0.5g cada vez, una vez por la mañana, mediodía y tarde respectivamente. Pacientes con síntomas leves y moderados, 0.5g por la mañana, mediodía y tarde respectivamente. Cuando se mejoran los síntomas significativamente, se toma 0.5g todas las noches o antes de acostarse cada dos días. Tras la administración, se debe acostarse sobre un lado por media hora. |
| 剂型、规格<br>Formulaciones y especificaciones | 片剂：每片 0.25g。栓剂：每个 0.5g。肠溶片：每片 0.25g。<br>Una tableta: 0.25g. Un supositorio: 0.5g. Una tableta con recubrimiento entérico: 0.25g. |

2.2　甲氧苄啶类 Trimetoprima

| **药品名称 Drug Names** | 甲氧苄啶 Trimetoprima |
|---|---|
| 适应证<br>Indicaciones | 常与磺胺药合用（多应用复方制剂）于治疗肺部感染、急慢性支气管炎、菌痢、尿路感染、肾盂肾炎、肠炎、伤寒、疟疾等，也与多种抗生素合用。本品单独可应用于大肠埃希菌、奇异变形杆菌、肺炎克雷伯杆菌、肠杆菌属、凝固酶阴性的金黄色葡萄球菌所致单纯性尿路感染。本品单用易引起细菌耐药，故不宜单独用。<br><br>Se usa frecuentemente en combinación con las sulfamidas(preparación compuesta de múltiples aplicaciones) para tratar infección pulmonar, bronquitis aguda y crónica, disentería, infección del tracto urinario, pielonefritis, enteritis, fiebre tifoidea, malaria, etc. También se usa en combinación con una variedad de antibióticos. Este medicamento solo se puede aplicar a las infecciones del tracto urinario no complicadas causadas por E. coli, proteus mirabilis, klebsiella pneumoniae, enterobacter y staphylococcus coagulasa - negativos.Este producto por sí solo puede conducir a la resistencia bacteriana, por lo que no debe ser utilizado solo. |
| 用法、用量<br>Administración y dosis | 口服，每次 0.1 ~ 0.2g，一日 0.2 ~ 0.4g。<br>Se toma por vía oral: 0.1 ~ 0.2g cada vez, 0.2 ~ 0.4g al día. |
| 剂型、规格<br>Formulaciones y especificaciones | 片剂：每片 0.1g。<br>Una tableta: 0.1g. |

**续 表**

| 2.3 硝基呋喃类 Nitrofuran | |
| --- | --- |
| **药品名称 Drug Names** | **呋喃妥因 Nitrofurantoin** |
| 适应证<br>Indicaciones | 本品主要应用于敏感菌所致的泌尿系统感染。一般地说，微生物对本品不易耐药，如停药后重新用药，仍可有效。但近年来耐药菌株有一定程度发展。必要时可与其他药物（如 TMP）联合应用以提高疗效。<br><br>Se usa para infección del sistema urinario debido a cepas susceptibles. En términos generales, los microorganismos tienen menos resistencia al producto y después de interrumpir la administración del medicamento sigue siendo válido el retratamiento. Pero en los últimos años, las cepas han tenido cierto desarrollo en la resistencia al medicamento y en casos necesarios puede usarse en combinación con otros fármacos(como por ejemplo TMP) con fin de mejorar la eficacia. |
| 用法、用量<br>Administración y dosis | 每次 0.1g，一日 0.2 ～ 0.4g，至尿内检菌阴性再继续用 3 日。但连续应用不宜超过 14 日。<br><br>0.1g cada vez, 0.2 ～ 0.4g al día. Si se prueban negativas bacterias en la orina, se sigue usando por tres días, y no conviene durar más de 14 días en el uso continuo. |
| 剂型、规格<br>Formulaciones y especificaciones | 肠溶片：每片 0.05g；0.1g。<br>Una tableta con recubrimiento entérico: 0.05g; 0.1g. |
| **药品名称 Drug Names** | **呋喃唑酮 Furazolidona** |
| 适应证<br>Indicaciones | 主要用于菌痢、肠炎，也可用于伤寒、副伤寒、梨形鞭毛虫病和阴道滴虫病。<br><br>Se usa principalmente para disentería y enteritis así como tifoidea, paratifoidea, giardia lamblia y tricomoniasis vaginal. |
| 用法、用量<br>Administración y dosis | 常用量 1 次 0.1g，一日 3 ～ 4 次，症状消失后再服 2 日。梨形鞭毛虫病疗程为 7 ～ 10 日。<br><br>Dosis habitual, 0.1g cada vez, 3 ～ 4 veces al día, se sigue tomando por dos días cuando desaparezcan los síntomas. El ciclo de tratamiento de giardia lamblia es de 7 ～ 10 días. |
| 剂型、规格<br>Formulaciones y especificaciones | 片剂：每片 0.1g。<br>Una tableta: 0.1g. |

| 2.4 喹诺酮类 Quinolonas | |
| --- | --- |
| **药品名称 Drug Names** | **吡哌酸 Ácido pipemídico** |
| 适应证<br>Indicaciones | 临床主要应用于敏感革兰阴性杆菌和葡萄球菌所致尿路、肠道和耳道感染，如尿道炎、膀胱炎、菌痢、肠炎、中耳炎等。<br><br>En clínica se usa para infecciones del tracto urinario, intestino y el canal auditivo debido a sensible bacterias Gram-negativas y estafilococo, tales como uretritis, cistitis, disentería, enteritis y la otitis media, etc. |
| 用法、用量<br>Administración y dosis | 成人口服：1 次 0.5g，一日 1.5 ～ 2g，分次给予，一般不超过 10 日。<br><br>Se toma por vía oral para adultos: 0.5g cada vez, 1.5 ～ 2g al día, dividido en varias veces, generalmente no sobrepasa 10 días. |
| 剂型、规格<br>Formulaciones y especificaciones | 片剂：每片 0.25g；0.5g。胶囊剂：每胶囊 0.25g。<br>Una tableta: 0.25g;0.5g. Una cápsula: 0.25g. |
| **药品名称 Drug Names** | **诺氟沙星 Norfloxacina** |
| 适应证<br>Indicaciones | 本品应用于敏感菌所致泌尿道、肠道、耳鼻喉科、妇科、外科和皮肤科等感染性疾病。<br><br>Se usa para infecciones del tracto urinario y intestino, infecciones ORL, infecciones ginecológicas, infecciones quirúrgicas e infecciones dermatológicas entre otras enfermedades infecciosas debido a cepas susceptibles. |
| 用法、用量<br>Administración y dosis | 口服，成人 1 次 0.1 ～ 0.2g，一日 3 ～ 4 次。空腹服药吸收较好。一般疗程为 3 ～ 8 日，少数病例可达 3 周。对于慢性泌尿道感染病例，可先用一般量 2 周，再减量为 200mg/d，睡前服用，持续数月。严重病例及不能口服者静脉滴注。用量：每次 200 ～ 400mg，每 12 小时 1 次。将一次量加于输液中，静脉滴注 1 小时。 |

**续　表**

| | |
|---|---|
| | Se toma por vía oral para adultos: 0.1 ～ 0.2g cada vez, 3 ～ 4 veces al día, mejor efecto con estómago vacío. Generalmente, el ciclo de tratamiento es de 3 ～ 8 días, raras veces puede alcanzar a tres semanas. En infecciones urinarias crónicas, se toma dosis habitual por dos semanas y la reduce a 200mg/d al acostarse durante meses. En casos graves o los pacientes que no pueden tomar por vía oral, se adopta infusión intravenosa. Dosis: 200 ～ 400mg cada vez, con intervalo de 12 horas. Se agrega una dosis en la infusión para gotear por una hora. |
| 剂型、规格<br>Formulaciones y especificaciones | 胶囊：每粒 100mg。输液：每瓶 200mg/100ml（尚有其他规格）。滴眼液：8ml（24mg）。软膏：1%。<br><br>Una cápsula: 100mg. Infusión: 200mg/100ml cada botella (también hay de otras especificaciones). Gotas para los ojos: 8ml(24mg). ungüento:1%. |
| 药品名称 Drug Names | 氧氟沙星 Ofloxacina |
| 适应证<br>Indicaciones | 主要用于上述革兰阴性菌所致的呼吸道、咽喉、扁桃体、泌尿道（包括前列腺）、皮肤及软组织、胆囊及胆管、中耳、鼻窦、泪囊、肠道等部位的急、慢性感染。<br><br>Se usa para infecciones agudas y crómicas del tracto respiratorio, la garganta, las amígdalas, el tracto urinario(incluyendo próstata), la piel y tejidos blandos, la vesícula biliar y los conductos biliares, el oído medio, los senos nasales, saco lagrimal y el intestino entre otras partes debido a bacterias Gram-negativas. |
| 用法、用量<br>Administración y dosis | 口服：每日 200 ～ 600mg，分 2 次服。根据病情适当调整剂量。抗结核用量为每日 0.3g，顿服。控制伤寒反复感染：每日 50mg，连用 3 ～ 6 个月。静脉滴注给药：每次 200 ～ 400mg，每 12 小时 1 次，以适量输液稀释，静脉滴注 1 小时。<br><br>Se toma por vía oral: 200 ～ 600mg al día, en dos veces. Se ajusta la dosis oportunamente según la gravedad. Dosis contra la tuberculosis: 0.3g al día, tomando tras comidas. Para controlar infecciones repetidas de tifoidea: 50mg al día durante 3 y 6 meses. Administración por infusión: 200 ～ 400mg cada vez, con intervalo de 12 horas, diluido en cantidad apropiada de infusión, una hora de goteo. |
| 剂型、规格<br>Formulaciones y especificaciones | 片剂：每片 100mg。注射液：每支 400mg/10ml（用前需稀释）。输液：每瓶 400mg/100ml（可直接输注）。<br><br>Una tableta: 100mg. Una inyección: 400mg/10ml(se debe diluirlo antes del uso). Infusión: 400mg/100ml cada botella(se puede inyectar directamente). |
| 药品名称 Drug Names | 左氧氟沙星 Levofloxacina |
| 适应证<br>Indicaciones | 主要用于上述革兰阴性菌所致的呼吸道、咽喉、扁桃体、泌尿道（包括前列腺）、皮肤及软组织、胆囊及胆管、中耳、鼻窦、泪囊、肠道等部位的急、慢性感染。<br><br>Se usa para infecciones agudas y crómicas del tracto respiratorio, la garganta, las amígdalas, el tracto urinario(incluyendo próstata), la piel y tejidos blandos, la vesícula biliar y los conductos biliares, el oído medio, los senos nasales, saco lagrimal y el intestino entre otras partes debido a bacterias Gram-negativas. |
| 用法、用量<br>Administración y dosis | 口服：每次 100mg，一日 2 次，根据感染严重程度可增量，最多每次 200mg，一日 3 次。静脉滴注，一日 200 ～ 600mg，分 1 ～ 2 次静脉滴注。<br><br>Se toma por vía oral: 100mg cada vez, dos veces al día, la dosis puede incrementarse según la gravedad de infecciones , la dosis máxma es de 200mg cada vez, tres veces al día. Infusión intravenosa, 200 ～ 600mg al día, en 1 ～ 2 veces. |
| 剂型、规格<br>Formulaciones y especificaciones | 片剂：每片 100mg；200mg；500mg。注射液：200mg（100ml）；300mg（100ml）；500mg（100ml）。<br>Una tableta: 100mg; 200mg; 500mg. Inyección: 200mg(100ml); 300mg(100ml); 500mg(100ml). |

**续 表**

| 药品名称 Drug Names | 依诺沙星 Enoxacina |
|---|---|
| 适应证<br>Indicaciones | 用于敏感菌所致的咽喉、支气管、肺、尿路、前列腺、胆囊、肠道、中耳、鼻旁窦等部位感染，也可用于脓皮病及软组织感染。<br><br>Se usa para infecciones de la garganta, el bronquio, el pulmón, el tracto urinario, la próstata, la vesícula biliar, intestino, el oído medio y los senos paranasales entre otras partes debido a cepas susceptibles. También se usa para pioderma e infección de tejidos blandos. |
| 用法、用量<br>Administración y dosis | 成人常用量一日 400～600mg（按无水物计量）。分 2 次给予。<br><br>La dosis habitual de adultos 400～600mg al día(se calcula por sustancia anhidra), dividida en dos veces. |
| 剂型、规格<br>Formulaciones y especificaciones | 片剂：每片100mg（标示量以无水物计量，相当于含水物108.5mg）；200mg（相当于含水物217mg）。<br><br>Una tableta: 100mg(calculado en anhidro, equivalente a 108.5mg del hidrato); 200mg(equivalente a 217mg del hidrato). |
| 药品名称 Drug Names | 环丙沙星 Ciprofloxacina |
| 适应证<br>Indicaciones | 适用于敏感菌所致的呼吸道、尿道、消化道、胆道、皮肤和软组织、盆腔、眼、耳、鼻、咽喉等部位的感染。<br><br>Se usa para infecciones del tracto respiratorio, tracto urinario, tracto gastrointestinal, tracto biliar, la piel y tejidos blandos, pelvis, los ojos, los oídos, las nariz y la garganta entre otras partes debido a cepas susceptibles. |
| 用法、用量<br>Administración y dosis | 口服：成人1次250mg，一日2次，重症者可加倍量。但一日最高量不可超过1500mg。肾功能不全者（肌酐消除率低于30ml/min）应减少服量。静脉滴注：1次100～200mg，一日2次，预先用等渗氯化钠或葡萄糖注射液稀释，滴注时间不少于30分钟。<br><br>Se toma por vía oral: adultos 250mg una vez, dos veces al día, la dosis puede duplicar para pacientes de síntomas graves. Pero la dosis diaria máxima no debe sobrepasar 1500mg. Los pacientes con insuficiencia renal(aclaramiento de creatinina inferior a 30ml/min) deben tomar menos dosis. Infusión intravenosa: 100～200mg cada vez, dos veces al día, diluido de antemano en solución isotónica de cloruro de sodio o inyección de glucosa, por al menos 30 minutos. |
| 剂型、规格<br>Formulaciones y especificaciones | 片剂：每片（标示量按环丙沙星计算）为250mg；500mg；750mg（含盐酸盐一水合物量分别为291mg、582mg和873mg）。注射液：每支100mg（50ml）；200mg（100ml）（含乳酸盐分别为127.2mg和254.4mg）。<br><br>Una tableta: (calculado en la dosis de ciprofloxacina) 250mg; 500mg; 750mg (pesos respectivos de monohidrato que incluye clorhidrato: 291mg, 582mg y 873mg). Una inyección: 100mg(50ml); 200mg(100ml) (que son 127.2mg y 254.4mg si se incluyen lactato).) |
| 药品名称 Drug Names | 洛美沙星 Lomefloxacina |
| 适应证<br>Indicaciones | 应用于上述敏感菌所致的下呼吸道、尿道感染。本品对链球菌、肺炎链球菌、洋葱假单胞菌、支原体和厌氧菌均无效。<br><br>Se usa para infecciones del tracto respiratorio inferior, tracto urinario debido a cepas susceptibles. No tiene eficacia para streptococcus, streptococcus pneumoniae, pseudomonas cepacia, mycoplasma y anaerobios. |
| 用法、用量<br>Administración y dosis | 口服：每日1次400mg，疗程10～14日。手术感染的预防，手术前2～6小时，1次服400mg。静脉滴注：每次200mg，一日2次，或每次400mg，一日1次。每100mg药物需用5%葡萄糖液或0.9%氯化钠液60～100ml稀释后缓慢滴注。肾功能不全者的用量，按血清肌酐值，依下式计算：男性：[体重（kg）×（140－年龄）]／[72×血清肌酐值（mg/dl）]女性：按男性结果×0.85。<br><br>Se toma por vía oral: 400mg 1 vez al día, ciclo de tratamiento 10～14 días. Prevención de infecciones quirúrgicas, 2～6 horas antes de la operación, 400mg de una vez. Infusión intravenosa: 200mg cada vez, dos veces al día, o 400mg 1 vez al día. Se necesita 60～100ml de 5% solución de glucosa o 0.9% solución de cloruro de sodio para diluir cada 100mg del medicamento y gotearlo lentamente. La dosis para pacientes de insuficiencia renal, por valores de creatinina sérica, se calcula de la forma siguiente: hombres: peso corporal(kg)×(140-edad)]／[72×valor de creatinina sérica(mg/dl)] mujeres: resultado de hombres×0.85. |

**续 表**

| | |
|---|---|
| 剂型、规格<br>Formulaciones y especificaciones | 薄膜衣片：每片400mg。注射液（盐酸盐或天冬氨酸盐）：每支100mg/2ml；每瓶200mg/100ml、400mg/250ml。<br>recubierto con película: 400mg. Inyección (clorhidrato oaspartato): 100mg/2ml) cada una o 200mg/100ml, 400mg/250ml cada botella. |
| 药品名称 Drug Names | 培氟沙星 Pefloxacina |
| 适应证<br>Indicaciones | 用于治疗革兰阴性菌和金黄色葡萄球菌引起的中度或重度感染。如：泌尿系统、呼吸道、耳鼻喉、生殖系统、腹部和肝、胆系统感染，脑膜炎、骨和关节感染，败血症和心内膜炎。<br>Se usa para infecciones moderadas o graves debido a bacterias Gram-negativas y staphylococcus aureus, tales como infecciones del tracto urinario, tracto respiratorio, el oído, las nariz, la garganta, sistema reproductivo, el abdomen, el sistema del hígado y vesícula biliar, meningitis, infecciones de huesos y articulaciones, septicemia y endocarditis. |
| 用法、用量<br>Administración y dosis | 口服：成人每日400～800mg，分2次给予。静脉滴注：一次0.4g，加入5%葡萄糖注射液250ml中，缓慢滴入，滴注时间不少于60分钟，每12小时一次。<br>Se toma por vía oral: adultos 400 ～ 800mg al día, dividido en dos veces. Infusión intravenosa: 0.4g cada vez, se agrega a 250ml de 5% inyección de glucosa y se gotea lentamente por al menos 60 minutos, cada 12 horas. |
| 剂型、规格<br>Formulaciones y especificaciones | 片剂：每片200mg。注射液（甲磺酸盐）：每支400mg（5ml）。<br>Una tableta: 200mg. Una inyección (mesilato): 400mg(5ml). |
| 药品名称 Drug Names | 芦氟沙星 Rufloxacina |
| 适应证<br>Indicaciones | 临床用于敏感菌引起的下呼吸道及尿道感染。如肺炎、急慢性支气管炎、急慢性肾盂肾炎、急性膀胱炎、尿道炎及皮肤软组织化脓性感染。<br>En clínica se usa para infecciones del tracto respiratorio inferior y tracto urinario debido a cepas susceptibles, tales como neumonía, bronquitis aguda y crónica, pielonefritis aguda y crónica, cistitis aguda, uretritis e infección séptica de la piel y los tejidos blandos. |
| 用法、用量<br>Administración y dosis | 成人每日1次，每次200mg，早餐后服。5～10日为一疗程。前列腺炎的疗程可达4周。<br>Adultos 1 vez al día, 200mg cada vez, se toma después del almuerzo. Ciclo de tratamiento: 5 ～ 10 días. El ciclo de tratamiento para prostatitis puede alcanzar a 4 semanas. |
| 剂型、规格<br>Formulaciones y especificaciones | 片剂：每片200mg。胶囊剂：每粒100mg。<br>Una tableta: 200mg. Una cápsula: 100mg. |
| 药品名称 Drug Names | 司帕沙星 Sparfloxacina |
| 适应证<br>Indicaciones | 临床用于敏感菌所致的咽喉、扁桃体、支气管、肺、胆囊、尿道、前列腺、肠道、子宫、中耳、鼻旁窦等部位感染，还可用于皮肤、软组织感染及牙周组织炎。<br>En clínica se usa para infecciones de garganta, amígdalas, bronquios, pulmón, vesícula biliar, uretra, próstata, intestino, útero, el oído medio y los senos paranasales entre otras partes debido a cepas susceptibles. También se aplica a infecciones de la piel y tejidos blandos y periodontitis. |
| 用法、用量<br>Administración y dosis | 口服：成人每次100～300mg，最多不超过400mg，一日1次。疗程一般为5～10日。<br>Se toma por vía oral: adultos 100 ～ 300mg cada vez, no sobrepasa 400mg, 1vez al día. Ciclo de tratamiento es generalmente 5 ～ 10 días. |
| 剂型、规格<br>Formulaciones y especificaciones | 胶囊剂：每粒100mg。<br>Una cápsula: 100mg. |
| 药品名称 Drug Names | 氟罗沙星 Fleroxacina |
| 适应证<br>Indicaciones | 用于敏感菌所致的呼吸系统、泌尿生殖系统、消化系统的感染，以及皮肤软组织、骨、关节、耳鼻喉、腹腔、盆腔感染。<br>Se usa para infecciones de sistema respiratorio, sistema genitourinario y sistema digestivo debido a cepas susceptibles. También se usa para infecciones de la piel y tejidos blandos, huesos, articulaciones, oídos, nariz y garganta, abdomen y pelvis. |

**续　表**

| | |
|---|---|
| 用法、用量<br>Administración y dosis | 口服：每日 0.4g，一次顿服。疗程视感染不同而定：复杂性尿路感染 1～2 周；呼吸道感染 1～3 周；皮肤、软组织感染 4 日～3 周；骨髓炎、化脓性关节炎 2～12 周；伤寒 1～2 周；沙眼衣原体尿道炎 5 日；单纯性尿路感染、细菌性痢疾、淋球菌尿道炎（宫颈炎）只用 1 次。静脉滴注：一次 200～400mg，一日 1 次，加入 5% 葡萄糖注射液 250ml 中，避光缓慢滴注（每 100ml 滴注至少 45～60 分钟）。<br><br>Se toma por vía oral: 0.4g al día, una vez cada comida. El ciclo de tratamiento se varía según infecciones diferentes: infecciones urinarias complicadas 1～2 semanas; infecciones respiratorias 1～3 semanas; infecciones de la piel y tejidos blandos 4 días a 3 semanas; osteomielitis, artritis séptica: 2～12 semanas; ifoidea 1～2 semanas; chlamydia trachomatis uretritis 5 días; infecciones no complicadas del tracto urinario, la disentería, gonorrea uretritis (cervicitis) sólo se tama una vez. Infusión intravenosa: 200～400mg 1 vez al día, se agrega a 250ml de 5% inyección de glucosa y se gotea lentamente y en la oscuridad(100 ml al menos por 45 a 60 minutos). |
| 剂型、规格<br>Formulaciones y especificaciones | 胶囊剂：每粒 200mg；400mg。<br>Una cápsula: 200mg; 400mg. |
| 药品名称 Drug Names | 莫西沙星 Moxifloxacina |
| 适应证<br>Indicaciones | 适用于敏感菌所致的呼吸道感染，包括慢性支气管炎急性发作，轻度或中度的社区获得性肺炎，急性鼻窦炎等。<br><br>Se usa para infecciones de tracto respiratorio debido a cepas susceptibles, tales como exacerbación aguda de la bronquitis crónica, neumonía adquirida en la comunidad de intensidad leve o moderada y sinusitis aguda, etc. |
| 用法、用量<br>Administración y dosis | 成人每日 1 次 400mg，连用 5～10 日，口服或静脉滴注。滴注时间为 90 分钟。<br>Adultos 400mg 1 vez al día, 5～10 días consecutivos, por vía oral o infusión intravenosa. La duración de goteo es de 90 minutos. |
| 剂型、规格<br>Formulaciones y especificaciones | 片剂 400mg。<br>注射液 250ml（莫西沙星 0.4g）。<br>Una tableta: 400mg.<br>Una inyección: 250ml (0.4g de moxifloxacina). |
| 药品名称 Drug Names | 加替沙星 Gatifloxacina |
| 适应证<br>Indicaciones | 用于敏感菌所致的慢性支气管炎急性发作、急性鼻窦炎、社区获得性肺炎、尿路感染、急性肾盂肾炎、女性淋球菌性宫颈感染。<br><br>Se usa para exacerbación aguda de la bronquitis crónica, sinusitis aguda, neumonía adquirida en la comunidad, infección del tracto urinario, pielonefritis aguda y infección gonocócica cervical femenino debido a cepas susceptibles. |
| 用法、用量<br>Administración y dosis | 静脉给药：成人每次 200～400mg，一日 1 次，疗程一般 5～10 日。治疗中由静脉给药改为口服给药时，无须调整剂量。治疗非复杂性淋球菌尿路或直肠感染和女性淋球菌性宫颈感染，400mg 单次给药。中度肝功能不全者，无须调整剂量；中、重度肾功能不全者，应减量使用。<br><br>Administración por vía intravenosa: adultos 200～400mg 1 vez al día, ciclo de tratamiento 5～10 días. En el tratamiento, cuando se administra por vía oral en vez de por vía intravenosa, no hace falta ajustar la dosis. En el tratamiento de infecciones del tracto urinario o rectal no complicadas por neisseria gonorrhoeae y infección gonocócica cervical femenino, 400mg, la dosis única. Para los pacientes con insuficiencia renal de gravedad moderada, no hace falta ajustar la dosis; los de gravedad moderada a severa, se debe reducir la dosis. |
| 剂型、规格<br>Formulaciones y especificaciones | 片剂：每片 100mg；200mg；400mg。注射液：100mg（100ml）；200mg（100ml）；400mg（40ml）。<br>Una tableta: 100mg; 200mg; 400mg. Una inyección: 100mg(100ml); 200mg(100ml); 400mg(40ml). |
| 药品名称 Drug Names | 帕珠沙星 Pazufloxacina |
| 适应证<br>Indicaciones | 用于敏感菌所致的呼吸道感染、泌尿道感染，妇科、外科、耳鼻喉科和皮肤科等感染性疾病。<br><br>Se usa para infecciones del tracto respiratorio, tracto urinario, infecciones ginecológicas, infecciones quirúrgicas, infecciones ORL e infecciones dermatológicas entre otras enfermedades infecciosas debido a cepas susceptibles. |

续　表

| 用法、用量<br>Administración y dosis | 静脉滴注，每次 300mg，滴注时间为 30 ～ 60 分钟，一日 2 次，疗程 7 ～ 14 日。肾功能不全者应调整剂量：肾清除率＞ 44.7ml/min，每次 300mg，一日 2 次；肾清除率为 13.6 ～ 44.7ml/min，每次 300mg，一日 1 次；透析患者用量为每次 300mg，每 3 日 1 次。<br><br>Infusión intravenosa, 300mg cada vez, el tiempo de la infusión 30 ～ 60 minutos, dos veces al día, ciclo de tratamiento 7 ～ 14 días. Los pacientes con insuficiencia renal deben ajustar la dosis: aclaramiento de creatinina de 13.6 ～ 44.7ml/min, 300mg cada vez, una vez al día; la dosis diaria de los pacientes en diálisis es 300mg cada vez, una vez cada 3 días. |
|---|---|
| 剂型、规格<br>Formulaciones y especificaciones | 甲磺酸帕珠沙星注射液：100mg（10ml）；150mg（10ml）；200mg（100ml）；300mg（100ml）。<br>Pazufloxacin mesilate inyección: 100mg(10ml); 150mg(10ml); 200mg(100ml); 300mg(100ml). |
| 药品名称 Drug Names | 托氟沙星 Tosufloxacina |
| 适应证<br>Indicaciones | 临床用于敏感菌引起的呼吸系统、泌尿系统、胃肠道、皮肤软组织感染，以及中耳炎、牙周炎、眼睑炎等。<br><br>En clínica se usa para infecciones del tracto respiratorio y tracto urinario, infección gastrointestinal, infección de la piel y tejidos blandos, así como otitis media, periodontitis y blefaritis, etc. debido a cepas susceptibles. |
| 用法、用量<br>Administración y dosis | 口服每次 75 ～ 150mg，一日 2 ～ 3 次，一般疗程 3 ～ 7 日；最多每日剂量 600mg，分 2 ～ 3 次服用，疗程 14 日。<br><br>Se toma por vía oral 75 ～ 150mg, 2 ～ 3 veces al día, ciclo de tratamiento general 3 ～ 7 días; la dosis diaria máxima 600mg, en 2 ～ 3 veces, ciclo de tratamiento 14 días. |
| 剂型、规格<br>Formulaciones y especificaciones | 托西酸托氟沙星片：每片 75mg；150mg；300mg。甲苯磺酸托氟沙星片：每片 150mg。<br>Tableta de tosilato tosufloxacina: 75mg; 150mg; 300mg. Tableta tosufloxacina toluenosulfónica: 150mg. |

2.5　硝基咪唑类 Nitroimidazol

| 药品名称 Drug Names | 甲硝唑 Metronidazol |
|---|---|
| 适应证<br>Indicaciones | 主要用于治疗或预防上述厌氧菌引起的系统或局部感染，如腹腔、消化道、女性生殖系、下呼吸道、皮肤及软组织、骨和关节等部位的厌氧菌感染，对败血症、心内膜炎、脑膜感染及使用抗生素引起的结肠炎也有效。治疗破伤风常与破伤风抗毒素（TAT）联用。还可用于口腔厌氧菌感染。<br><br>Se usa principalmente para tratar o prevenir infección sistémica o local debido a anaerobios, tales como infecciones por anaerobios de cavidad abdominal, tracto gastrointestinal, sistema reproductivo femenino, las vías respiratorias inferiores, la piel y tejidos blandos, huesos y articulaciones entre otras partes. También tiene efecto para la septicemia, endocarditis, meningitis así como colitis causada por antibióticos. Se usa en combinación con antitoxina tetánica(TAT)para tratar el tétanos. Puede ser utilizado para las infecciones por anaerobios orales. |
| 用法、用量<br>Administración y dosis | 厌氧菌感染：口服，1 次 0.2 ～ 0.4g，一日 0.6 ～ 1.2g；静脉滴注，1 次 500mg，8 小时 1 次，每次滴注 1 小时。一疗程 7 日。预防用药：用于腹部或妇科手术前一天开始服药，1 次 0.25 ～ 0.5g，一日 3 次。治疗破伤风：一日量 2.5g，分次口服或静脉滴注。<br><br>Infecciones por anaerobios: por vía oral, 0.2 ～ 0.4g cada vez, 0.6 ～ 1.2g al día; infusión intravenosa, 500mg cada vez, cada 8 horas, cada vez por una hora. El ciclo de tratamiento es de 7 días. Administración preventiva: se toma un día antes de la cirugía abdominal o ginecológica, 0.25 ～ 0.5g una vez, tres veces al día. Tratamiento de tétanos: dosis diaria de 2.5g, en varias veces por vía oral o infusión. |
| 剂型、规格<br>Formulaciones y especificaciones | 片剂：每片 0.2g。注射液：50mg（10ml）；100mg（20ml）；500mg（100ml）；1.25g（250ml）；500mg（250ml）。甲硝唑葡萄糖注射液：250ml，含甲硝唑 0.5g 及葡萄糖 12.5g。栓剂：每个 0.5g；1g。甲硝唑阴道泡腾片：每片 0.2g。 |

**续 表**

Una tableta：0.2g. Inyección：50mg（10ml）；100mg（20ml）；500mg（100ml）；1.25g（250ml）；500mg（250ml）. Inyección de metronidazol y glucosa：250ml，0.5g de metronidazol y 12.5g de glucosa. Un supositorio：0.5g；1g. Tableta efervescente vaginal metronidazol：0.2g.

| 药品名称 Drug Names | 替硝唑 Tinidazol |
| --- | --- |
| 适应证<br>Indicaciones | 用于厌氧菌的系统与局部感染，如腹腔、妇科、手术创口、皮肤软组织、肺、胸腔等部位感染以及败血症、肠道或泌尿生殖道毛滴虫病、梨形鞭毛虫病及肠道和肝阿米巴病。<br><br>Se usa para infección sistémica o local debido a anaerobios, tales como infección de cavidad abdominal, infección ginecológica, infecciones de heridas quirúrgicas, la piel y tejidos blandos, pulmón y cavidad torácica entre otras partes así como septicemia, tricomoniasis intestinal o genitourinario, giardia lamblia y amebiasis intestinal y hepático. |
| 用法、用量<br>Administración y dosis | 厌氧菌系统感染：口服每日2g；重症可静脉滴注，每日1.6g，1次或分为2次给予。手术感染的预防：术前12小时服2g，手术间或结束后输注1.6g（或口服2g）。非特异性阴道炎：每日2g，连服2日。急性齿龈炎：1次口服2g。泌尿生殖道毛滴虫病：1次口服2g，必要时重复1次；或每次0.15g，一日3次，连用5日。需男女同治以防再次感染。儿童1次50～75mg/kg，必要时重复1次。合并白念珠菌感染者须同时进行抗真菌治疗。梨形鞭毛虫病：1次2g。肠阿米巴病：每日2g，服2～3日。儿童每日50～60mg，连用5日。肝阿米巴病：每日1.5～2g，连用3日，必要时可延长至5～10日。应同时排出脓液。口服片剂应于餐间或餐后服用。静脉滴注每400mg（200ml）应不少于20分钟。<br><br>Infecciones sistémicas por anaerobios: por vía oral, 2g al día; en casos graves, se puede adoptar la infusión, 1.6g al día, administrado en una o dos veces. Prevención de infecciones quirúrgicas: se toma 2g 12 horas antes de la operación, y se inyecta 1.6g o se toma 2g durante y después de la operación. Vaginitis inespecífica: 2g al día, 2 días consecutivos. Gingivitis aguda: se toma 2g cada vez por vía oral. Tricomoniasis intestinal: se toma 2g cada vez por vía oral y en casos necesarios se repite una vez; o 0.15g cada vez, 3 veces al día, 5 días consecutivos. Se debe tratar a hombres y mujeres a la vez para evitar otra infección. Niños 50～75mg/kg una vez, puede duplicar la administración en casos necesarios. Los infectados también por Candida albicans deben adoptar terapia antifúngica a la vez. Giardia lamblia: 2g una vez. Amebiasis intestinal: 2g al día, durante 2～3 días. Niños 50～60mg al día, durante 5 días. Amebiasis hepático: 1.5～2g al día, 3 días consecutivos, en casos necesario, se extiende hasta 5～10 días y se descarga pus a la vez.Se toman tabletas orales durante o después de la comida. La infusión intravenosa de 400mg(200ml)no debe durar menos a 20 minutos. |
| 剂型、规格<br>Formulaciones y especificaciones | 片剂：每片0.25g；0.5g。注射液：每瓶400mg/200ml或800mg/400ml（含葡萄糖5.5%）。栓剂：每个0.2g。<br><br>Una tableta: 0.25g; 0.5g. Una inyección: 400mg/200ml o 800mg/400ml cada botella (que incluye 5.5% glucosa). Un supositorio: 0.2g. |
| 药品名称 Drug Names | 奥硝唑 Ornidazol |
| 适应证<br>Indicaciones | 用于由厌氧菌感染引起的多种疾病。男女泌尿生殖道毛滴虫、贾第鞭毛虫感染引起的疾病。还用于肠、肝阿米巴病。<br><br>Se usa para una variedad de enfermedades causadas por las infecciones anaeróbicas, tales como tricomoniasis urogenital masculino y femenino e infección causada por giardia así como amebiasis intestinal y hepático. |
| 用法、用量<br>Administración y dosis | 口服：预防术后厌氧菌感染，术前12小时服用1500mg，以后每次500mg，一日2次，至术后3～5日；治疗厌氧菌感染，每次500mg，一日2次；急性毛滴虫病，于夜间单次服用1500mg；慢性毛滴虫病，1次500mg，一日2次，共用5日；贾第鞭毛虫病，于夜间顿服1500mg，用药1～2日；阿米巴痢疾，于夜间顿服1500mg，用药3日；其他阿米巴病，1次500mg，一日2次。静脉滴注：预防术后厌氧菌感染，术前1～2小时给药1000mg，术后12小时给药500mg，24小时再给药500mg；治疗厌氧菌感染，初始剂量为500～1000mg，以后每12小时500mg，疗程3～6日。 |

| | |
|---|---|
| | Se toma por vía oral: para prevenir infecciones postoperarias causadas por anaerobios, 1500mg, 12 horas antes de la operación, en adelante 500mg cada vez, dos veces al día, 3 ～ 5 días tras la operación; para tratar infecciones postoperarias causadas por anaerobios, 500mg cada vcz, dos veces al día; tricomoniasis aguda, por la noche una dosis de 1500mg; tricomoniasis crónica, 500mg cada vez, dos veces al día, 5 días en total; giardiasis, 1500mg por la noche, administración de 1 ～ 2 días; disentería amebiana, 1500mg por la noche, administración de 3 días; otros amebiasis, 500mg una vez, dos veces al día. Infusión intravenosa: para prevenir infecciones postoperarias causadas por anaerobios, se administra 1000mg, 1 ～ 2 horas antes de la operación; 500mg, 12 horas después de la operación; 500mg 24 horas después; para tratar infecciones postoperarias causadas por anaerobios, la dosis inicial es de 500 ～ 1000mg, en adelante 500mg cada 12 horas, con un ciclo de tratamiento de 3 ～ 6 días. |
| 剂型、规格<br>Formulaciones y especificaciones | 片剂（胶囊剂）：每片（粒）0.25g。<br>注射液：0.25g（5ml）。<br>奥硝唑氯化钠（葡萄糖）注射液：0.25g（100ml）；0.5g（100ml）。<br>Una tableta (cápsula): 0.25g.<br>Una inyección: 0.25g(5ml).<br>Una inyección de ornidazol y cloruro de sodio (glucosa): 0.25g(100ml); 0.5g(100ml). |
| 药品名称 Drug Names | 塞克硝唑 Secnidazol |
| 适应证<br>Indicaciones | 主要用于由阴道毛滴虫引起的尿道炎和阴道炎，肠阿米巴病，肝阿米巴病及贾第鞭毛虫病。<br>Se usa principalmente para uretritis y vaginitis, amebiasis intestinal y hepático y giardiasis debido a trichomonas vaginalis. |
| 用法、用量<br>Administración y dosis | 口服，成人 2g，单次服用。治疗阴道滴虫病和尿道滴虫病，配偶应同时服用。肠阿米巴病：有症状的急性阿米巴病，成人 2g，单次服用；儿童 30mg/kg，单次服用；无症状的急性阿米巴病，成人一次 2g，一日 1 次，连服 3 日；儿童一次 30mg/kg，一日 1 次，连服 3 日。肝脏阿米巴病：成人一日 1.5g，一次或分次口服，连服 5 日；儿童一次 30mg/kg，一次或分次口服，连服 5 日。贾第鞭毛虫病：儿童 30mg/kg，单次服用。<br>Se toma por vía oral, 2g para adultos, dosis única. Para tratar tricomoniasis vaginal y tricomoniasis uretral, la pareja debe tomarlo a la vez. Amebiasis intestinal: los pacientes con síntomas de amebiasis agudo, 2g para adultos, dosis única; 30mg/kg para niños, dosis única; los pacientes sin síntomas de amebiasis agudo, 2g para adultos, 1 vez al día, 3 días consecutivos; 30mg/kg para niños, 1 vez al día, 3 días consecutivos. Amebiasis hepático: adultos 1.5g al día, en una o varias veces por vía oral, 5 días consecutivos; 30mg/kg para niños, en una o varias veces por vía oral, 5 días consecutivos. Giardiasis: 30mg/kg para niños, dosis única. |
| 剂型、规格<br>Formulaciones y especificaciones | 片剂（胶囊）：每片/粒 0.25g；0.5g。<br>Una tableta (cápsula): 0.25g; 0.5g. |

2.6　噁唑烷酮类 Oxazolonas

| 药品名称 Drug Names | 利奈唑胺 Linezolida |
|---|---|
| 适应证<br>Indicaciones | 主要用于控制耐万古霉素屎肠球菌所致的系统感染，包括败血症、肺炎及复杂性皮肤和皮肤组织感染等。<br>Se usa principalmente para infección sistémica por enterococcus faecium resistente a vancomicina, tales como septicemia, neumonía e infecciones complicadas de la piel y los tejidos blandos, etc. |
| 用法、用量<br>Administración y dosis | 口服与静滴剂量相同。成人和超过 12 岁儿童，每次 600mg，每 12 小时一次。治疗耐万古霉素肠球菌感染疗程 14 ～ 28 日。肺炎、菌血症及皮肤软组织感染疗程 10 ～ 14 日。儿童（出生至 11 岁者），每次 10mg/kg，每 12 小时一次，疗效欠佳可增至每 8 小时一次，口服或静脉给药。<br>La dosis por vía oral es igual a la de infusión intravenosa. Adultos y niños mayores a 12 años, 600mg cada vez, cada 12 horas. El ciclo de tratamiento para tratar infección por enterococcus faecium resistente a vancomicina es de 14 ～ 28 días. El curso de la neumonía, bacteremia e infección de los tejidos blandos de la piel es de 10 a 14 días. Niños (menores de 11 años),la dosis administrada es de 10mg/kg una vez cada 12 horas. Cuando el efecto no es bueno, una vez cada 8 horas, por vía oral o infusión intravenosa. |

**续 表**

| 剂型、规格<br>Formulaciones y<br>especificaciones | 片剂：每片 600mg。注射液：600mg（300ml）。<br>Una tableta: 600mg. Una inyección: 600mg(300ml). |
|---|---|

### 3. 抗结核药 Medicamentos anti-tuberculosis

| 药品名称 Drug Names | 异烟肼 Isoniacida |
|---|---|
| 适应证<br>Indicaciones | 主要用于各型肺结核的进展期、溶解播散期、吸收好转期，尚可用于结核性脑膜炎和其他肺外结核等。本品常需和其他抗结核病药联合应用，以增强疗效和克服耐药菌。此外，对痢疾、百日咳、麦粒肿等也有一定疗效。<br><br>Se usa principalmente para todo tipo de tuberculosis en la etapa progresiva, etapa expansiva y etapa de absorción. Se puede utilizar para la meningitis tuberculosa y otras tuberculosis extrapulmonar. Necesita frecuentemente combinar con otros medicamentos antituberculosos a fin de mejorar la eficacia y evitar la aparición de bacterias resistentes a los antibióticos. Además tiene cierto efecto para disentería, tos ferina y sty. |
| 用法、用量<br>Administración y dosis | 口服：成人 1 次 0.3g，1 次顿服；对急性粟粒性肺结核或结核性脑膜炎，1 次 0.2 ～ 0.3g，一日 3 次。静脉注射或静脉滴注：对较重度浸润结核，肺外活动结核等，1 次 0.3 ～ 0.6g，加 5% 葡萄糖注射液或等渗氯化钠注射液 20 ～ 40ml，缓慢推注；或加入输液 250 ～ 500ml 中静脉滴注。百日咳：一日按 10 ～ 15mg/kg，分为 3 次服。麦粒肿：一日按 4 ～ 10mg/kg，分为 3 次服。局部（胸腔内注射治疗局灶性结核等）：1 次 50 ～ 200mg。<br><br>Se toma por vía oral: adultos 0.3g una vez, dosis única; tuberculosis miliar aguda o meningitis tuberculosa, 0.2 ～ 0.3g una vez, tres veces al día. Inyección o infusión intravenosa: para infiltración de la tuberculosis de grado pesado, tuberculosis extrapulmonar, etc. 0.3 ～ 0.6g una vez, agregado por 20 ～ 40ml de 5% inyección de glucosa o inyección isotónica de cloruro de sodio, inyectado lentamente; o agregado por 250 ～ 500ml de infusión. La tos ferina: 10 ～ 15mg/kg al día, en tres veces. Pocilga: 4 ～ 10mg/kg al día, en tres veces. Parcial(inyección intrapleural en el tratamiento de la tuberculosis focal, etc.): 50 ～ 200mg al día. |
| 剂型、规格<br>Formulaciones y<br>especificaciones | 片剂：每片 0.05g；0.1g；0.3g。<br>注射液：每支 0.1g（2ml）。<br>Una tableta: 0.05g; 0.1g; 0.3g.<br>Una inyección: 0.1g(2ml). |
| 药品名称 Drug Names | 对氨基水杨酸钠 Aminosalicilato de sodio |
| 适应证<br>Indicaciones | 本品很少单独应用，常配合异烟肼、链霉素等应用，以增强疗效并避免细菌产生耐药性。也可用于甲状腺功能亢进症。对于甲亢合并结核患者较适用，在用碘剂无效而影响手术时，可短期服用本品为手术创造条件。本品尚有较强的降血脂作用。<br><br>Rara vez se usa por sí solo, y frecuentemente se combina con isoniacida y estreptomicina a fin de mejorar la eficacia y evitar la aparición de bacterias resistentes a los antibióticos. También se puede usar para hipertiroidismo. Se aplica a pacientes con tuberculosis hipertiroidismo y cuando se usa el yodo sin eficacia en una operación se lo puede aplicar para crear condiciones de la cirugía. Tiene fuerte efecto de reducción de lípidos en sangre. |
| 用法、用量<br>Administración y dosis | 口服：每次 2 ～ 3g，一日 8 ～ 12g，饭后服。小儿每日 200 ～ 300mg/kg，分 4 次服。静脉滴注：每日 4 ～ 12g（先从小剂量开始），以等渗氯化钠注射液或 5% 葡萄糖液溶解后，配成 3% ～ 4% 浓度滴注。小儿每日 200 ～ 300mg/kg。胸腔内注射：每次 10% ～ 20% 溶液 10 ～ 20ml（用等渗氯化钠注射液溶解）。甲亢手术前：一日 8 ～ 12g，分 4 次服，同时服用维生素 B、维生素 C。服药时间不可过长，以防毒性反应出现。<br><br>Se toma por vía oral: 2 ～ 3g cada vez, 8 ～ 12g al día, tras la comida. Niños 200 ～ 300mg/kg al día, en 4 veces. Infusión intravenosa: 4 ～ 12g al día(empieza por dosis pequeña), disuelto en la inyección isotónica de cloruro de sodio o 5% inyección de glucosa, ) preparado como infusión de concentración de 3% ～ 4%. Niños: 200 ～ 300mg/kg al día. Inyección intratorácica: 10 ～ 20ml de 10% ～ 20% solución (disuelto en inyección isotónica de cloruro de sodio). Antes de la cirugía de hipertiroidismo: 8 ～ 12g al día, en 4 veces, se toman vitamina B, C a la vez. El tiempo de administración no debe ser demasiado largo para evitar reacción tóxica. |

**续　表**

| | |
|---|---|
| 剂型、规格<br>Formulaciones y especificaciones | 片剂：每片 0.5g。<br>注射用对氨基水杨酸钠：每瓶 2g；4g；6g。<br>Una tableta: 0.5g.<br>Aminosalicilato de sodio para inyección: 2g; 4g; 6g cada botella. |
| **药品名称 Drug Names** | 利福平 Rifampicina |
| 适应证<br>Indicaciones | 主要应用于肺结核和其他结核病，也可用于麻风病的治疗。此外也可考虑用于耐甲氧西林金黄色葡萄球菌（MRSA）所致的感染。抗结核治疗时应与其他抗结核药联合应用。<br>Se usa principalmente para tuberculosis pulmonar y otras tuberculosis así como tratar la lepra. Además conside la posibilidad de tratar infecciones causadas por staphylococcus aureus resistente a la meticilina(MRSA). Debe combinar con otros medicamentos anti-TB en el tratamiento de tuberculosis. |
| 用法、用量<br>Administración y dosis | 肺结核及其他结核病：成人，口服，1 次 0.45～0.6g，一日 1 次，于早饭前服，疗程半年左右；1～12 岁儿童 1 次量为 10mg/kg，一日 2 次；新生儿 1 次 5mg/kg，一日 2 次。其他感染：一日量 0.6～1g，分 2～3 次给予，饭前 1 小时服用。沙眼及结膜炎：用 0.1% 滴眼剂，一日 4～6 次。治疗沙眼的疗程为 6 周。<br>Tuberculosis pulmonar, etc.: adultos, por vía oral, 0.45 ～ 0.6g cada vez, 1 vez al día, antes de almuerzo, medio año de ciclo de tratamiento; niño de 1 ～ 12 años de edad: una dosis de 10mg/kg, dos veces al día; recién nacidos: 5mg/kg una vez, dos veces al día. Otras infecciones: dosis diaria de 0.6 ～ 1g, dada en 2 ～ 3 veces, una hora antes de la comida. El tracoma y la conjuntivitis: colirio de 0,1%, 4 ～ 6 veces al día. El ciclo de tratamiento para tratar tracoma es de 6 semanas. |
| 剂型、规格<br>Formulaciones y especificaciones | 片（胶囊）剂：每片（粒）0.15g；0.3g；0.45g；0.6g。口服混悬液：20mg/ml。复方制剂：RIMACTAZIDE（含利福平及异烟肼）；RIMATAZIDE+Z（含利福平、异烟肼及吡嗪酰胺）。<br>Una tableta (cápsula): 0.15g; 0.3g; 0.45g; 0.6g. Suspensión por vía oral: 20mg/ml. Preparación compuesta: RIMACTAZIDE (que incluye rifampicina y isoniazida); RIMATAZIDE+Z (que incluye rifampicina, isoniazida y pirazinamida). |
| **药品名称 Drug Names** | 利福定 Rifandina |
| 适应证<br>Indicaciones | 用于各型肺结核和其他结核病，包括对多种抗结核药物已产生耐药性患者。亦用于麻风病及敏感菌感染性皮肤病等。<br>Se usa para todos tipos de tuberculosis pulmonar y otras tuberculosis, incluyendo pacientes con resistencia a múltiples medicamentos anti-TB. También se usa para la lepra e infecciones de la piel debido a cepas susceptibles, etc. |
| 用法、用量<br>Administración y dosis | 成人每日 150～200mg，早晨空腹一次服用。儿童按 3～4mg/kg，一次服用。治疗肺结核病的疗程为 6 个月～1 年。眼部感染采取局部用药（滴眼剂浓度 0.05%）。<br>Adultos 150 ～ 200mg al día, se toma de una vez con el estómago vacío por la mañana. Niños 3 ～ 4mg/kg, se toma de una vez. El ciclo de tratamiento para tratar tuberculosis pulmonar es de medio año a un año. En caso de infección ocular, se adopta tratamiento local(concentración de gotas para los ojos 0.05%). |
| 剂型、规格<br>Formulaciones y especificaciones | 胶囊：每粒 75mg；150mg。<br>Una cápsula: 75mg; 150mg. |
| **药品名称 Drug Names** | 利福喷丁 Rifapentina |
| 适应证<br>Indicaciones | 主要用于治疗结核病（常与其他抗结核药联合应用）。<br>Se usa principalmente para tratar tuberculosis(frecuentemente combina con otros medicamentos anti-TB). |
| 用法、用量<br>Administración y dosis | 1 次 600mg，每周只用 1 次（其作用约相当于利福平 600mg，一日 1 次）。必要时可按上量，每周 2 次。<br>600mg 1 vez a la semana(efecto equivalente a 600mg de rifampicina, 1 vez al día). En casos necesarios la dosis dos veces a la semana. |

**续　表**

| 剂型、规格<br>Formulaciones y especificaciones | 片（胶囊）剂：每片（粒）150mg；300mg。<br>Una tableta (cápsula): 150mg; 300mg. |
|---|---|
| **药品名称 Drug Names** | 利福霉素钠 Rifamicina de sodio |
| 适应证<br>Indicaciones | 用于不能口服用药的结核患者和耐甲氧西林金黄色葡萄球菌（MRSA）感染，以及难治性军团菌病。<br><br>Se usa para pacientes con tuberculosis que no puede tomar medicamentos por vía oral así como infecciones causadas por staphylococcus aureus resistente a la meticilina(MRSA) y enfermedad del legionario refractario. |
| 用法、用量<br>Administración y dosis | 肌内注射：成人1次250mg，每8～12小时1次。静脉注射（缓慢注射）：1次500mg，一日2～3次；小儿一日量10～30mg/kg。此外亦可稀释至一定浓度局部应用或雾化吸入。重症患者宜先静脉滴注，待病情好转后改肌内注射。用于治疗肾盂肾炎时，每日剂量在750mg以上。对于严重感染，开始剂量可酌增到一日1000mg。<br><br>Inyección intramuscular: adultos 250mg 1 vez, cada 8 ～ 12 horas. Inyección intravenosa (lenta): 500mg 1 vez, 2 ～ 3 veces al día; dosis diaria para niños: 10 ～ 30mg/kg. Además también se puede diluir hasta una concentración para aplicación local o inhalación. Los pacientes con síntomas graves convienen efectuar infusión intravenosa primero, y cuando mejoren un poco, pueden hacer inyección intramuscular. Para tratar pielonefritis, la dosis diaria es superior a 750mg. Para infecciones graves, la dosis inicial puede incrementarse a 1000mg al día según el caso. |
| 剂型、规格<br>Formulaciones y especificaciones | 注射用利福霉素钠：每瓶250mg。注射液：每支0.25g（5ml）（供静脉滴注用）；0.125g（2ml）（供肌内注射用）。<br><br>Rifamicina de sodio para inyección: 250mg cada botella. Una inyección: 0.25g(5ml)(para infusión); 0.125g(2ml)(para inyección intramuscular). |
| **药品名称 Drug Names** | 链霉素 Estreptomicina |
| 适应证<br>Indicaciones | 主要用于结核杆菌感染，也用于布氏杆菌病、鼠疫及其他敏感菌所致的感染。<br><br>Se usa principalmente para infección de tuberculosis, brucelosis, la plaga y otras infecciones debido a cepas susceptibles. |
| 用法、用量<br>Administración y dosis | 口服不吸收，只对肠道感染有效，现已少用。系统治疗需肌内注射，一般应用1次0.5g，一日2次，或1次0.75g，一日1次，1～2周为1个疗程。用于结核病，一日剂量为0.75～1g，1次或分成2次肌内注射。儿童一般一日15～25mg/kg，分2次给予；结核病治疗则一日20mg/kg，隔日用药。新生儿一日10～20mg/kg。用于治疗结核病时，常与异烟肼或其他抗结核药联合应用，以避免耐药菌株的产生。<br><br>No se absorbe por vía oral, sólo eficaz para infección intestinal, rara vez se utiliza ahora. Para el tratamiento sistémico se debe inyectar por vía intramuscular, 0.5g cada vez, dos veces al día, o 0.75g una vez al día, ciclo de tratamiento 1 ～ 2 semanas. Para tuberculosis, dosis diaria de 0.75 ～ 1g, dividida en una o dos veces por inyección intramuscular. Niños: 15 ～ 25mg/kg al día, dado en dos veces; el tratamiento de tuberculosis 20mg/kg al día, se administra cada dos días. Recién nacidos 10 ～ 20mg/kg al día. Para tratar tuberculosis, se combina con isoniazida u otros medicamentos anti-TB para evitar que aparezcan cepas resistentes. |
| 剂型、规格<br>Formulaciones y especificaciones | 注射用硫酸链霉素：每瓶0.75g；1g；2g；5g。<br>Estreptomicina para inyección: 0.75g; 1g; 2g; 5g cada botella. |
| **药品名称 Drug Names** | 乙胺丁醇 Etambutol |
| 适应证<br>Indicaciones | 为二线抗结核药，可用于经其他抗结核药治疗无效的病例，应与其他抗结核药联合应用。以增强疗效并延缓细菌耐药性的产生。<br><br>Es de la segunda línea de medicamentos antituberculosos. Se puede usar en casos sin eficacia de otros medicamentos anti-TB y se combina con otros fármacos anti-TB para mejorar la eficacia y postergar la ocurrencia de resistir a medicamentos de las cepas. |

**续 表**

| | |
|---|---|
| 用法、用量<br>Administración y dosis | 结核初治：一日 15mg/kg，顿服；或每周 3 次，每次 25～30mg/kg（不超过 2.5g）；或每周 2 次，每次 50mg/kg（不超过 2.5g）。结核复治，每次 25mg/kg，每日一次顿服，连续 60 日，继而按每次 15mg/kg，每日 1 次顿服。非典型分枝杆菌感染，按每次 15～25mg/kg，每日一次顿服。<br>El tratamiento inicial de la tuberculosis: 15mg/kg al día, dosis única; o 3 veces a la semana, 25～30mg/kg cada vez( no sobrepasa 2.5g); o dos veces a la semana, 50mg/kg cada vez( no sobrepasa 2.5g). Retratamiento de la tuberculosis: 25mg/kg cada vez, dosis única al día, 60 días consecutivos, y luego se administra 15mg/kg cada vez, dosis única al día. Infección por micobacterias atípicas, 15～25mg/kg cada vez, dosis única al día. |
| 剂型、规格<br>Formulaciones y especificaciones | 片剂：每片 0.25g。<br>Una tableta: 0.25g. |
| **药品名称 Drug Names** | **乙硫异烟胺 Etionamida** |
| 适应证<br>Indicaciones | 单独应用少，常与其他抗结核病药联合应用以增强疗效和避免病菌产生耐药性。<br>Rara vez se usa por sí solo, y frecuentemente se combina con otros medicamentos anti-TB a fin de mejorar la eficacia y evitar la aparición de bacterias resistentes a los medicamentos. |
| 用法、用量<br>Administración y dosis | 一日量 0.5～0.8g，一次服用或分次服（以一次服效果为好），必要时也可从小剂量（0.3g/d）开始。<br>Dosis diaria 0.5 ～ 0.8g, se administra en una o varias veces(efecto mejor en una vez), en casos necesarios, se puede empezar por dosis pequeña(0.3g/d). |
| 剂型、规格<br>Formulaciones y especificaciones | 肠溶片：每片 0.1g。<br>Una tableta con recubrimiento entérico: 0.1g. |
| **药品名称 Drug Names** | **丙硫异烟胺 Protionamida** |
| 适应证<br>Indicaciones | 本品仅对分枝杆菌有效，与其他抗结核药联合用于结核病经一线药物（如链霉素、异烟肼、利福平和乙胺丁醇）治疗无效者。<br>Sólo es eficaz para micobacterias y se combina con otros medicamentos anti-TB para pacientes sin efectos medicados con primera línea de fármacos(por ejemplo isoniacida, estreptomicina, rifampicina y etambutol). |
| 用法、用量<br>Administración y dosis | 口服，成人常用量，与其他抗结核药物合用，一次 250mg，一日 2～3 次。小儿常用量，与其他抗结核药合用，一次按体重口服 4～5mg/kg，一日 3 次。<br>Se toma por vía oral, dosis habitual de adultos, combinando con otros medicanmentos anti-TB, según el peso corporal, 4 ～ 5mg/kg, 3 veces al día. |
| 剂型、规格<br>Formulaciones y especificaciones | 肠溶片：每片 0.1g。<br>Una tableta con recubrimiento entérico: 0.1g. |
| **药品名称 Drug Names** | **吡嗪酰胺 Pirazinamida** |
| 适应证<br>Indicaciones | 与其他抗结核药联合用于经一线抗结核药（如链霉素、异烟肼、利福平和乙胺丁醇）治疗无效的结核病。本品仅对分枝杆菌有效。<br>Se combina con otros medicamentos anti-TB para pacientes con tuberculosis medicados con primera línea de fármacos(por ejemplo isoniacida, estreptomicina, rifampicina y etambutol) sin efectos.Sólo es eficaz para micobacterias. |
| 用法、用量<br>Administración y dosis | 口服。成人常用量，与其他抗结核药联合，每 6 小时按体重 5～8.75mg/kg，或每 8 小时按体重 6.7～11.7mg/kg 给予，最高每日 3g。治疗异烟肼耐药菌感染时可增加至每日 60mg/kg。<br>Se toma por vía oral. Dosis habitual de adultos, combinando con otros medicanmentos anti-TB, cada 6 horas, según el peso corporal, 5 ～ 8.75mg/kg, o cada 8 horas, según el peso corporal, 6.7 ～ 11.7mg/kg, dosis máxima al día 3g. En el tratamiento de infecciones resistentes a la isoniazida se puede incrementar a 60mg/kg al día. |

**续　表**

| 剂型、规格<br>Formulaciones y especificaciones | 肠溶片：每片 0.25g；0.5g。<br>Una tableta con recubrimiento entérico：0.25g；0.5g。 |
|---|---|

**4. 抗麻风病药及抗麻风病反应药 Medicamentos contra la lepra y contra la respuesta a lalepra**

| 药品名称 Drug Names | 氨苯砜 Dapsona |
|---|---|
| 适应证<br>Indicaciones | 主要用于治疗各型麻风。近年试用本品治疗系统性红斑狼疮、痤疮、银屑病、带状疱疹等。<br>Se usa principalmente para todos los tipos de lepra. En los últimos años tratan de usar este fármaco para lupus eritematoso sistémico, el acné, la psoriasis y el herpes zóster, etc. |
| 用法、用量<br>Administración y dosis | 治疗麻风病，口服，1 次 50～100mg，一日 100～200mg。可于开始每日 12.5～25mg，以后逐渐加量到每日 100mg。由于本品有蓄积作用，故每服药 6 日后停药一日，每服 10 周停药 2 周。必要时，可与利福平每日 600mg 联合应用。儿童剂量一日 1.4mg/kg。治疗红斑狼疮，一日 100mg，连用 3～6 个月；痤疮，一日 50mg；银屑病或变应性血管炎一日 100～150mg；带状疱疹，一日 3 次，1 次 25mg，连服 3～14 日；糜烂性扁平苔藓，一日 50mg，连用 3 个月。以上治疗中，均遵循服药 6 日，停药一日的原则。<br>Tratamiento de lepra, por vía oral, 50～100mg cada vez, 100～200mg al día. Se puede empezar por 12.5～25mg al día, incrementando en adelante gradualmente a 100mg al día. Como tiene efectos acumulativos, tras 6 días de administración, se interrumpe un día, tras 10 semanas de administración, se interrumpe 2 semanas. En casos necesarios, se puede combinar con 600mg de rifampicina. La dosis diaria para niños es de 1.4mg/kg. Para tratar lupus eritematoso, 100mg al día, 3～6 meses consecutivos; acné, 50mg al día; psoriasis o vasculitis alérgica: 100～150mg al día; herpes, 3 veces al día, 25mg cada vez, 3～14 días consecutivos; liquen plano erosivo, 50mg al día, 3 meses consecutivos. En los casos de arriba, se observa el principio de 6 días de administración con 1 día de interrupción. |
| 剂型、规格<br>Formulaciones y especificaciones | 片剂：每片 50mg；100mg。<br>Una tableta: 50mg; 100mg. |
| 药品名称 Drug Names | 醋氨苯砜 Acedapsona |
| 适应证<br>Indicaciones | 用于各型麻风病。<br>Se usa para todos los tipos de lepra. |
| 用法、用量<br>Administración y dosis | 肌内注射，1 次 0.225g，隔 60～75 日注射 1 次，疗程长达数年。为了防止长期单用本品导致细菌产生耐药性，可在用药期间加服氨苯砜 0.1～0.15g，每周 2 次。<br>Inyección intramuscular, 0.225g una vez, cada 60～75 días una inyección, ciclo de tratamiento por varios años. Para prevenir que por el uso a largo plazo las cepas aparezcan resistencia al medicamento, se puede tomar 0.1～0.15g de dapsone, dos veces a la semana durante la administración. |
| 剂型、规格<br>Formulaciones y especificaciones | 油注射液：每支 225mg（1.5ml）；450mg（3ml）；900mg（6ml）。为 40% 苯甲酸苄酯及 60% 蓖麻油的混悬剂。用前振摇均匀，用粗针头吸出，注入臀肌。<br>Inyección de aceite: 225mg(1.5ml); 450mg(3ml); 900mg(6ml). Es suspensión mixta de 40% benzoato de bencilo y 60% aceite de ricino. Sacudido de forma uniforme antes del uso, aspirado con aguja gruesa, se inyecta en glúteos. |
| 药品名称 Drug Names | 苯丙砜 Solasulfona |
| 适应证<br>Indicaciones | 主要用于治疗各型麻风。近年试用本品治疗系统性红斑狼疮、痤疮、银屑病、带状疱疹等。<br>Se usa principalmente para todos los tipos de lepra. En los últimos años tratan de usar este fármaco para lupus eritematoso sistémico, el acné, la psoriasis y el herpes zóster, etc. |
| 用法、用量<br>Administración y dosis | 肌内注射：每周 2 次，第 1～2 周每次 100～200mg，以后每 2 周递增 100mg/ 次，至第 14～16 周，每次量为 800mg，继续维持，每用药 10 周后，停药 2 周。口服：300mg/d，逐渐增量至 3g。每服药 10 周，停药 2 周。<br>Inyección intramuscular：dos veces a la semana，100～200mg cada vez durante la primera y la segunda semana，se incrementa 100mg/vez cada dos semanas en adelante，entre la catorce y quince semana，la dosis/vez es de 800mg，tras 10 semanas consecutivas de administración，se suspenden dos semanas. Se toma por vía oral：300mg/d，se incrementa gradualmente hasta 3g. Cada administración dura 10 semanas y se suspenden 2 semanas. |

**续　表**

| 剂型、规格<br>Formulaciones y especificaciones | 注射液：每支 2g（5ml）；4g（10ml）。片剂：每片 0.5g。<br>Una inyección: 2g(5ml); 4g(10ml). Una tableta: 0.5g. |
|---|---|
| **药品名称 Drug Names** | 氯法齐明 Clofazimina |
| 适应证<br>Indicaciones | 对于瘤型麻风和其他型麻风均有一定疗效，对耐砜类药物麻风杆菌感染也有效。可用于因用其他药物而引起急性麻风反应的病例。<br>Tiene cierto efecto para lepra lepromatosa y otros tipos de lepra, también eficaz para infección por bacilo de la lepra resistente a medicamentos sulfone. Se puede tratar reacción leprosa aguda por otros medicamentos. |
| 用法、用量<br>Administración y dosis | 口服。对麻风病，每日 100mg；对麻风反应，一日 200 ～ 400mg，麻风反应控制后，逐渐减量至每日 100mg。<br>Se toma por vía oral. Para tratar lepra, 100mg al día; reacción leprosa, 200 ～ 400mg al día, al ser controlada, se reduce la dosis hasta 100mg al día. |
| 剂型、规格<br>Formulaciones y especificaciones | 胶囊：每粒 50mg；100mg。胶丸（油蜡或聚乙二醇基质）：每丸 50mg。<br>Una cápsula: 50mg; 100mg. Una cápsul(de cera de aceite o polietileno glicol matriz): 50mg. |
| **药品名称 Drug Names** | 沙利度胺 Talidomida |
| 适应证<br>Indicaciones | 用于麻风结节性红斑。在 2006 年美国 FDA 批准用于治疗多发性骨髓瘤。中华医学会认可：除了可以治疗麻风结节性红斑外，在《临床诊疗指南·血液学分册》中沙利度胺可以治疗多发性骨髓瘤；在《临床诊疗指南·风湿学分册》中沙利度胺可以治疗强直性脊柱炎和白塞病。<br>Se usa para eritema nodoso leproso. En año 2006,la FDA aprobó su tratamiento del mieloma múltiple. Asociación Médica de China aprueba: a partir de tratar eritema nodoso leproso, en Volumen Hematología de Guías de Práctica Clínica talidomida puede tratar mieloma múltiple; en Volumen Reumatología de Guías de Práctica Clínica talidomida puede tratar espondilitis anquilosante y behcet. |
| 用法、用量<br>Administración y dosis | 口服每日 100 ～ 200mg，分 4 次服。对严重反应，可增至 300 ～ 400mg（反应得到控制即逐渐减量）。对长期反应者，需要较长期服药，每日或隔日服 25 ～ 50mg。移植后用药：一日 800 ～ 1600mg，分 4 次服，治疗可持续 2 ～ 700 日（平均为 240 日）。治疗完全有效的患者，再持续 3 个月以后逐渐减量（每 2 周减少 25%）；部分有效的患者，再观察到最大效应后还应再治疗 6 个月。<br>Se toma por vía oral, 100 ～ 200mg al día, en 4 tomas. Para reacciones graves, se puede incrementar a 300 ～ 400mg(al ser controladas la dosis puede reducirse). Para pacientes de reacciones a largo plazo, se deben administrar a largo plazo, 25 ～ 50mg al día o cada dos días. Administración después del trasplante: 800 ～ 1600mg al día, en 4 veces, el tratamiento puede durar 2 ～ 700 días(promedio de 240 días). Pacientes con tratamiento totalmente eficaz, deben seguir con la administración por 3 meses y luego reducir la dosis gradualmente(25% cada dos semanas); Pacientes con tratamiento parcialmente eficaz, al observar la mayor eficacia, deben seguir con la administración por 6 meses. |
| 剂型、规格<br>Formulaciones y especificaciones | 片剂：每片 25mg；50mg。<br>Una tableta: 25mg; 50mg. |

## 5. 抗真菌药 Antifúngicos

| **药品名称 Drug Names** | 两性霉素 B　Anfotericina B |
|---|---|
| 适应证<br>Indicaciones | 用于隐球菌、球孢子菌、荚膜组织胞浆菌、芽生菌、孢子丝菌、念珠菌、毛霉、曲霉等引起的内脏或全身感染。<br>Se usa para infección visceral o sistémica a causa de criptococosis, coccidioidomicosis, histoplasma capsulatum, blastomyces, sporothrix, candidiasis, enzima peludo y aspergillus. |

**续 表**

| | |
|---|---|
| 用法、用量<br>Administración y dosis | 临用前加灭菌注射用水适量使溶解（不可用氯化钠注射液溶解与稀释），再加入 5% 葡萄糖注射液（pH > 4.2）中浓度每 1ml 不超过 1mg。静脉滴注：开始用小剂量 1 ～ 2mg，逐日递增到一日 1mg/kg。每日给药一次，滴注速度通常为每分钟 1 ～ 1.5ml。疗程总量：白念珠菌感染约 1g，隐球菌脑膜炎约 3g。鞘内注射：对隐球菌脑膜炎，除静脉滴注外尚需鞘内给药。每次从 0.05 ～ 0.1mg 开始，逐渐递增至 0.5 ～ 1mg（浓度为 0.1 ～ 0.25mg/ml）。溶于注射用水 0.5 ～ 1ml 中，按鞘内注射法常规操作，共约 30 次，必要时可酌加地塞米松注射液以减轻反应。雾化吸入：适用于肺及支气管感染病例。一日量 5 ～ 10mg，溶于注射用水 100 ～ 200ml 中，分 4 次用。局部病灶注射：浓度 1 ～ 3mg/ml，3 ～ 7 日用 1 次，必要时可加普鲁卡因注射液少量；对真菌性脓胸和关节炎，可局部抽脓后，注入药 5 ～ 10mg，每周 1 ～ 3 次。局部外用：浓度 2.5 ～ 5mg/ml。腔道用药：栓剂 25mg。眼部用药：眼药水 0.25%；眼药膏 1%。口服：对肠道真菌感染一日 0.5 ～ 2g，分 2 ～ 4 次服用。<br><br>Antes de usarlo se agrega cierta cantidad de agua estéril de inyeccón para disolverlo(no se puede usar inyección de cloruro de sodio para disolverlo y diluirlo), más 5% inyección de glucosa(pH > 4.2), cuya concentración no excede 1mg cada 1ml. Infusión intravenosa: se empieza por dosis pequeña de 1 ～ 2mg, creciendo diariamente hasta 1mg/kg al día. Se administra 1 vez al día, con la velocidad general de 1 ～ 1.5ml/minuto. Dosis total del tratamiento: aproximadamente 1g para infección por Candida albicans, aproximadamente 3g para meningitis criptocócica. Inyección intratecal: para meningitis criptocócica, se necesita infusión intravenosa más inyección intratecal. Cada vez se empieza por 0.05 ～ 0.1mg, se incrementa gradualmente hasta 0.5 ～ 1mg (concentración de 0.1 ～ 0.25mg/ml). Se disuelve en 0.5 ～ 1ml de agua para inyección, se efectúa operación convencional de inyección intratecal, en total 30 veces, y se agrega inyección de dexametasona en casos necesarios para aliviar las reacciones. La inhalación: se aplica a infecciones pulmonales y bronquiales. Dosis diaria de 5 ～ 10mg, disuelta en 100 ～ 200ml de agua para inyección, dividida en 4 veces. Inyección de lesión local: concentración de 1 ～ 3mg/ml, 1 vez cada 3 ～ 7 días, se agrega inyección de procaína en casos necesarios; para empiema fungal y artritis, se puede extraer pus localmente y se inyecta 5 ～ 10mg del medicamento, 1 ～ 3 veces a la semana. Aplicación tópica: concentración de 2.5 ～ 5mg/ml. Aplicación de tractos: 25mg de supositorio. Aplicación para los ojos: 0.25% gotas; 1% pomada ocular. Se toma por vía oral: 0.5 ～ 2g al día para infecciones fúngicas intestinales, en 2 ～ 4 veces. |
| 剂型、规格<br>Formulaciones y especificaciones | 注射用两性霉素 B（脱氧胆酸钠复合物）：每支 5mg；25mg；50mg。<br>Anfotericina B para inyección (complejo de desoxicolato de sodio): 5mg; 25mg; 50mg. |
| 药品名称 Drug Names | 伊曲康唑 Itraconazol |
| 适应证<br>Indicaciones | 主要应用于深部真菌所引起的系统感染如类球孢子菌病、类球孢子菌病、组织胞浆菌病、芽生菌病、着色真菌病、孢子丝菌病等。也可用于念珠菌病和曲霉病。<br><br>Se usa principalmente para infección sistémica a causa de fúngica profunda, tales como paracoccidioidomicosis, paracoccidioidomicosis, histoplasmosis, blastomicosis, cromomicosis y esporotricosis, etc. También se puede aplicar a candidiasis y aspergilosis. |
| 用法、用量<br>Administración y dosis | 一般为一日 100 ～ 200mg，顿服，一般疗程为 3 个月，个别情况下疗程延长到 6 个月。短程间歇疗法：1 次 200mg，一日 2 次，连服 7 日为一个疗程。停药 2 一日，开始第 2 个疗程，指甲癣服 2 个疗程，趾甲癣服 3 个疗程，治愈率分别为 97% 和 69.4%。<br><br>Generalmente 100 ～ 200mg al día, dosis única, 3 meses de tratamiento, se extiende a 6 meses en casos particulares. Terapia intermitente: 200mg una vez, dos veces al día, 7 días consecutivos como un ciclo. Se suspenden 2 días para empezar el segundo ciclo, tiña de uñas dos ciclos, tiña de uñas de los pies 3 ciclos, y la tasa de curación puede alcanzar a 97% y 69.4% respectivamente. |
| 剂型、规格<br>Formulaciones y especificaciones | 片剂：每片 100mg；200mg。<br>注射液：25ml；250mg。<br>Una tableta: 100mg; 200mg.<br>Una inyección: 25ml; 250mg. |
| 药品名称 Drug Names | 氟康唑 Fluconazol |
| 适应证<br>Indicaciones | 应用于敏感菌所致的各种真菌感染，如隐球菌性脑膜炎、复发性口咽念珠菌病等。<br>Se usa para las infecciones fúngicas causadas por bacterias sensibles, tales como eningitis criptocócica y candidiasis orofaríngea recurrente, etc. |

> **续　表**

| | |
|---|---|
| 用法、用量<br>Administración y dosis | 念珠菌性口咽炎或食管炎：第一日口服 200mg，以后每日服 100mg，疗程 2 ～ 3 周（症状消失仍需用药），以免复发。 念珠菌系统感染：第 1 日 400mg，以后每日 200mg。疗程 4 周或症状消失后再用 2 周。隐球菌性脑膜炎第 1 日 400mg，以后每日 200mg。如患者反应正常，也可用一日 1 次 400mg，至脑脊液细菌培养阴性后 10 ～ 12 周。 肾功能不全者，减少用量。肌酐清除率 > 50ml/min 者用正常量；肌酐清除率为 21 ～ 50ml/min 者用 1/2 量；肌酐清除率为 11% ～ 20%ml/min 者用 1/4 量。 口服和静脉输注用量相同。静脉滴注速度约为 200mg/h。可加入到葡萄糖液、生理氯化钠液、乳酸钠林格液中滴注。<br><br>Faringitis o esofagitis por Candida: se toma 200mg el primer día, y 100mg/día después, 2 ～ 3 semanas de tratamiento(se debe seguir administrando cuando desaparezcan los síntomas), con el fin de evitar que se repita. Infección sistémica por Candida: se toma 400mg el primer día, y 200mg/día después, 4 semanas de tratamiento o al desaparecer los síntomas, se usa 2 semanas más. Meningitis criptocócica: se toma 400mg el primer día, y 200mg/día después. Si los pacientes revelan respuesta normal, también se puede usar 400mg/vez/día por 10 ～ 12 semanas al ser probado nagativo el cultivo bacteriano del líquido cefalorraquídeo. Los pacientes con insuficiencia renal, deben reducir la dosis. Los pacientes con aclaramiento de creatinina > 50ml/min, dosis normal; 21 ～ 50ml/min, la mitad; 11 ～ 20ml/min, 1/4. La dosis por vía oral y la por infusión intranenosa son iguales. La velocidad de infusión intranenosa es aproximadamente 200mg/h. Se puede agregar solución de glucosa, solución fisiológica de cloruro de sodio y ringer lactato a la infusión. |
| 剂型、规格<br>Formulaciones y especificaciones | 片剂（胶囊）：每片（粒）50mg；100mg；150mg 或 200mg。<br>注射剂：每瓶 200mg/100ml。<br><br>Una tableta (cápsula): 50mg; 100mg; 150mg o 200mg.<br>Una inyección: 200mg/100ml. |
| **药品名称 Drug Names** | 伏立康唑 Voriconazol |
| 适应证<br>Indicaciones | 用于治疗侵入性曲霉病，以及对氟康唑耐药的严重进入性念珠菌病感染及由足放线病菌属和镰刀菌属引起的严重真菌感染。主要用于进行性、致命危险的免疫系统受损的 2 岁以上患者。<br><br>Se usa para tratar aspergilosis invasiva, infecciones graves causadas por candidiasis invasora resistente a fluconazol e infecciones fúngicas graves causadas por scedosporium y fusarium. Se aplica principalmente a pacientes mayores a dos años con progresivo y fatal daño peligroso del sistema inmune. |
| 用法、用量<br>Administración y dosis | 负荷剂量：第 1 日静脉滴注 6mg/kg/ 次，12 小时 1 次；口服 400mg/ 次（体重 ≥ 40kg）或 200mg/ 次（体重 < 40kg），每 12 小时一次。 维持剂量：第 2 日起静滴 4mg/kg bid，或 200mg bid（体重 ≥ 40kg），或 100mg bid（体重 < 40kg）。均为 12 小时 1 次。治疗口咽、食管、白念珠菌病：口服，每次 200mg，一日 2 次；静脉注射，每次 3 ～ 6mg/kg，12 小时 1 次。<br><br>La dosis de carga: el primer día, infusión intravenosa 6mg/kg/vez, 12 horas una vez; por vía oral 400mg/vez(peso corporal ≥ 40kg) o 200mg/vez(peso corporal < 40kg), 12 horas una vez. Dosis de mantenimiento: Desde el segundo día infusión intravenosa 4mg/kg bid, o 200mg bid(peso corporal ≥ 40kg) o 100mg bid (peso corporal < 40kg). Cada 12 horas. Para tratar candidiasis orofaríngea, candidiasis esofágica y candidiasis: Se toma por vía oral, 200mg/vez, dos veces al día; inyección intravenosa, 3 ～ 6mg/kg cada vez, 12 horas una vez. |
| 剂型、规格<br>Formulaciones y especificaciones | 片剂：每片 50mg；200mg。 注射用伏立康唑：每支 200mg。<br>Una tableta: 50mg; 200mg. Voriconazol para inyección: 200mg. |
| **药品名称 Drug Names** | 氟胞嘧啶 Flucitosina |
| 适应证<br>Indicaciones | 用于念珠菌和隐球菌感染，单用效果不如两性霉素 B，可与两性霉素 B 合用，以增加疗效（协同作用）。<br><br>Se usa para infecciones causadas por candida y cryptococcus neoformans.La eficacia no es tan buena como anfotericina B y debe combinar con anfotericina B para mejorar la eficacia(efecto sinérgico). |

**续 表**

| 用法、用量<br>Administración y dosis | 口服：一日 4～6g，分 4 次服，疗程自数周至数月。静脉注射，一日 50～150mg/kg，分 2～3 次。单用本品时真菌易产生耐药性，宜与两性霉素 B 合用。<br><br>Se toma por vía oral: 4～6g al día, en 4 veces, el ciclo de tratamiento dura desde varias semanas hasta meses. Inyección intravenosa, 50～150mg/kg al día, dividida en 2～3 vece. Cuando se usa solo el medicamento el hongo es fácil de producir resistencia, se debe utilizar en combinación con anfotericina B. |
|---|---|
| 剂型、规格<br>Formulaciones y especificaciones | 片剂：每片 250mg；500mg。注射液：2.5g（250ml）。<br>Una tableta: 250mg; 500mg. Una inyección: 2.5g(250ml). |

| 药品名称 Drug Names | 特比奈芬 Terbinafina |
|---|---|
| 适应证<br>Indicaciones | 用于浅表真菌引起的皮肤、指甲感染，如毛癣菌、犬、小孢子菌、絮状表皮癣菌等引起的体癣、股癣、足癣、甲癣以及皮肤白念珠菌感染。<br><br>Se usa para infecciones de la piel y uñas causadas por hongos superficiales, tales como tiña corporal, tiña inguinal, tinea pedis, tinea e infección de la piel de candida albicans causadas por trichophyton, microsporum canis y epidermophyton floccosum. |
| 用法、用量<br>Administración y dosis | 口服，每日 1 次 250mg，足癣、体癣、股癣服用 1 周；皮肤念珠菌病 1～2 周；指甲癣 4～6 周，趾甲癣 12 周（口服对花斑癣无效）。外用（1% 霜剂）用于体癣、股癣、皮肤念珠菌病、花斑癣等，每日涂抹 1～2 次，疗程不定（1～2 周）。<br><br>Por vía oral, 250mg/vez/día, se toma por 1 semana para tratar tinea pedis, tiña corporal y tiña cruris; candidiasis en la piel 1～2 semanas; tiña de uñas 4～6 semanas, tiña de uñas de los pies 12 semanas (No tiene eficacia por vía oral para tratar versicolor). Uso cutáneo(1% crema) para tiña corporal, tiña cruris, candidiasis en la piel, versicolor, etc., 1～2 veces al día, ciclo de tratamiento indefinido(aproximadamente 1～2 semanas). |
| 剂型、规格<br>Formulaciones y especificaciones | 片剂：每片 125mg 或 250mg。霜剂：1%。<br>Una tableta: 125mg o 250mg. Crema: 1%. |

| 药品名称 Drug Names | 美帕曲星 Mepartricina |
|---|---|
| 适应证<br>Indicaciones | 用于白念珠菌阴道炎和肠道念珠菌病，也可用于阴道或肠道滴虫病。本品在肠道内与甾醇类物质结合成不吸收的物质，可用于治疗良性前列腺肿大。<br><br>Se usa para vaginitis causada por candida albicans y candidiasis intestinal. También se usa para tricomoniasis vaginal o intestinal. Este producto con esteroles en el intestino se convierte en material no absorbente, se puede utilizar para tratar el agrandamiento benigno de la próstata. |
| 用法、用量<br>Administración y dosis | 阴道或肠道念珠菌感染或滴虫病（用含十二烷基硫酸钠的复合片）：1 次 100 000U（2 片），每 12 小时 1 次，连用 3 日为 1 疗程。对于复杂性病例，疗程可酌情延长。宜食后服用。治疗前列腺肿大或肠道念珠菌病、滴虫病（用不含十二烷基硫酸钠的片剂）：一日 1 次，每次 100 000U。<br><br>Se usa para infección vaginal o intestinal por Candida o tricomoniasis (se toma tabletas compuestas que contienen dodecil sulfato de sodio): 100000 unidades 1 vez(2 tabletas), 12 horas 1 vez, 3 días consecutivos como un ciclo. En casos complicados, el ciclo puede extenderse correspondientemente. Conviene tomarse tras la comida. Para tratar agrandamiento de la próstata, candidiasis intestinal o tricomoniasis(se toma tabletas compuestas que contienen dodecil sulfato de sodio): 1 vez al día, 100000 unidades 1 vez. |
| 剂型、规格<br>Formulaciones y especificaciones | 肠溶片：每片 50 000U。阴道片：每片 25 000U。乳膏：供黏膜用。<br>Una tableta con recubrimiento entérico: 50000 unidades. Una tableta vaginal: 25000 unidades. Crema: se utiliza para la mucosa. |

| 药品名称 Drug Names | 阿莫罗芬 Amorolfina |
|---|---|
| 适应证<br>Indicaciones | 用于治疗皮肤及黏膜浅表真菌感染，如体癣、手癣、足癣、甲真菌病及阴道白念珠菌病等。<br><br>Se usa para tratar infecciones fúngicas superficiales de la piel y las membranas mucosas, tales como tinea corporis, tinea manus, tinea pedis, onicomicosis y candidiasis vaginal, etc. |
| 用法、用量<br>Administración y dosis | 甲真菌病：锉光病甲后将擦剂均匀涂抹于患处，每周 1～2 次。指甲感染一般连续用药 6 个月，趾甲感染持续用药 9～12 个月。皮肤浅表真菌感染：用 0.25% 乳膏局部涂抹，一日 1 次，至临床症状消失后继续治疗 3～5 日。阴道念珠菌病：先用温开水或 0.02% 高锰酸钾无菌溶液冲洗阴道或坐浴，再将 1 枚栓剂置于阴道深处。<br><br>Onicomicosis: se quitan uñas enfermas y se aplica linimento de manera uniforme a la zona afectada, 1～2 veces cada semana. Para infección de uñas generalmente se aplica por 6 meses consecutivos, infección de uñas de los pies se aplica por 9～12 meses consecutivos. Infección fúngica superficial de la piel: aplicación tópica de 0.25% pomada, 1 vez al día, cuando desaparezcan los síntomas clínicos, se sigue tratando por 3～5 días. Candidiasis vaginal: primero se usa agua caliente o 0.02% solución estéril de permanganato de potasio para limpiar la vagina o efectuar baño de asiento, y se pone 1 supositorio muy adentro de la vagina. |
| 剂型、规格<br>Formulaciones y especificaciones | 擦剂：每瓶 125mg（2.5ml）。<br>乳膏剂：每支 0.25%（5g）。<br>栓剂：每枚 25mg；50mg。<br>Linimento: 125mg(2.5ml) cada botella. Crema: 0.25%(5g). Un supositorio: 25mg; 50mg. |
| 药品名称 Drug Names | 醋酸卡泊芬净 Acetato de caspofungina |
| 适应证<br>Indicaciones | 用于治疗对其他治疗无效或不能耐受的侵袭性曲霉菌病；对疑似真菌感染的粒细胞缺乏伴发热患者的经验治疗；口咽及食管念珠菌病。侵袭性念珠菌病，包括中性粒细胞减少症及非中性粒细胞减少症患者的念珠菌血症。<br><br>Se usa para tratar la aspergilosis invasiva intolerante o sin otra terapia; como tratamiento empírico para sospechosa infección fúngica en pacientes neutropénicos con fiebre; así como tratar candidiasis orofaríngea y esofágica. Candidiasis invasora incluye neutropenia y candidemia en pacientes sin neutropenia. |
| 用法、用量<br>Administración y dosis | 第 1 日给予单次 70mg 负荷剂量，随后每日给予 50mg 的剂量。本品约需要 1 小时的时间经静脉缓慢输注给药。疗程取决于患者疾病的严重程度、被抑制的免疫功能恢复情况及对治疗的临床反应。对于治疗无临床反应而对本品耐受性良好的患者可以考虑将每日剂量加大到 70mg。<br><br>El primer día, se administra 70mg/vez como dosis de carga, y después, dosis de 50mg al día. El medicamento necesita 1 hora para administrarse por vía intravenosa. El ciclo de tratamiento depende de la gravedad de la enfermedad, la recuperación de la función inmunológica inhibida y la reacción clínica al tratamiento. Para tratar a pacientes sin reacciones clínicas y con buena tolerancia al medicamento, se puede considerar aumentar la dosis diaria hasta 70mg. |
| 剂型、规格<br>Formulaciones y especificaciones | 注射用醋酸卡泊芬净：50mg；70mg（以卡泊芬净计量）。<br>Acetato de caspofungin para inyección: 50mg; 70mg(calculado en caspofungin). |
| 药品名称 Drug Names | 米卡芬净 Micafungina |
| 适应证<br>Indicaciones | 用于治疗食管念珠菌感染，预防造血干细胞移植患者的念珠菌感染。<br>Se usa para tratar candidiasis esofágica y prevenir infección por candida en trasplante de progenitores hematopoyéticos. |
| 用法、用量<br>Administración y dosis | 治疗食管念珠菌病的推荐剂量为 150mg/d，预防造血干细胞移植患者的念珠菌感染的推荐剂量为 50mg/d。平均疗程分别为 15 日和 19 日。只能用生理盐水（可用 5% 葡萄糖注射液代替）配制和稀释。每 50mg 米卡芬净钠先加入 5ml 生理盐水溶解。为减少泡沫的产生，须轻轻转动玻璃瓶，不可用力振摇。随后将已溶解好的米卡芬净钠溶液加入到 100ml 生理盐水中滴注给药，给药时间至少 1 小时。 |

**续　表**

| | |
|---|---|
| | La dosis recomendada para tratar candidiasis esofágica es de 150mg/d, y la dosis recomendada para prevenir infecciones por Candida de los pacientes sometidos a trasplante de células madre hematopoyéticas es de 50mg/d. El ciclo de tratamiento de promedio es de 15 días y 19 días respectivamente. Sólo se usa solución salina fisiológica(5% inyección de glucosa como alternativa) para preparar y diluirlo. Cada 50mg de micafungina primero se diluye en 5ml de la solución salina fisiológica. Para reducir la formación de espuma, se debe girar suavemente el frasco de vidrio y no se puede agitarlo enérgicamente. Después se agrega la micafungina diluida a 100ml de la solución salina fisiológica para efectuar la infusión, cuyo período no deve ser menos a 1 hora. |
| 剂型、规格<br>Formulaciones y especificaciones | 米卡芬净钠冻干粉针：每瓶 50mg；100mg。<br>Polvo liofilizado de micafungina: 50mg; 100mg cada botella. |
| **药品名称 Drug Names** | **阿尼芬净 Anidulafungina** |
| 适应证<br>Indicaciones | 用于治疗食管念珠菌感染，念珠菌性败血症，念珠菌引起的腹腔脓肿及念珠菌性腹膜炎。<br>Se usa para tratar candidiasis esofágica, candida septicemia, absceso abdominal y peritonitis causada por candida albicans. |
| 用法、用量<br>Administración y dosis | 静脉给药：食管性念珠菌病，第一日 100mg，随后每日 50mg 疗程至少 14 日，且至少持续至症状消失后 7 日。念珠菌性败血症等，第一日 200mg，随后每日 100mg，疗程持续至最后一次阴性培养后至少 14 日。<br>Se administra por vía intravenosa: candidiasis esofágica, 100mg el primer día, y luego 50mg al día durante al menos 14 días como un ciclo de tratamiento, y dura al menos 7 días después de que desaparezcan los síntomas. Candida septicemia, etc., 200mg el primer día, y luego 100mg al día, el ciclo de tratamiento dura al menos 14 días tras el último cultivo negativo. |
| 剂型、规格<br>Formulaciones y especificaciones | 注射用阿尼芬净：每瓶 50mg；100mg。<br>Anidulafungina para inyección: 50mg; 100mg cada botella. |
| **药品名称 Drug Names** | **制霉菌素 Nistatina** |
| 适应证<br>Indicaciones | 口服用于治疗消化道念珠菌病。<br>Se toma por vía oral para tratar candidiasis gastrointestinal. |
| 用法、用量<br>Administración y dosis | 消化道念珠菌病：口服，成人 1 次 50 万～100 万 U，一日 3 次。小儿每日按体重 5 万～10 万 U/kg，分 3～4 次服。<br>Candidiasis gastrointestinal: por vía oral, adultos entre 0.5 y 1 millón unidades 1 vez, 3 veces al día. Niños: conforme al peso corporal 50000～100000 unidades/kg, en 3～4 veces. |
| 剂型、规格<br>Formulaciones y especificaciones | 片剂：50 万 U。软膏：每克 10 万 U。栓剂：每枚 10 万 U。<br>Una tableta: 500000 unidades. Una pomada: 100000 unidades por 1g. Un supositorio: 100000 unidades. |
| **药品名称 Drug Names** | **咪康唑 Miconazol** |
| 适应证<br>Indicaciones | 局部治疗念珠菌性外阴阴道病和革兰阳性细菌引起的双重感染。<br>Se usa para tratamiento local de candidiasis vulvovaginal e infecciones duales causadas por bacterias Gram positivas. |
| 用法、用量<br>Administración y dosis | 静脉给药：治疗深部真菌病一日常用量为 600～1800mg，分 3 次给予。局部用药：常作为全身用药的补充。<br>Administración por vía intravenosa: generalmente dosis diaria para tratar micosis profunda es de 600～1800mg, en 3 veces. Aplicación tópica: habitualmente como suplemento de la administración sistémica. |
| 剂型、规格<br>Formulaciones y especificaciones | 注射液：200mg。栓剂：100mg。霜剂：15g。<br>Una inyección: 200mg; Un supositorio: 100mg; Crema: 15g. |

**续　表**

| 6. 抗病毒药 Antivirales | |
|---|---|
| 药品名称 Drug Names | 阿昔洛韦 Aciclovir |
| 适应证<br>Indicaciones | 用于防治单纯疱疹病毒 HSV1 和 HSV2 的皮肤或黏膜感染，还可用于带状疱疹病毒感染。<br><br>Se usa para tratar y prevenir infección de piel o de las mucosas causada por virus del herpes simple HSV1 y HSV2. También se usa para infección por el virus de herpes zoster. |
| 用法、用量<br>Administración y dosis | 口服：1 次 200mg，每 4 小时 1 次或一日 1g，分次给予。疗程根据病情不同，短则几日，长者可达半年。肾功能不全者酌情减量。静脉滴注：1 次用量 5mg/kg，加入输液中，滴注时间为 1 小时，每 8 小时 1 次，连续 7 日。12 岁以下儿童 1 次按 250mg/ m² 用量给予。急性或慢性肾功能不全者，不宜用本品静脉滴注，因为滴速过快时可引起肾衰竭。国内治疗乙型肝炎的用法为 1 次滴注 7.5mg/kg，一日 2 次，溶于适量输液，维持滴注时间约 2 小时，连续应用 10 ～ 30 日。治疗生殖器疱疹，1 次 0.2g，一日 4 次，连用 5 ～ 10 日。<br><br>Se toma por vía oral: 200mg 1 vez, cada 4 horas o 1g al día, dividido en varias veces. El ciclo de tratamiento según la gravedad dura varios días como mínimo y como máximo medio año. Los pacientes con insuficiencia renal deben reducir la dosis correspondientemente. Infusión intravenosa: 5mg/kg cada dosis, al agregarse a la infusión, dura 1 hora, 8 horas 1 vez, 7 días consecutivos. A los niños menores de 12 años de edad, se administra 250mg/ m² 1 vez. A los pacientes con insuficiencia renal aguda o crónica, no les conviene administrarse por infusión intravenosa porque la velocidad excesiva puede causar insuficiencia renal. La dosis en China para tratar hepatitis B es 7.5mg/kg una infusión, 2 veces al día, disuelto en cierta cantidad de infusión, que dura aproximadamente 2 horas, aplicación continua de 10 ～ 30 días. Para tratar genital herpes, 0.2g 1 vez, 4 veces al día, 5 ～ 10 días consecutivos. |
| 剂型、规格<br>Formulaciones y especificaciones | 胶囊剂：每粒 200mg。 注射用阿昔洛韦（冻干制剂）：每瓶 500mg（标示量，含钠盐 549mg，折合纯品 500mg）。滴眼液：0.1%。眼膏：3%。霜膏剂：5%。<br><br>Una cápsula：200mg. Aciclovir para inyección （preparación liofilizada）：500mg cada botella（cantidad declarada，contiene 549mg de sodio；equivalente a 500mg de aciclovir）. Gotas para los ojos：0.1%. Ungüento para los ojos：3%. Cream：5%. |
| 药品名称 Drug Names | 更昔洛韦 Ganciclovir |
| 适应证<br>Indicaciones | 用于巨细胞病毒感染的治疗和预防，也可适用于单纯疱疹病毒感染。<br><br>Se usa para tratar y prevenir infección por citomegalovirus. También se usa para infección causada por virus del herpes simple. |
| 用法、用量<br>Administración y dosis | 诱导治疗：静脉滴注 5mg/kg（历时至少 1 小时），每 12 小时 1 次，连用 14 ～ 21 日（预防用药则为 7 ～ 14 日）；维持治疗：静脉滴注，5mg/kg，一日 1 次，每周用药 7 日；或 6mg/kg，一日 1 次，每周用药 5 日。口服，每次 1g，一日 3 次，与食物同服，可根据病情选用其中之一。输液配制：将 500mg 药物（钠盐），加 10ml 注射用水振摇，使其溶解，液体应澄明无色，此溶液在室温时稳定 12 小时，切勿冷藏。进一步可用 0.9% 氯化钠、5% 葡萄糖、林格或乳酸钠等输液稀释至含药量低于 10mg/ml，供静脉滴注 1 小时。<br><br>Terapia de inducción: infusión intravenosa 5mg/kg (que dura por lo menos 1 hora), 12 horas 1 vez, 14 ～ 21 días consecutivos (como prevención 7 ～ 14 días); tratamiento de mantenimiento: infusión intravenosa, 5mg/kg, 1 vez al día, se administra por 7 días una semana; o 6mg/kg, 1 vez al día, 5 días una semana. Por vía oral, 1g 1 vez, 3 veces al día, con la comida, uno de los cuales se puede seleccionar de acuerdo a la condición. Preparación de la infusión: se agrega 500mg del medicamento(sodio) a 10ml del agua para inyección, agitándose para disolverlo. El líquido debe ser transparente, la solución debe ser estable durante 12 horas a temperatura del ambiente y no refrigere. Además, se puede diluirlo con infusiones tales como 0.9% cloruro de sodio, 5% glucosa, Ringer o Ringer lactato a la concentración inferior a 10mg/ml, por vía intravenosa por 1 hora. |
| 剂型、规格<br>Formulaciones y especificaciones | 胶囊剂：每粒 250mg。 注射剂（冻干粉针）：每瓶 500mg。<br>Una cápsula：250mg. Una inyección （polvo liofilizado）：500mg cada botella. |

**续 表**

| 药品名称 Drug Names | 伐昔洛韦 Valaciclovir |
| --- | --- |
| 适应证<br>Indicaciones | 本品主要应用于治疗带状疱疹，也可用于治疗 HSV1 和 HSV2 感染。<br>Se usa principalmente para tratar zoster. También se usa para infección causada por HSV1 y HSV2. |
| 用法、用量<br>Administración y dosis | 口服，成人每日 0.6g，分 2 次服，疗程 7 ~ 10 日。<br>Se toma por vía oral, adultos 0.6g al día, en 2 veces, ciclo de tratamiento 7 ~ 10 días. |
| 剂型、规格<br>Formulaciones y<br>especificaciones | 片剂：每片 200mg；300mg。<br>Una tableta: 200mg; 300mg. |
| 药品名称 Drug Names | 泛昔洛韦 Famciclovir |
| 适应证<br>Indicaciones | 用于治疗带状疱疹和原发性生殖器疱疹。<br>Se usa para tratar zoster y herpes genital primario. |
| 用法、用量<br>Administración y dosis | 口服，成人一次 0.25g，每 8 小时 1 次，治疗带状疱疹的疗程为 7 日，治疗原发性生殖器疱疹的疗程为 5 日。<br>Se toma por vía oral, adultos 0.25g una vez, cada 8 horas, ciclo de tratamiento de 7 días para tratar Zoster, ciclo de tratamiento de 5 días para tratar herpes genital primario. |
| 剂型、规格<br>Formulaciones y<br>especificaciones | 片剂：每片 125mg；250mg；500mg。<br>Una tableta: 125mg; 250mg; 500mg. |
| 药品名称 Drug Names | 奥司他韦 Oseltamivir |
| 适应证<br>Indicaciones | 用于成人和 1 岁及 1 岁以上儿童的甲型和乙型流感的治疗（磷酸奥司他韦能够有效治疗甲型和乙型流感，但是乙型流感的临床应用数据尚不多）。用于成人和 13 岁及 13 岁以上青少年的甲型和乙型流感的预防。<br>Se usa para el tratamiento de la gripe A y B en adultos y niños de 1 o más años de edad(oseltamivir puede tratar con eficacia la gripe A y B, pero los datos clínicos de la gripe B no son muchos). Se usa para la prevención de la gripe A y B en adultos y adolescentes de 13 o más años de edad. |
| 用法、用量<br>Administración y dosis | 成人推荐量，每次 75mg，一日 2 次，共 5 日。肾功能不全者：肌酐清除率 < 30ml/min 者每日 75mg，共 5 日。肌酐清除率 < 10ml/min 者尚无研究资料，应慎重使用。<br>Dosis recomendada para adultos, 75mg cada vez, 2 veces al día, en total 5 días. Los pacientes con insuficiencia renal: aclaramiento de creatinina < 30ml/min, 75mg al día, en total 5 días. Aclaramiento de creatinina < 10ml/min, no hay datos de la investigación y deben ser utilizados con precaución. |
| 剂型、规格<br>Formulaciones y<br>especificaciones | 胶囊剂：每粒 75mg（以游离碱计量）。<br>Una cápsula: 75mg (calculado en álcali libre). |
| 药品名称 Drug Names | 扎那米韦 Zanamivir |
| 适应证<br>Indicaciones | 用于治疗流感病毒感染以及季节性预防社区内 A 和季节性预防社区 B 型流感。<br>Se usa para el tratamiento de la infección por el virus de la gripe así como prevención de la gripe estacional de tipo A y B dentro de la comunidad. |
| 用法、用量<br>Administración y dosis | 成人和 12 岁以上的青少年，一日 2 次，间隔约 12 小时。一日 10mg，分 2 次吸入，一次 5mg，经口吸入给药，连用 5 日。随后数日，两次的服药时间尽可能保持一致，剂量间隔 12 小时。季节性预防社区内 A 和 B 型流感：成人 10mg，每天 1 次，28 日，在流感暴发 5 日内开始治疗。<br>Adultos y adolescentes mayores a 12 años de edad, 2 veces al día, con intervalo de 12h. 10mg al día, se inhala 2 veces, 5mg 1 vez, por vía oral, 5 días consecutivos. Varios días después, las horas de administración deben ser lo más fijadas posibles, con intervalo de 12 horas. Prevención estacional de Gripe A y Gripe B dentro de la comunidad: adultos 10mg, 1 vez al día, 28 días, el tratamiento comienza 5 días dentro del brote de gripe. |

**续　表**

| | |
|---|---|
| 剂型、规格<br>Formulaciones y especificaciones | 吸入粉雾剂：每个泡囊含扎那米韦（5mg）和乳糖（20mg）的混合粉末。<br>Polvo para inhalación: cada vesícula contiene polvo mixto de zanamivir(5mg)y lactosa(20mg). |
| 药品名称 Drug Names | 阿巴卡韦 Abacavir |
| 适应证<br>Indicaciones | 本品常与其他药物联合用于艾滋病的治疗。<br>Se usa en combinación con otros medicamentos para tratar AIDS. |
| 用法、用量<br>Administración y dosis | 与其他抗反转录酶药物合用。成人：一次 300mg，一日 2 次。3 月龄至 16 岁儿童：一次 8mg/kg，一日 2 次。<br>Combina con otros fármacos antirretrovirales. Adultos: 300mg 1 vez, 2 veces al día. Niños entre 3 meses y 16 años de edad: 8mg/kg 1 vez, 2 veces al día. |
| 剂型、规格<br>Formulaciones y especificaciones | 片剂：300mg（以盐基计量）。口服液：20mg/ml。<br>Una tableta: 300mg(calculado en base). Líquido por vía oral: 20mg/ml. |
| 药品名称 Drug Names | 阿糖腺苷 Vidarabina |
| 适应证<br>Indicaciones | 有抗单纯疱疹病毒 HSV1 和 HSV2 作用，用以治疗单纯疱疹病毒性脑炎，也用以治疗免疫抑制患者的带状疱疹和水痘感染。但对巨细胞病毒则无效。本品的单磷酸酯有抑制乙肝病毒复制的作用。<br>Se usa para luchar contra virus del herpes simple HSV1 y HSV2, tratar encefalitis por el virus del herpes simple y tratar infecciones de la varicela y zoster en los pacientes inmunodeprimidos. Pero no tiene validez en citomegalovirus. El monofosfato del producto inhibir la replicación del VHB. |
| 用法、用量<br>Administración y dosis | 单纯疱疹病毒性脑炎：一日量为 15mg/kg，按 200g 药物、500ml 输液（预热至 35～40℃）的比率配液，作连续静脉滴注，疗程为 10 日。带状疱疹：10mg/kg 连用 5 日，用法同上。<br>Encefalitis por el virus del herpes simple: dosis diaria de 15mg/kg, preparar la solución con proporción de 200g medicamento, 500ml infusión (precalentada a 35～40℃ ), como infusión intravenosa, ciclo de tratamiento 10 días. Herpes zoster: 10mg/kg, 5 días consecutivos, administración igual que arriba. |
| 剂型、规格<br>Formulaciones y especificaciones | 注射液（混悬液）：200mg（1ml）；1000mg（5ml）。加入输液中滴注用。注射用单磷酸阿糖腺苷：每瓶 200mg。<br>Una inyección (suspensión): 200mg(1ml); 1000mg(5ml). Se agrega a la fusión para gotear. Monofosfato Vidarabina para inyección: 200mg cada botella. |
| 药品名称 Drug Names | 利巴韦林 Ribavirina |
| 适应证<br>Indicaciones | 用于呼吸道合胞病毒引起的病毒性肺炎与支气管炎，皮肤疱疹病毒感染。<br>Se usa para neumonía viral y la bronquitis causadas por el virus respiratorio sincitial así como la infección por el virus del herpes de la piel. |
| 用法、用量<br>Administración y dosis | 口服：一日 0.8～1g，分 3～4 次服用。肌内注射或静脉滴注：一日 10～15mg/kg，分 2 次，静脉滴注宜缓慢。用于早期出血热，每日 1g，加入输液 500～1000ml 中静脉滴注，连续应用 3～5 日。滴鼻：用于防治流感，用 0.5% 溶液（以等渗氯化钠溶液配制），每 1 小时 1 次。滴眼：治疗疱疹感染，浓度 0.1%，一日数次。<br>Se toma por vía oral: 0.8～1g al día, en 3～4 veces. Inyección intramuscular o infusión intravenosa: 10～15mg/kg al día, en 2 veces, la infusión intravenosa debe ser lenta. Para la fiebre hemorrágica precoz, se usa 0.5% solución (se prepara con solución isotónica de cloruro de sodio), 1 vez 1 hora. Gotas para los ojos: para tratar las infecciones por herpes, concentración de 0.1%, varias veces al día. |
| 剂型、规格<br>Formulaciones y especificaciones | 片剂：每片 50mg；100mg。颗粒剂：每袋 50mg；100mg。注射液：100mg（1ml）；250mg（2ml）。<br>Una tableta: 50mg; 100mg. Gránulos: 50mg; 100mg cada saco. Una inyección: 100mg(1ml); 250mg(2ml). |

**续　表**

| 药品名称 Drug Names | 齐多夫定 Zidovudina |
|---|---|
| 适应证<br>Indicaciones | 　　用于治疗获得性免疫缺陷综合征（AIDS）。患者有并发症（卡氏肺囊虫病或其他感染）时尚需应用对症的其他药物联合治疗。<br>　　Se usa para tratar síndrome de inmunodeficiencia adquirida(AIDS). Los pacientes con complicaciones (enfermedad carinii u otras infecciones) requieren la aplicación sintomática de otros fármacos en combinación. |
| 用法、用量<br>Administración y dosis | 　　成人常用量：1 次 200mg，每 4 小时 1 次，按时间给药。有贫血的患者：可按 1 次 100mg 给药。<br>　　Dosis habitual para adultos: 200mg 1 vez, cada 4 horas, se administra por el tiempo. Pacientes con anemia: se administra 100mg 1 vez. |
| 剂型、规格<br>Formulaciones y especificaciones | 　　胶囊剂：每粒 100mg。<br>　　Una cápsula: 100mg. |
| 药品名称 Drug Names | 拉米夫定 Lamivudina |
| 适应证<br>Indicaciones | 　　用于乙型肝炎病毒所致的慢性乙型肝炎，与其他抗反转录病毒药连用于治疗人类免疫缺陷病毒感染。<br>　　Se usa para hepatitis crónica causada por el virus de la hepatitis B y combina con otros fármacos antirretrovirales para tratar la infección del virus de inmunodeficiencia humana. |
| 用法、用量<br>Administración y dosis | 　　成人：慢性乙型肝炎，一日 1 次，100mg 口服；HIV 感染，推荐剂量一次 150mg，一日 2 次，或一次 300mg；一日 1 次。<br>　　Adultos: hepatitis B crónica, 1 vez al día, 100mg por vía oral; infección HIV, dosis recomendada 150mg 1 vez, 2 veces al día, o 300mg 1 vez; 1 vez al día. |
| 剂型、规格<br>Formulaciones y especificaciones | 　　片剂：每片 100mg；150mg。<br>　　Una tableta: 100mg; 150mg. |
| 药品名称 Drug Names | 阿德福韦酯 Adefovir dipivoxil |
| 适应证<br>Indicaciones | 　　用于乙型肝炎病毒感染，人类免疫缺陷病毒感染。<br>　　Se usa para infección por el virus de la hepatitis B e infección por el virus de la inmunodeficiencia humana. |
| 用法、用量<br>Administración y dosis | 　　成人口服：慢性乙型肝炎，一日 1 次，每次 10mg；HIV 感染，一日 1 次，每次 125mg，疗程 12 周。静脉滴注：HIV 感染，每次 1～3mg/kg，一日 1 次或每周 3 次，每次给药时间不少于 30 分钟。皮下注射剂量同静脉滴注。<br>　　Adultos por vía oral: hepatitis B crónica, 1 vez al día, 100mg cada vez; infección HIV, 1 vez al día, 125mg cada vez, ciclo de tratamiento 12 semanas. Infusión intravenosa: infección HIV, 1～3mg/kg 1 vez, 1 vez al día o 3 veces una semana, el tiempo de administración cada vez no debe ser inferior a 30 minutos. La dosis subcutánea debe ser igual a infusión intravenosa. |
| 剂型、规格<br>Formulaciones y especificaciones | 　　阿德福韦酯片（胶囊）：每片（粒）10mg。<br>　　Tableta de adefovir dipivoxil(cápsula): 10mg. |
| 药品名称 Drug Names | 恩替卡韦 Entecavir |
| 适应证<br>Indicaciones | 　　用于病毒复制活跃，血清转氨酶 ALT 持续升高或肝脏组织学显示有活动性病变的慢性成人乙型肝炎的治疗。<br>　　Se usa para el tratamiento de hepatitis B crónica en adultos con la replicación viral activa, el aumento contínuo de los niveles séricos de transaminasas ALT o muestra de la actividad de trastornos en la histología hepática. |
| 用法、用量<br>Administración y dosis | 　　口服，一日 1 次，每次 0.5mg。拉米夫定治疗时发生病毒血症或出现拉米夫定耐药突变的患者推荐剂量为一日 1 次，每次 1.0mg，空腹服用。<br>　　Se toma por vía oral: 1 vez al día, 0.5mg cada vez. En el tratamiento con lamivudina, si se produce viremia o aparecen mutaciones de resistencia a lamivudina, la dosis recomendada es de 1 vez al día, 1.0mg cada vez, con estómago vacío. |

续　表

| 剂型、规格<br>Formulaciones y especificaciones | 片剂：每片 0.5mg。<br>Una tableta: 0.5mg. |
|---|---|
| **药品名称 Drug Names** | **替比夫定 Telbivudina** |
| 适应证<br>Indicaciones | 用于有病毒复制证据，血清转氨酶（ALT 或 AST）持续升高或肝组织学显示有活动性病变的慢性成人乙型肝炎的患者。<br>Se usa para el tratamiento de hepatitis B crónica en adultos con la replicación viral activa, el aumento contínuo de los niveles séricos de transaminasas (ALT o AST) o muestra de la actividad de trastornos en la histología hepática. |
| 用法、用量<br>Administración y dosis | 成人和青少年（≥ 16 岁）推荐剂量为 600mg，一日 1 次口服，餐前或餐后均可，不受进食影响。<br>Adultos y adolescentes( ≥ 16 años de edad) dosis recomendada de 600mg, 1 vez al día por vía oral, antes o después de la comida, no afectada por la alimentación. |
| 剂型、规格<br>Formulaciones y especificaciones | 片剂：每片 600mg。<br>Una tableta: 600mg. |
| **药品名称 Drug Names** | **聚乙二醇干扰素 α-2a　Peginterferón alfa-2a** |
| 适应证<br>Indicaciones | 用于肝硬化代偿期或无肝硬化的慢性乙型或丙型肝炎的治疗。<br>Se usa para cirrosis descompensada o hepatitis crónica B o C sin cirrosis. |
| 用法、用量<br>Administración y dosis | 皮下注射，推荐剂量为一次 180μg，每周 1 次，共用 48 周。发生中度和重度不良反应的患者，应调整剂量，初始剂量一般减至 135μg，有些病例需减至 90μg 或 45μg。随不良反应的减轻，逐渐增加或恢复至常规剂量。<br>Vía subcutánea, dosis recomendada de 180μg 1 vez 1 semana, 48 semanas en total. Pacientes con reacciones adversas moderadas y graves deben ajustar la dosis, la dosis inicial generalmente se reduce a 135μg, en algunos casos a 90μg o 45μg. Con el alivio de las reacciones adversas, se incrementa gradualmente o se recupera a la dosis habitual. |
| 剂型、规格<br>Formulaciones y especificaciones | 注射液：每支 180μg（1ml）；135μg（1ml）。<br>Una inyección: 180μg(1ml); 135μg(1ml). |
| **药品名称 Drug Names** | **奈韦拉平 Nevirapina** |
| 适应证<br>Indicaciones | 常与其他药物联合应用于治疗 I 型 HIV 感染。单独用本品则病毒可迅速产生耐药性。<br>Combina frecuentemente con otros fármacos para tratar infección por el VIH de tipo I.Si se usa solo el virus puede producir rápidamente la resistencia. |
| 用法、用量<br>Administración y dosis | 成人：先导期剂量，每日 1 次 200mg，用药 14 日（以减少皮疹发生）；以后一日 2 次，每次 200mg。儿童：2 个月～ 8 岁，一日一次 4mg/kg，用药 14 日，以后一日 2 次，每次 7mg/kg；儿童：8 岁以上，一日一次 4mg/kg，用药 14 日，以后一日 2 次，每次 4mg/kg。所有患者的用量每日不超过 400mg。<br>Adultos: dosis en el período de piloto, 200mg 1 vez, 14 días de aplicación (para reducir la aparición de erupciones en la piel); en adelante 2 veces al día, 200mg cada vez. Niños: de 2 meses ～ 8 años de edad, 4mg/kg 1 vez al día, 14 días de aplicación, en adelante 2 veces al día, 200mg cada vez; niños: mayores a 8 años de edad, 4mg/kg 1 vez al día, 14 días de aplicación, en adelante 2 veces al día, 4mg cada vez. La dosis diaria para todos los pacientes no debe ser superior a 400mg. |
| 剂型、规格<br>Formulaciones y especificaciones | 片剂（胶囊剂）：每片（粒）200mg。<br>Una tableta (cápsula): 200mg. |
| **药品名称 Drug Names** | **司他夫定 stavudina** |
| 适应证<br>Indicaciones | 用于治疗 I 型 HIV 感染。<br>Se usa para tratar infección por el VIH de tipo I. |

| 续 表 | |
|---|---|
| 用法、用量<br>Administración y dosis | 成人：体重 ≥ 60kg 者，口服一次 40mg，一日 2 次（相隔 12 小时）；体重 < 60kg 者，口服一次 30mg，一日 2 次。儿童：体重 ≥ 30kg 者，按成人剂量；体重 < 30kg 者，一次 1mg/kg，一日 2 次。肾功能低下者，需根据其肌酐清除率调整剂量。<br><br>Adultos: con peso corporal ≥ 60kg, se toma por vía oral 40mg 1 vez, 2 veces al día (con intervalo de 12 horas); con peso corporal < 60kg, se toma por vía oral 30mg 1 vez, 2 veces al día. Niños: con peso corporal ≥ 30kg, dosis de adultos; con peso corporal < 30kg, 1mg/kg 1 vez, 2 veces al día. Los pacientes con insuficiencia renal deben ajustar la dosis según el aclaramiento de creatinina. |
| 剂型、规格<br>Formulaciones y especificaciones | 胶囊剂：每粒 20mg；30mg；40mg。<br>Una cápsula: 20mg; 30mg; 40mg. |
| 药品名称 Drug Names | 利托那韦 Ritonavir |
| 适应证<br>Indicaciones | 单独使用或与其他反转录酶抑制药联合用于治疗 HIV 感染。<br><br>Se usa solo o en combinación con otros fármacos inhibidores de la transcriptasa inversapara para tratar infección por HIV. |
| 用法、用量<br>Administración y dosis | 口服：成人初始剂量一次 300mg，一日 2 次，之后每 2～3 日每次用量增加 100mg，直至达推荐剂量每次 600mg，一日 2 次。2 岁以上儿童初始剂量一次 250mg/㎡，一日 2 次，之后每 2～3 日每次用量增加 50mg/㎡，直至达推荐剂量每次 400mg/㎡，一日 2 次。最大剂量不超过每次 600mg，一日 2 次。<br><br>Se toma por vía oral: adultos la dosis inicial de 300mg 1 vez, 2 veces al día, en adelante se incrementa 100mg cada 2～3 días 1 vez, hasta la dosis recomendada de 600mg 1 vez, 2 veces al día. Niños mayores a 2 años de edad la dosis inicial de 250mg 1 vez, 2 veces al día, en adelante se incrementa 50mg cada 2～3 días 1 vez, hasta la dosis recomendada de 400mg 1 vez, 2 veces al día. La dosis máxima no sobrepasa 600mg 1 vez, 2 veces al día. |
| 剂型、规格<br>Formulaciones y especificaciones | 软胶囊：每粒 100mg。<br>Una cápsula suave: 100mg. |
| 药品名称 Drug Names | 膦甲酸钠 Foscarnet de sodio |
| 适应证<br>Indicaciones | 主要用于免疫缺陷者（如艾滋病患者）发生的巨细胞病毒性视网膜炎的治疗。也可用于对阿昔洛韦耐药的免疫缺陷者（如 HIV 感染患者）的皮肤黏膜单纯疱疹病毒感染或带状疱疹病毒感染。<br><br>Se usa para tratar retinitis por citomegalovirus en inmunocomprometidos(i.e.paciente de SIDA). También se usa para tratar infección por el virus del herpes simple mucocutáneo o infección por el virus zoster en inmunocomprometidos resistentes a aciclovir (i.e.pacientes infectados por el VIH). |
| 用法、用量<br>Administración y dosis | 静脉滴注：初始剂量 60mg/kg，每 8 小时 1 次，至少需 1 小时恒速滴入，用 2～3 周；剂量、给药间隔、连续应用时间须根据患者的肾功能与用药耐受程度予以调节。维持量为每日 90～120mg/kg，静脉滴注 2 小时。<br><br>Infusión intravenosa: dosis inicial de 60mg/kg, 8 horas 1 vez, por lo menos se necesita 1 hora de velocidad constante para gotear, durante 2～3 semanas; la dosis, el intervalo y el tiempo de aplicación continua deben ajustarse según la función renal y la tolerancia del medicamento del paciente. La dosis de mantenimiento es de 90～120mg/kg al día y la infusión intravenosa dura 2 horas. |
| 剂型、规格<br>Formulaciones y especificaciones | 注射液：每瓶 600mg（250ml）；1200mg（500ml）。<br>Una inyección: 600mg(250ml);1200mg(500ml) cada botella. |
| 药品名称 Drug Names | 去羟肌苷 Didanosina |
| 适应证<br>Indicaciones | 用于 I 型 HIV 感染，常与其他抗反转录酶药物联合应用（鸡尾酒疗法）。<br><br>Se usa para tratar infección por el VIH de tipo I.Combina frecuentemente con otros fármacos inhibidores de la transcriptasa inversapara (terapia del cóctel).) |

**续　表**

| | |
|---|---|
| 用法、用量<br>Administración y dosis | 成人：体重≥ 60kg 者，一次 200mg，一日 2 次，或一日 400mg，一次顿服；体重＜ 60kg 者，一次 125mg，一日 2 次，或一日 250mg，一次顿服. 儿童：120mg/㎡，一日 2 次或一日 250mg，一次顿服。肾功能低下者应按肌酐清除率调整剂量。饭前 30 分钟服用，片剂应充分咀嚼或溶于 1 小杯水中、搅拌混匀后服用。<br><br>Adultos: con peso corporal ≥ 60kg, 200mg 1 vez, 2 veces al día, o 400mg al día, dosis única; con peso corporal ＜ 60kg, 125mg 1 vez, 2 veces al día, o 250mg al día, dosis única. Niños: 120mg/㎡, 2 veces al día, o 250mg al día, dosis única. Los pacientes con insuficiencia renal deben ajustar la dosis según el aclaramiento de creatinina. Se toma 30 minutos antes de la comida, y los comprimidos deben masticarse o disolverse en un vaso de agua, en que se agitan y se mezclan antes de la toma. |
| 剂型、规格<br>Formulaciones y especificaciones | 片剂：50mg；100mg。<br>Una tableta: 50mg; 100mg. |
| 药品名称 Drug Names | 茚地那韦 Indinavir |
| 适应证<br>Indicaciones | 和其他抗反转录病毒药物联合使用，用于治疗成人及儿童 HIV-1 感染。<br>Combina con otros fármacos antirretrovirales para tratar infección por el VIH-1 en adultos y niños. |
| 用法、用量<br>Administración y dosis | 推荐的开始剂量为 800mg，每 8 小时口服 1 次。与利福布汀联合治疗建议将利福布汀的剂量减半，而本药计量增加至每 8 小时 1g。与酮康唑合用，本药的剂量应减少至每 8 小时 600mg。肝功能不全患者，剂量应减至每 8 小时 600mg。3 岁以上（可口服胶囊的儿童）：本品的推荐剂量为每 8 小时口服 500mg/㎡。儿童剂量不能超过成人剂量（即每 8 小时 800mg）。<br><br>La dosis inicial recomendada es de 800mg, y se toma 1 vez cada 8 horas por vía oral. Se propone reducir la dosis de rifabutina a la mitad en el tratamiento combinado con rifabutina y incrementar la dosis de este medicamento a 1g cada 8 horas. En combinación con ketoconazol, la dosis debe reducirse a 600mg cada 8 horas. Para los pacientes con insuficiencia renal, la dosis debe reducirse a 600mg cada 8 horas. Los mayores a 3 años de edad(niños que pueden tomar cápsulas): la dosis recomendada es de 500mg/㎡ cada 8 horas por vía oral. La dosis de niños no debe sobrepasar la de adultos(i.e. 800mg cada 8 horas). |
| 剂型、规格<br>Formulaciones y especificaciones | 胶囊剂：每粒 200mg。<br>Una cápsula: 200mg. |
| 药品名称 Drug Names | 金刚烷胺 Amantadina |
| 适应证<br>Indicaciones | 用于亚洲 A- Ⅱ型流感感染发热患者。常用于震颤麻痹。<br>Se usa para infección de la gripe de tipo A- Ⅱ asiática en pacientes con fiebre. Se usa frecuentemente para parkinsonismo. |
| 用法、用量<br>Administración y dosis | 流感 A 病毒感染：成人：每日 200mg，分 1 ～ 2 次服用；儿童：新生儿与 1 岁内婴儿不用；1 ～ 9 岁，每日 4.4 ～ 8.8mg/kg，1 ～ 2 次，每日最大剂量不超过 150mg，9 ～ 12 岁，100 ～ 200mg/d。<br><br>La infección por el virus de la gripe A: adultos: 200mg al día, en 1 ～ 2 veces; niños: los recién nacidos y bebés menores a 1 año de edad no lo usan; de entre 1 y 9 años de edad, 4.4 ～ 8.8mg/kg al día, en 1 ～ 2 veces, la dosis diaria máxima no sobrepasa 150mg, de entre 9 y 12 años de edad, 100 ～ 200mg/d. |
| 剂型、规格<br>Formulaciones y especificaciones | 片（胶囊）剂：0.1g。<br>Una tableta (cápsula): 0.1g. |

7. 抗寄生虫病药 Medicamentos contra enfermedades parasitarias

7.1　抗疟药 Antimaláricos

| | |
|---|---|
| 药品名称 Drug Names | 氯喹 Cloroquina |
| 适应证<br>Indicaciones | 主要用于治疗疟疾急性发作，控制疟疾症状，还可用于治疗肝阿米巴病、华支睾吸虫病、肺吸虫病、结缔组织病等。另可用于光敏性疾病，如日晒红斑症。<br>Se usa para tratar el ataque agudo de malaria, controlar los síntomas de la malaria. También se usa para tratar amebiasis hepática, clonorquiasis, paragonimiasis y enfermedad del tejido conectivo, etc. Además se usa para enfermedades fotosensibles, como por ejemplo eritema solare. |

| | |
|---|---|
| 用法、用量<br>Administración y dosis | （1）控制疟疾发作：①口服：首剂 1g，6 小时后 0.5g，第 2、3 日各服 0.5g，如与伯氨喹合用，只需第一日服本品 1g。小儿首次 16mg/kg（高热其酌情减量，分次服），6～8 小时后及第 2～3 日各服 8mg/kg。②静脉滴注：恶性疟第一日 1.5g，第 2、3 日 0.5g。一般每 0.5～0.75g 氯喹用 5% 葡萄糖注射液或 0.9% 氯化钠注射液 500ml 稀释，静脉滴注速度为每分钟 12～20 滴，第一日量与 12 小时内全部输完。（2）疟疾症状抑制性预防：每周服 1 次，每次 0.5g，小儿每周 8mg/kg。(3) 抗阿米巴肝脓肿：每 1、2 日一日 2～3 次，每次服 0.5g，以后每日 0.5g，连用 2～3 周。<br><br>（4）治疗结缔组织病：对盘状红斑狼疮及类风湿关节炎，开始剂量一日 1～2 次，每次 0.25g，经 2～3 周后，如症状得到控制，改为一日 2～3 次，每次量不宜超过 0.25g，长期维持。对系统性红斑狼疮，用皮质激素治疗症状缓解后，可加用氯喹以减少皮质激素用量。<br><br>(1)Para controlar episodios de malaria: ① por vía oral: dosis inicial 1g, 6 horas después 0.5g, el segundo y el tercer día 0.5g respectivamente, si combina con primaquina, sólo se necesita tomar 1g el primer día. La dosis inicial para niños 16mg/kg (si se trata de fiebre, se reduce la dosis correspondientemente, en varias veces), 6～8 horas después así como el segundo y el tercer día, 8mg/kg respectivamente. ② infusión intravenosa: para falciparum malaria, el primer día 1.5g, el segundo y el tercer día 0.5g. Generalmente cada 0.5～0.75g de cloroquina se diluye en 500ml de 5% inyección de glucosa o 0.9% inyección de cloruro de sodio. La velocidad de infusión intravenosa es de 12～20 gotas cada minuto, y la dosis del primer día se agota dentro de 12 horas. (2) Para suprimir los síntomas de malaria como prevención: 1 vez cada semana, 0.5g cada vez, 8mg/kg cada semana para niños. (3) Para tratar el absceso hepático amebiano: el primer y el segundo día, 2～3 veces al día, 0.5g cada vez, 0.5g al día en adelante, durante 2～3 semanas consecutivas. (4) Para el tratamiento de la enfermedad del tejido conectivo: para el lupus eritematoso discóide y la artritis reumatoide, la dosis inicial de administración es de 0, 25 mg una vez al día, durante un curso de 2 a 3 semanas, si los síntomas se controlan, se convierte en 2～3 veces al día, la dosis de cada vez no debe sobrepasar 0.25g, mantenimiento a largo plazo. Para el Lupus Eritematoso Sistémico, después del tratamiento con corticosteroides para aliviar los síntomas, se puede añadir con cloroquina para reducir la cantidad de corticoides. |
| 剂型、规格<br>Formulaciones y especificaciones | 片剂：每片含磷酸氯喹 0.075g；0.25g。<br>注射液：每支 129mg（盐基 80mg）（2ml）；250mg（盐基 155mg）（2ml）。<br>Una tableta：contiene 0.075g；0.25g de fosfato de cloroquina；<br>Inyección:129mg（80mg de base）（2ml）；250mg（155mg de base）（2ml）. |
| **药品名称 Drug Names** | 羟氯喹 Hidroxicloroquina |
| 适应证<br>Indicaciones | 本品主要用于疟疾的预防和治疗，也用于类风湿关节炎和青少年类风湿关节炎，以及盘状红斑狼疮和系统性红斑狼疮的治疗。<br><br>Se usa principalmente para prevenir y tratar la malaria, artritis reumatoide y artritis reumatoide juvenil, así como lupus eritematoso discoide y lupus eritematoso sistémico. |
| 用法、用量<br>Administración y dosis | 治疗急性疟疾：成人口服，首次 800mg，以后每 6～8 小时 400mg，然后每 2 日 400mg；儿童首剂量 10mg/kg，6 小时后第 2 次服药 5mg/kg，第 2、3 日，每日一次 5mg/kg。预防疟疾：在进入疟疾流行区前一周，服 400mg，以后每周 1 次 400mg；儿童 5mg/kg。治疗风湿性关节炎和红斑狼疮：成人开始每日 400mg，分次服，维持量每日 200～400mg，每日剂量不超过 6.5mg/kg。青少年患者治疗 6 个月无效即应停药。<br><br>Para tratar malaria aguda: adultos por vía oral, 800mg la primera vez, 400mg cada 6～8 horas en adelante, luego 400mg cada 2 días; la dosis inicial para niños 10mg/kg, 6 horas después se toma 5mg/kg en la segunda vez, el segundo y el tercer día, 5mg/kg 1 vez al día. Para prevenir malaria: en la semana antes de que comience la epidemia de malaria, se toma 400mg, y 400mg cada semana en adelante; niños 5mg/kg. Para tratar artritis reumatoide y lupus eritematoso: adultos al principio 400mg al día, dividido en varias veces, dosis de mantenimiento 200～400mg al día, la dosis diaria no sobrepasa 6.5mg/kg. Los pacientes adolescentes tratados por 6 meses sin eficacia deben dejar de administrarse. |
| 剂型、规格<br>Formulaciones y especificaciones | 片剂：每片 100mg；200mg。<br>Una tableta: 100mg; 200mg. |

**续　表**

| 药品名称 Drug Names | 青蒿素 Artemisinina |
|---|---|
| 适应证<br>Indicaciones | 用于间日疟，恶性疟特别是抢救脑型疟有良效，其退热时间及疟原虫转阴时间都较氯喹短，对氯喹有抗药性的疟原虫，使用本品有效。<br><br>Se usa para plasmodium vivax malaria. Tiene buen efecto para falciparum malaria，sobre todo el tratamiento de la malaria cerebral. El tiempo de enfriamiento y el tiempo de eliminación del parásito duran menos en comparación con cloroquina. Se puede usar este medicamento para atacar. |
| 用法、用量<br>Administración y dosis | （1）口服：先服 1g，6～8 小时后再服 0.5g，第 2、3 日各服 0.5g，疗程 3 日，总量为 2.5g。小儿总剂量 15mg/kg，按上述方法 3 日内服完。（2）直肠给药：先服 0.6g，6 小时后再服 0.6g，第 2、3 日各服 0.4g。（3）深部肌内注射：第 1 次 200mg，6～8 小时后再给 100mg，第 2、3 日各肌内注射 100mg，总剂量 500mg（个别重症第 4 日再给 100mg）。或连用 3 日，每日肌内注射 300mg，总量 900mg。小儿 15mg/kg，按上述方法 3 日内注完。<br><br>(1)Por vía oral: 1g primero, 0.5g tras 6～8 horas, 0.5g el segundo y el tercer día respectivamente, el ciclo de tratamiento dura 3 días, y la dosis total es de 2.5g. La dosis total para niños es de 15mg/kg, y se toma según la forma arriba mencionada dentro de 3 días. (2)Por vía rectal: 0.6g primero, 0.6g tras 6 horas, 0.4g el segundo y el tercer día respectivamente. (3)Inyección intramuscular profunda: 200mg la primera vez, 100mg 6～8 horas después, 100mg por vía intramuscular el segundo y el tercer día respectivamente, dosis total de 500mg (en casos graves hasta el cuarto día se inyecta 100mg). O 3 días consecutivos, 300mg al día por vía intramuscular, dosis total de 900mg. Niños 15mg/kg, se termina dentro de 3 días según la forma arriba mencionada. |
| 剂型、规格<br>Formulaciones y especificaciones | 油注射液：每支 50mg（2ml）；100mg（2ml）；200mg（2ml）；300mg（2ml）。<br>水混悬注射液：每支 300mg（2ml）。<br>片剂：每片 50mg；100mg。<br>栓剂：每粒 400mg；600mg。<br>Una inyección de aceite: 50mg(2ml); 100mg(2ml); 200mg(2ml); 300mg(2ml).<br>Una inyección de suspensión mixta: 300mg(2ml).<br>Una tableta: 50mg; 100mg.<br>Un supositorio: 400mg; 600mg. |
| 药品名称 Drug Names | 青蒿素哌喹 Artemisinina y piperaquina |
| 适应证<br>Indicaciones | 用于恶性疟和间日疟。<br>Se usa para falciparum malaria y plasmodium vivax malaria. |
| 用法、用量<br>Administración y dosis | 口服，成人总剂量 8 片，每日早晚各一次，每次 2 片。<br>Se toma por vía oral, dosis total para adultos es de 8 tabletas, por la mañana y por la noche, 2 tabletas cada vez. |
| 剂型、规格<br>Formulaciones y especificaciones | 复方制剂，每片含青蒿素 6.25mg，哌喹 375mg。<br>Preparación compuesta, cada contiene 6.25mg de artemisinina y 375mg de piperaquina. |
| 药品名称 Drug Names | 双氢青蒿素 Dihidroarternisinina |
| 适应证<br>Indicaciones | 用于治疗各类疟疾，尤其适用于抗氯喹和哌喹的恶性疟和凶险型脑型疟疾的救治。<br>Se usa para todos los tipos de malaria, sobre todo falciparum malaria resistente a cloroquina y piperaquina así como severa malaria cerebral. |
| 用法、用量<br>Administración y dosis | 口服，一日 1 次，成人一日 60mg，首剂加倍；儿童按年龄递减；连用 5～7 日。<br>Se toma por vía oral, 1 vez al día, para adultos 60mg al día, y se duplica la dosis inicial; para niños la dosis se va reduciendo por edad descendente; 5～7 días consecutivos. |
| 剂型、规格<br>Formulaciones y especificaciones | 片剂：每片 20mg。复方制剂：每片含双氢青蒿素 40mg，磷酸氯喹 320mg。<br>Una tableta: 20mg. Preparación compuesta: que contiene 40mg de dihydroarteannuin y 320mg de fosfato de cloroquina. |

| 药品名称 Drug Names | 双氢青蒿素磷酸哌喹 Dihidroartemisinina y piperaquina fosfato |
|---|---|
| 适应证<br>Indicaciones | 用于恶性疟和间日疟。<br>Se usa para falciparum malaria y plasmodium vivax malaria. |
| 用法、用量<br>Administración y dosis | 　　口服，成人总剂量8片，每日早晚各1次，每次2片。年龄≥16岁者，首剂2片，第6～8小时服2片，第24小时服用2片，第32小时服用2片。年龄11～15岁者，首剂1.5片，第6～8小时服1.5片，第24小时服用1.5片，第32小时服用1.5片。年龄7～10岁者，首剂1片，第6～8小时服1片，第24小时服用1片，第32小时服用1片。<br>　　Se toma por vía oral，adultos dosis total de 8 tabletas，por la mañana y por la noche，2 tabletas cada vez。Edad ≥ 16 años，dosis inicial de 2 tabletas，entre la 6ª y la 8ª hora 2 tabletas，la 24ª hora 2 tabletas，La 32ª hora 2 tabletas。Edad entre 11 y 15 años，dosis inicial de 1.5 tabletas，entre la 6ª y la 8ª hora 1.5 tabletas，la 24ª hora 1.5 tabletas，La 32ª hora 1.5 tabletas。Edad entre 7 y 10 años，dosis inicial de 1 tableta，entre la 6ª y la 8ª hora 1 tableta，la 24ª hora 1 tableta，La 32ª hora 1 tableta。 |
| 剂型、规格<br>Formulaciones y especificaciones | 　　复方制剂：每片含双氢青蒿素40mg，磷酸哌喹320mg。<br>　　Preparación compuesta：que contiene 40mg de dihydroarteannuin y 320mg de fosfato de piperaquina。 |
| 药品名称 Drug Names | 蒿甲醚 Arteméter |
| 适应证<br>Indicaciones | 　　本品对恶性疟（包括抗氯喹恶性疟及凶险型疟）的疗效较佳，效果确切，显效迅速，近期疗效可达100%。用药后2日内，多数病例血中原虫转阴并退热。复燃率8%。较青蒿素低。与伯氨喹合用可进一步降低复燃率。临床还适用于急性上呼吸道感染的高热患者，进行对症处理，取得较好疗效。退热效应一般在肌内注射后半小时即开始出现，体温呈梯形逐渐下降，4～6小时左右再逐渐回升，无体温骤降的现象，退热作用稳定。本品肌内注射后，患者出汗少，不至引起老年人、儿童、虚弱患者发生虚脱等不良反应。<br>　　Tiene una mejor eficacia，el efecto exacto y en forma rápida para falciparum malaria。El efecto a corto plazo puede ser 100%。Dos días después del tratamiento，en la mayoría de los casos，el parásito queda eliminado en sangre y baja la fiebre。La tasa de recrudecimiento es del 8%，menor que artemisinina。Si combina con primaquina puede bajar la asa de recrudecimiento aún más。En clínica también se aplica a infección aguda del tracto respiratorio superior en los pacientes con fiebre alta y logra buenos efectos。Los efectos antipiréticos empiezan a aparecer dentro de media hora tras la inyección intramuscular，la temperatura corporal disminuye gradualmente de forma trapezoidal y luego aumenta gradualmente tras aproximádamente 4 ～ 6 horas，no hay momentos de caída drástica en temperatura corporal y el efecto antipirético resulta estable。Tras la inyección intramuscular，los pacientes tienen menos sudor así que no causa reacciones adversas como colapso etc. en los viejos，niños y pacientes frágiles。 |
| 用法、用量<br>Administración y dosis | 　　抗疟：肌内注射，第一日160mg，第2～5日各80mg。小儿首剂量按3.2mg/kg计量，以后按1.6mg/kg计量。口服，首剂160mg，第2日起一日一次，一次80mg，连服5～7日。退热：肌内注射160mg。<br>　　Para tratar malaria：inyección intramuscular，160mg el primer día，80mg entre el segundo y el quinto día respectivamente。La dosis inicial para niños se calcula en 3.2mg/kg，y 1.6mg/kg en adelante。Por vía oral，la dosis inicial de 160mg，desde el segundo día 1 vez al día，80mg 1 vez，5 ～ 7 días consecutivos。Para bajar la fiebre：por vía intramuscular，160mg。 |
| 剂型、规格<br>Formulaciones y especificaciones | 　　油注射液：每支80mg（1ml）。胶囊：每胶囊40mg。片剂：每片40mg。复方制剂：每片含蒿甲醚0.02g，本芴醇0.12g。<br>　　Inyección de aceite：80mg(1ml)。Una cápsula：40mg。Una tableta：40mg。Preparación compuesta：que contiene 0.02g de arteméter y 0.12g de lumefantrina。 |

**续　表**

| 药品名称 Drug Names | 奎宁 Quinina |
|---|---|
| 适应证<br>Indicaciones | 抑制或杀灭良性疟（间日疟、三日疟）及恶性疟原虫的红内期，能控制疟疾症状，有解热、子宫收缩的作用。<br><br>Se usa para inhibir o matar a parásito de la malaria benigna(malaria vivax o malaria quartana) así como plasmodium falciparum en su fase eritrocítica. Puede controlar los síntomas de la malaria, tener efecto antipirético y de contracciones uterinas. |
| 用法、用量<br>Administración y dosis | 成人常用量：严重病例（如脑型）可采用二盐酸奎宁按体重 5～10mg/kg（最高量 500mg），加入氯化钠注射液 500ml 中静脉滴注，4 小时滴完，12 小时后重复一次，病情好转后改为口服。<br><br>Dosis habitual para adultos: en casos graves (como por ejemplo malaria cerebral), se puede adoptar 5～10mg/kg de diclorhidrato de quinina según el peso corporal(la dosis máxima de 500mg), se agrega a 500ml de la inyección de cloruro de sodio para hacer la infusión intravenosa por 4 horas, y se repite una vez tras 12 horas. Cuando los síntomas se mejoren se toma por vía oral. |
| 剂型、规格<br>Formulaciones y especificaciones | 硫酸奎宁片：0.3g。盐酸奎宁片：0.33g；0.12g。二盐酸奎宁注射液：0.25g（1ml）；0.5g（1ml）；0.25g（10ml）。复方奎宁注射液：每支 2ml，含盐酸奎宁 0.136g，咖啡因 0.034g，乌拉坦 0.028g。<br><br>Tableta de sulfato de quinina: 0.3g. Tableta de clorhidrato de quinina: 0.33g; 0.12g. Quinina diclorhidrato inyección: 0.25g(1ml); 0.5g(1ml); 0.25g(10ml). Inyección de quinina Compuesto: 2ml, que contiene 0.136g de clorhidrato de quinina, 0.034g de cafeína y 0.028g de uretano. |
| 药品名称 Drug Names | 伯氨喹 Primaquina |
| 适应证<br>Indicaciones | 主要用于根治间日疟和控制疟疾传播，常与氯喹或乙胺嘧啶合用，对红内期作用较弱，对恶性疟红内期则完全无效，不能作为控制症状的药物应用。对某些疟原虫的红前期也有影响，但因需用剂量较大，已接近极量，不够安全，故也不能作为病因预防药应用。<br><br>Se usa para eliminar malaria vivax de forma radical y controlar la propagación de la malaria. Frecuentemente combina con cloroquina o pirimetamin., Tiene poco efecto para la fase eritrocítica y ningún efecto para la fase eritrocítica de falciparum malaria, y tampoco se puede aplicar para controlar síntomas. Afecta a determinado plasmodium en la fase exoeritrocítica, sin embargo, debido a la gran dosis requerida, casi cerca de la dosis máxima, no resulta seguro usarla y por lo tanto no se puede aplicar como medicina preventiva de la enfermedad. |
| 用法、用量<br>Administración y dosis | 成人常用量：口服，①根治间日疟：采用一次 13.2mg，一日 3 次，连服 7 日。②用于消灭恶性疟原虫配子体时采用一日 26.4mg，连服 3 日。<br><br>Dosis habitual para adultos: por vía oral, ① para eliminar malaria vivax de forma radical: 13.2mg 1 vez, 3 veces al día, 7 días consecutivos. ② para eliminar gametocitos de Plasmodium falciparum: 26.4mg al día, 3 días consecutivos. |
| 剂型、规格<br>Formulaciones y especificaciones | 片剂：每片含磷酸伯氨喹 13.2mg 或 26.4mg（相当于伯氨喹盐基 7.5mg 或 15mg）。<br><br>Una tableta: que contiene 13.2mg o 26.4mg de fosfato de primaquina (equivalente a 7.5mg o 15mg de primaquina base). |
| 药品名称 Drug Names | 乙胺嘧啶 Pirimetamina |
| 适应证<br>Indicaciones | 主要用于预防疟疾，也可用于治疗弓形虫病。最近发现本品有抗药性虫株产生，合并应用其他抗疟药及磺胺类药物等，可提高其抗疟效果。<br><br>Se usa para prevenir malaria y tratar toxoplasmosis. Últimamente decubrieron cepas resistentes al producto y se puede combinar con otros antimaláricos y las sulfamidas, etc. para mejorar la eficacia. |
| 用法、用量<br>Administración y dosis | （1）预防疟疾：成人每次服 25mg，每周 1 次，小儿 0.9mg/kg，最高限于成人剂量。<br>（2）抗复发治疗：成人每日服 25～50mg，连用 2 日，小儿酌减（多与伯氨喹合用）。<br>（3）治疗弓形虫病：每日 50mg 顿服，共 1～3 日（视耐受力而定），以后每日 25mg，疗程 4～6 周。小儿 1mg/kg，分 2 次服。1～3 日后 0.5mg/kg，分 2 次服，疗程 4～6 周。必要时，可重复 1～2 个疗程。<br><br>(1) Para prevenir malaria: adultos 25mg 1 vez 1 semana, niños 0.9mg/kg, la dosis máxima no sobrepasa la de adultos. |

**续 表**

|  | (2) La terapia anti-retroviral: adultos 25 ～ 50mg al día, 2 días consecutivos, niños menos dosis correspondientemente(en muchos caso combina con primaquina).<br>(3) Para tratar toxoplasmosis: 50mg al día, dosis única, 1 ～ 3 días en total(dependiendo de la tolerancia), 25mg al día en adelante, ciclo de tratamiento de 4 ～ 6 semanas. Niños 1mg/kg en 2 veces. Tras 1 ～ 3 días 0.5mg/kg en 2 veces, ciclo de tratamiento de 4 ～ 6 semanas. En casos necesarios, se puede repetir 1 ～ 2 ciclos. |
|---|---|
| 剂型、规格<br>Formulaciones y especificaciones | 片剂：每片 6.25mg。膜剂：每格 6.25mg。<br>Una tableta: 6.25mg. Una membrana: 6.25mg. |

## 7.2 抗阿米巴病药 Antiamebiana

| 药品名称 Drug Names | 双碘喹啉 Diiodohidroxiquinolina |
|---|---|
| 适应证<br>Indicaciones | 用于治疗轻型或无明显症状的阿米巴痢疾。与依米丁、甲硝唑合用，治疗急性阿米巴痢疾及较顽固病例。对肠外阿米巴如肝脓肿无效。<br>Se usa para tratar la disentería amebiana leve o sin síntomas obvios. Combina con emetina y metronidazol para tratar disentería amebiana aguda y los casos más obstinados. No tiene validez para ameba parenteral como el absceso hepático. |
| 用法、用量<br>Administración y dosis | 成人常规剂量：口服给药，一次 400 ～ 600mg，一日 3 次，连服 14 ～ 21 日，儿童常规剂量：口服给药，一次 5 ～ 10mg/kg，用法同成人，重复治疗需间隔 15 ～ 20 日。<br>Dosis habitual para adultos: por vía oral, 400 ～ 600mg 1 vez, 3 veces al día, 14 ～ 21 días consecutivos, dosis habitual para niños: por vía oral, 5 ～ 10mg/kg 1 vez, la forma igual que adultos, el tratamiento repetido debe tener un intervalo de 15 ～ 20 días. |
| 剂型、规格<br>Formulaciones y especificaciones | 双碘喹啉片：每片 200mg。<br>Una tableta de diiodohydroxyquinoline: 200mg. |
| 药品名称 Drug Names | 依米丁 Emetina |
| 适应证<br>Indicaciones | 适用于急性阿米巴痢疾急需控制症状者，肠外阿米巴病因其毒性大，已少用，由于消除急性症状效率较好，而根治作用低，故不适用于症状轻微的慢性阿米巴痢及无症状的带包囊者。此外，本品还可用于蝎子蜇伤。<br>Se aplica a los urgentemente necesitados de controlar síntomas de la disentería amebiana aguda. En caso de ameba parenteral, como es altamente tóxico se debe usar menos. Ya que tiene buen efecto para eliminar síntomas augdos pero no de forma radical no se aplica a disentería amebiana crónica con síntomas leves así como los con quistes sin ningún síntoma. Además puede tratar aguijón del escorpión. |
| 用法、用量<br>Administración y dosis | (1) 治阿米巴痢：体重 60kg 以下按每日 1mg/kg 计量（60kg 以上者，剂量仍按 60kg 计量），一日 1 次或分 2 次做深部皮下注射，连用 6 ～ 10 日为 1 疗程，如未愈，30 日后再用第二疗程。<br>(2) 治蝎子蜇伤：以本品 3% ～ 6% 注射液少许注入蜇孔内即可。<br>(1) Para tratar disentería amebiana: peso corporal menor a 60kg, calculado por 1mg/kg al día (mayor a 60kg, la dosis se calcula igual), 1 o 2 veces al día, inyección subcutánea profunda, 6 ～ 10 días consecutivos como un ciclo de tratamiento, si no se cura, se usa el segundo ciclo 30 días después. (2) Para tratar aguijón del escorpión: se inyecta 3% ～ 6% inyección del medicamento al agujero de sting. |
| 剂型、规格<br>Formulaciones y especificaciones | 注射液：每支 30mg（1ml）；60mg（1ml）。<br>Una inyección: 30mg(1ml);60mg(1ml). |

## 7.3 抗滴虫病药 Antitricomoniasis

| 药品名称 Drug Names | 甲硝唑 Metronidazol |
|---|---|
| 适应证<br>Indicaciones | 用于治疗厌氧杆菌引起的产后盆腔炎、败血症、牙周炎等。还可用于治疗贾第鞭毛虫病病、酒糟鼻。用于阑尾、结肠手术、妇产科手术，可降低或避免手术感染。也可用于治疗阿米巴痢和阿米巴肝脓肿，疗效与依米丁相仿。 |

**续　表**

| | |
|---|---|
| | Se usa para tratar enfermedad inflamatoria pélvica de postparto, septicemia y periodontitis, etc. debido a anaerobios. También puede tratar giardia y rosácea. Se aplica a cirugía de apéndice, cirugía de colon, y cirugía ginecológica así que disminuye o evita la posibilidad de infecciones quirógicas. También se puede usar para tratar la disentería amebiana y absceso hepático amebiano. Tiene efecto similar a emetina. |
| 用法、用量<br>Administración y dosis | （1）治滴虫病：成人一日 3 次，每次服 200mg，另每晚以 200mg 栓剂放入阴道内，连用 7～10 日，为保证疗效，需男女同治。<br>（2）治阿米巴病：成人一日 3 次，每次 400～800mg（大剂量宜慎用），5～7 日为一疗程。<br>（3）治贾第鞭毛虫病：常用量每次 400mg，一日 3 次口服，疗程 5～7 日。<br>（4）治疗由厌氧菌引起的产后盆腔感染、败血症、骨髓炎等：一般口服 200～400mg，一日 600～1200mg，也可静脉滴注。<br>（5）治酒糟鼻：口服 200mg，一日 2～3 次，配合 2% 甲硝唑霜外擦，一日 3 次，一疗程 3 周。<br><br>(1)Para tratar trichomoniasis: adultos 3 veces al día, 200mg cada vez, además, 200mg de supositorio en la vagina todas las noche, 7 días consecutivos, y para garantizar la eficacia, se debe tratar tanto a hombres como a mujeres.<br>(2)Para tratar Amebiasis: adultos 3 veces al día, 400～800mg cada vez,(dosis grande se usa con precaución), ciclo de tratamiento 5～7 días.<br>(3)Para tratar la giardiasis: dosis habitual es de 400mg cada vez, 3 veces al día por vía oral, ciclo de tratamiento 5～7 días.<br>(4)Para tratar infecciones pélvicas posparto, septicemia y osteomielitis, etc. debido a anaerobios: generalmente 200～400mg por vía oral, 600～1200mg al día, también por vía intravenosa.<br>(5)Para tratar rosácea: 200mg por vía oral, 2～3 veces al día, en combinación con 2% crema de metronidazol para uso externo, 3 veces al día, ciclo de tratamiento 3 semanas. |
| 剂型、规格<br>Formulaciones y especificaciones | 片剂：每片 200mg。阴道泡腾片：每片 200mg。栓剂：每个 0.5g；1g。注射液：50mg（10ml）；100mg（20ml）；500mg（100mg）；1.25g（250mg）；500mg（250ml）。甲硝唑葡萄糖注射液：甲硝唑 0.5g+ 葡萄糖 12.5g（250ml）。<br><br>Una tableta: 200mg. Una tableta efervescente vaginal: 200mg. Un supositorio: 0.5g; 1g. Una inyección: 50mg(10ml); 100mg(20ml); 500mg(100ml); 1.25g(250mg); 500mg(250ml). Inyección de metronidazol y glucosa: 0.5g de metronidazol + 12.5g(250ml) de glucosa. |

## 7.4　抗血吸虫病药 Antiesqnistosomiticos

| 药品名称 Drug Names | 吡喹酮 Praziquantel |
|---|---|
| 适应证<br>Indicaciones | 主要用于治疗血吸虫病。其特点为：剂量小（约为现用一般药物剂量的 1/10），疗程短（从现用药物的 20 日或 10 日缩短为 1～2 日）、不良反应轻、由较高的近期疗效。血吸虫病患者经本品治疗后，半年粪检虫卵转阴率为 97.7%～99.4%，由于本品对毛蚴、尾蚴也有杀灭效力，故也用于预防血吸虫感染。也有以本品治疗脑囊虫病。<br><br>Se usa para tratar la esquistosomiasis. Las características de su uso son: pequeña dosis(1/10 de la dosis normal), ciclo corto(reducido de 20 o 10 días de los medicamentos generales a 1 o 2 días), reacciones adversas leves y buen efecto a corto plazo. Tras el tratamiento del producto para los pacientes con la esquistosomiasis, la tasa negativa de examen fecal por medio año será de 97.7%～99.4%. Como puede eliminar miracidium y cercaria puede usarse para prevenir la esquistosomiasis. También se usa para tratar cisticercosis cerebral. |
| 用法、用量<br>Administración y dosis | 口服治疗血吸虫病：一次 10mg/kg，一日 3 次，急性血吸虫病连服 4 日，慢性血吸虫病连服 2 日。皮肤涂擦 1% 浓度吡喹酮，12 小时内对血吸虫尾蚴有可靠的防护作用。治脑囊虫病，每日 20mg/kg，体重＞60kg 者，以 60kg 计量，分 3 次服用，9 日为一疗程，总量 180mg/kg，疗程间隔 3～4 个月。<br><br>Por vía oral para tratar esquistosomiasis: 10mg/kg 1 vez, 3 veces al día, 4 días consecutivos paraesquistosomiasis aguda, 2 días consecutivos paraesquistosomiasis crónica. Se aplica 1% praziquantel en la piel como protección fiable de cercaria. Para tratar cisticercosis cerebral, 20mg/kg al día, los con peso corporal ＞60kg, calculado en 60kg, se administra en 3 veces, ciclo de tratamiento 9 días, dosis total 180mg/kg, intervalo de tratamientos 3～4 meses. |
| 剂型、规格<br>Formulaciones y especificaciones | 胶囊剂：每粒 25mg；50mg。片剂：每片 25mg。<br>Una cápsula: 25mg; 50mg. Una tableta: 25mg. |

### 7.5　抗其他吸虫病 Contra otros trematodos

| 药品名称 Drug Names | 硫氯酚 Bitionol |
|---|---|
| 适应证<br>Indicaciones | 对肺吸虫囊蚴有明显杀灭作用，临床用于肺吸虫病、牛肉绦虫病、姜片虫病。<br>Tiene obvio efecto letal para metacercarias de paragonimus. En clínica se usa para paragonimiasis, teniasis bovis y fasciolopsiasis. |
| 用法、用量<br>Administración y dosis | 口服：每日 50～60mg/kg（成人与小儿同）。对肺吸虫病及华支睾吸虫病可将全日量分 3 次服用，隔日服药，疗程总量 30～45g，对姜片虫病，可于睡前半空腹将 2～3g 药物 1 次服完；对牛肉绦虫病，可将总量（50mg/kg）分 2 次服用，间隔半小时，服完第二次药后，3～4 小时服泻药。<br>Por vía oral: 50～60mg/kg al día(adultos y niños). Para paragonimiasis y enfermedad clonorquiasis, se divide la dosis diaria en 3 veces, y se toma cada 2 días, la dosis del ciclo 30～45g, para fasciolopsiasis, se toma 2～3g de una vez media hora antes de acostarse con estómago vacío; para teniasis bovis, se divide la dosis total (50mg/kg) en 2 veces, con intervalo de media hora, después de la segunda administración, 3～4 horas después se toma lustramentum. |
| 剂型、规格<br>Formulaciones y especificaciones | 片剂：每片 0.25g。胶囊剂：每粒 0.5g。<br>Una tableta: 0.25g. Una cápsula: 0.5g. |

### 7.6　抗丝虫病 Antifilariasis

| 药品名称 Drug Names | 乙胺嗪 Dietilcarbamacina |
|---|---|
| 适应证<br>Indicaciones | 用于马来丝虫病和斑氏丝虫病的治疗。<br>Se usa para tratar malayan filariasis y bancroftian filariasis. |
| 用法、用量<br>Administración y dosis | （1）口服：1 次 0.1～0.2g，一日 0.3～0.6g，分 2～3 次服用，7～14 日为一疗程。<br>（2）大剂量短程疗法：治马来丝虫病可用本品 1.5g，一次顿服，或与一日内分 2 次服；治斑氏丝虫病总量 3g，与 2～3 日分服完，本法不良反应较重。<br>（3）预防：于流行区按每日 5～6mg/kg 服药，服 6～7 日，或按上量每周或每月服一日，直至总量达 70～90mg/kg 为止。<br>(1)Por vía oral: 0.1～0.2g 1 vez, 0.3～0.6g al día, en 2～3 veces, ciclo de tratamiento 7～14 días.<br>(2)Terapia de dosis grande a corto plazo: para tratar malayan filariasis, se usa 1.5g del medicamento, dosis única, o en 2 veces al día; para tratar bancroftian filariasis, dosis total de 3g, administrada en 2～3 días, con reacciones adversa grandes.<br>(3)Prevención: durante la epidemia se administra 5～6mg/kg al día, durante 6～7 días, o la misma dosis se toma 1 día cada semana o mes, hasta la dosis total alcanza a 70～90mg/kg. |
| 剂型、规格<br>Formulaciones y especificaciones | 片剂：每片 50mg；100mg。<br>Una tableta: 50mg; 100mg. |

### 7.7　抗利什曼原虫药 Medicamentos anti-Leishmania

| 药品名称 Drug Names | 葡萄糖酸锑钠 Estibogluconato sódico |
|---|---|
| 适应证<br>Indicaciones | 用于黑热病病因治疗，近期疗效可达 99%，2 年复发率低于 10%，复发病例可再用本品治疗。<br>Se usa para el tratamiento contra la causa de kala-azar. El efecto curativo a corto plazo puede ser de hasta el 99%. La tasa de recurrencia en dos años es inferior a 10%. En casos de recurrencia, se puede adoptarlo de nuevo para el tratamiento. |
| 用法、用量<br>Administración y dosis | 肌内或静脉注射。（1）一般成人 1 次 1.9g（6ml），一日 1 次，连用 6～10 日；或总剂量按体重 90～130mg/kg（以 50kg 为限），等分 6～10 次，一日 1 次。（2）小儿总剂量按体重 150～200mg/kg，分为 6 次，一日 1 次。（3）对敏感性较差的虫株感染者，可重复 1～2 个疗程，间隔 10～14 日。（4）对全身情况较差者，可每周注射 2 次，疗程 3 周或更长。（5）对近期曾接受锑剂治疗者，可减少剂量。 |

续　表

| | Inyección intramuscular o intravenosa. (1) Generalmente adultos 1.9g 1 vez (6ml), 1 vez al día, 6～10 días consecutivos; o la dosis total de 90 ～ 130mg/kg(límite de 50kg) se divide en 6 ～ 10 veces, 1 vez al día, de acuerdo al peso corporal. (2) La dosis total de niños de 150 ～ 200mg/kg se divide en 6 veces, 1 vez al día. (3) Para infectados de parásitos menos sensibles se puede repetir 1 ～ 2 ciclos de tratamiento, con intervalo de 10 ～ 14 días. (4) Para pacientes de mal estado general, se inyecta 2 veces 1 semana, ciclos de 3 semanas o más tiempo. (5) Para los pacientes que aceptaron la terapia de antimonio últimamente, se puede reducir la dosis. |
|---|---|
| 剂型、规格<br>Formulaciones y especificaciones | 注射液：每支 6ml，含葡萄糖酸锑钠 1.9g，约相当于五价锑 0.6g。<br>Una inyección: 6ml, que contiene 1.9g de estibogluconato sódico, aproximadamente equivalente a 0.6g de antimonio pentavalente. |

### 7.8　驱肠虫 Medicamentos Antihelmínticos

| 药品名称 Drug Names | 哌嗪 Piperazina |
|---|---|
| 适应证<br>Indicaciones | 用于肠蛔虫病、蛔虫所致的不全性肠梗阻和胆道蛔虫病较痛的缓解期。此外，亦可用于驱蛲虫。<br>Se usa para tratar obstrucción intestinal causada por ascariasis intestinal y ascárides así como el doloroso periodo de remisión de ascariasis biliar. Además se puede usar para exterminar oxiuros. |
| 用法、用量<br>Administración y dosis | （1）枸橼酸哌嗪：驱蛔虫，成人 3 ～ 3.5g，睡前一次服用，连服 2 日，小儿每日 100 ～ 160mg/kg，一日量不得超过 3g，连服 2 日，一般不必服泻药；驱蛲虫，成人每次 1 ～ 1.2g，一日 2 ～ 2.5g，连服 7 ～ 10 日，小儿一日 60mg/kg，分 2 次服用，每日总量不超过 2g，连服 7 ～ 10 日。<br>（2）磷酸哌嗪：驱蛔虫，一日 2.5 ～ 3g，睡前 1 次服用，连服 2 日，小儿每日 80 ～ 130mg/kg，一日量不得超过 2.5g，连服 2 日；驱蛲虫，每次 0.8 ～ 1g，一日 1.5 ～ 2g，连服 7 ～ 10 日，小儿一日 50mg/kg，分 2 次服，一日总量不超过 2g，连服 7 ～ 10 日。<br>(1)Citrato de piperazina: para exterminar ascárides, adultos 3 ～ 3.5g, se toma antes de acostarse, 2 días consecutivos, niños 100 ～ 160mg/kg al día, la dosis diaria no debe sobrepasar 3g, 2 días consecutivos, generalmente se hace falta tomar laxante; para exterminar oxiuros, adultos 1 ～ 1.2g, 2 ～ 2.5g al día, 7 ～ 10 días consecutivos, niños 60mg/kg, en 2 veces, la dosis diaria no debe sobrepasar 2g, 7 ～ 10 días consecutivos.<br>(2) Fosfato de piperazina: para exterminar ascárides, 2.5 ～ 3g al día, se toma de 1 vez antes de acostarse, 2 días consecutivos, niños 80 ～ 130mg/kg al día, la dosis diaria no debe sobrepasar 2.5g, 2 días consecutivos; para exterminar oxiuros, 0.8 ～ 1g 1 vez, 1.5 ～ 2g al día, 7 ～ 10 días consecutivos, niños 50mg/kg al día, en 2 veces, la dosis diaria no debe sobrepasar 2g, 7 ～ 10 días consecutivos. |
| 剂型、规格<br>Formulaciones y especificaciones | 枸橼酸哌嗪片：每片 0.25g；0.5g。<br>枸橼酸哌嗪糖浆：每 100ml 含本品 16g。<br>磷酸哌嗪片：每片 0.2g；0.5g。<br>Una tableta de citrato de piperazina: 0.25g; 0.5g.<br>Jarabe de citrato de piperazina: cada 100ml contiene 16g del medicamento.<br>Una tableta de fosfato de piperazina: 0.2g; 0.5g. |
| 药品名称 Drug Names | 左旋咪唑 Levamisol |
| 适应证<br>Indicaciones | 主要用于驱蛔虫及钩虫。由于本品单剂量有效率较高，故适于集体治疗，可于噻嘧啶合用治疗严重钩虫感染；与噻苯唑或恩波吡维铵合用治疗肠线虫混合感染；与枸橼酸乙胺嗪先后序贯应用于抗丝虫感染。<br>Se usa para expulsar ascárides y anquilostomas. Como la dosis unitaria tiene mayor eficiencia, conviene el tratamiento masivo, combinar con morantel para tratar anquilostomiasis grave, combinar con tiabendazol o embonato de pirvinio para tratar infección mixta de nematodos intestinales, combinar con dietilcarbamazina en orden secuencial para atacar la infección por filarias. |
| 用法、用量<br>Administración y dosis | （1）驱虫病：口服，①成人 1.5 ～ 2.5mg/kg，空腹或睡前顿服；②小儿剂量为 2 ～ 3mg/kg。<br>（2）驱钩虫：口服，1.5 ～ 2.5mg/kg，每晚 1 次，连服 3 日。<br>（3）治疗丝虫病：4 ～ 6mg/kg，分 3 次服，连服 3 日。<br>(1) Para exterminar parasitosis: por vía oral, ① adultos 1.5 ～ 2.5mg/kg, con estómago vacío o de una vez antes de acostarse; ② dosis para niños 2 ～ 3mg/kg.<br>(2) Para exterminar anquilostomas: por vía oral, 1.5 ～ 2.5mg/kg, 1 vez cada noche, 3 días consecutivos.<br>(3) Para tratar filariasis: 4 ～ 6mg/kg, en 3 veces, 3 días consecutivos. |

**续　表**

| 剂型、规格<br>Formulaciones y especificaciones | 片剂：每片 25mg；50mg。肠溶片：每片 25mg；50mg。颗粒剂：每 1g 含盐酸左旋咪唑 5mg。糖浆：0.8g（100ml）；4g（500ml）；16g（200ml）。搽剂：为左旋咪唑的 0.7% 二甲亚砜溶液或其硼酸酒精溶液。<br><br>Una tableta: 25mg; 50mg. Una tableta efervescente vaginal: 25mg; 50mg. Un gránulo: cada 1g contiene 5mg de clorhidrato de levamisol. Jarabe: 0.8g(100ml); 4g(500ml); 16g(200ml). Linimento: 0.7% sulfóxido de dimetilo o solución de alcohol de ácido bórico de levamisol. |
|---|---|
| **药品名称 Drug Names** | 阿苯达唑 Albendazol |
| 适应证<br>Indicaciones | 用于驱除蛔虫、蛲虫、钩虫、鞭虫，也可用于家畜的驱虫。<br><br>Se usa para expulsar ascárides, oxiuros, anquilostomas y tricúridos así como expulsar a parásitos para el ganado. |
| 用法、用量<br>Administración y dosis | 口服，驱钩虫、蛔虫、蛲虫、鞭虫，0.4g 顿服。2 周岁以上小儿，单纯蛲虫、单纯蛔虫感染，0.2g 顿服。治疗囊虫病：每天 15 ~ 20mg/kg，分 2 次服用。10 日为 1 个疗程。停药 15 ~ 20 日后，可进行第 2 疗程治疗。一般为 2 ~ 3 个疗程。必要时可重复治疗。其他寄生虫如粪类圆线虫等，每日服 400mg，连服 6 日。必要时重复给药 1 次。12 岁以下儿童；用量减半，服法同成人或遵医嘱。<br><br>Se toma por vía oral, para exterminar ascárides, oxiuros, anquilostomas y tricúridos, 0.4g dosis única. Niños mayores a 2 años, con infección simple de oxiuros y ascárides, 0.2g dosis única. Para tratar cisticercosis: 15 ~ 20mg/kg al día, en 2 veces. 10 días un ciclo de tratamiento. Tras 15 ~ 20 días interrumpida la administración, se puede efectuar el segundo ciclo de tratamiento. Generalmente son 2 ~ 3 ciclos. En casos necesarios, se puede repetir el tratamiento. Para otros parásitos tales como strongyloides stercoralis, etc., se toma 400mg al día, 6 días consecutivos. En casos necesarios, se puede repetir la administración. Niños menores a 12 años: dosis a la mitad, forma igual a adultos o seguir las recomendaciones del médico. |
| 剂型、规格<br>Formulaciones y especificaciones | 片（胶囊）剂：每片（粒）100mg；200mg。干糖浆：每袋 200mg。<br>Una tableta(cápsula): 100mg; 200mg. Jarabe seco: 200mg cada saco. |

8. 主要作用于中枢神经系统的药物 Medicamentos que actúa princepalmente en el sistema nervioso central

8.1　中枢神经系统兴奋药 Estimulantes del sistema nervioso central

| **药品名称 Drug Names** | 尼可刹米 Niketamida |
|---|---|
| 适应证<br>Indicaciones | 用于中枢性呼吸及循环衰竭、麻醉药及其中枢抑制药的中毒。<br><br>Se usa para fallo respiratorio y circulatorio central, así como intoxicación de narcóticos e inhibidores del sistema nervioso central. |
| 用法、用量<br>Administración y dosis | 常用量：皮下注射、肌内或静脉注射，每次 0.25 ~ 0.5g。必要时 1 ~ 2 小时重复用药。极量：皮下、肌内或静脉注射，一次 1.25g。6 个月以下，婴儿 75mg/ 次，一岁 125mg/ 次，4 ~ 7 岁 175mg/ 次。<br><br>Dosis habitual: inyección subcutánea, intramuscular o intravenosa, 0.25~0.5g cada vez. En casos necesarios, se puede repetir la administración dentro de 1~2 horas. Dosis máxima: por inyección subcutánea, intramuscular o intravenosa, 1.25g 1 vez. Bebés menores a 6 meses, 75mg/vez, de un año, 125mg/vez, de 4~7 años, 175mg/vez. |
| 剂型、规格<br>Formulaciones y especificaciones | 注射液：每支 0.375g（1.5ml）；0.5g（2ml）；0.25g（1ml）。<br>Una inyección: 0.375g(1.5ml); 0.5g(2ml); 0.25g(1ml). |
| **药品名称 Drug Names** | 洛贝林 Lobelina |
| 适应证<br>Indicaciones | 用于新生儿窒息、一氧化碳引起的窒息、吸入麻醉剂及其他中枢神经抑制药（如阿片、巴比妥类）的中毒及肺炎、白喉等疾病引起的呼吸衰竭。<br><br>Se usa para asfixia neonatal, asfixia por monóxido de carbono, intoxicación por la inhalación de narcóticos e inhibidor del sistema nervioso central(tales como opiáceos y barbitúricos) así como fallo respiratorio causado por neumonía y difteria entre otras enfermedades. |

**续　表**

| | |
|---|---|
| 用法、用量<br>Administración y dosis | 　皮下注射或肌内注射：常用量，成人 1 次 3 ～ 10mg（极量：1 次 20mg，1 日 50mg）；儿童 1 次 1 ～ 3mg。静脉注射：成人 1 次 3mg（极量：1 次 6mg，1 日 20mg）；儿童 1 次 0.3 ～ 3mg。必要时每 30 分钟可重复 1 次。静脉注射需缓慢。新生儿窒息可注入脐静脉，用量为 3mg。<br>　Inyección subcutánea o intramuscular: dosis habitual, adultos 3~10mg 1 vez (dosis máxima: 20mg 1 vez, 50mg al día); niños 1~3mg 1 vez. Inyección intravenosa: adultos 3mg 1 vez (dosis máxima: 6mg 1 vez, 20mg al día); niños 0.3~3mg 1 vez. En casos necesarios, se puede repetir la inyección cada 30 minutos. La inyección intravenosa debe ser lenta. Por la asfixia los recién nacidos pueden ser inyectados en la vena umbilical, con la dosis de 3mg. |
| 剂型、规格<br>Formulaciones y especificaciones | 　注射液：每支 3mg（1ml）；10mg（1ml）。<br>　Una inyección: 3mg(1ml); 10mg(1ml). |
| **药品名称 Drug Names** | 戊四氮 Pentetrazol |
| 适应证<br>Indicaciones | 　用于急性传染病、麻醉药及巴比妥类药物中毒时引起的呼吸抑制，急性循环衰竭。安全范围小，现已少用。<br>　Se usa para inhibición respiratoria e insuficiencia circulatoria aguda causadas por enfermedades infecciosas agudas e intoxicación de narcóticos y barbitúricos. El margen de seguridad es limitado. Ahora se lo usa menos. |
| 用法、用量<br>Administración y dosis | 　皮下注射、肌内注射、静脉注射，每次 0.05 ～ 0.1g，每 2 小时 1 次。极量 1 日 0.3g。<br>　Inyección subcutánea, intravenosa o intramuscular, 0.05~0.1g 1 vez cada 2 horas. Dosis máxima diaria 0.3g. |
| 剂型、规格<br>Formulaciones y especificaciones | 　注射液：每支 0.1g（1ml）；0.3g（3ml）。<br>　Una inyección: 0.1g(1ml); 0.3g(3ml). |
| **药品名称 Drug Names** | 贝美格 Bemegrida |
| 适应证<br>Indicaciones | 　用于解救巴比妥类、格鲁米特、水合氯醛等药物的中毒。应用于加速硫喷妥钠麻醉后的恢复。<br>　Se usa para la desintoxicación de barbitúricos, glutetimida e hidrato de cloral entre otras medicinas. Se aplica para acelerar la recuperación tras la anestesia de tiopental sódico. |
| 用法、用量<br>Administración y dosis | 　因本品作用迅速，多采用静脉滴注，作用维持 10 ～ 20 分钟。常用量 0.5%10ml（50mg），用 5% 葡萄糖注射液稀释静脉滴注。宜可静脉注射，每 3 ～ 5 分钟注射 50mg，至病情改善或出现中毒症状为止。<br>　Como tendrá efectos de forma muy rápida, se adopta frecuentemente la infusión intravenosa que dura 10~20 minutos. Dosis habitual 0.5% 10ml (50mg), se diluye en 5% inyección de glucosa para preparar infusión intravenosa. También puede ser por inyección intravenosa, 50mg cada 3~5minutos, hasta que los síntomas se mejoren o aparezcan los síntomas de intoxicación. |
| 剂型、规格<br>Formulaciones y especificaciones | 　注射液：每支 50mg（10ml）。<br>　Una inyección: 50mg(10ml). |
| **药品名称 Drug Names** | 咖啡因 Cafeína |
| 适应证<br>Indicaciones | 　（1）解救因急性感染中毒、催眠药、麻醉药、镇痛药中毒引起的呼吸、循环衰竭。<br>　（2）与溴化物合用，使大脑皮质兴奋、抑制过程恢复平衡，用于神经官能症。<br>　（3）与阿司匹林、对乙酰氨基酚制成复方制剂用于一般性头痛；与麦角胺合用治疗偏头痛。<br>　（4）用于小儿多动症（注意力缺陷综合征）。<br>　（5）治疗未成熟新生儿呼吸暂停或阵发性呼吸困难。<br>　(1) Se usa para la desintoxicación de infecciones agudas y el tratamiento de fallo respiratorio y circulatorio causado por toxicación de hipnóticos, narcóticos y analgésicos.<br>　(2) Combina con bromuro para neurosis excitando la corteza cerebral e inhibiendo el restablecimiento del equilibrio.<br>　(3) Prepara compuestos con aspirina y acetaminofeno para tratar dolor de cabeza y combina con ergotamina para tratar migraña.<br>　(4) Se usa para trastorno por déficit de atención e hiperactividad(TDAH)<br>　(5) Se usa para apnea del sueño o disnea paroxismal de los recién nacidos prematuros. |

**续　表**

| 用法、用量<br>Administración y dosis | （1）口服。常用量：1 次 0.1～0.3g，1 日 0.3～1.0g；极量：1 次 0.4g，一日 1.5g。<br>　　（2）解救中枢抑制：肌内注射或皮下注射安钠咖注射液（详见制剂项下）。常用量：皮下或肌内注射，1 次 1～2ml，一日 2～4ml；极量皮下或肌内注射，1 次 3ml，一日 12ml。<br>　　（3）调节大脑皮质活动：口服咖溴合剂，每日 10～15ml，1 日 3 次，餐后服。<br>　　(1)Se toma por vía oral. Dosis habitual: 0.1~0.3g 1 vez, 0.3~1.0g al día; dosis máxima: 0.4g 1 vez, 1.5g al día.<br>　　(2)Rescatar a la inhibición del sistema nervioso central: inyección de la cafeína y benzoato de sodio por vía intramuscular o subcutánea(vease preparación de la dosis). Dosis habitual: por vía intramuscular o subcutánea, 1~2ml 1 vez, 2~4ml al día; dosis máxima por vía intramuscular o subcutánea, 3ml 1 vez, 12mlal día.<br>　　(3)Regular la actividad cortical: se toma mezcla de bromuro de cafeína, 10~15ml, 3 veces al día, tras cada comida. |
|---|---|
| 剂型、规格<br>Formulaciones y especificaciones | 片剂：每片 30mg。<br>Una tableta: 30mg. |
| 药品名称 Drug Names | 甲氯芬酯 Meclofenoxato |
| 适应证<br>Indicaciones | 用于外伤性昏迷、新生儿缺氧、儿童遗尿症、意识障碍、老年性精神病、酒精中毒及某些中枢和周围神经症状。<br>Se usa para coma traumático,hipoxia neonatal, enuresis nocturna en niños, perturbación de conciencia, psicosis senil, alcoholismo y algunos de los síntomas nerviosos central y periférico. |
| 用法、用量<br>Administración y dosis | （1）口服，成人 1 次 0.1～0.3g，一日 0.3～0.9g；最大剂量可达一日 1.5g。儿童 1 次 100mg，一日 3 次。<br>　　（2）肌内注射或静脉滴注：成人 1 次 0.25g，一日 1～3 次。溶于 5% 葡萄糖溶液 250～500ml 中供静脉滴注。新生儿可注入脐静脉。小儿每次 60～100mg，一日 2 次。新生儿缺氧症，一次 0.06g，每 2 小时一次。<br>　　(1)Se toma por vía oral, adultos 1 vez 0.1~0.3g, 0.3~0.9g al día; la dosis máxima puede alcanzar 1.5g al día. Niños 100mg 1 vez, 3 veces al día.<br>　　(2)Inyección intramuscular o infusión intravenosa: adultos 0.25g 1 vez, 1~3 veces al día. Se diluye en 250~500ml de 5% solución de glucosa como infusión intravenosa. Los recién nacidos pueden ser inyectados en la vena umbilical. Niños 60~100mg cada vez, 2 veces al día. Anoxia neonatal, 0.06g 1 vez cada 2 horas. |
| 剂型、规格<br>Formulaciones y especificaciones | 胶囊剂：每粒 0.1g；注射用盐酸甲氯芬酯：每支 0.1g；0.25g。<br>Una cápsula: 0.1g; ácido clorhídrico de meclofenoxato para inyección: 0.1g; 0.25g. |
| 药品名称 Drug Names | 乙哌立松 Eperisona |
| 适应证<br>Indicaciones | 可用于改善下列疾病的肌紧张状态：颈肩腕综合征，肩周炎，腰痛症；也可用于改善下列疾病所致的痉挛性麻痹：脑血管障碍，痉挛性脊髓麻痹，颈椎病，手术后遗症（包括脑、脊髓肿瘤），外伤后遗症（脊髓损伤、头部外伤），肌萎缩性侧索硬化症，婴儿大脑性轻瘫，脊髓小脑变性症，脊髓血管障碍，亚急性脊髓神经症（SMON）及其他脑脊髓疾病。<br>Se usa para mejorar la tensión muscular de las siguientes enfermedades: síndrome cervicobraquial, periartritis escapulohumeral y lumbago; también se usa para mejorar la parálisis espástica de las siguientes enfermedades: trastornos cerebrovasculares, parálisis espinal espástica, espondilosis cervical, complicaciones quirúrgicas (incluyendo el cerebro, los tumores de la médula espinal), secuelas de trauma (lesión de la médula espinal, lesión en la cabeza), la esclerosis lateral amiotrófica, parálisis cerebral infantil, degeneración espinocerebelosa la enfermedad, trastornos vasculares de la columna vertebral, trastorno de la médula espinal subaguda (SMON), y otras enfermedades del cerebro y la médula espinal. |
| 用法、用量<br>Administración y dosis | 餐后口服。通常成人一次 50mg（1 片），一日 3 次。<br>Se toma por vía oral tras comidas. Generalmente para adultos 50mg cada vez(1 tableta), 3 veces al día. |

| 剂型、规格<br>Formulaciones y especificaciones | 片剂：每片 50mg。<br>Una tableta: 50mg. |
| --- | --- |
| 药品名称 Drug Names | 细胞色素 C　Citocromo C |
| 适应证<br>Indicaciones | 用于各种组织缺氧的急救或辅助治疗，如一氧化碳中毒、催眠药中毒、新生儿窒息、严重休克期缺氧、麻醉及肺部疾病引起的呼吸困难、高山缺氧、脑缺氧及心脏疾病引起的缺氧，但疗效有时不显著。<br><br>Se usa como primer auxilio o terapia adyuvante para todos los tipos de hipoxia tisular, tales como intoxicación por monóxido de carbono, intoxicación por hipnóticos, asfixia neonatal, hipoxia en síncope severo, dificultades respiratorias causadas por enfermedades pulmonares y anestesia, hipoxia en altas motañas, hipoxia cerebral así como hipoxia causado por enfermedades cardiacas, pero la eficacia a veces no es tan destacada. |
| 用法、用量<br>Administración y dosis | 静脉注射或滴注：成人每次 15～30mg，每日 30～60mg。儿童用量酌减。静脉注射时，加 25% 葡萄糖注射液 20ml 混匀后，缓慢注射。亦可用 5%～10% 葡萄糖注射液或生理盐水稀释后静脉滴注。粉针（冻干型）用 25% 葡萄糖注射液 20ml 或 5% 葡萄糖注射液或灭菌生理盐水溶解后滴注。<br><br>Inyección o infusión intravenosa: adultos 15~30mg cada vez, 30~60mg al día. La dosis para niños se reduce correspondientemente. En la inyección intravenosa se agrega 20ml de 25% inyección de glucosa para mezclarse e inyectarse lentamente. También se puede diluir en 5%~10% inyección de glucosa o solución salina fisiológica antes de la infusión. Diluido en 20ml de 25% inyección de glucosa o 5% inyección de glucosa o solución salina estéril por aguja de polvo(liofilizado) se efectúa la infusión. |
| 剂型、规格<br>Formulaciones y especificaciones | 注射液：每支 15mg（2ml）。注射用细胞色素 C：每支 15mg。<br>Una inyección: 15mg(2ml). Citocromo para inyección: 15mg. |

8.2　镇痛药 Medicamentos analgésicos

| 药品名称 Drug Names | 吗啡 Morfina |
| --- | --- |
| 适应证<br>Indicaciones | ①镇痛：现仅用于创伤、手术、烧伤等引起的剧痛。②心肌梗死。③心源性哮喘。④麻醉前给药。<br>① aliviar el dolor: se usa sólo para dolor agudo causado por la herida, la quirugía, y la quemadura entre otras. ② infarto de miocardio. ③ asma cardíaca. ④ antes de la administración de la anestesia. |
| 用法、用量<br>Administración y dosis | ①常用量：口服，1 次 5～15mg，一日 15～60mg；皮下注射，1 次 5～15mg，一日 15～40mg；静脉注射，5～10mg。②极量：口服，1 次 30mg，一日 100mg；皮下注射，1 次 20mg，一日 60mg；硬膜外腔注射，一次极量 5mg，用于手术后镇痛。<br><br>① Dosis habitual: por vía oral, 5~ 15mg 1 vez, 15~60mg al día; por inyección subcutánea, 5~ 15mg 1 vez, 15~40mg al día; por inyección intravenosa, 5~10mg. ② Dosis máxima: por vía oral, 30mg 1 vez, 100mg al día; inyección subcutánea, 20mg 1 vez, 60mg al día; inyección epidural, dosis máxima de 5mg, para la analgesia postoperatoria. |
| 剂型、规格<br>Formulaciones y especificaciones | 注射液：每支 5mg（0.5ml）；10mg（1.0ml）。片剂：每片 5mg；10mg。<br>Una inyección: 5mg(0.5ml); 10mg(1.0ml). Una tableta: 5mg；10mg. |
| 药品名称 Drug Names | 哌替啶 Petidina |
| 适应证<br>Indicaciones | ①各种剧痛，如创伤、烧伤、烫伤、术后疼痛等；②心源性哮喘；③麻醉前给药；④内脏剧烈绞痛（胆绞痛、肾绞痛需与阿托品合用）；⑤与氯丙嗪、异丙嗪等合用进行人工冬眠。<br><br>① se usa para dolor agudo causado por la herida, la quirugía, y la quemadura entre otras. ② asma cardíaca. ③ antes de la administración de la anestesia. ④ rigores de cólico (combinar con atropina para tratar cólico biliar y cólico renal).　⑤ combinar con clorpromazina y prometazina, etc. para realizar hibernación artificial. |

**续　表**

| | |
|---|---|
| 用法、用量<br>Administración y dosis | ①口服：一次 25～100mg，一日 200～400mg；极量：1 次 150mg，一日 600mg。②皮下注射或肌内注射：1 次 25～100mg，一日 100～400mg；极量：1 次 150mg，一日 600mg。2 次用要间隔不宜少于 4 小时。③静脉注射：成人以每次 0.3mg/kg 为限。④麻醉前肌内注射：成人以每 1kg 体重 1.0mg，术前 30～60 分钟给予。麻醉过程中静脉滴注，成人以每 1kg 体重 1.2～2.0mg 计算总量，配成稀释液，以每分钟 1mg 静脉滴注，小儿滴速减慢。⑤手术后镇痛及癌性镇痛：以每日 2.1～2.5mg/kg 计量为限，经硬膜外腔缓慢注入或泵入。<br><br>① Se toma por vía oral：25～100mg 1 vez，200～400mg al día；dosis máxima：150mg 1 vez，600mg al día. ② Inyección subcutánea o intramuscular：25～100mg 1 vez，100～400mg al día；dosis máxima：150mg 1 vez，600mg al día. El intervalo entre 2 veces no debe ser inferior a 4 horas. ③ Inyección intravenosa：adultos 0.3mg/kg 1 vez como máximo. ④ La inyección intramuscular antes de la anestesia：adultos cada 1kg de peso corporal se administra 1.0mg，30～60 minutos antes de la operación. Durante la anestesia，se efectúa la infusión intravenosa，se calcula la dosis total en 1.2～2.0mg cada 1kg del peso corporal para adultos y prepara la solución diluida para gotear 1mg cada minuto por vía intravenosa，con velocidad ralentizada para niños. ⑤ Analgesia postoperatoria y alivio del dolor por cáncer：calculado en 2.1～2.5mg/kg al día，por inyección o bombeo epidural lento. |
| 剂型、规格<br>Formulaciones y especificaciones | 片剂：每片 25mg；50mg。注射液：每支 50mg（1ml）；100mg（2ml）。<br>Una tableta: 25mg; 50mg. Una inyección: 50mg(1ml); 100mg(2ml). |
| 药品名称 Drug Names | 美沙酮 Metadona |
| 适应证<br>Indicaciones | 适用于创伤性、癌症剧痛、外科手术后和慢性疼痛。也用于阿片、吗啡及海洛因成瘾者的脱毒治疗。<br><br>Se aplica a dolores de lesión traumática，de cáncer，después de la cirugía y crónico. También se usa para desintoxicación de adictos de opio，morfina y heroína. |
| 用法、用量<br>Administración y dosis | （1）口服：成人每日 10～15mg，分 2～3 次服用。儿童每日按 0.7mg/kg 计量，分 4～6 次服用。极量：一次 10mg，一日 20mg。（2）肌内注射或皮下注射：每次 2.5～5mg，一日 10mg～15mg。三角肌注射血浆峰值高，作用出现快，因此可采用三角肌注射。极量：1 次 10mg，一日 20mg。<br><br>(1)Por vía oral：10~15mg al día para adultos；en 2~3 veces. 0.7mg/kg al día para niños，en 4~6 veces. Dosis máxima: 10mg 1 vez，20mg al día. (2)Por inyección intramuscular o subcutánea: 2.5~5mg 1 vez，10mg~15mgal día. Como inyección en el deltoides puede tener el valor plasmático máximo y producir efectos rápidamente se puede adoptarla. Dosis máxima: 10mg 1 vez，20mg al día. |
| 剂型、规格<br>Formulaciones y especificaciones | 片剂：每片 2.5mg；7.5mg；10mg。注射液：每支 5mg（1ml）7.5mg（2ml）。<br>Una tableta: 2.5mg; 7.5mg; 10mg. Una inyección: 5mg(1ml)7.5mg(2ml). |
| 药品名称 Drug Names | 芬太尼 Fentanilo |
| 适应证<br>Indicaciones | 适用于各种疼痛及外科、妇科等手术后和手术过程中的镇痛；也用于防止或减轻手术后的谵妄；还可与麻醉药合用，作为麻醉辅助用药，与氟哌利多配伍制成"安定镇痛剂"，用于大面积换药及进行小手术的镇痛。<br><br>Se usa para todos los tipos de dolores y aliviar dolores después de operaciones quirúrgica，ginecológica entre otras；también se usa para prevenir o aliviar delirios después de cirugías；puede combinar con narcóticos como fármaco adyuvantes de anestesia；preparar compuestos con droperidol como analgésico para aliviar dolor en apósito de zona amplia o en cirugía menor. |
| 用法、用量<br>Administración y dosis | ①麻醉前给药：0.05～0.1mg，于手术前 30～60 分钟肌内注射。②诱导麻醉：静脉注射 0.05～0.1mg，间隔 2～3 分钟重复注射，直至达到要求；危重患者、年幼及年老患者的用量减小至 0.025～0.05mg。③维持麻醉：当患者出现苏醒状时，静脉注射或肌内注射 0.025～0.05mg。④一般镇痛及术后镇痛：肌内注射 0.05～0.1mg。可控制手术后疼痛、烦躁和呼吸急迫，必要时可于 1～2 小时后重复给药。硬膜外腔注入镇痛，一般 4～10 分钟起效，20 分钟脑脊液浓度达峰值，作用持续 3～6 小时。⑤贴片：每 3 天用 1 贴，贴于锁骨下胸部皮肤。 |

|  | ① Administración antes de la anestesia: 0.05~0.1mg, 30~60 minutos antes de la cirugía por vía intramuscular. ② Inducción de la anestesia: 0.05~0.1mg por vía intravenosa, se repite la inyección con un intervalo de 2~3 minutos hasta alcanzar los requisitos; Para pacientes pesados, menores y mayores, la dosis se reduce al 0.025~0.05mg. ③ Mantenimiento de anestesia: cuando los pacientes se despiertan se inyecta 0.025~0.05mg por vía intravenosa o intramuscular. ④ Analgesia general y analgesia postoperatoria: 0.05~0.1mg por vía intramuscular. Puede controlar el dolor, la irritabilidad y la respiración urgente tras la operación. En casos necesarios se puede repetir la administración dentro de 1~2 horas. Analgesia por inyección epidural, por lo general tiene efectos dentro de 4 y 10 minutos, y la concentración del líquido cefalorraquídeo alcanza el pico dentro de 20 minutos. Los efecto puede durar entre 3 y 6 horas. ⑤ Parche: cada 3 días, en la piel del pecho subclavia. |
|---|---|
| 剂型、规格<br>Formulaciones y especificaciones | 注射液：每支 0.1mg（2ml）。贴片（多瑞吉）：每小时可释放芬太尼 25μg、50μg、75μg、100μg。复方芬太尼注射液：每 1ml 含芬太尼 0.1mg，异丙嗪 25mg。<br>Una inyección: 0.1mg(2ml). (Parche(durogesic): cada hora se libera 25μg, 50μg, 75μg y 100μg de fentanilo. Inyección de fentanil compuesto: cada 1ml contiene 0.1mg de fentanilo y 25mg de prometazina. |
| 药品名称 Drug Names | 阿芬太尼 Alfentanilo |
| 适应证<br>Indicaciones | 用于麻醉前、中、后的镇静与镇痛，适用于心脏冠状动脉血管旁路术的麻醉。<br>Se usa para la sedación y analgesia antes, durante y tras la anestesia. Se aplica a la anestesia para cirugía de bypass de la arteria coronaria. |
| 用法、用量<br>Administración y dosis | 静脉注射：按手术长短而决定极量。手术 10 分钟以内完成者 7～15μg/kg；60 分钟手术，40～80μg/kg；手术超过 60 分钟者，可改为每分钟 1μg/kg，连续静脉滴注，至手术结束前 10 分钟停止给药。<br>Inyección intravenosa: la dosis máxima depende de la duración quirúrgica. Dentro de 10 minutos, 7~15μg/kg; de 60 minutos, 40~80μg/kg; mayor a 60 minutos, 1μg/kg cada minuto, se administra la infusión intravenosa continuamente hasta 10 minutos antes del final de la operación. |
| 剂型、规格<br>Formulaciones y especificaciones | 注射液（盐酸盐）：每支 1mg（2ml）。<br>Una inyección (clorhidrato): 1mg(2ml). |
| 药品名称 Drug Names | 舒芬太尼 Sufentanilo |
| 适应证<br>Indicaciones | 用于麻醉前、中、后的镇静与镇痛，适用于心脏冠状动脉血管旁路术的麻醉。<br>Se usa para la sedación y analgesia antes, durante y tras la anestesia. Se aplica a la anestesia para cirugía de bypass de la arteria coronaria. |
| 用法、用量<br>Administración y dosis | 麻醉时间长约 2 小时，总剂量 2μg/kg，维持量 10～25μg。麻醉时间长 2～8 小时，总剂量 2～8μg/kg，维持量 10～50μg。心血管手术麻醉，5μg/kg。<br>Si la anestesia dura aproximadamente 2 horas, dosis total de 2μg/kg, dosis de mantenimiento 10~25μg. Si la anestesia dura aproximadamente 2~8 horas, dosis total de 2~8μg/kg, dosis de mantenimiento 10~50μg. Anestesia cirugía cardiovascular, 5μg/kg. |
| 剂型、规格<br>Formulaciones y especificaciones | 注射液：每支 50μg（2ml）；100μg（2ml）；250μg（2ml）。<br>Una inyección: 50μg(2ml); 100μg(2ml); 250μg(2ml). |
| 药品名称 Drug Names | 瑞芬太尼 Remifentanilo |
| 适应证<br>Indicaciones | 用于麻醉诱导和全身麻醉中维持镇痛。<br>Se usa para mantener analgesia durante la inducción de la anestesia y anestesia general. |
| 用法、用量<br>Administración y dosis | 10mg 加入 200ml 生理盐水。用于静脉麻醉时，剂量为 0.25～2.0μg/（kg·min），或间断注射 0.25～1.0μg/kg。<br>Se agrega 200ml de la solución salina fisiológica al 10mg del fármaco. Cuando se utiliza en la anestesia intravenosa, la dosis es de 0.25~2.0μg/(kg·min), o se inyecta 0.25~1.0μg/kg de forma intermitente. |

| 剂型、规格<br>Formulaciones y especificaciones | 注射用瑞芬太尼：每支 1mg；2mg；5mg。<br>Remifentanilo para inyección: 1mg; 2mg; 5mg. |
| --- | --- |
| 药品名称 Drug Names | 布桂嗪 Bucinazina |
| 适应证<br>Indicaciones | 临床上用于偏头痛、三叉神经痛、炎症性及外伤性疼痛、关节痛、痛经、癌症引起的疼痛等。<br>En clínica se usa para migraña, neuralgia del trigémino, dolor inflamatorio y traumático, dolor en las articulaciones, dismenorrea, dolor causado por el cáncer, etc. |
| 用法、用量<br>Administración y dosis | （1）口服：成人 1 次 30～60mg，一日 90～180mg；小儿每次 1mg/kg。疼痛剧烈时用量可酌增。<br>（2）皮下或肌内注射：成人 1 次 50～100mg，一日 1～2 次。<br>(1)Se toma por vía oral: adultos 30~60mg 1 vez, 90~180mg al día; niños 1mg/kg 1 vez. Se puede aumentar la dosis en dolor severo. (2)Inyección subcutánea o intramuscular: adultos 50~l00mg 1 vez, 1~2 veces al día. |
| 剂型、规格<br>Formulaciones y especificaciones | 片剂：每片 30mg；60mg。注射液：每支 50mg（2ml）；100mg（2ml）。<br>Una tableta: 30mg; 60mg. Una inyección: 50mg(2ml); 100mg(2ml). |
| 药品名称 Drug Names | 喷他佐辛 Pentazocina |
| 适应证<br>Indicaciones | 适用于各种慢性剧痛。<br>Se usa para todos los tipos de dolores agudos. |
| 用法、用量<br>Administración y dosis | 静脉注射、肌内注射或皮下注射，每次 30mg。口服，每次 25～50mg。必要时每 3～4 小时 1 次。<br>Inyección intravenosa, intramuscular o subcutánea, 30mg 1 vez. Por vía oral: 25~50mg 1 vez. En casos necesarios, cada 3~4 horas 1 vez. |
| 剂型、规格<br>Formulaciones y especificaciones | 片剂：每片 25mg；50mg。注射液：每支 15mg（1ml）；30mg（1ml）。<br>Una tableta: 25mg; 50mg. Una inyección: 15mg(1ml); 30mg(1ml). |
| 药品名称 Drug Names | 羟考酮 Oxicodona |
| 适应证<br>Indicaciones | 用于缓解中、重度疼痛。<br>Se usa para aliviar dolores leves y moderados. |
| 用法、用量<br>Administración y dosis | （1）一般镇痛，使用控释制剂，每 12 小时服用 1 次，用药剂量取决于患者的疼痛的严重程度和既往镇痛药用药史。首次服用阿片类或弱阿片类药物初始用药剂量一般为 5mg，每 12 小时服用 1 次。已接受口服吗啡治疗的患者，改用本品的每日用药剂量换算比例为：口服本品 10mg 相当于口服吗啡 20mg。应根据患者个体情况滴定用药剂量。调整剂量时，不改变用药次数，只调整每次剂量，调整幅度是在上次一次的用药剂量基础上增长 25%～50%。大多数患者的最高用药剂量为每 12 小时服用 200mg，少数患者可能需要更高的剂量。控释制剂必须整片吞服，不得掰开、咀嚼或研磨。如果掰开、咀嚼或研磨药片，会导致羟考酮的快速释放与潜在致死量的吸收。<br>（2）术后疼痛：使用本药复方胶囊，每次 1～2 粒，间隔 4～6 小时可重复用药一次。（3）癌症、慢性疼痛：使用本药复方胶囊，每次 1～2 粒，一日 3 次。儿童：口服，一次 0.05～0.15mg/kg，每 4～6 小时一次。一次用量最多 5mg。<br>(1)Dolor general, se utiliza dosificación de liberación controlada 1 vez cada 12 horas, y la dosis depende de la severidad del dolor del paciente y de la historia previa de medicación analgésica. La primera dosis inicial de opioides o opiáceos suaves es generalmente de 5 mg, 1 vez por 12 h. Los pacientes que ya reciben tratamiento con morfina oral al cambiar de fármaco toman en la proporción de dosis diaria como lo siguiente: la administración oral del 10 mg equivalente a 20 mg morfina oral. La dosis debe ajustarse en base a las circunstancias individuales de cada paciente. Al ajustar la dosis, no se debe cambiar la frecuencia de administración sino la cantidad de cada dosis, siendo un aumento de 25% a 50% sobre la base de la última dosis. La dosis máxima de la mayoría de los pacientes es de 200mg por 12h, y algunos pacientes pueden requerir más dosis. La dosificación de liberación controlada debe tragarse enteras piezas y no se puede romper aparte, masticar o moler. Si se rompen aparte, se mastican o se muelen pastillas puede causar una rápida liberación de la absorción de la oxicodona y potencialmente de dosis letal. (2)Dolor postoperario: se usan cápsulas del fármaco, 1~2 tabletas cada vez, se puede repetir la administración cada 4~6 horas. (3)Dolor crónico por cáncer: se usan cápsulas del fármaco, 1~2 tabletas cada vez, 3 veces al día. Niños: por vía oral, 0.05~0.15mg/kg cada vez, cada 4~6 horas. La dosis máxima es de 5mg. |

**续　表**

| 剂型、规格<br>Formulaciones y especificaciones | 片剂：5mg。控释片：5mg；10mg；20mg；40mg。复方胶囊剂：每粒含羟考酮 5mg、对乙酰氨基酚 500mg。<br>Una tableta: 5mg. Pastillas de liberación controlada: 5mg, 10mg; 20mg; 40mg. Combinación de Cápsulas: 5mg oxicodona y 500mg paracetamol cada pedazo. |
|---|---|
| **药品名称 Drug Names** | **地佐辛 Dezocina** |
| 适应证<br>Indicaciones | 用于术后痛、内脏及癌性疼痛。<br>Se usa para el dolor postoperatorio, el dolor visceral y el dolor de cáncer. |
| 用法、用量<br>Administración y dosis | 肌内注射：开始时 10mg，以后每隔 3～6 小时，2.5～10mg。静脉注射：开始 5mg，以后每隔 2～4 小时，2.5～10mg。<br>Inyección intramuscular: 10mg al principio, en adelante cada 3~6 horas, 2.5~10mg. Inyección intravenosa: 5mg al principio, en adelante cada 2~4 horas, 2.5~10mg. |
| 剂型、规格<br>Formulaciones y especificaciones | 注射液：每支 5mg（1ml）；10mg（1ml）。<br>Una inyección: 5mg(1ml); 10mg(1ml). |
| **药品名称 Drug Names** | **普瑞巴林 Pregabalina** |
| 适应证<br>Indicaciones | 用于治疗外周神经痛及辅助性治疗局限性部分癫痫发作。我国批准的适应证为：用于治疗带状疱疹后神经痛。<br>Se usa para el tratamiento de dolor neuropático periférico y el tratamiento adyuvante de las convulsiones parciales. La aplicación aprobada por el Estado es tratar neuralgia posherpética. |
| 用法、用量<br>Administración y dosis | 口服，每日剂量为 150～600mg，分 2～3 次给药。一般起始剂量为每次 75mg，一日 2 次。如果每日服用本品 300mg，2～4 周后疼痛仍未得到充分缓解、且可耐受本品的患者，剂量可增至每次 300mg，一日 2 次，或每次 200mg，一日 3 次（即 600mg/d）。由于不良反应呈剂量依赖性，且不良反应可导致更高的停药率，故剂量超过 300mg/d 仅应用于耐受 300mg/d 剂量的持续性疼痛患者。<br>Se toma por vía oral, dosis diaria de 150~600mg, dividida en 2~3 veces. Generalmente la dosis inicial es de 75mg cada vez, 2 veces al día. Si se toma 300mg al día, el dolor no se ha liberado completamente 2~4 semanas después, y el paciente puede tolerar el producto, la dosis puede incrementarse a 300 mg 1 vez, 2 veces al día o 200 mg 1 vez, 3 veces al día(es decir, 600 mg/d). Dado que las reacciones adversas dependen de la dosis y reacciones adversas pueden conducir a mayores tasas de interrupción, las dosis superiores a 300 mg/d se aplican sólo a los pacientes con intolerancia a 300mg/d con dolor persistente. |
| 剂型、规格<br>Formulaciones y especificaciones | 胶囊：每粒 75mg；150mg。<br>Una cápsula: 75mg; 150mg. |
| **药品名称 Drug Names** | **曲马多 Tramadol** |
| 适应证<br>Indicaciones | 用于中、重度急慢性疼痛，服后 0.5 小时生效，持续 6 小时。亦用于术后痛、创伤痛、癌性痛、心脏病突发性痛、关节痛、神经痛及分娩痛。<br>Se usa para dolores agudos y crónicos de intensidades moderada y severa, entra en vigor dentro de media hora y la eficacia dura 6 horas. También se usa para dolor postoperatorio, dolor de trauma, dolor por cáncer, dolor repentino de enfermedad cardiaca, dolor en las articulaciones, neuralgia y dolor del parto. |
| 用法、用量<br>Administración y dosis | 成人：口服，每次量不超过 100mg，24 小时不超过 400mg，连续用药不超过 48 小时，累计用量不超过 800mg。静脉、皮下、肌内注射，每次 50～100mg，1 日不超过 400mg。<br>Adultos: por vía oral, la dosis no sobrepasa 100mg cada vez, la dosis por 24 horas no sobrepasa 400mg, la administración continua no sobrepasa 48 horas, y la dosis acumulada no sobrepasa 800mg. Inyección intravenosa, intramuscular o subcutánea, 50~100mg 1 vez, la dosis diaria no sobrepasa 400mg. |

**续 表**

| 剂型、规格<br>Formulaciones y<br>especificaciones | 注射液：每支 50mg（2ml）；100mg（2ml）。胶囊剂：每粒 50mg。栓剂：每 1ml（40 滴）含药 100mg。缓释片：每片 100mg。<br>Una cápsula：50mg. Un supositorio：cada 1ml（40 gotas）contiene 100mg del medicamento. Una tableta de liberación sostenida：100mg. |
|---|---|
| **药品名称 Drug Names** | **四氢帕马丁 Tetrahidropalmatina** |
| 适应证<br>Indicaciones | 对胃肠、肝胆系统疾病的钝痛镇痛效果好，对外伤等剧痛效果差。以用于分娩镇痛及痛经。催眠、镇静效果较好，治疗剂量无成瘾性。1 次服用 100mg，服后 20 ～ 30 分钟入睡，持续 5 ～ 6 小时，无后遗作用，故可用于暂时性失眠。<br>Tiene mejor efecto de analgesia de dolor sordo para enfermedades de sistemas gastrointestinal y hepatobiliar, menos efecto para dolor de traumas entre otros. Se usa para analgesia de dolor de parto y dismenorrea. Tiene alta eficacia para hipnosis y sedación. La dosis para el tratamiento no es adictiva. Toma 100mg cada vez y hace conciliar el sueño dentro de 20~30 minutos y la eficacia dura 5~6 horas sin efectos secundarios por lo que puede aplicarse a insomnio temporal. |
| 用法、用量<br>Administración y dosis | ①镇痛：口服，每次 100 ～ 150mg，一日 2 ～ 4 次；皮下注射，每次 60 ～ 100mg。痛经：口服每次 50mg。②催眠：口服，每次 100 ～ 200mg。<br>① Alivio de dolor: por vía oral, 100~150mg 1 vez, 2~4 veces al día; inyección subcutánea, 60~100mg 1 vez. Dismenorrea: por vía oral, 50mg 1 vez. ② Hipnosis: por vía oral, 100~200mg 1 vez. |
| 剂型、规格<br>Formulaciones y<br>especificaciones | 片剂：每片 50mg。注射液：每支 60mg（2ml）；100mg（2ml）。<br>Una tableta: 50mg. Una inyección: 60mg(2ml); 100mg(2ml). |
| **药品名称 Drug Names** | **罗通定 Rotundina** |
| 适应证<br>Indicaciones | 用于因疼痛失眠的患者。亦可用于为胃溃疡和十二指肠溃疡的疼痛、月经痛，分娩后宫缩痛、紧张性失眠、痉挛性咳嗽等。<br>Se aplica a pacientes con insomnio causaado por dolores. También se usa par dolores causados por úlcera gástrica y úlcera duodenal, dismenorrea, dolor de la contraccion uterina del parto, insomnio por tensión nerviosa y tos espasmódica, etc. |
| 用法、用量<br>Administración y dosis | 镇痛：口服，每次 60 ～ 120mg，1 日 1 ～ 4 次；肌内注射，每次 60 ～ 90mg，1 日 1 ～ 4 次。催眠：成人于睡前服 1 次 30 ～ 90mg。<br>Alivio de dolor: por vía oral, 60~120mg 1 vez, 1~4 veces al día; inyección intramuscular, 60~90mg 1 vez, 1~4veces al día. Hipnosis: adultos 30~90mg 1 vez antes de acostarse. |
| 剂型、规格<br>Formulaciones y<br>especificaciones | 片剂：每片 30mg；60mg。注射液（硫酸罗通定）：每支 60mg（2ml）。<br>Una tableta: 30mg; 60mg. Una inyección (rotundine sulfúrico): 60mg(2ml). |
| **药品名称 Drug Names** | **麦角胺 Ergotamina** |
| 适应证<br>Indicaciones | 主要用于偏头痛，可使头痛减轻，但不能预防和根治。以用于其他神经性头痛。<br>Se usa principalmente para migraña, puede aliviar el dolor de cabeza pero no puede prevenir y curar de forma radical. También se usa para otros dolores de cabeza nerviosos. |
| 用法、用量<br>Administración y dosis | ①口服：每次 1 ～ 2mg，1 日不超过 6mg，1 周不超过 10mg。效果不及皮下注射。②皮下注射：每次 0.25 ～ 0.5mg，24 小时内不超过 1mg，本品早期给药效果好，头痛发作时用药效果差。<br>① Por vía oral: 1~2mg 1 vez, no sobrepasa 6mg al día, no sobrepasa 10mg en una semana. Los efectos no son tan buenos como inyección subcutánea. ② Inyección subcutánea: 0.25~0.5mg 1 vez, no sobrepasa 1mg dentro de 24 horas, tiene buenos efectos en la administración temprana, menos efectos para ataques del dolor de cabeza. |
| 剂型、规格<br>Formulaciones y<br>especificaciones | 片剂：每片 0.5mg；1mg。注射液：每支 0.25mg（ml）；0.5mg（1ml）。<br>Una tableta: 0.5mg; 1mg. Una inyección: 0.25mg(ml); 0.5mg(1ml). |

**续　表**

| 药品名称 Drug Names | 乙酰乌头碱 Acetilaconitina |
|---|---|
| 适应证<br>Indicaciones | 用于各种中度程度疼痛、肩关节周围炎、颈椎病、肩臂痛、腰痛、关节扭伤、风湿性关节炎、类风湿关节炎、坐骨神经痛、带状疱疹、小手术术后痛。<br><br>Se usa para todos los tipos de dolores moderados, periartritis, espondilosis cervical, dolor de hombro y brazo, dolor de espalda, esguinces, artritis reumatoide, artritis reumatoide, ciática, herpes zóster, dolor postoperatorio en operación menor. |
| 用法、用量<br>Administración y dosis | 口服：每次 0.3mg，一日 1～2 次，餐后服。每次量不超过 0.3mg，每月不宜超过 2 次，服药间隔 6 小时。1 个疗程 10 日，疗程间隔 3～5 日 。肌内注射：每次 0.3mg，一日 1～2 次，注射用水稀释至 2ml 后注射。小儿或老年人每日或隔日 1 次。2 个疗程宜间隔 3～5 日。<br><br>Por vía oral: 0.3mg 1 vez, 1~2 veces al día, tras las comidas. Cada dosis no sobrepasa 0.3mg y cada mes no sobrepasa 2 veces, con intervalo de administración de 6 horas. Un ciclo de tratamiento de 10 días, con intervalo de 3~5 días. Inyección intramuscular: 0.3mg 1 vez, 1~2 veces al día, se inyecta tras diluirse en 2ml de agua. Niños o viejos 1 vez al día o 1 vez cada 2 días. El intervalo entre los 2 ciclos conviene ser 3~5 días. |
| 剂型、规格<br>Formulaciones y especificaciones | 片剂：每片 0.3mg。注射液：每支 0.3mg（1ml）。<br>Una tableta: 0.3mg. Una inyección: 0.3mg(1ml). |
| 药品名称 Drug Names | 洛美利嗪 Lomerizina |
| 适应证<br>Indicaciones | 用于偏头痛的预防性治疗。<br>Se usa para el tratamiento preventivo de migraña. |
| 用法、用量<br>Administración y dosis | 成人 1 次 5mg，一日 2 次，早餐后及晚餐后或睡眠前服用。根据症状适量增减，但 1 日剂量不超过 20mg。<br><br>Adultos 5mg 1 vez, 2 veces al día, se toma tras el almuerzo, tras la cena o antes de acostarse. Se ajusta la dosis sobre la base de los síntomas, pero la dosis diaria no sobrepasa 20mg. |
| 剂型、规格<br>Formulaciones y especificaciones | 片剂（胶囊）：每片（粒）5mg。<br>Una tableta (cápsula): 5mg. |
| 药品名称 Drug Names | 齐考诺肽 Ziconotida |
| 适应证<br>Indicaciones | 用于需要鞘内治疗且对其他镇痛治疗（如应用全身性镇痛药或鞘内注射吗啡等）不耐受或疗效差的严重慢性疼痛患者。<br><br>Se usa para necesitados de la terapia intratecal o pacientes intolerantes o de menor eficacia de otros tratamientos analgésicos(como por ejemplo la aplicación de analgésicos sistémicos o inyección de morfina intratecal, etc.) con dolores crónicos y severos. |
| 用法、用量<br>Administración y dosis | 鞘内输注给药。起始剂量不宜超过 1 日 2.4mg（或 1 小时 0.1mg）。宜缓慢增量，即每周增加剂量不超过 2～3 次，每次增量不超过 1 日 2.4mg（或 1 小时 0.1mg），直至第 21 日时达到最大推荐剂量 1 日 19.2mg（或 1 小时 0.8mg）。<br><br>Infusión intratecal. La dosis inicial no conviene sobrepasar a 2.4mg al día(o 0.1mg por h). Conviene aumentarse lentamente, es decir, dosis semanal no aumenta más de 2 a 3 veces, cada aumento no sobrepasa a 2.4mg al día(o 0.1mg por 1h), hasta el día 21 alcanza la dosis recomendada máxima de 19.2mg al día (o 0.8mg por 1h). |
| 剂型、规格<br>Formulaciones y especificaciones | 5ml：500μg（100μg/ml）；20ml：500μg（25μg/ml）。<br>5ml:500μg(100μg/ml); 20ml:500μg(25μg/ml). |
| 药品名称 Drug Names | 他喷他多 Tapentadol |
| 适应证<br>Indicaciones | 用于各种急性和慢性疼痛。<br>Se usa para todos los tipos de dolores agudos y crónicos. |

| | |
|---|---|
| 用法、用量<br>Administración y dosis | 口服，每4～6小时1次，一次1片。<br>Se toma por vía oral, 4~6 horas 1 tableta 1 vez. |
| 剂型、规格<br>Formulaciones y especificaciones | 片剂：每片50mg；75mg；100mg。<br>Una tableta: 50mg; 75mg; 100mg. |
| 药品名称 Drug Names | 阿片全碱 Papaveretum |
| 适应证<br>Indicaciones | 同吗啡。用于各种疼痛及止泻，药效持久。<br>Igual que morfina. Se usa para todos los tipos de dolores y como antidiarreico con eficacia duradera. |
| 用法、用量<br>Administración y dosis | 皮下注射，每次6～12mg。口服，每次5～15mg，一日3次。极量：1次30mg。<br>Inyección subcutánea, 6~12mg 1 vez. Por vía oral, 5~15mg 1 vez, 3 veces al día. Dosis máxima: 30mg 1 vez. |
| 剂型、规格<br>Formulaciones y especificaciones | 片剂：每片5mg。注射液：20ml（1ml）。栓剂：20mg。<br>Una tableta: 5mg. Una inyección: 20ml(1ml). Un supositorio: 20mg. |
| 药品名称 Drug Names | 荷包牡丹碱 Dicentrine |
| 适应证<br>Indicaciones | 有一定镇痛、镇静作用。用于头痛、腰痛、牙痛、小手术后痛及神经衰弱。<br>Hay cierto efecto analgésico y sedante. Se usa para dolor de cabeza, espalda, los dientes así como dolor postoperatorio en operación menor y la neurastenia. |
| 用法、用量<br>Administración y dosis | 口服：1次20～60mg。<br>Se toma por vía oral: 20~60mg 1 vez. |
| 剂型、规格<br>Formulaciones y especificaciones | 片剂：每片20mg。<br>Una tableta: 20mg. |
| 药品名称 Drug Names | 山豆碱 Total Alcali de Sophora Tonkinesis |
| 适应证<br>Indicaciones | 用于慢性气管炎、哮喘、咽喉肿痛、关节痛等。<br>Se usa para bronquitis crónica, asma, dolor de garganta y dolor en las articulaciones, etc. |
| 用法、用量<br>Administración y dosis | 肌内注射每次2ml，一日2次。<br>Inyección intramuscular 2ml 1 vez, 2 veces al día. |
| 剂型、规格<br>Formulaciones y especificaciones | 注射液：10mg（2ml）。<br>Una inyección: 10mg(2ml). |
| 药品名称 Drug Names | 匹米诺定 Piminodina |
| 适应证<br>Indicaciones | 用于术前给药，胆囊炎合并胆石、胰腺炎、癌症等引起的剧痛。<br>Se usa antes de la operación y se aplica al dolor causado por colecistitis y colelitiasis, pancreatitis, cáncer, etc. |
| 用法、用量<br>Administración y dosis | 皮下注射或肌内注射：1次10～20mg，必要时每4小时1次。口服：1次25～50mg。有成瘾性。<br>Inyección intramuscular o subcutánea: 10~20mg 1 vez, si es necesario, puede ser cada 4 horas 1 vez. Por vía oral: 25~50mg 1 vez. Tiene adicción. |
| 剂型、规格<br>Formulaciones y especificaciones | 片剂：每片25mg；注射液：10mg（1ml）。<br>Una tableta: 25mg; una inyección: 10mg(1ml). |
| 药品名称 Drug Names | 西马嗪 Simazina |
| 适应证<br>Indicaciones | 用于术后、外伤性疼痛。<br>Se usa para dolor postoperatorio y dolor traumático. |

**续　表**

| | |
|---|---|
| 用法、用量<br>Administración y dosis | 口服：每次 0.4 ～ 0.8g。小儿酌减。<br>Se toma por vía oral: 0.4~0.8g 1 vez. Para niños la dosis se reduce correspondientemente. |
| 剂型、规格<br>Formulaciones y especificaciones | 片剂：每片 0.4g。<br>Una tableta: 0.4g. |
| **药品名称 Drug Names** | **千金藤啶碱 Estefolidina** |
| 适应证<br>Indicaciones | 用于血管性头痛、偏头痛、多动性运动障碍、儿童多动秽语综合征。<br>Se usa para cefalea vascular, migraña, discinesia hiperactividad, síndrome de hiperactividad infantil de tourette. |
| 用法、用量<br>Administración y dosis | 预防血管性头痛：1 次 25 ～ 75mg，一日 3 次，餐后服。治疗急性发作：1 次 15 ～ 100mg，顿服。治疗多动性运动障碍：25 ～ 100mg，一日 3 次，餐后服。儿童用量按成人量的 1/3 ～ 1/2 计量。<br>Para prevenir cefalea vascular: 25~75mg 1 vez, 3 veces al día, tras las comidas. Para tratar ataques agudos: 15~100mg 1 vez, dosis única. Para tratar discinesia hiperactividad: 25~100mg, 3 veces al día, tras las comidas. La dosis de niños se calcula en 1/3~1/2 la dosis de adultos. |
| 剂型、规格<br>Formulaciones y especificaciones | 片剂：每片 25mg。<br>Una tableta: 25mg. |
| **药品名称 Drug Names** | **高乌甲素 Lappaconitina** |
| 适应证<br>Indicaciones | 用于中度以上疼痛、术后疼痛、坐骨神经痛。<br>Se usa para dolores de intensidades mayores de moderadas, dolor postoperatorio y ciática. |
| 用法、用量<br>Administración y dosis | 口服：每次 5 ～ 10mg，一日 1 ～ 3 次。肌内注射或静脉滴注，每次 4mg，一日 1 ～ 2 次。<br>Se toma por vía oral: 5~10mg 1 vez, 1~3 veces al día. Inyección intramuscular o infusión intravenosa, 4mg 1 vez, 1~2 veces al día. |
| 剂型、规格<br>Formulaciones y especificaciones | 片剂：每片 5mg。注射液：4mg（2ml）。<br>Una tableta: 5mg. Una inyección: 4mg(2ml). |
| **药品名称 Drug Names** | **美西麦角 Metisergida** |
| 适应证<br>Indicaciones | 用于预防反复发作的偏头痛。对急性头痛发作无效。<br>Se usa para prevenir migraña recurrente. No tiene validez para ataques de migrañas agudos. |
| 用法、用量<br>Administración y dosis | 起始剂量 1 ～ 2mg，一日 2 次；每 3 ～ 4 周增加 1 ～ 2mg；疗程不宜超过 6 个月。宜间断用药，每半年停药 3 周以上。<br>Dosis inicial 1~2mg, 2 veces al día; cada 3~4 semanas se incrementa 1~2mg; el ciclo de tratamiento no debe sobrepasar 6 meses. Conviene administrarse de forma intermitente, más de 3 semanas de interrupción cada medio año. |
| 剂型、规格<br>Formulaciones y especificaciones | 片剂：每片 1mg。<br>Una tableta: 1mg. |
| **药品名称 Drug Names** | **氨酚氢可酮 Paracetamol y hidrocodona bitartrato** |
| 适应证<br>Indicaciones | 本品用于缓解中度到中重度头痛。<br>Se usa para aliviar dolores de cabeza moderado a severo. |
| 用法、用量<br>Administración y dosis | 每 4 ～ 6 小时 1 ～ 2 片，24 小时的总用药量不应超过 5 片。<br>1~2 tabletas cada 4~6 horas, la dosis total dentro de 24 horas no debe sobrepasar 5 tabletas. |
| 剂型、规格<br>Formulaciones y especificaciones | 片剂：每片含重酒石酸氢可酮 5mg、对乙酰氨基酚 500mg。<br>Una tableta: contiene 5mg de bitartrato de hidrocodona y 500mg de acetaminofeno. |

**续 表**

| 8.3 解热镇痛抗炎药 No esteroides antiinflamatorios | |
|---|---|
| 药品名称 Drug Names | 阿司匹林 Aspirina |

| 适应证<br>Indicaciones | ①用于发热、头痛、神经痛、肌肉痛、风湿热、急性风湿性关节炎及类风湿关节炎等，为风湿热，风湿性关节炎及类风湿关节炎首选药，可迅速缓解急性风湿性关节炎的症状。对急性风湿热伴有心肌炎者，可合用皮质激素。②用于痛风。③预防心肌梗死、动脉血栓、动脉粥样硬化等。④用于治疗胆道蛔虫病（有效率90%以上）。⑤粉剂外用可治足癣。⑥儿科用于皮肤黏膜淋巴结综合征（川崎病）的治疗。<br><br>① Se usa para fiebre, dolor de cabeza, neuralgia, dolor muscular, fiebre reumática, la artritis aguda y la artritis reumatoide, etc. Es la primera opción para la fiebre reumática, la artritis y la artritis reumatoide y puede aliviar los síntomas de la artritis reumatoide aguda rápidamente. Puede combinar con los corticosteroides para tratar pacientes de fiebre reumática con miocarditis. ② Se usa para gota. ③ Se usa para prevenir infarto de miocardio, rombosis arterial, aterosclerosis, etc. ④ Se usa para tratar ascariasis biliar (eficiencia de más del 90%). ⑤ Polvo tópico puede curar la tiña del pie. ⑥ En pediatría, se usa para tratar síndrome del nódulo linfático mucocutáneo (enfermedad de Kawasaki). |
|---|---|
| 用法、用量<br>Administración y dosis | （1）解热阵痛：①口服，每次0.3～0.6g，一日3次，或需要时服用。②直肠给药：1次0.3～0.6g，一日0.9～1.8g；儿童1～3岁，1次0.1g，一日1次；3～6岁，1次0.1～0.15g，一日1～2次；6岁以上，1次0.15～0.3g，一日2次。<br><br>（2）抗风湿：1次0.6～1g，一日3～4g。服时宜嚼碎，并可与碳酸钙或氢氧化铝或复方氢氧化铝（胃舒平）合用以减少对胃刺激。一疗程3个月左右。小儿1日0.1g/kg，分3次服，前3日先服半量以减少不良反应。<br><br>（3）抑制血小板聚集：预防心肌梗死、动脉血栓、动脉粥样硬化，一日1次，每次75～150mg。<br><br>（4）治疗胆道蛔虫病：每次1g，一日2～3次，连用2～3日。当阵发性绞痛停止24小时后即停药，然后再行常规驱虫。<br><br>（5）治疗X射线照射或放疗引起的腹泻：每次服0.6～0.9g，一日4次。<br><br>（6）预防旁路移植术后再狭窄：每次服50mg。<br><br>（7）治疗足癣：先用温开水或1∶5000的高锰酸钾溶液洗涤患处，然后用本品粉末撒布患处，一般2～4次可愈。<br><br>（8）用于小儿皮肤黏淋巴结综合征：开始每日按80～100mg/kg，分3～4次服，热退2～3日后改为每日30mg/kg，每3～4次服，连服2个月或更久。血小板增多、血液呈高凝状态期间，每日5～10mg/kg，1次顿服。<br><br>(1)Efecto analgésico y antipirético: ① por vía oral, 0.3~0.6g cada vez, 3 veces al día, o se toma en casos necesarios. ② por vía rectal: 0.3~0.6g cada vez, 0.9~1.8g al día; niños de 1~3 años de edad, 0.1g 1 vez al día, de 3~6 años de edad, 0.1~0.15g 1 vez, 1~2 veces al día; mayores a 6 años de edad, 0.15~0.3g 1 vez, 2 veces al día.<br><br>(2)Efecto antirreumático: 0.6~1g 1 vez, 3~4g al día. Cuando se toma deben masticarlo y combinarlo con carbonato de calcio o hidróxido de aluminio o compuesto de hidróxido de aluminio (Weishuping) para reducir la irritación estomacal. Un ciclo de tratamiento dura aproximadamente 3 meses. Niños 0.1g/kg al día, en 3 veces, se toma la mitad de la dosis en los primeros 3 días para reducir reacciones adversas.<br><br>(3)Para inhibir la agregación plaquetaria: como prevención de infarto de miocardio, trombosis arterial y aterosclerosis, 1 vez al día, 75~150mg 1 vez.<br><br>(4)Para tratar ascariasis biliar: 1g 1 vez, 2~3 veces al día, 2~3 días consecutivos. Se interrumpe la adminsitración 24 horas después de detener calambres paroxísticos, y luego se efectúa la desparasitación de rutina.<br><br>(5)Para tratar diarrea a causa de irradiación con rayos X o inducida por radioterapia: 0.6~0.9g 1 vez, 4 veces al día.<br><br>(6)Para prevenir la restenosis después de la derivación: 50mg 1 vez.<br><br>(7)Para tratar pedis: primero lavar la área afectada con agua caliente o solución de permanganato de potasio con relación de 1∶5000, a continuación, se extiende el polvo del producto en este área afectada, generalmente de 2 a 4 veces puede curarse.<br><br>(8)Para tratar síndrome del nódulo linfático mucocutáneo: a principio 80~100mg/kg al día, en 3~4 veces, 2~3 días después de bajar la fiebre se convierte en 30mg/kg al día, en 3~4 veces, 2 meses consecutivos o más tiempo. Cuando se aumentan las plaquetas y la sangre presenta el estado de hipercoagulabilidad, 5~10mg/kg al día, dosis única. |

**续　表**

| | |
|---|---|
| 剂型、规格<br>Formulaciones y especificaciones | 片剂：每片 0.05g；0.1g；0.2g；0.3g；0.5g。泡腾片：每片 0.3g；0.5g。放于温水 150～250ml 中，溶化后饮下。肠溶片（胶囊）：每片（粒）40mg；0.15g；0.3g；0.5g。对胃刺激小，适于长期大量服用。散剂：每袋 0.1g；0.5g。栓剂：每粒 0.1g；0.3g；0.45g；0.5g。<br><br>Una tableta: 0.05g; 0.1g; 0.2g; 0.3g; 0.5g. Efervescente: 0.3g; 0,5g. Se disuelve en 150~250ml de agua caliente. Tableta con recubrimiento entérico(cápsula): 40mg; 0.15g; 0.3g; 0.5g. Tiene menos irritación al estómago y adecuada para dosis a largo plazo. Polvo: 0.1g; 0.5g cada saco. Un supositorio: 0.1g; 0.3g; 0.45g; 0.5g. |
| 药品名称 Drug Names | 阿司匹林精氨酸盐 Aspirina arginina |
| 适应证<br>Indicaciones | 主要用于发热、头痛、神经痛、牙痛、肌肉痛及活动性风湿病、类风湿关节炎、创伤及术后疼痛。<br><br>Se usa para fiebre, dolor de cabeza, neuralgia, dolor de dientes, dolor muscular, reumatismo activo, artritis reumatoide, dolor traumático y dolor postoperario. |
| 用法、用量<br>Administración y dosis | 肌内注射：成人每次 1g，一日 1～2 次，或依病情按医嘱用药；儿童 10～25mg/kg。临时用，每瓶内加入 0.9% 氯化钠生理盐水或加入灭菌注射用水 2～4ml，溶解后注入。<br><br>Inyección intramuscular: adultos 1g 1 vez, 1~2 veces al día, o se administra de acuerdo a los síntomas y la instrucción del médico; niños 10~25mg/kg. Para uso temporal, se disuelve en 0,9% de NaCl solución salina o 2~4ml de agua estéril para la inyección antes de la inyección. |
| 剂型、规格<br>Formulaciones y especificaciones | 注射用阿司匹林精氨酸盐：每瓶 0.5g（相当阿司匹林 0.25g）；1g（相当于阿司匹林 0.5g）。<br><br>Aspirina-arginina para inyección: 0.5g cada botella(equivalente a 0.25g de aspirina); 1g(equivalente a 0.5g de aspirina). |
| 药品名称 Drug Names | 阿司匹林赖氨酸盐 Aspirina-DL-lisina |
| 适应证<br>Indicaciones | 主要用于发热及轻、中度的疼痛，如上呼吸道感染引起的发热、手术后痛、癌性疼痛、风湿痛、关节痛及神经痛等。<br><br>Se usa principalmente para fiebre y dolores leves y moderados, taoes como fiebre causada por infección del tracto respiratiorio superior, dolor postoperario, dolor por cáncer, dolor reumático, dolor de articulaciones y neuralgia, etc. |
| 用法、用量<br>Administración y dosis | 肌内注射或静脉滴注：每次 0.9～1.8g，一日 2 次；儿童 1 日 10～25mg/kg。以 0.9% 氯化钠注射液溶解后静脉滴注。<br><br>Inyección intramuscular o infusión intravenosa: 0.9~1.8g cada vez, 2 veces al día; niños 10~25mg/kg al día. Se diluye en 0.9% inyección de cloruro de sodio antes de la infusión intravenosa. |
| 剂型、规格<br>Formulaciones y especificaciones | 注射用阿司匹林赖氨酸盐：每瓶 0.9g（相当于阿司匹林 0.5g）；0.5g（相当于阿司匹林 0.28g）。<br><br>Aspirina-DL-lisina para inyección: 0.9g cada botella(equivalente a 0.5g de aspirina); 0.5g(equivalente a 0.28g de aspirina). |
| 药品名称 Drug Names | 美沙拉秦 Mesalazina |
| 适应证<br>Indicaciones | 适用于溃疡性结肠炎和克罗恩病。<br>Se usa para úlcera colitis y enfermedad de Crohn. |
| 用法、用量<br>Administración y dosis | 口服：可用一杯水漱服或在就餐时吞服。溃疡性结肠炎：急性期，每次 1～2 袋，一日 3～4 次（4g/d，8 袋）；缓解期，每次 1 袋，一日 3～4 次（2g/d，4 袋）。克罗恩病：缓解期，每次 1 袋，一日 3～4 次（2g/d，4 袋）。<br><br>Por vía oral: se toma con un vaso de agua o se traga al comer. Úlcera colitis: etapa aguda, 1~2 sacos cada vez, 3~4 veces al día(4g/d,8 sacos); período de remisión, 1 saco 1 vez, 3~4 veces al día(2g/d,4 sacos). Enfermedad de Crohn: período de remisión, 1 saco 1 vez, 3~4 veces al día(2g/d,4 sacos). |
| 剂型、规格<br>Formulaciones y especificaciones | 缓释颗粒剂：每袋 500mg。<br>Gránulos de liberación sostenida: 500mg cada saco. |

**续　表**

| 药品名称 Drug Names | 对乙酰氨基酚 Paracetamol |
|---|---|
| 适应证<br>Indicaciones | 用于感冒发热、关节痛、神经痛及偏头痛、癌性痛及手术后镇痛。本品还可用于对阿司匹林过敏、不耐受或不适于应用阿司匹林的患者（水痘、血友病以及其他出血性疾病等）。<br><br>Se usa para fiebre, dolor de las articulaciones, la neuralgia, la jaqueca, el dolor por cáncer y dolor post-operatorio. Éste también se puede usar para pacientes con alergia a la aspirina, intolerantes o del inadecuado uso de la aspirina.(varicela, hemofilia y otros trastornos hemorrágicos). |
| 用法、用量<br>Administración y dosis | 口服：1 次 0.3～0.6g，1 日 0.6～1.8g，一日量不宜超过 2g，一个疗程不宜超过 10 日；儿童 12 岁以下按每日 1.5g/㎡分次服（如按年龄计：2～3 岁，一次 160mg；4～5 岁，一次 240mg；6～8 岁，一次 320mg；9～10 岁，一次 400mg；11 岁，一次 480mg。每 4 小时或必要时服一次）。肌内注射：1 次 0.15～0.25g。直肠给药：1 次 0.3～0.6g，1 日 1～2 次。3～12 岁小儿，一次 0.15～0.3g，1 日 1 次。<br><br>Se toma por vía oral: 0.3~0.6g 1 vez, 0.6~1.8g al día, la dosis diaria no debe sobrepasar 2g, un ciclo de tratamiento no debe sobrepasar 10 días; niños menores a 12 años de edad, 1.5g/㎡ al día, en varias veces(si se calcula según la edad: de 2~3 años, 160mg 1 vez; de 4~5 años, 240mg 1 vez; de 6~8 años, 320mg 1 vez; de 9~10 años, 400mg 1 vez; de 11 años, 480mg 1 vez. Se toma cada 4 horas o en casos necesarios). Inyección intramuscular: 0.15~0.25g 1 vez. Por vía rectal: 0.3~0.6g 1 vez, 1~2 veces al día. Niños de 3~12 años, 0.15~0.3g 1 vez al día. |
| 剂型、规格<br>Formulaciones y especificaciones | 片剂：每片 0.3g；0.5g。胶囊剂：每粒 0.3g。咀嚼片：每片 80mg。泡腾冲剂：每袋 0.1g；0.5g。口服液：每支 0.25g（10ml）。栓剂：每粒 0.15g；0.3g；0.6g。注射液：每支 0.075g（1ml）；0.25g（2ml）。凝胶剂：每支 120mg（5g）。<br><br>Una tableta：0.3g；0.5g. Una cápsula：0.3g. Una tableta masticable：80mg. Gránulos efervescentes：0.1g；0.5g cada saco. Líquido por vía oral：0.25g（10ml）. Un supositorio：0.15g；0.3g；0.6g. Una inyección：.075g（1ml）；0.25g（2ml）. Un gel：120mg（5g）. |
| 药品名称 Drug Names | 吲哚美辛 Indometacina |
| 适应证<br>Indicaciones | ①急、慢性风湿性关节炎、痛风性关节炎及癌性疼痛。也可用于滑囊炎、腱鞘炎及关节囊炎等。还用于恶性肿瘤引起的发热或其他难以控制的发热。因本品不良反应较大，不宜作为治疗关节炎的首选药物，仅用于其他 NSAIDs 治疗无效的或不能耐受的患者。②抗血小板聚集，可防止血栓形成，但疗效不如阿司匹林。③治疗 Behcet 综合征，退热效果好；用于 Batter 综合征，效果尤其显著。④用于胆绞痛、输尿管结石症引起的绞痛；对偏头痛也有一定的疗效，也可用于月经痛。⑤本药滴眼液用于眼科手术及非手术因素引起的非感染性炎症。<br><br>① Se usa para artritis reumatoide aguda y crónica, la artritis gotosa y dolor por cáncer. También se puede utilizar para la bursitis, tenosinovitis y capsulitis, etc. También se aplica al calor causado por tumores malignos u otro calor no controlado. Debido a las reacciones adversas no conviene ser la primera opción para el tratamiento de la artritis, y sólo se aplica a los pacientes o intolerantes con NSAIDs sin otra terapia eficaz. ② Se usa en contra de agregación plaquetaria y para prevenir la trombosis, pero los efectos no son tan buenos como la aspirina. ③ Para el tratamiento del síndrome de Behcet, tine un buen efecto de enfriamiento; para el síndrome de bateador, el efecto es particularmente significativo. ④ Se usa para el cólico biliar, el cólico causado por litiasis ureteral;tiene cierto efecto para migraña y también se puede utilizar para el dolor menstrual. ⑤ Gotas para los ojos de este medicamento se usa para la cirugía ocular e inflamación no infecciosa causadas por factores no quirúrgicos. |
| 用法、用量<br>Administración y dosis | 口服。开始时每次服 25mg，1 日 2～3 次，饭时或饭后立即服用（可减少胃肠道不良反应）。治疗风湿性关节炎等症时，如未见不良反应，可逐渐增至 100～150mg，1 日最大量不超过 150mg，分 3～4 次服用，现已采用胶丸或栓剂剂型，使胃肠道不良反应发生率降低，栓剂且有维持药效较长的特点。直肠给药，1 次 50mg，1 日 50～100mg，一般连用 10 日为一个疗程。控释胶囊：一日 1 次，每次 75mg，或 1 次 25mg，一日 2 次。必要时 1 次 75mg，一日 2 次。小儿口服常用量：每日按 1.5～2.5mg/kg，分 3～4 次，有效后减至最低量。乳膏剂涂擦按摩患处，一日 2～3 次。经眼给药：眼科手术前：1 次 1 滴，术前 3、2、1 和 0.5 小时各滴一次。眼科手术后：1 次 1 滴，一日 1～4 次。其他非感染性炎症：1 次 1 滴，一日 4～6 次。 |

续　表

Se toma por vía oral. Al principio se toma 25mg cada vez, 2~3 veces al día, durante o de inmediato después de las comidas (puede reducir las reacciones adversas gastrointestinales). En el tratamiento de artritis reumatoide, etc. si no aparecen reacciones adversas, se puede incrementar la dosis a 100~150mg, la dosis diaria máxima no sobrepasa 150mg, en 3~4 veces, ahora se adopta forma farmacéutica como cápsula o supositorio para reducir las reacciones adversas gastrointestinales, y supositorios pueden obtener efectos duraderos. Por vía rectal, 50mg 1 vez, 50~100mg al día, generalmente un ciclo de 10 días. Cápsulas de liberación controlada: 1 vez al día, 75mg cada vez, o 25mg cada vez, 2 veces al día. En casos necesarios, 75mg 1 vez, 2 veces al día. La dosis habitual para niños por vía oral: 1.5~2.5mg/kg al día, en 3~4 veces, reducida a la dosis mínima si es eficaz. Cremas de masaje frota la zona afectada, 2~3 veces al día. Se administra por los ojos: antes de la cirugía ocular: 1 gota 1 vez, 3h,2h,1h y 0.5h antes de la cirugía respectivamente. Tras a cirugía ocular: 1 gota 1 vez, 1~4 veces al día. Inflamación no infecciosa: 1 gota 1 vez, 4~6 veces al día.

| 剂型、规格<br>Formulaciones y especificaciones | 肠溶片：每片 25mg。胶囊：25mg。胶丸：每丸 25mg。控释胶囊每粒 25mg；75mg。控释片：每片 25mg；50mg；75mg。贴片：每片 12.5mg。栓剂：每粒 25mg；50mg；100mg。乳膏剂：每支 100mg（10g）。滴眼液：8ml：40mg。<br><br>Una tableta con recubrimiento entérico: 25mg. Una cápsula: 25mg. Una píldora: 25mg. Una cápsula de liberación sostenida: 25mg; 75mg. Una parche: 12.5mg. Un supositorio: 25mg; 50mg; 100mg. Gotas para los ojos: 8ml：40mg. |
|---|---|
| **药品名称 Drug Names** | 双氯芬酸 Diclofenaco |
| 适应证<br>Indicaciones | 用于类风湿关节炎、神经炎、红斑狼疮及癌症、手术后疼痛，各种原因引起的发热。<br><br>Se usa para artritis reumatoide, neuritis, lupus y dolor por cáncer, dolor post-operatorio, y fiebre causada por una variedad de razones. |
| 用法、用量<br>Administración y dosis | 口服：成人，每日剂量为 100～150mg，分 2～3 次服用。对轻度患者及 14 岁以上的青少年酌减。此药最好在餐前用水整片送下。肌内注射深部注射，1 次 50mg，一日 1 次，必要时数小时在注射 1 次。外用：擦剂，根据疼痛部位大小，1～3ml 均匀涂于患处，一日 2～4 次，一日总量不超过 15ml。乳膏，根据疼痛部位大小，1 次 2～4g 涂于患处，并轻轻按摩，一日 3～4 次，一日总量不超过 30g。<br><br>Se toma por vía oral: adultos, dosis diaria de 100~150mg, en 2~3 veces. Para pacientes con síntomas leves y adolescentes mayores a 14 años de edad, la dosis se reduce correspondientemente. El fármaco se traga mejor antes de la comida con agua. Inyección intramuscular profunda, 50mg 1 vez al día, si es necesario se repite la inyección dentro de varias horas. Tópica: linimento, de acuerdo con el tamaño de la zona dolorosa, se aplica 2~4g cada vez de manera uniforme a la zona afectada 3~4 veces al día no exceda la cantidad total de 30g. |
| 剂型、规格<br>Formulaciones y especificaciones | 片剂：每片 25mg。擦剂：20ml：200mg。乳膏：25g：750mg。注射液：50mg（2ml）。<br>Una tableta: 25mg. Linimento: 20ml：200mg. Crema: 25g：750mg. Una inyección: 50mg(2ml). |
| **药品名称 Drug Names** | 萘普生 Naproxeno |
| 适应证<br>Indicaciones | 用于类风湿关节炎、骨关节炎、强直性脊柱炎、痛风、运动系统（如关节、肌肉及肌腱）的慢性变性疾病及轻、中度疼痛如痛经等。<br><br>Se usa para artritis reumatoide, osteoartritis, espondilitis anquilosante, gota, enfermedad crónica y degenerativa del sistema de movimiento (tales como las articulaciones, músculos y tendones), dolor leve y dolor moderado, tales como dismenorrea. |
| 用法、用量<br>Administración y dosis | 口服，开始每日剂量 0.5～0.75g，维持量每日 0.375～0.75g，分早晨和傍晚 2 次服用。轻、中度疼痛或痛经时，开始用 0.5g，必需时 6～8 小时在服 0.25g，日剂量不超过 1.25g。肌内注射，一次 100～200mg，一日一次。栓剂直肠给药，一次 0.25g，一日 0.5g。<br><br>Se toma por vía oral, al principio la dosis diaria de 0.5~0.75g, dosis de mantenimiento 0.375~0.75g al día, por la mañana y por la noche. Dolor leve, moderado o dismenorrea, al principio se usa 0.5g, si es necesario tras 6~8 horas se toma 0.25g, la dosis diaria no sobrepasa 1.25g. Inyección intramuscular, 100~200mg 1 vez al día. Los supositorios rectales, 0.25g 1 vez, 0.5g al día. |

**续 表**

| 剂型、规格<br>Formulaciones y especificaciones | 片（胶囊）剂：每片（粒）0.1g；0.125g；0.25g。缓释胶囊（片）：每粒（片）0.25g。注射液：每支 100mg（2ml）；200mg（2ml）。栓剂：每粒 0.25g。<br><br>Una tableta (cápsula): 0.1g; 0.125g; 0.25g. Una tableta de liberación sostenida: 0.25g. Una inyección: 100mg(2ml); 200mg(2ml). Un supositorio: 0.25g. |
|---|---|
| **药品名称 Drug Names** | 布洛芬 Ibuprofeno |
| 适应证<br>Indicaciones | 用于风湿性及类风湿关节炎及抗炎、镇痛、解热作用与阿司匹林、保泰松相似，比对乙酰氨基酚好。在患者不能耐受阿司匹林、保泰松等时，可试用。<br><br>Se usa para reumatismo y artritis reumatoide, y su efecto anti-inflamatorio, analgésico y antipirético es similar a la aspirina y fenilbutazona, mejor que acetaminofeno. Se puede probar en pacientes intolerantes a aspirina y fenilbutazona. |
| 用法、用量<br>Administración y dosis | 抗风湿，一次 0.4～0.8g，一日 3～4 次。镇痛，一次 0.2～0.4g，每 4～6 小时 1 次。成人最大限量每日 2.4g。<br><br>Contra reumatismo, 0.4~0.8g 1 vez, 3~4 veces al día. Aliviar el dolor, 0.2~0.4g 1 vez, cada 4~6 horas. La dosis máxima para adultos es de 2.4g al día. |
| 剂型、规格<br>Formulaciones y especificaciones | 片剂（胶囊）：每片（粒）0.1g；0.2g；0.3g。缓释胶囊：每粒 0.3g。颗粒剂：每袋 0.1g；0.2g。干混悬剂：每瓶 1.2g（34g）。糖浆剂：每支 0.2g（10ml）。口服液：每支 0.1g（10ml）。混悬剂：每瓶 2.0g（100ml）。擦剂：每瓶 2.5g（50ml）。栓剂：每粒 50mg；100mg。<br><br>Una tableta (cápsula): 0.1g; 0.2g; 0.3g. Una cápsula de liberación sostenida: 0.3g. Un supositorio: 0.1g; 0.2g cada saco. Una suspensión seca: 1.2g(34g)cada botella. Un jarabe: 0.2g(10ml). Líquido por vía oral: 0.1g(10ml). Una suspensión: 2.0g(100ml)cada botella. Un linimento: 2.5g(50ml)cada botella. Un supositorio: 50mg; 100mg. |
| **药品名称 Drug Names** | 酮洛芬 Ketoprofeno |
| 适应证<br>Indicaciones | 用于类风湿关节炎、风湿性关节炎、骨关节炎、强直性脊柱炎及痛风等。本品治疗关节炎时，连续用药 2～3 周可达最佳疗效。<br><br>Se usa para artritis reumatoide, reumatoide, osteoartritis, espondilitis y gota, etc. Cuando este medicamento trata artritis, puede obtener la mejor eficiencia tras tratamiento de 2~3 semanas consecutivas. |
| 用法、用量<br>Administración y dosis | 口服：每次 50mg，一日 150mg，分 3～4 次；每日最大用量 200mg，或每次 100mg，一日 2 次，为避免对胃肠道刺激，应餐后服用，整个胶囊吞服。<br><br>Se toma por vía oral: 50mg 1 vez, 150mg al día, en 3~4 veces; la dosis máxima al día es de 200mg, o 100mg 1 vez, 2 veces al día, para evitar la irritación gastrointestinal, se debe tomar después de una comida, y tragar cápsulas enteras. |
| 剂型、规格<br>Formulaciones y especificaciones | 肠溶胶囊：每粒 20mg；50mg。控释胶囊：每粒 20mg。缓释片：每片 75mg。搽剂：每支 0.3g（10ml）；0.9g（30ml）；1.5g（50ml）。<br><br>Una cápsula con recubrimiento entérico: 20mg; 50mg. Una cápsula de liberación sostenida: 20mg. Una tableta de liberación sostenida: 75mg. Un linimento: 0.3g(10ml); 0.9g(30ml); 1.5g(50ml). |
| **药品名称 Drug Names** | 芬布芬 Fenbuféno |
| 适应证<br>Indicaciones | 用于类风湿关节炎、风湿性关节炎、骨关节炎、强直性脊柱炎及痛风等。应用于牙痛、手术后疼痛、外伤疼痛等的镇痛。<br><br>Se usa para artritis reumatoide, reumatoide, osteoartritis, espondilitis y gota, etc. Se aplica a detener el dolor dental, dolor postoperario y dolor traumático, etc. |
| 用法、用量<br>Administración y dosis | 口服，成人一次 0.6～0.9g，一次或分次服用。多数患者晚上口服 0.6g 即可。分次服用时，每日总量不得超过 0.9g。<br><br>Se toma por vía oral, adultos 0.6~0.9g 1 vez, en 1 o varias veces. La mayoría de los pacientes toman por vía oral 0.6g por la noche. Si se toma en varias veces, la dosis total al día no sobrepasa 0.9g. |
| 剂型、规格<br>Formulaciones y especificaciones | 片剂：每片 0.15g；0.3g。胶囊剂：每粒 0.5g。<br><br>Una tableta: 0.15g; 0.3g. Una cápsula: 0.5g. |

**续　表**

| 药品名称 Drug Names | 吡洛芬 Pirprofeno |
| --- | --- |
| 适应证<br>Indicaciones | 用于风湿性关节炎、骨关节炎、强直性脊柱炎、非关节型风湿病、急性疼痛、术后痛及癌性痛等。<br><br>Se usa para reumatoide, osteoartritis, espondilitis, Reumatismo no articular, dolor agudo, dolor postoperatorio y dolor del cáncer, etc. |
| 用法、用量<br>Administración y dosis | 开始口服，每日 800mg，一次 2 次分服。症状改善后，每日 600mg 维持。类风湿关节炎、强直性脊柱炎开始 1000mg/d，分 3 次服，持续 1～2 周。镇痛：每次 200～400mg，一日 1200mg。肌内注射每次 400mg。数小时后可重复使用。<br><br>Se toma por vía oral, 800mg al día, dividida en 1 o 2 veces. Cuando los síntomas se mejoren, se toma 600mg al día como dosis de mantenimiento. Para reumatoide y espondilitis, al principio, 1000mg/d, en 3 veces, durante 1~2 semanas. Alivio de dolor: 200~400mg cada vez, 1200mg al día. Inyección intramuscular 400mg cada vez. Se puede repetirla dentro de varias horas. |
| 剂型、规格<br>Formulaciones y especificaciones | 片剂：每片 200mg。<br>Una tableta: 200mg. |

| 药品名称 Drug Names | 阿明洛芬 Alminoprofeno |
| --- | --- |
| 适应证<br>Indicaciones | 用于风湿性和类风湿关节炎、神经根痛、肌腱炎、创伤（骨折、挫伤、扭伤）、痛经、产后子宫绞痛、牙痛、中耳炎等。<br><br>Se usa para reumatismo y artritis reumatoide, dolor radicular, tendinitis, traumatismos (fractura, esguince, contusión), dismenorrea, uterinas posparto cólicos, dolor de muelas, otitis media, etc. |
| 用法、用量<br>Administración y dosis | 口服，成人每次 300mg，一日 2～3 次，可根据疗效酌情减量。治疗子宫绞痛时，一日 300～600mg 分 2 次餐前服。<br><br>Se toma por vía oral, adultos 300mg 1 vez, 2~3 veces al día, la dosis se puede reducir según los efectos. Al tratar uterinas posparto cólicos, 300~600mg al día, en 2 veces antes de la comida. |
| 剂型、规格<br>Formulaciones y especificaciones | 片剂：每片 150mg；300mg。<br>Una tableta: 150mg; 300mg. |

| 药品名称 Drug Names | 洛索洛芬 Loxoprofeno |
| --- | --- |
| 适应证<br>Indicaciones | 用于类风湿关节炎、变形性关节炎、腰痛、关节周围炎、颈肩腕综合征，以及手术后、外伤后和拔牙后的镇痛抗炎，急性上呼吸道炎症和解热镇痛。<br><br>Se usa para artritis reumatoide, osteoartritis, dolor de espalda, inflamación alrededor del síndrome de las articulaciones, el cuello y la muñeca, así como analgésico postoperatorio y anti-inflamatoria después de la extracción del diente después de un traumatismo, inflamación de las vías respiratorias y dolores agudos antipiréticas. |
| 用法、用量<br>Administración y dosis | 餐后服用。慢性炎症疼痛：成人一次 60mg，一日 3 次。急性炎症疼痛：顿服 60～120mg。可根据年龄、症状适当增减，一次最大剂量不超过 180mg。<br><br>Se toma después de la comida. Dolor inflamatorio crónico: adultos 60mg 1 vez, 3 veces al día. Dolor inflamatorio agudo: dosis única 60~120mg. La dosis se puede aumentar o reducir según la edad o síntomas, la dosis máxima no sobrepasa 180mg. |
| 剂型、规格<br>Formulaciones y especificaciones | 片剂：每片 60mg。胶囊：每粒 60mg。颗粒剂：2g ：60mg。<br>Una tableta: 60mg. Una cápsula: 60mg. Un gránulado: 2g ：60mg. |

| 药品名称 Drug Names | 吡罗昔康 Piroxicam |
| --- | --- |
| 适应证<br>Indicaciones | 用于治疗风湿性及类风湿关节炎。<br>Se usa para reumatismo y artritis reumatoide. |
| 用法、用量<br>Administración y dosis | 口服：抗风湿，一日 20mg，一日 1 次；抗痛风，一日 40mg，一日 1 次，连续 4～6 日。肌内注射：一次 10～20mg，一日 1 次。<br><br>Se toma por vía oral: antirreumático, 20mg al día, 1 vez al día; anti-gota, 40mg al día, 1 vez al día, 4~6 días consecutivos. Inyección intramuscular: 10~20mg 1 vez, 1 vez al día. |

**续 表**

| 剂型、规格<br>Formulaciones y<br>especificaciones | 片（胶囊）剂：每片（粒）10mg；20mg。注射液：每支 10mg（1ml）；20mg（2ml）。凝胶剂：<br>每支 50mg（10g）；60mg（12g）。搽剂：每支 0.5g（50ml）。软膏：每支 0.1g（10g）。<br>Una tableta: 10mg; 20mg. Una inyección: 10mg(1ml); 20mg(2ml). Un gel: 50mg(10g); 60mg(12g).<br>Un linimento: 0.5g(50ml). Una pomada: 0.1g(10g). |
| --- | --- |
| **药品名称 Drug Names** | 美洛昔康 Meloxicam |
| 适应证<br>Indicaciones | 用于类风湿关节炎和骨关节炎的对症治疗。<br>Se usa para el tratamiento sintomático de la artritis reumatoide y la osteoartritis. |
| 用法、用量<br>Administración y dosis | 类风湿性骨关节炎：成人一日 15mg，一日 1 次，根据治疗后反应，剂量可减至 7.5mg/d。骨<br>关节炎：7.5mg/d，如果需要，剂量可增至 15mg/d。严重肾衰竭者，剂量不应超过 7.5mg/d。<br>Para artritis reumatoide: adultos 15mg al día, 1 vez al día, según las reacciones tras el tratamiento, la<br>dosis puede reducirse a 7.5mg/d. Para osteoartritis: 7.5mg/d, si es necesario, la dosis se puede aumentar<br>a 15mg/d. Para los pacientes con insuficiencia renal, la dosis no debe sobrepasar 7.5mg/d. |
| 剂型、规格<br>Formulaciones y<br>especificaciones | 片剂：每片 7.5mg；15mg。<br>Una tableta: 7.5mg; 15mg. |
| **药品名称 Drug Names** | 氯诺昔康 Lorenxicam |
| 适应证<br>Indicaciones | 用于妇产科矫形手术后的急性疼痛，急性坐骨神经痛及腰痛。亦可用于慢性腰痛、关节炎、<br>类风湿关节炎和强直性脊柱炎。<br>Se usa para alivio del dolor agudo después de cirugía ortopédica obstétrica, la ciática aguda y<br>el lumbago. También se usa en alivio del lumbago crónico, la artritis, la artritis reumatoide y la<br>espondilitis anquilosante. |
| 用法、用量<br>Administración y dosis | 急性轻度或中度疼痛：每日剂量为 8 ～ 16mg，分 2 ～ 3 次服用；每日最大剂量为 16mg。<br>风湿性疾病引起的关节疼痛和炎症：每日剂量为 12mg，分 2 ～ 3 次服用；服用剂量不应超过<br>16mg。<br>Para dolor agudo leve o moderado：La dosis diaria es de 8 ～ 16 mg divididos en 2 ó 3 tomas y<br>no debe exceder a 16 mg diarios como máximo. Para dolor e inflamación causados por enfermedades<br>reumáticas: La dosis diaria de 12 mg divididos en 2 ó 3 veces en tomas, no debe exceder a 16 mg<br>diarios como máximo. |
| 剂型、规格<br>Formulaciones y<br>especificaciones | 片剂：4mg。<br>Tableta: 4 mg. |
| **药品名称 Drug Names** | 塞来昔布 Celecoxib |
| 适应证<br>Indicaciones | 用于急、慢性骨关节炎和类风湿关节炎。<br>Se usa para tratamiento de osteoartritis aguda y crónica y artritis reumatoide. |
| 用法、用量<br>Administración y dosis | 治疗关节炎，一日 200mg，分 2 次服或顿服；用于类风湿关节炎，剂量为一日 100mg 或<br>200mg，一日 2 次。<br>Para la artritis: La dosis diaria es de 200mg divididos en 2 tomas o en una sola toma. Para Artritis<br>reumatoide：La dosis diaria es de 100 ～ 200 mg divididos en 2 tomas. |
| 剂型、规格<br>Formulaciones y<br>especificaciones | 胶囊：每粒 100mg。<br>Cápsula: 100mg. |
| **药品名称 Drug Names** | 帕瑞昔布 Parecoxib |
| 适应证<br>Indicaciones | 用于术后疼痛的短期治疗。<br>Se usa para tratamiento a corto plazo del dolor postoperatorio. |

续　表

| 用法、用量<br>Administración y dosis | 成人，40mg/ 次，静注或深部肌内注射，随后视需要间隔 6 ～ 12 小时给药给予 20 ～ 40mg，总剂量不超过 80mg/d。<br><br>Para adultos：Se administra inyección intravenosa o intramuscular profunda de 40 mg cada vez. Dependiente de la necesidad, puede repetir el medicamento de 20 ～ 40mg cada 6 ～ 12 horas. La dosis total no excede a 80 mg diarios. |
|---|---|
| 剂型、规格<br>Formulaciones y especificaciones | 注射粉针：每瓶 20mg；40mg。<br>Polvo para inyección: 20 mg, 40 mg. |

| 药品名称 Drug Names | 尼美舒利 Nimesulida |
|---|---|
| 适应证<br>Indicaciones | 主要用于类风湿关节炎和骨关节炎、痛经、手术后疼和发热等。<br><br>Se usa principalmente para tratamiento de artritis reumatoide, la osteoartritis, dismenorrea, dolor y fiebre postoperatorio etc. |
| 用法、用量<br>Administración y dosis | 口服：成人，每次 100mg，一日 2 次，餐后服用。儿童常用剂量为 5mg/（kg・d），一日 2 ～ 3 次服用。老年人不需调整剂量。<br><br>Por vía oral. Para dultos y ancianos: la dosis es de 100 mg 2 veces al día tomados después de alimentos. Para niños: La dosis habitual es de 5mg/kg/d divididos en 2 ó 3 veces tomas. |
| 剂型、规格<br>Formulaciones y especificaciones | 片剂：每片 50mg；100mg。<br>Tableta: 50 mg, 100 mg. |

| 药品名称 Drug Names | 安乃近 Metamizol sódico |
|---|---|
| 适应证<br>Indicaciones | 主要用于解热、急性关节炎、头痛、风湿性痛、牙痛及肌肉痛等。<br><br>Se usa principalmente para alivio de fiebre, artritis aguda, cefalea, dolor reumático, odontalgia y mialgia. |
| 用法、用量<br>Administración y dosis | 口服：一次 0.25 ～ 0.5g，一日 0.75 ～ 1.25g。滴鼻：小儿退热常以 10% ～ 20% 滴鼻，5 岁以下，每次每侧鼻孔 1 ～ 2 滴，必要时重复用一次；5 岁以上适当加量。深部肌内注射：每次 0.25 ～ 0.5g；小儿每次 5 ～ 10mg/kg。<br><br>Por vía oral: 0.25 ～ 0.5g cada vez y 0.75 ～ 1.25g diarios. Por vía intranasal：Para fiebre en niños, se administra 1 ó 2 goteos de gota nasal a 10% ～ 20% en cada fosa para niños menores de 5 años y puede repetir la medicación cuando sea necesario. Para niños mayores de 5 años puede aumentar la dosis apropiadamente. Inyeccion I.M.profunda: 0.25 ～ 0.5g cada vez y para infantes, 5 ～ 10mg/kg cada vez. |
| 剂型、规格<br>Formulaciones y especificaciones | 片剂：每片 0.25g；0.5g。滴液：1ml ：200mg。注射液：每支 0.25g（1ml）；0.5g（2ml）。滴鼻剂：10% ～ 20%。<br>Tableta: 0.25g, 0.5g; Gotas: 1ml:200mg; Inyección: 0.25g(1ml)，0.5g (2 ml); Gota nasal: 10% ～ 20%. |

| 药品名称 Drug Names | 保泰松 Fenilbutazona |
|---|---|
| 适应证<br>Indicaciones | 用于类风湿关节炎、风湿性关节炎、强直性脊柱炎及急性痛风等。常需连续使用或与其他药物配合使用。亦用于丝虫病急性淋巴管炎。<br><br>Se usa para tratamiento de artritis reumatoide y reumática, espondilitis anquilopoyética y gota aguda etc. A menudo requerir el uso continuo o utilizado en conjunción con otros fármacos. También lo usa en tratamiento de filariasis linfangitis aguda. |
| 用法、用量<br>Administración y dosis | ①关节炎：开始一日量 0.3 ～ 0.6g，分 3 次餐后服用。一日量不宜超过 0.8g。1 周后如无不良反应，可继续服用递减至每日量 0.1 ～ 0.2g。②丝虫病急性淋巴管炎：每次服 0.2g，一日 3 次，总量 1.2 ～ 3g，急性炎症控制后，再用抗丝虫药治疗。<br><br>① Artristis: La dosis inicial es de 0.3 ～ 0.6g diarios divididos en 3 tomas después de alimentos. Dosis maxima no debe exceder a 0.8g diarios. Si no aparece reacciones adversas durante una semana, continua la medicación a dosis de 0.1 ～ 0.2g diarios reduciendo gradualmente. ② Filariasis linfangitis aguda: 0.2g 3 veces al dia. La dosis total es de 1.2 ～ 3g diarios. Después de controlarla inflamacion aguda, continua con medicación anti-filarial. |

| | |
|---|---|
| 剂型、规格<br>Formulaciones y especificaciones | 片（胶囊）剂：每片（粒）0.1g；0.2g。栓剂：25mg。注射液：600mg（3ml）。<br>Tableta o Cáptura: 0.1g, 0.2g; Supositorio: 25mg; Inyección: 600mg (3 ml). |
| 药品名称 Drug Names | 萘丁美酮 Nabumetona |
| 适应证<br>Indicaciones | 本品用于急、慢性关节炎及永动性软组织损伤、扭伤和挫伤、术后疼痛、牙痛、痛经等。<br>Se usa para tratamiento de artritis aguda y crónica, perpetuas lesiones,esguinces y contusiones en tejidos blandos, dolor posoperatorio, odontalgia y dismenorrea. |
| 用法、用量<br>Administración y dosis | 口服，每次1g，一日1次，睡前服。一次最大量为2g。一日2次服。体重不足50kg的成人，可以每日0.5g起始，逐渐上调至有效剂量。<br>Por vía oral: 1g una vez al dia antes de acostarse. Dosis maxima es de 2g diarios y deberia ser divididos en 2 tomas. Adultos con peso menor de 50 kg, comenza a 0.5g diarios y aumenta gradualmente hasta la dosis efectiva. |
| 剂型、规格<br>Formulaciones y especificaciones | 片剂：每片0.25g；0.5g；0.75g。胶囊剂：每粒0.2g；0.25g。分散片：每片0.5g。干混悬剂：0.5g。<br>Tableta: 0.25g, 0.5g y 0.75g; Cápsula: 0.2g y 0.25g; Comprimido dispersable: 0.5g; Suspensión: 0.5g. |
| 药品名称 Drug Names | 来氟米特 Leflunomida |
| 适应证<br>Indicaciones | 用于成人风湿性关节炎的治疗。<br>Se usa para tratamiento de artritis reumática en adultos. |
| 用法、用量<br>Administración y dosis | 由于半衰期较长建议间隔24小时给药。建议开始最初治疗的3日给予负荷量（50mg/d），之后给予维持剂量20mg/d。<br>El intervalo de dosificacion recomendado es de 24 horas debido a la larga vida media de la droga. Recomienda dosis inicial de 50 mg diarios en los primeros 3 días. Posteriormente se aplica dosis de mantenimiento de 20 mg diarios. |
| 剂型、规格<br>Formulaciones y especificaciones | 片剂：每片10mg；20mg；100mg。<br>Tableta: 10mg, 20mg y 100mg. |
| 药品名称 Drug Names | 复方骨肽 Ossotida Compuesto |
| 适应证<br>Indicaciones | 用于风湿、类风湿关节炎、骨质疏松、颈椎病等疾病的症状改善。同时用于骨折或骨科手术后骨愈合，可促进骨愈合和骨新生。<br>Se usa para mejoramiento de síntomas de artritis reumatoide y reumática, la osteoporosis, la espondilosis cervical, etc. También se usa para fomentar la consolidación ósea y su crecimiento después de la fractura o cirugía ortopédica. |
| 用法、用量<br>Administración y dosis | 肌内注射，一次30～60mg，一日一次；静脉滴注，一次60～150mg，一日一次，10～30日为一个疗程或遵遗嘱，亦可在痛点或穴位注射。<br>Inyección por I.M. de 30～60mg una vez al dia; Infusión por I.V. de 60～150mg una vez al dia. Un curso de tratamiento tardará 10 a 30 días o lo cumpli bajo consejo específico de médicos. También puede inyectarse en los puntos o en el punto donde duele. |
| 剂型、规格<br>Formulaciones y especificaciones | 注射液：每支30mg（2ml）；75mg（5ml）多肽物质。<br>Inyección: 30 mg (2ml), 75 mg (5ml) material peptídico. |
| 药品名称 Drug Names | 硫辛酸 Ácido Lipoico |
| 适应证<br>Indicaciones | 用于糖尿病周围神经病变引起的感觉异常。<br>Se usa para tratamiento de parestesia causada por neuropatía periférica diabética. |
| 用法、用量<br>Administración y dosis | 静脉注射应缓慢，最大速度为每分钟50mg（2ml）。本品也可加入生理盐水静脉滴注如250～500mg（10～20ml）加入100～250ml生理盐水中、静脉滴注时间为30分钟。<br>Lenta Inyección por I.V. a velocidad inferior a 50mg(2ml) por minuto. También puede ser infusión por I.V. diluidos en salina normal, por ejempro infusión por I.V. de 250～500mg (10～20ml) diluidos en 100～250ml de Normal Saline. Se administra la infusión en 30 minutos. |

**续　表**

| 剂型、规格<br>Formulaciones y especificaciones | 注射液：每支 0.6g（20ml）。<br>Inyección: 0.6g (20ml). |
|---|---|

| 药品名称 Drug Names | 氟比洛芬 Flurbiprofeno |
|---|---|
| 适应证<br>Indicaciones | 主要用于风湿性关节炎。<br>Se usa principalmente para tratamiento de la artritis reumática. |
| 用法、用量<br>Administración y dosis | 一日 150～200mg，分次服。<br>150～200mg diarios divididos en varias tomas. |
| 剂型、规格<br>Formulaciones y especificaciones | 片剂：每片 50mg；100mg。<br>Tableta: 50mg, 100mg. |

| 药品名称 Drug Names | 醋氯芬酸 Aceclofenaco |
|---|---|
| 适应证<br>Indicaciones | 用于类风湿关节炎及骨关节炎等症状。<br>Se usa para tratamiento de la artritis reumatoide y la osteoartritis. |
| 用法、用量<br>Administración y dosis | 每次 100mg，一日 2 次。<br>100 mg 2 veces al día. |
| 剂型、规格<br>Formulaciones y especificaciones | 片剂：每片 100mg。<br>Tableta: 100mg. |

## 8.4　抗痛风药 Medicamentos contra la gota

| 药品名称 Drug Names | 秋水仙碱 Colchicina |
|---|---|
| 适应证<br>Indicaciones | 用于痛风性关节炎的急性发作、预防复发性痛风性关节炎的急性发作、家族性地中海热。<br>Se usa para tratamiento del ataque agudo de artritis gotosa y prevención del ataque agudo de artritis gotosa recurrente y la fiebre mediterránea familiar. |
| 用法、用量<br>Administración y dosis | （1）急性期治疗：①口服：成人常用量为每 1～2 小时服 0.5～1mg，至关节症状缓解或出现恶心、呕吐、腹泻等胃肠道不良反应时停用。一般需要 3～5mg，不宜超过 6mg，症状可在 6～12 小时减轻，24～48 小时控制，以后 48 小时不需服用本品。此后每次给 0.5mg，一日 2～3 次（0.5～1.5mg/d），共 7 日。②静脉注射：用于急性痛风发作和口服用药胃肠道反应过于剧烈者。可将此药 1mg 用 0.9% 氯化钠注射液 20ml 稀释，缓慢注射（20～30 分钟）。24 小时剂量不超过 2mg，但应注意勿使药物外漏，视病情需要 6～8 小时后可在注射，有肾功能减退者 24 小时不超过 3mg。<br>（2）口服，口服每次 0.5～1mg，但疗程量酌定，要注意不良反应的出现，出现即停药。<br><br>(1)tratamiento en fase aguda: ① Por vía oral: La dosis habitual para adultos es de 0.5～1mg cada 1～2 horas hasta el alivio de la síntoma de artritis o aparición de reacciones adversas gastrointestinales como náuseas, vómitos y diarrea. Generalmente la síntoma puede mejorarse en 6～12 horas con medicamento de 3～5mg (y no debe exceer a 6mg) y controlarse en 24～48horas. Los siguientes 48 horas no toma este fármaco. Y después continua el medicamento durante 7 dias a dosis de 0.5mg 2 ó 3 veces al dia. ② Inyección por I.V.: Para pacientes que aguantan ataques de gota aguda o severas reacciones adversas gastrointestinales de administración oral, se aplica inyección por I.V. lenta de 20～30 minutos de la dilución de 1mg de dicha droga y 20ml de Cloruro de Sodio al 0.9%. La dosis total no excede a 2mg en 24 horas y puede repetir la medicación dentro de 6～8 horas según la necesidad. Para pacientes con empeoramiento de la función renal la dosis diara no excede a 3mg. Hay que tener precaución de la fuga de medicina.<br>(2)Por vía oral a una dosis de 0.5～1 mg cada vez. No hay definición exacta sobre la dosis total y debe dejar la medicación una vez que aparezca reacciones adversas. |
| 剂型、规格<br>Formulaciones y especificaciones | 片剂：每片 0.5mg；1mg。注射液：0.5mg/ml。<br>Tableta: 0.5mg, 1mg; Inyección: 0.5mg/ml. |

| 药品名称 Drug Names | 丙磺舒 Probenecida |
|---|---|
| 适应证<br>Indicaciones | 用于慢性痛风的治疗。<br>Se usa para tratamiento de gota crónica. |
| 用法、用量<br>Administración y dosis | ①慢性痛风：口服每次 0.25g，一日 2～4 次，1 周后可增至每次 0.5～1g，一日 2 次。每日最大剂量不超过 2g。②增强青霉素类的作用：每次 0.5g，一日 4 次。儿童：25mg/kg，每 3～9 小时 1 次。2～14 岁或体重在 50kg 以下儿童，首剂按体重 0.025g/kg，或按体表面积 0.7g/㎡，以后每次 0.01g/kg 或按体表面积 0.3g/㎡，一日 4 次。<br><br>① Gota crónica: Por vía oral a dosis de 0.25g 2～4 veces al día. Después de una semana puede cambiar a una dosis de 0.5～1g 2 veces al día. La dosis máxima diaria no excede a 2g. ② reforzar la eficacia de penicilina: 0.5g 4 veces al día. Para niños: 25 mg/kg cada 3～9 horas. Para niños de entre 2 y 14 años o con peso menor de 50 kg: aplica dosis inicial de 0.025g/kg ó 0.7g/㎡ subcutánea y después, la dosis cambia a 0.01g/kg ó 0.3g/㎡ subcutánea 4 veces al día. |
| 剂型、规格<br>Formulaciones y especificaciones | 片剂：每片 0.25g；0.5g。<br>Tableta; 0.25g, 0.5g. |
| 药品名称 Drug Names | 苯溴马隆 Benzbromarona |
| 适应证<br>Indicaciones | 用于反复发作的痛风性关节炎伴高尿酸血症即痛风湿患者。<br>Se usa para tratamiento de artritis gotosa recurrente con hiperuricemia (o gota) . |
| 用法、用量<br>Administración y dosis | 每次 25～100mg，一日一次，餐后服用，剂量逐渐增加，连用 3～6 个月。<br>inicialmente se toma 25～100mg una vez al dia después de alimentos y continue la medicación durante 3～6 meses mienstras aumenta la dosis gradualmente. |
| 剂型、规格<br>Formulaciones y especificaciones | 片剂：每片 50mg。<br>Tableta: 50mg. |
| 药品名称 Drug Names | 别嘌醇 Alopurinol |
| 适应证<br>Indicaciones | 用于慢性原发性或继发性痛风、痛风性肾病。<br>Se usa para tratamiento de gota crónica primaria o secuntaria y nefropatía gotosa. |
| 用法、用量<br>Administración y dosis | 用于降低血中尿酸浓度：开始每次 0.05g，一日 2～3 次，剂量渐增，2～3 周后增至每日 0.2～0.4g，分 2～3 次服，每日最大量不超过 0.6g。维持量：每次 0.1～0.2g，一日 2～3 次。儿童剂量每日 8mg/kg。治疗尿酸结石：口服每次 0.1～0.2g，一日 1～4 次或 300mg，一日 1 次。<br><br>Se usa para reducir la concentración de ácido úrico en la sangre: Dosis inicial es de 0.05g 2 ó 3 veces al día. Dentro de 2～3 semanas, aumenta gradualmente a 0.2～0.4g diarios divididos en 2 ó 3 tomas. La dosis máxima no excede a 0.6g diarios. Dosis de mantenimiento: 0.1～0.2g 2 ó 3 veces al día. Dosis para niños: 8mg/kg diadios. Para tratamiento de cálculos de ácido úrico: Por vía oral a dosis 0.1～0.2g cada 6-24 horas o 300mg una vez al dia. |
| 剂型、规格<br>Formulaciones y especificaciones | 片剂：每片 0.1g。<br>Tableta: 0.1g. |
| 药品名称 Drug Names | 非布司他 Febuxostat |
| 适应证<br>Indicaciones | 用于预防和治疗高尿酸血症及其引发的痛风。<br>Se usa para prevención y tratamiento de la hiperuricemia y la gota desencadenada. |
| 用法、用量<br>Administración y dosis | 本品服用剂量为一日 1 次 40mg 或 80mg，不推荐用于高尿酸血症的痛风患者。<br>40～80mg una vez al día y no recomendable para pacientes de gota causada por hiperuricemia. |
| 剂型、规格<br>Formulaciones y especificaciones | 片剂：每片 80mg；120mg。<br>Tableta: 80mg, 120mg. |

**续 表**

8.5　抗癫痫药 Medicamentos antiepilépticos

| 药品名称 Drug Names | 苯妥英钠 Fenitoína Sódica |
|---|---|
| 适应证<br>Indicaciones | ①主要用于复杂性癫痫发作、单纯部分性发作、全身强直阵挛性发作和癫痫持续状态。本品在脑组织中达有效浓度较慢，因此疗效出现缓慢，需要连续多次服药才有效。②治疗三叉神经痛和坐骨神经痛、发作性舞蹈手足徐动症、发作性控制障碍、肌强直症及隐性营养不良性大疱性表皮松解。③用于治疗室上性或室性期前收缩，室性心动过速，尤适用于强心苷中毒时的室性心动过速，室上性心动过速也可适用。<br><br>① Se usa principalmente en tratamiento de convulsiones complejas o parciales simples, convulsiones tónico-clónicas generalizadas y el estado epiléptico. El efecto del fármaco es lento y necesita medicamento continuo para que sea eficaz porque es lento optener concentración efectiva en el tejido cerebral. ② trastornos del control, miotonía e invisible epidermolisis bullosa distrófica. ③ Se usa también en tratamiento de latidos prematuros supraventriculares o ventriculares, taquicardia ventricular especialmente en intoxicación de glucósidos cardíacos. Es efectivo también para taquicardia supraventricular. |
| 用法、用量<br>Administración y dosis | ①口服抗癫痫：成人常用量，一次 50 ～ 100mg，一日 2 ～ 3 次，一日 100 ～ 200mg；极量：一次 300mg，一日 500mg。宜从小剂量开始，酌情增量，但需避免过量。体重在 30kg 以下的小儿，按每日 5mg/kg 给药，分 2 ～ 3 次服用，每日不宜超过 250mg。注射剂用于癫痫持续状态时，可用 150 ～ 250mg，加 5% 葡萄糖注射液 20 ～ 40ml，在 6 ～ 10 分钟缓慢静脉注射，每分钟不超过 50mg，必要时经 30 分钟在注射 100 ～ 150mg。②治疗三叉神经痛：口服，每次 100 ～ 200mg，一日 2 ～ 3 次。<br><br>① Uso antiepilépticos por vía oral: Dosis habitual para adultos es de 50 ~ 100mg 2 ó 3 veces al día y 100 ~ 200mg diarios. La dosis máxima no excede a 300mg cada vez y 500mg diarios. Debe empieza a dosis pequeña y aumentarla gradualmente mientras que hay que evitar uso excesivo. Para infantes con peso menor de 30kg, la dosis es de 5mg/kg diarios divididos en 2 ~ 3 tomas y la dosis máxima no excede a 250mg diarios. La inyección se usa en tratamiento del estado epiléptico a dosis de 150 ~ 250mg diluidos n 20 ~ 40ml solución de glucosa a 5%. Se administra lenta inyección por I.V. dentro de 6 ~ 10 minutos y la dosis no excede a 50mg cada minuto. En caso necesario puede repetir la medicación de 100 ~ 150mg durante 30 minutos. ② Para tratamiento de neuralgia del trigémino: por vía oral a dosis de 100 ~ 200mg 2 ó 3 veces al dia. |
| 剂型、规格<br>Formulaciones y especificaciones | 片剂：每片 50mg；100mg。注射剂：每支 100mg；250mg。<br>Tableta: 50mg, 100mg; Inyección: 100mg, 250mg. |
| 药品名称 Drug Names | 卡马西平 Carbamazepina |
| 适应证<br>Indicaciones | ①治疗癫痫：是单纯部分及复杂部分性发作的首选药，对复杂部分性发作疗效优于其他癫痫药。对典型或不典型失神发作、肌阵挛发作无效。②抗外周神经痛：包括三叉神经痛、舌咽神经痛、多发性硬化、糖尿病性周围性神经痛及疱疹后神经痛。亦可用于三叉神经痛缓解后的长期预防用药。对三叉神经痛、舌咽神经痛疗效较苯妥英钠好，用药后 24 小时即可奏效。③治疗神经源性尿崩症，可能是由于促进抗利尿激素的分泌有关。④预防或治疗狂躁抑郁症：临床使用证明本药对狂躁症及抑郁症均有明显治疗作用，也能减轻或消除精神分裂症患者狂躁、妄想症状。⑤抗心律失常作用：能对抗由地高辛中毒所致的心律失常。能使其完全或基本恢复正常心律。临床使用证明，对室性或室上性期前收缩均有效，可使症状消除，尤其是伴有慢性心功能不全者疗效更好。⑥酒精戒断综合征。<br><br>① Epilepsia: Es fármaco de elección para convulsiones parciales simples y complejas y es más eficaz para convulsión parcial compleja en comparación con otros fármacos. No tiene efecto en tratamiento de crisis de ausencias típicas o atípicas y convulsiones mioclónicas. ② Alivio del dolor neuropático periférico que incluye neuralgia del trigémino, neuralgia del glosofaríngeo, esclerosis múltiple, neuralgia periférica diabética y neuralgia post-herpética. También se usa a largo plaza como medicamento de prevención después de aliviar la neuralgia del trigémino. Tiene mejor eficacia en tratamiento de neuralgia del trigémino y la del glosofaríngeo en comparación con fenitoína. Se efectua dentro de 24 horas tras medicación. ③ Se usa en tratamiento de la diabetes insípida neurogénica que puede ser relacionada con el efecto de promoción de la secreción de la hormona antidiurética. ④ Se usa en prevención y tratamiento del síndrome maníaco depresivo: El uso clínico muestra que la droga tiene un efecto terapéutico significativo en tratamiento de la manía y la depresión así como reducir o eliminar |

**续 表**

| | |
|---|---|
| | los síntomas maníacos y delirantes para pacientes de esquizofrenia.　⑤ Tiene efecto antiarrítmico. Puede usarla en tratamiento de la arritmia causada por la intoxicación de digoxina y pacientes puede recuperarse. casi o completamente al rítmo cardiaco normal. El uso clínico muestra que es eficaz en tratamiento de latidos prematuros supraventriculares o ventriculares eliminando los síntomas. Es especialmente más eficaz para pacientes con insuficiencia cardíaca crónica. ⑥ Se usa en tratamiento del síndrome de abstinencia alcohólica. |
| 用法、用量<br>Administración y dosis | ①癫痫、三叉神经痛：口服，1 日 300～1200mg，分 2～4 次服用。开始 1 次 100mg，一日 2 次，以后一日 3 次。个别三叉神经痛患者剂量可达每日 1000～1200mg。疗程最短 1 周，最长 2～3 个月。②尿崩症：口服，每日 600～1200mg。③抗躁狂症：口服，每日剂量为 300～600mg，分 2～3 次服，最大剂量每日 1200mg。④心律失常：口服，每日 300～600mg，分 2～3 次服。⑤酒精戒断综合征：口服，一次 200mg，一日 3～4 次。<br><br>① Epilepsia y neuralgia del trigémino: por vía oral a dosis de 300-1200mg diarios divididos en 2～4 tomas. Dosis inicial es de 100mg 2 veces al día y luego aumentar a 3 veces al día. Algunos pacientes de neuralgia del trigémino puede tomar 1000～1200mg diarios y el curso de tratamiento tardará por lo mínimo 1 semana y puede prolongar hasta 2 ó 3 meses como máximo. ② Diabetes insípida: por vía oral a dosis de 600～1200mg diarios. ③ Anti-mania: por vía oral a dosis de 300～600mg diarios divididos en 2 ó 3 tomas. La dosis máxima no excede a 1200mg diarios. ④ Arritmia: por vía oral a dosis de 300～600mg diarios divididos en 2 ó 3 tomas. ⑤ Síndrome de abstinencia alcohólica: por vía oral a dosis de 200mg 3 ó 4 veces al día. |
| 剂型、规格<br>Formulaciones y especificaciones | 片剂：每片 100mg；200mg；400mg。缓释片：每片 200mg；400mg。咀嚼片：每片 100mg；200mg。胶囊剂：每粒 200mg。糖浆剂：20mg/ml。栓剂：125mg；250mg。<br><br>Tableta: 100mg, 200mg, 400mg; Tableta de liberación prolongada: 200mg, 400mg; Tableta masticable: 100mg, 200mg; Cápsula: 200mg; Jarabe: 20mg/ml; Supositorio: 125mg, 250mg. |
| 药品名称 Drug Names | 奥卡西平 Oxcarbazepina |
| 适应证<br>Indicaciones | 用于复杂性部分发作、全身强直阵挛性发作的但要治疗及难治性癫痫的辅助治疗。本品的优点是没有自身诱导，可代替卡马西平，用于对后者有过敏反应者。<br><br>Se usa idividualmente para tratamiento de convulsiones parciales complejas y convulsiones tonicoclónicas generalizadas, así como tratamiento adyuvante de epilepsia refractaria. La ventaja de dicha droga existe en que no tiene auto-inducción y puede ser alternativa de carbamazepina para pacientes a la que son alérgicos. |
| 用法、用量<br>Administración y dosis | 口服：开始剂量为 300mg/d，以后可逐渐增量至 600～2400mg/d，以达到满意的疗效。剂量超过 2400mg/d，神经系统不良反应增加。小儿从 8～10mg/（kg·d）开始，可逐渐增量至 600mg/d。以上每日剂量均应分 2 次服用。<br><br>Por vía oral: dosis inicial es de 300mg diarios y puede incrementar gradualmente a 600～2400mg diarios para tener efecto satisfecho. Cuando la dosis diaria excede a 2400mg, se ve más reacción adversa del sistema nervioso. Para niños empieza desde dosis diaria de 8-10mg/kg e incrementa gradualmente a 600mg diarios. Se administra divididos en 2 tomas. |
| 剂型、规格<br>Formulaciones y especificaciones | 片剂：每片 0.15g；0.3g；0.6g。<br>Tableta: 0.15g, 0.3g, 0.6g. |
| 药品名称 Drug Names | 托吡酯 Topiramato |
| 适应证<br>Indicaciones | 主要作为其他抗癫痫药的辅助治疗，用于单纯部分性发作、复杂部分性发作和全身强直阵挛性发作，尤其对 Lennox-Gastaut 综合征和 West 综合征（婴儿痉挛症）的疗效较好。本品远期疗效好，无明显耐受性，大剂量可用作单药治疗。<br><br>Se usa principalmente como adyuvante de otros fármacos antiepilépticos para tratamiento de convulsiones parciales simples y complejas así como convulsiones tónico-clónicas generalizadas. Tiene eficacia evidente para síntomas de Lennox-Gastaut y síntomas de WEST. La droga tiene buena eficacia en tratamiento a largo plazo y no hay tolerancia significativa. Puede utilizarse en monoterapia a grande dosis. |

**续　表**

| 用法、用量<br>Administración y dosis | 口服。成人：初始极量为每晚 25 ～ 50mg，然后每周增加 1 次，每次增加 25mg，直至症状控制为止。通常有效剂量为每日 200 ～ 300mg。2 岁以上儿童：初始剂量为每日 12.5 ～ 25mg，然后逐渐增加至 5 ～ 9mg/（kg·d），维持剂量为 100mg，分 2 次服。体重大于 43kg 的儿童，有效剂量范围与成人相当。<br><br>Por vía oral. Dosis para adultos: inicialmente es de 25 ~ 50mg por la noche e incrementar en 25mg cada una semana hasta que controle los síntomas. Dosis efectiva habitual es de 200 ~ 300mg diarios. Para niños mayores de 2 años: inicialmente es 12.5 ~ 25mg diarios e incrementar gradualmente a 5 ~ 9mg/kg diarios. La dosis de mantenimiento es de 100mg diarios divididos en 2 tomas. Para niños con peso mayor de 43kg tiene la dosis efectiva igual que los adultos. |
|---|---|
| 剂型、规格<br>Formulaciones y especificaciones | 片剂：每片 25mg；50mg；100mg。<br>Tableta: 25mg, 50mg,100mg. |
| **药品名称 Drug Names** | 乙琥胺 Etosuximida |
| 适应证<br>Indicaciones | 主要用于失神小发作，为首选药。<br>Se usa principalmente para tratamiento de crisis de ausencia como el fármaco de elección. |
| 用法、用量<br>Administración y dosis | 口服。剂量：开始量，3 ～ 6 岁为 1 次 250mg，一日 1 次。6 岁以上的儿童及成人，一次 250mg，1 日 2 次。以后可酌情增剂量。最大剂量：6 岁以下最大剂量可增为 1 日 1g，6 岁以上儿童及成人可增加为 1.5g。一般是每 4 ～ 7 日增加 250mg，至满意控制症状而不良反应最小为止。<br><br>Por vía oral: Dosis inicial para niños de 3 ~ 6 años es de 250mg una vez al día y para niños meyores de 6 años y adultos es de 250mg 2 veces al día. Puede aumentar la dosis según la necesidad. Dosis máxima para niños menores de 6 años no excede a 1g diarios y para niños mayores de 6 años y adultos no debe exceder a 1.5 g diarios. Generalmente agrega en 250mg cada 4 ~ 7 días hasta cuando tenga mejor controlado del síntoma y menor reacción adversa. |
| 剂型、规格<br>Formulaciones y especificaciones | 胶囊剂：每粒 0.25g。糖浆剂：5g/100ml。<br>Cápsula: 0.25g; Jarabe: 5g/100ml. |
| **药品名称 Drug Names** | 丙戊酸钠 Valproato de sodio |
| 适应证<br>Indicaciones | 主要用于单纯或复杂性失神发作、肌阵挛发作、全身强直阵挛发作（大发作，GTCS）的治疗。可使 90% 失神发作和全身强直阵挛发作得到良好控制，也用于单纯部分性发作、复杂部分性发作及部分性发作继发 GTCS。<br><br>Se usa principalmente para tratamiento de crisis de ausencias simples o complejas, crisis mioclónicas y convulsiones tónico-clónicas generalizadas (Crisis de gran mal, GTCS). Puede controlar bien el 90% de crisis de ausencias y GTCS. También se usa en tratamiento de convulsiones parciales simples y complejas y la convulsión generalizada secuntaria de la crisis parcial. |
| 用法、用量<br>Administración y dosis | 口服。成人 1 次 200 ～ 400mg，1 日 400 ～ 1200mg。儿童每日 20 ～ 30mg/kg，分 2 ～ 3 次服用。一般以从低剂量开始。如原服用其他抗癫痫药者，可合并应用，也可逐减少原药量，视情况而定。<br><br>Por vía oral. Dosis para adultos, 200 ~ 400mg cada vez y 400 ~ 1200mg darios. Dosis para niños es de 20 ~ 30mg/kg diarios divididos en 2 ~ 3 tomas. Generalmente comienza desde pequeña dosis. Para pacinetes que también está utilizando otros fármacos antiepilépticos puede tomar esta droga en conjunción o puede disminuir la dosis de ese fármaco según la necesidad. |
| 剂型、规格<br>Formulaciones y especificaciones | 片剂：每片 100mg；200mg。胶囊剂：每粒 200mg；250mg。肠溶片：每片 250mg；500mg。缓释片：每片 500mg。糖浆剂：200mg（5ml）；500mg（5ml）。<br>Tableta: 100mg, 200mg; Cápsula: 200mg, 250mg; Tableta con recubrimiento entérico: 250mg, 500mg; Tableta de liberación prolongada: 500mg; Jarabe: 200mg(5ml), 500mg(5ml). |
| **药品名称 Drug Names** | 拉莫三嗪 Lamotrigina |
| 适应证<br>Indicaciones | 本品用于成人和 12 岁以上儿童复杂部分性发作或全身强直阵挛性癫痫发作的辅助治疗。作为辅助治疗用于难治性癫痫时，可用于 2 岁以上儿童及成人。<br><br>Se usa como tratamiento adyuvante de convulsiones parciales complejas o convulsiones tónico-clónicas generalizadas para adultos y niños mayores de 12 años. En tratamiento adyuvante de epilepsia refractaria, puede administrarse en adultos e infantes mayores de 2 años. |

**续 表**

| | |
|---|---|
| 用法、用量<br>Administración y dosis | 口服。单独使用：成人初始剂量 25mg，一日 1 次；2 周后可增至 50mg，一日 1 次；在 2 周后，可酌情增加剂量，最大增加量为 50 ～ 100mg。此后，每隔 1 ～ 2 周，可增加剂量 1 次，直至达到最佳疗效，一般需经 6 ～ 8 周。通常有效维持量为 100 ～ 200mg/d，一次或分 2 次服用。儿童初始剂量 1mg/kg，维持剂量 3 ～ 6mg/kg。与丙戊酸合用：成人和 12 岁以上儿童：初始剂量 25mg，隔日 1 次，每 3 ～ 4 周开始改为 25mg，一日 1 次，在 2 周后，酌情增加剂量，最大增量为 0.5 ～ 1mg/kg。此后，每隔 1 ～ 2 周，可增加剂量 1 次，直至达到最佳疗效，通常有效维持量为 1 ～ 2mg/（kg·d），一次或分 2 次服用。与具诱导作用的抗癫痫药物合用：初始剂量 50mg，一日 1 次，，服药 2 周后可增至 100mg/d，分 2 次服，在 2 周后，可酌情增加剂量，最大增加量为 100mg，此后，每隔 1 ～ 2 周，可增加剂量 1 次，直至达到最佳疗效。通常有效维持量为 200 ～ 400mg/d，分 2 次服用。2 ～ 12 岁儿童：初始剂量 2mg/（kg·d），分 2 次服，2 周后增至 5mg/（kg·d），分 2 次服，在 2 周后，可酌情增加剂量，最大增加量为，2 ～ 3mg/kg，此后，每隔 1 ～ 2 周，可增加剂量 1 次，直至达到最佳疗效。维持剂量 10mg/（kg·d），最大剂量为 400mg/d。<br><br>Por vía oral. Uso individual: dosis inicial para adultos es de 25mg 1 vez al día y 2 semanas después puede aumentar a 50mg 1 vez al día. Puede aumentar la dosis gradualmente después de 2 semanas en 50-100mg según la situación. Luego puede aumentar la dosis cada 2 ~ 3 semanas hasta que consigue la mejor eficacia que generalmente tarda 6 ~ 8 semanas. La dosis habitual de mantenimiento es de 100 ~ 200mg diarios divididos en 1 ó 2 tomas. Dosis inicial para niños es de 1mg/kg y la de mantenimiento es de 3 ~ 6mg/kg. Uso en conjunción con el ácido valproico: dosis inicial para adultos y niños mayores de 12 años es de 25mg cada otro día. En la tercera o cuarta semana cambia a 25mg cada día. Dos semanas después puede aumentar la dosis en 0.5 ~ 1mg/kg como máximo. Se puede agregar la dosis a esta cantidad cada 2 ó 3 semanas hasta conseguir la mejor eficacia. La dosis habitual de mantenimiento es de 1 ~ 2mg/kg diarios divididos en 1 ó tomas. Uso en conjunción con fármacos antiepilépticos con efecto de inducción: Dosis inicial es de 50mg una vez al día y 2 semanas después puede aumentar a 100mg diarios divididos en 2 tomas. Después de 2 semanas puede aumentar la dosis en 100mg como máximo. Se puede agregar la dosis a esta cantidad cada 2 ~ 3 semanas hasta que consigue la mejor eficacia. Dosis habitual de mantenimiento es de 200 ~ 400mg diarios divididos en 2 tomas. Para niños de 2 ~ 12 años: la dosis inicial es de 2mg/kg diarios divididos en 2 tomas y dentro de 2 semanas aumenta a 5mg/kg diarios divididos en 2 tomas. Dos semanas después puede aumentar la dosis en 2 ~ 3mg/kgcomo máximo. Se puede agregar la dosis a esta cantidad cada 2 ~ 3 semanas hasta que consigue la mejor eficacia. Dosis habitual de mantenimiento es de 10mg/kg diarios y la máxima no excede a 400mg diarios. |
| 剂型、规格<br>Formulaciones y especificaciones | 片剂：每片 25mg；100mg；150mg；200mg。<br>Tableta: 25mg, 100mg, 150mg, 200mg. |

| 药品名称 Drug Names | 加巴喷丁 Gabapentina |
|---|---|
| 适应证<br>Indicaciones | 用于常规治疗无效的某些部分性癫痫辅助治疗，亦可用于治疗部分性癫痫发作继发全身性发作。<br><br>Se usa para tratamiento adyuvante de epilepsia parcial ineficaz de la terapia convencional y la convulsión generalizada secuntaria de la crisis parcial. |
| 用法、用量<br>Administración y dosis | 口服，成人每日 300mg，睡前服；第 2 日 600mg，分 2 次服；第 3 日 900mg，分 3 次服。此剂量随疗效而定，多数患者在 900 ～ 1800mg 有效。肾功能不全者需要减少剂量。停药应缓停。<br><br>Por vía oral. La dosis diaria para adultos en el primer día es de 300mg tomados antes de acostarse, en el segundo día es de 600mg diarios divididos en 2 tomas y el tercer día, 900mg diarios en 3 tomas. La dosis se cambia según el efecto y la mayoría de pacientes consiguen eficacia con dosis diaria de 900 ~ 1800mg. Para pacientes de disfunción renal tiene que disminuir la dosis. Debe dejar el medicamento gradualmente también. |
| 剂型、规格<br>Formulaciones y especificaciones | 胶囊剂：每粒 100mg；300mg；400mg。<br>Cápsula: 100mg, 300mg, 400mg. |

**续　表**

| 药品名称 Drug Names | 左乙拉西坦 Levetiracetam |
| --- | --- |
| 适应证<br>Indicaciones | 用于成人及 4 岁以上儿童癫痫患者部分性发作的治疗。<br>Se usa para tratamiento de epilepsia con convulsiones parciales para adultos y niños mayores de 4 años. |
| 用法、用量<br>Administración y dosis | 口服：成人和青少年体重≥ 50kg，起始剂量为每次 500mg，一日 2 次，最多可增至每次 1500mg，一日 2 次，每 2 ～ 4 周增加或减少每次 500mg，一日 2 次。4 ～ 11 岁儿童和青少年体重＜ 50kg，起始剂量为每次 10mg/kg，一日 2 次，最多可增至 30mg/kg，每 2 ～ 4 周增加或减少每次 10mg/kg，一日 2 次。肾功能不全者，根据肌酐清除率调整剂量。<br>Por vía oral. Para adultos y juventud con peso mayor de 50kg, la dosis inicial es de 500mg 2 veces al día. La dosis máxima no excede a 1500mg 2 veces al día. Incrementa o induce cada 2 ~ 4 semanas la dosis en 500mg y 2 veces al día. Para niños de 4-11 años y juventud con peso menor de 50kg, la dosis inicial es 10mg /kg 2 veces al día. La dosis máxima no excede a 30mg/kg. Incrementa o induce la dosis cada 2-4 semanas en 10mg/kg 2 veces al día. Para pacientes con disfunción renal puede cambiar la dosis según el aclaramiento de creatinina. |
| 剂型、规格<br>Formulaciones y especificaciones | 片剂：每片 0.25g；0.5g；1.0g。<br>Tableta: 0.25g, 0.5g, 1.0g. |
| 药品名称 Drug Names | 扑米酮 Primidona |
| 适应证<br>Indicaciones | 作用于苯巴比妥相似，但作用及毒性均较低。用于治疗癫痫大发作及精神运动性发作有效。<br>Tiene efecto similar a Fenobarbital pero con menor efecto y toxicidad. Se usa para tratamiento de convulsiones de gran mal y convulsión psicomotora. |
| 用法、用量<br>Administración y dosis | 口服：开始每次 0.05g，1 周后逐渐增至每次 0.25g，一日 0.5 ～ 0.75g。极量一日 1.5g。儿童一日 12.5 ～ 25mg/kg。分 2 ～ 3 次服用，宜从小剂量开始，逐渐增量。<br>Por vía oral: dosis inicial es de 0.05g cada vez y dentro de 1 semana aumenta gradualmente a 0.25g cada vez. Dosis diaria es de 0.5-0.75g y no debe exceder a 1.5g. Para niños la dosis diaria es de 12.5 ~ 25mg/kg divididos en 2 ó 3 tomas empezando con pequeña dosis inicial y agregándola gradualmente. |
| 剂型、规格<br>Formulaciones y especificaciones | 片剂：0.25g。<br>Tableta: 0.25g. |

8.6　镇静药、催眠药和抗惊厥 Los sedantes, hipnóticos y anticonvulsivos

| 药品名称 Drug Names | 咪达唑仑 Midazolam |
| --- | --- |
| 适应证<br>Indicaciones | 用于治疗失眠症，亦可用于外科手术或诊断检查时作诱导睡眠用。<br>Se usa en tratamiento de insomnio e inducción del sueño en cirugía o diagnósticos. |
| 用法、用量<br>Administración y dosis | 口服：治疗失眠症，每次 15mg，睡前服。肌内注射：术前 20 ～ 30 分钟注射，成人一般为 10 ～ 15mg（0.10 ～ 0.15mg/kg）。可单用，亦可与镇痛药合用。儿童剂量可稍高，为 0.15 ～ 0.2mg/kg。作儿童诱导麻醉，用本品 5 ～ 10mg（0.15 ～ 0.2mg/kg）与氯胺酮 50 ～ 100mg（8mg/kg）合用。静脉注射：术前准备，术前 5 ～ 10 分钟注射 2.5 ～ 5mg（0.05 ～ 0.1mg/kg），可单用或与抗胆碱药合用。用于诱导麻醉，成人为 10 ～ 15mg（0.15 ～ 0.2mg/kg），儿童为 0.2mg/kg。用于维持麻醉，小剂量静脉注射，剂量和时间间隔视患者个体差异而定。<br>Por vía oral: Para tratamiento de insomnio se toma 15mg antes de acostarse. Inyección por I.M.: Medicación tomada 20 ~ 30 minutos antes de cirugía a dosis de 10~15mg(0.10~0.15mg/kg)para adultos. Puede utilizarse individualmente o en conjunción con analgésicos. Dosis para niños puede ser un poco más que es de 0.15~0.2mg/kg. En inducción de la anestesia para niños, usan 5~10mg(0.15~0.2mg/kg) de este fármaco en conjunción con 50~100mg(8mg/kg) de ketamina. Inyección por I.V.: En preparación preoperatoria se toma 2.5~5mg(0.05~0.1mg/kg) con 5 ~ 10 minutos antes de cirugía. Puede usarse individualmente o en conjunción con anticolinérgicos. En inducción de la anestesia, dosis para adultos es de 10~15mg(0.15~0.2mg/kg) y para niños es de 0.2mg/kg. Para mantener la anestesia se usa inyección por I.V. a dosis pequeña. La dosis y el intervalo de medicación dependen de la condición de cada pacient. |

**续 表**

| 剂型、规格<br>Formulaciones y especificaciones | 片剂：每片 15mg。注射液：每支 5mg（1ml）；10mg（2ml）；15mg（3ml）。<br>Tableta: 15mg; Inyección: 5mg(1ml)；10mg(2ml)；15mg(3ml). |
|---|---|

| 药品名称 Drug Names | 苯巴比妥 Fenobarbital |
|---|---|

| 适应证<br>Indicaciones | 用于：①镇静：如焦虑不安、烦躁、甲状腺功能亢进、高血压、功能性恶心、小儿幽门痉挛症；②催眠：偶用于顽固性失眠症，但醒后往往有疲倦、嗜睡等后遗效应；③抗惊厥：常用其对抗中枢兴奋药中毒或高热、破伤风、脑炎、脑出血等病引起的惊厥；④抗癫痫：用于癫痫大发作和部分性发作的治疗，出现作用快，也可用于癫痫持续状态；⑤麻醉前给药；⑥与解热镇痛药配伍应用，以增强其作用；⑦治疗新生儿高胆红素血症。<br><br>Se usa en: ① Sedación: por ejempro para ansiedad, irritabilidad, hipertiroidismo, hipertensión, náusea funcional, espasmos pilórica infantil. ② Hipnotización: a veces se usa en insomnio intratable pero hay efectos residuales como fatiga y somnolencia. ③ Anticonvulsivo: Utilización habitual en intoxicación por droga estimulante del sistema nervioso central y convulsiones causadas por fiebre, tétanos, encefalitis y hemorragia cerebral. ④ Antiepiléptico: Utilización en tratamiento de convulsiones gran mal o parciales con la rápida acción. También se usa para el estado epiléptico. ⑤ Administración antes de anestesia. ⑥ Se utiliza junto con analgésicos antipiréticos para mejorar su función. ⑦ Se usa en el tratamiento de la hiperbilirrubinemia neonatal. |
|---|---|
| 用法、用量<br>Administración y dosis | ①口服：一般情况，常用量，1 次 15 ～ 150mg，一日 30 ～ 200mg；极量，1 次 250mg，1 日 500mg。小儿，用于镇静每次 2mg/kg，用于惊厥每次 3 ～ 5mg/kg，用于抗高胆红素血症每日 5 ～ 8mg/kg，分次口服。②皮下、肌内注射或缓慢静脉注射：常用量，1 次 0.1 ～ 0.2g，一日 1 ～ 2 次；极量，1 次 0.25g，一日 0.5g。③镇静、抗癫痫：口服，每次 0.015 ～ 0.03g，一日 3 次。④催眠：每次 0.03 ～ 0.09g，睡前口服 1 次。⑤抗惊厥：肌内注射其钠盐，每次 0.1 ～ 0.2g，必要时 4 ～ 6 小时后重复一次。⑥麻醉前给药：术前 0.5 ～ 1 小时肌内注射 0.1 ～ 0.2g。⑦癫痫持续状态：肌内注射 1 次 0.1 ～ 0.2g。<br><br>① Por vía oral. Dosis habitual es de 15 ~ 150mg cada vez y 30 ~200mg diarios. Dosis máxima no excede a 250mg cada vez y 500mg diarios. Para infantes se toman 2mg/kg cada vez para sedación, 3~5mg/kg cada vez para convulsiones y para hiperbilirrubinemia, 5~8mg/kg diarios divididos en varias tomas por vía oral. ② Inyección subcutánea, intramuscular o inyección lenta intravenosa: Dosis habitual es de 0.1~0.2g cada vez y 1 ~ 2 veces al día. Dosis máxima no excede a 0.25g cada vez y 0.5g diarios. ③ Para sedación y antiepilepsia: Por vía oral a una dosis de 0.015~0.03g cada vez y 3 veces al día. ④ Para hipnotización: Por vía oral antes de acostarse a una dosis de 0.03~0.09g. ⑤ Anticonvulsiones: Inyección por I.M. el fenobarbital sódico a una dosis de 0.1~0.2g cada vez y puede repetir la medicación dentro de 4 ~ 6 horas en caso necesario. ⑥ Administración antes de anestesia: Inyección I.M. de 0.1~0.2g 0.5 ~ 1 hora antes de cirugía. ⑦ Para el estado epiléptico: Inyección por I.M. de 0.1~0.2g. |
| 剂型、规格<br>Formulaciones y especificaciones | 片剂：每片 0.01g；0.015g；0.03g；0.1g。注射用苯巴比妥：每支 0.05g；0.1g；0.2g。鲁米托品片每片含苯巴比妥 15mg，硫酸阿托品 0.15mg。用于主动和神经功能失调所致头痛、呕吐、颤抖、胃肠道紊乱性腹痛等。一次 1 片，极量 1 次 5 片。<br><br>Tableta: 0.01g, 0.015g, 0.03g, 0.1g; Fenobarbital para inyección: 0.05g, 0.1g, 0.2g; Tableta de Lumitropine: incluye 15mg de Fenobarbital y 0.15mg de atropina sulfato. Se utiliza en alivio de cefalea, vómitos, temblores y dolor abdominal de trastornos gastrointestinales causados por disfunción autonómica. La dosis es de 1 tableta cada vez y por lo máximo 5 tabletas cada vez. |

| 药品名称 Drug Names | 异戊巴比妥 Amobarbital |
|---|---|

| 适应证<br>Indicaciones | 用于镇静、催眠、抗惊厥。<br>Se usa para sedación, hipnotización y anticonvulsiones. |
|---|---|
| 用法、用量<br>Administración y dosis | （1）口服：①成人，常用量：催眠，每次 0.1 ～ 0.2g，于睡前顿服，适用于难入睡者；镇静，每次 0.02 ～ 0.04g，一日 2 ～ 3 次。极量：1 次 0.2g，一日 0.6g。老年人或体弱患者，即便是给予常用量也可产生兴奋、神经错乱或抑郁，须减量。②小儿，常用量：催眠，个体差异大；镇静，每次 2mg/kg（或 60mg/m²），一日 3 次。<br>（2）肌内或缓慢静脉注射：①成人，常用量：催眠，每次 0.1 ～ 0.2g；镇静，每次 0.03 ～ 0.05mg，一日 2 ～ 3 次；抗惊厥（癫痫持续状态），缓慢静脉注射 0.3 ～ 0.5g。极量：1 次 0.25g，一日 0.5g。②小儿，常用量：催眠（或抗惊厥），肌内注射每次 3 ～ 5mg/kg（或 125mg/m²）；镇静，每日 6mg/kg，一日 2 ～ 3 次。 |

**续　表**

|  |  |
| --- | --- |
|  | (1) Por vía oral：　① Dosis habitual para adultos: En hipnotización para pacientes que tienen dificultad de dormirse, se toma 0.1 ~ 0.2g antes de acostarse. Para sedación la dosis es de 0.02~0.04g 2 ó 3 tomas al día. Dosis máxima no excede a 0.2g cada vez y 0.6g diarios. Para pacientes ancianos y debiles hay que disminuir la dosis porque puede causar exitación, insania o depresión con medicación a dosis habitual. ② Dosis habitual para infantes: Para hipnotización la dosis varian según cada paciente y hay gran diferencia. Para sedación la dosis es de 2mg/kg o 60mg/ ㎡ 3 veces al día.<br><br>(2) Inyección por I.M. o lenta inyección por I.V.:　① Dosis habitual para adultos: Para hipnotización la dosis es de 0.1~0.2g . Para sedación la dosis es de 0.03~0.05mg 2 ó 3 tomas al día. Para anticonvulsiones ( estado epiléptico), toma la lenta inyección por I.V. a dosis de 0.3~0.5g. Dosis máxima no excede a 0.25g cada vez y 0.5g diarios. ② Dosis habitual para infantes: Para hipnotización o anticonvulsiones, se administra inyección por I.M. a dosis de 3~5mg/kg o 125mg/ ㎡ cada vez, para sedación la dosis es de 6mg/kg diarios divididos en 2 ~ 3 tomas. |
| 剂型、规格<br>Formulaciones y especificaciones | 片剂：每片 0.1g 。注射用异戊巴比妥钠：每支 0.1g；0.25g。<br>Tableta: 0.1g; Amobarbital para inyección: 0.1g, 0.25g. |

| 药品名称 Drug Names | 司可巴比妥 Secobarbital |
| --- | --- |
| 适应证<br>Indicaciones | 主要适用于不易入睡的患者。也可用于抗惊厥。<br>Se usa principalmente para pacientes con dificultad de dormirse y también sirve como anticonvulsivo. |
| 用法、用量<br>Administración y dosis | 口服：成人常用量，催眠 0.1 ~ 0.2g，临睡前一次顿服；镇静 1 次 30 ~ 50mg，一日 3 ~ 4 次。成人极量 1 次 0.3g。尚可皮下注射（1 次量 0.1g）。<br>Por vía oral: Dosis habitual para adultos es de 0.1 ~ 0.2g para hipnosis tomados antes de acostarse, 30 ~ 50 mg 3 ó 4 veces al dia para sedación. Dosis máxima para adultos es de 0.3g cada vez. Inyección subcutánea aceptable(0.1g cada vez). |
| 剂型、规格<br>Formulaciones y especificaciones | 胶囊剂：每粒 0.1g；注射用司可巴比妥：每支 0.05g。<br>Cápsula: 0.1g: Secobarbital para Inyección: 0.05g. |

| 药品名称 Drug Names | 佐匹克隆 Zopiclona |
| --- | --- |
| 适应证<br>Indicaciones | 用于各种原因引起的失眠症，尤其适用于不能耐受次晨残余作用的患者。<br>Se usa para tratamiento de insomnio causado por variedad de razones, especialmente para los pacientes que no pueden tolerar los efectos residuales de la mañana siguiente. |
| 用法、用量<br>Administración y dosis | 睡前服 7.5mg。老年人、肝功能不全者，睡前服 3.75mg，必要时可增加至 7.5mg。<br>Por vía oral a dosis de 7.5 mg antes de acostarse, Para ancianos y pacientes con disfunción hepática se toma 3.75 mg antes de acostarse y puede aumentar hasta 7.5 mg en caso necesario. |
| 剂型、规格<br>Formulaciones y especificaciones | 片剂：每片 3.75mg；7.5mg。<br>Tableta: 3.75mg, 7.5 mg. |

| 药品名称 Drug Names | 唑吡坦 Zolpidem |
| --- | --- |
| 适应证<br>Indicaciones | 用于治疗短暂性、偶发性失眠症或慢性失眠的短期治疗。<br>Se usa para tratamiento a corto plazo de insomnio transitorio y ocasional, insomnio crónico. |
| 用法、用量<br>Administración y dosis | 常用量为 10mg，睡前服。偶发性失眠，一般用药 2 ~ 5 日。长期用药应不超过 4 周。老年人及肝功能不全者剂量减半，必要时可增至 10mg。<br>Dosis habitual es de 10mg antes de acostarse. Para insomnio ocasional se administra durante 2 ~ 5 dias. La medicación a largo plazo no debe exceder a 4 semanas. Para ancianos y pacientes con disfunción hepática, la dosis será la mitad de la habidual y puede aumentar hasta 10 mg si es necesario. |
| 剂型、规格<br>Formulaciones y especificaciones | 片剂：每片 10mg；5mg。<br>Tableta: 10 mg, 5mg. |

| 药品名称 Drug Names | 水合氯醛 Hidrato de cloral |
|---|---|
| 适应证<br>Indicaciones | 用于神经性失眠、伴有显著兴奋的精神病及破伤风痉挛、士的宁中毒等。<br><br>Se usa para tratamiento de insomnio por nervios, psicosis acompañada con excitación evidente, tetanospasmina e intoxicación por estricnina. |
| 用法、用量<br>Administración y dosis | 口服或灌肠。常用量，一次 0.5～1.5g，极量，一次 2g，一日 4g。睡前 1 次。口服 10% 溶液 5～15ml（一般服 10ml），以多量水稀释并添加胶浆剂（掩盖其不良臭味，避免刺激）后服用，或服用其合剂（加有淀粉、糖浆剂）以减少刺激。抗惊厥：多用灌肠法给药，将 10% 溶液 15～20ml 稀释 1～2 倍后 1 次灌入。<br><br>Por vía oral o enema. Dosis habitual es de 0.5~1.5g cada vez y la máxima no excede a 2g cada vez o 4g diarios. Se toma 1 vez antes de acostarse. Administración oral de 5～15ml (generalmente se toma 10ml) de la solución a 10% diluidos con gran cantidad de agua e hidrogel que se lo agrega para ocultar su mal olor y evitar la irritación, o también puede tomar su mezcla con almidón y jarabe para eliminar la irritación. Para uso anticonvulsivo habitualmente hace enema de 15～20ml de solución a 10% diluida a 1～2 veces de la cantidad de la solución. |
| 剂型、规格<br>Formulaciones y especificaciones | 水合氯醛合剂：有水合氯醛 65g，溴化钠 65g，淀粉 20g，枸橼酸 0.25g，薄荷水 0.5ml，琼脂糖浆 500ml，蒸馏水适量，共配成 1000ml。水合氯醛遇热易挥发分解，须调好其他成分防冷后再加入。如无琼脂糖浆时可用单糖浆代替。<br><br>Mezcla de hidrato de cloral: 1000ml que incluye 65g de hidrato de cloral, 65g de bromuro de sodio, 20g de almidón, 0.25g de citrato, 0.5ml de agua de menta, 500ml de jarabe de agarose y agua destilada. Como el hidrato de cloral se descompuesta facilmente cuando se calienta, hay que agregarlo después de que tenga listo otros compuestos. Si no hay jarabe de agorose puede usar almíbar simple como alternativa. |

| 药品名称 Drug Names | 扎来普隆 Zaleplón |
|---|---|
| 适应证<br>Indicaciones | 用于入睡困难的失眠症的短期治疗。临床研究结果显示扎来普隆能缩短入睡时间，但还未见其能增加睡眠时间和减少清醒次数。<br><br>Se usa en tratamiento a corto plazo de insomnio que tenga dificultad de dormirse. Los estudios clínicos muestra que el zaleplón puede acortar el tiempo para conciliar el sueño pero aún no se refleja el aumento del tiempo del sueño o reducción de despierto. |
| 用法、用量<br>Administración y dosis | 口服，一次 5～10mg（1～2 粒），睡前服用或入睡困难时服用。与所有的镇静催眠药一样，当清醒时，服用会导致记忆损伤、幻觉、协调障碍、头晕。体重较轻的患者，推荐剂量为一次 5mg（1 粒）。老年患者、糖尿病患者和轻、中度肝功能不全患者，推荐剂量为一次 5mg（1 粒）。每晚只服用一次。持续用药时间限制在 7～10 日。如果服药 7～10 日后失眠仍未减轻，医生应对患者失眠的原因重新评估。<br><br>Por vía oral a dosis de 5～10mg cada vez (1～2 tabletas). Se administra antes de acostarse o cuando no puede conciliar el sueño. Igual como otros sedantes-hipnóticos, si lo toman cuando está sobrio puede causar pérdida de memoria, alucinaciones, trastornos de coordinación y mareos. Para pacientes con menor peso,ancianos, diabéticos y los de disfunción hepática leve o moderada, la dosis recomendada es de 5mg (1 tableta). Se toma 1 vez cada noche y la medicación continua debe aplicarse en 7～10 días. Si lo continua después de este tiempo y no hay efecto en el alivio de insomnio, médicos deben reevaluar el razón del insomnio. |
| 剂型、规格<br>Formulaciones y especificaciones | 胶布剂：每粒 5mg。片剂、分散片：片剂 5mg。<br><br>Cinta: 5mg; Tableta y comprimidos dispersable: 5mg. |

| 药品名称 Drug Names | 艾司佐匹克隆 Eszopiclona |
|---|---|
| 适应证<br>Indicaciones | 用于失眠的短期治疗。<br><br>Se usa para tratamiento a corto plazo de insomnio. |
| 用法、用量<br>Administración y dosis | 常用量为睡前口服 2mg，可逐渐增量至 3mg。对于入睡困难的老年患者起始剂量推荐为 1mg，可逐渐增量至 2mg。对于易醒的老年患者起始剂量为 2mg。<br><br>Dosis habitual: administración oral de 2mg antes de acostarse y puede aumentarse gradualmente a 3mg. Para pacientes ancianos que tienen dificultad de dormirse recomienda una dosis inicial de 1mg y aumentar gradualmente a 2mg. Para ancianos que se despierta facilmente recomienda una dosis inicial de 2mg. |

**续　表**

| 剂型、规格<br>Formulaciones y especificaciones | 片剂：2mg，3mg。<br>Tableta::2mg,3mg. |
|---|---|
| **药品名称 Drug Names** | **溴化钾 Bromuro de potasio** |
| 适应证<br>Indicaciones | 常用于神经衰弱。癔症、神经性失眠、精神兴奋状态。<br>Se usa para tratamiento de neurastenia, síntomas histeria, insomnio por nervios y excitación mental. |
| 用法、用量<br>Administración y dosis | 口服：10% 溶液 5～10ml，一日 3 次。饭后服。不宜空腹服用。<br>Por vía oral a dosis de 5～10ml de la solución a 10%, 3 veces al día después de alimentos. No recomienda tomarla en ayunas. |
| 剂型、规格<br>Formulaciones y especificaciones | 溶液：10%。<br>Solución: 10%. |
| **药品名称 Drug Names** | **戊巴比妥钠 Pentobarbital sódico** |
| 适应证<br>Indicaciones | 同异戊巴比妥，用于催眠、麻醉前给药。<br>Igual como Amobarbital que se usa para hipnotización y administración antes de anestesia. |
| 用法、用量<br>Administración y dosis | 催眠：0.1～0.2g；麻醉前给药：手术当日清晨服 0.1g，必要时术前半小时再服 0.1g。极量：1 次 0.2g，一日 0.6g。<br>Para hipnotización: 0.1～0.2g; Administración antes de anestesia: 0.1g en la mañana del dia de cirugía. Y si es necesario, toma otro 0.1g media hora antes de la cirugía. |
| 剂型、规格<br>Formulaciones y especificaciones | 片剂：0.05g；0.1g。注射剂：0.1g；0.5g。<br>Tableta: 0.05g, 0.1g; Inyección: 0.1g, 0.5g. |

8.7　抗帕金森病药 Medicamentos contra la enfermedad de parkinson

| **药品名称 Drug Names** | **左旋多巴 Levodopa** |
|---|---|
| 适应证<br>Indicaciones | 改善肌强直和运动迟缓效果明显，持续用药对震颤、流涎、姿势不稳及吞咽困难亦有效。①帕金森病（原发性震颤麻痹）；脑炎后或合并有脑动脉硬化及中枢神经系统的一氧化碳与猛中毒后的症状性帕金森综合征（非药源性震颤麻痹综合征）。可减轻没震颤麻痹的症状，改善肌张力，使肢体活动更趋正常。对轻、中度病情者效果较好，重度或老年患者较差。②肝性脑病：可使患者清醒，症状改善。肝性脑病可能与中枢递质多巴胺异常有关，服用后，可改善中枢功能而奏效。亦有学者认为左旋多巴可提高大脑对氨的耐受性，但不能改善肝脏损伤和肝功能。③神经痛：早期服用可缓解神经痛。④高泌乳素血症：可抑制下丘脑的促甲状腺激素释放激素，兴奋泌乳素释放抑制因子，因而减少泌乳素的分泌，用于治疗高泌乳素血症，对乳溢症有一定疗效。⑤脱毛症：其机制可能是增加血液到组织的儿茶酚胺浓度，促进毛发生长。⑥促进小儿生长发育：可通过促进生长激素的分泌，加速小儿骨骼的生长发育。治疗垂体功能低下症。<br>Tiene efecto evidente en mejorar los síntomas de la rigidez muscular y bradicinesia. Su medicación a largo plaza es eficaz para tratamiento de temblores, salivación, inestabilidad postural y dificultad para tragar. ① Se usa para enfermedad de Parkinson (parkinsonismo primario), Parkinsonismo sintomático (Parkinsonismo no farmacológico) después de la encefalitis o asociado con arteriosclerosis cerebral y envenenamiento por monóxido y manganeso en el sistema nervioso central. Puede aliviar los síntomas de Parkinsonismo y mejorar el tono muscular para que la actividad física sea más normal. Es más eficacia para caso leve y moderado en comparación con caso severo y pacientes ancianos. ② Se usa para encefalopatía hepática: puede hacer despertar a los pacientes y mejorar los síntomas. La encefalopatía hepática puede ser relacionado con la anormalidad de Dopamina, un neurotransmisor central, así que es eficaz mediante mejorar la función central. También hay gente cree que la Levodopa puede mejorar la tolerancia cerebral al amonio pero no tiene efecto en mejorar el daño hepático y la función hepática. ③ Se usa para neuralgia: El uso temprano puede aliviar la neuralgia. ④ Se usa para hiperprolactinemia: Puede inhibir la secreción de hormona liberadora de tirotropina hipotalámica y hacer excitar factor inhibidor para reducir la secreción de prolactina. Se usa en tratamiento de hiperprolactinemia y tiene cierto efecto para el síndrome de galactorrea. ⑤ Se usa para alopecia: El mecanismo del fármaco puede ser aumentar la concentración de catecolamina en la sangre a los tejidos así que promueve el crecimiento del cabello. ⑥ Se usa para promover el crecimiento y desarrollo del niño: Puede acelerar el crecimiento y desarrollo de hueso del niño mediante la promoción de la secreción de hormona del crecimiento. También puede usarse en tratamiento de hipopituitarismo. |

| | |
|---|---|
| 用法、用量<br>Administración y dosis | ①治疗震颤麻痹：口服，开始时一日 0.25～0.5g，分 2～3 次服用。每服 2～4 日后，每日量增加 0.125～0.5g。维持量 1 日 3～6g，分 4～6 次服，连续用药 2～3 周见效。在剂量递增过程中，如出现恶心等，应停止增量，待症状消失后在增量。②治疗肝性脑病：1 日 0.3～0.4g，加入 5% 葡萄糖溶液 500ml 中静脉滴注，待完全清醒后，减量至 1 日 0.2g，继续 1～2 日后停药。或用本品 5g 加入生理盐水 100ml 中，鼻饲或灌肠。<br><br>① En tratamiento de parkinsonismo: Por vía oral. Dosis inicial es de 0.25～0.5g diarios divididos en 2 ó 3 tomas. En cada 2～4 días aumenta en 0.125～0.5g diarios. La dosis de mantenimiento es de 3～6g diarios divididos en 4～6 tomas. Se ve efecto dentro de 2 ó 3 semanas de medicación. Si al aumentar la dosis aparece acción adversa como náusea, debe dejar aumentarla y vuelve a agregar cuando desaparezca el síntoma. ② En tratamiento de encefalopatía hepática: Se administra infusión por I.V. a dosis de 0.3～0.4g diarios diluidos en 500ml de solución de glucosa a 5%. Cuando se despierta totalmente el paciente, reduce la dosis a 0.2g diarios y continua la medicación dentro de 1 ó 2 días. O puede administrarse también por nasogástrica o enema a dosis de 5g diluidos en 100ml de Normal Saline. |
| 剂型、规格<br>Formulaciones y especificaciones | 片剂：每片 50mg；100mg；250mg。胶囊剂：每粒 100mg；125mg；250mg。<br>Tableta: 50mg, 100mg, 250mg; Cápsula: 100mg, 125mg, 250mg. |
| **药品名称 Drug Names** | 卡比多巴 Carbidopa |
| 适应证<br>Indicaciones | ①主用与左旋多巴合用治疗各种原因引起的帕金森症，可获较好临床效果，但晚期重型患者的治疗较差。②本品与左旋多巴联合应用，治疗单眼弱视疗效好，尤其是对屈光参差性单眼弱视、弱视性质为中心注视的弱视。<br><br>① Tiene buen efecto clínico en tratamiento de enfermedad de Parkinson en conjunción con Levodopa pero no es muy eficaz para pacientes graves de dicha enfermedad avanzada. ② En combinación con Levodopa tiene eficacia en tratamiento de ambliopía monocular especialmente la ambliopía monocular anisometropía y la ambliopía con fijación central. |
| 用法、用量<br>Administración y dosis | 首次剂量，卡比多巴 10mg，左旋多巴 100mg，一日 4 次；以后每隔 3～7 日每日增加卡比多巴 40mg，左旋多巴 400mg，直至每日量卡比多巴 200mg，左旋多巴 2g 为限。多采用其复方制剂如患者先用左旋多巴，需停药 8 小时以上才能在合用二药。<br><br>Dosis inicial: 10 mg de carbidopa y 100mg de levodopa, 4 veces al día. Luego incrementar la dosis cada 3～7 días en 40mg de carbidopa y 400mg de levodopa. La dosis máxima diaria es de 200mg de carbidopa y 2g de levodopa. Siempre utiliza su preparación en compuesto. Generalmente pacientes puede tomar el carbidopa dentro de 8 horas si toman primero levodopa. |
| 剂型、规格<br>Formulaciones y especificaciones | 片剂：每片 25mg。<br>Tableta: 25mg. |
| **药品名称 Drug Names** | 苄丝肼 Benserazida |
| 适应证<br>Indicaciones | 一般苄丝肼与左旋多巴按 1：4 配伍应用，用于帕金森病和帕金森综合征，可减少左旋多巴的用量，增强其疗效并减其外周不良反应。对药物引起的帕金森症无效。<br><br>Se usa generalmente en conjunción con Levodopa a razón de 1：4 en tratamiento de enfermedad de parkinson y parkinsonismo. Puede disminuir la cantidad de Levodopa para mejorar la eficacia de Benserazida y reducir reacciones adversas perifericas relativas. No es eficaz para parkinsonismo causado por fármacos. |
| 用法、用量<br>Administración y dosis | 多与左旋多巴合用，开始时 1 次，苄丝肼 25mg 及左旋多巴 100ng，一日 2 次；然后每隔 1 周将苄丝肼增加 25mg/d 及左旋多巴 100mg/d，至每日剂量苄丝肼达 250mg 及左旋多巴达 100mg 为止。分 3～4 次服用。<br><br>Se usa generalmente en conjunción con Levodopa. Inicialmente se toma cada vez 25mg de Benserazida y 100mg de Levodopa y dos veces al día. Después agrega cada 2 semana en 25mg/d de Benserazida y 100mg/d de Levodopa hasta que la dosis diaria llega a 250mg de Benserazida y 100mg de Levodopa y se toman divididos en 3～4 veces. |

**续 表**

| 剂型、规格<br>Formulaciones y especificaciones | 多巴丝肼：每胶囊 125mg（含苄丝肼 25mg 及左旋多巴 100mg）；250mg（含苄丝肼 50mg 及左旋多巴 200mg）。<br>Levodopa y benserazida: cápsula 125mg(incluyendo 25mg de Benserazida y 100mg de Levodopa); cápsula 250mg (incluyendo 50mg de Benserazida y 200mg de Levodopa). |
|---|---|
| **药品名称 Drug Names** | 多巴丝肼 Levodopa y benserazida |
| 适应证<br>Indicaciones | 适用于原发性震颤麻痹（帕金森病）、脑炎后或合并有脑动脉硬化的症状性帕金森综合征。<br>Se usa para tratamiento de parkinsonismo primaria (enfermedad de Parkinson), síndrome parkinsonismo de encefalitis asociada con la arteriosclerosis cerebral. |
| 用法、用量<br>Administración y dosis | 口服，成人，第一周 1 次 125mg，2 次 / 日。以后每隔 1 周每日增加 125mg。一般日剂量不得超过 1g，分 3～4 次服用。<br>Por vía oral. Para adultos: dosis diaria de 250mg divididas en 2 tomas en la primera semana. Aumenta la dosis cada 2 semanas en 125mg y dosis diaria máxima no excede a 1g divididos en 3 ~ 4 tomas. |
| 剂型、规格<br>Formulaciones y especificaciones | 胶囊剂、片剂：① 125mg：左旋多巴 100mg 和苄丝肼 25mg；② 250mg：左旋多巴 200mg 和苄丝肼 50mg。控释片：125mg。分散片：125mg。<br>Cápsula/Tableta: ① 125mg: Levodopa 100mg y Benserazida 25mg, ② 250mg: Levodopa 200mg y Benserazida 50mg; Tableta de liberación controlada: 125mg; Comprimido dispersable：125mg. |
| **药品名称 Drug Names** | 溴隐亭 Bromocriptina |
| 适应证<br>Indicaciones | ①抗震颤麻痹，疗效优于金刚烷胺及苯海索，对僵直、少动亦效果好，对重症患者亦效果好，常用于左旋多巴疗效不佳或不能耐受患者，症状波动者，对左旋多巴复方制剂无效者。特点是显效快，持续时间长。②治疗慢性精神分裂症和躁狂症，尤其是以阴性症状为主的精神病理基础，是多巴胺功能降低所致。治疗抑郁症，通过增强多巴胺能神经元的活性而对抑郁症有效。治疗抗精神病药恶性综合征。③闭经或乳溢，用于各种原因所致催乳激素过高引起的闭经或乳溢，对垂体瘤诱发者，可作为手术或放射治疗的辅助治疗。④抑制生理性泌乳。⑤用于催乳激素过高的引起的经前期综合征，对周期性乳房痛和乳房结节，可使症状改善，但对非周期性乳房痛和月经正常几乎无效。⑥用于肢端肥大症，无功能性垂体肿瘤，垂体性甲状腺功能亢进。治疗库欣病：大多数库欣病由皮质素瘤引起，少数为下丘脑分泌促甲状腺激素释放激素异常。溴隐亭可以降低促皮质素，故可以治疗库欣病。⑦治疗女性不育症。⑧治疗男性性功能减退，对男性乳腺发育、阳痿、精液不足等有一定疗效。⑨治疗可卡因戒断综合征，可有效减轻可卡因的瘾欲和戒断的焦虑症状。⑩可用于 huntington 舞蹈症。<br><br>① Se usa en tratamiento de parkinsonismo y tiene mejor efecto que amantadina y trihexifenidilo. Es eficaz para rigidez y falta de ejercicio tanto leves como severos. Se usa habitualmente para pacientes que no puede conseguir buen efecto con medicación de levodopa, o intolerantes a este fármaco, o tiene síntomas fluctúan tras medicación, o los que no tiene eficacia desde compuesto levodopa. Se caracteriza por la rápida acción y larga duración. ② Se usa en tratamiento de esquizofrenia crónica y manía, especialmente esquizofrenia basica con síntomas negativos causados por la función reduida de la dopamina. También puede usarse en tratamiento de depresión mediante mejorar la actividad de las neuronas dopaminérgicas así como el síndrome neuroléptico maligno. ③ Se usa en tratamiento de amenorrea o galactorrea causados por la alta prolactina. Para pacientes de tumores hipofisarios, puede usar como medicación adyuvante en cirugía o radioterapia. ④ En inhibición de la lactancia fisiológica. ⑤ Se usa en tratamiento de Síndrome Premenstrual causado por la alta prolactina y puede mejorar síntomas del dolor cíclico del seno y los nódulos de mama. No tiene eficacia en dolor no cíclico en los senos o menstruación normal. ⑥ Se usa en tratamiento de acromegalia, tumor hipofisario no funcionante, e hipertiroidismo pituitaria. También se usa para enfermedad de Cushing que causada principalmente por tumor de corticotropina y otros casos menores, por la secreción hipotalámica inormal de GRH. La bromocriptina puede reducir la corticotropina que en este caso puede usarse para tratar la enfermedad de Cushing. ⑦ Se usa en tratamiento de la infertilidad femenina. ⑧ Se usa en tratamiento de la disfunción sexual masculina. Tiene cierta eficacia en tratamiento de ginecomastia, impotencia y falta de esperma. ⑨ Se usa en tratamiento de síndrome de abstinencia de la cocaína aliviando la adicción a la cocaína y síntomas de ansiedad en la abstinencia. ⑩ Se usa en tratamiento de corea de Huntington. |

**续 表**

| 用法、用量<br>Administración y dosis | ①震颤麻痹：开始每次 1.25mg，一日 2 次，2 周内逐渐加量，必要时每 2～4 周每日增加 2.5mg，以找到最佳治疗的最小剂量，每日剂量 20mg 为宜。②用于闭经或溢乳、抑制泌乳、不育症、肢端肥大等。<br><br>① En tratamiento de parkinsonismo: dosis inicial es de 1.25mg 2 veces al día y aumenta gradualmente la dosis en 2 semanas. Si es necesario puede aumentar en 2.5mg diarios cada 2 ~ 4 semanas para llegar a la dosis mínima con mejor eficacia. Dosis diaria recomendada es de 20mg. ② En tratamiento de amenorrea, galactorrea, supresión de la lactancia, esterilidad y acromegalia. |
|---|---|
| 剂型、规格<br>Formulaciones y especificaciones | 片剂：每片 2.5mg。<br>Tableta: 2.5mg. |
| 药品名称 Drug Names | 普拉克索 Pramipexol |
| 适应证<br>Indicaciones | 单独或与左旋多巴合用于治疗帕金森病，可明显减少静息时的震颤。晚期帕金森病用该药与左旋多巴共同的治疗时，可使患者对左旋多巴的治疗量减少 27%～30%，并可延长症状最佳控制时间平均每天 2 小时。<br><br>Se usa para tratamiento de enfermedad de Parkinson con utilizacion individual o en conjunción con Levodopa. Puede reducir significativamente el temblor de reposo. Para pacientes de enfermedad de Parkinson avanzada puede disminuir el medicamento de levodopa en 27% ~ 30% de la dosis y prolonga el tiempo de control óptimo de los síntomas a 2 horas por día. |
| 用法、用量<br>Administración y dosis | 按病情程度每次 1.5～4.5mg，一日 3 次。<br>Dosis de 1.5 ~ 4.5mg según la condición del paciente, 3 veces al día. |
| 剂型、规格<br>Formulaciones y especificaciones | 片剂：片剂 0.125mg；0.25mg；0.5mg；1mg；1.5mg。<br>Tableta: 0.125mg, 0.25mg, 0.5mg, 1mg, 1.5mg. |
| 药品名称 Drug Names | 司来吉兰 Selegilina |
| 适应证<br>Indicaciones | 适用于帕金森病，常作为左旋多巴、美多巴或信尼麦的辅助用药。<br>Se usa en tratamiento de la enfermedad de Parkinson y a menudo sirve como medicamento adyuvante de levodopa, madopar o sinemet. |
| 用法、用量<br>Administración y dosis | 口服，每日 10mg，早晨 1 次顿服；或每次 5mg，早、晚 2 次服用。<br>Por vía oral. Dosis diaria es de 10mg una vez en la mañana o divididos en 2 tomas en la mañana y en la noche. |
| 剂型、规格<br>Formulaciones y especificaciones | 片剂：每片 5mg。<br>Tableta: 5 mg. |
| 药品名称 Drug Names | 雷沙吉兰 Rasagilina |
| 适应证<br>Indicaciones | 用于治疗帕金森病，可单用或作为左旋多巴的辅助用药。<br>Se usa en tratamiento de la enfermedad de Parkinson y puede administrarse individualmente o como medicamento adyuvante de levodopa. |
| 用法、用量<br>Administración y dosis | 单药治疗：每次 1mg，一日 1 次。与左旋多巴联合治疗：起始剂量每次 0.5mg，一日 1 次，维持剂量为 0.5～1mg，一日 1 次。老年患者需调整剂量。<br><br>Uso individual: 1mg una vez al día; Uso adyuvante en conjunción con levodopa: dosis diaria inicial es de 0.5mg y la de mantenimiento es de 0.5 ~ 1mg. Para pacientes ancianos debe seguir con el consejo especifico de médicos. |
| 剂型、规格<br>Formulaciones y especificaciones | 片剂：0.5mg；1mg。<br>Tableta: 0.5mg, 1mg. |

续　表

| 药品名称 Drug Names | 苯海索 Trihexifenidilo |
|---|---|
| 适应证<br>Indicaciones | ①临床用于震颤麻痹，脑炎后或动脉硬化引起的震颤麻痹，对改善流涎有效，对缓解僵直、运动迟缓疗效较差，改善震颤明显，但总的治疗效果不及左旋多巴、金刚烷胺。主要用于轻症及不耐受左旋多巴的患者。常与左旋多巴合用。②药用利血平及吩噻嗪类引起的锥体外系反应。③肝豆状核变性。④畸形性肌张力障碍、癫痫、慢性精神分裂症、抗精神病药所致的静坐不能。<br><br>① Se usa clínicamente en tratamiento de enfermedad de Parkinson y parkinsonismo causado por encefalitis o arteriosclerosis. Es eficaz para mejorar la salivación y tiene efecto significativo en aliviar temblor. Tiene poca eficacia en aliviar la rigidez y bradicinesia. El efecto general de tratamiento no es tan bueno como levodopa y amantadina. Se usa principalmente en pacientes leves e intolerantes a levodopa. Habitualmente lo usa en conjunción con levodopa.　② Se usa en tratamiento de reacciones extrapiramidales inducidas por reserpina y fenotiazina.　③ Se usa en tratamiento de hepatolenticular degeneración.　④ Se usa en tratamiento de distonía muscular deformante, epilepsia, esquizofrenia crónica y acatisia causada por fármacos antipsicóticos. |
| 用法、用量<br>Administración y dosis | 常用量：口服，开始时一日 1～2mg，一日 2 次；逐日递增至一日 5～10mg，分次服用。对药物引起的锥体外系反应：口服开始第一日 1mg，并逐增剂量直至每日 5～10mg，一日 2 次。口服，一日最多不超过 10mg。<br><br>Dosis habitual: Por vía oral. Dosis inicial es de 1～2mg diarios divididos en 2 tomas y agrega gradualmente a 5～10mg diarios divididos en viarias tomas. En caso de reacciones extrapiramidales inducidas por fármacos: Por vía oral. Dosis inicial es de 1mg en el primer dia y agraga gradualmente a 5-10mg diarios divididos en 2 tomas. Dosis máxima por vía oral no excede a 10mg diarios. |
| 剂型、规格<br>Formulaciones y especificaciones | 片剂：每片 2mg。胶囊剂：每粒 5mg。<br>Tableta: 2 mg. Cápsula: 5mg. |
| 药品名称 Drug Names | 金刚烷胺 Amantadina |
| 适应证<br>Indicaciones | ①用于不能耐受左旋多巴治疗的震颤麻痹患者；②亚洲 A-Ⅱ型流感、病毒性感染发热患者；③脑梗死所致的自发性意识低下。<br><br>① Se usa en pacientes de parkinsonismo que no toleran el tratamiento con levodopa; ② Se usa en pacientes con fiebre por la infección del virus de la influenza asiática tipo A-Ⅱ; ③ Se usa en pacientes de baja conciencia espontánea dedibo al infarto cerebral. |
| 用法、用量<br>Administración y dosis | 口服：成人每次 100mg，早晚各 1 次，最大剂量每日 400mg。小儿用量酌减，可连用 3～5 日，最多 10 日。1～9 岁小儿每日 3mg/kg，最大用量不超过 150mg/d。<br><br>Por vía oral. Para adultos: dosis diaria de 100mg divididos en 2 tomas y la máxima no excede a 400mg. Para niños: la dosis se reduce y puede continuar la medicación dentro de 3～5 dias o 10 dias como máximo. Niños de entre 1～9 años administran dosis diaria de 3mg/kg y la dosis máxima no excede a 150mg/d. |
| 剂型、规格<br>Formulaciones y especificaciones | 片剂：每片 100mg。胶囊剂：每粒 100mg。糖浆剂：60ml：300mg。颗粒剂：6g：60mg；12g：140mg。<br>Tableta: 100mg; Cápsula: 100mg; Jarabe: 60ml:300mg; Gránulos: 6g:60mg 12g:140mg. |
| 药品名称 Drug Names | 美金刚 Memantina |
| 适应证<br>Indicaciones | ①用于震颤麻痹综合征。②能够改善阿尔茨海默病患者的认知、行为、日常活动和临床症状，可用于重度患者。<br><br>① Se usa para tratamiento del parkinsonismo.　② Se usa en pacientes de Alzheimerpuede para mejorar su cognición, el comportamiento, las actividades de la vida diaria y los síntomas clínicos relacionados. Se puede usar en pacientes graves. |
| 用法、用量<br>Administración y dosis | 口服或胃肠道给药，成人和 14 岁以上青年第 1 周，每日 10mg，分 2～3 次给药；以后每周增加 10mg/d。维持剂量：一次 10mg，一日 2～3 次。需要时还可增加。剂量因人而异。14 岁以下儿童的维持量为每日 0.5～1.0mg/kg。<br><br>Por vía oral o parenteral. Para adultos y juventud mayor de 14 años, dosis diaria es de 10mg divididos en 2 ó 3 tomas en la primera semana y aumenta la dosis cada semana en 10mg/d. Dosis de mantenimiento es de 10mg diarios divididos en 2 ó 3 tomas y puede agregar la dosis segun la necesidad y condición física de pacientes. Para pacientes menores de 14 años, dosis diaria de mantenimiento es del 0.5～1.0 mg/kg. |

**续　表**

| 剂型、规格<br>Formulaciones y especificaciones | 片剂：每片 10mg。滴剂：10mg。注射液：每支 10mg（2ml）。<br>Tableta: 10mg. Gota: 10mg. Inyección: 10mg (2ml). |
|---|---|

### 8.8　抗精神病药 Antipsicóticos

| 药品名称 Drug Names | 氯丙嗪 Clorpromazina |
|---|---|
| 适应证<br>Indicaciones | ①治疗精神病：用于控制精神分裂症或其他精神病的兴奋躁动、紧张不安、幻觉、妄想等症状，对忧郁症状及木僵症状的疗效较差。对Ⅱ型精神分裂症患者无效，甚至可以加重病情。②镇吐：几乎对各种原因引起的呕吐，如尿毒症、胃肠炎、癌症、妊娠及药物引起的呕吐均有效。也可治疗严重呃逆。但对晕动症呕吐无效。③低温麻醉及人工冬眠：用于低温麻醉时可以防止休克发生。人工冬眠时，与哌替啶、异丙嗪配成冬眠合剂用于创伤性休克、中毒性休克、烧伤、高热及甲状腺危象的辅助治疗。④与镇痛药合用，治疗癌症晚期患者的剧痛。⑤治疗心力衰竭。⑥试用于治疗巨人症。<br><br>① Se usa en tratamiento de psicosis controlando la esquizofrenia o otros síntomas de psicosis como por ejempro excitación y agitación, estado nervioso, alucinación y dilirios. La eficacia no es buena para depresión y estupor. No tiene efecto en esquizofrenia de tipo II hasta que puede empeorar la enfermedad.　② Se usa en tratamiento de vómitos causados por uremia, gastroenteritis, cáncer, gestación y fármacos.　③ Se usa en anestesia de hipotermia y la hibernación artificial. En anestesia de hipotermia lo usa para prevención de choque. En la hibernación artificial lo usa en conjunción con meperidina y prometazina para tratamiento de choque traumático, choque tóxico, quemaduras, fiebre alta y tratamiento adyuvante de la tormenta tiroidea. ④ Se usa en conjunción con sedantes para alivio del dolor violento de cáncer avanzada. ⑤ Se usa para tratamiento de insuficiencia cardíaca. ⑥ Puede usarse en tratamiento de gigantismo. |
| 用法、用量<br>Administración y dosis | ①口服：a.用于呕吐，1次12.5～25mg，一日2～3次；b.用于精神病，1日50～600mg。开始每日25～50mg，分2～3次服用，逐渐增加至每日300～450mg，症状减轻后再减至1日100～150mg。极量每次150mg，每日600mg。②肌内或静脉注射：a.用于呕吐，1次25～50mg；b.用于神经病，1次25～100mg。目前多采用静脉注射。极量每次100mg，每日400mg。c.治疗心力衰竭：肌内注射小剂量，每次5～10mg，一日1～2次，也可静脉滴注，速度每分钟0.5mg。<br><br>① Por vía oral. a. Para vómitos: 12.5～25mg 2 ó 3 veces al día. b. Para psicosis: 50～600mg diarios. Dosis inicial es de 25～50mg diarios divididos en 2 ó 3 tomas y agrega gradualmente a 300～450mg diarios. Cuando se alivia los síntomas reduce a 100～150mg diarios. Dosis máxima es de 150mg cada vez y 600mg diarios. ② Intramuscular e intravenosa: a. para el vómito, 25～50mg cada vez; b. Para la psicosis, 25～100mg cada vez, principalmente por vía intravenosa. El límite de administracíon es 100mg, 400mg por día. c. Para el tratamiento de la insuficiencia cardíaca, inyección intramuscular de 5 a 10mg una a dos veces al día; Por vía intravenosa, 0.5mg por minuto. |
| 剂型、规格<br>Formulaciones y especificaciones | 片剂：每片5mg；12.5mg；25mg；50mg。注射液：每支10mg（1ml）；25g（1ml）；50mg（2ml）。<br>Tableta: 5mg, 12.5mg, 25mg, 50mg; Inyección: 10mg (1ml), 25mg (1ml), 50mg (2ml). |
| 药品名称 Drug Names | 奋乃静 Perfenazina |
| 适应证<br>Indicaciones | ①用于治疗偏执性精神病、反应性精神病、症状性精神病，单纯性及慢性精神分裂症。②用于治疗恶心、呕吐、呃逆等症，神经症具有焦虑紧张症的患者，亦可用小剂量配合其他药物治疗。<br><br>① Se usa en tratamiento de psicosis paranoide, psicosis reactiva, psicosis sintomática y esquizofrenia simple y crónica.　② Alivio de síntomas de náusea, vómito e hipo. Para pacientes catatónicos con neurosis de ansiedad, puede aplicar dosis pequeña en combinación con otros fármacos. |
| 用法、用量<br>Administración y dosis | 口服：用于呕吐焦虑，1次2～4mg，一日2～3次；用于精神病，开始时1日6～12mg，逐日增量至一日30～60mg，分3次服。肌内注射：用于精神病，一次5～10mg，隔6小时1次或酌情调整；用于呕吐一次5mg。<br><br>Por vía oral: para vómito y ansiedad: 2～4mg 2 ó 3 tomas al día. Para psicosis, la dosis inicial es de 6～12mg diarios y agrega gradualmente a 30～60mg diarios, divididos en 3 tomas. Inyección por I.M.: en tratamiento de psicosis: 5～10mg cada vez y repetir la medicación cada 6 horas o puede cambiar el intervalo según la situación. En tratamiento de vómito toma 5mg cada vez. |

**续　表**

| 剂型、规格<br>Formulaciones y<br>especificaciones | 片剂：每片 2mg；4mg。注射液：每支 5mg（2ml）；5mg（1ml）。<br>Tableta: 2mg, 4mg; Inyección: 5mg (2ml), 5mg(1ml). |
|---|---|
| **药品名称 Drug Names** | 氟奋乃静 Flufenazina |
| 适应证<br>Indicaciones | 用于妄想、紧张型精神分裂症、痴呆和中毒性精神病。亦可用于控制恶心呕吐。其癸酸酯注射液有长效作用。<br>Se usa para tratamiento de delirio, esquizofrenia catatónica, la demencia y la psicosis tóxica. También se puede utilizar para controlar las náuseas y los vómitos. Su inyección decanoato tiene efecto de larga duración. |
| 用法、用量<br>Administración y dosis | 口服：成人常用剂量 1 次 2mg，一日 1～2 次；逐渐递增，日服总量可达 20mg。老年或体弱者从最小剂量开始，然后每日用量递增在 1～2mg。<br>Por vía oral. Dosis habitual para adultos es de 2mg, 1～2 veces al dia y puede aumentar gradualmente hasta 20mg diadios. Ancianos y pacientes debilitados toman dosis de 2mg diarios y luego la aumentan en 1～2mg cada dia. |
| 剂型、规格<br>Formulaciones y<br>especificaciones | 片剂：1 片 2mg；5mg。注射液：每支 2mg（1m）；5mg（1ml）；10mg（2ml）。<br>Tableta: 2mg, 5mg; Inyección: 2mg (1ml), 5mg (1 ml), 10 mg (2ml). |
| **药品名称 Drug Names** | 三氟拉嗪 Trifluoperazina |
| 适应证<br>Indicaciones | ①主要用于治疗精神病，对急、慢性精神分裂症，尤其对妄想型与紧张型较好。②用于镇吐。<br>① Se usa principalmente en el tratamiento de la psicosis. Tiene buena eficacia en tratamiento de esquizofrenia aguda y crónica, especialmente la paranoide y catatónica. ② Indicación antiemética. |
| 用法、用量<br>Administración y dosis | 口服，一次 5～10mg，一日 15～30mg。必要时可逐渐递增至每日 45mg。也用于镇吐，口服，一次 1～2mg，一日 2～4mg。<br>Por vía oral. Dosis de 5～10mg 3 veces al dia. Puede aumentar agradualmente a 45mg diarios en caso necesario. Tambien puede usar en tratamiento antiemético por vía oral a dosis diaria de 2～4mg divididos en 2 tomas. |
| 剂型、规格<br>Formulaciones y<br>especificaciones | 片剂：每片 1mg；5mg。<br>Tableta: 1mg, 5mg. |
| **药品名称 Drug Names** | 硫利达嗪 Tioridazina |
| 适应证<br>Indicaciones | 主要用于治疗精神分裂症,适用于伴有激动、焦虑、紧张的精神分裂症、躁狂症、更年期精神病。亦用于儿童多动症及行为障碍。因锥体外系反应少而广泛应用。<br>Se usa principalmente para el tratamiento de la esquizofrenia: la esquizofrenia acompañada con exitación, ansiedad y tensión, la manía y la psicosis de la menopausia. También se usa en los niños con TDAH (Trastorno por déficit de atención con hiperactividad) y trastornos conductuales. Se aplica ampliamente por su poca reacción extrapiramidal. |
| 用法、用量<br>Administración y dosis | 开始时口服每次 25～100mg，一日 3 次。然后根据病情及耐受情况逐渐递增至充分治疗剂量每次 100～200mg，一日 3 次。最多可达每日 800mg。老年或体质弱者，从小剂量开始逐渐增加，每日总量低于成年人。<br>Dosis oral inicial de 25～100mg, 3 veces al dia. Aumenta agradualmente a dosis terapéutica completa de 100～200mg cada, 3 veces al dia, 800mg horas según la condición y toleración del paciente. Para ancianos y pacientes debilitados, inicie dosis pequeña y aumenta gradualmente la dosis y la diaria es inferior a la de los adultos. |
| 剂型、规格<br>Formulaciones y<br>especificaciones | 片剂：每片 10mg；25mg；50mg；100mg；200mg。<br>Tableta: 10mg, 25mg, 50mg, 100mg, 200mg. |

**续 表**

| 药品名称 Drug Names | 氟哌啶醇 Haloperidol |
|---|---|
| 适应证<br>Indicaciones | 主要用于：①用于各种急、慢性精神分裂症。特别适合于急性青春型和伴有敌对情绪及攻击行动的偏执型精神分裂症，亦可用于对吩噻嗪类治疗无效的其他类型或慢性精神分裂症。②焦虑性神经症。③儿童抽动 - 秽语综合征，有称 Tourette 综合征（TS），小剂量本品治疗有效，能消除不自主的运动，又能减轻和消除伴存的精神症状。④呕吐及顽固性呃逆。<br><br>Se usa principalmente: ① en tratamiento de esquizofrenia aguda y crónica, especialmente esquizofrenia paranoide juvenil aguda y la que asocia con hostilidad y comportamiento de ataques. También se usa para esquizofrenia crónica o de otro tipo que no tiene efecto tras medicamento con las fenotiazinas. ② en tratamiento de neurosis de angustia. ③ en tratamiento de síndrome de Tourette infantil (o TS). Es eficaz con medicación a pequeña dosis y puede quitar movimiento involuntario así como aliviar y eliminar los síntomas psiquiátricos asociados. ④ en tratamiento de vómitos e hipo intratable. |
| 用法、用量<br>Administración y dosis | ①口服：用于精神病：成人开始剂量每次 2～4mg，一日 2～3 次；逐渐增至 8～12mg，一日 2～3 次。一般剂量每日 20～30mg。维持治疗每次 2～4mg，一日 2～3 次。儿童及老年人，剂量减半。用于呕吐和焦虑：每日 0.5～1.5mg。用于抽动 - 秽语综合征：一般剂量每次 1～2mg，一日 3 次。②肌内注射：每次 5～10mg，一日 2～3 次。③静脉注射：10～30mg 加入 25% 葡萄糖注射液在 1～2 分钟缓慢注入，每 8 小时 1 次。好转后可改口服。<br><br>① Por vía oral: En tratamiento de psicosis: dosis inicial para adultos es de 2 ~ 4mg por 2 ó 3 veces al día y aumenta gradualmente a 8 ~ 12mg por 2 ó 3 veces al día. La dosis habitual es de 20 ~ 30mg diarios. En mantenimiento de tratamiento la dosis es de 2 ~ 4mg por 2 ó 3 veces al día. Para infantes y ancianos, se aplica la mitad de la dosis habitual. En tratamiento de vómitos y ansiedad: 0.5 ~ 1.5mg diarios. En tratamiento de síndrome de Tourette infantil: dosis habitual es de 1 ~ 2mg por 3 veces al día. ② Inyección por I.M.: 5 ~ 10mg por 2 ó 3 veces al día. ③ Inyección por I.V.: 10 ~ 30mg diluidos en solución de glucosa a 25% y se administra lentamente dentro de 1 ó 2 minutos. Se aplica la medicación cada 8 horas. Cuando se mejore, cambia a administración oral. |
| 剂型、规格<br>Formulaciones y<br>especificaciones | 片剂：每片 2mg；4mg；5mg。注射液：每支 5mg（1ml）。<br>Tableta: 2mg, 4mg, 5mg; Inyección: 5mg (1ml). |
| 药品名称 Drug Names | 氟哌利多 Droperidol |
| 适应证<br>Indicaciones | ①治疗精神分裂症的急性精神运动性兴奋躁狂状态。②神经安定镇痛术：利用本药的安定作用及增强镇痛作用的特点，将其与镇痛药芬太尼一起静脉注射，使患者产生一种特殊麻醉状态，用于烧伤大面积换药，各种内镜检查及造影等。③麻醉前给药，具有较好的抗精神紧张、镇吐抗休克的作用等。<br><br>① Se usa en tratamiento del estado maníaco de excitación psicomotriz agudo. ② Se usa en neuroleptanalgesia: Por su efecto de sedación y mejoramiento del efecto analgésico, se administra en inyección por I.V. junto con el fármaco analgésico fentanilo para que el paciente esté en un estatus especial de anestesia durante el cambio de apósito para quemadura extensa y endoscopia y angiografía. ③ Se usa en medicación antes de anestesia por su buen efecto anti-estrés, antiemético y anti-choque. |
| 用法、用量<br>Administración y dosis | ①治疗精神分裂症：一日 10～30mg，分 1～2 次肌内注射。②神经安定镇痛术：每 5mg 加芬太尼 0.1mg，在 2～3 分钟缓慢静脉注射，5～6 分钟如未达一级麻醉状态，可追加半倍至 1 倍剂量。③麻醉前给药：手术前 0.5 小时肌内注射 2.5～5mg。<br><br>① En tratamiento de esquizofrenia: 10-30mg diarios divididos en 1 ~ 2 veces administrados en inyección por I.M.. ② En la neuroleptanalgesia: 5mg de droperidol con 0.1mg de fentanilo administrados en inyección lenta por I.V. dentro de 2 ó 3 minutos. Si en 5 ~ 6 minutos no consigue el mejor estado de anestesia, puede agregar media o la misma cantidad. ③ En medicación antes de anestesia: administración en inyección por I.M. a dosis de 2.5 ~ 5mg media hora antes de cirugía. |
| 剂型、规格<br>Formulaciones y<br>especificaciones | 注射液：每支 5mg（1ml）。<br>Inyección: 5mg (1ml). |

续 表

| 药品名称 Drug Names | 氯哌噻吨 Clopentixol |
| --- | --- |
| 适应证<br>Indicaciones | ①长期使用可预防精神分裂症复发，对慢性患者可改善症状；对幻觉、妄想、思维障碍、行为紊乱、兴奋躁动等效果较好。②对智力障碍伴精神运动性兴奋状态、儿童严重攻击性行为障碍、老年动脉硬化性痴呆疗效较好。<br><br>① Medicamento a largo plaza puede prevenir la recaída de esquizofrenia y alivio de síntomas para pacientes crónicos. Tiene buen efecto en tratamiento de alucinaciones, delirios, trastornos del pensamiento, trastorno de conportamiento, excitación y agitación.　② Tiene buen efecto en tratamiento del estado de excitación psicomotriz acompañado con atraso mental, trastornos graves de conportamiento agresivo infantil y demencia senil por arteriosclerosis. |
| 用法、用量<br>Administración y dosis | 口服：开始剂量每日 10mg，一日 1 次，以后可逐渐增至每日 80mg，分 2～3 次服；维持剂量每日 10～40mg。速效针剂：深部肌内注射 50～100mg，一般 72 小时注射 1 次，累计总量不超过 400mg。癸酸酯长效针剂：一般 200mg 肌内注射，每 2～4 周 1 次，根据情况调整。<br><br>Por vía oral. Dosis inicial es de 10mg una vez al día y puede aumentarla hasta 80mg diarios divididos en 2～3 tomas. La dosis de mantenimiento es de 10～40mg diarios. Inyección de acción rápida: Inyección por I.M. profunda a dosis de 50～100mg cada 72 horas y la dosis total no excede a 400mg. Inyección de decanoato de acción prolongada: dosis habitual es de 200mg en inyección por I.M. cada 2～4 semanas y puede ajustarlo según la necesidad. |
| 剂型、规格<br>Formulaciones y especificaciones | 片剂：每片 10mg。注射剂：速效针剂 50mg（1ml），长效针剂 200mg（1ml）。<br>Tableta: 10mg; Inyección de acción rápida: 50mg (1ml); inyección de acción prolongada: 200mg (1ml). |
| 药品名称 Drug Names | 氟哌噻吨 Flupentixol |
| 适应证<br>Indicaciones | ①用于急、慢性精神分裂症，对淡漠，意志减退，违拗症状及分裂症后抑郁效果较好；长效制剂用于维持治疗和慢性精神分裂症的治疗。②各种原因引起的抑郁或焦虑症状。③有癫痫、老年痴呆、精神发育迟滞及酒、药依赖伴发的精神症状。<br><br>① Se usa en tratamiento de esquizofrenia aguda y crónica y tiene buen efecto para indiferencia, hypobulia, síntomas negativismo y depresión por la esquizofrenia. Las formulaciones de acción prolongada se utiliza en tratamiento de mantenimiento y el de esquizofrenia crónica.　② Se usa en tratamiento de síntomas de depresión y ansiedad causados por distintos razones.　③ Se usa en tratamiento de síntomas psiquiátricos asociados con epilepsia, la enfermedad de Alzheimer, atraso mental y dependencia de alcohol y fármacos. |
| 用法、用量<br>Administración y dosis | ①用于精神病：口服，初始每次 5mg，一日 1 次，以后视情况可逐渐加量，必要时可增至每日 40mg；维持剂量每次 5～20mg，一日 1 次。深部肌内注射，起始剂量 10mg 注射一次，1 周后可酌情加量；治疗剂量每次 20～40mg，每 2 周注射一次；维持剂量每次 20mg，每 2～4 周注射一次。②用于治疗忧郁性神经症：口服，每次 1mg，一日 2 次。最大剂量为每日 3mg。<br><br>① En tratamiento de psicosis: por vía oral a dosis de 5mg una vez al día y puede aumentarla gradualmente según la necesidad hasta los 40mg diarios. Dosis de mantenimiento es de 5～20mg una vez al día. Inyección por I.M.profunda a dosis inicial de 10mg y aumenta la dosis una semana después según la necesidad. La dosis para tratamiento es 20～40mg cada 2 semanas, la dosis de mantenimiento es 20mg cada 2～4 semanas. ② En tratamiento de neurosis depresiva: Por vía oral a dosis de 1mg por 2 veces al día. La dosis máxima es de 3mg diarios. |
| 剂型、规格<br>Formulaciones y especificaciones | 片剂：每片 0.5mg；3mg；5mg。癸酸酯注射剂：每支 20mg（1ml）。<br>Tableta: 0.5mg, 3mg, 5mg; Inyección de decanoato: 20mg(1ml). |
| 药品名称 Drug Names | 氟哌噻吨美利曲辛 Flupentixol y melitraceno |
| 适应证<br>Indicaciones | ①用于治疗神经症。治疗多种焦虑抑郁状态。②用于治疗神经性头痛、偏头痛、紧张性头痛，某些顽固性疼痛及慢性疼痛等。<br><br>① Se usa en el tratamiento de trastornos neurológicos y trastornos deprecivos y ansioso. ② Se usa en el tratamiento de la cefalea neuropática, la migraña, cefalea tensional. |

**续 表**

| | |
|---|---|
| 用法、用量<br>Administración y dosis | 口服：一日2片，早晨单次顿服，或早晨中午各服1片。严重者一日3片，早晨2片，中午1片。维持剂量为一日1片，早晨服。<br><br>Por vía oral de 2 tabletas, una vez al día en la mañana o 2 veces divididas en la mañana y en el mediodía. Para pacientes graves, dosis diaria es de 3 tabletas: 2 en la mañana y 1 en el mediodía. Dosis de mantenimiento es de 1 tableta diaria tomada en la mañana. |
| 剂型、规格<br>Formulaciones y especificaciones | 片剂：每片含哌噻吨0.5mg和美利曲辛10mg。<br>Tableta: cada una incluye 0.5mg de flupentixol y 10mg de melitraceno. |

| 药品名称 Drug Names | 舒必利 Sulpirida |
|---|---|
| 适应证<br>Indicaciones | ①对淡漠、退缩、木僵、抑郁、幻觉和妄想症状的效果较好，适用于精神分裂症单纯型、偏执型、紧张型及慢性精神分裂症的孤僻、退缩、淡漠症状；对抑郁症状有一定疗效。②用于治疗呕吐、酒精中毒性精神病、智力发育不全伴有人格障碍、胃及十二指肠溃疡等。<br><br>① Tiene buen efecto en tratamiento de apatía, retraimiento, estupor, depresión, alucinaciones y delirios. Puede utilizar para esquizofrenia de tipo simple, paranoide y catatónico así como síntomas de apatía y retraimiento de esquizofrenia crónica. ② Se usa en tratamiento de vómitos, psicosis alcohólica, trastornos de la personalidad asociados con el retraso mental y úlceras gástricas y duodenales. |
| 用法、用量<br>Administración y dosis | ①治疗精神病：口服，开始每日300～600mg，可缓慢增至一日600～1200mg；肌内注射，每日200～600mg，分2次注射；静脉滴注，每日300～600mg，稀释后缓慢滴注，滴注时间不少于4小时。一般以口服为主，对拒药者或治疗开始1～2周可用注射给药，以后改为口服。②治疗呕吐：口服，每次100～200mg，一日2～3次。<br><br>① En tratamiento de psicosis: Por vía oral a dosis inicial de 300～600mg diarios y puede aumentar gradualment a 600～1200mg diarios; Inyección por I.M. a dosis de 200～600mg diarios divididos en 2 veces; Infusión lenta por I.V. de más de 4 horas a dosis de 300～600mg diarios tras dilución. Generalmente se administra oralmente y puede aplicarse por inyecciones para pacientes que rechaza al medicamento o pacientes ya llevan la medicación durante 1～2 semanas y después, cambia a tomarlo por vía oral. ② En tratamiento de vómitos: por vía oral a dosis de 100～200mg 2 ó 3 veces al día. |
| 剂型、规格<br>Formulaciones y especificaciones | 片剂：每片10mg；50mg；100mg；200mg。注射液：每支50mg（2ml）；100mg（2ml）。<br>Tableta: 10mg, 50mg, 100mg, 200mg; Inyección: 50mg (2ml), 100mg (2ml). |

| 药品名称 Drug Names | 氯氮平 Clozapina |
|---|---|
| 适应证<br>Indicaciones | 对精神分裂症的阳性或阴性症状有较好的疗效，适用于急性和慢性精神分裂的各种亚型，对偏执型、青春型效果好。也可减轻与精神分裂症有关的感情症状（如抑郁、负罪感、焦虑）。本品也用于治疗躁狂症或其他精神障碍的兴奋躁动和幻觉、妄想，适用于难治性精神分裂症。因导致粒细胞减少症，一般不宜作为首选药，而用于患者经历了其他两种抗精神病药充分治疗无效或不耐受其他药物治疗时。<br><br>Tiene buen efecto para tratamiento de síntomas postivos o negativos de esquizofrenia y es esficaz en tratamiento de subtipos de esquizofrenia aguda o crónica especialmente de tipo paranoide y juvenil. Se puede aliviar los síntomas emocionales asociados con la esquizofrenia (por ejempro sentimiento de depresión, culpa y ansiedad). Se utiliza también en tratamiento de manía u otros trastornos mentales como agitación, alucinaciones y delirios. Es eficaz para esquizofrenia refractaria. Como dará lugar a la neutropenia, generalmente no lo elije como fármaco preferido a menos de que no se vea ningún efecto tras medicación de otros antipsicóticos o aparezca intolerancia del paciente. |
| 用法、用量<br>Administración y dosis | 口服：开始一次25mg，一日1～2次；然后每日增加25～50mg，耐受性好，在开始治疗的2周末将一日总量增至300～450mg，均为一日分1～2次服用。肌内注射：每次50～100mg，一日2次。<br><br>Por vía oral a dosis inicial de 25mg 1 ó 2 veces al día. Aumenta la dosis en 25～50mg cada día y en las primeras dos semanas de tratamiento aumenta la dosis hasta 300～450mg diarios y divididos en 1 ó 2 tomas. Es un fármaco Bien tolerado. Inyección por I.M.: 50～100mg por 2 veces al día. |

续　表

| 剂型、规格<br>Formulaciones y especificaciones | 片剂：每片 25mg；50mg。<br>Tableta: 25mg, 50mg. |
|---|---|
| **药品名称 Drug Names** | 奥氮平 Olanzapina |
| 适应证<br>Indicaciones | 用于治疗严重阳性症状或阴性症状的精神分裂症和其他精神病的急性期及维持期。亦可用于缓解精神分裂症及相关疾病常见的继发性感情症状。<br><br>Se usa en tratamiento de esquizofrenia con síntomas graves positivos o negativos y otra psiquiátrica en la fase aguda y de mantenimiento. También puede aliviar la esquizofrenia y los relacionados síntomas emocionales secundarios. |
| 用法、用量<br>Administración y dosis | 口服，一日 10～15mg。可根据病情调整剂量一日 5～20mg。老年人、女性、非吸烟者、有低血压倾向者、严重肾功能损害者或中度肝功能损伤者，起始剂量为一日 5mg，如需加量，剂递增为每次 5mg，递增一次间隔至少 1 周。<br><br>Por vía oral a dosis de 10～15mg diarios. Puede ajustar la dosis a 5～20mg diarios según la situación . Para los ancianos, mujeres, no fumadores, pacientes con tendencia a la hipotensión, paciente con grave insuficiencia renal o lesión hepática moderada, la dosis inicial es de 5mg diarios. Si es necesario puede agregar la dosis en 5mg cada vez y el intervalo de ajuste de dosis es por lo menos 1 semana. |
| 剂型、规格<br>Formulaciones y especificaciones | 片剂：每片 2.5mg；5mg；7.5mg；10mg。<br>Tableta: 2.5mg, 5mg, 7.5mg, 10mg. |
| **药品名称 Drug Names** | 喹硫平 Quetiapina |
| 适应证<br>Indicaciones | ①用于各种精神分裂症，不仅对精神分裂症阳性症状有效，对阴性症状也有一定疗效。②也可以减轻与精神分裂症有关的感情症状如抑郁、焦虑及认知缺陷症状。<br><br>① Es eficaz en tratamiento de variedad de esquizofrenias de los síntomas positivos y negativos. ② Se usa en alivio de síntomas en sentimiento asociados con esquizofrenia, por ejempro depresión, ansiedad y déficits cognitivos. |
| 用法、用量<br>Administración y dosis | 口服，成人：起始剂量为 1 次 25mg，一日 2 次。每隔 1～3 日增加 25mg，逐渐加量至一日 300～600mg，分 2～3 次服用。老年人：用本品应慎重，推荐起始剂量为每日 25mg。每日增加剂量幅度为 25～50mg，直至有效剂量，有效剂量可以较一般成人低。<br><br>Por vía oral. Para adultos la dosis inicial es de 25mg 2 veces al día. Agrega 25mg cada 1～3 días hasta 300～600mg diarios y debe tomarlos divididos en 2～3 veces. Para ancianos: hay que utilizarlo con cuidado. La dosis inicial recomendada es 25mg diarios y agrega gradualmente en 25～50mg cada día hasta llegar a la dosis efectiva que puede ser menor que la de adultos. |
| 剂型、规格<br>Formulaciones y especificaciones | 片剂：每片 25mg；100mg；200mg。<br>Tableta: 25mg, 100mg, 200mg. |
| **药品名称 Drug Names** | 利培酮 Risperidona |
| 适应证<br>Indicaciones | 用于治疗急性和慢性精神分裂症状。特别是对阳性及阴性症状及其伴发的情感症状（如焦虑、抑郁等）有较好的疗效。也可减轻与精神分裂症有关的情感症状。对于急性期治疗有效患者，维持期治疗中，本品可继续发挥临床效果。<br><br>Se usa en tratamiento de síntomas agudos y crónicos de esquizofrenia, especialmente los síntomas positivos y negativos así como los emocionales asociados, por ejempro ansiedad, depresión etc. Puede aliviar los síntomas emocionales relacionados con esquizofrenia. Para pacientes que consigue efecto en fase aguda, puede seguir con esta medicación en tratamiento de mantenimiento por su eficacia clínica. |
| 用法、用量<br>Administración y dosis | 口服，宜从小剂量开始。初始剂量为每次 1mg，一日 2 次，剂量逐渐增至第 3 日为 3mg，以后每周调整一次剂量，最大疗效剂量为每日 4～6mg。老年患者起始剂量为每次 0.5mg，一日 2 次。<br><br>Por vía oral y empieza con dosis pequeña. La dosis inicial es de 1mg 2 veces al día. En el tercer día agrega la dosis a 3mg y ajusta la dosis cada semana. La dosis máxima no excede a 4～6mg diarios. Para los ancianos la dosis inicial es de 0.5mg y 2 veces al día. |

**续　表**

| 剂型、规格<br>Formulaciones y especificaciones | 片剂：每片 1mg；2mg。<br>Tableta: 1mg, 2mg. |
|---|---|
| **药品名称 Drug Names** | 帕潘立酮 Paliperidona |
| 适应证<br>Indicaciones | ①用于精神分裂症急性期治疗。②用于精神分裂症、双向情感障碍的躁狂期及孤独症的治疗。<br>① Se usa para tratamiento de esquizofrenia en etapa aguda.　② Se usa en tratamiento de la esquizofrenia y el trastorno bipolar en la fase maníaca y el autismo. |
| 用法、用量<br>Administración y dosis | 成人：口服，每次 6mg，一日 1 次，早晨服药。需要进行剂量增加时，推荐增量为每日增加 3mg。一日最大推荐剂量为 12mg。<br>Para adultos: administración oral a dosis de 6mg una vez al día tomados en la mañana. En caso necesario puede aumentar la dosis en 3mg cada día como recomendable. La dosis diaria máxima recomendable es del 12mg. |
| 剂型、规格<br>Formulaciones y especificaciones | 缓释片：3mg；6mg；9mg。<br>Tableta de liberación prolongada: 3mg, 6mg, 9mg. |
| **药品名称 Drug Names** | 齐拉西酮 Ziprasidona |
| 适应证<br>Indicaciones | ①主要用于精神分裂症治疗。也能改善分裂症状伴发的抑郁症状。②可用于情感性障碍的狂躁期治疗。<br>① Se usa principalmente en tratamiento de esquizofrenia y puede aliviar el síntoma depresivo asociado. ② Puede usrse en la fase maníaca de tratamiento de trastornos emocionales. |
| 用法、用量<br>Administración y dosis | 口服：初始治疗一日 2 次，每次 20mg，餐时口服。视病情可逐渐增加到一日 2 次，每次 80mg。调整剂量时间间隔一般应不少于 2 日。维持治疗一日 2 次，每次 20mg。肌内注射：用于精神分裂症患者的急性激越期治疗。每次 10～20mg，最大剂量为每日 40mg。如需长期使用，应改为口服。<br>Por vía oral. En primera fase de tratamiento, la dosis es de 20mg 2 veces al día, tomados acompañados con alimentos. Puede cambiar la dosis según la situación a 80mg 2 veces al día. El intervalo de ajuste de dosis es 2 días como mínimo. En tratamiento de mantenimiento, la dosis es de 20mg 2 veces al día. Inyección por I.M.: se usa en tratamiento de esquizofrenia en fase de agitación aguda a una dosis de 10～20mg cada vez y la dosis máxima es de 40mg diarios. Si tiene que aplicarla a largo plazo, debe tomarlo por vía oral. |
| 剂型、规格<br>Formulaciones y especificaciones | 片剂：20mg；60mg。胶囊剂：20mg；40mg；60mg；80mg。注射液：10mg（1ml）；20mg（1ml）。<br>Tableta: 20mg, 60mg; Cápsula: 20mg, 40mg, 60mg, 80mg; Inyección: 10mg (1ml), 20mg (1ml). |
| **药品名称 Drug Names** | 五氟利多 Penfluridol |
| 适应证<br>Indicaciones | 对精神分裂症各型和各病程均有疗效，控制幻觉、妄想及淡漠、退缩等症状疗效好。主要用于慢性精神分裂症患者的维持治疗，对急性患者也有效。<br>Es eficaz en tratamiento de variedad de esquizofrenias en su cualquier fase. Tiene buen efecto en controlar los síntomas de alucinaciones, delirios y apatía, retraimiento. Se usa principalmente en tratamiento de mantenimiento de esquizofrenia crónica y es eficaz también para casos agudos. |
| 用法、用量<br>Administración y dosis | 口服，每次 20～60mg，每周 1 次，重症或耐药患者可加至每周 120mg，1 次服或 2 次分服（一半在前半周，一半在后半周服）。<br>Por vía oral a dosis de 20～60mg cada semana. Para pacientes graves o tolerantes puede aumentar la dosis a 120mg cada semana, tomados 1 vez o divididos en 2 veces (1 vez en el primer mitad de la semana y otra en la segunda mitad). |
| 剂型、规格<br>Formulaciones y especificaciones | 片剂：每片 5mg；20mg。<br>Tableta: 5mg, 20mg. |

续　表

| 药品名称 Drug Names | 阿立哌唑 Aripiprazol |
| --- | --- |
| 适应证<br>Indicaciones | 用于治疗各类型的精神分裂症。国外临床试验表明，本品对精神分裂症的阳性和阴性症状均有明显疗效，也能改善伴发的情感症状，降低精神分裂症的复发率。<br><br>Se usa en tratamiento de todo tipo de esquizofrenias. Ensayos clínicos extranjeros muestran que este fármaco tiene eficacia evidente en tratamiento de síntomas positivos o negativos de esquizofrenia y puede mejorar síntomas emocionales asociados así como reducir recaída de la esquizofrenia. |
| 用法、用量<br>Administración y dosis | 口服，一日 1 次。推荐用法为第 1 周起始剂量每日 5mg，第 2 周为每日 10mg，第 3 周为每日 15mg，之后可根据个体的疗效耐受情况调整剂量。有效剂量范围每日 10 ～ 30mg，最大剂量不应超过每日 30mg。<br><br>Por vía oral una vez al día. Recomenda dosis inicial de 5mg diarios en la primera semana, 10mg diarios en la segunda y 15mg diarios en la tercera semana y luego puede ajustar la dosis según la condición del paciente. Dosis efectiva es de 10 ~ 30mg diarios y la máxima no excede a 30mg diarios. |
| 剂型、规格<br>Formulaciones y especificaciones | 片剂：每片 5mg；10mg。<br>Tableta: 5mg, 10mg. |
| 药品名称 Drug Names | 曲美托嗪 Trimetozina |
| 适应证<br>Indicaciones | 用于伴有恐惧、紧张和情绪激动的神经精神症状及儿童行为障碍；对于带有神经质综合征的患者，本品可有效地消除兴奋；在精神病的治疗上可作为一种维持治疗用药。<br><br>Se usa en tratamiento de síntomas neuropsiquiátricos asociados con pánico, tensión y excitación y trastornos infantiles de comportamiento. Puede eliminar la excitación para pacientes con síntomas neuróticos. Puede ser fármaco de mantenimiento en tratamiento de psicosis. |
| 用法、用量<br>Administración y dosis | 每次口服 300mg，一日 3 ～ 6 次。<br>Por vía oral: 300mg y 3 ~ 6 vecez al día. |
| 剂型、规格<br>Formulaciones y especificaciones | 片剂：每片 300mg。<br>Tableta: 300mg. |
| 药品名称 Drug Names | 癸氟奋乃静 Decanoato de flufenazina |
| 适应证<br>Indicaciones | 应用同氟奋乃静。对幻觉、妄想、木僵、淡漠、孤独和紧张性兴奋有较好疗效。对兴奋躁动和焦虑紧张也有效。对慢性精神分裂症可使淡漠和退缩减轻，改善与环境接触的反应。也可用于精神分裂症缓解期的维持治疗。<br><br>Indicación similar a flufenazina. Tiene buen efecto en tratamiento de alucinaciones, delirios, estupor, apatía, soledad y excitación catatónica. También es eficaz en tratamiento de agitación, ansiedad y tensión. En caso de esquizofrenia crónica, puede aliviar la apatía y la retirada y puede mejorar las reacciones al contactar con el entorno. Se usa también en el tratamiento de mantenimiento de esquizofrenia en remisión. |
| 用法、用量<br>Administración y dosis | 深部肌内注射，开始剂量 12.5mg，以后每 2 周肌注 25mg。剂量宜从小剂量开始，以后酌情增加或减少。<br><br>Inyección por I.M. profunda. Dosis inicial es de 12.5mg y luego 25mg cada 2 semanas. Empieza el medicamento a pequeña dosis y según la necesidad puede aumentar o disminuir la dosis. |
| 剂型、规格<br>Formulaciones y especificaciones | 注射液：每支 25mg（1ml）；25mg（2ml）。<br>Inyección: 25mg (1ml), 25mg (2ml). |

**续 表**

### 8.9 抗焦虑药 Anti-ansiolíticos

| 药品名称 Drug Names | 地西泮 Diazepam |
|---|---|
| 适应证<br>Indicaciones | ①焦虑症及各种功能性神经病。②失眠，尤其对焦虑性失眠疗效极佳。③癫痫：可与其他癫痫药合用，治疗癫痫大发作或小发作，控制癫痫持续状态时应静脉注射。④各种原因引起的惊厥，如癫痫、破伤风、小儿高热惊厥等。⑤脑血管意外或脊髓损伤性中枢性僵直或腰肌劳损、内镜检查等所致肌肉痉挛。⑥其他：偏头痛、肌紧张性头痛、呃逆、炎症引起的反射性肌肉痉挛、惊恐症、酒精戒断综合征，还可以治疗家族性、老年性和特发性震颤，可用于麻醉前给药。<br><br>① Se usa en tratamiento de ansiedad y neurologías funcionales.  ② Se usa en tratamiento de insomnio, especialmente eficaz para insomnio asociado con ansiedad.  ③ Se usa en tratamiento de epilepsia: puede administrarse junto con otros fármacos antiepilépticos para epilepsia de gran mal o las convulsiones. En cuanto a controlar el estado epiléptico se debe administrar por vía de inyección I.V.. ④ Se usa en tratamiento de convulsiones, por ejempro la epilepsia, tétanos, , convulsiones infantiles por la fiebre etc. ⑤ Se usa en tratamiento de espasmos musculares causados por accidente cerebrovascular, espondilitis por la lesión de la médula espinal, tensión muscular lumbar y endoscopias. ⑥ Se usa en tratamiento de otras enfermedades como espasmo muscular reactivo, trastorno de pánico y síndrome de abstinencia alcohólica causados por la migraña, cefalea tensional, el hipo y la inflamación, así como temblor familiar,senil y esencial. También se administra antes de anestesia. |
| 用法、用量<br>Administración y dosis | （1）口服：①抗焦虑：每次 2.5 ~ 10mg，一日 3 次。②催眠：每次 5 ~ 10mg，睡前服用。③麻醉前给药：1 次 10mg。④抗惊厥：成人每次 2.5 ~ 10mg，一日 2 ~ 4 次。6 个月以上儿童，每次 0.1mg/kg，一日 3 次。⑤缓解肌肉阵挛：每次 2.5 ~ 5mg，一日 3 ~ 4 次。（2）静脉注射：①成人基础麻醉：10 ~ 30mg。②癫痫持续状态：开始 5 ~ 10mg，每 5 ~ 10 分钟按需要重复，达 30mg 后必要时每 2 ~ 4 小时重复治疗。静脉注射要缓慢。<br><br>(1) Por vía oral: ① ansiolítico: 2.5 ~ 10mg por 3 veces al día. ② hipnotización: 5 ~ 10mg diarios antes de acostarse.  ③ administración antes de anestesia: 10mg cada vez.  ④ anticonvulsivo: Para adultos es de 2.5 ~ 10mg por 2 ~ 4 veces al día y para niños mayores de 6 meses es de 0.1mg/kg por 3 veces al día. ⑤ Alivio de mioclónica: 2.5 ~ 5mg por 3 ó 4 veces al día. (2) Inyección por I.V.: ① En anestesia básica de adultos: 10 ~ 30mg. ② Para el estado de epilepsia: dosis inicial es de 5 ~ 10mg cada vez y repetir el medicamento cada 5 ~ 10 minutos según la necesidad. Al llegar a 30mg en total puede cambiar a medicación repetida cada 2 ~ 4 horas. La inyección por I.V. debe administrarse lentamente. |
| 剂型、规格<br>Formulaciones y especificaciones | 片剂：每片 2.5mg；5mg。胶囊剂：每粒 10mg。注射液：每支 10mg（2ml）。<br>Tableta: 2.5mg, 5mg; Cápsula: 10mg; Inyección: 10mg (2ml). |

| 药品名称 Drug Names | 奥沙西泮 Oxazepam |
|---|---|
| 适应证<br>Indicaciones | 用于焦虑障碍，伴有焦虑的失眠，并能缓解急性酒精戒断症状 。<br>Se usa para tratamiento de trastorno de ansiedad, insomnio asociado con ansiedad y alivio de síntomas de abstinencia alcohólica aguda. |
| 用法、用量<br>Administración y dosis | 口服。焦虑和戒酒症状：每次 15 ~ 30mg，一日 3 ~ 4 次；老年人应当适当减量。失眠：1 次 15mg，睡前服用。<br>Por vía oral. Para síntomas de ansiedad y de abstinencia alcohólica: 15 ~ 30mg 3 ó 4 veces al día y reduce la dosis para pacientes ancianos. En tratamiento de insomnio: 15mg tomados antes de acostarse. |
| 剂型、规格<br>Formulaciones y especificaciones | 片剂：每片 10mg；15mg；30mg。<br>Tableta: 10mg, 15mg, 30mg. |

| 药品名称 Drug Names | 硝西泮 Nitrazepam |
|---|---|
| 适应证<br>Indicaciones | ①用于各种失眠的短期治疗，口服后 30 分钟左右起作用，维持睡眠 6 小时。②可用于治疗多种癫痫，尤其对阵挛性发作效果较好。<br><br>① Se usa en tratamiento a corto plazo de insomnio. Se efectua dentro de 30 minutos después de administración oral y puede mantener el sueño durante 6 horas. ② Se usa en tratamiento de epilepsias y es eficaz especialmente para alivio de convulsiones clónicas. |

**续　表**

| | |
|---|---|
| 用法、用量<br>Administración y dosis | 口服。催眠：成人 5～10mg，儿童 2.5～5mg，睡前 1 次服用；抗焦虑：每次 5mg，1 日 2～3 次；抗癫痫：每次 5～30mg，一日 3 次，可酌情增加。老年、体弱者减半。<br><br>Por vía oral. Para insomnio: 5～10mg para adultos y 2.5～5mg para niños, tomados antes de acostarse. Para ansiedad: 5mg 2 ó 3 veces al día. Para epilepsia: 5～30mg 3 veces al día y puede aumentar la dosis según la necesidad. Para ancianos y debiles la dosis es la mitad. |
| 剂型、规格<br>Formulaciones y especificaciones | 片剂：每片 5mg；10mg。<br>Tableta: 5mg, 10mg. |
| **药品名称 Drug Names** | 氟西泮 Flurazepam |
| 适应证<br>Indicaciones | 用于难以入睡、夜间屡醒及早醒的各种失眠。<br><br>Se usa en tratamiento de insomnio caracterizado por la dificultad en dormirse, repetidos despertares o despertar precoz. |
| 用法、用量<br>Administración y dosis | 口服：15～30mg，睡前 1 次服用，年老体弱者开始时每次服用 15mg，根据反应适当加量。<br><br>Por vía oral a dosis 15～30mg antes de acostarse. Para ancianos y pacientes debilitados, la dosis inicial es de 15mg y puede aumentar según la reacción. |
| 剂型、规格<br>Formulaciones y especificaciones | 片剂：每片 15mg。胶囊剂：每粒 5mg；15mg；30mg。<br>Tableta: 15mg; Cápsula: 5mg, 15mg, 30mg. |
| **药品名称 Drug Names** | 氯硝西泮 Clonazepam |
| 适应证<br>Indicaciones | ①主要用于治疗癫痫和惊厥，对各型癫痫均有效，尤以对小发作和肌阵挛发作疗效最佳。静脉注射治疗癫痫持续状态。②可用于治疗焦虑状态和失眠。③对舞蹈症亦有效。对药物引起的多动症、慢性多发性抽搐、僵人综合征、各类神经痛也有一定疗效。<br><br>① Se usa principalmente en tratamiento de epilepsia y convulsiones. Es eficaz para todo tipo de epilepsias especialmente para convulsiones y crisis mioclónicas. Administración de inyección por I.V puede curar el estado epiléptico.　② Puede usarse en tratamiento de ansiedad e insomnio.　③ Tiene efecto en tratamiento de corea y en alivio de ADHD inducido por fármacos, trastorno de tics múltiples motores crónicos, síndrome de la persona rígida y varios tipos de neuralgia. |
| 用法、用量<br>Administración y dosis | ①口服：成人，初始剂量每天 1mg，2～4 周逐渐增加到一日 4～8mg，分 3～4 次服用；儿童，5 岁以下初始剂量每天 0.25mg，5～12 岁每天 0.5mg，分 3～4 次服用，逐渐增加剂量到一日 1～3mg（5 岁以下）和 3～6mg（5～12 岁）。②肌内注射：1 次 1～2mg，一日 2～4mg。③静脉注射：癫痫持续状态，成人，一次 1～4mg；儿童，一次 0.01～0.1mg/kg，注射速度要缓慢。或将 4mg 溶于 500ml 生理盐水，以能够控制惊厥发作的速度而缓慢滴注。<br><br>① Por vía oral. Para adultos la dosis inicial es de 1mg diarios y aumenta a 4～8mg diarios divididos en 3～4 tomas dentro de 2～4 semanas. Para niños menores de 5 años la dosis inicial es de 0.25mg diarios y 0.5mg diarios para niños de entre 5 y 12 años. Se toma divididos en 3～4 veces y aumenta la dosis gradualmente a 1～3mg diarios para niños menor de 5 años y 3～6mg darios para niños de entre 5 y 12 años. ② Inyección por I.M.: 1～2mg cada vez y 2～4mg diarios. ③ Inyección por I.V.: en caso del estado epiléptico 1～4mg cada vez para adultos y para niños la dosis es de 0.01～0.1mg/kg cada vez . La inyección debe administrarse lentamente. O puede ser administración de infusión lenta para controlar las convulsiones a una dosis de 4mg diluidos en 500ml de Normal Saline. |
| 剂型、规格<br>Formulaciones y especificaciones | 片剂：每片 0.5mg；1mg；2mg。注射液：每支 1mg（1ml）；2mg（2ml）。<br>Tableta: 0.5mg, 1mg, 2mg; Inyección: 1mg (1ml), 2mg (2ml). |
| **药品名称 Drug Names** | 劳拉西泮 Lorazepam |
| 适应证<br>Indicaciones | ①主要用于严重焦虑症、焦虑状态及惊恐焦虑的急性期控制，适宜短期使用。可用于伴有精神抑郁的焦虑，但不推荐用于原发性抑郁症的患者。②失眠。③癫痫。④还可用于癌症化疗时止吐（限注射剂），治疗紧张性头痛，麻醉前及内镜检查前的辅助用药。 |

① Se usa principalmente en contro en fase aguda de ansiedad severa, el estado de ansiedad y pánico. Recomienda medicació a corto plazo. Puede usar en pacientes de ansiedad asociada con depresión pero no es recomendable para pacientes de depresión primaria. ② Tratamiento de insomnio. ③ Tratamiento de epilepsia. ④ Se usa también como antiemético en la quimioterapia del cáncer ( solamente por vía inyecdable ) y en tratamiento de cefalea tensional así como fármaco adyuvante antes de la anestesia y endoscopia.

| 用法、用量<br>Administración y dosis | ①焦虑症：口服，一次 1～2mg，一日 2～3 次。②失眠：睡前 1 小时一次服用 1～4mg。③麻醉前给药：术前 1～2 小时，口服 4mg 或肌内注射 2～4mg。④癫痫持续状态：肌内或静脉注射，1 次 1～4mg。⑤化疗止吐：在化疗前 30 分钟注射 1～2mg，预防呕吐发生。<br><br>① Tratamiento de ansiedad: por vía oral a una dosis de 1～2mg 2 ó 3 veces al día. ② Tratamiento de insomnio: 1～4mg tomados antes de acostarse. ③ Medicamento antes de anestesia: 4mg por vía oral o 2～4mg de inyección por I.V. administrados 1～2 horas antes de cirugía. ④ Tratamiento del estado epiléptico: 1～4mg de inyección por I.M. o I.V.. ⑤ Antiemético en la quimioterapia: 1～2mg de inyección 30 minutos antes de la quimioterapia para prevenir los vómitos. |
| :-- | :-- |
| 剂型、规格<br>Formulaciones y especificaciones | 片剂：每片 0.5mg；1mg；2mg。注射液：每支 2mg（2ml）；4mg（2ml）。<br>Tableta: 0.5mg, 1mg, 2mg; Inyección: 2mg (2ml), 4mg (2ml). |
| 药品名称 Drug Names | 氟硝西泮 Flunitrazepam |
| 适应证<br>Indicaciones | 用于催眠（主要用于严重失眠的短期治疗），麻醉前给药和诱导麻醉。<br><br>Se usa para la hipnotización, principalmente en el tratamiento a corto plazo de insomnio grave, administración antes de anestesia y la inducción de la anestesia. |
| 用法、用量<br>Administración y dosis | 催眠：口服，1～2mg，睡前一次服用。术前给药：肌内注射，1～2mg。诱导麻醉：缓慢静脉注射，1～2mg。<br><br>Para hipnotización: por vía oral a dosis 1～2 mg antes de acostarse; Administración preoperatoria: dosis 1～2mg vía Inyección por I.M. ; Inducción de anestesia: dosis 1～2mg vía lenta inyección por I.V. |
| 剂型、规格<br>Formulaciones y especificaciones | 片剂：每片 1mg；2mg。注射液：每支 2mg（2ml）。<br>Tableta: 1mg, 2mg; Inyección: 2mg (2ml). |
| 药品名称 Drug Names | 艾司唑仑 Estazolam |
| 适应证<br>Indicaciones | ①用于各种类型的失眠。催眠作用强，口服后 20～60 分钟可入睡，维持 5 小时。②用于焦虑、紧张、恐惧及癫痫大、小发作，亦可用于术前镇静。<br><br>① Se usa en tratamiento de insomnio. Tiene efecto significativo en hipnotización que puede conciliar el sueño dentro de 20～60 minutos y mantenerlo durante 5 horas.　② Se usa en alivio de ansiedad, tensión, pánico, crisis o convulsiones de gran mal. Se usa también en sedación preoperatoria. |
| 用法、用量<br>Administración y dosis | 口服。镇静、抗焦虑：1 次 1～2mg，一日 3 次；催眠：1 次 1～2mg，睡前服；抗癫痫：1 次 2～4mg，一日 3 次；麻醉前给药：1 次 2～4mg，术前 1 小时服用。<br><br>Por vía oral. Para sedación y uso ansiolítico: 1～2mg 3 veces al día. Para hipnotización: 1～2mg tomados antes de acostarse. Para uso antiepiléptico: 2～4mg 3 veces al día. Para medicación antes de la anestesia: 2～4mg tomados 1 hora antes de cirugía. |
| 剂型、规格<br>Formulaciones y especificaciones | 片剂：每片 1mg；2mg。<br>Tableta：1mg，2mg. |
| 药品名称 Drug Names | 阿普唑仑 Alprazolam |
| 适应证<br>Indicaciones | ①用于治疗焦虑症、抑郁症、失眠。可作为抗惊恐药。②能缓解急性酒精戒断症状。③对药源性顽固性呃逆有较好的治疗作用。<br><br>① Se usa en tratamiento de ansiedad, depresión e insomnio. Se puede utilizar como medicamento anti-pánico.　② Puede aliviar síntomas agudos de abstinencia alcohólica.　③ Tiene buen efecto en tratamiento de hipo intratable inducido por medicamentos. |

续　表

| 用法、用量<br>Administración y dosis | 口服。抗焦虑：一次 0.4mg，一日 3 次，以后酌情增减，量大剂量每日 4mg。抗抑郁：一般为一次 0.8mg，一日 3 次，个别患者可增至每日 10mg。镇静、催眠：0.4 ～ 0.8mg，睡前顿服。抗惊恐：每次 0.4mg，一日 3 次，必要时可酌情增量。老年人：初始剂量一次 0.2mg，一日 3 次，根据病情和对药物反应酌情增量。<br><br>Por vía oral. Antiolítoco: 0.4mg 3 veces al día y ajuste la dosis gradualmente según la necesidad. Dosis máxima no debe exceder a 4mg diarios. Antidepresivo: dosis habitual es de 0.8mg 3 veces al día. En caso necesario puede aumentar a 10mg diarios. Para sedación e hipnotización: 0.4~0.8mg tomados antes de acostarse. Anti-pánico: 0.4mg 3 veces al día y ajuste la dosis gradualmente según la necesidad. Para pacientes ancianos, la dosis inicial es de 0.2mg y 3 veces al día y debe ajustar la dosis según la condición del paciente y las reacciones tras medicación. |
|---|---|
| 剂型、规格<br>Formulaciones y especificaciones | 片剂：每片 0.25mg；0.4mg；0.5mg；1mg。<br>Tableta: 0.25mg, 0.4mg, 0.5mg, 1mg. |
| **药品名称 Drug Names** | 奥沙唑仑 Oxazolam |
| 适应证<br>Indicaciones | 用于焦虑症、神经症的治疗。亦可用于麻醉前给药。<br>Se usa en tratamiento de trastorno de ansiedad y neurosis así como administración antes de la anestesia. |
| 用法、用量<br>Administración y dosis | 口服。抗焦虑：一次 10 ～ 20mg，一日 3 次。镇静催眠：一次 15 ～ 30mg，睡前顿服。麻醉前给药：术前 1 小时给予 1 ～ 2mg/kg。<br><br>Por vía oral. Ansiolítico: 10 ~ 20mg 3 veces al dia y puede ajustar la dosis según necesidad y la máxima no debe exceder a 4mg diarios. Para sedación e hipnotización: 15 ~ 30mg tomados antes de acostarse. Administración antes de la anestesia: 1 ~ 2mg/kg, 1 hora antes de la cirugía. |
| 剂型、规格<br>Formulaciones y especificaciones | 片剂：每片 5mg；10mg；20mg。胶囊剂：每粒 10mg。<br>Tableta: 5mg, 10mg, 20mg; Vápsula: 10mg. |
| **药品名称 Drug Names** | 美沙唑仑 Mexazolam |
| 适应证<br>Indicaciones | 可用于神经症、身心疾病，自主神经失调等疾病时的紧张、焦虑、抑郁、易疲劳、睡眠障碍等的治疗。<br>Se usa en tratamiento del estrés, la ansiedad, la depresión, la fatiga, los trastornos del sueño provocados por la neurosis, enfermedades físicas y mentales, trastornos del sistema nervioso autónomo. |
| 用法、用量<br>Administración y dosis | 口服，每日 1.5 ～ 3mg，分 3 次服用，必要时根据年龄、症状适当调整剂量。老年人每日剂量为 1.5mg。<br>Por vía oral a dosis diaria de 1.5 ~ 3mg divididos en 3 tomas. En caso necesario puede ajustar la dosis según la edad y síntomas. Para ancianos la dosis diaria es de 1.5mg. |
| 剂型、规格<br>Formulaciones y especificaciones | 片剂：每片 0.5mg；1mg。<br>Tableta:0.5mg, 1mg. |
| **药品名称 Drug Names** | 谷维素 Orizanol |
| 适应证<br>Indicaciones | 用于自主神经失调（包括胃肠、心血管神经症）、周期性精神病、脑震荡后遗症、精神分裂症和周期型、更年期综合征、月经前期紧张症等，但疗效不够明显。<br>Se usa para tratamiento de trastornos del sistema nervioso autónomo (incluyendo neurosis gastrointestinales y cardiovasculares), psicosis periódica, secuelas de concusión cerebral, esquizofrenia, síndrome de la menopausia periódica y trastorno de estrés premenstrual. Pero los efectos no son evidentes. |
| 用法、用量<br>Administración y dosis | 口服：每次 10mg，一日 3 次。有时可用至每日 60mg。疗程一般 3 个月左右。<br>Por vía oral: 10mg 3 veces al día. Puede aumentar a 60mg diarios y el curso de tratamiento suele ser unos 3 meses. |
| 剂型、规格<br>Formulaciones y especificaciones | 片剂：每片 5mg；10mg。<br>Tableta: 5mg, 10mg. |

续　表

| 8.10　抗躁狂药 Antimaníacos |
|---|

| 药品名称Drug Names | 碳酸锂 Carbonato de litio |
|---|---|
| 适应证<br>Indicaciones | ①主要用于治疗躁狂症，对躁狂和抑郁交替发作的双相情感性精神障碍有很好的治疗和预防复发作用，对反复发作的抑郁症也有预防发作作用。一般于用药后 6～7 日症状开始好转。因锂盐无镇静作用，一般主张对严重急性躁狂患者先与氯丙嗪或氟哌啶醇合用，急性症状控制后再单用碳酸锂维持。②还可用于治疗分裂 - 情感性精神病，粒细胞减少，再生障碍性贫血，月经过多症，急性菌痢。<br><br>① Se usa principalmente en tratamiento de manía y tiene buen efecto en tratamiento y prevención de recaídas del trastorno bipolar con episodios alternativos de manía y depresión así como depresión de episodios repetidos. Generalmente se mejora tras medicación de 6 ó 7días. Porque el litio no tiene efecto de sedación, habitualmente se administra junto con clorpromazina o haloperidol para pacientes gravis de manía aguda y después de controlar los síntomas agudos puede usar el carbonato de litio para tratamiento de mantenimiento. ② Se usa también en tratamiento de psicosis esquizoafectivo, neutropenia, anemia aplásica, menorragia y disentería aguda. |
| 用法、用量<br>Administración y dosis | ①躁狂症：口服，一般以小剂量开始，每次 0.125～0.25g，一日 3 次。可逐渐加到每次 0.25～0.5g，一般不超过每日 1.5～2.0g。症状控制后维持量一般不超过每日 1g，分 3～4 次服用。预防复发时，需持续用药 2～3 年。②粒细胞减少、再生障碍性贫血：口服 10 日，每次 0.3g。一日 3 次。③月经过多症：月经第 1 日服 0.6g，以后每日服 0.3g，均分为 3 次服，共服 3 日，总量 1.2g 为 1 疗程。每一月经周期服 1 疗程。④急性菌痢：每次 0.1g，一日 3 次，首剂加倍。少数症状较重者，头 1～3 日每次剂量均可加倍，至症状及粪便明显好转后，以原剂量维持 2～3 日，再递减剂量，3～4 日停药。<br><br>① En tratamiento de manía: Por vía oral a dosis inicial pequeña de 0.125～0.25g por 3 veces al día y puede aumentar gradualmente a 0.25～0.5g cada vez. La dosis máxima no debe exceder a 1.5～2g diarios. Al controlar la enfermedad se aplica dosis de mantenimiento de 1g diarios como máxomo divididos en 3 ó 4 tomas. En la prevención de recaída debe seguir la medicción durante 2 ó 3 años. ② En tratamiento de neutropenia y anemia aplásica: se administra oralmente durante 10 días a una dosis de 0.3g por 3 veces al día. ③ En tratamiento de menorragia: En el primer día de la menstruación se toma 0.6g diarios y en los siguientes 2 días, 0.3g diarios. Se toma en 3 tomas divididas y la dosis total de un curso de tratamiento cada menstruación es de 1.2g. ④ En tratamiento de disentería aguda: 0.1g por 3 veces al día y debe duplicar la dosis en la primera toma. Para casos severos puede duplicar la dosis en los primeros 3 días hasta se ve mejoramiento evidente del síntoma o taburete. Sigue medicación a la dosis original dentro de 2 ó 3 días y la disminuye gradualmente hasta dejar la medicación en 3 ó 4 días. |
| 剂型、规格<br>Formulaciones y especificaciones | 片剂：每片 0.125g；0.25g；0.5g。缓释片剂：每片 0.3g。胶囊剂：每粒 0.25g；0.5g。<br>Tableta: 0.125g, 0.25g: Tableta de liberación prolongada: 0.3g; Cápsula: 0.25g, 0.5g. |

| 药品名称Drug Names | 卡马西平 Carbamazepina |
|---|---|
| 适应证<br>Indicaciones | 可用于急性躁狂发作，抑郁发作及双相情感性精神障碍的维持治疗。锂盐治疗无效或不能耐受时可考虑选用卡马西平代替。<br><br>Se usa en tratamiento de mantenimiento de episodio maníaco agudo, episodio depresivo y trastorno bipolar. Puede ser alternativa de litio cuando éste no se efectua o pacientes estén intolerantes. |
| 用法、用量<br>Administración y dosis | 抗躁狂症：口服，成人开始每日 400mg，分 2 次服用。以后隔 1～2 周每日量增加 200mg，分 3～4 次服。治疗量每日 600～1200mg，分 3～4 次服，与其他肝药酶诱导剂合用可达每日 1600mg。急性躁狂症，每日 600～1200mg，分 2 次服用。<br><br>Anti-mania: por vía oral y para adultos la dosis inicial es de 400mg diarios didividos en 2 tomas y aumenta la dosis en 200mg diarios cada 2～3 semanas y divididos en 3～4 tomas. Dosis para tratamiento es de 600～1200mg diarios divididos en 3～4 tomas y puede aumentar a 1600mg diarios cuando lo usa en conjunción con otros inductores de enzimas hepáticas. En tratamiento de manía aguda: 600-1200mg diarios divididos en 2 tomas. |
| 剂型、规格<br>Formulaciones y especificaciones | 片剂：每片 100mg；200mg；400mg。胶囊剂：每粒 200mg；300mg。<br>Tableta: 100mg, 200mg, 400mg; Cápsula: 200mg, 300mg. |

| 续　表 | |
|---|---|
| 药品名称 Drug Names | 丙戊酸钠 Valproato de sodio |
| 适应证<br>Indicaciones | 可用于急性躁狂发作的治疗，长期服用对双相情感性神经障碍的反复发作具有预防作用。<br><br>Se usa en tratamiento de episodio maníaco agudo. El medicamento a largo plazo tiene efecto de prevención del trastorno bipolar. |
| 用法、用量<br>Administración y<br>dosis | 治疗躁狂症：口服，小剂量开始，每次 200mg，一日 2～3 次，逐渐增加至每次 300～400mg，一日 2～3 次。最高剂量不超过每日 1600mg。6 岁以上儿童每日 20～30mg/kg，分 3～4 次服用。<br><br>En tratamiento de mania: por vía oral y empieza a dosis pequeña de 200mg 2 ó 3 veces al día. Gradualmente aumenta la dosis hasta 300～400mg 2 ó 3 veces al día. Dosis máxima no excede a 1600mg diarios. Para niños mayores de 6 años la dosis es de 20～30mg/kg diarios divididos en 3 ó 4 tomas. |
| 剂型、规格<br>Formulaciones y<br>especificaciones | 片剂：每片 200mg。<br>Tableta: 200mg. |

8.11 　抗抑郁药 Los antidepresivos

| 药品名称 Drug Names | 丙米嗪 Imipramina |
|---|---|
| 适应证<br>Indicaciones | ①用于各种类型的抑郁症治疗。对内源性抑郁症、反应性抑郁症及更年期抑郁症均有效，但疗效出现慢（多在 1 周后才出现效果）。对精神分裂症伴发的抑郁状态 则几乎无效或疗效差。②可用于惊恐发作的治疗，其疗效与 MAOIs 相当。③可用于小儿遗尿症。<br><br>① Se usa en tratamiento de varios tipos de depresión. Es eficaz para depresión endógena, reactiva y menopausia pero la acción es lenta que se efectua generalmente 1 semana después de medicamento. Para depresión asociada con la esquizofrenia se ve poco efecto. ② Puede usarse en tratamiento del ataque de pánico que tiene efecto similar a maois. ③ Se puede usar en tratamiento de enuresis infantil. |
| 用法、用量<br>Administración y<br>dosis | 口服。①治疗抑郁症、惊恐发作：成人每次 12.5～25mg，一日 3 次，老年体弱者一次量从 12.5mg 开始，逐渐增加剂量，极量一日 200～300mg。需根据耐受情况调整用量。②小儿遗尿：6 岁以上，一次 12.5～25mg，每晚 1 次。如在 1 周内未获满意效果，12 岁以下每日可增至 50mg，12 岁以上每日可增至 75mg。<br><br>Por vía oral. ① En tratamiento de la depresión y los ataques de pánico: 12.5～25mg cada vez para adultos y se administra 3 veces al día. Para ancianos y debiles la dosis inicial es de 12.5mg y aumenta la dosis gradualmente. La dosis máxima no debe exceder a 200～300mg diarios y puede ajustarla según la tolerancia del paciente. ② En tratamiento de enuresis infantil: para niños mayores de 6 años la dosis es 12.5～25mg cada día tomados por la noche. Si no tiene efecto dentro de 1 semana, puede aumentar a 50mg diarios para niños menores de 12 años y 75mg diarios para los mayores de 12 años. |
| 剂型、规格<br>Formulaciones y<br>especificaciones | 片剂：每片 10mg；25mg；50mg；75mg。胶囊剂：每粒 75mg；100mg；125mg。缓释胶囊：每粒 50mg。注射剂：每支 25mg（2ml）。<br>Tableta: 10mg, 25mg, 50mg, 75mg; Cápsula: 75mg, 100mg, 125mg; Cápsula de liberación prolongada: 50mg; Inyección: 25mg (2ml). |
| 药品名称 Drug Names | 氯米帕明 Clomipramina |
| 适应证<br>Indicaciones | ①用于治疗内源性、反应性、神经性、隐匿性抑郁症及各种抑郁状态；伴有抑郁症的精神分裂症。②对强迫性神经症具有较好的疗效。③对恐怖症、惊恐发作、继发性焦虑、慢性疼痛综合征、神经性厌食及发作性睡病均有一定疗效。<br><br>① Se usa en tratamiento de depresión y estado de depresivo de tipo endógeno, reactivo, neurológico y enmascarado, la esquizofrenia asociada con la depresión. ② Tiene buen efecto en tratamiento de trastorno obsesivo-compulsivo. ③ Es eficaz en tratamiento de fobia, ataque de pánico, ansiedad secundaria, síndrome de dolor crónico, anorexia nerviosa y narcolepsia. |

**续 表**

| 用法、用量<br>Administración y dosis | （1）治疗抑郁症、强迫症：①口服，成人初始每次25mg，一日3次（或服缓释片，75mg，每晚一次），1周内可见增至最适宜的治疗量。一日最大剂量为250mg。症状好转后，改为维持量，每日50～100mg（缓释片剂每日75mg）。老年患者，开始每日10mg，逐渐增加至30～50mg（约10日），然后改维持量以每日不超过75mg为宜。②静脉滴注：开始每日剂量每日25～50mg，用250ml葡萄糖注射液稀释，输入时间不低于2小时。通常剂量为每日100mg。<br>（2）治疗慢性痛性疾病：每日10～150mg，最好同时服用镇痛药。<br><br>(1) En tratamiento de depresión y trastorno obsesivo-compulsivo: ① Por vía oral: para adultos la dosis es de 25mg por 3 veces al día o si toma tableta de liberación prolongada la dosis es de 75mg una vez por la noche. Durante una semana puede aumentar a la dosis más efectiva para tratamiento. Por lo máximo no debe exceder a 250mg diarios. Cuando se ve mejoramiento, cambia a dosis de mantenimiento de 50 ~ 100mg diarios ó 75mg diarios de tableta de liberación prolongada. Para pacientes ancianos, inicie desde 10mg diarios y aumenta gradualmente a 30 ~ 50mg dentro de 10 días y luego cambia a dosis de mantenimiento no excedida a 75mg diarios. ② Infusión por I.V.: Dosis inicial es de 25 ~ 50mg diarios diluidos en 250ml de solución de glucosa. La infusión se administra durante más de 2 horas. Dosis habitual es de 100mg diarios.<br>(2) En tratamiento de enfermedad de dolor crónico: 10 ~ 150mg diarios y es mejor tomar analgésicos al mismo tiempo. |
| :--- | :--- |
| 剂型、规格<br>Formulaciones y especificaciones | 片剂：每片10mg；25mg；50mg。缓释片：每片75mg。胶囊剂：每粒25mg；50mg；75mg。注射剂：每支25mg（2ml）。<br>Tableta: 10mg, 25mg, 50mg; Tableta de liberación prolongada: 75mg; Cápsula: 25mg, 50mg, 75mg; Inyección: 25mg (2ml). |
| **药品名称 Drug Names** | 阿米替林 Amitriptilina |
| 适应证<br>Indicaciones | ①用于治疗各型抑郁症或抑郁状态。对内因性抑郁症和更年期抑郁症疗效较好，对反应性抑郁症及神经官能症的抑郁状态亦有效。对兼有焦虑和抑郁症状患者，疗效优于丙米嗪。与电休克联合使用于重症抑郁症，可减少电休克次数。②用于缓解慢性疼痛。③亦用于治疗小儿遗尿症、儿童多动症。<br><br>① Se usa en tratamiento de uba variedad de depresión o síntomas depresivos. Es eficaz para depresión endógena y menopáusica así como depresión reactiva y síntomas depresivos de neurosis. Tiene mejor efecto comparado con imipramina para pacientes de depresión y ansiedad. Se usa en conbinación con descarga eléctrica en tratamiento de depresión severa y puede reducir el uso de descarga eléctrica. ② Para alivio de dolor crónico. ③ Se usa también en tratamiento de enuresis infantil y TDAH infantil. |
| 用法、用量<br>Administración y dosis | ①治疗抑郁症、慢性疼痛：口服，每次25mg，一日2～4次，以后递增至每日150～300mg，分次服。维持量每日50～200mg。老年患者和青少年，每日50mg，分次或夜间1次服。静脉注射或肌内注射，成人每次20～30mg，一日3～4次。②治疗遗尿症：睡前1次口服，10～25mg。③治疗儿童多动症：7岁以上儿童每次10～25mg，一日2～3次。<br><br>① En tratamiento de depresión y dolor crónico: por vía oral a dosis de 25mg 2 ó 4 veces al día. Aumenta la dosis gradualmente a 150 ~ 300mg diarios en varias tomas. La dosis de mantenimiento es de 50 ~ 200mg diarios. Para ancianos y juventud, la dosis es de 50mg diarios una vez por la noche o divididamente. Inyección por I.V. o I.M.: la dosis para adultos es 20 ~ 30mg 3 ó 4 veces al día. ② En tratamiento de enuresis: 10 ~ 25mg una vez antes de acostarse. ③ En tratamiento de TDAH infantil: para niños mayores de 7 años la dosis es de 10 ~ 25mg 2 ó 3 veces al día. |
| 剂型、规格<br>Formulaciones y especificaciones | 片剂：每片10mg；25mg；50mg；75mg；100mg；150mg。缓释胶囊剂：每粒25mg；50mg；75mg。注射剂：每支20mg（2ml）；50mg（2ml）；100mg（10ml）。<br>Tableta: 10mg, 25mg, 50mg, 75mg, 100mg, 150mg; Cápsula de liberación prolongada: 25mg, 50mg, 75mg; Inyección: 20mg (2ml), 50mg(2ml), 100mg(10ml). |
| **药品名称 Drug Names** | 多塞平 Doxepina |
| 适应证<br>Indicaciones | ①用于治疗抑郁症和各种焦虑抑郁为主的神经症，亦可用于更年期精神病，对抑郁和焦虑的躯体性疾病和慢性酒精性精神病也有效。也可用于镇静及催眠。②本品外用膏剂用于治疗慢性单纯性苔藓、湿疹、过敏性皮炎、特应性皮炎等。<br><br>① Se usa en tratamiento de depresión y variedad de neurosis de ansiedad y depresión así como psicosis menopáusica. Es eficaz para enfermedades somaticas de depresión y ansiedad y psicosis alcohólica crónica. Puede usarse también en sedación e hipnotización. ② El ungüento tópico se utiliza en tratamiento de liquen simple crónico, eczema, dermatitis alérgica y atópica. |

**续　表**

| | |
|---|---|
| 用法、用量<br>Administración y<br>dosis | ①口服，初始剂量每次 25mg，一日 3 次，然后逐渐增至每日 150 ~ 300mg。宜在餐后服用，以减少胃部刺激。严重的焦虑性抑郁症可肌内注射，每次 25 ~ 50mg，一日 2 次。②局部外用：于患处涂布一薄层，一日 3 次，每次涂布面积不超过总面积的 5%，2 次使用应间隔 4 小时。建议短期敷用，不超过 7 ~ 8 日。<br><br>① Por vía oral. Dosis inicial es de 25mg 3 veces al día. Aumenta la dosis gradualmente a 150 ~ 300mg diarios. Debe tomarlos después de alimento para disminuir estímulo al estómago. Puede administrar inyección por I.M. en caso de severa depresión ansiosa a una dosis de 25 ~ 50mg 2 veces al día. ② Uso tópico: Recubierto con una capa 3 veces al día en la área afectada que debe ser menor de la 5% del cuerpo. El intervalo de medicación debe ser más de 4 horas. Recomienda medicación a corto plazo que será dentro de 7 ~ 8 días. |
| 剂型、规格<br>Formulaciones y<br>especificaciones | 片剂：每片 5mg；10mg；25mg；50mg；100mg。胶囊剂：每粒 10mg；25mg；50mg；75mg；100mg；150mg。注射剂：每支 25mg（1ml）；50mg（2ml）。盐酸多塞平乳膏：每支 10g。<br><br>Tableta: 5mg, 10mg,25mg, 50mg, 100mg; Cápsula: 10mg, 25mg, 50mg, 75mg, 100mg, 150mg; Inyección: 25mg(1ml), 50mg (2ml); Crema de Doxepina Clorhidrato: 10g. |
| 药品名称 Drug Names | 吗氯贝胺 Moclobemida |
| 适应证<br>Indicaciones | ①对双相、单相、激动型、阻滞型及各种亚型抑郁症均有效。对精神运动性阻滞和情绪抑郁症状的改善显著。用于对 TCAs 不适用或已不再有效的患者。②对睡眠障碍也有一定效果。<br><br>① Es eficaz para tratamiento de subtipos de depresión como la depresión bipolar, unipolar, agitada y retardada. Puede mejorar significativamente el retraso psicomotor y los síntomas de depresión emocional. Se puede utilizar para pacientes que no consigue efecto con TCAS. ② Tiene efecto también en tratamiento de trastorno del sueño. |
| 用法、用量<br>Administración y<br>dosis | 口服：每日 100 ~ 400mg，分次饭后服，可根据病情增减至每日 150 ~ 600mg。<br><br>Por vía oral. Dosis diaria de 100 ~ 400mg divididos en varias tomas después de alimentos. Según la necesidad puede disminuir la dosis a 150 ~ 600mg diarios. |
| 剂型、规格<br>Formulaciones y<br>especificaciones | 片剂：每片 75mg；100mg；150mg；300mg。胶囊剂：每粒 100mg。<br>Tableta: 75mg, 100mg, 150mg, 300mg; Cápsula: 100mg. |
| 药品名称 Drug Names | 氟西汀 Fluoxetina |
| 适应证<br>Indicaciones | ①用于治疗伴有焦虑的各种抑郁症，尤宜用于老年抑郁症。②用于治疗惊恐状态，对广泛性焦虑障碍也有一定疗效。③用于治疗强迫障碍，但药物剂量应相应加大。④适用于社交恐惧症、进食障碍。<br><br>① Se usa en tratamiento de depresión asociada con ansiedad especialmente la depresión senil. ② Se usa en tratamiento del estado de pánico y tiene efecto en tratamiento de trastorno de ansiedad generalizada. ③ Se usa en tratamiento de de trastorno obsesivo-compulsivo y debe aumentar la dosis adecuadamente. ④ Puede usarse en tratamiento de la fobia social y trastorno de la alimentación. |
| 用法、用量<br>Administración y<br>dosis | 口服。①治疗抑郁症：最初治疗建议每日 20mg，一般 4 周后才能显效。若未能控制症状，可考虑增加剂量，每日可增加 20mg。最大推荐剂量每日 80mg。维持治疗可以每日使用 20mg。②强迫症：建议初始剂量为每日晨 20mg，维持治疗可以每日 20 ~ 60mg。③暴食症：建议每日 60mg。④惊恐障碍：初始剂量每日 10mg，1 周后可逐渐增加至每日 20mg，如果症状没有有效控制，可适当增加剂量至每日 60mg。<br><br>Por vía oral. ① En tratamiento de depresión: Recomienda 20mg diarios al iniciar el tratamiento y generalmente se efectua durante 4 semanas. Si no puede controlar los síntomas puede aumentar la dosis en 20mg cada día. La dosis máxima recomedada es de 80mg diarios y la de mantenimiento es de 20mg diarios. ② En tratamiento de trastorno obsesivo-compulsivo: la dosis inicial recomendada es de 20mg diarios una vez tomados en la mañana y la de mantenimiento es de 20 ~ 60mg diarios. ③ En caso de bulimia, la dosis recomendada es de 60mg diarios. ④ En caso de trastorno de pánico, la dosis inicial es de 10mg diarios y después de 1 semana agrega gradualmente a 20mg diarios. Si no está controlado el síntoma aumenta la dosis hasta los 60mg diarios. |

**续 表**

| 剂型、规格<br>Formulaciones y<br>especificaciones | 片剂：每片 10mg；20mg。肠溶片：90mg。胶囊剂：每粒 5mg；10mg；20mg；40mg；60mg。<br>Tableta: 10mg, 20mg; Tabletas con recubrimiento entérico: 90mg; Cápsula: 5mg, 10mg, 20mg, 40mg, 60mg. |
|---|---|
| 药品名称 Drug Names | 氟伏沙明 Fluvoxamina |
| 适应证<br>Indicaciones | ①用于治疗各类抑郁症，特别是持久性抑郁症状及自杀风险大的患者。②还可治疗强迫症和心身性疾病。<br>① Se usa en tratamiento de todo tipo de depresión especialmente los síntomas depresivos persistentes y pacientes de gran riesgo de suicidio. ② También puede usarse en tratamiento de trastorno obsesivo-compulsivo y psicosomático. |
| 用法、用量<br>Administración y<br>dosis | 口服。①抗抑郁：初始剂量每日 50～100mg，睡前服。每4～7日增加 50mg，剂量可视病情调整，剂量超过每日 150mg 时应分次服用，饭时或饭后服。维持期用药，以 1 日 50～100mg 为宜。②强迫症：初始剂量每日 100～300mg。最大剂量为每日 300mg。<br>Por vía oral. ① Uso antidepresivo: Dosis inicial es de 50～100mg diarios tomados antes de acostarse. Agrega 50mg cada 4～7 días y puede ajustar la dosis según la necesidad. Cuando la dosis diaria excede a 150mg debe tomarlos divididamente acompañado o después de alimentos. Dosis de mantenimiento es 50～100mg diarios. ② En tratamiento de trastorno obsesivo-compulsivo: Dosis inicial es de 100~300mg diarios y no excede a 300mg diarios. |
| 剂型、规格<br>Formulaciones y<br>especificaciones | 片剂：每片 50mg；100mg；200mg。胶囊剂：每粒 20mg。肠溶片：90mg。<br>Tableta: 50mg, 100mg, 200mg; Cápsula: 20mg; Tabletas con recubrimiento entérico: 90mg. |
| 药品名称 Drug Names | 帕罗西汀 Paroxetina |
| 适应证<br>Indicaciones | ①用于治疗抑郁症。适合治疗伴有焦虑症和抑郁症患者，作用比 TCAs 快，而且远期疗效比丙米嗪好。②亦可用于惊恐障碍、社交恐怖症及强迫症的治疗。<br>① Se usa en tratamiento de depresión y es eficaz para pacientes de depresión acompañada con ansiedad. Tiene acción más rápida que TCAs y mejor efecto que imipramina en tratamiento a largo plazo. ② Se usa también en tratamiento de trastorno de pánico, fobia social y trastorno obsesivo-compulsivo. |
| 用法、用量<br>Administración y<br>dosis | 口服。通常一日剂量范围在 20～50mg，一般从 20mg 开始，一日 1 次，早餐时顿服。连续用药 3 周。以后根据临床反应增减剂量，每次增减 10mg，间隔不得少于 1 周。最大推荐剂量为每日 50mg（治疗强迫症可 60mg）。老年人或肝、肾功能不全者可从每日 10mg 开始，每日最高剂量不超过 40mg。对于肌酐清除率 < 30ml/min 的患者，推荐剂量每日 20mg。<br>Por vía oral. Dosis habitual es de entre 20 y 50mg diarios. Empieza desde 20mg una vez al día tomados en el desayuno y la medicación continua durante 3 semanas. Luego según la respuesta clínica puede aumentar o disminuir la dosis en 10mg con intervalo de más de 1 semana. La dosis máxima recomendada es de 50mg diarios y en caso de trastorno obsesivo-compulsivo, (puede ser 60mg diarios). Para pacientes ancianos y de insuficiencia hepática y renal empieza la administración a 10mg diarios y no excede a 40mg diarios. Para pacientes con clearance de creatinina menor de 30 ml/min, la dosis recomendada es de 20mg diarios. |
| 剂型、规格<br>Formulaciones y<br>especificaciones | 片剂：每片 20mg；30mg。<br>Tableta: 20mg, 30mg. |
| 药品名称 Drug Names | 舍曲林 Sertralina |
| 适应证<br>Indicaciones | 用于治疗抑郁症、强迫症、心境恶劣、性欲倒错等。预防抑郁症复发。<br>Se usa en tratamiento de depresión, trastorno obsesivo-compulsivo, distimia, parafilias y en prevención de recaída de depresión. |
| 用法、用量<br>Administración y<br>dosis | 口服。开始每日 50mg，一日 1 次，与食物同服，早晚均可。数周后增加 50mg。调整剂量时间间隔不能短于 1 周。常用剂量为每日 50～100mg，最大剂量为每日 200mg（此剂量不得连续服用超过 8 周以上）。需长期服用者，需用最低有效量。 |

**续　表**

| | |
|---|---|
| | Por vía oral. Dosis inicial es de 50mg una vez al día acompañado con alimentos. Puede tomarlos en la mañana o en la noche. Dentro de unas semanas agrega 50mg y el intervalo de ajustar dosis debe ser más de 1 semana. La dosis habitual es de 50 ~ 100mg diarios y no excede a 200mg diarios, (dosis que no puede aplicarse durante más de 8 semanas continuas. Para medicación a largo plazo debe aplicar a la dosis efectiva más pequeña). |
| 剂型、规格<br>Formulaciones y<br>especificaciones | 片剂：每片 50mg；100mg。胶囊剂：每粒 50mg；100mg。<br>Tableta: 50mg, 100mg; Cápsula: 50mg, 100mg. |
| **药品名称 Drug Names** | 西酞普兰 Citalopram |
| 适应证<br>Indicaciones | ①用于内源性或非内源性抑郁症。②焦虑性神经症、广场恐惧症、强迫症、经前期心境障碍神经症。③酒精依赖性行为障碍、痴呆的行为问题。④卒中后病理性哭泣。<br>① Se usa en tratamiento de depresión endógena o no endógena. ② Se usa en tratamiento de neurosis de angustia, agorafobia, trastorno obsesivo-compulsivo y trastorno disfórico premenstrual. ③ Se usa en tratamiento de trastornos del comportamiento por alcoholismo y demencia. ④ Se usa en tratamiento del llanto patológico después del accidente cerebrovascular. |
| 用法、用量<br>Administración y<br>dosis | 口服。每日 20 ~ 60mg，一日 1 次，晨起或晚间顿服。推荐初始剂量为每日 20mg，再根据患者症状控制情况酌情增减，逐渐达到稳定控制病情的最小有效剂量。计量调整间隔时间不能少于 1 周，一般为 2 ~ 3 周。通常需要经过 2 ~ 3 周的治疗方可判定疗效。为防止复发，治疗至少持续 6 个月。肝功能不全及年龄超过 65 岁的老人：推荐剂量较常量减半。<br>Por vía oral. La dosis diaria es de 20 ~ 60mg una vez tomados en la mañana o en la noche. La dosis inicial recomendada es de 20mg diarios y aumentarla gradualmente según la necesidad hasta la dosis efectiva más pequeña para mantener el tratamiento. El intervalo de ajustar la dosis debe ser más de 1 semana que generalmente será 2 ó 3 semanas. Habitualmente puede determinar la eficacia tras medicación de 2 ~ 3 semanas. Para prevenir la recaída, el tratamiento siempre dura más de 6 meses. Para pacientes ancianos y de insuficiencia hepática, recomenda reducir a la mitad de a dosis habitual. |
| 剂型、规格<br>Formulaciones y<br>especificaciones | 片剂：每片 10mg；20mg；30mg；40mg。口服液：每支 20mg（10ml）。<br>Tableta: 10mg, 20mg, 30mg, 40mg; Solución oral: 20mg (10ml). |
| **药品名称 Drug Names** | 艾司西酞普兰 Escitalopram |
| 适应证<br>Indicaciones | ①用于内源性或非内源性抑郁症。②焦虑性神经症、广场恐惧症、强迫症、经前期心境障碍神经症。③酒精依赖性行为障碍、痴呆的行为问题。④卒中后病理性哭泣。<br>① Se usa en tratamiento de depresión endógena o no endógena. ② Se usa en tratamiento de neurosis de angustia, agorafobia, trastorno obsesivo-compulsivo y trastorno disfórico premenstrual. ③ Se usa en tratamiento de trastornos del comportamiento por alcoholismo y demencia. ④ Se usa en tratamiento del llanto patológico después del accidente cerebrovascular. |
| 用法、用量<br>Administración y<br>dosis | 口服。治疗抑郁症：一日 10mg，一日 1 次。根据患者的临床情况最大剂量可增至每日 20mg。通常 2 ~ 4 周可控制抑郁症状，症状缓解后需巩固维持治疗至少 6 个月。伴或不伴恐怖症的患者：初始剂量为每日 5mg，持续 1 周后可考虑增加至每日 10mg。根据患者的个体反应，剂量可增至每日 20mg。老年患者：推荐半量使用本品，最大剂量也不应超过每日 20mg。肝功能不全者或 CYP2C19 慢代谢者：建议起始剂量每日 5mg，持续 2 周后，可根据患者的个体反应，剂量增加至每日 10mg。<br>Por vía oral. En tratamiento de depresión: la dosis es de 10mg una vez al día y según la respuesta clínica del paciente la dosis máxima puede llegar a 20mg diarios. Generalmente puede controlar los síntomas depresivos dentro de 2 ~ 4 semanas y debe continuar con tratamiento de mantenimiento después del alivio de los síntomas durante 6 meses por lo menos. En cuanto a pacientes asociados con o sin fóbicos: la dosis inicial es de 5mg diarios y después de medicación de 1 semana puede aumentarla a 10mg diarios e incluso 20mg según la condición del paciente. Para pacientes ancianos recomienda la mitad de la dosis habitual y la máxima no debe exceder a 20mg diarios. Para pacientes de insuficiencia hepática o metabolizadores lentos de CYP2C19: la dosis inicial recomendada es de 5mg diarios y después de medicamento de 2 semanas puede aumentar a 10mg según la condición del paciente. |

**续 表**

| 剂型、规格<br>Formulaciones y especificaciones | 片剂：每片 5mg；10mg。<br>Tableta: 5mg, 10mg. |
| --- | --- |

## 8.12 抗脑血管病药 Medicamentos contra la enfermedad cerebrovascular

| 药品名称 Drug Names | 尼莫地平 Nimodipina |
| --- | --- |
| 适应证<br>Indicaciones | ①用于急性脑血管病恢复期的血液循环改善。各种原因的蛛网膜下腔出血后的脑血管痉挛，及其所致的缺血性神经障碍高血压、偏头痛等。②也被用作缺血性神经元保护和血管性痴呆的治疗。③对突发性耳聋也有一定疗效。<br><br>① Se usa en mejoramiento de circulación de la sangre de la recuperación de la enfermedad cerebrovascular aguda y tratamiento de vasoespasmo cerebral e hipertensión y migraña causados por trastornos neurológicos isquémicos asociados con la hemorragia subaracnoidea. ② Se usa también en protección neuronal de la isquemia y tratamiento de demencia vascular. ③ Tiene cierta eficacia en tratamiento de sordera súbita. |
| 用法、用量<br>Administración y dosis | 口服：①治疗缺血性脑血管病：片剂，每次 30～40mg，一日 3 次；缓释剂，每次 60mg，一日 2 次。连用 1 个月。②治疗突发性聋：片剂，每次 10～20mg，一日 3 次；缓释剂，每次 60mg，一日 1 次。5 日一个疗程，可用 3～4 个疗程。③治疗轻、中度高血压：每次 40mg，一日 3 次。④治疗偏头痛：片剂，每次 40mg，一日 3 次；缓释剂，每次 60mg，一日 2 次，12 周为 1 个疗程。⑤老年性认知功能减退或血管性痴呆：每次 30～40mg，一日 3 次，连服 2 个月。⑥蛛网膜下腔出血所致脑血管痉挛：片剂，每次 40～60mg，一日 2～3 次，发病当日即可服用；缓释剂每次 60mg，一日 2 次。连用 3～4 周 1 个疗程。如需手术，术前停药，术后可继续服用。静脉滴注：治疗蛛网膜下腔出血，滴速 0.5μg/（kg•min），随时检测血压，病情稳定后改口服，成人每次 20～30mg，一日 2 次。<br><br>Por vía oral: ① En tratamiento de enfermedad Cerebrovascular Isquémica: Tabletas: 30～40mg por 3 veces al día; Tableta de liberación prolongada: 60mg por 2 veces al día y se administra durante 1 mes. ② En tratamiento de sordera súbita: Tabletas: 10～20mg por 3 veces al día; Tableta de liberación prolongada: 60mg una vez al día. Un curso de tratamiento es de 5 días y puede repetir hasta 3 ó 4 cursos. ③ En tratamiento de hipertensión leve y moderada: 40mg por 3 veces al día. ④ En tratamiento de migraña: Tabletas: 40mg por 3 veces al día; Tableta de liberación prolongada: 60mg por 2 veces al día y un curso de tratamiento es de 12 semanas. ⑤ En tratamiento de disfunción cognitiva senil o demencia vascular: 30~40mg por 3 veces al día y se administra durante 2 meses. ⑥ En tratamiento de vasoespasmo cerebral causado por la hemorragia subaracnoidea: Tabletas: 40～60mg por 2 ó 3 veces al día y puede administrarse en el primer día de la aparición del síntoma; Tableta de liberación prolongada: 60mg por 2 veces al día. Se administra durante 3 ó 4 semanas como un curso de tratamiento. Si necesita cirugía hay que dejar la medicación y puede retomarlos después de la cirugía. Infusión I.V. para tratamiento de hemorragia subaracnoidea: 0.5μg/(kg•min) y al mismo tiempo tenga observado la presión arterial. Cuando tenga controlado la enfermedad puede seguir medicación por vía oral a dosis de 20～30mg por 2 veces al día para adultos. |
| 剂型、规格<br>Formulaciones y especificaciones | 片剂：每片 10mg；20mg；30mg。胶囊剂：20mg；30mg。控释片：每片 60mg。缓释片：每片 60mg。缓释胶囊：每粒 60mg。注射剂：每支 2mg（10ml）；4mg（20ml）；8mg（40ml）；10mg（50ml）；25mg（50ml）；20mg（100ml）。<br><br>Tableta: 10mg, 20mg, 30mg; Cápsula: 20mg, 30mg; Tableta de liberación controlada: 60mg; Tableta de liberación prolongada: 60mg; Cápsula de liberación prolongada: 60mg; Inyección: 2mg(10ml), 4mg(20ml), 8mg(40ml), 10mg (50ml), 25mg (50ml), 20mg (100ml). |
| 药品名称 Drug Names | 桂利嗪 Cinarizina |
| 适应证<br>Indicaciones | ①用于脑血栓形成、脑梗死、短暂性缺血发作、脑动脉硬化、脑出血恢复期、蛛网膜下腔出血恢复期、脑外伤后遗症、前庭性眩晕与平衡障碍（包括晕动病等）、冠状动脉硬化及供血障碍，以及由于末梢循环不良引起的疾病（如间歇性跛行及 Raynaud 病等）。②有文献报道，本品还可用于治疗慢性荨麻疹、老年性皮肤瘙痒等过敏性皮肤病。还可以治疗顽固性呃逆。<br><br>① Se usa en tratamiento de trombosis cerebral, infarto cerebral, ataque isquémico transitorio, arteriosclerosis cerebral, recuperación de hemorragia cerebral y hemorragia subaracnoidea, secuelas de la lesión cerebral traumática, vértigo vestibular y trastornos del equilibrio (incluyendo la enfermedad de movimiento), enfermedad arterial coronaria y trastornos de la sangre, enfermedades causados por mala circulación periférica por ejempro claudicación intermitente y enfermedad de Raymaud. ② Se ha informado de que se puede usar en tratamiento de enfermedades alérgicas de la piel por ejempro urticaria crónica y prurito senil así como hipo intratable. |

**续　表**

| 用法、用量<br>Administración y dosis | 口服：一般每次 25 ～ 50mg，一日 3 次，饭后服。晕动病患者于乘车船前 1 ～ 2 小时，1 次服用 30mg；乘车船期间每 6 ～ 8 小时服用 1 次（根据头晕等症状情况）。静脉注射：1 次 20 ～ 40mg，缓慢注入。<br><br>Por vía oral: dosis habitual es de 25 ~ 50mg por 3 veces al día después de alimentos. Para pacientes de enfermedad de movimiento, se administra 30mg 1 ó 2 horas antes de tomar vehículo o barco y durante el recorrido repetir la medicación cada 6 ~ 8 horas según la necesidad. Inyección lenta por I.V.: 20 ~ 40mg cada vez. |
|---|---|
| 剂型、规格<br>Formulaciones y especificaciones | 片剂：每片 15mg；25mg。胶囊剂：每粒 25mg；75mg。注射剂：每支 20mg（20ml）。<br>Tableta: 15mg, 25mg; Cápsula: 25mg, 75mg; Inyección: 20mg (20ml). |
| 药品名称 Drug Names | 氟桂利嗪 Flunarizina |
| 适应证<br>Indicaciones | ①脑动脉缺血性疾病，如脑动脉硬化、短暂性脑缺血发作、脑血栓形成、脑栓塞和脑血管痉挛。②有前庭刺激或脑缺血引起的头晕、耳鸣、眩晕。③血管性偏头痛的防治。④癫痫辅助治疗。⑤周围血管病：间歇性跛行、下肢静脉曲张及微循环障碍、足踝水肿等。<br><br>① Se usa en tratamiento de enfermedad isquémica del sistema arterial cerebral, por ejempro arteriosclerosis cerebral, ataque isquémico transitorio, trombosis verebral, embolia cerebral y vasoespasmo cerebral. ② Se usa en alivio de mareos, tinnitus y vértigos causados por estimulación vestibular o isquemia cerebral. ③ Se usa en prevención y tratamiento de migraña vascular. ④ Se usa en tratamiento adyuvante de epilepsia. ⑤ Se usa en tratamiento de enfermedad vascular periférica, por ejempro claudicación intermitente, várices de las extremidades inferiores, trastorno de microcirculación y edema del tobillo. |
| 用法、用量<br>Administración y dosis | 口服。脑动脉硬化、脑梗死恢复期：每日 5 ～ 10mg，一日 1 次，睡前服用。中枢性和外周性眩晕者、椎动脉供血不足者：每日 10 ～ 30mg，2 ～ 8 周为一个疗程。特发性耳鸣者：每次 10mg，每晚一次，10 日为 1 个疗程。偏头痛预防：每次 5 ～ 10mg，一日 2 次。间歇性跛行：每日 10 ～ 20mg。<br><br>Por vía oral. En tratamiento de arteriosclerosis cerebral y recuperación de infarto cerebral: 5-10mg una vez al día tomados antes de acostarse. En tratamiento de vértigos centrales y periféricos e insuficiencia de la arteria vertebral: 10 ~ 30mg diarios y un curso de tratamiento tarda 2 ~ 8 semanas. En caso de tinnitus idiopático: 10mg una vez por la noche y un curso de tratamiento tarda 10 días. En prevención de migraña: 5 ~ 10mg por 2 veces al día. En caso de claudicación intermitente: 10 ~ 20mg diarios. |
| 剂型、规格<br>Formulaciones y especificaciones | 片剂：每片 5mg。胶囊剂：每粒 5mg。滴丸：每丸 1.25mg。<br>Tableta: 5mg; Cápsula: 5mg; Píldora: 1.25mg. |
| 药品名称 Drug Names | 降纤酶 Defibrasa |
| 适应证<br>Indicaciones | ①急性脑梗死，短暂性脑缺血发作（TIA），以及脑梗死再复发的预防。②心肌梗死，不稳定型心绞痛及心肌梗死再复发的预防。③四肢血管病，包括股动脉栓塞，血栓闭塞性脉管炎，雷诺病。④血液呈高黏状态、高凝状态、血栓前状态。⑤突发性耳聋。⑥肺栓塞。<br><br>① Se usa en prevención del infarto cerebral agudo, ataque isquémico transitorio (TIA) y recurrencia de infarto cerebral. ② Se usa en prevención del infarto de miocardio, angina inestable y recurrencia de infarto de miocardio. ③ Se usa en tratamiento de enfermedades vasculares en las extremidades, por ejempro embolización de la arteria femoral, tromboangeítis obliterante y enfermedad de Raynaud. ④ Se usa cuando la sangre esté en estado de alta viscosidad, estado de hipercoagulabilidad, estado protrombótico. ⑤ Se usa en tratamiento de sordera súbita. ⑥ Se usa en tratamiento de embolia pulmonar. |
| 用法、用量<br>Administración y dosis | 静脉滴注：急性发作期，1 次 10U，一日 1 次，连用 3 ～ 4 日。非急性发作期，首次 10U，维持量 5 ～ 10U，每日或隔日 1 次，2 周为 1 个疗程。<br><br>Infusión por I.V.: En etapa exacerbación aguda: 10U una vez al día y medicamento continua por 3 ó 4 días. En etapa no exacerbación aguda: Dosis inicial de 10U y 5 ~ 10U en tratamiento de mantenimiento. Se administra una vez al día o cada otro día y el curso de tratamiento tarda 2 semanas. |

**续 表**

| 剂型、规格<br>Formulaciones y especificaciones | 注射剂（冻干制剂）：每支 5U；10U。<br>Inyección (preparación liofilizada): 5U, 10U. |
|---|---|
| **药品名称 Drug Names** | 巴曲酶 Defibrina |
| 适应证<br>Indicaciones | 用于急、慢性缺血性脑血管病（以急性效果明显），突发性耳聋，慢性动脉闭塞症，振动病，末梢循环障碍。也用于中、轻度高血压病。<br><br>Se usa en tratamiento de enfermedad Cerebrovascular isquémica aguda y crónica, especialmente en etapa aguda por su eficacia significativa, sordera súbita, enfermedad arterial oclusiva crónica, vibración y trastornos de la circulación periférica.  Se usa también en hipertensión leve y moderada. |
| 用法、用量<br>Administración y dosis | 静脉滴注：首次剂量 10BU，以后维持剂量为 5BU，隔日 1 次。用 100～250ml 生理盐水稀释，1～1.5 小时滴完。给药前血纤溶酶原超过 400mg/dl 或重度突发性耳聋患者剂量应加倍。通常治疗急性缺血性脑血管病一疗程 3 次，治疗突发性耳聋必要时可延长至 3 周，治疗慢性动脉闭塞症可延长至 6 周，但在延长期每次剂量改为 5BU，隔日 1 次。<br><br>Infusión por I.V.: Dosis inicial es de 10BU y la de mantenimiento es de 5BU. Se administra cada otro día diluidos en 100 ~ 250ml de Normal Saline y la infusión terminará en 1 ~ 1.5 horas. Hay que aumentar la dosis para pacientes que tiene el plasminógeno sobrepasado a 400mg/dl o pacientes de sordera súbita severa. Habitualmente el curso de tratamiento de la enfermedad Cerebrovascular isquémica aguda es de 3 medicaciones y puede extenderse a 3 semanas en caso de sordera súbita. Si es de enfermedad arterial oclusiva crónica el tratamiento será de 6 semanas y durante el período extendido se aplica a dosis de 5BU cada otro día. |
| 剂型、规格<br>Formulaciones y especificaciones | 注射剂：每支 5BU（0.5ml）；10BU（1ml）。<br>Inyección: 5BU(0.5ml), 10BU(1ml). |
| **药品名称 Drug Names** | 倍他司汀 Betahistina |
| 适应证<br>Indicaciones | 主要用于梅尼埃综合征、血管性头痛及脑动脉硬化，并可用于治疗急性缺血性脑血管疾病，如脑血栓、脑栓塞、一过性脑供血不足等；对高血压所致直立性眩晕、耳鸣等亦有效。<br><br>Se usa principalmente en tratamiento de síndrome de Meniere, cefalea vascular y arteriosclerosis cerebral así como enfermedad cerebrovascular isquémico aguda, por ejempro trombosis cerebral, embolia cerebral e insuficiencia cerebral transitoria. Es eficaz también para mareo ortostático y tinnitus causados por hipertensión. |
| 用法、用量<br>Administración y dosis | 盐酸倍他司汀片：口服，成人每次 4～8mg，一日 2～4 次，最大日量不得超过 48mg。甲磺酸倍他司汀片：口服，成人每次 2～6mg，一日 3 次，餐后服用。盐酸倍他司汀注射液：肌内注射，每次 2～4mg，一日 2 次；静脉滴注，每次 20mg，一日 1 次。将本品溶于 2ml 5% 葡萄糖溶液或 0.9% 氯化钠溶液中，在溶于静脉滴注液 500ml 中缓慢静脉滴注。<br><br>Tableta de Betahistina de hidrocloruro: por vía oral a una dosis de 4-8mg por 2 ~ 4 veces al día para adulos. La dosis máxima no excede a 48mg diarios. Tableta de Betahistina de mesilato: por vía oral a una dosis de 2 ~ 6mg por 3 veces al día para adulos después de alimentos. Inyección de Betahistina de hidrocloruro: inyección por I.M. a una dosis de 2 ~ 4mg por 2 veces al día e infusión por I.V. a una dosis de 20mg una vez al día diluidos con 2ml de solución de glucosa o de cloruro de sodio y luego diluidos en 500ml de solución de infusión. Se administra lentamente. |
| 剂型、规格<br>Formulaciones y especificaciones | 片剂（盐酸盐）：每片 4mg。片剂（甲磺酸盐）：每片 6mg。注射液：每支 2mg（2ml）；4mg（4ml）。<br>Tableta (de hidrocloruro): 4mg; Tableta (de mesilato): 6mg; Inyección: 2mg(2ml), 4mg(4ml). |
| **药品名称 Drug Names** | 罂粟碱 Papaverina |
| 适应证<br>Indicaciones | 用于脑血栓形成、脑栓塞、肺栓塞、肢端动脉痉挛及动脉栓塞性疼痛。还可用于调节冠脉血流，缓解胃肠道痉挛和咳嗽治疗。海绵体注射用于勃起障碍治疗。<br><br>Se usa en tratamiento de trombosis cerebral, embolia cerebral, embolia pulmonar, espasmo arterial de las extremidades y dolor de la embolización de la arteria. También puede usarse en regulación del flujo sanguíneo coronario, alivio de los espasmos gastrointestinales y tratamiento de la tos. La inyección intracavernosa se aplica en tratamiento de disfunción eréctil. |

**续　表**

| 用法、用量<br>Administración y dosis | 成人常用量：口服，每次 30 ～ 60mg，一日 3 次。肌内注射，每次 30mg，一日 90 ～ 120mg。静脉注射，每次 30 ～ 120mg，3 小时 1 次，应缓慢注射，不少于 1 ～ 2 分钟，以免发生心律失常及足以致命的窒息等。用于心脏停搏时，2 次给药要相隔 10 分钟。海绵体注射：推荐 1 次 30mg，每周连续 2 次或不超过 3 次。儿童：肌内或静脉注射，一次按体重 1.5mg/kg，一日 4 次。<br><br>Dosis habitual para adultos: por vía oral es de 30 ~ 60mg por 3 veces al día. Inyección por I.M. es de 30mg cada vez y 3 ó 4 veces al día. Inyección por I.V. es de 30 ~ 120mg cada 3 horas. Debe administrarse lentamente en 1 ~ 2 minutos por lo menos para evitar arritmia o asfixia letal. En caso de paro cardíaco debe aplicar la medicación con intervalo de 10 minutos. En inyección por intracavernosa, recomiendan 30mg cada vez y 2 ~ 3 veces cada semana. Para infantes, la dosis es de 1.5mg/kg por 4 veces al día en inyecciones por I.M. o I.V.. |
|---|---|
| 剂型、规格<br>Formulaciones y especificaciones | 片剂：每片 30mg。注射剂：每支 30mg（1ml）。<br>Tableta: 30mg; Inyección: 30mg (1ml). |
| **药品名称 Drug Names** | 己酮可可碱 Pentoxifilina |
| 适应证<br>Indicaciones | 用于脑血管障碍或脑卒中后引起的后遗症,伴有间歇性跛行的慢性闭塞性脉管炎,血管性头痛;也可用于血管性痴呆的预防和治疗（但目前国际上临床研究结论尚不肯定）。<br><br>Se usa en tratamiento de secuelas de trastornos cerebrovasculares y apoplejía, obliterante crónica acompañada con claudicación intermitente y cefalea vascular. También se usa en prevención y tratamiento de demencia vascular pero no hay conclusión definitiva según los estudios clínicos internacional actuales. |
| 用法、用量<br>Administración y dosis | ①口服：每次 100 ～ 400mg，一日 3 次，建议餐后即时服用。控释片，每次 400mg，一日 1 次。口服用药治疗缺血性脑血管病后遗症或血管性痴呆等，需连续 2 ～ 8 周可产生治疗效果。②静脉滴注：每次 200 ～ 400mg，溶于 250 ～ 500ml 静脉滴注液中缓慢滴注，90 ～ 180 分钟滴完，每次 1 ～ 2 次。配制好的药物需在 24 小时内使用。<br><br>① Por vía oral a dosis de 100 ~ 400mg por 3 veces al día tomados después de alimentos. De tableta de liberación prolongada la dosis es de 400mg una vez al día. La administración oral se efectua después de medicación continua de 2 ~ 8 semanas en tratamiento de secuelas de trastornos cerebrovasculares y demencia vascular. ② Infusión por I.V.: 200 ~ 400mg cada vez diluidos en 250 ~ 500ml de solución de infusión y se administra lentamente detro de 90 ~ 180 minutos y 1 ~ 2 veces al día. Medicamentos deben utilizarse dentro de 24 horas cuando estén preparados. |
| 剂型、规格<br>Formulaciones y especificaciones | 片剂（肠溶片）：每片 100mg。控释片：每片 400mg。注射液：每支 100mg（5ml）；300mg（15ml）。<br>Tableta (con recubrimiento entérico):100mg; Tableta de liberación controlada: 400mg; Inyección: 100mg(5ml), 300mg (15ml). |
| **药品名称 Drug Names** | 丁咯地尔 Buflomedil |
| 适应证<br>Indicaciones | ①适用于慢性脑血管供血不足引起的症状：眩晕、耳鸣、智力减退、记忆力或注意力减退、定向障碍等。②外周性血管疾病：间歇性跛行、雷诺综合征、血栓闭塞性脉管炎等。<br><br>① Se usa en tratamiento de síntomas causados por insuficiencia cerebrovascular crónica: vértigos, tinnitus, deterioro mental, pérdida de memoria o atención y desorientación. ② Se usa en tratamiento de enfermedad vascular periférica: claudicación intermitente, síndrome de Raynaud y tromboangeítis obliterante. |
| 用法、用量<br>Administración y dosis | 口服：片剂，每次 150 ～ 300mg，一日 2 ～ 3 次。每日最大剂量为 600mg；缓释片，每次 600mg，一日 1 次。肌内注射或静脉注射：每日 200 ～ 400mg。静脉滴注：每日 200 ～ 400mg，分 2 次，加于静脉滴注液 250 ～ 500ml 中缓慢滴注。轻中度肾功能不全者，用量减半，片剂，每次 150mg，一日 2 次，每日最大推荐剂量为 300mg；不推荐使用缓释片。肝功能不全者考虑减量使用。 |

**续　表**

| | |
|---|---|
| | Por vía oral. Tabletas：150 ~ 300mg　cada vez y 2 ~ 3 veces al día. Dosis máxima no excede a 600mg diarios. Tableta de liberación prolongada：600mg una vez al día. Inyección por I.M. o I.V.：200 ~ 400mg diarios. Infusión por I.V.：200 ~ 400mg diarios divididos en 2 veces. Se administra lentamente diluidos en 250 ~ 500ml de solución de infusión. Para pacientes de disfunción renal leve o medorada，la dosis será la mitad de la habitual：150mg por 2 veces al día de tabletas y la dosis máxima no excede a 300mg diarios. No recomienda tomar tableta de liberación prolongada. Para pacientes de disfunción hepática，debe considerar si hay que reducir la dosis según la necesidad. |
| 剂型、规格<br>Formulaciones y especificaciones | 片剂：每片 150mg；300mg。缓释片：600mg。注射液：每支 50mg（5ml）；100mg（10ml）。粉针剂：每支 50mg；100mg；200mg。<br><br>Tableta: 150mg, 300mg; Tableta de liberación prolongada: 600mg; Inyección: 50mg(5ml), 100mg(10ml); Polvo para inyección: 50mg, 100mg, 200mg. |
| 药品名称 Drug Names | 尼麦角林 Nicergolina |
| 适应证<br>Indicaciones | 用于急、慢性脑血管疾病和代谢性脑供血不足，急、慢性外周血管障碍，老年性耳聋和视网膜疾病等。也用于血管性痴呆，尤其在早期治疗时对认知、记忆等有改善，并能减轻疾病严重程度。<br><br>Se usa en tratamiento de enfermedad cerebrovascular aguda o crónica, insuficiencia cerebral metabólica, trastornos vasculares periféricos agudos y crónicos, sordera senil y enfermedades de la retina. También puede usarse para demencia vascular mejorando la cognitiva y memoria en el tratamiento precoz mientras reduciendo la gravedad de la enfermedad. |
| 用法、用量<br>Administración y dosis | 口服：每次 10 ~ 20mg，一日 3 次。片剂勿嚼服，可与食物同服。肌内注射：每次 2 ~ 4mg，一日 1 ~ 2 次。静脉注射：每次 2 ~ 4mg，溶于 100ml 的静脉滴注液中缓慢滴注，一日 1 ~ 2 次。<br><br>Por vía oral: 10 ~ 20mg por 3 veces al día. No se puede masticar las tabletas y puede tomarlas acompañadas con alimentos. Inyección por I.M.: 2 ~ 4mg y 1-2 veces al día. Infusión lenta por I.V.: 2 ~ 4mg diluidos en 100ml de solución de infusión, 1 ~ 2 veces al día. |
| 剂型、规格<br>Formulaciones y especificaciones | 片剂：每片 10mg。胶囊剂：每粒 15mg。注射剂：2mg（1ml）；2.5mg（1ml）；4mg（2ml）；8mg（2ml）；8mg（5ml）。<br><br>Tableta: 10mg; Cápsula: 15mg; Inyección: 2mg (1ml), 2.5mg (1ml), 4mg (2ml), 8mg (2ml), 8mg (5ml). |
| 药品名称 Drug Names | 川芎嗪 Ligustrazina |
| 适应证<br>Indicaciones | 适用于脑供血不足、脑栓塞、脉管炎、冠心病、心绞痛、突发性耳聋等。<br><br>Se usa en tratamiento de insuficiencia cerebral, embolia cerebral,tromboangeítis obliterante, enfermedad coronaria, angina y sordera súbita. |
| 用法、用量<br>Administración y dosis | 口服：每次 100mg，一日 3 次，30 日为一疗程。肌内注射：每次 40 ~ 50mg，一日 1 ~ 2 次，缓慢推注，15 日为一疗程。静脉滴注：每日 50 ~ 100mg，稀释于 250 ~ 500ml 静脉滴注液中缓慢滴注，15 日为一疗程。<br><br>Por vía oral: 100mg por 3 veces al día y un curso de tratamiento tarda 30 días. Inyección por I.M.: 40 ~ 50mg cada vez y 1 ~ 2 veces al día. Se administra lentamente y un curso de tratamiento tarda 15 días. Infusión lenta por I.V. : 50 ~ 100mg diarios diluidos en 250 ~ 500ml de solución de infusión y un curso de tratamiento tarda 15 días. |
| 剂型、规格<br>Formulaciones y especificaciones | 片剂：每片 50mg。注射用川芎嗪（盐酸盐）：每支 40mg；注射用川芎嗪（磷酸盐）：每支 50mg。<br><br>Tableta: 50mg; Ligustrazina para inyección (de clorhidrato): 40mg; Ligustrazina para inyección (de fosfato): 50mg. |
| 药品名称 Drug Names | 丁苯酞 Butilftalida |
| 适应证<br>Indicaciones | 适用于治疗轻、中度急性缺血性脑卒中及急性缺血性脑卒中患者神经功能缺损的改善。<br><br>Se usa en tratamiento de accidente cerebrovascular isquémico agudo leve o moderado y mejoramiento del déficit neurológico de accidente cerebrovascular isquémico agudo. |

续　表

| 用法、用量<br>Administración y dosis | ①可与复方丹参注射液联合使用。空腹口服。一次 2 粒（0.2g），一日 3 次，10 日为一疗程。本品应在患者病发后 48 小时内开始服用。②静脉滴注，一日 2 次，每次 25mg，每次滴注，时间不少于 50 分钟；2 次用要间隔不少于 6 小时，疗程 14 日。<br>① Se puede usar con inyección del compuesto Dan Shen. Por vía de oral en ayunas a dosis de 0.2g por 3 veces al día y un curso de tratamiento tarda 10 días. Debe administrarse dentro de 48 horas tras la aparición de los síntomas asociados. ② Infusión por I.V. a una dosis de 25mg por 2 veces al día y la infusión tardará más de 50 minutos y el intervalo de medicación será más de 6 horas. Un curso de tratamiento tarda 14 días. |
|---|---|
| 剂型、规格<br>Formulaciones y especificaciones | 胶囊：每粒 0.1g。丁苯肽氯化钠注射：丁苯肽 25mg 与氯化钠 0.9g（100ml）。<br>Cápsula: 0.1g; Inyección de Butyphthalide y cloruro de sodio: 100ml, incluyendo 25mg de Butyphthalide y 0.9g de cloruro de sodio. |

| 药品名称Drug Names | 奥扎格雷 Ozagrel |
|---|---|
| 适应证<br>Indicaciones | 用于缺血性脑卒中急性期，蛛网膜下腔出血术后的脑血管痉挛收缩和伴随的脑缺血症状。<br>Se usa en etapa aguda del accidente cerebrovascular isquémico así como el vasoespasmo cerebral y los asociados síntomas isquémicos cerebrales después de cirugía de la hemorragia subaracnoidea. |
| 用法、用量<br>Administración y dosis | ①缺血性脑卒中急性期：每次 40～80mg，溶于 500ml 静脉滴注液中连续静脉滴注，一日 1～2 次，1～2 周为一疗程。②蛛网膜下腔出血术后并发的脑血管痉挛及伴随而产生的脑缺血症状：每次 80mg，一日 1 次，溶于适量滴注液中，24 小时持续静脉滴注，可连续用药 2 周。<br>① En tratamiento del accidente cerebrovascular isquémico en etapa aguda: 40～80mg cada vez diluidos en 500ml de solución de infusión. Se administra 1 ó 2 veces al día y un curso de tratamiento tarda 1～2 semanas. ② En tratamiento del vasoespasmo cerebral y los asociados síntomas isquémicos cerebrales después de cirugía de la hemorragia subaracnoidea: 80mg una vez al día diluidos en solución de infusión. Se administra la infusión continuamente durante todo el día y puede seguir la medicación durante 2 semanas. |
| 剂型、规格<br>Formulaciones y especificaciones | 注射用奥扎格雷：20mg（2ml）；40mg（2ml）。奥扎格雷钠氯化钠（或葡萄糖）注射液：250ml（奥扎格雷钠 80mg）。<br>Ozagrel para inyección: 20mg(2ml), 40mg (2ml); Inyección de Ozagrel y cloruro de sodio (o glucosa): 250ml, (incluyendo 80mg Ozagrel). |

| 药品名称Drug Names | 曲克芦丁 Troxerutina |
|---|---|
| 适应证<br>Indicaciones | 用于闭塞性脑血管病引起的偏瘫、失语、冠心病梗死前综合征、中心视网膜炎、血栓性静脉炎、静脉曲张、雷诺综合征、血管通透性升高引起的水肿、淋巴水肿、烧伤及创伤水肿、动脉硬化。<br>Se usa en tratamiento de hemiplejía y afasia causadas por enfermedad cerebro vascular, síndrome preinfarto de la enfermedad coronaria, retinitis central, tromboflebitis, varice, síndrome de Raynaud, edema y linfedema causados por el aumento de la permeabilidad vascular, edema en quemaduras y edema traumático y arteriosclerosis. |
| 用法、用量<br>Administración y dosis | 口服：每次 200～300mg，一日 3 次。肌内注射：每次 100～200mg，一日 2 次。静脉滴注：每次 400mg，一日 1 次，20 天为一疗程，可用 1～3 个疗程，每疗程间隔 3～7 日。<br>Por vía oral, 200～300mg cada vez y 3 veces al día. Inyección por I.M.: 100～200mg cada vez y 2 veces al día. Infusión por I.V.:400mg una vez al día y un curso de tratamiento tarda 20 días. Puede repetir hasta 3 cursos con intervalo de 3～7 días entre cada curso. |
| 剂型、规格<br>Formulaciones y especificaciones | 片剂：每片 100mg。注射液：每支 100mg（2ml）；200mg（2ml）。<br>Tableta: 100mg; Inyección: 100mg (2ml), 200mg (2ml). |

| 药品名称Drug Names | 维生素 E 烟酸酯 Niacina de Vitamina E |
|---|---|
| 适应证<br>Indicaciones | 用于动脉硬化、脑震荡及轻微脑挫伤和脑外伤后遗症、头痛头晕、中心性视网膜炎等血管障碍性疾病，也可用于脂质代谢异常。<br>Se usa en tratamiento de trastornos vasculares: arteriosclerosis, conmoción cerebral, secuelas de leve contusión cerebral y lesion cerebral traumática, cefalea y mareo, retinitis central. También puede usarse en el Anormal de Metabolismo Lipídico. |

**续 表**

| 用法、用量<br>Administración y dosis | 口服，每次 0.1 ~ 0.2g，一日 3 次，餐后服。老年人可做适当调整。<br><br>Por vía oral, 0.1 ~ 0.2g cada vez y 3 veces al día, tomados después de alimentos. Para ancianos puede ajustar la dosis. |
|---|---|
| 剂型、规格<br>Formulaciones y especificaciones | 片剂：每片 0.1g。胶囊：每粒 0.1g。胶丸：每粒 0.1g。<br><br>Tableta: 0.1g; Cápsula: 0.1g; Cápsulas blandas: 0.1g. |
| **药品名称 Drug Names** | **灯盏花素 Breviscapina** |
| 适应证<br>Indicaciones | ①用于缺血性脑血管病，如脑供血不足、椎基底动脉供血不足、脑出血后遗症。②亦用于冠心病、心绞痛、高血压、高黏滞血症等心血管疾病。<br><br>① Se usa en tratamiento de Enfermedad Cerebrovascular Isquemica, por ejempro insuficiencia cerebral, insuficiencia de la arteria vertebrobasilar y secuelas de hemorragia cerebral.　② Se usa en tratamiento de enfermedades cardiovasculares: enfermedad coronaria, angina, hipertensión e hiperviscosidad. |
| 用法、用量<br>Administración y dosis | 口服：每次 40mg，一日 3 次。肌内注射：每次 2ml，一日 2 次，15 日为一疗程。静脉滴注：每次 4 ~ 8ml，一日 1 次，加入 500ml 静脉滴注液中稀释应用，10 日为一疗程。<br><br>Por vía oral, 40mg cada vez y 3 veces al día. Inyección por I.M.: 2ml cada vez y 2 veces al día, un curso de tratamiento tarda 15 días. Infusión por I.V.: 4 ~ 8ml una vez al día diluidos en 500ml de solución de infusión, un curso de tratamiento tarda 10 días. |
| 剂型、规格<br>Formulaciones y especificaciones | 片剂：每片 20mg。注射剂：每支 5mg（2ml）；20mg（5ml）。<br><br>Tableta: 20mg; Inyección: 5mg (2ml), 20mg (5ml). |
| **药品名称 Drug Names** | **地芬尼多 Difenidol** |
| 适应证<br>Indicaciones | 用于治疗各种原因引起的眩晕症（如椎基底动脉供血不足、梅尼埃病等）、恶心呕吐、自主神经功能紊乱、晕车晕船、运动病及外科麻醉手术后的呕吐等。<br><br>Se usa en tratamiento de vértigos causados por, como ejempro, la insuficiencia de la arteria vertebrobasilar o la enfermedad de Meniere, náuseas y vómitos, trastornos del sistema nervioso autónomo, cinetosis y mareo en barco, Motion Sickness y vómitos después de la anestesia quirúrgica. |
| 用法、用量<br>Administración y dosis | 口服：成人每次 25 ~ 50mg，一日 3 次；6 个月以上儿童，每次 0.9mg/kg，一日 3 次。肌内注射：每次 10 ~ 20mg，眩晕发作剧烈者可每次 20 ~ 40mg。<br><br>Por vía oral. Para adultos la dosis es de 25 ~ 50mg cada vez y 3 veces al día, para infantes mayores de 6 meses, la dosis es de 0.9mg/kg cada vez y 3 veces al día. Inyección por I.M.: 10 ~ 20mg cada vez y para pacientes de vértigo grave puede toar 20 ~ 40mg cada vez. |
| 剂型、规格<br>Formulaciones y especificaciones | 片剂：每片 25mg。注射液：每支 10mg（1ml）。<br><br>Tableta: 25mg; Inyección: 10mg (1ml). |
| **药品名称 Drug Names** | **长春西汀 Vinpocetina** |
| 适应证<br>Indicaciones | ①用于改善脑梗死、脑出血后遗症及脑动脉硬化引起的各种症状，如记忆障碍、眩晕、头痛、失语、抑郁症等。②还可用于各种眼底血液循环不良所致的视力障碍；听力损伤、耳鸣前庭功能障碍。③各种颅脑手术后脑功能的康复治疗。<br><br>① Se usa en mejoramiento de secuelas de hemorragia e infarto cerebral y síntomas causados por arteriosclerosis cerebral, por ejempro trastornos de memoria,vértigos, cefalea, afasia y depresión.　② Se usa también en tratamiento de discapacidad visual causada por una variedad de mala circulación sanguínea del fondo de ojo, discapacidad auditiva, tinnitus y disfunción vestibular.　③ Se usa en tratamiento de rehabilitación de funciones cerebrales después de cirugía cerebral. |
| 用法、用量<br>Administración y dosis | 口服：每次 5 ~ 10mg，一日 3 次，餐时口服。静脉滴注：起始剂量每日 20mg，一日 1 次；以后根据病情可增至每日 30mg，一日 1 次。<br><br>Por vía oral. 5 ~ 10mg cada vez y 3 veces al día, tomados acompañado con comidas. Infusión por I.V.: dosis inicial es de 20mg diarios una vez al día y puede aumentar la dosis a 30mg diarios una vez al día según la necesidad. |

续　表

| | |
|---|---|
| 剂型、规格<br>Formulaciones y especificaciones | 片剂：每片 5mg。注射液：20mg（2ml）。长春西汀葡萄糖注射液：100ml（长春西汀 10mg）；200ml（长春西汀 10mg）；250ml（长春西汀 10mg）。<br>Tableta: 5mg; Solució inyectable: 20mg (2ml); Inyección de glucosa Vinpocetina: 100ml con 10mg de Vinpocetina, 200ml con 10mg de Vinpocetina, 250ml con 10mg de Vinpocetina. |
| **药品名称Drug Names** | 依达拉奉 Edaravona |
| 适应证<br>Indicaciones | 用于改善急性脑梗死所致的神经症状、日常生活活动能力和功能障碍。<br>Indicación para la mejora de los síntomas neurológicos y difunción en actividades de vida diaria causados por el infarto cerebral agudo. |
| 用法、用量<br>Administración y dosis | 静脉滴注：一次 30mg，加入适量生理盐水中稀释后静滴，30 分钟内滴完，一日 2 次，14 日为一疗程。尽可能在发病 24 小时内开始给药。<br>Infusión por I.V. dentro de 30 minutos de 30mg de dicha droga diluciendo con Normal Saline, 2 veces al dia y un curso de tratamiento sera de 14 días. Recomienda empezar el medicamento dentro de 24horas de la aparición de los síntomas. |
| 剂型、规格<br>Formulaciones y especificaciones | 注射液：每支 10mg（5ml）；30mg（20ml）。<br>Inyección: 10mg (5ml), 30mg (2ml). |
| **药品名称Drug Names** | 血塞通 XueSaiTong |
| 适应证<br>Indicaciones | ①用于缺血性脑血管病、冠心病心绞痛，中医证见脑络瘀阻、卒中偏瘫、心脉瘀阻、胸痹心痛。②还可用于治疗视网膜血管阻塞、眼前房出血、青光眼；急性黄疸型肝炎、病毒性肝炎；外伤、软组织损伤及骨折恢复期。<br>① Se usa en tratamiento de enfermedad cerebrovascular isquémico, enfermedad coronaria, angina,estancamiento en redes cerebrales, apoplejía y hemiplejía, estasis sanguínea sistólica y obstrucción torácica。　② Se usa también en tratamiento de enfermedad oclusiva vascular retiniana, hipema, glaucoma, hepatitis ictérica aguda, hepatitis viral y en recuperación de trauma, lesión de los tejidos blandos y fractura. |
| 用法、用量<br>Administración y dosis | 口服：一次 50～100mg，一日 3 次。肌内注射：一次 100mg。一日 1～2 次。静脉滴注：一次 200～400mg，以 5%～10%utaotang 注射液 250～500ml 稀释后缓缓滴注，一日 1 次。静脉注射：每次 200mg，以 25%～50% 葡萄糖注射液 40～60ml 稀释后缓缓注射，一日 1 次。15 日为一疗程。停药 1～3 日后可进行第二疗程。<br>Por vía oral a una dosis de 50～100mg por 3 veces al día. Inyección por I.M. a dosis de 100mg cada vez y 1 o 2 veces al día. Infusión lenta por I.V. a dosis de 200～400mg diluidos en 250～500ml de solución glucosa a 5%～10% y se administra una vez al día. Inyección lenta por I.V. a dosis de 200mg una vez al día diluidos en 40～60ml de solución glucosa a 25%～50%. Un curso de tratamiento tarda 15 días y después de 1～3 días sin medicamento puede seguir con el otro curso. |
| 剂型、规格<br>Formulaciones y especificaciones | 片剂：每片 50mg。胶囊剂：每粒 60mg。注射液：每支 100mg（2ml）。<br>Tableta: 50mg; Cápsula: 60mg; Inyección: 100mg (2ml). |
| **药品名称Drug Names** | 七叶皂苷钠 Aescinato sódico |
| 适应证<br>Indicaciones | ①用于各种病因引起的脑水肿、创伤或手术所致肿胀。②也可用于静脉回流障碍、下肢静脉曲张、血栓性静脉炎、慢性静脉功能不全，下肢动脉阻塞性疾病，运动系统创伤造成的软组织血肿、水肿。③用于周围神经炎性疾病，如格林巴利综合征、多发性神经炎等。<br>① Se usa en tratamiento de edema cerebral e hinchazón por trauma y cirugía.　② Se usa también para trastornos venosos, varices en miembro inferior, tromboflebitis, insuficiencia venosa crónica, enfermedad arterial oclusiva de miembros inferiores y hematoma y edema de tejidos blandos causadoas por traumatismos del aparato locomotor. ③ Se usa en enfermedades del sistema nervioso periférico, por ejempro síndrome de Guillain-Barré y polineuritis. |
| 用法、用量<br>Administración y dosis | ① 静脉给药：一日 5～10mg 溶于 250ml 滴注液中静脉滴注；或 5～10ml 溶于 10～20ml10% 葡萄糖溶液或 0.9% 氯化钠溶液中，静脉注射。儿童 3 岁以下一日 0.05～0.1mg/kg 体重；3～10 岁一日 0.1～0.2mg/kg 体重。重症患者可多次给药，但一日总量不得超过 20mg。疗程 7～10 日。②口服：每次 30～60mg，一日 2 次，餐时或餐后口服，20 日为一疗程。 |

**续　表**

| | |
|---|---|
| | ① Administración intravenosa: infusión por I.V. a una dosis de 5 ~ 10mg diarios diluidiso en 250ml de solución de infusión, ó inyección por I.V. a una dosis de 5 ~ 10mg diluidos en 10 ~ 20ml de solución glocosa a 10% o solución de cloruro de sodio a 0.9%. Para niños menores de 3 años la dosis es de 0.05 ~ 0.1mg/kg diarios y para niños de entre 3 y 10 años la dosis es de 0.1 ~ 0.2mg/kg diarios. Para pacientes severos puede repetir la medicación y la dosis total no debe exceder a 20mg. Un curso de tratamiento tarda 7 ~ 10 días. ② Administración oral a una dosis de 30 ~ 60mg por 2 veces al día acompañados o después de alimentos. Un curso de tratamiento tarda 20 días. |
| 剂型、规格<br>Formulaciones y especificaciones | 片剂：每片 30mg。注射剂：每支 5mg；10mg；25mg。<br>Tableta: 30mg; Inyección: 5mg, 10mg, 25mg. |
| 药品名称 Drug Names | 葛根素 Puerarina |
| 适应证<br>Indicaciones | 可用于辅助治疗冠心病、心绞痛、心肌梗死，缺血性脑血管病，视网膜动、静脉阻塞，青光眼，突发性耳聋，小儿病毒性心肌炎、糖尿病。<br>Se usa en tratamiento adyuvante de enfermedad coronaria, angina, infarto de miocardio, enfermedad cerebrovascular isquémica, oclusión de la arteria o la vena retiniana, glaucoma, sordera súbita, miocarditis viral en la infancia y diabetes. |
| 用法、用量<br>Administración y dosis | ①静脉滴注：每次 0.4 ~ 0.6g，一日 1 次，10 ~ 20 日为一疗程，可连续使用 2 ~ 3 个疗程。最大用药剂量为 1.0g。②滴眼：一次 1 ~ 2 滴，闭目 3 ~ 5 分钟。首日 3 次，以后为一日 2 次。<br>① Infusión por I.V. a dosis de 0.4 ~ 0.6g una vez al día. Un curso de tratamiento tarda 10 ~ 20 días y puede repetir la medicación a 2 o 3 cursos. La dosis máxima es de 1g. ② Administración de gota oftalmológica a una dosis de 1 ~ 2 gotas cada vez y cerrar los ojos dentro de 3 ~ 5 minutos. 3 veces en el primer día de medicamento y luego cambia a 2 veces al día. |
| 剂型、规格<br>Formulaciones y especificaciones | 注射液：每支 100mg（2ml）；400mg（8ml）。粉针剂：每支 200mg。葛根素氯化钠注射液：100ml（葛根素 200mg）。葛根素滴眼液：50mg（5ml）。<br>Inyección: 100mg(2ml), 400mg(8ml); Polvo para inyección: 200mg; Inyección de Cloruro de sodio: 100ml (incluyendo 200mg) de puerarin; Gota oftalmológica de puerarin: 50mg (5ml). |

8.13　抗老年痴呆药和改善脑代谢药 Los medicamentos contra la demencia y para mejorar metabolismo del cerebro

| 药品名称 Drug Names | 加兰他敏 Galantamina |
|---|---|
| 适应证<br>Indicaciones | ①适用于治疗轻、中度阿尔茨海默病（AD），有效率 50% ~ 60%，疗效与他克林相当，但没有肝毒性。用药后 6 ~ 8 周治疗效果开始明显。②用于重症肌无力、脊髓灰质炎后遗症、儿童脑性麻痹、多发性神经炎、脊神经根炎及拮抗氯筒箭毒碱。<br>① Se usa en tratamiento de enfermedad de Alzheimer leve y moderada. La 50%~60% de los pacientes consiguen efecto tras la medicación. Tiene efecto similar a tacrina pero no tiene ninguna toxicidad hepática. La eficacia se ve evidente tras medicación de 6~8 semanas. ② Se usa en tratamiento de miastenia gravis, secuelas de poliomielitis, parálisis cerebral infantil, polineuritis, radiculitis y antagonización cloruro de tubocurarina. |
| 用法、用量<br>Administración y dosis | 口服：每次 10 ~ 20mg，一日 3 次。小儿每日 0.5 ~ 1mg/kg，分 3 次服。皮下或肌内注射：每次 2.5 ~ 10mg，一日 1 次。小儿每次 0.05 ~ 0.1mg/kg，一日 1 次。每个疗程 8 ~ 10 周。用于抗氯筒箭毒碱时肌内注射起始剂量 5 ~ 10mg，5 或 10 分钟后按需要可逐渐增加至每次 10 ~ 20mg。<br>Por vía oral. 10 ~ 20mg por 3 veces al día. Para infantes la dosis es de 0.5 ~ 1mg/kg diarios divididos en 3 tomas. Inyección subcutánea o por intramuscular: 2.5 ~ 10mg una vez al día y para infantes es de 0.05 ~ 0.1mg/kg una vez al día. Un curso de tratamiento tarda 8 ~ 10 semanas. Cuando se usa en antagonización de cloruro de tubocurarina, se administra inyección por I.M. a una dosis inicial de 5 ~ 10mg y según la necesidad puede aumentar a 10 ~ 20mg cada vez después de 5 ó 10 minutos. |
| 剂型、规格<br>Formulaciones y especificaciones | 口崩片：每片 5mg。分散片：每片 2.5mg。注射剂：每支 1mg（1ml）；2.5mg（1ml）；5mg（1ml）。<br>Tableta de desintegración oral: 5mg; Comprimidos dispersables: 2.5mg; Inyección: 1mg(1ml), 2.5mg(1ml), 5mg(1ml). |

续　表

| 药品名称 Drug Names | 美金刚 Memantina |
|---|---|
| 适应证<br>Indicaciones | 用于治疗中至重度的阿尔茨海默病（AD），以及震颤麻痹综合征的治疗。<br><br>Se usa en tratamiento de la enfermedad de Alzheimer mediada o severa y el parkinsonismo. |
| 用法、用量<br>Administración y<br>dosis | 口服。成人或 14 岁以上青少年：在治疗的前 3 周按每周递增 5mg 的方法逐渐达到维持剂量，即治疗第 1 周每日 5mg（晨服），第 2 周每日 10mg，分 2 次服用；第 3 周每日 15mg（早上 10mg，下午 5mg）；第 4 周开始维持剂量每日 20mg，分 2 次服。片剂可空腹服用，也可随食物同服。14 岁以下小儿：维持量每日 0.55 ～ 1.0mg/kg。中度肾功能损害者，应将剂量减至每日 10mg；不推荐严重肾衰竭患者使用。<br><br>Por vía oral. Para adultos y juventudes mayores de 14 años: en los primeros 3 semanas de tratamiento, la dosis se aumenta gradualmente desde 5mg diarios una vez en (la mañana) en la primera semana hasta 10mg diarios divididos en 2 tomas en la segunda semana y luego en la tercera semana, 15mg diarios divididos en 2 tomas (10mg en la mañana y 5mg en la tarde). En la cuarta semana se aplica la dosis de mantenimiento de 20mg diarios divididos en 2 tomas. Puede tomar las tabletas en ayunas o acompañadas con alimentos. Para infantes menores de 14 años: la dosis de mantenimiento es de 0.55 ～ 1.0mg/kg diarios. Dosis para pacientes de disfunción renal mediada será 10mg diarios. No recomiendan esta medicación para pacientes de disfunción renal severa. |
| 剂型、规格<br>Formulaciones y<br>especificaciones | 片剂：每片 5mg；10mg。胶囊：每粒 10mg。<br>Tableta: 5mg, 10mg; Cápsula: 10mg. |

| 药品名称 Drug Names | 吡拉西坦 Piracetam |
|---|---|
| 适应证<br>Indicaciones | 由衰老、脑血管病、脑外伤、CO 中毒等引起的记忆和轻中度脑功能障碍。亦可用于儿童发育迟缓。<br><br>Se usa en tratamiento de trastornos de la memoria y disfunción cerebral leve y moderada causados por senectud, enfermedad cerebrovascular, lesión cerebral traumática e intoxicación por CO. También lo usa en tratamiento del retraso del crecimiento en los niños. |
| 用法、用量<br>Administración y<br>dosis | ①口服：成人，每次 0.8 ～ 1.2g，一日 2 ～ 3 次，4 ～ 8 周为一个疗程。儿童、老年人，剂量酌减。②肌内注射：每次 1g，一日 2 ～ 3 次。③静脉注射：每次 4 ～ 6g，一日 2 次。④静脉滴注：用于改善脑代谢，每次 4 ～ 8g，用 250ml 滴注射液稀释后静脉滴注，一日 1 次。<br><br>① Por vía oral. Para adultos la dosis es de 0.8 ～ 1.2g cada vez y 2 ～ 3 veces al día. Un curso de tratamiento tarda 4 ～ 8 semanas. Para pacientes infantiles y ancianos disminuye la dosis según la condición. ② Inyección por I.M.: la dosis es de 1g cada vez y 2 ～ 3 veces al día. ③ Inyección por I.V.: 4 ～ 6g cada vez y 2 veces al día. ④ Infusión por I.V. para mejorar el metabolismo cerebral: 4 ～ 8g una vez al día diluidos en 250ml de solución de infusión. |
| 剂型、规格<br>Formulaciones y<br>especificaciones | 片剂：每片 0.4g。分散片：每片 0.8g。胶囊：每粒 0.2g；0.4g。注射剂：每支 1g（5ml）；2g（10ml）；4g（20ml）。氯化钠注射液：250ml（吡拉西坦 8g，氯化钠 2.25g）。<br>Tableta: 0.4g; Comprimido dispersable: 0.8g; Cápsula: 0.2g, 0.4g; Inyección: 1g(5ml), 2g(10ml), 4g(20ml); Inyección de Cloruro de Sodio: 250ml(que incluye 8g de Aniraceram y 2.25g de Cloruro de sodio). |

| 药品名称 Drug Names | 茴拉西坦 Aniracetam |
|---|---|
| 适应证<br>Indicaciones | 用于治疗脑血管疾病后的记忆功能减退和血管性痴呆，中、老年记忆减退（健忘症），对帕金森病症状有改善作用，用于脑梗死后遗症的情绪不稳定和抑郁状态。<br><br>Se usa en tratamiento de disfunción de la memoria y demencia vascular asociadas con enfermedades cerebrovasculares, pérdida de la memoria en edad mediana y tercera (amnesia). Puede mejorar síntomas de la enfermedad de Parkinson. Se usa para la inestabilidad emocional y estado de depresión asociados con secuelas de infarto cerebral. |
| 用法、用量<br>Administración y<br>dosis | 口服：每次 0.2g，一日 3 次。70 岁以上老人，每次 0.1g，一日 3 次。1 ～ 2 个月为一个疗程。可根据病情调整用量和疗程。<br><br>Por vía oral a una dosis de 0.2g por 3 veces al día. Para ancianos mayores de 70 años, la dosis es de 0.1g por 3 veces al día. Un curso de tratamiento tarda 1 ～ 2 meses. Puede ajustar la dosis y curso de tratamiento según la necesidad. |

**续 表**

| | |
|---|---|
| 剂型、规格<br>Formulaciones y especificaciones | 胶囊：每粒 0.1g。片剂：每片 0.05g。<br>Cápsula: 0.1g; Tableta: 0.05g. |
| **药品名称 Drug Names** | **奥拉西坦 Oxiracetam** |
| 适应证<br>Indicaciones | 用于轻中度血管性痴呆、老年性痴呆及脑外伤等症引起的记忆与智能障碍、大脑功能不全。<br>Se usa en tratamiento de demencia vascular leve y moderada, enfermedad de Alzheimer así como la disfunción cerebral, trastornos de memoria y atraso mental causados por lesión cerebral traumática. |
| 用法、用量<br>Administración y dosis | 口服：每次 0.8g，一日 2 次；重症每日 2～8g。静脉滴注：每次 4g，一日 1 次，可酌情减量，用前加入到 100～250ml 静脉滴注液中，摇匀。对功能缺失的治疗通常疗程为 2 周，对记忆与智能障碍的治疗通常疗程为 3 周。<br>Por vía oral a dosis de 0.8g y 2 veces al día. Si es caso severo, la dosis es de 2～8g diarios. Infusión por I.V. La dosis es de 4g una vez al día y puede reducir la dosis según la necesidad. Antes de la administración, los diluye y sacuden en 100～250ml de líquidos intravenosos. El tratamiento de disfunción tarda generalmente 2 semanas y de trastornos de memoria y atraso mental, tarda 3 semanas. |
| 剂型、规格<br>Formulaciones y especificaciones | 片剂：每片 0.4g。注射液：每支 1g（5ml）。<br>Tableta: 0.4g; Inyección: 1g (5ml). |
| **药品名称 Drug Names** | **银杏叶提取物 Extracto de Ginkgo biloba** |
| 适应证<br>Indicaciones | 主要用于脑部、外周血管及冠状动脉血管障碍的患者，包括脑卒中、痴呆症、急慢性脑功能不全及其后遗症。对于阿尔茨海默病、血管性痴呆及缓和性痴呆等患者应用本品后，智力可有所提高，但对明显痴呆者作用仍不佳。<br>Se usa en tratamiento de trastornos ceberales, trastornos vasculares periféricos y enfermedades vasculares coronarias, por ejempro apoplejía, demencia, disfunción cerebral aguda y crónica y las secuelas relacionadas. Es eficaz en mejorar la inteligencia para pacientes de enfermedad de Alzheimer y demencia vascular. El efecto no es bueno para pacientes de demencia aparente. |
| 用法、用量<br>Administración y dosis | 口服：每次 1～2 片，一日 3 次。静脉滴注：1～2 支，加入 250ml 或 500ml 输液剂中静脉滴注，一日 1～2 次。本品不同厂家说明书所列剂量并不一致，主要成分的配比也不同，所以需要根据具体说明书使用药物。<br>Administración oral: 1～2 tabletas por 3 veces al día. Administración de infusión por I.V.: 1～2 unidades diluidas en 250～500ml de solución de infusión, medicación 1～2 veces al día. Según distintas inducciones del cármaco, la dosis y la razón de componentes son diferentes y debe aplicar la medicación según la inducciones. |
| 剂型、规格<br>Formulaciones y especificaciones | 片剂：每片 40mg。注射剂：①金纳多：每支 5ml（含银杏叶提取物 17.5mg）。②舒血宁：2ml（含总黄酮醇苷 1.68mg；银杏内酯 A0.12mg）；5ml（含总黄酮醇苷 4.2mg；银杏内酯 A0.30mg）。<br>Tableta: 40mg; Inyección: ① de Ginaton: 5ml (incluyendo 17.5mg del extrato de Ginkgo Biloba). ② de Shuxuening: 2ml (incluyendo 1.68mg de Glucósidos Flavonol y 0.12mg de Ginkgólido A), 5ml (incluyendo 4.2mg de Glucósidos Flavonol y 0.3mg de Ginkgólido A). |
| **药品名称 Drug Names** | **阿米三嗪 / 萝巴新 Almitrina y Raubasina** |
| 适应证<br>Indicaciones | 用于治疗亚急性或慢性脑功能不全，如记忆力下降、缺血性听觉、前庭、视觉障碍；脑血管意外后的功能恢复。<br>Se usa para tratamiento de disfunción cerebral subaguda o crónica, por ejempro la pérdida de la memoria, trastornos isquémicos auditivoa, vestibulares y visuales, la recuperación funcional después de accidentes cerebrovasculares. |
| 用法、用量<br>Administración y dosis | 口服，每次 1 片，一日 2 次（早、晚服）。维持量每日一次，每次 1 片，餐后服。<br>Por vía oral: 2 tabletas diarias dividas en 2 tomas en la mañana y en la noche. Dosis de mantenimiento es de 1 tableta diaria después de alimento. |
| 剂型、规格<br>Formulaciones y especificaciones | 片剂：每片含二甲磺酸阿米三嗪 30mg，萝巴新 10mg。<br>Tableta: cada una incluye 30mg de Dimethanesulphonate Almitrina y 10mg de Raubasina. |

续　表

| 药品名称 Drug Names | 吡硫醇 Piritinol |
|---|---|
| 适应证<br>Indicaciones | 用于脑震荡综合征、脑外伤后遗症、脑炎及脑膜炎后遗症等引起的头痛、头晕、失眠、记忆力减退、注意力不集中、情绪变化等症状的改善，也可用于脑动脉硬化、老年痴呆等精神症状。<br><br>Se usa en alivio del cefalea, vértigos, insomnio, pértida de memoria y atención y cambios del estado de ánimo causados por el síndrome post conmoción cerebral, secuelas de la lesión cerebral traumática, encefalitis y secuelas de la meningitis. Se usa también en tratamiento de arteriosclerosis cerebral y enfermedad de Alzheimer. |
| 用法、用量<br>Administración y dosis | 口服：成人每次 100 ～ 200mg，一日 3 次。小儿每次 50 ～ 100mg，一日 3 次。静脉滴注：每次 200 ～ 400mg，一日 1 次，用 250ml 静脉滴注液稀释后使用。<br><br>Por vía oral: Para adultos la dosis es de 100 ~ 200mg por 3 veces al día y para infantes la dosis es de 50 ~ 100mg por 3 veces al día. Infusión por I.V.: 200 ~ 400mg una vez al día diluidos en solución de infusión. |
| 剂型、规格<br>Formulaciones y especificaciones | 片剂：每片 100mg；200mg。胶囊剂：每粒 100mg。注射剂：每支 100mg（1ml）；200mg（2ml）。盐酸吡硫醇葡萄糖注射液：250ml（盐酸吡硫醇 200mg，葡萄糖 5g）。<br><br>Tableta: 100mg, 200mg; Cápsula: 100mg; Inyección: 100mg(1ml), 200mg(2ml); Inyección de glucosa y Piritinol Clorhidrato: 250ml (incluyendo 200mg de Piritinol Clorhidrato y 5g de glucosa). |
| 药品名称 Drug Names | 小牛血去蛋白提取物 Derivados de desproteiniza-ción de la sangre de ternero |
| 适应证<br>Indicaciones | ①用于脑卒中、脑外伤、周围血管病及腿部溃疡。②亦可用于皮移植术、烧伤、烫伤、糜烂、创伤、压疮的伤口愈合；放射所引起的皮肤、黏膜损伤。③各种病因引起的角膜溃疡，角膜损伤，酸或碱引起的角膜灼伤，大泡性角膜炎，神经麻痹性角膜炎，角膜和结膜变性等。<br><br>① Se usa en tratamiento de apoplejía, lesión cerebral traumática, enfermedad vascular periférica y úlceras en las piernas. ② Se usa también en  cicatrización de heridas de injertos de piel, quemaduras, erosión, heridas, úlceras de decúbito y lesión de la mucosa y piel inducida por radiaciones.　③ También se usa en tratamiento de úlceras y lesiones corneales, quemaduras corneales causadas por ácidos o álcalis, queratitis bullosa, queratitis por parálisis del nervio,  degeneración de la córnea y la conjuntiva,  etc. |
| 用法、用量<br>Administración y dosis | 口服：每次 1 ～ 2 片，一日 3 次。整片吞服，一疗程 4 ～ 6 周。静脉注射或缓慢肌内注射：初期每日 10 ～ 20ml，进一步治疗剂量每天 5ml。静脉注射：10 ～ 50ml 加入静脉注射液 250ml 中滴注。皮肤外用：在保证创口或创面清洁的情况下外用。轻者可一日一次，涂于创面处；重者可每日 2 ～ 6 次，或酌情增加次数。眼科外用：滴于眼部患处，每次 1 滴，一日 3 ～ 4 次，或视病情而定。口腔外用：涂抹于患处每日 3 ～ 5 次，其中 1 次在睡前使用。<br><br>Por vía oral: 1 ~ 2 tabletas por 3 veces al día. Un curso tarda 4 ~ 6 semanas. Inyección por I.V. o I.M. lenta: dosis inicial de 10 ~ 20ml diarios y luego 5ml diarios. Infusión por I.V.: 10 ~ 50ml diluidos en 250ml de solución de infusión. Uso exterior en la piel: Se usa cuando esté limpia la herida. Para pacientes leves se usa una vez al día y se es caso severo, se usa 2 ~ 6 veces al día y puede aumentar la medicación en caso necesario. Uso exterior oftálmico: 1 gota por 3 ó 4 veces al día y puede ajustar la dosis según la necesidad. Uso exterior oral: 3 ~ 5 veces al día y entre ellas, una vez se usa antes de acostarse. |
| 剂型、规格<br>Formulaciones y especificaciones | 片剂：每片 200mg。注射剂：每支 80mg（2ml）；200mg（5ml）；400mg（10ml）。软膏：10%（20g：2.0g）。眼凝胶制剂：20%（5g：1g）。口腔膏：5%（5g：0.25g）。<br><br>Tabletas: 200mg; Inyección: 80mg(2ml), 200mg(5ml), 400mg(10ml); Crema: 10% (20g：2.0g); Gel contorno de ojos: 20%(5g：1g); Pasta oral：5%(5g：0.25g). |
| 药品名称 Drug Names | 胞磷胆碱 Citicolina |
| 适应证<br>Indicaciones | 主要用于急性颅脑外伤和脑手术所引起的意识障碍，以及脑卒中而致偏瘫的患者，也可用于耳鸣及神经性耳聋。对颅内出血引起意识障碍效果较差。<br><br>Se usa principalmente en lesión cerebral traumática aguda y trastorno de conciencia causado por cirugía cerebral, hemiplejia causado por la apoplejía,tinnitus y sordera nerviosa. La eficacia no es muy buena para tratar del trastorno de conciencia causado por hemorragia intracraneal. |

**续 表**

| | |
|---|---|
| 用法、用量<br>Administración y dosis | 　　静脉滴注：一日 0.25 ～ 0.5g，用 5% 或 10% 葡萄糖注射液稀释后缓缓滴注，每 5 ～ 10 日为一疗程。单纯静脉注射：每次 0.1 ～ 0.2g。肌内注射：一日 0.1 ～ 0.3g，分 1 ～ 2 次注射，脑出血急性期不宜大剂量应用。一般不采用肌内注射，若用时应经常更换注射部位。口服：每次 0.2g，一日 3 次。用于维持期治疗可为一次 0.1g，一日 3 次口服。<br><br>　　Infusión por I.V.: 0.25 ～ 0.5g diarios diluidos en solución de glucosa a 5% ～ 10%. Se administra lentamente y un curso de tratamiento tarda 5 ～ 10 días. Inyección simple por I.V.: 0.1 ～ 0.2g cada vez. Inyección por I.M.: 0.1 ～ 0.3g diarios divididos en 1 ó 2 veces y no recomienda aplicación de dosis grande en etapa aguda de hemorragia cerebral. Habitualmente no se administra inyección por I.M. y en caso de se obliga de esta aplicación debe cambiar de menudo lugar de la inyección. Por vía oral: 0.2g por 3 veces al día. En tratamiento de mantenimiento la dosis es de 0.1g por 3 veces al día. |
| 剂型、规格<br>Formulaciones y especificaciones | 　　注射剂：每支 0.2g（2ml）；0.25g（2ml）。片剂：每片 0.2g。胶囊剂：每粒 0.1g。<br><br>　　Inyección: 0.2g (2ml); 0.25g (2ml); Tableta: 0.2g; Cápsula: 0.1g. |
| **药品名称 Drug Names** | 单唾液酸四己糖神经节苷脂 Gangliosidos monosialicos de tetrahexosina |
| 适应证<br>Indicaciones | 　　用于脑脊髓创伤、脑血管意外，可用于帕金森病。<br><br>　　Se usa en tratamiento de traumatismo craneoencefálico y de la medula espinal y accidente cerebrovascular. Puede usarse para enfermedad de Parkinson. |
| 用法、用量<br>Administración y dosis | 　　每日 20 ～ 40mg，一次或分次肌内注射或缓慢静脉注射。急性期：每日 100mg，静脉滴注；2 ～ 3 周后改为维持量，每日 20 ～ 40mg，一般 6 周。对帕金森病，首剂量 500 ～ 1000mg，静脉滴注；第二日起每日 200mg，皮下、肌内注射或静脉滴注，一般用至 18 周。<br><br>　　Dosis diaria es de 20 ～ 40mg administrados una vez o varias veces en inyección por I.M. o I.V.. En etapa aguda: la dosis es de 100mg diarios en infusión por I.V. y después de 2 o 3 semanas cambia a dosis de mantenimiento de 20 ～ 40mg diarios que durará generalmente 6 semanas. En cuanto a enfermedad de Parkinson, la dosis inicial es de 500-1000mg en infusiión por I.V. y desde el segundo día cambia a dosis de 200mg diarios en inyección subcutánea, o por I.M. o infusión por I.V. El tratamiento tardará generalmente 18 semanas. |
| 剂型、规格<br>Formulaciones y especificaciones | 　　注射液：每支 20mg（2ml）；100mg（5ml）。粉针剂：每支 40mg；100mg。<br>　　Inyección: 20mg(20ml), 100mg(50ml); Polvo para inyección: 40mg, 100mg. |
| **药品名称 Drug Names** | 脑蛋白水解物 Hidrolizados de proteínas del cerebro |
| 适应证<br>Indicaciones | 　　适用于尤以注意及记忆障碍的器质性脑病性综合征，原发性痴呆如老年性痴呆，血管性痴呆（如多发梗死性痴呆），混合性痴呆，卒中、颅脑手术后的脑功能障碍，神经衰弱及衰竭症状。<br><br>　　Se usa en tratamiento de síndrome orgánico cerebral especialmente trastornos de atención y memoria, demencia primaria ( por ejempro la enfermedad de Alzheimer), demencia vascular (tales como demencia multi-infarto), demencia mixta, disfunción cerebral asociada con apoplejía y cirugía cerebral, neurastenia y agotamiento nervioso. |
| 用法、用量<br>Administración y dosis | 　　成人常用 10 ～ 30ml 稀释于 5% 葡萄糖或生理盐水 250ml 中缓慢滴注，60 ～ 120 分钟滴完，一日 1 次，每疗程注射 10 ～ 20 次，依病情而定。轻微病例或经大剂量用药后为保持疗效者，可用肌内注射、皮下注射或静脉注射，每次 1 ～ 5ml；皮下注射不超过每次 2ml，肌内注射不超过每次 5ml；静脉注射不超过每次 10ml。应用 10 ～ 20 次，以后每周 2 ～ 3 次，可重复几个疗程，直至临床表现不再改善为止。<br><br>　　Para adultos habitualmente se administra infusión lenta dentro de 60 a 120 minutos a una dosis de 10-30ml diarios diluidos en 250ml de solución de glucosa o Normal Saline a 5%. Un curso de tratamiento incluye 10 ～ 20 medicaciones y puede ajustar según la necesidad. Para pacientes leves o tras medicamento de gran dosis y necesita tratamiento de mantenmiento, puede administrarse inyección por I.M. o I.V. o subcutánea a una dosis de 1 ～ 5ml: Si es inyección subcutánea la dosis no excede a 2ml, si es inyección por I.M. la dosis no excede a 5ml y si es inyección por I.V. la dosis no debe exceder a 10ml. Se aplica 10 ～ 20 veces y luego se administra 2 ó 3 veces cada semana y puede repetir varios cursos hasta que no se ve mejoramiento clínico. |

**续　表**

| 剂型、规格<br>Formulaciones y especificaciones | 注射液：每支 2ml；5ml；10ml。<br>Inyección: 2ml, 5ml, 10ml. |
|---|---|
| 药品名称 Drug Names | 赖氨酸 Lisina |
| 适应证<br>Indicaciones | ①用于颅脑损伤综合征、脑血管病、记忆力减退等。②赖氨酸缺乏引起的小儿食欲缺乏、营养不良及脑发育不全等。<br>① Se usa en tratamiento de síndrome de lesión cerebral traumática, enfermedades cerebrovasculares y pérdida de memoria. ② Se usa en tratamiento de anorexia, desnutrición y disgenesia cerebral infantiles causadas por deficiencia de lisina. |
| 用法、用量<br>Administración y dosis | 口服：每次 3g，一日 1 次，10～15 日为一疗程。静脉滴注：一日 1 次，每次 3g，稀释于 250ml 静脉滴注液中缓慢滴注，20 次为一疗程。<br>Por vía oral a dosis de 3g una vez al día y un curso de tratamiento tarda 10～15 días. Lenta infusión por I.V. a dosis de 3g una vez al día diluidos en 250ml de solución intravenosa y un curso de tratamiento tarda 20 días. |
| 剂型、规格<br>Formulaciones y especificaciones | 散剂：每袋 3g。注射液：每支 3g（10ml）。<br>Polvo: 3g; Inyección: 3g(10ml). |

8.14　麻醉药及其辅助用药 Anestésicos y auxiliares anestésicos

| 药品名称 Drug Names | 恩氟烷 Enflurano |
|---|---|
| 适应证<br>Indicaciones | 应用于符合全身麻醉，（此时浓度 0.5% 即足够，3% 为极限），可与多种静脉全身麻醉药和全身麻醉辅助用药联用或合用。<br>Se usa en anestesia general con aplicación de solución a 0.5% y como máximo a 3%. Puede usarse junto con fármacos de anestesia total intravenosa y fármaco adyuvante de anestesia general. |
| 用法、用量<br>Administración y dosis | 使用量应根据患者的具体情况而定。<br>La dosis administrada debe determinarse en función de las circunstancias específicas del paciente. |
| 剂型、规格<br>Formulaciones y especificaciones | 液体剂：100ml；150ml；250ml。<br>Agtente líquido: 100ml, 150ml, 250ml un perfume. |
| 药品名称 Drug Names | 异氟烷 Isoflurano |
| 适应证<br>Indicaciones | 可用于各种手术的麻醉。<br>Se usa en anestesia de todo tipo de cirugía. |
| 用法、用量<br>Administración y dosis | 成人诱导麻醉时吸入气体内浓度一般为 1.5%～3%；维持麻醉时气体内浓度为 1%～1.5%。麻醉较深时对循环及呼吸系统均有抑制作用。骨骼肌松弛作用亦较好。<br>En inducción de anestesia para adultos, la concentración del gas aspirado es 1.5%～3%; En el mantenimiento de anestesia la concentración es de 1%～1.5%. Durante anestesia profunda inhibirá sistemas circulatorio y respiratorio. Tiene buen efecto como relajante muscular esquelética. |
| 剂型、规格<br>Formulaciones y especificaciones | 液体剂：每瓶 100ml；250ml。<br>Agtente líquido: 100ml, 250ml un perfume. |
| 药品名称 Drug Names | 七氟烷 Sevoflurano |
| 适应证<br>Indicaciones | 作为全身麻醉药应用。<br>Se usa en anestesia general. |

955

| | |
|---|---|
| 用法、用量<br>Administración y<br>dosis | 麻醉诱导时，以 50% ~ 70% 氧化亚氮与本品 2.5% ~ 4% 吸入。使用睡眠量的静脉麻醉时，本品的诱导量通常为 0.5% ~ 5%。麻醉维持，应以最低有效浓度维持外科麻醉状态，常为 4% 以下。<br><br>En la inducción de anestesia, inhala gas con dicho fármaco a 2.5% ~ 4% y óxido nitroso a 50% ~ 70%. En anestesia intravenosa a cantidad para inducir el sueño, la dosis de inducción de dicho fármaco es habitualmente 0.5% ~ 5%. En mantenimiento de anestesia debe administrar a la mínima concentración efectiva que generalmente es menor de 4%. |
| 剂型、规格<br>Formulaciones y<br>especificaciones | 吸入用七氟烷：120ml；250ml。<br>Sevoflurano para inhalación: 120ml, 250ml. |
| **药品名称 Drug Names** | 硫喷妥钠 Tiopental Sódico |
| 适应证<br>Indicaciones | 常用于静脉麻醉、诱导 麻醉、基础麻醉、抗惊厥及复合麻醉等。<br><br>Se usa en anestesia intravenosa, inducción de anestesia, anestesia básico, uso anticonvulsivos y anestesia combinada. |
| 用法、用量<br>Administración y<br>dosis | ①静脉麻醉：一般多用 5% 或 2.5% 溶液，缓慢注入。成人，一次 4 ~ 8mg/kg，经 30 秒左右即进入麻醉，神志完全消失，但肌肉松弛不完全，也不能随意调节，麻醉深度，故多用于小手术。如患者有呼吸快、发声、移动等现象，即为苏醒的表现，可再注射少量以持续麻醉。极量：一次 1g（即 5% 溶液 20ml）。②基础麻醉：用于小儿、甲状腺功能亢进症及精神紧张患者。成人，肌内注射，每次 0.5g，以 2.5% 溶液，做深部肌内注射。③诱导麻醉：一般用 2.5% 溶液缓慢静脉注射，1 次 0.3g（1 次不超过 0.5g），继以乙醚吸入。④抗惊厥：每次静脉注射 0.05 ~ 0.1g。<br><br>① En anestesia intravenosa: inyección lenta de solución a 5% o 2.5%, para adultos la dosis es de 4 ~ 8mg/kg. Dentro de 30 minutos estará en anestesia sin ninguna conciencia pero la relajación muscular no es completa. No se puede ajustar la dosis arbitrariamente. Debido a su efecto de anestesia profunda siempre se usa en cirugías simples. Si hay fenómenos como respiración rápida, voz, monimiento, el paciente se está despertando y puede inyectar un poco más para mantener la anestesia. La dosis máxima no excede a 1g cada vez, es decir 20ml de la solución al 5%. ② En anestesia básica: Se usa en pacientes infantil, de hipertiroidismo o de estrés mental. Para adultos se administra inyección por I.M. profunda a dosis de 0.5g de solución a 2.5%. ③ En inducción de anestesia: Se administra lenta inyección por I.V. de solución al 2.5% con dosis de 0.3g cada vez (la dosis no puede exceder a 0.5g cada vez) y luego seguido por inhalación de éter. ④ Uso anticonvulsivos: Se administra inyección por I.V. a dosis de 0.05 ~ 0.1g. |
| 剂型、规格<br>Formulaciones y<br>especificaciones | 注射用硫喷妥钠：每支 0.5g；1g（含无水碳酸钠 6%）。<br>Tiopental Sódico para inyección: 0.5g, 1g (6% de la cantidad es de carbonato sódico anhidro). |
| **药品名称 Drug Names** | 氯胺酮 ketamina |
| 适应证<br>Indicaciones | ①各种小手术或诊断操作时，可单独使用本品进行麻醉。对于需要肌肉松弛的手术，应加用肌肉松弛剂；对于内脏牵引较重的手术，应配合其他药物以减少牵引反应。②作为其他全身麻醉的诱导剂使用。③辅助麻醉性能较弱的麻醉剂进行麻醉，或与其他全身或局部麻醉复合使用。<br><br>① Se puede utilizar individualmente en cirugías pequeñas o procesos diagnósticos. Si en la cirugía necesita relajar músculos debe agregar relajantes musculares y en la que tiene fuerte tracción visceral, debe agregar otros fármacos para reducir estas tracciones. ② Utilización como inductor de otras anestesias generales. ③ Adyuvante en anestesia con otros fármacos de leve desempeño anestésico o uso compuesto junto con otros fármacos en anestesias generales o parciales. |
| 用法、用量<br>Administración y<br>dosis | ①成人常用量：全身麻醉诱导，静脉注射 1 ~ 2mg/kg，注射应较慢（60 秒以上）。全身麻醉维持，一次静脉注射 0.5 ~ 1mg/kg。②极量：静脉注射每分钟 4mg/kg；肌内注射，一次 13mg/kg。<br><br>① Dosis habitual para adultos: Para inducción de anestesia se aplica inyección por I.V. de 1 ~ 2mg/kg a velocidad lenta que dura más de 60 segundos. Para anestesia general se aplica inyección por I.V. de solo 1 vez de 0.5 ~ 1mg/kg. ② Dosis máxima: 4mg/kg cada minuto en inyección por I.V. y 13mg/kg cada vez en inyección por I.M.. |

**续　表**

| 剂型、规格<br>Formulaciones y<br>especificaciones | 注射液：100mg（2ml）；100mg（1ml）；200mg（20ml）。<br>Inyección: 100mg (2ml), 100mg (1ml), 200mg (2ml). |
|---|---|
| **药品名称 Drug Names** | **依托咪酯 Etomidato** |
| 适应证<br>Indicaciones | 可用于诱导麻醉。<br>Se usa para la inducción de la anestesia. |
| 用法、用量<br>Administración y<br>dosis | 成人：0.3mg/kg，于 15 ～ 60 秒静脉注射完毕。<br>Adulto: Inyección por I.V. dentro de 15 ~ 60 segundos a dosis de 0.3mg/kg. |
| 剂型、规格<br>Formulaciones y<br>especificaciones | 注射液：每支 20mg（10ml）。<br>Inyección: 20mg (10ml). |
| **药品名称 Drug Names** | **羟丁酸钠 Hidroxibutirato sódico** |
| 适应证<br>Indicaciones | 常用于全身麻醉或诱导麻醉，以及局部麻醉、腰椎麻醉的辅助用药，适用于老年人、儿童及脑、神经外科手术，外伤、烧伤患者的麻醉。<br>Se usa principalmente en anestesia general o inducción de la anestesia, fármaco adyuvante en anestesia parcial y espinal. Puede usar en cirugía cerebral y neurocirugía para ancianos e infantiles así como anestesia para pacientes de trauma y quemadura. |
| 用法、用量<br>Administración y<br>dosis | （1）诱导麻醉：一次静脉注射，成人 60mg/kg；注射速度 1g/min。<br>（2）维持麻醉：静脉注射，一次 12 ～ 80mg/kg。<br>（3）极量：一次总量 300mg/kg。<br>(1) Inducción de anestesia: Inyecciín por I.V. de solo 1 vez a una dosis de 60mg/kg y velocidad de 1g/min para adultos.<br>(2) Mantenimiento de anestesia: Inyección por I.V. de 12 ~ 80mg/kg cada vez.<br>(3) Dosis máxima: 300mg/kg cada vez. |
| 剂型、规格<br>Formulaciones y<br>especificaciones | 注射液：每支 2.5g（10ml）。<br>Inyección: 2.5g (10ml). |
| **药品名称 Drug Names** | **丙泊酚 Propofol** |
| 适应证<br>Indicaciones | 用于全身麻醉的诱导和维持。常与硬膜外或脊髓麻醉同时应用，也常与镇痛药、肌松药及吸入性麻醉药同用。适用于门诊患者。<br>Se usa en la inducción y mantenimiento de anestesia. Habitualmente se usa en anestesia epidural o espinal o junto con analgésicos, relajantes musculares y anestésicos inhalados. Se usa en pacientes ambulatorios. |
| 用法、用量<br>Administración y<br>dosis | 静脉注射。诱导麻醉：每 10 秒钟注射 40mg，直至产生麻醉。大多数成人用量 2 ～ 2.5mg/kg。维持麻醉：常用量为每分钟 0.1 ～ 0.2mg/kg。<br>Inyección por I.V.. Para inducción de anestesia la dosis es de 40mg cada 10 segundos hasta que tiene efecto de anestesia. Habitualmente la dosis para adultos es aproximadamente 2 ~ 2.5mg/kg. Para mentenimiento de anestesia: dosis habitual es de 0.1 ~ 0.2mg/kg cada minuto. |
| 剂型、规格<br>Formulaciones y<br>especificaciones | 注射液：每支 200mg（20ml）；500mg（50ml）；1g（100ml）。丙泊酚中 / 长链脂肪乳注射液：200mg（20ml）。<br>Inyección: 200mg(20ml), 500mg(50ml), 1g(100ml); Inyección de propofol en emulsión grasa de cadena media y larga: 200mg(20ml). |
| **药品名称 Drug Names** | **普鲁卡因 Procaína** |
| 适应证<br>Indicaciones | 主要用于浸润麻醉、蛛网膜下腔阻滞麻醉、神经传导阻滞麻醉和用于治疗某些损伤和炎症，可使发炎损伤部位的症状得到一定的缓解（封闭疗法）。还可用于纠正四肢血管舒缩功能障碍。<br>Se usa principalmente en anestesia de infiltración, anestesia espinal, anestesia por bloqueo de nervio y en tratamiento de ciertas lesiones e inflamaciones aliviando los síntomas mediante terapia de bloqueo. Tanbién puede usarse en tratamiento de disfunción vasomotora en limbs. |

**续 表**

| | |
|---|---|
| 用法、用量<br>Administración y dosis | （1）浸润麻醉，溶液浓度多为 0.25% ～ 0.5%（口腔科有时用其 4% 的溶液），每次用量 0.05 ～ 0.25g，每小时不可超过 1.5g。其麻醉时间短，可加入少量肾上腺素 [1 ：（100 000 ～ 200 000）] 以延长作用的时间。<br>　　（2）蛛网膜下腔阻滞麻醉，一次量不宜超过 0.15g，用 5% 溶液，约可麻醉 1 小时，主要用于腹部以下需时不长的手术。<br>　　（3）"封闭疗法"，将 0.25% ～ 0.5% 溶液注射于与病变有关的神经周围或病变部位。<br>　　(1) En anestesia de infiltración, generalmente se usa solución a 0.25% ~ 0.5% y a veces se usa la 4% en estomatología. La dosis es de 0.05 ~ 0.25g cada vez y no excede a 1.5g cada hora. La anestesia dura poco tiempo y puede agregar un poco de epinefrina a proporción de 1:100000 ~ 1:200000 para prolongar el efecto de anestesia.<br>　　(2) En la anestesia espinal: Se usa la solución a 5% y la dosis no debe exceder a 0.15g cada vez. La anestesia durará 1 hora aproximadamente y se aplica principalmente en cirugías no largas y en zona bajo abdomen.<br>　　(3) En terapia de bloqueo, se administra inyección de solución a 0.25%~0.5% en la lesión o nervios periféricos asociados con la lesión. |
| 剂型、规格<br>Formulaciones y especificaciones | 注射液：每支 100mg（20ml）；50mg（20ml）；100mg（10ml）；40mg（2ml）。注射用盐酸普鲁卡因：每支 150mg；1g。<br>Inyección: 100mg(20ml), 50mg(20ml), 100mg(10ml), 40mg(2ml). Procaína clorhidrato para inyección: 150mg, 1g. |
| **药品名称Drug Names** | 丁卡因 Tetracaína |
| 适应证<br>Indicaciones | 用于黏膜表面麻醉、神经阻滞麻醉、硬膜外麻醉和蛛网膜下隙麻醉。<br>Se usa en anestesia mucosa en la superficie, anestesia por bloqueo de nervio, anestesia epidural y anestesia subaracnoidea. |
| 用法、用量<br>Administración y dosis | ①黏膜麻醉：眼科用 0.5% ～ 1% 溶液，鼻喉科用 1% ～ 2% 溶液，总量不得超过 20ml。应用时应于每 3ml 中加入 0.1% 盐酸肾上腺素溶液 1 滴。浸润麻醉用 0.025% ～ 0.03% 溶液。②神经阻滞用 0.1% ～ 0.3% 溶液。③蛛网膜下隙麻醉时用 10 ～ 15ml 与 脑脊液混合后注入。④硬膜外麻醉用 0.15% ～ 0.3% 溶液，与利多卡因合用时最高浓度为 0.3%。极量：浸润麻醉、神经传导阻滞，一次 0.1g。<br>　　① En anestesia mucosa: en oftalmología se administra la solución a 0.5% ~ 1%, en rinología y laringología se administra la solución a 1% ~ 2% y la dosis total no excede a 20ml. En la aplicación hay que agregar 1 gota de solución de clorhidrato de epinefrina a 0.1% en cada 3ml de esa solución. En anestesia de infiltración se administra la solución a 0.025% ~ 0.03%. ② En el bloqueo de nervio se administra la solución a 0.1% ~ 0.3%. ③ En anestesia subaracnoidea se administra a dosis de 10 ~ 15ml mezclados con el líquido cefalorraquídeo. ④ En anestesia epidural se administra la solución a 0.15% ~ 0.3% y cuando se usa con Lidocaína la concentración máxima de la solución no excede a 0.3%. Dosis máxima en anestesia de infiltración y por bloqueo de nervio no debe exceder a 0.1g cada vez. |
| 剂型、规格<br>Formulaciones y especificaciones | 注射液：每支 50mg（5ml）。注射用盐酸丁卡因：10mg；15mg；20mg；50mg。盐酸丁卡因凝胶：1.5g；70mg。<br>Inyección: 50mg (5ml). Tetracana Clorhidrato para inyección: 10mg, 15mg, 20mg, 50mg. Gel de Tetracana Clorhidrato: 1.5g:70mg. |
| **药品名称Drug Names** | 利多卡因 Lidocaína |
| 适应证<br>Indicaciones | 主要用于阻滞麻醉及硬膜外麻醉。也用于室性心律失常，如室性心动过速及频发室性期前收缩。<br>Se usa principalmente en anestesia por bloqueo y anestesia epidural, así como tratamiento de arritmias ventriculares por ejempro la taquicardia ventricular y contracciones ventriculares prematuras de manera frecuente. |
| 用法、用量<br>Administración y dosis | （1）局部麻醉：阻滞麻醉用 1% ～ 2% 溶液，每次用量不宜超过 0.4g。表面麻醉用 2% ～ 4% 溶液，喷雾或蘸药贴敷，一次不超过 100mg，也可以 2% 胶浆剂抹于食管、咽喉气管或导尿管的外壁；妇女做阴道检查时可用棉签蘸 5 ～ 7ml 于局部。尿道扩张术或膀胱镜检查时用量 200 ～ 400mg。气雾剂或喷雾剂 2% ～ 4%，供做内镜检查用，每次 2%10 ～ 30ml，4%5 ～ 15ml。浸润麻醉用 0.25% ～ 0.5% 溶液，每小时用量不超过 0.4g。硬膜外麻醉用 1% ～ 2% 溶液，每次用量不超过 0.5g。<br>　　（2）心律失常。 |

**续　表**

| | |
|---|---|
| | (1) En anestesia tópica: se administra la solución a 1% ~ 2% en anestesia por bloqueo y la dosis no debe exceder a 0.4g. En anestesia de superficie se usa solución a 2% ~ 4% de spray o aderezo y la dosis no excede a 100mg diarios. También puede administrarse en pared esofágica, traqueal, de la garganta o del catéter usando el mucílago a 2%. Cuando las mujeres hacen examen vaginal, puede administrarse parcialmente a dosis de 5 ~ 7ml con un hisopo de algodón。En caso de dilatación de la uretra o en la cistoscopia, la dosis es de 200 ~ 400mg. En la endoscopia puede usar la solución a 2% ~ 4% de aerosal o spray a una dosis de 10 ~ 30ml de la solución a 2% o 5 ~ 15ml de la solución a 4%. En la anestesia de infiltración se usa solución a 0.25% ~ 0.5% y la dosis no excede a 0.4g cada hora. En anestesia epidural se usa solución a 1% ~ 2% y la dosis no excede a 0.5g cada vez.<br>(2) Se usa en tratamiento de arritmias. |
| 剂型、规格<br>Formulaciones y especificaciones | 注射液：每支 0.1g（5ml）；0.4g（20ml）。胶浆剂：2%。盐酸利多卡因气雾剂：2%；4%。<br>Inyección: 0.1g (5ml), 0.4g(20ml). Mucílago: 2%. Aerosal de Tetracana Clorhidrato: 2%, 4%. |
| 药品名称 Drug Names | 布比卡因 Bupivacaína |
| 适应证<br>Indicaciones | 浸润麻醉用；神经传导阻滞麻醉。<br>Se usa en anestesia de infiltración，anestesia por bloqueo de nervio. |
| 用法、用量<br>Administración y dosis | 浸润麻醉用 0.1% ~ 0.25% 溶液；神经传导阻滞用 0.5% ~ 0.75% 溶液。一次极量 200mg，一日极量 400mg。<br>Para anestesia de infiltración: solución al 0.1% ~ 0.25%, Para anestesia por bloqueo de nervio: solución al 0.5% ~ 0.75%. Dosis máxima es de 200mg cada vez y 400mg al dia. |
| 剂型、规格<br>Formulaciones y especificaciones | 注射液：每支 12.5mg（5ml）；25mg（5ml）；37.5mg（5ml）。<br>Inyección: 12.5mg (5ml), 25mg (5ml), 37.5mg (5ml). |
| 药品名称 Drug Names | 罗哌卡因 Ropivacaína |
| 适应证<br>Indicaciones | 用于区域组织麻醉和硬膜外麻醉；也可用于区域组织镇痛，如硬膜外术后或分娩镇痛。<br>Para La anestesia regional y epidural. También se usa en la analgesia regional, como la analgesia epidural después de la cirugía o la analgesia en el parto. |
| 用法、用量<br>Administración y dosis | 区域组织麻醉和硬膜外麻醉：0.5% ~ 1% 溶液。一次最大剂量为 200mg。区域组织镇痛：0.2% 溶液。<br>Para anestesia regional y epidural: solución al 0.5% ~ 1%, dosis máxima no excede a 200mg. Para analgesia regional: solución al 0.2%. |
| 剂型、规格<br>Formulaciones y especificaciones | 注射液：20mg（10ml）；40mg（20ml）；75mg（10ml）；150mg（20ml）；100mg（10ml）；200mg（200ml）。<br>Inyección: 20mg (10ml), 40mg (20ml), 75mg (10ml), 150mg (20ml), 100mg (10ml), 200mg (20ml). |
| 药品名称 Drug Names | 达克罗宁 Diclonina |
| 适应证<br>Indicaciones | 对黏膜穿透力强，作用迅速，可做表面麻醉。对皮肤有镇痛、止痒及杀菌作用，可用于火烧、擦伤、痒疹、虫咬伤、痔瘘、溃疡、压疮及镜检前的准备。<br>Debido a la fuerte y rápida penetración de mucosa, puede utilizarse en anestesia superficial. Puede aliviar el dolor, pización de la piel y tiene efecto en esterilización, por lo cual se indica en quemadura, abrasiones, erupciones, picaduras de insectos, hemorroides, úlceras, úlceras de decúbito y preparación de microscopía. |
| 用法、用量<br>Administración y dosis | 多制成 1% 的软膏、乳膏或 0.5% 的溶液供用。<br>Siempre lo producen en pomada y crema a 1% o solución a 0.5%. |
| 剂型、规格<br>Formulaciones y especificaciones | 软膏：1%；乳膏：1%；溶液：0.5%。<br>Pomada: 1%; Crema: 1%; La solución: 0.5%. |

**续　表**

| 药品名称 Drug Names | 泮库溴铵 Bromuro de Pancuronio |
|---|---|
| 适应证<br>Indicaciones | 主要用作外科手术麻醉的辅助用药（气管插管和肌松）。<br><br>Se usa principalmente como adyuvante de la anestesia quirúrgico ( intubación endotraqueal y relajación muscular). |
| 用法、用量<br>Administración y dosis | 静脉注射。成人常用量 40 ～ 100μg/kg。与乙醚、氟烷合用时应酌减剂量。<br><br>Inyección por I.V.. Dosis habitual para adultos: 40~100mg/kg. Disminuye la dosis cuando lo usa junto con éter, halotano. |
| 剂型、规格<br>Formulaciones y especificaciones | 注射液：每支 4mg（2ml）。<br>Inyección: 4mg (2ml). |
| 药品名称 Drug Names | 罗库溴铵 Bromuro de Rocuronio |
| 适应证<br>Indicaciones | 用于气管插管，也可用于各种手术中肌松的维持。<br>Se usa en la intubación endotraguea y mantenimiento de relajación musculares en cirugías. |
| 用法、用量<br>Administración y dosis | 插管：0.6mg/kg 单次静脉注射。维持量：0.15mg/kg，单次静脉注射；每分钟 5 ～ 10μg/kg 连续静脉滴注。吸入麻醉下应适当减量。<br><br>Para intubación: Inyección por I.V. a dosis de 0.6mg/kg de una vez. Para mantenimiento: 0.15mg/kg en inyección por I.V. de una vez o 5 ~ 10mg/kg/min en infusión por I.V.. En anestesia por inhalación debe reducir la dosis apropiadamente. |
| 剂型、规格<br>Formulaciones y especificaciones | 注射液：每支 50mg（5ml）；100mg（10ml）。<br>Inyección: 50mg (5ml); 100mg (10ml). |
| 药品名称 Drug Names | 维库溴铵 Bromuro de Vecuronio |
| 适应证<br>Indicaciones | 为中效非去极化型肌松药。肌松效应及用途等均似于泮库溴铵，但稍强，持续时间为泮库溴铵的 1/3 ～ 1/2。<br><br>Es relajante muscular no despolarizante con intermedia duración. Tiene el efecto y utilización como relajante muscular similar a Bromuro de Pancuronio pero el efecto es más fuerte mientras que la duración es la 1/3 ó 1/2 de la de Bromuro de Pancuronio. |
| 用法、用量<br>Administración y dosis | 静脉注射，常用量为 70 ～ 100μg/kg。<br>Inyección I.V.. Dosis habitual: 70~100μg/kg. |
| 剂型、规格<br>Formulaciones y especificaciones | 注射用维库溴铵：每支 4mg，以所附溶剂溶解后应用。<br>bromuro de vecuronio para inyección: 4mg, al usar tiene que diluirlo con la solución adjuntada. |
| 药品名称 Drug Names | 阿库氯铵 Cloruro de Alcuronio |
| 适应证<br>Indicaciones | 为去极化型肌松药，其特点与泮库溴铵相似，其效应比筒箭毒碱强 1.5 ～ 2 倍。静脉注射后肌松起效快（30 秒），2 ～ 3 分钟达高峰，维持 20 ～ 30 分钟。停药后恢复亦快。<br><br>Es relajante muscular despolarizante, tiene caracteristicas similares a Bromuro de Pancuronio. Su efectp es de 1,5 a 2 veces más fuerte que el Tubocurarina. Tarda 30 segundos tras la inyección I.V. para tener efecto de rejalar el músculo, alcanza al pico dentro de 2 ~ 3 minutos y dura 20 ~ 30 minutos. Se recupera en breve al dejar el medicamento. |
| 用法、用量<br>Administración y dosis | 静脉注射：首次剂量为 150μg/kg，随后为 300μg/kg，间隔 15 ～ 25 分钟注射一次。<br><br>Inyección I.V.: Dosis inicial de 150mg/kg y luego aumenta a 300mg/kg. Se aplica la medicación cada 15 ~ 25 minutos. |
| 剂型、规格<br>Formulaciones y especificaciones | 注射液：每支 10mg（2ml）。<br>Inyección: 10mg (2ml). |

**续　表**

| 药品名称 Drug Names | 哌库溴铵 Bromuro de Pipecuronio |
|---|---|
| 适应证<br>Indicaciones | 为长效非去极化型肌松药，是泮库溴铵的衍生物，作用类似泮库溴铵，肌松持续时间为 20 分钟。也可用作外科手术麻醉的辅助用药。<br><br>Es relajante muscular no despolarizante con larga duración. Tiene efecto similar a bromuro de pancuronio siendo derivado de este fármaco. El efecto de relajar músculos dura 20 inutos. Puede utilizar como adyuvante en anestesia de cirugía. |
| 用法、用量<br>Administración y<br>dosis | 气管插管在静脉注射后 3 分钟，用药量为静脉注射 0.08 ～ 0.1mg/kg；肾功能不全者用药量不超过 0.04mg/kg。<br><br>La intubación traqueal se aplica 3 minutos después de la inyección por I.V.. La dosis de inyección por I.V. es de 0.08 ~ 0.1mg/kg y para pacientes de disfunción renal la dosis méxima no excede a 0.04mg/kg. |
| 剂型、规格<br>Formulaciones y<br>especificaciones | 注射剂：每支 4mg（附有溶剂）。<br>Inyección: 4mg (con solución adjuntada). |
| 药品名称 Drug Names | 阿曲库铵 Atracurio |
| 适应证<br>Indicaciones | 为非去极化型肌松药。作用与筒箭毒碱相同，起效快（1 分钟）、持续时间短（15 分钟）。大剂量可促使组胺释放。用于各种手术时需肌松或控制呼吸情况。<br><br>Es relajante muscular despolarizante. Tiene efecto igual como Tubocurarina. Se caracteriza por el rápido efecto (1 minuto) y corta duración (15 minutos). Cuando lo usa en grande dosis puede inducir la liberación de histamina. Utilización para relajación muscular o controlar la respiración en cirugías. |
| 用法、用量<br>Administración y<br>dosis | 静脉注射起始剂量 0.3 ～ 0.6mg/kg，然后可以静脉滴注每分钟 5 ～ 10μg/kg 维持。<br><br>Dosis inicial de inyección por I.V. es de 0.3 ~ 0.6mg/kg y dosis de mantenimiento en infusión por I.V. es de 5 ~ 10μg/kg cada minuto. |
| 剂型、规格<br>Formulaciones y<br>especificaciones | 注射液：每支 25mg（2.5ml）；50mg（5ml）。<br>Inyección: 25mg (2.5ml), 50mg (5ml). |
| 药品名称 Drug Names | 顺阿曲库铵 Cisatracurio |
| 适应证<br>Indicaciones | ①其效能为阿曲库铵的 4 ～ 5 倍；②消除半衰期约为 24 分钟；③作用持续时间 45 ～ 75 分钟；④无组胺释放作用，无心血管不良反应。<br><br>① Tiene efecto de 4-5 veces que el Atracurio. ② La vida media de eliminación es de aproximadamente 24 minutos. ③ El efecto dura 45 ~ 75 minutos. ④ No hay efecto sobre la liberación de histamina y no causará reacciones adversas cardiovasculares. |
| 用法、用量<br>Administración y<br>dosis | 成人用量为 0.05mg/kg，常用气管插管用量为 0.15 ～ 0.20mg/kg，插管时间在静脉注射后 150 秒左右。<br><br>Dosis para adultos es de 0.05mg/kg, dosis habidual en intubación traqueal es de 0.15 ~ 0.2mg/kg. Se aplica la intubación traqueal 150 segundos después de la infusión. |
| 剂型、规格<br>Formulaciones y<br>especificaciones | 注射液：每支 10mg（5ml）；20mg（10ml）；40mg（20ml）。<br>Inyección: 10mg (5ml), 20mg (10ml), 40mg (20ml). |
| 药品名称 Drug Names | 琥珀胆碱 Succinilcolina |
| 适应证<br>Indicaciones | 为速效肌肉松弛药；也用于需快速气管内插管。<br>Es relajante muscular de acción rápida y se utiliza también en la intubación traqueal rápida. |
| 用法、用量<br>Administración y<br>dosis | 成人静脉注射一次 1 ～ 2mg/kg。多用其 2% ～ 5% 溶液。注射后 1 分钟即出现肌肉松弛，持续 2 分钟。如需继续维持其作用，可用其 0.1% ～ 0.2% 溶液，以每分钟 2.5mg 的速度静脉注射；亦可静脉滴注，静脉滴注液可用生理盐水或 5% 葡萄糖液稀释至 0.1% 浓度。极量，静脉注射一次 250mg。 |

**续 表**

| | Inyección por I.V. para adultos: 1 ~ 2mg/kg cada vez y se usa más la solución a 2% ~ 5%. Tiene acción rápida dentro de 1 minutos y dura 2 minutos tras la inyección. Si necesita mentener el efecto, utiliza la solución a 0.1% ~ 0.2% en inyección por I.V. a velocidad de 2.5mg/min, o infusión por I.V. de dilución a 0.1% con Normal Saline o de solución de glucosa a 5%. La dosis máxima de inyección por I.V es de 250mg cada vez. |
|---|---|
| 剂型、规格<br>Formulaciones y especificaciones | 注射液：每支 50mg（1ml）；100mg（2ml）。<br>Inyección: 50mg (1ml), 100mg (2ml). |

9. 主要作用于自主神经系统的药物 Medicamento que actúan princepalmente sobre el sistema nervioso autónomo

9.1　拟胆碱药和抗胆碱药 Medicamentos similares a los colinérgicos y anticolinérgicos

| 药品名称 Drug Names | 卡巴胆碱 Carbachol |
|---|---|
| 适应证<br>Indicaciones | 主要用于治疗青光眼。<br>Se usa principal en tratamiento del glaucoma. |
| 用法、用量<br>Administración y dosis | 局部用药。0.75% ~ 3% 溶液滴眼，用于对毛果芸香碱无反应或不能耐受者。成人两眼分别滴入 1 ~ 2 滴，4 ~ 8 小时一次。给药后需用手指压迫内眦 1 ~ 2 分钟，以减少吸收，减少全身不良反应。在白内障手术时起缩瞳作用并减少后眼压上升，可用 0.01%0.5ml 滴眼。<br><br>Medicación parcial. Para pacientes que no consiguen efecto o no tienen tolerancia a la pilocarpina: 1 ~ 2 gotas en los ojos cada 4 ~ 8 horas para los adultos. Presionan 1 ~ 2 minutos los cantos internos para reducir la absorción y reacciones adversas.　En cirugía de cataratas, lo utiliza como miótico y reducir la elevación de la presión intraocular a una dosis de 0.5ml de la gota a 0.01%. |
| 剂型、规格<br>Formulaciones y especificaciones | 滴眼液：0.25%；1.5%；2.25%；3%。注射液：每支 0.1mg（1ml）。<br>Gota oftalmológica: 0.25%, 1.5%, 2.25%; 3%. Inyección: 0.1mg (1ml). |
| 药品名称 Drug Names | 毛果芸香碱 Pilocarpina |
| 适应证<br>Indicaciones | 治疗原发性青光眼，包括开角型与闭角型青光眼。滴眼后，缩瞳作用于 10 ~ 30 分钟出现，维持 4 ~ 8 小时；最大降眼压作用约 75 分钟内出现，维持 4 ~ 14 小时；可缓解或消除青光眼症状。也可用于唾液腺功能。<br><br>Se usa para tratamiento del glaucoma primario de ángulo abierto o cerrado. Tras tomar la gota oftalmológica, el efecto miótico aparece en 10 a 30 minutos y dura 4 ~ 8 horas; el efecto máximo de reducir la presión intraocular ocurre en 75 minutos y dura 4 ~ 14 horas; puede aliviar o eliminar los síntomas de glaucoma. También tiene efecto en el sistema de la glándula salival. |
| 用法、用量<br>Administración y dosis | 滴眼液配成 0.5% ~ 4% 毛果芸香碱（常用 1% 及 2%，增加浓度可增加药效，但超过 4% 时，药效无明显增加）。滴眼后 10 ~ 15 分钟开始缩瞳，30 ~ 50 分钟作用最强，约持续 24 小时，睫状肌痉挛作用约持续 2 小时。滴药后 10 ~ 15 分钟开始降眼压，持续 4 ~ 8 小时，故应每日滴眼 3 ~ 4 次。<br><br>Gota oftalmológica: solición a 0.5% ~ 4% utilizando la Pilocarpina (la solución habitual es a 1% ~ 2%, la elevación de concentración aumenta la eficacia y cuando la concentración llega a 4% o más, no hay mucha diferencia en eficacia.). El efecto miótico aparece en 10 ~ 15 minutos y dentro de 30 ~ 50 minutos llega a su máximo efecto y dura 24 horas. En caso del espasmo del músculo ciliar, el efecto dura 2 horas y dentro de 10 ~ 15 minutos empieza a reducir la presión intraocular y dura 4 ~ 8 horas, así que toma la gota 3 ~ 4 veces al día. |
| 剂型、规格<br>Formulaciones y especificaciones | 滴眼液：1%；2%。片剂：（SALAGEN）：每片 5mg。注射液：每支 10mg（1ml）。<br>Gota oftalmológica: 1%, 2%; Tableta (Salagen): 5mg; Inyección: 10mg (1ml). |
| 药品名称 Drug Names | 毒扁豆碱 Fisostigmina |
| 适应证<br>Indicaciones | 主要用其 0.2% ~ 0.5% 溶液点眼，用于治疗原发性闭角型青光眼，药效比毛果芸香碱强而持久。它对中枢神经系统的作用是小剂量时兴奋，大剂量时抑制，故已较少做全身给药，只用于眼科。 |

续　表

| | |
|---|---|
| | Se usa la solución a 0.2% ~ 0.5% como gota oftalmológica en tratamiento de glaucoma primario de ángulo cerrado y tiene duración más larga y efecto más fuerte que la pilocarpina. Sobre el sistema nervioso central, tiene efecto de excitación con pcqueña dosis y efecto de inhibición con grande dosis. Así que en pocas veces lo usa en medicación general sino que sólo en oftalmología. |
| 用法、用量<br>Administración y dosis | 注射液，皮下注射或肌内注射，一次 0.5mg 或遵医嘱。 眼膏，晚上临睡前点眼，涂于眼睑内，一般白天用毛果芸香碱，晚上用本品。或遵医嘱。<br><br>Inyección: Se administra subcutánea o intramuscular a una dosis de 0.5mg o según consejo del médico. Crema oftalmologico: Se aplica en el párpado antes de acostarse y durante el día siempre usa pilocarpina. O se administra según consejos del médico. |
| 剂型、规格<br>Formulaciones y especificaciones | 水杨酸毒扁豆碱滴眼剂：有水杨酸毒扁豆碱 0.25g，硼酸 1.8g，亚硫酸氢钠 0.1g，蒸馏水加至 100ml 配制；或由水杨酸毒扁豆碱 0.46g。氯化钠 0.8g，依地酸二钠 0.1g，尼泊金乙酯 0.03g（加热溶解），蒸馏水加至 100ml 配成。<br><br>Gota oftalmológica de salicilato de fisostigmina: 100ml compuestos por 0.25g de salicilato de fisostigmina, 1.8g de ácido bórico, 0.1g de bisulfito de sodio y agua destilada. 100ml compuestos por 0.46g de salicilato de fisostigmina, 0.8g de cloruro de sodio, 0.1g de edetato disódico, 0.03g de etilparabeno (disuelto calentado) y agua destilada. |
| 药品名称 Drug Names | 新斯的明 Neostigmina |
| 适应证<br>Indicaciones | 多用于重症肌无力及腹部手术后的肠麻痹。<br>Se usa para la miastenia grave y parálisis intestinal después de la cirugía abdominal. |
| 用法、用量<br>Administración y dosis | 口服其溴化物，一次 15mg，一日 45mg；极量：一次 30mg，一日 100mg。皮下注射、肌内注射其甲硫酸盐，每日 1 ~ 3 次，每次 0.25 ~ 1.0mg；极量：一次 1mg，一日 5mg。以 0.05% 眼药水用于青少年假性近视眼，一日 2 次，每次 1 ~ 2 滴，3 个月为 1 疗程。<br><br>Administración oral de Neostigmina de bromuro a dosis 15mg cada vez y 45 mg diarios. Dosis máxima es 30mg cada vez y 100mg diarios. Inyección subcutánea y intramuscular, utiliza la neostigmina de sulfato a una dosis de 0.25 ~ 1.0mg y 1 ~ 3 veces al día. La dosis máxima es de 1mg cada vez y 5mg diarios. Para seudomiopía adolescente, utiliza la gota oftalmológica a 0.05%, 1 ~ 2 gotas y 2 veces al día, un curso de tratamiento tarda 3 meses. |
| 剂型、规格<br>Formulaciones y especificaciones | 片剂：每片 15mg。注射液：每支 0.5mg（1ml）；1mg（2ml）。<br>Tableta: 15mg; Inyección: 0.5mg (1ml), 1mg (2ml). |
| 药品名称 Drug Names | 溴吡斯的明 Bromuro de piridostigmina |
| 适应证<br>Indicaciones | 用于：①重症肌无力；②术后腹气胀或尿潴留；③对抗非去极化型肌松药的肌松作用。<br>Se usa para tratamiento de la miastenia grave, distensión abdominal postoperatoria o retención urinaria y utilización contra los efectos relajantes musculares no-despolarizantes. |
| 用法、用量<br>Administración y dosis | （1）重症肌无力：口服，一次 60mg，一日 3 次；皮下或肌内注射，每日 1 ~ 5mg，或根据病情而定。<br>（2）术后腹气胀或尿潴留：肌内注射，一次 1 ~ 2mg。<br>（3）对抗非去极化型肌松药的肌松：静脉注射，一次 2 ~ 5mg。<br><br>(1) Para la miastenia grave: por vía oral de 60mg y 3 veces al día, inyección subcutánea y intramuscular de 1 ~ 5mg diarios o cambia la dosis según la necesidad.<br>(2)Para la distensión abdominal postoperatoria o retención urinaria: Inyección por I.V. de 1 ~ 2mg.<br>(3)Utilización contra los efectos relajantes musculares no-despolarizantes: Inyección por I.V. de 2 ~ 5mg. |
| 剂型、规格<br>Formulaciones y especificaciones | 片剂：每片 60mg；缓释片：180mg。注射剂：每支 5mg（1ml）；10mg（2ml）。<br>Tableta: 60mg; Tableta de liberación prolongada: 180mg; Inyección: 5mg (1ml), 10mg (2ml). |

| 药品名称 Drug Names | 石杉碱甲 Huperzina A |
| --- | --- |
| 适应证<br>Indicaciones | 可用于重症肌无力及良性记忆障碍。对阿尔茨海默病和脑器质性病变引起的记忆障碍也有所改善。<br><br>Se usa para tratamiento de la miastenia grave y trastornos benignos de memoria. Puede mejorar los trastornos de memoria causados por la enfermedad de Alzheimer y enfermedad orgánica cerebral. |
| 用法、用量<br>Administración y<br>dosis | （1）重症肌无力：肌内注射，每次 0.2 ～ 0.4mg，每日 1 ～ 2 次。<br>（2）记忆功能减退：口服，一次 0.1 ～ 0.2mg，一日 2 次。因个体差异，一般应从小剂量开始。每日最多不超过 0.45mg。<br><br>(1) Para la miastenia grave: se administra inyección por I.V. de 0.2 ~ 0.4mg y 1 ó 2 veces al día.<br>(2)Para trastornos de la memoria: por vía oral de 0.1 ~ 0.2mg y 2 veces al día. La dosis se ajusta depende de la condición del paciente y comienza siempre a dosis pequeña. La dosis máxima no excede a 0.45mg diarios. |
| 剂型、规格<br>Formulaciones y<br>especificaciones | 片剂：每片 0.05mg。<br>Tableta: 0.05mg. |
| 药品名称 Drug Names | 多奈哌齐 Donepezil |
| 适应证<br>Indicaciones | 可用轻、中度阿尔茨海默病的治疗。<br>Se usa para tratamiento de la enfermedad de Alzheimer leve o moderada. |
| 用法、用量<br>Administración y<br>dosis | 口服，一日 1 次，每次 5 ～ 10mg。<br>Por vía oral a dosis diaria de 5 ~ 10mg. |
| 剂型、规格<br>Formulaciones y<br>especificaciones | 片剂：每片 5mg；10mg。<br>Tableta: 5mg, 10mg. |
| 药品名称 Drug Names | 加兰他敏 Galantamina |
| 适应证<br>Indicaciones | 本品可用于重症肌无力，进行性肌营养不良，脊髓灰质炎后遗症，儿童脑型麻痹，因神经系统疾病所致感觉或运动障碍，多发性神经炎等。<br><br>Se usa para tratamiento de la miastenia grave, distrofia muscular progresiva, secuelas de poliomielitis, parálisis cerebral infantil, discapacidades motoras y sensoriales causadas por trastornos neurológicos y polineuritis. |
| 用法、用量<br>Administración y<br>dosis | （1）肌内注射或皮下注射：每次 2.5 ～ 10mg，小儿每次 0.05 ～ 0.1mg/kg，一日 1 次，1 个疗程 2 ～ 6 周。<br>（2）口服：每次 10mg，一日 3 次。小儿每日 0.5 ～ 1mg/kg，分 3 次服用。<br><br>(1) Inyección subcutánea y intramuscular a dosis de 2.5 ~ 10mg cada vez y para niños la dosis es de 0.05 ~ 0.1mg/kg. Se administra 1 vez al día y un curso de tratamiento tarda 2 ~ 6 semanas.<br>(2) Por vía oral: 10mg y 3 veces al día. Para niños la dosis es 0.5 ~ 1mg/kg diarios didivídos en 3 tomas. |
| 剂型、规格<br>Formulaciones y<br>especificaciones | 注射液：1mg（1ml）；2.5mg（1ml）；5mg（1ml）。片剂：5mg。<br>Inyección: 1mg (1ml), 2.5mg (1ml), 5mg (1ml); Tableta: 5mg. |
| 药品名称 Drug Names | 阿托品 Atropina |
| 适应证<br>Indicaciones | 临床上的用途主要是：①抢救感染中毒性休克。②治疗锑剂引起的阿 - 斯综合征。③治疗有机磷农药中毒。④缓解内脏绞痛，包括胃肠痉挛引起的疼痛、肾绞痛、胆绞痛、胃及十二指肠溃疡。⑤用于麻醉前给药，可减少麻醉过程中支气管黏液分泌，预防术后引起肺炎，并可消除吗啡对呼吸的抑制。⑥眼科用药，用于角膜炎、虹膜睫状体炎。 |

**续　表**

| | |
|---|---|
| | La indicación principal en clínica: ① En tratamiento de choque tóxico y séptico. ② En tratamiento de síndrome de Adams causado por antimonio. ③ En tratamiento de intoxicación por plaguicidas organofosforados. ④ En alivio de cólico visceral, por ejempro dolor provocado por el espasmo gastrointestinal, cólico renal, cólico biliar, úlceras gástricas y duodenales. ⑤ En administración antes de anestesia para reducir la secreción de moco bronquial durante la anestesia, prevenir la neumonía posoperatoria y emilinar la inhibición de la morfina sobre la respiración. ⑥ En medicación oftalmológica para tratamiento de queratitis e iridociclitis. |
| 用法、用量 Administración y dosis | ①感染中毒性休克：成人每次 1～2mg，小儿每次 0.03～0.05mg/kg，静脉注射，每 15～30 分钟 1 次，2～3 次后加情况不见好转可逐渐增加用量，至情况好转后即减量或停药。②锑剂引起的阿 - 斯综合征：发现严重心律失常时，立即静脉注射 1～2mg（用 5%～25% 葡萄糖液 10～20ml 稀释），同时肌内注射或皮下注射 1mg，15～30 分钟后再静脉注射 1mg。如患者无发作，可根据心律及心率情况改为每 3～4 小时 1 次皮下注射或肌内注射 1mg，48 小时后如不再发作，可逐渐减量，最后停药。③有机磷农药中毒：a. 与碘解磷定等合用时：对中度中毒，每次皮下注射 0.5～1mg，隔 30～60 分钟 1 次；对严重中毒，每次静脉注射 1～2mg，隔 15～30 分钟 1 次，病情稳定后，逐渐减量并改用皮下注射。b. 单用时：对轻度中毒，每次皮下注射 0.5～1mg，隔 30～120 分钟 1 次；对中度中毒，每次皮下注射 1～2mg，隔 15～30 分钟 1 次；对重度中毒，即刻静脉注射 2～5mg，以后每次 1～2mg，隔 15～30 分钟 1 次，根据病情逐渐减量和延长间隔时间。④缓解内脏绞痛：每次皮下注射 0.5mg。⑤用于麻醉前给药：皮下注射：0.5mg。⑥用于眼科：用 1%～3% 眼药水滴眼或眼膏涂眼。滴时按住内眦部，以免流入鼻腔吸收中毒。<br><br>① En tratamiento de choque tóxico y séptico: 1～2mg cada vez pra adultos y 0.03～0.05mg/kg cada vez para infantes. Se administra inyección por I.V. cada 15～30 minutos. Si no se mejora tras 2 ó 3 veces de medicación puede aumentar gradualmente la dosis hasta se ve mejoramiento y luego reducir la dosis o dejar la medicación. ② En tratamiento de síndrome de Adams causado por antimonio: En caso de que aparecza arritmia severa, hay que inyectar de inmediata por I.V. a dosis de 1～2mg diluidos en 10～20ml de solución de glucosa y mientras tanto se administra inyección por I.M. o subcutánea a dosis de 1mg. Después de 15～30 minutos repite la inyección por I.V. de 1mg. Si pacientes no tienen convulsiones, puede cambiar a 1mg cada 3 ó 4 horas en inyección por I.M. o subcutánea según el ritmo cardiaco. Si no tienen convulciones dentro de 48 horas puede reducir la dosis gradualmente hasta que dejen la medicación. ③ En tratamiento de intoxicación por plaguicidas organofosforados: a. Se usa en conjunción con Yoduro de Pralidoxima: Para intoicicación moderada se administra 0.5～1mg cada 30～60 minutos en inyección subcutánea. Para intoicicación severa se administra 1～2mg cada 15～30 minutos en inyección por I.V. y cuando esté controlada reduce la dosis gradualmente y cambia a inyección subcutánea. b. Se usa individualmente: Para intoicicación leve se administra 0.5～1mg cada 30～120 minutos por inyección subcutánea. Para intoicicación moderada se administra 1～2mg cada 15～30 minutos. Para intoicicación severa se administra 2～5mg de inmediata en inyección por I.V. y luego 1～2mg cada 15～30 minutos. Puede ajustar la dosis y el intervalo de medicación según la necesidad. ④ En alivio de cólico visceral: Se administra 0.5mg en inyección subcutánea. ⑤ En administración antes de anestesia: Se administra 0.5mg en inyección subcutánea. ⑥ En medicación oftalmológica: Gota o crema oftalmológica a 1%～3%. Al usar la gota debe mantener pulsado el canto para evitar la intoxicación por absorción en la cavidad nasal. |
| 剂型、规格 Formulaciones y especificaciones | 片剂：每片 0.3g。注射液：每支 0.5mg（1ml）；1mg（2ml）；5mg（1ml）。滴眼剂：取硫酸阿托品 1g，氯化钠 0.29g，无水磷酸二氢钠 0.4g，无水磷酸氢二钠 0.47g，羟胺乙酯 0.03g，蒸馏水加至 100ml 配成。<br><br>Tableta: 0.3g; Inyección: 0.5mg(1ml), 1mg(2ml), 5mg(1ml); Gota oftalmológica: 100ml que incluye 1g de ttropina sulfato, 0.29g de cloruro de sodio, 0.4g de fosfato monosódico anhidro, 0.47g de fosfato disódico anhidro, 0.03g de hidroxilamina etílico y agua destilada. |
| **药品名称 Drug Names** | 东莨菪碱 Escopolamina |
| 适应证 Indicaciones | 临床用作镇静药，用于全身麻醉前给药、晕动病、震颤麻痹、狂躁性精神病、有机磷农药中毒等。由于本品既兴奋呼吸又对大脑皮质呈镇静作用，故用于抢救极重型流行性乙型脑炎呼吸衰竭（常伴有剧烈频繁的抽搐）亦有效。<br><br>Se usa clínicamente como un sedante en administración antes de anestesia, enfermedad de movimiento, parkinsonismo, psicosis maníaco e intoxicación por plaguicidas organofosforados. Porque este fármaco tiene efecto excitante en respiración y al mismo tiene es sedante sobre la corteza cerebral, es eficaz en rescate de insuficiencia respiratoria de encefalitis epidémica B muy severa que siempre asociada con violentas convulsiones frecuentes. |

**续　表**

| 用法、用量<br>Administración y dosis | 　口服：一次 0.3～0.6mg，一日 0.6～1.2mg；极量一次 0.6mg，一日 1.8mg。皮下注射：一次 0.2～0.5mg；极量一次 0.5mg，一日 1.5mg。抢救乙型脑炎呼吸衰竭：以 1ml 含药 0.3mg 的注射液直接静脉注射或稀释于 10% 葡萄糖溶液 30ml 内做静脉注射，常用量为 0.02～0.04mg/kg，用药间歇时间一般为 20～30 分钟，用药总量最高达 6.3mg。<br><br>　Por vía oral: 0.3 ~ 0.6mg cada vez y 0.6 ~ 1.2mg diarios. Dosis máxima es 0.6mg cada vez y 1.8mg diarios. Inyección subcutánea: 0.2 ~ 0.5mg cada vez. Dosis máxima es de 0.5mg cada vez y 1.5mg diarios. En rescate de insuficiencia respiratoria de encefalitis epidémica B: inyección por I.V. de inyección a 0.3mg:1ml ó diluidos en 30ml de solución de glucosa a 10%. Dosis habitual es de 0.02 ~ 0.04mg/kg y con intervalo de 20 ~ 30 minutos. Dosis máxima no excede a 6.3mg. |
|---|---|
| 剂型、规格<br>Formulaciones y especificaciones | 　片剂：每片 0.3mg。注射液：每支 0.3mg（1ml）；0.5mg（1ml）。晕动片：每片含东莨菪碱 0.2mg、苯巴比妥钠 30mg、阿托品 0.15mg。<br><br>　Tableta: 0.3mg; Inyección: 0.3mg(1ml), 0.5mg(1ml); Pastillas para el mareo: incluye 0.2mg de escopolamina, 30mg de fenobarbital y 0.15mg de atropina. |
| **药品名称 Drug Names** | 山莨菪碱 Anisodamina |
| 适应证<br>Indicaciones | 　适用于下列疾病：①感染中毒性休克：如暴发型流行性脑脊髓膜炎、中毒性痢疾等。②血管性疾病：脑血栓、脑栓塞、瘫痪、脑血管痉挛、血管神经性头痛、血栓闭塞性脉管炎等。③各种神经痛：如三叉神经痛、坐骨神经痛等。④平滑肌痉挛：胃、十二指肠溃疡，胆道痉挛等。⑤眩晕病。⑥眼底疾病：中心性视网膜炎、视网膜色素变性、视网膜动脉血栓等。⑦突发性耳聋：配合新针疗法可治疗其他耳聋。<br><br>　Se usa ① En tratamiento de choque tóxico y séptico, por ejempro meningitis meningocócica fulminante y disentería tóxica. ② En tratamiento de enfermedades vasculares, por ejempro trombosis cerebral, embolia cerebral, parálisis, vasoespasmo cerebral, cefalea angioneurótica y tromboangeítis obliterante. ③ En tratamiento de neuralgias, por ejempro neuralgia del trigémino y ciática. ④ En tratamiento de espasmo del músculo liso, úlcera estomacal, úlcera duodenal y espasmo biliar. ⑤ En tratamiento de vértigos. ⑥ En tratamiento de enfermedades de la retina: retinitis central, retinitis pigmentosa y trombo de la arteria de la retina. ⑦ En tratamiento de sordera súbita y con otra terapia de la acupuntura puede tratar de otros sordos. |
| 用法、用量<br>Administración y dosis | 　(1) 肌内注射或静脉注射：成人一般一次 5～10mg，一日 1～2 次；也可经稀释后静脉注射。用于：①抢救感染中毒性休克：根据病情决定剂量。成人静脉注射每次 10～40mg，小儿 0.3～2mg/kg，需要时每隔 10～30 分钟可重复给药，情况不见好转可加量。病请好转可逐渐延长间隔时间，直至停药。②治疗脑血栓：加入 5% 葡萄糖液中静脉注射，每日 30～40mg。③一般慢性疾病：每次肌内注射 5～10mg，一日 1～2 次，可连用 1 个月以上。④治疗严重三叉神经痛：有时需加大剂量至每次 5～20mg，肌内注射。⑤治疗血栓闭塞性脉管炎：每次静脉注射 10～15mg，一日 1 次。<br><br>　(2) 口服：一日 3 次，一次 5～10mg。皮肤或黏膜局部使用，无刺激性。<br><br>　(1) Inyección por I.M. o I.V.: 5 ~ 10mg para adultos por 1 ó 2 veces al día. O puede inyectar por I.V. tras dilución. Lo administra en ① rescate de choque tóxico y séptico y puede ajustar la dosis según la necesidad. Para adultos se adiministra inyección por I.V. a 10 ~ 40mg cada vez. Para infantes, 0.3 ~ 2mg/kg y puede repetir la medicación cada 10 ~ 30 minutos en caso necesario. Si no se mejora, puede aumentar la dosis y en caso contrario puede prolongar el invervalo de medicación hasta que la dejen. ② Trombo cerebral: Se administra inyección por I.V. de 30 ~ 40mg diarios diluidos en solución de glucosa a 5%. ③ Enfermedades Crónicas: Se administra inyección por I.M. a 5 ~ 10mg por 1 ó 2 veces al día. Puede administrarse continuamente durante 1 mes. ④ Grave neuralgia del trigémino: a veces hay que aumentar la dosis a 5 ~ 20mg cada vez en inyección por I.M.. ⑤ Tromboangeítis obliterante: 10 ~ 15mg una vez al día por inyección I.V.<br>　(2) Por vía oral: 5 ~ 10mg por 3 veces al día. Se administra parcialmente en la piel o mucosas y no tiene efecto irritante. |
| 剂型、规格<br>Formulaciones y especificaciones | 　氢溴酸山莨菪碱片剂：每片 5mg。注射液：每支 1ml（10mg）；1ml（20mg）。<br><br>　Tableta de anisodamina bromhidrato: 5mg; Inyección: 1ml(10mg), 1ml(20mg). |

**续　表**

| 药品名称 Drug Names | 托吡卡胺 Tropicamida |
|---|---|
| 适应证<br>Indicaciones | 散瞳药，主要用于散瞳检查眼底和散瞳验光。<br>Es midriático y se usa para el examen dilatado de fondo de los ojos y optometría dilatada. |
| 用法、用量<br>Administración y<br>dosis | 本品 0.5% 溶液滴眼 1～2 次，滴入结膜囊，一次一滴，间隔 5 分钟滴第二次，即可满足散瞳检查的需要。<br>Dosis: Solución de gota a 0.5%, 1 gota en el saco conjuntival. Dentro de 5 minutos repite la medicación y luego puede hacer los tres examenes. |
| 剂型、规格<br>Formulaciones y<br>especificaciones | 滴眼液：每支 12.5mg（5ml）；25mg（5ml）；15mg（6ml）；30mg（6ml）。<br>Gota oftalmológica: 12.5mg(5ml), 25mg(5ml), 15mg(6ml), 30mg(6ml). |
| 药品名称 Drug Names | 颠茄 Belladona |
| 适应证<br>Indicaciones | 用于胃及十二指肠溃疡、轻度胃肠、肾和胆绞痛等。<br>Se usa para tratamiento de úlceras gástricas y duodenales, calambres leves gastrointestinales, renales y cólicos biliares. |
| 用法、用量<br>Administración y<br>dosis | （1）酊剂：每次服 0.3～1ml。极量：一次 1.5ml，一日 4.5ml。<br>（2）片剂：每次服 10～30mg，一日 30～90mg。极量：一次 50mg，一日 150mg。<br>(1) Tintura: dosis administrada oral de 0.3 ~ 1ml cada vez. Dosis máxima no excede a 1.5ml cada vez y 4.5ml diarios.<br>(2) Tableta: 10 ~ 30mg cada vez y 30 ~ 90mg diarios. Dosis máxima no excede a 50mg cada vez y 150mg diarios. |
| 剂型、规格<br>Formulaciones y<br>especificaciones | 酊剂：含生物碱 0.03%；浸膏：含生物碱 1%。片剂：每片含颠茄浸膏 10mg。<br>Tintura: contiene 0,03% de alcaloides. Extracto: contiene 1% de alcaloides. Tableta: contiene 10mg de extracto de Belladona. |
| 药品名称 Drug Names | 后马托品 Homatropina |
| 适应证<br>Indicaciones | 用于散瞳检查眼底和散瞳验光。也可用于弱视和斜视的压抑疗法。<br>Se usa para el examen dilatado de fondo de los ojos, optometría dilatada y en terapia de supresión de ambliopía y estrabismo. |
| 用法、用量<br>Administración y<br>dosis | 滴眼液滴入结膜囊，一次一滴。眼膏涂在结膜囊，一次少许。用药次数根据患者的年龄和使用目的以及瞳孔变化而决定。<br>1 gota o un poco de crema en el saco conjuntival cada vez. La frecuencia de medicación depende de la edad de paciente y el propósito del uso, así como los cambios pupilares. |
| 剂型、规格<br>Formulaciones y<br>especificaciones | 氢溴酸后马托品滴眼剂：1%～5%。眼膏：2%。<br>Gota oftalmológica de Bromhidrato Homatropina: 1% ~ 5%; Crema oftalmológica：2% |

9.2　拟肾上腺素药和抗肾上腺素药 Medicamentos adrenérgicos y para los receptores antiepinefrérgicos

| 药品名称 Drug Names | 萘甲唑啉 Nafazolina |
|---|---|
| 适应证<br>Indicaciones | 用于过敏性及炎症性鼻充血、急慢性鼻炎、眼充血等，对细菌性，过敏性结膜炎也有效，并能减轻眼睑痉挛。对麻黄碱有耐受性者，可选用本品。<br>SE usa para tratamiento de congestión nasal alérgica e inflamatoria, rinitis aguda y crónica, enrojecimiento de los ojos etc. Utilización también para conjuntivitis bacteriana y alérgica aliviando el blefaroespasmo. Es eficaz para pacientes intolerantes a la efedrina. |
| 用法、用量<br>Administración y<br>dosis | 治鼻充血，用其 0.05%～0.1% 溶液，每侧鼻孔滴 2～3 滴；治疗充血用其滴眼液，一次 1～2 滴。<br>Para congesticón nasal: 2 ~ 3 gotas en cada lado de la nariz de la gota a 0.05% ~ 0.1%. Para enrojecimiento de ojos: 1 ~ 2 gotas cada vez. |

**续　表**

| | |
|---|---|
| 剂型、规格<br>Formulaciones y especificaciones | 滴鼻剂：每瓶 0.05%（10ml）；0.1%（10ml）。盐酸萘甲唑林滴眼液：1.2mg（10ml）。<br>Gota nasal: 0.05%(10ml), 0.1%(10ml); Gota oftalmológica de Clorhidrato de nafazolina: 1.2mg (10ml). |
| **药品名称 Drug Names** | **米多君 Midodrina** |
| 适应证<br>Indicaciones | 主要用于各种原因引起的低血压，压力性尿失禁、射精功能障碍。<br>Se usa principalmente para tratamiento de hipotensión, incontinencia urinaria de esfuerzo y disfunción eyaculatoria. |
| 用法、用量<br>Administración y dosis | 口服：初始剂量为 1 次 2.5mg，一日 2～3 次。必要时可逐渐增加到一次 10mg，一日 3 次的维持剂量。<br>Por vía oral: La dosis inicial es de 2.5mg y 2～3 veces al día. En caso necesario aumenta gradualmente a la dosis de mantenimiento de 10mg y 3 veces al día. |
| 剂型、规格<br>Formulaciones y especificaciones | 盐酸米多君片：2.5mg。<br>Comprimidos de hidrocloruro de midodrina: 2.5mg. |
| **药品名称 Drug Names** | **拉贝洛尔 Labetalol** |
| 适应证<br>Indicaciones | 用于治疗轻度和重度高血压和心绞痛。采用静脉注射能治疗高血压危象。<br>Se usa para tratamiento de la hipertensión leve y severa y la angina. Se administra inyección por I.V. para tratamiento de las crisis hipertensivas. |
| 用法、用量<br>Administración y dosis | 口服：初始剂量为 1 次 100mg，一日 2～3 次。必要时可逐渐增加到一次 200mg，一日 3～4 次。通常对轻、中、重度高血压患者的每日剂量相应为 300～800mg、600～1200mg、1200～2400mg，加用利尿剂时可适当减量。静脉注射：一次 100～200mg。<br>Por vía oral: La dosis inicial es de 100mg y 2～3 veces al día. En caso necesario aumenta gradualmente a 200mg y 3～4 veces al día. Habitualmente para pacientes de hipertensión leve, moderada y severa la dosis diaria es respectivamente de 300～800mg, 600～1200mg, 1200～1400mg. Si al mismo tiempo utiliza diuréticos, puede reducir la dosis. Inyección por I.V.: 100～200mg cada vez. |
| 剂型、规格<br>Formulaciones y especificaciones | 片剂：每片 100mg；200mg。注射液：每支 50mg（5ml）。<br>Tableta: 100mg, 200mg; Inyección: 50mg (5ml). |
| **药品名称 Drug Names** | **卡维地洛 Carvedilol** |
| 适应证<br>Indicaciones | 可用于原发性高血压及心绞痛。<br>Se usa para tratamiento de la hipertensión esencial y la angina. |
| 用法、用量<br>Administración y dosis | 口服：初始剂量为 25mg/d，一次服用；可根据需要逐渐增剂量至 50mg，分 1～2 次服下；最大日剂量不超过 100mg。<br>Por vía oral: La dosis inicial es de 25mg una vez al día. En caso necesario aumenta gradualmente a 50mg diarios divididos en 1～2 tomas. Dosis máxima no excede a 100mg diarios. |
| 剂型、规格<br>Formulaciones y especificaciones | 片剂：每片 6.25mg；10mg；12.5mg；20mg。胶囊：10mg。<br>Tableta: 6.25mg, 10mg, 12.5mg, 20mg; Cápsula: 10mg. |
| **药品名称 Drug Names** | **酚妥拉明 Fentolamina** |
| 适应证<br>Indicaciones | 用于血管痉挛性疾病，如肢端动脉痉挛症（即雷诺病）、手足发绀症等、感染中毒性休克及嗜铬细胞瘤的诊断试验等。用于室性期前收缩亦有效。<br>Se usa en tratamiento de enfermedades vasoespásticas, por ejempro enfermedad de Raynaud y acrocyanosis, exámenes de diagnóstico del choque tóxico y séptico y feocromocitoma. Es eficaz también en tratamiento de latidos ventriculares prematuros. |

续　表

| 用法、用量<br>Administración y dosis | （1）治疗血管痉挛性疾病：肌内注射或静脉注射。每次 5～10mg，20～30 分钟后按需要可重复给药。<br>（2）抗休克：以 0.3mg 每分钟的剂量进行静脉滴注。<br>（3）室性期前收缩：开始 2 日，每次口服 50mg，一日 4 次；如无效，则以后 2 日将剂量增加至每次 75mg，一日 4 次；如仍无效，可增至一日 400mg；如在无效，即应停用。无论何种剂量，一旦有效，就按该剂量继续服用 7 日。<br>（4）诊断嗜铬细胞瘤：静脉注射 5mg。注射后 30 分钟测血压一次，可连续测 10 分钟，如在 2～4 分钟血压降低 4.67/3.3kPa（35/25mmHg）以上为阳性结果。<br>（5）做阴茎海绵体注射，可使阴茎海绵窦平滑肌松弛、扩张而勃起，可用于治疗勃起障碍，一次注射 1mg。<br><br>(1) En tratamiento de enfermedades vasoespásticas: Se administra inyecciones por I.M. o I.V. a una dosis de 5 ~ 10mg y puede repetir la medicación dentro de 20 ~ 30 minutos según la necesidad.<br>(2) Anti-choque: Infusión por I.V. a una dosis de 0.3mg/min.<br>(3) En tratamiento de latidos ventriculares prematuros: En los primeros 2 días se administra oralmente 50mg por 4 veces al día. Si no se ve eficacia aumenta la dosis a 75mg por 4 veces al día en los siguientes 2 días. Si tampoco tiene efecto aumenta a 400mg diarios y en caso de que a esta dosis no hay efectos, hay que dejar la medicación inmediatamente. Si consigue eficacia a cualquier dosis debe continuar la medicación en 7 días a la dosis efectiva.<br>(4) En exámen de diagnóstico de feocromocitoma: Se administra inyección por I.V. a una dosis de 5mg y después de 30 minutos media la presión arterial durante 10 minutos continuos. Si durante 2 ~ 4 minutos la presión arterial baja en más de 4.67/3.3kPa (35/25mmHg), el resultado es positivo.<br>(5) La inyección intracavernosa puede hacer erección al músculo liso cavernoso por relajarse y expandirse. Se usa en tratamiento de la disfunción eréctil con administración de 1mg cada vez. |
|---|---|
| 剂型、规格<br>Formulaciones y especificaciones | 片剂：每片 25mg。甲磺酸酚妥拉明注射液：每支 5mg（1ml）；10mg（1ml）。<br>Tableta: 25mg; Inyección de mesilato de fentolamina: 5mg(1ml), 10mg(1ml). |
| 药品名称 Drug Names | 妥拉唑林 Tolazolina |
| 适应证<br>Indicaciones | 用于血管痉挛性疾病如肢端动脉痉挛症、手足发绀、闭塞性血栓静脉炎等。<br>Se usa para tratamiento de enfermedades vasoespásticas por ejempro síndrome de Raynaud, acrocyanosis, tromboflebitis oclusiva etc. |
| 用法、用量<br>Administración y dosis | 口服，一次 15mg，一日 45～60mg；肌内注射或皮下注射，一次 25mg。<br>Por vía oral: 15mg cada vez y diariamente 35 ~ 60mg. Inyección intramuscular o subcutánea: 25mg cada vez. |
| 剂型、规格<br>Formulaciones y especificaciones | 片剂：每片 25mg。注射液：25mg（1ml）。<br>Tableta: 25mg; Inyección: 25mg (1ml). |
| 药品名称 Drug Names | 酚苄明 Fenoxibenzamina |
| 适应证<br>Indicaciones | 用于周围血管疾病，也可用于休克及嗜铬细胞瘤引起的高血压。早泄治疗。<br>Se usa para tratamiento de enfermedades vasculares periféricas, choque, hipertensión causada por feocromocitoma y eyaculación precoz. |
| 用法、用量<br>Administración y dosis | 口服：用于血管痉挛性疾病，开始一日 1 次，10mg，一日 2 次，隔日增 10mg；维持量一次 20mg，一日 2 次。用于早泄，一次 10mg，一日 3 次。静脉注射：每日 0.5～1mg/kg。静脉滴注（抗休克）：0.5～1mg/kg，加入 5% 葡萄糖液 250～500ml 中静脉滴注（2 小时滴完），一日总量不超过 2mg/kg。<br><br>Por vía oral: Para enfermedades vasoespásticas: La dosis inicial 10mg una vez al día y luego 2 veces al día y aumenta la dosis en 10mg diarios cada 2 días. La dosis de mantenimiento es de 20mg y 2 veces al día. Para eyaculación precoz, la dosis de 10mg y 3 veces al día. Inyección por I.V.: 0.5 ~ 1mg/kg diarios. Infusión de uso anti-choque: 0.5 ~ 1mg/kg diluidos con 250 ~ 500ml de solución de glucosa a 5%, la infusión se terminará dentro de 2 horas. Dosis máxima no excede a 2mg/kg diarios. |

**续　表**

| 剂型、规格<br>Formulaciones y<br>especificaciones | 片剂：每片 5mg；10mg。注射液：每支 10mg（1ml）。<br>Tableta: 5mg, 10mg; Inyección: 10mg (1ml). |
|---|---|
| **药品名称 Drug Names** | **普萘洛尔 Propranolol** |
| 适应证<br>Indicaciones | 　　用于治疗多种原因所致的心律失常，如房性及室性期前收缩（效果较好）、窦性及室上性心动过速、心房颤动等，但室性心动过速应慎用。锑剂中毒引起的心律失常，当其他药物无效时可使用本品。此外，也可用于心绞痛、高血压、嗜铬细胞瘤（术前准备）等。治疗心绞痛时，常与硝酸酯类合用，可提高疗效，互相抵消不良反应。对高血压有一定疗效，不易引起直立性低血压的影响的特点。<br><br>　　Se usa en tratamiento de arritmias, por ejempro latidos prematuros auriculares y ventriculares, taquicardia sinusal y supraventricular, fibrilación auricular. Pero en caso de taquicardia ventricular, hay que usarlo con cuidado. Si es arritmia causada por envenenamiento de antimonio y no tiene eficacia con otros fármacos, puede usar el propranolol. Además se puede usar en tratamiento de angina, hipertensión y feocromocitoma (preparación preoperatoria). En tratamiento de angina siempre se usa junto con nitratos para mejorar la eficacia y se anulan entre sí las reacciones adversas. Tiene eficacia en tratamiento de hipertensión y hay poca posibilidad de hipotensión ortostática. |
| 用法、用量<br>Administración y<br>dosis | 　　（1）口服：①心律失常：每日 10 ～ 30mg，分 3 次服，根据心律、心率及血压变化及时调整。②嗜铬细胞瘤：术前 3 日服用，一日 60mg，分 3 次服。③心绞痛：每日 40 ～ 80mg，分 3 ～ 4 次服，从小剂量开始逐渐加至 80mg 以上。剂量过小常无效。④高血压：每次 5mg，一日 4 次，1 ～ 2 周后加 1/4 量，严密监控下可加至一日 100mg。<br>　　（2）静脉滴注：宜慎用。对麻醉中的心律失常以 1mg/min 的速度静脉滴注，一次 2.5 ～ 5mg，稀释于 5% ～ 10% 葡萄糖液 100ml 内滴注。严密监控血压、心律和心率变化，随时调整速度。如心率转慢，立即停药。<br><br>　　(1) Por vía oral:　① En tratamiento de arritmia: 10 ~ 30mg diarios divididos en 3 tomas y puede ajustar la dosis según la frecuencia cardíaca y cambios de la presión arterial.　② En tratamiento de feocromocitoma: Se toma 3 días antes de cirugía a una dosis de 60mg diarios divididos en 3 tomas. ③ En tratamiento de angina: 40 ~ 60mg diarios divididos en 3 ó 4 tomas y aumenta la dosis gradualmente hasta 80mg. Siempre no es eficaz la administración a pequeña dosis. ④ En tratamiento de hipertensión: 5mg por 4 veces al día y dentro de 1 ó 2 semanas aumenta en 1/4 de la dosis y bajo estricta observación puede aumentar hasta 100mg diarios.<br>　　(2) Infusión por I.V.: Debe administrarse con cuidado. En tratamiento de arritmia durante la anestesia, se administra a velocidad de 1mg/min de 2.5 ~ 5mg diluidos en 100ml de solución de glucosa a 5% ~ 10%. Debe ajustar la velocidad cuando observa estrictamente la presión arterial y la frecuencia cardíaca. Si se ralentiza el ritmo cardiaco hay que dejar la medicación inmediatamente. |
| 剂型、规格<br>Formulaciones y<br>especificaciones | 片剂：每片 10mg。注射液：每支 5mg（5ml）。<br>Tableta: 10mg; Inyección: 5mg (5ml). |
| **药品名称 Drug Names** | **噻吗洛尔 Timolol** |
| 适应证<br>Indicaciones | 　　治疗高血压病、心绞痛、心动过速及青光眼。①对轻中度高血压疗效较好，无明显不良反应，可与利尿剂同用。②心肌梗死患者长期服用本品可降低发病率和死亡率。对青光眼起效快，不良反应小、耐受性好。滴后 20 分钟，眼压下降，经 1 ～ 2 小时达最大效应，作用持续 24 小时。对瞳孔大小、对光反应及视力无影响。<br><br>　　Se usa para tratamiento de hipertensión, angina, taquicardia y glaucoma.　① Tiene buena eficacia en tratamiento de hipertensión leve o moderada y no hay reacciones adversas significativas. Puede usar en conjunción con diuréticos.　② Para pacientes de infarto de miocardio puede reducir la morbilidad y mortalidad con medicación a largo plazo. En cuanto al glaucoma tiene eficacia rápida y poca reaación adversa y buena tolerancia. 20 minutos después de la medicación la presión intraocular se reduce y dentro de 1 ~ 2 horas consigue mejor efecto y durará 24 horas. No influye al tamaño de la pupila, la reacción a la luz y la visión. |
| 用法、用量<br>Administración y<br>dosis | 　　口服：每次 5 ～ 10mg，一日 2 ～ 3 次。滴眼：0.25% 滴眼剂，一次 1 滴，一日 2 次。如效果不佳，可改用 5% 滴眼剂，一次 1 滴，一日 2 次。<br>　　Por vía oral: 5 ~ 10mg y 2 ~ 3 tomas al día. Gota oftalmológica a 0.25%: 1 gota y 2 veces al día. Si no es muy eficaz, cambia a tomar Gota oftalmológica a 5%: 1 gota y 2 veces al día. |

**续　表**

| 剂型、规格<br>Formulaciones y especificaciones | 片剂：每片 2.5mg；5mg。滴眼剂：12.5mg（5ml）；25mg（5ml）。<br>Tableta: 2.5mg, 5mg; Gota oftalmológica: 12.5mg(5ml), 25mg(5ml). |
|---|---|
| **药品名称 Drug Names** | 索他洛尔 Sotalol |
| 适应证<br>Indicaciones | 用于高血压，也可用于心绞痛、心律失常。<br>Se usa para tratamiento de hipertensión así como la angina y arritmia. |
| 用法、用量<br>Administración y dosis | 高血压：初始 1 日 80mg，分 2 次服用，需要时可加至一日 160～600mg。心绞痛和心律失常：口服，一日 160mg，一日 1 次（清晨）服用。<br>Tratamiento de hipertensión: dosis inicial de 80mg diarios divididos en 2 tomas y en caso necesario puede aumentar a 160～600mg diarios. Tratamiento de angina y arritmia: dosis oral de 160mg diarios tomados en la madrugada. |
| 剂型、规格<br>Formulaciones y especificaciones | 片剂：每片 20mg；40mg；80mg；160mg；200mg。<br>Tableta: 20mg, 40mg, 80mg, 160mg, 200mg. |
| **药品名称 Drug Names** | 阿替洛尔 Atenolol |
| 适应证<br>Indicaciones | 用于高血压、心绞痛及心律失常。对青光眼有效。<br>Se usa para tratamiento de hipertensión, la angina y arritmia. Es eficaz para tratamiento de glaucoma. |
| 用法、用量<br>Administración y dosis | 口服：一日 1 次 100mg 用于心绞痛，一日 1 次 100mg，或每次 25～50mg，一日 2 次。用于高血压每次 50～100mg，一日 1～2 次。青光眼用 4% 溶液滴剂。<br>Por vía oral. Dosis diaria de 100mg. Para tratamiento de angina: dosis es 100mg diarios o 25～50mg cada vez y 2 tomas al día. Para tratamiento de hipertensión la dosis es 50～100mg vada vez y 1～2 tomas al día. Para tratamiento de glaucoma, utiliza gota de solución a 4%. |
| 剂型、规格<br>Formulaciones y especificaciones | 片剂：每片 12.5mg；25mg；50mg；100mg。<br>Tableta: 12.5mg, 25mg, 50mg, 100mg. |
| **药品名称 Drug Names** | 美托洛尔 Metoprolol |
| 适应证<br>Indicaciones | 用于各型高血压及心绞痛。静脉注射对心律失常、特别是室上性心律失常也有效。<br>Se usa para tratamiento de hipertensión y angina. Tiene eficacia en tratamiento de arritmia especialmente la arritmia supraventricular por inyección I.V. |
| 用法、用量<br>Administración y dosis | （1）口服：剂量需个体化。一般用于高血压，一日 1 次 100mg 维持量为一日 1 次，100～200mg，必要时加至每日 400mg，早晚分服。用于心绞痛，一日 100～150mg，分 2～3 次服，必要时加至每日 150～300mg。<br>（2）静脉注射：用于心律失常。开始为 5mg（每分钟 1～2mg）每隔 5 分钟重复注射，直至有效，一般总量为 10～15mg。<br>(1)Por vía oral. La dosis cambia según la necesidad. Uso principalmente para tratar la hipertensión a dosis 100mg diarios en 1 toma y la dosis de mantenimiento es de 100～200mg diarios en 1 toma y puede aumentar a 400mg diarios divididos en 2 tomas en la mañana y la noche. En caso de angina la dosis es 100～150mg diarios divididos en 2～3 tomas y puede aumentar a 150～300mg diarios en caso necesario.<br>(2)Inyección por I.V.: Para tratamiento de la arritmia, la dosis inicial es de 5mg (velocidad 1～2mg por minuto) y repetir la medicación cada 5 minutos hasta que sea efectiva. Dosis total habitual es de 10～15mg. |
| 剂型、规格<br>Formulaciones y especificaciones | 片剂：25mg；50mg；100mg。胶囊剂：每粒 50mg。缓释片：每片 100mg；200mg。<br>Tableta: 25mg, 50mg, 100mg; Cápsula: 50mg; Tableta de liberación prolongada: 100mg, 200mg. |

**续 表**

| 药品名称 Drug Names | 比索洛尔 Bisoprolol |
|---|---|
| 适应证<br>Indicaciones | 用于高血压及心绞痛。<br>Se usa para tratamiento de hipertensión y angina. |
| 用法、用量<br>Administración y dosis | 一日 5 ~ 20mg，一次口服。大多数一日口服 10mg 即可。<br>Por vía oral a dosis diaria 5 ~ 20mg. Para mayoría de pacientes basta los 10mg diarios. |
| 剂型、规格<br>Formulaciones y especificaciones | 片剂：每片 2.5mg；5mg。胶囊：2.5mg；5mg；10mg。<br>Tableta: 2.5mg, 5mg; Cápsula: 2.5mg, 5mg, 10mg. |

| 药品名称 Drug Names | 倍他洛尔 Betaxolol |
|---|---|
| 适应证<br>Indicaciones | 用于高血压、开角型青光眼的治疗。<br>Se usa para tratamiento de hipertensión y glaucoma de ángulo abierto. |
| 用法、用量<br>Administración y dosis | 高血压：口服，一日 1 次 20mg，在 7 ~ 14 日达良效，如需要可加至一日 1 次 40mg。老年患者酌减。用于开角型青光眼：0.5% 滴眼剂一日 2 次。<br>Para tratamiento de la hipertensión: por vía oral a dosis 20mg diarios y puede tener eficacia dentro de 7 ~ 14 días. Si es necesario puede aumentar a 40mg diarios. Para ancianos disminuye la dosis. Para tratamiento de glaucoma de ángulo abierto, utiliza la gota oftalmológica a 0.5% y 2 veces al día. |
| 剂型、规格<br>Formulaciones y especificaciones | 片剂：每片 20mg。滴眼剂：0.25%；0.5%；1%。<br>Tableta: 20mg; Gota oftalmológica: 0.25%, 0.5%, 1%. |

| 药品名称 Drug Names | 艾司洛尔 Esmolol |
|---|---|
| 适应证<br>Indicaciones | 用于轻度高血压和心绞痛。<br>Se usa para tratamiento de hipertensión leve y angina. |
| 用法、用量<br>Administración y dosis | 口服，一日 1 次，100 ~ 200mg。<br>Por vía oral: dosis diaria 100 ~ 200mg. |
| 剂型、规格<br>Formulaciones y especificaciones | 片剂：200mg；注射剂：200mg（2ml）。<br>Tableta: 200mg; Inyección: 200mg(2ml). |

**10. 主要作用于心血管系统的药物 Medicamento que actúan princepalmente sobre el sistema cardiovascular**

**10.1　钙通道阻滞药 Medicamentos para bloquear los canales de calcio**

| 药品名称 Drug Names | 维拉帕米 Verapamilo |
|---|---|
| 适应证<br>Indicaciones | 用于抗心律失常和抗心绞痛。对于阵发性室上性心动过速最有效；对房室交界区心动过速疗效也很好；也可用于心房颤动、心房扑动、房性期前收缩。<br>Se usa para en motivo antiarrítmico y antianginoso. Es eficaz especialmente para la taquicardia supraventricular paroxística y buena en tratamiento de la taquicardia ectópica de la unión AV. Utilización también en tratamiento de la fibrilación y aleteo auricular y contracción auricular prematura . |
| 用法、用量<br>Administración y dosis | 口服：一次 40 ~ 120mg，一日 3 ~ 4 次。维持剂量每次 40mg，一日 3 次。稀释后缓慢静脉注射或静脉滴注，0.075 ~ 0.15mg/kg，症状控制后改用片剂口服维持。<br>Por vía oral. 40 ~ 120mg cada vez y 3 ~ 4 tomas al día. Dosis de mantenimiento es 40mg y 3 tomas al día. Inyección o infusión lenta por I.V.: dilución de 0.075 ~ 0.15mg/kg y cuando controla el síntoma, cambia a mantener el medicamento por vía oral de tabletas. |
| 剂型、规格<br>Formulaciones y especificaciones | 片剂：每片 40mg。<br>注射液：每支 5mg（2ml）。<br>Tableta: 40mg;<br>Inyección: 5mg (2ml). |

**续　表**

| 药品名称 Drug Names | 硝苯地平 Nifedipina |
|---|---|
| 适应证<br>Indicaciones | 用于预防和治疗冠心病和心绞痛，特别是变异型心绞痛和冠状动脉痉挛所致的心绞痛，对呼吸功能没有不良影响，故适用于患有呼吸道阻塞性疾病的心绞痛患者，其疗效优于 β 受体拮抗剂。还适用于各种类型的高血压，对顽固性、重度高血压也有较好疗效。由于能降低后负荷，对顽固性充血性心力衰竭亦有良好疗效，宜于长期服用。<br><br>Se usa para prevención y tratamiento de enfermedades coronaria y angina, especialmente angina variante y angina causada por espasmo de la arteria coronaria. No hay efecto negativa en la función respiratoria, por lo que pacientes de angina con enfermedad pulmonar obstructiva puede utilizarlo. Tiene mejor efecto comparado con antagonista de los receptores β. También se utiliza en tratamiento de hipertensiones de viarios tipos especialmente para hipertensión intratable y severa. Como puede reducir la poscarga, es eficaz para insuficiencia cardíaca congestiva refractaria y buena para medicación a largo plazo. |
| 用法、用量<br>Administración y<br>dosis | 口服：一次 5～10mg，一日 15～30mg。急用时可舌下含服。对慢性心力衰竭，每 6 小时 20mg，咽部喷药，每次 1.5～2mg（喷 3～4 次）。<br><br>Por vía oral: 5～10mg cada vez y 15～30mg diarios. En caso emergente puede utilizarla por vía oral sublingual. En cuanto a insuficiencia cardíaca crónica, 20mg cada 6 horas. De rociar la garganta con el spray, la dosis es de 1.5～2mg cada vez (rocie 3～4 veces). |
| 剂型、规格<br>Formulaciones y<br>especificaciones | 片剂：普通片每片 5mg；10mg。控释片：每片 20mg。胶丸剂：每丸 5mg。胶囊剂：每粒 5mg；10mg。喷雾剂：每瓶 100mg。<br><br>Tableta normal: 5mg, 10mg; Tableta de liberación prolongada: 20mg; Cápsula blanda: 5mg; Cápsula: 5mg, 10mg; Spray: 100mg |
| 药品名称 Drug Names | 尼卡地平 Nicardipina |
| 适应证<br>Indicaciones | 用于治疗高血压、脑血管疾病、脑血栓形成或脑出血后遗症及脑动脉硬化症等。<br><br>Se usa para tratamiento de hipertensión, enfermedades cerebrovasculares, trombosis cerebral o secuelas de hemorragia cerebral y arteriosclerosis cerebral. |
| 用法、用量<br>Administración y<br>dosis | 口服：每次 20mg，一日 60mg。静脉滴注：高血压急症时以每分钟 0.5μg/kg 速度开始，根据血压监测调节滴速。<br><br>Por vía oral: 60mg diarios divididos en 3 tomas. Infusión por I.V.: dosis inicial 0.5mg/kg por minuto en tratamiento de emergencia hipertensiva y ajusta la velocidad según el monitoreo de la presión arterial. |
| 剂型、规格<br>Formulaciones y<br>especificaciones | 片剂：普通片每片 10mg；20mg；40mg。缓释片：每片 10mg。盐酸尼卡地平注射液：5ml：5mg（以尼卡地平计算）。<br><br>Tableta normal: 10mg, 20mg, 40mg; Tableta de liberación prolongada: 10mg; Inyección de clorhidrato de nicardipina: 5ml:5mg (calculado en base de la cantidad de nicardipina) |
| 药品名称 Drug Names | 尼群地平 Nitrendipina |
| 适应证<br>Indicaciones | 用于冠心病及高血压，尤其是患有这两种疾病的患者，也可用于充血性心力衰竭。<br><br>Se usa para tratamiento de enfermedades coronaria y hipertensión, especialmente para pacientes de las dos enfermedades. Utilización también en tratamiento de Insuficiencia Cardíaca Congestiva. |
| 用法、用量<br>Administración y<br>dosis | 口服，1 次 10mg，一日 30mg。<br><br>Por vía oral: dosis diaria de 30mg divididos en 3 tomas. |
| 剂型、规格<br>Formulaciones y<br>especificaciones | 片剂：每片 10mg。<br><br>Tableta: 10mg. |
| 药品名称 Drug Names | 尼莫地平 Nimodipina |
| 适应证<br>Indicaciones | 用于脑血管疾病，如脑血管灌注不足、脑血管痉挛、蛛网膜下腔出血、脑卒中和偏头痛等。对突发性耳聋也有一定疗效。<br><br>Se usa para tratamiento de enfermedades cerebrovasculares por ejempro Hipoperfusión cerebral, Vasoespasmo cerebral, Hemorragia subaracnoidea, apoplejía y migraña. También es eficaz en tratamiento de Sordera súbita. |

**续　表**

| 用法、用量<br>Administración y<br>dosis | 口服：一日剂量 40 ～ 60mg，分 2 ～ 3 次服用。<br>Por vía oral a dosis diaria 40 ~ 60mg divididos en 2 ~ 3 veces. |
|---|---|
| 剂型、规格<br>Formulaciones y<br>especificaciones | 片剂：20mg。<br>Tableta: 20mg. |

| 药品名称 Drug Names | 非洛地平 Felodipina |
|---|---|
| 适应证<br>Indicaciones | 用于高血压病、缺血性心脏病和心力衰竭患者。<br>Se usa para tratamiento de hipertensión, cardiopatía isquémica e insuficiencia cardíaca. |
| 用法、用量<br>Administración y<br>dosis | 一日剂量 20mg，分次服。<br>Por vía oral a dosis diaria de 20mg divididos en varias tomas. |
| 剂型、规格<br>Formulaciones y<br>especificaciones | 片剂：每片 5mg；10mg。<br>Tableta: 5mg, 10mg. |

| 药品名称 Drug Names | 氨氯地平 Amlodipina |
|---|---|
| 适应证<br>Indicaciones | 用于治疗高血压，单独应用或与其他抗高血压药合用均可；也可用于稳定型心绞痛患者，尤其是对硝酸盐和 β 受体拮抗剂无效者。<br>Se usa para tratamiento de hipertensión tanto como medicamento individual o junto con otros fármacos antihipertensivos. Utilización también para pacientes con angina estable, especialmente para los que no consiguen eficacia tras medicamento de nitratos y antagonistas de los receptores β. |
| 用法、用量<br>Administración y<br>dosis | 口服，开始时 1 次 5mg，一日 1 次，以后可根据患者的临床反应，可将剂量增加，最大可增至每日 10mg。<br>Por vía oral: La dosis inicial es de 5 mg diarios. Según la respuesta clínica de pacients puede aumentar la dosis a 10 mg diarios como máxima. |
| 剂型、规格<br>Formulaciones y<br>especificaciones | 片剂：每片 2.5mg；5mg；10mg。<br>Tableta: 2.5mg, 5mg, 10mg. |

| 药品名称 Drug Names | 左氨氯地平 Levamlodipina |
|---|---|
| 适应证<br>Indicaciones | 用于治疗高血压，单独应用或与其他抗高血压药合用均可；也可用于稳定型心绞痛患者，尤其是对硝酸盐和 β 受体拮抗剂无效者。<br>Se usa para tratamiento de hipertensión tanto como medicamento individual o junto con otros fármacos antihipertensivos. Utilización también para pacientes con angina estable, especialmente para los que no consiguen eficacia tras medicamento de nitratos y antagonistas de los receptores β. |
| 用法、用量<br>Administración y<br>dosis | 口服，开始时 1 次 2.5mg，一日 1 次；根据患者的临床反应，可将剂量增加，最大可增至每日 5mg，一日 1 次。<br>Por vía oral a dosis inicial de 2.5 mg diarios. Según la respuesta clínica de pacients puede aumentar la dosis a 5mg diarios como máxima. |
| 剂型、规格<br>Formulaciones y<br>especificaciones | 片剂：每片 2.5mg。<br>Tableta: 2.5mg. |

| 药品名称 Drug Names | 西尼地平 Cilnidipina |
|---|---|
| 适应证<br>Indicaciones | 用于治疗高血压，可单独应用，或与其他降压药合用。<br>Se usa para tratamiento de hipertensión tanto como medicamento individual o junto con otros fármacos antihipertensivos. |

| 续　表 | |
|---|---|
| 用法、用量<br>Administración y<br>dosis | 口服：1 次 5 ～ 10mg，一日 1 次，必要时可增至 20mg，一日 1 次。早餐后服用。根据患者的临床反应，可将剂量增加，最大可增至每次 10mg。<br><br>Por vía oral: 5 ~ 10mg diarios, en caso necesario puede aumentar a 20mg diarios. Tómala después de desayuno. Según la respuesta clínica del paciente puede aumentar la dosis a 10mg cada vez como máximo. |
| 剂型、规格<br>Formulaciones y<br>especificaciones | 片剂：每片 5mg。<br>Tableta: 5mg. |
| 药品名称Drug Names | 拉西地平 Lacidipina |
| 适应证<br>Indicaciones | 用于治疗高血压。<br>Se usa para tratamiento de hipertensión. |
| 用法、用量<br>Administración y<br>dosis | 开始时一日 1 次，每次 4mg，如效果不佳可增至一日 1 次，每次 6mg。肝功能不全患者，开始时需减半量。<br><br>Dosis inicial: 4 mg diarios. Si no es eficaz, aumenta la dosis a 6mg diarios. Para pacientes de insuficiencia hepática, debe disminuir la dosis inicial a la mitad. |
| 剂型、规格<br>Formulaciones y<br>especificaciones | 片剂：每片 2mg；4mg。<br>Tableta: 2mg, 4mg. |
| 药品名称Drug Names | 地尔硫䓬 Diltiazem |
| 适应证<br>Indicaciones | 用于室上性心律失常、典型心绞痛、变异型心绞痛、老年人高血压等。<br>Se usa para tratamiento de arritmia supraventricular, angina típica y variante, la hipertensión en los ancianos. |
| 用法、用量<br>Administración y<br>dosis | 口服，常用量，1 次 30 ～ 60mg，一日 90 ～ 180mg。用于心律失常：口服，1 次 30 ～ 60mg，一日 4 次；起始剂量为 250μg/kg，于 2 分钟静脉注射；必要时 15 分钟后再给 350μg/kg。以后的剂量应根据患者的情况个体化制订。在心房颤动或心房扑动患者，最初输注速率 5 ～ 10mg/h，必要时可增至最大 15mg/h（增幅 5mg/h）。静脉输注最多可维持 24 小时。用于心绞痛：每 6 ～ 8 小时 30 ～ 60mg。用于高血压：一日剂量 120 ～ 240mg，分 3 ～ 4 次服用。<br><br>Por vía oral: dosis habitual de 30 ~ 60mg cada vez y 90 ~ 180mg diarios. En caso de tratamiento de arritmia: administración oral a dosis 30 ~ 60mg y 4 veces al día. Inyección por I.V. dentro de 2 minutos a dosis inicial de 250μg/kg y si es necesario puede repetir la inyección a dosis de 350μg/kg. La dosis siguiente depende de la situación de cada paciente. En caso de fibrilación oaleteo auricular, la velocidad inicial es de 5 ~ 10mg/hora y puede aumentar hasta 15mg/h en caso necesario. El medicamento de inyección dura 24 horas a la máxima. En caso de angina la dosis es de 30 ~ 60mg cada 6 ~ 8 horas y si es hipertensión la dosis es 120 ~ 240mg diarios divididos en 3 ~ 4 tomas. |
| 剂型、规格<br>Formulaciones y<br>especificaciones | 片剂：普通片每片 30mg；60mg；90mg。缓释片：每片 30mg；60mg；90mg。缓释胶囊：90mg。注射用盐酸地尔硫䓬：10mg；50mg。<br>Tableta normal: 30mg, 60mg, 90mg; Tableta de liberación prolongada: 30mg, 60mg, 90mg; Cápsula de liberación prolongada: 90mg; clorhidrato de diltiazem para inyección: 10mg, 50mg. |
| 药品名称Drug Names | 桂利嗪 Cinarizina |
| 适应证<br>Indicaciones | 用于脑血栓形成、脑栓塞、脑动脉硬化、脑出血恢复期、蛛网膜下腔出血恢复期、脑外伤后遗症、内耳眩晕症、冠状动脉粥样硬化、由于末梢循环不良引起的疾病等。<br><br>Se usa para tratamiento de trombosis cerebral, embolia pulmonar, arteriosclerosis cerebral, medicamento para recuperacion de una hemorragia cerebral y subaracnoidea, tratamiento de secuelas de la lesión cerebral, vértigo de oído interno, aterosclerosis coronaria y enfermedades causadas por la mala circulación periférica. |
| 用法、用量<br>Administración y<br>dosis | 口服：每次 25 ～ 50mg，一日 3 次，餐后服。静脉注射：1 次 20 ～ 40mg，缓慢注入。<br>Por vía oral: 25 ~ 50mg y 3 veces al día después de alimentos. Inyección lenta por I.V.: 20 ~ 40mg. |

**续 表**

| 剂型、规格<br>Formulaciones y especificaciones | 片剂及胶囊剂：每片（粒）25mg。<br>注射液：每支 20mg（20ml）。<br>Tableta y Cápsula: 25mg; Inyección: 20mg (20ml). |
|---|---|
| 药品名称Drug Names | 氟桂利嗪 Flunarizina |
| 适应证<br>Indicaciones | 药理及应用同桂利嗪相似，有扩血管作用。此外，对注意力减弱、记忆力障碍、易激动及平衡功能障碍、眩晕等均有一定疗效。用于老年患者。<br>Farmacología y aplicaciones similares a Cinnarizine como un vasodilatador. Además puede utilizar para tratamiento de atenuación de atención, trastornos de la memoria, irritabilidad, disfunción de equilibrio y vértigo. Utilización para ancianos. |
| 用法、用量<br>Administración y dosis | 1 次 5～10mg，一日 10mg（以氟桂利嗪计量），在一般情况下，可于晚上顿服。<br>Dosis: 5～10mg cada vez y 10mg diarios. Generalmente se toma por la noche de solo 1 vez. |
| 剂型、规格<br>Formulaciones y especificaciones | 胶囊剂：每粒 5mg（以氟桂利嗪计量）。<br>Cápsula: 5mg de flunarizina. |
| 药品名称Drug Names | 利多氟嗪 Lidoflazina |
| 适应证<br>Indicaciones | 用于心绞痛。<br>Se usa para tratamiento de angina. |
| 用法、用量<br>Administración y dosis | 口服，1 次 60mg，一日 3 次。<br>Por vía oral: 60mg y 3 veces al día. |
| 剂型、规格<br>Formulaciones y especificaciones | 片剂：每片 60mg。<br>Tableta: 60mg. |

10.2　治疗慢性心功能不全的药物 Medicamentos para el tratamiento de la insuficiencia cardíacacrónica

| 药品名称Drug Names | 洋地黄毒苷 Digitoxina |
|---|---|
| 适应证<br>Indicaciones | 用于维持治疗慢性心功能不全。<br>Se usa para tratamiento de mantenimiento de la disfunción cardiaca crónica. |
| 用法、用量<br>Administración y dosis | 主要采用口服，不宜口服者可以肌内注射，必要时静脉注射。全效量：成人 0.7～1.2mg；于 48～72 小时分次服用。小儿 2 岁以下 0.03～0.04mg/kg，2 岁以上 0.02～0.03mg/kg。维持量：成人一日 0.05～0.1mg，小儿为全效量的 1/10，一日 1 次。<br>Administración principal por vía oral y para pacientes que no puede tomarlo por vía oral puede utilizarlo en inyección por I.M. y en caso necesario puede ser inyección por I.V.. Dosis efectiva completa: 0.7～1.2 mg para adultos y divididos en varias tomas dentro de 48～72 horas. 0.03～0.04mg/kg para niño menor de 2 años y 0.02～0.03mg/kg para niño mayor de 2 años. Dosis de mantenimiento para adultos es de 0.05～0.1mg y para niños sera 1/10 de la dosis efectiva completa y la toma de 1 vez al día. |
| 剂型、规格<br>Formulaciones y especificaciones | 片剂：每片 0.1mg。<br>注射液：每支 0.2mg（1ml）。<br>Tableta: 0.1mg; Inyección: 0.2mg (1ml). |
| 药品名称Drug Names | 地高辛 Digoxina |
| 适应证<br>Indicaciones | 用于各种急性和慢性心功能不全和室上性心动过速、心房颤动和心房扑动等。<br>Se usa para tratamiento de la disfunción cardiaca aguda o crónica, taquicardia supraventricular, fibrilación y aleteo auricular . |

**续　表**

| 用法、用量<br>Administración y dosis | 全效量：成人口服 1～1.5mg；于 24 小时内分次服用。小儿 2 岁以下 0.06～0.08mg/kg，2 岁以上 0.04～0.06mg/kg。不宜口服者也可静脉注射，临用前以 10% 或 25% 葡萄糖注射液稀释后应用，常用量静脉注射 1 次 0.25～0.5mg；极量，1 次 1mg。维持量：成人每日 0.125～0.5mg，分 1～2 次服用；小儿为全效量的 1/4。<br><br>Dosis efectiva completa: Administración oral para adultos: 1～1.5mg divididos en varias tomas al día. Para niño menor de 2 años: 0.06～0.08mg/kg. Para niño mayor de 2 años: 0.04～0.06mg/kg. Pacientes que no puede tomarlo por vía oral lo pueden utilizar en inyección por I.V. diluidos con solución de glucosa a 10%～25% y la dosis habidual es de 0.25～0.5mg cada vez y la dosis máxima es de 1mg cada vez. Dosis de mantenimiento: Para adultos es de 0.125～0.5mg diarios divididos en 1～2 veces y para niños la dosis es el 1/4 de la dosis efectiva completa. |
| --- | --- |
| 剂型、规格<br>Formulaciones y especificaciones | 片剂：每片 0.25mg。注射液：0.5mg（2ml）。<br>Tableta: 0.25mg; Inyección: 0.5mg (2ml). |
| **药品名称 Drug Names** | **毛花苷 C Lanatosida C** |
| 适应证<br>Indicaciones | 用于急性和慢性心力衰竭。<br>Se usa para tratamiento de la insuficiencia cardíaca aguda y crónica. |
| 用法、用量<br>Administración y dosis | 缓慢全效量：口服，1 次 0.5mg，一日 4 次。维持量：一般为一日 1mg，以 2 次服用。静脉注射：成人常用量，全效量 1～1.2mg，首次剂量 0.4～0.6mg；2～4 小时后可再给予 0.2～0.4mg，用葡萄糖注射液稀释后缓慢注射。<br><br>Dosis efectiva completa lenta: administración oral de 0.5mg y 4 tomas al día. Dosis de mantenimiento: dosis habidual de 1mg y 2 veces al día. Inyección por I.V.: dosis habidual de adultos de efecto completo: 1～1.2mg, dosis inicial es de 0.4～0.6mg, dentro de 2～4 horas repite la inyección lenta de 0.2～0.4mg diluidos con solución de glucosa. |
| 剂型、规格<br>Formulaciones y especificaciones | 片剂：每片 0.5mg。注射液：0.4mg（2ml）。<br>Tableta: 0.5mg; Inyección: 0.4mg (2ml). |
| **药品名称 Drug Names** | **去乙酰毛花苷 Deslanósida** |
| 适应证<br>Indicaciones | 用于急性心力衰竭及心房颤动及心房扑动等。<br>Se usa para tratamiento de la insuficiencia cardíaca aguda, fibrilación auricular y El aleteo auricular. |
| 用法、用量<br>Administración y dosis | 静脉注射 成人常用量：用葡萄糖注射液稀释后缓慢注射，1 次 0.4～0.8mg。全效量 1～1.6mg，于 24 小时内分次注射。儿童每日 20～40μg/kg，分 1～2 次给药。然后改用口服毛花苷丙维持治疗。<br><br>Inyección lenta por I.V.: adultos: 0.4～0.8 mg cada vez dilucidos con solución glucosa. Dosis efectiva completa: 1～1.6mg inyectados en varias veces dentro de 24 horas. Niños: 20～40μg/kg diarios divididos en 1～2 veces. Después mantener el tratamiento con administración oral de lanatoside. |
| 剂型、规格<br>Formulaciones y especificaciones | 注射液：每支 0.2mg（1ml）；0.4mg（2ml）。<br>Inyección: 0.2mg (1ml), 0.4mg (2ml). |
| **药品名称 Drug Names** | **毒毛花苷 K　Strofantin K** |
| 适应证<br>Indicaciones | 用于急性心力衰竭。动脉硬化性心脏病患者发生心力衰竭时，如心率不快可选用本品。<br>Se usa para tratamiento de la insuficiencia cardíaca aguda. Utilización también para pacientes de enfermedad cardíaca arteriosclerótica cuando sucede la insuficiencia cardíaca. |
| 用法、用量<br>Administración y dosis | 静脉注射：首剂 0.125～0.25mg，加入等渗葡萄糖注射液 20～40ml 内缓慢注入（时间不少于 5 分钟），1～2 小时后重复 1 次，总量每日 0.25～0.5mg。病情转好后，可改用洋地黄苷口服制剂，给予适当的全效量。<br><br>Inyección por I.V.: dosis primera de 0.125～0.25mg con 20～40ml de solución isotónica de glucosa. La inyección se aplica en más de 5 minutos. Dentro de 1～2 horas repetir la medicación. Dosis diaria es 0.25～0.5mg. Cuando se mejora, cambia a administración oral de glucósidos digitálicos a dosis efectiva comleta. |

**续　表**

| | |
|---|---|
| 剂型、规格<br>Formulaciones y especificaciones | 注射液：每支 0.25mg（1ml）。<br>Inyección: 0.25mg (1ml). |
| 药品名称 Drug Names | 氨力农 Amrinona |
| 适应证<br>Indicaciones | 用于对洋地黄、利尿药、血管舒张药治疗无效或效果欠佳的各种原因引起的急性、慢性顽固性充血性心力衰竭的短期治疗。<br><br>Se usa para tratamiento a corto plazo de insuficiencia cardíaca congestiva refractaria aguda o crónica que no consigue eficacia significativa tras tratamiento condigitálicos, diuréticos y vasodilatadores. |
| 用法、用量<br>Administración y dosis | 静脉注射负荷量：0.75mg/kg，2～3分钟缓慢静注，继之以每千克5～10μg/min维持静脉滴注，单次剂量最大不超过2.5mg/kg。每日最大量＜10mg/kg。疗程不超过2周。<br><br>Inyección por I.V. en primeros 2～3 minutos de dosis máxima 0.75 mg/kg y luego infusión por I.V. a 5～10mg/kg por minuto y la dosis máxima no exede a 2.5mg/kg cada vez. Dosis diaria máxima no excede a 10mg/kg y el curso de tratamiento no supera a 2 semanas. |
| 剂型、规格<br>Formulaciones y especificaciones | 注射液：每支 50mg（2ml）；100mg（2ml）。<br>Inyección: 50mg (2ml), 100mg (2ml). |
| 药品名称 Drug Names | 米力农 Milrinona |
| 适应证<br>Indicaciones | 用于对洋地黄、利尿药、血管舒张药治疗无效或效果欠佳的各种原因引起的急性、慢性顽固性充血性心力衰竭的短期治疗。<br><br>Se usa para tratamiento a corto plazo de insuficiencia cardíaca congestiva refractaria aguda o crónica que no consigue eficacia significativa tras tratamiento condigitálicos, diuréticos y vasodilatadores. |
| 用法、用量<br>Administración y dosis | 静脉滴注：每分钟12.5～75μg/kg。一般开始10分钟以50μg/kg，然后以每分钟0.375～0.75μg/kg维持。每日最大剂量不超过1.13mg/kg。<br><br>Infusión por I.V.: 12.5～75μg/kg por minuto. Habitualmente la dosis en los primeros 10 minutos es de 50μg/kg por minuto y luego mantener la dosis a 0.375～0.75μg/kg por minuto. Dosis diaria no excede a 1.13mg/kg. |
| 剂型、规格<br>Formulaciones y especificaciones | 注射液：每支 10mg（10ml）。<br>Inyección: 10mg (10ml). |

10.3　抗心律失常药 Antiarritmias

| | |
|---|---|
| 药品名称 Drug Names | 奎尼丁 Quinidina |
| 适应证<br>Indicaciones | 主要用于阵发性心动过速、心房颤动和期前收缩等。<br>Se usa para tratamiento de taquicardia paroxística, fibrilación y aleteo auricular, latidos prematuros. |
| 用法、用量<br>Administración y dosis | （1）口服：第一天，每次0.2g，每2小时1次，连续5次；如无效而又无明显毒性反应，第二天增至每次0.3g、第三天每次0.4g，每2小时1次，连续5次。每日总量一般不宜超过2g。恢复正常心律后，改维持量，每日0.2～0.4g。若连服3～4日无效或有毒性反应者，应停药。<br>（2）静脉注射：在十分必要时采用静脉注射并须在心电图观察下进行。每次0.25g，以5%葡萄糖液稀释至50ml缓慢静脉注射。<br><br>(1) Por vía oral. En el primer día la dosis es 0.2g cada 2 horas y la repite 5 veces consecutivas. Si no es eficaz y no hay toxicación evidente, en el segundo día aumenta a 0.3g cada vez y en el tercer día, 0.4g, la toma cada 2 horas y 5 veces consecutivas al día. Dosis diaria no excede a 2g. Después de recuperar el ritmo cardíaco normal, toma dosis de mantenimiento de 0.2～0.4g diarios y si no es eficaz y no hay toxicación evidente tras la toma consecutiva en 3～4 días, debe dejar el medicamento.<br>(2) Inyección por I.V.: lo toma cuando es definitivamente necesaria y hay que aplicarlo bajo observación del electrocardiograma. Lenta inyección de 0.25g cada vez diluidos a 50ml con solución de glucosa a 5%. |

**续　表**

| | |
|---|---|
| 剂型、规格<br>Formulaciones y<br>especificaciones | 片剂：每片 0.2g。<br>葡萄糖酸奎尼丁注射液：每支 0.5g（10ml）。<br>Tableta: 0.2g; Inyección de gluconato de quinidina: 0.5g (10ml). |
| **药品名称 Drug Names** | 普鲁卡因胺 Procainamida |
| 适应证<br>Indicaciones | 用于阵发性心动过速、频发期前收缩（对室性期前收缩疗效较好）、心房颤动和心房扑动，常与奎尼丁交替使用。<br><br>Se usa para tratamiento de taquicardia paroxística, frecuentes latidos prematuros especialmente eficaz para latido ventricular prematuro, fibrilación y aleteo auricular. Siempre se usa indistintamente con quinidina. |
| 用法、用量<br>Administración y<br>dosis | （1）口服：一日 3～4 次，每次 0.5～0.75g，心律正常后逐渐减至一日 2～6 次，每次 0.25g。<br>（2）静脉滴注：每次 0.5～1g，溶于 5%～10% 葡萄糖溶液 100ml 内，开始 10～30 分钟，点滴速度可适当加快，于 1 小时内滴完。无效者，1 小时后再给一次，24 小时内总量不超过 2g。<br>（3）静脉注射：每次 0.1～0.2g。<br>（4）肌内注射：每次 0.25～0.5g。<br><br>(1) Por vía oral. 0.5～0.75g y 3～4 veces al día y después de recuperar el ritmo cardíaco normal, toma dosis de mantenimiento de 0.25g y 2～6 veces al día.<br>(2) Infusión por I.V.: dilución de 0.5～1g de dicha droga con 100ml de solución de glucosa a 5%～10%. En los primeros 10～30minutos puede aumentar la velocidad y terminar la infusión dentro de 1 hora. Si no se ve efecto puede repetir la medicación 1 hora después. Dosis diaria no excede a 2g.<br>(3) Inyección por I.V.: 0.1～0.2g.<br>(4) Inyección por I.M.: 0.25～0.5g. |
| 剂型、规格<br>Formulaciones y<br>especificaciones | 片剂：每片 0.125g；0.25g。　　注射液：每支 0.1g（1ml）；0.2g（2ml）；0.5g（5ml）；1g（10ml）。<br>Tableta: 0.125g, 0.25g; Inyección: 0.1g (1ml), 0.2g (2ml), 0.5g(5ml), 1g(10ml). |
| **药品名称 Drug Names** | 丙吡胺 Disopiramida |
| 适应证<br>Indicaciones | 用于房性期前收缩、阵发性房性心动过速、心房颤动、室性期前收缩等，对室上性心律失常的疗效似较好。<br><br>Se usa para tratamiento de extrasístoles auriculares, taquicardia auricular paroxística, fibrilación auricular, latido ventricular prematuro. Tiene buena eficacia para tratamiento de arritmias supraventriculares. |
| 用法、用量<br>Administración y<br>dosis | 口服，每次 0.1～0.15g，一日 0.4～0.8g。最大剂量不超过 800mg/d。静脉注射，每次 1～2mg/kg，最大剂量每次不超过 150mg，用葡萄糖注射液 20ml 稀释后在 5～10 分钟注完。必要时，可在 20 分钟后重复一次。静脉滴注，每次 100～200mg，以 5% 葡萄糖注射液 500ml 稀释，一般滴注量为每小时 20～30mg。<br><br>Por vía oral, 0.1～0.15g cada dia y la dosis diaria es 0.4～0.8g. Dosis máxima no excede a 800mg diarios. En inyección por I.V.de dilución de 20ml de solución de glucosa, lleva una dosis de 1.2mg/kg y la máxima no excede a 150mg cada vez. La inyección debe terminarse dentro de 5～10 minutos y puede repetirlo después de 20minutos si es necesario. En infusión por I.V. de dilución de 500ml de solución de glucosa a 5%, la dosis habitual es 20～30mg por hora. |
| 剂型、规格<br>Formulaciones y<br>especificaciones | 片剂：每片 100mg。注射液：每支 50mg（2ml）；100mg（2ml）。<br>Tableta: 100mg; Inyección: 50mg (2ml), 100mg (2ml). |
| **药品名称 Drug Names** | 利多卡因 Lidocaina |
| 适应证<br>Indicaciones | 本品适用于心肌梗死、洋地黄中毒、锑剂中毒、外科手术等所致的室性期前收缩、室性心动过速和心室颤动。<br><br>Se usa para tratamiento de infarto de miocardio, intoxicación digitalina y de antimonio, síntomas de latido ventricular prematuro,taquicardia ventricular y fibrilación ventricular causadas por cirugía. |

**续　表**

| 用法、用量<br>Administración y<br>dosis | 静脉注射，1～2mg/kg，继以0.1%溶液静脉滴注，每小时不超过100mg。也可肌内注射，4～5mg/kg，60～90分钟重复一次。<br><br>Inyección por I.V.: 1～2mg/kg y luego continua con infusión por I.V. de solución a 0.1%, dosis no excede a 100mg/hora. Inyección por I.M.: 4～5mg/kg en cada 1～1.5 horas. |
|---|---|
| 剂型、规格<br>Formulaciones y<br>especificaciones | 注射液：每支0.1g（5ml）；0.4g（20ml）。<br><br>Inyección: 0.1g (5ml), 0.4g (20ml). |

| 药品名称 Drug Names | 苯妥英钠 Fenitoína Sódica |
|---|---|
| 适应证<br>Indicaciones | 用于洋地黄中毒苷所引起的室上性和室性心律失常及对利多卡因无效的心律失常。<br><br>Se usa para tratamiento de taquicardia supraventriculares y ventricular por la intoxicación digitalina y arritmia que no tiene eficacia tras tomar Lidocaína. |
| 用法、用量<br>Administración y<br>dosis | 口服：每次0.1～0.2g，一日2～3次。口服极量：每次0.3g，一日0.5g。静脉注射：每次0.125～0.25g，缓慢注入，一日总量不超过0.5g。<br><br>Por vía oral: 0.1～0.2g y 2～3 tomas al día. Dosis oral máxima no excede a 0.3g cada vez y 0.5g diarios. Lenta inyección por I.V.: 0.125～0.25g cada vez y dosis máxima no excede a 0.5g diarios. |
| 剂型、规格<br>Formulaciones y<br>especificaciones | 片剂：每片0.05g；0.1g。<br>注射用苯妥英钠：每支0.125g；0.25g。<br><br>Tableta: 0.05g, 0.1g; Fenitoína sódica para inyección: 0.125g, 0.25g. |

| 药品名称 Drug Names | 美西律 Mexiletina |
|---|---|
| 适应证<br>Indicaciones | 用于急、慢性室性心律失常，如室性早期前收缩、室性心动过速、心室颤动及洋地黄苷中毒引起的心律失常。<br><br>Se usa de tratamiento de arritmia ventriculares aguda o crónica, por ejempro arritmia causada por latido ventricular prematuro, taquicardia ventricular, fibrilación ventricular y Intoxicación por digitoxina. |
| 用法、用量<br>Administración y<br>dosis | （1）口服：每次50～200mg，一日150～600mg，或每6～8小时1次。以后可酌情减量维持。<br>　　（2）静脉注射、静脉滴注：开始量100mg，加入5%葡萄糖注射液20ml中，缓慢静脉注射（3～5分钟）。如无效，可在5～10分钟后再给50～100mg一次。然后以1.5～2mg/min的速度静脉滴注，3～4小时后滴速减至0.75～1mg/min，并维持24～48小时。<br><br>(1) Por vía oral: 50～200mg cada vez y 150～600mg diarios o una toma cada 6～8 horas, luego puede disminuir la dosis gradualmente según la necesidad.<br>(2) Inyección o infusión por I.V.: dosis inicial 100mg de dicha droga con 20ml de solución de glucosa a 5%. Se administra la inyección lentamente que tarda 3～5 minutos. So no es eficaz, puede dar 50～100mg más después de 5～10 minutos. Luego toma infusión a velocidad 1.5～2 mg/min y disminuir a 0.75～1mg/min después de 3～4 horas y mantenerlo dentro de 24～48 horas. |
| 剂型、规格<br>Formulaciones y<br>especificaciones | 片剂：每片50mg；100mg；250mg。<br>胶囊剂：每粒50mg；100mg；400mg。<br>注射液：100mg（2ml）。<br><br>Tableta: 50mg, 100mg, 250mg; Cápsula: 50mg, 100mg, 400mg; Inyección: 100mg (2ml). |

| 药品名称 Drug Names | 普罗帕酮 Propafenona |
|---|---|
| 适应证<br>Indicaciones | 用于预防或治疗室性或室上性异位搏动，室性或室上性心动过速，预激综合征，电转复律后室颤发作等。经临床试用，疗效确切，起效迅速，作用时间持久，对冠心病、高血压所引起的心律失常有较好的疗效。<br><br>Se usa para tratamiento o prevención de extrasístoles y taquicardia ventriculares o supraventricular, síndrome de preexcitación, fibrilación ventricular tras la cardioversión eléctrica. Según el ensayo clínico, tiene efecto bueno y rápido con larga duración que es eficaz para tratamiento de arritmia causada por enfermedad coronaria e hipertensión. |

**续　表**

| | |
|---|---|
| 用法、用量<br>Administración y dosis | 口服：1 次 100～200mg，一日 3～4 次。治疗量，一日 300～900mg，分 4～6 次服用。维持量，一日 300～600mg，分 2～4 次服用。由于其局部麻醉作用，宜在饭后与饮料或食物同时吞服，不得嚼碎。必要时可在严密监护下缓慢静脉注射或静脉滴注，1 次 70mg，每 8 小时 1 次。一日总量不超过 350mg。<br><br>Por vía oral, 100～200mg y 3～4 veces al día. Dosis para tratamiento: 300～900 mg diarios divididos en 4～6 tomas. Dosis de mantenimiento: 300～600mg divididos en 2～4 tomas. Debido a su anestésico parcial, debe tragarlo después de alimentos o junto con bedida o comida y no se puede masticar. En caso necesario puede ser medicación en inyección o infusión lenta por I.V. bajo observación excricta. La dosis de 70mg cada 8 horas y no excede a 350mg diarios. |
| 剂型、规格<br>Formulaciones y especificaciones | 片剂：每片 50mg；100mg；150mg。<br>注射液：每支 17.5mg（5ml）；35mg（10ml）。<br>Tableta：50mg，100mg，150mg；Inyección：17.5mg（5ml），35mg（10ml）. |
| **药品名称 Drug Names** | 恩卡尼 Encainida |
| 适应证<br>Indicaciones | 用于室性期前收缩、室性心动过速及心室颤动。也可用于室上性心动过速，对折返性心动过速，尤其是预激综合征有效。<br><br>Se usa para tratamiento de latido ventricular prematuro, La taquicardia ventricular y fibrilación ventricular. También es eficaz en tratamiento de taquicardia supraventricular, la taquicardia por reentrada y síndrome de preexcitación. |
| 用法、用量<br>Administración y dosis | 口服，每次 25～75mg，一日 3～4 次。静脉注射，以 0.5～1mg/kg，于 15～20 分钟注完。小儿口服一日剂量 60～120mg/m² 或 2～7.5mg/kg，分 3～4 次服用。通常从小剂量开始，在严密观察下逐渐增量。<br><br>Por vía oral: 25～75mg y 3～4 tomas al día. Inyección por I.V.: 0.5～1mg/kg y se administra dentro de 15～20 minutos. Para niños la dosis oral es 60～120mg/m² diarios ó 2～7.5mg/kg diarios divididos en 3～4 tomas. Habitualmente comienza con pequeña dosis y aumentarla gradualmente bajo la observación excrita. |
| 剂型、规格<br>Formulaciones y especificaciones | 胶囊剂：每粒 25mg；35mg；50mg。<br>注射液：25mg（1ml）；50mg（2ml）。<br>Cápsula：25mg，35mg，50mg；Inyección：25mg（1ml），50mg（2ml）. |
| **药品名称 Drug Names** | 氟卡尼 Flecainida |
| 适应证<br>Indicaciones | 用于室上性心动过速、房室结或房室折返心动过速、心房颤动、儿童顽固性交界性心动过速及伴有预激综合征者。对其他抗心律失常药物无效的病例，氟卡尼常有效。<br><br>Se usa para tratamiento de taquicardia supraventricular, nodal auriculoventricular o taquicardia por reentrada atrioventricular, fibrilación auricular, Taquicardia intratable de la unión en niños y pacientes con síndrome de preexcitación. Siempre es eficaz para casos que no consigue efecto de otros fármacos antiarrítmicos. |
| 用法、用量<br>Administración y dosis | 口服：成人开始时每次 100mg，一日 2 次，然后每隔 4 日，每次增加 50mg，最大剂量每次 200mg，一日 2 次；儿童每次 50～100mg，一日 2 次。静脉滴注：成人 2mg/kg，于 15 分钟滴完；儿童 2mg/kg，于 10 分钟内滴完。<br><br>Por vía oral: Adultos: dosis inicial 100mg y 2 veces al día y aumentar en 50mg cada vez en cada 5 dias. Dosis máxima no excede a 200mg cada vez y 2 tomas al día. Niños: 50～100mg y 2 veces al día. Infusión por I.V.: Para adultos: infusión dentro de 15 minutos a dosis de 2mg/kg; Para niños: infusión dentro de 10 minutos a dos de 2mg/kg. |
| 剂型、规格<br>Formulaciones y especificaciones | 片剂：每片 100mg。<br>注射液：50mg（5ml）；100mg（10ml）。<br>Tableta：100mg；Inyección：50mg（5ml），100mg（10ml）. |

**续 表**

| 药品名称 Drug Names | 胺碘酮 Amiodarona |
|---|---|
| 适应证<br>Indicaciones | 用于室性和室上性心动过速和期前收缩、阵发性心房扑动和心动颤动，预激综合征等。也可用于伴有充血性心力衰竭和急性心肌梗死的心律失常患者。对其他抗心律失常药物如丙吡胺、维拉帕米、奎尼丁、β 受体拮抗剂无效的顽固性阵发性心动过速常能奏效。此外，还用于慢性冠脉功能不全和心绞痛。<br><br>Se usa para tratamiento de taquicardia supraventriculares y ventricular, latido prematuro, aleteo auricular y fibrilación paroxística, y síndrome de preexcitación. Utilización también para pacientes de arritmia asociada con la insuficiencia cardíaca congestiva y el infarto agudo de miocardio. Es eficaz para taquicardia paroxística refractaria que no se ve efecto de otros fármacos antiarrítmicos, por ejempro la disopiramida, verapamilo, quinidina y antagonista de los receptores β. Además se usa en tratamiento de insuficiencia coronaria crónica y angina. |
| 用法、用量<br>Administración y<br>dosis | 口服：每次 0.1～0.2g，一日 1～4 次；或开始每次 0.2g，一日 3 次。餐后服。3 天后改用维持量，每次 0.2g，一日 1～2 次。<br><br>Por vía oral: 0.1～0.2g y 1～4 veces al día, o toma una dosis inicial de 0.2g y 3 veces al día y 3 días después cambia a dosis de mantenimiento de 0.2g y 1～2 veces al día. |
| 剂型、规格<br>Formulaciones y<br>especificaciones | 片剂：每片 0.2g。<br>胶囊剂：每粒 0.1g；0.2g。<br>注射液：150mg（3ml）。<br>Tableta: 0.2g; Cápsula: 0.1g, 0.2g; Inyección: 150mg (3ml). |

| 药品名称 Drug Names | 依地酸二钠 Edetato disódico |
|---|---|
| 适应证<br>Indicaciones | 常用于洋地黄苷中度所致的心律失常。<br>Se usa para tratamiento de la arritmia causada por la intoxicación de glucósidos digitálicos |
| 用法、用量<br>Administración y<br>dosis | 静脉注射：每次 1～3g，以 50% 的葡萄糖注射液 20～40ml 稀释后注入。静脉滴注：每次 4～6g，用 5%～10% 葡萄糖注射液 500ml 稀释后在 1～3 小时滴完。<br><br>Inyección por I.V.: 1～3g cada vez diluidos con 20～40ml de solución de glucosa a 50%. Infusión por I.V.: 4～6mg cada vez diluidos con 500ml de solución de glucosa a 5%～10% y se administra lentamente dentro de 1～3 horas. |
| 剂型、规格<br>Formulaciones y<br>especificaciones | 注射液：每支 1g（5ml）。<br>Inyección: 1g (5ml). |

| 药品名称 Drug Names | 门冬氨酸钾镁 Aspartato de magnesio y aspartato potasio |
|---|---|
| 适应证<br>Indicaciones | 用于期前收缩、阵发性心动过速、心绞痛、心力衰竭等。此外，还可用于急性黄疸型肝炎、肝细胞功能不全、其他急慢性肝病、低钾血症等。<br><br>Se usa para tratamiento de latido prematuro, taquicardia paroxística, angina e insuficiencia cardíaca. Utiización también en tratamiento de hepatitis ictericia aguda, insuficiencia hepática, otras enfermedades hepáticas aguda o crónica y hipopotasemia. |
| 用法、用量<br>Administración y<br>dosis | 静脉滴注：一日量 10～20ml，用时以 10 倍量的输液稀释后缓慢滴注。<br>Infusión por I.V.: lenta infusión de 10～20ml diarios dilucidos con fluido de 10 veces la cantidad. |
| 剂型、规格<br>Formulaciones y<br>especificaciones | 注射液：每支 10ml，含钾盐及镁盐各 500mg。<br>Inyección: 10ml y incluye 500mg de potasio y 500mg de magnesio. |

10.4 防治心绞痛药 Medicamentos para prevenir y tratar la angina

| 药品名称 Drug Names | 硝酸甘油 Nitroglicerina |
|---|---|
| 适应证<br>Indicaciones | 用于防治心绞痛。<br>Se usa para prevención de angina. |

续　表

| | |
|---|---|
| 用法、用量<br>Administración y dosis | 　根据不同的临床需求，硝酸甘油可以通过舌下含服给药、黏膜给药、口服给药、透皮给药或静脉途径给药。①用于治疗急性心绞痛：可给予硝酸甘油片舌下含服、舌下喷雾给药或黏膜给药。片剂（每片 0.3 ～ 0.6mg）置于舌下，必要时可重复含服。喷雾给药则可每次将 0.4 ～ 0.8mg（1 ～ 2 揿）喷至舌下，然后闭嘴，必要时可喷 3 次。硝酸甘油黏膜片应置于上唇和齿龈之间，1 次 1 ～ 2mg。②用于稳定型心绞痛的长期治疗：通常透皮剂的形式给予。将膜敷贴于皮肤上，药物以恒速进入皮肤。作用时间长，几乎可达 24 小时。③用于控制性降压或治疗心力衰竭：静脉滴注，开始剂量按每分钟 5μg，可每 3 ～ 5 分钟增加 5μg 以达到满意效果。如在 20μg/min 时无效可以 10μg/min 递增，以后可 20μg/min，一但有效则剂量渐减小和给药间期延长。<br>　Según diferentes necesidades clínicas, puede tomarla por administración sublingual, mucosal, oral, transdérmica o vía inyección intravenosa. ① Para tratamiento de angina aguda: administración sublingual de tableta, aerosol o mucosa. Dosis: tableta sublingual: 0.3 ~ 0.6mg y puede repetir utilización en caso necesario; aerosol sublingual: 0.4 ~ 0.8mg (1 ~ 2 pulse) y puede aumentar a 3 veces en caso necesario; mucosa sublingual: 1 ~ 2mg cada vez y debe ser colocado entre el labio superior y la encía. ② Para tratamiento a largo plazo de angina estable: administración transdérmica, coloca la mucosa en la piel y el fármaco entra en la piel a velocidad constante y tiene larga duración hasta 24 horas. ③ Para tratamiento de la hipotensión controlada o insuficiencia cardíaca: En infusión intravenosa: dosis inicial 5mg cada minuto y puede aumentar en 5μg cada 3 ~ 5 minutos para ser más eficaz. Si no se ve efecto evidencial cuando llega a 20mg/min puede aumentar gradualmente la dosis en 10mg/min y luego 20mg/min. Una vez que tiene eficacia, disminuye gradualmente la dosis y prolongar el intervalo de medicación. |
| 剂型、规格<br>Formulaciones y especificaciones | 　片剂：每片 0.3mg；0.5mg；0.6mg。缓释硝酸甘油片：每片含 2.5mg。注射液：1mg（1ml）；2mg（1ml）；5mg（1ml）；10mg（1ml）。硝酸甘油膜：每格含硝酸甘油 0.5mg。<br>　Tableta: 0.3mg, 0.5mg, 0.6mg; Tableta de liberación prolongada: incluye 2.5mg de nitroglicerina; Inyección: 1mg (1ml), 2mg(1ml), 5mg (1ml), 10mg(1ml); Parche：cada incluye 0.5mg de nitroglicerina. |
| 药品名称 Drug Names | 戊四硝酯 Tetranitrato de pentaeritritolo |
| 适应证<br>Indicaciones | 　用于预防心绞痛的发作。<br>　Se usa para prevención de angina |
| 用法、用量<br>Administración y dosis | 　口服：一日 3 ～ 4 次，每次 10 ～ 30mg。<br>　Por vía oral: 10 ~ 30mg y 3 ~ 4 veces al día. |
| 剂型、规格<br>Formulaciones y especificaciones | 　片剂：每片 10mg；20mg。复方制剂：每片含戊四硝醇 20mg、硝酸甘油 0.5mg。<br>　Tableta: 10mg, 20mg; Preparación en compuesto: 20mg de Tetranitrato de pentaeritritilo y 0.5mg de nitroglicerina. |
| 药品名称 Drug Names | 硝酸异山梨酯 Dinitrato de Isosorbida |
| 适应证<br>Indicaciones | 　急性心绞痛发作的防治。<br>　Se usa para tratamiento y prevención de angina aguda. |
| 用法、用量<br>Administración y dosis | 　片剂：急性心绞痛发作时缓解心绞痛，舌下给药，1 次 5mg；预防心绞痛发作，口服，一日 2 ～ 3 次，1 次 5 ～ 10mg，一日 10 ～ 30mg；治疗心力衰竭，口服 1 次 5 ～ 20mg，6 ～ 8 小时一次。外用乳膏：1 次 0.6g，均匀涂抹在心前区约 5cm×5cm，一日 1 次。缓释片：一日 2 次，1 次 1 片。静脉滴注：每小时 2mg，剂量须根据患者反应而调节，且必须密切监测患者脉搏、心率及血压。喷雾吸入：每次 1.25 ～ 3.75mg。<br>　Tableta: para alivio del dolor de angina aguda, medicación sublingual y 5mg cada vez; para prevención de angina, dosis oral de 5 ~ 10mg y 2 ~ 3 veces al día, la dosis diaria es 10 ~ 20mg; para tratamiento de insuficiencia cardíaca, dosis oral de 5 ~ 20mg cada 6 ~ 8 horas al día. Crema tópica: 0.6g diarios y embadurna uniformemente en la zona precordial en un superficie de 5cm×5cm. Tableta de liberación prolongada: 1 tableta y 2 veces al día. Infusión por I.V.: 2mg cada hora y cambia la dosis según la respuesta del paciente y debe observa estrictamente el pulso, el rítmo cardíaco y la presión arterial del paciente. Spray: 1.25 ~ 3.75mg cada vez. |

**续　表**

| 剂型、规格<br>Formulaciones y especificaciones | 普通片：每片 2.5mg；5mg；10mg。缓释片：每片 20mg；40mg。注射液：10mg（10ml）。喷雾剂：250mg/200 次。乳膏：1.5g（10g）。<br><br>Tableta normal: 2.5mg, 5mg, 10mg; Tableta de liberación prolongada: 20mg, 40mg; Inyección: 10mg(10ml); Spray: 250mg/200veces; Crema: 1.5g(10g). |
|---|---|
| **药品名称 Drug Names** | 单硝酸异山梨酯 Mononitrato de isosorbida |
| 适应证<br>Indicaciones | 用于冠心病的长期治疗和预防心绞痛发作，也用于心肌梗死后的治疗。<br><br>Se usa para tratamiento a largo plazo de enfermedad coronaria, prenvencion de angina y tratamiento después del infarto de miocardio. |
| 用法、用量<br>Administración y dosis | 口服，一日 20mg，每日 2 次，必要时可增至一日 3 次，饭后服。缓释片：1 次 1 片，一日 2 次，不宜嚼碎。<br><br>Por vía oral: 20mg y 2 veces al día y en caso necesario puede aumentar a 3 veces al día. Se toma después de alimentos. Tableta de liberación prolongada: 1 tableta y 2 veces al día, no se puede masticar. |
| 剂型、规格<br>Formulaciones y especificaciones | 普通片：每片 20mg；40mg；60mg。<br>缓释片：每片 40mg。<br>Tableta: 20mg, 40mg, 60mg; Tableta de liberación prolongada: 40mg. |
| **药品名称 Drug Names** | 曲美他嗪 Trimetazidina |
| 适应证<br>Indicaciones | 用于冠脉功能不全、心绞痛、陈旧性心肌梗死等。对伴有严重心功能不全者，可与洋地黄苷并用。<br><br>Se usa para tratamiento de La insuficiencia coronaria, angina y Infarto de miocardio antiguo. Para pacientes con grave insuficiencia cardíaca, puede tomarla junto con glucósidos digitálicos. |
| 用法、用量<br>Administración y dosis | 口服：1 次 2～6mg，一日 3 次，饭后服；总剂量每日不超过 18mg。常用维持量为 1 次 1mg，一日 3 次。静脉注射：1 次 8～20mg，加于 25% 葡萄糖注射液 20ml 中。静脉滴注：8～20mg，加于 5% 葡萄糖注射液 500ml 中。<br><br>Por vía oral: 2～6mg y 3 veces al día después de alimentos. La dosis diaria no excede a 18mg. Dosis habitual de mantenimiento es de 1mg y 3 veces al día. Inyección por I.V.: 8～20mg diluidos con 20ml de solución inyectable de glucosa a 25%. Infusión por I.V.: 8～20mg diluidos con 500 ml de solución inyectable de glucosa a 5%. |
| 剂型、规格<br>Formulaciones y especificaciones | 片剂：每片 2mg；3mg。注射液：每支 4mg（2ml）。<br>Tableta: 2mg, 3mg; Inyección: 4mg (2ml). |
| **药品名称 Drug Names** | 双嘧达莫 Dipiridamol |
| 适应证<br>Indicaciones | 弥散性血管内凝血，血栓栓塞性疾病。防止冠心病发展。<br><br>Se usa para tratamiento de coagulación intravascular diseminada (DIC) y enfermedad tromboembólica, prevención del empeoramiento de enfermedad coronaria. |
| 用法、用量<br>Administración y dosis | 口服：每次 25～100mg，一日 3 次，饭前 1 小时服。在症状改善后，可改为每日 50～100mg，分 2 次服用。<br><br>por Vía oral: 25～100mg y 3 veces al día, tomada 1 hora antes de alimentos. Cuando se mejora puede cambiar a 50～100mg diarios divididos en 2 tomas. |
| 剂型、规格<br>Formulaciones y especificaciones | 片剂：每片 25mg。<br>Tableta: 25mg. |
| **药品名称 Drug Names** | 丹参酮 ⅡA 磺酸钠 Tanshinon ⅡA Sulfonato sódico |
| 适应证<br>Indicaciones | 用于冠心病心绞痛、胸闷及心肌梗死，对室性期前收缩也可使用。对冠心病患者的疗效与复方丹参注射液相似。<br><br>Se usa para tratamiento de enfermedad coronaria, angina, opresión en pecho y infarto de miocardio. También es usado en tratamiento de contracciones ventriculares prematuras. Tiene eficacia similar como la solución inyectable Dan Shen en el tratamiento de enfermedad coronaria. |

**续　表**

| 用法、用量<br>Administración y dosis | 　　肌内注射、静脉注射或静脉滴注：一日 1 次 40～80mg。注射用 25% 葡萄糖注射液 20ml 稀释，静脉滴注用 5% 葡萄糖注射液 250～500ml 稀释。<br>　　Inyección por I.M. o I.V. o infusion por I.V. : 40～80mg diarios. Para inyecciones, usa la dilución con 20ml de inyección de glucosa a 25%. Para infusión, usa la dilución con 250～500ml de inyección de glucosa a 5%. |
|---|---|
| 剂型、规格<br>Formulaciones y especificaciones | 　　注射液：每支 10mg（2ml）。<br>　　Inyección: 10mg (2ml). |

| 药品名称 Drug Names | 川芎嗪 Ligustrazina |
|---|---|
| 适应证<br>Indicaciones | 　　适用于闭塞性血管疾病、脑血栓形成、脉管炎、冠心病、心绞痛等。对缺血性脑血管病的急性期、恢复期及其后遗症，如脑供血不足、脑血栓形成、脑栓塞、脑动脉硬化等均有较好疗效，能改善这些疾病引起的偏瘫、失语、吞咽困难、肢体麻木、无力、头痛、头晕、失眠、耳鸣、步态不稳、记忆力减退等症状。<br>　　Se usa para tratamiento de enfermedad vascular oclusiva, trombosis cerebral, tromboangeítis obliterante, enfermedad coronaria y angina. Tiene buena eficacia en tratamiento de enfermedad cerebrovascular isquémica en la etapa aguda y la recuperación así como tratamiento de lassecuelas, por ejempro, insuficiencia cerebral, trombosis cerebral, embolia cerebral y arteriosclerosis cerebral. Puede mejorar las síntomas causada por estas enfermedades tales como la hemiplejía, afasia, disfagia, entumecimiento, debilidad, cefalea, mareo, insomnio, tinnitus, aarcha inestable y pérdida de la memoria. |
| 用法、用量<br>Administración y dosis | 　　口服：磷酸盐片剂一次 2 片，一日 3 次，1 个月为 1 疗程。肌内注射：盐酸盐注射液，每次 2ml，一日 1～2 次。磷酸盐注射液，每次 2～4ml，一日 1～2 次，15 日为 1 疗程，宜缓慢注射。静脉滴注：盐酸盐注射液，每日 1 次 2～4ml，或磷酸盐注射液每日 1 次 4～6ml，均稀释于 5%～10% 葡萄糖注射液（或氯化钠注射液、低分子右旋糖酐注射液）250～500ml 中缓慢滴注，宜在 3～4 小时滴完，10～15 日为 1 疗程。<br>　　Por vía oral: 2 tabletas de ligustrazine fosfato y 3 veces al día, un curso de tratamiento tarda 1 mes. Inyección por I.M.: solución de clorhidrato 2ml y 1～2 veces al día, solución de fosfato 2～4ml y 1～2 veces al día. Un curso de tratamiento tarda 15 días y recomienda inyección lenta. Infusión por I.M.: solución de clorhidrato 2～4ml o solución de fosfato 4～6ml diluidos con 250～500ml de solución de glucosa o de Cloruro de Sodio o dextrano, lenta infusión dentro de 3～4 horas, un curso de tratamiento tarda 10～15 días. |
| 剂型、规格<br>Formulaciones y especificaciones | 　　片剂：每片含川芎嗪磷酸盐 50mg。注射液：盐酸盐注射液，每支 40mg（2ml）；磷酸盐注射液，每支 50mg（2ml）。<br>　　Tableta: cada una incluye 50mg de ligustrazine fosfato. Inyección: de clorhidrato 40mg(2ml), de fosfato 50mg(2ml). |

| 药品名称 Drug Names | 葛根素 Puerarina |
|---|---|
| 适应证<br>Indicaciones | 　　用于辅助治疗冠心病、心绞痛、心肌梗死，视网膜动、静脉阻塞、突发性耳聋、血性脑血管病、小儿病毒性心肌炎、糖尿病等。眼科用于原发性开角型青光眼、高眼压症、原发性闭角型青光眼、继发性青光眼。<br>　　Se usa para tratamiento adyuvante de enfermedad coronaria, angina, infarto de miocardio, oclusión de la vena retiniana, o oclusión de la arteria retiniana, sordera súbita, enfermedad cerebrovascular hemorrágico, miocarditis viral en niños y la diabetes. En oftalmología, se utiliza en tratamiento de glaucoma primario de ángulo abierto, hipertensión ocular, glaucoma primario de ángulo cerrado y glaucoma secundario. |
| 用法、用量<br>Administración y dosis | 　　静脉滴注：每次 200～600mg，加入 5% 葡萄糖注射液 250～500ml 中静脉滴注，一日一次，10～20 日为一疗程，可连续使用 2～3 个疗程。超过 65 岁的老人连续使用总剂量不超过 5g。葛根素葡萄糖注射液：静脉滴注，每次 0.4～0.6g，一日 1 次，15 日为一疗程。滴眼液：1%，一次 1～2 滴，滴入眼睑内，闭目 3～5 分钟。首日 3 次，以后一日 2 次，早晚各一次。偶有一过性异物感或刺激感。 |

**续　表**

| | Infusión por I.V.: 200 ~ 600mg diluidos con 250 ~ 500ml de solución inyectable de glucosa a 5%, una vez al día y un curso de tratamiento tarda 10 ~ 20 días y puede continuar con 2 ~ 3 cursos. Para ancianos mayores de 65 años la dosis total de uso consecutivo no excede a 5g. En caso de inyección de purarin, la infusión por I.V. se aplica a 0.4 ~ 0.6g diarios y un curso de tratamiento tarda 15 días. Gota oftalmología: 1% y 1 ~ 2 gotas cada vez, instilación en párpados y tener los ojos cerrados en 3 ~ 5 minutos. En el primer día lo utiliza 3 veces y luego 2 veces al día tomados en la mañana y en la noche. Ocasionalmente causará sensación de cuerpo extraño o irritación. |
|---|---|
| 剂型、规格<br>Formulaciones y especificaciones | 注射液：每支 100mg（2ml）；250mg（5ml）。注射用葛根素：每支 0.1g。葛根素葡萄糖注射液：每瓶 0.2g（100ml）；0.25g（100ml）；0.3g（150ml）；0.3g（250ml）；0.5g（250ml）。各种规格均含 5% 葡萄糖液。<br><br>Inyección: 100mg (2ml), 250mg (5ml); Puerarin para inyección: 0.1g; Inyección de purarin: 0.2g(100ml),0.25g(100ml),0.3g(150ml), 0.3g(250ml),0.5g(250ml), todo incluye glucosa a 5%. |
| 药品名称 Drug Names | 愈风宁心片 YuFengNingXin comprimidos |
| 适应证<br>Indicaciones | 具有增加脑血流量及冠脉血流量的作用。可用于缓解高血压症状（颈项强痛）、治疗心绞痛及突发性耳聋，有一定疗效。<br><br>Se usa para aumentar el flujo sanguíneo cerebral y flujo sanguíneo coronario. Puede se usa para alivio de síntomas de la hipertensión (dolor en el cuello), tratamiento de angina y Sordera súbita. |
| 用法、用量<br>Administración y dosis | 每次 5 片，一日 3 次。<br>5 tabletas y 3 veces al día. |
| 剂型、规格<br>Formulaciones y especificaciones | 片剂：每片含总黄酮 60mg。<br>Tableta: cada una incluye 60mg de flavonoide. |
| 药品名称 Drug Names | 银杏叶提取物 Extracto de hoja de Ginkgo |
| 适应证<br>Indicaciones | 用于治疗冠心病心绞痛、脑血管痉挛、脑供血不全、记忆力衰退等。也适用于支气管哮喘、老年性痴呆等病。<br><br>Se usa para tratamiento de enfermedad coronaria, angina, vasoespasmo cerebral, Insuficiencia cerebrovascular y pérdida de la memoria. También se usa en tratamiento de asma bronquial y enfermedad de Alzheimer. |
| 用法、用量<br>Administración y dosis | 口服：每次 20 ~ 40mg，一日 3 次。肌内注射：每次 7 ~ 15mg，一日 1 ~ 2 次。静脉滴注：每日 87.5 ~ 175mg。<br><br>Por vía oral: 20 ~ 40mg y 3 veces al día. Inyección por I.M.: 7 ~ 15mg y 1 ~ 2veces al día. Infusión por I.V.: 87.5 ~ 175mg diarios. |
| 剂型、规格<br>Formulaciones y especificaciones | 常用的制剂有片剂、缓释糖衣片、口服液、强化滴剂、酊剂、注射液及静脉滴注剂等。<br><br>uso en formulaciones de tabletas, tabletas de liberacioón prolongada recubiertas de azúcar, solución oral, gotas, tinturas, inyecciones y solución de infusión por I.V.. |
| 药品名称 Drug Names | 地奥心血康 DiAoXinXuekang |
| 适应证<br>Indicaciones | 用于冠心病、心绞痛，能改善症状。<br>Se usa para alivio de síntomas de enfermedad coronaria y angina. |
| 用法、用量<br>Administración y dosis | 口服，一次 0.2g，一日 3 次，有效后可改为 1 次 0.1g，一日 3 次。<br>Por vía oral: dosis 0.2g diarios divididos en 3 tomas. Cuando tenga efecto puede cambiar a 0.1mg diarios divididos en 3 tomas. |
| 剂型、规格<br>Formulaciones y especificaciones | 常用其胶囊、片剂、颗粒和软胶囊（均为 0.1g）。口服液每支 0.1g（10ml）。<br>Cápsula/Tableta/Gránulos: 0.1g; Solución oral: 0.1g(10ml). |

**续　表**

| 药品名称 Drug Names | 辅酶Ⅰ Coenzima Ⅰ |
|---|---|
| 适应证<br>Indicaciones | 用于冠心病，可改善冠心病的胸闷、心绞痛等症状。<br><br>Se usa para tratamiento de enfermedad coronaria, alivio de síntomas relativas como opresión en el pecho y la angina. |
| 用法、用量<br>Administración y<br>dosis | 肌内注射：一日 1 次 5mg，溶于 0.9% 氯化钠注射液 2ml，14 日为一疗程。大多应用 2 个疗程。<br><br>Inyección por I.M.: solución de 5mg de dicha droga con 2ml solución de Cloruro de Sodio a 0.9%. Un curso de tratamiento tarda 14 días y la medicación suele tardar 2 cursos. |
| 剂型、规格<br>Formulaciones y<br>especificaciones | 注射用辅酶Ⅰ：每支 5mg。<br>Inyección de Nadide: 5mg. |

10.5　周围血管舒张药 Vasodilatadores periféricos

| 药品名称 Drug Names | 二氢麦角碱 Dihidroergotoxina |
|---|---|
| 适应证<br>Indicaciones | 主要与异丙嗪、哌替啶等配成冬眠合剂应用。也可用于动脉内膜炎、肢端动脉痉挛症、血管痉挛性偏头痛等。<br><br>Se usa principalmente para hacer cóctel lítico junto con prometazina, petidina etc. Indicación también para tratamiento de Meningitis Arterial, síndrome de Raynaud y Migraña por el Vasoespasmo. |
| 用法、用量<br>Administración y<br>dosis | 肌内注射或皮下注射，每日或隔日 1 次，每次 0.3 ~ 0.6mg；亦可舌下给药（含片），每 4 ~ 6 小时 1 次，每次 0.5 ~ 2mg。不宜口服。<br><br>Inyección intramuscular o subcutánea: dosis 0.3 ~ 0.6mg cada 1´o 2 días. Por vía sublingual (comprimidos): 0.5 ~ 2mg cada 4 ~ 6 horas. No puede tomarlo por vía oral. |
| 剂型、规格<br>Formulaciones y<br>especificaciones | 含片：每片 0.25mg；0.5mg。　注射液：每支 0.3mg（1ml）。<br>Tableta sublingual：0.25mg, 0.5mg; Inyección: 0.3mg (1ml). |

| 药品名称 Drug Names | 烟酸 Ácido nicotínico |
|---|---|
| 适应证<br>Indicaciones | 烟酸可用于治疗糙皮病，但因易于产生面部潮红等不良反应，而烟酰胺则无，故一般选用后者。此外，烟酸还有较强的周围血管扩张作用，口服后数分钟即见效，可维持数分钟至 1 小时，用于治疗血管性偏头痛、头痛、脑动脉血栓形成、肺栓塞、内耳眩晕症、冻伤、中心性视网膜脉络膜炎等。大剂量（一日 2 ~ 6g）可降低血脂（主要是三酰甘油），适用于Ⅳ、Ⅲ、Ⅴ型高脂血症，亦可用于Ⅱ型患者。烟酰胺无扩张血管及降血脂作用。<br><br>Se usa para tratamiento de pelagra pero causa facilmente reacciónes adversas como enrojacimiento facial, por lo cual se usa más la nicotinamida que no hay dicha reacción. Además el Ácido Nicotñinico es un fuerte vasodilatador y se ve efecto dentro de unos minutos tras medicamento y puede mantener el efecto hasta una hora, también se utiliza en tratamiento de migraña vascular, cefalea, trombosis de la arteria cerebral, embolia pulmonar, vértigos en oídos internos, quemadura por frío y choroiditis de la retina central. Con dosis grande de 2 ~ 6g diarios puede reducir los lípidos sanguíneos (principalmente triglicéridos) y hiperlipidemia de tipo IV, III, V y II. La Nicotinamida no es eficaz para la dilatación de los vasos sanguíneos y reducción de lípidos sanguíneos. |
| 用法、用量<br>Administración y<br>dosis | （1）口服：一次 50 ~ 200mg，一日 3 ~ 4 次，餐后服。用于降血脂，一日 3 ~ 6g，分 3 ~ 4 次于餐后服用。<br>（2）静脉注射或肌内注射：一次 10 ~ 50mg，一日 1 ~ 3 次。用于脑血管疾病：一次 50 ~ 200mg，加于 5% ~ 10% 葡萄糖注射液 100 ~ 200ml 中静脉滴注，一日 1 次。<br><br>(1) Por vía oral: 50 ~ 200mg y 3 ~ 4 veces al día después de alimentos. En caso hipolipemiante, la dosis es de 3 ~ 6g diarios didividos en 3 ~ 4 tomas después de alimentos.<br>(2) Inyección por I.V. o I.M.: 10 ~ 50mg y 1 ~ 3 veces al día. Si son enfermedades cerebrovasculares, la dosis es 50 ~ 200mg diluidos con 100 ~ 200ml de solución de glucosa a 5% ~ 10% y se administra infusión por I.V. una vez al día. |
| 剂型、规格<br>Formulaciones y<br>especificaciones | 片剂：每片 50mg；100mg。注射液：每支 20mg（2ml）；50mg（1ml）；100mg（2ml）；50mg（5ml）。<br>Tableta: 50mg, 100mg; Inyección: 20mg (2ml), 50mg (1ml), 100mg (2ml), 50mg (5ml). |

续　表

| 药品名称 Drug Names | 烟酸肌醇酯 Nicotinato de inositol |
|---|---|
| 适应证<br>Indicaciones | 用于高脂血症、冠心病、各种末梢血管障碍性疾病（如闭塞性动脉硬化症、肢端动脉痉挛症、冻伤、血管性偏头痛等）的辅助治疗。<br><br>Se usa en terapia adyuvante de hiperlipidemia, enfermedad coronaria y otros trastornos vasculares periféricos, por ejempro Arteriosclerosis obliterante, síndrome de Raynaud, Frostbite y Migraña vascular. |
| 用法、用量<br>Administración y dosis | 口服：一日 3 次，一次 0.2 ~ 0.6g。连续服用 1 ~ 3 个月。<br>Por vía oral: 0.2 ~ 0.6g y 3veces al dia. Medicamento continuo de 1 ~ 3 meses. |
| 剂型、规格<br>Formulaciones y especificaciones | 片剂：每片 0.2g。<br>Tableta: 0.2g. |
| 药品名称 Drug Names | 维生素 E 烟酸酯 Niacina de Vitamina E |
| 适应证<br>Indicaciones | 用于治疗脑动脉硬化、脑卒中、脑外伤后遗症、脂质代谢异常、高血压、冠心病及循环障碍引起的各种疾病。其不良反应小，无烟酸样面部潮红等不良反应。<br><br>Se usa para tratamiento de arteriosclerosis cerebral, apoplejía, secuelas de la lesión cerebral, anormal metabolismo lipídico, hipertensión, enfermedad coronaria u otras enfermedades causadas por trastornos circulatorios. Tiene poca reacción adversa, no tiene efecto secundario de enrojecimiento facial como toma la niacina. |
| 用法、用量<br>Administración y dosis | 口服：每次 100 ~ 200mg，一日 3 次，餐后服用。<br>Por vía oral: 100 ~ 200mg y 3 veces al dia después de alimentos. |
| 剂型、规格<br>Formulaciones y especificaciones | 胶囊剂：每粒 100mg。<br>Cápsula: 100mg. |
| 药品名称 Drug Names | 罂粟碱 Papaverina |
| 适应证<br>Indicaciones | 主要用于脑血栓形成、肺栓塞、肢端动脉痉挛症及动脉栓塞性疼痛等。对高血压、心绞痛、幽门痉挛、胆绞痛、肠绞痛、支气管哮喘等在一般剂量下疗效不显著。<br><br>Se usa para tratamiento de trombosis cerebral, embolia pulmonar, síndrome de Raynaud y dolor del embolización de las arterias. No tiene efecto evidencial con dosis habitual para hipertensión, angina, espasmo pilórico, cólico biliar, cólico y asma bronquial. |
| 用法、用量<br>Administración y dosis | 口服：常用量，每次 30 ~ 60mg，一日 3 次；极量，一次 200mg，一日 600mg。肌内注射或静脉滴注：每次 30mg，一日 90 ~ 120mg，一日量不宜超过 300mg。<br><br>Por vía oral: La dosis habitual es de 30 ~ 60mg y 3 veces al dia. Dosis máxima no excede a 200mg cada vez y 600mg diarios. Administración de inyección intramuscular o infusión intravenosa: 30mg cada vez y dosis diaria es de 90 ~ 120mg. La máxima no excede a 300mg diarios. |
| 剂型、规格<br>Formulaciones y especificaciones | 片剂：每片 30mg。注射液：每支 30mg（1ml）。<br>Tableta: 30mg; Inyección: 30mg (1ml). |
| 药品名称 Drug Names | 西地那非 Sildenafil |
| 适应证<br>Indicaciones | 用于治疗勃起功能障碍（ED）。<br>Se usa para tratamiento de Disfunción Eréctil. |
| 用法、用量<br>Administración y dosis | 一般剂量为 50mg，在性活动前约 1 小时（或 0.5 ~ 4 小时）服用。基于药效和耐药性，剂量可增至 100mg（最大推荐剂量）或降至 25mg。每日最多服用 1 次。<br><br>Dosis habitual por vía oral: 50mg tomada 1 hora (ó 0.5 ~ 4 horas) antes de actividades sexuales. Depende del efecto y la tolerancia a la droga puede aumentar la dosis a 100mg como máximo o disminuir a 25mg. Una toma al día como máximo. |

续 表

| 剂型、规格<br>Formulaciones y especificaciones | 片剂：25mg；50mg；100mg。<br>Tableta: 25mg, 50mg, 100mg. |
|---|---|
| **药品名称 Drug Names** | 环扁桃酯 Ciclandelato |
| 适应证<br>Indicaciones | 用于脑血管意外及其后遗症、脑动脉硬化症、脑外伤后遗症、肢端动脉痉挛症、手足发绀、闭塞性动脉内膜炎、内耳眩晕症等。<br><br>Se usa para tratamiento de accidente cerebrovascular y sus secuelas, Arteriosclerosis cerebral, secuelas de la lesión cerebral, síndrome de Raynaud, cianosis en las manos y pies, Meningitis arterial oclusiva y vértigo del oído interno. |
| 用法、用量<br>Administración y dosis | 一次服 100～200mg，一日 3～4 次。症状改善后，可减量至一日 300～400mg。对脑血管疾病一般每次服 200～400mg，一日 3 次。<br><br>Por vía oral: 100～200mg y 3～4 veces al día. Cuando se mejora el síntoma puede disminuir la dosis a 300～400mg diarios. Dosis habidual para enfermedades cerebrovasculares: 200～400mg y 3 veces al día. |
| 剂型、规格<br>Formulaciones y especificaciones | 胶囊剂：每粒 100mg。<br>Cápsula: 100mg. |
| **药品名称 Drug Names** | 长春西汀 Vinpocetina |
| 适应证<br>Indicaciones | 用于治疗由于大脑血液循环障碍引起的精神性或神经性症状如记忆力障碍、失语症、行动障碍、头晕、头痛等，高血压性脑病、大脑血管痉挛、大脑动脉内膜炎、进行性脑血管硬化。眼科用于因视网膜和脉络膜血管硬化及血管痉挛引起的斑点退化。耳科用于治疗老年性耳聋、眩晕等。<br><br>Se usa para tratamiento de los síntomas psiquiátricos o neurológicos causado por trastornos de la circulación sanguínea cerebral, por ejempro trastornos de la memoria, afasia, Problemas de movilidad, Mareos y cefalea, y tratamiento de Encefalopatía hipertensiva, Vasoespasmo cerebral, meningitis en arteria cerebral y la esclerosis vascular cerebral progresiva. En oftalmología, se utiliza para tratamiento de la degeneración macular causada por la esclerosis vascular de la retina y la coroides. En otología, utilización para tratamiento de presbiacusia y vértigo. |
| 用法、用量<br>Administración y dosis | 急性病例可用注射剂，每次 10mg，一日 3 次，静脉滴注或静脉注射，用时以 0.9% 氯化钠注射液稀释到 5 倍体积。然后口服片剂，一日 3 次，每次 1～2 片。对慢性患者，一日 3 次，每次 1～2 片。维持剂量时一次 1 片，一日 3 次。<br><br>Para casos agudos puede utilizar la inyección de 10mg y 3 veces al dia en infusión o inyección por I.V. diluidos con 5 cantidad dela inyección de Cloruro de Sodio a 0.9%. Luego cambia a tomar tabletas por vía oral de 1～2 tabletas y 3 veces al día. Para casos crónicos, dosis oral de 1～2 tabletas y 3 veces al día. Dosis de mantenimiento es 1 tableta y 3 veces al día. |
| 剂型、规格<br>Formulaciones y especificaciones | 片剂：每片 5mg。注射液：每支 10mg（2ml）。<br>Tableta: 5mg; Inyección: 10mg (2ml). |
| **药品名称 Drug Names** | 倍他司汀 Betahistina |
| 适应证<br>Indicaciones | 用于内耳眩晕症，对脑动脉硬化、缺血性脑血管病、头部外伤或高血压所致的体位性眩晕、耳鸣等亦可用。<br><br>Se usa para alivio del Vértigo del oído interno y vértigo ortostático y Tinnitus causados por Arteriosclerosis cerebral, enfermedad cerebrovascular isquémica, traumatismo craneal o la hipertensión. |
| 用法、用量<br>Administración y dosis | 口服每次 4～8mg，一日 2～4 次。肌内注射一次 2～4mg，一日 2 次。<br>Por vía oral: 4～8mg y 2～4 veces al dia. Por vía I.M.: 2～4mg y 2 veces al dia. |
| 剂型、规格<br>Formulaciones y especificaciones | 片剂：每片 4mg；5mg。注射液：每支 2mg（2ml）；4mg（2ml）。<br>Tableta: 4mg, 5mg; Inyección: 2mg (2ml), 4mg (2ml). |

| 药品名称 Drug Names | 地芬尼多 Difenidol |
|---|---|
| 适应证<br>Indicaciones | 用于各种原因引起的眩晕症如椎基底动脉供血不全、梅尼埃病、自主神经功能紊乱、晕车晕船等。<br><br>Se usa para tratamiento de vértigos causados por Insuficiencia vertebrobasilar, enfermedad de Meniere, disfunción autonómica, la cinetosis etc. |
| 用法、用量<br>Administración y dosis | 口服：一日 3 次，每次 25 ~ 50mg。<br>Por vía oral: 25 ~ 50mg y 3 veces al dia. |
| 剂型、规格<br>Formulaciones y especificaciones | 片剂：每片 25mg。<br>Tableta: 25mg. |
| 药品名称 Drug Names | 血管舒缓素 Kallidinogenasa |
| 适应证<br>Indicaciones | 用于脑动脉硬化症、闭塞性动脉内膜炎、闭塞性血管炎、四肢慢性溃疡、肢端动脉痉挛症、手足发绀、老年性四肢冷感、中央视网膜炎、眼底出血等。由于易被消化酶破坏，口服作用时间短，效力不及注射。<br><br>Se usa para tratamiento de Arteriosclerosis cerebral, Meningitis arterial oclusiva, Vasculitis oclusiva, úlcera crónica en las extremidades, síndrome de Raynaud, cianosis en manos y pies, apatía senil en las extremidades, retinitis central y hemorragia retiniana. Susceptible al daño de las enzimas digestivas, tiene menor eficacia la administrción oral en comparación con la inyectable. |
| 用法、用量<br>Administración y dosis | ①口服，每次 1 片（含 10U），空腹时服。②注射临用时溶解（10U/1.5ml）后进行肌内注射或皮下注射，一次量 10 ~ 20U，每日 1 ~ 2 次。轻症每日 10U，以 3 周为一疗程。眼科亦可作眼结膜下注射，每次 5U。<br><br>① Por vía oral: 1 comprimido cada vez y toma en ayunas. ② Inyección intramuscular o subcutánea: solución a 10 unidades/1.5ml, cada vez 10 ~ 20unidades y 2 veces al dia. Para casos leves, dosis diaria es de 10 unidades y un curso de tratamiento tarda 3 semanas. Para enfermedades oftalmológicas, puede tomar inyección conjuntival de 5 unidades cada vez. |
| 剂型、规格<br>Formulaciones y especificaciones | 片剂：每片 10U。<br>注射用血管舒缓素：每支 10U。<br>Tableta: 10 unidades; Kallidinogenase para inyección: 10 U. |
| 药品名称 Drug Names | 二氢麦角胺 Dihidroergotamina |
| 适应证<br>Indicaciones | 用于偏头痛急性发作及血管性头痛等。<br>Se usa para alivio de los ataques agudos de migraña y cefalea vascular. |
| 用法、用量<br>Administración y dosis | 因口服吸收不佳，治偏头痛多采用注射，肌内注射一次 1 ~ 2mg，一日 1 ~ 2 次。口服一次 1 ~ 3mg，一日 2 ~ 3 次。<br><br>Debido a la mala absorción de la administración oral, generalmente es más recomendable la inyección. Inyección por I.M.: 1 ~ 2mg cada vez y 1 ~ 2 veces al dia. Por vía oral: 1 ~ 3mg cada vez y 2 ~ 3 veces al dia. |
| 剂型、规格<br>Formulaciones y especificaciones | 片剂：1mg。注射液：1mg（1ml）。<br>Tableta: 1mg; Inyección: 1mg (1ml). |
| 药品名称 Drug Names | 尼麦角林 Nicergolina |
| 适应证<br>Indicaciones | 用于脑血管疾病及下肢闭塞性动脉内膜炎等。<br>Se usa para enfermedad cerebrovascular y extremidad inferior arterial oclusiva meningitis. |
| 用法、用量<br>Administración y dosis | 口服：一次 5mg，一日 3 次；肌内注射或静脉注射：一次 2.5 ~ 5mg。<br>Por vía oral: dosis 15mg diarios divididos en 3 veces. Inyección I.M. O I.V..: 2.5 ~ 5mg cada vez. |

**续　表**

| 剂型、规格<br>Formulaciones y<br>especificaciones | 片剂：5mg。注射液：2.5mg（1ml）。<br>Tableta:5mg; Inyección: 2.5mg (1ml). |
|---|---|
| **药品名称 Drug Names** | 长春胺 Vincamina |
| 适应证<br>Indicaciones | 用于脑血管障碍、脑栓塞、脑血栓形成及出血后遗症等。对脑动脉硬化症的疗效比二氢麦角碱和罂粟碱强，需长期应用方可见效。<br>Se usa para tratamiento de los trastornos cerebrovasculares, embolia cerebral y secuelas de la trombosis y hemorragia cerebral. Tiene mejor eficacia en tratamiento de arteriosclerosis cerebral en comparación con dihydroergotoxine y papaverina y necesita medicamento a largo plazo. |
| 用法、用量<br>Administración y<br>dosis | 口服：一次 5～20mg，一日 2～3 次；肌内注射：一次 5～15mg，一日 2～3 次。<br>Por vía oral: 5 ~ 20mg cada vez y 2 ~ 3 veces al dia. Inyección por I.M,: 5 ~ 15mg cada vez y 2 ~ 3 veces al dia. |
| 剂型、规格<br>Formulaciones y<br>especificaciones | 片剂：5mg。注射液：5mg（2ml）。<br>Tableta:5mg; Inyección: 5mg (2ml). |

10.6　降血压药 Antihipertensivos

| **药品名称 Drug Names** | 可乐定 Clonidina |
|---|---|
| 适应证<br>Indicaciones | 本品预防偏头痛亦有效。亦能降低眼压，可用于治疗开角型青光眼。<br>Se usa para prevención de la migraña, reducir la presión intraocular y tratamiento del glaucoma de ángulo abierto. |
| 用法、用量<br>Administración y<br>dosis | （1）治疗高血压：口服，常用量，每次服 0.075～0.15mg，一日 3 次。可逐渐增加剂量，通常维持剂量为一日 0.2～0.8mg。极量，一次 0.6mg。缓慢静脉注射：每次 0.15～0.3mg，加于 50% 葡萄糖注射液 20～40ml 中（多用于三期高血压及其他危重高血压病）注射。<br>（2）预防偏头痛：一日 0.1mg，分 2 次服，8 周为一疗程（第 4 周以后，一日量可增至 0.15mg）。<br>（3）治青光眼：用 0.25% 液滴眼。低血压患者慎用。<br>(1) En tratamiento de hipertensión: Por vía oral y la dosis habitual es de 0.075 ~ 0.15mg y 3 veces al dia. Puede aumentar la dosis agradualmente. Dosis de mantenimiento es de 0.2 ~ 0.8mg diarios y la dosis máxima no excede a 0.6mg cada vez. Inyección lenta por I.V.: solución de 0.15 ~ 0.3mg de dicha droga con 20 ~ 40ml de inyección de glucosa al 50% (uso princial en tratamiento del tercer etapa de hipertensión u otras hipertensiónes graves).<br>(2) En prevención de migraña: 0.1mg diarios divididos en 2 tomas. Un curso de tratamiento tarda 8 semanas y desde la quinta semana puede aumentar la dosis diaria a 0.15mg.<br>(3) En tratamiento de glaucoma：gotas a 0.25%. Pacientes con hipotensión ten precaución al utilizarla. |
| 剂型、规格<br>Formulaciones y<br>especificaciones | 片剂：每片 0.075mg；0.15mg。贴片：每片 2mg。注射液：每支 0.15mg（1ml）。滴眼液：12.5mg（5ml）。<br>Tableta: 0.075mg, 0.15mg; Parche: 2mg; Inyección: 0.15mg (1ml); Gota oftalmológica：12.5mg (5ml). |
| **药品名称 Drug Names** | 哌唑嗪 Prazosina |
| 适应证<br>Indicaciones | 用于治疗轻、中度高血压，常与 β 受体拮抗剂或利尿剂合用，降压效果更好。由于本品既能扩张容量血管，降低前负荷，又能扩张阻力血管，降低后负荷，可用于治疗中、重度慢性充血性心力衰竭及心肌梗死后心力衰竭。对常规疗法（洋地黄类、利尿剂）无效或效果不显著的心力衰竭患者也有效。<br>Se usa para tratamiento de hipertensión leve y moderada y siempre se usa junto con antagonista de los receptores β y diuréticos para conseguir mejor efecto antihipertensivo. Como puede reducir la precarga ampliando la capacidad de los vasos sanguíneo y reducir la poscarga extendiendo la capacidad de los vasos de resistencia, se usa en el tratamiento de insuficiencia cardiaca congestiva crónica en etapa moderada y grave. Es eficaz para pacientes de insuficiencia cardiaca que no consiguen efectos válidos de la terapia convencional. |

**续 表**

| | |
|---|---|
| 用法、用量<br>Administración y dosis | 口服：开始每次 0.5～1mg，一日 1.5～3mg，以后逐渐增至一日 6～15mg。对充血性心力衰竭，维持量通常为一日 4～20mg，分次服用。<br>Por vía oral: La dosis inicial 0.5～1mg cada vez y dosis diaria de 1.5～3mg. Incrementa gradualmente la dosis hasta 6～15mg diarios. Para insuficiencia cardíaca congestiva, la dosis de mantenimiento es 4～20mg diarios divididas en varias tomas |
| 剂型、规格<br>Formulaciones y especificaciones | 片剂：每片 0.5mg；1mg；2mg；5mg。<br>Tableta: 0.5mg, 1mg, 2mg, 5mg. |
| 药品名称 Drug Names | 特拉唑嗪 Terazosina |
| 适应证<br>Indicaciones | 用于高血压，也可用于良性前列腺增生。<br>Se usa para tratamiento de hipertensión y también se usa en la hiperplasia prostática benigna. |
| 用法、用量<br>Administración y dosis | 口服：开始时，一次不超过 1mg，睡前服用，以后可根据情况逐渐增量，一般为一日 8～10mg；一日最大剂量 20mg。用于前列腺肥大，一日剂量为 5～10mg。<br>Por vía oral: La dosis inicial no excede a 1mg y debe tomarlos antes de acostarse. Luego puede incrementar la dosis según la necesidad. La dosis diaria habitual es de 8～10mg y la máxima no excede a 20mg diarios. Para hipertrofia prostática，la dosis diaria es 5～10mg. |
| 剂型、规格<br>Formulaciones y especificaciones | 片剂：每片 0.5mg；1mg；2mg；5mg；10mg。<br>Tableta: 0.5mg, 1mg, 2mg, 5mg, 10mg. |
| 药品名称 Drug Names | 多沙唑嗪 Doxazosina |
| 适应证<br>Indicaciones | 用于高血压。<br>Se usa para tratamiento de hipertensión. |
| 用法、用量<br>Administración y dosis | 开始时，口服一日 1 次 0.5mg，根据情况可每 1～2 周逐渐增加剂量至一日 2mg，然后再增量至一日 4～8mg。<br>Por vía oral: La dosis inicial es de 0.5mg al dia y según la situación, puede aumentar la dosis cada 1～2 semanas a 2mg diarios e incluso a 4～8mg diarios. |
| 剂型、规格<br>Formulaciones y especificaciones | 常用甲磺酸盐的片剂：每片 0.5mg；1mg；2mg；4mg；8mg。<br>Tableta de metanosulfonato común: 0.5mg, 1mg, 2mg, 4mg, 8mg. |
| 药品名称 Drug Names | 乌拉地尔 Urapidilo |
| 适应证<br>Indicaciones | 用于各类型的高血压（口服）。可与利尿降压药、β 受体拮抗药合用；也用于高血压危象及手术前、中、后对高血压升高的控制性降压（静脉注射）。<br>Se usa para tratamiento de hipertensión (vía oral). Puede usar con medicamentos antihipertensivos y diuréticos, antagonista de los receptores β. Utilización también en hipotensión controlada (por vía intravenosa) antes o durante o después de la cirugía y la crisis hipertensiva. |
| 用法、用量<br>Administración y dosis | 口服：开始时一次 60mg，早晚各服 1 次，如血压逐渐下降，可减量为每次 30mg。维持量一日 30～180mg。<br>静脉注射：一般剂量为 25～50mg，如用 50mg，应分 2 次给药，其间隔为 5 分钟。<br>静脉滴注：将 250mg 溶于输液 500ml 中，开始滴速为 6mg/min，维持剂量滴速平均为 120mg/h。<br>Por vía oral: La dosis inicial es de 60mg en la mañana y en la noche. Si la presión arterial baja gradualmente puede disminuir la dosis a 30mg cada vez. Dosis diaria de mantenimiento es del 30～180mg. Inyección intravenosa: dosis habidual es de 25～50mg. Si necesita aplicar 50mg, debe dividirla en 2 tomas y con 5 minutos de intervalo. Infusión intravenosa: solución 250mg:500ml a velocidad inicial de 6mg/minuto y la de mantenimiento es del 120mg/hora. |
| 剂型、规格<br>Formulaciones y especificaciones | 缓释胶囊剂：每胶囊 30mg；60mg。注射液：每支 25mg（5ml）；50mg（10ml）。<br>Cápsulas de liberación prolongada: 30mg, 60mg; Inyección: 25mg (5ml), 50mg (10ml). |

**续　表**

| 药品名称 Drug Names | 利血平 Reserpina |
|---|---|
| 适应证<br>Indicaciones | 对于轻度至中等度的早期高血压，疗效显著（精神紧张病例疗效尤好），长期应用小剂量，可将多数患者的血压稳定于正常范围内，但对严重和晚期病例，单用本品疗效较差，常与肼屈嗪、氢氯噻嗪等合用，以增加疗效。<br><br>Tiene efecto significativo en el tratamiento de hipertensión leve y moderada en etapa temprana (especialmente para alivio de estrés mental). Pequeña dosis para medicamento a largo plazo. Para la mayoría de os pacientes puede mantener la presión arterial en un rango normal pero para casos graves y avanzados, el efecto de dicha utilización sola es mala y para que tiene más eficacia siempre lo usa junto con hidralazina y hidroclorotiazida. |
| 用法、用量<br>Administración y dosis | 作为降压药，每日口服 0.25～0.5mg，一次顿服或 3 次分服。如长期应用，须酌减剂量只求维持药效即可。作为安定药，每日量 0.5～5mg。亦可肌内注射或静脉注射。<br><br>Indicación antihipertensiva: por vía oral 0.25～0.5mg tomada en una sóla vez o divididos en 3 veces. Si es medicación a largo plazo, debe reducir la dosis de mantenimiento. Indicación antipsicótica: dosis diaria 0.5～5mg. También puede utilizarse en inyección por I.M. o I.V.. |
| 剂型、规格<br>Formulaciones y especificaciones | 片剂：每片 0.25mg。<br>注射液：每支 1mg（1ml）。<br>Tableta: 0.25mg;<br>Inyección: 1mg (1ml). |
| 药品名称 Drug Names | 肼屈嗪 Hidralazina |
| 适应证<br>Indicaciones | 现多用于肾性高血压及舒张压较高的患者。单独使用效果不甚好，且易引起不良反应，故多与利血平、氢氯噻嗪、胍乙啶或普萘洛尔合用以增加疗效。<br><br>Se usa principalmente en alvivio de hipertensión renal y alta presión arterial diastólica. Efecto de utilización individual no es bueno y facilmente atrae reacciones adversas, por lo que para que sea mas eficaz, siempre usa junto con reserpina, hidroclorotiazida, guanetidina o propranolol. |
| 用法、用量<br>Administración y dosis | 口服或静脉注射、肌内注射。一般开始时用小量，每次 10mg，一日 3～4 次，用药 2～4 日。以后用量逐渐增加。维持量，一日 30～200mg，分次服用。<br><br>Por vía oral o inyecciones por I.V. o I.M.. La dosis inicial es de 10mg, 3～4 veces al dia y la medicación tarda 2～4 días. Incrementa gradualmente la dosis después. Dosis de mantenimiento 30～200mg diarios divididos en varias tomas. |
| 剂型、规格<br>Formulaciones y especificaciones | 片剂：每片 10mg；25mg；50mg。缓释片：每片 50mg。注射液：每支 20mg（1ml）。<br>Tableta：10mg，25mg, 50mg; Tableta de liberación prolongada: 50mg; Inyección: 20mg (1ml). |
| 药品名称 Drug Names | 双肼屈嗪 Dihidralazina |
| 适应证<br>Indicaciones | 现多用于肾性高血压及舒张压较高的患者。单独使用效果不甚好，且易引起不良反应，故多与利血平、氢氯噻嗪、胍乙啶或普萘洛尔合用以增加疗效。<br><br>Se usa principalmente en alvivio de hipertensión renal y alta presión arterial diastólica. Efecto de utilización individual no es bueno y facilmente atrae reacciones adversas, por lo que para que sea mas eficaz, siempre usa junto con reserpina, hidroclorotiazida, guanetidina o propranolol. |
| 用法、用量<br>Administración y dosis | 口服：一次 12.5～25mg，一日 25～50mg。发生耐受性后，可加大到每次 50mg，一日 3 次。<br><br>Por vía oral: 12.5～25mg cada vez y la dosis diaria es 25～50mg. Después de aparecer tolerancia a la droga, puede aumentar a 50mg y 3 veces al dia. |
| 剂型、规格<br>Formulaciones y especificaciones | 片剂：每片 12.5mg；25mg。　　注射用双肼屈嗪：25mg。<br>Tableta: 12.5mg, 25mg; Inyección de Dihidralazina：25mg. |
| 药品名称 Drug Names | 硝普钠 Nitroprusiato sódico |
| 适应证<br>Indicaciones | 用于其他降压药无效的高血压危象，疗效可靠，且由于其作用持续时间较短，易于掌握。用于心力衰竭，能使衰竭的左心室排血量增加，心力衰竭症状得以缓解。<br><br>Se usa para la crisis hipertensiva que otros fármacos antihipertensivos son ineficaces, es eficaz y fiable, y la duración de la acción es más corta y fácil de dominar. Se usa para la insuficiencia cardíaca, puede aumentar la fila de sangre del ventrículo izquierdo insuficiente, para aliviar los síntomas de la insuficiencia cardíaca. |

**续 表**

| | |
|---|---|
| 用法、用量<br>Administración y dosis | 临用前，先用 5% 葡萄糖注射液溶解，再用 5% 葡萄糖注射液 250 ～ 1000ml 稀释。静脉滴注，每分钟 1 ～ 3μg/kg。开始时速度可略快，血压下降后可减慢。但用于心力衰竭、心源性休克时，开始宜缓慢，以 10 滴 / 分为宜，以后再酌情加快速度。用药不宜超过 72 小时。<br><br>Antes de su uso, primero disoluciona con la inyección de glucosa de 5%, y luego usa la inyección de glucosa de 5% de 250 ~ 1000 ml para la dilución. Inyección de goteo vía intravenosa, 1 ~ 3 μg/kg por cada minuto. Al comenzar, la velocidad puede ser un poco más rápido, con la disminución de la presión arterial puede ser lento. Pero cuando se usa para la insuficiencia cardiaca, shock cardiogénico, debe inyectar lentamente, con 10 gotas / minutos, luego, puede acelerar el ritmo según la situación. La utilización de la medicación no debe ser más de 72 horas. |
| 剂型、规格<br>Formulaciones y especificaciones | 注射用硝普钠：每支 50mg。<br><br>Para la inyección se usa Nitroprusiato Sódico: cada una de 50 mg. |

| 药品名称 Drug Names | 卡托普利 Captopril |
|---|---|
| 适应证<br>Indicaciones | 用于治疗各种类型高血压，特别是常规疗法无效的高血压。由于本品通过降低血浆血管紧张素Ⅱ和醛固酮水平，而使心脏前、后负荷减轻，故可用于顽固性慢性心力衰竭，对洋地黄、利尿剂和血管扩张剂无效的心力衰竭患者也有效。<br><br>Se usa para el tratamiento de diversos tipos de hipertensión, en particular la hipertensión que no es válido con la terapia convencional. Debido a este producto a través de reducir los niveles plasmáticos de angiotensina II y de la aldosterona, se reduce la carga del corazón antes y después, así que pueden utilizarse para insuficiencia cardiaca crónica refractarios, es eficaz para los pacientes que no tienen efectos válidos con glucósidos digitálicos, diuréticos y vasodilatadores. |
| 用法、用量<br>Administración y dosis | 口服：一次 25 ～ 50mg，一日 75 ～ 150mg。开始时每次 25mg，一日 3 次（饭前服用）；渐增至每次 50mg，一日 3 次。每日最大剂量为 450mg。儿童，开始每日 1mg/kg，最大 6mg/kg，分 3 次服用。<br><br>Por vía oral: una vez de 25 ~ 50 mg, un día de 75 ~ 150 mg. Al comenzar, cada vez es de 25 mg, tres veces al día (antes de las comidas); gradualmente se aumenta a cada vez de 50 mg, tres veces al día. La dosis diaria máxima es de 450 mg. Para los niños, al comenzar, es de 1 mg / kg al día, y la máxima es de 6 mg / kg que se divide en tres veces. |
| 剂型、规格<br>Formulaciones y especificaciones | 片剂：12.5mg；25mg；50mg；100mg。复方卡托普利片：每片含卡托普利 10mg，氢氯噻嗪 6mg。<br><br>Tabletas:12.5mg；25mg；50mg 100mg. Tableta de compuesto de Captopril: Cada tableta contiene 10 mg de Captopril, 6mg de hidroclorotiazida. |

| 药品名称 Drug Names | 依那普利 Enalapril |
|---|---|
| 适应证<br>Indicaciones | 用于高血压及充血性心力衰竭的治疗。<br>Se usa para el tratamiento de la hipertensión y la insuficiencia cardíaca congestiva. |
| 用法、用量<br>Administración y dosis | 口服 10mg，一日服 1 次，必要时也可静脉注射以加速起效。可根据患者情况增加至日剂量 40mg。<br><br>Por vía oral: 10 mg, 1 vez al día, en caso necesario, también se puede inyectar por vía intravenosa para acelerar la acción. De acuerdo con la condición de los pacientes puede aumentar la dosis diaria hasta 40mg. |
| 剂型、规格<br>Formulaciones y especificaciones | 片剂：每片 5mg；10mg；20mg。<br>Tabletas: Cada tableta de 5 mg; 10 mg; 20mg. |

| 药品名称 Drug Names | 贝那普利 Benazepril |
|---|---|
| 适应证<br>Indicaciones | 用于各型高血压和充血性心力衰竭患者。对正在服用地高辛和利尿药的充血性心力衰竭患者可使心排血量增加，全身和肺血管阻力、平均动脉压、肺动脉压及右心房压下降。<br><br>Se usa para los pacientes de todo tipo de la hipertensión y la insuficiencia cardíaca congestiva. Para los pacientes con insuficiencia cardíaca congestiva que están tomando medicamentos de digoxina y diuréticos, se puede aumentar la frecuencia cardíaca de corazón, y reducir la resistencia vascular pulmonar y sistémica, la presión arterial media, la presión arterial pulmonar y la presión de aurícula derecha. |

**续　表**

| 用法、用量<br>Administración y<br>dosis | 用于降血压，口服，开始剂量为一日 1 次 10mg，然后可根据病情渐增剂量至每日 40mg，一次或分 2 次服用。严重肾功能不全者或心力衰竭患者或服用利尿药的患者，初始剂量为一日 5mg，充血性心力衰竭患者，每日剂量为 2.5 ~ 20mg。<br><br>Para la reducción de la presión arterial, por vía oral, al comenzar, la dosis es de 10 mg una vez al día, y luego según la gravedad de la enfermedad, puede aumentar gradualmente la dosis a 40 mg al día que se tome de una vez o 2 veces. Para los pacientes con insuficiencia renal grave o los pacientes con insuficiencia cardiaca o los que está tomando diuréticos, la dosis diaria inicial es de 5 mg al día, para los pacientes con insuficiencia cardíaca congestive, la dosis diaria es de 2,5 ~ 20mg. |
|---|---|
| 剂型、规格<br>Formulaciones y<br>especificaciones | 片剂：每片 5mg；10mg；20mg。<br>Tabletas: Cada tableta de 5 mg; 10 mg; 20mg. |
| **药品名称 Drug Names** | 培哚普利 Perindopril |
| 适应证<br>Indicaciones | 用于治疗高血压。<br>Se usa para el tratamiento de la hypertension. |
| 用法、用量<br>Administración y<br>dosis | 口服，一日 1 次 4mg，可根据病情增至一日 8mg。老年患者及肾功能低下患者酌情减量。<br>Por vía oral, 4 mg 1 vez al día, de acuerdo con la enfermedad aumenta a 8 mg al día. Para los pacientes de edad avanzada y pacientes con disfunción renal deben tomar con reducciones apropiadas. |
| 剂型、规格<br>Formulaciones y<br>especificaciones | 片剂：每片 2mg；4mg。<br>Tabletas: Cada tableta de 2 mg; 4mg. |
| **药品名称 Drug Names** | 氯沙坦 Losartán |
| 适应证<br>Indicaciones | 用于高血压和充血性心力衰竭患者的治疗。<br>Se usa para el tratamiento de la hipertensión y la insuficiencia cardíaca congestiva. |
| 用法、用量<br>Administración y<br>dosis | 口服，一日 1 次，10 ~ 100mg；一般维持量一日 1 次 50mg，剂量增加，抗高血压效果不再增加。<br>Por vía oral, 1 vez al día, cada vez de 10 ~ 100 mg; la dosis de mantenimiento general es de 50 mg de 1 vez al día, al aumentar la dosis, el efecto de antihipertensivo ya no importa. |
| 剂型、规格<br>Formulaciones y<br>especificaciones | 氯沙坦钾，片剂：50mg，100mg；胶囊：50mg。<br>Losartán potásico, tabletas: 50 mg, 100 mg; cápsula: 50 mg. |
| **药品名称 Drug Names** | 缬沙坦 Valsartán |
| 适应证<br>Indicaciones | 用于治疗高血压。<br>Se usa para el tratamiento de la hypertension. |
| 用法、用量<br>Administración y<br>dosis | 常口服其胶囊剂，每粒含 80mg 或 160mg，每次 80mg，一日 1 次，亦可根据需要增加至每次 160mg，或加用利尿药。也可与其他降压药合用。<br>A menudo se toma sus cápsulas por vía oral, cada cápsula es de 80 mg o 160 mg, cada vez de 80 mg, una vez al día, y se puede aumentar hasta 160 mg de cada vez, o combinar con diuréticos según sea necesario. También se puede utilizar en combinación con otros fármacos antihipertensivos. |
| 剂型、规格<br>Formulaciones y<br>especificaciones | 胶囊：80mg；160mg。<br>Cápsulas: 80 mg; 160mg. |
| **药品名称 Drug Names** | 厄贝沙坦 Irbesartán |
| 适应证<br>Indicaciones | 用于治疗原发性高血压。<br>Se usa para el tratamiento de la hipertensión esencial. |
| 用法、用量<br>Administración y<br>dosis | 口服每次 150mg，一日 1 次，对血压控制不佳者可加至 300mg 或合用小剂量噻嗪类利尿药。<br>Por vía oral cada vez de150 mg, una vez al día, para los pacientes con la presión arterial mal controlada, se puede aumentar a 300 mg o combinar con fármacos de diuréticos tiazídicos de bajas dosis. |

| | |
|---|---|
| 剂型、规格<br>Formulaciones y especificaciones | 片剂：每片 150mg。<br>Tabletas: Cada tableta de 150 mg. |
| 药品名称 Drug Names | 坎地沙坦 Candesartán |
| 适应证<br>Indicaciones | 用于高血压治疗。<br>Se usa para el tratamiento de la hipertensión. |
| 用法、用量<br>Administración y dosis | 口服，每次 8～16mg，一日 1 次。也可与氨氯地平、氢氯噻嗪合用。中、重度肝、肾功能不全患者应适当调整剂量。<br>Por vía oral, cada vez de 8～16 mg, una vez al día. También puede combinar con amlodipino, hidroclorotiazida. Los pacientes con disfunción de hígado y riñón moderada a severa deben ajustar la dosis apropiadamente. |
| 剂型、规格<br>Formulaciones y especificaciones | 片剂：4mg，8mg；胶囊：4mg，8mg；分散片：4mg。<br>Tableta: 4mg, 8mg; Cápsula: 4mg, 8mg; Tableta de dispersión: 4mg. |
| 药品名称 Drug Names | 替米沙坦 Telmisartán |
| 适应证<br>Indicaciones | 用于原发性高血压的治疗。<br>Se usa para el tratamiento de la hipertensión esencial. |
| 用法、用量<br>Administración y dosis | 一日 1 次，一次 1 片，40mg/片。<br>Una vez al día, cada vez 1 tableta, de 40 mg / tableta. |
| 剂型、规格<br>Formulaciones y especificaciones | 片剂：每片 40mg。<br>Tabletas: Cada tableta de 40mg. |
| 药品名称 Drug Names | 吲达帕胺 Indapamida |
| 适应证<br>Indicaciones | 对轻、中度原发性高血压具有良好效果。单独服用降压效果显著，不必加用其他利尿剂。可与 β 受体拮抗剂合并应用。<br>Tiene buenos resultados para el tratamiento de hipertensión esencial de nivel leve a moderado. El efecto antihipertensivo de uso individual es significativo, y no hay la necesidad de combinar con otros diuréticos. En las aplicaciones pueden ser combinados con el antagonista del receptor β. |
| 用法、用量<br>Administración y dosis | 口服：一次 2.5mg，一日 1 次，维持量可 2 日一次 2.5mg。<br>Por vía oral: una vez de 2.5mg, una vez al día, la dosis de mantenimiento puede ser de una vez de 2.5mg por dos días. |
| 剂型、规格<br>Formulaciones y especificaciones | 片剂：每片 2.5mg。<br>Tabletas: Cada tableta de 2.5mg. |
| 药品名称 Drug Names | 甲基多巴 Metildopa |
| 适应证<br>Indicaciones | 用于中、重度、恶性高血压。<br>Se usa para la hipertensión moderada, grave, y maligna. |
| 用法、用量<br>Administración y dosis | 每次服 250mg，一日 3 次。<br>Se toma cada vez de 250 mg, 3 veces al día. |
| 剂型、规格<br>Formulaciones y especificaciones | 片剂：250mg。<br>Tabletas: 250 mg. |

| 药品名称 Drug Names | 胍乙啶 Guanetidina |
|---|---|
| 适应证<br>Indicaciones | 用于中、重度舒张压高的高血压。<br>Se usa para la presión arterial diastólica moderada y grave. |
| 用法、用量<br>Administración y<br>dosis | 开始每日 10mg，以后视病情每隔 5 ～ 7 日递增 10mg，分次服用。一般一日不超过 100mg。<br>Al comienzo, es de10 mg al día, después, dependiendo de la condición de enfermedad, se incrementa gradualmente la dosis de 10 mg con intervalo de 5 ~ 7 días, y se toma en dosis divididas. Generalmente Día no exceda 100 mg. |
| 剂型、规格<br>Formulaciones y<br>especificaciones | 片剂：10mg；25mg。<br>Tabletas: 10 mg; 25 mg. |
| 药品名称 Drug Names | 倍他尼定 Betanidina |
| 适应证<br>Indicaciones | 用于中、重度舒张压高的高血压。<br>Se usa para la presión arterial diastólica moderada y grave. |
| 用法、用量<br>Administración y<br>dosis | 开始：一次 10mg，一日 3 次；维持：20 ～ 200mg/d。<br>Al comienzo: una vez 10 mg, 3 veces al día; en dosis de mantenimiento: 20 ~ 200 mg / d. |
| 剂型、规格<br>Formulaciones y<br>especificaciones | 片剂：10mg；50mg。<br>Tabletas: 10 mg; 50 mg. |
| 药品名称 Drug Names | 异喹胍 Debrisoquina |
| 适应证<br>Indicaciones | 用于中、重度舒张压高的高血压。<br>Se usa para la presión arterial diastólica moderada y grave. |
| 用法、用量<br>Administración y<br>dosis | 开始：一次 10mg，一日 1 ～ 2 次；维持：40 ～ 120mg/d。<br>Al comienzo: una vez 10 mg, 1 ~ 2 veces al día; en dosis de mantenimiento: 40 ~ 200 mg / d. |
| 剂型、规格<br>Formulaciones y<br>especificaciones | 片剂：10mg；20mg。<br>Tabletas: 10 mg; 20 mg. |
| 药品名称 Drug Names | 西拉普利 Cilazapril |
| 适应证<br>Indicaciones | 用于治疗各种程度原发性高血压和肾性高血压，也可与洋地黄和（或）利尿剂合用作为治疗慢性心力衰竭的辅助药物。<br>Se usa para el tratamiento de diversos grados de hipertensión esencial y la hipertensión renal, y también puede combinar con digital y (o) diuréticos que se sirve como medicamento auxiliar para el tratamiento de la insuficiencia cardíaca crónica. |
| 用法、用量<br>Administración y<br>dosis | 口服：一日 1 次 2.5 ～ 5mg。<br>Por vía oral: Una vez al día de 2.5 ~ 5 mg. |
| 剂型、规格<br>Formulaciones y<br>especificaciones | 片剂：2.5mg；5mg。<br>Tabletas: 2.5 mg; 5 mg. |
| 药品名称 Drug Names | 喹那普利 Quinapril |
| 适应证<br>Indicaciones | 高血压、充血性心力衰竭。<br>Se usa para el tratamiento de la hipertensión, insuficiencia cardíaca congestiva. |

**续　表**

| 用法、用量<br>Administración y dosis | 口服：一日 10 ～ 80mg，1 次或分 2 次服用。<br>Por vía oral: 10 ~ 80 mg al día, de 1 vez o 2 veces. |
|---|---|
| 剂型、规格<br>Formulaciones y especificaciones | 片剂：10mg。<br>Tableta: 10mg. |
| **药品名称 Drug Names** | **雷米普利 Ramipril** |
| 适应证<br>Indicaciones | 用于治疗原发性高血压。<br>Se usa para el tratamiento de la hipertensión esencial. |
| 用法、用量<br>Administración y dosis | 口服：一日 1 次 2.5 ～ 5mg。<br>Por vía oral: Una vez al día de 2.5 ~ 5 mg. |
| 剂型、规格<br>Formulaciones y especificaciones | 片剂：1.25mg，2.5mg，5mg。<br>Tableta: 1.25mg, 2.5mg, 5mg. |
| **药品名称 Drug Names** | **咪达普利 Imidapril** |
| 适应证<br>Indicaciones | （1）原发性高血压；<br>（2）肾实质性病变所致继发性高血压。<br>(1) Hipertensión esencial;<br>(2) Hipertensión arterial secundaria causada por lesiones parenquimatosas renales. |
| 用法、用量<br>Administración y dosis | 口服：一日 1 次 5 ～ 10mg。<br>Por vía oral: Una vez al día de 5 ~ 10 mg. |
| 剂型、规格<br>Formulaciones y especificaciones | 片剂：5mg；10mg。<br>Tabletas: 5 mg; 10 mg. |
| **药品名称 Drug Names** | **赖诺普利 Lisinopril** |
| 适应证<br>Indicaciones | 用于高血压和充血性心力衰竭。<br>Se usa para la hipertensión y la insuficiencia cardíaca congestiva. |
| 用法、用量<br>Administración y dosis | 口服：一日 1 次 5 ～ 20mg。最多一日不超过 80mg。<br>Por vía oral: Una vez al día de 5 ~ 20 mg. La dosis máxima al día no debe exceder 80 mg. |
| 剂型、规格<br>Formulaciones y especificaciones | 片剂：5mg；10mg；20mg。<br>Tabletas: 5 mg; 10 mg; 20mg. |
| **药品名称 Drug Names** | **福辛普利 Fosinopril** |
| 适应证<br>Indicaciones | 适用于治疗高血压和心力衰竭。治疗高血压时，可单独使用作为初始治疗药物，或与其他抗高血压药物联合使用。治疗心力衰竭时，可与利尿剂合用。<br>Se usa para el tratamiento de la hipertensión y la insuficiencia cardíaca. En el tratamiento de la hipertensión, se puede utilizar individualmente como terapia inicial, o en combinación con otros fármacos antihipertensivos. En el tratamiento de la insuficiencia cardíaca, se puede combinar con diuréticos. |
| 用法、用量<br>Administración y dosis | 口服：一日 1 次 5 ～ 40mg。最大剂量一日 80mg。<br>Por vía oral: Una vez al día de 5 ~ 40 mg. La dosis máxima al día no debe exceder 80 mg. |

**续　表**

| 剂型、规格<br>Formulaciones y especificaciones | 片剂：10mg；20mg。<br>Tabletas: 10 mg; 20 mg. |
| --- | --- |

## 10.7　抗休克的血管活性药 Medicamento vasoactivo contra el choque

| 药品名称 Drug Names | 去甲肾上腺素 Noradrenalina (Norepinefrina) |
| --- | --- |
| 适应证<br>Indicaciones | 临床上主要用它的升压作用，静脉滴注用于各种休克（但出血性休克禁用），以升高血压，保证对重要器官（如脑）的血液供应。<br><br>Su función clínica principalmente es el aumento de su presión arterial, La infusión intravenosa se aplica para una variedad de shock (pero es deshabilitada para el shock hemorrágico) para aumentar la presión arterial, garantizar el suministro de sangre a los órganos vitales (como el cerebro). |
| 用法、用量<br>Administración y dosis | （1）静脉滴注：临用前稀释，每分钟滴入 4～10μg，根据病情调整剂量。可用 1～2mg 加入生理盐水或 5% 葡萄糖注射液 100ml 内静脉滴注，根据情况掌握滴注速度，待血压升至所需水平后，减慢滴速，以维持血压正常范围。如效果不佳，应换用其他升压药。对危急病例可用 1～2mg 稀释到 10～20ml，徐徐注射入静脉，同时根据血压以调节其剂量，待血压回升后，再用滴注法维持。<br>（2）口服：治上消化道出血，每次服注射液 1～3ml（1～3mg），一日 3 次，加入适量冷盐水服下。<br><br>(1) La infusión intravenosa: Antes de la aplicación hace la dilución con gotas de 4 ~ 10μg por cada minuto, puede ajustar la dosis de acuerdo a la enfermedad. Es disponible de 1 ~ 2 mg en la solución salina normal o inyección de glucosa de 5% de 100 ml en la infusión intravenosa de goteo, dependiendo de las circunstancias se capta la velocidad de infusión de goteo, después de que la presión arterial se eleva hasta el nivel requerido, se reduce la velocidad de goteo, con el fin de mantener el rango normal de la presión arterial. Si es ineficaz, debería sustituirse por otros vasopresores. Para casos de emergencia, es disponible de usar 1 ~ 2mg con la dilución hasta 10 ~ 20 ml, lentamente se inyecta en la vena, y de acuerdo a la presión de la sangre puede ajustar la dosis, hasta que la presión arterial se vuelve a aumentar, sigue manteniendo por goteo.<br>(2) Por vía oral: se usa para el tratamiento de la hemorragia gastrointestinal, cada vez toma una inyección de 1 ~ 3 ml (1 ~ 3 mg), tres veces al día, añadiendo una cantidad correcta de solución salina fría. |
| 剂型、规格<br>Formulaciones y especificaciones | 注射液：每支 2mg（1ml）（以重酒石酸盐计量）；10mg（2ml）（以重酒石酸盐计量）。<br>Inyección: Cada 2 mg (1 ml) (Medida por sal de bitartrato); 10 mg (2 ml) (Medida por sal de bitartrato). |

| 药品名称 Drug Names | 去氧肾上腺素 Fenilefrina |
| --- | --- |
| 适应证<br>Indicaciones | 用于感染中毒性及过敏性休克、室上性心动过速、防治全身麻醉及腰椎麻醉时的低血压。眼科用于散瞳检查，特点是作用时间短，不麻痹调节功能，不引起眼压升高。<br><br>Se usa para la infección de la toxicidad, shock anafiláctico, taquicardia ventricular, y para la prevención y el tratamiento de la hipotensión de anestesia general y la anestesia lumbar. En caso de los ojos, se usa para el examen de la vista con dilatación, que se caracteriza por la corta duración de la acción, no hay parálisis en la función de ajuste y no causa aumento de la presión intraocular. |
| 用法、用量<br>Administración y dosis | （1）肌内注射或静脉滴注：①常用量：肌内注射，一次 2～5mg；静脉滴注，一次 10～20mg。稀释后缓慢滴注。②极量：肌内注射，一次 10mg；静脉滴注，每分钟 0.1mg。<br>（2）滴眼：用于散瞳检查，用 2%～5% 溶液滴眼。<br><br>(1) Inyección intramuscular o infusión intravenosa: ① Dosis habitual: Inyección intramuscular, una vez de 2 ~ 5 mg; Infusión intravenosa, una vez de 10 ~ 20 mg. Despúes de ser diluida, hace la infusión lentamente. ② Dosis máxima: Inyección intramuscular, una vez de 10mg; Infusión intravenosa, 0,1 mg por minuto.<br>(2) Goteo para ojo: se usa para el examen de ojos dilatados, con una solución de 2% ~ 5% para el goteo de ojos. |
| 剂型、规格<br>Formulaciones y especificaciones | 注射液：每支 10mg（1ml）。滴眼剂：为 2%～5% 溶液。<br>Inyección: Cada de 10 mg (1 ml). Gotas para los ojos: Solución de 2% ~ 5%. |

**续 表**

| 药品名称 Drug Names | 甲氧胺 Metoxamina |
|---|---|
| 适应证<br>Indicaciones | 用于外科手术，以维持或恢复动脉压，尤其适用于做脊椎麻醉造成的血压降低。又用于大出血、创伤及外科手术所引起的低血压、心肌梗死所致休克及室上性心动过速。<br><br>Se usa en la cirugía, para mantener o restablecer la presión arterial, sobre todo se aplica para la disminución de la presión arterial causada por la anestesia espinal. Y se usa para la hipotensión causada por sangrado, trauma y cirugía, shock causada por el infarto de miocardio y taquicardia supraventricular. |
| 用法、用量<br>Administración y<br>dosis | （1）肌内注射、静脉注射或静脉滴注：①常用量：肌内注射，一次 10～20mg；静脉注射：一次 5～10mg；静脉滴注，一次 20～60mg，稀释后缓慢滴注。②极量：肌内注射，一次 20mg，一日 60mg；静脉注射：一次 10mg。<br>（2）对急症病例或收缩压降至 8kPa（60mmHg）甚至更低的病例，缓慢静脉注射 5～10mg，注射一次量不超过 10mg，并严密观察血压变动。静脉注射后，继续肌内注射 15mg，以维持较长药效。<br>（3）对室上性心动过速病例，用 10～20mg，以 5% 葡萄糖注射液 100ml 稀释，做静脉滴注。也可用 10mg 加入 5%～10% 葡萄糖注射液 20ml 中缓缓静脉注射。注射时应观察心率及血压，当心率突然减慢时，应停注。<br>（4）对处理心肌梗死的休克病例，开始肌内注射 15mg，接着静脉滴注，静脉滴注液为 5%～10% 葡萄糖注射液 500ml 内含本品 60mg，滴速应随血压反应而调整，每分钟不宜超过 20 滴。<br><br>(1) Inyección intramuscular, inyección intravenosa o infusión intravenosa: ① Dosis habitual: Inyección intramuscular, una vez de 10～20 mg; Inyección intravenosa: una vez de 5～10 mg; Infusión intravenosa, una vez de 20～60 mg, después de la dilución, hace la infusión lentamente. ② Dosis máxima: Inyección intramuscular, una vez de 20 mg, 60 mg al día; Inyección intravenosa: una vez de 10 mg.<br>(2) Para casos de emergencia, o caso que la presión arterial sistólica se redujo a 8 kPa (60 mmHg) o el caso de presión aún más baja, la inyección intravenosa lenta es de 5～10 mg, la cantidad de inyección de una vez no puede ser más de 10 mg y debe mantener una estrecha observación de los cambios de la presión arterial. Después de la inyección intravenosa, continúa la inyección intramuscular de 15 mg, para mantener una eficacia con duración más larga.<br>(3) Para el caso de taquicardia supraventricular, usa 10～20 mg para hace la dilución con inyección de glucosa de 5% de 100ml y realiza la infusión intravenosa. También es disponible de usar10mg en la inyección de glucosa de 5%～10% de 20 ml para la inyección intravenosa lentamente. Durante la inyección, debe observar la frecuencia cardíaca y la presión arterial, cuando de repente se ralentiza la frecuencia cardíaca, se debe parar la inyección.<br>(4) Para casos de tratamiento de shock de infarto de miocardio, comienza la inyección intramuscular de15mg, y enseguida hace la infusión intravenosa, la solución de infusión intravenosa es de 500ml inyección de glucosa de 5%～10% que contiene Metoxamina de 60 mg, la velocidad de goteo debe ser ajustada con la respuesta de la presión arterial y no debe exceder 20 gotas por minuto. |
| 剂型、规格<br>Formulaciones y<br>especificaciones | 注射液：每支 10mg（1ml）；20mg（1ml）。<br>Inyección: Cada de 10 mg (1 ml); 20 mg (1 ml). |
| 药品名称 Drug Names | 间羟胺 Metaraminol |
| 适应证<br>Indicaciones | 用于各种休克及手术时低血压。在一般用量下，不致引起心律失常，因此也可用于心肌梗死性休克。<br><br>Se usa para todo tipo de shocks y la hipotensión en la cirugía. En la dosis habitual, no se causa arritmias, por lo tanto, también puede ser utilizado para el shock de infarto de miocardio. |
| 用法、用量<br>Administración y<br>dosis | （1）肌内注射或静脉滴注：①常用量：肌内注射一次 10～20mg；静脉滴注，一次 10～40mg，稀释后缓慢滴注，如以 15～100mg 加入 0.9% 氯化钠注射液或 5%～10% 葡萄糖注射液 250～500ml 中静脉滴注，每分钟 20～30 滴，用量及滴速随血压情况而定。②极量：静脉滴注一次 100mg（每分钟 0.2～0.4mg）。<br>（2）局部鼻充血可用 0.25%～0.5% 的等渗缓冲液（pH=6）每小时喷入或滴入 2～3 滴，每日不超过 4 次，一疗程为 7 日。 |

**续　表**

| | |
|---|---|
| | (1) Inyección intramuscular o infusión intravenosa: ① Dosis habitual: inyección intramuscular de una vez de 10 ~ 20 mg; Infusión intravenosa, una vez de 10 ~ 40 mg, de ser diluida, hace goteo lentamente, tal como en 15 ~ 100 mg se agrega inyección de cloruro de sodio de 0,9% o inyección de glucosa de 5% ~ 10% de 250 ~ 500 ml para la infusión intravenosa, de 20 ~ 30 gotas por minuto, la dosificación y la velocidad de goteo se ajuste de acuerdo con las condiciones de presión de la sangre. ② Dosis máxima: infusión intravenosa de una vez de 100 mg (0.2 ~ 0.4 mg por minuto). <br> (2) Para descongestionantes nasales tópicos, es disponible de tampón isotónico de 0,25% ~ 0,5% (pH = 6) o se inyecta en rociado o en el goteo de 2 ~ 3 gotas por hora, no debe ser más de cuatro veces al día, un curso de tratamiento es siete días. |
| 剂型、规格 <br> Formulaciones y especificaciones | 注射液：每支 10mg（1ml）（以间羟胺计量）；50mg（5ml）（以间羟胺计量）。 <br> Inyección: Cada una de 10 mg (1 ml) (Medida por Metaraminol); 50 mg (5 ml) (Medida por Metaraminol). |
| 药品名称Drug Names | 肾上腺素 Adrenalina (Epinefrina) |
| 适应证 <br> Indicaciones | 用于抢救过敏性休克、心脏骤停、支气管哮喘急性发作。与局部麻醉药合用延长其药效。 <br> Se usa para el rescate del shock anafiláctico, paro cardiaco, exacerbación aguda de asma bronquial. Puede usar en combinación con anestésicos locales para extender su eficacia. |
| 用法、用量 <br> Administración y dosis | 常用量：皮下注射，一次 0.25 ~ 1mg；心室内注射，一次 0.25 ~ 1mg。极量：皮下注射，一次 1mg。 <br> Dosis habitual: inyección subcutánea, una vez de 0.25 ~ 1mg; Inyección intraventricular, una vez de 0.25 ~ 1mg. Dosis máxima: por vía subcutánea, una vez de 1mg. |
| 剂型、规格 <br> Formulaciones y especificaciones | 注射液：1mg（1ml）。 <br> Inyección: Cada una de 10 mg (1 ml). |
| 药品名称Drug Names | 多巴胺 Dopamina |
| 适应证 <br> Indicaciones | 用于各种类型休克，包括中毒性休克、心源性休克、出血性休克、中枢性休克，特别对伴有肾功能不全、心排出量降低、周围血管阻力增高而已补足血容量的患者更有意义。 <br> Se usa para todo tipo de shocks, incluyendo shock tóxico, shock cardiogénico, shock hemorrágico, shock central, en particular tiene efectos más significados para los pacientes con la disfunción renal, disminución del gasto cardíaco, resistencia vascular periférica aumentada y el volumen de sangre conformada. |
| 用法、用量 <br> Administración y dosis | 静脉注射，一次 20mg，稀释后缓慢滴注；极量，每分钟 20μg/kg。将 20mg 加入 5% 葡萄糖注射液 200 ~ 300ml 中静脉滴注，开始每分钟 20 滴左右（即每分钟滴入 75 ~ 100μg），以后根据血压情况，可加快速度或加大浓度。 <br> La inyección intravenosa, una vez de 20 mg, de ser diluida, hace la infusión de gotas lentamente; Dosis máxima, 20μg/kg por minuto. Pone 20mg en la inyección de glucosa de 5% de 200 ~ 300 ml para la infusión intravenosa, al comienzo, es alrededor de 20 gotas por minuto (es decir, gotas de75 ~ 100 μg por minuto), y luego, de acuerdo con la presión arterial, puede acelerar la velocidad o aumentar la concentración. |
| 剂型、规格 <br> Formulaciones y especificaciones | 注射液：每支 20mg（2ml）。 <br> Inyección: Cada una de 20 mg (2 ml). |
| 药品名称Drug Names | 多巴酚丁胺 Dobutamina |
| 适应证 <br> Indicaciones | 用于心排血量低和心率慢的心力衰竭患者，其改善左心室功能的作用优于多巴胺。 <br> Se usa para los pacientes con insuficiencia cardiaca de bajo gasto cardíaco y lenta tasa de del corazón, la función en mejora de ventricular izquierda era mejor que la Dopamina. |
| 用法、用量 <br> Administración y dosis | 静脉滴注：250mg 加入 5% 葡萄糖注射液 250 或 500ml 中滴注，每分钟 2.5 ~ 10μg/kg。 <br> Infusión intravenosa: 250 mg en inyección de glucosa de 5% de 250 o 500 ml para la infusión, 2.5 ~ 10 μg/kg por minuto. |

**续　表**

| 剂型、规格<br>Formulaciones y especificaciones | 注射液：每支 20mg（按多巴酚丁胺计）（2ml）；200mg（按多巴酚丁胺计）（2ml）。<br>Inyección: Cada de 20 mg (Medida por Dobutamina) (2 ml), 200 mg (Medida por Dobutamina) (20 ml). |
| --- | --- |
| **药品名称 Drug Names** | 血管紧张素胺 Angiotensinamida |
| 适应证<br>Indicaciones | 用于外伤或手术后休克和全身麻醉或腰椎麻醉时所致的低血压症等。<br>Se usa para trauma o shock después de cirugía y la hipotensión causada por la anestesia general o anestesia espinal. |
| 用法、用量<br>Administración y dosis | 静脉滴注：一次 1 ~ 1.25mg，溶解于 5% 葡萄糖或 0.9% 氯化钠注射液 500ml 中，滴速一般每分钟 3 ~ 10μg，应经常测定血压，随时调整滴速。<br>La infusión intravenosa: Cada vez de 1 ~ 1.25mg, disuelto en glucosa de 5% o inyección de cloruro de sodio de 0,9% de 500ml, por goteo generalmente es 3 ~ 10μg por minuto, se debe medir la presión arterial a menudo, para ajustar la tasa de goteo en cualquier momento. |
| 剂型、规格<br>Formulaciones y especificaciones | 注射用血管紧张素胺：每支 1mg。<br>La amida angiotensina para inyección: Cada de 1 mg. |

10.8　调节血脂药及抗动脉粥样硬化药 Medicamentos reguladores de lípidos y contra la aterosclerosis

| **药品名称 Drug Names** | 氯贝丁酯 Clofibrato |
| --- | --- |
| 适应证<br>Indicaciones | 用于动脉粥样硬化及其继发症，如冠状动脉病、脑血管疾病、周围血管病及糖尿病所致动脉疾病等。<br>Se usa para la aterosclerosis y la enfermedad secundaria, por ejemplo la enfermedad arterial coronaria, enfermedad cerebrovascular, enfermedad vascular periférica y enfermedad arterial inducida por la diabetes. |
| 用法、用量<br>Administración y dosis | 口服，一次 0.25 ~ 0.5g，一日 3 次，饭后服。<br>Por vía oral, una vez de 0.25 ~ 0.5 g, 3 veces al día, se toma después de las comidas. |
| 剂型、规格<br>Formulaciones y especificaciones | 胶囊剂：每粒 0.25g；0.5g。<br>Cápsulas: Cada de 0.25 g; 0.5 g. |
| **药品名称 Drug Names** | 非诺贝特 Fenofibrato |
| 适应证<br>Indicaciones | 用于高胆固醇血症、高三酰甘油血症及混合性高脂血症，疗效确切，且耐受性好。<br>Se usa para hipercolesterolemia, hipertrigliceridemia e hiperlipidemia mixta, es eficaz y bien tolerada. |
| 用法、用量<br>Administración y dosis | 口服：一次 100mg，一日 2 ~ 3 次。<br>Por vía oral: una vez de 100 mg, 2 ~ 3 veces al día. |
| 剂型、规格<br>Formulaciones y especificaciones | 胶囊（片）剂：每粒（片）100mg；200mg；300mg。<br>Cápsulas (tabletas) ; cada cápsula (tableta) de 100mg; 200mg; 300mg. |
| **药品名称 Drug Names** | 洛伐他汀 Lovastatina |
| 适应证<br>Indicaciones | 用于原发性高胆固醇血症（Ⅱa 及 Ⅱb 型）。也用于合并有高胆固醇血症和高三酰甘油血症，而以高胆固醇血症为主的患者。<br>Se usa para hipercolesterolemia primaria (tipo Ⅱa y Ⅱb). También se utiliza para la hipercolesterolemia y la hipertrigliceridemia combinada, y los pacientes con la enfermedad principal de hipercolesterolemia. |

**续 表**

| 用法、用量<br>Administración y dosis | 口服，开始剂量一日1次20mg，晚餐时服用，必要时于4周内调整剂量，最大剂量一日80mg，1次或分2次服用。<br>Por vía oral, Al comienzo, cada día 1 vez de 20 mg, se toma en la cena, si es necesario, puede ajustar la dosis dentro de las 4 semanas, la dosis máxima es de 80 mg al día que se toma de 1 veces o 2 veces. |
| --- | --- |
| 剂型、规格<br>Formulaciones y especificaciones | 片剂：每片10mg；20mg；40mg。<br>Tabletas: cada tableta de 10 mg; 20 mg;40 mg. |

| 药品名称Drug Names | 辛伐他汀 Simvastatina |
| --- | --- |
| 适应证<br>Indicaciones | 用于原发性高胆固醇血症（Ⅱa及Ⅱb型）。也用于合并有高胆固醇血症和高三酰甘油血症，而以高胆固醇血症为主的患者。<br>Se usa para hipercolesterolemia primaria (tipo Ⅱa y Ⅱb). También se utiliza para la hipercolesterolemia y la hipertrigliceridemia combinada, y los pacientes con la enfermedad principal de hipercolesterolemia. |
| 用法、用量<br>Administración y dosis | 口服，一日1次10mg，晚餐时服，必要时于4周内增量至一日1次40mg。<br>Por vía oral, una vez de 10mg al día, se toma en la cena. Si es necesario, puede incrementar la dosis de una vez de 40 mg al día dentro de 4 semanas. |
| 剂型、规格<br>Formulaciones y especificaciones | 片剂：每片10mg；20mg。<br>Tabletas: cada tableta de 10 mg; 20 mg. |

| 药品名称Drug Names | 普伐他汀 Pravastatina |
| --- | --- |
| 适应证<br>Indicaciones | 用于原发性高胆固醇血症（Ⅱa及Ⅱb型）。也用于合并有高胆固醇血症和高三酰甘油血症，而以高胆固醇血症为主的患者。<br>Se usa para hipercolesterolemia primaria (tipo Ⅱa y Ⅱb). También se utiliza para la hipercolesterolemia y la hipertrigliceridemia combinada, y los pacientes con la enfermedad principal de hipercolesterolemia. |
| 用法、用量<br>Administración y dosis | 口服，一日10mg，分2次服用，可根据情况增量至一日20mg。<br>Por vía oral, 10 mg al día, se toma en 2 veces, puede incrementar la dosis a 20 mg al día de acuerdo con la situación. |
| 剂型、规格<br>Formulaciones y especificaciones | 片剂：每片5mg；10mg。<br>Tabletas: cada tableta de 5 mg;10 mg. |

| 药品名称Drug Names | 氟伐他汀 Fluvastatina |
| --- | --- |
| 适应证<br>Indicaciones | 用于饮食控制无效的高胆固醇血症。<br>Se usa para hipercolesterolemia que no es válida con el control de dieta. |
| 用法、用量<br>Administración y dosis | 用量：口服一日1次20mg，晚间服用。<br>Dosis: por vía oral 1 vez de 20 mg al día, se toma por la noche. |
| 剂型、规格<br>Formulaciones y especificaciones | 胶囊剂：每粒20mg；40mg。<br>Cápsulas: cada cápsula de 20 mg; 40 mg. |

| 药品名称Drug Names | 阿托伐他汀 Atorvastatina |
| --- | --- |
| 适应证<br>Indicaciones | 用于原发性高胆固醇血症、混合型高脂血症或饮食控制无效杂合于家族型高胆固醇血症患者。<br>Se usa para los pacientes con la hipercolesterolemia primaria, hiperlipidemia mixta o hipercolesterolemia familiar de control de la dieta ineficaz. |
| 用法、用量<br>Administración y dosis | 口服：一日10mg，如需要，4周后可增至每日80mg。<br>Por vía oral, 10 mg al día, si es necesario, puede incrementar la dosis de 80 mg al día despúes de 4 semanas. |

**续 表**

| 剂型、规格<br>Formulaciones y especificaciones | 片剂：每片 10mg；20mg；40mg。<br>Tabletas: cada tableta de 10 mg; 20 mg;40 mg. |
|---|---|
| **药品名称 Drug Names** | **瑞舒伐他汀 Rosuvastatina** |
| 适应证<br>Indicaciones | 用于高脂血症和高胆固醇血症。<br>Se usa para la hiperlipidemia e hipercolesterolemia. |
| 用法、用量<br>Administración y dosis | 口服，一日 5～40mg，开始治疗时应从 10mg 开始，需要时增至 20～40mg，不宜开始时直接用 40mg。<br>Por vía oral, 5～40 mg al día, al comienzo, el tratamiento debe inciar desde 10 mg. Si es necesario, puede incrementar a 20～40 mg. No es apropiado el uso directo de 40 mg al inicio. |
| 剂型、规格<br>Formulaciones y especificaciones | 片剂：每片 5mg；10mg；20mg。<br>Tabletas: cada tableta de 5 mg;10 mg; 20 mg. |
| **药品名称 Drug Names** | **普罗布考 Probucol** |
| 适应证<br>Indicaciones | 用于Ⅱa 型高脂血症，与其他降脂药物可用于Ⅱb 和Ⅲ、Ⅳ型高脂血症。<br>Se usa para la hiperlipidemia de tipo Ⅱa, y se puede utilizar con otros fármacos anti-hipolipemiantes para el tratamiento de hiperlipidemia de tipo Ⅱb, Ⅲ y Ⅳ. |
| 用法、用量<br>Administración y dosis | 口服，一次 500mg，一日 2 次，早、晚餐时服用。<br>Por vía oral, cada vez de 500 mg, 2 veces al día, se toma en el desayuno y la cena. |
| 剂型、规格<br>Formulaciones y especificaciones | 片剂：每片 500mg。<br>Tabletas: cada tableta de 500 mg. |
| **药品名称 Drug Names** | **考来烯胺 Colestiramina** |
| 适应证<br>Indicaciones | 用于Ⅱ型高脂血症、动脉粥样硬化及肝硬化、胆石病引起的瘙痒。其缺点是用量大，约 2% 的患者产生胃肠道反应。<br>Se usa para la picazón causada por la hiperlipidemia de tipo Ⅱ, la aterosclerosis y la cirrosis del hígado, cálculos biliares. La desventaja es la aplicación de una gran cantidad, y aproximadamente el 2% de los pacientes tienen reacciones gastrointestinales. |
| 用法、用量<br>Administración y dosis | （1）治疗动脉粥样硬化：一日 3 次，每次服粉剂 4～5g。<br>（2）止痒：开始时一日量 6～10g，维持量每日 3g，分 3 次服。<br>(1)Tratamiento de la aterosclerosis: tres veces al día, cada vez se toma una porción de polvo de 4～5 g.<br>(2) Tratamiento de picazón: al inicio, la cantidad es de 6～10 g al día, la cantidad de mantenimiento es de 3 g diaria, y se toma en 3 veces. |
| 剂型、规格<br>Formulaciones y especificaciones | 散剂：每包 4g。<br>Polvo: Cada paquete de 4g. |
| **药品名称 Drug Names** | **依折麦布 Ezetimiba** |
| 适应证<br>Indicaciones | 治疗原发性高端固醇血症。<br>Se usa para el tratamiento con esteroides de final hiperlipidemia primaria. |
| 用法、用量<br>Administración y dosis | 一日 1 次，一次 10mg，可单独服用或他汀类联合应用。<br>Una vez al día, cada vez de 10 mg, se puede tomar solo o en combinación con otros medicamentos estatinos. |
| 剂型、规格<br>Formulaciones y especificaciones | 片剂：每片 10mg。<br>Tabletas: cada tableta de 100 mg. |

**续　表**

| 药品名称Drug Names | 血脂康 XueZhiKang |
|---|---|
| 适应证<br>Indicaciones | 治疗动脉粥样硬化及原发性高脂血症。<br>Se usa para el tratamiento de la aterosclerosis y la hiperlipidemia primaria. |
| 用法、用量<br>Administración y<br>dosis | 口服 2 粒 / 次，一日 2 次。<br>Por vía oral, 2 pastillas/vez, 2 veces al día. |
| 剂型、规格<br>Formulaciones y<br>especificaciones | 胶囊（丸）：0.3g/ 粒。<br>Cápsulas (pastillas): 0.3g / pastilla. |
| 药品名称Drug Names | 心脑康 XinNaoKang |
| 适应证<br>Indicaciones | 用于治疗动脉粥样硬化、冠心病、心绞痛、高脂血症、高血压、脑动脉硬化、偏瘫（脑出血和脑血栓形成）等。亦可作为动脉粥样硬化症的预防用药。<br>Se usa para el tratamiento de la aterosclerosis, enfermedad cardíaca coronaria, angina de pecho, la hiperlipidemia, la hipertensión, la arteriosclerosis cerebral, hemiplejia (hemorragia cerebral y trombosis cerebral) etc. La aterosclerosis se puede utilizar como el medicamento de prevención para aterosclerosis. |
| 用法、用量<br>Administración y<br>dosis | 口服：每次 2 粒，一日 3 次，饭后服用，1 个月为一疗程，一般以连用 2 ～ 3 个疗程为宜。偏瘫患者每次 3 粒，一日 3 次，连服至症状好转或基本痊愈。<br>Por vía oral: Cada vez dos cápsulas, tres veces al día, se toma después de las comidas, el curso de tratamiento es de un mes, por lo general es aprópiado que se toma 2 ~ 3 cursos de tratamiento continuos. Para los pacientes hemipléjicos, debe tomar 3 cápsulas cada vez, tres veces al día, se toma cotinuamente hasta que los síntomas básicos están mejorados o básicamente curados. |
| 剂型、规格<br>Formulaciones y<br>especificaciones | 软胶囊剂：每粒 415mg。<br>Cápsulas blandas: Cada de 415 mg. |

11. 主要作用于呼吸系统的药物 Medicamentos que actúan princepalmente sobre el sistema respiretorio

11.1　祛痰药 Expectorantes

| 药品名称Drug Names | 氯化铵 Cloruro de Amónio |
|---|---|
| 适应证<br>Indicaciones | 用于急性呼吸道炎症时痰黏稠不易咳出者。常与其他复方制剂合用。纠正代谢性碱中毒。其酸化尿液作用可使一些需要在酸性尿液中显效的药物产生作用。也可增加汞剂的利尿作用及四环素和青霉素的抗菌作用；还可促进碱性药物的排泄。<br>Se usa para los pacientes que tiene la inflamación respiratoria aguda y esputo pegajoso que es difícil de expectorar. A menudo, se usa en combinación con otro medicamento de compuesto. Puede corregir la alcalosis metabólica. Tiene la función de acidificación de la orina, así que juega su papel para algunas drogas que se accionan en la orina ácida. También puede fortalecer los efectos de la diuresis y la tetraciclina y la penicilina antibacterial; También puede promover la excreción de medicamentos básicos. |
| 用法、用量<br>Administración y<br>dosis | ①祛痰：口服，成人一次 0.3 ～ 0.6g，一日 3 次。②治疗代谢性碱中毒或酸化尿液：静脉滴注，每日 2 ～ 20g，每小时不超过 5g。<br>① Expectorante: Por vía oral, para adultos, una vez de 0.3 ~ 0.6 g, 3 veces al día. ② Tratamiento de la alcalosis metabólica o la acidificación de la orina: goteo intravenoso, 2 ~ 20 g al día, no debe exceder de 5 g por hora. |
| 剂型、规格<br>Formulaciones y<br>especificaciones | 片剂：每片 0.3mg。注射液：每支 5g（500ml）。<br>Tabletas: Cada tableta de 0.3 mg. Inyección: Cada de 5 g (500 ml). |
| 药品名称Drug Names | 溴己新 Bromhexina |
| 适应证<br>Indicaciones | 用于慢性支气管炎、哮喘、支气管扩张、矽肺等有白色痰液不易咳出的患者，脓性痰患者需加用抗生素控制感染。 |

**续 表**

| | |
|---|---|
| | Se usa para los pacientes con bronquitis crónica, asma, bronquiectasias, la silicosis, etc, que tienen esputo blanco y difíciles de expectorar. Para los pacientes de esputo purulento requirieron la adición de antibióticos para controlar la infección. |
| 用法、用量<br>Administración y dosis | 口服：成人一次 8 ～ 16mg。肌内注射：一次 4 ～ 8mg，一日 2 次。静脉注射：一日 4 ～ 8mg，加入 5% 葡萄糖氯化钠溶液 500ml 中。气雾吸入：一次 2ml，一日 2 ～ 3 次。<br><br>Por vía oral: Para adultos una vez de 8 ~ 16 mg. Inyección intramuscular: una vez de 4 ~ 8 mg, 2 veces al día. Inyección intravenosa: 4 ~ 8 mg al día, con glucosa de solución de cloruro sódico de 5% de 500ml. Inhalación: una vez de 2 ml, 2 ~ 3 veces al día. |
| 剂型、规格<br>Formulaciones y especificaciones | 片剂：每片4mg；8mg。注射液：每支 0.2%，2mg（1ml）；4mg（2ml）。气雾剂：0.2% 溶液。<br><br>Tabletas: cada tableta de 4 mg; 8 mg. Inyección: Cada una de 0.2%, 2 mg (1 ml); 4 mg (2 ml). Aerosol: solución de 0.2%. |
| **药品名称Drug Names** | **氨溴索 Ambrosol** |
| 适应证<br>Indicaciones | 用于急慢性支气管炎及支气管哮喘、支气管扩张、肺气肿、肺结核、肺尘埃沉着病、术后的咳痰困难等。注射药可用于术后肺部并发症的预防及早产儿、新生儿呼吸窘迫综合征的治疗。本品高剂量有降低血浆尿酸浓度和促进尿酸排泄的作用。可用于治疗痛风。<br><br>Se usa para la bronquitis aguda y crónica y asma bronquial, bronquiectasias, enfisema, tuberculosis, neumoconiosis, dificultades de expectoración postoperatorias, etc. Las drogas inyectables se pueden utilizar para la prevención de complicaciones pulmonares postoperatorias y el tratamiento del síndrome de dificultad respiratoria neonatal de bebés prematuros. Este producto con una alta dosis puede reducir las concentraciones de ácido úrico de plasma y promover la excreción de ácido úrico. Se usa para el tratamiento de la gota. |
| 用法、用量<br>Administración y dosis | 口服：成人及 12 岁以上儿童，每次 30mg，一日 3 次。长期使用剂量可减半。静脉注射、肌内注射及皮下注射：成人每次 15mg，一日 2 次。亦可加入生理盐水或葡萄糖溶液中静脉滴注。<br><br>Por vía oral: Adultos y niños mayores de 12 años, cada vez de 30 mg, 3 veces al día. Para el uso a largo plazo puede reducirse la dosis a la mitad. Inyección intravenosa, intramuscular y subcutánea: para adultos cada vez de 15 mg, 2 veces al día. En el caso de la inyección por vía intravenosa podría unirse en una solución salina o solución de glucosa. |
| 剂型、规格<br>Formulaciones y especificaciones | 片剂：每片 15mg；30mg。胶囊剂：每粒 30mg。缓释胶囊：每粒 75mg。口服溶液剂：每支 15mg（5ml）；180mg（60ml）；300mg（100ml）；600mg（100ml）。气雾剂：每瓶 15mg（2ml）。注射液：每支 15mg（2ml）。<br><br>Tabletas: Cada tableta de 15 mg; 30 mg. Cápsulas: Cada de 30 mg. Cápsulas Suelte: Cada de 75mg. Solución oral: Cada de 15 mg (5 ml), 180 mg (60 ml), 300 mg (100 ml), 600 mg (100 ml). Aerosol: Cada botella de 15 mg (2 ml). Inyección: Cada de 15 mg (2 ml). |
| **药品名称Drug Names** | **乙酰半胱氨酸 Acetilcisteína** |
| 适应证<br>Indicaciones | ①用于术后、急慢性支气管炎、支气管扩张、肺结核、肺炎、肺气肿等引起的黏稠分泌物过多所致的咳痰困难。②用于乙酰氨基酚中毒的解毒及环磷酰胺引起的出血性膀胱炎的治疗。<br><br>① Se usa para el tratamiento de difícil de expectoración causada por las excesivas secreciones pegajosas después de la cirugía, la bronquitis aguda y crónica, la bronquiectasias, la tuberculosis, la neumonía, enfisema, etc.. ② Se usa para la desintoxicación de envenenamiento por acetaminofeno y el tratamiento de la cistitis hemorrágica inducida por ciclofosfamida. |
| 用法、用量<br>Administración y dosis | （1）喷雾吸入：仅用于非紧急情况下，临用下溶解于氯化钠液中成 10% 溶液，每次 1 ～ 3ml，一日 2 ～ 3 次。<br>（2）气管滴入：急救时 5% 溶液经气管插管或气管套管直接滴入，每次 0.5 ～ 2ml，一日 2 ～ 4 次。<br>（3）气管注入：急救时 5% 溶液用 1ml 注射器自气管的甲状软骨环骨膜处注入管腔内，每次 0.5 ～ 2ml（婴儿每次 0.5ml，儿童每次 1ml，成人每次 2ml）。<br>（4）口服：成人每次 200mg，一日 2 ～ 3 次。<br><br>(1) Inhalación de rocíe: Sólo se usa para situaciones no emergentes. Para su aplicación se disuelve en una solución de cloruro de sodio de 10%, cada vez de 1 ~ 3 ml, 2 ~ 3 veces al día. |

**续　表**

| | |
|---|---|
| | (2) Instilación intratraqueal: En primeros auxilios, use la solución al 5% para la instilación directa a través de tubo de intubación o tubo de traqueotomía, cada vez de 0.5 ~ 2 ml, 2 ~ 4 veces al día.<br>(3) Inyección intratraqueal: En primeros auxilios,use la solución dc 5% cn la jeringa de 1 ml y se inyecta en el lumen desde el periostio del anillo de cartílago tiroides, cada vez de 0.5 ~ 2 ml (para bebé cada vez de 0.5 ml, para niños cada vez de 1 ml, para adultos cada vez de 2 ml.)<br>(4) Por vía oral: para adultos cada vez de 200 mg, 2 ~ 3 veces al día. |
| 剂型、规格<br>Formulaciones y especificaciones | 片剂：每片 200mg；500mg。喷雾剂：每瓶 0.5g；1g。颗粒剂：每袋 100mg。泡腾片：每片 600mg。<br><br>Tabletas: cada tableta de 200 mg; 500mg. Rocíe: cada botella de 0.5 g; 1g. Gránulos: cada bolso de 100mg. Tabletas efervescentes: Cada tableta de 600 mg. |
| **药品名称Drug Names** | 羧甲司坦 Carbocisteína |
| 适应证<br>Indicaciones | 用于慢性支气管炎、支气管哮喘等引起的痰液黏稠、咳痰困难和痰阻气管等。亦可用于术后咳痰困难和肺炎合并症。用于小儿非化脓性中耳炎，有预防耳聋效果。<br><br>Se usa para el tratamiento de esputo pegajoso, dificultades de expectoración y bloqueo de tráquea por la flema causada por bronquitis crónica, asma bronquial. Puede ser utilizado para el tratamiento de dificultad de expectoración y complicaciones de la neumonía después de la cirugía. Se usa para la otitis media no supurativa de niños, y tiene efecto para la prevención de la sordera. |
| 用法、用量<br>Administración y dosis | 口服，成人每次 0.25 ~ 0.5g，一日 3 次。儿童 1 日 30mg/kg。<br><br>Por vía oral, para adultos cada vez de 0.25 ~ 0.5g, 3 veces al día. Para niños, 30mg/kg al día. |
| 剂型、规格<br>Formulaciones y especificaciones | 口服液：每支 0.2g（10ml）；0.5g（10ml）。糖浆剂：2%（20mg/ml）。片剂：每片 0.25g。泡腾剂：每包 0.25g。<br><br>Líquidos por vía oral: Cada uno de 0.2 g (10 ml); 0.5 g (10 ml). Jarabe: 2% (20mg/ml). Tabletas: Cada tableta de 0.25g. Tabletas efervescentes: Cada paquete de 0.25 g. |
| **药品名称Drug Names** | 标准桃金娘油 Gelomirtol |
| 适应证<br>Indicaciones | 用于急、慢性支气管炎、鼻窦炎、支气管扩张、肺结核、矽肺及各种原因引起的慢性阻塞性肺疾病。亦可用于支气管造影术后，可促进造影剂的排除。<br><br>Se usa para el tratamiento de la enfermedad pulmonar obstructiva crónica causada por bronquitis aguda y crónica, sinusitis, bronquiectasia, tuberculosis, silicosis y por otras razones. Puede ser utilizado para la angiografía bronquial después de la cirugía, puede promover la exclusión del medicamento de radiografía. |
| 用法、用量<br>Administración y dosis | 口服。成人：每次 300mg，一日 2 ~ 3 次；4 ~ 10 岁儿童：每次 120mg，一日 2 次。<br><br>Por vía oral. Para adultos: cada vez de 300 mg, 2 ~ 3 veces al día; para niños de edad de 4 ~ 10 años: cada vez de 120 mg, 2 veces al día. |
| 剂型、规格<br>Formulaciones y especificaciones | 胶囊剂：每粒 120mg；300mg。<br><br>Cápsulas: Cada de 120 mg; 300 mg. |
| **药品名称Drug Names** | 碘化钾 Yoduro de Potasio |
| 适应证<br>Indicaciones | 为刺激性祛痰剂，可使痰液变稀，易于咳出，并可增加支气管分泌。配成含碘食盐，预防地方性甲状腺肿。<br><br>Es farmacia expectorante estimulado, pueden ser fácilmente entresacar la mucosidad, fácil de expectorar, aumentar la secreción bronquial. Se combina en la sal como la sal yodada para prevenir el bocio endémico. |
| 用法、用量<br>Administración y dosis | 口服，每次 6 ~ 10ml，一日 3 次。<br><br>Por vía oral, cada vez de 6 ~ 10 ml, 3 veces al día. |

**续 表**

| 剂型、规格<br>Formulaciones y especificaciones | 合剂：每100ml含碘化钾5g。<br>Compuesto: cada 100ml contiene 5g de yoduro de potasio. |
|---|---|

| 药品名称 Drug Names | 美司钠 Mesna |
|---|---|
| 适应证<br>Indicaciones | 用于慢性支气管炎、肺炎、肺癌患者痰液黏稠、术后肺不张等所致咳痰困难者。<br>Se usa para los pacientes con dificultades de la expectoración causada por la bronquitis crónica, la neumonía, y los pacientes con cáncer de pulmón de la viscosidad del esputo, atelectasia postoperatoria. |
| 用法、用量<br>Administración y dosis | 雾化吸入或气管内滴入，每次20%溶液1～2ml。局部刺激作用，可引起咳嗽及支气管痉挛。不宜与红霉素、四环素、氨茶碱合用。<br>Inhalación de atomización o instilación intratraqueal, cada solución de 20% de 1～2 ml. Tiene efecto de irritación local. Puede causar tos y broncoespasmo. No debe ser combinada con eritromicina, tetraciclina, teofilina. |
| 剂型、规格<br>Formulaciones y especificaciones | 气雾剂：0.2g/ml。溶液剂：10%水溶液。<br>Aerosol: 0.2g/ml. Soluciones: solución acuosa al 10%. |

11.2 镇咳药 Anti-tusivos

| 药品名称 Drug Names | 可待因 Codeína |
|---|---|
| 适应证<br>Indicaciones | ①各种原因引起的剧烈干咳和刺激性咳嗽，尤适用于伴有胸痛的剧烈咳嗽。由于本品能抑制呼吸道腺体分泌和纤毛运动，故对少量痰液的剧烈咳嗽，应与祛痰药并用。②用于中度疼痛的镇痛。③局部麻醉或全身麻醉时的辅助用药，具有镇静作用。<br>① Se usa para tos severa y tos irritativa causada por diversas razones, especialmente para el dolor en el pecho acompañado con tos severa. Dado que el producto puede inhibir la secreción glandular y el movimiento ciliar respiratorio, por lo tanto, en caso de tos con una pequeña cantidad de mucosidad, debe ser usada junto con medicamentos expectorantes. ② Tiene efecto analgésico para el dolor moderado. ③ Es medicamento adyuvante para anestesia local o anestesia general y tiene efecto sedante. |
| 用法、用量<br>Administración y dosis | （1）成人：①常用量：口服或皮下注射，一次15～30mg，1日30～90mg。缓释片剂一次1片（45mg），一日2次；②极量：一次100mg，一日250mg。<br>（2）儿童：镇痛，口服，每次0.5～1.0mg/kg，一日3次，或一日3mg/kg；镇咳，为镇痛剂量的1/3～1/2。<br>(1) Para adultos: ① Dosis habitual: por vía oral o por vía subcutánea, una vez de 15～30 mg, 30～90 mg al día. Una tabletas de liberación prolongada de una vez (45 mg), 2 veces al día; ② Dosis máxima: 100 mg cada vez: 250mg al día.<br>(2) Para niños: analgésico, se toma por vía oral, cada 0.5～1.0mg/kg, tres veces al día, o 3mg/kg al día; antitusivos, es de1/3～1/2 de dosis analgésicas. |
| 剂型、规格<br>Formulaciones y especificaciones | 片剂：每片15mg；30mg。缓释胶囊：每粒45mg。糖浆剂：0.5%，10ml，100ml。注射液：每支15mg（1ml）；30mg（1ml）。<br>Tabletas: cada tableta de 15 mg; 30mg. Cápsulas de liberación prolongada: cada cápsula de 45 mg. Jarabe: 0.5%,10ml,100ml. Inyección: cada una de 15 mg (1ml); 30 mg (1ml). |

| 药品名称 Drug Names | 福尔可定 Folcodina |
|---|---|
| 适应证<br>Indicaciones | 用于剧烈干咳和中度疼痛。<br>Se usa para la tos seca severa y el dolor moderado. |
| 用法、用量<br>Administración y dosis | 口服：常量，一次5～10mg，一日3～4次；极量，一日60mg。<br>Por vía oral:, Dosis habitual: una vez de 5～10 mg, 3～4 veces al día; Dosis máxima: 60mg al día. |
| 剂型、规格<br>Formulaciones y especificaciones | 片剂：每片5mg；10mg；15mg；30mg。<br>Tabletas: Cada tableta de 5mg;10mg;15mg;30mg. |

续　表

| 药品名称 Drug Names | 喷托维林 Pentoxiverina |
| --- | --- |
| 适应证<br>Indicaciones | 用于上呼吸道感染引起的无痰干咳和百日咳等，对小儿疗效优于成人。<br>Se usa para la tos ferina sin flema causada por las infecciones del tracto respiratorio superior y tos de cien días, los efectos en niños son mejores que en adultos. |
| 用法、用量<br>Administración y dosis | 口服，成人，每次 25mg，一日 3～4 次。<br>Por vía oral: adultos, cada vez de 25 mg, 3 ~ 4 veces al día. |
| 剂型、规格<br>Formulaciones y especificaciones | 片剂：每片 25mg。滴丸：每丸 25mg。冲剂：每袋 10g。糖浆剂：0.145%；0.2%；0.25%。<br>Tabletas: Cada tableta de 25mg. Goteo de pastillas: Cada pastilla de 25 mg. Gránulos: cada bolsa de 10 g. Jarabes: 0.145%; 0.2%; 0.25%. |

| 药品名称 Drug Names | 右美沙芬 Dextrometorfano |
| --- | --- |
| 适应证<br>Indicaciones | 用于干咳，适用于感冒、急、慢性支气管炎、支气管哮喘、咽喉炎、肺结核及其他上呼吸道感染时的咳嗽。<br>Se usa para la tos seca y es aplicable para tos causada por resfriados, bronquitis aguda y crónica, asma bronquial, laringitis, tuberculosis y otras infecciones del tracto respiratorio superior. |
| 用法、用量<br>Administración y dosis | 口服，成人，每次 10～30mg，一日 3 次。一日最大剂量 120mg。<br>Por vía oral, adultos, cada vez de 10 ~ 30 mg, 3 veces al día. Dosis máxima es de 120 mg al día. |
| 剂型、规格<br>Formulaciones y especificaciones | 片剂：每片 10mg；15mg。分散片：每片 15mg；30mg。胶囊剂：每粒 15mg。颗粒剂：每袋 7.5mg；15mg。糖浆剂：每瓶 15mg（20ml）；150mg（100ml）。注射剂：每支 5mg。<br>Tabletas: Cada tableta de 10 mg; 15 mg. Tabletas sueltas: Cada una de15 mg; 30 mg. Cápsulas: Cada cápsula de 15 mg. Gránulos: cada bolsa de 7.5 mg; 15 mg. Jarabes: cada botella de15 mg (20 ml); 150 mg (100 ml). Inyección: Cada una de 5 mg. |

11.3　平喘药 Medicamentos para el asma

| 药品名称 Drug Names | 麻黄碱 Efedrina |
| --- | --- |
| 适应证<br>Indicaciones | ①预防支气管哮喘发作和缓解轻度哮喘发作，对急性重度哮喘发作效果不佳。②用于蛛网膜下腔麻醉或硬膜外麻醉引起的低血压及慢性低血压。③治疗各种原因引起的鼻黏膜充血、肿胀引起的鼻塞。<br>① Se usa para la prevención del asma bronquial y el alivio de los ataques de asma leves, tiene pobres efectos sobre la crisis de asma aguda grave.　② Se usa para la hipotensión y la hipotensión crónica inducida por la anestesia subaracnoidea o anestesia epidural. ③ Se usa para el tratamiento de inflamación nasal causada por diversas causas de la congestión nasal,.hinchazón nasal, |
| 用法、用量<br>Administración y dosis | （1）支气管哮喘：口服：成人，常用量一次 15～30mg，一日 45～90mg；极量，一次 60mg，一日 150mg。皮下或肌内注射：成人，常用量一次 15～30mg，一日 45～60mg；极量，一次 60mg，一日 150mg。<br>（2）蛛网膜下隙麻醉或硬膜外麻醉时维持血压：麻醉前皮下或肌内注射 20～50mg。慢性低血压症，每次口服 20～50mg，一日 150mg。<br>（3）解除鼻黏膜充血、水肿：以 0.5%～1% 溶液滴鼻。<br>(1) Asma bronquial: Por vía oral: adultos, la dosis habitual de una vez es de 15 ~ 30 mg, 45 ~ 90 mg al día; dosis máxima, una vez de 60 mg, 150 mg al día. Inyección subcutánea o intramuscular: adultos, la dosis habitual de una vez es de 15 ~ 30mg, 45 ~ 60 mg al día; dosis máxima, una vez de 60 mg, 150 mg al día.<br>(2) En la anestesia subaracnoidea o anestesia epidural se mantiene la presión arterial: antes de la anestesia, hace la inyección subcutánea o intramuscular de 20 ~ 50 mg. Para hipotensión crónica, se toma por vía oral de 20 ~ 50 mg, 150 mg al día.<br>(3) Puede aliviar la congestión nasal, edema: hace goteo por vía intranasal con una solución de 0.5% ~ 1%. |

**续 表**

| 剂型、规格<br>Formulaciones y<br>especificaciones | 片剂：每片 15mg；25mg；30mg。注射液：每支 30mg（1ml）；50mg（1ml）。滴鼻剂：0.5%<br>（小儿）；1%（成人）；2%（检查、手术或止血时用）。<br><br>Tabletas: Cada tableta de 15 mg; 25 mg; 30 mg. Inyección: Cada una de 30 mg (1 ml), 50 mg (1 ml).<br>Gotas nasales: 0.5% (niños); 1% (para adultos), el 2% (para examen, cirugía o sangrado). |
|---|---|

| 药品名称 Drug Names | 异丙肾上腺素 Isoproterenol(Isoprenalina) |
|---|---|

| 适应证<br>Indicaciones | （1）支气管哮喘：适用于控制哮喘发作，常气雾吸入给药，作用快而强，但持续时间短。<br>（2）心搏骤停：治疗各种原因及溺水、电击、手术意外和药物中毒等引起的心搏骤停。必要时可与肾上腺素和去甲肾上腺素配合使用。<br>（3）房室传导阻滞。<br>（4）抗休克：心源性休克和感染性休克。对中心静脉压高、心排血量低者，应在不足血容量的基础上使用本品。<br><br>(1) Asma bronquial: Se aplica para el control de asma, a menudo se hace por inhalación del aerosol, tiene efecto rápido y fuerte, pero de corta duración.<br>(2) Paro cardíaco: se usa para tratamiento de detención cardíaca causada por diversas causas y ahogamiento, descargas eléctricas, accidentes quirúrgicos y la intoxicación de medicamentos, etc. Se combina con la epinefrina y la norepinefrina en conjunción, si es necesario.<br>(3) Bloqueo auriculoventricular.<br>(4) Anti-shock: Shock cardiogénico y shock séptico. Para los pacientes que tienen presión venosa central alta, gasto cardíaco bajo, debe utilizar este medicamento en base de la insuficiencia de volumen de sangre. |
|---|---|
| 用法、用量<br>Administración y<br>dosis | （1）支气管哮喘：舌下含服，成人常用量一次 10～15mg，一日 3 次；极量，一次 20mg，一日 60mg。气雾剂吸入，常用量，一次 0.1～0.4mg；极量，一次 0.4mg，一日 2.4mg。重复使用的间隔时间不宜少于 2 小时<br>（2）心搏骤停：心腔内注射 0.5～1mg。<br>（3）房室传导阻滞：Ⅱ度者采用舌下含服，每次 10mg，每 4 小时一次；Ⅲ度者如心率低于 40 次/分时，可用 0.5～1mg 溶 5% 葡萄糖液 200～300ml 缓慢静脉滴入。<br>（4）抗休克：以 0.5～1mg 加入 5% 葡萄糖液 200ml 中，静脉滴注，滴速 0.5～2μg/分，根据心率调整滴速，使收缩压维持在 12kPa（90mmHg）脉压维持在 2.7kPa（20mmHg）以上，心率 120 次/分以下。<br><br>(1) Asma bronquial: se toma por vía sublingual. La dosis habitual de adultos de una vez es 10 ~ 15 mg, 3 veces al día; Dosis máxima: una vez de 20 mg, 60 mg al día. Inhalación de aerosoles, dosis habitual de una vez de 0.1 ~ 0.4 mg; dosis máxima, una vez de 0.4 mg, 2.4 mg al día. El tiempo de intervalos de uso de repetición no debe ser menos de dos horas.<br>(2) Paro cardíaco: la inyección intracardiaca es de 0.5 ~ 1 mg.<br>(3) Bloqueo auriculoventricular: Para los pacientes de grado Ⅱ se toma por vía sublingual, cada vez de 10 mg, cada 4 horas una vez; Para los pacientes de grado Ⅲ, tales como la frecuencia cardíaca de menos de 40 latidos / min, puede hacer lentamente la infusión intravenosa con 0,5 ~ 1 mg disuelto en la solución de glucosa al 5% de 200 ~ 300 ml.<br>(4) Anti-shock: utilice 0.5 ~ 1 mg para agregar en la solución de glucosa al 5% de 200 ml. Infusión intraveno, la tasa de goteo es 0.5 ~ 2 μg / min, puede ajustar el ritmo de goteo en base del ritmo cardíaco, y se mantiene la presión arterial sistólica en 12 kPa (90 mmHg), la presión del pulso por encima de 2.7 kPa (20 mmHg ), la frecuencia cardíaca menos de 120 latidos / min. |
| 剂型、规格<br>Formulaciones y<br>especificaciones | 片剂：每片 10mg。纸片：每片 5mg。气雾剂：浓度为 0.25%，每瓶可喷吸 200 次左右，每揿约 0.175mg。注射液：每支 1mg（2ml）。<br><br>Tabletas: Cada tableta de 10mg. Papel: Cada papel de 5mg. Aerosol: la concentración es de 0.25%, y cada botella de spray puede absorber alrededor de 200 veces, cada vez la porción es de 0.175mg. Inyección: Cada una de 1 mg (2 ml). |

| 药品名称 Drug Names | 沙丁胺醇 Salbutamol |
|---|---|

| 适应证<br>Indicaciones | 用于防治支气管哮喘，哮喘型支气管和肺气肿的支气管痉挛。防止发作多用气雾吸入，预防可用口服。<br><br>Se usa para la prevención y tratamiento de asma bronquial, asma bronquial y broncoespasmo enfisema. Para detener las convulsiones, se usa la inhalación de aerosol, y para la prevención se utilice por vía oral. |
|---|---|

续　表

| | |
|---|---|
| 用法、用量<br>Administración y<br>dosis | 口服：成人，每次 2～4mg，一日 3 次。气雾吸入：每次 0.1～0.2mg，必要时每 4 小时重复一次，但 24 小时内不宜超过 8 次，粉雾吸入，成人每次吸入 0.4mg，一日 3～4 次。静脉注射：一次 0.4mg，用 5% 葡萄糖液 20ml 或氯化钠液 20ml 稀释后，缓慢注射。静脉滴注：一次 0.4mg，用 5% 葡萄糖液 100ml 稀释后滴入。肌内注射：一次 0.4mg，必要时可重复注射。<br><br>Por vía oral: Para adultos, cada vez de 2～4 mg, 3 veces al día. Inhalación aerosol: Cada vez de 0.1～0.2 mg, si es necesario, se repite cada 4 horas, pero no debe ser más de 8 veces en 24 horas. Inhalación de polvo seco, para adultos cada vez de 0.4 mg, 3～4 veces al día. Inyección intravenosa: una dosis de 0.4 mg, con una solución de glucosa al 5% de 20 ml o cloruro de sodio de 20 ml, después de la dilución, hace la inyección lentamente. Infusión intravenosa: una vez de 0.4 mg, con una solución de glucosa al 5% de de 100 ml, después de la dilución se hace la infusión. Inyección intramuscular: cada vez de 0.4 mg, cuando sea necesario, puede hacer las inyecciones repetidas veces. |
| 剂型、规格<br>Formulaciones y<br>especificaciones | 片（胶囊）剂：每片（粒）0.5mg；2mg。缓释片（胶囊）剂：每粒 4mg；8mg。气雾剂：溶液型 0.2%（g/g），每瓶 20mg（200 揿）每揿 0.1mg。粉雾剂胶囊：每粒 0.2mg；0.4mg，用粉物吸入器吸入。注射液：每支 0.4mg（2ml）。糖浆剂：4mg（1ml）。<br><br>Tabletas (cápsulas): Cada tableta (cápsula) es de 0.5mg; 2mg. Tabletas de liberación (cápsulas): Cada una de 4 mg; 8 mg. Aerosol: solución al 0.2% (g / g), cada botella de 20 mg (una porción de 200) cada porción de 0.1 mg. Cápsulas de inhalación de polvo seco: Cada cápsula de 0.2mg; 0.4mg, con un inhalador de polvo para su uso. Inyección: Cada dosis de 0.4 mg (2 ml). Jarabes: 4 mg (1 ml). |
| 药品名称 Drug Names | 福莫特罗 Formoterol |
| 适应证<br>Indicaciones | 用于慢性哮喘于慢性阻塞性肺疾病的维持治疗与预防发作，因其为长效制剂，特别适用于哮喘夜间发作患者，疗效尤佳。能有效预防运动型哮喘的发作。<br><br>Se utiliza en el tratamiento de mantenimiento y la prevención de los episodios de asma crónica de la enfermedad pulmonar obstructiva crónica, debido a que es una formulación de acción prolongada, es muy apropiado especialmente para los pacientes de asma nocturna, y tiene mucha eficacia. Puede prevenir con eficacia las acciones de asma del movimiento. |
| 用法、用量<br>Administración y<br>dosis | 口服：成人每次 40～80μg，一日 2 次。气雾吸入：成人每次 4.5～9μg，一日 2 次。<br><br>Por vía oral: Para adultos cada vez de 40～80μg, 2 veces al día. Inhalación aerosol: Para adultos cada vez de 4.5～9μg, dos veces al día. |
| 剂型、规格<br>Formulaciones y<br>especificaciones | 片剂：每片 20μg；40μg。干糖浆：20mg（0.5g）；气雾剂：每瓶 60 喷（每喷含本品 9μg）。片剂：每片含本品 20μg。干粉吸入剂：每瓶 60 喷（每喷含本品 4.5μg）；每瓶 60 喷（每喷含本品 9μg。<br><br>Tabletas: cada tableta de 20μg; 40μg. Jarabe seco: 20 mg (0.5 g); Aerosol: cada botella del aerosol de 60 veces (cada aspersión contiene una porción de formoterol de 9μg). Tabletas: Cada tableta contiene formoterol de 20 mg. Polvo seco de inhalador: cada botella de 60 aspersiones (cada aspersión aerosol contiene formoterol de 4.5μg); cada botella de 60 aspersiones (cada aerosol contiene la formoterol de 9μg. |
| 药品名称 Drug Names | 丙卡特罗 Procaterol |
| 适应证<br>Indicaciones | 用于防治支气管哮喘，喘息性支气管炎和慢性阻塞性肺疾病所致喘息症状。<br><br>Se usa para la prevención y el tratamiento de la respiración sibilante causada por asma bronquial, bronquitis asmática y enfermedad pulmonar obstructiva crónica. |
| 用法、用量<br>Administración y<br>dosis | 口服，成人，每晚睡前一次服 50μg，或每次 25～50μg，早晚（睡前）各服一次。<br><br>Por vía oral, para adultos, Se toma por vía oral una vez de 50μg cada noche antes de dormir, o cada vez de 25～50 μg, se toma una vez respectivamente por la matañana y por la noche (antes de acostarse). |
| 剂型、规格<br>Formulaciones y<br>especificaciones | 片剂（胶囊）剂：每片（粒）含本品 25μg；50μg。口服液：0.15mg（30ml）。气雾剂：2mg，每揿含 10μg。<br><br>Tabletas (cápsulas): Cada tableta (cápsula) contiene el procaterol de 25μg; 50μg. Líquidos por vía oral: 0.15 mg (30 ml). Aerosol: 2 mg, cada porción contiene 10μg. |
| 药品名称 Drug Names | 沙美特罗 Salmeterol |
| 适应证<br>Indicaciones | 用于哮喘、喘息性支气管炎和可逆性气管阻塞。<br><br>Se usa para el asma, bronquitis asmática y la obstrucción reversible de vías respiratorias. |

**续 表**

| 用法、用量<br>Administración y dosis | 粉物吸入：成人，每次 50μg，一日 2 次；儿童，每次 25μg，一日 2 次。气雾吸入：剂量用法同上。<br>Inhalación de polvo seco: Para adultos, cada vez de 50 μg, 2 veces al día; Para niños, 25μg cada vez, 1 ~ 2 veces al día. Inhalación de aerosol: El uso de dosis es lo mismo como lo anterior. |
|---|---|
| 剂型、规格<br>Formulaciones y especificaciones | 粉雾剂胶囊：每粒含本品 50μg。气雾剂：λ 每喷含本品 25μg。<br>Cápsulas de inhalación de polvo seco: Cada cápsula contiene salmeterol de 50μg. Aerosol: λ cada porción contiene salmeterol de 25μg. |
| 药品名称 Drug Names | 班布特罗 Bambuterol |
| 适应证<br>Indicaciones | 用于支气管哮喘、慢性喘息性支气管炎、阻塞性肺气肿及其他伴有支气管痉挛的肺部疾病。<br>Se usa para el asma bronquial, bronquitis asmática crónica, enfisema y otras enfermedades pulmonares asociadas con broncoespasmo. |
| 用法、用量<br>Administración y dosis | 每晚睡前口服一次，成人 10mg，12 岁以下儿童 5mg。<br>Se toma por vía oral una vez cada noche antes de dormir, para adultos es de 10 mg, para los niños menores de 12 años es de 5mg. |
| 剂型、规格<br>Formulaciones y especificaciones | 片剂（胶囊）：每片（粒）10mg；20mg。口服液：10mg（10ml）。<br>Tabletas (cápsulas): Cada tableta (cápsula) de 10mg; 20mg. Líquidos por vía oral: 10 mg (10 ml). |
| 药品名称 Drug Names | 异丙托溴铵 Bromuro de ipratropio |
| 适应证<br>Indicaciones | ①用于缓解慢性阻塞性肺疾病（COPD）引起的支气管痉挛、喘息症状。②防治哮喘、尤适用于因用 β 受体激动药产生肌肉震颤、激动过速而不能耐受此类药物的患者。<br>① Se usa para el alivio de broncoespasmo, sibilancias causadas por la enfermedad pulmonar obstructiva crónica (EPOC). ② Se usa para la prevención y el tratamiento del asma, especialmente para los pacientes con temblores musculares, agitación y taquicardia producidos por el fármaco de estimulación de los receptores β quienes no pueden tolerar este tipo de medicamentos. |
| 用法、用量<br>Administración y dosis | 气雾吸入：成人一次 40 ~ 80μg，一日 3 ~ 4 次。雾化吸入：成人，一次 100 ~ 500μg（14 岁以下 50 ~ 250μg），用生理盐水稀释到 3 ~ 4ml，至雾化器中吸入。<br>Inhalación de aerosol : para adultos cada vez de 40 ~ 80μg, 3 ~ 4 veces al día. Inhalación de atomización: para adultos, cada vez de 100 ~ 500μg (para personas de edad de menor de 14 años, es de 50 ~ 250μg), De ser diluida en la solución salina de 3 ~ 4 ml, se hace la inhalación por el nebulizador. |
| 剂型、规格<br>Formulaciones y especificaciones | 气雾剂：每喷 20μg，40μg；每瓶 200 喷（10ml）。吸入溶液剂：2ml：异丙托溴铵 500μg。雾化溶液剂：50μg（2ml）；250μg（2ml）；500μg（2ml）；500μg（20ml）<br>Aerosol: Cada pulverización de 20 μg, 40μg; cada botella de spray es de 200 pulverizaciones (10 ml). Soluciones para inhalación: 2 ml: bromuro de ipratropio de 500μg. Soluciones de atomización: 50 μg (2 ml); 250μg (2 ml); 500μg (2 ml); 500μg (20 ml). |
| 药品名称 Drug Names | 噻托溴铵 Bromuro de tiotropio |
| 适应证<br>Indicaciones | 用于治疗慢性阻塞性肺疾病及支气管哮喘，对于急性哮喘发作无效。<br>Se usa para el tratamiento de la enfermedad pulmonar obstructiva crónica y asma bronquial, y no es válido para el ataque de asma agudo. |
| 用法、用量<br>Administración y dosis | 噻托溴铵粉吸入剂（胶囊）：每粒 18μg，每次吸入 1 粒，一日 1 次。<br>Polvo para inhalación de bromuro de tiotropio (cápsulas); cada cápsula es de 18μg, cada vez en la inhalación es de 1 cápsula. 1 vez al día. |
| 剂型、规格<br>Formulaciones y especificaciones | 粉雾剂：18μg。<br>Inhalación de polvos: 18μg. |

| 药品名称 Drug Names | 氨茶碱 Aminofilina |
|---|---|
| 适应证<br>Indicaciones | 用于①支气管哮喘和喘息性支气管炎，与 β 受体激动剂合用可提高疗效。在哮喘持续状态，常选用本品与肾上腺皮质激素配伍进行治疗；②治疗急性心功能不全和心源性哮喘；③胆绞痛。<br><br>Se usa para ① Asma bronquial y bronquitis asmática, en combinación con agonistas β puede mejorar el resultado. En el estado asmático, este producto suele elegir la compatibilidad con el tratamiento con glucocorticoides; ② Tratamiento de la insuficiencia cardíaca aguda y asma cardíaco; ③ Cólico biliar. |
| 用法、用量<br>Administración y<br>dosis | 口服：成人，常用量，一次 0.1 ～ 0.2g，一日 0.3 ～ 0.6g；极量，一次 0.5g，一日 1g。肌内注射或静脉注射：成人，常用量，一次 0.25 ～ 0.5g，一日 0.5 ～ 1g；极量，一日 0.5g。以 50% 葡萄糖注射液 20 ～ 40mg 稀释后缓慢静脉注射（不少于 10 分钟）。静脉滴注：以 5% 葡萄糖注射液 500ml 稀释后滴注。直肠给药：栓剂或保留灌肠，一次 0.3 ～ 0.5g，一日 1 ～ 2 次。<br><br>Por vía oral: adultos, dosis habitual, cada vez de 0.1 ~ 0.2 g, 0.3 ~ 0.6g al día; dosis máxima, 0.5g por cada vez, 1g al día. Inyección intramuscular o inyección intravenosa: para adultos, la dosis habitual es 0.25 ~ 0.5 g por cada vez, 0.5 ~ 1g al día; Dosis máxima, 0.5 g al día. Después de la dilución de inyección de glucosa al 50% de 20 ~ 40 mg, hace la inyección intravenosa lenta (no menos de 10 minutos). Infusión intravenosa: Después de la dilución de inyección de glucosa al 5% de 500 ml, hace la infusión. Administración rectal: utilice supositorios o enemas de retención, 0.3 ~ 0.5 g por cada vez, 1 ~ 2 veces al día. |
| 剂型、规格<br>Formulaciones y<br>especificaciones | 片剂：每片 0.05g；0.1g；0.2g。肠溶片：每片 0.05g；0.1g。注射液：①肌内注射用每支 0.125g（2ml）；0.25g（2ml）；0.5g（2ml）。②静脉注射用每支 0.25g（10ml）。栓剂：每粒 0.25g。缓释片每片 0.15g；0.2g。<br><br>Tabletas: Cada tableta de 0.05 g; 0.1 g; 0.2 g. Tabletas con recubrimiento entérico: Cada tableta de 0.05 g; 0.1 g. Inyección: ① inyección intramuscular cada de 0.125 g (2 ml); 0.25 g (2 ml); 0.5 g (2 ml). ② inyección intravenosa Cada de 0.25 g (10 ml). Supositorios: cada de 0.25 g. Tabletas de liberación sostenida, cada de 0.15 g; 0.2g. |
| 药品名称 Drug Names | 多索茶碱 Doxofilina |
| 适应证<br>Indicaciones | 适用于支气管哮喘、喘息性支气管炎及其他伴支气管痉挛的肺部疾病。<br><br>Se usa para el asma bronquial, bronquitis asmática y otras enfermedades pulmonares asociadas con broncoespasmo. |
| 用法、用量<br>Administración y<br>dosis | 口服：一日 2 片或每 12 小时 1 ～ 2 粒胶囊，或一日 1 ～ 3 包散剂冲服。急症可先注射 100mg，然后每 6 小时静脉注射一次，也可每日静脉滴注 300mg。<br><br>Por vía oral: cada día 2 tabletas o cada 12 horas 1 ~ 2 cápsulas o 1 ~ 3 paquetes de polvo al día. En caso emergente puede inyectar primero 100 mg, y luego cada 6 horas se inyecta por vía intravenosa una vez, y se puede inyectar por goteo intravenosa una vez al día de 300 mg. |
| 剂型、规格<br>Formulaciones y<br>especificaciones | 片剂：每片 200mg；300mg；400mg。胶囊剂：每粒 200mg；300mg。散剂：每包 200mg。注射液：每支 100mg（10ml）。葡萄糖注射液：每瓶 0.3g 与葡萄糖 5g（100ml）。<br><br>Tabletas: Cada tableta de 200 mg, 300 mg, 400 mg. Cápsulas: Cada cápsula de 200 mg; 300 mg. Polvo suelto: Cada paquete de 200mg. Inyección: Cada dosis de100 mg (10 ml). Inyección de glucosa: cada botella de 0.3 g y glucosa de 5 g (100 ml). |
| 药品名称 Drug Names | 二羟丙茶碱 Diprofilina |
| 适应证<br>Indicaciones | 用于支气管哮喘、喘息性支气管炎，尤适用于伴有心动过速的哮喘患者。亦可用于心源性肺水肿引起的喘息。<br><br>Se usa para el asma bronquial, bronquitis asmática, especialmente para los pacientes de asma con taquicardia. Y puede utilizarse para el respiro ocasionado por el edema pulmonar cardiogénico. |
| 用法、用量<br>Administración y<br>dosis | 口服：一次 0.1 ～ 0.2g，一日 3 次。极量，一次 0.5g，一日 1.5g。肌内注射：一次 0.25 ～ 0.5g，静脉滴注：用于严重哮喘发作，一日 0.5 ～ 1g，加于 5% 葡萄糖液 1500 ～ 2000ml 中滴入。直肠给药：一次 0.25 ～ 0.5g。<br><br>Por vía oral: Cada vez de 0.1 ~ 0.2 g, 3 veces al día. Dosis máxima, una vez de 0.5 g, 1.5 g al día. Inyección intramuscular: Cada vez de 0.25 ~ 0.5 g, Infusión intravenosa: se usa para ataque de asma severo, 0.5 ~ 1 g al día, en una solución de glucosa al 5% de 1500 ~ 2000ml para hacer la infusión. La administración de dosis rectal: Cada vez de 0.25 ~ 0.5 g. |

**续 表**

| 剂型、规格<br>Formulaciones y<br>especificaciones | 片剂：每片 0.1g；0.2g。注射液：每支 0.25g（2ml）。葡萄糖注射液：每瓶 0.25g 与葡萄糖 5g（100ml）。栓剂：每粒 0.25g。<br><br>Tabletas: Cada tableta de 0.1 g; 0.2 g. Inyección: Cada 0.25 g (2 ml). Inyección de glucosa: a 5 g de glucosa 0.25 g botella (100 ml). Supositorios: cada pastilla de 0.25 g. |
|---|---|

| 药品名称 Drug Names | 色甘酸钠 Cromoglicato sódico |
|---|---|

| 适应证<br>Indicaciones | ①支气管哮喘：可用于预防各型哮喘发作。对外源性哮喘疗效显著，特别是对已知抗原的年轻患者疗效更佳，对内源性哮喘和慢性哮喘亦有一定疗效，约50%患者的症状改善或完全控制。对依赖肾上腺皮质激素的哮喘患者，经本品后可减少或完全停用肾上腺皮质激素。运动性哮喘患者预先给药几乎可防止全部病例发作。一般因于接触抗原前1周给药，但运动性哮喘可在运动前15分钟给药。β肾上腺素受体激动剂合用可提高疗效。②过敏性鼻炎，季节性花粉症，春季角膜、结膜炎、过敏性湿疹及某些皮肤瘙痒症。③溃疡性结肠炎和直肠炎：本品灌肠后可改善症状，内镜检查和活检均可见炎症及损伤减轻。<br><br>① Asma bronquial: se puede utilizar para la prevención de diversos tipos de ataques de asma. Tiene efecto significativo para el asma exógeno, especialmente para los pacientes jóvenes con antígenos conocidos se acciona con mejor eficacia, en caso de asma endógeno y el asma crónica tienen un cierto efecto, para alrededor de la mitad de los pacientes hay mejoría de los síntomas o bajo control total. Para los pacientes de asma dependientes de hormona adrenocorticotrópica, después del uso del presente producto puede reducir o parar por completo del uso de las hormonas suprarrenales. Para los pacientes de asma inducida por el ejercicio, si recibe el tratamiento previo, casi puede prevenir la producción de todos los casos, convulsiones. Generalmente debe hace tomar el medicamento una semana antes de la exposición al antígeno, pero para el asma inducida por el ejercicio puede tomarse 15 minutos antes del ejercicio. La combinación con agonistas de receptores de β-adrenérgicos puede aumentar su eficacia. ② Rinitis alérgica, fiebre del heno estacional, córnea de primavera, conjunctivitis, eccema atópico y algunos pruritos. ③ Colitis ulcerosa y la proctitis: Este producto puede mejorar los síntomas después de la enema, en el examen microscópico y la biopsia se observan el alivio de inflamación y las lesiones. |
|---|---|

| 用法、用量<br>Administración y dosis | （1）支气管哮喘：粉物吸入，每次20mg，一日4次；症状减轻后，一日40～60mg；维持量，一日20mg。气雾吸入，每次2.5～7mg，一日3～4次，每日最大剂量32mg。<br>（2）过敏性鼻炎：干粉吸入或吹入鼻腔，每次10mg，一日4次。<br>（3）季节性花粉症和春季角膜、结膜炎：滴眼，2%溶液，一次2滴，一日数次。<br>（4）过敏性湿疹、皮肤瘙痒症：外用5%～10%软膏。<br>（5）溃疡性结肠炎、直肠炎：灌肠，每次200mg。<br><br>(1) Asma bronquial: Inhalación de polvo seco, cada vez de 20 mg, 4 veces al día, después de alivio de los síntomas, 40 ~ 60 mg; dosis de mantenimiento, el día de 20mg. Inhalación, cada 2.5 ~ 7 mg, 3 ~ 4 veces al día, la dosis diaria máxima es de 32 mg.<br>(2) Rinitis alérgica: Inhalación de polvo seco o insuflación nasal, cada vez de 10 mg, 4 veces al día.<br>(3) Fiebre del heno estacional y la córnea de la primavera, la conjuntivitis, colirio: goteo para los ojos, en solución al 2%, 2 veces al día.<br>(4) Eccema atópica, prurito: Ungüento tópico de uso exterior de 5% ~ 10%.<br>(5) Colitis ulcerosa, proctitis: Enema, cada vez de 200 mg. |
|---|---|

| 剂型、规格<br>Formulaciones y especificaciones | 粉雾剂胶囊：每粒20mg，装于专用喷雾器内吸入。气雾剂：每瓶700mg（200揿），每揿3.5mg。软膏：5%～10%。滴眼剂：0.16g/8ml（2%）。<br><br>Cápsulas de inhalación de polvo seco: Cada cápsula de 20mg, conservadas en un inhalador de aerosol especializado. Aerosol: cada botella de 700mg (200 porciones), cada porción de 3,5 mg. Ungüento: 5% ~ 10%. Gotas para los ojos: 0.16g/8ml (2%). |
|---|---|

| 药品名称 Drug Names | 酮替芬 Ketotifeno |
|---|---|

| 适应证<br>Indicaciones | ①支气管哮喘，对过敏性、感染性和混合性哮喘均有预防发作效果。②哮喘性支气管炎、过敏性咳嗽。③过敏性鼻炎、过敏性结膜炎及过敏性皮炎。<br><br>① Hay efectos de prevención para asma bronquial, episodios alérgicos, infecciosos y asmas mixtas. ② Bronquitis asmática, tos alérgica. ③ Rinitis alérgica, conjuntivitis alérgica y dermatitis atópica. |
|---|---|

| | |
|---|---|
| 用法、用量<br>Administración y dosis | （1）口服：①片剂，成人及儿童均为每次 1mg，一日 2 次，早、晚服用；②小儿可服其口服溶液，一日 1 ～ 2 次（一次量：4 ～ 6 岁，2ml；6 ～ 9 岁，2.5ml；9 ～ 14 岁，3ml）。<br>（2）滴鼻：一次 1 ～ 2 滴，一日 1 ～ 3 次。<br>（3）滴眼：滴入结膜囊，一日 2 次，一次 1 滴，或每 8 ～ 12 小时滴 1 次。<br>(1) Por vía oral: ① tabletas, tanto para adultos como para niños son cada vez de 1 mg, 2 veces al día, se toma por la mañana y por la noche; ② Para bebés pueden servir el líquido por vía oral, 1 ~ 2 veces al día (la dosis de una vez: 4 ~ 6 años de edad, 2 ml; 6 ~ 9 años de edad, 2.5 ml; 9 ~ 14 años de edad, 3 ml).<br>(2) Gotas intranasal: una vez de 1 ~ 2 gotas, 1~3 veces al día.<br>(3) Gotas para los ojos: instilación al saco conjuntival, 2 veces al día, una vez de una gota o cada 8 - 12 horas 1 gota. |
| 剂型、规格<br>Formulaciones y especificaciones | 片剂：每片 0.5mg；1mg。胶囊剂：每粒 0.5mg；1mg。口服溶液：1mg（5ml）。滴鼻液：15mg（10ml）。滴眼液：2.5mg（5ml）。<br>Tabletas: Cada tableta de 0.5mg; 1mg. Cápsulas: Cada cápsula de 0.5mg; 1mg. Líquido por vía oral: 1 mg (5 ml). Gotas intranasales: 15 mg (10 ml). Gotas para los ojos: 2.5 mg (5 ml). |
| 药品名称 Drug Names | 氮䓬司汀 Azelastina |
| 适应证<br>Indicaciones | 用于治疗支气管哮喘、过敏性鼻炎或过敏性结膜炎。<br>Se usa para el tratamiento de asma bronquial, rinitis alérgica o conjuntivitis alérgica. |
| 用法、用量<br>Administración y dosis | 支气管哮喘：口服，成人一次 2 ～ 4mg，6 ～ 12 岁儿童一次 1mg，一日 2 次。过敏性鼻炎：口服，一次 1mg，一日 2 次，在早餐后及睡前各服 1 次；喷鼻，一次 1 喷，一日 2 ～ 4 次。过敏性结膜炎：滴眼，一次 1 滴，一日 2 ～ 4 次。<br>Asma bronquial: Por vía oral, para adultos cada vez de 2 ~ 4 mg, para niños de 6 ~ 12 años de edad cada vez de 1 mg, 2 veces al día. Rinitis alérgica: Por vía oral, cada vez de 1 mg, 2 veces al día, se toma cada porción después del desayuno y antes de acostarse; Pulverización nasal, una vez de una pulverización, 2 ~ 4 veces al día. Conjuntivitis alérgica: gotas para los ojos, una vez de1 gota, 2 ~ 4 veces al día. |
| 剂型、规格<br>Formulaciones y especificaciones | 片剂：每片 1mg；2mg。颗粒剂：0.2%。喷鼻剂：10mg（10ml）。滴眼液：2.5mg（5ml）。<br>Tabletas: Cada tableta de 1mg; 2mg. Gránulos: 0.2%. Aerosol nasal: 10 mg (10 ml). Gotas para los ojos: 2.5 mg (5 ml). |
| 药品名称 Drug Names | 倍氯米松 Beclometasona |
| 适应证<br>Indicaciones | ①本品吸入给药可用于慢性哮喘患者；②鼻喷用于过敏性鼻炎；③外用治疗过敏所致炎症性皮肤病如湿疹、神经性或接触性皮炎、瘙痒症等。<br>① Este producto de uso de inhalación puede ser utilizado para los pacientes con asma crónica; ② Aerosol nasal se usa para la rinitis alérgica; ③ El tratamiento tópico puede curar enfermedades inflamatorias de la piel causadas por las alergias, tales como eczema, dermatitis de contacto o neurológica, prurito. |
| 用法、用量<br>Administración y dosis | 气雾吸入，成人开始剂量每次 50 ～ 200μg，一日 2 次或 3 次，每日最大剂量 1mg。儿童用量依年龄酌减，每日最大剂量 0.8mg。长期吸入的维持量应个体化，以减至最低剂量又能控制症状为准。粉雾吸入，成人每次 200μg，一日 3 ～ 4 次。儿童每次 100μg，一日 2 次或遵医嘱。<br>Inhalación de aerosol, para adultos, la dosis inicial es cada vez de 50 ~ 200μg, 2 o 3 veces al día, la dosis máxima diaria es de 1 mg. La dosis de niños se reduce de acuerdo con la edad, la dosis máxima diaria es de 0.8 mg. La dosis de mantenimiento a largo plazo de inhalación debe ser individualizada, tanto para minimizar la dosis como para controlar los síntomas. Inhalación de polvo, para adultos, cada vez de 200μg, 3 ~ 4 veces al día. Para niños cada vez de 100 μg, 2 veces al día o según las indicaciones. |
| 剂型、规格<br>Formulaciones y especificaciones | 气雾剂：每瓶 200 喷（每喷 50μg；80μg；100μg；200μg；250μg）；每瓶 80 喷（每喷 250μg）。粉雾剂胶囊：每粒 50μg；100μg；200μg。喷鼻剂：每瓶 10mg（每喷 50μg）。软膏剂：2.5mg/10g。霜剂：2.5mg/10g。<br>Aerosoles: cada botella de 200 pulverizaciones (cada pulverización de 50 μg; 80μg; 100 μg; 200μg; 250μg); cada botella de 80 pulverizaciones (cada pulverización de 250μg). Cápsulas de inhalación de polvo seco: Cada cápsula de 50 μg; 100 μg; 200μg. Aerosol nasal: cada botella de 10 mg (50 μg por pulverización). Ungüento: 2.5mg/10g. Crema: 2.5mg/10g. |

**续　表**

| 药品名称 Drug Names | 布地奈德 Budesonida |
|---|---|
| 适应证<br>Indicaciones | ①用于肾上腺皮质激素依赖性或非依赖性支气管哮喘及喘息性支气管炎患者，可有效地减少口服肾上腺皮质激素的用量，有助于减轻肾上腺皮质激素的不良反应。②用于慢性阻塞性肺病。<br><br>① Se usa para los pacientes con hormona adrenocorticotrópica de c arácter dependiente o asma bronquial y bronquitis asmáticas de no dependiente. Puede reducir efectivamente la cantidad de dosis de glucocorticoides por vía oral y ayudar a mitigar los efectos adversos de la hormona corticotropina. ② Se usa para la enfermedad pulmonar obstructiva crónica. |
| 用法、用量<br>Administración y dosis | 气雾吸入：成人，开始剂量每次 200～800μg，一日 2 次，维持量因人而异，通常为每次 200～400μg，一日 2 次；儿童，开始剂量每次 100～200μg，一日 2 次，维持量也应个体化，以减至最低剂量又能控制症状为准。<br><br>Inhalación de aerosol: adultos, la dosis inicial es de 200 ~ 800 μg, 2 veces al día, La dosis de mantenimiento se varía, por lo general cada vez de 200 ~ 400 μg, 2 veces al día; Para los niños, la dosis inicial es cada vez de 100 ~ 200μg, 2 veces al día, la dosis de mantenimiento debe ser individualizada, tanto para minimizar la dosis como para controlar los síntomas. |
| 剂型、规格<br>Formulaciones y especificaciones | 气雾剂：每瓶 10mg（100 喷，200 喷），每喷 100μg，50μg；每瓶 20mg（100 喷），每喷 200μg；每瓶 60mg（300 喷），每喷 200μg。粉雾剂：每瓶 20mg；40mg，每喷 200μg。<br><br>Aerosol: Botella de 10 mg (100 por pulverización, 200 por pulverización), cada botella de 100 μg, 50 μg; cada botella de 20 mg (100 por pulverización), cada botella de 200μg; cada botella de 60 mg (300 por pulverización), cada botella de 200μg. La inhalación de polvo seco: cada botella de 20 mg; 40 mg, cada pulverización de 200μg. |
| 药品名称 Drug Names | 氟替卡松 Fluticasona |
| 适应证<br>Indicaciones | 雾化吸入用于慢性持续性哮喘的长期治疗，亦可治疗过敏性鼻炎。<br><br>La inhalación de atomización se usa para el tratamiento a largo plazo de asma crónica persistente, y también la rinitis alérgica. |
| 用法、用量<br>Administración y dosis | （1）支气管哮喘：雾化吸入，成人和 16 岁以上青少年起始剂量：①轻度持续，一日 200～500μg，分 2 次给予；②中度持续，一日 500～1000μg，分 2 次给予；③重度持续，一日 1000～2000μg，分 2 次给予。16 岁以下儿童起始剂量，根据病情及身体发育情况酌情给予，一日 100～400μg；5 岁以下 1 日 100～200μg。维持量亦应个体化，以减至最低剂量又能控制症状为准。<br><br>（2）过敏性鼻炎：鼻喷，一次 50～200μg，一日 2 次。<br><br>(1) Asma bronquial: Inhalación de atomización, la dosis inicial para adultos y adolescentes mayores de 16 años: ① leve persistente, 200 ~ 500μg al día, divida en 2 veces; ② moderado persistente, 500 ~ 1000 μg al día, divida en 2 veces; ③ severa persistente, 1000 ~ 2000μg al día, divida en 2 veces. La dosis inicial para los niños menores de 16 años de edad, se toma de acuerdo a la condición física y el desarrollo de las facultades discrecionales, 100 ~ 400 μg al día; para los niños menores de 5 años de edad, 100 ~ 200μg al día. La dosis de mantenimiento debe ser individualizada, tanto para minimizar la dosis como para controlar los síntomas.<br>(2) Rinitis alérgica: aerosol nasal, 50 ~ 200μg cada vez, 2 veces al día. |
| 剂型、规格<br>Formulaciones y especificaciones | 气雾剂：每瓶 60 喷；120 喷（每喷 25μg；50μg；125μg；250μg）。喷鼻剂：每瓶 120 喷（每喷 50μg）。<br><br>Aerosol: cada botella de 60 pulverizaciones; 120 pulverizaciones (25μg; 50 μg; 125μg, 250μg por pulverización). Aerosol nasal: cada botella de 120 pulverizaciones (50 μg por pulverización). |
| 药品名称 Drug Names | 曲安奈德 Acetónido de triamcinolona |
| 适应证<br>Indicaciones | 用于支气管哮喘。<br>Se usa para el asma bronquial. |
| 用法、用量<br>Administración y dosis | 常用气雾吸入：成人每日 0.8～1.0mg，儿童每日 0.4mg，分 4 次给药。<br>Inhalación de aerosol haibtual: para adultos 0.8 ~ 1.0 mg diariamente, para niños 0.4 mg diariamente, se divide en 4 veces para su uso. |

续　表

| 剂型、规格<br>Formulaciones y especificaciones | 鼻喷雾剂：每支 6ml ［6.6mg，120 喷（55μg/ 喷）］ 。<br>Aerosol nasal: Cada una de 6 ml [6.6 mg, 120 de pulverizaciones (55μg / pulverización)]. |
|---|---|
| **药品名称 Drug Names** | **糠酸莫米松 Furoato de mometasona** |
| 适应证<br>Indicaciones | 用于预防和治疗各种过敏性鼻炎，亦可试用于支气管哮喘。<br>Se usa para la prevención y tratamiento de diversas rinitis alérgica, y también está en prueba para el asma bronquial. |
| 用法、用量<br>Administración y dosis | 成人常用量：每侧鼻孔 2 喷，每喷 50μg，一日 1 次，一日总量 200μg。症状控制后，剂量减至一日总量 100μg 以维持疗效。12 岁以下儿童：每侧鼻孔 1 喷，每喷 50μg，一日 1 次，一日总量 100μg。维持量酌减。<br>Dosis habitual para adultos: 2 pulverizaciones en cada lado de la fosa nasal, 50 μg por cada pulverización, 1 vez al día, 200μg de dosis total al día. Con el control de los síntomas, la dosis total diaria se reduce a 100 μg para mantener la eficacia. Para los niños menores de 12 años de edad: 1 pulverización en cada lado de la fosa nasal, 50 μg por cada pulverización, 1 vez al día, 100 μg de dosis total al día. La dosis de mantenimiento se reduce de acuerdo con las circunstancias. |
| 剂型、规格<br>Formulaciones y especificaciones | 喷鼻剂：每支 60 喷，每喷 50μg。<br>Aerosol nasal: cada de 60 pulverizaciones, 50 μg por cada pulverización. |
| **药品名称 Drug Names** | **扎鲁司特 Zafirlukast** |
| 适应证<br>Indicaciones | 用于①慢性轻至中度支气管哮喘的预防和治疗，尤其适于对阿司匹林敏感或有阿司匹林哮喘的患者或伴有上呼吸道疾病（如鼻息肉、过敏性鼻炎）者，但不宜用于治疗急性哮喘；②激素抵抗型哮喘或拒绝使用激素的哮喘患者；③严重哮喘时加用本品以维持控制哮喘发作或用以减少激素用量。<br>Se usa ① para la prevención y el tratamiento del asma bronquial crónica leve a moderada, especialmente es adecuado para los pacientes de la aspirina o sensible a la aspirina o asma asociado con el tracto respiratorio superior (por ejemplo, pólipos nasales, rinitis alérgica), pero no es bueno para el tratamiento de la asma aguda; ② los pacientes con asma resistente a esteroides o quienes rechazan el uso de hormonas en asma; ③ para asma grave puede agregar este producto con el fin de mantener el control del asma o para reducir el uso de la cantidad de hormonas. |
| 用法、用量<br>Administración y dosis | 口服：成人及 12 岁以上儿童，每次 20mg，一日 2 次，餐前 1 小时或餐后 2 小时服，用于预防哮喘时，应持续用药。<br>Por vía oral: Adultos y niños mayores de 12 años de edad, 20 mg por cada vez, 2 veces al día, se toma en 1 hora antes o 2 horas después de la comida, cuando se utiliza para prevenir el asma deben continuar a largo plazo el medicamento. |
| 剂型、规格<br>Formulaciones y especificaciones | 片剂：每片 20mg；40mg。<br>Tabletas: cada tableta de 20 mg; 40mg. |
| **药品名称 Drug Names** | **孟鲁司特钠 Montelukast sódico** |
| 适应证<br>Indicaciones | 用于预防支气管哮喘和支气管哮喘的长期治疗。也用于治疗阿司匹林敏感的哮喘，预防运动性哮喘。对激素已耐药的患者本品亦有效。<br>Se usa para la prevención de asma bronquial y el tratamiento a largo plazo de del asma crónico. También se usa para el tratamiento del asma sensible a la aspirina, la prevención del asma inducida por el ejercicio. Para los pacientes con hormona-resistente, este producto tiene acciones efectivas. |
| 用法、用量<br>Administración y dosis | 口服：成人 10mg，一日 1 次，每晚睡前服。6 ～ 14 岁儿童 5mg，一日 1 次。2 ～ 6 岁儿童 4mg，一日 1 次。<br>Por vía oral: para adultos 10mg, 1 vez al día, se toma cada noche antes de acostarse. Para niños de 6 ～ 14 años de edad 5mg, 1 vez al día. Para niños de 2 ～ 6 años 4mg, 1 vez al día. |
| 剂型、规格<br>Formulaciones y especificaciones | 片剂：每片 4mg；5mg。包衣片：10mg。<br>Tabletas: Cada una de 4mg; 5mg. Tabletas recubiertas: 10 mg. |

**续　表**

| 药品名称 Drug Names | 普仑司特 Pranlukast |
|---|---|
| 适应证<br>Indicaciones | 用于支气管哮喘的预防和治疗。<br>Se usa para la prevención y el tratamiento del asma bronquial. |
| 用法、用量<br>Administración y dosis | 口服，成人一次 225mg，一日 2 次（餐后服）。<br>Por vía oral, para adultos 225 mg por cada vez, 2 veces al día (después de la comida). |
| 剂型、规格<br>Formulaciones y especificaciones | 胶囊剂：每粒 112.5mg。<br>Cápsulas: Cada cápsula de 112.5mg. |
| 药品名称 Drug Names | 吡嘧司特 Pemirolast |
| 适应证<br>Indicaciones | 用于预防或减轻支气管哮喘发作，不能迅速缓解急性哮喘发作。<br>Se utiliza para prevenir o aliviar el asma bronquial, no puede aliviar rápidamente los ataques agudos de asma. |
| 用法、用量<br>Administración y dosis | 口服：成人常用量每次 10mg，一日 2 次，早、午或临睡前服用。<br>Por vía oral: dosis habitual de adultos es cada vez de 10 mg, 2 veces al día, se toma por la mañana, por la tarde o antes de acostarse. |
| 剂型、规格<br>Formulaciones y especificaciones | 片剂：一片 10mg。<br>Tabletas: Cada tableta de 10mg. |
| 药品名称 Drug Names | 阿桔片 Combinaciones opiata y platycodon grandiflorum comprimidos |
| 适应证<br>Indicaciones | 镇咳、祛痰。<br>Antitusivo, expectorante. |
| 用法、用量<br>Administración y dosis | 一次 3～4 片，一日 3 次。<br>Cada vez de 3 ~ 4 tabletas, 3 veces al día. |
| 剂型、规格<br>Formulaciones y especificaciones | 片剂：300mg。<br>Tabletas:300mg. |
| 药品名称 Drug Names | 川贝枇杷糖浆 ChuanBeiPiPa jarabe |
| 适应证<br>Indicaciones | 化痰止咳。<br>Puede eliminar la flema y aliviar la tos. |
| 用法、用量<br>Administración y dosis | 一次 10ml，一日 3 次。<br>Cada vez de 10 ml, 3 veces al día. |
| 剂型、规格<br>Formulaciones y especificaciones | 糖浆：100ml，120ml，150ml。<br>Jarabe: 100ml, 120ml, 150ml. |
| 药品名称 Drug Names | 复方鲜竹沥液 FuFangXianZhuLi solución |
| 适应证<br>Indicaciones | 清热化痰，止咳。<br>Puede compensar el calor, eliminar la flema y aliviar la tos. |
| 用法、用量<br>Administración y dosis | 一次 20ml，一日 2～3 次。<br>Cada vez de 20 ml, 2 ~ 3 veces al día. |

**续　表**

| 剂型、规格<br>Formulaciones y especificaciones | 口服溶液：10ml，20ml，30ml。<br>Solución oral: 10ml, 20ml, 30ml. |
|---|---|
| **药品名称 Drug Names** | 急支糖浆 JiZhi jarabe |
| 适应证<br>Indicaciones | 清热化痰。用于外感风热咳嗽。<br>Puede compensar el calor, eliminar la flema para el tratamiento de la tos de calor y viento. |
| 用法、用量<br>Administración y dosis | 一次 20～30ml，一日 3～4 次。<br>Cada vez de 20 ~ 30 ml, 3 ~ 4 veces al día. |
| 剂型、规格<br>Formulaciones y especificaciones | 糖浆：100ml，200ml。<br>Jarabe: 100ml, 200ml. |

12. 主要作用于消化系统的药物 Medicamento que actúan principalmente sobre el sistema digestivo

12.1　抗酸药 Anti-ácidos

| **药品名称 Drug Names** | 氢氧化铝 Hidróxido de aluminio |
|---|---|
| 适应证<br>Indicaciones | 主要用于胃酸过多、胃及十二指肠溃疡、反流性食管炎及上消化道出血等。由于铝离子在肠内与磷酸盐结合成不溶解的磷酸铝自粪便排出，故尿毒症患者服用大剂量氢氧化铝后可减少磷酸盐的吸收，减轻酸血症（但同时应注意上述不良反应）。<br><br>Se utiliza principalmente para la hiperacidez, úlceras gástricas y duodenales, esofagitis por reflujo y hemorragia digestiva alta. A medida que los iones de aluminio y fosfato en el intestino combinan en fosfato de aluminio que es insoluble en las heces, por lo que los pacientes urémicos que toman gran dosis de hidróxido de aluminio pueden reducir la absorción de sal de fosfato, y aliviar la acidosis (pero hay que observar las reacciones adversas arriba mencionadas). |
| 用法、用量<br>Administración y dosis | 口服，一次 0.6～0.9g，一日 1.8～2.7g。现多用氢氧化铝凝胶。治胃酸过多和溃疡病等，一次 4～8ml，一日 12～24ml，饭前 1 小时和睡前服；病情严重时剂量可加倍。<br><br>Por vía oral, 0.6 ~ 0.9g por cada vez, 1.8 ~ 2.7 g al día. Ahora se usa más gel de hidróxido de aluminio. Para el tratamiento de hiperacidez y la úlcera, debe tomar 4 ~ 8 ml por cada vez, 12 ~ 24 ml al día, se toma 1 hora antes de las comidas y antes de acostarse; en condición seria, la dosis puede ser duplicada. |
| 剂型、规格<br>Formulaciones y especificaciones | 片剂：每片 0.3g。<br>Tabletas: Cada tableta de 0.3g. |
| **药品名称 Drug Names** | 铝碳酸镁 Hidrotalcito |
| 适应证<br>Indicaciones | 主要用于胃及十二指肠溃疡、反流性食管炎、急慢性胃炎和十二指肠球炎等。也用于胃酸过多引起的胃部不适，如胃灼痛、胃灼热、反酸及腹胀、恶心、呕吐等的对症治疗。<br><br>Se utiliza principalmente para las úlceras gástricas y duodenales, esofagitis por reflujo, gastritis aguda y crónica y duodenal van mucho más. También se utiliza para causar hiperacidez estomacal, como acidez estomacal, acidez estomacal, reflujo ácido y distensión abdominal, náuseas, vómitos y otros tratamientos sintomáticos. |
| 用法、用量<br>Administración y dosis | 一般一日 3 次，一次 1.0g，餐后 1 小时服用。十二指肠球部溃疡 6 周为一疗程，胃溃疡 8 周为一疗程。<br><br>Generalmente es 3 veces el día, 1.0 g por cada vez, se toma una hora después de la comida. Para el tratamiento de úlcera duodenal seis semanas es un curso, para la úlcera péptica ocho semanas es un curso. |
| 剂型、规格<br>Formulaciones y especificaciones | 片剂（咀嚼片）：每片 0.5g。<br>Tabletas (masticables): Cada tableta de 0.5g. |

**续 表**

| 药品名称 Drug Names | 碳酸钙 Carbonato de calcio |
|---|---|
| 适应证<br>Indicaciones | 用于胃酸过多引起的反酸、胃灼热等症状。适用于胃、十二指肠溃疡及反流性食管炎的治疗。也用于补充机体钙缺乏，如各种机体对钙需求量增加的情况，可作为骨质疏松症的辅助治疗。另外，本品也用于治疗肾衰竭患者的高磷血症，同时纠正轻度代谢性酸中毒。作为磷酸盐结合剂，治疗继发性甲状旁腺功能功能亢进纤维性骨炎所致的高磷血症。<br><br>Se usa para el reflujo ácido, acidez estomacal y otros síntomas causados por el exceso de ácido en el estómago. Se usa para el tratamiento de la úlcera de estómago y esofagitis por reflujo. También se utiliza para complementar la deficiencia de calcio en el cuerpo, tales como la demanda de incrementación de calcio de diversos organismo, se puede utilizar para el tratamiento adyuvante de la osteoporosis. Además, este elemento también se utiliza para el tratamiento de la hiperfosfatemia en los pacientes con insuficiencia renal, mientras que tiene efecto de corrección de la acidosis metabólica leve. Como aglutinantes de fosfato, tiene acciones para la hiperfosfatemia causada por osteítis de hiperparatiroidismo secundario de hipertiroidismo. |
| 用法、用量<br>Administración y dosis | 用于中和胃酸，每次 $0.5 \sim 1g$，一日 $3 \sim 4$ 次，餐后 $1 \sim 1.5$ 小时服用可维持缓冲时间长达 $3 \sim 4$ 小时，如餐后即服，因随食物一起排空而失去作用。用于高磷血症，每日 1.5g，最高每日可用至 13g，进餐时服用或与氢氧化铝合用。用于补钙，每日 $1 \sim 2g$，分 $2 \sim 3$ 次与食物同服，老年人可适当补充维生素 D。<br><br>Se utiliza para neutralizar el ácido del estómago, $0.5 \sim 1$ g por cada vez, $3 \sim 4$ veces al día, se toma en $1 \sim 1.5$ horas despúes de la comida para mantener una reserva de hasta $3 \sim 4$ horas, y si se toma inmediatamente después de la comida, va a ser vaciado junto con la comida y se pierde su efecto. Para hiperfosfatemia, 1.5 g al día, la dosis máxima diaria es de 13g, se toma con las comidas o en combinación con hidróxido de aluminio. Para el suplemento de calcio, $1 \sim 2$ g al día, se toma en $2 \sim 3$ veces junto con la comida, para los ancianos es apropiado suplementar vitamina D. |
| 剂型、规格<br>Formulaciones y especificaciones | 片剂：每片 0.5g（相当于元素钙 200mg）。<br>Tabletas: Cada tableta de 0.5 g (equivalente a 200 mg de calcio elemental). |

12.2 胃酸分泌抑制剂 Inhibidores de la secreción de ácido gástrico

| 药品名称 Drug Names | 西咪替丁 Cimetidina |
|---|---|
| 适应证<br>Indicaciones | 用于治疗十二指肠溃疡、胃溃疡、上消化道出血等。治疗十二指肠溃疡愈合率为74%（对照组为37%），愈合时间大多在4周左右。对胃溃疡疗效不及十二指肠溃疡。另据报道，还可用于治疗带状疱疹和包括生殖器在内的其他疱疹性感染。<br><br>Se usa para el tratamiento de la úlcera duodenal, úlcera gástrica, sangrado gastrointestinal superior. Tiene una tasa de74% (37% en el grupo control) para la curación de tratamiento de úlcera duodenal, el tiempo de curación es de aproximadamente 4 semanas. Tiene menos efectos en la úlcera gástrica que en la úlcera duodenal. Según otro informe, también se usa para el tratamiento del herpes zoster y otras infecciones de herpes, con genital incluido. |
| 用法、用量<br>Administración y dosis | （1）口服，每次 $200 \sim 400mg$，一日 $800 \sim 1600mg$，一般于餐后及睡前各服一次，疗程一般为 $4 \sim 6$ 周。亦有主张 1 次 400mg，一日 2 次的疗法。另外，也有报道夜间一次给予双倍剂量（800mg）的疗法。<br>（2）注射：用葡萄糖注射液或葡萄糖氯化钠注射液稀释后静脉滴注，每次 $200 \sim 600mg$；或用上述溶液 20ml 稀释后缓慢静脉注射，每次 200mg，$4 \sim 6$ 小时一次。一日剂量不宜超过 2g。也可直接肌内注射。<br><br>(1) Por vía oral, cada una de $200 \sim 400$ mg, 800 días $\sim 1600$mg, generalmente se toma respectivamente después de la comida y antes de acostarse. El curso del tratamiento es por lo general de $4 \sim 6$ semanas. También puede ser una vez de 400 mg, dividido en 2 veces al día. Por otra parte, se informó también hay una menera de uso de ofrecer una dosis doble (800 mg) por la noche.<br>(2) Inyección: hace la inyección intravenosa con la glucosa o cloruro de sodio diluida, $200 \sim 600$ mg por cada vez; o hace la inyección intravenosa lenta después de la dilución de la solución de arriba mencionada de 20 ml, 200 mg por cada vez, $4 \sim 6$ horas por cada vez. La dosis diaria no debe superar 2 g. Puede también ser directamente inyectado por vía intramuscular. |

**续　表**

| | |
|---|---|
| 剂型、规格<br>Formulaciones y especificaciones | 片剂：每片 0.2g；0.8g。胶囊剂：每粒 0.2g。注射液：每支 0.2g（2ml）。<br>Tabletas: Cada tableta de 0.2 g; 0.8 g. Cápsulas: Cada cápsula de 0.2g. Inyección: Cada una de 0.2 g (2 ml). |
| **药品名称 Drug Names** | 雷尼替丁 Ranitidina |
| 适应证<br>Indicaciones | 用于治疗十二指肠溃疡、良性胃溃疡、术后溃疡、反流性食管炎及卓 - 艾综合征等。静脉注射可用于上消化道出血。<br>Se usa para el tratamiento de la úlcera duodenal, úlcera gástrica benigna, úlcera postoperatoria, esofagitis por reflujo y síndrome de Zollinger-Ellison. La inyección intravenosa se puede utilizar para la hemorragia gastrointestinal superior. |
| 用法、用量<br>Administración y dosis | 口服：一日 2 次，每次 150mg，早晚饭时服。维持剂量每日 150mg，于餐前顿服。用于反流性食管炎的治疗，一日 2 次，每次 150mg，共用 8 周。对卓 - 艾综合征，开始一日 3 次，每次 150mg，必要时剂量可加至每日 900mg。对慢性溃疡病有复发史患者，应在睡前给予维持剂量。治疗上消化道出血，可用本品 50mg 肌内注射或缓慢静脉注射（1 分钟以上），或以每小时 25mg 的速率间歇静脉滴注 2 小时。以上方法一般一日 2 次或每 6～8 小时 1 次。<br>Por vía oral: 2 veces al día, 150 mg por cada vez, se toma en el desayuno y la cena. La dosis de mantenimiento diaria es de 150 mg, se toma antes de la comida. Se usa para el tratamiento de la esofagitis por reflujo, dos líneas al día, 150mg por cada vez, en total se usa ocho semanas. Para el síndrome de Zollinger-Ellison, en el principio, se toma tres veces al día, 150 mg por cada vez, se puede añadir la dosis diaria necesaria a 900 mg. Para los pacientes con historia de la recurrencia de enfermedad de la úlcera crónica, la dosis de mantenimiento deben administrarse antes de acostarse. Se usa para el tratamiento de la hemorragia gastrointestinal,hace la inyección intramuscular o inyección intravenosa lenta de 50 mg del presente elemento (por lo menos más de un minuto o), o 25 mg por hora de infusión intravenosa a una velocidad de intermitentes de 2 horas. Generalmente los métodos anteriores son de 2 veces al día o 6～8 horas por cada vez. |
| 剂型、规格<br>Formulaciones y especificaciones | 片（胶囊）剂：每片（粒）150mg。泡腾颗粒：0.15g/1.5g。糖浆剂：1.5g/100ml。注射液：每支 50mg（2ml）；50mg（5ml）。<br>Tabletas (cápsulas): Cada tableta (cápsula) de 150mg. Granulado efervescente: 0.15g/1.5g. Jarabe: 1.5g/100ml. Inyección: Cada de 50 mg (2 ml), 50 mg (5 ml). |
| **药品名称 Drug Names** | 枸橼酸铋雷尼替丁 Citrato de bismuto y ranitidina |
| 适应证<br>Indicaciones | 用于胃及十二指肠溃疡。与抗生素合用可协同根除幽门螺杆菌，预防十二指肠溃疡的复发。<br>Se usa para las úlceras gástricas y duodenales. Puede usar en combinación con antibióticos para erradicar sinérgicamente la helicobacter pylori, y prevenir la recurrencia de la úlcera duodenal. |
| 用法、用量<br>Administración y dosis | 成人一次 1 粒，一日 2 次，餐前服。治疗胃溃疡 8 周一疗程，治疗十二指肠溃疡 4 周为一疗程。轻至中度肾功能损害及肝功能不全者无需改变剂量。<br>Para adultos una tableta por cada vez, 2 veces al día se toma antes de las comidas. El curso de tratamiento de la úlcera es de 8 meses, y el curso de tratamiento de las úlceras duodenales es de cuatro semanas. Para los pacientes con insuficiencia renal y disfunción hepática de nivel leve a moderada no necesitan el cambio de la dosis. |
| 剂型、规格<br>Formulaciones y especificaciones | 胶囊剂：每粒含枸橼酸铋雷尼替丁 350mg。<br>Cápsulas: Cada cápsula contiene 350 mg de citrato de bismuto de ranitidina. |
| **药品名称 Drug Names** | 法莫替丁 Famotidina |
| 适应证<br>Indicaciones | 口服用于胃及十二指肠溃疡、吻合口溃疡，反流性食管炎；口服或静脉注射用于上消化道出血（消化性溃疡、急性应激性溃疡，出血性胃炎所致），卓 - 艾综合征。<br>Se toma por vía oral para la úlcera gástrica y duodenal, úlcera anastomótica, esofagitis por reflujo; Se toma por vía oral o se inyecta por vía intravenosa para la hemorragia digestiva alta (causada por úlcera péptica, úlcera de estrés aguda, gastritis hemorrágica), y el síndrome de Zollinger-Ellison. |

**续　表**

| | |
|---|---|
| 用法、用量<br>Administración y dosis | 口服，一次 20mg，一日 2 次（早餐后，晚餐后或临睡前），4 ～ 6 周为一疗程，溃疡愈合后维持量减半，睡前服。肾功能不全者应调整剂量。缓慢静脉注射或静脉滴注 20mg（溶于生理盐水或葡萄糖注射液 20ml 中），一日 2 次（间隔 12 小时），疗程 5 日，一旦病情许可，应迅速将静脉给药改为口服给药。<br><br>Por vía oral, cada 20 mg, 2 veces al día (después del desayuno, después de la cena o antes de irse a dormir), de 4 a 6 semanas para un curso de tratamiento, la curación de la úlcera después de la dosis de mantenimiento reducido a la mitad antes de acostarse. Dosis Insuficiencia renal debe ajustarse. Slow inyección intravenosa o infusión intravenosa de 20 mg (disuelto en solución salina o la inyección de glucosa en 20 ml), 2 veces al día (cada 12 horas), el tratamiento durante cinco días, una vez que las condiciones lo permiten, deberá, sin demora intravenosa para la administración oral. |
| 剂型、规格<br>Formulaciones y especificaciones | 片剂：每片 10mg；20mg。分散片：每片 20mg。胶囊剂：每粒 20mg。散剂：10%（100mg/g）。注射液：每支 20mg（2ml）；每瓶 20mg/100ml。<br><br>Tabletas: Cada tableta de 10 mg; 20 mg. Tabletas dispersables: cada tableta de 20 mg: Cápsulas: Cada cápsula de 20mg. Polvo: 10% (100 mg / g). Inyección: Cada una de 20 mg (2 ml), cada botella de 20mg/100ml. |
| 药品名称 Drug Names | 奥美拉唑 Omeprazol |
| 适应证<br>Indicaciones | 主要用于十二指肠溃疡和卓 - 艾综合征，也可用于胃溃疡和反流性食管炎；静脉注射可用于消化性溃疡急性出血的治疗。与阿莫西林和克拉霉素或与甲硝唑与克拉霉素合用，以杀灭幽门螺杆菌。<br><br>Se utiliza principalmente para úlcera duodenal y síndrome de Zollinger-Ellison, también se puede utilizar para la úlcera y la esofagitis de reflujo, la inyección intravenosa se puede utilizar para el tratamiento de la hemorragia de úlcera péptica aguda. Se usa en combinación con metronidazol, claritromicina, amoxicilina y claritromicina para matar Helicobacter pylori. |
| 用法、用量<br>Administración y dosis | 可口服或静脉给药。治疗十二指肠溃疡，一日 1 次，每次 20mg，疗程 2 ～ 4 周。治疗卓 - 艾综合征，初始剂量为一日 1 次，每次 60mg，90% 以上患者用每日 20 ～ 120mg 即可控制症状，如剂量大于每日 80mg，则应分 2 次给药，治疗反流性食管炎，剂量为每日 20 ～ 60mg，治疗消化性溃疡出血，静脉注射，一次 40mg，每 12 小时一次，连用 3 日。<br><br>Puede tomar por vía oral o se inyecta por vía intravenosa. Para el tratamiento de la úlcera duodenal, 1 vez al día, 20 mg por cada vez, un curso de tratamiento es de 2 ~ 4 semanas. Para el tratamiento del síndrome de Zollinger-Ellison, la dosis diaria inicial es de 1 vez al día, 60 mg por cada vez, para 90% de los pacientes, con una dosis diaria de 20 ~ 120 mg puede controlar los síntomas. Si la dosis diaria es mayore de 80 mg, debe administrarse en 2 veces. Para el tratamiento la esofagitis por reflujo, la dosis diaria es de 20 ~ 60 mg. Para el tratamiento de la hemorragia por úlcera péptica, hace la inyección intravenosa, 40 mg por cada vez, una vez por cada 12 horas, se usa continuamente tres días. |
| 剂型、规格<br>Formulaciones y especificaciones | 胶囊剂：每粒 20mg。肠溶片：每片 20mg。注射用奥美拉唑：每支 40mg。<br><br>Cápsulas: Cada cápsula de 20mg. Tabletas con recubrimiento entérico: Cada tableta de 20mg. Inyección con Omeprazol: Cada una de 40mg. |
| 药品名称 Drug Names | 兰索拉唑 Lansoprazol |
| 适应证<br>Indicaciones | 用于胃溃疡、十二指肠溃疡、吻合口溃疡及反流性食管炎、卓 - 艾综合征等。<br><br>Se usa para la úlcera gástrica, úlcera duodenal, úlcera anastomótica y la esofagitis por reflujo, síndrome de Zollinger-Ellison. |
| 用法、用量<br>Administración y dosis | 成年人一般一日口服 1 次，一次 1 粒（片）。胃溃疡、吻合口溃疡、反流性食管炎 8 周为一疗程。十二指肠溃疡 6 周为一疗程。<br><br>Generalmente para adultos la dosis por vía oral es 1 vez al día, una tableta (pastilla) por cada vez. Para la úlcera gástrica, úlcera anastomótica, esofagitis por reflujo ocho semanas es un curso de tratamiento. para el tratamiento de la úlcera duodenal, seis semanas es un curso. |

**续　表**

| 剂型、规格<br>Formulaciones y especificaciones | 片（胶囊）剂：每片（粒）30mg。<br>Tabletas (cápsulas): Cadatableta (cápsula) de 30mg. |
|---|---|
| **药品名称 Drug Names** | **泮托拉唑 Pantoprazol** |
| 适应证<br>Indicaciones | 主要用于胃及十二指肠溃疡、胃 - 食管反流性疾病、卓 - 艾综合征等。<br>Se utiliza principalmente para las úlceras gástricas y duodenales, el estómago, la enfermedad de reflujo esofágico, y el síndrome de Zollinger-Ellison. |
| 用法、用量<br>Administración y dosis | 一般患者一日服用 1 片（40mg），早餐前或早餐间用少量水送服，不可嚼碎。个别对其他药物无反应的病例可一日服用 2 次；老年患者及肝功能受损者，一日剂量不得超过 40mg。十二指肠溃疡疗程 2 周，必要时再服 2 周；胃溃疡及反流性食管炎疗程 4 周，必要时再服 4 周。总疗程不超过 8 周。　静脉滴注：一日 1 次 40mg，疗程依需要而定，但一般不超过 8 周。<br>Generalmente los pacientes toman una pastilla (40 mg) al día, se toma antes del desayuno o en el desayuno con una pequeña cantidad de agua, no pueden masticar. Para algunos pacientes individuales que no responden a otros medicamentos se pueden tomar dos veces al día; Para los pacientes ancianos y los con insuficiencia hepática, la dosis diaria no debe ser superior de 40 mg. Un curso del tratamiento de úlcera duodenal es de dos semanas, si es necesario, se sirve dos semanas más; Un curso del tratamiento de la úlcera gástrica y esofagitis por reflujo es de 4 semanas, si es necesario, se sirve cuatro semanas más. El curso total no debe ser más de ocho semanas. Infusión intravenosa: 1 vez de 40 mg al día, el curso del tratamiento puede ser ajustado según la necesidad, pero generalmente no debe ser más de ocho semanas. |
| 剂型、规格<br>Formulaciones y especificaciones | 片（肠溶）剂：每片 40mg。注射用泮托拉唑：每支 40mg。<br>Tabletas (con cubierta entérica): Cada tableta de 40mg. Inyección con Pantoprazol: Cada una de 40mg. |
| **药品名称 Drug Names** | **雷贝拉唑 Rabeprazol** |
| 适应证<br>Indicaciones | 用于治疗活动性十二指肠溃疡、活动性良性胃溃疡、弥散性或溃疡性胃 - 食管反流症。<br>Se usa para el tratamiento de la úlcera duodenal activa, la úlcera gástrica benigna activa, estómago difuso o la enfermedad de reflujo de estómago-esofágico ulcerosa. |
| 用法、用量<br>Administración y dosis | 活动性十二指肠溃疡：一次 10 ～ 20mg，一日 1 次，连服 2 ～ 4 周；活动性良性胃溃疡：一次 20mg，一日 1 次，连服 4 ～ 6 周；胃 - 食管反流症：一次 20mg，一日 1 次，连服 6 ～ 10 周。均早晨服用，片剂必须整片吞服。<br>Para la úlcera duodenal activa: 10 ~ 20 mg por cada vez, una vez al día, se toma continuamente 2 ~ 4 semanas; Para la úlcera gástrica benigna activa: 20 mg por cada vez, una vez al día, se toma continuamente 4 ~ 6 semanas; Para la enfermedad por reflujo de estómago - esofágico: 20 mg por cada vez, una vez al día, se toma continuamente 6 ~ 10 semanas. Deben tomar por la mañana, y las tabletas deben tragarse enteras. |
| 剂型、规格<br>Formulaciones y especificaciones | 片（肠溶）剂：每片 10mg；20mg。<br>Tabletas (con cubierta entérica): Cada tableta de 10 mg; 20 mg. |
| **药品名称 Drug Names** | **艾司奥美拉唑 Esomeprazol** |
| 适应证<br>Indicaciones | 用于食管反流性疾病。①治疗糜烂性反流性食管炎。②已经治愈的食管炎患者长期维持治疗，以防止复发。③为食管反流性疾病的症状控制。本品联合适当的抗菌疗法，用于根除幽门螺杆菌，使幽门螺杆菌感染相关的消化性溃疡愈合，并防止其复发。<br>Se usa para la enfermedad de reflujo esofágico. ① tratamiento de la esofagitis erosiva por reflujo. ② para los pacientes de esofagitis quienes se han curado, se usa en el curso de mantenimiento a largo plazo para prevenir la recurrencia. ③ control de los síntomas de la enfermedad de reflujo esofágico. Este elemento puede ser combinado con la terapia antimicrobiana para la erradicación de Helicobacter pylori, y curar la úlcera péptica causada por la infección por Helicobacter pylori y evitar su recurrencia. |

**续　表**

| | |
|---|---|
| 用法、用量<br>Administración y<br>dosis | （1）治疗糜烂性反流性食管炎：一次 40mg，一日 1 次，连服 4 周。对于食管炎未治愈或症状持续的患者，建议再治疗 4 周。<br><br>（2）已经治愈的食管炎患者长期维持治疗，以防止复发：一次 20mg，一日 1 次。<br><br>（3）胃食管反流性疾病的症状控制：无食管炎的患者一次 20mg，一日 1 次，如用药 4 周后症状未得到控制，应对患者做进一步检查，症状消除后，可采用即时疗法（即需要时口服 20mg，一日 1 次）。<br><br>（4）联合适当的抗菌疗法，用于根除幽门螺杆菌：采用联合用药方案，本品一次 20mg，阿莫西林一次 1g，克拉霉素一次 500mg，均为一日 2 次，共用 7 日。老年人和轻度肾功能损害者，无须调整剂量；轻中度肝功能损害的患者无须调整剂量。严重肝功能损害的患者，一日用量为 20mg。本品对酸不稳定，口服制剂均为肠溶制剂，服用时应整片（粒）吞服，不应嚼碎或压碎，至少应于餐前 1 小时服用。<br><br>(1) Tratamiento de la esofagitis por reflujo erosivo: 40mg por cada vez, 1 vez al día, se toma continuamente 4 semanas. Para los pacientes con síntomas de esofagitis no curados o síntomas persistidos, se recomenda que recibe otro curso de tratamiento de 4 semanas.<br><br>(2) Para los pacientes con esofagitis que se han curado puede mantener el tratamiento a largo plazo para prevenir la recurrencia: 20 mg por cada vez, 1 vez al día.<br><br>(3) Control de síntomas de la enfermedad por reflujo gastroesofágico: para los pacientes sin esofagitis, 20 mg por cada vez, una vez al día, si se toma la medicina después de 4 semanas, los síntomas no estácontrolados, los pacientes debe recibir un examen más profunda, después de la eliminación de los síntomas, puede usar un tratamiento inmediato (es decir, si hay la necesidad, se toma por vía oral 20 mg al día).<br><br>(4) Tratamiento de combinación con antimicrobiana para la erradicación de Helicobacter pylori: el uso de combinación, 20 mg del presente producto de una vez, amoxicilina de 1 g de una vez, claritromicina de 500 mg de una vez, 2 veces al día, y se toma en total 7 días. Los ancianos y las personas con insuficiencia renal leve, no hay necesidad de ajuste de dosis; los pacientes con insuficiencia hepática leve a moderada no hay necesidad de ajuste de dosis. Para los pacientes con insuficiencia hepática grave, la dosis es de 20 mg al día. Este producto es lábil a los ácidos, los medicamentos orales son preparaciones con cubierta entérica, debe tomar toda la pieza (tableta) de ingestión, sin masticarse o triturar, y se toma por lo menos 1 hora antes de las comidas. |
| 剂型、规格<br>Formulaciones y<br>especificaciones | 片（肠溶）剂：每片 20mg；40mg（以埃索美拉唑计量）。<br><br>Tabletas (con cubierta entérica): Cada tableta de 20 mg; 40 mg (Medida por Esomeprazol). |
| 药品名称 Drug Names | 丙谷胺 Proglumida |
| 适应证<br>Indicaciones | 用于治疗胃溃疡和十二指肠溃疡、胃炎等。由于本品抑制胃酸分泌的作用较弱，临床已不再单独用于治疗溃疡病，但其利胆作用较受重视。也可用于非甾体抗炎药合用，预防后者对胃黏膜的损害。<br><br>Se usa para el tratamiento de las úlceras gástricas y duodenales, gastritis, etc. Como el producto es débil en el efecto de la inhibición de secreción de ácido gástrico, no se utiliza clínicamente solo para tratamiento de la enfermedad de la úlcera, pero tiene un efecto significativo para colerético. También puede ser utilizado junto con los medicamentos anti-inflamatorios no esteroideos, para prevenir el daño a la mucosa gástrica. |
| 用法、用量<br>Administración y<br>dosis | 口服，一次 0.4g，一日 3～4 次，餐前 15 分钟给药，连续服 30～60 日（可根据胃镜或 X 线检查结果决定用药期限）。<br><br>Por vía oral, 0,4 g por cada vez, 3～4 veces al día, se toma 15 minutos antes de la comida, y se toma consecutivamente 30～60 días (puede decidir el curso de tratamiento de acuerdo a resultados de la endoscopia o radiografías). |
| 剂型、规格<br>Formulaciones y<br>especificaciones | 片（胶囊）剂：每片（粒）0.2g。<br><br>Tabletas (cápsulas): Cada tableta (cápsula) de 0.2g. |

**续　表**

### 12.3　胃黏膜保护剂 Protectores de mucosa gástrica

| 药品名称 Drug Names | 枸橼酸铋钾 Citrato de potasio bismuto |
|---|---|
| 适应证<br>Indicaciones | 　　用于胃及十二指肠溃疡的治疗，也用于复合溃疡、多发溃疡、吻合口溃疡和糜烂性胃炎等。本品与抗生素合用，可根除幽门螺杆菌。用于幽门螺杆菌相关的胃、十二指肠溃疡及慢性胃炎、胃ＭＡＬＴ淋巴瘤、早期胃癌术后、胃食管反流病及功能性消化不良等。也可与抑制胃酸分泌药（质子泵抑制剂和 H$_2$ 受体拮抗剂）组成四联方案，作为根除幽门螺杆菌失败的补救治疗。<br>　　Se usa para el tratamiento de las úlceras gástricas y duodenales, sino también para las úlceras complejas, múltiples úlceras, úlcera anastomótica y gastritis erosiva. Este producto se utiliza en combinación con los antibióticos pueden erradicar Helicobacter pylori. Se usa para Helicobacter pylori gástrica y úlcera duodenal asociada y la gastritis crónica, linfoma MALT gástrico, enfermedad por reflujo gástrico postoperatorio temprano y dispepsia funcional. También puede combinar con los medicamento de inhibición de la secreción de ácido gástrico y las drogas (inhibidores de bomba de protones y los antagonistas de los receptores H$_2$) están en forma de un medicamento cuádruple como la terapia de rescate de Helicobacter pylori no erradicada. |
| 用法、用量<br>Administración y dosis | 　　颗粒剂：一次一袋，一日 3 ～ 4 次，餐前半小时和睡前服用。片剂或胶囊剂：一次 2 片（粒），一日 2 次，早餐前半小时与睡前用温水送服，忌用含碳酸饮料（如啤酒等）；服药前、后半小时，不要喝牛奶或服用抗酸剂和其他碱性药物，疗程 4 ～ 8 周，然后停用含铋药物 4 ～ 8 周，如有必要，可再继续服用 4 ～ 8 周。<br>　　Gránulos: un paquete por una vez, 3 ~ 4 veces al día, se toma media hora antes de las comidas y antes de acostarse. Tabletas o cápsulas: dos tabletas (cápsulas) por una vez, 2 veces al día, se toma media hora antes del desayuno y antes de acostarse con agua tibia, se prohibe el uso de las bebidas carbonatadas (como la cerveza, etc); media hora antes y despúes de tomar el medicamento, no tome leche o medicamentos de antiácidos y otros medicamentos básicos, un curso de tratamiento es de 4 ~ 8 semanas, y luego pare el uso de medicamentos que contienen bismuto por 4 ~ 8 semanas, si es necesario, luego puede continuar a tomar el medicamento de cuatro - ocho semanas. |
| 剂型、规格<br>Formulaciones y especificaciones | 　　颗粒剂：每袋 1.2g，含本品 300mg。片（胶囊）剂：每片（粒）120mg。<br>　　Gránulos: cada paquete de 1.2 g, que contiene el Citrato de Potasio Bismuto de 300mg. Tabletas (cápsulas): Cada tableta (cápsula) de 120mg. |
| 药品名称 Drug Names | 胶体果胶铋 Pectina de bismuto coloidal |
| 适应证<br>Indicaciones | 　　用于胃及十二指肠溃疡，也可用于慢性浅表性胃炎、慢性萎缩性胃炎和消化道出血的治疗。本品与抗生素合用，可根除幽门螺杆菌。用于幽门螺杆菌相关的胃、十二指肠溃疡及慢性胃炎、胃 MALT　淋巴瘤、早期胃癌术后、胃食管反流病及功能性消化不良等。也可与抑制胃酸分泌药（质子泵抑制剂和 H$_2$ 受体拮抗药）组成四联方案，作为根除幽门螺杆菌失败的补救治疗。<br>　　Se usa para las úlceras gástricas y duodenales, también se puede utilizar para la gastritis crónica superficial, gastritis atrófica crónica y la hemorragia gastrointestinal. Este producto se utiliza en combinación con los antibióticos para erradicar Helicobacter pylori. Se usa para úlceras gástricas y duodenales asociada con la Helicobacter pylori y la gastritis crónica, linfoma MALT gástrico, cáncer temprano gástrico postoperatorio, la enfermedad por reflujo gastroesofágico y la dispepsia funcional. También puede combinar con los medicamento de inhibición de la secreción de ácido gástrico y las drogas (inhibidores de bomba de protones y los antagonistas de los receptores H$_2$) están en forma de un medicamento cuádruple como la terapia de rescate de Helicobacter pylori no erradicada. |
| 用法、用量<br>Administración y dosis | 　　治疗消化性溃疡和慢性胃炎：一次 3 ～ 4 粒，一日 4 次，于三餐前半小时各服一次，睡前加服 1 次。疗程一般为 4 周。治疗消化道出血：将胶囊内药物倒出，用水冲开搅匀服用，日剂量一次服用，儿童用量酌减。<br>　　Tratamiento para la úlcera péptica y la gastritis crónica: 3 ~ 4 tabletas por cada vez, 4 veces al día, se toma media hora antes de las comidas y se toma respectivamente una vez, antes de acostarse una vez más. Un curso del tratamiento es generalmente de cuatro semanas. Para el tratamiento de la hemorragia digestiva: vierte la droga en la cápsula y pone en el agua y revuelva para el servicio, la dosis diaria es una vez, la cantidad para niños debe ser reducida. |

**续　表**

| 剂型、规格<br>Formulaciones y especificaciones | 胶囊剂：每粒 50mg。<br>Cápsulas: Cada cápsula de 50mg. |
|---|---|
| 药品名称 Drug Names | 胶体酒石酸铋 Tartrato de bismuto coloidal |
| 适应证<br>Indicaciones | 用于治疗慢性结肠炎、溃疡性结肠炎、肠功能紊乱及与幽门螺杆菌有关的消化性溃疡和慢性胃炎。<br>Se usa para el tratamiento de la colitis crónica, la colitis ulcerosa, trastornos intestinales y gastritis crónica y úlcera péptica asociada con Helicobacter pylori. |
| 用法、用量<br>Administración y dosis | 口服，一次 165mg（3 粒），一日 3 ~ 4 次，儿童用量酌减。一般 4 周为一疗程。<br>Por vía oral, 165 mg (3 tabletas) por cada vez, 3 ~ 4 veces al día, la cantidad de niños debe ser reducida. Generalmente un curso de tratamiento es de cuatro semanas. |
| 剂型、规格<br>Formulaciones y especificaciones | 胶囊剂：每粒 55mg（以铋计量）。<br>Cápsulas: Cada cápsula de 55 mg (medido por bismuto). |
| 药品名称 Drug Names | 米索前列醇 Misoprostol |
| 适应证<br>Indicaciones | 用于胃及十二指肠溃疡。对十二指肠溃疡，口服本品 200μg 一日 4 次，4 周后愈合率为 54%，对照组口服西咪替丁 300mg 一日 4 次，4 周后愈合率为 61%，疗效略低于西咪替丁，但本品在保护胃黏膜不受损伤方面比西咪替丁更为有效。<br>Se usa para las úlceras y duodenal. Para la úlcera duodenal, se toma por vía oral de 200μg de 4 veces al día, la tasa de curación después de cuatro semanas es del 54%, en el grupo de comparación, se toma 300 mg de cimetidina 4 veces al día, la tasa de curación después de cuatro semanas es del 61%, la eficacia se observa ligeramente inferior que la de cimetidina, pero el presente producto no se daña la mucosa gástrica y tiene una protección más eficaz que la cimetidina. |
| 用法、用量<br>Administración y dosis | 一次 200μg，一日 4 次，于餐前和睡前口服。疗程 4 ~ 8 周。<br>200μg por cada vez, 4 veces al día, se toma antes de las comidas y antes de acostarse. Un curso de tratamiento es de 4 ~ 8 semanas. |
| 剂型、规格<br>Formulaciones y especificaciones | 片剂：每片 200μg。<br>Tabletas: Cada tableta de 200μg. |
| 药品名称 Drug Names | 硫糖铝 Sucralfato |
| 适应证<br>Indicaciones | 用于胃及十二指肠溃疡，也用于胃炎。<br>Se usa para las úlceras gástricas y duodenales, y también para la gastritis. |
| 用法、用量<br>Administración y dosis | 口服，一次 1g，一日 3 ~ 4 次，餐前 1 小时及睡前服用。<br>Por vía oral, 1 g por cada vez, 3 ~ 4 veces al día, se toma una hora antes de las comidas y antes de acostarse. |
| 剂型、规格<br>Formulaciones y especificaciones | 片剂：每片 0.25g；0.5g。分散片：每片 0.5g。胶囊剂：每粒 0.25g。悬胶剂：每袋 5ml（含硫糖铝 1g）。<br>Tabletas: Cada tableta de 0.25 g; 0.5 g. Tabletas dispersables: Cada tableta de 0.5 g. Cápsulas: Cada cápsula de 0.25g. Pegamento colgante: cada paquete de 5ml (incluyendo 1 g de sucralfato). |
| 药品名称 Drug Names | 麦滋林 -S　Marzulena-S |
| 适应证<br>Indicaciones | 用于胃炎、胃溃疡和十二指肠溃疡，可明显缓解临床症状，并有较好的预防溃疡复发的作用。<br>Se usa para la gastritis, úlceras gástricas y duodenales, puede aliviar significativamente los síntomas y prevenir la recurrencia de la úlcera con un mejor efecto. |

**续　表**

| | |
|---|---|
| 用法、用量<br>Administración y dosis | 成人一般一日 1.5 ～ 2.5g，分 3 ～ 4 次口服，剂量可随年龄与症状适当增减。<br>Para adultos generalmente es de 1.5 ~ 2.5g por cada día, divididos en 3 ~ 4 veces al día para tomar por vía oral, la dosis se puede aumentar o disminuir según la edad y los síntomas. |
| 剂型、规格<br>Formulaciones y especificaciones | 颗粒剂：1g 内含水溶性薁 3mg 和 L- 谷酰胺 990mg。<br>Gránulos: en 1g contiene 3mg de azuleno soluble y 990 mg de L-glutamina. |
| **药品名称 Drug Names** | 替普瑞酮 Teprenona |
| 适应证<br>Indicaciones | 用于胃溃疡，也用于急性胃炎和慢性胃炎的急性加重期。<br>Se usa para la úlcera gástrica, y también para la gastritis aguda y exacerbación aguda de la gastritis crónica. |
| 用法、用量<br>Administración y dosis | 餐后 30 分钟内口服，一日 3 次，一次 1 粒胶囊（50mg）或颗粒剂 0.5g（含本品 50mg）。<br>Se toma por vía oral dentro de 30 minutos después de la comida, 3 veces al día, cada vez de una cápsula (50 mg) o gránulos de 0,5 g (que contiene Teprenone de 50mg). |
| 剂型、规格<br>Formulaciones y especificaciones | 胶囊剂：每粒 50mg。颗粒剂：100mg（含本品）/g。<br>Cápsulas: Cada cápsula de 50mg. Gránulos: 100 mg (que contiene teprenone) / g. |
| **药品名称 Drug Names** | 吉法酯 Gefarnato |
| 适应证<br>Indicaciones | 用于治疗胃及十二指肠溃疡，急慢性胃炎，结肠炎，胃痉挛等。<br>Se usa para el tratamiento de las úlceras gástricas y duodenales, gastritis aguda y crónica, colitis, espasmos del estómago. |
| 用法、用量<br>Administración y dosis | 口服，对一般肠胃不适、胃酸过多、胃胀及消化不良等，可根据病情一次 1 ～ 2 片，一日 3 次。治疗消化性溃疡及急慢性胃炎，一次 2 片，一日 3 次，餐后服用；症状较轻者疗程 4 ～ 5 周，重症者疗程 2 ～ 3 个月。儿童剂量酌减。<br>Por vía oral, en general se usa para el tratamiento de estómago indispuesto, hiperacidez, la hinchazón y la indigestión, de acuerdo con la enfermedad, puede ser 1 ~ 2 tabletas por cada vez, 3 veces al día. Para el tratamiento deúlcera péptica y gastritis agudo y crónico, se toma dos tabletas por cada vez, tres veces al día, después de las comidas; Para los pacientes con síntomas leves, el curso de tratamiento es de 4 ~ 5 semanas, para pacientes con síntomas severos un curso es de 2 ~ 3 meses. Las dosis para niños puede ser reducida. |
| 剂型、规格<br>Formulaciones y especificaciones | 片剂：每片 0.4g。<br>Tabletas: Cada tableta de 0.4 g. |
| **药品名称 Drug Names** | 甘草锌 Licorzinc |
| 适应证<br>Indicaciones | 用于口腔、胃、十二指肠及其他部位的溃疡症，还可用于促进刀口、创伤和烧伤的愈合。儿童厌食、异食癖、生长发育不良、肠病性肢端皮炎及其他儿童、成人锌缺乏症也可用本品治疗。本品还可用于青春期痤疮。<br>Se usa para la cavidad oral, el estómago, el duodeno y otras partes con la enfermedad de la úlcera, se puede utilizar para promover la curación de heridas de incisión y quemaduras. Tiene efectos para anorexia de niños, pica, falta de crecimiento y desarrollo, y enteropatía acrodermatitis, la deficiencia de zinc de niños y de adultos. También pueden utilizar este producto para el acné adolescente. |
| 用法、用量<br>Administración y dosis | （1）治疗消化性溃疡：片剂 1 次 0.5g，或颗粒剂 1 次 10g，一日 3 次，疗程 4 ～ 6 周。必要时可减半再服 1 个疗程巩固疗效。<br>（2）治疗青春期痤疮，口腔溃疡及其他病症：片剂 1 次 0.25g，或颗粒剂 1 次 5g，一日 2 ～ 3 次。治疗青春期痤疮疗程 4 ～ 6 周。愈后一日服药 1 次，片剂 0.25g，或颗粒剂 5g，服 4 ～ 6 周，以减少复发。<br>（3）保健营养性补锌，一日片剂 0.25g 即可，1 次或分 2 次服用；或颗粒剂 1 次 1.5g，一日 2 ～ 3 次。<br>（4）儿童用量每日按 0.5 ～ 1.5mg（以元素锌计）/kg 计算，分 3 次服用。 |

|  | (1) Tratamiento de la úlcera péptica: una vez de tableta de 0.5g o una vez de gránulos de 10g, 3 veces al día, un curso de tratamiento de cuatro - seis semanas. Si es necesario, puede reducir la dosis a la mitad y luego se sirve un curso más para la consolidación del efecto. <br> (2)Tratamiento del acné juvenil, úlceras en la boca y otros síntomas: Una vez de tableta de 0.25g o gránulos de 1 5g, 2 ~ 3 veces al día. Un curso del tratamiento del acné de los adolescentes es de 4 a 6 semanas. De ser curado, toma el medicamento una vez al día, tabletas de 0.25 g o gránulos de 5g, se toma 4 ~ 6 semanas, para reducir la recurrencia. <br> (3) Para salud y nutrición de complementación de zinc, 0.25 g de tableta al día, se toma de una vez o se divide en 2 veces, o gránulos 1.5g de una vez, 2 ~ 3 veces al día. <br> (4) Dosis diaria para los niños es de 0,5 ~ 1,5 mg (medido por cinc elemental) / kg, tres veces al día. |
|---|---|
| 剂型、规格 <br> Formulaciones y especificaciones | 片剂：每片 0.25g（相当于含锌 12.5mg，甘草酸 87.5mg）。 <br> 颗粒剂：每小袋 1.5g（相当于含元素锌 3.6 ~ 4.35mg）。 <br> Tabletas: Cada tableta de 0.25 g (equivalente a 12.5 mg de zinc, ácido regaliz 87.5mg). Gránulos: Cada paquete de 1,5 g (equivalente de zinc elemental de 3.6 ~ 4.35mg). |
| 药品名称 Drug Names | 瑞巴派特 Rebamipida |
| 适应证 <br> Indicaciones | 主要用于胃溃疡，但不宜单独用于 Hp 感染。也用于改善急性胃炎及慢性胃炎急性加重期的胃黏膜病变（如糜烂、出血、充血、水肿等）。 <br> Se utiliza principalmente para las úlceras de estómago, pero no es conveniente usar solamente para la infección por Hp. También se utiliza para mejorar la gastritis aguda y exacerbación aguda de la gastritis crónica, lesión de la mucosa gástrica en período de exacerbación aguda de la gastritis crónica (tales como la erosión, la hemorragia, edema, etc). |
| 用法、用量 <br> Administración y dosis | 口服，一般一次 0.1g，一日 3 次，早、晚及睡前服用。 <br> Por vía oral, generalmente 0.1 g por cada vez, 3 veces al día, se toma por la mañana, por la tarde y antes de acostarse. |
| 剂型、规格 <br> Formulaciones y especificaciones | 片剂：一片 0.1g。 <br> Tabletas: Cada tableta de 0.1 g. |
| 药品名称 Drug Names | 复方铝酸铋 Compuestas de aluminato de bismuto |
| 适应证 <br> Indicaciones | 用于胃及十二指肠溃疡、慢性浅表性胃炎、十二指肠球炎、胃酸过多症及功能性消化不良等。 <br> Se usa para las úlceras gástricas y duodenales, gastritis crónica, la inflamación duodenal, hiperacidez y dispepsia funcional. |
| 用法、用量 <br> Administración y dosis | 成人一日 3 次，一次 1 ~ 2 片，餐后嚼碎服。疗程为 1 ~ 3 个月；以后可减量维持防止复发。 <br> Para adultos 3 veces al día, cada vez de 1 ~ 2 tabletas, debe masticar para tomar despúes de la comida. Un curso del tratamiento es de 1 ~ 3 meses, y más tarde puede reducir la dosis para evitar la reducción de la recurrencia. |
| 剂型、规格 <br> Formulaciones y especificaciones | 复方片剂，每片含铝酸铋 200mg、甘草浸膏粉 300mg、重质碳酸镁 400mg、碳酸氢钠 200mg、弗朗鼠李皮 25mg、茴香 10mg。 <br> Tabletas compuestas, cada tableta contiene aluminio de bismuto de 200 mg, 300 mg de polvo de extracto de regaliz, fuertecarbonato de magnesio de 400mg, sodio de bicarbonato de 200 mg, cuero de francis espino cerval de 25mg, hinojo de 10mg. |

12.4　胃肠解痉药 Medicamento para aliviar los espasmos gastrointestinales

| 药品名称 Drug Names | 丁溴东莨菪碱 Butilbromuro de escopolamino |
|---|---|
| 适应证 <br> Indicaciones | （1）用于胃、十二指肠、结肠纤维内镜检查的术前准备，内镜逆行胰胆管造影和胃、十二指肠、结肠的气钡低张造影或计算机腹部体层扫描（CT 扫描）的术前准备，可有效减少或抑制胃肠道蠕动。 <br> （2）用于治疗各种病因引起的胃肠道痉挛、胆绞痛、肾绞痛或胃肠道蠕动亢进等。 <br> (1) Se usa para la preparación preoperatoria del estómago, el duodeno, el colon fibra de endoscopia, la colangiopancreatografía retrógrada endoscópica y radiografía del estómago, el duodeno, el bario del colon hipotónica angiografía abdominal o preparación previa a la cirugía de tomografía computarizada (CT), puede reducir efectivamente o inhibir la motilidad gastrointestinal. <br> (2) Se usa para el tratamiento de espasmos gastrointestinales, cólicos biliares, renales motilidad cólica o gastrointestinal, o el hipertiroidismo causadas por diversas causas, etc. |

**续　表**

| 用法、用量<br>Administración y<br>dosis | 口服：1 次 10mg，一日 3 次。肌内注射、静脉注射或静脉滴注（溶于葡萄糖注射液、0.9% 路华纳注射液中滴注）：一次 20 ～ 40mg；或 1 次 20mg，间隔 20 ～ 30 分钟后再用 20mg。<br>Por vía oral: Una vez de 10 mg, 3 veces al día. La inyección intramuscular, inyección intravenosa o infusión intravenosa (hace la infusión de inyección en inyección solubles de glucosa, cloruro de sodio al 0,9%): 20 ～ 40 mg por cada vez, o una vez de 20mg, con un intervalo de 20 ~ 30 minutos usa otra vez de 20 mg. |
| --- | --- |
| 剂型、规格<br>Formulaciones y<br>especificaciones | 注射液：每支 20mg（1ml）。胶囊剂：每粒 10mg。片剂：每片 10mg。<br>Inyección: Cada una de 20 mg (1 ml). Cápsulas: Cada cápsula de10mg. Tabletas: Cada tableta de 10mg. |

| 药品名称 Drug Names | 曲美布汀 Trimebutina |
| --- | --- |
| 适应证<br>Indicaciones | 用于慢性胃炎引起的胃肠道症状，如腹部胀满感、腹痛和嗳气等；也用于肠道易激综合征。<br>Se usa para la gastritis crónica causada por síntomas gastrointestinales, tales como plenitud abdominal, dolor abdominal, y eructos, etc; también para el síndrome del intestino irritable. |
| 用法、用量<br>Administración y<br>dosis | 治疗慢性胃炎，通常成人一次 100mg，一日 3 次。可根据年龄、症状适当增减剂量。治疗肠易激综合征，一般一次 100 ～ 200mg，一日 3 次。<br>Tiene tratamiento para la gastritis crónica, generalmente para adultos 100 mg por cada vez, 3 veces al día. Puede aumentar o disminuir la dosis de acuerdo a la edad. Para síndrome del intestino irritable e. El tratamiento del síndrome de colon irritable, por lo general 100 ~ 200 mg por cada vez, 3 veces al día. |
| 剂型、规格<br>Formulaciones y<br>especificaciones | 片剂：每片 100mg；200mg。<br>Tabletas: Cada tableta de 100 mg, 200 mg. |

| 药品名称 Drug Names | 溴丙胺太林 Bromuro de Propantelina |
| --- | --- |
| 适应证<br>Indicaciones | 用于胃及十二指肠溃疡的辅助治疗，也用于胃炎、胰腺炎、胆汁排泄障碍、遗尿和多汗症。<br>Se usa para el tratamiento adyuvante de las úlceras gástricas y duodenales, pero también para la gastritis, la pancreatitis, trastornos de excreción biliar, la incontinencia urinaria, y la hiperhidrosis |
| 用法、用量<br>Administración y<br>dosis | 一次 15mg，一日 3 ～ 4 次，餐前服，睡前 30mg；治疗遗尿可于睡前口服 15 ～ 45mg。<br>15 mg por cada vez, 3 ~ 4 veces al día, se toma antes de las comidas, 30 mg antes de acostarse; Para el tratamiento de la enuresis puede tomar 15 ~ 45 mg antes de acostarse por vía oral. |
| 剂型、规格<br>Formulaciones y<br>especificaciones | 片剂：15mg。<br>Tabletas: 15 mg. |

12.5　助消化药 Medicamentos para ayudar con la digestión

| 药品名称 Drug Names | 多酶 Multienzimá |
| --- | --- |
| 适应证<br>Indicaciones | 用于多种消化酶缺乏的消化不良症。<br>Se usa para la indigestión digestivo causada por una variedad de deficiencia de la enzima. |
| 用法、用量<br>Administración y<br>dosis | 口服，一次 1 ～ 2 片，一日 3 次，餐前服。<br>Por vía oral, 1 ~ 2 por cada vez, 3 veces al día, se toma antes de las comidas. |
| 剂型、规格<br>Formulaciones y<br>especificaciones | 13mg（胃蛋白酶）～ 300mg（胰酶）。<br>13 mg (pepsina) ~ 300mg (tripsina). |

| 药品名称 Drug Names | 复方慷彼申片 Comprimidos compuestos de combizim |
| --- | --- |
| 适应证<br>Indicaciones | 用于各种原因所致的消化不良症。<br>Se usa para la indigestión causada por una variedad de motivos. |

| 用法、用量<br>Administración y<br>dosis | 口服：一次 1 片，一日 3 次，饭时或餐后服用。<br>Por vía oral, 1 tableta por cada vez, 3 veces al día, se toma durante la comida o antes de las comidas. |
|---|---|
| 剂型、规格<br>Formulaciones y<br>especificaciones | 肠溶片剂：24mg（米曲菌酶提取物）～ 220mg（胰酶）。<br>Tabletas con recubrimiento entérico: 24 mg (m extractos enzimáticos aspergilosis) ~ 220mg (tripsina). |
| 药品名称Drug Names | 干酵母 Levadura seca |
| 适应证<br>Indicaciones | 用于营养不良、消化不良、食欲缺乏、腹泻及胃肠胀气。<br>Se usa para la desnutrición, indigestión, pérdida de apetito, diarrea y flatulencia. |
| 用法、用量<br>Administración y<br>dosis | 口服：一次 0.5 ～ 4g，嚼碎服。剂量过大可引起腹泻。<br>Por vía oral: 0.5 ~ 4g por cada vez, debe masticar para su uso. Una dosis excesiva puede causar diarrea. |
| 剂型、规格<br>Formulaciones y<br>especificaciones | 片剂：每片 0.2g；0.3g；0.5g。<br>Tabletas: Cada tableta de 0.2 g; 0.3 g; 0.5 g. |

12.6　促胃肠动力药 Medicamento que estimula el movimiento gastrointestinal

| 药品名称 Drug Names | 甲氧氯普胺 Metoclopramida |
|---|---|
| 适应证<br>Indicaciones | （1）因脑部肿瘤手术、肿瘤放疗及化疗、脑外伤后遗症、急性颅脑损伤以及药物所引起的呕吐。<br>（2）胃胀气性消化不良、食欲缺乏、嗳气、恶心、呕吐。<br>（3）海空作业引起的呕吐及晕车。<br>（4）可增加食管括约肌压力，从而减少全身麻醉时胃肠道反流所致吸入性肺炎的发生率；可减轻钡剂检查时的恶心、呕吐反应，促进钡剂通过；十二指肠插管前服用，有助于顺利插管。<br>（5）对糖尿病性胃轻瘫，胃下垂等。<br>（6）可减轻偏头痛引起的恶心，并可能由于提高胃通过率而促进麦角胺的吸收。<br>（7）其催乳作用可试用于乳量严重不足的产妇。<br>（8）胆道疾病和慢性胰腺炎的辅助治疗。<br><br>(1) Secuelas debido a la cirugía del tumor cerebral, la radioterapia y la quimioterapia, la lesión cerebral traumática, lesión cerebral aguda y vómitos inducidos por fármacos.<br>(2) Dispepsia, flatulencia, pérdida de apetito, eructos, náuseas y vómitos.<br>(3) Vómitos y el mareo causado por las operaciones marítimas y aéreas.<br>(4) Puede aumentar la presión del esfínter esofágico, reduciendo así el reflujo gastrointestinal causado por la incidencia de la neumonía por aspiración durante la anestesia general; Puede aliviar las náuseas y vómitos en el examen de comida de bario, promover el paso de bario; se toma antes de la intubación duodenal para ayudar a la intubación suave.<br>(5) Puede usar para la gastroparesia diabética, gastroptosis.<br>(6) Puede aliviar las náuseas causadas por la migraña y aumentar la tasa de paso de estómago para promover la absorción de ergotamina.<br>(7) Su papel de la prolactina puede ser probado en las puérperas con una grave escasez de leche materna.<br>(8) Tiene tratamiento adyuvante para la enfermedad del tracto biliar y pancreatitis crónica. |
| 用法、用量<br>Administración y<br>dosis | ① 口服：一次 5 ～ 10mg，一日 10 ～ 30mg。餐前半小时服用。② 肌内注射：1 次 10 ～ 20mg。每日剂量一般不超过 0.5mg/kg，否则易引起锥体外系反应。<br>① Por vía oral: 5 ~ 10mg por cada vez, 10 ~ 30 mg al día. Se toma una media hora antes de la comida. ② Inyección intramuscular: una vez de 10 ~ 20 mg. La dosis diaria no debe exceder de 0.5mg/kg, al contrario es fácil de causar reacciones extrapiramidales. |
| 剂型、规格<br>Formulaciones y<br>especificaciones | 片剂：每片 5mg。注射液：每支 10mg（1ml）。<br>Tabletas: Cada tableta de 5mg. Inyección: Cada una de10 mg (1 ml). |

**续　表**

| 药品名称 Drug Names | 多潘立酮 Domperidona |
|---|---|
| 适应证<br>Indicaciones | （1）由胃排空延缓、反流性胃炎、慢性胃炎、反流性食管炎引起的消化不良症状；其他消化系统疾病引起的呕吐。<br>（2）胃轻瘫，尤其是糖尿病性胃轻瘫可缩短胃排空时间，使胃潴留症状消失。<br>（3）各种原因引起的恶心呕吐；抗帕金森综合征药物引起的胃肠道症状及多巴胺受体激动药所致的恶心呕吐。偏头痛、痛经、颅外伤及颅内病灶、放射治疗以及左旋多巴非甾体抗炎药等引起的恶心呕吐。检查和治疗措施引起的恶心呕吐；儿童因各种原因引起的急性和持续性呕吐等。对细胞毒性药物引起的呕吐只在不太严重时有效。<br>（4）可作为消化性溃疡的辅助治疗药物，用于消除胃窦部潴留。<br><br>(1) Se usa para el tratamiento de retraso del vaciado gástrico, gastritis por reflujo, gastritis crónica, indigestión y otros síntomas de la esofagitis por reflujo causado; el vómito causado por otras enfermedades digestivas.<br>(2) Gastroparesia, especialmente para diabéticos gástrica gastroparesia que se puede acortar el tiempo de vaciado de estómago, para que se desaparecen los síntomas de retención gástrica.<br>(3) Náuseas y vómitos causados por diversas razones, los síntomas gastrointestinales causados por el medicamento de anti-parkinsoniano y agonistas de náuseas y vómitos inducidos por fármacos de receptor de dopamina. Náuseas y vómitos causados por migraña, dismenorrea, lesiones extracraneales lesiones intracraneales, la radioterapia y la levodopa medicamentos anti-inflamatorios no esteroideos. náuseas y vómitos inducidos por el examen y tratamiento; Vómitos agudas y persistentes de niño debido a diversas causas. Para vómitos inducida por fármacos citotóxicos, tiene efecto sólo cuando no vómitos no son severos.<br>(4) Se puede utilizar como un tratamiento auxiliar de la úlcera péptica, para la eliminación de la retención de antro gástrico. |
| 用法、用量<br>Administración y<br>dosis | （1）肌内注射：一次 10mg，必要时可重复给药。<br>（2）口服：一次 10 ～ 20mg，一日 3 次，餐前服。<br>（3）直肠给药：一次 60mg，一日 2 ～ 3 次。栓剂最好在直肠空时插入。<br><br>(1) Inyección intramuscular: 10 mg por cada vez, puede ofrecer inyecciones con repetidas veces cuando sea necesario.<br>(2) Por vía oral: 10 ~ 20 mg por cada vez, 3 veces al día antes de las comidas.<br>(3) Administración rectal: 60 mg por cada vez, 2 ~ 3 veces al día. Es mejor insertar el supositorio al recto vacío. |
| 剂型、规格<br>Formulaciones y<br>especificaciones | 片剂：每片 10mg。栓剂：每粒 60mg。注射液：每支 10mg（2ml）。滴剂：10mg/ml。混悬液：1mg/ml。<br><br>Tabletas: Cada tableta de 10mg. Supositorios: Cada uno de 60mg. Inyección: Cada una de 10 mg (2 ml). Gotas: 10mg/ml. Líquido suspendido: 1mg/ml. |
| 药品名称 Drug Names | 西沙必利 Cisaprida |
| 适应证<br>Indicaciones | （1）可增加胃肠动力，用于胃轻瘫综合征，或上消化道不适，X 线、内镜检查阴性的症候群，特征为早饱、餐后饱胀、食量减低、胃胀、过多的嗳气、食欲缺乏、恶心、呕吐或类似溃疡的主诉（上腹部灼痛）。<br>（2）胃 - 食管反流：包括食管炎的治疗及维持治疗。<br>（3）与运动功能失调有关的假性肠梗阻导致的推进性蠕动不足和胃肠内容物滞留。<br>（4）可恢复结肠的推进性运动，作为慢性便秘患者的长期治疗。<br><br>(1) Puede aumentar la motilidad gastrointestinal, se usa para el síndrome de la gastroparesia, o indigestión de gastrointestinal superior, de rayos X, el síndrome de endoscopia negativo, caracterizado por la sensación de saciedad temprana, plenitud posprandial, la reducción del apetito, distensión excesiva, eructos, anorexia, náuseas, vómitos o úlceras similares (quemadura abdominal superior).<br>(2) Reflujo de estómago - esofágico: incluyendo el tratamiento y mantenimiento de esofagitis y la terapia.<br>(3) La motilidad propulsora inadecua y contenido gastrointestinal varados causados por pseudo-obstrucción intestinal asociada con trastornos de movimiento.<br>(4) Puede restaurar el movimiento de promoción de colon, sirve como un tratamiento a largo plazo para los pacientes con estreñimiento crónico. |

续 表

| 用法、用量<br>Administración y dosis | 　　口服，根据病情，一日总量为 15 ～ 40mg，分 2 ～ 4 次给药。食管炎的维持治疗：一次 10mg，一日 2 次，早餐前和睡前服用；或一次 20mg，一日 1 次，睡前服用。病情严重者剂量可加倍。<br><br>　　Por vía oral, de acuerdo con la enfermedad, la dosis total diaria es de 15 ~ 40 mg, dividida en 2 ~ 4 veces. Para el tratamiento de mantenimiento de la esofagitis: 10 mg por cada vez, 2 veces al día, se toma antes del desayuno y antes de dormir, o 20 mg por cada vez, una vez al día, se toma antes de acostarse. Para los pacientes con casos más graves, la dosis puede ser duplicada. |
|---|---|
| 剂型、规格<br>Formulaciones y especificaciones | 　　片剂：每片 5mg；10mg。胶囊剂：每粒 5mg。干混悬剂：100mg。<br><br>　　Tabletas: Cada tableta de 5mg, 10mg. Cápsulas: Cada cápsula de 5mg. Líquido suspedido seco: 100 mg. |

| 药品名称 Drug Names | 莫沙必利 Mosaprida |
|---|---|
| 适应证<br>Indicaciones | 　　（1）慢性胃炎或功能性消化不良引起的消化道症状，如上腹部胀满感、腹胀、上腹部疼痛；嗳气、恶心、呕吐；胃烧灼感等。<br>　　（2）胃食管反流病和糖尿病胃轻瘫。<br>　　（3）胃大部切除术患者的胃功能障碍。<br><br>　　(1) Para síntomas gastrointestinales causadas por gastritis crónica o dispepsia funcional, tales como plenitud abdominal, distensión abdominal, dolor abdominal, eructos, náuseas, vómitos, sensación de ardor de estómago.<br>　　(2) La enfermedad por reflujo gastroesofágico y la gastroparesia diabética.<br>　　(3) Disfunción gástrica de pacientes con gastrectomía. |
| 用法、用量<br>Administración y dosis | 　　一次 5mg，一日 3 次，餐前服用。<br>　　Cada vez de 5 mg, 3 veces al día, se toma antes de las comidas. |
| 剂型、规格<br>Formulaciones y especificaciones | 　　片剂：每片 5mg。<br>　　Tabletas: Cada tableta de 5mg. |

12.7　止吐药和催吐药 Antieméticos y eméticos

| 药品名称 Drug Names | 昂丹司琼 Ondansetrón |
|---|---|
| 适应证<br>Indicaciones | 　　用于治疗由化疗和放疗引起的恶心、呕吐，也可用于预防和治疗手术后引起的恶心呕吐。<br><br>　　Se usa para el tratamiento de náuseas y vómitos causados por la quimioterapia y de la radioterapia, también se puede utilizar para prevenir y tratar las náuseas y vómitos causados por la cirugía. |
| 用法、用量<br>Administración y dosis | 　　（1）治疗由化疗和放疗引起的恶心呕吐：①成人：给药途径和剂量应视患者情况因人而异，剂量一般为 8 ～ 32mg，为避免治疗 24 小时后出现恶心呕吐，均应让患者持续服药，每次 8mg，一日 2 次，连服 5 日。②儿童：5mg/m$^2$ 静脉注射，12 小时后再口服 4mg，化疗后应持续给予病儿口服 4mg，一日 2 次，连服 5 日。③老年人：可依成年人给药法给药，一般不需调整。<br>　　（2）预防或治疗手术后呕吐：①成人：一般可于麻醉诱导同时静脉滴注 4mg，或于麻醉前 1 小时口服 8mg，之后每隔 8 小时口服 8mg，共 2 次。已出现术后恶心呕吐时，可缓慢静脉滴注 4mg 进行治疗。②肾衰竭患者：不需调整剂量、用药次数或用药途径。③肝衰竭患者：由于主要自肝脏代谢，对中度或严重肝衰竭患者，每日用药剂量不应超过 8mg。<br><br>　　(1) Se usa para el tratamiento de las náuseas y vómitos causados por la quimioterapia y la radioterapia: ① Para adultos:La vía de administración y la dosis deben variar según la condición del paciente, generalmente la dosis es de 8 ~ 32 mg, Para prevenir las náuseas y los vómitos dentro de 24 horas después del tratamiento, el paciente debe seguir tomando 8 mg por cada vez, 2 veces al día, en 5 días continuos. ② Para niños: 5mg/m$^2$ de inyección por vía intravenosa, después de 12 horas recibe la administración oral de 4 mg, después de la quimioterapia, se debe dar a los niños enfermos continuar la administración oral de 4mg, 2 veces al día, en 5 días continuos. ③ Para ancianos: según el método de dosificación de adultos, se ofrece la administración, en general, no hay la necesidad de ajustes. |

续　表

| | (2) Puede prevenir y tratar vómitos despúes de la cirugía: ① Para adultos: generalmente se usa para la inducción de anestesia y al mismo tiempo, la inyección por vía intravenosa de 4 mg, o se toma por vía oral de 8 mg una hora antes anestesia, y se toma por vía oral de 8 mg por un intevalo de 8 horas, y en total 2 veces. Cuando se han producido náuseas y vómitos postoperatorios, puede usar el tratamiento de infusión intravenosa de 4mg. ② Para lacientes de insuficiencia renal: no hay la necesidad de ajustar la dosis, veces de medicación o vía de administración. ③ Para los pacientes con insuficiencia hepática: Principalmente es debido a metabolismo auto-hepática, se usa paraacientes con insuficiencia hepática grave o moderada, la dosis diaria no debe ser superior a 8 mg. |
|---|---|
| 剂型、规格<br>Formulaciones y especificaciones | 注射液：每支 4mg（1ml）；8mg（2ml）。片剂：每片 4mg；8mg。<br>Inyección: Cada una de 4 mg (1 ml), 8 mg (2 ml). Tabletas: Cada tableta de 4 mg; 8 mg. |
| 药品名称 Drug Names | 托烷司琼 Tropisetrón |
| 适应证<br>Indicaciones | 主要用于预防和治疗癌症化疗引起的恶心、呕吐。<br>Se utiliza principalmente para la prevención y tratamiento del cáncer inducido por la quimioterapia náuseas y vómitos. |
| 用法、用量<br>Administración y dosis | 一日 5mg，总疗程 6 日。第一日，静脉给药，在化疗前将本品 5mg 溶于 100ml 生理盐水、林格液或 5% 葡萄糖注射液中静脉滴注或缓慢静脉注射，第 2～6 日，口服给药，一日一次，一次 1 粒胶囊（5mg），于进食前至少 1 小时服用，或于早上起床后立即用水送服。疗程 2～6 日，轻症者可适当缩短疗程。<br>5mg por cada día, un curso total es de seis días. El primer día, administrado por vía intravenosa, antes de la quimioterapia, usa 5mg de este producto disuelto en 100 ml de solución salina, solución de Ringer o solución de glucosa al 5% y hace el goteo por vía intravenosa o hace la inyección intravenosa lentamente, En 2～6 días, se toma la medicina por vía oral, una vez al día, una cápsula (5 mg) por cada vez, se toma por lo menos 1 hora antes de la comida, o se toma por la mañana inmediatamente después de levantarse con el agua. Un curso de tratamiento es de 2～6 días, para pacientes con condiciones leves pueden acortar el curso apropiadamente. |
| 剂型、规格<br>Formulaciones y especificaciones | 注射液：每支 5mg（1ml）。胶囊剂：每粒 5mg。<br>Inyección：Cada inyección de 5 mg （1 ml）. Cápsulas；Cada cápsula de 5mg. |
| 药品名称 Drug Names | 格拉司琼 Granisetrón |
| 适应证<br>Indicaciones | 用于预防和治疗化疗、放疗及手术后引起的恶心和呕吐。<br>Se usa para la prevención y el tratamiento de náuseas y vómitos causados por la quimioterapia, la radioterapia y post-operativa. |
| 用法、用量<br>Administración y dosis | 将本品以注射用生理盐水 20～50ml 稀释后，于化疗或放疗前一日 1 次静脉滴注，成人剂量一次 40μg/kg，或给予标准剂量 3mg，如症状未见改善，可再增补一次；对老年患者及肾功能不全患者一般不需调整剂量。每一疗程可连续使用 5 日。<br>Este producto será inyectado despúes de ser diluido en la solución salina de 20～50 ml, hace la antes de la infusión intravenosa una vez al día antes antes de la quimioterapia o la radioterapia, la dosis para adultos es 40μg/kg por cada vez, o se ofrece una dosis estándar de 3 mg, si los síntomas no se observan mejorados, puede suplementar otra vez; para los pacientes de edad avanzada y los pacientes de insuficiencia renal por lo general no es necesario ajustar la dosis. Un curso puede utilizarse de forma continua durante cinco días. |
| 剂型、规格<br>Formulaciones y especificaciones | 注射液：每支 3mg（3ml）。片（胶囊）剂：每片（粒）1mg。<br>Inyección：Cada inyección de 3 mg （3 ml）. Tabletas （cápsulas）：Cada tableta （cápsula） de 1mg. |
| 药品名称 Drug Names | 阿扎司琼 Azasetrón |
| 适应证<br>Indicaciones | 用于化疗及放疗引起的消化系统症状，如恶心、呕吐等。<br>Se usa para los síntomas gastrointestinales inducidos por la quimioterapia radioterapia, tales como náuseas y vómitos. Se usa para los síntomas gastrointestinales inducidos por la quimioterapia y radioterapia, tales como náuseas y vómitos. |

续　表

| 用法、用量<br>Administración y<br>dosis | 成人一般用量为 10mg，一日一次静脉注射。<br>Generalmente la dosis para adultos es de 10 mg, una vez al día por vía intravenosa. |
|---|---|
| 剂型、规格<br>Formulaciones y<br>especificaciones | 注射剂：每支 10mg（2ml）。<br>Inyección: cada una de 10 mg (2 ml). |

| 药品名称 Drug Names | 地芬尼多 Difenidol |
|---|---|
| 适应证<br>Indicaciones | 用于各种原因引起的眩晕、恶心、呕吐等症状。<br>Se usa para mareos, náuseas, vómitos y otros síntomas causados por varias razones. |
| 用法、用量<br>Administración y<br>dosis | 口服：一次 25～50mg，一日 3 次；肌内注射：一次 20～40mg，一日 4 次。儿童（6 个月以上）：每次 0.9mg/kg，一日 3 次。<br>Por vía oral: 25～50 mg por cada vez, 3 veces al día; Inyección intramuscular: 20～40 mg por cada vez, 4 veces al día. Para los niños (de mayor de 6 meses o más): 0.9mg/kg por cada vez, tres veces al día. |
| 剂型、规格<br>Formulaciones y<br>especificaciones | 片剂：25mg。注射液：10mg/1ml。<br>Tabletas: 25 mg. Inyección: 10mg/1ml. |

12.8　泻药 Laxativo

| 药品名称 Drug Names | 硫酸镁 Sulfato de magnesio |
|---|---|
| 适应证<br>Indicaciones | （1）导泻，肠内异常发酵，亦可与驱虫剂并用；与药用炭合用，可治疗食物或药物中毒。<br>（2）阻塞性黄疸及慢性胆囊炎。<br>（3）惊厥、子痫、尿毒症、破伤风、高血压脑病及急性肾性高血压危象等。<br>（4）也用于发作频繁而其他治疗效果不佳的心绞痛患者，对伴有高血压的患者效果较好。<br>（5）外用热敷消炎去肿。<br><br>(1) Para la catarsis, la fermentación intestinal anormal, también puede usar en combinación con repelente de insectos; en combinación con carbón medicinal,y puede tratar la intoxicación por alimentos.<br>(2) Ictericia obstructiva y colecistitis crónica.<br>(3) Convulsiones, eclampsia, uremia, tétanos, encefalopatía hipertensiva y hipertensiva renal aguda, etc.<br>(4) también es utilizado para los pacientes con angina de las convulsiones frecuentes y que otros tratamientos no tienen mucho efecto, pero tienen efectos mejores para los pacientes con hipertensión.<br>(5) Uso caliente tópico antiinflamatorio para la hinchazón. |
| 用法、用量<br>Administración y<br>dosis | （1）导泻：一次口服 5～20g，清晨空腹服，同时饮 100～400ml 水，也可用水溶解后服用。<br>（2）利胆：每次 2～5g，一日 3 次，餐前或两餐间服。也可服用 33% 溶液，每次 10ml。<br>（3）抗惊厥、降血压等：肌内注射，一次 1g，10% 溶液，每次 10ml；静脉滴注，一次 1～2.5g，将 25% 溶液 10ml 用 5% 葡萄糖注射液稀释成 1% 浓度缓慢静脉滴注。<br><br>(1) Catarsis: Por vía oral 5～20 g por cada vez, se toma por la mañana con el estómago vacío, y debe beber 100～400 ml de agua, se pueden disolverlo en el agua.<br>(2) Vesícula biliar: 2～5 g por cada vez, 3 veces al día, se toma antes de las comidas o entre las comidas. puede tomar la solución al 33%, 10ml por cada vez.<br>(3) Para anticonvulsivos, la presión arterial, etc: Inyección intramuscular, 1 g por cada vez, solución al 10%, 10 ml por cada vez; Infusión intravenosa, 1～2,5 g por cada vez, 25% de solución de 10 ml se diluyó lentamente a la glucosa al 5% y use la inyección de concentración de 1% para el goteo intravenoso. |
| 剂型、规格<br>Formulaciones y<br>especificaciones | 注射液：每支 1g（10ml）；2.5g（10ml）。<br>Inyección: cada una de 1 g (10ml); 2.5g (10ml). |

**续　表**

| 药品名称 Drug Names | 甘油 Glicerina |
|---|---|
| 适应证<br>Indicaciones | 用于便秘、降眼压和颅内压。<br>Se usa para el estreñimiento, disminución de la presión intraocular y la presión intracraneal. |
| 用法、用量<br>Administración y<br>dosis | （1）便秘：使用栓剂，一次 1 粒塞入肛门（成人用大号栓、小儿用小儿栓），对小儿及年老体弱者较为适宜。也可用本品 50% 溶液灌肠。<br>（2）降眼压和降颅内压：口服 50% 甘油溶液（含 0.9% 氯化钠），一次 200ml，一日服 1 次，必要时一日服 2 次，但要间隔 6 ～ 8 小时。<br>(1) Estreñimiento: utilice los supositorios, un upositorio por cada vez insertado en el ano (para los adultos con supositorio grande, para los niños con supositorio pediátrico), es apropiado para los niños y los ancianos y enfermos. Puede usar la s olución al 50% para el enema.<br>(2) Para la reducción de la presión intraocular y la presión intracraneal: toma por vía oral la solución de glicerol al 50% (que contiene cloruro de sodio al 0.9%), 200 ml por cada vez, 1 vez durante el día, 2 veces al día cuando sea necesario, pero debe mantener un intervalo de 6 ~ 8 horas. |
| 剂型、规格<br>Formulaciones y<br>especificaciones | 栓剂：含甘油约 90%，大号每个约重 3g，小号每个约重 1.5g。<br>甘油溶液：包括 10% 甘油生理盐水溶液、10% 甘油葡萄糖溶液、10% 甘油甘露醇溶液和 50% 甘油盐水溶液。<br>Supositorio: que contiene aproximadamente 90% de glicerol, cada supositorio grande tiene un peso de aproximadamente 3 g, cada supositorio pediátrico tiene peso de aproximadamente 1.5 g. Solución de glicerol: comprende 10% de solución salina fisiológica de glicerol, 10% de solución de glicerol, 10% de glicerol y 50% de solución de glicerol de sal de manitol. |
| 药品名称 Drug Names | 开塞露 Glicerina enema |
| 适应证<br>Indicaciones | 本品为治疗便秘的直肠用溶液剂。<br>Este producto se usa para el tratamiento de soluciones rectales de estreñimiento. |
| 用法、用量<br>Administración y<br>dosis | 用时将容器顶端刺破，外面涂油脂少许，徐徐插入肛门，然后将药液挤入直肠内，引起排便。成人用量每次 20ml（1 支）。<br>Para su uso, hay que pinchar la parte superior del recipiente, engrasar el exterior un poco, se inserta lentamente en el ano, y luego exprimir el líquido en el interior del recto, causando intestinal. La dosis de adultos es 20 ml (1 sucursal) por cada vez. |
| 剂型、规格<br>Formulaciones y<br>especificaciones | 每支 20ml。<br>Cada una de 20ml. |
| 药品名称 Drug Names | 硫酸钠 Sulfato de sodio |
| 适应证<br>Indicaciones | 为容积性泻药。<br>Es medicamento de laxantede volumen. |
| 用法、用量<br>Administración y<br>dosis | 散剂：一次 5 ～ 20g，溶于 250ml 水，清晨空腹服用；肠溶胶囊：一次 5g，一日 1 ～ 3 次。排便后即可停药，如 12 小时后未排便，可追加服药 1 ～ 2 次。<br>olvo: 5 ~ 20g por cada vez, disuelto en 250 ml de agua, se toma por la mañana con el estómago vacío; Cápsulas con recubrimiento entérico: 5g por cada vez, 1 ~ 3 veces al día. después de la evacuación intestinal puede parar el medicamento. Si no hay evacuación intestinal después de 12 horas, se puede añadir la medicación de 1 ~ 2 veces. |
| 剂型、规格<br>Formulaciones y<br>especificaciones | 散剂：500g。<br>肠溶胶囊：1g/ 粒。<br>Polvo: 500g. Cápsulas con recubrimiento entérico: 1 g / cápsula. |
| 药品名称 Drug Names | 液状石蜡 Líquido de parafina |
| 适应证<br>Indicaciones | 使粪便稀释变软，同时润滑肠壁，使粪便易于排出。<br>Puede diluir, ablandar taburete, mientras que realizar la lubricación de la pared intestinal, fácil de descargar heces. |

续 表

| 用法、用量<br>Administración y<br>dosis | 一次 15～30ml，睡前服用。<br>15 - 30 ml por cada vez, se toma antes de acostarse. |
|---|---|
| 剂型、规格<br>Formulaciones y<br>especificaciones | 原液：500ml。<br>Líquido puro: 500ml. |

## 12.9 止泻药 Anti-diarreico

| 药品名称 Drug Names | 双八面体蒙脱石 Esmectita dioctahédrica |
|---|---|
| 适应证<br>Indicaciones | 用于急慢性腹泻，尤以对儿童急性腹泻疗效为佳，但在必要时应同时治疗脱水，也用于食管炎及与胃、十二指肠、结肠疾病有关的疼痛的对症治疗。<br>Se usa para la diarrea aguda y crónica, especialmente tiene un mejor efecto para la diarrea aguda de los niños, pero si es necesario, debe realizar el tratamiento de la deshidratación, pero también puede usar para el tratamiento sintomático de la esofagitis y el estómago, el duodeno, enfermedades del colon relacionados con el dolor. |
| 用法、用量<br>Administración y<br>dosis | 成人一次 1 袋，一日 3 次，治疗急性腹泻首剂应加倍。食管炎患者宜于餐后服用，其他患者于餐前服用，将本品溶于半杯温水中送服。<br>Para adultos, 1 bolsa por cada vez, 3 veces al día, la primera dosis del tratamiento de la diarrea aguda se debe doblar. Para los pacientes con esofagitis debe tomar el medicamento después de las comidas, y para otros pacientes, debe tomar el medicamento antes de las comidas, se disolverá el presente producto en medio vaso de agua caliente para el uso. |
| 剂型、规格<br>Formulaciones y<br>especificaciones | 散剂：每小袋内含双八面体蒙脱石 3g、葡萄糖 0.749g、糖精钠 0.007g、香兰素 0.004g。<br>Polvo: Cada bolsa contiene 3g de montmorillonita dioctaédrica, 0.749g de glucosa, 0.007 g de sacarina de sodio, 0.004 g de vainillina. |
| 药品名称 Drug Names | 鞣酸蛋白 Tannalbin |
| 适应证<br>Indicaciones | 用于急性胃肠炎非细菌性腹泻。<br>Se usa para la diarrea gastroenteritis aguda no bacteriana. |
| 用法、用量<br>Administración y<br>dosis | 一日 3 次，每次 1～2g，空腹服。<br>Tres veces al día, 1 ~ 2 g por cada vez, se toma con el estómago vacío. |
| 剂型、规格<br>Formulaciones y<br>especificaciones | 片剂：0.25g；0.5g。<br>Tabletas: 0.25g; 0.5g. |
| 药品名称 Drug Names | 碱式碳酸铋 Subcarbonato de bismuto |
| 适应证<br>Indicaciones | 用于腹泻、慢性胃肠炎、胃及十二指肠溃疡。<br>Se usa para la diarrea, gastroenteritis crónica, úlceras gástricas y duodenales. |
| 用法、用量<br>Administración y dosis | 一日 3 次，每次 0.3～0.9g，餐前服。<br>Tres veces al día, 0.3 ~ 0.9g por cada vez, se toma antes de las comidas. |
| 剂型、规格<br>Formulaciones y<br>especificaciones | 片剂：0.3g。<br>Tabletas: 0.3g. |

## 12.10 微生态药物 Medicamentos microecológica

| 药品名称 Drug Names | 地衣芽孢杆菌活菌 Licheniformis de bacillus viables |
|---|---|
| 适应证<br>Indicaciones | 用于细菌与真菌引起的急慢性腹泻及各种原因所致的肠道菌群失调的防治。<br>Se usa para el tratamiento y la prevención de la diarrea aguda y crónica causada por bacterias y hongos, y desequilibio de la flora intestinal causado por una variedad de razones. |

**续　表**

| | |
|---|---|
| 用法、用量<br>Administración y dosis | 口服：每次 0.5g，一日 3 次，小儿减半或遵医嘱。<br>Por vía oral: 0.5 g por cada vez, 3 veces al día, para los niños se reduce la dosis a la mitad o según las indicaciones. |
| 剂型、规格<br>Formulaciones y especificaciones | 胶囊剂：每粒 0.25g（含 2.5 亿活菌）。<br>Cápsulas: Cada cápsula de 0.25 g (incluye 250 millones de células viables). |
| 药品名称 Drug Names | 嗜酸乳杆菌 Lactobacillus |
| 适应证<br>Indicaciones | 用于急慢性腹泻的对症治疗。<br>Se usa para el tratamiento sintomático de la diarrea aguda y crónica. |
| 用法、用量<br>Administración y dosis | 胶囊剂：成人及儿童一日 2 次，一次 2 粒，成人首剂量加倍；婴儿一日 2 次，一次 1～2 粒，首剂量 2 粒。散剂：成人及儿童一日 2 次，一次 1 袋，成人首剂量加倍；婴儿一日 2 次，一次 1 袋。胶囊剂可用水吞服亦可倒出内容物混合于水中饮服。<br>Cápsulas: Para adultos y niños, 2 veces al día, dos cápsula por cada vez, la primera dosis de adultos debe ser de dosis doble; Para bebés, 2 veces al día, 1～2 cápsulas por cada vez, la primera dosis debe ser de dos cápsulas. Polvo: Para adultos y niños, 2 veces al día, cada vez de una bolsa, la primera dosis de adultos debe ser de dosis doble; Para bebés, 2 veces al día, cada vez de una bolsa. Las cápsulas pueden tragarse con agua o vierte su contenido y se mezcla en agua para su uso. |
| 剂型、规格<br>Formulaciones y especificaciones | 胶囊剂：每胶囊含灭活冻干的嗜酸乳杆菌 50 亿和中和后冻干的培养基 80mg。散剂：每小袋含灭活冻干的嗜酸乳杆菌 50 亿和中和后冻干的培养基 160mg.<br>Cápsulas: Cada cápsula contiene 5000 millones de lactobacillus acidophilus y 80 mg de liofilizada inactivada después de medio liofilización. Polvo: Cada cápsula contiene 5000 millones de lactobacillus acidophilus y 160 mg de liofilizada inactivada después de medio liofilización. |
| 药品名称 Drug Names | 复合乳酸菌 Lactobacilos compuestos |
| 适应证<br>Indicaciones | 用于各种原因引起的肠道菌群紊乱、急慢性腹泻、肠易激综合征、抗生素相关性腹泻的治疗。亦可用于预防或减少抗生素及化疗药物所致的肠道菌群紊乱的辅助治疗。<br>Se usa para el tratamiento de la flora intestinal para diversas causas por diversas enfermedades, diarrea aguda y crónica, síndrome del intestino irritable, diarrea asociada a antibióticos. Se pueden utilizar para prevenir o reducir los antibióticos, y el tratamiento adyuvante de la flora intestinal inducidos por la quimioterapia. |
| 用法、用量<br>Administración y dosis | 口服：一次 1～2 粒，一日 1～3 次，根据病情和年龄可适当增减。<br>Por vía oral: 1～2 cápsulas por cada vez, 1～3 veces al día, de acuerdo con la condición y la edad pueden aumentar o disminuir. |
| 剂型、规格<br>Formulaciones y especificaciones | 胶囊剂：每粒 0.33g（含活乳酸菌 2 万个以上）。<br>Cápsulas: Cada cápsula de 0.33 g (que contienen los lactobacilos vivos 20.000 o más. |
| 药品名称 Drug Names | 双歧杆菌嗜酸乳杆菌肠球菌三联活菌 Bifidobacterium, lactobacillus y enterococcos combinados vivos |
| 适应证<br>Indicaciones | 用于肠道菌群失调引起的腹泻、腹胀等，也用于慢性腹泻和轻中型急性腹泻，以调节肠道功能；对缓解便秘也有较好疗效，还可作为肝硬化、急慢性肝炎及肿瘤化疗等的辅助用药。<br>Se usa para la diarrea, hinchazón causadas por la flora intestinal, y también para la diarrea crónica y diarrea aguda leve a moderada, para regular la función intestinal; para aliviar el estreñimiento y también tiene un buen efecto, y también se usa como el medicamento adyuvante para cirrosis, hepatitis aguda y crónica y quimioterapia de cáncer. |
| 用法、用量<br>Administración y dosis | 口服：一次 420～630mg，一日 2～3 次，餐后服用。小于 1 岁儿童每次 105mg；1～6 岁一次 210mg；6～13 岁一次 210～420mg。婴幼儿可取胶囊内药粉用温开水调服。<br>Por vía oral: 420～630 mg por cada vez, 2～3 veces al día, se toma después de las comidas. Para niños de menos de 1 año de edad, 105 mg por cada vez;Para niños de1～6 años, 210 mg por cada vez; Para niños de 6～13 años de edad, 210～420 mg por cada vez. Para niños de brazos, puede vertir el polvo dentro de la cápsula y se mezcla en el agua tibia para el uso. |

| 剂型、规格<br>Formulaciones y especificaciones | 胶囊剂：每粒210mg。散剂：每包1g；2g。<br>Cápsulas: Cada cápsula de 210 mg. Polvo: Cada paquete de 1g; 2g. |
|---|---|
| 药品名称 Drug Names | 枯草杆菌肠球菌二联活菌 Bacillus subtilis y enterococos faecium combinadas vivas |
| 适应证<br>Indicaciones | 治疗和预防抗生素相关性腹泻、旅行者腹泻及其他腹泻；也可用于肠易激综合征（ＩＢＳ）及炎性肠病的辅助治疗。<br>Tiene tratamiento y prevención para la diarrea asociada a antibióticos, diarrea del viajero y otra diarrea; también se pueden usar para el síndrome del intestino irritable（ＩＢＳ）y la terapia adyuvante para la enfermedad intestinal inflamatoria. |
| 用法、用量<br>Administración y dosis | 12岁以上儿童及成人：口服，一次1～2粒，一日2～3次。<br>Para los niños mayores de 12 años y los adultos: Por vía oral, 1～2 cápsulas por cada vez, 2～3 veces al día. |
| 剂型、规格<br>Formulaciones y especificaciones | 胶囊（肠溶）剂：每粒250mg。<br>Cápsulas (entérica): Cada cápsula de 250mg. |
| 药品名称 Drug Names | 乳酶生 Lactasina |
| 适应证<br>Indicaciones | 用于消化不良、肠发酵、小儿饮食不当引起的腹泻等。<br>Se usa para la indigestión, la fermentación intestinal, la diarrea de los niños causados por una dieta inadecuada, etc. |
| 用法、用量<br>Administración y dosis | 一次0.3～1.0g，一日3次，餐前服。<br>0.3～1.0 g por cada vez, 3 veces al día, se toma antes de las comidas. |
| 剂型、规格<br>Formulaciones y especificaciones | 片剂：0.15g；0.3g。<br>Tabletas: 0.15g; 0.3g. |

12.11　治疗肝性脑病药 Medicamentos para el tratamientode la encefalopatía hepática

| 药品名称 Drug Names | 乳果糖 Lactulosa |
|---|---|
| 适应证<br>Indicaciones | 用于肝性脑病的辅助治疗，也用于内毒素血症和治疗便秘。<br>Se usa para el tratamiento adyuvante de la encefalopatía hepática, también se utiliza para el tratamiento de la endotoxemia y estreñimiento. |
| 用法、用量<br>Administración y dosis | 治疗肝性脑病和内毒素血症：开始一次10～20mg，一日2次，后改为一次3～5g，一日2～3次；以每日排软便2～3次为宜。治疗肝性脑病时可将本品200g加入700ml水或生理盐水中，保留灌肠30～60分钟，每4～6小时一次。本品与新霉素合用可提高对肝性脑病的疗效。治疗便秘：一次5～10mg，一日1～2次，应根据个人反应调节，如48小时未见效果，可适当增加剂量。<br>Tiene tratamiento de la encefalopatía hepática y endotoxemia: al inicio, 10～20 mg por cada vez, 2 veces al día, posteriormente cambia a 3～5 g por cada vez, 2～3 veces al día, mejor con descarga de heces blandas de 2～3 veces al día. Cuando se trata de la encefalopatía hepática, utilice 200g de este producto y puede ser añadido a 700 ml de agua o solución salina, mantiene derramar al enema por 30 - 60 minutos, 4～6 horas por cada vez. Este producto se utiliza en combinación con neomicina, y puede mejorar la eficacia para el tratamiento de la encefalopatía hepática. Para el estreñimiento: 5～10 mg por cada vez, 1～2 veces al día, y se debe ajustar de acuerdo con la respuesta individual, si dentro de 48 horas no se observa efecto, puede incrementar la dosis. |
| 剂型、规格<br>Formulaciones y especificaciones | 乳果糖粉：每袋5g；100g；500g。乳果糖颗粒：每袋10g。乳果糖口服液：5g(10ml)；50g(100ml)。乳果糖糖浆：60%。<br>Polvo de lactulosa: cada paquete de 5g; 100g; 500g. Partículas Lactulosa: cada paquete de 10 g. Lactulosa oral: 5 g (10 ml), 50 g (100 ml). Jarabe de lactulosa: 60%. |

**续　表**

| 药品名称 Drug Names | 谷氨酸钠 Glutamato de sodio |
|---|---|
| 适应证<br>Indicaciones | 用于肝性脑病及酸血症。<br>Se usa para la encefalopatía hepática y acidosis. |
| 用法、用量<br>Administración y<br>dosis | 肝性脑病：每次静脉滴注 11.5g，用 5% 葡萄糖注射液 750 ～ 1000ml 或 10% 葡萄糖注射液 250 ～ 500ml 稀释，于 1 ～ 4 小时滴完，滴注过快可引起流涎、潮红、呕吐等。必要时可于 8 ～ 12 小时后重复给药，一日量不宜超过 23g。酸血症：用量根据病情决定。<br><br>Para encefalopatía hepática: 11.5 g de infusión intravenosa por cada vez, diluido en la inyección de glucosa al 5% de 750 ~ 1000 ml o en la inyección de glucosa al 10% de 250 ~ 500 ml, y se finaliza la infusión dentro de 1 ~ 4 horas. Si el goteo es demasiado rápido puede causar la salivación excesiva, enrojecimiento y vómitos. Cuando sea necesario, puede ofrecer la administración después de un intervalo de 8 ~ 12 horas de una vez repetida, la dosis diaria no debe exceder de 23g. Para acidosis: la cantidad es determinada de acuerdo a la condición de la enfermedad. |
| 剂型、规格<br>Formulaciones y<br>especificaciones | 注射液：每支 5.75g/20ml。<br>Inyección: Cada una de 5.75g/20ml. |
| 药品名称 Drug Names | 支链氨基酸 Aminoácidos de cadena ramificada |
| 适应证<br>Indicaciones | 支链氨基酸 3H 注射液、六合氨基酸注射液主要用于支 / 芳比失调引起的肝性脑病及各种肝病引起的氨基酸代谢紊乱。14 氨基酸 -800 主要用于肝功能不全合并蛋白营养缺乏症和肝性脑病。<br><br>Inyección de aminoácidos 3H de cadena ramificada, y inyección de aminoácidos LIUHE se utilizan principalmente para encefalopatía hepática causado por el desequilibrio en la proporción aromático/cadena ramificada y el trastorno de metabolismo de los aminoácidos causado por una variedad de enfermedades hepáticas. El amino ácidos 14 -800 se usa principalmente para la disfunción del hígado, deficiencias nutricionales de proteína y encefalopatía hepática. |
| 用法、用量<br>Administración y<br>dosis | 静脉滴注：一日 2 次，一次 250ml，与等量 10% 葡萄糖注射液串联后作缓慢滴注（不宜超过 3ml/min）。如疗效显著者（完全清醒），后阶段剂量可减半。疗程一般为 10 ～ 15 日。中心静脉滴注：每日量以 0.68 ～ 0.87g/kg 计，成人剂量相当于一日 500 ～ 750ml，与 25% ～ 50% 高渗葡萄糖注射液等量混匀后，经中心静脉缓慢滴注，低速不得超过 40 滴 / 分。<br><br>Infusión intravenosa: 2 veces al día, 250 ml por cada vez, con una cantidad igual de 10% de inyección de glucosa y después de la integración en serie hace la infusión lenta (no debe exceder de 3ml/min). Si la eficacia fueron significativamente (completamente despierta), la dosis puede reducirse a la mitad en la etapa posterior. El curso de tratamiento es de 10 ~ 15 días. Infusión venosa central: La dosis diaria es medida por 0,68 ~ 0.87g/kg, la dosis diaria del adulto es equivalente a 500 ~ 750 ml, con mezcla la inyección de glucosa hipertónica de 25% ~ 50%, hace la infusión intravenosa por la venosa central en una baja velocidad que no debe exceder de 40 gotas / min. |
| 剂型、规格<br>Formulaciones y<br>especificaciones | 注射液：250ml-10.65g（总氨基酸）。<br>Inyección: 250ml-10.65g (aminoácidos total). |
| 药品名称 Drug Names | 谷氨酸钾 Glutamato de potasio |
| 适应证<br>Indicaciones | 用于肝性脑病、酸血症，常与谷氨酸钠合用，以维持电解质平衡。<br>Se usa para la encefalopatía hepática, la acidosis, a menudo se usa en combinación con glutamato de sodio para mantener el equilibrio de electrolitos. |
| 用法、用量<br>Administración y<br>dosis | 静脉滴注：一次 6.3g，其余用法、注意同谷氨酸钠。<br>Infusión intravenosa: 6.3 g por cada vez, otros usos y notas son lo mismo con lo de glutamato de sodio. |
| 剂型、规格<br>Formulaciones y<br>especificaciones | 注射液：6.3g（20ml）。<br>Inyección: 6.3 g (20 ml). |

**续　表**

| 药品名称 Drug Names | 精氨酸 Arginina |
|---|---|
| 适应证<br>Indicaciones | 用于肝性脑病，适用于忌钠患者。也适用于其他原因引起血氨过高所致的精神症状。<br>Se usa para la encefalopatía hepática, aplicable para los pacientes de prohibición de sodio. También se aplica a psicosis causada por amoniaco de la sangre demasiado alto inducido por en otras razones. |
| 用法、用量<br>Administración y dosis | 静脉滴注：一次 15～20g，以 5% 葡萄糖液 500～1000ml 稀释，滴注宜慢（每次 4 小时以上）。用其盐酸盐，可引起高氯性酸血症，肾功能不全者禁用。滴注太快可引起流涎、潮红、呕吐等。<br>La infusión intravenosa: 15～20g por una vez, solución de glucosa de 5% de 500～1000ml diluida para la infusión lenta (debe ser más de 4 horas por cada vez). Con la sal clorhidrato, puede causar la acidosis de cloruro alto, se prohíbe a utilizar los pacientes con insuficiencia renal. Si la velocidad de goteo es demasiado rápida, puede causar salivación, enrojecimiento, vómitos. |
| 剂型、规格<br>Formulaciones y especificaciones | 注射液：5g（20ml）。<br>Inyección: 5 g (20 ml). |

| 药品名称 Drug Names | 谷氨酸 Glutámico ácido |
|---|---|
| 适应证<br>Indicaciones | 可预防肝性脑病；减少癫痫小发作发作次数；治疗胃酸不足。<br>Puede prevenir la encefalopatía hepática, reducir las acciones de convulsiones episodias; tratar la insuficiencia de ácido estomacal. |
| 用法、用量<br>Administración y dosis | 预防肝性脑病：每次 2.5～5g，一日 4 次；用于癫痫小发作：一次 2～3g，一日 3～4 次；治疗胃酸不足：一次 0.3g，一日 3 次。肾功能不全或无尿患者慎用。不宜与碱性药物合用。与抗胆碱药合用有可能减弱后者的药效。<br>Prevención de la encefalopatía hepática: 2.5～5 g por cada vez, 4 veces al día; se usa para las convulsiones episodias: 2～3 g por cada vez, 3～4 veces al día; Tratamiento de la deficiencia de ácido gástrico: 0.3 g por una vez, 3 veces al día. Los pacientes con insuficiencia renal o nada de orina deben usar con precaución. No debe combinarse con medicamentos básicos. Y si se combina con los fármacos anticolinérgicos pueden debilitar la eficacia de este último. |
| 剂型、规格<br>Formulaciones y especificaciones | 片剂：每片 0.3g；0.5g。<br>Tabletas: Cada tableta de 0.3 g; 0.5 g. |

## 12.12　治疗肝炎辅助用药 Medicamentos auxiliares para el tratamiento de la hepatitis

| 药品名称 Drug Names | 联苯双酯 Bifendato |
|---|---|
| 适应证<br>Indicaciones | 用于迁延性肝炎及长期单项丙氨酸氨基转移酶异常者。对肝炎主要症状如肝区痛、乏力、腹胀等的改善有一定疗效，但对肝脾大的改变无影响。<br>Se usa para la hepatitis persistente y anomalías de alanina aminotransferasa simples crónicas a largo plazo. Tiene un cierto efecto para el mejoramiento de los síntomas principales de la hepatitis, tales como dolor de hígado, fatiga, distensión abdominal, pero no tiene efecto en los cambios en el agrandamiento del hígado y el bazo. |
| 用法、用量<br>Administración y dosis | 口服，一日量 75～150mg。多采用一日 3 次，每次服 25mg。<br>Por vía oral, la cantidad es de 75～150 mg. Frecuentemente se usa tres veces al día, 25 mg por cada vez. |
| 剂型、规格<br>Formulaciones y especificaciones | 片剂：每片 25mg。滴丸：每丸 1.5mg，口服，一次 7.5～15mg，一日 22.5～45mg。<br>Tabletas: Cada tableta de 25mg. Pastillas de goteo: cada pastilla de 1.5 mg, por vía oral, 7.5～15 mg por cada vez, 22.5～45 mg al día. |

| 药品名称 Drug Names | 门冬氨酸钾镁 Aspartato de potasio y magnesio |
|---|---|
| 适应证<br>Indicaciones | 用于急性黄疸型肝炎、肝细胞功能不全，也可用于其他急慢性肝病。本品还可用于低钾血症、洋地黄中毒引起的心律失常、心肌炎后遗症、慢性心功能不全、冠心病等。 |

|  | Se usa para la hepatitis ictericia aguda, disfunción hepatocelular, también se puede utilizar para otra enfermedad hepática aguda y crónica. Este producto también se puede utilizar para la hipopotasemia, arritmia causada por la intoxicación digitálica, secuelas miocarditis, insuficiencia cardíaca crónica, la enfermedad cardíaca coronaria, etc. |
| --- | --- |
| 用法、用量<br>Administración y dosis | 注射液：一般为成人 10 ~ 20ml，加入 5% 或 10% 葡萄糖注射液 250 ~ 500ml 中缓慢静脉滴注，一日 1 次。儿童用量酌减。对重症黄疸患者，一日可用 2 次。对低血钾患者可适当加大剂量。口服：一般为一次 1 片，一日 3 次。由于各制品的含量有所不同，应用前须详阅产品说明书，并按其规定使用。<br><br>Inyección: Generalmente para los adultos es de 10 ~ 20 ml, con inyección de glucosa de 5% o 10% de 250 ~ 500 ml y se hace la infusión intravenosa lenta, 1 vez al día. La dosis de niños debe ser reducida. Para los pacientes con ictericia severa, es disponible dos veces al día. Para los pacientes con hipopotasemia es apropiado aumentar la dosis. Por vía oral: generalmente es una tableta por cada vez, tres veces al día. Dado que el contenido de cada producto es diferente, antes de la aplicación debe leer la especificación del producto detalladamente, y luego usar según sus disposiciones. |
| 剂型、规格<br>Formulaciones y especificaciones | 片剂：含门冬氨酸 252mg，钾 36.1mg，镁 11.8mg。口服液：含无水 L- 门冬氨酸钾 451mg（钾 103mg），无水门冬氨酸镁 403.6mg（镁 34mg），按门冬氨酸计为 723mg，每支 5ml 或 10ml。门冬氨酸钾镁注射液：每支 10ml（每 1ml 含无水 L- 门冬氨酸 85mg、钾 11.4mg、镁 4.2mg）。注射用门冬氨酸钾镁：每瓶含无水 L- 门冬氨酸 850mg、钾 114mg、镁 42mg。<br><br>Tabletas: con 252 mg de aspartato, 36.1mg de potasio, 11.8mg de magnesio. Líquido por vía oral: que contiene 451mg de potasio anhidro deácido L-aspártico (103 mg de potasio), 403.6mg aspartato de magnesio de anhidro (34 mg de magnesio), medida de acuerdo con aspartato, es de 723mg, cada una es de 5 ml o 10 ml. Inyección de potasio aspartato de magnesio de: Cada una contiene10 ml (cada 1 ml contiene 85 mg de anhidro-L-aspártico ácido, 11.4mg de potasio, 4.2 mg de magnesio). La inyección de aspartato de magnesio y potasio: cada botella que contiene 850 mg de anhidro ácido L-aspártico, 114 mg de potasio, 42 mg de magnesio. |

| 药品名称 Drug Names | 水飞蓟宾 Silibinina |
| --- | --- |
| 适应证<br>Indicaciones | 慢性迁延性肝炎、慢性活动性肝炎、初期肝硬化、中毒性肝损伤等。<br>La hepatitis crónica persistente, hepatitis activa crónica, cirrosis temprana, daño hepático tóxico, etc. |
| 用法、用量<br>Administración y dosis | 口服，一次 70 ~ 140mg，一日 3 次，餐后服。维持量可减半。<br>Por vía oral, cada 70 ~ 140 mg, 3 veces al día después de la comida. La dosis de mantenimiento puede reducirse a la mitad. |
| 剂型、规格<br>Formulaciones y especificaciones | 水飞蓟宾片：35mg，38.5mg。水飞蓟宾胶囊剂：每粒 35mg，140mg。水飞蓟宾葡甲胺片：50mg（相当于水飞蓟宾 35.6mg）。<br>Tabletas silibinina: 35mg, 38.5mg. Cápsulas silibinina: Cada cápsula de 35 mg, 140 mg. Tabletas de meglumina silibinina: 50mg (equivalente a 35.6mg de silibinina). |

| 药品名称 Drug Names | 牛磺酸 Taurina |
| --- | --- |
| 适应证<br>Indicaciones | 可用于急慢性肝炎、脂肪肝、胆囊炎等，也可用于支气管炎、扁桃体炎、眼炎等感染性疾病。感冒、酒精戒断症状、关节炎、肌强直等可试用本品治疗。<br><br>Puede ser utilizado para la hepatitis aguda y crónica, hígado graso, la colecistitis, etc, también se puede utilizar para la bronquitis, amigdalitis, oftalmia y otras enfermedades infecciosas. Para los síntomas del resfriado, abstinencia de alcohol, artritis, rigidez muscular, etc, se pueden probar usando este medicamento. |
| 用法、用量<br>Administración y dosis | 治疗急慢性肝炎，成人每次服 0.5g，一日 3 次；儿童每次 0.5g，一日 2 次。<br>Tratamiento de la hepatitis aguda y crónica, adulto por 0.5 g de servir, 3 veces al día; niño cada 0.5 g, 2 veces al día |
| 剂型、规格<br>Formulaciones y especificaciones | 片（胶囊）剂：每片（粒）0.5g。冲剂：每袋含牛磺酸 0.5g。<br>Tabletas (cápsulas): Cada tableta (cápsula) de 0.5g. Gránulos: cada paquete contiene 0,5 g de taurina. |

**续 表**

| 药品名称 Drug Names | 促肝细胞生长因子 Factores de promoción de crecimiento de hepatocitos |
|---|---|
| 适应证<br>Indicaciones | 用于亚急性重型肝炎（病毒性；肝功能衰竭早期或中期）的辅助治疗。<br><br>Se usa para la terapia adyuvante de la hepatitis severa sub-aguda (viral; insuficiencia hepática principios o mediados). |
| 用法、用量<br>Administración y dosis | 口服，一次 100～150mg，一日 3 次，疗程 3 个月，可连续使用 2～4 个疗程；肌内注射，一次 40mg，一日 2 次；必要时也可将本品 80～120mg 加入 10% 葡萄糖注射液中静脉点滴，一日 1 次。疗程视病情而定，一般为 1 个月。<br><br>Por vía oral, 100～150 mg por cada vez, tres veces al día, un curso de tratamiento es de 3 meses, puede usar de manera continua 2～4 cursos; Inyección intramuscular, 40 mg por cada vez, 2 veces al día, si es necesario, puede agregar el producto de 80～120 mg en glucosa al 10% para la inyección intravenosa, una vez al día. El curso del tratamiento depende de la enfermedad, por lo general es de un mes. |
| 剂型、规格<br>Formulaciones y especificaciones | 颗粒剂：每袋 50mg。注射用促肝细胞生长素：20mg。<br>Gránulos: cada bolsa de 50 mg. Inyección de Factores de Promoción de Crecimiento de Hepatocitos: 20 mg. |
| 药品名称 Drug Names | 甘草酸二铵 Glicirrato dediamina |
| 适应证<br>Indicaciones | 用于伴有 ALT 升高的慢性肝炎。<br><br>Se usa para la terapia adyuvante de la hepatitis severa sub-aguda (viral; insuficiencia hepática principios o mediados). |
| 用法、用量<br>Administración y dosis | 口服，一次 150mg，一日 3 次；静脉滴注，30ml 用 10% 葡萄糖注射液 250ml 稀释后缓慢静脉滴注，一日 1 次。<br><br>Por vía oral, 150 mg por cada vez, tres veces al día; Infusión intravenosa, andir 30 ml en 250 ml do inyección de glucosa al 10%, mezclar bien, infusión intravenosa lenta una vez al dia. |
| 剂型、规格<br>Formulaciones y especificaciones | 胶囊：每粒 50mg。注射液：每支 50mg（10ml）。<br>Gránulos: cada bolsa de 50 mg. Inyección: 50mg(10ml). |
| 药品名称 Drug Names | 硫普罗宁 Tiopronina |
| 适应证<br>Indicaciones | 用于：①脂肪肝、早期肝硬化、急慢性肝炎、酒精及药物引起的肝炎。②重金属中毒。③降低化疗及放疗的不良反应，升高白细胞，并可预防化疗、放疗所致二次肿瘤的发生。<br><br>Se usa para: ① hígado graso, cirrosis temprana, hepatitis aguda y crónica, y el alcohol de la hepatitis inducida por medicamentos. ② Intoxicación por metales pesados. ③ Puede reducir los efectos adversos de la quimioterapia y la radioterapia, aumentar las células blancas de la sangre, y prevenir la quimioterapia, tumores secundarios inducidos por la terapia de radiación. |
| 用法、用量<br>Administración y dosis | ①肝病治疗：餐后口服，一次 1～2 片，一日 3 次，连服 12 周，停药 3 个月后继续下一疗程；急性病毒性肝炎初期每次 2～4 片，一日 3 次，连服 1～3 周，以后一次 1～2 片，一日 3 次。②重金属中毒：一次 1～2 片，一日 2 次。③化疗及放疗引起的白细胞减少症：餐后口服，化疗及放疗前一周开始服用，一次 2～4 片，一日 2 次，连服 3 周。<br><br>① Enfermedad hepática: se toma postprandial por vía oral, 1～2 veces por cada vez, 3 veces al día, 12 semanas continuas, después de la interrupción del tratamiento de tres meses, se continúa el siguiente curso; En el tratamiento de hepatitis aguda temprana, se toma 2～4 tabletas por cada vez, 3 veces al día, y se toma de manera continua 1～3 semanas, posteriormente 1～2 tabletas por cada vez, 3 veces al día. ② Para intoxicación por metales pesados: 1～2 tabletas por cada vez, 2 veces al día. ③ Para la leucopenia causada por la quimioterapia y la radioterapia: se toma por vía oral postprandial y una semana antes de la quimioterapia o la radioterapia, 2～4 veces por cada vez, 2 veces al día, 3 semanas continuas. |
| 剂型、规格<br>Formulaciones y especificaciones | 片剂：每片 0.1g。<br>Tabletas: cada tableta de 0.1 g. |

| 药品名称 Drug Names | 葡醛内酯 Glucurolactona |
| --- | --- |
| 适应证<br>Indicaciones | 用于急慢性肝炎、肝硬化；本品又有一定的解毒作用，可用于食物或药物中毒。<br>Se usa para la hepatitis, la cirrosis hepática aguda y crónica; Este producto tiene un cierto efecto de desintoxicación y se puede utilizar para alimentos o medicamentos. |
| 用法、用量<br>Administración y dosis | 口服：一日 3 次，每次 0.1 ~ 0.2g。肌内或静脉注射：一日 1 ~ 2 次，每次 0.1 ~ 0.2g。<br>Por vía oral: tres veces al día, 0.1 ~ 0.2g por cada vez. Inyección intramuscular o intravenosa: 1 ~ 2 veces al día, 0.1 ~ 0.2g por cada vez. |
| 剂型、规格<br>Formulaciones y especificaciones | 片剂：0.05g；0.1g。注射液：0.1g（2ml）。<br>Tabletas: 0.05 g; 0.1 g. Inyección: 0.1 g (2 ml). |

| 药品名称 Drug Names | 辅酶 A　Coenzima A |
| --- | --- |
| 适应证<br>Indicaciones | 用于白细胞减少症、原发性血小板减少性紫癜、功能性低热等，对脂肪肝、肝性脑病、急慢性肝炎、冠脉硬化、慢性动脉炎、心肌梗死、慢性肾功能减退引起的肾病综合征、尿毒症等可作为辅助治疗药。<br>Se usa para leucopenia, púrpura trombocitopénica idiopática, la fiebre de funcionalidad, se usa como la terapia adyuvante para hígado graso, encefalopatía hepática, hepatitis aguda y crónica, esclerosis coronaria, la arteritis crónica, infarto de miocardio, el síndrome nefrótico integral causado por disfunción renal crónica, y la uremia. |
| 用法、用量<br>Administración y dosis | 静脉滴注：一日 1 ~ 2 次或隔日 1 次，每次 50 ~ 100U；肌内注射：一日 1 次，每次 50 ~ 100U。一般以 7 ~ 14 日为 1 疗程。<br>Infusión intravenosa: 1 ~ 2 veces al día o cada dos días, 50 ~ 100 unidades por cada vez; Inyección intramuscular: 1 vez al día, 50 ~ 100 unidades por cada vez. Generalmente un curso de tratamiento es de 7 ~ 14 días. |
| 剂型、规格<br>Formulaciones y especificaciones | 注射用辅酶 A：50U；100U。<br>Coenzima A inyectable: 50 unidades; 100 unidades. |

12.13　利胆药 Medicamento que favorece la vesícula biliar

| 药品名称 Drug Names | 熊去氧胆酸 Acido ursodesoxicólico |
| --- | --- |
| 适应证<br>Indicaciones | 用于不宜手术治疗的胆固醇型胆结石。应用时，仔细选择病例十分重要。对胆囊功能基本正常，结石直径在 5mm 以下，X 线能透过，非钙化型的浮动胆固醇型结石有较高的治愈率。结石的大小与溶石成功率密切相关，直径小于 5mm 者为 70%，5 ~ 10mm 者约为 50%。由于表面积 / 体积的比值较大，故较小的结石对治疗反应较好。本品不能溶解胆色素结石、混合结石及不透过 X 线的结石。对中毒性肝障碍、胆囊炎、胆道炎和胆汁性消化不良等也有一定的治疗效果。<br>Se usa para el tratamiento de cálculos biliares de colesterol que no son adecuados para la cirugía. En su aplicación, es muy importante la selección cuidadosa de los pacientes. Tienen una tasa de curación más alta para los casos que funciones biliares son normales, el diámetro de la piedra de la vesícula es menos de 5 mm, los rayos X son permeables, y la piedar es de tipo de no calcificada de colesterol flotante. El tamaño de la piedra está estrechamente relacionado con la tasa de éxito de disulción de la piedra , si el diámetro de la piedra es menos de 5 mm, la tasa es 70%, si el diámetro es entre aproximadamente 5 ~ 10 mm, la tasa es 50%. Debido a la gran proporción de área de superficie / volumen, por lo que las piedras más pequeñas tienen mejores respuestas al tratamiento. Este producto no puede disolver los cálculos de pigmentos biliares, cálculos de pigmentos mezclados y las piedras no permeables por rayos X. también tienen un efecto terapéutico para el trastorno hepático tóxico, colecistitis, colangitis y dispepsia biliar. |
| 用法、用量<br>Administración y dosis | 口服，利胆，1 次 50mg，一日 150mg。早、晚进餐时分次给予。疗程最短为 6 个月，6 个月后超声波检查及胆囊造影无改善者可停药；如结石已有部分溶解，则继续服药直至结石完全溶解。如治疗中有反复胆绞痛发作，症状无改善甚至加重，或出现明显结石钙化时，则宜终止治疗，并进行外科手术。溶胆石，一日 450 ~ 600mg，分 2 次服用。 |

**续 表**

| | Por vía oral, vesícula biliar, 50 mg por cada vez, 150 mg al día. Se toma en el desayuno y la cena. El curso más corto es de seis meses, después de seis meses si en el examen de la ecografía de la vesícula biliar y la angiografía no hay mejoramiento puede interrumpir el medicamento; si la piedra h sido disuelta parcialmente, sigue tomando los medicamentos hasta que la piedra esté completamente disuelta. Si durante el tratamiento hay episodios de cólico biliar de repetidas veces, los síntomas no mejoran e incluso , agravan, o aparece de manera significativa las piedras calcificadas, es deseable terminar el tratamiento, y realiza la cirugía. Para disolver cálculos biliares, 450 ~ 600 mg al día, dividida en 2 veces para su uso. |
|---|---|
| 剂型、规格<br>Formulaciones y especificaciones | 片剂：每片 50mg。<br>Tabletas: Cada tableta de 50mg. |

12.14　治疗炎性肠病药 Medicamentos para el tratamiento de la enfermedad inflamatoria intestinal

| 药品名称 Drug Names | 美沙拉秦 Mesalazina |
|---|---|
| 适应证<br>Indicaciones | 用于治疗溃疡性结肠炎、克罗恩病（Crohn 病）；栓剂用于治疗溃疡性直肠炎。<br>Se usa para el tratamiento de la colitis ulcerosa, la enfermedad de Crohn (enfermedad de Crohn); Los supositorios se usan para el tratamiento de la proctitis ulcerosa. |
| 用法、用量<br>Administración y dosis | ①口服：溃疡性结肠炎急性发作，一次 1g，一日 4 次。维持治疗，一次 0.5g，一日 3 次。克罗恩病，一次 1g，一日 4 次。儿童及老年人用量应酌减。②直肠给药：一次 1g，一日 1 ~ 2 次。<br>① Por vía oral: para la exacerbación aguda de la colitis ulcerosa, 1 g por cada vez, 4 veces al día. En el tratamiento de mantenimiento, 0.5 g por cada vez, 3 veces al día. La enfermedad de Crohn, 1 g por cada vez, 4 veces al día. La dosis para los niños y ancianos deben ser reducida. ② Administración rectal: 1 g por cada vez, 1 ~ 2 veces al día. |
| 剂型、规格<br>Formulaciones y especificaciones | 片剂：每片 0.25g；0.4g；0.5g。缓释片：每片 0.5g。缓释颗粒：每袋 0.5g。肠溶片：每片 0.5g。栓剂：每粒 1g。<br>Tabletas: Cada tableta de 0.25 g; 0.4 g; 0.5 g. Tabletas de liberación prolongada: Cada tableta de 0.5 g. Gránulos de liberación: cada paquete de 0.5g. Tabletas con recubrimiento entérico: Cada tableta de 0.5 g. Supositorios: Cada supositorio de 1g. |

| 药品名称 Drug Names | 柳氮磺吡啶 Sulfasalazina |
|---|---|
| 适应证<br>Indicaciones | 主要用于炎症性肠炎，即 Crohn 病和溃疡性结肠炎。<br>Se utiliza principalmente para la enfermedad inflamatoria del intestino, enfermedad de Crohn y la colitis ulcerosa. |
| 用法、用量<br>Administración y dosis | 口服。成人常用量：初剂量为一日 2 ~ 3g，分 3 ~ 4 次口服，无明显不适量，可渐增至一日 4 ~ 6g。待肠病症状缓解后逐渐减量至维持量，一日 1.5 ~ 2g。小儿初剂量为一日 40 ~ 60mg/kg，分 3 ~ 6 次口服，病情缓解后改为维持量一日 30mg/kg，分 3 ~ 4 次口服。<br>Por vía oral. Dosis habitual para adultos: la dosis inicial diaria es de 2 ~ 3 g, divida en 3 ~ 4 veces al día por vía oral, si no hay fenómenos anormales obviamente, puede incrementar gradualmente la dosis hasta 4 ~ 6 g al día. Después del alivio de los síntomas intestinales, se puede reducir la dosis para el mantenimiento de 1.5 ~ 2g al día. La dosis pediátrica inicial es de 40 ~ 60mg/kg, divida en 3 ~ 6 veces al día por vía oral, después del alivio de los síntomas, puede mantener la dosis de 30mg/kg al día, divida en 3 ~ 4 veces al día por vía oral. |
| 剂型、规格<br>Formulaciones y especificaciones | 片剂（胶囊剂）：每片（粒）0.25g。栓剂：每粒 0.5g。<br>Tabletas (cápsulas): Cada tableta (cápsula) de 0.25 g. Supositorios: Cada supositorio de 0.5g. |

| 药品名称 Drug Names | 奥沙拉秦 Olsalazina |
|---|---|
| 适应证<br>Indicaciones | 用于治疗急慢性溃疡性结肠炎与节段性回肠炎，并用于缓解期的长期维持治疗。<br>Se usa para el tratamiento de la colitis ulcerosa aguda y crónica y la enfermedad de Crohn, y se usa para el mantenimiento de tratamiento a largo plazo en el período de la remisión. |

续　表

| 用法、用量<br>Administración y dosis | 口服，治疗开始时一日 1g，分次服用，根据患者反应逐渐提高剂量至一日 3g，分 3 ～ 4 次服用。儿童为一日 20 ～ 40mg/kg。长期维持治疗，成人一日 1g，分 2 次服用；儿童一日 15 ～ 30mg/kg。本品随食物同服。<br><br>Por vía oral, la dosis al inicio es 1g al día en dosis divididas, de acuerdo con la respuesta del paciente puede aumentar gradualmente la dosis a 3 g por cada día, dividos en tres - cuatro veces al día. La dosis para niños es de 20 ~ 40mg/kg. es terapia de mantenimiento a largo plazo, para adultos 1 g al día, divida en 2 veces; Para los niños es 15 ~ 30mg/kg al día. Este producto puede comer junto con la comida. |
|---|---|
| 剂型、规格<br>Formulaciones y especificaciones | 胶囊剂：每粒 250mg。<br>Cápsulas: Cada cápsula de 250mg. |

12.15　其他消化系统用药 Otros medicamentos para el sistema digestivo

| 药品名称 Drug Names | 奥曲肽 Octreotida |
|---|---|
| 适应证<br>Indicaciones | 用于：①门静脉高压引起的食管静脉曲张破裂出血。②应激性溃疡及消化道出血。③重型胰腺炎及内镜逆行胰胆管造影（ＥＲＣＰ）术后急性胰腺炎并发症。④缓解由胃、肠及胰内分泌系统肿瘤所引起的症状。⑤突眼性甲状腺肿和肢端肥大症。⑥胃肠道瘘管。<br><br>Se usa para：① hemorragia de ruptura de varices esofágicas causada por la hipertensión portal. ② subrayar úlceras y sangrado gastrointestinal. ③ pancreatitis grave y la colangiopancreatografía retrógrada endoscópica (ERCP) de la pancreatitis aguda postoperatorias. ④ aliviar los síntomas de cáncer de estómago, intestino y sistema endocrino pancreático. ⑤ enfermedad de tiroides exoftálmico hinchado y la acromegalia. ⑥ fístula gastrointestinal. |
| 用法、用量<br>Administración y dosis | （1）预防胰腺手术后并发症：手术前 1 小时，0.1mg 皮下注射；以后 0.1mg 皮下注射，一日 3 次，连续 7 日。<br>（2）治门静脉高压引起的食管静脉曲张出血：静脉注射开始 0.1mg，以后 0.5mg，每 2 小时 1 次静脉滴注。<br>（3）应激性溃疡及消化道出血：皮下注射 0.1mg，一日 3 次。<br>（4）重型胰腺炎：皮下注射 0.1mg，一日 4 次，疗程 3 ～ 7 日。<br>（5）胃肠道瘘管和消化道内分泌系统肿瘤的辅助治疗：皮下注射 0.1mg，一日 3 次，疗程 10 ～ 14 日。<br>（6）突眼性甲状腺肿和肢端肥大症：皮下注射 0.1mg，一日 3 次；肢端肥大症疗程和剂量需视疗效而定，有时可长达数月。<br><br>(1) Prevención de complicaciones de la cirugía de páncreas: una hora antes de la cirugía, la inyección subcutánea de 0.1 mg; posteriormente 0.1 mg de inyección subcutánea, 3 veces al día, 7 días continuas.<br>(2) tratamiento de hemorragia de ruptura de varices esofágicas causada por la hipertensión portal: inyección intravenosa al inicio 0.1mg, después, 0.5 mg, una infusión intravenosa por cada dos horas.<br>(3) úlceras por estrés y hemorragia gastrointestinal: 3 0.1 mg de inyección por vía subcutánea, 3 veces diariamente.<br>(4) pancreatitis severa: 0.1 mg de inyección subcutánea, 4 veces al día, un curso de tratamiento de 3 ~ 7 días.<br>(5) terapia adyuvante de fístula gastrointestinal y cáncer de sistema endocrino gastrointestinall: 0,1 mg de inyección subcutánea, 3 veces al día, un curso de tratamiento de 10 ~ 14 días.<br>(6) enfermedad de tiroides exoftálmico hinchado y la acromegalia: inyección subcutánea de 0.1 mg, 3 veces al día; El curso de tratamiento y la dosis para la acromegalia depende de la eficacia, a veces puede durar varios meses. |
| 剂型、规格<br>Formulaciones y especificaciones | 注射液：每支 0.1mg（1ml）。<br>Inyección: Cada inyección de 0.1 mg (1 ml). |
| 药品名称 Drug Names | 生长抑素 Somatostatina |
| 适应证<br>Indicaciones | 用于严重急性上消化道出血，如胃出血、十二指肠出血、胃和十二指肠溃疡出血、出血性胃炎、食管静脉曲张破裂出血等；预防胰腺术后及 ERCP 术后的并发症，急性胰腺炎，胰腺、胆囊和肠道瘘管的辅助性治疗；治疗类风湿关节炎引起的严重疼痛。 |

| | |
|---|---|
| | Se usa para la hemorragia digestiva aguda grave, hemorragia duodenal, hemorragia de úlcera gástrica y hemorragia duodenal, hemorrágica gastritis, hemorragia por varices esofágicas;puede prevenir la cirugía pancreática y enfermedades de ERCP postoperatorias, es la terapia adyuvante de pancreatitis aguda, el páncreas, la vesícula biliar y fístula intestinal; puede tratar el dolor severo causado por la artritis reumatoide. |
| 用法、用量<br>Administración y dosis | （1）治疗上消化道出血，以 3mg 溶于 500ml0.9% 氯化钠或 5% 葡萄糖注射液中，连续 12 小时静脉滴注。某些病例可在连续滴注前给予 250μg 缓慢（不少于 3 分钟）静脉注射。为避免再出血，在止血后用同一剂量维持治疗 48 ～ 72 小时，总疗程不应超过 120 小时，延长静脉滴注时间并不加强效果。<br><br>（2）预防胰腺术后并发症，在手术开始时以 250μg/h 速度连续静脉滴注，术后连续静脉滴注 5 日。<br><br>（3）预防 ERCP 术后并发症，术前 1 小时以 250μg/h 速度连续静脉滴注，持续 12 小时。<br><br>（4）急性胰腺炎：以 250μg/h 速度连续静脉滴注 5 ～ 7 日。<br><br>（5）胰腺、胆囊及肠道瘘管的辅助性治疗，以 250μg/h 速度连续静脉滴注，直到瘘管闭合之后 2 日，在此期间应结合全胃肠外营养治疗，疗程应不超过 20 日。<br><br>（6）治疗类风湿关节炎引起的严重疼痛，以 750μg 溶于 2ml0.9% 氯化钠注射液中作关节腔内注射，每隔 7 日或 15 日重复一次，连续 4 ～ 6 次。<br><br>(1) tratamiento de la hemorragia gastrointestinal superior, use 3 mg para disolver en el cloruro de sodio al 0.9 % de 500ml o el la inyección de glucosa al 5%, hace la infusión intravenosa por 12 horas consecutivas. Para algunos casos antes de la infusión continua se pueden hacer inyección intravenosa de 250μg lentamente (no menos de 3 minutos ). Para evitar el sangrado, después de la hemostasia, use la misma dosis para el mantenimiento de tratamiento por 48 ～ 72 horas , el curso total no debe ser superior a 120 horas, con el tiempo prolongado de la infusión intravenosa no se mejora el efecto.<br><br>(2) prevención de complicaciones postoperatorias de páncreas, al inicio de la cirugía debe hacer la infusión intravenosa continua por una velocidad de 250μg/h, después de la cirugía, hace la infusión intravenosa continua por 5 días.<br><br>(3) prevención de las complicaciones post- ERCP , una hora antes de la cirugía hace la infusión intravenosa continua por una velocidad de 250μg/h y mantiene 12 horas.<br><br>(4) pancreatitis aguda : hace la infusión intravenosa por una velocidad de 250μg/h de 5 ～ 7 días continuos.<br><br>(5) la terapia adyuvante de páncreas, vesícula biliar y fístula intestinal, hace la infusión intravenosa continua por una velocidad de 250μg/h, hasta dos días después del cierre de la fístula, durante este período, deben combinarse con la terapia de nutrición parenteral total , el curso del tratamiento no debe ser superar a 20 días.<br><br>(6) Tratamiento del dolor severo causado por la artritis reumatoide, use 750μg para disolver en la inyección de cloruro de sodio al 0.9 % de 2ml para la inyección intra -articular, repite por un intervalo de cada 7 días o 15 días, y por 4 ～ 6 veces continuas. |
| 剂型、规格<br>Formulaciones y especificaciones | 注射用生长抑素：每支 250μg；750μg；3mg。<br>Somatostatina inyectable: Cada una de 250μg, 750μg; 3 mg. |
| 药品名称 Drug Names | 抑肽酶 Aprotinina |
| 适应证<br>Indicaciones | 用于预防和治疗急性胰腺炎、纤维蛋白溶解所引起的出血、弥散性血管内凝血。也用于抗休克治疗。腹腔手术后，直接注入腹腔可预防术后肠粘连。<br><br>Se usa para la prevención y tratamiento de la pancreatitis hemorrágica aguda, fibrinolítico inducido por la coagulación intravascular diseminada. También se utiliza en la terapia anti-shock. Después de la cirugía abdominal, se puede inyectar directamente en la cavidad abdominal para prevenir las adherencias postoperatorias. |
| 用法、用量<br>Administración y dosis | 第 1 ～ 2 日，一日 8 万～ 12 万 U，首剂用量应大些，缓慢静脉注射（每分钟不超过 2ml）。维持剂量宜采用静脉滴注，一日 2 万～ 4 万 U。由纤维蛋白溶解引起的出血，应立即静脉注射 8 万～ 12 万 U，以后每 2 小时 1 万 U，直至出血停止。预防剂量：手术前一日开始，每日 2 万 U，共 3 日。治疗肠瘘及连续渗血也可局部应用。预防术后肠粘连，在手术切口闭合前，腹腔直接注入 2 万～ 4 万 U，注意勿与伤口接触。 |

续　表

| | En el 1 ~ 2 días, la dosis es 80.000 ~ 120.000 U al día, la primera dosis debería ser más grande, hace la inyección intravenosa lentamente (no debe exceder de 2 ml por minuto). La dosis de mantenimiento se debe utilizar por vía intravenosa de 20.000 ~ 40.000 U al día. El sangrado causada por la fibrinólisis, debe hacer inmediatamente la inyección intravenosa de 80.000 ~ 120.000 U, a continuación, cada dos horas 10.000 U, hasta que el sangrado se detenga. La dosis profiláctica: Un día antes de la cirugía, usa 20.000 U al día, en total de 3 días. También se puede aplicar tópicamente para el tratamiento de la fístula intestinal y sangrado continuo. Para la prevención de la adherencia intestinal postoperatoria, antes de cerrar la incisión, se inyecta directamente en la cavidad abdominal 20.000 ~ 40.000 U, debe ser cuidado de no tocar la herida. |
|---|---|
| 剂型、规格<br>Formulaciones y especificaciones | 注射抑肽酶：每支 1 万 U；5 万 U；10 万 U；50 万 U。<br>La aprotinina inyectable: Cada 10.000 U; 50.000 U; 100.000 U; 500 .000 U. |
| 药品名称 Drug Names | 加贝酯 Gabexato |
| 适应证<br>Indicaciones | 用于急性轻型（水肿型）胰腺炎；也可用于急性出血性坏死型胰腺炎的辅助治疗。<br>Se usa para la pancreatitis aguda (edematosa); también se puede utilizar para ayudar en el tratamiento de la pancreatitis necrotizante hemorrágica aguda |
| 用法、用量<br>Administración y dosis | 仅供静脉滴注。每次 100mg，治疗开始 3 日，每日用量 300mg，症状减轻后改为每日 100mg，疗程 6 ~ 10 日。先以 5ml 注射用水注入冻干粉针瓶内，待溶解后注入 5% 葡萄糖注射液或林格氏液 500ml 中，供静脉滴注用。滴注速度不宜过快，应控制在 1mg/（kg·h）以内，不宜超过 2.5mg/（kg·h）。<br>Sólo se suministra para la infusión intravenosa. 100mg por cada vez, En los primeros tres días del tratamiento, la cantidad de la dosis es de 300 mg al día, de ser aliviados los síntomas, la dosis es de 100 mg al día, el curso de tratamiento es de 6 ~ 10 días. Primero, use agua para inyección de 5 ml para inyectar a la botella de polvo liofilizado, de ser disuelta, hace la inyección de dextrosa al 5% o 500 ml de solución de Ringer para uso intravenoso. No debe ser demasiado rápido la velocidad de goteo y debe ser controlada dentro de 1 mg / (kg · h), y no debe exceder de 2.5 mg / (kg · h). |
| 剂型、规格<br>Formulaciones y especificaciones | 注射用加贝酯：每支 0.1g。<br>Gabexate Inyectable: Cada una de 0.1g. |
| 药品名称 Drug Names | 二甲硅油 Dimeticona |
| 适应证<br>Indicaciones | 用于胃肠道胀气及急性肺气肿。<br>Se usa para la flatulencia gastrointestinal y enfisema aguda. |
| 用法、用量<br>Administración y dosis | （1）消胀气：一次 0.1 ~ 0.2g，一日 3 次，嚼碎服。<br>（2）抢救急性肺水肿：使用气雾剂，用时将瓶倒置，距患者口鼻约 15cm 处，揿压瓶帽，在吸气时（或呼气终末时）连续喷入或与给氧同时进行，直至泡沫减少、症状改善为止。必要时可反复适用。<br>(1) Para eliminar la flatulencia: 0.1 ~ 0.2 g por cada vez, 3 veces al día, masticar para su uso.<br>(2) Para tratamiento de edema agudo de pulmón: uso de aerosoles, cuando se utiliza, ponga la botella con boca hacia abajo con una distancia de la boca y la nariz del paciente por unos 15 cm, pulse la tapa de la botella con presión, cuando se aspira, (o en el momento cuando se termina la expiración) debe inyectar continuamente o llevar a cabo simultáneamente con la inspiración de oxígeno hasta que la espuma es reducida, los síntomas están mejorados. Se puede aplicar por varias veces, si es necesario. |
| 剂型、规格<br>Formulaciones y especificaciones | 片剂：每片含二甲硅油 25mg 或 50mg，另含氢氧化铝 40mg 或 80mg，为分散剂。二甲硅油气雾剂：每瓶总量 18g，内含二甲硅油 0.15g，此外，尚含适量薄荷脑及抛射剂氟利昂（F12）。二甲硅油散：含二甲硅油 6%，为抗泡沫药。<br>Tabletas: cada tableta contiene 25 mg de simeticona o 50 mg, 40 mg o 80 mg de hidróxido de aluminio, como un dispersante. Aerosol de simeticona: una botella de 18 g en total, que contiene 0.15 g de simeticona, además contiene una cantidad apropiada de mentol y Freón propelente (F12). Polvo de Simeticona: contiene simeticona de 6%, como agentes anti-espumantes. |

13. 主要作用于血液及造血系统的药物 Medicamentos que actúan principalmente sobre el sistema sanguíneo y el sistema hematopoyético

13.1 促凝血药 Medicamentos que promueven la coagulación de la sangre

| 药品名称 Drug Names | 亚硫酸氢钠甲萘醌 Bisulfito de menadiona de sodio |
|---|---|
| 适应证<br>Indicaciones | （1）止血：用于阻塞性黄疸、胆瘘、慢性腹泻、广泛性切除所致肠吸收功能不全者，早产儿、新生儿低凝血酶原血症，香豆素类或水杨酸类过量及其他原因所致凝血酶原过低等引起的出血。亦可用于预防长期口服广谱抗生素类药物引起的维生素 K 缺乏症。<br>（2）镇痛：用于胆石症、胆道蛔虫症引起的胆绞痛。<br>（3）解救杀鼠药"敌鼠钠"（diphacin）中毒：此时宜用大剂量。<br>(1) Hemorragia: Para la disfunción absorción intestinal causada por la ictericia obstructiva, fístula biliar, diarrea crónica, escisión amplia, la enfermedad de hiperlipidemia primaria de trombina baja de los niños prematuros, y recién nacidos, la hemorragia debido a la protrombina baja inducida por la sobredosis de cumarina o ácido salicílico y otras causas de. Puede ser utilizado para la prevención de la deficiencia de vitamina K debido al uso por vía oral de los medicamentos antibióticos de amplio espectro a largo plazo.<br>(2) Analgesia: se usa para el cólico biliar causada por colelitiasis, ascariasis biliar.<br>(3) Desintoxicación de rodenticidas "Difacinona sodio" (Diphacin): En este caso debe usar dosis de gran cantidad. |
| 用法、用量<br>Administración y dosis | （1）止血：成人口服，一次 2～4mg，一日 6～20mg；肌内注射，一次 2～4mg，一日 4～8mg。防止新生儿出血，可在产前 1 周给妊娠期妇女肌内注射，一日 2～4mg。<br>（2）胆绞痛：肌内注射，一次 8～16mg。<br>(1) Hemorragia: por vía oral, para adultos, 2～4mg por cada vez, 6～20 mg al día; Inyección intramuscular: 2～4 mg por cada vez, 4～8 mg al día. Para prevenir el sangrado neonatal, puede hacer la inyección intramuscular para las mujeres embarazadas con una semana antes de prenatal, 2～4 mg diariamente.<br>(2) Cólico biliar: Inyección intramuscular, 8～16 mg por cada vez. |
| 剂型、规格<br>Formulaciones y especificaciones | 片剂：每片 2mg。注射液：每支 2mg（1ml）；4mg（1ml）。<br>Tabletas: Cada tableta de 2 mg. Inyección: Cada una de 2 mg (1 ml), 4 mg (1 ml). |
| 药品名称 Drug Names | 植物甲萘醌（维生素 $K_1$）Fitomenadiona (Vitamina $K_1$) |
| 适应证<br>Indicaciones | （1）止血：用于阻塞性黄疸、胆瘘、慢性腹泻、广泛性切除所致肠吸收功能不全者，早产儿、新生儿低凝血酶原血症，香豆素类或水杨酸类过量及其他原因所致凝血酶原过低等引起的出血。亦可用于预防长期口服广谱抗生素类药物引起的维生素 K 缺乏症。<br>（2）镇痛：用于胆石症、胆道蛔虫症引起的胆绞痛。<br>（3）解救杀鼠药"敌鼠钠"（diphacin）中毒：此时宜用大剂量。<br>(1) Hemorragia: Para la disfunción absorción intestinal causada por la ictericia obstructiva, fístula biliar, diarrea crónica, escisión amplia, la enfermedad de hiperlipidemia primaria de trombina baja de los niños prematuros, y recién nacidos, la hemorragia debido a la protrombina baja inducida por la sobredosis de cumarina o ácido salicílico y otras causas de. Puede ser utilizado para la prevención de la deficiencia de vitamina K debido al uso por vía oral de los medicamentos antibióticos de amplio espectro a largo plazo.<br>(2) Analgesia: se usa para el cólico biliar causada por colelitiasis, ascariasis biliar.<br>(3) Desintoxicación de rodenticidas "Difacinona sodio" (Diphacin): En este caso debe usar dosis de gran cantidad. |
| 用法、用量<br>Administración y dosis | 肌内注射或静脉注射：一次 10mg，一日 1～2 次，或根据具体病情而定；口服：一次 10mg，一日 3 次。<br>Inyección intramuscular o intravenosa: 10 mg por cada vez, 1~2 veces al día, o puede ajustar de acuerdo con las condiciones específicas; Por vía oral: 10 mg por cada vez, 3 veces al día. |
| 剂型、规格<br>Formulaciones y especificaciones | 片剂：10mg。<br>注射液：10mg（1ml）；2mg（1ml）。<br>Tabletas: 10 mg. Inyección: 10 mg (1 ml); 2 mg (1 ml). |

**续　表**

| 药品名称 Drug Names | 氨基己酸 Acido aminocaproico |
| --- | --- |
| 适应证<br>Indicaciones | 用于纤溶性出血、如脑、肺、子宫、前列腺、肾上腺、甲状腺等外伤或手术出血。术中早期用药或术前用药，可减少手术中渗血，并减少输血量。亦用于肺出血、肝硬化出血及上消化道出血。<br><br>Se usa pra la hemorragia fibrinolítica, tales como hemorragia por traumatismo o cirugía del cerebro, de pulmón, de útero, de próstata, de suprarrenales, de tiroides,etc. Utilice la medicación temprana en la cirugía o antes de la cirugía, puede reducir el sangrado y reducir la cantidad de transfusión de sangre. También se utiliza para la hemorragia pulmonar, cirrosis hepática y hemorragia de gastrointestinal superior. |
| 用法、用量<br>Administración y dosis | 静脉滴注，初用量 4 ~ 6g，以 5% ~ 10% 葡萄糖注射液或生理盐水 100ml 稀释，15 ~ 30 分钟滴完，维持量为每小时 1g，维持时间依病情而定，一日量不超过 20g，可连用 3 ~ 4 日。口服，成人，每次 2g，依病情服用 7 ~ 10 日或更久。<br><br>Infusión intravenosa, la dosis inicial es de 4 ~ 6 g, use la inyección de glucosa al 5% ~ 10% o solución salina de 100 ml, de ser diluidas, termina el goteo dentro de 15 ~ 30 minutos. La dosis de mantenimiento es de 1 g por cada hora. El tiempo de mantenimiento depende de la enfermedad, la cantidad diaria no debe exceder de 20 g, se puede utilizar 3 ~ 4 días continuos. Por vía oral, para adultos, 2g por cada vez, dependiendo de la enfermedad puede tomar 7 ~ 10 días o más. |
| 剂型、规格<br>Formulaciones y especificaciones | 片剂：每片 0.5g。注射液：每支 1g（10ml）；2g（10ml）。<br>Tabletas: Cada tableta de 0,5 g. Inyección: Cada una de 1 g (10 ml); 2g (10 ml). |
| 药品名称 Drug Names | 氨甲苯酸 Acido aminonetilbenzoico |
| 适应证<br>Indicaciones | 用于纤维蛋白溶解过程亢进所致的出血，如肺、肝、胰、前列腺、肾上腺等手术时的异常出血，妇产科和产后出血及肺结核咳血或痰中带血、血尿、前列腺肥大出血、上消化道出血等，对一般慢性渗血效果较显著，但对癌症出血及创伤出血无止血作用。此外，尚可用于链激酶或尿激酶过量引起的出血。<br><br>Se usa para hemorragia causado por el hipertiroidismo del proceso fibrinolítico, por ejemplo sangrados anormales durante la cirugía de los pulmones, hígado, páncreas, próstata, adrenal y otros casos, la hemorragia de obstetricia y posparto y hemoptisis tuberculosis o esputo con sangre, orina con sangre, sangrado de la próstata agrandada , hemorragia de gastrointestinal superior, tiene el efecto significativo para la hemorragia crónica general, no funciona para el sangrado y el trauma del cáncer, y hemorragia de trauma. Además, se pueden ser utilizando para el sangrado excesivo causado por la estreptoquinasa o uroquinasa. |
| 用法、用量<br>Administración y dosis | 静脉注射，每次 0.1 ~ 0.3g，用 5% 葡萄糖注射液或 0.9% 氯化钠注射液 10 ~ 20ml 稀释后缓慢注射，一日最大用量 0.6g。<br><br>Inyección intravenosa, 0.1 ~ 0.3g por cada vez, use la inyección de glucosa al 5% o cloruro de sodio al 0.9% de 10 ~ 20 ml después de ser diluida, hace la inyección lentamente, la dosis diaria máxima es de 0.6 g. |
| 剂型、规格<br>Formulaciones y especificaciones | 片剂：每片 0.125g；0.25g。注射液：每支 0.05g（5ml）；0.1g（10ml）。<br>Tabletas: Cada tableta de 0.125 g; 0.25 g. Inyección: Cada una de 0.05 g (5 ml), 0.1 g (10 ml). |
| 药品名称 Drug Names | 血凝酶 Hemocoagulasa |
| 适应证<br>Indicaciones | 可用于治疗和防治多种原因引起的出血。<br>Se usa para el tratamiento y prevención de la hemorragia causada por diversas razones. |
| 用法、用量<br>Administración y dosis | 静脉注射、肌内注射，也可局部使用。成人：一次 1.0 ~ 2.0kU，紧急情况下，立即静脉注射 1.0kU，同时肌内注射 1.0kU。各类外科手术：手术前 1 小时，肌内注射 1.0kU；或手术前 15 分钟，静脉注射 1.0kU。手术后每日肌内注射 1.0kU，连用 3 日，或遵医嘱。<br><br>La inyección intravenosa, inyección intramuscular, o se puede utilizar parcialmente. Adultos: 1,0 ~ 2.0kU por cada vez, en situaciones de emergencia, debe hacer inyección intravenosa inmediata de 1.0kU, al mismo tiempo la inyección intramuscular de 1.0kU. Se usa para las cirugías de varios tipos: Una hora antes de la cirugía, hace la inyección intramuscular de 1.0kU, o 15 minutos antes de la cirugía, hace la inyección intravenosa de 1.0kU. Después de la cirugía, hace la inyección intramuscular diaria de 1.0kU, por tres días continuos, o según las indicaciones del doctor. |

| 剂型、规格<br>Formulaciones y<br>especificaciones | 注射用凝血酶（REPTILASE）每支 0.5kU；1kU；2kU。<br>Trombina inyectable (REPTILASE) cada inyección de 0.5kU; 1kU; 2kU. |
|---|---|
| **药品名称 Drug Names** | **酚磺乙胺 Etamsilato** |
| 适应证<br>Indicaciones | 用于预防和治疗外科手术出血过多，血小板减少性紫癜或过敏性紫癜及其他原因引起的出血，如脑出血、胃肠道出血、泌尿道出血、眼底出血、牙龈出血、鼻出血和皮肤出血等。<br><br>Se usa para la prevención y tratamiento de la hemorragia excesiva causada por la cirugía o hemorragia debido a la reducción de púrpura trombocitopénica o la púrpura alérgica y otras causas, tales como la hemorragia cerebral, hemorragia gastrointestinal, hemorragia del tracto urinario, hemorragia retiniana, sangrado de las encías, sangrado de la nariz y sangrado de la piel, etc. |
| 用法、用量<br>Administración y<br>dosis | （1）预防手术出血：术前 15～30 分钟静脉注射或肌内注射，一次 0.25～0.5g，必要时 2小时后再注射 0.25g，一日 0.5～1.5g。<br>（2）治疗出血：成人，口服，每次 0.5～1g，一日 3 次。肌内注射或静脉注射每次 0.25～0.5g，一日 2 次或 3 次。也可与 5% 葡萄糖注射液或生理盐水混合静脉滴注，每次 0.25～0.75g，一日 2 次或 3 次，必要时可根据病情增加剂量。<br><br>(1) prevención de la hemorragia quirúrgica: 15～30 minutos antes de la cirugía hace la inyección intravenosa o inyección intramuscular, 0.25 g～0.5 g por cada vez, si es necesario, después de dos horas, hace la inyección de 0.25 g, 0.5～1.5 g al día.<br>(2) tratamiento de sangrado: adultos, por vía oral, 0.5～1 g por cada vez, tres veces al día. La inyección intramuscular o inyección intravenosa de 0.25～0.5 g por cada vez, 2 veces o tres veces al día. También puede ser mezclado con 5% de inyección de dextrosa o solución salina por vía intravenosa de 0.25～0.75 g por cada vez, 2～3 veces al día, si es necesario, se puede aumentar la dosis de acuerdo con la enfermedad. |
| 剂型、规格<br>Formulaciones y<br>especificaciones | 片剂：每片 0.25g；0.5g。注射液：每支 0.25g（2ml）；0.5g（5ml）；1.0g（5ml）。<br>Tabletas: Cada tableta de 0.25 g; 0.5 g. Inyección: Cada una de 0.25 g (2 ml); 0.5 g (5 ml); 1.0 g (5 ml). |
| **药品名称 Drug Names** | **卡巴克络 Carbazocromo** |
| 适应证<br>Indicaciones | 用于毛细血管通透性增加所致的出血，如特发性紫癜、视网膜出血、慢性肺出血、肠胃出血、鼻出血、咯血、血尿、痔出血、子宫出血、脑出血等。<br><br>Se usa para la hemorragia debido al aumento de la permeabilidad capilar, tales como la púrpura idiopática, hemorragia retiniana, hemorragia pulmonar crónica, hemorragia gastrointestinal, epistaxis, hemoptisis, hematuria, sangrado de las hemorroides, hemorragia de útero, hemorragia cerebral. |
| 用法、用量<br>Administración y<br>dosis | （1）卡络柳钠片：口服，每次 2.5～5mg，一日 3 次。卡落柳钠注射液：肌内注射，每次 5～10mg，一日 2～3 次。不可静脉注射。<br>（2）注射用卡络磺钠：肌内注射，每次 20mg，一日 2 次；静脉注射，每次 25～50mg，一日 1 次；静脉滴注，每次 60～80mg，加入输液中滴注。<br><br>(1) Tabletas de carbazocromo de sodio: por vía oral, 2.5～5 mg por cada vez, 3 veces al día. Inyección de carbazocromo de sodio: Inyección intramuscular, 5～10 mg por cada vez, 2～3 veces al día. No puede inyectar por vía intravenosa.<br>(2) Inyección de carbazocromo de sulfonato de sodio: Inyección intramuscular, 20 mg por cada vez, 2 veces al día, la inyección intravenosa, 25～50 mg por cada vez, una vez al día; Inyección intravenosa, 60～80 mg por cada vez, agrega en la infusión para el goteo. |
| 剂型、规格<br>Formulaciones y<br>especificaciones | 卡络柳钠片：每片 2.5mg；5mg。卡络柳钠注射液：每支 5mg（1ml）；10mg（2ml）。注射用卡络磺钠：20mg。<br>Tabletas de carbazocromo de sodio: 2.5 mg por cada tableta; 5 mg. Inyección carbazocromo de sodio: Cada inyección de 5 mg (1 ml); 10 mg (2 ml). Inyección de carbazocromo sulfonato de sodio: 20 mg. |

**续　表**

| 药品名称 Drug Names | 重组人凝血因子Ⅷ　Factor Ⅷ de coagulación humano recombinante |
| --- | --- |
| 适应证<br>Indicaciones | 用于纠正和预防凝血因子Ⅷ缺乏或因患获得性因子Ⅷ抑制物增多症而引起的出血。主要用于治疗甲型血友病。<br><br>Se usa para el tratamiento correctivo y preventivo de la hemorragia causada por la deficiencia de factor Ⅷ de coagulación o la enfermedad de aumento de inhibidor del factor Ⅷ . Se usa principalmente para el tratamiento de la hemofilia. |
| 用法、用量<br>Administración y<br>dosis | 静脉滴注：①轻度关节出血：一次 8 ～ 10U/kg，一日 1 ～ 2 次，连用 1 ～ 4 日；使 F Ⅷ c 水平提高到正常水平的 15% ～ 20%。②中度关节，肌肉出血：一次 15U/kg，一日 2 次，需用 3 ～ 7 日，使 F Ⅷ c 水平提高到正常水平的 30%。③大出血或严重外伤而无出血证据：一次 25U/kg，一日 2 次，至少用 7 日；使 F Ⅷ c 水平提高到正常水平的 50%。④外科手术或严重外伤伴出血：40 ～ 50U/kg 于术前 1 小时开始输注，使 F Ⅷ c 水平达到正常水平的 80% ～ 100%，随后使 F Ⅷ c 水平维持在正常水平的 30% ～ 60%，为 10 ～ 14 日。⑤预防出血：体重大于 50kg，一日 500U；小于 50kg 者，一日 250U。使 F Ⅷ c 水平达到到正常水平的 5% ～ 10%。⑥抗 F Ⅷ c 抗体生成伴出血：首剂 5000 ～ 10 000U/h，维持剂量为 300 ～ 1000U/h，使体内 F Ⅷ c 水平维持在 30 ～ 50U/ml，如联合应用血浆交换术，宜追加本品 40U/kg，以增强疗效。<br><br>Infusión intravenosa: ① sangrado leve de las articulaciones: 8 ~ 10U/kg por cada vez, 1 ~ 2 veces al día, con uso de 1 ~ 4 días continuos; puede aumentar el nivel del Factor Ⅷ c a un nivel normal entre 15% y 20%. ② sangrado de moderado de las articulaciones, sangrado muscular: 15U/kg por cada vez, 2 veces al día, se necesita tomar 3 ~ 7 días, puede aumentar el nivel Factor  Ⅷ c al nivel normal de 30%.  ③ sangrado o hemorragia severa de trauma sin evidencia: 25U/kg por cada vez, 2 veces al día, con uso de por lo menos siete días, puede aumentar el nivel F Ⅷ c al nivel normal de 50%. ④ sangrado severo de la cirugía o trauma: hace la transfusión de 40 ~ 50U/kg una hora antes de la cirugía, para que el nivel de F Ⅷ c alcanzan de 80% ~ 100% del nivel normal, a continuación, se mantiene el nivel de F Ⅷ c a 30% ~ 60% de los niveles normales por alrededor de 10 ~ 14 días. ⑤ prevenir el sangrado: Para pacientes de peso superior a 50 kg, la primera dosis es de 500U al día; Para pacientes de peso menos de 50 kg, es 250U al día. Así el nivel F Ⅷ c llega a un 50% ~ 10% de los niveles normales. ⑥ hemorragia generada por la producción de anticuerpos de F Ⅷ c: la primera dosis es de 5000 ~ 10000u / h, la dosis de mantenimiento es de 300 ~ 1000U / h, por lo que los niveles de F Ⅷ c en el cuerpo se mantiene a 30 ~ 50 U, Si se usa la combinación de cirugía de intercambio de plasma, es conveniente añadir este producto de 40U/kg, para mejorar el efecto. |
| 剂型、规格<br>Formulaciones y<br>especificaciones | 人凝血因子Ⅷ：每瓶 100U；200U；250U；300U；400U；500U；750U；1000U。<br>Factor de coagulación humano Ⅷ : cadda botella  de 100U; 200U 250U; 300U 400U; 500U; 750U; 1000U. |
| 药品名称 Drug Names | 重组人血小板生成素 Trombopoietina humana recombinante |
| 适应证<br>Indicaciones | 用于治疗实体瘤化疗后所致的血小板减少症，适用对象为血小板低于 $50 \times 10^9$/L 且医生认为有必要升高血小板治疗的患者。<br><br>Se usa para el tratamiento de la reducción de plaquetas de sangre causada después de la quimioterapia de tumores sólidos. Es conveniente para los pacientes con plaquetas menos de $50 \times 10^9$/L y que el médico considera que es necesario aumentar la terapia de plaquetas, |
| 用法、用量<br>Administración y<br>dosis | 恶性实体肿瘤化疗时，可于给药结束后 6 ～ 24 小时皮下注射本品，剂量为每日 300U/kg，一日 1 次，连用 14 日。<br><br>En la quimioterapia de tumores sólidos malignos , es disponible de ofrecer el medicamento en 6 ~ 24 horas después de la administración para hace la inyección subcutánea, una dosis diaria es de 300U/kg, una vez por cada día, con uso continuo de 14 días. |
| 剂型、规格<br>Formulaciones y<br>especificaciones | 注射液：7500U（1ml）；15 000U（1ml）。<br>Inyección: 7500U (1 ml); 15 000U (1 ml). |
| 药品名称 Drug Names | 重组人白细胞介素 -11　Interleucina-11 humana recombinante |
| 适应证<br>Indicaciones | 用于实体瘤和白血病放、化疗后血小板减少症的预防和治疗及其他原因引起的血小板减少症的治疗。 |

**续 表**

| | |
|---|---|
| | Se usa para la prevención y el tratamiento de la reducción de plaquetas de sangre después de la quimioterapia los tumores sólidos y leucemia y la reducción de plaquetas de sangre inducida por otras causas. |
| 用法、用量<br>Administración y<br>dosis | 应用剂量为25μg/kg，于化疗结束后24～48小时起或发生血小板减少症后皮下注射，一日一次，疗程一般为7～14日。血小板计数恢复后应及时停药。<br>La aplicación de dosis es de 25μg/kg, en 24 a 48 horas después de la finalización de la quimioterapia o de la trombocitopenia de reducción de plaquetas de sangre, hace la inyección subcutánea, una vez al día, y un curso de tratamiento es generalmente 7～14 días. Después de la recuperación del recuento de plaquetas debe suspender de inmediato el medicamento. |
| 剂型、规格<br>Formulaciones y<br>especificaciones | 注射用重组人白细胞介素 -11：每支 1.5mg；3.0mg。<br>Interleucina humana recombinante-11 inyectable: Cada inyección de 1.5 mg; 3.0 mg. |
| **药品名称 Drug Names** | 云南白药 YunNanBaiYao |
| 适应证<br>Indicaciones | 缩短凝血时间，具有止血作用。<br>Puede acortar el tiempo de coagulación, y tiene el efecto de hemostasia. |
| 用法、用量<br>Administración y<br>dosis | 成人一次服0.2～0.3g，重症可酌加，但一次不宜超过0.5g，每隔4小时服1次。若初服无反应，可连续服用。小儿2岁以上者，一次服0.03g；5岁以上者，一次服0.06g。<br>Para adultos la porción es de 0.2～0.3g por cada vez, si es grave la enfermedad puede aumentar la dosis, pero no debe ser más de 0.5 g por cada vez, cada 4 horas se toma una vez. Si no hay respuesta al inicio, puede tomar de manera continua. Para niños de 2 años de edad o mayores, debe tomar 0.03 g por cada vez; para niños de 5 años de edad o mayores, debe tomar 0.06 g por cada vez. |
| 剂型、规格<br>Formulaciones y<br>especificaciones | 胶囊：250mg；气雾剂：85g。<br>Cápsula: 250mg; Aerosol: 85g. |
| **药品名称 Drug Names** | 氨甲环酸 Acido tranexámico |
| 适应证<br>Indicaciones | 用于各种出血性疾病、手术时异常出血等。<br>Se usa para una variedad de trastornos de la coagulación, hemorragia anormal durante la cirugía. |
| 用法、用量<br>Administración y<br>dosis | 口服，一次 1.0～1.5g，一日 2～6g。静脉注射或静脉滴注：一次 0.25～0.5g，一日 0.75～2g。静脉注射以 25% 葡萄糖注射液稀释，静脉滴注液以 5%～10% 葡萄糖注射液稀释。<br>Por vía oral, 1.0～1.5 g por cada vez, 02～6 g al día. La inyección intravenosa o infusión intravenosa: 0.25～0.5 g por cada vez, 0.75～2g al día. La inyección intravenosa se diluye con 25% de glucosa, la infusión intravenosa se diluye con 5%～10% de la inyección de glucosa. |
| 剂型、规格<br>Formulaciones y<br>especificaciones | 片剂：0.125g；0.25g。胶囊：0.25g。注射液：0.1g（2ml）；0.2g（2ml）；0.25g（5ml）；0.5g（5ml）；1.0g（10ml）。注射用氨甲环酸：0.2g；0.4g；0.5g；1.0g。<br>Tabletas: 0.125 g; 0.25 g. Cápsulas: 0.25 g. Inyección: 0.1 g (2 ml); 0.2 g (2 ml); 0.25 g (5 ml); 0.5 g (5 ml); 1.0 g (10 ml). ácido tranexámico inyectable: 0.2 g; 0.4 g; 0.5 g; 1.0 g. |
| **药品名称 Drug Names** | 鱼精蛋白 Protamina |
| 适应证<br>Indicaciones | 用于因注射肝素过量而引起的出血，以及自发性出血如咳血。<br>Se usa para el sangrado excesivo causado por la heparina, y hemorragia espontánea, como tos con sangre. |
| 用法、用量<br>Administración y<br>dosis | ①抗肝素过量：静脉注射，用量应与最后一次作用肝素量相当（本品 1mg 中可中和肝素 100U），但一次不超过 50mg。②抗自发性出血：静脉滴注，一日 5～8mg/kg，分 2 次，间隔 6 小时。每次以生理盐水 300～500ml 稀释。连用不宜超过 3 日。注射宜缓慢（10 分钟内注入量以不超过 50mg 为度）。 |

续　表

|  | ① Sobredosis de anti-heparina: Inyección intravenosa, la cantidad de dosis debe ser la cantidad equivalente con la última acción de heparina (1mg en este producto puede neutralizar la heparina de 100 unidades), pero no debe ser más de 50 mg por una vez. ② Anti-hemorragia espontánea: Infusión intravenosa, 5 ~ 8mg/kg al día, dividida en 2 veces, con un intervalo de 6 horas. Cada vez se diluye solución salina de 300 ~ 500 ml. Se utiliza no más de 3 días. La inyección debe ser lenta (El volumen de inyección en 10 minutos no debe exceder de 50 mg.) |
| --- | --- |
| 剂型、规格<br>Formulaciones y especificaciones | 硫酸鱼精蛋白注射液：50mg（5ml）；100mg（10ml）。　　注射用硫酸鱼精蛋白：50mg。<br>Inyección de sulfato de protamina: 50 mg (5 ml); 100 mg (10 ml). Inyección de sulfato de protamina: 50 mg. |
| 药品名称 Drug Names | 凝血酶 Trombina |
| 适应证<br>Indicaciones | 局部止血药。可用于局部出血及消化道出血。<br>Es agente hemostático tópico. Puede ser utilizado para el sangrado local y sangrado gastrointestinal. |
| 用法、用量<br>Administración y dosis | 局部出血：以干燥粉末或溶液（50 ~ 250U/ml）喷洒或喷雾于创伤表面。消化道出血：以溶液（10 ~ 100U/ml）口服或局部灌注。严禁注射。<br>Hemorragia parcial: Use polvo seco o una solución (50 ~ 250U/ml) para rociar o pulverizar sobre la superficie de la herida. Hemorragia digestiva: toma la solución (10 ~ 100 U/ml) por vía oral o hace la infusión tópica.Se prohibe la inyección. |
| 剂型、规格<br>Formulaciones y especificaciones | 凝血酶冻干粉剂：200U；500U；1000U；2000U；5000U；10 000U。<br>Polvo liofilizado de trombina: 200U; 500U; 1000U; 2000U; 5000U; 10 000U. |
| 药品名称 Drug Names | 凝血酶原复合物 Protrombina compleja |
| 适应证<br>Indicaciones | 用于手术、急性肝坏死、肝硬化等所致出血的防治。<br>Se usa para la prevención y tratamiento de la hemorragia debido a la cirugía, necrosis hepática aguda, la cirrosis. |
| 用法、用量<br>Administración y dosis | 本品仅供静脉滴注，且用前新鲜配制。每瓶加注射用水 25ml 使溶，按输血法过滤，滴速不超过 60 滴 / 分。<br>Este producto se administra solamente mediante infusión por vía intravenosa, y antes de su uso, debe preparar reciéntemente. En cada botella agrega 25 ml de agua para la inyección soluble, se filtra a través de transfusiones, la velocidad de goteo no debe exceder de 60 gotas / min. |
| 剂型、规格<br>Formulaciones y especificaciones | 注射剂（冻干粉）：200U；400U。<br>Inyección (polvo liofilizado):200 U; 400U. |

13.2　抗凝血药 Anticoagulantes

| 药品名称 Drug Names | 枸橼酸钠 Citrato de sodio |
| --- | --- |
| 适应证<br>Indicaciones | 仅用于体外抗凝血。<br>Solo para anticoagulación in vitro. |
| 用法、用量<br>Administración y dosis | 输血时预防凝血，每 100ml 全血加入 2.5% 输血用枸橼酸钠注射液 10ml。<br>Prevención de la coagulación durante la transfusión. 10ml de citrato de sodio para transfusión al 2.5% por 100ml de sangre total. |
| 剂型、规格<br>Formulaciones y especificaciones | 注射液：2.35% ~ 2.65%。<br>Inyección: 2.35% ~ 2.65%. |

**续 表**

| 药品名称 Drug Names | 肝素钠 Sodio de heparina |
|---|---|
| 适应证<br>Indicaciones | （1）预防血栓形成和栓塞，如深部静脉血栓、心肌梗死、肺栓塞、血栓静脉炎及术后血栓形成等。<br>（2）治疗各种原因引起的弥散性血管内凝血（DIC），如细菌性脓毒血症、胎盘早期剥离、恶性肿瘤细胞溶解所致的 DIC，但蛇咬伤所致的 DIC 除外。早期应用可防止纤维蛋白原和其他凝血因子的消耗。<br>（3）其他体外抗凝血，如心导管检查、心脏手术外循环、血液透析等。<br><br>(1) prevención de la trombosis y embolia, tales como trombosis venosa profunda, infarto de miocardio, embolia pulmonar, tromboflebitis y trombosis postoperatoria, etc.<br>(2) tratamiento de la coagulación intravascular diseminada (DIC) causada por diversas razones, tales como la sepsis bacteriana, desprendimiento de la placenta, la DIC inducida por la lisis de células malignas, excepto la DIC causada por las mordeduras de serpientes. La aplicación temprana impide el consumo del fibrinógeno y otros factores de la coagulación.<br>(3) otros anticoagulantes in vitro, como el cateterismo cardiaco, la cirugía cardiaca fucra dcl círculo, la hemodiálisis. |
| 用法、用量<br>Administración y<br>dosis | （1）静脉注射：成人首剂 5000U 加入 100ml0.9% 氯化钠注射液中，在 30 ～ 60 分钟滴完。需要时可每隔 4 ～ 6 小时重复静脉滴注 1 次，每次 5000U，总量可达 25 000U/d。为维持恒定血药浓度，也可每 24 小时 10 000 ～ 20 000U 加入 1000ml0.9% 氯化钠注射液中静脉滴注，速度 20 滴 / 分。用于体外循环时，375U/kg；体外循环超过 1 小时者，每 1kg 体重加 125U。<br>（2）静脉注射或深部肌内注射（或皮下注射）：每次 5000 ～ 10 000U。<br><br>(1) Inyección intravenosa: La primera dosis para adultos es de 5000U añadida 100ml de inyección de cloruro sódico al 0.9%, debe terminar el goteo dentro de 30 ～ 60 minutos. Cuando sea necesario, repite una infusión intravenosa de 5000 U por cada 4 ～ 6 horas, con una cantidad total de 25 000U / d. Para mantener una concentración de sangre constante, también puede hacer la infusión intravenosa de 10 000 ～ 20 000U por cada 24 horas, con 1000ml de inyección de cloruro de sodio al 0.9%, la velocidad es de 20 gotas / min. Cuando se utiliza para la circulación extracorpórea, es de 375u/kg; Para los pacientes con circulación extracorpórea por más de una hora, por cada 1 kg de peso corporal, añade 125u más.<br>(2) Inyección intravenosa o inyección intramuscular profunda (o inyección subcutánea): 5000 - 10 000U por cada vez. |
| 剂型、规格<br>Formulaciones y<br>especificaciones | 注射液：每支 1000U（2ml）；5000U（2ml）；12 500U（2ml）。<br>Inyección: Cada una de 1000u (2 ml); 5000U (2 ml); 12 500U (2 ml). |
| 药品名称 Drug Names | 肝素钙 Cálcica de heparina |
| 适应证<br>Indicaciones | 用于预防和治疗血栓 - 栓塞性疾病及血栓形成。本品具有较明显的抗醛固酮活性，故亦适于人工肾、人工肝和体外循环使用。<br><br>Se utiliza para la prevención y tratamiento de enfermedades tromboembólicas y trombosis.Tiene un efecto antialdosterona más evidente, por lo que también es adecuado para riñones artificiales, hígado artificial y circulación extracorpórea. |
| 用法、用量<br>Administración y<br>dosis | ①用于血栓 - 栓塞意外：皮下注射，首次 0.01ml/kg，5 ～ 7 小时后以 APTT 检测剂量是否合适，12 小时 1 次，每次注射后 5 ～ 7 小时进行新的检查，连续 3 ～ 4 日。②用于内科预防：皮下注射，首剂 0.005ml/kg，注射后 5 ～ 7 小时以 APTT 检测调整合适剂量，一次 0.2ml，一日 2 ～ 3 次，或一次 0.3ml，一日 2 次。③用于外科预防：皮下注射，术前 0.2ml，术后每 12 小时 0.2ml，至少持续 10 日。<br><br>① Para accidentes tromboembolíticos: inyección subcutánea, la primera dosis de 0,01 ml/kg ajuste la dosis adecuada de acuerdo con los resultados del APTT 5 a 7 horas después de la administración,una vez cada 12 horas. El APTT debe realizarse 5 a 7 horas después de cada administración para probar si la dosis administrada es adecuada. Administración continua durante 3 a 4 días. ② Para la prevención interna: inyección subcutánea, la primera dosis de 0,005 ml/Kg, ajuste la dosis adecuada de acuerdo con los resultados del APTT después de 5 a 7 horas después de la administración.0,2 ml por dosis,2 ～ 3 veces al día, o 0,3 ml por dosis,2 veces al día. ③ Para la prevención quirúrgica: inyección subcutánea, 0,2 ml antes de la operación, 0, 2 ml después de la operación cada 12 horas, por lo menos 10 días de administración continua. |

**续　表**

| 剂型、规格<br>Formulaciones y especificaciones | 注射液：2500U（0.3ml）。<br>Inyección: 2500U (0.3ml). |
|---|---|
| **药品名称 Drug Names** | 低分子量肝素 Heparina de bajo peso molecular |
| 适应证<br>Indicaciones | （1）预防深部静脉血栓形成和肺栓塞。<br>（2）治疗已形成的急性深部静脉血栓。<br>（3）在血液透析或血液滤过时，防止体外循环系统中发生血栓或血液凝固。<br>（4）治疗不稳定型心绞痛及非 ST 段抬高心肌梗死。<br>(1) prevención de la trombosis venosa profunda y la embolia pulmonar.<br>(2) tratamiento de de la trombosis aguda venosa profunda que se han formado.<br>(3) Durante la hemodiálisis o la hemofiltración, puede prevenir la trombosis o coagulación de la sangre en el sistema de derivación cardiopulmonar.<br>(4) tratamiento de la angina inestable y infarto de miocardi de elevación no segmento ST. |
| 用法、用量<br>Administración y dosis | （1）本品给药途径为腹壁皮下注射或静脉注射或遵医嘱。<br>（2）血透时预防血凝块形成。<br>(1) La administración de este producto es vía subcutánea abdominal o inyección intravenosa o según las indicaciones.<br>(2). Puede prevenir la formación de coágulos durante la hemodiálisis. |
| 剂型、规格<br>Formulaciones y especificaciones | 针剂：5000U。<br>Inyección de aguja: 5000 U. |
| **药品名称 Drug Names** | 华法林 Warfarina |
| 适应证<br>Indicaciones | （1）防治血栓栓塞性疾病，可防止血栓形成与发展，如治疗血栓栓塞性静脉炎，降低肺栓塞的发病率和死亡率，减少外科大手术、风湿性心脏病、髋关节固定术、人工置换心脏瓣膜手术等的静脉血栓发生率。<br>（2）心肌梗死的治疗辅助用药。<br>(1)Tiene prevención y tratamiento de la enfermedad tromboembólica, puede prevenir la formación y el desarrollo de trombosis, tales como el tratamiento de flebitis tromboembólica, reducir la morbilidad y la mortalidad de la embolia pulmonar , reducir la incidencia de la trombosis venosa en la cirugía mayor, de la enfermedad reumática del corazón, la fijación de la cadera, de corazón prostética cirugía valvular.<br>(2) tratamiento adyuvante del infarto de miocardio. |
| 用法、用量<br>Administración y dosis | 口服，第一日 5～20mg，次日起用维持量，一日 2.5～7.5mg。<br>Por vía oral, 5～20 mg del primer día, a partir del día siguiente empieza a tomar la dosis de mantenimiento de 2.5～7.5 mg por cada día. |
| 剂型、规格<br>Formulaciones y especificaciones | 片剂：每片 2.5mg；5mg。<br>Tabletas:cada tableta de 2.5 mg; 5mg. |
| **药品名称 Drug Names** | 利伐沙班 Rivaroxaban |
| 适应证<br>Indicaciones | 用于髋关节或膝关节置换手术成年患者，以预防静脉血栓形成（VTE）。<br>Se usa para los pacientes adultos de cirugía de reemplazo de cadera o de rodilla para prevenir la formación de trombosis venosa (VTE). |
| 用法、用量<br>Administración y dosis | 口服，10mg，一日 1 次。如伤口已止血，首次用药时间应于手术后 6～10 小时进行。<br>Por vía oral, 10 mg, una vez al día. Si la herida ya se ha sangrado, debe tomar la primera dosis entre 6 y 10 horas después de la cirugía. |
| 剂型、规格<br>Formulaciones y especificaciones | 片剂：每片 10mg。<br>Tabletas: Cada tableta de 10mg. |

**续 表**

| 药品名称 Drug Names | 重组链激酶 Estreptokinasa recombinante |
|---|---|
| 适应证<br>Indicaciones | 用于治疗血栓栓塞性疾病，如深静脉血栓、周围动脉栓塞、急性肺栓塞、血管外科手术后的血栓形成、导管给药所致血栓形成、新鲜心肌梗死、中央视网膜动静脉栓塞等。<br><br>Se usa para el tratamiento de enfermedades tromboembólicas tales como trombosis venosa profunda, trombosis arterial periférica, embolia pulmonar, trombosis vascular después de la cirugía, la administración del catéter debido a la trombosis, infarto de miocardio, fresco, trombosis de la vena central de la retina, etc. |
| 用法、用量<br>Administración y<br>dosis | 一般推荐本品 150 万 U 溶解于 5% 葡萄糖 100ml，静脉滴注 1 小时。<br><br>Este producto se recomienda generalmente 1 500 000 U disuelto en glucosa al 5% de 100 ml, infusión intravenosa por 1 hora. |
| 剂型、规格<br>Formulaciones y<br>especificaciones | 注射用冻干链激酶：每支 10 万 U；15 万 U；20 万 U；25 万 U；30 万 U；50 万 U；75 万 U；150 万 U。<br><br>Estreptoquinasa liofilizada inyectable: Cada una de 100 000 U; 150 000 U; 200 000 U; 250 000 U; 300 000 U; 500 000 U; 750 000 U; 1500 000 U. |
| 药品名称 Drug Names | 尿激酶 Uroquinasa |
| 适应证<br>Indicaciones | 用于急性心肌梗死、肺栓塞、脑血管栓塞、周围动脉或静脉栓塞、视网膜动脉或静脉栓塞等。也可用于眼部炎症、外伤性组织水肿、血肿等。<br><br>Se usa para infarto agudo de miocardio, embolia pulmonar, embolia cerebral, arteriopatía periférica o trombosis venosa, arterial o trombosis venosa de la retina. También se puede utilizar para la inflamación ocular, edema traumático, hematoma. |
| 用法、用量<br>Administración y<br>dosis | ①肺栓塞：初次剂量 3 万～4 万 U，间隔 24 小时重复给药一次，最多使用 3 次。②心肌梗死：建议 0.9% 氯化钠注射液配制后，按 6000U/ 分钟的给药速度冠状动脉内连续滴注 2 小时，滴注前应先行静脉给予肝素 2500～10 000U。<br><br>① Embolia pulmonar: dosis inicial de 30 000～40 000 U, repitió el intervalo de dosificación de 24 horas de tiempo, con un máximo de tres veces. ② Infarto de miocardio: Se recomienda que con la preparación de cloruro de sodio al 0,9%, la velocidad es 6,000 unidades / min, hace la infusión continua de la arteria intracoronaria por dos horas, antes de la infusión, debe ofrecer heparina de 2500～10 000 unidades por vía intravenosa. |
| 剂型、规格<br>Formulaciones y<br>especificaciones | 注射用尿激酶：每瓶 1 万 U；5 万 U；10 万 U；20 万 U；25 万 U；50 万 U；150 万 U；250 万 U。<br><br>Uroquinasa inyectable: cada botella de 10 000 U; 50 000 U; 100 000 U; 200 000 U; 250 000 U; 500 000 U; 1500 000 U; 2500 000 U. |
| 药品名称 Drug Names | 阿替普酶 Alteplasa |
| 适应证<br>Indicaciones | 用于急性心肌梗死和肺栓塞的溶栓治疗。<br>Se usa para la terapia trombolítica en el infarto agudo de miocardio y la embolia pulmonar. |
| 用法、用量<br>Administración y<br>dosis | （1）静脉注射：将本品 50mg 溶于灭菌注射用水中，使溶液浓度为 1mg/ml，给予静脉注射。<br>（2）静脉滴注：将本品 100mg 溶于 0.9% 氯化钠注射液 500ml 中，在 3 小时内按以下方式滴完，即：前 2 分钟先注入 10mg，以后 60 分钟内滴入 50mg，最后剩余时间内滴完所余 40mg。<br><br>(1) Inyección intravenosa: 50 mg de este producto se disuelve en agua estéril para inyección, y la concentración de la solución es de 1mg/ml y hace la inyección intravenosa.<br>(2) infusión intravenosa: 100 mg de este producto se disuelve en inyección de cloruro de sodio al 0,9% de 500ml, dentro de tres horas debe finalizar el goteo de la siguiente forma: en los dos primeros minutos, inyecta 10mg,en los siguientes 60 minutos, instila 50 mg, en el tiempo remanente, inyecta el resto de 40mg. |
| 剂型、规格<br>Formulaciones y<br>especificaciones | 注射用：每瓶 20mg；50mg。<br>Inyección: cada botella de 20mg; 50mg. |

**续　表**

| 药品名称 Drug Names | 瑞替普酶 Reteplasa |
|---|---|
| 适应证<br>Indicaciones | 用于成人由冠状动脉梗死引起的急性心肌梗死的溶栓疗法，能改善心功能。<br><br>Se usa para el tratamiento trombolítico de adultos para el infarto agudo de miocardio causado por infarto coronario, y puede mejorar la función del corazón. |
| 用法、用量<br>Administración y dosis | 10MU 缓慢静脉注射 2～3 分钟以上，间隔 30 分钟后可重复给药（10MU）1 次，目前尚无 2 次以上重复给药的经验。<br><br>Hace la inyección intravenosa lenta de 10MU por 2～3 minutos, después de un intervalo de 30 minutos, puede repetir la dosis (10 MU) por una veces, actualmente no hay experiencia de administración de más de dos veces. |
| 剂型、规格<br>Formulaciones y especificaciones | 注射用：每支 5.0MU。<br>Inyección: Cada una de 5.0MU. |
| 药品名称 Drug Names | 巴曲酶 Defibrina |
| 适应证<br>Indicaciones | 用于急性缺血性脑血管病，突发性耳聋，慢性动脉闭塞症如闭塞性血栓脉管炎、闭塞性动脉硬化症和末梢循环障碍等。<br><br>Se usa para la enfermedad cerebrovascular isquémica aguda, sordera súbita, enfermedad arterial oclusiva crónica, tales como la vasculitis trombo oclusivo, arteriosclerosis obliterante y trastornos circulatorios periféricos. |
| 用法、用量<br>Administración y dosis | 静脉滴注：成人首次 10 巴曲霉单位（BU），以后隔日 1 次，5BU。使用前用 100～200ml 的 0.9% 氯化钠注射液静脉滴注 1 小时以上。通常疗程为 1 周，必要时可增至 3～6 周。<br><br>Infusión intravenosa: la primera dosis para adultos es de 10 unidades de barras adultos aspergillus (BU), después 5BU por cada dos días. Antes del uso, utilice inyección de cloruro de sodio al 0,9% de 100～200 ml para hacer la infusión intravenosa por más de 1 hora. Típicamente el curso de tratamiento dura una semana, si es necesario, se puede aumentar a 3～6 semanas. |
| 剂型、规格<br>Formulaciones y especificaciones | 注射液：每支 10BU（1ml）；5BU（0.5ml）。<br>Inyección: Cada una de 10BU (1 ml); 5BU (0.5 ml). |
| 药品名称 Drug Names | 蚓激酶 Lumbroquinasa |
| 适应证<br>Indicaciones | 用于缺血性脑血管病中纤维蛋白原增高及血小板聚集率增高的患者。<br><br>Se usa para los pacientes con aumento de fibrinógeno y aumento de la agregación plaquetaria de la enfermedad cerebrovascular isquémica. |
| 用法、用量<br>Administración y dosis | 口服：一次 2 粒，一日 3 次，餐前半小时服用。3～4 周为一疗程，也可连续服用。<br><br>Por vía oral: dos cápsulas por una vez, tres veces al día, una media hora antes de la comida. 3～4 semanas es un curso de tratamiento, también se pueden tomar de forma continua. |
| 剂型、规格<br>Formulaciones y especificaciones | 肠溶胶囊：每粒 30 万 U。<br>Cápsulas con recubrimiento entérico: Cada cápsula de 300 mil unidades. |

13.3　血浆代用品 Sustitutos del plasma

| 药品名称 Drug Names | 右旋糖酐 40 Dextrano 40 |
|---|---|
| 适应证<br>Indicaciones | ①各种休克：用于失血、创伤、烧伤及中毒性休克，还可早期预防因休克引起的弥散性血管内凝血。②体外循环时，还可代替部分血液预充心肺机。③血栓性疾病如脑血栓形成、心绞痛和心肌梗死、血栓闭塞性脉管炎、视网膜动静脉血栓、皮肤缺血性溃疡等。④肢体再植和血管外科手术，可预防术后血栓形成，并可改善血液循环，提高再植成功率。<br><br>① diversos shocks: para las shocks de pérdida de sangre, traumatismos, quemaduras y shock tóxico, y también la prevención temprana de la coagulación intravascular diseminada causada por shock. ② Durante la CPB, también puede sustituir parte de las máquinas de cardio sangre precargadas. ③ enfermedades trombóticas, tales como trombosis cerebral, angina de pecho e infarto de miocardio, tromboangeítis obliterante, trombosis de la vena retiniana, úlceras cutáneas isquémicas, etc. ④ reimplantación de extremidades y cirugía vascular, pueden prevenir la trombosis postoperatoria, pueden mejorar la circulación sanguínea, mejorar la tasa de éxito de la reimplantación. |

**续 表**

| | |
|---|---|
| 用法、用量<br>Administración y dosis | 静脉滴注（10% 溶液），一次 250 ~ 500ml，成人和儿童每日不超过 20ml/kg。抗休克时滴注速度为 20 ~ 40ml/min，在 15 ~ 30 分钟注入 500ml。对冠心病和脑血栓患者应缓慢静脉滴注。疗程视病情而定，通常每日或隔日 1 次，7 ~ 14 次为 1 疗程。<br><br>Infusión intravenosa (solución al 10%), 250 ~ 500 ml por cada vez, la dosis diaria para adultos y niños no debe exceder de 20ml/kg. Cuando la velocidad de infusión anti-shock es de 20 ~ 40ml/min, debe inyectar500ml dentro de 15 ~ 30 minutos. Para los pacientes con enfermedad coronaria y de trombosis cerebrales deben reducir la velocidad de goteo intravenoso. El curso de tratamiento depende de la situación de la enfermedad, por lo general es una vez para todos los días o una vez por cada dos días, 7 ~ 14 veces es un curso de tratamiento. |
| 剂型、规格<br>Formulaciones y especificaciones | 右旋糖酐 40（低分子右旋糖酐）葡萄糖注射液：每瓶 10g（100ml）；25g（250ml）；50g（500ml）；6g（100ml）；15g（250ml）；30g（500ml）。均含葡萄糖 5%。<br>右旋糖酐 40（低分子右旋糖酐）氯化钠注射液：每瓶 10g（100ml）；25g（250ml）；50g（500ml）；6g（100ml）；15g（250ml）；30g（500ml）。均含氯化钠 0.9%。<br><br>Inyección de glucosa de Dextrano 40 (dextrano de bajo molecular)：cada botella de 10g（100 ml）；25g（250ml）；50g（500ml）；6g（100ml）；15g（250ml）；30g（500ml）. Contiene glucosa de 5%. Inyección de Cloruro de Sodio de Dextrano 40 (dextrano de bajo molecular)：cada botella de 10 g（100 ml）；25g（250ml）；50g（500ml）；6g（100ml）；15g（250ml）；30g（500ml）. Contiene cloruro sódico al 0.9%. |
| **药品名称 Drug Names** | 右旋糖酐 70 Dextrano 70 |
| 适应证<br>Indicaciones | 用于防治低血容量休克如出血性休克、手术中休克、烧伤性休克。也可用于预防手术后血栓形成和血栓性静脉炎。<br><br>Se usa para la prevención y el tratamiento de shock hipovolémico, como shock hemorrágico, shock quirúrgico, shock de quemaduras. También se puede utilizar para la prevención de trombosis y la cirugía tromboflebitis. |
| 用法、用量<br>Administración y dosis | 静脉滴注，每次 500ml，每分钟注入 20 ~ 40ml。每日最大量不超过 1000 ~ 1500ml。<br>Infusión intravenosa: 500ml por cada vez, inyección de 20 ~ 40 ml por minuto. La dosis máxima diaria no debe ser superior a 1000 ~ 1500 ml. |
| 剂型、规格<br>Formulaciones y especificaciones | 右旋糖酐 70（中分子右旋糖酐）葡萄糖注射液：每瓶 30g（500ml），含葡萄糖 5%。右旋糖酐 70（中分子右旋糖酐）氯化钠注射液：每瓶 30g（500ml），含氯化钠 0.9%。<br><br>Inyección de Glucosa de Dextrano 70 (dextrano molecular): cada botella de 30 g (500 ml), que contiene glucosa al 5%. Inyección de Cloruro de Sodio de Dextrano 70 (dextrano molecular): cada botella de 30 g (500 ml), que contiene cloruro de sodio al 0.9%. |
| **药品名称 Drug Names** | 右旋糖酐 10 Dextrano 10 |
| 适应证<br>Indicaciones | 用于急性失血性休克、创伤及烧伤性休克、急性心肌梗死、心绞痛、脑血栓形成、脑供血不全、血栓闭塞性脉管炎、雷诺病等。此外，术前有低血容量及硬膜外麻醉后所致的低血压者均可使用本品升压。<br><br>Se usa para shock hemorrágico agudo, trauma, quemaduras y descargas, infarto agudo de miocardio, angina de pecho, trombosis cerebral, insuficiencia cerebral, trombosis obliterante, enfermedad de Raynaud. Además, los pacientes de hipovolemia preoperatoria y pacientes de hipotensión debido a la anestesia epidural puede usar este producto para impulsar la presión arterial. |
| 用法、用量<br>Administración y dosis | 静脉滴注：速度为 5 ~ 15ml/min，血压上升后，可酌情减慢。每次 500 ~ 1000ml（参见药品说明书）。<br><br>Infusión intravenosa: la velocidad es de 5 ~ 15ml/min, de ser aumentada la presión arterial, puede reducir la velocidad cuando sea necesario. 500 ~ 1000ml por cada vez (véase las instrucciones del medicamento). |
| 剂型、规格<br>Formulaciones y especificaciones | 右旋糖酐 10（小分子右旋糖酐）葡萄糖注射液：每瓶 30g（500ml）；50g（500ml），均含葡萄糖 5%。<br>右旋糖酐 10（小分子右旋糖酐）氯化钠注射液：每瓶 30g（500ml）；50g（500ml），均含氯化钠 0.9%。 |

**续　表**

| | Inyección de glucosa de dextrano 10 (dextrano molécula pequeña): cada botella de 30g (500 ml); 50 g (500 ml), que contiene glucosa al 5%. Inyección de Cloruro de Sodio de Dextrano 10 (dextrano de molécula pequeña): cada botella de 30g (500 ml); 50 g (500 ml), que contiene cloruro de sodio al 0.9%. |
|---|---|
| 药品名称 Drug Names | 琥珀酰明胶 Gelatina succinilato |
| 适应证<br>Indicaciones | 　用于各种原因引起的低血容量休克的早期治疗，如失血、创伤或手术、烧伤、败血症、腹膜炎、胰腺炎或挤压伤等引起的休克。也可用于体外循环或预防麻醉时出现的低血压。<br><br>　Se usa para el tratamiento temprano de shock hipovolémico por una variedad de causas, tales como shocks causado por la pérdida de sangre, trauma o cirugía, quemaduras, sepsis, peritonitis, pancreatitis, o lesiones por aplastamiento. También se puede utilizar para la hipotensión causada por la circulación extracorpórea o prevenir la anestesia. |
| 用法、用量<br>Administración y dosis | 　静脉输注的剂量和速度取决于患者的实际情况。严重急性失血时可在 5 ～ 10 分钟输入 500ml，直至低血容量症状缓解。快速输入时应加温液体但不超过 37℃。大量输注时应确保维持血细胞比容不低于 25%。大出血者，本品可于血液同时使用。可经同一输液器输注本品和血液。成人少量出血，可在 1 ～ 3 小时输注 500 ～ 1000ml。<br><br>　La dosis intravenosa y la velocidad depende de la situación real del paciente. Para pérdida de sangre aguda severa, puede inyectar 500ml dentro de 5 ～ 10 minutos, hasta que se alivien los síntomas de volumen de sangre de nivel bajo. Durante la inyección rápida, debe calentar el líquido, pero no debe ser más de 37 ℃ . Durante la inyección de gran cantidad, asegúrese de que el mantenimiento de hematocrito no debe ser inferior a 25%. Por pacientes de sangrado grave, este producto se puede utilizar de forma simultánea en la sangre. Este producto se puede introducir a través de la misma infusión y sangre. Para adultos de poco sangrado , introduzca 500 ~ 1000ml dentro de 1 ~ 3 horas. |
| 剂型、规格<br>Formulaciones y especificaciones | 　注射液：每瓶 500ml。<br>　Inyección: cada botella de 500 ml. |
| 药品名称 Drug Names | 羟乙基淀粉 200/0.5 Almidón hidroxietil 200/0.5 |
| 适应证<br>Indicaciones | 　用于预防和治疗各种原因引起的血容量不足和休克，如手术、创伤、感染、烧伤等；急性等容血液稀释，减少手术中对供血的需要，节约用血；治疗性血液稀释，改善血流动力学指标，使红细胞聚集减少，血细胞和血液黏稠度下降，改善微循环。据报道，本品还有防止和堵塞毛细血管漏的作用，在毛细血管通透性增加的情况下使用本品，可减少白蛋白渗漏，减轻组织水肿，减少炎症介质产生，对危重患者更有利。<br><br>　Se usa para la prevención y tratamiento de la deficiencia del volumen de sangre y shock causada por diversas causas, tales como la cirugía, trauma, infecciones, quemaduras, etc; para la hemodilución normovolémica aguda y reducir la necesidad del suministro de sangre en la cirugía, para la conservación de la sangre; tratamiento de hemodilución terapéutica, mejorar la reología de la sangre, para que se reduzca la agregación de los glóbulos rojos, se disminuye los glóbulos y la viscosidad sanguínea, mejorar la microcirculación. Según los informes, este producto tiene el papel de prevención y bloqueo de extravasación capilar, si usa este producto en el caso del aumento de la permeabilidad capilar, se puede reducir la pérdida de albúmina, reducir el edema, reducir los mediadores de la inflamación, y es más favorable para pacientes en estado crítico. |
| 用法、用量<br>Administración y dosis | 　静脉滴注。由于能有过敏反应发生，开始的 10 ～ 20ml 应缓慢滴注，每日用量和滴注速度取决于失血量、血液浓缩程度，每日总量不应大于 33ml/kg（6% 浓度），在心肺功能正常的患者，其血细胞比容应不低于 30%。①治疗和预防容量不足或休克（容量替代治疗）：使用不同浓度中分子羟乙基淀粉溶液最大剂量 6% 的为 33ml/kg，10% 的为 20ml/kg。②急性等容血液稀释（ANH）：手术前即刻开展 ANH，按 1 : 1 比例，每日剂量（2 ～ 3）×500ml（6%），采血量：（2 ～ 3）×500ml（自体血），输注速度 1000ml/（15 ～ 30 分钟），采血速度 1000ml/（15 ～ 30 分钟）。③治疗性血液稀释：治疗可分为等容血液稀释（放血）和高容血液稀释（不放血），按药物不同浓度，给药剂量每日可分为低（250ml）、中（500ml）、高（1000ml）3 种，滴注速度：0.5 ～ 2 小时 250ml，4 ～ 6 小时 500ml，8 ～ 24 小时 1000ml，建议治疗 10 日。 |

| | |
|---|---|
| | Infusión intravenosa. Debido a que se produce una reacción alérgica, el inicio de la 10 ~ 20 ml debe reducir la velocidad de infusión, la tasa de dosis y la infusión diaria depende de la cantidad de pérdida de sangre, nivel en sangre de la concentración, el total diaria no debe exceder 33ml/kg (concentración de 6%), para pacientes con función pulmonar normal, el hematocrito no debe ser inferior a 30%.　① Tratamiento y prevención de la deficiencia del volumen o shock (terapia de reemplazo de volumen): utilice solución de almidón de hidroxietilo de diferentes concentraciones al 6% de la dosis máxima de 33ml/kg, el al10% es 20ml/kg. ② Hemodilución normovolémica aguda ( ANH ) : antes de la cirugía, lleva inmediatamente la ANH , 01:01 , la dosis diaria es ( 2 ~ 3 ) × 500 ml ( 6 % ), el volumen de sangre : ( 2 ~ 3 ) × 500 ml ( sangre autóloga ) , la velocidad de infusión es 1000 ml / ( 15 ~ 30 min ) , la velocidad de la sangre es 1000ml / ( 15 ~ 30 min ) . ③ Hemodilución terapéutica : el tratamiento se puede dividir en hemodilución normovolémica ( sangre ) y hemodilución alta (sin sangre ) , de acuerdo con diferentes concentraciones del fármaco , la dosis diaria se pueden dividir en tres clases de bajo (250 ml ) , medio (500 ml ) , alto( 1000 ml ). La velocidad de infusión es: 250 ml en 0.5 ~ 2 horas, 500 ml en 4 ~ 6 horas , 1000ml en 8 ~ 24 horas, se recomienda que el curso de tratamiento dura 10 días. |
| 剂型、规格<br>Formulaciones y especificaciones | 6% 中分子羟乙基淀粉 200/0.5 氯化钠注射液：每瓶 500ml。10% 中分子羟乙基淀粉 200/0.5 氯化钠注射液：每瓶 500ml。<br><br>Inyección de Cloruro de Sodio de almidón hidroxietil molecular 200/0.5 al 6%: cada botella de 500 ml. Inyección de Cloruro de Sodio de almidón hidroxietil molecular 200/0.5 al 10%: cada botella de 500 ml. |

| 药品名称 Drug Names | 羟乙基淀粉 130/0.4　Almidón hidroxietil 130/0.4 |
|---|---|
| 适应证<br>Indicaciones | 用于治疗和预防血容量不足、急性等容血液稀释（ＡＮＨ）。<br><br>Se usa para el tratamiento y prevención de la hipovolemia, la hemodilución normovolémica aguda (ANH). |
| 用法、用量<br>Administración y dosis | 同中分子羟乙基淀粉 200/0.5，每日最大剂量按体重 33ml/kg，据患者需要可持续使用数日，治疗持续时间取决于低血容量程度及血流动力学参数和稀释效果。在欧洲已批准用于 0 ~ 2 岁儿童，每日最大剂量 50ml/kg。国内儿童用药正在研究中。<br><br>Lo mismo como el almidón hidroxietil molecular 200/0.5. La dosis máxima diaria es 33ml/kg por peso corporal, de acuerdo con las necesidades del paciente es sostenible el uso de varios días, la duración del tratamiento depende del grado de hipovolemia y parámetros hemodinámicos y los efectos de dilución. Ha sido aprobado en Europa el uso para los niños de 0 ~ 2 años de edad, la dosis diaria máxima de 50ml/kg. En china, La medicación infantil está en estudio. |
| 剂型、规格<br>Formulaciones y especificaciones | 6% 中分子羟乙基淀粉 130/0.4 氯化钠注射液：每瓶 250ml；500ml。<br><br>Inyección de cloruro de sodio de almidón hidroxietil molecular 130/0.4 al 6%: cada botella de 250ml; 500ml. |

| 药品名称 Drug Names | 包醛氧淀粉 Almidón de oxígeno aldehído |
|---|---|
| 适应证<br>Indicaciones | 用于各种原因造成的氮质血症。<br><br>Se usa para la azotemia causada por diversas razones. |
| 用法、用量<br>Administración y dosis | 口服：餐后用温开水送服。一日 2 ~ 3 次，一次 5 ~ 10g，或遵医嘱。<br><br>Por vía oral: toma la medicación con agua tibia después de la comida. 2 ~ 3 veces al día, 5 ~ 10g por cada vez, o según las indicaciones. |
| 剂型、规格<br>Formulaciones y especificaciones | 胶囊：每粒 0.625g。粉剂：每袋 5g。<br><br>Cápsulas: Cada cápsula de 0.625 g. Polvo: cada paquete de 5g. |

| 药品名称 Drug Names | 聚维酮 Polividona |
|---|---|
| 适应证<br>Indicaciones | 用于外伤性出血及其他原因引起的血容量减少。<br><br>Se usa para la disminución de volumen de sangre causada por el sangrado traumático y otras causas. |
| 用法、用量<br>Administración y dosis | 视病情而定，一般为 500 ~ 1000ml 静脉滴注。<br><br>Dependiendo de la enfermedad, por lo general la infusión intravenosa es 500 ~ 1000ml. |

**续　表**

| 剂型、规格<br>Formulaciones y especificaciones | 注射液：3.5%（250ml）。<br>Inyección: 3.5% (250 ml). |
|---|---|
| **药品名称 Drug Names** | 羟乙基淀粉 40Almidón hidroxietil 40 |
| 适应证<br>Indicaciones | 为血容量扩充剂。用于各种手术、外伤的失血，中毒性休克等的补液。<br>Es el expansor de volumen de sangre. Se usa para la pérdida de sangre por una variedad de cirugías traumas, la infusión de fluidos causada por el shock tóxico. |
| 用法、用量<br>Administración y dosis | 视病情而定，一般为 500 ～ 1000ml 静脉滴注。<br>Dependiendo de la enfermedad, por lo general la infusión intravenosa es 500 ~ 1000ml. |
| 剂型、规格<br>Formulaciones y especificaciones | 注射液：6%（500ml）。<br>Inyección: 6% (500 ml). |
| **药品名称 Drug Names** | 人血白蛋白 Albúmina humana |
| 适应证<br>Indicaciones | 用于失血性休克、脑水肿、流产等引起的白蛋白缺乏、肾病等。<br>Se usa para ladeficiencia de albúmina y enfermedad renal inducida por shock hemorrágico, el edema cerebral, el aborto, etc. |
| 用法、用量<br>Administración y dosis | 静脉注射或静脉滴注：用量视病情而定。<br>Inyección intravenosa o infusión intravenosa: la cantidad depende de la enfermedad. |
| 剂型、规格<br>Formulaciones y especificaciones | 注射液：5%；10%；20%；25%。冻干粉：5g；10g。<br>Inyección: 5%; 10%; 20%; 25%. Polvo liofilizado: 5g; 10g. |

### 13.4　抗贫血药 Medicamentos antianemia

| **药品名称 Drug Names** | 硫酸亚铁 Sulfato ferroso |
|---|---|
| 适应证<br>Indicaciones | 用于慢性失血（月经过多、慢性消化道出血、子宫肌瘤出血、钩虫病失血等）、营养不良、妊娠、儿童发育期等引起的缺铁性贫血。用药后贫血症状迅速改善，用药 1 周左右即可见网织红细胞增多，血红蛋白每日可增加 0.1% ～ 0.3%，4 ～ 8 周可恢复至正常。<br>Se usa para la anemia por deficiencia de hierro causada por el sangrado crónico (menorragia, sangrado gastrointestinal crónico, sangrado uterino fibromas, pérdida anquilostomiasis sangre, etc), la desnutrición, el embarazo, el desarrollo infantil y otras causas. Los síntomas de anemia se mejoran rápidamente después del tratamiento, con el uso de la medicación de alrededor de una semana se ve el aumento de reticulocitos, el incremento diario de hemoglobina es de 0.1% ~ 0.3%, en cerca de 4 ~ 8 semanas puede volver a la normalidad. |
| 用法、用量<br>Administración y dosis | 口服，成人，每次 0.3g，一日 3 次，餐后服用。<br>Por vía oral, para adultos, 0,3 g por cada vez, 3 veces al día, se toma después de las comidas. |
| 剂型、规格<br>Formulaciones y especificaciones | 硫酸亚铁片：每片 0.3g。硫酸亚铁缓释片：每片 0.25g；0.45g。<br>Tabletas de sulfato ferroso: Cada tableta de 0.3 g. Tabletas de liberación sostenida de sulfato ferroso: Cada tableta de 0.25 g; 0.45 g. |
| **药品名称 Drug Names** | 葡萄糖酸亚铁 Gluconato ferroso |
| 适应证<br>Indicaciones | 用于各种原因引起的缺铁性贫血，如营养不良、慢性失血、月经过多、妊娠、儿童生长期等所致的缺铁性贫血。<br>Su usa para la anemia de deficiencia de hierro causada por diversas causas, tales como la desnutrición, la pérdida crónica de sangre, menorragia, el embarazo, crecimiento de los niños, etc. |

**续 表**

| | |
|---|---|
| 用法、用量<br>Administración y<br>dosis | 口服：预防，成人，一次 0.3g，一日 1 次；儿童：一次 0.1g，一日 2 次。治疗，成人，一次 0.3 ~ 0.6g，一日 3 次；儿童：一次 0.1 ~ 0.2g，一日 3 次。<br><br>Por vía oral: Prevención, para adultos, 0.3 g por cada vez, una vez al día; para niños: 0.1 g por cada vez, 2 veces al día. Tratamiento para adultos, 0.3 ~ 0.6 g por cada vez, 3 veces al día; para niños: 0.1 ~ 0.2 g por cada vez, 3 veces al día. |
| 剂型、规格<br>Formulaciones y<br>especificaciones | 片剂（糖衣片）：每片 0.1g；0.3g。胶囊剂：每粒 0.25g；0.3g；0.4g。糖浆：每瓶 0.25g（10ml）；0.3g（10ml）。<br><br>Tabletas (tabletas recubiertos): cada tableta de 0.1g; 0.3g. Cápsulas: Cada cápsula de 0.25 g; 0.3 g; 0.4 g. Jarabe: cada botella de 0.25 g (10 ml); 0.3 g (10 ml). |
| **药品名称 Drug Names** | 蔗糖铁 Hierro sacarosa |
| 适应证<br>Indicaciones | 主要用于治疗口服铁不能有效缓解的缺铁性贫血。<br><br>Principalmente se usa para el tratamiento la anemia de deficiencia de hierro que no se aliviaeficazmente por el tratamiento por vía oral. |
| 用法、用量<br>Administración y<br>dosis | 本品只能与 0.9%w/v 生理盐水混合使用。应以滴注或缓慢注射的方式给药，或直接注射到透析器的静脉端给药。<br><br>Este producto sólo funciona con la mezcla de solución salina de 0,9% w / v. La infusión se debe administrar por goteo o inyección lenta, o la inyección directa al lado de la vena de la administración dializador. |
| 剂型、规格<br>Formulaciones y<br>especificaciones | 蔗糖铁注射液：5ml ： 100mg（铁元素）。<br>Inyección de Hierro Sacarosa: 5 ml ： 100 mg (elemento de hierro). |
| **药品名称 Drug Names** | 叶酸 Ácido fólico |
| 适应证<br>Indicaciones | 巨幼红细胞性贫血，尤适用于营养不良或婴儿期、妊娠期叶酸需要增加所致的巨幼红细胞贫血。用于治疗恶性贫血时，虽可纠正异常血常规，但不能改善神经损害症状，故应以维生素 $B_{12}$ 为主，叶酸为辅。也用于妊娠期和哺乳期妇女的预防用药。<br><br>La anemia megaloblástica, especialmente para la anemia megaloblástica causada por desnutrido o el aumento de ácido fólico durante la infancia o el embarazo. Cuando se utiliza en el tratamiento de la anemia perniciosa, aunque puede corregir la sangre anormal, no puede mejorar el daño síntomas neurológicos, por lo tanto debe ser principalmente la vitamina $B_{12}$, con suplemento de ácido fólico. También se utiliza como profilaxis para las mujeres durante el embarazo y el período de lactancia. |
| 用法、用量<br>Administración y<br>dosis | 口服：成人，一次 5 ~ 10mg，一日 5 ~ 30mg。肌内注射：一次 10 ~ 20mg。妊娠期和哺乳期妇女的预防用药：口服一次 0.4mg，一日 1 次。<br><br>Por vía oral: Adultos, 5 ~ 10 mg por cada vez, 5 ~ 30 mg al día. La inyección intramuscular: 10 ~ 20 mg por cada vez. Medicamento preventivo para los las mujeres con embarazo y en periodo de lactancia profilaxis: 0.4 mg de una vez por vía oral, una vez al día. |
| 剂型、规格<br>Formulaciones y<br>especificaciones | 叶酸片：每片 0.4mg；5mg。注射液：每支 15mg（1ml）。复方叶酸注射液：每支 1ml，含叶酸 5mg、维生素 $B_{12}$ 30μg。<br><br>Tabletas de ácido fólico: cada tableta de 0.4 mg; 5mg. Inyección: Cada inyección de15 mg (1 ml). Inyección compuesta de Ácido fólico: Cada inyección de 1 ml que contiene 5 mg de ácido fólico, 30μg de vitamina $B_{12}$. |
| **药品名称 Drug Names** | 氰钴胺（维生素 $B_{12}$）Cianocobalamina (Vitamina $B_{12}$) |
| 适应证<br>Indicaciones | 用于治疗恶性贫血，亦与叶酸合用用于治疗各种巨幼红细胞性贫血、抗叶酸药引起的贫血及脂肪泻、全胃切除或胃大部切除。尚用于神经系统疾病（如神经炎、神经萎缩等）、肝脏疾病（肝炎、肝硬化等）等。<br><br>Se usa para el tratamiento de la anemia perniciosa, también se usa en combinación con ácido fólico para el tratamiento de la anemia megaloblástica de una variedad, anemia causada por fármaco anti-folato, esteatorrea, gastrectomía total o subtotal. Se usa para los trastornos neurológicos (tales como neuritis, atrofia), enfermedades de hígado (hepatitis, cirrosis, etc.), etc. |

**续 表**

| 用法、用量<br>Administración y dosis | 肌内注射，成人，一日内 0.025 ～ 0.1mg 或隔日 0.05 ～ 0.2mg。用于神经系统疾病时，用量可酌增。<br>Inyección intramuscular, para adultos, 0.025 ~ 0.1 mg al día o 0.05 ~ 0.2 mg por cada dos días. Cuando se utiliza en los trastornos neurológicos, la dosis se puede aumentar según la situación. |
|---|---|
| 剂型、规格<br>Formulaciones y especificaciones | 注射液：每支 0.05mg（1ml）；0.1ng（1ml）；0.25mg（1ml）；0.5mg（1ml）；1mg（1ml）．<br>Inyección: Cada inyección de 0.05 mg (1 ml); 0.1 ng (1 ml); 0.25 mg (1 ml); 0.5 mg (1 ml); 1 mg (1 ml). |

| 药品名称 Drug Names | 腺苷钴胺 Cobamamida |
|---|---|
| 适应证<br>Indicaciones | 主要用于巨幼红细胞型贫血、营养不良性贫血、妊娠期贫血，亦用于神经性疾病如多发性神经炎、神经根炎、三叉神经痛、坐骨神经痛、神经麻痹、营养性神经疾病及放射线和药物引起的白细胞减少症。<br>Principalmente se usa para la anemia megaloblástica, la desnutrición, la anemia, la anemia durante el embarazo, y también para los trastornos neurológicos como neuritis múltiple, radiculitis, neuralgia, ciática, parálisis, trastornos neurológicos y la trombocitopenia de leucocito causada por la radiación y medicación. |
| 用法、用量<br>Administración y dosis | 口服，一人，一次 0.5 ～ 1.5mg，一日 1.5 ～ 4.5mg。肌内注射，一日 0.5 ～ 1mg。<br>Por vía oral, para adultos, 0.5 ~ 1.5 mg por cada vez, 1.5 días ~ 4.5 mg al día. Inyección intramuscular, 0.5 ~ 1mg al día. |
| 剂型、规格<br>Formulaciones y especificaciones | 片剂：每片 0.25mg。注射液：每支 0.5mg（1ml）。冻干粉针：0.5mg；1.0mg；1.5mg。<br>Tabletas: cada tableta de 0.25 mg. Inyección: Cada inyección de 0.5 mg (1 ml). Polvo liofilizado: 0.5 mg; 1.0 mg; 1.5 mg. |

| 药品名称 Drug Names | 甲钴胺 Mecobalamina |
|---|---|
| 适应证<br>Indicaciones | 用于治疗缺乏维生素 $B_{12}$ 引起的巨幼细胞性贫血，也用于周围神经病。<br>Se usa para el tratamiento de la anemia megaloblástica causada por la deficiencia de vitamina $B_{12}$, y también para la neuropatía periférica. |
| 用法、用量<br>Administración y dosis | 肌内注射或静脉注射。①成人巨红细胞性贫血：通常一次 500μg，一日 1 次，隔日 1 次。给药约 2 个月后，可维持治疗，一次 500μg，每 1 ～ 3 个月 1 次。②周围神经病：通常，成人一次 500μg，一日 1 次，一周 3 次，可按年龄、症状酌情增减。<br>Inyección intramuscular o inyección intravenosa. ① anemia de células gigantes de adultos: generalmente es 500μg por una vez, una vez al día, una vez por cada dos días. Aproximadamente dos meses después de la administración, se puede mantener el tratamiento, 500μg por una vez, cada 1 ~ 3 meses una vez. ② Neuropatía periférica: normalmente, para adultos es un 500μg por una vez, una vez al día, tres veces por una semana, de acuerdo a la edad y los síntomas, se puede ajustar la dosis apropiadamente. |
| 剂型、规格<br>Formulaciones y especificaciones | 注射液：1ml ：500μg。<br>Inyección: 1 ml ：500μg |

| 药品名称 Drug Names | 重组人促红细胞生成素 Eritropoyetina humana recombinante |
|---|---|
| 适应证<br>Indicaciones | 用于慢性肾衰竭和晚期肾病所致的贫血，也用于多发性骨髓瘤相关的贫血和骨髓增生异常综合征（MDS）及骨癌引起的贫血。对结缔组织病（类风湿关节炎和系统性红斑狼疮）所致的贫血也有效。<br>Su usa para la anemia causada por insuficiencia renal crónica y enfermedad renal en etapa terminal, y también para la anemia relacionado con mieloma múltiple y síndrome mielodisplásico (MDS) y la anemia debida a cáncer de huesos. También es efectiva para la enfermedad de la anemia causada por el tejido conectivo (artritis reumatoide y el lupus eritematoso sistémico). |

**续 表**

| | |
|---|---|
| 用法、用量<br>Administración y dosis | 可静脉注射或皮下注射，剂量应个体化，一般开始剂量为 50 ～ 150U/kg，每周 3 次。治疗过程中需视血细胞比容或血红蛋白水平调整剂量或调节维持量。建议以血细胞比容 30% ～ 33% 或血红蛋白 100 ～ 120g/L 为指标，调节维持剂量。<br><br>Inyección intravenosa o Inyección subcutánea, la dosis debe ser individualizada, por lo general la dosis inicial es de 50 ～ 150 unidades / kg, 3 veces a la semana. En el curso del tratamiento debe ajustar la dosis o mantenerla dosis depende del nivel de hematocrito o hemoglobina. Se sugiere que la escala de hematocrito es 30% ～ 33% o hemoglobina de 100 ～ 120 g / L como un índice para ajustar la dosis de mantenimiento. |
| 剂型、规格<br>Formulaciones y especificaciones | 重组人促红细胞生成素注射液（CHO 细胞）：每支 2000U（1ml）；4000U（1ml）；10 000U（1ml）。<br>注射用重组人促红细胞生成素（CHO 细胞）：每支 2000U；4000U；10 000U。<br><br>Inyección de Eritropoyetina Humana Recombinante (células CHO): Cada inyección de 2000U (1 ml); 4000U (1 ml); 10 000U (1 ml). Eritropoyetina humana recombinante inyectable (células CHO): Cada una de 2000U; 4000U; 10 000U. |
| **药品名称 Drug Names** | 琥珀酸亚铁 Succinato ferroso |
| 适应证<br>Indicaciones | 用于缺铁性贫血的预防和治疗。<br>Se usa para la prevención y el tratamiento de la anemia de deficiencia de hierro. |
| 用法、用量<br>Administración y dosis | 预防：普通成人一日 0.1g；妊娠期妇女一日 0.2g；儿童一日 0.03 ～ 0.06g。治疗：成人一次 0.1 ～ 0.2g，一日 3 次；儿童一次 0.05 ～ 0.1g，一日 1 ～ 2 次餐后服。<br><br>Prevención: para adultos 0.1 g al día; Para las mujeres embarazadas 0.2 g al día; Para niños, 0.03 ～ 0.06 g al día. Tratamiento: para adultos 0.1 ～ 0.2 g por cada vez, 3 veces al día; Para niños, 0.05 ～ 0.1 g por cada vez, 1 o 2 veces al día que se toma después de la comida. |
| 剂型、规格<br>Formulaciones y especificaciones | 片剂：0.1g。胶囊剂：0.1g。<br>Tableta: 0.1 g. Cápsulas: 0.1g. |
| **药品名称 Drug Names** | 富马酸亚铁 Fumarato ferroso |
| 适应证<br>Indicaciones | 用于治疗缺铁性贫血。<br>Se usa para el tratamiento de la anemia de deficiencia de hierro. |
| 用法、用量<br>Administración y dosis | 口服，一次 0.2 ～ 0.4g，一日 3 次，疗程：轻症 2 ～ 3 周，重症 3 ～ 4 周。<br><br>Por vía oral, 0.2 ～ 0.4 g por cada vez, 3 veces al día. Curso de tratamiento: 2 ～ 3 semanas para síntomas leves, 3 ～ 4 semanas para síntomas graves. |
| 剂型、规格<br>Formulaciones y especificaciones | 片剂：0.2g；0.05g。胶囊剂：0.2g。<br>Tabletas：0.2 g；0.05 g. Cápsulas：0.2 g. |
| **药品名称 Drug Names** | 枸橼酸铁铵 Citrato de amonio férrico |
| 适应证<br>Indicaciones | 适用于儿童及不能吞服药片的患者。由于含铁量低，不适于重症贫血病例。<br><br>Es adecuado para los niños y los pacientes que no pueden tragar pastillas. Debido al bajo contenido de hierro, no es adecuado para los casos de anemia severa. |
| 用法、用量<br>Administración y dosis | 口服，一次 0.5 ～ 2g，一日 3 次，餐后服。<br>Por vía oral, 0.5 ～ 2 g por cada vez, 3 veces al día, se toma después de la comida. |
| 剂型、规格<br>Formulaciones y especificaciones | 溶液：10%。<br>Solución: 10%. |
| **药品名称 Drug Names** | 右旋糖酐铁 Hierro dextrano |
| 适应证<br>Indicaciones | 适用于不能耐受口服铁制剂的缺铁性贫血患者或者需要迅速纠正缺铁者。<br><br>Se aplica para los pacientes de la anemia por deficiencia de hierro que no tolera los preparados de hierro por vía oral o aquellos que necesitan corregir rápidamente la deficiencia de hierro. |

**续　表**

| 用法、用量<br>Administración y dosis | 深部肌内注射：每日 1ml。<br>Inyección intramuscular profunda: 1 ml al día. |
|---|---|
| 剂型、规格<br>Formulaciones y especificaciones | 注射液：每毫升含元素铁 25mg。<br>Inyección: Cada un ml de la inyección contiene 25 mg de hierro elemental. |

| 药品名称 Drug Names | 山梨醇铁 Hierro sorbitol |
|---|---|
| 适应证<br>Indicaciones | 适用于不能耐受口服铁制剂的缺铁性贫血患者或者需要迅速纠正缺铁者。<br>Se aplica para  los pacientes de la anemia por deficiencia de hierro que no tolera los preparados de hierro por vía oral o aquellos que necesitan corregir rápidamente la deficiencia de hierro. |
| 用法、用量<br>Administración y dosis | 深部肌内注射，一次 1.5～2ml（相当于铁 75～100mg）。<br>Inyección intramuscular profunda, 1.5～2 ml por cada vez (equivalente a 75～100 mg de Fe. |
| 剂型、规格<br>Formulaciones y especificaciones | 注射剂 :100mg<br>inyección: 100 mg |

| 药品名称 Drug Names | 亚叶酸钙 Folinato de calcio |
|---|---|
| 适应证<br>Indicaciones | 常用作氨蝶呤及甲氨蝶呤过量时的解毒剂。此外,尚可用于巨幼红细胞性贫血及白细胞减少症。<br>Se utiliza como metotrexato y el antídoto para la sobredosis de metotrexato. Puede usar para la anemia megaloblástica y leucopenia. |
| 用法、用量<br>Administración y dosis | 肌内注射：①抗叶酸代谢药中度中毒，一次 6～12mg，每 6 小时 1 次，共 4 次。②巨幼红细胞性贫血：一日 1mg，一日 1 次。③白细胞减少症：一次 3～6mg，一日 1 次。静脉滴注：抗叶酸代谢药重度中毒：75mg 于 12 小时内滴注完毕，随后改为肌内注射。<br>Inyección intramuscular:　① intoxicación moderada de metabolito antifolate, 6～12 mg por cada vez, cada 6 horas una vez, en total, 4 veces. ② anemia megaloblástica: 1mg al día, una vez al día. ③ leucopenia: 3～6 mg por cada vez, una vez al día. Infusión intravenosa: intoxicación grave de antifolato metabolito: debe finalizar la infusión de 75 mg en 12 horas, y luego cambia a la inyección intramuscular. |
| 剂型、规格<br>Formulaciones y especificaciones | 注射用冻干粉：3mg；5mg。<br>Polvo liofilizado para inyección: 3 mg; 5mg. |

13.5　促进白细胞增生药 Medicamentos para promover la proliferación de leucocitos

| 药品名称 Drug Names | 维生素 $B_4$（腺嘌呤）　Vitamina $B_4$（Adenina） |
|---|---|
| 适应证<br>Indicaciones | 用于各种原因如放射治疗、苯中毒、抗肿瘤药和抗甲状腺药物等引起的白细胞减少症，也用于急性粒细胞减少症。<br>Se usa para la enfermedad de reduccion de leucopenia causada por una variedad de razones, tales como la terapia de radiación, intoxicación por benceno, drogas contra el cáncer y drogas anti-tiroides, y también para la neutropenia aguda. |
| 用法、用量<br>Administración y dosis | 口服，成人，一次 10～20mg，一日 3 次。肌内注射或静脉注射，一日 20～30mg。<br>Por vía oral, para adultos, 10～20 mg por cada vez, 3 veces al día. Inyección intramuscular o intravenosa, 20～30 mg al día. |
| 剂型、规格<br>Formulaciones y especificaciones | 片剂：每片 10mg；25mg。注射用维生素 $B_4$：每支 20mg。<br>Tabletas: Cada tableta de 10 mg; 25 mg. Vitamina $B_4$ Inyectable: Cada una de 20mg. |

| 药品名称 Drug Names | 苦参总碱 Sophora de alcaloides |
|---|---|
| 适应证<br>Indicaciones | 用于肿瘤放疗、化疗及其他原因引起的白细胞减少症（包括再生障碍性贫血、慢性放射病、慢性肝炎等）。<br>Se usa para la radioterapia del cáncer, la quimioterapia y otras causas leucopenia (incluyendo anemia aplásica, enfermedad por radiación crónica, hepatitis crónica, etc |

**续 表**

| 用法、用量<br>Administración y dosis | 肌内注射，每次 0.2g，一日 2 次。<br>Inyección intramuscular, 0.2 g por cada vez, 2 veces al día. |
|---|---|
| 剂型、规格<br>Formulaciones y especificaciones | 注射液：0.2g（1ml）。<br>Inyección: 0.2 g (1 ml). |

| 药品名称 Drug Names | 鲨肝醇 Batilol |
|---|---|
| 适应证<br>Indicaciones | 用于各种原因引起的粒细胞减少。<br>Se usa para la reducción de granulocitos causada por una variedad de causas. |
| 用法、用量<br>Administración y dosis | 一日 50 ～ 150mg，分 3 次口服。<br>Cada día de 50 ~ 150 mg, 3 veces al día por vía oral. |
| 剂型、规格<br>Formulaciones y especificaciones | 片剂：25mg；50mg。<br>Tabletas: 25 mg; 50 mg. |

| 药品名称 Drug Names | 利可君 Leucogen |
|---|---|
| 适应证<br>Indicaciones | 用于防治各种原因引起的白细胞较少、再生障碍性贫血。<br>Se utiliza para la prevención y el tratamiento de la deficiencia de leucocito y anemia aplásica causadas por una variedad de causas. |
| 用法、用量<br>Administración y dosis | 口服，一次 20mg，一日 3 次。<br>Por vía oral, 20mg por cada vez, 3 veces al día. |
| 剂型、规格<br>Formulaciones y especificaciones | 片剂：10mg；20mg。<br>Tabletas: 10mg; 20 mg. |

| 药品名称 Drug Names | 肌苷 Inosina |
|---|---|
| 适应证<br>Indicaciones | 用于治疗各种原因所致的白细胞较少、血小板减少等。<br>Se usa para el tratamiento de la deficiencia de leucocito y reducción de trombocitopenia causada por una variedad de razones. |
| 用法、用量<br>Administración y dosis | 口服：一次 200 ～ 600mg，一日 3 次。静脉注射或静脉滴注：一次 200 ～ 600mg，一日 1 ～ 2 次。<br>Por vía oral: un 200 ~ 600 mg, 3 veces al día. Inyección intravenosa o infusión intravenosa: 200 ~ 600 mg por cada vez, 1 ~ 2 veces al día. |
| 剂型、规格<br>Formulaciones y especificaciones | 片剂：200mg。注射液：100mg（2ml）；200mg（5ml）。<br>Tabletas: 200 mg. Inyección: 100 mg (2 ml); 200 mg (5 ml). |

| 药品名称 Drug Names | 氨肽素 Aminopolipeptida |
|---|---|
| 适应证<br>Indicaciones | 用于原发性血小板减少性紫癜、过敏性紫癜、白细胞减少症和再生障碍性贫血。<br>Se usa para la púrpura trombocitopénica idiopática, púrpura de irritabilidad, leucopenia y anemia aplásica. |
| 用法、用量<br>Administración y dosis | 口服：成人一次 1g，一日 3 次；小儿酌减。用药至少 4 周，有效者可连续服用。<br>Por vía oral: Para adultos, 1g por una vez, tres veces al día, Para los niños se puede reducir la dosis. El curso de la medicación dura por lo menos cuatro semanas, los pacientes con eficacia puede seguir el uso continuamente. |
| 剂型、规格<br>Formulaciones y especificaciones | 片剂：0.2g。<br>Tabletas:0.2g. |

**续 表**

### 13.6 抗血小板药物 Antiplaquetarios

| 药品名称 Drug Names | 阿司匹林 Aspirina |
|---|---|
| 适应证<br>Indicaciones | 可用于预防心、脑血管疾病的发作及人工心脏瓣膜或其他手术后的血栓形成。临床研究发现在男性患者预防脑卒中的效果似乎较女性患者为佳,这可能与女性的血小板环氧酶对阿司匹林的耐受性较高有关。<br><br>Se puede usar para prevenir los ataques al corazón y las enfermedades cerebrovasculares y válvulas cardíacas artificiales o la formación de coágulos de sangre después de la cirugía. En los estudios clínicos encontraron que la prevención del ictus en pacientes masculinos es mejor que las pacientes de sexo femelino. Puede estar relacionado con la mayor tolerancia ciclooxigenasa de las plaquetas a la aspirina para las mujeres. |
| 用法、用量<br>Administración y dosis | 用于防治短暂性脑缺血和卒中:成人常用量,每次 75 ~ 300mg,一日 1 次。预防用,一般一日 75 ~ 150mg;治疗用,一般一日 300mg。用于缺血性心脏病,可预防心肌梗死,减少心律失常的发生率和死亡率。<br><br>Para la prevención y el tratamiento de la isquemia cerebral transitoria y accidente cerebrovascular: la dosis habitual de adultos es 75 ~ 300 mg por cada vez, una vez al día. Para uso preventivo, generalmente es 75 ~ 150 mg al día; Para uso terapéutico, generalmente es 300 mg al día. Para la enfermedad isquémica del corazón, puede prevenir el infarto de miocardio y reducir la incidencia de arritmias y la mortalidad. |
| 剂型、规格<br>Formulaciones y especificaciones | 肠溶片:每片 25mg;40mg;100mg。<br>Tabletas con recubrimiento entérico: Cada tableta de 25 mg; 40 mg; 100 mg. |
| 药品名称 Drug Names | 双嘧达莫 Dipiridamol |
| 适应证<br>Indicaciones | 用于血栓栓塞性疾病及缺血性心脏病。<br>Se usa para la enfermedad tromboembólica y enfermedad isquémica del corazón. |
| 用法、用量<br>Administración y dosis | 单独应用疗效不及与阿司匹林合用者。单独应用时,一日口服 3 次,一次 25 ~ 100mg;与阿司匹林合用时其剂量可减少至一日 100 ~ 200mg。<br><br>Su aplicación individual no es mejor que la aplicación combinada con aspirina. Cuando se aplica su uso individual, debe tomar por vía oral 3 veces al día, 25 ~ 100 mg por cada vez; Si en combinación con aspirina, la dosis diaria se puede reducir hasta 100 ~ 200 mg al día. |
| 剂型、规格<br>Formulaciones y especificaciones | 片剂:每片 25mg。<br>Tabletas: 25 mg por cada tableta. |
| 药品名称 Drug Names | 氯吡格雷 Clopidogrel |
| 适应证<br>Indicaciones | 用于预防和治疗因血小板高聚集引起的心、脑及其他动脉循环障碍疾病,如近期发作的脑卒中、心肌梗死和确诊的外周动脉疾病。<br><br>Se usa para la prevención y el tratamiento de enfermedades de corazón, el cerebro y otros trastornos de la circulación arterial debido a la alta agregación de plaquetas, tales como el accidente cerebrovascular reciente atacado, infarto de miocardio, y la enfermedad arterial periférica exterior diagnosticado. |
| 用法、用量<br>Administración y dosis | 一日一次,每次 75mg。<br>Una vez al día, 75mg por cada vez. |
| 剂型、规格<br>Formulaciones y especificaciones | 片剂:每片 25mg。<br>Tabletas: 25 mg por cada tableta. |

续　表

| 药品名称 Drug Names | 替罗非班 Tirofibán |
| --- | --- |
| 适应证<br>Indicaciones | 用于急性冠脉综合征、不稳定型心绞痛和非 Q 波心肌梗死、急性心肌梗死和急性缺血性心脏猝死等，包括可用药控制的患者和需做 PTCA、血管成形术或动脉粥样硬化血管切除术的患者。替罗非班可减少急性冠脉综合征和冠脉内介入治疗后冠心病事件发生率，改善患者症状和预后。<br><br>Se usa para el síndrome coronario agudo, angina inestable y infarto de miocardio no onda Q, infarto agudo de miocardio y muerte cardíaca isquémica aguda, etc, incluyendo pacientes de control de drogas y pacientes con necesidad de hacer la PTCA, pacientes con cirugía de angioplastia o resección vascular de la aterosclerosis. Tirofibán puede reducir los síndromes coronarios agudos y la incidencia de episodios de cardiopatía coronaria después de la intervención coronaria percutánea, mejorar los síntomas y el pronóstico. |
| 用法、用量<br>Administración y dosis | 与肝素合用，静脉给药。开始 30 分钟给药速度为 0.4μg/（kg·min），然后减为维持量 0.1μg/（kg·min），2 ～ 5 日为一疗程。患者至少给药 48 小时，此期间不进行手术治疗（除非患者发病为顽固性心肌缺血或新的心肌梗死）。<br><br>Se usa en combinación con la heparina, administrada por vía intravenosa. En los primeros 30 minutos, la tasa de administración es de 0.4μg / (kg · min), y después se reduce a una dosis de mantenimiento de 0.1μg / (kg · min). 2 ~ 5 días es un curso de tratamiento. Debe dar la medicación a los pacientes por lo menos 48 horas, durante el cual no se realiza la cirugía (a menos que el paciente tiene la isquemia miocárdica o infarto de miocardio refractario nuevo). |
| 剂型、规格<br>Formulaciones y especificaciones | 注射液：每瓶 5mg（100ml）。<br>Inyección: 5 mg (100 ml ) por cada botella. |
| 药品名称 Drug Names | 奥扎格雷 Ozagrel |
| 适应证<br>Indicaciones | 用于治疗急性血栓性脑梗死及伴发的运动障碍，改善蛛网膜下腔出血手术后血管痉挛及其并发的脑缺血症状。<br><br>Se usa para el tratamiento de infarto trombótico agudo y los trastornos del movimiento asociados, puede mejorar el vasoespasmo después de la cirugía de la hemorragia subaracnoidea síntomas concurrentes de la isquemia cerebral. |
| 用法、用量<br>Administración y dosis | 常用制剂为奥扎格雷钠注射液，每支 20mg。以生理盐水或葡萄糖注射液稀释后静脉滴注，一日 80mg。如与其他抗血小板药合用时，本品剂量宜酌减。<br><br>Su preparación común es de la inyección de ozagrel, cada inyección de 20 mg. Después de ser diluida con solución salina o inyección glucosa, hace la infusión intravenosa, 80 mg al día. Cuando se combina con otros medicamentos anti-plaquetas, la dosis de este producto debe ser reducida. |
| 剂型、规格<br>Formulaciones y especificaciones | 注射用奥扎格雷：20mg；40mg。奥扎格雷注射液：每支 20mg（1ml）；40mg（2ml）。<br>Ozagrel Inyectable: 20 mg; 40 mg. Inyección de Ozagrel: Cada una de 20 mg (1 ml), 40 mg (2 ml). |
| 药品名称 Drug Names | 曲克芦丁 Troxerutina |
| 适应证<br>Indicaciones | 用于脑血栓形成和脑栓塞所致的偏瘫、失语及心肌梗死前综合征、动脉硬化、中心性视网膜炎、血栓性静脉炎、静脉曲张、血管通透性高引起的水肿等。<br><br>Se usa para hemiplejía y afasia provocada por la trombosis cerebral y embolia cerebral y síndrome de ex infarto de miocardio, aterosclerosis, la retinitis central, tromboflebitis, venas varicosas, el edema causada por la alta permeabilidad vascular. |
| 用法、用量<br>Administración y dosis | 口服：一次 300mg，一日 2 ～ 3 次。肌内注射：一次 100 ～ 200mg，一日 2 次，20 日为一疗程，可用 1 ～ 3 个疗程，每疗程间隔 3 ～ 7 日。静脉滴注：一次 400mg，一日 1 次，用 5% ～ 10% 葡萄糖注射液稀释。<br><br>Por vía oral. 300 mg por cada vez, 2 ~ 3 veces al día. Inyección intramuscular: 100 ~ 200 mg por cada vez, 2 veces al día, 20 días es un curso, es disponible de 1 ~ 3 cursos de tratamiento, entre cada curso hay un intervalo de 3 ~ 7 días. Infusión intravenosa: 400 mg por cada vez, una vez al día, se diluye con la inyección de glucosa al 5% ~ 10%. |
| 剂型、规格<br>Formulaciones y especificaciones | 片剂：每片 100mg。注射液：每支 100mg（2ml）。<br>Tabletas: Cada tableta de 100 mg. Inyección: Cada una de 100 mg (2 ml). |

**续　表**

| 药品名称 Drug Names | 氯贝丁酯 Clofibrato |
|---|---|
| 适应证<br>Indicaciones | 能降低血小板的黏附作用，它能降低血小板对 ADP 和肾上腺素导致聚集的敏感性，并可抑制 ADP 诱导的血小板聚集。它还可延长血小板寿期。可单独应用或与抗凝剂合用于缺血性心脏病的患者。<br><br>Puede reducir la adhesión de las plaquetas, y puede reducir la sensibilidad de plaquetas a ADP y la agregación provocada por la epinefrina, e inhibir la agregación plaquetaria inducida por ADP. También se puede extender el tiempo de vida de la plaqueta. Puede ser utilizado solo o combinado con anticoagulantes para pacientes con cardiopatía isquémica. |
| 用法、用量<br>Administración y dosis | 口服。一日 3 次，一次 0.25 ～ 0.5g。<br>Por vía oral. 3 veces al día, 0.25 ~ 0.5g por cada vez. |
| 剂型、规格<br>Formulaciones y especificaciones | 胶囊：0.25g；0.5g。<br>Cápsulas: 0.25 g; 0.5 g. |

## 14. 主要作用于泌尿系统的药物 Medicamento que actúa principalmente en el sistema urinario

### 14.1　利尿药 Diuréticos

| 药品名称 Drug Names | 呋塞米 Furosemida |
|---|---|
| 适应证<br>Indicaciones | （1）水肿性疾病：包括心脏性水肿、肾性水肿（肾炎、肾病及各种原因所致的急、慢性肾衰竭）、肝硬化腹水、功能障碍或血管障碍所引起的周围性水肿，尤其是应用其他利尿药效果不佳时，应用本品仍可能有效。静脉给药或与其他药物合用，可治疗急性肺水肿和急性脑水肿等。<br>（2）高血压：不作为原发性高血压的首选药，但当噻嗪类药物疗效不佳，尤其当伴有肾功能不全或出现高血压危象时，尤为适用。<br>（3）预防急性肾衰竭：用于各种原因导致的肾脏血流灌注不足，例如失水、休克、中毒、麻醉意外及循环功能不全等，及时应用可减少急性肾小管坏死的机会。<br>（4）高钾血症及高钙血症。<br>（5）抗利尿激素分泌过多症（SIADH）。<br>（6）稀释性低钠血症，尤其时当血钠浓度低于 120mmol/L 时。<br>（7）急性药物中毒：用本品可加速毒物排泄。<br><br>(1) Enfermedad de edemas: incluyen edema cardíaco, edema renal (insuficiencia renal aguda y crónica nefritis, enfermedad renal y por todas las causas), cirrosis hepática, edema periférico causadas por la disfunción o trastornos vasculares, especialmente caundo en aplicaciones de otros diuréticos tienen resultados pobres, con el uso de este producto puede resultar válido. La administración intravenosa o en combinación con otros fármacos, puede tratar el edema pulmonar agudo y el edema cerebral aguda.<br>(2) Hipertensión: no es la primera elección como el medicamento esencial de hipertensión, pero cuando los medicamentos tiofeno tiene pobre eficacia, sobre todo cuando se acompaña de insuficiencia renal o crisis hipertensiva, es particularmente aplicable este medicamento.<br>(3) Prevención de la hipoperfusión del flujo sanguíneo renal provocada por diversas causas, tales como deshidratación, shock, intoxicación, accidentes de anestesia y la insuficiencia circulatoria. Con la aplicación oportuna puede reducir el riesgo de necrosis tubular aguda.<br>(4) Hiperpotasemia e hipercalcemia.<br>(5) Enfermedad de la secreción excesiva de la hormona antidiurética (SIADH).<br>(6) Hiponatremia de dilución, sobre todo cuando la concentración de sodio sérico es inferior a 120 mmol / L.<br>(7) Intoxicación aguda: puede acelerar la velocidad de excreción de toxinas. |
| 用法、用量<br>Administración y dosis | 成人：水肿：①口服，开始一日 20 ～ 40mg，一日 1 ～ 2 次，必要时 6 ～ 8 小时后追加 20 ～ 40mg，直至出现满意的利尿效果。最大剂量虽可达一日 600mg，但一般应控制在 100mg 以下，分 2 ～ 3 次服用。以防过度利尿和发生不良反应。部分患者剂量可减至 20 ～ 40mg，隔日 1 次，或 1 周中连续服药 2 ～ 4 日，一日 20 ～ 40mg。②肌内注射或静脉注射，一次 20 ～ 40mg，隔日一次，根据需要亦可一日 1 ～ 2 次，必要时可每 2 小时追加剂量。一日量视需要可增至 120mg。静脉注射宜用氯化钠注射液稀释后缓慢注射，不宜与其他药物混合。 |

|  | Adultos: Edema: ① Por vía oral. Al inicio, 20 ~ 40 mg al día, 1 ~ 2 veces por cada día, si es necesario, toma una dosis adicional de 20 ~ 40 mg después de6 a 8 horas, hasta que haya un efecto diurético satisfactoria. La dosis máxima diaria puede ser 600 mg, pero en general debería ser controlada debajo de 100 mg, 2 ~ 3 veces al día para evitar la aparición de reacciones adversas y micción excesiva. Para algunos pacientes, la dosis se puede reducir a 20 ~ 40 mg al día, una vez por cada dos días, o toma la medicación de 2 ~ 4 veces continuas dentro de una semana, 20 ~ 40 mg al día. ② Inyección intramuscular o intravenosa, 20 ~ 40mg por cada vez, una vez por cada dos días, si es necesario también los días 1 o 2 veces, si es necesario,puede ser 1 ~ 2 veces al día, y puede agregar la dosis por cada 2 horas. La dosis diaraia se puede aumentar hasta 120mg cuando sea necesario. Para la inyección intravenosa lenta se prefiere la inyección de cloruro de sodio diluido, sin mezclar con otras drogas. |
|---|---|
| 剂型、规格<br>Formulaciones y especificaciones | 片剂：每片20mg。注射液：每支20mg（2ml）。<br>Tabletas: Cada tableta de 20mg. Inyección: Cada una de 20 mg (2 ml). |
| **药品名称Drug Names** | 布美他尼 Bumetanida |
| 适应证<br>Indicaciones | （1）水肿性疾病：包括心脏性水肿、肾性水肿（肾炎、肾病及各种原因所致的急、慢性肾衰竭）、肝硬化腹水、功能障碍或血管障碍所引起的周围性水肿，尤其是应用其他利尿药效果不佳时，应用本品仍可能有效。静脉给药或与其他药物合用，可治疗急性肺水肿和急性脑水肿等。<br>（2）高血压：不作为原发性高血压的首选药，但当噻嗪类药物疗效不佳，尤其当伴有肾功能不全或出现高血压危象时，尤为适用。<br>（3）预防急性肾衰竭：用于各种原因导致的肾脏血流灌注不足，例如失水、休克、中毒、麻醉意外及循环功能不全等，及时应用可减少急性肾小管坏死的机会。<br>（4）高钾血症及高钙血症。<br>（5）抗利尿激素分泌过多症（SIADH）。<br>（6）稀释性低钠血症，尤其时当血钠浓度低于120mmol/L时。<br>（7）急性药物中毒：用本品可加速毒物排泄。<br>(1) Enfermedad de edemas: incluyen edema cardíaco, edema renal (insuficiencia renal aguda y crónica nefritis, enfermedad renal y por todas las causas), cirrosis hepática, edema periférico causadas por la disfunción o trastornos vasculares, especialmente caundo en aplicaciones de otros diuréticos tienen resultados pobres, con el uso de este producto puede resultar válido. La administración intravenosa o en combinación con otros fármacos, puede tratar el edema pulmonar agudo y el edema cerebral aguda.<br>(2) Hipertensión: no es la primera elección como el medicamento esencial de hipertensión, pero cuando los medicamentos tiofeno tiene pobre eficacia, sobre todo cuando se acompaña de insuficiencia renal o crisis hipertensiva, es particularmente aplicable este medicamento.<br>(3) Prevención de la hipoperfusión del flujo sanguíneo renal provocada por diversas causas, tales como deshidratación, shock, intoxicación, accidentes de anestesia y la insuficiencia circulatoria. Con la aplicación oportuna puede reducir el riesgo de necrosis tubular aguda.<br>(4) Hiperpotasemia e hipercalcemia.<br>(5) Enfermedad de la secreción excesiva de la hormona antidiurética (SIADH).<br>(6) Hiponatremia de dilución, sobre todo cuando la concentración de sodio sérico es inferior a 120 mmol / L.<br>(7) Intoxicación aguda: puede acelerar la velocidad de excreción de toxinas. |
| 用法、用量<br>Administración y dosis | （1）成人：①水肿：口服，一次0.5～2mg，一日1次，必要时可一日2～3次，总量有时可高达一日10mg；肌内或静脉注射，起始0.5～1mg，必要时每隔2～3小时重复，最大剂量为一日10mg。②急性肺水肿及左心衰：将本品2～5mg加入500ml氯化钠注射液中静脉滴注，30～60分钟滴完。也可肌内注射或静脉注射，一次1～2mg，必要时间隔20分钟再给药1次。<br>（2）儿童：口服，一次0.01～0.02mg/kg，必要时4～6小时1次；肌内或静脉注射：剂量同口服。<br>(1) Adultos: ① Edema: Por vía oral, 0.5 ~ 2 mg por cada vez, una vez al día. Si es necesario, puede ser 2 ~ 3 veces al día, a veces la dosis total puede ser de 10 mg al día; Inyección intramuscular o intravenosa, la dosis inicial es de 0.5 ~ 1 mg, si es necesario, repete por cada 2 ~ 3 horas, la dosis máxima de 10 mg al día. ② Edema aguda pulmonar e insuficiencia ventricular izquierda: Utilice 2 ~ 5 mg de este producto en la inyección de cloruro de sodio de 500ml para la infusión intravenosa, y termina el goteo dentro de 30 ~ 60 minutos. Puede hacer la inyección intramuscular o inyección intravenosa, 1~ 2 mg por cada vez, con un intervalo necesario de 20 minutos para dar el medicamento otra vez.<br>(2) Para niños: Por vía oral, 0.01 ~ 0.02 mg por cada vez, si es necesario,una vez por cada 4 ~ 6 horas; Hace la inyección intramuscular o intravenosa: Toma la misma dosis por vía oral. |

续　表

| 剂型、规格<br>Formulaciones y<br>especificaciones | 片剂：每片 1mg。注射液：每支 0.5mg（2ml）。<br>Tabletas: Cada tableta de 1mg. Inyección: Cada inyección de 0.5 mg (2 ml). |
|---|---|
| 药品名称Drug Names | 托拉塞米 Torasemida |
| 适应证<br>Indicaciones | ①各种原因所致水肿：如，由于原发或继发性肾脏疾病及何种原因所致急、慢性肾衰竭、充血性心力衰竭，以及肝硬化等所致的水肿；与其他药合用治疗急性脑水肿等。②急、慢性心力衰竭。③原发或继发性高血压。④急、慢性肾衰竭，本品可增加尿量，促进尿钠排出。⑤肝硬化腹水。⑥急性毒物或药物中毒。本品通过强效、迅速的利尿作用，配合充分的液体补充，不仅可以加速毒性物质和药物的排泄，而且由于其肾脏保护作用，还可减轻有毒物质对近曲小管上皮细胞的损害。<br><br>① Edema causada por diversas razones: por ejemplo, edema debido a la enfermedad de riñón primaria o secundaria y insuficiencia renal aguda y crónica de alguna causa, insuficiencia cardiaca congestiva, y cirrosis hepática; terapia de combinación con otros fármacos edema cerebral aguda. ② Insuficiencia cardíaca aguda y crónica. ③ Hipertensión primaria o secundaria. ④ Insuficiencia renal aguda y crónica, el uso de este producto se puede aumentar la producción de orina, promover la excreción de sodio en orina. ⑤ Cirrosis hepática. ⑥ Venenos agudos o envenenamiento. A través de efecto diurético potente y rápido, con reposición de líquidos adecuada, este medicamento no sólo puede acelerar la excreción de sustancias tóxicas y estupefacientes, sino también tiene efecto protector renal, para mitigar los daños de las sustancias tóxicas en los túbulos proximales células epiteliales. |
| 用法、用量<br>Administración y<br>dosis | （1）心力衰竭：口服或静脉注射（用 5% 葡萄糖注射液或氯化钠注射液稀释），初始剂量一般为一次 5～10mg，一日 1 次，递增至一次 10～20mg，一日 1 次。<br>（2）急性或慢性肾衰竭：口服，开始 5mg，可增加至 20mg，均为一日 1 次。需要时可静脉注射，一次 10～20mg，一日 1 次。必要时可由初始剂量逐渐增加为每日 100～200mg。<br>（3）肝硬化腹水：口服，开始 5～10mg，一日 1 次；以后可增加至一次 20mg，一日 1 次，但最多不超过 40mg。静脉注射同口服，一日剂量不超过 40mg。<br>（4）高血压：口服，开始每日 2.5mg 或 5mg，需要时可增至每日 10mg，单用或与其他降压药合用。<br><br>(1) Insuficiencia cardíaca: Por vía oral o inyección intravenosa (con inyección de dextrosa al 5% o inyección de sodio dilución cloruro para diluir), generalmente la dosis inicial es de 5～10mg por cada vez, una vez al día, se puede incrementar gradualmente a 10～20 mg por cada vez, una vez al día.<br>(2) Insuficiencia renal aguda o crónica: Por vía oral, la dosis inicial es de 5mg, puede aumentar a 20 mg, una vez al día. Cuando sea necesario, puede hacer la inyección intravenosa, 10～20 mg por cada vez, una vez al día. Cuando es necesario, la dosis inicial puede incrementarse gradualmente a 100～200 mg al día.<br>(3) Cirrosis hepática: Por vía oral. La dosis inicial es de 5～10 mg, una vez al día, y posteriormente puede aumentar a 20 mg por cada vez, una vez al día, pero la dosis máxima no debe ser más de 40 mg. Inyección intravenosa con dosis por vía oral, la dosis diaria no exceda de 40 mg.<br>(4) Hipertensión: Por vía oral, la dosis inicial es de 2,5 mg o 5 mg al día, Cuando sea necesario, puede aumentar hasta 10 mg al día, se usa solo o en combinación con otros fármacos antihipertensivos. |
| 剂型、规格<br>Formulaciones y<br>especificaciones | 片剂：每片 2.5mg；5mg；10mg；20mg。注射液：每支 10mg（1ml）；20mg（2ml）。<br>Tabletas: Cada tableta de 2.5 mg; 5mg; 10mg; 20mg. Inyección: Cada inyección de 10 mg (1 ml), 20 mg (2 ml). |
| 药品名称Drug Names | 氢氯噻嗪 Hidroclorotiazida |
| 适应证<br>Indicaciones | （1）各种水肿性疾病：排泄体内过多的钠和水，减少细胞外液容量，消除水肿。常见的适应证包括充血性心力衰竭、肝硬化腹水、肾病综合征、急慢性肾炎水肿、慢性肾衰竭早期、肾上腺皮质激素和雌激素治疗所致的钠、水潴留。<br>（2）高血压：可单独或与其他降压药联合应用，主要用于治疗原发性高血压。<br>（3）肾性尿崩症、中枢性尿崩症：单独用于肾性尿崩症，与其他抗利尿剂联合亦可用于中枢性尿崩症。<br>（4）肾结石：主要用于预防含钙成分形成的结石。 |

**续　表**

| | |
|---|---|
| | (1) Enfermedades de edema de diversos tipos: puede excretar el exceso de sodio y agua en el cuerpo para la reducción de volumen de fluido extracelular, eliminar el edema. Las indicaciones comunes incluyen insuficiencia cardíaca congestiva, cirrosis, síndrome nefrótico, edema causado por nefritis aguda y crónica, insuficiencia renal crónica temprana, hormona adrenocorticotrópica y estrógeno terapia de retención de sodio y agua.<br>(2) Hipertensión: se puede utilizar solo o en combinación con otros fármacos antihipertensivos, sobre todo para el tratamiento de la hipertensión esencial.<br>(3) Insípida nefrogénica la diabetes, la diabetes insípida central: se usa solo para la diabetes insípida nefrogénica. En combinación con otros medicamentos anti-diurético puede ser utilizado para la diabetes insípida central.<br>(4) Piedras en el riñón: principalmente se utiliza para prevenir la formación de piedra de cálculos de calcio. |
| 用法、用量<br>Administración y dosis | 成人口服：①治疗水肿性疾病：一次 25 ～ 50mg，一日 1 ～ 2 次，或隔日治疗，或每周连服 3 ～ 5 日。为预防电解质紊乱及血容量骤降，宜从小剂量（12.5 ～ 25mg/d）用起，以后根据利尿情况逐渐加重。②心源性水肿：开始用小剂量，一日 12.5 ～ 25mg，以免因盐及水分排泄过快而引起循环障碍或其他症状；同时注意调整洋地黄用量，以免由于钾的丢失而导致洋地黄中毒。③肝性腹水：最好与螺内酯合用，以防血钾过低诱发肝性脑病。④高血压：常与其他药合用，可减少后者剂量，减少不良反应。开始一日 50 ～ 100mg，分 1 ～ 2 次服用，并按降压效果调整剂量，1 周后为每日 25 ～ 50mg 的维持量。⑤尿崩症：成人口服：一次 25mg，一日 3 次；或一次 50mg，一日 2 次。<br><br>儿童口服：一日按体重 1 ～ 2mg/kg，或按体表面积 30 ～ 60mg/m2，分 1 ～ 2 次服用，并按疗效调整剂量。小于 6 个月的婴儿，剂量可达一日 3mg/kg。<br><br>Para adultos: por vía oral: ① tratamiento de la enfermedad del edema : 25 ~ 50 mg por cada vez , 2 veces al día , o tratamiento por cada dos días, 3 ~ 5 días continuos en una semana. Para evitar el desequilibrio electrolítico y la caída del volumen de sangre , debería empezar por dosis pequeña ( 12.5 ~ 25 mg / d ), y posteriormente se aumenta gradualmente de acuerdo a la situación diurético. ② Edema cardiogénico: debe comenzar con una dosis pequeña , 12.5 ~ 25 mg al día , a fin de evitar los trastornos circulatorios o otros síntomas causados por la excreción exceso de sal y de agua; teniendo cuidado de ajustar la dosis de la digital , con el fin de evitar la toxicidad digitalis causada por la pérdida de potasio. ③ Ascitis de hígado : Es mejor se usa en combinación con espirolactona para prevenir la encefalopatía hepática inducida por la hipocaliemia. ④ Hipertensión : Se usa a menudo en combinación con otros fármacos , que pueden reducir la dosis para aliviar las reacciones adversas . Al inicio, 50 ~ 100 mg al día, dividida en 1 ~ 2 veces, y luego ajuste la dosis de acuerdo con el efecto antihipertensivo , después de una semana, la dosis diaria de mantenimiento es de 25 ~ 50 mg. ⑤ Insípida : Para adultos por vía oral.: 25 mg por cada vez, 3 veces al día, o 50 mg por cada vez, 2 veces al día .<br><br>Para niños, por vía oral: de acuerdo al peso es de 1 - 2mg/kg al día o de acuerdo a la superficie corporal es de 30 ~ 60mg/ m² , dividida en 1 ~ 2 veces al día, se ajuste la dosis de acuerdo con la eficacia. Para los bebés menores de seis meses, la dosis puede alcanzar a 3mg/kg al día. |
| 剂型、规格<br>Formulaciones y especificaciones | 片剂：每片 10mg；25mg；50mg。<br>Tabletas: Cada tableta de 10 mg; 25 mg; 50 mg. |
| **药品名称 Drug Names** | 吲达帕胺 Indapamida |
| 适应证<br>Indicaciones | 作用与氢氯噻嗪相似，但比后者利尿作用强 10 倍。可用于慢性肾衰竭。<br>Su función es similar con la hidroclorotiazida, pero su efecto diurético es 10 veces fuerte que el último. Puede ser utilizado en la insuficiencia renal crónica. |
| 用法、用量<br>Administración y dosis | 水肿，口服，一次 2.5mg，必要时 5mg，一日 1 次；降压，一次 2.5mg，一日 1 次，维持量可每 2 日 2.5 ～ 5mg。<br>Edema, por vía oral, 2.5 mg por una vez, cuando sea necesario, 5mg, una vez al día; Reducción de presión arterial, 2.5mg por una vez, una vez al día, la dosis de mantenimiento es de 2.5 ~ 5mg por cada dos días. |
| 剂型、规格<br>Formulaciones y especificaciones | 片剂：2.5mg。<br>Tabletas: 2.5mg. |

| 续　表 | |
|---|---|
| **药品名称 Drug Names** | 螺内酯 Espironolactona |
| 适应证<br>Indicaciones | ①治疗与醛固酮升高有关的顽固性水肿，故对肝硬化和肾病综合征的患者较有效，而对充血性心力衰竭效果较差（除非因缺钠而引起的继发性醛固酮增多者外）。也可用于特发性水肿的治疗。单用本品时利尿效果往往较差，故常与噻嗪类、髓袢利尿药合用，既能增强利尿效果，又可防止低血钾。②治疗高血压，可作为原发性或继发性高血压的辅助用药，尤其是应用于有排钾离子作用的利尿药时。③原发性醛固酮增多症的诊断与治疗。④低钾血症的预防，与噻嗪类利尿药合用，增强利尿效果并预防低钾血症。<br><br>① Tratamiento del edema refractario relacionado con la elevación de aldosterona, por lo tanto es más eficaz para los pacientes con cirrosis y síndrome nefrótico y es menos eficaz para la insuficiencia cardíaca congestiva (excepto para los pacientes con el aumento de aldosteronismo secundario causado por la falta de sodio). También se puede utilizar para el tratamiento del edema idiopático. Con el uso individual, el efecto diurético es a menudo pobre, por lo tanto, a menudo se usa en combinación con una tiazida, diuréticos de asa, para mejorar el efecto diurético, y también para evitar la hipopotasemia. ② Tratamiento de la hipertensión, puede ser utilizado como medicamento adyuvante de hipertensión primaria o secundaria, especialmente cuando se aplica con diuréticos que tienen papel de la excreción de potasio. ③ diagnóstico y tratamiento de la enfermedad de aldosteronismo primario. ④ Puede prevenir la hipocalemia, y se usa en combinación con los diuréticos tiazídicos y fortalecer el efecto diurético y prevenir la hipocaliemia. |
| 用法、用量<br>Administración y<br>dosis | 成人口服。①治疗水肿：一次 20～40mg，一日 3 次。用药 5 日后，如疗效满意，继续用原量。②治疗高血压：开始一日 40～80mg，分 2～4 次服用，至少 2 周，以后酌情调整剂量。本品不宜与血管紧张素转换酶抑制剂合用，以免增加发生高钾血症的机会。③治疗原发性醛固酮增多症：手术前患者一日用量 100～400mg，分 2～4 次服用。不宜手术的患者，则选用较小剂量维持。④诊断原发性醛固酮增多症：长期试验，一日 400mg，分 2～4 次服用，连续 3～4 周。短期试验，一日 400mg，分 2～4 次服用，连续 4 日。老年人对本药较敏感，开始用量宜偏小。<br>儿童口服，治疗水肿性疾病，开始一日按体重 1～3mg/kg 或按体表面积 30～90mg/m²，单次或分 2～4 次服用，连用 5 日后酌情调整剂量。最大剂量一日 3～9mg/kg 或 90～270mg/m²。<br><br>Para adultos por vía oral.. ① Tratamiento del edema: 20～40 mg por cada vez, 3 veces al día. Con 5 días de tratamiento, si los resultados son satisfactorios, siguen utilizando la cantidad original. ② Tratamiento de la hipertensión: Al inicio, 40～80 mg por cada día, dividida en 2～4 veces al día, dura por lo menos dos semanas, y después, puede ajustar la dosis según la situación. Este producto no debe ser utilizado en combinación con un inhibidor de la enzima convertidora de la angiotensina, para evitar el aumento de la probabilidad de hiperpotasemia. ③ Tratamiento de aldosteronismo primario: Se usa para los pacientes antes de la cirugía, la dosis diaria es de 100～400 mg, dividida en 2～4 veces al día. Los pacientes que no es conveniente para la cirugía, debe utilizar una dosis de cantidad menor para su mantenimiento. ④ Diagnóstico de aldosteronismo primario: Para prueba a largo plazo, 400 mg al día, dividida en 2～4 veces al día dura 3～4 semanas. Para prueba a corto plazo, 400 mg al día, 2～4 veces al día, dura cuatro días consecutivos. Las personas de edad avanzada son más sensibles al fármaco, la dosis debe empezar poco a poco.<br>Para tratamiento oral de los niños de la enfermedad edema, que comienza de acuerdo con el peso de 1～3mg/kg o superficie corporal de 30～90 mg / m², de una sola vez o dividida en 2～4 veces al día, con el uso de 5 días consecutivos, puede ajustar la dosis. La dosis máxima diaria es de 3～9mg/kg o 90～270 mg / m². |
| 剂型、规格<br>Formulaciones y<br>especificaciones | 片剂：每片 20mg。胶囊剂：每粒 20mg（微粒制剂 20mg 与普通制剂 100mg 的疗效相仿）。<br>Tabletas: Cada tableta de 20mg. Cápsulas: Cada cápsula de 20 mg (formulación de 20 mg y la eficacia de las partículas ordinarias formulación de 100 mg es similar). |
| **药品名称 Drug Names** | 氨苯蝶啶 Triamtereno |
| 适应证<br>Indicaciones | 用于治疗各类水肿，如心力衰竭、肝硬化及慢性肾炎引起的水肿或腹水，以及糖皮质激素治疗过程中发生的水钠潴留。常与排钾利尿药合用。亦用于对氢氯噻嗪或螺内酯无效的病例。<br><br>Se usa para el tratamiento de diversos tipos de edema, tales como el edema o ascitis inducida por la insuficiencia cardiaca, cirrosis y nefritis crónica, y la retención de sodio que se producen proceso de tratamiento con glucocorticoides. A menudo se usa en combinación con diuréticos de excreción de potasio. También se utiliza en los casos que la hidroclorotiazida o espironolactona son inválidas. |

| | |
|---|---|
| 用法、用量<br>Administración y dosis | 口服，成人，开始一次 25～50mg，一日 2 次，餐后服，最大剂量每日不宜超过 300mg。维持阶段可改为隔日疗法。与其他利尿剂合用时，两者均应减量。儿童，开始一日按体重 2～4mg/kg 或按体表面积 120mg/m²，分 2 次服，每日或隔日疗法。以后酌情调整剂量。最大剂量不超过每日 6mg/kg 或 300mg/m²。<br><br>Por vía oral., para adultos, al inicio es de 25 ~ 50 mg por cada vez, 2 veces al día, se toma después de la comida, la dosis máxima diaria no debe exceder de 300 mg. En la fase de mantenimiento del tratamiento se puede cambiar por cada dos días. Cuando se combina con otros diuréticos, ambas dosises deben ser reducidas. Para los niños se comienzan de acuerdo con el peso de 2 ~ 4mg/kg o superficie corporal 120 mg / m² al día, dividida en 2 veces para todos los días o cada dos días. Posteriormente puede ajustar la dosis de acuerdo con la situación. La dosis máxima diaria no exceda de 6mg/kg o 300 mg/m². |
| 剂型、规格<br>Formulaciones y especificaciones | 片剂：每片 50mg。<br>Tabletas: Cada tableta de 50mg. |
| 药品名称 Drug Names | 阿米洛利 Amilorida |
| 适应证<br>Indicaciones | 本品同氨苯蝶啶，主要用于治疗水肿性疾病，亦可用于难治性低钾血症的辅助治疗。氨苯蝶啶和螺内酯均大部分经肝脏代谢，当肝功能严重损害时，剂量不易控制，此时则可应用不经肝脏代谢的本品。另外，本品可增加氢氯噻嗪和利尿酸等利尿药的作用，并减少钾的丢失，故一般不单独应用。<br><br>El producto es lo mismo con Triamtereno, principalmente para el tratamiento de la enfermedad del edema, se puede utilizar como tratamiento adyuvante de la hipopotasemia refractario. El triamtereno y espironolactona se metabolizan principalmente en el hígado, caundo hay daño hepático severo, la dosis es difícil de controlar, entonces puede aplicar este producto que no es metabolismo hepático. Además, este producto puede aumentar los efectos diuréticos de hidroclorotiazida y ácido úrico, y reducir la pérdida de potasio, por lo tanto, generalmente, no se aplica individualmente. |
| 用法、用量<br>Administración y dosis | 口服：开始一次 2.5～5mg，一日 1 次；必要时可增加剂量，但每日不宜超过 20mg。<br><br>Por vía oral: al inicio es 2.5 ~ 5 mg por una vez, una vez al día; Puede aumentar la dosis, si es necesario, pero la dosis diaria no puede ser más de 20 mg. |
| 剂型、规格<br>Formulaciones y especificaciones | 片剂：每片含 2.5mg；5mg。<br>Tabletas: Cada tableta contiene 2.5 mg; 5mg. |
| 药品名称 Drug Names | 乙酰唑胺 Acetazolamida |
| 适应证<br>Indicaciones | 用于治疗青光眼、心脏性水肿、脑水肿，亦用于癫痫小发作。<br><br>Se usa para el tratamiento de glaucoma, edema cardíaco, edema cerebral, sino también para las convulsiones. |
| 用法、用量<br>Administración y dosis | （1）青光眼：一般口服给药，①开角型青光眼，首量 0.25g，一日 1～3 次。维持剂量根据患者对药物的反应而定，尽量适用较小剂量使眼压得到控制，一般 1 次 0.25g，一日 2 次就可使眼压控制在正常范围。②继发性青光眼和手术前降眼压，一次 0.25g，一般一日 2～3 次。③闭角型青光眼急性发作，首次 0.5g，以后一次 0.125～0.25g，一日 2～3 次维持。④青光眼急性发作时的抢救或某些恶心、呕吐不能口服的患者，可静脉或肌内注射本品。将本品 0.5g 溶于 5～10ml 灭菌注射用水静脉注射，或溶于 2.5ml 灭菌注射用水肌内注射；也可静脉注射 0.25g 或肌内注射 0.25g 交替使用。对于一些急性发作的青光眼患者，可在 2～4 小时重复上述剂量，但继续治疗应根据患者情况改为口服给药。<br>（2）脑水肿：口服，一次 0.25g，一日 2～3 次。<br>（3）心源性水肿：口服，一次 0.25～0.5g，一日 1 次，早餐后服用药效最佳。<br>（4）癫痫小发作：其作用可能与抑制脑组织中的碳酸酐酶有关。口服，一次 0.5～1g，一日 1 次。与其他药物合用时则不超过 0.25g。儿童：①青光眼：口服，一日 5～10mg/kg，分 2～3 次服用；②青光眼急性发作：静脉或肌内注射，一次 5～10mg/kg，每 6 小时 1 次。 |

续　表

(1) Glaucoma: La administración en general es por vía oral. ① Glaucoma de ángulo abierto, la primera dosis es de 0.25g, 1 ~ 3 veces al día. La dosis de mantenimiento puede ser ajustada según la respuesta del paciente a los fármacos. Trata de aplicar una dosis menor para el control de la presión intraocular, por lo general es 0.25 g por cada vez, dos veces al día puede controlar la presión intraocular en el rango normal. ② Glaucoma secundario y hipotensor ocular antes de la cirugía, 0.25 g por una vez, en general 2 ~ 3 veces al día. ③ Ataque agudo de glaucoma de ángulo cerrado, la primera dosis es de 0.5g, y después 0.125 ~ 0.25 g por cada vez, 2 ~ 3 veces al día para mantener. ④ Para los pacientes en salvamento o náuseas durante el ataque del glaucoma agudo, que vomita y no puede tomar por vía oral, puede hacer inyección intravenosa o intramuscular de este producto. 0.5 g de este producto se disuelve en 5 ~ 10 ml de agua estéril para inyección por vía intravenosa, se disuelve en 2.5 ml de agua estéril para inyección intramuscular; y puede hacer inyección intravenosa de 0.25 g o inyección intramuscular de 0.25 g de manera intercambiable. Para algunos pacientes con ataque agudo de glaucoma, se puede repetir la dosis dentro de dos - cuatro horas, pero la continuación del tratamiento debe ser cambiado para administración oral de acuerdo con la condición del paciente.

(2) Edema cerebral: Por vía oral, 0.25 g por una vez, 2 ~ 3 veces al día.

(3) Edema cardiogénico: Por vía oral, 0.25 ~ 0.5 g por una vez, una vez al día. El efecto es mejor cuando se toma después del desayuno.

(4) Convulsiones: su papel puede estar relacionado con la anhidrasa carbónica en la inhibición de tejido cerebral. Por vía oral, 0.5 ~ 1g por una vez, una vez al día. Cuando se combina con otros fármacos no debe ser más de 0.25 g. Para niños: ① Glaucoma: por vía oral, 5 ~ 10mg/kg al día, dividida en 2 ~ 3 veces; ② Glaucoma agudo: Inyección intravenosa o intramuscular, 5 ~ 10mg/kg por una vez, una vez por cada 6 horas.

| | |
|---|---|
| 剂型、规格<br>Formulaciones y especificaciones | 片剂：每片 0.25g。注射用乙酰唑胺：每支 500mg。<br>Tabletas: Cada tableta 0.25g. La acetazolamida inyectable: Cada una de 500mg. |

14.2　脱水药 Drogas para deshidratación

| 药品名称 Drug Names | 甘露醇 Manitol |
|---|---|
| 适应证<br>Indicaciones | ①治疗各种原因引起的脑水肿，降低颅内压，防止脑疝；②降低眼压；当在应用其他降眼压药无效或青光眼的术前准备时应用；③预防急性肾小管坏死：在大面积烧伤、严重创伤、广泛外科手术时，常因肾小球滤过率降低及血容量减少而出现少尿、无尿，极易发生肾衰竭，应及时用本品预防；④作为其他利尿药的辅助药，治疗某些伴有低钠血症的顽固性水肿（因本品排水多于排钠，故不适用于全身性水肿的治疗）；⑤鉴别肾前性因素或急性肾衰竭引起的少尿；⑥对于某些药物过量或毒物引起的重度，可促进上述物质的排泄，防止肾毒性；⑦术前肠道准备；⑧作清洗剂，应用于经尿道内做前列腺切除术。<br><br>① Tratamiento del edema cerebral causado por varias razones,reducción de la presión intracraneal, prevención de la hernia; ② Reducir la presión intraocular: Cuando la aplicación de otras drogas de presión intraocular no es válida o antes de la cirugía de glaucoma; ③ Prevención de la necrosis tubular aguda: En las cirugías de las quemaduras de grandes áreas, un trauma severo, cirugía extensa, a menudo debido a la reducción de la tasa de filtración glomerular y la hipovolemia y oliguria, anuria, puede ocurrir fácilmente la insuficiencia renal, es oportuno el uso de este producto para la prevención; ④ Como fármacos adyuvantes de otros diuréticos, puede tratar el edema refractario asociada con hiponatremia (debido a que este producto puede eliminar más agua que el sodio, por lo tanto no es aplicable para el tratamiento de edema generalizado); ⑤ Identificación de oliguria causada por factores prerrenales o insuficiencia renal aguda; ⑥ Su usa para el envenenamiento causado por la sobredosis severa de ciertos medicamentos o venenos, puede promover la excreción de las sustancias para prevenir la toxicidad renal; ⑦ preparación intestinal preoperatoria; ⑧ se usa como agentes de limpieza, que es aplicable para la resección transuretral de la próstata. |
| 用法、用量<br>Administración y dosis | （1）利尿：静脉滴注，按体重 1 ~ 2g/kg，一般为 20% 溶液 250 ~ 500ml，并调整剂量使尿量维持在每小时 30 ~ 50ml。<br>（2）脑水肿、颅内高压和青光眼：静脉滴注，按体重 1.5 ~ 2g/kg，配成 15% ~ 20% 浓度于 30 ~ 60 分钟滴完（当患者衰弱时，剂量可减为 0.5g/kg）。<br>（3）预防急性肾小管坏死：先给予 12.5 ~ 25g，10 分钟内静脉滴注，若无特殊情况，再给 50g，1 小时内静脉滴注，若尿量能维持在每小时 50ml 以上，则可继续应用 5% 溶液静滴；若无效则立即停药。同时需注意补足血容量。 |

|  | （4）鉴别肾前性少尿和肾性少尿：按体重 0.2g/kg，以 20% 浓度于 3 ～ 5 分钟静脉滴注。如用药 2 ～ 3 小时以后尿量仍低于 30 ～ 50ml/h，最多再试用一次，若仍无反应则应停药。心功能减退或心力衰竭者，慎用或不宜使用。<br><br>（5）药物或毒物中毒：50g 以 20% 溶液静脉滴注，调整剂量使尿量维持在每小时 100 ～ 500ml。<br><br>（6）术前肠道准备：口服，于术前 4 ～ 8 小时以 10% 溶液 1000ml 于 30 分钟内口服完毕。<br><br>(1) Diurético: Infusión intravenosa, de acuerdo con el peso 1 ~ 2g/kg, en general, es solución al 20% de 250 ~ 500 ml, y puede ajustar la dosis para que la orina se mantiene a 30 ~ 50 ml por hora.<br><br>(2) Edema cerebral, hipertensión intracraneal y glaucoma: Infusión intravenosa, de acuerdo con el peso 1.5 ~ 2g/kg, denominado la concentración de 15% a 20% dentro de 30 a 60 minutos para terminar el goteo (cuando el paciente es débil, la dosis se puede reducir a 0,5 g / kg).<br><br>(3) Prevención de la necrosis tubular aguda: primero se ofrece 12.5 ~ 25 g, dentro de 10 minutos hace la infusión intravenosa, si no hay circunstancias excepcionales, ofrece otra vez de 50 g, dentro de 1 hora hace la infusión intravenosa, si la orina se puede mantener a 50 ml por hora o más, puede continuar la aplicación de una solución al 5% por vía intravenosa; Si no es válido, puede inmediatamente suspenderlo. Al mismo tiempo, es necesario prestar atención a completar el volumen de sangre.<br><br>(4) Identificación prerrenal oliguria y oliguria renal: de acuerdo con el peso es de 0.2g/kg, por una concentración de 20% y hace la infusión intravenosa dentro de 3 ~ 5 minutos. Si después de 2 ~ 3 horas del uso del medicamento, la orina es todavía inferior a 30 ~ 50 ml / h, puede volver a intentarlo, si sigue sin haber respuesta debe ser interrumpido. Para pacientes con la disfunción cardíaca o insuficiencia cardíaca, se deben usar con precaución o no usarlo.<br><br>(5) Envenenamiento de drogas o tóxico: 50g de solución al 20% por vía intravenosa, puede ajustar la dosis para mantener la orina en 100 ~ 500 ml por hora.<br><br>(6) Preparación del intestino antes de la cirugía: por vía oral, 4 ~ 8 horas antes de la cirugía, use la solución al 10% de 1000ml para tomar por vía oral dentro de 30 minutos. |
|---|---|
| 剂型、规格<br>Formulaciones y especificaciones | 注射液：每瓶 10g（50ml）；20g（100ml）；50g（250ml）；100g（500ml）；150g（3000ml）。<br>Inyección: cada botella de 10g (50 ml), 20 g (100 ml), 50 g (250 ml), 100 g (500 ml), 150g (3000ml). |
| 药品名称 Drug Names | 甘油果糖 Glicerina fructosa |
| 适应证<br>Indicaciones | ①由脑血管疾病、脑外伤、脑肿瘤、颅内炎症及其他原因引起的急、慢性颅内压增高，脑水肿症；②改善下列疾病的意识障碍、神经障碍和自觉症状，如脑梗死（脑栓死、脑血栓）、脑内出血、蛛网膜下腔出血、头部外伤、脑脊髓膜炎等；③脑外科手术术前缩小脑容积；④脑外科手术后降颅内压；⑤青光眼患者降低眼压或眼科手术缩小眼容积。<br><br>① El aumento de la presión intracraneal aguda y crónica, la enfermedad de edema cerebral inducidas por de la enfermedad cerebrovascular, traumatismo cerebral, tumores cerebrales, inflamación cerebral y otras causas; ② Puede mejorar la conciencia, trastornos neurológicos y los síntomas de las siguientes enfermedades, tales como infarto cerebral (perno de muerte cerebral, trombosis cerebral), hemorragia intracerebral, hemorragia subaracnoidea, traumatismo craneal, meningitis, etc; ③ Reducción del volumen del cerebro antes de la cirugía cerebral; ④ Reducción de la presión intracraneal después de la cirugía del cerebro; ⑤ Reducción de la presión intraocular o reducción del volumen de ojos en la cirugía oftálmica ocular para los pacientes con glaucoma. |
| 用法、用量<br>Administración y dosis | 静脉滴注。①治疗颅内压增高、脑水肿：成人一次 250 ～ 500ml，一日 1 ～ 2 次；儿童用量为 5 ～ 10ml/kg。每 500ml 需滴注 2 ～ 3 小时，连续给药 1 ～ 2 周。②脑外科手术时缩小脑容积：一次 500ml，静脉滴注时间为 30 分钟。③降低眼压或眼科手术时缩小眼容积：一次 250 ～ 500ml，静脉滴注时间为 45 ～ 90 分钟。<br><br>Infusión intravenosa. ① Tratamiento de aumento de la presión intracraneal, edema cerebral: la dosis para adultos es de 250 ~ 500 ml por cada vez, 1 ~ 2 veces al día, la dosis para niños es de 5 ~ 10ml/kg. Cada 500 ml necesita 2 ~ 3 horas para la infusión y el suministro de medicamento debe ser 1 ~ 2 semanas de forma continua. ② Reducción del volumen de cerebro durante la cirugía cerebral: 500 ml por cada vez. La infusión intravenosa dura 30 minutos. ③ Reducción de presión intraocular o reducción de volumen de ojos en la cirugía ocular: 250 ~ 500 ml por cada vez, El tiempo de infusión intravenosa es de 45 ~ 90 minutos. |
| 剂型、规格<br>Formulaciones y especificaciones | 注射液：每瓶 250ml；500ml（每 1ml 中含甘油 100mg、果糖 50mg、氯化钠 9mg）。<br>Inyección: cada botella de 250 ml; 500 ml (cada 1 ml contiene 100 mg de glicerol, 50 mg de fructosa, 9 mg de cloruro de sodio). |

**续　表**

### 14.3　治疗尿崩症用药 Medicamentos para el tratamiento de la diabetes insípida

| 药品名称 Drug Names | 鞣酸加压素 Tanina vasopresina |
|---|---|
| 适应证<br>Indicaciones | ①中枢性尿崩症、头部手术或外伤所致的暂时性尿崩症的治疗。②用于中枢性尿崩症、肾性尿崩症的鉴别诊断试验。③食管静脉曲张破裂出血及咯血。<br><br>① Tratamiento de diabetes insípida temporal causado por diabete insípida central, cirugía de cabeza o trauma.　② Prueba para el diagnóstico diferencial de la diabetes insípida central, diabetes insípida nefrogénica. ③ Hemorragia y hemoptisis de ruptura de varices esofágicas. |
| 用法、用量<br>Administración y dosis | （1）中枢性尿崩症：①成人，加压素注射液 3mg 皮下或肌内注射，一日 2 ～ 3 次。②儿童，加压素注射液 1 ～ 1.5mg 皮下或肌内注射，一日 2 ～ 3 次。<br>（2）中枢性尿崩症的诊断：禁水 - 加压素试验时，皮下注射加压素注射液 3mg，继续禁水 2 小时测血和尿渗透压、尿量、尿比重、血压、脉率等。儿童酌情减量。<br>（3）食管静脉曲张破裂出血及咯血：加压素注射液 3mg 稀释后缓慢静脉注射，或 6 ～ 12mg 加入 200 ～ 500ml 的 5% 葡萄糖注射液中缓慢静脉滴注。<br><br>(1) Diabetes insípida central: ① Para adultos, inyección de vasopresina de 3 mg por vía subcutánea o por vía intramuscular, 2 ~ 3 veces al día. ② Para niños, inyección de vasopresina de 1 ~ 1.5 mg por vía subcutánea o por vía intramuscular, 2 ~ 3 veces al día.<br>(2) Diagnóstico de diabetes insípida central: cuando en la prueba de la prohibición de agua – vasopresina, hace la inyección de vasopresina de 3mg por vía subcutánea, continúe prohibir agua por dos horas y examina sangre y orina, la osmolaridad, la producción de orina, la gravedad específica de la orina, presión arterial, frecuencia del pulso, etc . Para niños, puede reducir la dosis apropiadamente.<br>(3) Hemorragia por ruptura de varices esofágicas y hemoptisis: De ser diluida la inyección de vasopresina de 3mg, hace la intravenosa lentamente, o en 6 ~ 12 mg agrega 200 ~ 500 ml de inyección de glucosa goteo al 5% para el intravenoso lento. |
| 剂型、规格<br>Formulaciones y especificaciones | 注射液：每支 6mg（1ml）；12mg（1ml）。<br>Inyección: Cada una de 6 mg (1 ml), 12 mg (1 ml). |
| 药品名称 Drug Names | 垂体后叶粉 Polvo de pituitaria posterior |
| 适应证<br>Indicaciones | 治疗尿崩症。<br>Hay tratamiento para la diabetes insípida. |
| 用法、用量<br>Administración y dosis | 用特制小匙（每匙装量为 30 ～ 40mg）取出本品 1 小匙，以小指头抹在鼻黏膜上；亦可将取出的粉剂倒在纸上，卷成卷纸，用左手压住左鼻孔，用右手将纸卷插入右鼻孔内，抬头轻轻将粉刺吸进鼻腔内。一日 3 ～ 4 次。<br><br>Con una cuchara especial (alrededor de 30 ~ 40 mg por cada cuchara) saca este producto de una cucharadita y con el dedo meñique, lo puso en la mucosa nasal; Se puede colocar el polvo sacado en un papel, y enrolla el papel en un rollo, mantenga pulsada la fosa nasal izquierda con la mano izquierda, y use la mano derecha para rodar el rollo en la fosa nasal derecha, levanta la cabeza para aspirar el acné suavemente en la cavidad nasal. Es de 3 ~ 4 veces al día. |
| 剂型、规格<br>Formulaciones y especificaciones | 鼻吸入粉剂：每瓶 1g（附小匙）。<br>Polvo para inhalación nasal: cada botella de 1 g (con un cucharadita adjuntada). |
| 药品名称 Drug Names | 去氨加压素 Desmopresina |
| 适应证<br>Indicaciones | ①中枢性尿崩症及颅外伤或手术所致的暂时性尿崩症：用后可减少尿排出，增加尿渗透压，减低血浆渗透压，减少尿频和夜尿（一般对肾源性尿崩症无效）。②治疗 5 岁以上患有夜间遗尿症的患者。③肾尿液浓缩功能试验：有助于对肾功能的鉴别，对于诊断不同部位的尿道感染尤其有效。④对于轻度血友病及 I 型血管性血友病患者，在进行小型外科手术时可控制出血或预防出血。⑤因尿毒症、肝硬化及先天的或用药诱发的血小板功能障碍而引起的出血时间过长和不明原因的出血，用本品可使出血时间缩短或恢复正常。 |

| | |
|---|---|
| | ① Diabetes insípida central y diabetes insípida temporal debido al trauma craneal o cirugía: Después de su uso puede reducir la orina, aumentar la osmolaridad urinaria, minimizar la osmolaridad del plasma, reducir la frecuencia urinaria y nocturia (generalmente no es válido para diabetes insípida nefrogénica). ② Tratamiento de la enuresis nocturna para los pacientes mayores de 5 años. ③ Para pruebas de función de concentración de orina del riñón: Puede ayudar a identificar la función renal, particularmente es eficaz para el diagnóstico de las infecciones del tracto urinario en las diferentes partes. ④ Para los pacientes de hemofilia leve y de von Willebrand tipo Ⅰ, pueden controlar el sangrado o prevenir el sangrado durante los procedimientos quirúrgicos. ⑤ Para el sangrado prolongado y sangrado inexplicable causados por uremia, cirrosis y congénito o disfunción plaquetaria inducida por fármacos puede usar este producto para acortar el tiempo de sangrado o recuperar a la normalidad. |
| 用法、用量<br>Administración y<br>dosis | （1）中枢性尿崩症①鼻腔给药：a. 鼻喷剂：成人开始 10μg，睡前喷鼻，以后根据尿量每晚递增 2.5μg，直至获得良好睡眠。b. 成人开始一次 10μg，逐渐调整到最适剂量，一日 3～4 次，儿童用量酌减。②口服：因人而异，区分调整。③静脉注射。<br><br>（2）夜间遗尿症：鼻腔给药或口服。<br><br>（3）肾尿液浓缩功能试验：鼻腔给药或肌内、皮下注射。<br><br>（4）治疗性控制出血或手术前预防出血：静脉滴注。<br><br>(1) Diabetes insípida central ① administración intranasal: a. spray nasal: La dosis inicial para adultos es de 10μg, spray nasal antes de acsotarse, de acuerdo a la cantidad de orina puede incrementar 2.5μg por cada noche, hasta que se consiga una buena noche de sueño. b. La dosis inicial para adultos es de 10μg, y se ajuste gradualmente a la dosis óptima, 3 ~ 4 veces al día. La cantidad de niños puede ser reducida. ② Por vía oral: se varía depende de cada individuo, puede ajustar de acuerdo con las diferencias. ③ Inyección intravenosa.<br>(2) Enuresis nocturna: la administración nasal o por vía oral.<br>(3) Pruebas de función de concentración de orina del riñón: administración intranasal o inyección intramuscular, inyección subcutánea.<br>(4) Control terapéutico de sangrado o prevención de sangrado antes de la cirugía: infusión intravenosa. |
| 剂型、规格<br>Formulaciones y<br>especificaciones | 片剂：每片 100μg；200μg。鼻喷雾剂：每支 250μg（2.5ml，每喷 0.1ml，含 10μg）。滴鼻液：每支 250μg（2.5ml）。注射液：每支 4μg（1ml）。<br><br>Tabletas: Cada tableta de 100 μg; 200μg. Los aerosoles nasales: Cada uno de 250μg (2.5 ml, 0.1 ml por cada aerosol, conteniendo 10μg). Nasal Drops: Cada una de 250μg (2.5 ml). Inyección: Cada una de 4μg (1 ml). |

## 15. 主要作用于生殖系统的药物 Medicamento que actúan princepalmente en el sistema reproducetivo

## 15.1 子宫收缩药及引产药 Medicamentos para la contracción uterina y drogas de aborto

| 药品名称 Drug Names | 垂体后叶素 Pituitrina |
|---|---|
| 适应证<br>Indicaciones | 产后出血、产后子宫复原不全、促进宫缩引产（由于有升高血压作用，现产科已少用）、肺出血、食管及胃底静脉曲张破裂出血和尿崩症等。<br><br>Se usa para la hemorragia posparto, la recuperación incompleta del útero después del parto, promoción de contracciones parto inducido (debido al efecto de aumento de la presión arterial, ahora se usa menos en obstetricia), hemorragia pulmonar, de esófago y la hemorragia de ruptura de varices gástricas y la diabetes insípida. |
| 用法、用量<br>Administración y<br>dosis | （1）一般应用：肌内注射，每次 5～10U。<br>（2）肺出血：可静脉注射或静脉滴注。<br>（3）产后出血：必须在胎儿和胎盘均已分娩出之后方可肌内注射 10U，如作预防性应用，可在胎儿前肩娩出后立即静脉注射 10U。<br>（4）临产阵缩弛缓不正常者（偶亦用于催生，但须谨慎）：将 5～10U 本品以 5% 葡萄糖注射液 500ml 稀释后缓慢静脉滴注，并严密观察宫缩情况，适时调整滴速。<br>（5）尿崩症：肌内注射，常用量为每次 5U，一日 2 次。<br>（6）消化道出血：可用本品静脉滴注，其用量和溶媒同肺出血，每分钟 0.1～0.5U。 |

| 续　表 | |
|---|---|
| | (1) Aplicación General: inyección intramuscular, 5 ~ 10U por cada vez.<br>(2) Hemorragia pulmonar: inyección intravenosa o infusión intravenosa.<br>(3) Hemorragia posparto: después del nacimiento del feto y la placenta puede hacer la inyección intramuscular de 10U. Si es utilizado como las aplicaciones profilácticas, puede hacer la inyección intravenosa de 10U después de la expulsión del feto antes de que el hombro.<br>(4) para los pacientes de contracción de matriz flácida no normal (aunque a veces también se usa para el nacimiento, debe tener mucho cuidado): 5 ~ 10U del producto, de ser diluida en la inyección glucosa al 5% de 500 ml, haga la infusión intravenosa y tenga una observación minuciosa de las contracciones,puede ajustar la velocidad del goteo.<br>(5) Insípida: inyección intramuscular, la dosis habitual 5U por cada vez, 2 veces al día.<br>(6) Sangrado gastrointestinal: Puede hacer la infusión intravenosa de este producto, la cantidad y el medio de disolución es lo mismo con hemorragia pulmonar, 0.1 ~ 0.5U por minuto. |
| 剂型、规格<br>Formulaciones y especificaciones | 注射液：每支 5U（1ml）；10U（1ml）。<br>Inyección: Cada una de 5U (1 ml); 10U (1 ml). |
| 药品名称 Drug Names | 缩宫素 Oxitocina |
| 适应证<br>Indicaciones | 用于引产、催产、产后出血和子宫复原不全；滴鼻用于促排乳；催产素激惹试验。<br>Se usa para la hemorragia de la inducción del trabajo de parto, de la oxitocina, la hemorragia post-parto y la recuperación uterina incompleta; Use secreción nasal para la promoción de la leche; Se usa para la prueba de provocación con oxitocina. |
| 用法、用量<br>Administración y dosis | （1）引产或催产：静脉滴注。<br>（2）防治产后出血或促进子宫复原：将本品 5 ~ 10U 加于 5% 葡萄糖注射液中静脉滴注，每分钟滴注 0.02 ~ 0.04U，胎盘排出后可肌内注射 5 ~ 10U。<br>（3）子宫出血：肌内注射，1 次 5 ~ 10U。肌内注射极量，1 次 20U。<br>（4）催乳：在哺乳前 2 ~ 3 分钟，用滴鼻液，每次 3 滴或少量喷于一侧或双侧鼻孔内。<br>（5）催产素激惹试验：试验剂量同引产，用稀释后的缩宫素作静脉滴注，直到 10 分钟出现 3 次有效宫缩。<br>(1) Inducción o Oxitocina: infusión intravenosa.<br>(2) Prevención de la hemorragia posparto o fortalecimiento de la recuperación del útero: Agrega 5 ~ 10U de este producto en 5% de solución de glucosa por vía intravenosa, infusión de 0.02 ~ 0.04U por minuto, después de sacar la placenta, hace la inyección intramuscular de 5 ~ 10U.<br>(3) Sangrado: inyección intramuscular de 1 5 ~ 10U por una vez. La dosis máxima de inyección intramuscular es de 20U por una vez.<br>(4) Prolactina: 2 ~ 3 minutos antes de la lactancia materna, use gotas nasales, 3 gotas o aerosol de una pequeña cantidad en una o ambas fosas nasales.<br>(5) Prueba de provocación con oxitocina: La dosis de prueba con oxitocina es lo mismo con la inducción, use la oxitocina diluida para hace la infusión intravenosa, hasta que en 10 minutos hay contracciones eficaces de tres veces. |
| 剂型、规格<br>Formulaciones y especificaciones | 注射液：每支 2.5U（0.5ml）；5U（1ml）；10U（1ml）。滴鼻液：每支 40U（1ml）。鼻喷雾剂：每瓶 200U（5ml）（每喷 0.1ml，相当于 4U）。<br>Inyección: Cada de 2.5 U (0.5 ml); 5U (1 ml); 10U (1 ml). Nasal Drops: Cada de 40U (1 ml). Los aerosoles nasales: cada botella de 200U (5 ml) (0.1 ml por pulverización, equivalente a 4U). |
| 药品名称 Drug Names | 米非司酮 Mifepristona |
| 适应证<br>Indicaciones | 本品除用于抗早孕、催经止孕外,尚可用于中期妊娠引产（与前列腺素合用）、死胎引产、扩宫颈。<br>Este producto se utiliza, además de anti-embarazo, recordatorios de terminar el embarazo, se puede utilizar para aborto trimestre (combinado con prostaglandina), muerte fetal, aborto, la expansión del cuello uterino. |
| 用法、用量<br>Administración y dosis | （1）中期妊娠引产（在妊娠 13 ~ 24 周用人工方法终止妊娠）①与米索前列醇配伍；②与卡前列甲酯配伍。<br>（2）宫内死胎引产：口服，一次 200mg，一日 2 次或每日 1 次 400 ~ 600mg，连服 2 日，一般在 72 小时后排出死胎。 |

|  | （3）扩宫颈：口服，1 次 100 ～ 200mg。宫内手术前软化和扩张宫颈：于术前 48 小时口服 600mg。<br><br>(1) Aborto trimestre (embarazo entre 13 ~ 24 semanas, haga la interrupción del embarazo por métodos artificiales) ① se combina con Misoprostol; ② se combina con metilo y carboprost.<br>(2) Inducción de muerte fetal intrauterino: por vía oral, 200 mg por una vez, 2 veces al día o una vez de 400 ~ 600 mg al día, toma dos días consecutivos, por lo general en después de 72 horas descarga el feto muerto.<br>(3) Expansión del cuello uterino: por vía oral, 100 ~ 200 mg por una vez. Ablandamiento y dilatación del cuello uterino antes de la cirugía intrauterina: 48 horas antes de la cirugía toma 600 mg por vía oral |
|---|---|
| 剂型、规格<br>Formulaciones y especificaciones | 片剂：每片 25mg；200mg。<br>Tabletas: Cada tableta de 25mg; 200mg. |
| 药品名称 Drug Names | 地诺前列酮 Dinoprostona |
| 适应证<br>Indicaciones | 可用于中期妊娠引产、足月妊娠引产和治疗性流产，对妊娠毒血症（先兆子痫、高血压）、妊娠合并肾疾患者、过期妊娠、死胎不下、水泡状胎块、羊膜早破、高龄初产妇等均可应用。<br><br>Puede ser utilizado para aborto trimestre, la inducción del parto al término del embarazo y el aborto terapéutico, puede ser usado para los pacientes con la toxemia del embarazo (pre-eclampsia, hipertensión), enfermedad renal con el embarazo, el embarazo prolongado, parto muerto alto, mola hidatidiforme, rotura prematura de membranas, primípara ancianos, etc. |
| 用法、用量<br>Administración y dosis | （1）催产：普通阴道栓，一次 3mg，置于阴道后穹窿深处，6 ～ 8 小时后若产程无进展，可再放置一次。<br>（2）引产①静脉滴注法②宫腔内羊膜腔外注射法（中期妊娠引产）③阴道内给药法④宫颈内给药法。<br>（3）产后出血：将本品注射液 5mg 用所吸附的稀释液稀释后溶于氯化钠注射液中，缓慢静脉滴注（开始宜慢，以后可酌情加快）。<br><br>(1) Oxitocina: Supositorio vaginal normal, 3mg por cada vez, localizado en el fondo de la bóveda, si no hay progreso de producción después de 6 a 8 horas en la vagina, se puede colocar una vez más.<br>(2) Aborto ① Goteo intravenoso ② Inyección amniótico intrauterino (aborto trimestre) ③ administración vaginal dentro de la vagina ④ administración cervical dentro de la cerviz<br>(3) Hemorragia posparto: después de la dilución de 5mg de este producto; se disuelve en la inyección de cloruro de sodio para hacer la infusión intravenosa lenta (debe ser lento al principio, después, puede acelerar la velocidad de acuerdo con la situación). |
| 剂型、规格<br>Formulaciones y especificaciones | 注射液：每支 2mg（1ml）。阴道栓：每粒 3mg；20mg。控释阴道栓（普贝生）：每粒 10mg。<br>凝胶剂：普比迪，每支 0.5mg/3g；普洛舒定，每支 1mg/3g；2mg/3g。<br>Inyección: Cada una de 2 mg (1 ml). Supositorio vaginal: Cada uno de 3 mg; 20 mg. Supositorio vaginal de liberación controlada (Propess): Cada uno de 10 mg. Geles: Prepidil, cada una de 0.5mg/3g; Prostin, cada una de 1mg/3g; 2mg/3g. |
| 药品名称 Drug Names | 米索前列醇 Misoprostol |
| 适应证<br>Indicaciones | 本品单用于中期引产，效果不佳，一般均与米非司酮联合应用，不良反应比卡前列甲酯栓轻。<br>Si este producto se utiliza solamente en la inducción a medio plazo, el efecto no es bueno, por lo general, se usa en combinación con mifepristona y tiene menos reacciones adversas que carboprost perno metilo. |
| 用法、用量<br>Administración y dosis | 中期妊娠引产：①先顿服米非司酮 200mg，36 小时后在阴道后穹窿放置米索前列醇 3 片（600μg）。②在服用米非司酮 36 ～ 48 小时后，一次口服米索前列醇 500μg。<br>Aborto trimestre: ① primero toma la mifepristona de 200mg, después de 36 horas, coloque misoprostol de 3 tabletas (600μg) en el fondo de saco posterior. ② 36 ~ 48 horas después de tomar la mifepristona, debe toma una vez de 500μg de misoprostol por vía oral. |

**续　表**

| 剂型、规格 Formulaciones y especificaciones | 片剂：每片 200µg。<br>Tabletas: cada tableta de 200µg. |
|---|---|
| 药品名称 Drug Names | 依沙吖啶 Etacridina |
| 适应证 Indicaciones | ①中期妊娠引产，终止 12～26 周妊娠。②用于外科创伤、黏膜感染等消毒。<br>① la interrupción del embarazo trimestre,la terminación de gestación de 12～26 semanas. ② Se usa para la desinfección de trauma quirúrgico, infecciones de las mucosas, etc. |
| 用法、用量 Administración y dosis | （1）羊膜腔内注射：由下腹壁向羊膜腔内注射本品 1% 溶液 5～10ml（含药 50～100mg）。每周用量不超过 100mg。妊娠 20 在 20 周以内者用 50mg，在 20 周以上者用 100mg。<br>（2）羊膜腔外注射：先冲洗阴道，一日一次，冲洗 3 日。在消毒的情况下，将橡皮导尿管送入羊膜腔外，经导尿管注入药液 50ml（取本品 1% 的注射液 10ml，加注射用水 40ml，含药 100mg）。注药后将导尿管折叠结扎放入阴道，保留 24 小时后取出。<br>（3）外用灭菌：用 0.1%～0.2%（用片剂溶解配制而成）溶液，局部洗涤、湿敷。<br>(1) Inyección intra-amniótico: inyección intra-amniótico de este producto al 1% de solución de 5～10 ml (que contiene fármaco de 50～100 mg) hacia la pared abdominal. La cantidad semanal no debe ser más de 100 mg. Para los pacientes de embarazo de 20 semanas o en menos de 20 semanas, debe utilizar 50 mg. Para los pacientes de embarazo de más de 20 semanas, la cantidad es de100 mg.<br>(2) Inyección amniótico: Primero hay que lavar la vagina, una vez al día por tres días. En condiciones estériles, coloque el catéter de caucho en la parte exterior de la cavidad amniótica, a través del catéter puede inyectar el líquido de 50 ml (1% de este producto de 10 ml, agrega agua de inyección de 40 ml, contiene el fármaco de 100 mg). Después de la inyección, dobla el catéter de inyección y coloca dentro de la vagina, mantiene por 24 horas y después eliminalo.<br>(3)Esterilización externa: Líquido al 0.1%～0.2% (se prepara mediante la disolución de tabletas), lava parcialmente y deposita en forma húmeda. |
| 剂型、规格 Formulaciones y especificaciones | 片剂：每片 100mg。注射用依沙吖啶：每支 100mg。<br>Tabletas: Cada tableta de 100 mg. Inyección de etacridina: Cada una de 100 mg. |

15.2 退乳药物 Antilactantes

| 药品名称 Drug Names | 溴隐亭 Bromocriptina |
|---|---|
| 适应证 Indicaciones | ①分娩后、自发性、肿瘤性、药物等引起的闭经；②高泌乳素血症引起的月经紊乱、不孕、继发性闭经、排卵减少；③抑制泌乳，预防分娩后和早产后的泌乳；④产后的乳房充血、高泌乳素血症引起的特殊的乳房触痛、乳房胀痛和烦躁不安；⑤高泌乳素血症引起男性性功能低下（如阳痿和精子减少引起的不育）；⑥肢端肥大症的辅助治疗。<br>① amenorrea después del parto, con espontaneidad, con cáncer, causada por drogas, etc; ② trastornos menstruales, infertilidad, amenorrea secundaria, la reducción de la ovulación inducidas por hiperprolactinemia ; ③ suprimir la lactancia, prevenir la secreción de la leche después del parto y del parto prematuro; ④ especial sensibilidad en los senos, sensibilidad en los senos y la irritabilidad causada por la congestión del senos, , la hiperprolactinemia después del parto; ⑤ disfunción sexual masculina causada por la hiperprolactinemia (tales como la impotencia y infertilidad causada por la disminución de esperma); ⑥ tratamiento adyuvante de la acromegalia. |
| 用法、用量 Administración y dosis | （1）产后回乳：口服，如为预防性用药，分娩后 4 小时开始服用 2.5mg，以后改为一日 2 次，1 次 2.5mg，连用 14 日；如已有乳汁分泌，则一日用 2.5mg，2～3 日后改为一日 2 次，一次 2.5mg，连用 14 日。<br>（2）高泌乳素血症引起的闭经溢乳、不孕症：口服，常用起始量为一次 1.25mg，一日 2～3 次；若症状未得到控制，可逐渐增量至一次 2.5mg，一日 2～3 次，餐后服用，直至月经恢复正常，再继续用药几周，完全停止则需 12～13 周，以防复发。<br>（3）产后乳房充血：轻者可口服，一次 2.5mg，如需要又没停止泌乳，则 6～12 小时后可重复一次。短时间用药不会抑制泌乳。<br>（4）男性高泌乳素血症引起的性功能低下：口服，1 次 1.25mg，一日 2～3 次，逐渐增加至一日 5～10mg，分 3 次服用。 |

|  |  |
|---|---|
|  | （5）肢端肥大症：开始一日 2.5mg，经 7 ～ 14 日后根据临床反应可逐渐增至一日 10 ～ 20mg，分 4 次与食物同服。<br><br>（6）垂体泌乳素瘤：口服，起始量为一日 1.25mg，维持量为一日 5 ～ 7.5mg，最大量为每日 15mg。<br><br>(1) Leche espalda postparto: por vía oral, es como medicación preventiva, cuatro horas después del parto puede empezar a tomar 2.5 mg, más tarde cambia a 2 veces al día, 2.5 mg por una vez, en total 14 días consecutivos; Si hay secreción de leche, el uso es de 2.5 mg al día, después de 2 ~ 3 días cambia a 2 veces al día, una vez de 2.5 mg, en total 14 días consecutivos.<br><br>(2) Hiperprolactinemia galactorrea Amenorrea inducida infertilidad: por vía oral, la dosis inicial es de 1.25 mg por una vez, 2 ~ 3 veces al día; Si los síntomas no están bajo control, puede aumentar gradualmente hasta una vez de 2.5 mg, 2 ~ 3 veces al día, se toma después de la comida, hasta que la menstruación vuelva a la normalidad, y luego debe continuar a usar por un par de semanas, con 12 ~ 13 semanas puede suspender la dosis para evitar la recurrencia.<br><br>(3) Congestión del pecho después del parto: Para casos leves, puede tomar por vía oral, 2.5 mg por una vez. Si hay la necesidad y no detiene la lactancia, después de 6 ～ 12 horas puede repetir por otra vez. El uso del medicamentos a corto plazo no inhibe la lactancia.<br><br>(4) Disfunción sexual inducida por la hiperprolactinemia masculina: por vía oral, una vez de 1.25mg, 2 o 3 veces al día, aumentando gradualmente a 1 5 ～ 10 mg al día, dividida en 3 veces.<br><br>(5) Acromegalia: La dosis inicial es de 2.5 mg, después de 7 ～ 14 días basada en la respuesta clínica, se puede aumentar gradualmente a 10 ～ 20 mg al día, dividida en cuatro veces para tomar junto con la comida.<br><br>(6) Hipófisis prolactinoma: por vía oral, la dosis inicial es de 1.25 mg al día, la dosis diaria de mantenimiento es de 5 ～ 7.5 mg, la cantidad máxima diaria es de15 mg. |
| 剂型、规格<br>Formulaciones y especificaciones | 片剂：每片 4mg。<br>Tabletas: Cada tableta de 4 mg. |

16. 主要作用于内分泌系统的药物 Medicamentos que actúan principalmente en el sistema endocrino

16.1　肾上腺皮质激素和促肾上腺皮质激素 Adrenocorticosteroid y adrenocorticotrophic hormone

| 药品名称 Drug Names | 氢化可的松 Hidrocortisona |
|---|---|
| 适应证<br>Indicaciones | 用于结缔组织病、系统性红斑狼疮、严重的支气管哮喘、皮肌炎、血管炎等过敏性疾病，急性白血病、恶性淋巴瘤等病症。<br><br>Se usa para la enfermedad del tejido conectivo, lupus eritematoso sistémico, asma bronquial grave, dermatomiositis, vasculitis y otras enfermedades alérgicas, leucemia aguda, linfoma y otras enfermedades. |
| 用法、用量<br>Administración y dosis | 氢化可的松注射液：每次 100 ～ 200mg，与 0.9% 氯化钠注射液或 5% 葡萄糖注射液 500ml 混合均匀后作静脉滴注。注射用氢化可的松琥珀酸钠：50mg 或 100mg。临用时，以生理盐水或 5% 葡萄糖注射液稀释后静脉滴注或肌内注射。醋酸氢化可的松片：一日 1 ～ 2 次，每次 1 片。醋酸氢化可的松眼膏：一日 2 ～ 3 次。　醋酸氢化可的松滴眼液：用前摇匀。<br><br>Hidrocortisona inyectable: 100 ~ 200 mg por cada vez, mezcla con el 0,9% de cloruro de sodio o el 5% de la inyección de glucosa de 500 ml para hacer la infusión intravenosa. Inyección de succinato sódico de hidrocortisona: 50 mg o 100 mg. Para su uso, después de diluida con la solución salina o inyección dextrosa al 5%, hace la inyección intravenosa o intramuscular. Tabletas de acetato de hidrocortisona: 1 ~ 2 veces al día, una tableta por cada vez. Pomada de acetato de hidrocortisona: 2 ~ 3 veces al día. Gotas de ojo de acetato de hidrocortisona: Debe agitar bien antes de usar. |
| 剂型、规格<br>Formulaciones y especificaciones | 氢化可的松注射液：10mg（2ml）；25mg（5ml）；50mg（10ml）；100mg（20ml）（为氢化可的松的稀乙醇溶液）。醋酸氢化可的松注射液：125mg（5ml）（为醋酸氢化可的松的无菌混悬液）。注射用氢化可的松琥珀酸钠：50mg 或 100mg（按氢化可的松计算）。醋酸氢化可的松片：每片 20mg。醋酸氢化可的松软膏：1%。醋酸氢化可的松眼膏：0.5%。醋酸氢化可的松滴眼液：3ml ： 15mg。 |

**续　表**

| | Inyección de hidrocortisona: 10 mg (2 ml); 25 mg (5 ml); 50 mg (10 ml); 100 mg (20 ml) (solución de etanol como hidrocortisona diluir). Inyección de hidrocortisona de acetato: 125 mg (5 ml) (es suspensión estéril de hidrocortisona de acetato). Succinato de hidrocortisona sódico para inyección: 50 mg o 100 mg (calculado por hidrocortisona). Tabletas de hidrocortisona de acetato: Cada tableta de 20mg. Ungüento de hidrocortisona de acetato : 1%. Ungüento de ojos de hidrocortisona de acetato: 0.5%. Gotas de ojos de hidrocortisona de acetato: 3 ml: 15 mg. |
|---|---|
| **药品名称 Drug Names** | 泼尼松 Prednisona |
| 适应证<br>Indicaciones | 用于结缔组织病、系统性红斑狼疮、严重的支气管哮喘、皮肌炎、血管炎等过敏性疾病，急性白血病、恶性淋巴瘤等病症。<br><br>Se usa para la enfermedad del tejido conectivo, lupus eritematoso sistémico, asma bronquial grave, dermatomiositis, vasculitis y otras enfermedades alérgicas, leucemia aguda, linfoma y otras enfermedades. |
| 用法、用量<br>Administración y dosis | （1）补充替代疗法口服，1 次 5～10mg，一日 10～60mg，早晨起床后服用 2/3，下午服用 1/3。<br>（2）抗炎口服，一日 5～60mg。<br>（3）自身免疫性疾病口服，一日 40～60mg，病情稳定后可逐渐减量。<br>（4）过敏性疾病，口服一日 20～40mg，病情症状减轻后减量，每隔 1～2 日减少 5mg。<br>（5）防止器官移植排异反应，一般在术前 1～2 日开始每日口服 100mg，术后 1 周改为每日 60mg，以后逐渐减量。<br>（6）治疗急性白血病、恶性肿瘤等，每日口服 60～80mg，症状缓解后减量。<br>(1) Terapias orales complementarias y alternativas, por vía oral. 5～10 mg por cada vez, 10～60 mg al día, toma 2/3 en la mañana después de levantarse, en la tarde toma 1/3.<br>(2) Antiinflamatorio, por vía oral, 5～60 mg al día.<br>(3) Enfermedades autoinmunes por vía oral, 40～60 mg al día, después de que la condición está estable, puede disminuir la dosis.<br>(4) Enfermedades alérgicas, por vía oral, 20～40 mg al día, después del alivio de los síntomas de la enfermedad, puede reducir la dosis de 5mg por cada 1～2 días.<br>(5) Prevenir el rechazo de trasplante de órgano, por lo general en 1～2 días antes de la cirugía se inicia la administración por vía oral de 100 mg al día, después de una semana, cambia a 60 mg al día, y luego se reduce gradualmente.<br>(6) Tratamiento de la leucemia aguda, tumores malignos,etc. La administración por vía oral diaria es de 60～80 mg, después del alivio de los síntomas, puede reducir la dosis. |
| 剂型、规格<br>Formulaciones y especificaciones | 醋酸泼尼松片：每片 5mg。醋酸泼尼松眼膏：0.5%。<br>Tabletas de Prednisona: Cada tableta de 5 mg. Ungüento de Prednisona: 0.5%. |
| **药品名称 Drug Names** | 泼尼松龙 Prednisolona |
| 适应证<br>Indicaciones | 用于过敏性和自身免疫性疾病。<br>Se usa para las enfermedades alérgicas y autoinmunes. |
| 用法、用量<br>Administración y dosis | 口服：成人开始一日 15～40mg，需用时可用到 60mg 或一日 0.5～1mg/kg，发热患者分三次服用，体温正常者每日晨起一次顿服。病情稳定后应逐渐减量，维持量 5～10mg，视病情而定。小儿开始用量 1mg/kg。肌内注射：一日 10～30mg。静脉滴注：1 次 10～25mg，溶于 5%～10% 葡萄糖溶液 500ml 中应用。关节腔或软组织内注射（混悬液）：1 次 5～50mg，用量依关节大小而定，应在无菌条件下操作，以防引起感染。滴眼：一次 1～2 滴，一日 2～4 次，治疗开始的 24～48 小时，剂量可酌情加大至每小时 2 滴，注意不宜过早停药。<br>Por vía oral: La dosis inicial para adultos es de 15～40 mg al ía, caundo sea necesario, puede usar 60 mg o 0.5～1mg/kg al día. Los pacientes con fiebre toman tres veces, Los pacientes con temperatura corporal normal toma una vez por la mañana. Después de la condición estable, debe disminuir gradualmente, con la dosis de mantenimiento de 5～10 mg, dependiendo de la enfermedad. La dosificación pediátrica inicial es de 1mg/kg. Inyección intramuscular: 10～30 mg al día. Infusión intravenosa: 10～25 mg por cada vez, disuelto en la solución de glucosa al 5%～10% de 500 ml para las aplicaciones. Inyección en el tejido blando o intra-articular (suspensión): 5～50 mg por cada vez, la cantidad depende del tamaño de la articulación, debe operar bajo condiciones asépticas para prevenir la infección. Goteo de ojos: 1～2 gotas por cada vez, 2～4 veces al día, el tratamiento se inicia entre 24～48 horas, la dosis puede aumentarse a 2 gotas por cada hora, Cuidado que no es conveniente la retirada prematura. |

**续 表**

| 剂型、规格<br>Formulaciones y especificaciones | 醋酸泼尼松龙片：每片5mg。醋酸泼尼松龙注射液（混悬液）：125mg（5ml）。泼尼松龙磷酸钠注射液：20mg（1ml）。泼尼松龙软膏：0.25%～0.5%。 泼尼松龙眼膏：0.25%。泼尼松龙滴眼液：1%。<br><br>Tabletas de acetato de prednisolona: Cada tableta de 5mg. Inyección de acetato de prednisolona (suspensión): 125 mg (5 ml). Inyección de Prednisolona Sodio Fosfato: 20 mg (1 ml). Pomada de prednisolona: 0.25% a 0.5%. Prednisolona ungüento: 0.25%. Gotas de prednisolona: 1%. |
|---|---|
| **药品名称 Drug Names** | **甲泼尼龙 Metilprednisolona** |
| 适应证<br>Indicaciones | 用于抗炎治疗风湿性疾病、肌原疾病、皮肤疾病、过敏状态、眼部疾病、胃肠道疾病、呼吸道疾病、水肿状态；免疫抑制治疗、休克、内分泌失调等。<br><br>Se usa para el tratamiento de enfermedades inflamatorias reumáticas, enfermedades miogénicas, enfermedades de la piel, enfermedad alérgica, trastornos oculares, enfermedades gastrointestinales, enfermedades respiratorias, edema de estado; el tratamiento inmunosupresor, shock, trastornos endocrinos, etc. |
| 用法、用量<br>Administración y dosis | 口服：开始一日16～24mg，分2次服用，维持量一日4～8mg。关节腔内及肌内注射：一次10～40mg。用于危重病情作为辅助疗法时，推荐剂量时30mg/kg体重，将已溶解的药物与5%葡萄糖注射液、生理盐水注射液或者两者混合后至少静脉输注30分钟。此剂量可于48小时内，每4～6小时重复一次。冲击疗法：一日1g，静脉注射，使用1～4日；或每月1g，静脉注射，使用6个月。系统性红斑狼疮：一日1g，静脉注射，使用3日。多发性硬化症：一日1g，静脉注射，使用3日或5日。肾小球肾炎、狼疮性肾炎：一日1g，静脉注射，使用3、5或7日。<br><br>Por vía oral: Al inicio, la dosis es de 16 ~ 24 mg al día, divida en 2 veces, la dosis de mantenimiento es 4 ~ 8 mg al día. inyección intraarticular e inyección intramuscular: 10 ~ 40 mg por cada vez. Cuando se utiliza como una terapia adjunta en estado crítico, es recomendable ofrecer la dosis de acuerdo con el peso del cuerpo de 30mg/kg, pone el fármaco disuelto en la inyección de glucosa al 5%, la solución salina o la mezcla de ambas para hacer la infusión intravenosa por al menos 30 minutos. Esta dosis puede ser utilizada dentro de 48 horas, repite una vez por cada 4 ~ 6 horas. Terapia de shock: 1 g al día, inyección intravenosa, usando 1 ~ 4 días, o 1g mensualmente, inyección intravenosa, usando 6 meses. Lupus eritematoso sistémico: 1 g al día, inyección intravenosa, utilizando 3 días. Esclerosis múltiple: 1 g al día, inyección intravenosa, usando 3 días o 5 días. Glomerulonefritis, nefritis lúpica: 1 g al día, inyección intravenosa, usando 3, 5 o 7 días. |
| 剂型、规格<br>Formulaciones y especificaciones | 片剂：每片2mg；4mg。甲泼尼龙醋酸酯混悬注射液（局部注射）：每支20mg（1ml）；40mg（1ml）。甲泼尼龙琥珀酸钠注射液：每支相当于甲泼尼龙40mg；125mg；500mg。<br><br>Tabletas: 2 mg; 4mg por cada tableta. Inyección de suspensión de acetato de metilprednisolona (inyección local): Cada una de 20 mg (1 ml), 40 mg (1 ml). Inyección de Metilprednisolona Succinato Sódico: Cada equivalente a metilprednisolona de 40 mg; 125 mg; 500mg. |
| **药品名称 Drug Names** | **曲安西龙 Triamcinolona** |
| 适应证<br>Indicaciones | 用于类风湿关节炎、其他结缔组织炎症、支气管哮喘、过敏性皮炎、神经性皮炎、湿疹等，尤其适用于对皮质激素禁忌的伴有高血压或水肿的关节炎患者。<br><br>Se usa para la artritis reumatoide, otra inflamación del tejido conectivo, asma bronquial, dermatitis atópica, neurodermatitis, eczema, especialmente para los pacientes con hipertensión o edema artritis quienes son prohibidos del uso de la corticosteroide. |
| 用法、用量<br>Administración y dosis | （1）口服：开始时一次4mg，一日2～4次。维持量为一次1～4mg，一日1～2次，通常维持量不超过8mg。<br>（2）肌内注射：每1～4周一次40～80mg。<br>（3）皮下注射：一次5～20mg。<br>（4）关节腔内注射：每1～7周一次5～40mg。<br><br>(1) Por vía oral.: Al inicio es de 4 mg por cada vez, 2~4 veces al día. La dosis de mantenimiento es de 1 ~ 4 mg por cada vez, 1 ~ 2 veces al día, por lo general no debe ser más de 8 mg.<br>(2) Inyección intramuscular: cada 1 ~ 4 semanas por una vez de 40 ~ 80 mg.<br>(3) Inyección subcutánea: 5 ~ 20mg por cada vez.<br>(4) Inyección intra-articular: cada 1 ~ 7 semanas por una vez de 5 ~ 40 mg. |

**续　表**

| 剂型、规格<br>Formulaciones y<br>especificaciones | 片剂：每片1mg；2mg；4mg。　曲安西龙双醋酸酯混悬注射液：每支125mg（5ml）；200mg（5ml）.<br>　Tabletas: Cada tableta de 1mg; 2mg;; 4mg. inyección de suspensión de triamcinolona y diacetato: Cada una de 125 mg (5 ml); 200 mg (5 ml). |
| --- | --- |
| 药品名称 Drug Names | 曲安奈德 Acetónido de triamcinolona |
| 适应证<br>Indicaciones | 用于各种皮肤病（如神经性皮炎、湿疹、牛皮癣等）、支气管哮喘、过敏性鼻炎、关节痛、肩周围炎、腱鞘炎、急性扭伤、慢性腰腿痛及眼科炎症等。鼻喷雾剂用于治疗常年性过敏性鼻炎或季节性过敏性鼻炎。<br><br>　Se usa para diversas enfermedades de la piel (como neurodermatitis, eczema, psoriasis, etc), el asma bronquial, rinitis alérgica, dolor articular, inflamación alrededor del hombro, tenosinovitis, esguinces agudos, dolor lumbar crónico y la inflamación de los ojos. El aerosol nasal es usa para el tratamiento de la rinitis alérgica perenne o rinitis alérgica estacional. |
| 用法、用量<br>Administración y<br>dosis | （1）支气管哮喘：肌内注射，成人每次1ml（40mg），每3周1次，5次为一疗程，患者症状较重者可用80mg；6～12岁儿童减半，在必要时3～6岁幼儿可用成人剂量的1/3。穴位或局部注射，成人一次1ml（40mg），在扁桃体穴或颈前甲状软骨旁注射，每周1次，5次为一疗程，注射前先用少量普鲁卡因局麻。<br>　（2）过敏性鼻炎：肌内注射，一次1ml（40mg），每3周1次，5次为一疗程；下鼻甲注射，鼻腔先喷1%利多卡因表面麻醉后，在双下鼻甲前端各注入本品0.5ml，每周1次，4～5次为一疗程。<br>　（3）各种关节病：一次10～20mg，加0.25%利多卡因液10～20ml，用5号针头，一次进针直至病灶，每周2～3次或隔日一次，症状好转后每周1～2次，4～5次为一疗程。<br>　（4）皮肤病：直接注入皮损部分，通常每一部位用0.2～0.3mg，视患部大小而定，每处每次不超过0.5mg，必要时每隔1～2周重复使用。局部外用：一日2～3次，一般早晚各一次。治疗皮炎、湿疹时，疗程2～4周。<br>　（5）鼻腔内用药：用前须振摇5次以上；12岁以上的儿童、成人及老人，推荐剂量为每鼻孔2喷（共220μg），一日1次。症状得到控制时，可降低剂量至每鼻孔1喷（共110μg），一日1次。如3周后症状无改善应看医生。<br><br>(1) Asma bronquial : Inyección intramuscular, para adultos 1 ml (40 mg ) por cada vez , una vez por cada 3 semanas, 5 veces es un curso de tratamiento, para los pacientes con síntomas graves es de 80mg; para niños de 6 ~ 12 años de edad debe reducir la dosis a la mitad, cuando sea necesario, la dosis para niños de 3 ~ 6 años de edad es de 1/ 3 de la dosis de adultos. Inyección en puntos o local, para adultos,1 ml (40 mg ) por cada vez, hace las inyecciones en punto de amígdala o antes del cuello al lado cartílago tiroides , una vez por cada semana , 5 veces es un curso de tratamiento, antes de la inyección debe hacer anestesia local con una pequeña cantidad de procaína.<br>(2) Rinitis alérgica : Inyección intramuscular , 1 ml (40 mg ) por cada vez , una vez por cada 3 semanas , 5 veces es un curso; Inyección cornete inferior, primero hace el aerosol nasal de lidocaína al 1 %, después de anestesia tópica, en frente de los cornetes inferiores, inyecta este producto de 0.5 ml, 1 veces por cada semana , cuatro ~ cinco veces es un curso de tratamiento.<br>(3) Diversas enfermedades de las articulaciones : 10 ~ 20 mg por cada vez, más de una solución de lidocaína al 0.25 % de 10 ~ 20 ml, con la quinta aguja , una aguja de una vez hasta la lesión, 2 ~ 3 veces por cada semana o una vez por cada dos días, una semana después de que los síntomas se mejoran, es 1 ~ 2 veces por cada semana, 4 ~ 5 veces es un curso de tratamiento.<br>(4) Dermatología : Inyección directa en las partes de la piel dañada, por lo general es 0.2 ~ 0.3 mg por cada área, dependiendo del tamaño de la zona afectada , cada parte cada vez no debe ser más de 0.5 mg, si es necesario, repite el uso por cada 1 ~ 2 semanas . Uso tópico: 2 ~ 3 veces al día, generalmente una vez por la mañana y una vez por la noche. Tratamiento de dermatitis, eczema , un curso de tratamiento es 2 ~ 4 semanas.<br>(5) Administración intranasal : antes de su uso debe agitar más de cinco veces; La dosis recomendable para los niños mayores de 12 años de edad, adultos y ancianos , es de 2 pulverizaciones para cada fosa nasal ( en total 220μg), una vez al día. Cuando se han controlado los síntomas, la dosis se puede reducir a 1 pulverización en cada fosa nasal (en total 110μg) , una vez al día. Si los síntomas no han sido mejorados después de tres semanas, debe consultar a un médico. |

**续　表**

| 剂型、规格<br>Formulaciones y especificaciones | 注射液（混悬剂）：每支 40mg（1ml）。复方曲安奈德霜：每支 5g；10g；15g；20g。鼻喷雾剂：每支 6ml［6.6mg，120 喷（55µg/ 喷）］。<br><br>Inyección (suspensión): Cada una de 40 mg (1 ml). Crema de acetónido de triamcinolona compuesto: Cada una de 5g; 10g; 15g; 20g. Aerosol nasal: Cada una de 6 ml [6,6 mg, 120 de pulverizaciones (55µg / pulverización)]. |
|---|---|
| **药品名称 Drug Names** | 布地奈德 Budesónida |
| 适应证<br>Indicaciones | 用于支气管哮喘的症状和体征的长期控制。粉吸入剂用于需适用糖皮质激素维持治疗以控制基础炎症的支气管哮喘、慢性阻塞性肺疾病患者。鼻喷雾剂用于季节性和常年性过敏性鼻炎、血管运动性鼻炎；预防鼻息肉切除术后鼻息肉的再生，对症治疗鼻息肉。<br><br>Para el control a largo plazo de los síntomas y signos de asma bronquial. La inhalación de polvo es para tratar del paciente que necesita controlar la inflamación subyacente del asma bronquial y la enfermedad pulmonar obstructiva crónica con aplicación de corticosteroides.El aerosol nasal es para la rinitis alérgica estacional y perenne y la rinitis vasomotora. Prevención de regeneración de pólipos nasales postoperatorias y servirá para tratar los pólipos nasales. |
| 用法、用量<br>Administración y dosis | 剂量应个体化，成人初始剂量为 200 ~ 1600µg/d，分 2 ~ 4 次给药（较轻微的病例 200 ~ 800µg/d，较严重的 800 ~ 1600µg/d）。一般一次 200µg，早晚各一次，病情严重时一日 4 次。7 岁以上儿童：200 ~ 800µg/d，分 2 ~ 4 次使用。2 ~ 7 岁儿童：200 ~ 400µg/d，分成 2 ~ 4 次使用。维持剂量成人一日 100 ~ 600µg，儿童 100 ~ 800µg；当哮喘控制后可减至最低有效维持剂量。鼻喷，成人及 6 岁以上儿童，起始剂量为一日 256µg，次剂量可早晨一次喷入和早晚 2 次喷入（即早晨每个鼻孔内喷入 2 喷；或早晚 2 次，每个鼻孔内喷 1 喷）。<br><br>La dosis debe ser individualizada.La dosis inicial para adultos es 200 ~ 1600µg/d,divida en 2 a 4 dosis al día(Los casos leves tienen el tosis de 200 ~ 800 µg/d , más grave 800 ~ 1600µg / d). Normalmente 200 µg/d cada vez, una por la mañana y una por la noche, y 4 dosis al día si es grave. Para los niños mayores de 7 años:200 ~ 800µg/d, dividida en 2 a 4 dosis. Para niños de 2 a 7 años:200 ~ 400µg/d, dividida en 2 a 4 dosis. Dosis de mantenimiento para adultos: 100 ~ 600µg/ d, y de niños: 100 ~ 800µg.Una vez controlado el asma, la dosis se puede reducir a la mínima de mantenimiento eficaz. la aplicación del aerosol nasal: para los adultos y niños mayores de 6 años de edad , la dosis inicial es 256µg al día.Una dosis puede ser inyectado por una vez en la mañana o por dos veces en la mañana y en la noche (es decir, rociar dos sprays en cada fosa nasal por la mañana o un spray en cada fosa nasal en la mañana y otro spray en la noche). |
| 剂型、规格<br>Formulaciones y especificaciones | 气雾剂：10ml：10mg（50µg/ 喷，200 喷 / 瓶）；10ml：20mg（100µg/ 喷，200 喷 / 瓶）；5ml：20mg（200µg/ 喷，100 喷 / 瓶）。<br>雷诺考特鼻喷雾剂（白色或类白色黏稠混悬液）：64µg/ 喷（120 喷 / 支，药液浓度 1.28mg/ ml）.<br>粉吸入剂：0.1mg/ 吸（200 吸 / 支）。<br>细微颗粒混悬液：0.5mg/2ml；1mg/2ml。<br><br>Aerosol: 10 ml:10 mg (50 µg/spray, 200 sprays/botella); 10 ml :20 mg (100µg/spray, 200 sprays/ botella); 5ml:20mg (200µg/spray, 100 sprays/botella).<br>Spray nasal Rhinocort ( suspensión viscosa de color blanco o casi blanco): 64µg sprays/ (120 sprays, solución de concentración: 1.28mg/ml )<br>Polvo para inhalación : 0.1 mg/inhalación ( 200 inhalaciones)<br>Suspensión de partículas finas : 0.5mg/2ml; 1mg/2ml |
| **药品名称 Drug Names** | 氟替卡松 Fluticasona |
| 适应证<br>Indicaciones | 用作持续性哮喘的长期治疗，季节性过敏性鼻炎（包括枯草热）和常年性过敏性鼻炎的预防和治疗。外用可缓解炎症性和瘙痒性皮肤病。吸入剂适用于 12 岁及以上患者预防用药维持治疗哮喘。<br><br>Se utiliza para el tratamiento a largo plazo de asma persistente, la prevención y el tratamiento de la rinitis alérgica estacional ( incluyendo fiebre del heno) y rinitis alérgica perenne.Utilizando tópicamente puede aliviar la inflamación y picor de la piel.La inhalación se aplica para el mantenimiento de tratamiento y prevención para pacientes mayores de 12 años. |

**续　表**

| | |
|---|---|
| 用法、用量<br>Administración y dosis | 　　成人，老年患者和 12 岁以上儿童：一日 1 次，每个鼻孔各 2 喷，以早晨用药为好，某些患者需一日 2 次，每个鼻孔各 2 喷。当症状得到控制时，维持剂量为一日 1 次，每个鼻孔各 1 喷。若症状复发，可相应增加剂量，每日最大剂量为每个鼻孔不超过 4 喷。4 ～ 11 岁儿童：一日 1 次，每个鼻孔各 1 喷。某些患者需一日 2 次，每个鼻孔各 1 喷，最大剂量为每个鼻孔不超过 2 喷。湿疹 / 皮炎：成人及 1 岁以上儿童，一日 1 次涂于患处。其他适应证，一日 2 次。吸入剂：轻度哮喘：100 ～ 250μg，一日 2 次；中度哮喘：250 ～ 500μg，一日 2 次；重度哮喘：500 ～ 1000μg，一日 2 次。<br><br>　　Para adultos y los mayores de 12 años: una vez al día, 2 sprayes en cada foso nasal, mejor se usa por la mañana.Graves pacientes necesitan 2 dosis al día. Una vez está controlado el síntoma, la dosis de mantenimiento es una vez al dia, un spray en cada foso nasal. Si los síntomas se repiten , la dosis puede aumentarse en consecuencia, la dosis diaria máxima no debe ser más de cuatro sprays en cada fosa nasal.Para niños de 4 a 11 años: una vez al día, un spray en cada foso nasal.Pacientes graves necesitan 2 veces al día, un spray en cada foso nasal. Eczema / Dermatitis: para adultos y niños mayores de 1 año, se aplica a la zona afectada una vez al día.Otras indicaciones: 2 veces al día. Aerosol para inhalación: asma leve: 100 ～ 250μg , 2 veces al día; asma moderada: 250 ～ 500μg , 2 veces al día ; asma severa : 500 ～ 1000μg , 2 veces al día. |
| 剂型、规格<br>Formulaciones y especificaciones | 　　鼻喷剂：50μg×120 喷。吸入气雾剂：125μg×60 喷 / 支，250μg×60 泡 / 盒。乳膏：15g ： 7.5mg（0.05%）；30g ： 15mg（0.05%）。<br>　　Aerosol nasal: 50μg × 120 sprays . Aerosol para inhalación : 125μg × 60 aerosol / support, 250μg × 60 burbuja / caja. Crema : 15 g ： 7.5 mg ( 0.05 % ) ; 30 g ： 15 mg ( 0.05 % ) . |
| 药品名称 Drug Names | 莫米松 Mometasona |
| 适应证<br>Indicaciones | 　　用于治疗成人及 12 岁以上儿童的季节性或常年性鼻炎。对于中至重度季节性过敏性鼻炎的患者，建议在花粉季节开始前 2 ～ 4 周使用本品作预防治疗。也用于对皮脂类固醇有效的皮肤病如异位性皮炎。<br><br>　　Se aplica para el tratamiento de rinitis estacional o perenne a los adultos y niños mayores de 12 años. Para los pacientes con moderada y severa rinitis alérgica estacional, se recomienda aplicar este producto dos a cuatro semanas antes de la temporada de polen para la prevención y el tratamiento. Se aplica también para enfermedades de la piel para las cuales los corticosteroides son eficaces, tales como la dermatitis atópica. |
| 用法、用量<br>Administración y dosis | 　　鼻喷剂：成人（包括老年患者）和 12 岁以上儿童，常用推荐剂量为每侧鼻孔 2 喷（每喷为 50μg），一日 1 次（总量为 200μg）。当症状被控制时，可减至每侧鼻孔 1 喷（总量为 100μg），如果症状未被有效控制，则可增至每侧鼻孔 4 喷（400μg），在症状控制后减少剂量。乳膏：一日 1 次，涂于患处。<br><br>　　Aerosol nasal: adultos (los ancianos incluidos) y niños mayores de 12 años,la dosis comúnmente recomendada es de 2 inhalaciones en cada lado de la nariz ( cada pulverización es 50μg ) y una vez al día (un total de 200μg ). Cuando se controlan los síntomas , la dosis se puede reducir a un spray a cada lado de la nariz (un total de 100μg) , si los síntomas no se controlan con eficacia, podría ser aumentada a 4 sprays a cada lado de la nariz ( 400 μg ) , reduciendo la dosis al controlarse los síntomas. Crema: se aplica una vez al día en la zona afectada. |
| 剂型、规格<br>Formulaciones y especificaciones | 　　鼻喷剂：50μg×60 揿 / 支；50μg×120 揿 / 支。<br>　　乳膏：5g ： 5mg。<br>　　Aerosol: 50μg×60 sprays/support; 50μg×120sprays/support.<br>　　crema: 5g ： 5mg. |
| 药品名称 Drug Names | 地塞米松 Dexametasona |
| 适应证<br>Indicaciones | 　　用于过敏性与自身免疫性炎症性疾病。多用于结缔组织病、活动性风湿病、类风湿关节炎、红斑狼疮、严重支气管哮喘、严重皮炎、溃疡性结肠炎、急性白血病等，也用于某些严重感染及中毒、恶性淋巴瘤的综合治疗。片剂还用于某些肾上腺皮质疾病的诊断。<br><br>　　Se utiliza para las enfermedades inflamatorias alérgicas y autoinmunes. Se aplica más frecuentemente para la enfermedad del tejido conectivo, el reumatismo activo, la artritis reumatoide, el lupus, el asma bronquial grave, dermatitis severa, la colitis ulcerosa, la leucemia aguda y entre otras. También se aplica en ciertas infecciones e intoxicaciones graves, el tratamiento integral de linfoma maligno. Las tabletas también se utiliza para diagnosticar ciertas enfermedades de la corteza suprarrenal. |

续 表

| | |
|---|---|
| 用法、用量<br>Administración y dosis | 口服，一日 0.75～3mg，每日 2～4 次；维持剂量每日 0.75mg。一般剂量静脉注射每次 2～20mg；静脉滴注时，应以 5% 葡萄糖注射液稀释，可 2～6 小时重复给药至病情稳定，但大剂量连续给药一般不超过 72 小时。还可用于缓解恶性肿瘤所致的脑水肿，首剂静脉推注 10mg，随后每 6 小时肌内注射 4mg，一般 12～24 小时患者可有所好转，2～4 日后逐渐减量，5～7 日停药。对不宜手术的脑肿瘤，首剂可静脉推注 50mg，以后每 2 小时重复给予 8mg，数日后再减至一日 2mg，分 2～3 次静脉给予。用于鞘内注射每次 5mg，间隔 1～3 周注射一次；关节腔内注射一般每次 0.8～4mg，按关节腔大小而定。<br><br>Se toma oralmente 2 a 4 veces al día y 0.75 a 3 mg al día; la diaria dosis de mantenimiento es de 0.75 mg. La dosis general para intravenosa es cada vez 2～20mg; el producto para intravenosa debe diluirse con 5 % glucosa. Se puede aplicar con repetición cada 2 a 6 horas hasta que llegue a una condición estable. pero el periodo de aplicación de gran dosis no debe continuar más de 72 horas. Para el alivio del edema cerebral causado por cáncer, se aplica la inyección intravenosa con la primera dosis de 10 mg, seguido de la inyección intramuscular de 4 mg cada seis horas. Generalmente después de 12 a 24 horas el paciente puede ser mejorado , reduciendo la dosis gradualmente después de 2 a 4 días y deteniendo la aplicación después de 5 a 7 días. Para los tumores cerebrales inoperables, la primera dosis de inyección intravenoso puede ser de 50 mg , después añade 8 mg cada dos horas, reduciéndola a 2 mg por día unos días más tarde, divida en 2 a 3 veces. En cuanto a la inyección intratecal, se aplica cada vez 5 mg con intervalos de 1 a 3 semanas. Para la inyección intra-articular se aplica cada vez 0.8～4 mg, de acuerdo con el tamaño de la cavidad de la articulación. |
| 剂型、规格<br>Formulaciones y especificaciones | 醋酸地塞米松片：每片 0.75mg。<br>地塞米松磷酸钠注射液：2mg（1ml）；5mg（1ml）。<br><br>Tabletas de Acetato de Dexametasona: 0.75mg.<br>Inyección de Fosfato de Sodio Dexametasona：2mg(1ml); 5mg(1ml). |
| **药品名称 Drug Names** | 倍他米松 Betametasona |
| 适应证<br>Indicaciones | 用于治疗活动性风湿病、类风湿关节炎、红斑性狼疮、严重支气管哮喘、严重皮炎、急性白血病等，也可用于某些感染的综合治疗。<br><br>Se utiliza para tratar el reumatismo activo, la artritis reumatoide, el lupus eritematoso sistémico, el asma bronquial grave, la dermatitis severa, la leucemia aguda, y entre otros. También se usa para tratar ciertas infecciones integrales. |
| 用法、用量<br>Administración y dosis | 口服，成人开始一日 0.5～2mg，分次服用。维持量为一日 0.5～1mg。肌内注射、静脉注射或静脉滴注用倍他米松磷酸钠：用于危急患者的抢救。<br><br>Se toma oralmente : adultos comienzan por una dosis de 0.5～2 mg diariamente, dividida en varias veces. Dosis diaria de mantenimiento es de 0.5～1 mg. Betametasona fosfato sódico de inyección intramuscular y intravenosa, o de la transfusión intravenosa se usa para rescatar a los pacientes en crisis. |
| 剂型、规格<br>Formulaciones y especificaciones | 片剂：每片 0.5mg。倍他米松醋酸酯注射液：每支 1.5mg（1ml）。<br><br>Comprimidos: 0.5mg cada comprimido, Inyección de Betametasona Acetato: 1.5mg cada support (1ml). |
| **药品名称 Drug Names** | 氟氢可的松 Fludrocortisona |
| 适应证<br>Indicaciones | 可与糖皮质类固醇一起用于原发性肾上腺皮质功能减退症的替代治疗。也适用于低肾素低醛固酮综合征和自主神经病变所致直立性低血压等。因本品内服易致水肿，多供外用局部涂敷治疗皮脂溢性湿疹、接触性皮炎、肛门、阴部瘙痒等症。<br><br>Puede ser una terapia de reemplazo en conjunción con glucocorticoides para el tratamiento del síndrome de insuficiencia suprarrenal primaria.También se aplica a tratar la hipotensión postural causada por sídrome de bajas renina y aldosterona y síndrome de neuropatía autónoma.A modo que este producto tomado por vía oral puede causar edema , se aplica por vía tópica con más frecuencia para tratar el eczema seborreica, la dermatitis de contacto y pruritos anal y genital y entre otros. |
| 用法、用量<br>Administración y dosis | 替代治疗：成人口服，一日 0.1～0.2mg，分 2 次。局部皮肤涂敷一日 2～4 次。<br><br>Terapia de reemplazo: por vía oral para adultos diariamente 0.1～0.2 mg , dividido en 2 veces. De forma tópica en la piel 2～4 veces al día. |

**续　表**

| 剂型、规格<br>Formulaciones y<br>especificaciones | 片剂：每片 0.1mg。醋酸氟氢可的松软膏：0.025%。<br>Tabletas: Cada tableta es de 0.1 mg.　Fludrocortisona acetato pomada: 0.025%. |
|---|---|
| **药品名称 Drug Names** | **氯倍他索 Clobetasol** |
| 适应证<br>Indicaciones | 治疗皮肤炎症和瘙痒症，如神经性皮炎、接触性皮炎、脂溢性皮炎、湿疹、局限性瘙痒症、盘状红斑狼疮等。<br>El tratamiento de la inflamación y prurito, por ejemplo, neurodermatitis, dermatitis de contacto, dermatitis seborreica, eczema prurito, limitaciones, lupus eritematoso discoide, etc. |
| 用法、用量<br>Administración y<br>dosis | 外用：涂患处，一日 2～3 次，待病情控制后，改为一日 1 次。<br>Por vía tópica: revestir 2 o 3 veces al día, hasta que la enfermedad está controlada, reduzca a una vez al día. |
| 剂型、规格<br>Formulaciones y<br>especificaciones | 软膏：0.05%。霜剂：0.025%。<br>Ungüento: 0.05%. Crema: 0.025%. |
| **药品名称 Drug Names** | **氟轻松 Fluocinolona** |
| 适应证<br>Indicaciones | 湿疹（特别是婴儿湿疹）、神经性皮炎、皮肤瘙痒症、接触性皮炎、牛皮癣、盘状红斑狼疮、扁平苔藓、外耳炎、日光性皮炎等。<br>Para el Tratamiento de eczema (en particular el eczema infantil), neurodermatitis, prurito, dermatitis de contacto, psoriasis, lupus eritematoso discoide, Liquen plano, otitis externa, la dermatitis solar etc.. |
| 用法、用量<br>Administración y<br>dosis | 皮肤洗净后局部外用，薄薄涂于患处，可轻揉促其渗入皮肤，一日 3～4 次。<br>Lavar la piel antes de la aplicación por vía tópica a la piel, sobe suavemente para mejor absorción. Aplique 3 a 4 veces al día. |
| 剂型、规格<br>Formulaciones y<br>especificaciones | 醋酸氟轻松软膏、乳膏：0.025%。<br>Ungüento o crema: 0.025%. |
| **药品名称 Drug Names** | **倍氯米松 Beclometasona** |
| 适应证<br>Indicaciones | 外用可治疗各种炎症皮肤病如湿疹、过敏性皮炎、神经性皮炎、接触性皮炎、牛皮癣、瘙痒等。气雾剂可用于预防和治疗常年性及季节性的过敏性鼻炎和血管舒缩性鼻炎。<br>El uso por vía tópica es para diversas inflamación de la piel tales como eczema, dermatitis alérgica, neurodermatitis, dermatitis de contacto, psoriasis, urticaria y entre otros. El aerosol se utiliza para la prevención y el tratamiento de la rinitis alérgica estacional y perenne y rinitis vasomotora. |
| 用法、用量<br>Administración y<br>dosis | 乳膏或软膏用于皮肤病：一日 2～3 次，涂于患处，必要时包扎之。气雾剂用于治疗哮喘：成人，一日 3～4 次，每次 2 揿，严重者一日 12～16 揿，根据病情好转情况逐渐减量；儿童，一日 2～4 次，一日 1～2 揿。鼻气雾剂，用于防止过敏性鼻炎，鼻腔喷雾给药，成人，一次每鼻孔 2 揿，一日 2 次，也可一次每鼻孔 1 揿（50μg），一日 3～4 次。一日总量不可超过 8 揿（400μg）。<br>Crema o ungüento para enfermedades de la piel: 2 a 3 veces al día, aplicarse a la zona afectada, vendarlo si es necesario. Aerosol para el tratamiento del asma: Adultos, 3 a 4 veces al día, 2 presiones para cada vez. Para los graves, aplique 12 a 16 presiones al día. reduciendo la dosis gradualmente de acuerdo con las condiciones de gravedad. Para los niños, 2 a 4 veces al día y 1 o 2 presiones para una vez. Se usa el aerosol nasal para prevenir la rinitis alérgica. Para adultos, cada vez aplique 2 presiones en cada orificio nasal, dos veces al día. O se puede aplicar una presión en cada orificio nasal (50 µg), 3 a 4 veces al día. En suma no se puede aplicar más de 8 presiones al día (400µg). |
| 剂型、规格<br>Formulaciones y<br>especificaciones | 软膏：0.025%。鼻气雾剂、喷雾剂：50μg/揿（200 揿 / 支），250μg/揿（80 揿 / 支），50μg/揿（200 揿、支）。<br>Ungüento: 0.025%. Aerosoles nasales: 50µg / presión (200 presiones), 250µg/ presión (80 presiones), 50 µg/ presión (200 presión). |

**续 表**

| 药品名称 Drug Names | 哈西奈德 Halcinonida |
|---|---|
| 适应证<br>Indicaciones | 用于银屑病和湿疹性皮炎。用于银屑病，具有疗程短、不良反应少的特点。<br>Se utiliza para la psoriasis y dermatitis eczema.Tiene menos efectos secundarios y periodo de aplicación más corto para tratar la psoriasis. |
| 用法、用量<br>Administración y dosis | 一日 2～3 次，涂于患处。<br>2 a 3 veces al día, aplicada a la zona afectada. |
| 剂型、规格<br>Formulaciones y especificaciones | 乳膏、软膏：0.1%。<br>crema o Ungüento: 0.1% |

| 药品名称 Drug Names | 可的松 Cortisona |
|---|---|
| 适应证<br>Indicaciones | 主要用于肾上腺皮质功能减退症的替代治疗。<br>Se utiliza principalmente para la terapia de reemplazo de la hipofunción suprarrenal. |
| 用法、用量<br>Administración y dosis | 口服：成人，一日剂量 25～37.5mg，清晨服 2/3，午后服 1/3. 当患者有应激状况时（如发热、感染）可适当加量，增到一日 100mg，肌内注射：一日 25mg，有应激状况适当加量，有严重应激时，应改用氢化可的松静脉滴注。<br>Por vía oral: adultos, 25～37.5 mg al día. una 2/3 para la mañana y la 1/3 para la tarde. Cuando el paciente tiene condiciones de estrés (como fiebre, infección) pueden aumentar la dosis diaria a 100 mg. Inyección intramuscular : 25 mg diario, aumentando la dosis si hay estrés, cuando hay un estrés severo, debe usar hidrocortisona a través de inyección intravenosa. |
| 剂型、规格<br>Formulaciones y especificaciones | 醋酸可的松注射液（混悬液）：每瓶 125mg（5ml）。醋酸可的松片：每片 5mg；25mg。<br>Acetato de cortisona (suspensión) para inyección: cada botella 125 mg (5 ml) . Tabletas de acetato cortisona: cada una 5mg y 25mg. |

16.2 雄激素及同化激素 Andrógenos y hormonas de asimilación de proteínas

| 药品名称 Drug Names | 丙酸睾酮 Propionato de testosterona |
|---|---|
| 适应证<br>Indicaciones | 原发性或继发性男性性功能低减，男性青春期发育迟缓；绝经期后女性晚期乳腺癌的姑息治疗等。<br>Tratamiento para la reducción primaria o secundaria de la función sexual masculina y el retraso en el desarrollo de la pubertad para los hombres. Y Tratamiento paliativo para el cáncer de mama metastásico para las mujeres posmenopáusicas. |
| 用法、用量<br>Administración y dosis | （1）成人常用量深部肌内注射，每次 25～50mg，每周 2～3 次。儿童常用量，每次 12.5～25mg，每周 2～3 次，疗程不超过 4～6 个月。<br>（2）功能性子宫出血，配合黄体酮使用肌内注射，每次 25～50mg，一日 1 次，共 3～4 次。<br>（3）绝经妇女晚期乳腺癌姑息性治疗，每次 50～100mg，每周 3 次，共用 2～3 个月。<br>(1) Dosis habitual para adultos por via de inyección intramuscular profunda: 25～50 mg cada vez,2～3 veces a la semana. Dosis habitual para niños: 12.5～25 mg cada vez, 2～3 veces a la semana , y el tratamiento no dura más de 4 a 6 meses.<br>(2) Para sangrado uterino disfuncional , se usa con inyecciones intramusculares de progesterona , cada vez 25～50 mg , una vez al día, en suma se aplica 3 a 4 veces.<br>(3) Para el tratamiento paliativo del cáncer de mama avanzado a mujeres posmenopáusicas, cada vez se aplica 50～100 mg, 3 veces a la semana , y el tratamiento dura dos o tres meses. |
| 剂型、规格<br>Formulaciones y especificaciones | 注射剂（油溶液）：每支 10mg（1ml）；25mg（1ml）；50mg（1ml）。<br>Inyección (solución de aceite): 10 mg (1 ml); 25 mg (1 ml); 50 mg (1 ml). |

续　表

| 药品名称 Drug Names | 苯丙酸诺龙 Nandrolona fenilpropionato |
|---|---|
| 适应证<br>Indicaciones | 慢性消耗性疾病、严重灼伤、手术前后骨折不易愈合和骨质疏松症、早产儿、儿童发育不良等。尚可用于不可手术的乳腺癌、功能性子宫出血、子宫肌瘤等。<br><br>Tratamiento para enfermedades crónicas de agotamiento, quemaduras graves y osteoporosis. Mejorar la curación de la fractura antes y después de la operación. Tratar los niños prematuros y los que tienen insuficiente desarrollo físico. Tratamiento para el cáncer de mama, hemorragia uterina funcional y leiomioma uterino sin recurrir a la cirugía. |
| 用法、用量<br>Administración y dosis | 深部肌内注射：成人每次 25mg，每 1～2 周一次，儿童每次 10mg，婴儿每次 5mg。女性转移性乳腺癌姑息性治疗，每周 25～100mg，疗程的长短视疗效及不良反应而定。<br><br>Inyección intramuscular profunda: cada vez 25 mg para adultos, una vez cada una o dos semanas, cada vez 10mg para niños, cada vez 5 mg para infantes. Para el tratamiento paliativo de cáncer de mama metastásico a las mujeres: cada semana 25～100 mg, dependiendo la duración de tratamiento de la eficacia y de los efectos secundarios. |
| 剂型、规格<br>Formulaciones y especificaciones | 注射液（油溶液）：每支 10mg（1ml）；25mg（1ml）。<br>Inyección (solución de aceite): 10 mg (1 ml); 25 mg (1 ml) |
| 药品名称 Drug Names | 司坦唑醇 Estanozolol |
| 适应证<br>Indicaciones | 预防和治疗遗传性血管神经性水肿、慢性消耗性疾病、重病及手术后体弱消瘦、年老体弱、骨质疏松症、小儿发育不良、再生障碍性贫血、白细胞减少症、血小板减少症、高脂血症等。还用于防治长期使用皮脂激素引起的肾上腺皮质功能减退。<br><br>La prevención y el tratamiento de edema angioneurótico hereditaria,enfermedades crónicas de agotamiento, debilidad y pérdida de peso después de cirugía o enfermedad grave,debilidad de los ancianos,osteoporosis, la displasia de los niños, anemia aplásica,leucopenia, trombocitopenia, hiperlipidemia, etc.. También se utiliza para la prevención y el tratamiento de la insuficiencia suprarrenal provocada por el uso de la hormona del sebo a largo plazo. |
| 用法、用量<br>Administración y dosis | 口服：成人，开始时每次 2mg，一日 2～3 次（女性酌减）。如治疗效果明显，可每隔 1～3 个月减量，直至一日 2mg 维持量。儿童，一日 1～2mg，仅在发作时应用。<br><br>Por vía oral: Para adultos, al comienzo se aplica 2mg cada vez, 2 o 3 veces al día (reducir la dosis para mujeres). Si el efecto del tratamiento es obvio, se puede reducir la dosis entre cada 1 a 3 meses, hasta que la dosis se mantiene en 2 mg por día. Para los menores, 1～2 mg al día, sólo se aplica cuando aparece los síntomas. |
| 剂型、规格<br>Formulaciones y especificaciones | 片剂：每片 2mg。<br>Tabletas: cada una 2mg. |
| 药品名称 Drug Names | 达那唑 Danazol |
| 适应证<br>Indicaciones | 治疗子宫内膜异位症，尚用于纤维性乳腺炎、男性乳房发育、乳腺痛、痛经、腹痛等，可使肿块消失、软化或缩小，使疼痛消失或减轻。还用于性早熟、自发性血小板减少性紫癜、血友病和 Christmas 病（凝血因子Ⅸ缺乏）、遗传性血管性水肿、系统性红斑狼疮等。<br><br>Se utiliza para el tratamiento de endometriosis, mastitis fibrosos, ginecomastia, dolor de mama, dismenorrea, dolor abdominal, etc. Puede hacer desaparecer, suavizar o reducir la masa, hacer desaparecer o aliviar el dolor. Se puede aplicar para tratar precoz sexual, púrpura trombocitopénica espontánea, hemofilia y la enfermedad Chrismas (deficiencia de factor IX de coagulación de la sangre), angioedema hereditario, lupus eritematoso sistémico, etc. |
| 用法、用量<br>Administración y dosis | （1）子宫内膜异位症：口服，从月经周期第 1～3 日开始服用，一日 2 次，每次 200～400mg，总量一日不超过 800mg，连续 3～6 个月为一疗程，必要时可继续到第 9 个月。<br>（2）纤维性乳腺炎：口服，每次 50～200mg，一日 2 次，连用 3～6 个月。<br>（3）男性乳房发育：口服，每日 200～600mg。<br>（4）性早熟：口服，一日 200～400mg。<br>（5）血小板减少性紫癜：口服，每次 200mg，一日 2～4 次。 |

|  | （6）血友病：口服，一日 600mg，连用 14 日。<br><br>（7）遗传性血管性水肿：口服，开始每次 200mg，一日 2 ～ 3 次。急性发作时，剂量可提高到 200mg。<br><br>（8）红斑狼疮：每天 400 ～ 600mg。<br><br>(1)Para endometriosis:a partir del primer al tercer día del ciclo menstrual empieza a tomar por vía oral 2 veces al día, 200 ~ 400 mg cada vez. La dosis diaria no exceda de 800 mg. Se aplica durante 3 ~ 6 meses consecutivos como un ciclo de tratamiento, cuando necesario puede continuar el uso hasta nueve meses.<br><br>(2)Para mastitis fibrosos: por vía oral, cada vez 50 ~ 200 mg, 2 veces al día, se aplica durante 3 a 6 meses.<br><br>(3)Para ginecomastia: por vía oral, 200 ~ 600 mg al día.<br><br>(4)Para pubertad precoz: por vía oral, 200 ~ 400 mg al día.<br><br>(5) Para púrpura trombocitopénica: por vía oral, una vez 200 mg, 2 a 4 veces al día.<br><br>(6)Para hemofilia: 600 mg al día por por por vía oral, aplicando durante 14 días consecutivos.<br><br>(7) Para angioedema hereditario: por vía oral, al comienzo cada vez 200 mg, 2 a 3 veces al día. Cuando sucede un ataque agudo, la dosis se puede incrementar a 200 mg.<br><br>(8) Para eritematoso: 400 ~ 600 mg al día. |
|---|---|
| 剂型、规格<br>Formulaciones y especificaciones | 胶囊剂：每粒 100mg；200mg。<br><br>Cápsulas: cada una 100mg; 200mg. |

### 16.3 雌激素及其类似合成药物 Estrógenos y drogas sintéticas similares

| 药品名称 Drug Names | 雌二醇 Estradiol |
|---|---|
| 适应证<br>Indicaciones | 卵巢功能不全或卵巢激素不足引起的各种症状，主要是功能性子宫出血、原发性闭经、绝经期综合征以及前列腺癌等。<br><br>Se utiliza para tratamiento de insuficiencia ovárica o una variedad de síntomas debido a deficiencia hormonal ovárica, tales como hemorragia uterina funcional, amenorrea, síndrome de la menopausia, y cáncer de próstata, etc. |
| 用法、用量<br>Administración y dosis | 肌内注射：每次 0.5 ～ 1.5mg，每周 2 ～ 3 次。口服，一日 1 片。<br><br>Por vía de inyección intramuscular: Cada vez 0.5 ~ 1.5 mg, 2 a 3 veces a la semana. Por vía oral, una tableta al día. |
| 剂型、规格<br>Formulaciones y especificaciones | 注射液：每支 2mg（1ml）。凝胶：每支 80g；0.06%。片剂：每片 1mg。微粒化 17β 雌二醇片：每片 1mg；2mg。控释贴片：周效片，每片 2.5mg；3 ～ 4 日效片：每片 4mg。<br><br>Inyección: 2 mg (1 ml). Gel: cada tubo 80 g; 0.06%.　Tabletas: Cada tableta 1mg. Tabletas de estradiol 17β micronizado: Cada tableta 1mg; 2mg. Parche de liberación controlada: parche de efecto semanal, cada parche 2.5 mg; parche de efecto de 3 a 4 días: cada parche 4 mg. |
| 药品名称 Drug Names | 苯甲酸雌二醇 Estradiol benzoato |
| 适应证<br>Indicaciones | 卵巢功能不全、闭经、绝经期综合征、退奶及前列腺癌等。<br><br>Se utiliza para tratamiento de insuficiencia ovárica, amenorrea, síndrome de la menopausia,retirada de leche y cáncer de próstata, etc. |
| 用法、用量<br>Administración y dosis | （1）绝经期综合征：肌内注射，每次 1 ～ 2mg，每 3 日一次。<br><br>（2）子宫发育不良：肌内注射，每次 1 ～ 2mg，每 2 ～ 3 日一次。<br><br>（3）子宫出血：肌内注射，每次 1mg，一日 1 次，1 周后继续用黄体酮。<br><br>(1)Para síndrome de la menopausia: por vía de inyección intramuscular, cada vez 1 ~ 2 mg, una vez entre cada tres días.<br><br>(2) Para hipoplasia uterina: por vía de inyección intramuscular, cada vez 1 ~ 2 mg, una vez entre cada 2 ó 3 días.<br><br>(3)Para sangrado uterino: por vía de inyección intramuscular, cada vez 1 mg, una vez al día, continuando con el uso de progesterona después de una semana. |

**续　表**

| 剂型、规格<br>Formulaciones y especificaciones | 注射液：每支 1mg（1ml）；2mg（1ml）。<br>Inyección: 1 mg (1 ml), 2 mg (1 ml). |
|---|---|
| **药品名称 Drug Names** | **戊酸雌二醇 Valerato de estradiol** |
| 适应证<br>Indicaciones | 口服缓解绝经后更年期症状、卵巢切除后及非癌性疾病、放疗性去势的雌激素缺乏引起的症状，外用于治疗扁平疣。<br>De forma oral se utiliza para aliviar los síntomas de la menopausia y los de la deficiencia de estrógenos causados por escisión de ovario, enfermedades no cancerosas y castración de radioterapia. De forma tópica se utiliza para tratar las verrugas. |
| 用法、用量<br>Administración y dosis | 肌内注射：每次 5～10mg，每 1～2 周一次，平均替代治疗剂量为每 2 周 5～20mg，用于卵巢功能不全，每次 5～20mg，每个月 1 次。口服，一日 1～2mg，连续 21 日，停服 1 周后开始下一疗程。<br>Por vía de inyección intramuscular: Cada vez 5～10 mg, una vez entre cada 1 a 2 semanas, la dosis promedio de la terapia de reemplazo es 5～20 mg entre cada 2 semanas. para la disfunción ovárica, cada vez 5～20 mg, una veces al mes. Por vía oral, 1～2 mg al día durante 21 días consecutivos. Iniciar el siguiente ciclo de tratamiento después de dejar el uso durante una semana. |
| 剂型、规格<br>Formulaciones y especificaciones | 注射液：每支 5mg（1ml）；10mg（1ml）。片剂：每片 0.5mg；1mg；2mg。<br>Inyección: 5 mg (1 ml), 10 mg (1 ml). Tabletas: Cada tableta 0.5mg 1mg, 2mg. |
| **药品名称 Drug Names** | **炔雌醇 Etinilestradiol** |
| 适应证<br>Indicaciones | 月经紊乱，如闭经、月经过少、功能性子宫出血、绝经期综合征，子宫发育不全、前列腺癌等。也做口服避孕药中常用的雌激素成分。<br>Se utiliza para tratamiento de trastorno menstrual como amenorrea y oligomenorrea, hemorragia uterina funcional, síndrome de la menopausia, hipoplasia del útero y cáncer de próstata. |
| 用法、用量<br>Administración y dosis | 口服：每次 0.0125～0.05mg，每晚服用 1 次，用于前列腺癌每次 0.05～0.5mg，一日 3 次。<br>Por vía oral: Cada vez 0.0125～0.05mg, una vez a cada noche. Para el cáncer de próstata: cada vez 0,05～0.5 mg, 3 veces al día. |
| 剂型、规格<br>Formulaciones y especificaciones | 片剂：每片 5μg；12.5μg；50μg；500μg。<br>Tabletas: cada tableta 5μg；12.5μg；50μg；500μg. |
| **药品名称 Drug Names** | **雌三醇 Estriol** |
| 适应证<br>Indicaciones | 绝经后妇女因雌激素缺乏而引起的泌尿生殖道萎缩和萎缩性阴道炎（及老年性阴道炎），表现为外阴或阴道干燥、瘙痒、灼热、阴道分泌物异常及性交疼痛或尿频、尿急、尿失禁等症状。<br>Se aplica a atrofia urogenital y vaginitis atrófica (y vaginitis senil) con síntomas como sequedad, quemazón y picor vaginal o vulval, anomalía de secreción vaginal, dolores sexuales y síntomas de frecuencia, urgencia y incontinencia urinarias, etc. |
| 用法、用量<br>Administración y dosis | 阴道给药，常用剂量为一日 2mg，连续治疗 1 周，以后每周放置 1 粒维持或遵医嘱。绝经后妇女阴道手术前后，在手术前 2 周，每日使用 1 次 0.5g 软膏，术后 2 周内每周用药 2 次。可疑宫颈涂片辅助诊断检查前 1 周内，每 2 日用药 1 次，每次用 0.5g 乳膏。<br>Se aplica por vía vaginal, la dosis habitual es de 2mg al día durante una semana. Después se coloca un supositorio durante una semana o consulte al médico. Para las mujeres posmenopáusicas se aplica antes y después de la cirugía vaginal. Dos semanas antes de la cirugía, se aplica el ungüento 0,5 g en una vez para cada día. Dentro de 2 semanas después de la operación, se aplica dos veces a la semana. Dentro una semana antes del examen para el diagnóstico auxiliar de frotis cervicales sospechoso, se aplica el medicamento una vez entre cada dos días, cada vez se usa 0.5 g de crema. |
| 剂型、规格<br>Formulaciones y especificaciones | 栓剂：每枚 0.5mg；1mg；2mg。乳膏：15g：15mg。<br>Supositorio: 0.5mg; 1mg, 2mg. Crema: 15g：15 mg |

**续 表**

| 药品名称Drug Names | 尼尔雌醇 Nilestriol |
|---|---|
| 适应证<br>Indicaciones | 用于雌激素缺乏引起的绝经期或更年期综合征，如潮热、出汗、头痛、目眩、疲劳、烦躁易怒、神经过敏、外阴干燥、老年性阴道炎等。<br><br>Se utiliza para síndromes de menopausia por falta de estrógeno, tales como sofocos, sudación, dolor de cabeza, mareos, cansancio, irritabilidad, nerviosismo, vulva seco, vaginitis senil, etc. |
| 用法、用量<br>Administración y<br>dosis | 口服：一次 5mg，每个月 1 次。症状改善后维持量为每次 1～2mg，每个月 2 次，3 个月为一疗程。<br><br>Por vía oral: cada vez 5mg, una veces al mes. Al mejorar los síntomas, se aplica con la dosis de mantenimiento de 1 ~ 2 mg para cada vez, y 2 veces al mes, siendo tres meses como un ciclo de tratamiento. |
| 剂型、规格<br>Formulaciones y<br>especificaciones | 片剂：每片 1mg；2mg；5mg。<br>Tabletas: cada tableta 1mg 2mg, 5mg. |
| 药品名称Drug Names | 己烯雌酚 Dietilstilbestrol |
| 适应证<br>Indicaciones | 卵巢功能不全或垂体功能异常引起的各种疾病、闭经、子宫发育不全、功能性子宫出血、绝经期综合征、老年性阴道炎等。也用于不能进行手术的晚期前列腺癌。<br><br>Se aplica a enfermedades a causa de la insuficiencia ovárica y la función anormal de la pituitaria, tales como amenorrea, útero hipoplasia, hemorragia uterina funcional, síndrome de la menopausia, vaginitis senil, etc. También se utiliza para tratar el cáncer de próstata avanzado para la que no se puede realizar la cirugía. |
| 用法、用量<br>Administración y<br>dosis | （1）闭经：口服小剂量刺激垂体前页分泌促性腺激素，每日不超过 0.25mg。<br>（2）用于人工月经周期：每日服 0.25mg，连用 20 日，待月经后再用同法治疗，共 3 个周期。<br>（3）用于月经周期延长及子宫发育不全：每日服 0.1～0.2mg，持续半年，经期停服。<br>（4）治疗功能性子宫出血：每晚服 0.5～1mg，连服 20 日。<br>（5）用于绝经期综合征：每日服 0.25mg，症状控制后改为每日 0.1mg。<br>（6）老年性阴道炎：阴道塞药，每晚塞入 0.2～0.4mg，共用 7 日。<br>（7）配合手术用于前列腺癌：一日 3mg，分 3 次服，连用 2～3 个月，维持量每日 1mg。<br>（8）用于因子宫发育不良及子宫颈分泌物黏稠所致不育症：以小剂量促使宫颈黏液稀薄，精子宜透入，于月经后每日 0.1mg，共 15 日，疗程 3～6 个月。<br>（9）用于稽留流产（妊娠 7 个月内死胎经 2 个月或以上仍未娩出）：每次服 5mg，每日 3 次，5～7 日为一疗程，停药 5 日，如无效，可重复一疗程。<br><br>(1) Para amenorrea : Dosis baja por vía oral para estimular la pituitaria anterior con motivo de mejorar la secreción de la gonadotropina: no supere 0.25 mg al día.<br>(2)Para el ciclo menstrual artificial : 0.25mg al día por vía oral en 20 días consecutivos hasta la menstruación. Después se aplica el mismo tratamiento con el mismo método repetiéndolo para tres ciclos en total.<br>(3) Para prolongar ciclo  menstrual y tratar uterina hipoplasia: 0.1 ~ 0.2 mg al día en seis meses consecutivos, dejándolo durante la menstruación.<br>(4) Tratamiento del sangrado uterino disfuncional : 0.5 ~ 1 mg a cada noche en 20 días consecutivos.<br>(5) Para el síndrome de la menopausia : 0.25mg al día. Al estar controlado el síndrome, reduzca la dosis a 0.1mg al día.<br>(6)vaginitis senil: se aplica el supositorio vaginal , 0.2 ~ 0.4 mg a cada noche en 7 días consecutivos.<br>(7) Tratamiento del cáncer de próstata durante la terapia cirugía: 3 mg al día dividida en 3 veces en 2 a 3 meses consecutivos. La dosis de mantenimiento diaria es de 1 mg.<br>(8) Para la infertilidad debido a hipoplasia uterina y viscosas secreciones cervicales: diluir la secreción cervical mejorando la penetración del esperma. Se aplica 0.1 mg al día después de la menstruación en 15 días consecutivos, con un ciclo de tratamiento 3 a 6 meses.<br>(9) Para aborto retenido ( después de más de 2 meses no se entrega el parto muerto menores de 7 meses): cada vez 5 mg, 3 veces al día. se aplica 5 a 7 días como un ciclo de tratamiento. Repita el ciclo de tratamiento si no tiene efecto. |
| 剂型、规格<br>Formulaciones y<br>especificaciones | 片剂：每片 0.5mg；1mg；2mg。注射液：每支 0.5mg（1ml）；1mg（1ml）；2mg（1ml）。<br>Tabletas: Cada tableta 0.5mg; 1mg; 2mg. Inyección: 0.5 mg (1 ml); 1 mg (1 ml); 2 mg (1 ml). |

续　表

### 16.4　孕激素类 Progestinas

| 药品名称 Drug Names | 黄体酮 Progesterona |
| --- | --- |
| 适应证<br>Indicaciones | 　　用于习惯性流产、痛经、经血过多或血崩症、闭经等。口服大剂量也用于黄体酮不足所致疾患，如经前综合征、排卵停止所致月经紊乱、良性乳腺病、围绝经期激素替代疗法。<br><br>　　Se aplica al aborto habitual, dismenorrea, menorragia o metrorragia, amenorrea, etc. Por vía oral de gran cantidad también se utiliza para tratar enfermedades causadas por insuficiencia de progesterona así como síndrome premenstrual, trastornos menstruales debidos a la deja de ovulación y enfermedades benignas de mama. Además se aplica para la terapia de sustitución hormonal premenopáusica. |
| 用法、用量<br>Administración y dosis | 　　（1）习惯性流产：肌内注射，一次 10～20mg，一日 1 次，或每周 2～3 次，一直用到妊娠第 4 个月。<br>　　（2）先兆流产：肌内注射，一般一日 20～50mg，待疼痛及出血停止后减为一日 10～20mg。<br>　　（3）痛经：在月经之前 6～8 日每天肌内注射 5～10mg，共 4～6 日，疗程可重复若干次，对子宫发育不全所致的痛经，可与雌激素配合使用。<br>　　（4）经血过多和血崩症：肌内注射，一日 10～20mg，5～7 日为一疗程，可重复 3～4 个疗程，每疗程间隔 15～20 日。<br>　　（5）闭经：先肌内注射雌激素 2～3 周后，立即给予本品，每日肌内注射 3～5mg，6～8 日为一疗程，总剂量不宜超过 300～350mg，疗程可重复 2～3 次。<br>　　（6）功能性出血：肌内注射，一日 5～10mg，连用 5～10 日，如在用药期间月经来潮，应立即停药。<br><br>　　(1) Para aborto habitual: Por vía de inyección intramuscular, cada vez 10～20 mg, una vez al día o dos a tres veces a la semana durante los primeros cuatro meses de embarazo.<br>　　(2) Para aborto incipiente: Por vía de inyección intramuscular, generalmente 20～50 mg al día, reduciendo la dosis a 10～20 mg al día después de la desaparición del dolor y el sangrado.<br>　　(3) Para dismenorrea: Antes de la menstruación se aplican 6 a 8 inyecciones intramusculares de 5～10 mg al día en 4 a 6 días. El tratamiento se puede repetir varias veces. En cuanto a la dismenorrea debido a hipoplasia uterina, puede ser utilizado en conjunción con estrógeno.<br>　　(4) Para menorragia y metrorragia: Por vía de inyección intramuscular, 10～20 mg al día, aplicándose en 5～7 días para un ciclo de tratamiento que se puede repetir tres a cuatro veces. Entre ciclos hay un intervalo de 15 a 20 días.<br>　　(5) Para amenorrea: se aplica por vía de inyección intramuscular después de la aplicación de estrógeno durante 2 a 3 semanas. Se aplica 3～5 mg cada día, y 6～8 días para un ciclo de tratamiento que se puede repetir 2～3 tres veces con la dosis máxima de 300～350 mg.<br>　　(6) Para sangrado funcional: por vía de inyección intramuscular, cada día 5～10 mg, se aplica en 5 a 10 días consecutivos. Se debe suspender el uso de este producto en el periodo de menstruación. |
| 剂型、规格<br>Formulaciones y especificaciones | 　　注射液：每支 10mg（1ml）；20mg（1ml）。胶囊：每粒 100mg。<br>　　Inyección: 10 mg (1 ml); 20 mg (1 ml). Cápsulas: 100mg. |
| 药品名称 Drug Names | 甲羟孕酮 Medroxiprogesterona |
| 适应证<br>Indicaciones | 　　痛经、功能性闭经、功能性子宫出血、先兆流产或习惯性流产、子宫内膜异位症等。大剂量可用作长效避孕针，肌内注射 1 次 150mg，可避孕 3 个月。<br><br>　　Se utiliza para tratamiento de dismenorrea, amenorrea funcional, hemorragia funcional, aborto incipiente o habitual, endoetriosis, etc. Cuando se utiliza a gran cantidad de forma de inyección, se aplica para el anticonceptivo a largo plazo, siendo el efecto de 3 meses a recibir una inyección intramuscular de 150mg. |
| 用法、用量<br>Administración y dosis | 　　（1）功能性闭经：一日口服 4～8mg，连用 5～10 日。<br>　　（2）子宫内膜癌或肾癌：口服，一次 100mg，一日 3 次，肌内注射，起始 0.4～1g，1 周后可重复一次，待病情改善或稳定后，剂量改为 400mg，每月 1 次。<br>　　（3）避孕：肌内注射，每 3 个月一次 150mg，于月经来潮第 2～7 日注射。<br>　　(1) Para amenorrea funcional: Se aplica por vía oral 4～8 mg al día en 5 a 10 días consecutivos. |

|  | (2) Para cáncer endometrial o cáncer de riñón: Por vía oral, cada vez 100 mg, 3 veces al día. Por vía de inyección intramuscular, la dosis inicial es de 0.4 ~ 1 g, se puede repetir la aplicación una vez después de una semana. Después de el mejoramiento o estabilización de la enfermedad, la dosis se reduce a 400 mg cada vez y una vez al mes.<br><br>(3) Para anticoncepción: Por vía de inyección intramuscular, una vez de 150 mg  para tres meses. Se aplica entre el  segundo y el séptimo día de la menstruación. |
|---|---|
| 剂型、规格<br>Formulaciones y especificaciones | 片剂：每片 2mg；4mg；10mg。　注射液：100mg；150mg。<br>Tabletas: Cada una 2 mg; 4 mg; 10 mg. Inyección: 100mg; 150mg. |

| 药品名称 Drug Names | 炔孕酮 Etisterona |
|---|---|
| 适应证<br>Indicaciones | 功能性子宫出血、月经异常、闭经、痛经等。也用于防止先兆性流产和习惯性流产，但由于维持妊娠作用较弱，效果并不佳。如与雌激素炔雌醇合用，则疗效较好。<br><br>Se aplica a hemorragia uterina funcional, menstruación anormal,amenorrea, dismenorrea,etc. También se utiliza para prevenir el aborto incipiente y habitual.Tiene mejor efecto aplicándose junto con estrógeno etinilestradiol. |
| 用法、用量<br>Administración y dosis | 口服：一次 10mg，一日 3 次。舌下含服：一次 10 ～ 20mg，一日 2 ～ 3 次。<br><br>Por vía oral: cada vez 10 mg, 3 veces al día. Por vía sublingual: cada vez 10 ~ 20 mg, 2 a 3 veces al día. |
| 剂型、规格<br>Formulaciones y especificaciones | 片剂：每片 5mg；10mg；25mg。<br>Tabletas: Cada una 5mg; 10mg; 25mg. |

| 药品名称 Drug Names | 屈螺酮 Drospirenona |
|---|---|
| 适应证<br>Indicaciones | 女性避孕。<br>Anticoncepción femenina. |
| 用法、用量<br>Administración y dosis | 必须按照包装所表明的顺序，每天约在同一时间用少量液体送服。一日 1 片，连服 21 日。停药 7 日后开始服用下一盒药，其间通常会出现撤退性出血。<br><br>Debe seguir las instrucciones en el empaquete indicando el orden de aplicación. Se toma por vía oral una tableta a la misma hora cada día con una pequeña cantidad de líquido, y se repite en 21 días consecutivos. Comience a tomar la otra caja de la medicina 7 días después de la retirada, en la ocurriría generalmente sangrado de retirada . |
| 剂型、规格<br>Formulaciones y especificaciones | 复方制剂（优思明）：每片含屈螺酮 3mg 和炔雌醇 0.03mg。<br><br>Tabletas compuestas (Yasmín): Cada tableta contiene 3mg de drospirenona y 0.03mg de etinil estradiol |

## 16.5　促性腺激素 Gonadotropina

| 药品名称 Drug Names | 绒毛膜促性腺激素 Gonadotropina coriónica |
|---|---|
| 适应证<br>Indicaciones | （1）青春期隐睾症的诊断和治疗。<br>（2）垂体功能低下所致的男性不育。<br>（3）垂体促性腺激素不足所致的女性无排卵性不孕症。<br>（4）用于体外受精以获取多个卵母细胞。<br>（5）女性黄体功能不足、功能性子宫出血、妊娠早期先兆流产、习惯性流产。<br>(1)El diagnóstico y el tratamiento de criptorquidismo de la pubertad.<br>(2)Varones infértiles debido al hipopituitarismo.<br>(3)La infertilidad de anovulación debido a la deficiencia de la hormona gonadotropina.<br>(4)Para obtener ovocitos con motivo de fertilización en vitro.<br>(5)La insuficiencia lútea, hemorragia uterina funcional,aborto incipiente y habitual. |

续　表

| | |
|---|---|
| 用法、用量<br>Administración y<br>dosis | （1）促排卵：于绝经后促性腺激素末次给药后一日或氯米芬末次给药后 5 ～ 7 日肌内注射一次 5000 ～ 10 000U，连续治疗 3 ～ 6 周期，如无效，应停药。<br><br>（2）黄体功能不足：于经期第 15 ～ 17 日排卵之日起，隔日注射一次 1500U，连用 5 次，剂量可根据患者的反应作调整，妊娠后需维持原剂量直至 7 ～ 10 孕周。<br><br>（3）功能性子宫出血：肌内注射一次 1000 ～ 3000U。<br><br>（4）青春期前隐睾症，肌内注射一次，1000 ～ 5000U，每周 2 ～ 3 次。<br><br>（5）男性性功能减退症：肌内注射一次 1000 ～ 4000U，每周 2 ～ 3 次，持续数周至数月。<br><br>（6）先兆流产或习惯性流产：肌内注射一次 1000 ～ 5000U。<br><br>(1)Promover la ovulación: el día después de la última aplicación de gonadotropina o  5 a 7 días después de la última aplicación de clomifeno se aplica por vía de la inyección intramuscular una vez 5000 a 10 000 unidades en el tratamiento continuo postmenopáusica durante 3 a 6 ciclos. Si no tiene efecto, debe suspenderlo.<br><br>(2)Para insuficiencia lútea: después de 15 a 17 días a partir del primer día de la menstruación en la ovulación, se aplica 1.500 unidades una vez cada dos días, repitiéndose cinco veces. La dosis puede ajustarse según la respuesta del paciente, después del embarazo, la dosis inicial se debe mantener hasta la séptima a décima semana de embarazo.<br><br>(3) Para sangrado uterino disfuncional: una vez por vía de inyección intramuscular  de 1000 a 3000 unidades.<br><br>(4) Para criptorquidia antes de la pubertad,  por vía de inyección intramuscular, una vez 1000 a 5000 unidades, dos a tres veces a la semana.<br><br>(5) Para síndrome de disfunción sexual masculina: por vía de inyección intramuscular, una vez 1000 ~ 4000 unidades, 2 a 3 veces a la semana, aplicándose en varias semanas o hasta varios meses.<br><br>(6) Para aborto incipiente o aborto habitual, por vía de inyección intramuscular, una vez 1000 ~ 5000 unidades. |
| 剂型、规格<br>Formulaciones y<br>especificaciones | 注射用绒促性素：每支 500U；1000U；2000U；5000U。<br><br>Gonadotropina coriónica para inyección: cada una 500 unidades; 1000 unidades; 2000 unidades; 5000 unidades. |
| 药品名称 Drug Names | 尿促性素 Menotropina |
| 适应证<br>Indicaciones | ①与绒促性素或氯米芬配合使用以治疗无排卵性不孕症。②用于原发性或继发性闭经，男性精子缺乏症以及卵巢功能试验等。<br><br>① El tratamiento de la infertilidad de anovulación junto con el uso de Coriogonadotropina o Citrato de clomifeno. ② Para amenorrea primaria y secundaria,falta de esperma. Y se utiliza para pruebas de la función de ovario. |
| 用法、用量<br>Administración y<br>dosis | 肌内注射：用于诱导排卵，开始一日 75 ～ 150U，连用 7 ～ 12 日，至雌激素水平增高后，再肌内注射绒促性素，经 12 小时即排卵。用于男性性功能低下，开始 1 周给予 HCG 每次 2000U，共 2 ～ 3 次，以产生适当的男性特征。然后肌内注射本品，每次 75 ～ 150U，每周 3 次，同时给予 HCG 每次 2000U，每周 2 次。至少治疗 4 个月。<br><br>Por vía de inyección intramuscular, se utiliza para inducir la ovulación. Al inicio se aplica 75 a 150 unidades por día en 7 a 12 días consecutivos hasta los niveles de estrógeno se eleve. A continuación se aplica HCG por vía de inyección intramuscular. La ovulación comienza en12 horas. Para la disfunción sexual masculina, al inicio aplique HCG 2000 unidades repitiendo 2 a 3 veces durante la primera semana para producir apropiada masculinidad. Luego se aplica este producto por vía de inyección intramuscular, cada vez 75 a 150 unidades, tres veces a la semana, mientras se usa HCG 2000 unidades para cada vez, dos veces a la semana, continuándose en 4 meses por lo menos. |
| 剂型、规格<br>Formulaciones y<br>especificaciones | 注射用尿促性素：每支 75U；150U。<br><br>HMG para inyección: cada una 75 unidades; 150 unidades. |
| 药品名称 Drug Names | 普罗瑞林 Protirelina |
| 适应证<br>Indicaciones | 用于诊断 Graves 病、甲状腺功能减退症及促甲状腺素性突眼等。<br><br>Para el diagnóstico de la enfermedad de Graves, hipotiroidismo y exoftalmos tirotropina, etc. |

**续 表**

| | |
|---|---|
| 用法、用量<br>Administración y dosis | 静脉注射本品 200～500μg，观察血中促甲状腺激素水平的变化，正常人于注射后 15～30 分钟达峰值，为基础值的 2～3 倍以上。<br><br>Por vía de inyección intravenosa se aplica 200～500μg, observando los niveles de hormona estimulante del tiroides en la sangre. Para personas normales los niveles alcanza al máximo 15 a 30 minutos después de la inyección, más de 2 a 3 veces mayor que el valor básico. |
| 剂型、规格<br>Formulaciones y especificaciones | 注射用普罗瑞林：0.5mg。<br>Protirelina para inyección: 0.5 mg. |
| **药品名称 Drug Names** | 亮丙瑞林 Leuprorelina |
| 适应证<br>Indicaciones | 子宫内膜异位症，对伴有月经过多、下腹痛、腰痛及贫血等的子宫肌瘤，可使肌瘤缩小和（或）症状改善，绝经前乳腺癌且雌激素受体阳性患者；前列腺癌、中枢性性早熟症。<br><br>Para la endometriosis, cáncer de mama antes de la menopausia, los pacientes de receptor estrogénico positivo, cáncer de próstata, pubertad precoz central. Y para mejorar el leiomioma uterino acompañado de menorragia, dolor abdominal, dolor de espalda y anemia. |
| 用法、用量<br>Administración y dosis | 前列腺癌、绝经前乳腺癌，皮下注射，每次 3.75mg，每 4 周一次。子宫内膜异位症：通常成人皮下注射，每次 3.75mg，每 4 周一次，对体重低于 50kg 时，可以使用 1.88mg 的制剂。初次给药于经期开始后的第 1～5 日。子宫肌瘤：通常成人皮下注射每次 1.88mg，每 4 周一次，对体重过重或子宫明显增大的患者，应注射 3.75mg。初次给药于经期开始后的 1～5 日。中枢性性早熟症：通常皮下注射 30μg/kg，每 4 周一次，根据患者症状可增量至 90μg/kg。<br><br>Para cáncer de próstata y cáncer de mama antes de la menopausia, se aplica por vía subcutánea, cada vez 3.75 mg, una vez entre cada cuatro semanas. Para endometriosis, por vía subcutánea generalmente para los adultos, cada vez 3.75 mg, una vez entre cada cuatro semanas, para las mujeres con peso corporal inferior a 50 kg, se puede utilizar el producto de 1.88mg con su uso inicial después del primer al quito día desde el período menstrual. Para los fibromas uterinos, generalmente por vía subcutánea a los adultos, cada vez 1.88mg, una vez entre cada cuatro semanas. Para paciente sobrepeso o cuyo útero es grande, debe aplicar el producto de 3.75mg con su uso inicial después del primer al quito día desde el período menstrual. Para pubertad precoz central: por lo general se aplica por vía subcutánea, cada vez 30μg/kg, una vez entre cada cuatro semanas, de acuerdo a los síntomas del paciente la dosis puede ser incrementada gradualmente a 90μg/kg. |
| 剂型、规格<br>Formulaciones y especificaciones | 注射用亮丙瑞林微球：3.75mg/ 瓶。<br>Microesferas de leuprolida para inyección: 3.75 mg / botella. |
| **药品名称 Drug Names** | 戈舍瑞林 Goserelina |
| 适应证<br>Indicaciones | 前列腺癌：本品适用于可用激素治疗的前列腺癌。<br>乳腺癌：适用于可用激素治疗的绝经前期及围绝经期妇女的乳腺癌。<br>子宫内膜异位症：缓解症状包括减轻疼痛并减少子宫内膜损伤的大小和数目。<br>Cáncer de próstata disponible de tratamiento hormonal.<br>Cáncer de mama disponible de tratamiento hormonal para mujeres premenopáusicas y perimenopáusicas.<br>La endometriosis : para aliviar los síntomas, incluyendo el alivio del dolor y reducir el tamaño y el número de lesiones de endometrio. |
| 用法、用量<br>Administración y dosis | 腹部皮下注射植入剂：每 28 日一次，每次 3.6mg，如果必要可使用局部麻醉。子宫内膜异位症者治疗不应超过 6 个月。<br><br>Implantes subcutáneos abdominales: cada vez 3.6 mg, una vez en 28 días, aplicando anestésico local si es necesario. Para el tratamiento de la endometriosis la aplicación no debe exceder a 6 meses. |
| 剂型、规格<br>Formulaciones y especificaciones | 缓释植入剂：每支 3.6mg。<br>Implante de liberación sostenida: cada uno 3.6mg. |

**续　表**

| 药品名称 Drug Names | 丙氨瑞林 Alarelina |
|---|---|
| 适应证<br>Indicaciones | 子宫内膜异位症。<br>Para la endometriosis. |
| 用法、用量<br>Administración y dosis | 皮下或肌内注射，从月经来潮的第 1～2 日开始治疗，每次 150μg，一日 1 次，或遵医嘱。制剂在临用前用 2ml 灭菌生理盐水溶解。对子宫内膜异位症，3～6 个月为一疗程。<br>Por vía de inyección subcutánea o intramuscular, comience el tratamiento 1 a 2 días después de la menstruación, cada vez 150μg, una vez al día, o se aplica según las indicaciones de médico. Antes de su utilización disuelva en solución salina estéril de 2ml. Para la endometriosis, 3 a 6 meses es un ciclo de tratamiento. |
| 剂型、规格<br>Formulaciones y especificaciones | 注射用阿拉瑞林：每支 25μg；150μg。<br>Alarelin para inyección: 25μg; 150μg. |
| 药品名称 Drug Names | 曲普瑞林 Triptorelina |
| 适应证<br>Indicaciones | 临床主要用于前列腺癌，还用于促排卵，治疗妇女不育症。<br>Se utiliza principalmente para el cáncer de próstata clínico, y también para la inducción de la ovulación, tratamiento de la infertilidad de las mujeres. |
| 用法、用量<br>Administración y dosis | 缓释剂型仅可肌内注射，一次一支，每 4 周一次。皮下注射：一日 1 次 0.1mg。用于促排卵：于月经周期第 2 日开始，一日 1 次，0.1mg，连续 10～12 日。<br>Formas de dosificación de liberación sostenida sólo se aplica por vía de inyección intramuscular, cada vez una inyección, una vez en cuatro semanas. Por vía de inyección subcutánea: una vez 0.1mg para un día. Para la inducción de la ovulación: desde el segundo día después del ciclo menstrual se aplica una vez al día, cada vez 0.1 mg, durante 10 a 12 días consecutivos. |
| 剂型、规格<br>Formulaciones y especificaciones | 粉针剂：每支 0.1mg。<br>Polvo para inyección: 0.1mg. |

16.6　短效口服避孕药 Píldoras anticonceptivas de acción corta por vía oral

| 药品名称 Drug Names | 炔诺酮 Noretindrona |
|---|---|
| 适应证<br>Indicaciones | 除作为口服避孕药外，还可用于功能性子宫出血、妇女不育症、痛经、闭经、子宫内膜异位症、子宫内膜增生过长等。<br>No sólo sirve como anticonceptivos orales, sino también para la hemorragia uterina disfuncional, la infertilidad femenina, dismenorrea, amenorrea, endometriosis, hiperplasia endometrial, etc. |
| 用法、用量<br>Administración y dosis | 口服，一次 1.25～5mg，每日 1～2 次。<br>Por vía oral, cada vez 1.25～5 mg, 1 o 2 veces al día. |
| 剂型、规格<br>Formulaciones y especificaciones | 复方炔诺酮片（避孕片一号）：每片含炔诺酮 0.6mg 和炔雌醇 0.035mg。<br>Tabletas de noretindrona compuesto (tabletas anticonceptivas número uno): Cada tableta contiene 0.6 mg de noretindrona y 0.035mg de etinilestradiol. |
| 药品名称 Drug Names | 甲地孕酮 Megestrol |
| 适应证<br>Indicaciones | 主要用作短效口服避孕药，也可作肌内注射长效避孕药，还可用于治疗痛经、闭经、功能性子宫出血、子宫内膜异位症及子宫内膜腺癌等。由于其抗雌激素活性，近亦用于乳腺癌的姑息治疗。<br>Se utiliza principalmente para anticonceptivos orales de acción corta, se sirve de los anticonceptivos de acción prolongada de forma de inyección intramuscular, también para el tratamiento de la dismenorrea, amenorrea, sangrado uterino disfuncional, la endometriosis y el adenocarcinoma de endometrio.Debido a su actividad anti-estrogénica, se utiliza en el tratamiento paliativo de cáncer de mama. |

| | |
|---|---|
| 用法、用量<br>Administración y dosis | （1）用作短效口服避孕药：从月经周期第 5 日起，每天口服一片甲地孕酮片、膜或纸片，连服 22 日为一周期，停药后 2～4 日来月经，然后于第 5 日继续服下一个月的药。<br><br>（2）治疗功能性子宫出血：口服甲地孕酮片、膜或纸片，每 8 小时一次，每次 2mg，然后将剂量每 3 日递减一次，直至维持量每天 4mg，连服 20 日，流血停止后，每天加服炔雌醇 0.05mg 或己烯雌酚 1mg，共 20 日。<br><br>（3）闭经：口服，每次一片甲地孕酮片和炔雌醇 0.05mg，共 20 日，连服 3 个月。<br><br>（4）痛经和子宫内膜增生过长：于月经第 5～7 日开始，每日口服一片，共 20 日。<br><br>（5）子宫内膜异位症：每次一片，每日 2 次，共 7 日，然后每日 3 次，每次 1 片，共 7 日，再后，一日 2 次，每次 2 片，共 7 日，最后每天 20mg，共 6 周。<br><br>（6）子宫内膜癌：口服，一日 4 次，每次 10～80mg，连续 2 个月。<br><br>（7）乳腺癌：口服，一日 4 次，每次 40mg，连续 2 个月为一疗程。<br><br>(1) Se utiliza como anticonceptivo oral de acción corta: Desde el quinto día del ciclo menstrual, se toma cada día una tableta o un formador de película o una tableta de papel en 22 días consecutivos como un ciclo, 2 a 4 días después de la deja de su uso comienza la menstruación, continuando con un nuevo ciclo a parir del quinto día de la menstruación.<br><br>(2) Tratamiento del sangrado uterino disfuncional : tableta o formador de película o tableta de papel , cada vez 2 mg, una vez a cada 8 horas, reduciendo la dosis entre cada 3 días hasta la dosis de mantenimiento de 4 mg al día durante 20 días consecutivos. Al detenerse el sangrado, se aplica el uso adicional de etinil estradiol 0.05mg o dietilestilbestrol 1mg para cada día, en 20 días consecutivos.<br><br>(3) Para amenorrea: Por vía oral, cada vez una tableta de acetato de megestrol y 0,05 mg de etinilestradiol, en 20 días y hasta tres meses.<br><br>(4) Para dismenorrea y la hiperplasia endometrial: se inició después de los primeros 5～7 días de la menstruación, aplicándose una tableta por vía oral diariamente en 20 días .<br><br>(5) Para endometriosis: cada vez una tableta, dos veces al día durante 7 días; y luego cada vez una tableta, tres veces al día y durante 7 días; y después cada vez dos tabletas y dos veces al día y durante 7 días; por último 20mg para cada día en 6 semanas.<br><br>(6) Para cáncer endometrial: Por vía oral, 4 veces al día, cada vez 10～80 mg, en 2 meses consecutivos.<br><br>(7) cáncer de mama: por vía oral, 4 veces al día, cada vez 40 mg, aplicándose en 2 meses consecutivos como un ciclo de tratamiento. |
| 剂型、规格<br>Formulaciones y especificaciones | 片剂：每片 1mg；4mg。<br>膜剂：每片 1mg；4mg。<br>纸片：每片 1mg；4mg。<br><br>Tabletas: Cada tableta 1mg；4mg.<br>Formadores de película: 1 mg, 4 mg.<br>Tableta de papel: 1mg；4mg. |
| 药品名称 Drug Names | 炔诺孕酮 Norgestrel |
| 适应证<br>Indicaciones | 主要以炔雌醇组成复方作为短效口服避孕药，也可通过剂型改变用作长效避孕药，还可用于治疗痛经、月经不调。<br><br>Anticonceptivo oral de acción corta compuesto principalmente de etinilestradiol. También se puede utilizar como anticonceptivo de acción prolongada cambiando la dosis. Además se aplica para el tratamiento de dismenorrea y menstruación irregular. |
| 用法、用量<br>Administración y dosis | （1）用作短效口服避孕药：口服复方炔诺孕酮一号片或滴丸，从月经第 5 日开始，一日服 1 片（丸），连服 22 日，不能间断，服完后 3～4 日即来月经，并于月经的第 5 日再服下一个月的药。<br><br>（2）用作探亲避孕药：于探亲当晚开始服炔诺孕酮探亲避孕药，一日 1 片，服法同炔诺酮。<br><br>（3）用作房事后避孕药：房事后 72 小时内口服 2 片事后避孕药，12 小时后再服 2 片。<br><br>(1) Anticonceptivo oral de acción corta: tome tableta o píldora del goteo de norgestrel número uno a partir del quinto día desde el inicio de la menstruación, aplicando una tableta(o píldora)al día durante 22 días sin interrupción. 3～4 días después comenzaría la menstruación. Aplique otro ciclo desde el quinto día de la menstruación.<br><br>(2) Anticonceptivo antes del contacto sexual: empiece a tomar una tableta a la noche antes del contacto sexual, una tableta al día, refiriendo al uso de noretindrona.<br><br>(3) Anticonceptivo de emergencia: se toma 2 tabletas entre 72 horas después del contacto sexual, y otras dos en 12 horas. |

**续　表**

| 剂型、规格<br>Formulaciones y<br>especificaciones | 复方炔诺酮一号片（复甲一号）：每片含炔诺孕酮 0.3mg 和炔雌醇 0.03mg。<br>Tabletas noretisterona compuestas número uno: cada tableta contiene 0.3 mg de norgestrel y 0.03mg dc ctinilcstradiol. |
|---|---|

## 16.7　抗早孕药 Drogas antiembarazo

| 药品名称 Drug Names | 米非司酮 Mifepristona |
|---|---|
| 适应证<br>Indicaciones | 除用于抗早孕、催经止孕、胎死宫内引产外，还用于妇科手术操作，如宫内节育器的放置和取出、取内膜标本、宫颈管发育异常的激光分离及宫颈扩张和刮宫术。<br>Se utiliza no sólo para anti-embarazo, instar menstruación terminando embarazo y la inducción de fetal muerte, sino también para procedimientos quirúrgicos ginecológicos, tales como la colocación y extracción del DIU, tomar muestras de endometrio, separación de displasia cervical por láser, dilatación cervical y curetaje. |
| 用法、用量<br>Administración y<br>dosis | 停经≤ 49 日的健康早妊娠期妇女，于空腹或进食后 1 小时口服，①顿服 200mg；②每次 25mg，一日 2 次，连续 3 日，服药后禁食 1 小时。<br>Para mujeres sanas en el embarazo temprano dentro de 49 días después de la menopausia, se aplica con el estómago vacío o 1 hora después de comer ① 200mg cada vez y 3 veces al día; ② cada vez 25 mg, 2 veces al día durante tres días, comer después de 1 hora de su aplicación. |
| 剂型、规格<br>Formulaciones y<br>especificaciones | 片剂：每片 25mg；200mg。<br>Tabletas: 25mg; 200mg. |

## 16.8　高血糖素 Glucagón

| 药品名称 Drug Names | 高血糖素 Glucagón |
|---|---|
| 适应证<br>Indicaciones | 用于低血糖症，在一时不能口服或静脉注射葡萄糖时特别有用。用于心源性休克有效。<br>Para la hipoglucemia, especialmente útil en el momento de no poder usar glucosa por vía oral o intravenosa. Tiene efecto para el shock cardiogénico. |
| 用法、用量<br>Administración y<br>dosis | 肌内注射、皮下注射或静脉注射，用于低血糖症，每次 0.5 ~ 1.0mg，5 分钟左右即可见效。用于心源性休克，连续静脉滴注，每小时 1 ~ 12mg。<br>Para la hipoglucemia por vía intramuscular, subcutánea o intravenosa, cada vez 0.5 ~ 1.0mg, puede ser eficaz en alrededor de 5 minutos. Para el shock cardiogénico, por vía de la infusión intravenosa continua, cada hora 1 ~ 12 mg. |
| 剂型、规格<br>Formulaciones y<br>especificaciones | 注射用高血糖素：每支 1mg；10mg。<br>Glucagón para inyección: 1 mg; 10 mg. |

## 16.9　胰岛素 Insulina

| 药品名称 Drug Names | 胰岛素 Insulina |
|---|---|
| 适应证<br>Indicaciones | 用于糖尿病患者，控制血糖，特别是餐后血糖。<br>Para los pacientes con diabetes al controlar la glucosa en sangre, en particular la postprandial. |
| 用法、用量<br>Administración y<br>dosis | 餐前 30 分钟皮下注射，用药后 30 分钟内须进食含糖类的食物，一日 3 ~ 4 次。<br>Se aplica 3 a 4 veces al día por inyección subcutánea 30 minutos antes de las comidas. Hay que comer los alimentos que contienen hidratos de carbono dentro de 30 minutos después de su aplicación. |
| 剂型、规格<br>Formulaciones y<br>especificaciones | 注射液：重组人胰岛素注射液：每瓶 400U（10ml）。笔芯：300U（3ml）。生物合成人胰岛素注射液：每瓶 400U（10ml）。笔芯：300U（3ml）。胰岛素（猪）注射液：每瓶 400U（10ml）。<br>Inyección: insulina humana recombinante para inyección: 400U cada botella (10 ml). Recambio: 300U (3 ml). Insulina humana biosintética para inyección: 400U cada botella (10 ml). Recambio: 300U (3 ml). Insulina (porcinos) para inyección: 400U cada botella (10 ml). |

**续 表**

| 药品名称 Drug Names | 门冬胰岛素 Insulina aspartico |
| --- | --- |
| 适应证<br>Indicaciones | 用于控制餐后血糖，也可与中效胰岛素合用控制晚间或晨起高血糖。<br>Se utiliza para controlar la glucosa en sangre postprandial, también se puede utilizar en combinación con insulina de acción intermedia para controlar el alto nivel de azúcar en la sangre en la noche o temprano por la mañana. |
| 用法、用量<br>Administración y dosis | 于 3 餐前 15 分钟至进餐开始时皮下注射一次，根据血糖情况调整剂量。<br>Se aplica por vía de inyección subcutánea a los 15 minutos antes de cada comida, ajustando la dosis de acuerdo con la glucosa en sangre. |
| 剂型、规格<br>Formulaciones y especificaciones | 注射液：300U（3ml）。<br>Inyección: 300U(3ml). |
| 药品名称 Drug Names | 赖脯胰岛素 Insulina lispro |
| 适应证<br>Indicaciones | 用于控制餐后血糖，也可与中效胰岛素合用控制晚间或晨起高血糖。<br>Se utiliza para controlar la glucosa en sangre postprandial, también se puede utilizar en combinación con insulina de acción intermedia para controlar el alto nivel de azúcar en la sangre en la noche o temprano por la mañana. |
| 用法、用量<br>Administración y dosis | 于 3 餐前 15 分钟至进餐开始时皮下注射一次，根据血糖情况调整剂量。<br>Se aplica por vía de inyección subcutánea a los 15 minutos antes de cada comida, ajustando la dosis de acuerdo con la glucosa en sangre. |
| 剂型、规格<br>Formulaciones y especificaciones | 注射液：300U（3ml）。<br>Inyección: 300U(3ml). |
| 药品名称 Drug Names | 低精蛋白锌胰岛素 Isophane insulina |
| 适应证<br>Indicaciones | 用于糖尿病控制血糖，一般与短效胰岛素配合使用，提供胰岛素的日基础用量。<br>Para control de glucosa en sangre para la diabetes. Se utiliza por lo general en combinación con insulina de acción corta, ofreciendo la dosis diaria básica. |
| 用法、用量<br>Administración y dosis | 于睡前或早餐前每日一次给药或者早晚一日 2 次给药，以控制空腹血糖。<br>Se aplica una vez antes de dormir o el desayuno o dos veces a la mañana y a la noche para controlar la glucemia en ayunas. |
| 剂型、规格<br>Formulaciones y especificaciones | 注射液：每瓶 400U（10ml）。笔芯：300U（3ml）。<br>Inyección：400U cada botella（10 ml）. Recambio：300U (3 ml). |
| 药品名称 Drug Names | 精蛋白锌胰岛素 Insulina protamina zinc |
| 适应证<br>Indicaciones | 用于糖尿病控制血糖，一般与短效胰岛素配合使用，提供胰岛素的日基础用量。<br>Para control de glucosa en sangre para la diabetes. Se utiliza por lo general en combinación con insulina de acción corta, ofreciendo la dosis diaria básica. |
| 用法、用量<br>Administración y dosis | 于早餐前 0.5 小时皮下注射一次，剂量根据病情而定，每日用量一般为 10～20U。<br>Se aplica una vez por vía de inyección subcutánea media hora antes de desayuno, la dosis varía de acuerdo con la enfermedad, siendo generalmente 10～20U al día. |
| 剂型、规格<br>Formulaciones y especificaciones | 注射液：每瓶 400U（10ml）。<br>Inyección：400U cada botella(10ml). |
| 药品名称 Drug Names | 甘精胰岛素 Insulina glargina |
| 适应证<br>Indicaciones | 用于基础胰岛素替代治疗，一般也和短效胰岛素或口服降糖药配合使用。<br>Se utiliza para la terapia de reemplazo de insulina basal, en general se usa en combinación con insulina de acción rápida o los hipoglucemiantes orales. |

续　表

| 用法、用量<br>Administración y dosis | 每日傍晚注射一次，满足糖尿病患者的基础胰岛素需要量。<br>Por vía de inyección, una vez al día al atardecer para cumplir con los requerimientos de insulina básica de los pacientes diabéticos. |
|---|---|
| 剂型、规格<br>Formulaciones y especificaciones | 注射液：300U（3ml）。<br>Inyección: 300U(3ml). |

| 药品名称 Drug Names | 地特胰岛素 Insulina detemir |
|---|---|
| 适应证<br>Indicaciones | 用于治疗糖尿病。<br>Para el tratamiento de diabetes. |
| 用法、用量<br>Administración y dosis | 与口服降糖药联合治疗：起始剂量为 10U 或 0.1～0.2U/kg，一日 1 次，皮下注射，以后根据早餐前平均自测血糖浓度进行个体化的调整。<br>La terapia de combinación con hipoglucemiantes orales: la dosis inicial es de 10U o 0.1～0.2U/kg, una veces al día, por vía subcutánea, después se reajusta individualizadamente de acuerdo con las auto-prueba los niveles promedio de glucosa en la sangre antes del desayuno. |
| 剂型、规格<br>Formulaciones y especificaciones | 注射液：300U（3ml）。<br>Inyección: 300U(3ml). |

| 药品名称 Drug Names | 预混胰岛素 Insulina premix |
|---|---|
| 适应证<br>Indicaciones | 用于糖尿病控制血糖。<br>Para controlar la glucosa en la sangre tratando de diabetes. |
| 用法、用量<br>Administración y dosis | 于早餐前 0.5 小时皮下注射一次，剂量根据病情而定，每日用量一般为 10～20U。有时需要于晚餐前再注射一次。<br>Por vía de inyección subcutánea media hora antes de desayuno, la dosis de acuerdo a la enfermedad, la dosis diaria es generalmente 10～20U. A veces es necesario inyectar una vez adicional antes de la cena. |
| 剂型、规格<br>Formulaciones y especificaciones | 注射液：每瓶 400U（10ml）。笔芯：300U（3ml）。<br>Inyección：400U cada botella （10 ml）. Recambio：300U （3 ml）. |

16.10　口服降糖药 Hipoglucemiantes orales

| 药品名称 Drug Names | 甲苯磺丁脲 Tolbutamida |
|---|---|
| 适应证<br>Indicaciones | 一般用于成年后发病，单用饮食控制无效而胰岛功能尚存的轻、中度糖尿病患者，对胰岛素抵抗患者，可加用本品。对胰岛素依赖型患者及酸中毒昏迷者无效，不能完全代替胰岛素。<br>Generalmente se usa para pacientes diabéticos leve o moderada que se enfermen después de la edad adulta, que no puedan controlar la enfermedad con dieta y tengan una parte de función de islote. Para los pacientes con resistencia a la insulina, se pueden aplicar este producto. No tiene efecto para los pacientes dependientes de la insulina y en coma por acidosis, no puede sustituir completamente a la insulina. |
| 用法、用量<br>Administración y dosis | 餐前服药效果较好，如有胃肠反应，进餐时服药可减少反应。口服，一日剂量 1～2g，分次服用，一日 2～3 次，从小剂量开始，每 1～2 周加量一次。<br>Mejor antes de comida. Si tienen reacciones gastrointestinales, pueden tomar el medicamento a la comida. Por vía oral, cada día 1～2g, dividido en dos a tres veces al día. Comience con dosis pequeña, incrementando la dosis entre cada 1 a 2 semanas. |
| 剂型、规格<br>Formulaciones y especificaciones | 片剂：每片 0.5g。<br>Tabletas：cada una 0.5g. |

| 药品名称 Drug Names | 格列本脲 Glibenclamida |
|---|---|
| 适应证<br>Indicaciones | 用于饮食不能控制的轻、中度 2 型糖尿病。<br>Para diabetes tipo 2 leve y moderada que no puede ser controlada con dieta. |

**续 表**

| | |
|---|---|
| 用法、用量<br>Administración y dosis | 开始时每日剂量 2.5～5mg，早餐前 1 次服，或一日 2 次，早晚餐前各一次，然后根据情况每周增加 2.5mg，一般每日量为 5～10mg，最大不超过 15mg。<br><br>Al comienzo la dosis diaria es de 2.5～5 mg. Se toma una vez antes del desayuno y dos veces al día antes del desayuno y la cena. Luego aumente 2.5 mg a cada semana según las circunstancias. La dosis diaria en general es del 5～10 mg sin exceder al 15 mg. |
| 剂型、规格<br>Formulaciones y especificaciones | 片剂：每片 2.5mg。<br>Tabletas: cada una 2.5g |
| 药品名称 Drug Names | 格列吡嗪 Glipizida |
| 适应证<br>Indicaciones | 本品主要用于单用饮食控制治疗未能达到良好控制的轻、中度非胰岛素依赖型患者；对胰岛素抵抗患者可加用本品，但用量应在 30～40U 以下者。<br><br>Este producto se utiliza principalmente para pacientes leves y moderados, no dependientes de la insulina, y que no pueden controlar la enfermedad con dieta. Para los pacientes con resistencia a la insulina pueden aplicar este producto, pero la cantidad debe ser menos de 30～40U. |
| 用法、用量<br>Administración y dosis | 一般一日 2.5～20mg，先从小量 2.5～5mg 开始，餐前 30 分钟服用，一日剂量超过 15mg 时，应分成 2～3 次餐前服用。<br><br>Generalmente 2.5～20 mg al día 30 minutos antes de comida, comenzando con una pequeña dosis de 2.5～5mg. Cuando la dosis diaria es superior a 15 mg, se debe dividir en 2 o 3 veces antes de las comidas. |
| 剂型、规格<br>Formulaciones y especificaciones | 片剂：每片 2.5mg；5mg。控释片：每片 5mg。<br>Tabletas: cada una 2.5 mg; 5mg. Tabletas de liberación: Cada una 5 mg. |
| 药品名称 Drug Names | 格列齐特 Gliclazida |
| 适应证<br>Indicaciones | 成人 2 型糖尿病。<br>Para diabetes tipo 2 de edad adulta. |
| 用法、用量<br>Administración y dosis | 开始时一日 2 次，一日 40～80mg，早晚 2 餐前服用；连服 2～3 周，然后根据血糖调整用量，一般剂量一日 80～240mg，最大日剂量不超过 240mg。<br><br>Al comienzo se aplica 40～80 mg en 2 veces al día. Tome antes del desayuno y la cena en 2 a 3 semanas consecutivas. Reajuste la dosis según la glucosa en sangre, siendo la dosis generalmente 80～240 mg al día y no superior a 240 mg. |
| 剂型、规格<br>Formulaciones y especificaciones | 片剂：每片 80mg。缓释片：每片 30mg。<br>Tabletas: Cada una 80mg. Tabletas de liberación prolongada: Cada una 30mg. |
| 药品名称 Drug Names | 格列喹酮 Gliquidona |
| 适应证<br>Indicaciones | 2 型糖尿病合并轻至中度肾病者，但严重肾功能不全时应改用胰岛素治疗。<br>Para pacientes diabéticos tipo 2 con enfermedad renal de leve a moderada. Los con insuficiencia renal grave debe recurrir a la terapia con insulina. |
| 用法、用量<br>Administración y dosis | 口服，开始时 15mg，应在餐前 30 分钟服用。1 周后按需调整，必要时逐步加量，一般日剂量为 15～20mg，日剂量为 30mg 以内者，可于早餐前一次服用，更大剂量应分 3 次，分别与 3 餐前服用，最大日剂量不超过 180mg。<br><br>Por vía oral, al comienzo se aplica 15 mg 30 minutos antes de las comidas. Una semana después ajuste la dosis según la situación, aumentándola gradualmente. En general, la dosis diaria es 15～20 mg. Al ser menor a 30 mg la dosis diaria, podría tomarla por una vez antes del desayuno. Cuando la dosis es mayor, se debe dividir en tres veces antes de cada comida. La dosis diaria máxima no debe exceder a 180 mg. |
| 剂型、规格<br>Formulaciones y especificaciones | 片剂：每片 30mg。<br>Tabletas：cada una 30mg. |

**续 表**

| 药品名称Drug Names | 格列美脲 Glimepirida |
|---|---|
| 适应证<br>Indicaciones | 成人 2 型糖尿病。<br>Para diabetes tipo 2 de edad adulta. |
| 用法、用量<br>Administración y<br>dosis | 开始用量一日 1mg，一次顿服，如不能满意控制血糖，每隔 1 ～ 2 周逐步增加剂量至每日 2mg、3mg、4mg，最大推荐剂量为每日 6mg。<br>Comience con 1mg al día, una vez a la comida. Si no puede conseguir el control satisfactorio de la glucosa en sangre, aumente la dosis gradualmente entre cada 1 a 2 semanas hasta 2 mg , 3 mg, 4 mg al día. La dosis diaria máxima recomendada es 6 mg. |
| 剂型、规格<br>Formulaciones y<br>especificaciones | 片剂：每片 1mg；2mg。<br>Tabletas: cada una 1mg; 2mg. |
| 药品名称Drug Names | 二甲双胍 Metformina |
| 适应证<br>Indicaciones | （1）首选用于单纯饮食控制及体育锻炼治疗无效的 2 型糖尿病，特别是肥胖的 2 型糖尿病。<br>（2）与胰岛素合用可减少胰岛素用量，防止低血糖发生。<br>（3）与磺酰脲类降血糖药合用具协同作用。<br>(1) Preferido para la diabetes tipo 2 incontrolable con dieta y terapia de ejercicio, sobre todo para diabetes tipo 2 de obesos.<br>(2) La combinación con insulina puede reducir la dosis de insulina para prevenir la hipoglucemia.<br>(3) Tiene efecto sinérgico con fármacos hipoglucemiantes de sulfonilurea. |
| 用法、用量<br>Administración y<br>dosis | （1）普通片：开始时一次 0.25g，一日 2 ～ 3 次，以后可根据病情调整剂量。口服，一次 0.5g，一日 1 ～ 1.5g，最大剂量不超过 2g。餐中服药可减轻胃肠反应。<br>（2）缓释片：开始时一日 1 次，每次 0.5g，晚餐时服用。后根据血糖调整剂量。日最大剂量不超过 2g。<br>(1) Tableta ordinaria: al comienzo una vez de 0.25 g, 2 a 3 veces al día, reajustando la dosis de acuerdo con la gravedad de enfermedad. Por vía oral, cada vez 0.5 g, 1~ 1.5 g al día, la dosis máxima no supera 2 g. La aplicación durante comidas puede reducir las reacciones gastrointestinales.<br>(2) Tabletas de liberación prolongada: Al inicio cada vez 0.5g, una vez al día, tomándose durante la cena y reajustando la dosis de acuerdo con la glucosa en la sangre. La dosis máxima diaria no excede de 2g. |
| 剂型、规格<br>Formulaciones y<br>especificaciones | 片剂：每片 0.25g；0.5g；0.85g。缓释片：0.5g。<br>Tabletas: Cada una 0.25 g; 0.5 g; 0.85 g. Tabletas de liberación prolongada: 0.5g. |
| 药品名称Drug Names | 苯乙双胍 Fenformina |
| 适应证<br>Indicaciones | 用于单纯饮食控制不满意的 2 型糖尿病患者，尤其是肥胖者和伴高胰岛素血症者。与磺酰脲类降血糖药合用具协同作用。<br>Se utiliza para diabetes tipo 2 incontrolable con dieta, especialmente para pacientes obesos y con hiperinsulinemia. Tiene efecto sinérgico con fármacos hipoglucemiantes de sulfonilurea. |
| 用法、用量<br>Administración y<br>dosis | 口服：成人开始时一次 25mg，一日 2 次，餐前服，数日后可再增加 25mg，但最多每日不超过 75mg。<br>Por vía oral: Para adultos comiencen a cada vez 25 mg, 2 veces al día, antes de las comidas, aumentando la dosis en 25 mg después de unos días sin exceder un máximo de 75 mg diarios. |
| 剂型、规格<br>Formulaciones y<br>especificaciones | 片剂：每片 25mg。<br>Tabletas: cada una 25mg. |

**续 表**

| 药品名称 Drug Names | 瑞格列奈 Repaglinida |
|---|---|
| 适应证<br>Indicaciones | 用于饮食控制、降低体重与运动不能有效控制高血糖的 2 型糖尿病。与二甲双胍合用对控制血糖有协同作用。<br><br>Para diabetes tipo 2 que no puede ser controlada eficazmente con dieta, pérdida de peso y ejercicios. Tiene un efecto sinérgico en combinación con metformina para el control de glucosa en sangre. |
| 用法、用量<br>Administración y<br>dosis | 服药时间应在餐前 30 分钟内服用,剂量依个人血糖而定。推荐起始剂量为 0.5mg,最大的推荐单次剂量为 4mg,但最大日剂量不应超过 16mg。<br><br>Se toma dentro de los 30 minutos antes de una comida, definiendo la dosis en función de la glucosa en sangre. La dosis inicial recomendada es 0.5 mg, y la dosis máxima recomendada de una vez de aplicación es 4 mg, pero la dosis máxima diaria no debe exceder los 16 mg. |
| 剂型、规格<br>Formulaciones y<br>especificaciones | 片剂:每片 0.5mg;1mg;2mg。<br>Tabletas: cada una 0.5mg;1mg;2mg. |
| 药品名称 Drug Names | 那格列奈 Nateglinida |
| 适应证<br>Indicaciones | 用于饮食控制、降低体重与运动不能有效控制高血糖的 2 型糖尿病。与二甲双胍合用对控制血糖有协同作用。<br><br>Para diabetes tipo 2 que no puede ser controlada eficazmente con dieta, pérdida de peso y ejercicios. Tiene un efecto sinérgico en combinación con metformina para el control de glucosa en sangre. |
| 用法、用量<br>Administración y<br>dosis | 本品可单独应用,也可与二甲双胍合用,起始剂量一日 3 次,一次 60mg,餐前 15 分钟服药。常用剂量为餐前 60 ~ 120mg,并根据 HbAlc 检测结果调整剂量。<br><br>Se puede utilizar solo, también se puede utilizar en combinación con metformina. La dosis de partida es cada vez 60mg y tres veces al día, tomada 15 minutos antes de cada comida. La dosis habitual es 60 ~ 120 mg antes de las comidas, reajustándose según los resultados de pruebas de HbAlc. |
| 剂型、规格<br>Formulaciones y<br>especificaciones | 片剂:每片 30mg;60mg;120mg。<br>Tabletas: cada una 30mg;60mg;120mg. |
| 药品名称 Drug Names | 罗格列酮 Rosiglitazona |
| 适应证<br>Indicaciones | 本品仅适用于其他降糖药无法达到血糖控制目标的 2 型糖尿病患者。<br>Este producto sólo se puede aplicar a pacientes con diabetes tipo 2 que no pueden lograr los objetivos de control glucémico con otros fármacos antidiabéticos. |
| 用法、用量<br>Administración y<br>dosis | 单独用药:初始剂量为一日 4mg,单次或分 2 次口服,12 周后如空腹血糖下降不满意,剂量可加至一日 8mg,单次或分 2 次口服。<br><br>Se aplica solo: la dosis inicial es 4 mg al día, dividida en una vez o dos veces por vía oral. Si después de 12 semanas la reducción de glucemia en ayunas no es satisfactoria, la dosis diaria se puede incrementar hasta 8 mg, dividida en 1 o 2 veces al día. |
| 剂型、规格<br>Formulaciones y<br>especificaciones | 片剂:每片 2mg;4mg;8mg。<br>Tabletas: cada una 2mg;4mg;8mg. |
| 药品名称 Drug Names | 吡格列酮 Pioglitazona |
| 适应证<br>Indicaciones | 用于 2 型糖尿病,可于饮食控制和体育锻炼联合以改善血糖控制,可单独使用。当饮食控制、体育锻炼和单药治疗不能满意控制血糖时,也可与磺脲、二甲双胍或胰岛素合用。<br><br>Para la diabetes tipo 2, utilizado en combinación con dieta y ejercicio físico para mejorar el control glucémico. También se puede utilizar en combinación con sulfonilurea, metformina, o insulina cuando no pueden lograr el control satisfactorio por la dieta, el ejercicio, y la aplicación de monoterapia. |
| 用法、用量<br>Administración y<br>dosis | 口服,单药治疗初始剂量可为 15mg 或 30mg,一日 1 次;反应不佳时,可加量直至 45mg,一日 1 次。<br><br>La dosis inicial en monoterapia por vía oral puede ser 15mg o 30 mg, una vez al día; cuando no tienen suficiente eficacia, puede aumentar la dosis hasta 45 mg, una vez al día. |

**续　表**

| 剂型、规格<br>Formulaciones y<br>especificaciones | 片剂：每片 15mg。<br>Tabletas: cada una 15mg. |
|---|---|
| **药品名称 Drug Names** | **阿卡波糖 Acarbosa** |
| 适应证<br>Indicaciones | 可与其他口服降血糖药或胰岛素联合应用于胰岛素依赖型或非胰岛素依赖型的糖尿病。<br>Se aplica en combinación con otros agentes hipoglucémicos o insulina para las diabetes insulina-dependientes y no insulina-dependientes. |
| 用法、用量<br>Administración y<br>dosis | 口服剂量需个体化。一般维持量为一次 50 ～ 100mg，一日 3 次，餐前即刻吞服，或与第一口主食一起咀嚼服用。开始时从小剂量 25mg，一日 3 次，6 ～ 8 周后加量至 50mg，必要时可加至 100mg，一日 3 次，一日量不宜超过 300mg。<br>La dosis por vía oral debe ser individualizada. La dosis de mantenimiento en general es 50 ～ 100 mg, 3 veces al día antes de las comidas o se toma masticando con el primer bocado. Comience con dosis pequeña de 25 mg , 3 veces al día. 6 a 8 semanas después incremente la dosis a 50 mg o hasta 100 mg si es necesario, 3 veces al día , la dosis diaria no debe exceder a 300 mg. |
| 剂型、规格<br>Formulaciones y<br>especificaciones | 片剂：每片 50mg；100mg。<br>Tabletas: cada una 50mg; 100mg. |
| **药品名称 Drug Names** | **伏格列波糖 Voglibosa** |
| 适应证<br>Indicaciones | 改善糖尿病餐后高血糖。<br>Mejorar la diabetes hiperglucemia postprandial. |
| 用法、用量<br>Administración y<br>dosis | 口服，成人一次 200μg，一日 3 次，餐前服，疗效不明显时根据临床观察可将一次量增至 300μg。<br>Por vía oral, cada vez 200μg para adultos, tres veces al día antes de las comidas. Cuando no tiene obvio efecto, se puede aumentar la dosis a 300μg en función de la observación clínica. |
| 剂型、规格<br>Formulaciones y<br>especificaciones | 片剂：每片 200μg。<br>Tabletas: cada una 200μg. |
| **药品名称 Drug Names** | **西格列汀 Sitagliptina** |
| 适应证<br>Indicaciones | 用于经生活方式干预无法达标的 2 型糖尿病患者。可采用单药治疗或与其他口服降糖药联合治疗。<br>Para pacientes de diabetes tipo 2 quienes no pueden lograr efecto satisfactorio a través de intervención del estilo de vida. Puede ser utilizado como monoterapia o terapia de combinación con otros agentes hipoglucemiantes orales. |
| 用法、用量<br>Administración y<br>dosis | 本品单药治疗的推荐剂量为 100mg，一日 1 次。本品可与或不与食物同服。<br>La dosis recomendada de este producto como monoterapia es 100mg, una vez al día. Se puede utilizar con o sin comida. |
| 剂型、规格<br>Formulaciones y<br>especificaciones | 每片 100mg。<br>Cada tableta 100mg. |

16.11　甲状腺激素类药物 Medicamentos de hormona tiroidea

| **药品名称 Drug Names** | **左甲状腺素 Levotiroxina** |
|---|---|
| 适应证<br>Indicaciones | 适用于甲状腺激素缺乏的替代治疗。<br>Para la terapia de reemplazo de la falta de hormona tiroidea. |

**续　表**

| | |
|---|---|
| 用法、用量<br>Administración y dosis | 　　口服一般开始剂量一日 25 ～ 50μg，每 2 周增加 25μg，直到 100 ～ 150μg，成人维持量为一日 75 ～ 125μg，高龄患者、心功能不全者及严重黏液性水肿患者开始剂量应减为每日 12.5 ～ 25μg，以后每 2 ～ 4 周递增 25μg，不必要求达到完全替代剂量，一般一日 75 ～ 100μg 即可。婴儿及儿童甲状腺功能减退症，每日完全替代剂量为：6 个月以内 6 ～ 8μg/kg；6 ～ 12 个月，6μg/kg；1 ～ 5 岁 5μg/kg，6 ～ 12 岁，4μg/kg。静脉注射适用于黏液性水肿昏迷，首次剂量宜较大，200 ～ 400μg，以后一日 50 ～ 100μg，直到患者清醒改为口服。<br><br>　　Dosis inicial por vía oral diaria es 25 ~ 50μg, aumentándola en 25μg cada dos semanas, hasta 100 ~ 150μg al día. La dosis de mantenimiento para adultos es 75 ~ 125μg. Para pacientes de edad avanzada, o los con disfunción cardíaca o con severa mixedema, la dosis de partida debe reducirse al 12.5 ~ 25μg al día, incrementando la dosis en 25μg cada 2 a 4 semanas, sin necesariamente alcanzar dosis de reemplazo completa, siendo la dosis generalmente 75 ~ 100μg al día. Para los bebés y niños con hipotiroidismo, la dosis diaria de reemplazo completo es: 6 ~ 8μg/kg para los de 6 meses o menos; para los de 6 ~ 12 meses, 6μg/kg ; para los de 1 ~ 5 años, 5μg/kg; Para los de 6 ~ 12 años de edad, 4μg / kg. Por vía intravenosa se aplica para tratar el coma por mixedema, siendo necesario que la primera dosis sea grande, de 200 ~ 400μg, después 50 ~ 100 μg al día hasta que el paciente despierte. Luego se aplica por vía oral. |
| 剂型、规格<br>Formulaciones y especificaciones | 　　片剂：每片 25μg；50μg；100μg。注射液：每支 100μg（1ml）；200μg（2ml）；500μg（5ml）。<br>Tabletas: Cada una 25μg; 50μg; 100μg. Inyección: Cada 100 μg (1 ml); 200μg (2 ml); 500μg (5 ml). |

| 药品名称 Drug Names | 甲状腺片 Tabletas de tiroxina |
|---|---|
| 适应证<br>Indicaciones | 　　主要用甲状腺功能减退症的治疗。包括甲减引起的呆小病及黏液性水肿等。<br>　　Se utiliza principalmente en el tratamiento del hipotiroidismo, incluyendo cretinismo causado por el hipotiroidismo, la mixedema y entre otros. |
| 用法、用量<br>Administración y dosis | 　　常用量开始时一日 10 ～ 20mg，逐渐加量，维持量一般为一日 40 ～ 80mg。<br>　　La dosis inicial es 10~20 mg al día, aumentando gradualmente hasta la dosis de mantenimiento es por lo general 40 ~ 80 mg al día. |
| 剂型、规格<br>Formulaciones y especificaciones | 　　片剂：每片 10mg；40mg；60mg。<br>Tabletas: Cada una 10 mg; 40 mg; 60 mg. |

| 药品名称 Drug Names | 促甲状腺素 Tirotropina |
|---|---|
| 适应证<br>Indicaciones | 　　用于 TSH 试验及甲状腺癌诊断。<br>　　Se utiliza para la prueba de TSH y el diagnóstico del cáncer de tiroides. |
| 用法、用量<br>Administración y dosis | 　　① TSH 试验：每日肌内注射 2 次，每次 10μg，共 3 日。②提高甲状腺癌转移病灶吸 [131]I：甲状腺全切除后。每日肌内注射 10μg，共 7 日。使转移病灶吸 [131]I 率提高后再给予治疗量碘。<br>　　① Prueba de TSH: inyección intramuscular, 2 veces al día, cada vez 10μg, totalmente en 3 días. ② Mejorar la tasa de absorción de [131]I de metástasis del cáncer de tiroides: se aplica 10μg al día por vía de inyección intramuscular en 7 días totalmente después de la tiroidectomía total. . Después de aumentar la tasa de absorción de metástasis [131]I se da el yodo de cantidad terapéutica. |
| 剂型、规格<br>Formulaciones y especificaciones | 　　注射液：每支 10μg（6ml）。<br>Inyección:10μg(6ml). |

16.12　抗甲状腺药 Medicamentos contra la tiroides

| 药品名称 Drug Names | 丙硫氧嘧啶 Propiltiouracilo |
|---|---|
| 适应证<br>Indicaciones | 　　①甲状腺功能亢进的内科治疗。②甲状腺危象的治疗。③术前准备。<br>　　① Tratamiento médico del hipertiroidismo. ② Tratamiento de la tormenta tiroidea. ③ Preparación preoperatoria. |

**续　表**

| | |
|---|---|
| 用法、用量<br>Administración y<br>dosis | （1）成人甲状腺功能亢进：口服常用量300～450mg/天，分3次口服，极量一次0.2g，一日0.6g。小儿开始剂量每日按4mg/kg分次口服，维持量酌减。<br>（2）甲状腺危象：一日0.4～0.8g，分3～4次服用，疗程不超过1周。<br>（3）甲状腺功能亢进的术前准备：术前服用本品一次100mg，一日3～4次，使甲状腺功能恢复到正常或接近正常，然后加服2周碘剂再进行手术。<br>(1) Para hipertiroidismo adulto: la dosis habitual por vía oral es 300 ~ 450 mg / día, divida en 3 veces; la dosis máxima es 0.2 g, 0.6 g al día. La dosis inicial pediátrica es 4mg/kg dividida en varias veces, reduciendo la dosis de mantenimiento.<br>(2) Para tormenta tiroidea: 0.4 ~ 0.8 g al día, dividida en 3 a 4 veces, sin aplicarse más de una semana.<br>(3) preparación preoperatoria para hipertiroidismo: se toma este producto una vez 100mg, 3 a 4 veces al día, de modo que la función tiroidea vuelve a ser normal o casi normal, a continuación, se añade yodo en dos semanas antes de la cirugía. |
| 剂型、规格<br>Formulaciones y<br>especificaciones | 片剂：每片50mg；100mg。<br>Tabletas: Cada una 50mg; 100mg. |
| 药品名称 Drug Names | 甲巯咪唑 Metiamazol |
| 适应证<br>Indicaciones | ①甲状腺功能亢进的内科治疗。②甲状腺危象的治疗。③术前准备<br>① Tratamiento médico del hipertiroidismo. ② Tratamiento de la tormenta tiroidea. ③ Preparación preoperatoria. |
| 用法、用量<br>Administración y<br>dosis | 成人：开始时一日30mg，可按病情轻重调节为一日15～40mg，一日最大量60mg，分次口服，病情控制后逐渐减量，维持量：一日5～15mg，疗程一般12～18个月。小儿：开始剂量为每日0.4mg/kg，分3次口服。维持量约减半或按病情轻重调节。<br>Para adultos: al inicio 30 mg al día, reajustando la dosis a 15 ~ 40 mg al día de acuerdo con la gravedad. La dosis máxima es 60 mg al día, divididas en varias veces. Al controlar la enfermedad, reduzca gradualmente la dosis, siendo la dosis de mantenimiento 5 ~ 15 mg al día. El ciclo de tratamiento es generalmente 12 a 18 meses. Para el uso pediátrico: la dosis inicial es 0.4mg/kg al día, dividida en 3 veces por vía oral. La dosis de mantenimiento es aproximadamente la mitad o reajuste según la gravedad. |
| 剂型、规格<br>Formulaciones y<br>especificaciones | 片剂：每片5mg。<br>Tabletas: cada una 5mg. |

17. 主要影响变态反应和免疫功能的药物 Medicamentos que afectan principalmente a reacciones alérgicas y la función inmune

17.1　抗变态反应药物 Medicamentos antialérgicos

| | |
|---|---|
| 药品名称 Drug Names | 苯海拉明 Difenhidramina |
| 适应证<br>Indicaciones | ①主要用于Ⅰ型和Ⅳ型变态反应，对毛细血管通透性增加所致渗出、水肿、分泌物增多的疾病疗效较好，尤其适用于皮肤黏膜的过敏性疾病，如过敏性药疹、过敏性湿疹、血管性神经水肿和荨麻疹等。对平滑肌痉挛所致支气管哮喘的效果较差，需与氨茶碱、麻黄碱等合用。②镇静安眠和手术前给药。③抗帕金森和药物所致锥体外系症状。④防晕止吐：可用于乘船乘车所致晕动病，以及放射病术后及药物引起的恶心呕吐。⑤乳膏外用，治虫咬、神经性皮炎、瘙痒症等。<br>① Utilizado principalmente para alergia tipos Ⅰ y Ⅳ, y tiene mejor efecto para la exudación, la enfermedad de edema, aumento de las secrecionesal debido al aumento de la permeabilidad capilar. Especialmente eficaz para las enfermedades alérgicas de la piel y la mucosa tales como erupción alérgica, eczema atópico, edema vascular y urticaria nervios. Tiene pobre efecto para asma bronquial causada por el espasmo del músculo liso, mejor aplicando en combinación con con teofilina, efedrina, etc. ② Sedante e hipnóticos y aplicación antes de la cirugía. ③ Anti-Parkinson y para síntomas extrapiramidales inducidos por fármacos. ④ anticorona antiemético: Para mareo en coche y barco, náuseas y vómitos causados por la cirugía de radiación y por los medicamentos. ⑤ cremas tópicas, para picaduras de insectos, neurodermatitis, prurito, etc. |
| 用法、用量<br>Administración y<br>dosis | 可口服、肌内注射及局部应用。不能皮下注射，因有刺激性。成人：口服，一次25～50mg，一日2～3次。饭后服。肌内注射，一次12.5～25mg，一日3～4次；或一日5mg/kg，分次给药；或一日150mg/m²，分次给药。 |

续 表

| | |
|---|---|
| | Por vía oral, intramuscular y tópica. No se usa por vía subcutánea debido a su irritación. Para adultos: por vía oral, una vez 25 ~ 50 mg, 2 o 3 veces al día, después de las comidas. Por vía de inyección intramuscular, una vez 12.5 ~ 25 mg, 3 a 4 veces al día, o 5mg/kg al día, en dosis divididas; o 150mg / m$^2$ al día, en dosis divididas. |
| 剂型、规格<br>Formulaciones y especificaciones | 片剂：每片 25mg；50mg。注射液：每支 20mg（1ml）。乳膏：每支 20g。<br>Tabletas: cada una 25 mg; 50 mg. Inyección: 20 mg (1 ml). Crema: Cada tubo 20 g. |
| 药品名称 Drug Names | 异丙嗪 Prometazina |
| 适应证<br>Indicaciones | ①抗过敏：适用于各种过敏症（如哮喘、荨麻疹等）。②镇吐抗眩晕：可用于一些麻醉和手术后的恶心呕吐，乘车、船等引起的眩晕症等。③镇静催眠：可在外科手术和分娩时与哌替啶合用，缓解患者紧张情绪，或用于晚间催眠药。亦可与氯丙嗪等配成冬眠注射液用于人工冬眠。<br><br>① Alergia: se utiliza para todo tipo de alergias (como asma, urticaria, etc.) ② Antiemético y anti-vértigo: para náuseas y vómitos causados por la anestesia y la cirugía y mareos en coche y barco. ③ Sedante e hipnóticos: en combinación con petidina durante el parto y la cirugía para aliviar la tensión de los pacientes, o se usa como hipóticos de la noche. También se combina con la inyección de la clorpromazina para la hibernación hibernación artificial. |
| 用法、用量<br>Administración y dosis | ①抗过敏：成人，口服，一次 6.25 ~ 12.5mg，一日 3 次，饭后及睡前服用，必要时睡前 25mg；儿童，口服，每次按体重 0.125mg/kg 或按体表面积 7.5 ~ 15mg/m$^2$，每 4 ~ 6 小时 1 次，或睡前按体重 0.25 ~ 0.5mg/kg 或按体表面积 7.5 ~ 15mg/m$^2$；按年龄计算，每日量 5 岁 5 ~ 15mg，6 岁以上 10 ~ 15mg，可一日 1 次或分次服用。肌内注射，每次按体重 0.125mg/kg 或按体表面积 3.75mg/m$^2$，每 4 ~ 6 小时肌内注射 1 次。②止吐：成人，口服，开始时一次 12.5 ~ 25mg，必要时可每 4 ~ 6 小时服 12.5 ~ 25mg，通常 24 小时不超过 100mg。③抗眩晕：成人，旅行前口服，一次 12.5 ~ 25mg，必要时一日 2 次；儿童，口服，剂量减半。④镇静催眠：成人，口服，一次 12.5 ~ 25mg，睡前服用。儿童，口服，5 岁 6.25mg，6 ~ 12 岁 6.25 ~ 12.5mg。<br><br>① Alergia: Para adultos, por vía oral, una vez 6.25 ~ 12.5 mg, tres veces al día, después de las comidas y antes de acostarse. Si es necesario, 25mg antes de irse a la cama; Para niños, por vía oral, de acuerdo con el peso corporal cada vez 0.125mg/kg o según la superficie corporal cada vez 7.5 ~ 15mg / m$^2$, una vez entre cada 4 a 6 horas. O se aplica antes de acostarse según el peso 0.25 ~ 0.5mg/kg o según la superficie corporal 7.5 ~ 15 mg / m$^2$; en función de la edad, la cantidad diaria para los 5 años de edad es 5 ~ 15 mg, mayores de 6 años de edad,10 ~ 15 mg, pudiendo ser dosis de solo una vez s o divididas. Por vía de inyección intramuscular, según el peso cada vez 0.125mg/kg o según la superficie corporal cada vez 3.75 mg / m$^2$, una vez entre cada 4 a 6 horas. ② Antiemético: para adultos, por vía oral, al inicio una vez 12.5 ~ 25 mg,o 12.5 ~ 25 mg entre cada 4 a 6 horas si es necesario; por lo general no exceda de 100 mg en 24 horas. ③ anti-vértigo: Para adultos, se aplica por vía oral antes de viajar una vez 12.5 ~25mg, 2 veces al día si es necesario; para los niños, la dosis reduce a la mitad. ④ Sedantes e hipnóticos: para adultos, por vía oral, una vez 12.5 ~ 25 mg antes de la hora de acostarse; Para los niños, por vía oral, 6.25mg para los de 5 años, y 6.25 ~ 12.5 mg para los de 6 ~ 12 años . |
| 剂型、规格<br>Formulaciones y especificaciones | 片剂：每片 12.5mg；25mg。注射液：每支 25mg（1ml）；50mg（2ml）。<br>Tabletas: Cada una 12.5 mg; 25 mg. Inyección: 25 mg (1 ml), 50 mg (2 ml). |
| 药品名称 Drug Names | 去氯羟嗪 Decloxizina |
| 适应证<br>Indicaciones | 用于支气管哮喘、急慢性荨麻疹、皮肤划痕症、血管神经性水肿、接触性皮炎、光敏性皮炎、季节性花粉症、过敏性鼻炎及结膜炎等。<br><br>Para el asma bronquial, urticaria aguda y crónica, enfermedad por arañazo de piel, angioedema, dermatitis de contacto, dermatitis de fotosensibilidad, fiebre del heno estacional, rinitis alérgica y conjuntivitis. |
| 用法、用量<br>Administración y dosis | 口服：一日 3 次，一次 25 ~ 50mg。<br>Por vía oral, 3 veces al día, cada vez 25~50mg. |

**续　表**

| 剂型、规格<br>Formulaciones y<br>especificaciones | 片剂：每片 25mg；50mg。<br>Tabletas: cada una 25 mg; 50 mg. |
|---|---|
| **药品名称 Drug Names** | 阿伐斯汀 Acrivastina |
| 适应证<br>Indicaciones | 用于过敏性鼻炎及荨麻疹等。<br>Para la rinitis alérgica y la urticaria. |
| 用法、用量<br>Administración y<br>dosis | 成人及 12 岁以上儿童口服：一次 8mg，一日不超过 3 次。<br>Para adultos y niños mayores de 12 años, por vía oral: cada vez 8 mg , no se excede tres veces al día. |
| 剂型、规格<br>Formulaciones y<br>especificaciones | 胶囊剂：每粒 8mg。<br>Cápsulas: Cada una 8 mg. |
| **药品名称 Drug Names** | 左卡巴斯汀 Levocabastina |
| 适应证<br>Indicaciones | 用于局部治疗的滴眼剂和喷鼻剂，缓解过敏性鼻炎，预防包括鼻炎及结膜炎在内的过敏反应。<br>Gotas oculares y aerosol nasal para aliviar la rinitis alérgica y prevenir reacciones alérgicas incluyendo la rinitis y conjuntivitis. |
| 用法、用量<br>Administración y<br>dosis | （1）喷鼻: 成人及 12 岁以上儿童常用量为每个鼻孔喷 2 下，一日 2 次。必要时可增至每次喷 2 下，一日 3 ～ 4 次。连续用药直至症状消除。<br>（2）滴眼：每次 1 滴，一日 2 ～ 4 次。<br>(1) Aerosol nasal: para adultos y niños mayores de 12 años, la dosis usualmente utilizada es cada vez 2 pulverizaciones en cada orificio nasal, y dos veces al día. Puede aumentar la dosis si es necesario, aplicando cada vez en cada orificio nasal 2 pulverizaciones, 3 o 4 veces al día, continuando hasta que los síntomas eliminen.<br>(2) Gotas oculares: cada vez una gota para cada ojo, 2 a 4 veces al día. |
| 剂型、规格<br>Formulaciones y<br>especificaciones | 喷鼻剂（微悬浮液）：每支 10ml（0.5g/ml）。滴眼剂：0.5mg/kg。<br>Aerosol nasal (micro-suspensión): 10 ml (0.5g/ml). Gotas oculares: 0.5mg/kg. |
| **药品名称 Drug Names** | 咪唑斯汀 Mizolastina |
| 适应证<br>Indicaciones | 本品用于长效 $H_1$ 受体拮抗药，适用于季节性过敏性鼻炎、花粉症、常年性过敏性鼻炎及荨麻疹等皮肤过敏症状。<br>Este producto se utiliza como antagonista de los receptores H1 de acción prolongada para tratar la rinitis alérgica estacional, rinitis alérgica, rinitis alérgica perenne y la urticaria y otras alergias en la piel. |
| 用法、用量<br>Administración y<br>dosis | 口服，成人（包括老年人）和 12 岁以上儿童，推荐剂量为一次 10mg，一日 1 次。<br>Por vía oral, para adultos (incluidos los ancianos) y niños de 12 años de edad, la dosis recomendada es cada vez 10 mg, una vez al día. |
| 剂型、规格<br>Formulaciones y<br>especificaciones | 片剂：每片 10mg。<br>Tabletas: cada una 10mg. |
| **药品名称 Drug Names** | 赛庚啶 Ciproheptadina |
| 适应证<br>Indicaciones | 用于荨麻疹、湿疹、过敏性和接触性皮炎、皮肤瘙痒、鼻炎、偏头痛、支气管哮喘等。皮肤瘙痒通常在服药后 2 ～ 3 日消失。对库欣病、肢端肥大症也有一定疗效。<br>Se utiliza para la urticaria, eczema, dermatitis atópica y de contacto, prurito, rinitis, migraña, asma bronquial. Por lo general el picazón en la piel desaparece al cabo de 2 a 3 días después de la aplicación. Tiene cierto efecto para la enfermedad de Cushing y acromegalia. |

**续 表**

| | |
|---|---|
| 用法、用量<br>Administración y dosis | （1）口服，成人，一次 2～4mg，一日 3 次。儿童，口服，2～6 岁，一次 2mg，一日 2～3 次，7～14 岁，一次 4mg，一日 2～3 次，极量：一次 0.2mg/kg。作为食欲增进剂应用时，用药时间不超过 6 个月。<br>（2）乳膏外用。<br><br>(1) Se aplica por vía oral, para los adultos, una vez 2～4 mg, 3 veces al día. Para niños de 2 a 6 años de edad, por vía oral, una vez 2mg, 2 a 3 veces al día; para los de 7 a 14 años de edad, una vez 4mg, 2 a 3 veces al día, observando la dosis máxima: cada vez 0.2mg/kg. Cuando se aplica como promotor de apetito, la duración de la medicación debe exceder a seis meses.<br>(2) La crema se aplica por vía tópica. |
| 剂型、规格<br>Formulaciones y especificaciones | 片剂：每片 2mg。糖浆剂：4mg/kg。霜剂：每支 10g（0.5%），20g（0.5%）。乳膏剂：0.5%。<br>Tabletas: Cada una 2 mg. Jarabe: 4mg/kg. Crema: Cada una 10 g (0.5%), 20 g (0.5%). Crema: 0.5%. |
| **药品名称 Drug Names** | **氯雷他定 Loratadina** |
| 适应证<br>Indicaciones | 用于过敏性鼻炎、急性或慢性荨麻疹、过敏性结膜炎、花粉症及其他过敏性皮肤病。<br>Se utiliza para la rinitis alérgica, urticaria aguda o crónica, conjuntivitis alérgica, fiebre del heno y otras enfermedades alérgicas en la piel. |
| 用法、用量<br>Administración y dosis | 口服，成人及 12 岁以上儿童，一次 10mg，一日 1 次，空腹服用。日夜均有发作者，可一次 5mg，每日晨、晚各一次。儿童，口服，2～12 岁，体重大于 30kg 者，一次 5mg，一日一次。复方氯雷他定片：成人及 12 岁以上儿童，一次 1 片，一日 2 次。<br><br>Se administra por vía oral.Adultos y niños mayores de 12 años:10 mg cada vez, una vez al día, con el estómago vacío.Para los que tiene síntomas durante día y noche,5 mg 2 veces al día.Niños:por vía oral, 2 a 12 años de edad, que pesen más de 30 kg, 3 mg cada vez, una vez al día.Tabletas de loratadina Compuesto: Adultos y niños mayores de 12 años,una tableta 2 veces por día. |
| 剂型、规格<br>Formulaciones y especificaciones | 片剂：每片 10mg。胶囊剂：每粒 10mg。颗粒剂：5mg。糖浆剂：60mg/60ml。<br>Tabletas: 10mg por cada tableta. Cápsulas:10mg por cada cápsula. Gránulos: 5 mg. Jarabes: 60mg/60ml. |
| **药品名称 Drug Names** | **西替利嗪 Cetirizina** |
| 适应证<br>Indicaciones | 用于季节性和常年性过敏性鼻炎、结膜炎及过敏反应所致的瘙痒和荨麻疹。<br>Se utiliza para la rinitis alérgica estacional y perenne, conjuntivitis y reacciones alérgicas causadas por la comezón y la urticaria. |
| 用法、用量<br>Administración y dosis | 口服，成人及 12 岁以上儿童，一次 10～20mg，一日 1 次，或早晚各服 5mg。肾功能损害者需减量。儿童，2～6 岁者，一日 5mg；7～11 岁者，一日 10mg。<br><br>Se administra por vía oral, adultos y niños mayores de 12 años, 10～20 mg una vez al día, o 5mg 2 veces por la mañana y por la noche.Se requiere reducir la dosis para pacientes con disfunción renal.Los niños de 2 a 6 años de edad, 5 mg al día, 7～11 años, 10 mg al día. |
| 剂型、规格<br>Formulaciones y especificaciones | 片剂：每片 10mg。胶囊剂：每粒 10mg。分散片：每片 10mg。口服液：10mg/10ml。<br>Tabletas: 10mg por cada tableta. Cápsulas:10mg por cada cápsula.Comprimidos dispersables:10mg por cada comprimido.Líquido oral: 10mg/10ml. |
| **药品名称 Drug Names** | **依巴斯汀 Ebastina** |
| 适应证<br>Indicaciones | 用于季节性和常年性过敏性鼻炎和慢性荨麻疹、湿疹、皮炎、痒疹、皮肤瘙痒等。<br>Se utiliza para la rinitis alérgica estacional y perenne y la urticaria crónica, eczema, dermatitis, erupciones, picazón en la piel. |
| 用法、用量<br>Administración y dosis | （1）常年性过敏性鼻炎：成人，一日一次，每次 10mg；儿童（12～17），一日 1 次，每次 5mg。<br>（2）季节性过敏性鼻炎：成人，一日 1 次，每次 10mg，早上服用效果更好。如严重过敏患者可日服 20mg，但应从小剂量开始。儿童（2～15 岁），一日 1 次，每次 2.5～5mg。 |

**续　表**

| | |
|---|---|
| | (1) La rinitis alérgica perenne:Adultos,10mg una vez al día.Niños de edad de 12 a 17,5mg una vez al día.<br><br>(2) La rinitis alérgica estacional:Adultos,10mg una vez al día,se aconseja tomarlo por la mañana.Los pacientes alérgicos severos pueden tomar 20mg al día, pero debe comenzar con una dosis baja.Niños de edad de 2 a 15,2.5~5mg cada vez al día. |
| 剂型、规格<br>Formulaciones y especificaciones | 片剂：每片 10mg。<br>Tabletas:10mg por cada tableta. |
| **药品名称Drug Names** | 地氯雷他定 Desloratadina |
| 适应证<br>Indicaciones | 用于治疗慢性特发性荨麻疹、常年过敏性鼻炎及季节过敏性鼻炎。<br>Se utiliza para el tratamiento de la urticaria idiopática crónica, la rinitis alérgica perenne y rinitis alérgica estacional. |
| 用法、用量<br>Administración y dosis | （1）慢性特发性荨麻疹、常年过敏性鼻炎及季节过敏性鼻炎：成人口服，一日 1 次，一次 5mg。<br>（2）慢性特发性荨麻疹、常年过敏性鼻炎：儿童，口服，12 岁以上，一次 5mg，一日 1 次；6～11 岁者，一次 2.5mg，一日 1 次；12 个月～5 岁者，一次 1.25mg，一日 1 次；6～11 个月者，一次 1mg，一日 1 次。<br>（3）季节性过敏性鼻炎：儿童口服，12 岁以上者，一次 5mg，一日 1 次；6～11 岁者，一次 2.5mg，一日 1 次；2～5 岁者，一次 1.25mg，一日 1 次。<br>（4）肝、肾功能不全患者，在开始治疗时可隔日服用 5mg。<br>(1) Urticaria idiopática crónica, rinitis alérgica perenne y rinitis alérgica estacional: Adulto,por vía oral,5mg una vez al día.<br>(2) La urticaria crónica idiopática, rinitis alérgica perenne: Niños,por vía oral, mayores a 12, 5mg una vez al día; 6 a 11 años de edad, 2.5 mg una vez al día.<br>(3) Rinitis alérgica estacional:Niños,por vía oral, 12 años o más, 5mg una vez al día; 6 a 11 años de edad, 2.5 mg una vez al día; 2 a 5 años edad, 1.25 mg una vez al día.<br>(4) Pacientes con disfunción hepática y renal,debe tomar 5mg cada dos días al inicio del tratamiento. |
| 剂型、规格<br>Formulaciones y especificaciones | 片剂：每片 5mg。<br>Tableta:5mg por cada tableta. |
| **药品名称Drug Names** | 氮䓬斯汀 Azelastina |
| 适应证<br>Indicaciones | 口服或喷鼻可控制季节性或非季节性鼻炎及非过敏性血管收缩性鼻炎症状。滴眼剂可用于治疗过敏性结膜炎。<br>Se administra por vía oral o nasal para controlar la rinitis estacional o no estacional y los síntomas de la rinitis vasomotora no alérgica.Se utiliza las gotas para los ojos para el tratamiento de la conjuntivitis alérgica. |
| 用法、用量<br>Administración y dosis | （1）过敏性鼻炎（季节性或非季节性）：①成人及 12 岁以上儿童，经鼻给药：每次每鼻孔 1 喷（每喷 0.137mg），一日 2 次，作用持续时间 12 小时。在花粉季节连续用药对控制鼻部症状优于临时用药。对于非季节性过敏性鼻炎，可长期用药 6 个月，安全性和疗效良好。口服：每次 1～2mg，一日 2 次。或遵医嘱。② 5～11 岁儿童，经鼻给药：每次每鼻孔 1 喷，一日 2 次。口服：6 岁以上儿童，每次 1～2mg，一日 2 次。或遵医嘱。<br>（2）血管收缩性鼻炎：成人及 12 岁以上每次每鼻孔 1 喷（0.137mg），一日 2 次，或遵医嘱。<br>（3）过敏性结膜炎：成人滴患眼，每次 1 滴，一日 2 次。有报道 1 个疗程可用 8 个月。儿童滴眼剂只能用于 3 岁以上儿童。每次 1 滴，一日 2 次。有报道 1 个疗程可用至 8 个月。或遵医嘱。<br>（4）治疗和预防哮喘：成人或 6 岁以上儿童，口服，每次 1～4mg，一日 2 次；或每次 8mg，每日 1 次，睡前服。睡前服可用于控制哮喘夜间和晨起发作。遵医嘱。<br>（5）肝功能不全和老年患者无须调整剂量。<br>12 meses a 5 años, 1.25mg una vez al dia; 6 a 11 meses, 1mg una vez al dia. |

续 表

|  | (1) La rinitis alérgica (estacional y no estacional): ① Adultos y niños mayores de 12 años,se administra por vía nasal: se administra como una dosis de 0.137mg en cada una de las fosas nasales,2 veces al día, 12 horas de duración de la acción.Se aconseja la medicación continua durante la temporada de polen para los síntomas nasales por ser más eficaz que la medicación temporal.Para la rinitis alérgica no estacional,se puede administrar en un plazo de 6 meses,ya que la eficacia y seguridad son verificadas. Se administra por vía oral:1~2mg dos veces al día,o bajo prescripción médica.<br><br>(2) La rinitis vasomotora: Adultos y niños mayores de 12 años,se administra por vía nasal: se administra como una dosis de 0.137mg en cada una de las fosas nasales,2 veces al día o siga indicaciones del doctor.<br><br>(3) La conjuntivitis alérgica:Adultos,se pone al ojo afectado una gota (0.05%)cada vez,2 veces al día.Según reportado,un curso de tratamiento es disponible en ocho meses.Gotas para los ojos del niño sólo se pueden utilizar para niños mayores de 3 años.una gota (0.05%)cada vez,2 veces al día.Según reportado,un curso de tratamiento es disponible en ocho meses.O siga indicaciones del doctor.<br><br>(4) Tratamiento y prevención del asma: Adultos o niños mayores de 6 años,por vía oral, cada vez 1 ~ 4 mg, 2 veces al día, o cada vez 8 mg, 1 veces al día, antes de acostarse para controlar los ataques por la noche o temprano por la mañana,o siga indicaciones del doctor.<br><br>(5) No se requiere ajuste de la dosis en pacientes ancianos, en pacientes con disfunción hepática. |
|---|---|
| 剂型、规格<br>Formulaciones y especificaciones | 片剂：每片 0.5mg；1mg。颗粒剂：2mg/g。喷鼻剂：10mg/10ml。滴眼剂：2.5mg/5ml。<br>Tableta:0.5mg;1mg por cada tableta;Gránulos: 2 mg / g. Aerosol nasal: 10mg/10ml. Gotas para los ojos: 2.5mg/5ml |
| **药品名称 Drug Names** | 溴苯那敏 Bromfeniramina |
| 适应证<br>Indicaciones | 可用于慢性荨麻疹。<br>Se utiliza para la urticaria crónica. |
| 用法、用量<br>Administración y dosis | 口服：一日 3 ～ 4 次，一次 4 ～ 8mg。<br>Se administra por vía oral:4~8mg 3 o 4 veces al día. |
| 剂型、规格<br>Formulaciones y especificaciones | 片剂：4mg；缓释片：12mg。<br>Tabletas: 4mg; tabletas de liberación sostenida: 12mg. |
| **药品名称 Drug Names** | 氯苯那敏 Clorfeniramina |
| 适应证<br>Indicaciones | 用于过敏性鼻炎、感冒和鼻窦炎及过敏性皮肤疾患如荨麻疹、过敏性药疹或湿疹、血管神经性水肿、虫咬所致皮肤瘙痒。<br>Se utiliza para la rinitis alérgica, resfriados y sinusitis,así como trastornos alérgicos de la piel tales como urticaria, erupción alérgica o eccema, edema angioneurótico, picazón de la piel causada por picaduras de insectos. |
| 用法、用量<br>Administración y dosis | 口服，成人一次量 4mg，一日 3 次。肌内注射，一次 5 ～ 20mg。<br>Por vía oral, una cantidad de 4 mg, 3 veces al día. Por vía intramuscular, 5~20mg cada vez. |
| 剂型、规格<br>Formulaciones y especificaciones | 片剂：每片 4mg。胶囊剂：每粒 8mg。注射液：每支 10mg（1ml）；20mg（2ml）。<br>Comprimidos:4mg por cada comprimido. Cápsulas:8mg por cada cápsula. Inyección: Cada 10mg (1ml);20mg (2ml). |
| **药品名称 Drug Names** | 茶苯海明 Dimenhidrinato |
| 适应证<br>Indicaciones | 有镇吐、防晕作用、可用于妊娠、晕动症、放射线治疗及术后引起的恶心、呕吐。<br>Tiene efecto antiemético o antivertiginoso, ya que se utiliza para la prevención y control de náuseas y vómitos inducidos por el embarazo, el mareo, la radioterapia y la cirugía. |
| 用法、用量<br>Administración y dosis | 一次 25 ～ 50mg，一日 3 次。<br>25~50mg 3 veces al día. |

续　表

| 剂型、规格<br>Formulaciones y especificaciones | 片剂：25mg；50mg。<br>Comprimidos: 25 mg; 50 mg. |
|---|---|
| 药品名称 Drug Names | 色甘酸钠 Cromoglicato sódico |
| 适应证<br>Indicaciones | 　　用于预防过敏性哮喘的发作，改善主观症状，增加患者对运动的耐受能力，对于依赖皮质激素的患者，服用本品后可使之减量或完全缓解。患有慢性难治性哮喘的儿童应用本品大部分或完全缓解。与异丙肾上腺素合用，较单用时的效率显著增高。但本品起效较慢，需连续用药数天后才能见效。如已发病，用药多无效。对变态反应作用不明显的慢性哮喘也有疗效。用于过敏性鼻炎和季节性花粉症，能迅速控制症状。软膏外用于慢性过敏性湿疹及某些皮肤瘙痒症也有显著疗效。2% ～ 4% 滴眼液适用于花粉症、结膜炎和春季角膜炎结膜炎。<br><br>　　Se utiliza para la prevención de los ataques de asma alérgica ,la mejora de los síntomas subjetivos, y el aumento de la tolerancia al ejercicio en pacientes.Para los pacientes dependientes de corticosteroides,este medicamento les permite la reducción o remisión completa.También se logra una remisión mayor o completa después del tratamiento en los niños con asma refractaria crónica.Se obtiene un aumento significativo de eficacia en combinación con isoproterenol.El efecto no se surge notablemente hasta que se efectúe una continua administración durante varios días con el fin de lograr mayor eficacia y es posible que sea ineficaz si los síntomas de la enfermedad empiezan a presentar.Este medicamento tiene efecto evidente sobre el asma alérgica crónica,también puede controlar rápidamente los síntomas de rinitis alérgica estacional y la fiebre del heno.La pomada tópica presenta efecto significativo sobre el eczema atópico y cierto prurito crónico,y gotas para los ojos de 2% a 4% se puede utilizar para la fiebre del heno y conjuntivitis así como conjuntivitis y queratitis vernal. |
| 用法、用量<br>Administración y dosis | 　　（1）支气管哮喘：干粉喷雾吸入：成人，一次 20mg，一日 4 次。症状减轻后，一日 2 ～ 3 次；维持量一日 20mg。5 岁以上儿童用量同成人。<br>　　（2）过敏性鼻炎：干粉鼻吸入：一次 10mg，一日 4 次；2% 或 4% 溶液滴鼻或喷雾，每次用药量约含色甘酸钠 5mg，一日 6 次。<br>　　（3）食物过敏：成人，一次 200mg，一日 4 次，饭前服。2 岁以上儿童，一次 100mg，一日 4 次。如 2 ～ 3 周效果不佳，剂量可增加，每日不超过 40mg/kg，症状控制后可减量。<br>　　（4）滴眼：2% 或 4% 滴眼剂滴眼，一日数次。<br>　　（5）外用：5% ～ 10% 软膏，涂患处，一日 2 次。<br><br>　　(1) La asma bronquial: por vía de inhalación de polvo seco: Adulto, una vez 20 mg, 4 veces al día. Después del alivio de los síntomas,2 o 3 veces al día,dosis de mantenimiento es de 20 mg al día. Los niños menores de 5 años de edad se utiliza la misma dosis de los pacientes adultos.<br>　　(2) La rinitis alérgica: por vía de inhalación de polvo seco,10mg 4 veces al día;Solución intranasal de 2% o 4% o pulverizar,se administra cada vez una dosificación que contiene 5 mg de sodio cromolyn, 6 veces al día.<br>　　(3) Las alergias alimentarias: adultos, 200 mg 4 veces al día, antes de las comidas.Niños menores de 2 años de edad, 100 mg 4 veces al día.Si el efecto de la administración no es satisfactorio,se aconseja aumentar la dosis de no más de 40mg/kg al día y se puede reducir la dosis una vez que se logre un control de los síntomas.<br>　　(4) Las gotas para ojos:Se puede administrar las gotas para ojos de 2% o 4% varias veces al día.<br>　　(5) Por vía tópica: pomada de 5% a 10%,se aplica sobre la zona afectada 2 veces al día. |
| 剂型、规格<br>Formulaciones y especificaciones | 气雾剂：每瓶总量约 14g，内含色甘酸钠 0.7g，每揿含药量 3.5mg。胶囊剂：每粒 20mg。软膏：5% ～ 10%。滴眼剂：2%（8ml）；4%（8ml）。<br>Aerosol: el contenido de cada botella es de aproximadamente 14 g,que contiene que contiene 0.7g de sodio cromolyn, cada dosis contiene 3,5 mg de prensa. Capsula: 20mg por cápsula. Pomada: 5% ~ 10 %. Gotas para oios: 2% (8ml), 4%（8ml）. |
| 药品名称 Drug Names | 酮替芬 Ketotifeno |
| 适应证<br>Indicaciones | 　　（1）用于多种类型支气管哮喘，均有明显疗效，对过敏性哮喘疗效尤为明显，混合性次之，感染型约 50% 以上有效。对过敏性哮喘效果优于色甘酸钠。<br>　　（2）也可用于过敏性鼻炎、过敏性结膜炎、花粉症、急慢性荨麻疹、药物、食物或昆虫所致变态反应的预防和治疗。 |

|  | （1）Tiene un efecto significativo contra varios tipos de asma bronquial como el asma alérgica y mezclado,en el caso de asma infectado se comprueba eficaz para la mayoría de los pacientes.El efecto es más evidente que el cromoglicato contra el asma alérgica.<br>（2）Se utiliza para la prevención y el tratamiento de la rinitis alérgica, conjuntivitis alérgica, fiebre del heno, urticaria aguda y crónica, y la alergia inducida por drogas, alimentos o insectos. |
|---|---|
| 用法、用量<br>Administración y dosis | 口服：成人，一次 1mg，早、晚各服一次；若困意明显，可只在睡前服 1 次。<br><br>Se administra por vía oral:Adulto,1 mg dos veces por la mañana y por la noche. Si se siente con mucho sueño se aconseja tomarlo una vez al día antes de irse a dormir. |
| 剂型、规格<br>Formulaciones y especificaciones | 片剂：每片 1mg。胶囊剂：每粒 1mg。口服液：每支 1mg/5ml。滴眼液：2.5mg/5ml。滴鼻液：15mg/10ml。分散片：每片 1mg。鼻吸入粉雾剂：15.5mg/14g。<br><br>Tabletas: 1 mg por cada tableta.Cápsulas:1mg por cada cápsula. Líquido Oral:1mg/5ml. Gotas para ojos: 2.5mg/5ml. Gotas nasales: 15mg/10ml. Tableta:1 ¡mg por cada tableta. Polvo para inhalación nasal: 15.5mg/14g. |

### 17.2　免疫抑制药 Medicamentos inmunosupresores

| 药品名称 Drug Names | 环孢素 Ciclosporina |
|---|---|
| 适应证<br>Indicaciones | 主要用于肾、肝、心、肺、骨髓移植的抗排异反应，可与肾上腺皮质激素或其他免疫抑制剂合用，也可用于治疗类风湿关节炎、系统性红斑狼疮、肾病型慢性肾炎、自身免疫性溶血性贫血、银屑病、葡萄膜炎等自身免疫性疾病。<br><br>Se utiliza principalmente medicinas anti-rechazo para el trasplante de riñón,hígado, corazón, pulmón y médula ósea y se puede combinar con corticosteroides suprarrenales u otros agentes inmunosupresores,así como el tratamiento de la artritis reumatoide, el lupus eritematoso sistémico, nefritis enfermedad renal crónica, anemia hemolítica autoinmune, la psoriasis, uveítis enfermedades autoinmunes. |
| 用法、用量<br>Administración y dosis | （1）器官移植：①口服：于移植前 12 小时起一日服 8～10mg/kg，维持术后 1～2 周，根据血药浓度减至一日 2～6mg/kg，分 2 次服。②静脉注射：仅用于不能口服的患者，于移植前 4～12 小时每日给予 3～5mg/kg，以 5% 葡萄糖或生理盐水稀释至 1∶20 至 1∶100 的浓度于 2～6 小时缓慢滴注。<br>（2）自身免疫性疾病：口服，初始剂量为一日 2.5～5mg/kg，分 2 次服；症状缓解后改为最小剂量维持，但成人不应超过一日 5mg/kg，儿童不应超过 6mg/kg。<br><br>（1）El trasplante de órganos：① Por vía oral: 12 horas antes del trasplante se administra 8 ～10mg/kg al día y sigue aplicándose hasta 1 a 2 semanas después de la operación, dependiendo de la concentración plasmática se reduce a un diario de 2～6mg/kg, 2 veces el servicio.Según las concentraciones de plasma se reduce hasta 2～6mg/kg 2 veces al día. ② Inyección intravenosa:para los pacientes incapaces de realizar la administración oral, 4 a 12 horas antes del trasplante se les aplica 3～5mg/kg a diario, se diluye el medicamento con 5% de dextrosa o solución salina a una concentración de 1∶20 a 1∶100 y se les aplica la infusión de forma lenta en 2~6 horas.<br>（2）Enfermedades autoinmunes: por vía oral, la dosis inicial es de 2,5 a 5mg/kg al día, dividida en 2 dosis; Después de la remisión de los síntomas, se mantiene la dosis míninma, no más de 5mg/kg por día para adultos y 6mg/kg por día para niños. |
| 剂型、规格<br>Formulaciones y especificaciones | 胶囊剂：每粒 25mg；100mg。微乳化软胶囊：每粒 10mg；25mg；50mg；100mg。口服液：100mg/ml（50ml）。微乳化口服液：100mg/ml（50ml）。静脉滴注浓缩液：250mg/5ml；500mg/10ml。<br><br>Cápsulas: 25 mg por cada cápsula; 100 mg. Microemulsionamiento cápsulas blandas: 10 mg por cada cápsula; 25 mg; 50 mg; 100 mg.Líquido Oral: 100mg/ml (50 ml). Microemulsión Líquido oral: 100mg/ml (50 ml). Intravenosa concentrado para infusión: 250mg/5ml; 500mg/10ml. |
| 药品名称 Drug Names | 他克莫司 Tacrolimus |
| 适应证<br>Indicaciones | 主要用于器官移植的抗排异反应，尤其适用于肝移植，还可用于肾、心、肺、胰、骨髓及角膜移植等。<br><br>Se utiliza para el tratamiento de reacción anti-rechazo en trasplantes de órganos, especialmente para el trasplante de hígado,así como el de riñón, corazón, pulmón, páncreas, médula ósea y córnea. |

<table>
<tr><td colspan="2">续　表</td></tr>
</table>

| | |
|---|---|
| 用法、用量<br>Administración y dosis | 开始采用一日 0.05 ～ 0.1mg/kg（肾移植），或 0.01 ～ 0.05mg/kg（肝移植）持续静脉滴注。能进行口服时，改为口服胶囊，开始剂量为一日 0.15 ～ 0.3mg/kg，分 2 次服；在逐渐减至维持剂量，一日 0.1mg/kg，分 2 次服，亦可根据病情调整剂量，通常低于首次免疫抑制剂量。本品外用皮肤涂布可用于其他免疫抑制药疗效不佳或无法耐受的中重度特应性皮炎。<br><br>Se aconseja a comenzar con un dosis de 0.05 ～ 0.1 mg en trasplante de riñón, o 0.01 ～ 0.05 mg en trasplante de hígado por vía de infusión intravenosa continua.Cuando se puede administrar por vía oral, se administra cápsulas con un dosis inicial de 0.15 ～ 0.3mg/kg 2 veces diariamente dosis inicial de 0.15 ～ 0.3mg/kg, 2 veces al día y se reduce gradualmente hasta 0.1mg/kg 2 veces al día.Se puede ajustar la dosis conforme a la enfermedad, generalmente menos de Las primeras dosis inmunosupresoras.El revestimiento de la piel se aplica para el tratamiento de dermatitis atópica moderada o severa en que otros fármacos inmunosupresores falten eficacia o tolerancia. |
| 剂型、规格<br>Formulaciones y especificaciones | 胶囊剂：每粒 0.5mg；1mg；5mg。注射液：每支 5mg（1ml），用时稀释在 5% 葡萄糖或生理盐水中缓慢静脉滴注。外用软膏剂：3mg/10g；10mg/10g。<br><br>Cápsulas:0.5mg;1 mg;5mg por cada cápsula;Inyección: Cada unidad 5 mg (1 ml), por vía de lenta infusión intravenosa diluyéndose con 5% de glucosa o solución salina.Pomada tópica: 3mg/10g; 10mg/10g. |
| 药品名称 Drug Names | 吗替麦考酚酯 Micofenolato mofetil |
| 适应证<br>Indicaciones | 主要用于预防和治疗肾、肝、心脏及骨髓移植的排异反应。也可用于不能耐受其他免疫抑制剂或疗效不佳的类风湿关节炎、全身性红斑狼疮、原发性肾小球肾炎、牛皮癣等自身免疫性疾病。<br><br>Se utiliza para la prevención y el tratamiento de  reacción anti-rechazo en trasplantes de Riñón, hígado, corazón y médula ósea.También puede ser utilizado para artritis reumatoide, lupus eritematoso sistémico, glomerulonefritis primaria, psoriasis y otras enfermedades autoinmunesotros en que otros fármacos inmunosupresores falten eficacia o tolerancia. |
| 用法、用量<br>Administración y dosis | 用于器官移植：空腹口服，成人一日 1.5 ～ 2.0g，小儿 30mg/kg，分 2 次服，首剂量应在器官移植后 72 小时内服用；静脉注射，主要用于口服不能耐受者，每次注射时间多于 2 小时。用于自身免疫病：成人一日 1.5 ～ 2.0g，维持量 0.25 ～ 0.5g，一日 2 次，空腹服用。<br><br>Para el trasplante de órganos:se administra en ayunas por vía oral, adulto 1.5 ～ 2.0g diario, niños 30mg/kg, 2 veces, la primera dosis debe tomarse dentro de las 72 horas después del trasplante;Por vía de infusión intravenosa,se aplica para los pacientes que no pueden administrarse por vía oral,cada inyección durará más de 2 horas.Para la enfermedad autoinmunes: adulto diariamente 1.5 ～ 2.0 g, con un dosis de mantenimiento de 0.25 ～ 0.5 g, 2 veces al día, con el estómago vacío. |
| 剂型、规格<br>Formulaciones y especificaciones | 胶囊剂：每粒 250mg。片剂：每片 500mg。注射剂：每支 500mg。<br><br>Cápsulas:250mg por cada cápsula. Tabletas:500 mg por cada tableta. Inyección: 500mg por cada unidad. |
| 药品名称 Drug Names | 来氟米特 Leflunomida |
| 适应证<br>Indicaciones | 用于治疗风湿性关节炎、系统性红斑狼疮等自身免疫性疾病，亦可用于器官移植抗排异反应。<br><br>Se utiliza para el tratamiento de la artritis reumatoide, el lupus eritematoso sistémico y otras enfermedades autoinmunes, así como el tratamiento de reacciones anti-rechazo en trasplante de órganos. |
| 用法、用量<br>Administración y dosis | 口服，成人常用量：①类风湿关节炎、系统性红斑狼疮及银屑病关节炎，一次 20mg，一日 1 次；病情控制后可以一日 10 ～ 20mg 维持。②韦格纳肉芽肿病，一日 20 ～ 40mg 维持。③器官移植，负荷剂量一日 200mg，维持剂量一日 40 ～ 60mg。<br><br>Se administra por vía oral,la dosis para adultos: ① la artritis reumatoide, la artritis psoriásica y lupus eritematoso sistémico,20mg una vez al día;Al lograr un control de la enfermedad se puede ajustar la dosificación mantenida a 10~20mg. ② La granulomatosis de Wegener:20 ～ 40 mg para el mantenimiento. ③ Trasplante de órganos: la dosis de carga  es de 200mg al día, la dosis de mantenimiento de 40 ～ 60mg al día. |
| 剂型、规格<br>Formulaciones y especificaciones | 片剂：每片 10mg；20mg；100mg。<br>Tabletas: Cada tableta de 10 mg; 20 mg; 100mg. |

**续　表**

| 药品名称Drug Names | 泼尼松 Prednisona |
| --- | --- |
| 适应证<br>Indicaciones | 糖皮质激素对Ⅰ、Ⅱ、Ⅲ、Ⅳ型变态反性疾病具有程度不同的治疗效果。①在Ⅰ型变态反应疾病中，糖皮质激素应用广泛，可全身给药或局部给药，如用于过敏性鼻炎、异位性皮炎、过敏性哮喘等。②糖皮质激素用于治疗Ⅱ型的自身免疫性疾病往往有效，是寻常性天疱疮、自身免疫性溶血性贫血的首选药物，如泼尼松可使 60% ～ 80% 的自身免疫性溶血性贫血缓解。③糖皮质激素广泛应用于治疗免疫复合物疾病（Ⅲ型变态反应性疾病），主要是依靠其抗炎作用，但仅仅可缓解症状，无消除病因作用。对系统性红斑狼疮，糖皮质激素往往可降低抗核抗体的浓度及减少狼疮红细胞的出现，而且某些证据表明，对肾损伤的患者应用大剂量的糖皮质激素能改善肾功能并延长患者生命。④糖皮质激素是Ⅳ型变态反应性疾病的强力抑制剂，临床上用于移植器官或组织的排异反应、接触性皮炎等等。<br><br>Los glucocorticoides tiene distintos grados de efetos de tratamiento sobre metamorfosis de tipo Ⅰ , Ⅱ , Ⅲ , Ⅳ . ① En las enfermedades alérgicas de tipo I,los corticosteroides se han logrado un uso amplio y pueden ser administrados por vía sistémica o tópica,como para el tratamiento de la rinitis alérgica, la dermatitis atópica y el asma alérgica. ② Los corticosteroides que se utilizan para el tratamiento de enfermedades autoinmunes del tipo Ⅱ suelen ser eficaces, ya que es el medicamento preferido para el tratamiento de Pénfigo vulgar y Anemia hemolítica autoinmune,por ejemplo la prednisona puede aliviar 60% a 80% de los síntómas de la anemia hemolítica autoinmune. ③ Los corticosteroides se utilizan ampliamente en el tratamiento de enfermedades por inmunes-complejos( Ⅲ tipo de enfermedades alérgicas),lo que se basa principalmente en su efecto antiinflamatorio,sin embargo,éste medicamento sólo puede aliviar los síntomas en vez de eliminar la causa de la enfermedad. Para el lupus eritematoso sistémico,los corticosteroides pueden reducir en gran medida tanto la concentración de anticuerpos anti-nucleares como la apariencia de los eritrocitos de lupus.Ciertas evidencias han verificado que grandes dosis de corticosteroides pueden mejorar la función renal y prolongar la vida de los pacientes con fallo renal. ④ Los glucocorticoides son inhibidores fuertes contra las enfermedades alérgicas de tipo Ⅳ ,por lo que se utilizan para el tratamiento de reacciones anti-rechazo en trasplantes de órganos o tejidos y Dermatitis de contacto como un método clínico. |
| 用法、用量<br>Administración y dosis | 口服：一般一日 20 ～ 60mg，如疗效不明显可逐渐增至每日 100mg，维持量为一日 10mg。用于肾、肝、心脏等器官移植：一般术后一日 4mg/kg，加硫唑嘌呤一日 5mg/kg；维持剂量一日 10 ～ 20mg，加硫唑嘌呤一日 1 ～ 2mg/kg。<br><br>Se administra por vía oral: 20 ～ 60 mg diario, si no se logra un efecto significativo se puede aumentar la dosis gradualmente a 100 mg al día,y la dosis diaria de mantenimiento es de 10 mg.Para el tratamiento de trasplante de riñones,hígado, corazón y otros órganos:4mg/kg al día después de la operación,si se administra con la azatioprina la dosis será de 5mg/kg;la dosis de mantenimiento es de 10~20mg al día y 1~2mg/kg al día con la azatioprina. |
| 剂型、规格<br>Formulaciones y especificaciones | 片剂：每片 5mg。<br>Tableta:5mg por cada tableta. |
| 药品名称Drug Names | 硫唑嘌呤 Azatioprina |
| 适应证<br>Indicaciones | 主要用于器官移植时的排异反应,多与皮质激素并用,或加用淋巴细胞球蛋白（ALG），疗效好。也广泛用于类风湿关节炎、系统性红斑狼疮，自身免疫性溶血性贫血、特发性血小板减少性紫癜、活动性慢性肝炎、溃疡性结肠炎、重症肌无力、硬皮病等自身免疫性疾病。对慢性肾炎及肾病综合征，其疗效似不及环磷酰胺。由于其不良反应较多且严重，对上述疾病治疗不作为首选，通常是在单用糖皮质激素不能控制时才使用。<br><br>Se utiliza para el tratamiento de reacciones anti-rechazo en trasplantes de órganos y se usa con los Corticosteroides o con Globulina Linfocitos(ALG),lo que da buen efecto.También se puede utilizar para el tratamiento de enfermedades autoinmunes como la artritis reumatoide, lupus eritematoso sistémico, anemia hemolítica autoinmune, púrpura trombocitopénica idiopática, hepatitis activa crónica, la colitis ulcerosa, miastenia grave, esclerodermia. Para el tratamiento de Nefritis crónica y síndrome nefrótico, su eficacia no se muestra tan notable como ciclofosfamida. Debido a las reacciones adversas y graves, no se aconseja su uso como medicamento preferido para el tratamiento de estas enfermedades,y suele usarse cuando Glucocorticoides no se pueden lograr un control de los síntomas de la enfermedad. |

**续　表**

| | |
|---|---|
| 用法、用量<br>Administración y dosis | 口服：一日 1～3mg/kg，一般一日 100mg，一次服用，可连服数月。用于器官移植：一日 2～5mg/kg，维持量一日 0.5～3mg/kg。<br><br>Se administra por vía oral:1~3mg/kg al día,por lo común 100mg una vez al día y el tratamiento se puede durar en un plazo de unos meses.Para el trasplante de órganos: 2～5mg/kg, la dosis diaria de mantenimiento es de 0.5～3mg/kg. |
| 剂型、规格<br>Formulaciones y especificaciones | 片剂：每片 25mg；50mg；100mg。注射液：50mg（以硫唑嘌呤计量）。<br>Tabletas: 25 mg por cada tableta; 50 mg; 100mg. Inyección: 50 mg(Medido por azatioprina) |
| **药品名称 Drug Names** | 羟基脲 Hidroxicarbamida |
| 适应证<br>Indicaciones | 用于顽固性银屑病和脓疱性银屑病均有效，能减轻全身性脓疱性银屑病的脓疱、发热和中毒症状。短期用药，其毒性作用较甲氨蝶呤小，对有肝脏损伤不宜用甲氨蝶呤或用甲氨蝶呤无效的严重银屑病患者，可选用本品治疗。<br><br>Se utiliza para el tratamiento de Psoriasis obstinada y Psoriasis pustulosa, y puede reducir síntomas de pústulas, fiebre y síntomas de intoxicación.Si se aplica a corto plazo, sus efectos tóxicos son menos en comparación con Metotrexato,así que para los pacientes con psoriasis severa y con fallo renal y hepático,este medicamento puede ser utilizado para recibir mayor eficacia. |
| 用法、用量<br>Administración y dosis | 口服：每日 0.5～1.5g，4～8 周为 1 个疗程。<br>Por vía oral:0.5～1.5g al día, el plazo de tratamiento es de 4~8 semanas. |
| 剂型、规格<br>Formulaciones y especificaciones | 片剂：每片 400mg；500mg。胶囊剂：每粒 250mg；400mg；500mg。<br>Tableta:400mg;500mg por tableta;Cápsula:250mg；400mg；500mg por cada cápsula. |
| **药品名称 Drug Names** | 甲氨蝶呤 Metotrexato |
| 适应证<br>Indicaciones | 本品原为抗肿瘤药，经剂量、用法调整后用作免疫抑制药。主要用于类风湿关节炎、银屑病关节炎、红斑狼疮、脊柱关节病的周围关节炎、多肌炎、多发性肉芽肿等自身免疫性疾病。甲氨蝶呤间歇疗法治疗多发性肉芽肿起效较皮质激素、烷化剂或硫唑嘌呤迅速，故急性患者应首选本品。用于皮质激素无效的多肌炎、皮肌炎见见肌力改善、皮疹消退。根据报道甲氨蝶呤特别适用于顽固的进行性多发性肌炎和顽固的进行性眼色素层炎，治疗 1～2 周后可使麻痹或失明的患者恢复一定功能。其作用机制不明，可能与其抗炎作用有关。应用免疫抑制量的甲氨蝶呤后 24 小时内再给适量的甲酰四氢叶酸，可对抗甲氨蝶呤的毒性，但几乎不影响其免疫抑制作用。<br><br>Este producto se utiliza originalmente como antineoplásico y tras el ajuste de la dosis y la forma de uso se puede utilizar como inmunosupresores.Se emplea para el tratamiento de la artritis reumatoide, la artritis psoriásica, el lupus, Espondiloartropatía artritis periférica，Polimiositis y múltiples granulomas,etc.El efecto surge más rápido que los corticosteroides, agentes alquilantes o azatioprina en el tratamiento de múltiples granulomas si se toma la terapia intermitente,por lo tanto,será el medicamento más preferido para los pacientes con infarto agudo.Se observan mejoras en la fuerza de músculos y en erupciones cutáneas para el tratamiento de Polimiositis, Dermatomiositis cuando la aplicación de corticosteroides no haya logrado efecto.Según datos,el metotrexato tiene una eficacia notable para el tratamiento de polimiositis progresiva obstinada y Uveítis progresiva,ya que los pacientes con parálisis o ceguera que reciben tratamiento en un plazo de 1 o 2 semanas pueden restaurar ciertas funciones.Su mecanismo de acción es desconocido, y puede estar relacionado con los efectos anti-inflamatorios.Si se aplica leucovorina dentro de 24 horas después del uso de Metotrexato de una dosis de inmunosupresión,se reducerá la toxicidad del metotrexato pero casi no afecta a sus efectos inmunosupresores. |
| 用法、用量<br>Administración y dosis | 口服：初始剂量一次 7.5mg，1 周 1 次；可酌情增加至 20mg，1 周一次，分 2 次服。肌内注射：每次 10mg，1 周一次。静脉注射：每次 10～15mg，每周 1 次。银屑病，口服，一次 0.25～5mg，一日 1 次，6～7 日为一疗程。<br><br>Por vía oral: La dosis inicial es de 7.5 mg una vez a la semana, la dosis podrá ser discrecionalmente ajustada a 20mg dos veces a la semana.Por vía de inyección intramuscular:10 mg una vez por semana. Contra Psoriasis, por vía oral,0.25~5mg,una vez al día y el tratamiento es de 6 a 7 días. |

| | |
|---|---|
| 剂型、规格<br>Formulaciones y<br>especificaciones | 片剂：每片 2.5mg；5mg；10mg。注 射 液：每 支 5mg；10mg；20mg；25mg；50mg；100mg。<br>Tabletas: 2.5 mg; 5mg; 10mg por cada tableta.Líquido de inyección: 5 mg; 10 mg; 20 mg; 25 mg; 50 mg; 100 mg por cada unidad. |
| 药品名称 Drug Names | 环磷酰胺 Ciclofosfamida |
| 适应证<br>Indicaciones | 用于各种自身免疫性疾病，对严重类风湿关节炎及全身系统性红斑狼疮，大部分病例有效；对儿童肾病综合征，其疗效较硫唑嘌呤好，可长期缓解。可单独用药，但与皮质激素并用则疗效较佳，且不良反应较少。对多发性肉芽肿亦常用。与皮质激素并用则疗效较佳，且不良反应较少。与皮质激素并用于治疗天疱疮疗效也较好。此外，也用于治疗溃疡性结肠炎、特发性血小板减少性紫癜等自身免疫性疾病。也用于器官移植时抗排异反应，通常是与泼尼松、抗淋巴细胞球蛋白并用，其效果与硫唑嘌呤、泼尼松、抗淋巴细胞球蛋白的效果相似，且可避免硫唑嘌呤对肝脏可能产生的不良影响。<br><br>Se utiliza para el tratamiento de una variedad de enfermedades autoinmunes y el tratamiento es eficaz para la mayoría de los casos de la artritis reumatoide grave y el lupus eritematoso sistémico;Para el tratamiento de el síndrome nefrótico en niños,su eficacia es mejor que la azatioprina,ya que se puede lograr la remisión de síntomas a largo plazo.Se puede administrar solo,por otra parte,su uso combinado con los corticosteroides será más eficaz mientras que se reduce reacciones adversas.Además,el tratamiento con los dos medicamentos juntos contra el pénfigo se recibirá mejor efecto.También se utiliza para el tratamiento de la colitis ulcerosa, la púrpura trombocitopénica idiopática y otras enfermedades autoinmunes.Para el tratamiento de reacciones anti-rechazo en el trasplante de órganos suele aplicarse junto con prednisona,globulina anti-linfocito,su efecto es parecido al de la azatioprina, prednisonala globulina anti-linfocito, y se puede reducir posibles efectos adversos de la azatioprina sobre el hígado. |
| 用法、用量<br>Administración y<br>dosis | 自身免疫性疾病：口服，一日 2 ～ 3mg/kg，一日 1 次或隔日一次，连用 4 ～ 6 周。器官移植：口服，一日 50 ～ 150mg；静脉注射，一次 0.2g，一日或隔日 1 次，总量 8 ～ 10g 为一疗程。<br><br>Contra las enfermedades autoinmunes:se administra por vía oral,2~3mg/kg una vez al día o cada dos día,en un plazo de 4 a 6 semanas.En el trasplante de órganos:se administra por vía oral,50 a 150mg al día;Por vía intravenosa,0.2g al día o cada dos días,la dosificación total para un curso es de 8 a 10 g. |
| 剂型、规格<br>Formulaciones y<br>especificaciones | 片剂：50mg。注射剂：100mg；200mg。滴眼液：1%。<br>Tableta:50mg. Inyección:100mg; 200mg. Gotas para oios: 1%. |
| 药品名称 Drug Names | 苯丁酸氮芥 Clorambucil |
| 适应证<br>Indicaciones | 对于切特综合征、红斑狼疮病有较好疗效。尚用于治疗类风湿关节炎并发的脉管炎、伴有寒冷凝集素的自身免疫性溶血性贫血及依赖皮质激素的肾病综合征，与泼尼松龙并用于频发的肾病综合征。用于硬皮病可迅速组织其发展，使皮肤溃疡痊愈，肺功能改善。<br><br>Tiene un buen efecto para el tratamiento de síndrome de Chet y la enfermedad de lupus.También para el tratamiento de la artritis reumatoide complicado por vasculitis,la anemia hemolítica autoinmune acompañada por crioaglutininas,así como el síndrome nefrótico dependientes de corticosteroides.Se puede aplicar contra la esclerodermia para organizar rápidamente sus desarrollo, hacer curar las úlceras cutáneas curan y mejorar la función pulmonar. |
| 用法、用量<br>Administración y<br>dosis | 口服：一日 3 ～ 6mg，早饭前 1 小时或晚饭后 2 小时服用，连服数周，待疗效或骨髓抑制出现后减量，总量一般为 300 ～ 500mg。<br><br>Poe vía oral: 3 ～ 6 mg al día , 1 hora antes del desayuno o 2 horas después de la cena,el tratamiento puede durar varias semanas y se puede reducir la dosis tras la aparición de la eficacia o la aparición de la supresión de la médula ósea.La dosis total es generalmente de 300 ～ 500 mg. |
| 剂型、规格<br>Formulaciones y<br>especificaciones | 片剂：每片 1mg；2mg。纸型片：每格 2mg。<br>Tabletas: 1mg por cada tableta;2mg.Comprimidos de matriz: 2mg cada celular. |

**续　表**

## 17.3　免疫增强药 Inmunoestimulante

| 药品名称 Drug Names | 香菇多糖 Lentinan |
|---|---|
| 适应证<br>Indicaciones | 用于急慢性白血病、胃癌、肺癌、乳腺癌等肿瘤的辅助治疗，提高患者免疫功能，减轻放射治疗和化学治疗的副作用。亦可用于治疗乙型病毒性肝炎。<br><br>Se utiliza para el tratamiento ayudante de la leucemia aguda y crónica, cáncer de estómago, cáncer de pulmón, cáncer de mama y otros tumores,puede mejorar la Mejora la función inmune en pacientes y reducir los efectos secundarios de la radioterapia y la quimioterapia.También puede ser utilizado para el tratamiento de la hepatitis B. |
| 用法、用量<br>Administración y dosis | 口服：成人一次 12.5mg，一日 2 次；儿童一次 5～7.5mg，一日 2 次。静脉注射或静脉滴注：一次 2mg，每周 1 次。一般 3 个月为 1 疗程。<br><br>Por vía oral:adultos 12.5mg 2 veces al día;Niños 5~7.5mg,2 veces al día.Inyección o infusión intravenosa:2mg una vez a la semana,El tratamiento dura generalmente de 2 a 10 semana. |
| 剂型、规格<br>Formulaciones y especificaciones | 片剂：每片 2.5mg。注射剂：每支 1mg。<br>Tableta:2.5mg por tableta.Líquido de inyección:1mg por cada unidad. |
| 药品名称 Drug Names | 重组人白细胞介素 -2　Interleucina 2 recombinante humana |
| 适应证<br>Indicaciones | 用于肾细胞癌、黑色素瘤，控制癌性胸腔积液、腹水及其他晚期肿瘤；先天或后天免疫缺陷症，如艾滋病等；细菌、真菌及病毒感染，如慢性活动性乙型肝炎、慢性活动性 EB 病毒感染、麻风病、肺结核、白念珠菌感染等。<br><br>Se utiliza para el tratamiento de carcinoma de células renales, melanoma, el control del cáncer de mama, ascitis, y otros tumores avanzados;Síndrome de inmunodeficiencia congénita o adquirida, como el SIDA;Infecciones bacterianas, fúngicas y virales,tales como hepatitis crónica activa, infección por el virus EB crónica activa, la lepra, la tuberculosis, la infección por Candida albicans. |
| 用法、用量<br>Administración y dosis | 皮下注射：每日 20 万～40 万 U/m²，加入无菌注射用水 2ml，一日 1 次，每周连用 4 日，4 周为一疗程。肌内注射：慢性乙型肝炎每次 20 万 U，隔日一次。静脉滴注：20 万～40 万 U/m²，加入生理盐水 500ml，一日一次，每周连用 4 日，4 周为 1 疗程。腔内注射：癌性胸腔积液、腹水时先抽取胸腔内积液，在将本品 40 万～50 万 /m² 加入生理盐水 20ml 注入，每周 1～2 次，3～4 周为一疗程。瘤内或瘤周注射：10 万～30 万 U/m²，加至 3～5ml 注射用生理盐水中，分多点注射到瘤内或瘤周。每周 2 次，连用 2 周为一疗程。<br><br>Por vía subcutánea:200 000～400 000 U / m² al día y se añade 2 ml de agua estéril para inyección,una vez cada cuatro días,un plazo de 4 semanas para el tratamiento.Por vía intramuscular:contra la hepatitis B crónica 200 000 U una vez cada dos días.Por vía intravenosa:200 000～400 000 U/m²,se añade 500 ml de solución salina,una vez cada cuatro días, un plazo de 4 semanas para el tratamiento.Por vía intrapleural:para el cáncer de mama, ascitis,primero se tiene que extraer el derrame pleural,luego se aplica la inyección con el medicamento de 400 000～500 000U/m² diluido con 20 ml de solución salina,1 a 2 veces cada semana,un plazo de 3 a 4 semanas para el tratamiento.Por via peritumoral o intratumoral: 100 000 y 300 000 U / m²,se añade a la solución salina fisiológica para inyección de 3~5ml y se aplica la inyección multipunto.2 veces cada semana,un plazo de 2 semanas para el tratamiento. |
| 剂型、规格<br>Formulaciones y especificaciones | 注射剂：每支 2.5 万 U；5 万 U；10 万 U；20 万 U；50 万 U；100 万 U；200 万 U。<br>Líquidao de inyección：25 000U；50 000 U；100 000U；200 000U；500 000U；1 000 000U；2 000 000U. |
| 药品名称 Drug Names | 重组人白细胞介素 -11　Interleucina-11 recombinante humana |
| 适应证<br>Indicaciones | 用于实体瘤、非髓性白细胞病化疗后Ⅲ、Ⅳ度血小板减少症的治疗。<br>Se utiliza para el tratamiento de los tumores sólidos, enfermedad leucocitos no mieloide después de la quimioterapia Ⅲ , Ⅳ grado de trombocitopenia. |
| 用法、用量<br>Administración y dosis | 皮下注射，一次 25～50μg/kg（以 1ml 注射用水稀释），一日 1 次，7～14 日为 1 个疗程。于化疗结束后 24～48 小时开始或发生血小板减少症后给药，血小板计数恢复后应及时停药。 |

**续　表**

| | |
|---|---|
| | Por vía subcutánea, una vez 25 ~ 50μg/kg (diluido con 1 ml de agua para inyección 1 ml),Una vez al día, 7 a 14 días para el tratamiento.Empieza a las 24 y 48 horas después del la quimioterapia o la aparición de síntomas de la trombocitopenia,y debe interrumpirse inmediatamente después de la recuperación del recuento de plaquetas. |
| 剂型、规格<br>Formulaciones y especificaciones | 注射用粉针剂：每支 0.75mg（600 万 U）；1.5mg（1200 万 U）；3mg（2400 万 U）。<br>Polvo para inyección:0.75mg por cada unidad(6 000 000 U);1.5 mg por cada unidad(12 000 000 U);3 mg por cada unidad((24 000 000 U). |
| 药品名称 Drug Names | 重组人干扰素 Interferón recombinante humana (rh IFN)) |
| 适应证<br>Indicaciones | 干扰素可用于肿瘤、病毒感染及慢性活动性乙型肝炎等。<br>El interferón puede ser utilizado para el tratamiento del cáncer, infecciones virales, y de la hepatitis B crónica activa. |
| 用法、用量<br>Administración y dosis | 各种不同干扰素制剂的用法不同，简介于下，详见说明书。<br>Como el uso varia conforme a diferentes tipos de preparaciones de interferón,se aconseja consultar la Instrucción a continuación. |
| 剂型、规格<br>Formulaciones y especificaciones | 详见下述干扰素 α、β、γ 各亚型内容。<br>Vea a continuación  contenidos sobre cada subtipos de interferón α, β, γ. |
| 药品名称 Drug Names | 重组人干扰素 α-2a　Interferón α-2a recombinante humana (rh IFN α-2a)) |
| 适应证<br>Indicaciones | 用于治疗：①某些病毒性疾病：乙型肝炎、丙型肝炎、尖锐湿疣、带状疱疹、小儿病毒性肺炎和上呼吸道感染、慢性宫颈炎等。②某些恶性肿瘤：毛细胞白血病、慢性粒细胞白血病、多发性骨髓瘤、非霍奇金淋巴瘤、卡波西肉瘤、肾癌、喉乳头状瘤、黑色素瘤、蕈样肉芽肿、膀胱癌、基底细胞癌等。<br>Se utiliza para el tratamiento de:1.Enfermedades virales: hepatitis B, hepatitis C, verrugas genitales, herpes zoster, la neumonía viral en los niños y la infección del tracto respiratorio superior, cervicitis crónica,etc.2.tumores malignos:Leucemia de células pilosas, leucemia mielógena crónica, mieloma múltiple, linfoma no Hodgkin, sarcoma de Kaposi, cáncer de riñón, papiloma de laringe, melanoma, micosis fungoides, carcinoma de vejiga, carcinoma de células basales. |
| 用法、用量<br>Administración y dosis | 皮下或肌内注射给药，剂量和疗程如下：<br>①慢性活动性乙型肝炎：每次 500 万 U，一周 3 次，共用 6 个月。1 个月后病毒复制标志物如未见下降，剂量可增加至患者能耐受水平；如疗程 3 ~ 4 个月后症状未获改善，则应停止治疗。②急、慢性丙型肝炎：起始剂量为一次 300 万 ~ 500 万 U，一周 3 次，持续 3 个月。对血清谷丙转氨酶（ALT）正常的患者给予维持治疗：一次 300 万 U，一周 3 次，持续 3 个月。ALT 异常者停止使用。③多发性骨髓瘤：起始剂量为一次 300 万 U，一周 3 次，可根据患者的耐受性，逐周增加至最大耐受量（900 万 ~ 1800 万 U）。④毛细胞白血病：起始剂量为一次 300 万 U，一日 1 次，持续 16 ~ 24 周。如患者难以忍受，则剂量减为一次 150 万 U，一周 3 次。⑤慢性粒细胞白血病：采用逐渐增加剂量给药方案，即第 1 ~ 3 日，每日 300 万；第 4 ~ 6 日，每日 600 万 U；第 7 ~ 84 日，每日 900 万 U。治疗 8 ~ 12 周后，时视其疗效决定是否继续治疗。⑥非霍奇金淋巴瘤：作为肿瘤化疗的辅助用药，推荐剂量为：一次 300 万 U，一周 3 次，至少持续 12 周。⑦尖锐湿疣：皮下或肌内注射，一次 100 万 ~ 300 万 U，一周 3 次，使用 1 ~ 2 个月。⑧宫颈糜烂：非月经期睡前用手指将一枚栓剂放入阴道贴近子宫颈处，隔日一次，9 次为一疗程。<br>Se administra por vía subcutánea o inyección intramuscular, la dosis y la duración del tratamiento son las siguientes: ① contra la hepatitis B crónica activa: 5 000 000 U tres veces a la semana, por 6 meses en total.Si no se observa ningún disminución de los marcadores de la replicación viral,se puede ajustar la dosis hasta el nivel tolerable para los pacientes.Si el tratamiento de 3 a 4 meses no registra una mejora en las condiciones,éste debe ser detenido. ② Contra la hepatitis C aguda y crónica: una dosis inicial de 3 000 000 ~ 500 000 000 U, tres veces a la semana durante 3 meses.Para los pacientes con un nivel normal de Alanina aminotransferasa sérica (ALT),se les da un terapia de mantenimiento:3 000 000 U tres veces a la semana durante ③ meses.Para los pacientes anormales de ALT el uso debe ser detenido. ④ Contra |

**续·表**

| | Mieloma múltiple:Una dosis inicial de 3 000 000 U, 3 veces a la semana durante 3 meses.Se puede incrementar la dosis de modo progresivo hasta la dosis de máxima tolerancia (9 000 000~18 000 000 U)de acuerdo con la tolerancia del paciente. ④ Contra la lcuccmia de células pilosas:Una dosis inicial de 3 000 000 U, una vez al día  durante 16 a 24 semanas.Si surge intorelancia,se ajusta la dosis a 1 500 000 U 3 veces a la semana. ⑤ Contra la leucemia mieloide crónicas:se incrementa la dosis de modo progresivo,en los primeros días 3 000 000 U al día;desde el cuarto día al sexto día, 6 000 000 U al día;Del séptimo día al 84 días,9 000 000 U al día;Tras 8 a 12 semanas, se decidirá si debe continuar el tratamiento en función de su eficacia. ⑥ Contra el linfoma no Hodgkin:se administra como medicamiento adyuvante para la quimioterapia,la dosis recomendada es: 3 000 000 U tres veces a la semana durante al menos 12 semanas. ⑦ Contra la condiloma: por vía subcutánea o intramuscular, 1 000 000 a 3 000 000 U 3 veces a la semana durante 1 a 2 meses. ⑧ Contra la Erosión cervical:se coloca antes de dormir un supositorio con los dedos dentro de la vagina cerca del cuello uterino y debe evitar su uso durante el período menstrual.Se aplica cada dos días durante 9 meses. |
|---|---|
| 剂型、规格<br>Formulaciones y especificaciones | 注射剂：每支 100 万 U；300 万 U；450 万 U；500 万 U；600 万 U；900 万 U；1800 万 U。栓剂：每支 6 万 U；50 万 U。<br><br>Inyección:1.000.000 U;3.000.000 U;4.500.000 U;5.000.000 U;6.000.000 U;9.000.000 U;18.000.000 U por cada unidad. Supositorios: 60 000U, 500 000U por eada unidad. |
| **药品名称 Drug Names** | 聚乙二醇干扰素 α -2a Peginterferón alfa-2a |
| 适应证<br>Indicaciones | 用于治疗慢性丙型肝炎，适用于无肝硬化和非肝硬化代偿期的患者。<br><br>Se utiliza para el tratamiento de la hepatitis C crónica,Aplicable a los pacientes no cirróticos y no cirróticos con descompasada. |
| 用法、用量<br>Administración y dosis | 皮下注射，一次 180μg（1ml），每周 1 次，共 48 周。可根据发生的不良反应调整剂量，可减至 45 ～ 90μg 乃至 135μg，不良反应减轻后可增加或恢复之规定剂量。<br><br>Por vía subcutánea,180ug (1 ml) una vez a la semana durante 48 semanas.Se aconseja ajustar la dosis de acuerdo con la aparición de reacciones adversas hasta 45 ～ 90μg a 135μg.Y puede incrementarla a la dosis indicada al eliminar las efectos secundarios. |
| 剂型、规格<br>Formulaciones y especificaciones | 注射剂：每支 45μg/1ml；90μg/ml；135μg/1ml；180μg/1ml。注射剂（预充式注射器）：每支 135μg/0.5ml；180μg/0.5ml。<br><br>Líquido de inyección:45μg/1ml;90μg/ml;135μg/1ml;180μg/1ml por cada unidad.Inyección en jeringa precargada:135μg/0.5ml:180μg/0.5ml por cada unidad. |
| **药品名称 Drug Names** | 重组人干扰素 α -1b Interferón α -1b recombinante humana(rh IFN α -1b) |
| 适应证<br>Indicaciones | 用于病毒性疾病和某些恶性肿瘤。①已批准用于临床治疗的有：慢性乙型肝炎、丙型肝炎和毛细胞白血病。②已有临床实验结果和文献的有：带状疱疹、尖锐湿疣、流行性出血热和小儿呼吸道合胞病毒性肺炎等病毒性疾病，以及慢性粒细胞白血病、黑色素瘤、淋巴瘤、肝细胞瘤、肺癌、直肠癌、膀胱癌、多发性骨髓瘤等恶性肿瘤。③滴眼液可用于眼部病毒性疾病。<br><br>Se utiliza para el tratamiento de enfermedades virales y algunos tipos de cáncer:　① Con la calificación para el tratamiento clínico:La hepatitis B crónica, la hepatitis C y la leucemia de células pilosas. ② con los resultados de los ensayos clínicos y la literatura:enfermedades virales como Zoster viral del herpes, verrugas genitales, fiebre hemorrágica epidémica y neumonía por virus sincicial respiratorio pediátrico;La leucemia mielógena crónica, melanoma, linfoma, hepatoma, cáncer de pulmón, cáncer colorrectal, cáncer de vejiga, el mieloma múltiple y otras neoplasias malignas. ③ Las gotas para ojos se aplica para el tratamiento de virales oculares. |
| 用法、用量<br>Administración y dosis | 皮下或肌内注射给药，一次 30 ～ 50μg，隔日或一日 1 次，疗程不超过 6 个月或视病情而定。<br><br>Por vía subcutánea o intramuscular, 30 ～ 50 μg cada día o cada dos días.La duración del tratamiento depende de la evolución de la enfermedad, un curso de no más de seis meses |
| 剂型、规格<br>Formulaciones y especificaciones | 注射剂：每支 10μg（100 万 U）；20μg（200 万 U）；30μg（300 万 U）；50μg（500 万 U）。滴眼液：20 万 U/2ml。<br><br>Inyección:10 μg (1 000 000 U); 20μg (2 000 000 U); 30μg (3 000 000 U); 50 μg (5 000 000 U). Gotas para ojos: 200 000 U/2ml. |

**续　表**

| 药品名称 Drug Names | 重组人干扰素 α-2b　Interferón α-2b recombinante humana (rh IFN α-2b) |
|---|---|
| 适应证<br>Indicaciones | 用于：①慢性活动性乙型、丙型、丁型病毒性肝炎、带状疱疹、尖锐湿疣等病毒性疾病；②毛细血管性白血病、慢性粒细胞性白血病、多发性骨髓瘤、非霍奇金淋巴瘤、艾滋病相关的喉乳头状瘤或卡波西肉瘤、肾细胞癌、卵巢癌、恶性黑色素瘤等恶性肿瘤。<br><br>Se utiliza para el tratamiento de: ① Activa crónica hepatitis B, hepatitis C, hepatitis tipo D,Herpes zoster, verrugas genitales y otras enfermedades virales. ② Capilares leucemia, leucemia mielógena crónica, mieloma múltiple, linfoma no Hodgkin,Sarcoma o laríngeo Papiloma de Kaposi relacionado con el SIDA,carcinoma de células renales, cáncer de ovario, melanoma maligno y otros tumores malignos. |
| 用法、用量<br>Administración y<br>dosis | 推荐的给药途径、剂量及疗程如下：①慢性乙型、丙型肝炎：皮下注射，一次 300 万~500 万 U，每日或隔日 1 次，3~6 个月为一疗程。②慢性丁型肝炎：皮下注射，一次 300 万 U，一周 3 次，至少使用 3~4 个月。③毛细胞性白血病或喉乳头状瘤：皮下注射，一次 300 万 U，一周 3 次（隔日 1 次）。④慢性粒细胞白血病：单药治疗：皮下注射，一次 400 万~500 万 U，一日 1 次，至白细胞计数得到控制后，给予最大耐受量维持治疗；与阿糖胞苷合用：先用本药一次 500 万 U，一日 1 次，2 周后加用阿糖胞苷。若以上方案 8~12 周未见效应停止治疗。⑤多发性骨髓瘤：皮下注射，一次 300 万~500 万 U，一周 3 次（隔日 1 次）。⑥非霍奇金淋巴瘤：皮下注射，一次 500 万 U，一周 3 次（隔日一次），与化疗药合用。⑦艾滋病相关的卡波西肉瘤：皮下注射，一次 300 万 U，一周 3~5 次，也可每天 100 万~1200 万。⑧肾细胞癌：皮下注射或静脉给药，单药治疗，一次 300 万~400 万 U，可以一周 3 次、5 次或一日一次。⑨转移性类癌瘤：皮下注射，一次 300 万 U，一周 3 次，每日或隔日 1 次。⑩恶性黑色素瘤：诱导治疗，可先静脉给药，剂量为一次 2000 万 U，一周 5 次，共 4 周，然后皮下注射，一次 1000 万 U，一周 3 次，共 48 周。⑪尖锐湿疣：皮下注射，一次 100 万~300 万 U，一周隔日注射 3 次，1~2 个月为一疗程。<br><br>Véase a continuación la dosis,el tratamiento y la vía de administración recomendada: ① Contra Hepatitis B y tipo C crónica:Por vía subcutánea,3 000 000 U ~ 5 000 000 U,cada día o cada dos días durante tres a seis meses. ② Hepatitis d crónica: inyección subcutánea de 300 000U, 3 veces a la semana, durante al menos 3 a 4 meses. ③ Contra Leucemia de células pilosas o papiloma laríngeo:Por vía subcutánea,3 000 000 U 3 veces a la semana (cada dos días). ④ Contra la leucemia mieloide crónica:mediante monoterapia: por vía subcutánea 4 000 000 ~ 5 000 000 U al día hasta lograr un control de conteo de glóbulos blancos,se aplica el tratamiento de mantenimiento con dosis máxima tolerada;En combinación con citarabina: primero con este medicamiento 5 000 000 U al día durante 2 semanas,y por siguiente se añade Citarabina.Si el tratamiento no surge un efeto notable debe detenerse. ⑤ Contra Mieloma múltiple: por vía subcutánea,3 000 000 ~ 500 000 000 U tres veces a la semana (días alternos). ⑥ Contra linfoma no Hodgkin: por vía subcutánea,5 000 000 U tres veces a la semana (días alternos)combinado con las drogas de quimioterapia. ⑦ Contra Sarcoma de Kaposi relacionada con el SIDA : por vía subcutánea,3 000 000 U 3 a 5 veces a la semana, también puede ser de 1 000 000~ 1 200 000U al día. ⑧ Contra Carcinoma de células renales:por vía subcutánea o intravenosa,mediante monoterapia,3 000 000 a 4 000 000 U, puede ser tres veces a cinco veces a la semana, o una vez al día. ⑨ Contra Tumores carcinoides metastásicos: por vía subcutánea, 3 000 000 U tres veces a la semana, todos los días o cada dos días. ⑩ Contra el melanoma maligno: mediante la terapia de inducción,se puede administrar por vía intravenosa,la dosis es de 20 000 000 U 5 veces a la semana durante 4 semanas.luego se administra por vía subcutánea,10 000 000 U 3 veces a la semana durante 48 semanas. ⑪Contra Verrugas genitales: por vía subcutánea,1 000 000 a 3 000 000 U tres veces cada dos días durante una semana, el tratamiento dura 1 a 2 meses. |
| 剂型、规格<br>Formulaciones y<br>especificaciones | 注射用粉针剂：每支 100 万 U；300 万 U；500 万 U；1000 万 U；1800 万 U；3000 万 U。注射液（多剂量笔）：180 万 U/1ml。栓剂：每支 50 万 U。<br><br>Polvo para inyección:1 000 000 U;3 000 000 U;5 000 000 U;10 000 000 U;18 000 000 U; 30 000 000 U por cada unidad.Líquido de inyección (pluma de dosis múltiples): 1 800 000 U/1ml.).Supositorios:500 000 U por cada unidad. |
| 药品名称 Drug Names | 重组人干扰素 β　Interferon β recombinante humana(rh IFN β ) |
| 适应证<br>Indicaciones | （1）用于病毒性疾病的治疗，对 RNA、DNA 病毒均敏感，皮下或静脉注射给药用于治疗慢性活动性肝炎、新生儿巨细胞病毒性脑炎。外涂、滴鼻、病灶局部给药用于防治流感 A2 和 B 病毒、鼻病毒所致的感冒、带状疱疹、甚至起疱疹等。<br>（2）用于多发性硬化疾病。<br>（3）用于肿瘤性胸腔积液、毛细胞白血病、宫颈上皮肿瘤、或乳腺及子宫内膜肿瘤的甾体激素受体诱导治疗。 |

**续　表**

(1) Se utiliza para el tratamiento de enfermedades virales y es sensible para ARN, virus de ADN,ya que la administración subcutánea o intravenosa puede ser utilizado para el tratamiento de la hepatitis crónica activa, la encefalitis neonatal citomegalovirus. La administración recubiertos, intranasal, sobre álesiones tópicas puede aplicarse para la prevención y el tratamiento de Virus de la gripe A2 y B, resfriados causadas por rinovirus, herpes zoster y otros herpes.

(2) Contra la esclerosis múltiple.

(3) Se utiliza para La terapia de inducción del receptor de la hormona esteroide contra el derrame pleural, la leucemia de células peludas, neoplasia intraepitelial cervical o de mama y el cáncer de endometrio.

| 用法、用量<br>Administración y dosis | ①多发性硬化疾病：皮下注射，每次 44ug，每周 3 次。②生殖器疱疹、带状疱疹：肌内注射，一次 200 万 U，一日 1 次，连续 10 日。③扁平或尖锐湿疣：皮下或病灶局部注射，每日 100 万～ 300 万 U，连用 5 日为一疗程，每次 1 ～ 3 个疗程。或肌内注射，一日 200 万 U，连续 10 日。④慢性乙型肝炎：肌内注射，一次 500 万 U，每周 3 次，连续 6 个月。慢性丙型或丁型肝炎：前 2 个月每次 600 万 U，每周 3 次；后改为每次 300 万 U，每周 3 次，连续 3 ～ 6 个月。⑤宫颈上皮肿瘤：病灶内注射，300 万 U，一日 1 次，连续 5 日。后改为隔日一次，连续 2 周。⑥肿瘤性胸腔积液：胸椎穿刺后将 500 万 U 的本品注入胸膜腔。若 7 ～ 15 日后又出现胸腔积液，再次胸穿，注入本品 1000 万 U。若 15 日后再复发，用 50ml 生理盐水稀释 2000 万 U 药物注入胸腔。⑦毛细胞白血病：静脉内缓慢注入，诱导剂量每日 600 万 U，连续 7 日为一疗程，共 3 周（隔周）。维持剂量 600 万 U，每周 2 次，连续 24 周。⑧乳腺肿瘤和子宫内膜肿瘤：肌内注射，每次 200 万～ 600 万 U，每周 3 次（隔天），共 2 周。此方案在激素治疗期每间隔 4 周可重复使用。<br><br>① Contra Esclerosis múltiple: Por vía subcutánea,44ug 3 veces a la semana. ② Contra el herpes genital, herpes zoster: por vía intramuscular,2 000 000 una vez al día durante 10 días consecutivos. ③ Contar las verrugas planas o genitales:mediante La inyección subcutánea o sobre área de lesiones localizadas, 1 000 000 U a 3 000 000 U durante 5 días,1~3 curso de tratamiento.O vía intramuscular, de 2 000 000 U al día durante 10 días consecutivos. ④ Contra Hepatitis B crónica:por vía intramuscular,5 000 000 U 3 veces a la semana durante seis meses.5.Contra Neoplasia intraepitelial cervical: por vía intralesional, 3 000 000 U una vez al día durante. ⑤ días consecutivos. Más tarde se cambia a cada dos días durante 2 semanas. ⑥ Contra Derrame pleural neoplásico: se inyecta 5 000 000 U del medicamiento en la cavidad pleural tras el toracocentesis. ⑦ .Contra Leucemia de células pilosas: mediante inyección intravenosa lenta para inducir una dosis diaria de 6 000 000 U. Un curso 7 días consecutivos durante un total de 3 semanas (en intervalos de semanas) con una dosis de mantenimiento de 6 000 000U dos veces por semana durante 24 semanas. ⑧ Tumor de mama y tumor endometrial: inyección intramuscular, 2 000 000 ~ 6 000 000U cada vez, 3 veces por semana (en días alternados) durante 2 semanas. Se puede repetir el tratamiento cada 4 semanas durante el período de tratamiento hormonal. |
| --- | --- |
| 剂型、规格<br>Formulaciones y especificaciones | 注射用冻干粉：每安瓿 11μg/2ml（300 万 U）。注射液（预装式注射器）：22μg/0.5ml（600 万 U）；44μg/0.5ml（1200 万 U）。<br><br>Polvo liofilizado para inyección: 11μg/2ml por cada ampolla (3 000 000 U). Líquido de inyección (jeringa precargada): 22μg/0.5ml (6 000 000 U); 44μg/0.5ml (12 000 000 U). |
| **药品名称 Drug Names** | 重组人干扰素 γ（rh IFN γ）Interferon γ recombinantehumana (rh IFN γ) |
| 适应证<br>Indicaciones | 用于类风湿关节炎、迁延性肝病及肝纤维化的治疗。<br><br>Se utiliza para el tratamiento de la artritis reumatoide, Hepatitis crónica persistente y la fibrosis hepática. |
| 用法、用量<br>Administración y dosis | ①类风湿关节炎：皮下注射，初始剂量为一次 50 万 U，一日 1 次，连续 3 ～ 4 日，如无不良反应，将剂量加至每日 100 万 U；第二个月改为一次 150 万～ 200 万 U，隔日 1 次，总疗程为 3 个月。②肝纤维化：皮下注射，前 3 个月，一次 50 万 U，一日 1 次，后 6 个月，一次 100 万 U，隔日 1 次。<br><br>① Para el tratamiento de Artritis reumatoide:Por vía subcutánea,la dosis inicial es de 500 000 U,una vez al día,3 a 4 días consecutivos.Si no hay reacciones adversas, se añadió la dosis diaria a 1 000 000 U;El segundo mes se ajusta la dosis a 1 500 000 U a 2 000 000 U una vez cada dos días durante 3 meses. ② Contra fibrosis hepática:Por vía subcutánea,los primeros 3 meses,500 000 U una vez al día;Por los siguientes 6 meses,1 000 000 U cada dos días. |

**续 表**

| | |
|---|---|
| 剂型、规格<br>Formulaciones y especificaciones | 注射剂：每支 50 万 U；100 万 U；200 万 U。<br>Inyección: 500 000 U;100 000 U; 200 000 U por cada unidad. |
| 药品名称Drug Names | 人免疫球蛋白 Inmunoglobulina humana |
| 适应证<br>Indicaciones | 用于免疫缺陷疾病和传染性肝炎、麻疹、水痘、腮腺炎、带状疱疹等病毒感染和细菌感染的防治，也用于哮喘、过敏性鼻炎、湿疹等内源性过敏性疾病。<br><br>Se utiliza para la prevención y el tratamiento de las enfermedades de inmunodeficiencia y infecciones virales y bacterianas como la hepatitis infecciosa, sarampión, varicela, paperas, herpes zoster,así como enfermedades alérgicas endógenos como el asma, la rinitis alérgica, el eccema. |
| 用法、用量<br>Administración y dosis | 肌内注射：①预防麻疹：0.05～0.15ml/kg 或儿童 5 岁以下 1.5～3ml，成人不超过 6ml，预防效果 1 个月。②预防甲型肝炎：0.05～0.15ml/kg 或儿童 1.5～3ml，成人每次 3ml，预防效果 1 个月。③预防乙型肝炎：成人一次 200U，儿童 100U，必要时隔 3～4 周再注射一次。母亲为乙肝表面抗原或核心抗原双阳者，婴儿出生 24 小时内注射 100U，阻断预防。<br><br>Por vía intramuscular: ① Contra el sarampión:0.05~0.15ml/kg o 1.5~3ml para los niños menores de 5 años de edad,para adultos la dosis no superan los 6 ml,el efecto preventivo se logra en un mes. ② prevención de la hepatitis A: 0.05～0.15ml/kg,3 ml cada vez para adultos,1.5~3ml para niños,3 ml cada adulto,el efecto preventivo se logra en un mes. ③ Contra la hepatitis B:200 U para adultos, 100 U para niños,se aplica la inyección cada 3 a 4 semanas si es necesario.Si la madre lleva Antígeno de superficie de la hepatitis B o antígeno Core de doble positivo ,se debe realizar la inyección de 100 U para la prevención de bloqueo a su bebe dentro de las 24 horas de su nacimiento. |
| 剂型、规格<br>Formulaciones y especificaciones | 注射液（10%）：每支 150mg/1.5ml，300mg/3ml，500mg/5ml。注射冻干粉：每支 150mg；300mg；500mg。注射液：每支 100U；200U；400U。<br><br>Líquido de inyección (10%): 150mg/1.5ml;300mg/3ml;500mg/5ml por cada unidad.Polvo liofilizado para inyección:150 mg; 300 mg; 500 mg por cada unidad. inyección: 100U, 200U, 400U, por cada unidad. |
| 药品名称Drug Names | 静脉注射用人免疫球蛋白 Inmunoglobulina humana para uso intravenoso |
| 适应证<br>Indicaciones | 用于原发性和继发性免疫球蛋白缺乏症如 X 连锁低免疫球蛋白血症、重症感染、艾滋病；自身免疫性疾病如原发性血小板减少性紫癜、川崎病、重症系统性红斑狼疮等。<br><br>Sw utiliza para el tratamiento de la deficiencia primaria y secundaria de la inmunoglobulina como Inmunoglobulina ligada a X bajo la hiperlipidemia, infecciones graves y el SIDA;También contra las enfermedades autoinmunes como la púrpura trombocitopénica idiopática, enfermedad de Kawasaki, grave lupus eritematoso sistémico. |
| 用法、用量<br>Administración y dosis | （1）免疫球蛋白缺乏或低下症：按体重一日 400mg/kg，维持量为 200～400mg/kg，用药间隔视血清 IgG 水平定。<br>（2）特发性血小板减少性紫癜：开始一日 400mg/kg，连续 5 日，维持量一次 400mg/kg，每周一次或视血小板计数而定。<br>（3）川崎病：发病 10 日内使用。儿童一次 2.0g/kg，一次静脉滴注。<br>（4）严重感染：一日 200～400mg/kg，连续 3～5 日。<br><br>(1) Contra la deficiencia de inmunoglobulina o hipotiroidismo:400mg/kg al día,la dosis de mantenemiento es de 200 a 400mg/kg,y el nivel de intervalo de dosificación depende del nivel de IgG en suero.<br>(2) Contra la púrpura trombocitopénica idiopática:se comienza por 400mg/kg al día y la dosis de mantenimiento es de 400mg/kg una vez a la semana o Dependiendo del recuento de plaquetas.<br>(3) Contra la enfermedad de Kawasaki:se administra dentro de la aparición de síntomas,para niños 2.0g/kg cada vez por vía intravenosa.<br>(4) Contra infecciones graves: 200～400mg/kg al día,por 3～5 días consecutivos. |
| 剂型、规格<br>Formulaciones y especificaciones | 注射液（pH4）每瓶 1g；1.25g；2.5g；4g。<br>El líquido de inyección(PH4) :1g;1.25g;2.5g;4g cada botella. |

**续　表**

| 药品名称 Drug Names | 乌苯美司 Ubenimex |
|---|---|
| 适应证<br>Indicaciones | 竞争性抑制氨肽酶 B 及亮氨酸肽酶。可刺激骨髓细胞再生及分化。<br>Inhibe de forma competitiva aminopeptidasa B y peptidasa leucina. Puede incentivar la regeneración y diferenciación de las células de médula ósea. |
| 用法、用量<br>Administración y dosis | 口服，一日 30 ～ 100mg，1 次或分 2 次服。也可每周服 2 ～ 3 日，10 个月为 1 个疗程。<br>Por vía oral,30~100mg al día, por una vez o dos veces.También se puede tomar 2~3  días cada semana.10 meses constituye un curso de tratamiento. |
| 剂型、规格<br>Formulaciones y especificaciones | 片剂：每片 10mg。胶囊剂：每粒 10mg；30mg。<br>Tabletas: cada una 20mg. Cápsulas: cada una 10mg;30mg. |

| 药品名称 Drug Names | 白芍总苷 Glucósido total de peoniaceae |
|---|---|
| 适应证<br>Indicaciones | 免疫调节药，改善类风湿关节炎患者症状。<br>Fármacos inmunomoduladores que pueden aliviar los síntomas de los pacientes con artritis reumatoide. |
| 用法、用量<br>Administración y dosis | 口服，一次 300mg，一日 2 ～ 3 次。<br>Por vía oral, 300mg cada vez y 2~3 veces al día. |
| 剂型、规格<br>Formulaciones y especificaciones | 胶囊剂：每粒 300mg。<br>Cápsulas: cada una 300mg. |

18. 维生素类，酶和生化制剂，调节水、电解质和酸碱平衡及营养类药物 Vitaminas, Agentes enzimáticos y bioquímicos, medicamentos que regulacion el equilibrio de agua y electrolitos y ácidobase, y medicamentos para la nutrición

18.1　维生素类 Vitaminas

| 药品名称 Drug Names | 维生素 A　　Vitamina A(Retinol) |
|---|---|
| 适应证<br>Indicaciones | 用于：①维生素 A 缺乏症：如夜盲症、眼干燥症、角膜软化症和皮肤粗糙等。②用于补充需要，如妊娠、哺乳期妇女和婴儿等。③有学者认为对预防上皮癌、食管癌的发生有一定意义。<br>Se utiliza: ① contra la deficiencia de vitamina A: la ceguera nocturna, el síndrome del ojo seco, la queratomalacia y piel áspera etc.. ② para suplir necesidades para las mujeres en embarazo o lactancia y los bebés etc.. ③ puede prevenir en cierta medida el cáncer epitelial y el esofágico. |
| 用法、用量<br>Administración y dosis | （1）严重维生素 A 缺乏症：口服，成人一日 10 万 U，3 日后改为一日 5 万 U，给药 2 周，然后一日 1 万～ 2 万 U，再用药 2 个月。吸收功能障碍或口服困难者可用肌内注射，成人一日 5 万～ 10 万 U，3 日后改为每日 5 万 U，给药 2 周；1 ～ 8 岁儿童，一日 0.5 万～ 1.5 万 U，给药 10 日；婴儿，一日 0.5 万～ 1 万 U，给药 10 日。<br>（2）轻度维生素 A 缺乏症：一日 1 万～ 2.5 万 U，分 2 ～ 3 次口服。<br>（3）补充需要：成人每日 5000U，哺乳期妇女每日 5000U，婴儿一日 600 ～ 1500U，儿童每日 2000 ～ 3000U。<br>(1) Grave deficiencia de vitamina A: por vía oral, los adultos toman 100,000U al día, tras 3 días 50,000U al día con duración de 2 semanas, y después 10,000~20,000U al día para 2 meses. Para los pacientes con disfunción de absorción o con dificultades de tomarla por vía oral, se puede utilizar mediante inyección intramuscular: para los adultos 50,000~100,000U al día, tras 3 días 50,000U al día con duración de 2 semanas;para los niños de 1 a 8 años, 5,000~15,000U al día para 10 días; para los bebés, 5,000~10,000U al día con duración de 10 días.<br>(2) Leve deficiencia de vitamina A: por vía oral,10,000~25,000U al día por 2~3 veces.<br>(3) Para suplir necesidades: los adultos toman 5,000U al día; las mujeres en lactancia, 5000U al día; los bebés 600~1500U al día; y los niños 2000~3000U al día. |
| 剂型、规格<br>Formulaciones y especificaciones | 胶丸剂：每丸 5000U；2.5 万 U。<br>Cápsulas: cada una 5 000U; 25 000U. |

**续　表**

| 药品名称 Drug Names | 维生素 D　Vitamina D |
| --- | --- |
| 适应证<br>Indicaciones | 维生素 D 缺乏，防治佝偻病、骨软化症和婴儿手足搐搦症。<br>Contra la deficiencia de vitamina D, el raquitismo, la osteomalacia y la tetania de bebés. |
| 用法、用量<br>Administración y<br>dosis | （1）治疗佝偻病：口服一日 2500～5000U，1～2 个月后待症状开始消失时即改用预防量。若不能口服者、重症的患者，肌内注射一次 30 万～60 万 U，如需要，1 个月后再肌内注射 1 次，2 次总量不超过 90 万 U。用大剂量维生素 D 时如缺钙，应口服 10% 氯化钙，一次 5～10ml，一日 3 次，用 2～3 日。<br>（2）婴儿手足搐搦症：口服一日 2000～5000U，1 个月后改为每日 400U。<br>（3）预防维生素 D 缺乏症：用母乳喂养的婴儿一日 400U，妊娠期必要时一日 400U。<br><br>(1) El raquitismo: tome por vía oral,2500~5000U al día. Después de 1~2 meses, tome la dosis de prevención cuando los síntomas empiecen a desaparecer. Para los enfermos graves o los que no puedan tomarla por vía oral, se puede tomar mediante la inyección intramuscular, 300.000~600,000U una vez. Si necesita, inyecte otra vez después de 1 mes. La dosis total de dos veces no se puede sobrepasar 900,000U. Si carece de calcio cuando toma gran dosis de vitamina D, debe 10% de cloruro cálcico por vía oral, 5~10ml cada vez, 3 veces cada día, para 2~3 días.<br>(2) La tetania de bebés: por vía oral, 2000~5000U al día durante un mes y después 400U al día.<br>(3) Prevención de la deficiencia de vitamina D: para los bebés amamantados con leche materna 400U al día, 400U al día durante el embarazo si es necesario. |
| 剂型、规格<br>Formulaciones y<br>especificaciones | 维生素 $D_2$ 胶丸：每粒含 1 万 U。维生素 $D_2$ 片：每片 5000U；10000U。维生素 $D_2$ 胶性钙注射液：每支 1ml；10ml。每 1ml 含 D25 万 U，胶性钙 0.5mg。维生素 $D_3$ 注射液：每支 15 万 U（0.5ml）；30 万 U（1ml）；60 万 U（1ml）。用前及用时需服钙剂。维生素 AD 胶丸：每粒含维生素 A 3000U，维生素 D 300U。浓维生素 AD 胶丸：每粒含维生素 A 1 万 U，维生素 D 1000U。维生素 AD 滴剂：每 1g 含维生素 A 5000U，维生素 D 500U；每 1g 含维生素 A 5 万 U，维生素 D 5000U；每 1g 含维生素 A 9000U，维生素 D 3000U。<br><br>Cápsulas de vitamina $D_2$: cada una contiene 10 000U. Tabletas de vitamina $D_2$: cada una 5000U; 10 000U. Inyecciones de calcio glue de vitamina $D_2$: cada una 1ml;10ml. 1ml contiene 250 000U y 0.5mg de calcio glue. Inyecciones de vitamina $D_3$: cada una 150 000U(0.5ml);300 000U(1ml);600 000U(1ml). Antes y en el momento de tomarla se necesita tomar calcio. Cápsulas de vitamina AD: cada una contiene 10 000U de vitamina A y 1000U de vitamina D. Gotas de vitamina AD: cada gramo contiene 5000U de vitamina A y 500U de vitamina D; 50 000U de vitamina A y 5000U de vitamina D;9000U de vitamina A y 3000U de vitamina D. |
| 药品名称 Drug Names | 骨化三醇 Calcitriol |
| 适应证<br>Indicaciones | 应用于甲状腺功能低下症及血液透析患者的肾性营养不良，骨质疏松症，维生素 D 依赖性佝偻病（肾小管缺乏 1-α 羟化酶）。<br>Se utiliza contra el hipotiroidismo, la malnutrición renal de los enfermos de hemodiálisis, la osteoporosis y el raquitismo dependiente de vitamina D(Los túbulos renales carecen de hidroxilasa 1-α). |
| 用法、用量<br>Administración y<br>dosis | 口服剂量应根据患者的血钙浓度来决定。①血液透析患者的肾性营养不良：如患者血钙浓度正常或略低，口服，一日 0.25μg。如 2～4 周生化指标及病情无明显改变，则一日剂量可达到 0.5μg。每周应测 2 次血钙浓度，随时调整剂量。大多数血透患者用量在一日 0.5～1μg。②甲状腺功能低下：儿童 1～5 岁，一日 0.25～0.75μg；6 岁以上和成人，一日 0.5～2μg（用量须个体化）。<br><br>La dosis para tomar por vía oral depende de la concentración de calcio en la sangre.　① La malnutrición renal de los enfermos de hemodiálisis: si la concentración de calcio en la sangre del paciente es normal o levemente baja, tome por vía oral, 0.25μg al día. Si los marcadores bioquímicos y las condiciones de los pacientes no tienen cambios obvios en 2~4 semanas, se puede tomar 0.5μg al día. Se debe medir la concentración de calcio en la sangre dos veces a la semana y ajustar la dosis según el resultado. La mayoría de los enfermos de hemodiálisis deben tomar 0.5~1μg al día.　② El hipotiroidismo: para los niños 1~5 años, 0.25~0.75μg al día; para los mayores de 6 años y los adultos, 0.5~2μg al día ( La dosis ha de ser individualizada ). |
| 剂型、规格<br>Formulaciones y<br>especificaciones | 胶囊剂：每粒 0.25μg；0.5μg。<br>Cápsulas: cada una 0.25μg;0.5μg. |

**续 表**

| 药品名称 Drug Names | 阿法骨化醇 Alfacalcidol |
|---|---|
| 适应证<br>Indicaciones | 用于慢性肾衰竭合并骨质疏松症、甲状腺功能低下及抗维生素 D 的佝偻病患者。<br><br>Se utiliza para los enfermos de la crónica osteoporosis fusionada con la insuficiencia renal, el hipotiroidismo y el raquitismo resistente a la vitamina D. |
| 用法、用量<br>Administración y<br>dosis | （1）慢性肾衰竭合并骨质疏松：成人，口服，一次 0.5 ～ 1.0μg，一日 1 次。<br>（2）甲状腺功能低下和抗维生素 D 的佝偻病：成人，口服，一日 1.0 ～ 4.0μg，一日 2 ～ 3 次。<br>(1) La crónica osteoporosis fusionada con la insuficiencia renal: para los adultos, por vía oral, 0.5~1.0μg cada vez, una vez al día.<br>(2) El hipotiroidismo y el raquitismo resistente a la vitamina D: para los adultos, por vía oral, 1.0~4.0μg al día en 2~3 veces. |
| 剂型、规格<br>Formulaciones y<br>especificaciones | 胶囊剂：每粒 0.25μg；0.5μg；1.0μg。<br>Cápsulas: cada una 0.25μg;0.5μg;1.0μg |
| 药品名称 Drug Names | 维生素 B₁　Vitamina B₁ (Thiamina) |
| 适应证<br>Indicaciones | 用于脚气病防治及各种疾病的辅助治疗（如全身感染、高热、糖尿病、多发性神经炎、小儿麻痹后遗症及小儿遗尿症、心肌炎、食欲缺乏、消化不良、甲状腺功能亢进和妊娠期等）。对解除某些药物如链霉素、庆大霉素等引起的听觉障碍有帮助。<br><br>Se utiliza para la prevención del beriberi y la terapia ayudante de diversas enfermedades (así como la infección sistémica, fiebre, diabetes, polineuritis, las secuelas de la poliomielitis y la enuresis infantil, miocarditis, pérdida de apetito, la indigestión, el hipertiroidismo y el embarazo, etc.). Sirve para eliminar los problemas de audición causados por algunos fármacos como estreptomicina, gentamicina, etc |
| 用法、用量<br>Administración y<br>dosis | 成人每日的最小必需量为 1mg，孕妇及小儿因发育关系需要较多。在治疗脚气病及消化不良时可根据病情调整。成人 1 次 10 ～ 20mg，一日 3 次，口服；或 1 次 50 ～ 100mg，一日 1 次，肌内注射。儿童 1 次 5 ～ 10mg，一日 3 次，口服；或 1 次 10 ～ 20mg，一日 1 次，肌内注射。不宜静脉注射。<br><br>La dosis mínima para los adultos es 1mg al día y las embarazadas y los niños necesitan más debido a que están en desarrollo. Se puede ajustarla según la condición del paciente cuando trata el beriberi y la indigestión. Los adultos la toman por vía oral 10~20mg cada vez, 3 veces al día; o 50~100mg cada vez mediante la inyección intramuscular, una vez al día. Los niños la toman por vía oral 5~10mg cada vez, 3 veces al día; o 10~20mg cada vez mediante la inyección intramuscular, una vez al día. No se puede tomar mediante inyección intravenosa. |
| 剂型、规格<br>Formulaciones y<br>especificaciones | 片剂：每片 5mg；10mg。注射液：每支 10mg（1ml）；25mg（1ml）；50mg（2ml）；100mg（2ml）。<br>Tabletas: cada una 5mg;10mg. Inyecciones: cada una 10mg(1ml);25mg(1ml);50mg(2ml);100mg(2ml). |
| 药品名称 Drug Names | 维生素 B₂　Vitamina B₂ (Riboflavina) |
| 适应证<br>Indicaciones | 用于口角炎、唇炎、舌炎、眼结膜炎和阴囊炎等的防治。<br><br>Se utiliza para la prevención de la queilitis comisural, queilitis, glositis, conjuntivitis e inflamación del escroto, etc.. |
| 用法、用量<br>Administración y<br>dosis | 成人每日的需要量为 2 ～ 3mg。治疗口角炎、舌炎、阴囊炎等时，一次可服 5 ～ 10mg，一日 3 次，或皮下注射或肌内注射 5 ～ 10mg，一日 1 次，连用数周，至病势减退为止。<br><br>La dosis necesaria para los adultos es 2~3mg al día. Cuando se usa para tratar la queilitis comisural, glositis e inflamación del escroto, etcétera, se puede tomar 5~10mg una vez, 3 veces al día; o se puede tomar 5~10mg una vez, mediante inyecciones subcutáneas o intramusculares, una vez al día y se utiliza durante varias semanas consecutivas hasta que se cure la enfermedad. |
| 剂型、规格<br>Formulaciones y<br>especificaciones | 片剂：每片 5mg；10mg。注射液：每支 1mg（2ml）；5mg（2ml）；10mg（2ml）。<br>Tabletas: cada una 5mg;10mg.Inyecciones: cada una 1mg(2ml);5mg(2ml);10mg(2ml). |

**续 表**

| 药品名称 Drug Names | 烟酸 Ácido nicotínico |
|---|---|
| 适应证<br>Indicaciones | 用于预防和治疗因烟酸缺乏引起的糙皮病等。也用作血管扩张药，及治疗高脂血症。对于严格控制或选择饮食或接受肠道外营养的患者，因营养不良体重骤减，妊娠期、哺乳期妇女，以及服用异烟肼者，严重烟瘾、酗酒、吸毒者，烟酸的需要量均需增加。<br><br>Se utiliza para la prevención y curación de la pelagra causada por la deficiencia del ácido nicotínico, etc.. Se usa también como los vasodilatadores y para tratar la hiperlipidemia. La dosis necesaria se debe aumentar para los pacientes que controlan rigurosamente o eligen comidas, los que absorben la nutrición parenteral, los que pierden peso brúscamente debido a malnutrición, las mujeres en lactancia o embarazo, los que toman isoniazidas y los que tienen adicciones graves al alcohol, cigarrillos y drogas. |
| 用法、用量<br>Administración y dosis | （1）推荐膳食每日摄入量：出生至3岁5～9mg，4～6岁12mg，7～10岁12mg，男性青少年及成人15～20mg，女性青少年及成人13～15mg，孕妇17mg，哺乳期妇女20mg。<br>（2）糙皮病：成人口服：1次50～100mg，一日5次；静注：1次25～100mg，一日2次或多次。儿童口服：1次25～50mg，一日2～3次；静脉缓慢注射：一日300mg。<br>（3）抗高血脂：成人口服，缓释片或缓释胶囊，推荐1～4周一次0.5g，一日1次；5～8周为一次1g，一日1次；8周后，根据患者的疗效和耐受性逐渐增加，如有必要，最大剂量可加至2g。应在少量低脂肪饮食就睡前服用。须整片（粒）吞服。维持剂量：每日1～2g。女性患者的剂量低于男性患者。<br><br>(1) La diaria ingesta alimentaria recomendada: para los niños del nacimiento a los 3 años, 5~9mg; los de 4~6 años, 12mg; los de 7~10 años 12mg; los adolescentes y adultos masculinos, 15~20mg; las femeninas, 13~15mg; las embarazadas, 17mg; las mujeres en lactancia, 20mg.<br>(2) La pelagra: Para los adultos: por vía oral, 50~100mg cada vez, 5 veces al día; mediante la inyección intravenosa, 25~100mg cada vez, dos o más veces al día. Para los niños: por vía oral, 25~50mg cada vez, 2~3 veces al día; mediante la inyección intravenosa lenta, 300mg al día.<br>(3) Contra la hiperlipidemia: los adultos toman por vía oral tabletas o cápsulas de liberación sostenida y se recomienda 0.5g cada vez , una vez al día en las primeras 4 semanas; 1g cada vez entre las 5~8 semanas, una vez al día; se aumenta gradualmente según la eficacia y la tolerancia del enfermo después de 8 semanas y si es necesario se puede aumentar la dosis máxima a 2g. Se debe tomar antes de dormir tras pequeñas cantidades de dieta baja en grasas.Se debe tragar toda la pastilla o cápsula. La dosis de mantenimiento: 1~2g al día. Las enfermas debe tomar menos que los enfermos. |
| 剂型、规格<br>Formulaciones y especificaciones | 片剂、胶囊剂：每片50mg；100mg。注射液：50mg/ml；100mg/ml。<br>Tabletas o cápsulas: cada una 50mg;100mg.Inyecciones: 50mg/ml;100mg/ml. |
| 药品名称 Drug Names | 维生素 $B_6$   Vitamina $B_6$ (Pyridoxina) |
| 适应证<br>Indicaciones | 用于：①防治因大量或长期服用异烟肼、肼屈嗪等引起的周围神经炎、失眠、不安；减轻抗癌药和放射治疗引起恶心、呕吐或妊娠呕吐等。②治疗因而惊厥或给孕妇服用以预防婴儿惊厥。③白细胞减少症。④局部涂搽治疗痤疮、酒糟鼻、脂溢性湿疹等。<br><br>Se utiliza: ① contra la neuritis periférica,el insomnio y la ansiedad causados por el uso de grandes cantidades o de largo plazo de la isoniazida e hidralazina etc.; para aliviar la náusea, el vómito y el vómito del embarazo causados por medicamentos anticancerosos y radioterapias. ② contra la convulsión de bebés o la toman las embarazadas para prevenir la convulsión de bebés. ③ contra la leucopenia. ④ contra el acné, la rosácea, eczema seborreica etc. mediante la aplicación local. |
| 用法、用量<br>Administración y dosis | 口服：一次10～20mg，一日3次（缓释片一次50mg，一日1～2次）。皮下注射、肌内注射、静脉注射：一次50mg，一日1～2次）。皮下注射、肌内注射、静脉注射：一次50～100mg，一日1次。治疗白细胞减少症时，以50～100mg，加入5%葡萄糖注射液20ml中，作静脉注射，一日1次。<br><br>Por vía oral: 10~20mg cada vez, 3 veces al día (para las tabletas de liberación sostenida, 50mg cada vez, 1~2 veces al día). Mediante inyecciones subcutáneas, intramusculares e intravenosas: 50mg cada vez, 1~2 veces al día. Mediante inyecciones subcutáneas, intramusculares e intravenosas: 50~100mg cada vez, una vez al día. Al tratar la leucopenia, inyecte 50~100mg de este fármaco a 20ml de solución de dextrosa al 5% y utilícelo mediante inyección intravenosa, una vez al día. |

**续 表**

| | |
|---|---|
| 剂型、规格<br>Formulaciones y especificaciones | 片剂：每片 10mg。维生素 B₆ 缓释片：每片 50mg。注射液：每支 25mg（1ml）；50mg（1ml）；100mg（22ml）。霜剂：每支含 12mg。<br>Tabletas: cada una 10mg.Tabletas de liberación prolongada de Vitamina B₆: cada una 50mg. Inyecciones: cada una 25mg(1ml);50mg(1ml);100mg(22ml). Crema: cada una 12mg. |
| **药品名称 Drug Names** | 干酵母 Levaduras secas |
| 适应证<br>Indicaciones | 用于防止脚气病、多发性神经炎、糙皮病等。<br>Se utiliza para la prevención del beriberi, la polineuritis, la pelagra etc. |
| 用法、用量<br>Administración y dosis | 每次服 0.5～4g，一日 3 次，服时嚼碎。<br>Se toma mediante masticación 0.5~4g cada vez, 3 veces al día. |
| 剂型、规格<br>Formulaciones y especificaciones | 片剂：0.3g；0.5g。<br>Tabletas: 0.3g;0.5g. |
| **药品名称 Drug Names** | 维生素 C Vitamina C (Ácido ascórbico) |
| 适应证<br>Indicaciones | 用于：①坏血病的预防及治疗。②急慢性传染病时，消耗量增加，宜适当补充。病后恢复期，创伤愈合不良者，也应适当补充。③克山病患者在发生心源性休克时，可用大剂量治疗。④用于肝硬化、急性肝炎和砷、汞、铅、苯等慢性中毒时的肝脏损害。⑤其他：用于各种贫血、过敏性皮肤病、口疮、促进伤口愈合等。<br>Usos: ① Se utiliza para la prevención y curación del escorbuto. ② Cuando se usa contra los contagios crónico y agudo, de gasta más y se debe aumentar apropiadamente.Para los enfermos que tienen mala cicatrización en el período de recuperación después de la curación, se necesita aumentar debidamente también. ③ Se puede tomar enorme dosis para curar los pacientes con enfermedad de Keshan en shock cardiogénico. ④ Se utiliza contra la cirrosis, hepatitis aguda y el daño hepático causado por la intoxicación crónica por arsénico, mercurio, plomo, benceno, etc.. ⑤ Los demás: se utiliza contra la anemia, dermatosis alérgica, afta y fomenta la cicatrización de heridas, etc.. |
| 用法、用量<br>Administración y dosis | （1）一般应用：口服（饭后）一次 0.05～0.1g，一日 2～3 次；亦可静脉注射或肌内注射，或以 5%～10% 葡萄糖液稀释进行静脉滴注，一日 0.25～0.5g（小儿 0.05～0.3g），必要时可酌增剂量。<br>（2）克山病：首剂 5～10g，加入 25% 葡萄糖注射液中，缓慢静脉注射。<br>（3）口疮：将本品 1 片（0.1g）压碎，撒于溃疡面上，令患者闭口片刻，一日 2 次，一般 3～4 次即可治愈。<br>(1) Aplicación general: por vía oral(después de la comida), 0.05~0.1g cada vez, 2~3 veces al día; También se puede tomar mediante iyección intravenosa o intramuscular, o se utiliza mediante inyección intravenosa después de dilución con solución de glucosa al 5%~10%, 0.25~0.5g al día(para los niños 0.05~0.3g), y se puede aumentar la dosis debidamente si es necesario.<br>(2) La enfermedad de Keshan: envase 5~10g de este producto en la inyección de glucosa al 25% y inyecte por vía intravenosa lentamente.<br>(3) Afta: aplaste una tableta (0.1g) en polvo, espolvoréelo sobre la superficie de la úlcera y haga al enfermo a cerrar la boca por un rato, 2 veces al día. Se puede curar después de 3~4 veces generalmente. |
| 剂型、规格<br>Formulaciones y especificaciones | 片剂：每片 20mg；25mg；50mg；100mg；250mg。咀嚼片剂：每片 100mg。泡腾片：每片 500mg。注射液：每支 100mg（2ml）；250mg（2ml）；500mg（2ml）；2.5g（20ml）。<br>Tabletas: cada una 20mg;25mg;50mg;100mg;250mg. Tabletas masticables: cada una 100mg.Tabletas efervescentes: cada una 500mg. Inyecciones: cada una 100mg(2ml);250mg(2ml);500mg(2ml);2.5g(20ml). |
| **药品名称 Drug Names** | 维生素 E Vitamina E (Tocoferol) |
| 适应证<br>Indicaciones | 用于：①未进食强化奶或有严重脂肪吸收不良母亲所生的新生儿、早产儿、低出生体重儿。②未成熟儿、低出生体重儿常规应用于预防维生素 E 缺乏。③进行性肌营养不良的辅助治疗。④维生素 E 需要量增加的情况，如甲状腺功能亢进、吸收功能不良综合征、肝胆系统疾病等。 |

**续 表**

| | Usos: ① Pueden utilizarla los recién nacidos, niños prematuros, niños con bajo peso al nacer de las mujeres que no han tomado la leche fortificada o que sufren grave malabsorción de grasa. ② Se suele utilizar para la prevención de deficiencia de vitamina E para los niños prematuros y los con bajo peso al nacer. ③ Tratamiento adyuvante de la distrofia muscular. ④ En los casos de que se necesite mayor cantidad de vitamina E, por ejemplo, el hipertiroidismo, el síndrome de absorción deficiente y las enfermedades del sistema hepatobiliar, etc.. |
|---|---|
| 用法、用量<br>Administración y dosis | 口服或肌内注射：一次 10～100mg，一日 1～3 次。<br>Por vía oral o mediante inyección intramuscular: 10~100mg una vez, 1~3 veces al día. |
| 剂型、规格<br>Formulaciones y especificaciones | 片剂：每片5mg；10mg；100mg。胶丸：每丸5mg；10mg；50mg；100mg；200mg。粉剂：每克粉剂中含维生素 E0.5mg。注射液：每支 5mg（1ml）；50mg（1ml）。<br>Tabletas: cada una 5mg;10mg;100mg.Cápsulas: cada una 5mg;10mg;50mg;100mg;200mg.Polvo: cada gramo de polvo contiene Vitamina E 0.5mg. Inyecciones: cada una 5mg(1ml);50mg(1ml). |

## 18.2　酶类和其他生化制剂 Enzimas y otros agentes bioquímicos

| 药品名称 Drug Names | 胰蛋白酶 Tripsina |
|---|---|
| 适应证<br>Indicaciones | 临床上主要用于脓胸、血胸、外科炎症、溃疡、创伤性损伤、瘘管等所产生的局部水肿、血肿、脓肿等，虹膜睫状体炎、急性泪囊炎、视网膜周围炎、眼外伤等。喷雾吸入，用于呼吸道疾病。因对蛇毒蛋白（蛇毒的主要毒成分）有水解作用，故有将本品用于治疗毒蛇咬伤，曾试用于竹叶青、银环蛇、眼镜蛇、蝮蛇等毒蛇咬伤的各型病例。<br><br>Se utiliza principalmente contra el edema local, hematoma y absceso, etc. causados por el empiema, hemotórax, inflamación quirúrgica, úlceras, lesiones traumáticas y fístula, etc. y contra la iridociclitis, dacriocistitis aguda, inflamación de la retina y la lesión en el ojo, etc.. Puede tratar las enfermedades respiratorias mediante la inhalación del aerosol. Como tiene efecto de hidrólisis sobre las proteínas del veneno de víbora (el ingrediente principal del veneno), se puede utilizar para curar la mordedura de serpientes y se han aplicado a los heridos mordidos por muchos tipos de víboras, así como trimeresurus, serpiente coral, cobra y agkistrodonhalys, etc.. |
| 用法、用量<br>Administración y dosis | （1）一般应用：一次 5000U，一日 1 次，肌内注射，用量斟酌情况决定。为防止疼痛，可加适量普鲁卡因。局部用药视情况而定，可配成溶液剂（pH7.4～8.2，微碱性时活性最强）、喷雾剂、粉剂、软膏等，用于体腔内注射、患部注射、喷涂、湿敷、涂搽等。<br>（2）滴眼：0.25% 溶液，一日4～6次。冲洗泪道：0.25%～0.5%溶液（内加2%普鲁卡因少量），一次／日。眼浴 1：5000～1：10 000 溶液 10～20ml，1 次 10～20ml，一次 10～15 分钟，一日 1 次，或隔日 1 次。球后注射 1 次 1～2.5mg，隔日 1 次。肌内注射 1 次 2.5～5mg。一日 1～2 次。<br>（3）治蛇毒：取注射用结晶胰蛋白酶 2000～6000U，加 0.25%～0.5% 盐酸普鲁卡因（或注射用水）4～20ml 稀释，以牙痕为中心，在伤口周围做浸润注射，或在肿胀部位上方作环状封闭 1～2 次。如病情需要，可重复使用。若伤肢肿胀明显，可于注射 30 分钟后，切开伤口排毒减压（严重出血者例外），也可在肿胀部位针刺排毒。如伤口已坏死、溃疡，可用其 0.1% 溶液湿敷患处。<br><br>(1) Aplicación general: 5 000U a la vez, una vez al día, mediante inyección intramuscular, la dosis se determina según la condición del enfermo. Para evitar el dolor, se puede envasar procaina debidamente. La dosis de la aplicación local se determina según la situación, se pueden preparar como soluciones (PH7.4~8.2, las ligeramente alcalinas son más activas), aerosoles, polvos, ungüentos, etc., y se utilizan mediante inyecciones en cavidades corporales, en las partes enfermas, rociada, aplicación mojada, embadurnamiento, etc.<br>(2) Gotas para los ojos: soluciones al 0.25%, 4~6 al día. Enjuague del conducto lacrimal: soluciones al 0.25%~0.5% ( con una pequeña cantidad de procaína al 2%), una vez al día. Baño ocular: soluciones de 1 : 5000~1 : 10 000, 10~20ml y 10~15 minutos a la vez, una vez al día o una vez a dos días. Inyección intravítrea: 1~2.5mg a la vez, una vez a dos días. Inyección intramuscular: 2.5~5mg a la vez, 1~2 veces al día.<br>(3) contra el veneno de víbora: tome 2000~6000U de tripsina cristalina para inyección, dilúyala con 4~20ml de procaína clorhidrato al 0.25%~0.5% (o agua para inyección) y inyecte de infiltración alrededor de la herida, tomando como el centro las marcas de dientes, o haga bloqueos anulares 1~2 veces en la parte superior de la hinchazón. Se puede reutilizar si es necesario. Si el miembro lesionado tiene hinchazón grave, se puede transpirar toxinas y bajar la presión, haciendo una incisión en la herida (excepto los de hemorragias graves), después de 30 minutos tras la inyección. También se puede hacer la acupuntura en la hinchazón para transpirar toxinas. Si la herida ya es necrósica o ulcerada, se puede aplicar de manera mojada la solución al 0.1% en la parte afectada. |

**续　表**

| 剂型、规格<br>Formulaciones y<br>especificaciones | 注射用胰蛋白酶：每支 1.25 万 U；2.5 万 U；5 万 U；10 万 U（附灭菌缓冲液 1 瓶）。<br>Inyecciones de tripsina: cada una 12 500U; 25 000U; 50 000U; 100 000U (con una botella de solución estéril). |
|---|---|
| 药品名称Drug Names | 糜蛋白酶 Quimotripsina |
| 适应证<br>Indicaciones | 主要用于创伤或手术后创口愈合、抗炎及防止局部水肿、积血、扭伤血肿、乳房手术后水肿、中耳炎、鼻炎、角膜溃疡、泪道疾病、眼外伤、眼睑水肿、出血和玻璃体积血、慢性支气管炎、支气管扩张、肺脓肿及毒蛇咬伤等。<br><br>Se utiliza principalmente para la cicatrización de traumas o heridas quirúrgicas, contra la inflamación y prevenir el edema local, hematocele, hematoma de esguince, edema después de la cirugía de mama, otitis media, rinitis, úlceras corneales, enfermedades lagrimales, trauma ocular, edema palpebral, hemorragia y hematocele del humor vítreo, bronquitis crónica, bronquiectasia, absceso pulmonar y mordedura de víboras, etc.. |
| 用法、用量<br>Administración y<br>dosis | （1）肌内注射：以 0.9% 氯化钠注射液 5ml 溶解 4000U 后注射。<br>　（2）经眼用药：本品对眼球睫状韧带有选择性松弛作用，故可用于白内障摘除，使晶状体比较容易移去。眼科注入后房，一次 800U，以 0.9% 氯化钠注射液配成 1：5000 溶液，由瞳孔注入后房，经 2～3 分钟，在晶状体浮动后以生理盐水冲洗前后方中遗留的本品。<br>　（3）喷雾吸入：每次 5mg，以 0.9%% 氯化钠注射液配成 0.5mg/ml 浓度溶液使用。<br>　（4）用于处理软组织炎症或创伤，800U 糜蛋白酶溶于 1ml0.9% 氯化钠注射液注于创面。<br>　（5）毒蛇咬伤：糜蛋白酶 10～20mg 用注射用水 4ml 稀释后，以蛇牙痕迹为中心区域向后位浸润注射，并在伤口中心区域注射 2 针，再在肿胀上方 3cm 做环状封闭 1～2 层，根据不同部位 0.3～0.7ml，至少 10 针，最多 26 针。<br><br>(1) Inyección intramuscular: disuelva 4000U con inyección de cloruro sódico al 0.9% y después inyéctela.<br>　(2) Aplicación en los ojos: tiene efecto relajante selectivo sobre el ligamento ciliar del ojo, de modo que se puede utilizar en la extracción de cataratas para facilitar la eliminación del cristalino. Inyecte en la parte trasera de los ojos, 800U a la vez, prepare solución 1：5000 con inyecciones de cloruro sódico al 0.9% e inyéctela en la parte trasera a través de la pupila. Tras 2~3 minutos, después de que el cristalino flote, lave las partes trasera y delantera de los ojos con el suero fisiológico para eliminar los residuos de este producto.<br>　(3) La inhalación del aerosol: utilícela después de preparar la solución de concentración 0.5mg/ml con el cloruro sódico al 0.9%, 5mg a la vez.<br>　(4) Cuando se utiliza para tratar la inflamación o el trauma de los tejidos blandos, se debe disolver 800U de la quimotripsina en 1ml de inyección del cloruro sódico al 0.9% e inyectarla en la superficie del trauma.<br>　(5) Las mordeduras de víboras: diluya 10~20mg de la quimotripsina con 4ml de agua para inyección, inyecte de infiltración alrededor de la herida, tomando como el centro las marcas de dientes de víboras y haga dos inyecciones en el centro de la herida. Después haga bloqueos anulares 1~2 veces en la parte de 3cm superior a la hinchazón, con 0.3~0.7ml según las partes, 10 inyecciones al menos y 26 a lo más. |
| 剂型、规格<br>Formulaciones y<br>especificaciones | 注射用糜蛋白酶：每支 800U；4000U。<br>Inyecciones de quimotripsina: cada una 800U; 4000U. |
| 药品名称Drug Names | 抑肽酶 Aprotinina |
| 适应证<br>Indicaciones | 用于各型胰腺炎的治疗与预防；能抑制纤维蛋白溶酶，阻止胰脏中其他活性蛋白酶原的激活及胰蛋白酶原的活化，用于治疗和预防各种纤维蛋白溶解所引起的急性出血；能抑制血管舒张素，从而抑制其舒张血管、增加毛细血管通透性、降低血压的作用，用于各种严重休克状态。此外，在腹腔手术后直接注入腹腔，能预防肠粘连。<br><br>Se utiliza para la prevención y curación de todos los tipos de pancreatitis; puede inhibir la plasmina y prevenir la activación de otros originales de proteasa y del tripsinógeno en los páncreas, y se usa para prevenir y curar la hemorragia aguda causada por todos los tipos de fibrinólisis; puede inhibe el vasodilatador, de este modo cumple sus funciones de inhibirlo de dilatar los vasos sanguíneos, aumentar la permeabilidad capilar y bajar la presión arterial y se utiliza en todos tipos de graves estados de choque. Además, inyéctala directamente en las cavidades abdominales después de la cirugía en esta parte y puede evitar la adherencia intestinal. |

**续 表**

| 用法、用量<br>Administración y<br>dosis | （1）第1、2日每日注射5万～12万U，首剂用量应大一些，缓慢静脉注射（每分钟不超过2ml）。维持剂量应采用静脉滴注，一般一日4次，每日总量2万～4万U。<br>（2）对由纤维蛋白溶解引起的急性出血，立即静脉注射5万～10万U，以后每2小时1万U，直至出血停止。<br>（3）预防剂量：手术前1日开始，每日注射2万U，共3日。治疗肠瘘及连续渗血也可局部使用。<br>（4）预防术后肠粘连：在手术切后闭合前，腹腔内直接注入2万～4万U，注意勿与伤口接触。<br>（5）用于体外循环心脏直视手术。<br><br>(1) Se inyecta 50 000 ~120 000U en los 2 primeros días. La primera dosis debe ser mayor y se inyecta por vía intravenosa lentamente (no puede sobrepasar 2ml al minuto). La dosis de mantenimiento se debe tomar mediante infusión intravenosa, 20.000~40.000U en total divididos en 4 veces al día generalmente.<br>(2) Cuando trata la hemorragia aguda causada por la fibrinólisis, de debe tomar 50 000~100 000U inmediatamente mediante inyección intravenosa y después 10 000U cada 2 horas hasta que la hemorragia se detenga.<br>(3) La dosis de prevención: Inyecte 20 000U al día desde el día anterior de la cirugía, con duración de 3 días. Se puede aplicar localmente para tratar la fístula intestinal y sangría continua.<br>(4) Para evitar la adherencia intestinal: Inyecte directamente 20 000~40 000U en las cavidades abdominales antes de cerrar la incisión quirúrgica y tenga cuidado de no tocar la incisión.<br>(5) Se aplica en la cirugía a corazón abierto de circulación extracorpórea. |
|---|---|
| 剂型、规格<br>Formulaciones y<br>especificaciones | 注射液：每支5万U（5ml）；10万U（5ml）；50万U（5ml）。<br>Inyecciones: cada una 50 000U (5ml); 100 000U (5ml); 500 000U (5ml). |
| **药品名称 Drug Names** | 玻璃酸酶 Hialuronidasa |
| 适应证<br>Indicaciones | 一些以缓慢速度进行静脉滴注的药物如各种氨基酸、水解蛋白等，在与本品合用的情况下可改为皮下注射或肌内注射，使吸收加快。<br><br>Algunos fármacos que se toman mediante lenta infusión intravenosa así como todos los tipos del aminoácido y proteína hidrolizada, etc. Cuando se toman junto con este producto, se pueden utilizar por vía de inyecciones subcutáneas o intramusculares para que se absorba más rápido. |
| 用法、用量<br>Administración y<br>dosis | ①临用时将本品粉末溶于生理盐水中，常用量50或150国际U，配成每ml含0.7U、1.5U或2.0U的注射液，先注射于灌注部位。②皮下注射大量的某些抗生素（如链霉素）或其他化疗药物（如异烟肼等）以及麦角制剂时，合用本品，可使扩散加速，减轻痛感。③以150U溶解在25～50ml局部麻醉药中，如加入肾上腺素，可加速麻醉，并减少麻醉药的用量。④与胰岛素合用，可防止注射局部浓度过高而出现的脂肪组织萎缩。胰岛素休克疗法中用本品100～150U，促使胰岛素吸收量增加，注射较小量即可达血中有效浓度，因而减少其危险性。⑤球后注射促进玻璃体浑浊或出血的吸收，1次100～300U/ml，1次/日。⑥结膜下注射促使球后血肿的吸收，1次50～100U/0.5ml，1日或隔日1次。⑦滴眼预防结膜化学烧伤后睑球粘连，治疗外伤性眼眶出血、外伤性视网膜水肿，150U/ml，每2小时滴眼一次。⑧关节腔内注射，一次2ml，一周1次，连续3～5周。<br><br>① En la aplicación clínica, se disuelve el polvo de este producto en suero fisiolósico. la dosis normal es 50 o 150U, se prepara inyecciones de las que cada mililitro contiene 0.7U, 1.5U o 2.0U y se inyecta anteriormente en la parte de la perfusión. ② Cuando se toman mediante inyección subcutánea grandes cantidades de algunos antibióticos (así como la estreptomicina) u otros medicamentos de quimioterapia (como la isoniazida, etc.) y preparados del cornezuelo, la aplicación de este producto puede acelerar la proliferación y aliviar el dolor. ③ La solución de 150U en 25~50ml de anestésico local (por ejemplo, añade la epinefrina) puede acelerar la anestesia y reducir la dosis del anestésico. ④ Cuando se utiliza junto con la insulina, puede prevenir la atrofia del tejido adiposo causada por la demasiado alta concentración local en la inyección. Utilizar 100~150U de este producto en la terapia de choque de insulina puede promover una mayor absorción de la insulina. De modo que puede llegar una concentración en sangre efectiva con la inyección de una pequeña cantidad y reducir el riesgo. ⑤ La inyección intravítrea puede promover la absorción de opacidad del vítreo o de la sangre, 100~300U/ml a la vez, una vez al día. ⑥ La inyección subconjuntival puede promover la absorción de la hematoma, 50~100U/0.5ml a la vez, una vez al día o a dos días. ⑦ Utilizar las gotas para los ojos puede prevenir la adherencia del párpado y el globo del ojo después de las quemaduras químicas de la conjuntiva, tratar la hemorragia traumática orbital y el edema retiniano traumático, 150U/ml, una vez a dos horas. ⑧ La inyección intraarticular, 2ml a la vez, una vez a la semana, para 3~5 semanas consecutivas. |

续　表

| 剂型、规格<br>Formulaciones y especificaciones | 注射用玻璃酸酶：每支 150U；1500U。<br>Inyecciones de hyaluronidase: cada una 150U; 1500U. |
|---|---|
| 药品名称 Drug Names | 三磷酸腺苷 Adenosína trifosfato |
| 适应证<br>Indicaciones | 用于心力衰竭、心肌炎、心肌梗死、脑动脉硬化、冠状动脉硬化、心绞痛、阵发性心动过速、急性脊髓灰质炎、进行性肌萎缩性疾患、肝炎、肾炎、视疲劳、眼肌麻痹、视网膜出血、中心性视网膜炎、视神经炎、视神经萎缩等。本品不易透过细胞膜，能否发挥其生理效应，值得怀疑。其能量注射液为本品与辅酶 A 等配制的复方注射液，用于肝炎、肾炎、心力衰竭等。<br><br>Se utiliza contra la insuficiencia cardíaca, miocarditis, infarto de miocardio, arteriosclerosis cerebral, enfermedad de la arteria coronaria, angina de pecho, taquicardia paroxística, la poliomielitis aguda, enfermedad de atrofia muscular progresiva, la hepatitis, nefritis, fatiga visual, parálisis de los músculos oculares, hemorragia retiniana , retinitis central, neuritis óptica y atrofia óptica, etc.. Es difícil para este producto penetrar la membrana, por eso es dudoso que pueda cumplir sus funciones fisiológicas. La inyección compuesta de este producto y la coenzima A, etc. constituye la inyección de energía y se aplica contra la hepatitis, nefritis e insuficiencia cardíaca, etc.. |
| 用法、用量<br>Administración y dosis | 肌内注射或静脉注射，每次 20mg，一日 1 ～ 3 次。肌内注射多用注射液，静脉注射多用注射用三磷腺苷，另附有缓冲液溶解，再以 5% ～ 10% 葡萄糖注射液 10 ～ 20ml 稀释后缓慢静脉注射，也可用 5% ～ 10% 葡萄糖注射液稀释后静脉滴注。1% 生理盐水溶液滴眼，治疗弥漫性表层角膜炎和角膜外伤。<br><br>Tome 20mg a la vez, 1~3 veces al día, mediante inyecciones intramuscular o intravenosa. Se suelen aplicar las inyecciones por vía intramuscular y las inyecciones del adenosín trifosfato por vía intravenosa. Además se disuelve con tampón, se diluye con 10~20ml de inyección de glucosa al 5%~10% y después se toma mediante inyección o infusión intravenosa lenta. Se puede curar la queratitis superficial difusible y la lesión corneal mediante gotas del suero fisiológico al 1% para los ojos. |
| 剂型、规格<br>Formulaciones y especificaciones | 注射液：每支 20mg（2ml）。注射用三磷腺苷：每支 20mg；另附磷酸缓冲液 2ml。<br>Inyecciones: cada una 20mg(2ml). Inyecciones del adenosín trifosfato : cada una 20mg; además junto con 2ml de tampón fosfato. |

18.3　调节水、电解质和酸碱平衡用药 Medicamentos que regulan el equilibrio de agua, electrolitos y ácido-base

| 药品名称 Drug Names | 氯化钠 Cloruro sódico |
|---|---|
| 适应证<br>Indicaciones | 氯化钠注射液可补充血容量和钠离子，用于各种缺盐性失水症（如大面积烧伤、严重吐泻、大量发汗、强利尿药、出血等引起）。在大量出血而又无法进行输血时，可输入氯化钠注射液以维持血容量进行急救。还用于慢性肾上腺皮质功能不全（艾迪生病）治疗过程中补充氯化钠，一日约 10g。此外，生理盐水可用于洗伤口、洗眼、洗鼻及产科水囊引产等。<br><br>La inyección del cloruro sódico puede suplir la volemía e iones de sodio y se puede aplicar a todos tipos de la deshidratación con falta de sal (como los causados por quemaduras extensas, graves vómitos y diarrea, sudación, los diuréticos fuertes y sangría, etc.). Cuando no puede hacerse una transfusión frente a la hemorragia, se puede mantener la volemía mediante inyecciones del cloruro sódico para los primeros auxilios. Se también utiliza en el tratamiento de la insuficiencia corticosuprarrenal crónica (enfermedad de Addison) para suplir el cloruro sódico, 10g al día. Además el suero puede usarse para lavar las heridas, los ojos, las narices y para el aborto de vejigas obstétrico, etc.. |
| 用法、用量<br>Administración y dosis | （1）口服：用于轻度急性胃肠患者恶心、呕吐不严重者。<br>（2）高渗性失水：高渗性失水时，患者脑细胞和脊髓液渗透浓度升高，若对其治疗则会使血浆和细胞外液钠浓度和渗透浓度下降过快，可致脑水肿。一般认为，在治疗开始的 48 小时内，血浆钠浓度每小时下降应不超过 0.5mmol/L。<br>（3）等渗性失水：原则给予等渗溶液，如 0.9% 氯化钠注射液或复方氯化钠注射液，但上述溶液氯浓度明显高于血浆，单独大量使用可致高氯血症，故可将 0.9% 氯化钠注射液和 1.25% 碳酸氢钠或 1.86%（1/6M）乳酸钠以 7：3 的比例配制后补给。后者氯浓度为 107mmol/L，并可纠正代谢性酸中毒。<br>（4）低渗性失水：严重低渗性失水时，脑细胞内溶质减少以维持细胞容积。若治疗使血浆和细胞外液钠浓度和渗透浓度迅速回升，可致脑细胞损伤。一般认为，当血钠低于 120mmol/L 时， |

**续　表**

治疗使血钠上升速度在每小时 0.5mmol/L，不超过每小时 1.5mmol/L（稀释性低钠血症不需补钠）。当急性血钠低于 120mmol/L 或出现中枢神经系统症状时，可给予 3% 氯化钠注射液静脉滴注。一般要求在 6 小时内将血钠浓度提高至 120mmol/L 以上。参考补钠量为 3% 氯化钠 1ml/kg，可提高血钠 1mmol/L。待血钠回升至 120～125mmol/L 以上，可改用等渗溶液。慢性缺钠补钠速度要慢，剂量要少，使血钠浓度逐日回升至 130mmol/L。

　　（5）低氯性碱中毒：给予 0.9% 氯化钠注射液或复方氯化钠注射液（林格液）500～1000ml，以后根据碱中毒情况决定用量。

　　（6）外用：用生理氯化钠溶液洗涤伤口、冲洗眼部。

　　(1) Por vía oral: se utiliza para los enfermos con leve enfermedad gastrointestinal aguda los con náuseas y vómitos no graves.

　　(2) La deshidratación hipertónica: En el caso de la deshidratación hipertónica, la concentración osmótica de las células del cerebro y líquido cefalorraquídeo de los enfermos se aumenta. En este caso, el tratamiento puede hacer que la concentración de sodio y la osmótica en el plasma y fuera de las células bajen demasiado rápido, de modo que puede inducir edema cerebral. En general se considera que en las primeras 48 horas desde el comienzo del tratamiento la velocidad de baja de la concentración de sodio en el plasma no puede sobrepasar 0.5mmol/L a la hora.

　　(3) La deshidratación isotónica: en principio, se debe aplicar solución isotónica a los enfermos, así como inyección del cloruro sódico al 0.9% o inyección compuesta del cloruro sódico. No obstante, es obvio que la concentración de cloro en dichas soluciones es mayor que la en el plasma y el uso solo de grandes cantidades puede inducir la hipercloremia. Por eso se puede aplicar después de preparar la inyección del cloruro sódico al 0.9% con bicarbonato de sodio al 1.25% o lactato de sodio al 1.86% (1/6M) en proporción de 7:3. La preparación tiene una concentración del cloruro de 107mmol/L y puede corregir la acidosis metabólica.

　　(4) La deshidratación hipotónica: en el caso de grave eshidratación hipotónica, los solutos en las células cerebrales se reducen para mantener el volumen celular. El tratamiento puede provacar que la concentración de sodio y la osmótica en el plasma y fuera de las células aumenten rapidamente e inducir la lesión de las células del cerebro. En general se considera que cuando la hiponatremia es inferior a 120mmol/L, el tratamiento para aumentarla debe mantener una velocidad de 0.5mmol/L a la hora y no puede sobrepasar 1.5mmol/L a la hora (los enfermos con la hiponatremia dilucional no necesitan suplir sodio). Cuando la hiponatremia aguda es inferior a 120mmol o se descubre síntomas del sistema nervioso central, se puede aplicar inyección del cloruro sódico al 3% mediante infusión intravenosa. Generalmente se demanda que la hiponatremia llegue a ser superior a 120mmol/L dentro de 6 horas. La dosis de suplimento de sodio referente es 1ml/kg de cloruro sódico al 3% y puede aumentar la hiponatremia en 1mmol/L. Después de que la hiponatremia aumente superior a 120~125mmol/L, se puede sustituir con la solución isotónica. Para la deficiencia de sodio crónica, se debe suplir sodio lentamente con una dosis pequeña y aumentar la hiponatremia a 130mmol/L de día en día.

　　(5) La alcalosis hipoclorémica: se aplica 500~1000ml de inyección de cloruro sódico al 0.9% o de inyección compuesta de cloruro sódico (Solución de Riger) y después la dosis se determina según la situación de la alcalosis.

　　(6) Uso exterior: lave las heridas y los ojos con la solución de cloruro de sodio fisiológico.

| 剂型、规格<br>Formulaciones y especificaciones | 注射液：为含 0.9% 氯化钠的灭菌水溶液。每支（瓶）2ml；10ml；250ml；500ml；1000ml。浓氯化钠注射液：每支 1g（1ml），0.3g（10ml）。临用前稀释。复方氯化钠注射液（林格液）：灭菌溶液，每 100ml 中含氯化钠 0.85g，氯化钾 0.03g，氯化钙 0.033g，比生理盐水成分完全，可替代生理盐水用。葡萄糖氯化钠注射液：每 1000ml 中含葡萄糖 5% 及氯化钠 0.9%。每瓶 250ml；500ml；1000ml。口服补液盐：①每包 14.75g（大包中含氯化钠 1.75g，葡萄糖 11g；小包中含氯化钾 0.75g，碳酸氢钠 1.25g）。②每包 13.95g（氯化钠 1.75g，葡萄糖 10g，枸橼酸钠 1.45g，氯化钾 0.75g）。治疗和预防轻度急性腹泻。<br><br>Inyecciones: solución acuosa estéril que contiene cloruro sódico al 0.9%, cada una 2ml; 10ml; 250ml; 500ml; 1000ml. Inyecciones de cloruro sódico concentradas: cada una 1g(1ml),0.3g(10ml). Hay que diluirla antes de aplicarla. Inyecciones compuestas de cloruro sódico (Solución de Riger): solución estéril, cada 100ml contiene 0.85g de cloruro sódico, 0.03g de cloruro potásico y 0.033g de cloruro cálcico. Tiene ingredientes más completos que el suero fisiológico y puede sustituir este. Inyecciones de cloruro sódico y glucosa: cada 1000ml contiene glucosa 5% y cloruro sódico 0.9%. Una botella contiene 250ml; 500ml; 1000ml. Sales de rehidratación oral: ① Cada bolsa pesa 14.75g (la bolsa grande contiene 1.75g de cloruro sódico y 11g de glucosa; la pequeña contiene 0.75g de cloruro sódico y 1.25g de bicarbonato de sodio). ② Cada bolsa pesa 13.95g (cloruro sódico 1.75g, glucosa 10g, citrato de sodio 1.45g, cloruro potásico 0.75g). Puede prevenir y curar la aguda diarrea leve. |

**续　表**

| | |
|---|---|
| 药品名称 Drug Names | 氯化钾 Cloruro potásico |
| 适应证<br>Indicaciones | 用于低钾血症（多由严重吐泻不能进食、长期应用排钾利尿剂或肾上腺皮质激素所引起）的防治，亦可用于强心苷中毒引起的阵发性心动过速或频发室性期前收缩。<br><br>Se utiliza para la prevención de la hipopotasemia (en la mayoría de los casos causada por vómitos graves, diarrea, incapacidad de comer, la aplicación a largo plazo de los diuréticos ahorradores de potasio o de la corticotropina), y se también usa contra la taquicardia paroxística o la contracción ventricular externo frecuente causadas por la intoxicación de los glucósidos cardíacos. |
| 用法、用量<br>Administración y<br>dosis | 补充钾盐大多采用口服，一次 1g，一日 3 次。血钾过低，病情危急或吐泻严重口服不易吸收时，可用静脉滴注，每次用 10%～15% 液 10ml，用 5%～10% 葡萄糖注射液 500ml 稀释或根据病情酌定用量。<br><br>Para suplir la potasa, se toma mayoritariamente por vía oral, 1g a la vez, 3 veces al día. Cuando el enfermo sufre la hipopotasemia, en estado crítico o no puede absorberlo mediante toma oral debido a graves vómitos y diarrea, se puede aplicar vía infusión intravenosa, 10ml de la inyección al 10%~15% a la vez y se diluye con 500ml de la inyección de glucosa al 5%~10% o se determina la dosis según la condición del enfermo. |
| 剂型、规格<br>Formulaciones y<br>especificaciones | 片剂：每片 0.25g；0.5g。控释片（SLOW-K）：每片 0.6g。微囊片（PEL-K）：每片 0.75g。氯化钾口服液：100ml ：10g。注射液：：每支 1g（10ml）。复方氯化钾注射液：内含氯化钾 0.28%、氯化钠 0.42% 及乳酸钠 0.63%，可用于代谢性酸血症及低血钾。用量视病情而定，一般每日量 500～1000ml，静脉滴注。<br><br>Tabletas: cada una 0.25g;0.5g. Tabletas de liberación controlada(SLOW-K): cada una 0.6g. Microcápsulas en comprimidos(PEL-K)：cada una 0.75g. Líquido oral del cloruro potásico: 100ml ：10g. Inyecciones: cada una 1g (10ml). Inyecciones compuestas del cloruro potásico: cloruro potásico 0.28%, cloruro sódico 0.42%, lactato sódico 0.63% y se puede utilizar contra la acidemia metabólica y la hipopotasemia. La dosis se determina según la condición del enfermo. En general, se toma 500~1000ml al día vía infusión intravenosa. |
| 药品名称 Drug Names | 门冬氨酸钾镁 Aspartato de magnesio y potasio |
| 适应证<br>Indicaciones | 用于低钾血症、低钾及洋地黄中毒引起的心律失常、病毒性肝炎、肝硬化和肝性脑病的治疗。<br><br>Se utiliza contra la hipopotasemia, arritmia causada por la intoxicación de hipopotasemia y digital, hepatitis viral, cirrosis y encefalopatía hepática. |
| 用法、用量<br>Administración y<br>dosis | 口服：一次 1～2 片，一日 3 次。静脉滴注：心律失常、心肌梗死，一次 10～20ml，加入 5%～10% 葡萄糖液 50～100ml 中缓慢滴注，4～6 小时后有必要可重复。<br><br>Por vía oral: 1~2 tabletas a la vez, 3 veces al día. Infusión intravenosa: en caso de la arritmia y el infarto de miocardio, envase 10~20ml en solución de glucosa al 5%~10%, tómela vía infusión lenta y puede repetir este proceso después de 4~6 horas si es necesario. |
| 剂型、规格<br>Formulaciones y<br>especificaciones | 片剂：（钾 0.9mmol+ 镁 0.4mmol）；注射剂：[ 钾（2.7～3.1）mmol+ 镁（1.5～1.9）mmol]/10ml。<br><br>Tabletas: (0.9mmol de potasio + 0.4mmol de magnesio); Inyecciones: [(2.7~3.1)mmol de potasio + (1.5~1.9)mmol de magnesio]/10ml. |
| 药品名称 Drug Names | 枸橼酸钾 Citrato potásico |
| 适应证<br>Indicaciones | 用于低钾血症。<br>Se utiliza contra la hipopotasemia. |
| 用法、用量<br>Administración y<br>dosis | 一次 10～20ml<br>10~20ml a la vez. |
| 剂型、规格<br>Formulaciones y<br>especificaciones | 10% 合剂口服。<br>Preparación compuesta al 10%, por vía oral. |

**续 表**

| 药品名称 Drug Names | 氯化钙 Cloruro de cálcio |
|---|---|
| 适应证<br>Indicaciones | 本品可用于血钙降低引起的手足搐搦症及肠绞痛、输尿管绞痛、荨麻疹、渗出性水肿、瘙痒性皮肤病、镁盐中毒、佝偻病、软骨病、孕妇及哺乳期妇女钙盐补充，高血钾等。<br><br>Se puede utilizar contra la tetania causada por la baja de calcio sérico, el cólico, cólico ureteral, urticaria, edema exudativo, picazón de la piel, la intoxicación de magnesio, el raquitismo, la osteomalacia, la hiperpotasemia y para suplir calcio y cloruro sódico a las mujeres en lactancia, etc.. |
| 用法、用量<br>Administración y<br>dosis | （1）成人：①治疗低钙血症，500～1000mg（含 Ca 离子 136～272mg）缓慢静脉注射，速度不超过每分钟 50mg，根据反应和血钙浓度，必要时 1～3 日后重复。②心脏复苏：静脉或心室腔内注射，每次 200～400mg。应避免注入心肌内。③治疗高钾血症：先静脉注射 500mg，每分钟速度不超过 100mg，以后酌情用药。<br><br>（2）小儿：①治疗低钙血症，按体重 25mg/kg（含 Ca 离子 6.8mg）缓慢静脉注射。但一般情况下本品不用于小儿，因刺激性较大。②心脏复苏心室内注射，一次 10mg/kg，间隔 10 分钟可重复注射。<br><br>(1) Para los adultos: ① Se toma 500~1000mg (contiene 136~272mg de iones de calcio) mediante inyección intravenosa lenta para curar la hipocalcemia y la velocidad no puede sobrepasar a 50mg al minuto. Según la reacción y la concentración de calcio en la sangre, se puede repetir este proceso después de 1~3 días si es necesario. ② Recuperación cardíaca: vía inyecciones intravenosa o en las cavidades ventriculares, 200~400mg a la vez. Se debe evitar la inyección en los músculos cardíacos. ③ Contra la hiperpotasemia: primero tome 500mg vía inyección intravenosa, la velocidad no puede sobrepasar 100mg al minuto y después la dosis se determina según la condición del enfermo.<br><br>(2) Para los niños: ① Para curar la hipocalcemia, se toma según el peso 25mg/kg (contiene 6.8mg de iones de calcio), vía inyección intravenosa lenta. No obstante, generalmente no se aplica este producto a los niños, porque es demasiado estimulante. ② Se inyecta en las cavidades ventriculares para la recuperación cardíaca, 10mg/kg a la vez, y se puede reutilizar con intervalo de 10 minutos. |
| 剂型、规格<br>Formulaciones y<br>especificaciones | 注射液：每支 0.3g（10ml）；0.5g（10ml）；0.6g（20ml）；1g（20ml）。氯化钙葡萄糖注射液：为含氯化钙 5% 及葡萄糖 25% 的灭菌溶液，用于因血钙降低而至的手足搐搦、荨麻疹、血清反应等，1 次量 10～20ml，静脉注射，每日或隔日 1 次。禁用于肌内注射，以免引起组织坏死。氯化钙溴化钠注射液：每支 5ml，含氯化钙 0.1g，溴化钠 0.25g。每次静脉注射 5ml（重症可用 10ml），一日 1～2 次。静脉注射时宜缓慢，以免引起全身发热反应。禁用于肌内注射。<br><br>Inyecciones: cada una 0.3g(10ml);0.5g(10ml);0.6g(20ml);1g(20ml). Inyecciones de glucosa de cloruro cálcico: solución esterilizante con cloruro cálcico 5% y glucosa 25%. Se utiliza contra la tetania causada por la baja de calcio sérico, la urticaria y la reacción contra el suero, etc.. Se toma mediante inyección intravenosa, 10~20ml a la vez, una vez al día o a dos días. Se prohibe utilizar vía inyección intramuscular para evitar la necrosis de los tejidos. Inyecciones de cloruro cálcico y bromuro sódico: cada una 5ml, con 0.1g de cloruro cálcico y 0.25g de bromuro sódico. Se toma 5ml a la vea mediante inyección intravenosa (para los enfermos graves se puede utilizar 10ml), 1~2 veces al día. La inyección intravenosa se debe hacer lentamente para evitar la reacción de fiebre de todo el cuerpo. Se prohibe la inyección intramuscular. |
| 药品名称 Drug Names | 碳酸钙 Carbonato de cálcio |
| 适应证<br>Indicaciones | 用于低钙血症和高磷血症。<br>Se utiliza contra la hipocalcemia e hiperfosfatemia. |
| 用法、用量<br>Administración y<br>dosis | （1）低钙血症：成人口服，一次 1.25～1.5g，一日 1～3 次，进食时或进食后服用。尤其慢性肾衰竭患者伴高磷血症。<br><br>（2）制酸：成人口服：一次 0.5～2g，一日 3～4 次。<br><br>（3）高磷血症：成人口服：一日 3～12g，分次在进食时服用。每日 2g 以上钙时即可发生高钙血症，故应密切监测血清钙浓度。<br><br>(1) La hipocalcemia: para los adultos, por vía oral, 1.25~1.5g a la vez, 1~3 veces al día, al comer o después de comer. Especialmente los enfermos con fallo renal crónico acompañado por hiperfosfatemia.<br><br>(2) Inhibe del ácido: para los adultos, por vía oral, 0.5~2g a la vez, 3~4 veces al día.<br><br>(3) La hiperfosfatemia: para los adultos, por vía oral, 3~12g al día, divido en varias veces al comer. Cuando se absorbe más de 2g al día, es posible la hiperfosfatemia, por eso hay que mantener una estrecha monitorización de la concentración de calcio en suero. |

续　表

| | |
|---|---|
| 剂型、规格<br>Formulaciones y especificaciones | 片剂：0.5g（相当于 200mg 钙）。<br>Tabletas: 0.5g(equivalente a 200 mg de calcio). |
| **药品名称 Drug Names** | **葡萄糖酸钙 Gluconato de calcio** |
| 适应证<br>Indicaciones | 本品可用于血钙降低引起的手足搐搦症以及肠绞痛、输尿管绞痛，荨麻疹、渗出性水肿、瘙痒性皮肤病，镁盐中毒，佝偻病、软骨病、孕妇及哺乳期妇女钙盐补充，高血钾等。<br><br>Se puede utilizar contra la tetania causada por la baja de calcio sérico, el cólico, cólico ureteral, urticaria, edema exudativo, picazón de la piel, la intoxicación de magnesio, el raquitismo, la osteomalacia, la hiperpotasemia y para suplir calcio y cloruro sódico a las mujeres en lactancia, etc.. |
| 用法、用量<br>Administración y dosis | （1）口服：成人一次 0.5 ～ 2g，一日 3 次；儿童一次 0.5 ～ 1g，一日 3 次。<br>（2）静脉注射：每次 10% 注射液 10 ～ 20ml（对小儿手足搐搦症，每次 5 ～ 10ml）。加等量 5% ～ 25% 葡萄糖注射液稀释后缓慢静脉注射（每分钟不超过 2ml）。<br>(1) Por vía oral: para los adultos 0.5~2g a la vez, 3 veces al día; para los niños 0.5~1g a la vez, 3 veces al día.<br>(2) Inyección intravenosa: 10~20ml de inyección al 10% cada vez (5~10ml cada vez en contra de la tetania de los niños). Dilúyala con la misma cantidad de inyección de glucosa al 5%~25% y después tómela por inyección intravenosa lenta (no puede sobrepasar 2ml al minuto). |
| 剂型、规格<br>Formulaciones y especificaciones | 片剂：每片 0.1g；0.5g。含片：每片 0.1g；0.15g；0.2g。口服液：每支 1g（10ml）。注射液：每支 1g（10ml）。<br>Tabletas: cada una 0.1g;0.5g. Pastillas: cada una 0.1g;0.15g;0.2g. Líquido oral: cada una 1g(10ml). Inyecciones: cada una 1g(10ml). |
| **药品名称 Drug Names** | **乳酸钙 Lactato de calcio** |
| 适应证<br>Indicaciones | 用于防治钙缺乏症如手足搐搦症、骨发育不全、佝偻病，以及结核病、妊娠和哺乳期妇女的钙盐补充。<br><br>Se utiliza para la prevención y curación de la deficiencia del calcio, por ejemplo, la tetania, la osteogénesis imperfecta, el raquitismo, la tuberculosis y suple calcio y cloruro sódico a las mujeres en embarazo o lactancia. |
| 用法、用量<br>Administración y dosis | 每 1g 乳酸钙含钙为 130mg。成人：口服，一日 1 ～ 2g，分 2 ～ 3 次口服。小儿：按体重一日 45 ～ 65mg/kg，分 2 ～ 3 次口服。<br><br>Cada gramo de lactato de calcio contiene 130mg de calcio. Para los adultos: por vía oral, 1~2g al día, dividido en 2~3 veces. Para los niños: 45~65mg/kg al día según el peso, 2~3 veces por vía oral. |
| 剂型、规格<br>Formulaciones y especificaciones | 片剂：每片 0.25g；0.5g。<br>Tabletas: cada una 0.25g;0.5g. |
| **药品名称 Drug Names** | **硫酸镁 Sulfato de magnesio** |
| 适应证<br>Indicaciones | （1）可预防和治疗低镁血症，特别是急性低镁血症伴有肌肉痉挛、手足搐搦。<br>（2）先兆子痫和子痫、早产子宫肌肉痉挛等。<br>（3）导泻、利胆。<br>(1) Se puede prevenir y curar la hipomagnesemia, especialmente la hipomagnesemia acompañada por calambres musculares y tetania.<br>(2) Se usa contra la preeclampsia, eclampsia y espasmos musculares del útero prematuro, etc.<br>(3) Tiene la función de catarsis y beneficia a la vesícula biliar. |
| 用法、用量<br>Administración y dosis | （1）防止低镁血症：成人轻度镁缺乏，1g 硫酸镁，肌内注射或溶于 500ml5% 葡萄糖注射液内缓慢滴注，一日总量 2g。重度镁缺乏，一次按体重 0.25mmol/kg 硫酸镁，也可静脉滴注，将 2.5g 硫酸镁溶于 5% 葡萄糖注射液或氯化钠注射液 500ml 中，缓慢滴注 3 小时。严密观察呼吸等生命体征。<br>（2）全静脉内营养，按体重每日 0.125 ～ 0.25mmol 镁 /kg 添加。儿童全静脉内营养，按体重一日 0.125mmol 镁 /kg 添加。 |

**续 表**

（3）治疗先兆子痫和子痫，肌内注射：每次 1～2.5g 硫酸镁，根据病情决定剂量，最多每日肌注 6 次，并监测心电图、肌腱反射、呼吸和血压。静脉注射：将 1～2g 硫酸镁，以 5% 葡萄糖液稀释，推注速度每分钟不超过 150mg，静注硫酸镁可使血镁浓度突增至接近中毒浓度，必须严格掌握剂量，并严密观察呼吸、肌腱反射和心电图。静脉滴注：4g 硫酸镁加入 5% 葡萄糖注射液或氯化钠注射液 250ml 内，滴注速度每分钟不超过 4ml。

（4）抗惊厥：儿童按体重 20～40mg/kg，配成 20% 注射液肌内注射。慎用，不作为首选药物。

（5）导泻：成人口服：1 次 5～20g，用水 200～400ml 溶解后顿服。

（6）利胆：成人口服：1 次 2～5g，一日 3 次，用水配成 33% 溶液服用。

(1) Para prevenir la hipomagnesemia: para los adultos con leve deficiencia de magnesio, se inyecta por vía intramuscular 1g de sulfato de magnesio, o se diluye en 500ml de inyección de glucosa al 15% y después se toma mediante lenta infusión, 2g en total al día. Para los con grave deficiencia de magnesio, 0.25mmol/kg de sulfato de magnesio a la vez según el peso del enfermo,también se puede tomar mediante infusión intravenosa: diluya 2.5g de sulfato de magnesio en inyección de glucosa al 5% o en 500ml de inyección de cloruro sódico y después dedique 3 horas a la infusión lenta. Observa minuciosamente los signos vitales así como la respiración, etc..

(2) Nutrición intravenosa total: se suple 0.125~0.25mmol/kg del magnesio al día, para los niños, 0.125mmol/kg al día según el peso del niño.

(3) Contra la preeclampsia y eclampsia, inyección intramuscular: 1~2.5g de sulfato de magnesio a la vez, la dosis concreta se determina según la condición del enfermo. Se inyecta por vía intramuscular 6 veces a lo más al día y deben moritonizar el electrocardiograma, los reflejos tendinosos, la respiración y la presión arterial. Infusión intravenosa: se disuelve 4g de sulfato de magnesio en la solución de glucosa al 5% o en 250ml de la inyección de cloruro sódico y la velocidad no puede sobrepasar 4ml al minuto.

(4) Contra las convulsiones: para los niños, 20~40mg/kg según el peso y se prepara la inyección al 20% para inyectarla por vía intramuscular. Utilícela con precaución y no debe ser el fármaco de primera elección.

(5) Catarsis: para los adutos, 5~20g a la vez. Disuélvalo con 200~400ml de agua y después tómelo de una vez.

(6) Para beneficiar a la vesícula biliar: prepare solución al 33% con agua y tome 2~5g a la vez, 3 veces al día.

| 剂型、规格<br>Formulaciones y especificaciones | 注射剂：1g/10ml；2.5g/10ml。口服粉剂，按需要取用，配成溶液服用。<br>Inyecciones: 1g/10ml;2.5g/10ml. Polvo oral: se prepara solucón y se toma según la necesidad. |
|---|---|

| 药品名称 Drug Names | 乳酸钠溶液 Solución de lactato sódico |
|---|---|
| 适应证<br>Indicaciones | 可用于纠正代谢性酸血症。由于作用不及碳酸氢钠迅速，现已渐少用。但在高钾血症或普鲁卡因等引起的心律失常伴有酸血症者，仍以应用本品为宜。<br><br>Se puede utilizar para curar la acidemia metabólica. Como no funciona tan rápido como el bicarbonato sódico, se usa menos ahora. No obstante, deben utilizar este fármaco todavía los pacientes con arritmia acompañada por la acidemia, causada por la hiperpotasemia o procaína. |
| 用法、用量<br>Administración y dosis | 静脉滴注：每次 11.2% 液 5～8ml/kg，先用半量，以后根据病情再给其余量。用时须以 5%～10% 葡萄糖液 5 倍量稀释（成为 1.87%，即 1/6 克分子溶液）后静脉滴注。成人每次量一般为 1.87% 液 500～2000ml。<br><br>Infusión intravenosa: 5~8ml/kg de solución al 11.2% cada vez. Primero se utiliza la mitad de la dosis y después se aplica el resto según la condición del enfermo. Al mismo tiempo hay que diluirla con 5 veces de solución de glucosa al 5%~10% (1.87%, 1/6g solución molecular) y después témola por infusión intravenosa. La dosis para los adultos suele ser 500~2000ml de solución 1.87%. |
| 剂型、规格<br>Formulaciones y especificaciones | 注射液：每支 1.12g（10ml）；2.24g（20ml）；5.6g（50ml）。<br>Inyecciones: cada una 1.12g(10ml);2.24g(20ml);5.6g(50ml). |

**续　表**

| 药品名称 Drug Names | 葡萄糖 Glucosa |
|---|---|
| 适应证<br>Indicaciones | 用于：①腹泻、呕吐、重伤大失血等，体内损失大量水分时，可静脉滴注含本品 5%～10% 的溶液 200～1000ml，同时静脉滴注适宜生理盐水，以补充体液的损失及钠的不足。②不能摄取饮食物的重病患者，可注射本品或灌肠，以补助营养。③血糖过低症或胰岛素过量，静脉注射 50% 溶液 40～100ml，以保护肝脏。对糖尿病的酮中毒须与胰岛素同用。④降低眼压及因颅压增加引起的各种病症如脑出血、颅骨骨折、尿毒症等，25%～50% 溶液静脉注射，因其高渗压作用，将组织（特别是脑组织）内液体进入循环系统内由肾排出。注射时切勿注于血管之外，以免刺激组织。⑤高钾血症。<br><br>Usos: ① contra diarrea, vómitos, pérdida de sangre causada por heridas graves, etc. cuando pierde gran cantidad de agua el cuerpo, se puede tomar 200~1000ml de la solución con 5%~10% de este producto vía infusión intravenosa y se debe tomar al mismo tiempo una determinada cantidad de suero de la misma manera para compensar la pérdida de fluidos corporales y la deficiencia de sodio. ② Los enfermos graves que son incapaz de absorber comidas pueden inyectar este producto o hacer lavativas para suplir nutrición. ③ Para tratar el síndrome de hipoglucemia o la sobredosis de insulina, se debe tomar mediante inyección intravenosa de 40~100ml de la solución al 50% para proteger el hígado. En el caso de la intoxicación de ceto de la diabetes, se utiliza de la misma manera que el caso de insulina. ④ Se puede inyectar la solución al 25%~50% por vía intravenosa para aliviar las enfermedades causadas por el aumento de la presión intraocular e intracraneal, así como la hemorragia cerebral, fracturas de cráneo, uremia, etc. Debido a su efecto de la presión hipertónica, puede introducir el fluido de los tejidos (especialmente el tejido cerebral) en el sistema circulatorio y hacerlo excretarse por los riñones. No inyectes fuera de los vasos sanguíneos, para evitar estimular los tejidos. ⑤ Contra la hiperpotasemia. |
| 用法、用量<br>Administración y dosis | （1）补充热量：患者因为某些原因进食减少或不能进食，一般可给予 10%～25% 葡萄糖注射液静脉滴注，并同时补充体液。<br>（2）全静脉营养疗法：葡萄糖是此疗法中最重要的能量供给物质。在非蛋白质热能中，葡萄糖与脂肪供给热量之比为 2∶1。<br>（3）低血糖症：轻者口服，重者可先给予 50% 葡萄糖注射液 20～40ml 静脉滴注。<br>（4）饥饿性酮症：轻者口服，可先给予 5%～25% 葡萄糖注射液静脉滴注，每日 100g 葡萄糖可基本控制病情。<br>（5）失水：等渗性失水给予 5% 葡萄糖注射液静脉滴注。<br>（6）高钾血症：应用 10%～25% 注射液，每 2～4g 葡萄糖加正规胰岛素 1U，可降低血清钾浓度。但此疗法仅使细胞外钾离子进入细胞内，体内总钾含量不变。如不采取排钾措施，仍有再次出现高钾血症的可能。<br>（7）组织脱水：高渗溶液（一般采用 50% 注射液）快速静脉注射 20～50ml，但作用短暂。应注意防止高血糖，目前少用。用于调节腹膜透析液渗透压时，50% 葡萄糖注射液 20ml 即 10g 葡萄糖可使 1L 透析渗透压提高 55mOsm/（kg·H$_2$O）。<br>（8）葡萄糖耐量试验：空腹口服葡萄糖 1.75g/kg，于服后 0.5、1、2、3 小时抽血测血糖。血糖浓度正常上限分别为 6.9mmol/L、11.1mmol/L、10.5mmol/L、8.3mmol/L、6.9mmol/L。<br><br>(1) Para suplir el calor: para los enfermos que come menos o que no pueden comer, en general se puede aplicar mediante infusión intravenosa de solución de glucosa al 10%~25% y suolir fluidos corporales al mismo tiempo.<br>(2) La terapia de nutrición intravenosa total: la glucosa es el elemento más importante en esta terapia para suplir energía.En el caso del calor no proteico, la glucosa puede suplir calor dos veces el de grasa.<br>(3)La hipoglucemia: para los enfermos leves se toma por vía oral y para los graves, primero, se puede tomar 20~40ml de inyección de glucosa al 5% vía infusión intravenosa.<br>(4) Cetosis por inanición: para los enfermos leves se toma por vía oral, para los graves, primero, se puede tomar inyección de glucosa al 5%~25% vía infusión intravenosa y 100g de glucosa al día puede controlar la enfermedad en general.<br>(5) Deshidratación: contra la deshidratación isotónica se toma inyección de glucosa al 5% vía infusión intravenosa.<br>(6) Hiperpotasemia: se debe tomar inyección al 10%~25%. Se puede añadir una unidad de insulina regular a cada 2~4g de glucosa, lo cual puede bajar la concentración de potasio en suero. Pero esta terapia sólo hace que los iones de potasio extracelulares entren en las células, sin modificar el volumen total de potasio en el cuerpo. Si no toman medidas para eliminar potasio, es posible que la hiperpotasemia ataque al enfermo otra vez. |

**续 表**

| | |
|---|---|
| | (7) La deshidratación de los tejidos: inyecte rápido 20~50ml de solución hipertónica (se aplica inyección al 50% generalmente) por vía intravenosa. Pero sólo tiene efecto a corto plazo. Se debe evitar la hiperglucemia, por eso se utiliza raramente ahora. Cuando se usa para ajustar la presión osmótica de solución de diálisis peritoneal, 20ml (10g) de inyección de glucosa al 50% puede mejorar 1L de la presión osmótica de diálisis en 55mOsm/(kg · $H_2O$). <br><br>(8) La prueba de tolerancia a la glucosa: tome 1.75g/kg de glucosa por vía oral antes de comer y después extraiga sangre tras 0.5, 1, 2, 3 horas para medir la concentración de azúcar en la sangre. Los límites superiores de los niveles normales de azúcar en la sangre son 6.9mmol/L, 11.1mmol/L, 10.5mmol/L, 8.3mmol/L, 6.9mmol/L respectivamente. |
| 剂型、规格<br>Formulaciones y especificaciones | 粉剂：每袋 250g；500g。注射液：每支（瓶）50g（1000ml）；100g（1000ml）；50g（500ml）；25g（500ml）；12.5g（250ml）；25g（250ml）；1g（20ml）；5g（20ml）；10g（20ml）；2g（10ml）；0.5g（10ml）。<br><br>Polvo: cada bolsa de 250g;500g. Inyeccion: cada una 50g(1000ml);100g(1000ml);50g(500ml);25g(500ml);12.5g(250ml);25g(250ml);1g(20ml);5g(20ml);10g(20ml);2g(10ml);0.5g(10ml). |
| **药品名称 Drug Names** | 果糖 Fructosa |
| 适应证<br>Indicaciones | 对糖尿病、肝病患者供给能力、补充体液。此外，能加速乙醇代谢，用于急性中毒的辅助治疗。<br><br>Suministra fuerzas y suple fluidos corporales a los enfermos con diabetes y enfermedades hepáticas. Por lo demás, puede acelerar el metabolismo del alcohol y se utiliza en el tratamiento adyuvante de las intoxicaciones agudas. |
| 用法、用量<br>Administración y dosis | 用以静脉注射或静脉滴注，用量视病情而定。常用量为每次 500 ～ 1000ml。<br><br>Se utiliza mediante inyección o infusión intravenosa y la dosis se determina según la condición del enfermo. La dosis normal: 500~1000ml una vez. |
| 剂型、规格<br>Formulaciones y especificaciones | 注射液：每瓶 12.5g（250ml）；25g（250ml；500ml）；50g（500ml）。<br>Inyecciones: una botella de 12.5g(250ml);25g(250ml;500ml);50g(500ml). |
| **药品名称 Drug Names** | 口服补液盐 Sales de rehidratación oral |
| 适应证<br>Indicaciones | 用于补充水、钠和钾丢失的失水。治疗急性腹泻。<br><br>Tratamiento de la deshidratación en caso del déficit de agua, sodio y potasio. Tratamiento de la diarrea aguda. |
| 用法、用量<br>Administración y dosis | 每份必须加水 500ml 溶解混匀后服用。<br>（1）预防和治疗因腹泻、呕吐、经皮肤和呼吸道等液体丢失引起的轻、中度失水，可补充水、钾和钠，重度失水需静脉补液。①轻度失水：成人口服：开始时 50ml/kg，4 ～ 6 小时饮完，以后酌情调整剂量。儿童口服：开始时 50ml/kg，4 小时内饮完，直至腹泻停止。②中度失水：成人口服：开始时 50ml/kg，6 小时内饮完，其余应以静脉补液。儿童应以静脉补液为主。<br>（2）急性腹泻：①轻度腹泻，口服：成人一日 50ml/kg。②重度腹泻，应以静脉滴注为主，直至腹泻停止。<br><br>Se debe mezclar debidamente cada dosis con 500ml de agua antes administrarla.<br>(1) Prevención y tratamiento de la deshidratación leve o moderada a causa de diarreas, vómitos, o por vía cutánea y respiratoria. Reposición del déficit de agua, sodio y potasio. En el caso de la deshidratación severa, hay que emprender la rehidratación intravenosa. ① La deshidratación leve: los adultos: por vía oral, la dosis inicial: 50ml/kg en 4 ~ 6 horas; después se administra en dependencia de la situación. Los niños: por vía oral, la dosis inicial: 50ml/kg en 4 horas hasta que cesen las diarreas. ② La deshidratación moderada: Los adultos: por vía oral, la dosis inicial: 50ml/kg en 6 horas y también se emprender la rehidratación intravenosa. Los niños: rehidratación principalmente por vía intravenosa.<br>(2)Diarrea aguda: ① La diarrea leve, por vía oral: 50ml/kg al día para los adultos. ② La diarrea grave: principalmente rehidratación intravenosa hasta que cesen los vómitos. |
| 剂型、规格<br>Formulaciones y especificaciones | 口服补液盐 I：口服补液盐：每包总重 14.75g（大包中含氯化钠 1.75g，葡萄糖 11g；小包中含氯化钾 0.75g，碳酸氢钠 1.25g）（为500ml用量）。口服补液盐 II，每包总重 13.95g（氯化钠 1.75g，葡，萄糖 10g，枸橼酸钠 1.45g，氯化钾 0.75g）（为500ml用量）。<br><br>Sal de rehidratación oral I: 14.75g/sobre (cada sobre grande contiene cloruro de sodio 1.75g, glucosa 11g; cada sobre pequeño contiene cloruro de potasio 0.75g, bicarbonato de sodio1.25) (contenido para una disolución de 500ml) Sal de rehidratación oral II: 13.95g/sobre (cloruro de sodio 1.75g, glucosa 10g, citrato de sodio 1.45g, cloruro de potasio 0.75g) (contenido para una disolución de 500ml). |

**续　表**

| 药品名称 Drug Names | 腹膜透析液 Solución de diálisis peritoneal |
|---|---|
| 适应证<br>Indicaciones | 腹膜透析液可用于：①急性或慢性肾衰竭；②药物中毒；③顽固性心力衰竭；④电解质紊乱和酸碱平衡失调；⑤急性出血性胰腺炎和广泛化脓性腹膜炎等。<br><br>Contra: ① Falla renal aguda o crónica; ② Envenenamiento por fármacos; ③ Insuficiencia cardíaca refractaria; ④ Desequilibrio de electrolitos y ácido-base; ⑤ Pancreatitis hemorrágica aguda y peritonitis purulenta generalizada, etc. |
| 用法、用量<br>Administración y<br>dosis | （1）治疗急、慢性肾衰竭伴水潴留者，用间歇性腹膜透析每次 2L，留置 1～2 小时，一日交换 4～6 次。无水潴留者，用连续不卧床腹膜透析（CAPD），一般一日 4 次，每次 2L，日间每次间隔 4～5 小时，夜间一次留置 9～12 小时，以增加中分子尿毒症毒素清除。一般每日透析液量为 8L。<br>　　（2）治疗急性左心衰竭，酌情用 2.5% 或 4.25% 葡萄糖透析液 2L；后者留置 30 分钟，可脱水 300～500ml；前者留置 1 小时，可脱水 100～300ml。<br>　　（3）儿童：每次交换量一般为 50mg/kg 体重。<br>（1）Para los enfermos de falla renal aguda o crónica con retención de agua, la administración se realiza a través de la diálisis peritoneal intermitente, cada vez 2L, con períodos de equilibrio de 1～2 horas, por intercambio 4～6 veces al día. Para los enfermos sin retención de agua, la administración se realiza a través de la diálisis peritoneal continua ambulatoria (DPCA), generalmente 4 veces al día, cada vez 2L, con intercambios diurnos de 4～5 horas e intercambio nocturno de 9～12 horas (intercambio nocturno) para eliminar mejor toxinas urémicas medias. Normalmente se administran 8L de la solución al día.<br>（2）Para el tratamiento de la insuficiencia cardíaca izquierda aguda, se administran en dependencia de la situación 2L de solución de diálisis de glucosa a 2.5% o 4.25%; El tiempo de equilibrio del último es 30 minutos y se puede deshidratar 300～500 ml; El tiempo de equilibrio del primero es una hora y se puede deshidratar 100～300ml.<br>（3）Los niños: la dosis de intercambio es 50mg/kg cada vez, en términos generales. |
| 剂型、规格<br>Formulaciones y<br>especificaciones | （1）腹膜透析液（乳酸盐）：①含 1.5% 葡萄糖（1L，1.5L，2L，2.5L，5L，6L）；②含 2.5% 葡萄糖（1L，1.5L，2L，2.5L，5L，6L）；③含 4.25% 葡萄糖（1L，1.5L，2L，2.5L，5L，6L）；④含葡萄糖 4.0%（1000ml）。<br>　　（2）腹膜透析液（乳酸盐）（低钙）：①含葡萄糖 4.0%（2000ml）；②含葡萄糖 2.5%（1000ml）；③含葡萄糖 2.5%（2000ml）；④含葡萄糖 1.5%（2000ml）。<br>（1）Solución de diálisis peritoneal(lactato): ① Contiene 1.5% de glucosa(1L, 1.5L, 2L, 2.5L, 5L, 6L); ② Contiene 2.5% de glucosa(1L, 1.5L, 2L, 2.5L, 5L, 6L); ③ Contiene 4.25% de glucosa(1L, 1.5L, 2L, 2.5L, 5L, 6L); ④ Contiene 4% de glucosa (1000ml).<br>（2）Solución de diálisis peritoneal(lactato)(bajo calcio): ① Contiene 4.0% de glucosa (2000ml); ② Contiene 2.5% de glucosa (1000ml); ③ Contiene 2.5% de glucosa (2000ml); ④ Contiene 1.5% de glucosa (2000ml). |

18.4　营养药 Medicamentos nutriacionales

| 药品名称 Drug Names | 安素 Ensure |
|---|---|
| 适应证<br>Indicaciones | 用于乳糖不耐受患者，无法进固体饮食的外伤、慢性病、年老体弱、产妇、术前后及某些必须限制饮食的患者等。<br><br>Para pacientes con intolerancia a la lactosa, los con traumas o enfermedades crónicas, los frágiles, las embarazadas que no pueden digerir alimentos sólidos, y los que deben restringir su dieta antes o después de una operación. |
| 用法、用量<br>Administración y<br>dosis | 口服或鼻饲：取 5 量匙（约 55g）本品，加入开水溶解稀释至 250ml，按 1ml 标准稀释液提供 1 卡热量计算决定患者一日用量。<br><br>Por vía oral o por sonda nasogástrica: servir 5 medidas (alrededor de 55g) del polvo Ensure, agregar agua hasta 250ml. Al mezclarse como se indica, proporciona aproximadamente 1.0 kcal/ml, según lo cual se determina la dosis al día. |
| 剂型、规格<br>Formulaciones y<br>especificaciones | 粉剂：每罐 400g。<br>En polvo, 400g/lata. |

**续 表**

| 药品名称Drug Names | 肠内营养乳剂 (TP)　Emulsión nutricional enteral（TP） |
|---|---|
| 适应证<br>Indicaciones | 用于有胃肠功能的营养不良或摄入障碍、重症或手术后需要补充营养的患者。<br><br>Para pacientes con malnutrición por mala función gastrointestinal, los con trastornos de la ingestión, los que necesita suplementos nutricionales posterior a enfermedades graves o la hospitalización. |
| 用法、用量<br>Administración y<br>dosis | 通过管饲或口服使用，应按照患者的体重和营养状况计算每日用量。①对作为唯一营养来源的患者：推荐剂量为一日 30ml/kg（30kcal/kg）。②作为补充营养的患者：根据患者需要推荐剂量为一日 500～1000ml。③管饲给药时，应逐渐增加给药速度，第一日的速度约为 20ml/h，以后每日逐增至最大滴速 150ml/h。通过重力或泵调整输注速度。<br><br>Por vía oral o por sonda, la dosis diaria depende del peso y situación nutricional del paciente. ① Para pacientes que tienen la emulsión como la única fuente nutricional: se recomienda la dosis diaria de 30ml/kg (30kcal/kg). ② Para pacientes que tienen la emulsión como suplemento nutricional: se recomienda la dosis diaria de 500～1000ml según su necesidad. ③ Cuando se administra por vía de sonda, hay que ir creciendo la velocidad de administración. La del primer día es aproximadamente 20ml/h, y se aumenta cada día hasta la máxima de 150ml/h. Se puede ajustar la velocidad de infusión a través de la gravitación o la bomba. |
| 剂型、规格<br>Formulaciones y<br>especificaciones | 乳剂：500ml。<br>Emulsión; 500ml. |
| 药品名称Drug Names | 水解蛋白 Hidrolizado de proteínas |
| 适应证<br>Indicaciones | 用于各种原因的蛋白质缺乏和衰弱患者以及对一般蛋白质消化吸收障碍的病例。用量视病情酌定。<br><br>Pacientes desprovistos de proteán por cualquier causa y los frágiles, y los tienen dificultad para digerir y absorber proteína normal. La dosis depende de la condición de la enfermedad. |
| 用法、用量<br>Administración y<br>dosis | 口服：一次 1～5g/kg。静脉滴注：一般每次用 5% 溶液 500ml。<br><br>Por vía oral: cada vez 5g/kg. Por goteo intravenoso: normalmente cada vez se administran 500ml de la disolución a 5%. |
| 剂型、规格<br>Formulaciones y<br>especificaciones | 注射用水解蛋白：每瓶 500g。注射液：每瓶 25g（500ml）。<br>Hidrolizado de proteínas para inyección: 500g/botella. Inyección: 25g/botella (500ml). |
| 药品名称Drug Names | 复方氨基酸 (18AA)　Aminoácidos compuestos (18AA) |
| 适应证<br>Indicaciones | 用于营养不良或有发生营养不良危险的患者，分解代谢旺盛疾病的营养支持和蛋白质消耗或丢失过多或合成障碍引起的低蛋白血症。<br><br>Para pacientes que sufren malnutrición o que tiene riesgo de sufrirla. Ofrece apoyo nutricional a los pacientes con enfermedades originadas en anormalmente rápido metabolismo y catabolismo. Contra hipoproteinemia causada por el excesivo consumo o pérdida de proteínas o trastornos de la síntesis de proteínas. |
| 用法、用量<br>Administración y<br>dosis | 静脉滴注，250～500ml/ 次，1～4 次 / 日，滴速 40～50 滴 / 分。<br><br>Por goteo intravenoso, cada vez 250～500ml, 1～4 veces al día, a la velocidad de 40～50 gotas/minuto. |
| 剂型、规格<br>Formulaciones y<br>especificaciones | 250ml ：12.5g（总氨基酸）；500ml ：25g（总氨基酸）；500ml ：60g（总氨基酸）。<br>250ml ：12.5g (aminoácidos total); 500ml ：25g (aminoácidos total); 500ml ：60g (aminoácidos total). |
| 药品名称Drug Names | 复方氨基酸 (9AA)　Aminoácidos compuestos (9AA) |
| 适应证<br>Indicaciones | 用于急性和慢性肾功能不全患者的肠道外支持；大手术、外伤或脓毒血症引起的严重肾衰竭。<br><br>Ofrece apoyo parenteral a  pacientes con insuficiencia renal aguda o crónica; Contra insuficiencia renal grave causada por cirugías mayores, traumas o septicemia. |

**续　表**

| 用法、用量<br>Administración y dosis | 静脉滴注：成人一日 250～500ml，缓慢滴注。小儿用量遵医嘱。进行透析的急、慢性肾衰竭患者一日 1000ml，最大剂量不超过 1500ml。滴速不超过每分钟 15 滴。<br><br>Por goteo intravenoso: los adultos: 250～500ml al día, a una velocidad lenta. Dosis pediátrica según la prescripción médica. Para los pacientes con insuficiencia renal aguda o crónica que se someten a diálisis, 1000ml al día, y 1500ml como máximo. La velocidad no supera 15 gotas/minuto. |
|---|---|
| 剂型、规格<br>Formulaciones y especificaciones | 注射液：每瓶 250ml。<br>Inyección: 250ml/botella. |
| **药品名称 Drug Names** | 复方 α- 酮酸　Compuesto α cetoácido |
| 适应证<br>Indicaciones | 配合低蛋白质和高热量饮食，预防和治疗因慢性肾功能不全而造成蛋白质代谢失调引起的损害，延缓肾病进展。<br><br>Coordinación de una dieta baja en proteínas y alta en calorías, prevención y tratamiento de los perjuicios de trastornos metabólicos de proteínas originados en la insuficiencia renal crónica. Disminuir el progreso de la enfermedad renal. |
| 用法、用量<br>Administración y dosis | 口服：慢性肾功能不全，一般每次 4～8 片，一日 3 次，饭时服用；代偿期：每次 4～6 片，一日 3 次，服药期间配合低蛋白、高热量饮食。蛋白质摄入量为一日 0.5～0.6g/kg，高热量饮食为一日 146.44～167.36kJ/kg；失代偿期：每次 4～8 片，一日 3 次，配合低蛋白、高热量饮食。蛋白质摄入量为一日 0.3～0.4g/kg，高热量饮食为 146.44～167.36kJ/kg。<br><br>Por vía oral: para la insuficiencia renal crónica, normalmente 4～8 tabletas cada vez, 3 veces al día, administración durante una comida; Periodo de compensación: 4～6 tabletas cada vez, 3 veces al día, combinado con una dieta baja en proteínas y alta en calorías. El consumo diario de proteínas es 0.5～0.6/kg. Las calorías recomendables son 146.44~167.36kJ/kg al día; Periodo de descompensación: 4～8 tabletas cada vez, 3 veces al día, combinado con una dieta baja en proteínas y alta en calorías. El consumo diario de proteínas es 0.3~0.4/kg. Las calorías recomendables son 146.44～167.36kJ/kg al día. |
| 剂型、规格<br>Formulaciones y especificaciones | 片剂：0.63g<br>Tabletas:0.63g. |
| **药品名称 Drug Names** | 复方氨基酸 (3AA)　Aminoácidos compuestos (3AA) |
| 适应证<br>Indicaciones | 用于：①急性、亚急性、慢性重症肝炎以及肝硬化、慢性活动肝炎等；②促进胰岛素的分泌；③胆固醇合成的前体；④供给合成蛋白质的必需氨基酸原料；⑤促进蛋白质的合成；⑥抑制蛋白质的分解。<br><br>Utilizado para: ① Contra la hepatitis severa aguda, subaguda y crónica, la cirrosis hepática, la hepatitis crónica activa, etc.; ② Promover la secreción de insulina; ③ Precursores de la biosíntesis de colesterol; ④ Ofrecer los aminoácidos esenciales para la síntesis de proteínas; ⑤ Promover la síntesis de proteínas; ⑥ Inhibir la degradación de proteínas. |
| 用法、用量<br>Administración y dosis | 静脉滴注：一日 250～500ml，或用 5%～10% 葡萄糖注射液适量混合后，缓慢静脉滴注，每分钟不超过 40 滴。一般昏迷期可酌加量，疗程根据病情遵医嘱。<br><br>Administración intravenosa gota a gota: 250~550ml al día, o mezclar la inyección con una cantidad apropiada de la inyección de glucosa al 5%~10% y administrar la disolución gota a gota lentamente, a la velocidad menos de 40 gotas/minuto. Normalmente se puede aumentar la dosis en el estado de coma, y el curso de tratamiento según la enfermedad y la prescripción médica. |
| 剂型、规格<br>Formulaciones y especificaciones | 注射液：每瓶 250m。<br>Inyección: 250ml/botella. |
| **药品名称 Drug Names** | 复方氨基酸 (15AA)　Aminoácidos compuestos (15AA) |
| 适应证<br>Indicaciones | 用于大面积烧伤、创伤及严重感染等应激状态下肌肉分解代谢亢进、消化系统功能障碍、营养恶化及免疫功能下降患者的营养支持，亦用于手术后患者，改善其营养状态。<br><br>Soporte nutricional para pacientes con hipercatabolismo muscular, disfunción digestiva, deterioro nutricional o disminución de la función inmune bajo estrés como quemaduras extensas, traumas e infección grave. |

续　表

| 用法、用量<br>Administración y dosis | 静脉滴注一日 250～500ml，用适量 5%～10% 葡萄糖注射液混合后缓慢滴注。滴速不宜超过每 1 分钟 20 滴。<br><br>Por goteo intravenoso: 250～500ml al día, mezclar la inyección con una cantidad apropiada de la inyección de glucosa al 5%～10% y administrar la disolución gota a gota lentamente, a la velocidad menos de 20 gotas/minuto. |
|---|---|
| 剂型、规格<br>Formulaciones y especificaciones | 每瓶 250ml（总氨基酸 20g）。<br>250ml/botella (aminoácidos total 20g). |
| 药品名称Drug Names | 脂肪乳 Emulsión de grasas |
| 适应证<br>Indicaciones | 适用于需要高热量的患者（如肿瘤及其他恶性病）、肾损害、禁用蛋白质的患者和由于某种原因不能经胃肠道摄取营养的患者，以补充适当热量和必需脂肪酸。<br><br>Ofrecer calorías y ácidos grasos esenciales para pacientes con alta necesidad calórica (como los con tumores o enfermedades malignas) o con daño renal, los que no pueden consumir proteínas, o no pueden absorber nutrición por vía gastrointestinal. |
| 用法、用量<br>Administración y dosis | 静脉滴注：第一日脂肪量不应超过 1g/kg，以后剂量可酌增，但脂肪量不得超过 2.5g/kg，静脉滴注速度最初 10 分钟为 20 滴 / 分，如无不良反应出现，以后可逐渐增加，30 分钟后维持 40～60 滴 / 分。<br><br>Por goteo intravenoso: El primer día, la cantidad de grasa tiene que ser menos de 1g/kg y se puede aumentar la dosis según la situación sin superar 2.5g/kg. La velocidad inicial de administración es 20gotas/minuto. Si no se observan reacciones adversas, se puede aumentar poco a poco, y se mantiene en 40～60gotas/minuto después de 30 minutos. |
| 剂型、规格<br>Formulaciones y especificaciones | 注射乳剂：每瓶 100ml（10g）；100ml（20g）；100ml（30g）；250ml（25g）；250ml（50g）。<br>Emulsión inyectable: cada botella 100ml(10g),100ml (20g), 100ml (30g), 250ml (25g), 250ml (50g). |
| 药品名称Drug Names | ω-3 鱼油脂肪乳 Emulsión grasa de aceite de pescado ω-3 |
| 适应证<br>Indicaciones | 用于全身炎症反应综合征较严重但又需要肠外营养的患者。<br>Para pacientes con grave síndrome de respuesta inflamatoria sistémica y que necesita nutrición parenteral. |
| 用法、用量<br>Administración y dosis | 按体重一日 1～2ml/kg，即按体重一日 0.1～0.2g 鱼油 /kg，70kg 患者每日用量不超过 140ml。最大输注速率按体重不超过每小时 0.5ml/kg。必须与其他类型脂肪乳剂同时输注时，推荐打的鱼油量应占其中的 10%～20%。<br><br>La dosis depende del peso del paciente, 1～2ml/kg, o 0.1～0.5g de aceite de pescado/kg. Para los pacientes de más de 70 kg, la dosis no debe superar 140ml cada día. La velocidad máxima de perfusión no supera 0.5ml/kg/hora. Si es necesario inyectar la emulsión con otro tipo de emulsión inyectable, es recomendable el porcentaje 10%～20% del aceite de pescado. |
| 剂型、规格<br>Formulaciones y especificaciones | 注射剂：50ml；100ml。<br>Inyección: 50ml; 100ml. |
| 药品名称Drug Names | 多种微量元素（Ⅰ）　Múltiples elementos traza(I) |
| 适应证<br>Indicaciones | 本品用于新生儿和婴儿全肠外营养时补充电解质和微量元素日常需求。<br>Satisfacer la necesidad diaria de electrolitos y oligoelementos para los recién nacidos y los bebés durante la nutrición parenteral total. |
| 用法、用量<br>Administración y dosis | 新生儿和婴儿：一般每日用本品 4ml/kg，可根据病儿对电解质和微量元素需要的不同而调节用量。<br><br>Los recién nacidos y los bebés: normal dosis diaria de 4ml/kg. Se puede ajustar la dosis de acuerdo a la necesidad de electrolitos y oligoelementos de los niño/as enfermo/as. |

**续　表**

| 剂型、规格<br>Formulaciones y especificaciones | 注射液：每支 10ml。<br>Inyección: cada una 10ml. |
|---|---|
| **药品名称 Drug Names** | 多种微量元素注射液（Ⅱ）　Múltiples elementos traza(II) |
| 适应证<br>Indicaciones | 　一般饮食摄入不会引起微量元素的缺乏和过量，但长期肠外营养，可造成微量元素摄入不足，本品可满足成人，每日对所含微量元素的生理需要。仅用于 15kg 儿童及成人长期肠外全营养时补充电解质和微量元素。妊娠期妇女对微量元素的需要量轻度增高，本品也适用于妊娠期妇女。<br>　La normal ingesta dietética  no causará una falta o un exceso de elementos traza, pero la nutrición parenteral a largo plazo puede provocar la falta de estos elementos. En este caso, este producto puede satisfacer la diaria necesidad fisiológica de los oligoelementos de los adultos. Solamente para satisfacer la necesidad de electrolitos y oligoelementos de los niños de más de 15 kilos y los adultos durante la nutrición parenteral a largo plazo. La necesidad de oligoelementos de las embarazadas aumenta ligeramente así que este producto también es adecuado para ellas. |
| 用法、用量<br>Administración y dosis | 　成人推荐剂量为一日 10ml。加于复方氨基酸注射液或葡萄糖注射液 500ml 内滴注，滴注时间为 6～8 小时。配制好的输液必须在 24 小时内输注完毕，以免被污染。<br>　La dosis recomendable para los adultos es 10ml al día. Se administra por goteo añadiéndose a 500ml de una inyección de aminoácidos o de glucosa. El tiempo de goteo es 6～8 horas. La inyección preparada se debe administrar dentro de 24 horas para evitar la contaminación. |
| 剂型、规格<br>Formulaciones y especificaciones | 注射液：每支 10ml。<br>Inyección: cada una 10ml. |
| **药品名称 Drug Names** | 脂溶性维生素（Ⅰ）　Vitaminas loposoluble (I) |
| 适应证<br>Indicaciones | 　为长期肠外全营养患者补充需要的脂溶性维生素 A、维生素 D、维生素 E、维生素 K。<br>　Ofrecer las vitaminas solubles en grasa A, D, E, K a los pacientes con nutrición parenteral total a largo plazo. |
| 用法、用量<br>Administración y dosis | 　本品适用于 11 岁以下儿童及婴儿，一日 1ml/kg 体重，一日最大剂量 10ml。使用前在无菌条件下，将本品加入到脂肪乳注射液内（100ml 或以上量），轻轻摇匀后输注，并在 24 小时内用完。<br>　Adecuado para los niños y bebés menores de once años. La dosis diaria es 1ml/kg, y la máxima, 10ml. Antes de la administración, se debe mezclar debidamente este producto con una inyección de emulsión de grasa (más de 100 ml inclusivo) en condiciones estériles y administrar la disolución dentro de 24 horas. |
| 剂型、规格<br>Formulaciones y especificaciones | 注射液：每支 10ml。<br>Inyección: cada una 10ml. |
| **药品名称 Drug Names** | 脂溶性维生素（Ⅱ）　Vitaminas liposoluble (II) |
| 适应证<br>Indicaciones | 　为长期肠外全营养患者补充需要量的脂溶性维生素 A、维生素 D、维生素 E、维生素 K。<br>　Ofrecer las vitaminas solubles en grasa A, D, E, K a los pacientes con nutrición parenteral total a largo plazo. |
| 用法、用量<br>Administración y dosis | 　静脉滴注：将本品 1 支（10ml）加到脂肪乳注射剂内，轻摇混合后输注。11 岁以上儿童及本人用成人注射液，一日 10ml。<br>　Por goteo intravenoso: añadir una inyección (10ml) a la inyección de emulsión de grasa, mezclarlas bien, y administrar la inyección mezclada. Adecuada para los adultos y los niños mayores de 11 años. Dosis diaria: 10ml. |
| 剂型、规格<br>Formulaciones y especificaciones | 注射液：每支 10ml。<br>Inyección: cada una 10ml. |

**续 表**

| 药品名称 Drug Names | 水溶性维生素 Vitaminas soluble agua |
|---|---|
| 适应证<br>Indicaciones | 用于长期肠外全营养患者补充水溶性维生素。<br>Ofrecer las vitaminas solubles en agua a los pacientes con nutrición parenteral total a largo plazo. |
| 用法、用量<br>Administración y<br>dosis | 10kg 以上儿童及成人，一日 1 瓶，10kg 以下儿童每日按每千克体重给予 1/10 瓶。本品用注射用水或葡萄糖注射液 10ml 溶解后再稀释于同一类型药液中静脉滴注。<br><br>Para niños de más de 10 kilos y adultos, 1 botella al día. Para niños de menos de 10 kilos, se administra al día 1/10 de una botella para cada kilo. Disolver este producto en 10ml de agua para inyección o de una inyección de glucosa, diluir la disolución en un líquido del mismo tipo para administrarla por goteo intravenoso. |
| 剂型、规格<br>Formulaciones y<br>especificaciones | 冻干粉：每瓶含硝酸硫胺 3.1mg，核黄素磷酸钠 4.9mg，烟酰胺 40mg，盐酸吡多辛 4.9mg，泛酸钠 16.5mg，维生素 C 钠 113mg，生物素 60μg，叶酸 0.4mg，维生素 B$_{12}$ 5.0μg。<br><br>Polvo liofilizado:Cada vial contiene nitrato de tiamina 3.1mg, fosfato de riboflavina de sodio 4.9mg, nicotinamida 40mg, hidrocloruro de piridoxing 4.9mg, pantothenato de sodio 16.5mg, vitamina C sodio 113mg, biotina 60μg, ácido fólico 0.4mg, vitamina B$_{12}$5.0μg. |

### 19. 专科用药 Medicamentos especiallizados

### 19.1 老年病用药 Medicamentos para lageriatria

| 药品名称 Drug Names | 帕米膦酸二钠 Pamidronato disódico |
|---|---|
| 适应证<br>Indicaciones | （1）用于治疗恶性肿瘤患者骨转移疼痛和高钙血症。<br>（2）治疗骨质疏松症和骨质愈合不良。<br>（3）也用于甲状旁腺功能亢进症。<br>(1)Tratamiento del dolor por metástasis en los huesos y la hipercalcemia de pacientes con cáncer.<br>(2)Tratamiento de la osteoporosis y mala curación del hueso.<br>(3)Tratamiento del hiperparatiroidismo. |
| 用法、用量<br>Administración y<br>dosis | （1）用于治疗骨质疏松症：每月 1 次 30mg 静滴，连续 6 个月，改为预防量；每 3 个月 1 次 30mg 静滴，连续 2 年。<br>（2）治疗癌症骨转移性疼痛：一次用药 30～60mg，静脉缓慢滴注 4 小时以上，浓度不得超过 15mg/125ml，滴速不得大于 15～30mg/2h。<br>（3）治疗高钙血症：当血钙浓度＜ 3.0、3.0～3.5、3.5～4.0、＞ 4.0mmol/L，或＜ 12.0、12.0～14.0、14.0～16.0、＞ 16.0mg，用本品剂量为 15～30mg、30～60mg、60～90mg、90mg.<br>（4）治疗变形性骨炎及骨愈合不良：一日 30～60mg，连续 1～3 日；或每日 30mg，连续 6 周。<br>（5）预防癌症骨转移，每 4 周静滴 30～60mg。<br>(1)Tratamiento de la osteoporosis: cada mes 30mg por infusión, y se administra durante seis meses, después se aplica dosis de intervención de 30mg por infusión cada tres meses durante dos años.<br>(2)Tratamiento del dolor por metástasis en los huesos: 30～60mg cada vez por goteo intravenoso lento durante más de cuatro horas. La concentración de la disolución debe ser menos de 15mg/126ml y la velocidad de goteo menos de 15～30mg/2horas.<br>(3)Tratamiento de la hipercalcemia: concentración de calcio＜ 3.0, 3.0～3.5, 3.5～4.0, ＞4.0 mmol/L, o＜ 12.0, 12.0～14.0, 14.0～16.0, ＞ 16.0mg, la dosis e 15～30, 30～60, 60～90, 90mg.<br>(4)Tratamiento de la osteítis deformante y la mala curación del hueso: 30～60mg al día, durante 1～3 días; o 30mg al día, durante seis semanas.<br>(5)Prevención de la metástasis ósea del cáncer: 30～60mg por infusión cada cuatro semanas. |
| 剂型、规格<br>Formulaciones y<br>especificaciones | 片剂：每片 150mg。注射液：每支 15mg（5ml）。<br>Tabletas: cada una 150mg. Inyección: cada una 15mg(5ml). |

| 药品名称 Drug Names | 阿仑膦酸钠 Alendronato sódico |
|---|---|
| 适应证<br>Indicaciones | 用于治疗绝经后妇女骨质疏松症，预防髋部和脊柱骨折，也适用于男性骨质疏松症及增加骨质。<br>Tratamiento de la osteoporosis y prevención de fracturas de columna y cadera en mujeres posmenopáusicas. También apropiado para la osteoporosis y aumentar la densidad ósea en hombres. |

续　表

| | |
|---|---|
| 用法、用量<br>Administración y dosis | 口服，一日 1 次 10mg，或每周一次 70mg，早餐前 30 分钟用至少 200ml 白开水送服，不要咀嚼或吮吸药片。<br><br>Por vía oral, 10mg una vez al día, o 70mg una vez a la semana. Administrarlo con más de 200 ml de agua 30 minutos antes del desayuno. No masticar o chupar las tabletas. |
| 剂型、规格<br>Formulaciones y especificaciones | 片剂：每片 10mg；70mg。<br>Tabletas: cada una 10mg, 70mg. |
| 药品名称 Drug Names | 伊班膦酸钠 Ibandronato sódico |
| 适应证<br>Indicaciones | 用于伴有或不伴有骨转移的恶性肿瘤引起的高钙血症。<br>Contra la hipercalcemia causada por el cáncer con o sin metástasis óseas. |
| 用法、用量<br>Administración y dosis | 缓慢静脉滴注，滴注时间不得少于 2 小时。严格按照血钙浓度，治疗前适当给予 0.9% 氯化钠注射液进行水化治疗。中、重度单剂量给 2 ～ 4mg。<br><br>Por goteo intravenoso lento. La duración del goteo debe ser más de dos horas. Estrictamente de acuerdo con la concentración de calcio, aplicar la terapia de hidratación con la inyección de cloruro de sodio al 0.9% antes del tratamiento. |
| 剂型、规格<br>Formulaciones y especificaciones | 注射液：每支 1mg（1ml）。<br>Inyección: cada una 1mg(1ml). |
| 药品名称 Drug Names | 利塞膦酸钠 Risedronato sódico |
| 适应证<br>Indicaciones | （1）用于治疗绝经后妇女骨质疏松症，预防髋部和脊柱骨折，也适用于男性骨质疏松症，糖皮质激素诱导的骨质疏松症。<br>（2）治疗佩吉特病。<br><br>(1)Tratamiento de la osteoporosis y prevención de fracturas de columna y cadera en mujeres posmenopáusicas. También apropiado para la osteoporosis y la osteoporosis inducida por glucocorticoides en hombres.<br>(2) Tratamiento de la enfermedad de Paget. |
| 用法、用量<br>Administración y dosis | 口服，餐前 30 分钟直立服用，200ml 左右清水送服，服后 30 分钟内不应躺下。一日 1 次，一次 5mg。绝经后骨质疏松症：15mg/ 片，一日一次；35mg/ 片，1 周一次；75mg/ 片，1 个月连服 2 片；150mg/ 片，一个月一次。治疗男性骨质疏松症：15mg/ 片，一日一次。治疗 Paget 病：30mg/ 片，一日一次，连服 2 个月。<br><br>Por vía oral, administrar las tabletas de pie, 30 minutos antes de una comida, con 200 ml de agua y no acostarse dentro de 20 minutos. 5 mg una vez al día. Contra la osteoporosis en mujeres posmenopáusicas: 15mg/tableta, una vez al día; 35mg/tableta, una vez a la semana; 75mg/tableta, 2 tabletas una vez al mes; 150mg/tableta, una tableta una vez al mes. Contra la osteoporosis masculina: 15mg/tableta, una vez al día. Contra la enfermedad de Paget: 30mg/tableta, una vez al día durante dos meses. |
| 剂型、规格<br>Formulaciones y especificaciones | 片剂：每片 5mg；15mg；30mg；35mg；75mg；150mg<br>Tabletas: cada una 5mg, 15mg, 30mg, 35mg, 75mg, 150mg. |
| 药品名称 Drug Names | 降钙素 Calcitonina |
| 适应证<br>Indicaciones | （1）用于治疗绝经后妇女骨质疏松症，老年骨质疏松症。<br>（2）用于治疗恶性肿瘤患者骨转移疼痛和高钙血症。<br>（3）各种骨代谢疾病所致的骨痛。<br>（4）也用于甲状旁腺功能亢进症，缺乏动力或维生素 D 中毒导致的应变性骨炎。<br>（5）治疗佩吉特病。<br>（6）高钙血症和高钙血症危象。 |

**续　表**

|  |  |
|---|---|
|  | (1)Tratamiento de la osteoporosis en mujeres posmenopáusicas y la osteoporosis senil.<br>(2)Tratamiento del dolor por metástasis en los huesos y la hipercalcemia de pacientes con cáncer.<br>(3)Tratamiento de dolor causado por todo tipo de enfermedades metabólicas óseas.<br>(4)Tratamiento de hiperparatiroidismo，la enfermedad de Paget causada por la falta de motivación o la intoxicación por vitamina D.<br>(5)Tratamiento de la enfermedad de Paget.<br>(6)Tratamiento de la hipercalcemia y su crisis. |
| 用法、用量<br>Administración y dosis | （1）绝经后或老年骨质疏松症：①皮下或肌内注射，一日 50～100U；或隔日 100U。②鼻内用药，每次 100U，一日 1～2 次；或每次 50U，一日 2～4 次；或隔日 200U。12 周为一疗程。治疗期间，应日服钙元素 0.5～1.0g，维生素 D 400U。<br>（2）Paget 病：①皮下或肌内注射，一日 100U，改善后，隔日或每日注射 50U，必要时日剂量增至 200U。②鼻内用药：每次 100U，一日 2 次；或每次 50U，一日 4 次，少数病例可能需要每次 200U，一日 2 次。<br>（3）高钙血症：危象紧急处理每日 5～10U／kg，溶于 500ml 生理盐水中，静脉滴注至少 6 小时或日剂量分 2～4 次缓慢静脉注射，同时补液。慢性症状每日 5～10U/kg，1 次或 2 次皮下或肌内注射。也可一日 200～400U，分数次鼻内给药。<br>（4）痛性神经营养不良症：①皮下或肌内注射，一日 100U，持续 2～4 周，然后每次 100U，每周 3 次，维持 6 周以上。②鼻内给药，每日 200U，分 2～4 次给药，持续 2～4 周，然后每次 200U，每周 3 次，持续 6 周以上。<br><br>(1)Contra la osteoporosis en mujeres posmenopáusicas y la osteoporosis senil: ① Por vía intramuscular o subcutánea, 50-100U al día; O 100U cada otro día. ② Por vía intranasal, cada vez 100U, 1～2 veces al día; O cada vez 50U, 2～4 veces al día; O 200U cada otro día. 12 semanas constituyen un periodo de tratamiento. Durante el tratamiento, se debe consumir diariamente 0.5～1.0g de calcio y 400 unidades de vitamina D.<br>(2)Contra la enfermedad de Paget: ① Por vía intramuscular o subcutánea, 100U al día. Si aparece mejoramiento, 50U cada día o cada otro día. Cuando sea necesario, se puede aumentar la dosis hasta 200U. ② Por vía intranasal, cada vez 100U, 2 veces al día; O cada vez 50U, 4 veces al día. En unos cuantos casos, se pueden administrar 200U cada vez, 2 veces al día.<br>(3)Contra la hipercalcemia: en el tratamiento de emergencia de crisis, 5～10U/kg al día, disolver la calcitonina en 500 ml de solución salina normal y administrar la disolución por goteo intravenoso durante por lo menos seis horas, o dividir la dosis diaria en 2～4 porciones y administrar la disolución por inyección intravenosa junto con la infusión de fluidos. Contra las síntomas crónicas, 5～10U/kg al día, 1～2 veces por vía intramuscular o subcutánea, o 200～400U al día por vía intranasal por varias veces.<br>(4)Distrofia simpática refleja: ① Por vía intramuscular o subcutánea, 100U al día durante las primeras 2～4 semanas, y después 100U cada vez, 3 veces a la semana durante más de 6 semanas. ② Por vía intranasal, 200U al día, por 2～4 veces, en las primeras 2～4 semanas, y después 200U cada vez, 3 veces a la semana durante más de 6 semanas. |
| 剂型、规格<br>Formulaciones y especificaciones | 注射液：每支 1ml；2ml。喷鼻剂：每瓶 2ml。<br>Inyección: cada una 1ml; 2ml. Aerosol nasal: 2ml. |
| 药品名称 Drug Names | 骨化三醇 Calcitriol |
| 适应证<br>Indicaciones | （1）绝经后或老年骨质疏松症。<br>（2）肾性骨营养不良。<br>（3）特发性、假性或术后甲状旁腺功能低下。<br>（4）维生素 D 依赖型佝偻病，低血磷性抗维生素 D 型佝偻病。<br><br>(1)La osteoporosis en mujeres posmenopáusicas y la osteoporosis senil.<br>(2)La osteodistrofia renal.<br>(3)El hipoparatiroidismo postoperatorio, idiopático o pseudo-hipoparatiroidismo.<br>(4)Raquitismo vitamina D dependiente, raquitismo hipofosfatémico resistente a la vitamina D. |

| 续　表 | |
|---|---|
| 用法、用量<br>Administración y<br>dosis | ①绝经后或老年骨质疏松症：推荐剂量为每次 0.25μg，一日 2 次，最大剂量可至每次 0.5μg，一日 2 次。用药后第 1、3、6 个月应监测血钙及血肌酐，正常以后，可每 6 个月检测一次。调整剂量期间，需每周检测血钙。②肾性骨营养不良症：最初剂量为 0.25μg，每日口服一次，连服 2～4 周。对血清钙正常或偏低者，口服 0.25μg，每 2 日一次即可。注射剂的剂量为开始每次 0.5μg（0.01μg/kg），每周 3 次。如用药后 2～4 周患者时间鞣化指标和临床症状无明显改善，可每隔 2～4 周将用量增高 0.25μg/d。在此期间，应每周监测血钙至少 2 次。③甲状旁腺功能低或佝偻病患者：初始剂量 0.25μg，每晨服用。如生化指标和临床症状无明显改善，可每隔 2～4 周提高药物剂量。<br><br>① Contra la osteoporosis en mujeres posmenopáusicas y la osteoporosis senil: la dosis recomendable es 0.25μg cada vez, dos veces al día. La dosis máxima puede llegar a 0.5μg cada vez y dos veces al día. Después de empezar la administración, se debe monitorear el calcio sérico y la creatinina sérica en el primer, el tercer y el sexto mes. Cuando sean normales, se puede monitorearlos cada seis meses. Durante el periodo en el que se ajusta la dosis, se debe detectar el calcio sérico cada semana. ② Contra la osteodistrofia renal: la dosis inicial es 0.25μg, una vez al día por vía oral durante 2～4 semanas. Para las personas con el calcio sérico normal o relativamente bajo, una vez 0.25μg cada dos días, por vía oral. La dosis de inyección inicial es cada vez 0.5μg(0.01μg/kg), tres veces a la semana. Después de 2～4 semanas, si los indicadores bioquímicos y los síntomas clínicos del paciente no se mejoran, se puede aumentar la dosis en 0.25μg/d cada 2～4 semanas. En este proceso, se debe monitorear el calcio sérico dos veces por lo menos. ③ Contra el hipoparatiroidismo y el raquitismo: la dosis inicial es 0.25μg, se administra por la mañana. Si los indicadores bioquímicos y los síntomas clínicos no se mejoran, se puede aumentar la dosis cada 2～4 semanas. |
| 剂型、规格<br>Formulaciones y<br>especificaciones | 胶囊剂：每粒 0.25μg。注射剂：每支 1μg（1ml）；2μg（1ml）。<br>Cápsulas: 0.25μg/cápsula. Inyección: cada una 1μg(1ml), 2μg(2ml). |
| 药品名称 Drug Names | 阿法骨化醇 Alfacalcidol |
| 适应证<br>Indicaciones | 用于：预防骨质疏松症、佝偻病和软骨病、肾源性骨病、甲状旁腺功能减退症。<br>Para la prevención de osteoporosis, raquitismo, osteomalacia, osteodistrofia renal e hipoparatiroidismo. |
| 用法、用量<br>Administración y<br>dosis | 口服。骨质疏松症：成人，初始剂量一日 0.5μg，维持量为一日 0.25～0.5μg。其他指征患者：成人或体重 20kg 以上儿童初始剂量每日 1μg，老年人一日 0.5μg，维持剂量为一日 0.25～1μg。<br>Por vía oral. La osteoporosis: para adultos, la dosis inicial es 0.5μg al día, la dosis de mantenimiento es 0.25～0.5μg al día. Pacientes de otras enfermedades indicadas: para adultos o niños de más de 20 kilos, la dosis inicial es 1ug al día, para los de edad avanzada, 0.5μg al día, y la dosis de mantenimiento es 0.25～1μg al día. |
| 剂型、规格<br>Formulaciones y<br>especificaciones | 胶囊剂：每粒 0.25μg。片剂：每片 0.25μg；0.5μg。<br>Cápsulas: 0.25μg/cápsula. Tabletas: cada una 0.25μg, 0.5μg. |
| 药品名称 Drug Names | 碳酸钙 Carbonato de calcio |
| 适应证<br>Indicaciones | 用于预防和治疗钙缺乏症，以及妊娠和哺乳期妇女、绝经期妇女钙的补充。<br>Para la prevención y tratamiento de la deficiencia de calcio. Suplir calcio para mujeres en embarazo, lactancia o menopáusia. |
| 用法、用量<br>Administración y<br>dosis | 口服，一日 1～3 次，分次服。可根据个人情况酌情进行补充。<br>Por vía oral, 1～3 veces al día, administración por veces y según la situación individual. |
| 剂型、规格<br>Formulaciones y<br>especificaciones | 片剂：0.75g。咀嚼片：每片 1.25g。<br>Tabletas: 0.75g. Tabletas masticables: 1.25g/tableta. |

**续 表**

| 药品名称 Drug Names | 替勃龙 Tibolona |
| --- | --- |
| 适应证<br>Indicaciones | 用于绝经后引起的多种症状。<br>Para los síntomas de la menopausia. |
| 用法、用量<br>Administración y dosis | 口服，一日一次 2.5mg，最好固定时间服用，症状消除后可一日服半量，连续服用 3 个月或更长时间。<br>Por vía oral, 2.5mg una vez por día a la misma hora todos los días. Cuando desaparecen los síntomas, se puede disminuir la dosis a la mitad durante tres meses o más tiempo. |
| 剂型、规格<br>Formulaciones y especificaciones | 片剂：每片 2.5mg。<br>Tabletas: 2.5mg/tableta. |
| 药品名称 Drug Names | 雌二醇 Estradiol |
| 适应证<br>Indicaciones | 卵巢功能不全或卵巢激素不足引起的各种症状，主要是功能性子宫出血、原发性闭经、绝经期综合征及前列腺癌等。<br>Se utiliza para tratamiento de insuficiencia ovárica o una variedad de síntomas debido a deficiencia hormonal ovárica, tales como hemorragia uterina funcional, amenorrea, síndrome de la menopausia, y cáncer de próstata, etc. |
| 用法、用量<br>Administración y dosis | 肌内注射：每次 0.5～1.5mg，每周 2～3 次。口服，一日 1 片。<br>Por vía de inyección intramuscular: Cada vez 0,5～1,5 mg, 2 a 3 veces a la semana. Por vía oral, una tableta al día. |
| 剂型、规格<br>Formulaciones y especificaciones | 注射液：每支 2mg（1ml）。凝胶：每支 80g；0.06%。片剂：每片 1mg。微粒化 17β 雌二醇片：每片 1mg；2mg。控释贴片：周效片，每片 2.5mg；3～4 日效片：每片 4mg。<br>Inyección: 2 mg (1 ml). Gel: cada tubo 80 g; 0,06%. Tabletas: Cada tableta 1mg. Tabletas de estradiol 17β micronizado: Cada tableta 1mg; 2mg. Parche de liberación controlada: parche de efecto semanal, cada parche 2,5 mg; parche de efecto de 3 a 4 días: cada parche 4 mg. |
| 药品名称 Drug Names | 雷洛昔芬 Raloxifeno |
| 适应证<br>Indicaciones | 主要用于预防绝经后妇女的骨质疏松症。<br>Principalmente para la prevención de la osteoporosis posmenopáusica. |
| 用法、用量<br>Administración y dosis | 口服，一日 60mg，不受仅是限制。老年人无须调整剂量。由于疾病的必然过程，本品需要长期使用。<br>Por vía oral, 60mg al día a cualquier hora. No hace falta ajustarse la dosis para personas de la tercera edad. Es necesario tomar este medicamento a largo plazo por el proceso inevitable de la enfermedad. |
| 剂型、规格<br>Formulaciones y especificaciones | 片剂：每日 60mg。<br>Tabletas: 60mg/día. |
| 药品名称 Drug Names | 氨基葡萄糖 Glucosamina |
| 适应证<br>Indicaciones | 用于治疗和预防全身部位的骨关节炎。可缓解和消除骨关节炎的疼痛、肿胀等症状，改善关节活动功能。<br>Para el tratamiento y la prevención de la osteoartritis de todo el cuerpo. Puede aliviar y eliminar síntomas como el dolor y la hinchazón de la osteoartritis, y mejorar el funcionamiento de las articulaciones. |
| 用法、用量<br>Administración y dosis | 口服，每次 1～2 粒，一日 3 次，一般疗程 4～12 周，如有必要可延长服药时间。每年重复治疗 2～3 次。<br>Por vía oral, 1～2 cápsulas cada vez, tres veces al día. El tratamiento normalmente dura 4~12 semanas y se puede prolongar cuando sea necesario. Se repite el tratamiento 2-3 veces cada año. |

**续　表**

| | |
|---|---|
| 剂型、规格<br>Formulaciones y<br>especificaciones | 胶囊剂：每粒 0.24mg。<br>Cápsulas: 0.24mg/cápsula. |
| **药品名称 Drug Names** | 酚苄明 Fenoxibenzamina |
| 适应证<br>Indicaciones | （1）用于前列腺增生引起的尿潴留。<br>（2）嗜铬细胞瘤的治疗和术前准备。<br>（3）周围血管痉挛性疾病。<br>(1)Contra la retención urinaria causada por la hiperplasia de próstata.<br>(2)Para el tratameinto y preparación preoperatoria de la feocromocitoma.<br>(3)Contra la enfermedad vascular periférica con espasmos. |
| 用法、用量<br>Administración y<br>dosis | 开始每次 10mg，一日 2 次，以后隔日加量 10mg，直至获得临床效果或出现轻微不良反应。以每次 20 ～ 40mg，一日 2 ～ 3 次维持。<br>　La dosis inicial es 10mg cada vez, dos veces al día y se aumenta en 10mg cada otro día hasta aparecer efectos clínicos o reacciones adversas leves. La dosis de mantenimiento es 20 ~ 40mg cada vez, 2 ~ 3 veces al día. |
| 剂型、规格<br>Formulaciones y<br>especificaciones | 片剂：每片 10mg。<br>Tabletas: 10mg/tableta. |
| **药品名称 Drug Names** | 特拉唑嗪 Terazosina |
| 适应证<br>Indicaciones | （1）用于改善良性前列腺增生患者的排尿症状。<br>（2）还用于治疗慢性、非细菌性前列腺炎和前列腺痛，女性膀胱颈梗阻，结肠手术拔出导尿管前服用，预防急性尿潴留的发生。<br>（3）用于治疗高血压，可单独使用或与其他药合用。<br>(1)Para mejorar los síntomas urinarios de pacientes con hiperplasia benigna de próstata.<br>(2)Para el tratamiento de la prostatitis crónica no bacteriana y el dolor en la próstata, la obstrucción del cuello vesical en la mujer. Para la prevención de la retención urinaria aguda, se administra antes de sacarse el catéter en la cirugía de colon.<br>(3)Para la prevención de hipertensión, se puede administrar solo o en combinación con otros medicamentos. |
| 用法、用量<br>Administración y<br>dosis | （1）良性前列腺增生：口服，每次 2mg，一日一次，每晚睡前服用。<br>（2）高血压：初始剂量为睡前服用 1mg，且不应超过，以尽量减少首次低血压事件的发生。1 周后，每日单剂量可加倍以达到预期效果。常用维持剂量为一日 2 ～ 10mg。<br>　(1)Contra la hiperplasia benigna de próstata: por vía oral, 2mg una vez al día, se administra a la hora de acostarse.<br>　(2)Contra la hipertensión: la dosis inicial es 1mg al día y se administra a la hora de acostarse. No se puede superar esta dosis al principio para evitar la aparición de hipotensión. Después de una semana, la dosis diaria se puede multiplicar para alcanzar resultados esperados. La dosis de mantenimiento es frecuentemente entre 2 a 10mg al día. |
| 剂型、规格<br>Formulaciones y<br>especificaciones | 片剂：每片 1mg；2mg；5mg。胶囊剂：每粒 2mg。<br>Tabletas: 1mg, 2mg, 5mg/tableta. Cápsulas: 2mg/cápsula. |
| **药品名称 Drug Names** | 坦洛新 Tamsulosina |
| 适应证<br>Indicaciones | 主要用于治疗前列腺增生而导致的异常排尿症状，适用于轻、中度患者及未导致排尿障碍者，如已发生严重尿潴留患者不宜单独服用此药。<br>　Principalmente para el tratamiento de los síntomas urinarios anormales causados por la hiperplasia de próstata. La tamsulosina es apropiada para casos leves y moderados, y pacientes sin trastornos de la micción. No es recomendable que sólo administren este medicamento los pacientes con retención urinaria severa. |

**续　表**

| | |
|---|---|
| 用法、用量<br>Administración y dosis | 口服，一次 0.2mg，一日 1 次，餐后服。<br>Por vía oral, 0.2mg una vez al día después de una comida. |
| 剂型、规格<br>Formulaciones y especificaciones | 缓释胶囊剂：每粒 0.2mg。<br>Cápsulas de liberación prolongada: 0.2mg/cápsula. |

| 药品名称 Drug Names | 非那雄胺 Finasterida |
|---|---|
| 适应证<br>Indicaciones | （1）用于治疗良性前列腺增生，使增大的前列腺缩小，其逆转过程需要 3 个月以上；可以改善排尿症状，使最大尿流率增加；减少发生尿潴留和手术概率。<br>（2）可以治疗男性秃发，能促进头发增长并防止继续脱发。<br>(1)Para el tratamiento de la hiperplasia benigna de próstata reduciendo la próstata agrandada. Este proceso de reversión lleva más de tres meses. Puede mejorar los síntomas urinarios, aumentar la velocidad máxima del flujo urinario, disminuir la posibilidad de la retención urinaria y la cirugía.<br>(2)Para el tratamiento de la calvicie masculina, puede promover el crecimiento del cabello y evitar su pérdida. |
| 用法、用量<br>Administración y dosis | 口服。①治疗良性前列腺增生：一次 5mg，一日 1 次，6 个月为一疗程。空腹或与食物同时服用均可。肾功能程度不全者、老年人不需要调整剂量。②治疗脱发：一次 1mg，一日 1 次，睡前服用。一般连续服用 3 个月或更长时间才达到效果。<br>Por vía oral. ① Para el tratamiento de la hiperplasia benigna de próstata: 5mg una vez al día. Un período de tratamiento lleva seis meses. Se puede administrar con el estómago vacío o con alimentos. No hace falta ajustar la dosis para las personas con insuficiencia renal o de tercera edad. ② Para el tratamiento de la alopecia: 1mg una vez al día. Se administra a la hora de acostarse. Normalmente se consiguen resultados esperados después de más de tres meses consecutivos. |
| 剂型、规格<br>Formulaciones y especificaciones | 片剂：每片 1mg；5mg。<br>Tabletas: 1mg, 5mg/tableta. |

| 药品名称 Drug Names | 舍尼通 Cernilton |
|---|---|
| 适应证<br>Indicaciones | 用于良性前列腺增生，慢性、非细菌性前列腺炎及前列腺疼痛等。<br>Para el tratamiento de la hiperplasia benigna de próstata, la prostatitis crónica no bacteriana y el dolor en la próstata. |
| 用法、用量<br>Administración y dosis | 口服，一次 1 片，一日 2 次，早晚各一片，疗程 3 ～ 6 个月。衰老或肾功能不全者无须改变剂量。<br>Por vía oral, cada vez una tableta, dos veces al día, por la mañana y por la noche. No hace falta ajustar la dosis para las personas con insuficiencia renal o de tercera edad. |
| 剂型、规格<br>Formulaciones y especificaciones | 片剂：每片含 p5 70mg，E A10 4mg。<br>Tabletas: cada una contiene 70mg de p5, 4mg de EA10. |

| 药品名称 Drug Names | 前列通片 QianLieTong comprimidos |
|---|---|
| 适应证<br>Indicaciones | 用于急性前列腺炎、前列腺增生引起的尿潴留、尿血、尿频等症。<br>Contra la prostatitis aguda, y la retención urinaria, la hematuria y la micción frecuente causadas por la hiperplasia de próstata. |
| 用法、用量<br>Administración y dosis | 口服：大片每次服 4 片，或小片每次 6 片，一日 3 次。30 ～ 45 日为 1 个疗程。<br>Por vía oral: cada vez 4 tabletas grandes o 6 tabletas pequeñas, tres veces al día. Un período de tratamiento lleva 30 a 45 días. |
| 剂型、规格<br>Formulaciones y especificaciones | 片剂：340mg；胶囊：250mg，380mg，400mg。<br>Comprimido: 340 mg; cápsula: 250 mg, 380 mg, 400 mg. |

**续　表**

| 药品名称 Drug Names | 谷丙甘氨酸 Ácido glutámico alanina y glicina |
| --- | --- |
| 适应证<br>Indicaciones | 用于治疗前列腺增生引起的尿频、排尿困难及尿潴留症。尤适用于心肺功能不全和不宜手术的高龄患者。本品为氨基酸制剂，适合老年患者使用。<br>Para el tratamiento de la micción frecuente, la disuria y la retención urinaria. Especialmente apropiado para los pacientes de edad avanzada inoperables o con ineficiencia cardiopulmonar. Este medicamento es una preparación de aminoácidos, apropiada para pacientes de tercera edad. |
| 用法、用量<br>Administración y dosis | 口服，一次 2 片，一日 3 次，或根据病情适当增减。<br>Por vía oral, cada vez dos tabletas, tres veces al día. Se puede ajustar la dosis de acuerdo con la enfermedad. |
| 剂型、规格<br>Formulaciones y especificaciones | 片剂：每片 0.41g。<br>Tabletas: 0.41g/tableta. |
| 药品名称 Drug Names | 吡诺克辛 Pirenoxina |
| 适应证<br>Indicaciones | 用于治疗初期老年性白内障、轻度糖尿病性白内障或并发性白内障等。<br>Para el tratamiento de la catarata senil temprana, la catarata diabética leve, la catarata complicada, etc. |
| 用法、用量<br>Administración y dosis | 滴眼，用前充分摇匀，一次 1～2 滴，一日 3～5 次。<br>Gotas oftálmicas. Agite la botella antes de la administración. 1～2 gotas cada vez, 3～5 veces al día. |
| 剂型、规格<br>Formulaciones y especificaciones | 滴眼剂：每瓶装有密封的药片 1 片；每瓶内装溶剂 15ml。<br>Gotas oftálmicas: cada botella contiene una tableta sellada y 15ml de disolución. |

19.2　消毒防腐收敛药 Medicamentos esterilización estéril, antisepticcos y astringentes

| 药品名称 Drug Names | 过氧乙酸 Ácido peracético |
| --- | --- |
| 适应证<br>Indicaciones | 用于空气、环境消毒和预防消毒。<br>Para la desinfección del aire y el medio ambiente y la desinfección de prevención. |
| 用法、用量<br>Administración y dosis | 用前按比例稀释。最常用为稀释 500 倍，即用 20% 的本品 2ml 加水 998ml 制得，含过氧乙酸 0.04%。①空气消毒：1∶200 液对空气喷雾，每立方米空间含药 30ml。②预防性消毒：食具、毛巾、水果、蔬菜等用 1∶500 液洗刷浸泡，禽蛋用 1∶1000 液浸泡，时间为 5 分钟，密封 50～60 分钟。<br>Diluir la solución proporcionalmente antes del uso. La dilución más frecuente es 1:500 v/v, que equivale a 2 ml de la solución concentrada al 20% en 998 ml de agua, que contiene 0.04% del ácido peracético. ① Desinfección del aire: pulverizar en el aire la disolución de 1∶200, cada metro cúbito con 30ml. ② Desinfección de prevención: para utensilios, toallas, frutas y verduras, lavé y remójelos con la disolución de 1∶500. Para los huevos: remójelos con la disolución de 1∶1000 durante cinco minutos, y séllelos durante 50~60 minutos. |
| 剂型、规格<br>Formulaciones y especificaciones | 溶液：16%～20%。<br>Solución: 16%~20%. |
| 药品名称 Drug Names | 聚维酮碘 Povidona yodada |
| 适应证<br>Indicaciones | 用于皮肤、黏膜的窗口消毒，也用于化脓性皮炎、皮肤真菌感染、小面积烧烫伤及念珠菌阴道炎、细菌性阴道炎、混合感染性阴道炎、老年性阴道炎等。<br>Para la desinfección de las heridas en la piel y en las membranas mucosas. También se puede utilizar contra la dermatitis supurativa, infecciones de la piel por hongos, quemaduras pequeñas, vaginitis por Cándida, vaginitis bacteriana, vaginitis infecciosa mixta, vaginitis senil, etc. |

**续　表**

| 用法、用量<br>Administración y dosis | （1）外科手术消毒，0.5% 溶液刷洗 5 分钟。注射部位消毒，30 分钟以上。<br>（2）术野皮肤消毒，0.5% 溶液均匀涂抹 2 次。<br>（3）黏膜创伤或感染，用 0.1%～0.025% 溶液冲洗或软膏涂抹病患部位。<br>（4）皮肤感染 0.5% 溶液局部涂擦或软膏涂抹患处。<br>（5）阴道或直肠给药，每晚睡前 1 次，一次 1 支软膏或 1 个栓剂，7～10 日为一疗程。<br><br>(1)Desinfección quirúrgica: lavar con la solución al 0.5% por más de cinco minutos. Desinfección de los sitios de inyección debe durar más de treinta minutos.<br>(2) Desinfección de la piel del campo quirúrgico: aplicar frotando 2 veces con la solución al 0.5%.<br>(3) Infección o heridas en las membranas mucosas: enjugar con la solución al 0.1% ~ 0.25% o aplicar frotando la parte afectada con la pomada.<br>(4)Infección de la piel: aplicar frotando en la parte afectada con la solución al 0.5% o la pomada.<br>(5)La administración vaginal y rectal: una vez al día a la hora de acostarse. Cada vez con una pomada o un supositorio. Un periodo de tratamiento dura 7 ~ 10 días. |
|---|---|
| 剂型、规格<br>Formulaciones y especificaciones | 溶液：0.5%；1%；5%。软膏、乳膏或凝胶：10%。栓剂：每个 0.29g。<br>Solución: 0.5%, 1%, 5%. Pomada, crema o gel: 10%. Supositorios: cada uno 0.29g. |
| 药品名称 Drug Names | 氯己定 Clorhexidina |
| 适应证<br>Indicaciones | 用于皮肤、创面、妇产科、泌尿外科的消毒及卫生用品的消毒，也用于急性坏死性溃疡性牙龈炎、牙科术后口腔感染，预防和治疗癌肿和白血病患者的口腔感染、义齿引起的创伤性磨损继发细菌和真菌感染、滤泡性口炎等。<br><br>Para la desinfección de piel, heridas, obstetricia, ginecología, urología y productos para la higiene. También se puede utilizar contra la gingivitis ulceronecrotizante aguda y la infección bucal postoperatoria, prevención y tratamiento de la infección bucal de pacientes con cáncer o leucemia, la infección por hongos y bacteriana secundaria por desgaste traumático causadas por dentaduras, estomatitis folicular, etc. |
| 用法、用量<br>Administración y dosis | （1）手术消毒：以 1：5000 水溶液泡手 3 分钟。<br>（2）术野消毒：用 0.5% 乙醇（70%）溶液，其功效约与碘酊相当，但无皮肤刺激、亦不染色，因而特别适于面部、会阴部及儿童的术野消毒。<br>（3）创伤伤口消毒：用 1：2000 水溶液冲洗。<br>（4）含漱：以 1：5000 溶液漱口，对咽峡炎及口腔溃疡有效。<br>（5）烧伤、烫伤：用 0.5% 乳膏或气雾剂。<br>（6）分娩时产妇外阴及周围皮肤消毒，会阴镜检的润滑：用 1% 乳膏涂抹。<br>（7）器械消毒：消毒用 1：1000 水溶液，贮存用 1：5000 水溶液，加入 0.1% 亚硝酸钠浸泡，隔 2 周换一次。<br>（8）房间、家具等消毒：用 0.02% 溶液膀胱冲洗。<br>（9）滴眼液防腐：用 0.01% 溶液。<br>（10）伤口护理：用贴剂，清洁患处后，将中间护创贴在创伤处，两端用胶带固定。<br><br>(1)Desinfección quirúrgica: remojar las manos por tres minutos en la solución acuosa de 1：5000.<br>(2)Desinfección del campo quirúrgico: con la solución de etanol (70%) al 0.5%, que tiene la misma función de yodo pero no irrita ni tiñe la piel. Es particularmente adecuado para la desinfección del campo quirúrgico de la cara, el perineo y los niños.<br>(3)Desinfección de heridas: enjugar con la solución acuosa de 1：2000.<br>(4)Gargarismo: con la solución de 1：5000, eficaz para anginas y úlceras en la boca.<br>(5)Quemaduras y escaldaduras: con la crema o el aerosol al 0.5%.<br>(6)Desinfección de la vulva y la piel alrededor en el parto y la lubricación para la endoscopia perineal: aplicar frotando con la crema al 1%.<br>(7)Desinfección de instrumentos: para la desinfección se utiliza la solución acuosa de 1：1000, para guardarlos: en la solución acuosa de 1：5000 con el nitrito de sodio al 0.1%, y se cambia la solución cada dos semanas.<br>(8)Desinfección de la habitación y muebles: enjugar con la solución al 0.02%.<br>(9)Antisepsia de gotas oftálmicas: con la solución al 0.01%.<br>(10) Cuidado de las heridas: con parche. Ponga el parche en la herida fijando ambos extremos con cinta. |

**续　表**

| | |
|---|---|
| 剂型、规格<br>Formulaciones y<br>especificaciones | 制剂：葡萄糖酸氯己定含漱剂：0.016g（200ml）；0.04g（500ml）。葡萄糖酸氯己定溶液：50g（250ml）。稀葡萄糖酸氯己定溶液：12.5g（250ml）。醋酸氯己定片：每片 5mg。醋酸氯己定霜：1%。醋酸氯己定软膏：1%。<br><br>Preparación: gárgaras de gluconato de clorhexidina: 0.016g (200ml), 0.04g (500ml). Solución de gluconato de clorhexidina: 50g (250ml).Solución diluida de gluconato de clorhexidina: 12.5g(250ml). Tabletas de acetato de clorhexidina: 5mg/tableta. Crema de acetato de clorhexidina: 1%. Pomada de acetato de clorhexidina: 1%. |
| 药品名称 Drug Names | 戊二醛 Glutaraldehido |
| 适应证<br>Indicaciones | 用于器械消毒，也可用于治疗寻常疣、甲癣和多汗症。<br><br>Para la desinfección de instrumentos, y el tratamiento de verrugas comunes, onicomicosis e hiperhidrosis. |
| 用法、用量<br>Administración y<br>dosis | （1）碱性戊二醛水溶液或异丙醇溶液（浓度为 2%，pH 为 7.5 ～ 8.5）：对细菌繁殖体的作用时间为 10 ～ 20 分钟，对细菌芽孢为 4 ～ 12 小时。10% 溶液用于治疗寻常疣、甲癣和多汗症，局部涂擦，一日 1 ～ 2 次。配制好的 2% 碱性水溶液在室温下经 14 日后，杀菌作用即明显减退。<br>　　（2）酸性强化戊二醛液：是在 2% 戊二醛溶液中加入某些非离子型化合物作为强化剂配制而成。所加强化剂有稳定作用，又有协同增效作用。国外商品名为 Sonacide。国内曾用 0.25% 聚氧乙烯脂肪醇醚作为强化剂配制。此溶液因仍保持酸性（pH3.4），故稳定，室温下放置 18 个月，杀菌效能不减。同时加强药物表面活性，协同增效。杀菌力与碱性戊二醛相似，用法也相同。唯一缺点易导致金属生锈。<br>　　（3）人造心脏瓣膜消毒液：为其 0.65% 溶液，pH（7.4）与血液相似，系磷酸盐缓冲液。<br>　　（4）戊二醛气体：用于密封空间内表面的熏蒸消毒，因其不易在物体表面聚合，故优于甲醛。<br><br>(1) Solución acuosa de glutaraldehído alcalino o solución de isopropanol (la concentración es 2%, y el valor de pH es 7.5 ～ 8.5.): el tiempo de actuación dura 10 ～ 20 minutos para propágulos de bacterias, y dura 4 ～ 12 horas para esporas bacterianas. La solución al 10% se utiliza para el tratamiento de verrugas comunes, onicomicosis e hiperhidrosis. Se aplica frotando localmente una a dos veces al día. Disminuirá significativamente la función desinfectante de la preparada solución acuosa alcalina al 2% después de 14 días a temperatura ambiente.<br>(2) Solución ácida de glutaraldehído: se prepara añadiendo ciertos compuestos no iónicos como potenciador en la solución de glutaraldehído al 2%. El potenciador añadido, llamado Sonacide, ejerce funciones de estabilización y sinergias. En China se usaba éter graso del alcohol-polioxietileno al 0.25% como potenciador de preparación. Esta solución de acidez de pH 3.4, es estable y se puede conservar durante 18 meses a temperatura ambiente sin disminuir su eficacia desinfectante. Al mismo tiempo, puede aumentar la tensión superficial del medicamento con sinergías. Su capacidad bactericida es similar a la de glutaraldehído alcalino con la misma forma de aplicación. Causa fácilmente la oxidación de los metales, que es su único defecto.<br>(3)Desinfectante de válvulas cardíacas artificiales: solución al 0.65%, con un valor de pH (7.4) similar al de la sangre. Es un tampón fosfato.<br>(4) Gas de glutaraldehído: para la fumigación de la superficie de un espacio cerrado. Es mejor que formaldehído porque no tiene riesgo de polimerización en la superficie de materias. |
| 剂型、规格<br>Formulaciones y<br>especificaciones | 溶液：20%；25%，稀释后使用。<br>Disolución: 20%, 25%. Uso después de dilución. |
| 药品名称 Drug Names | 洗消净 Solución de hipoclorito de sodio y dodecilsulfato sódico |
| 适应证<br>Indicaciones | 适用范围广泛，可供器械、用具、衣物及排泄物消毒。<br>Adecuado para varios tipos de desinfección: la de instrumentos, aparatos, ropa y excrementos. |
| 用法、用量<br>Administración y<br>dosis | 取本品 50ml，用 10kg 水稀释，将被洗涤物品放在其中刷洗，即可达到消毒洗净的目的。也可浸泡 3 ～ 5 分钟，然后再刷洗，配制本品可用自来水，最适水温为 40℃ 左右。<br><br>Diluya 50ml de la solución con 10kg de agua, y lave las cosas con la disolución. De esta manera se desinfectan fácilmente. También puede remojar las cosas por tres a cinco minutos y luego lavarlas con agua. La preparación se puede realizar con agua corriente y la temperatura óptima es aproximadamente 40℃ . |

**续 表**

| 剂型、规格<br>Formulaciones y<br>especificaciones | 溶液：次氯酸钠溶液（含氯量不低于 5%）和 40% 十二烷基磺酸钠溶液等量混合配制。<br>La Solución:Se prepara mezclando una solución de hipoclorito de sodio (con un contenido de cloro no inferior al 5%) y una solución de dodecilsulfonato de sodio al 40% en cantidades iguales. |
|---|---|
| **药品名称 Drug Names** | **苯酚 Fenol** |
| 适应证<br>Indicaciones | 常用于消毒痰、脓、粪便和医疗器械。液化苯酚用于涂拭阑尾残端。<br>De uso común en la desinfección de sputo, pus, excrementos y dispositivos médicos. El fenol licuado se aplica en la apendicitis del muñón. |
| 用法、用量<br>Administración y<br>dosis | 外用消毒防腐剂。本品对人有腐蚀性、毒性，可引起新生儿黄疸，不宜长期使用。<br>Desinfectante y antiséptico tópico. Este producto es corrosivo y tóxico para las personas y puede causar la ictericia en recién nacidos. No es recomendable el uso a largo plazo. |
| 剂型、规格<br>Formulaciones y<br>especificaciones | 溶液 1% ~ 5%<br>Solución al 1% ~ 5%. |
| **药品名称 Drug Names** | **鱼石脂 Ictamol** |
| 适应证<br>Indicaciones | 有抑菌、消炎、抑制分泌和消肿等作用，可用于疖肿及外耳道炎等。<br>Funciones antibacteriana, anti-inflamatoria y de inhibición de la secreción y la hinchazón. Contra el furúnculo, la otitis externa, etc. |
| 用法、用量<br>Administración y<br>dosis | 外用涂擦，一日 2 次。滴耳，一日 3 次，一次 2 滴。<br>Uso externo: aplique la pomada dos veces al día. Gotas óticas: tres veces al día, cada vez dos gotas. |
| 剂型、规格<br>Formulaciones y<br>especificaciones | 10% 软膏；鱼石脂甘油滴耳剂。<br>Pomada al 10%; Gotas óticas de ictiol y glicerina. |
| **药品名称 Drug Names** | **乙醇 Etanol** |
| 适应证<br>Indicaciones | 75% 用于杀菌消毒。50% 用于防压疮。25% ~ 50% 擦浴用于高热患者物理退热。还可用于小面积烫伤的湿敷浸泡。在配制剂时用作溶剂。<br>Alcohol al 75%: desinfección. Alcohol al 50%: prevención de úlceras. Alcohol al 25% ~ 50%: se puede bajar la fiebre alta frotándose el cuerpo. También para compresas húmedas en quemaduras pequeñas. Puede servir de solvente en la preparación. |
| 用法、用量<br>Administración y<br>dosis | 用作消毒剂时注意浓度，过高或过低均影响杀菌效果。不宜用于伤口或破损的皮肤面。<br>Al usar el alcohol para la desinfección, cuide con la concentración, que afecta el efecto bactericida cuando es demasiado alta o baja. Es inadecuado para la herida en la piel. |
| 剂型、规格<br>Formulaciones y<br>especificaciones | 各种不同浓度的乙醇溶液。<br>Utilizar solución de alcohol de diferentes concentraciones. |
| **药品名称 Drug Names** | **甲紫 Metilrosanilina** |
| 适应证<br>Indicaciones | 有较好的杀菌作用，且无刺激性。用于皮肤革兰阳性菌和皮肤黏膜念珠菌病。<br>Tiene buen efecto bactericida sin irritación. Contra la bacteria Gram-positiva en la piel y la Candidiasis mucocutánea. |
| 用法、用量<br>Administración y<br>dosis | 外用涂擦。据报道，有一定致癌作用，故在伤口处禁用。<br>Uso externo. Según informes, tiene ciertos efectos carcinogénicos, por lo que es contraindicado su uso en las heridas. |
| 剂型、规格<br>Formulaciones y<br>especificaciones | 1% 溶液；1% 糊。<br>Solución al 1%; Pasta al 1%. |

**续 表**

| 药品名称 Drug Names | 依沙吖啶 Etacridina |
|---|---|
| 适应证<br>Indicaciones | 有消毒防腐作用，用于有感染及糜烂渗液的皮肤或创面。<br>Tiene efecto bactericida. Para piel o heridas con infección, erosión o exudado. |
| 用法、用量<br>Administración y dosis | 外用冲洗、湿敷。<br>Uso externo: lavadura, compresas húmedas. |
| 剂型、规格<br>Formulaciones y especificaciones | 0.1% 溶液。<br>Solución al 0.1%. |

| 药品名称 Drug Names | 高锰酸钾 Permanganato de potasio |
|---|---|
| 适应证<br>Indicaciones | 有强氧化作用，可除臭消毒，但作用短暂表浅。冲洗感染创面及膀胱炎用 0.1% ～ 0.5% 溶液，清除皮损表面的脓性分泌物和恶臭、湿敷治疗湿疹 0.025% ～ 0.01% 溶液，眼科用 0.01% ～ 0.02% 溶液，洗胃 1 : 1000 ～ 1 : 5000，坐浴 0.02%，水果、食具消毒 0.1%。<br><br>Con oxidación fuerte. Para desodorización y desinfección, pero el efecto dura poco. Solución al 0.1% ~ 0.5%: para lavar las heridas infectadas y contra la cistitis. Solución al 0.025% ~ 0.01%: para eliminar las secreciones purulentas de rupturas en la piel y el hedor, y para el tratamiento de la eczema con compresas húmedas. Solución al 0.01% ~ 0.02% para la oftalmología. Solución de 1 : 1000 ~ 1 : 5000 para el lavado gástrico. Solución al 0.02% para el baño. Solución al 0.1% para la desinfección de utensilios. |
| 用法、用量<br>Administración y dosis | 溶液应新配，久置或加热可迅速失效。其褐色斑可以用过氧化氢溶液或草酸溶液拭去。<br><br>Es necesario el uso inmediato de la solución preparada, que después de un largo tiempo o calentamiento pierde rápido su efecto. Se pueden eliminar las mancha marrones con la solución de peróxido o de ácido oxálico. |
| 剂型、规格<br>Formulaciones y especificaciones | 外用片：100mg。<br>Tabletas de uso externo: 100mg. |

| 药品名称 Drug Names | 过氧化氢溶液 Solución de peróxido de hidrógeno |
|---|---|
| 适应证<br>Indicaciones | 为强氧化剂，具有消毒、防腐、除臭及清洁作用，用于清洗创面、溃疡、脓窦、耳内脓液；涂擦治疗面部褐斑；在换药时可以去痂皮和黏附在伤口的敷料；稀释至 1% 浓度用于扁桃体炎、口腔炎、白喉等含漱。<br><br>Oxidante fuerte. Para desinfección, antisepsia, desodorización y limpieza. Puede lavar heridas, úlceras, pus, seno y pus en orejas; También para el tratamiento de manchas marrones en la piel; Puede eliminar la costra y la vendaje en heridas al cambiar la última; La solución diluida al 1% es un gargarismo adecuado para amigdalitis, estomatitis, difteria, etc. |
| 用法、用量<br>Administración y dosis | 除用于恶臭不洁的创面外，尤适用于厌氧菌感染及破损伤口、气性坏疽的创面，用 3% 溶液冲洗或湿敷，根据情况每日多次使用。<br><br>Además de ser adecuada para el tratamiento de heridas sucias con hedor, la solución es particularmente eficaz con infecciones por anaerobios, heridas abiertas, y heridas de gangrenà gaseosa. Lave o aplique compresa húmeda en las heridas con la solución al 3% varias veces al día según la situación. |
| 剂型、规格<br>Formulaciones y especificaciones | 本品为过氧化氢的 3% 水溶液。<br>Solución acuosa de peróxido de hidrógeno al 3%. |

| 药品名称 Drug Names | 呋喃西林 Furacilina |
|---|---|
| 适应证<br>Indicaciones | 有广谱抗菌活性，但对假单胞菌属疗效甚微，对真菌和病毒无效。表面消毒用 0.001% ～ 0.01% 水溶液，冲洗、湿敷患处，冲洗腔道或用于滴耳、滴鼻。<br><br>Con actividad antimicrobiana de amplio espectro. Pero es poco eficaz para pseudomonas, e ineficaz para hongos y virus. Solución acuosa al 0.001% ~ 0.01% para la desinfección superficial, lavar y aplicar compresas húmedas en la parte afectada y lavar orificios. También puede hacer gotas óticas y nasales. |

| 用法、用量<br>Administración y<br>dosis | （1）对本品过敏者禁用。<br>（2）口服毒性较大，目前仅供外用。<br>(1)Está contraindicado el uso por las personas alérgicas al producto.<br>(2)Es tóxico tomarlo por vía oral. Sólo para el uso externo. |
|---|---|
| 剂型、规格<br>Formulaciones y<br>especificaciones | 溶液：0.02%；0.2%。<br>La solución: 0.02%, al 0.2%. |
| 药品名称 Drug Names | 苯扎溴铵 Bromuro de benzalconio |
| 适应证<br>Indicaciones | 阳离子活性的广谱杀菌剂，杀菌力强，对皮肤和局部组织无刺激性，对金属、橡胶制品无腐蚀作用。1：1000～1：2000 溶液广泛用于手、皮肤、黏膜、器械等的消毒。可长期保存效力不减。<br>Desinfectante de amplio espectro con activos cationes, con fuerte bactericida, sin irritación de la piel o del tisular local, ni efecto corrosivo de metales o productos de caucho. La solución de 1：1000～1：2000 se utiliza ampliamente para la desinfección de manos, piel, mucosa, instrumentos, etc. Puede conservar su eficacia por largo tiempo. |
| 用法、用量<br>Administración y<br>dosis | （1）不可与普通肥皂配伍。<br>（2）泡器械加 0.5% 亚硝酸钠。<br>（3）不适用于膀胱镜、眼科器械、橡胶、铝制品及排泄物消毒。<br>(1)Está prohibido su uso junto con el jabón.<br>(2)Para remojar los instrumentos, añada el nitrito de sodio al 0.5%.<br>(3)No es adecuado para la desinfección de cistoscopia, instrumentos de la oftalmología, caucho, productos de aluminio y excrementos. |
| 剂型、规格<br>Formulaciones y<br>especificaciones | 溶液：1：1000～1：2000。<br>La solución de 1：1000～1：2000. |

### 19.3　皮肤科用药 Medicamentos dermatológicos

| 药品名称 Drug Names | 莫匹罗星 Mupirocina |
|---|---|
| 适应证<br>Indicaciones | 用于多种病菌引起的皮肤感染和湿疹、皮炎、糜烂、溃疡等继发性感染。报道称，本品预防或治疗给药，对降低皮肤外科手术后伤口化脓十分有效。<br>Para el tratamiento de infecciones de la piel causadas por una variedad de bacterias y eczema, dermatitis, erosiones, úlceras y otras infecciones secundarias. Según un informe, este producto es muy eficaz para prevenir o reducir las heridas purulentas después de cirugías de piel. |
| 用法、用量<br>Administración y<br>dosis | 涂于患处，也可用敷料包扎或覆盖，一日 3 次，5 日为一疗程。必要时可重复一疗程。<br>Aplique la pomada sobre la parte afectada. También puede envolver o cubrirla con venda. Tres veces al día. Un periodo de tratamiento dura cinco días. Si es necesario, se puede administrar por otro periodo. |
| 剂型、规格<br>Formulaciones y<br>especificaciones | 软膏：2%。<br>Pomada: 2%. |
| 药品名称 Drug Names | 夫西地酸 Ácido fusídico |
| 适应证<br>Indicaciones | 对与皮肤感染有关的革兰阳性球菌，尤其对葡萄球菌高度敏感，对耐药金葡菌也有效，对革兰阴性菌有一定作用。与其他抗菌素无交叉耐药性。<br>Con alta sensibilidad con cocos gram positivos relacionados con infecciones de la piel, sobre todo con el estafilococo. También es eficaz para staphylococcus aureus resistente a la meticilina. Tiene ciertos efectos sobre las bacterias gram negativas. Sin resistencia cruzada con otros antibióticos. |
| 用法、用量<br>Administración y<br>dosis | 涂于患处，并缓和摩擦。也可用敷料包扎，一日 2～3 次，7 日为一疗程，必要时可重复一疗程。<br>Aplique la crema sobre la parte afectada frotando suavemente. También puede vendarla. Dos a tres veces al día. Un periodo de tratamiento dura siete días. Si es necesario, se puede administrar por otro periodo. |

**续　表**

| 剂型、规格<br>Formulaciones y especificaciones | 乳膏：2%。<br>Crema: 2%. |
|---|---|
| **药品名称 Drug Names** | 环吡酮胺 Ciclopirox Olamina |
| 适应证<br>Indicaciones | 外用于治疗各种皮肤浅表或黏膜的癣菌病。<br>Para el tratamiento de todo tipo de tiña en la superficie de la piel o la mucosa. |
| 用法、用量<br>Administración y dosis | 涂患处，一日 2 次，甲癣，先用温水泡软灰指甲，再削薄病甲，涂药包扎。疗程一般 1～4 周（甲癣 13 周）。阴道栓用于治疗阴道念珠菌感染。<br>Aplique sobre la parte afectada, dos veces al día. Para la onicomicosis: primero ablande las uñas afectadas con agua caliente, adelgácelas, aplique el producto y véndelas. El periodo de tratamiento dura una a cuatro semanas normalmente (Para la onicomicosis dura 13 semanas.). El supositorio vaginal se usa contra la candidiasis vaginal. |
| 剂型、规格<br>Formulaciones y especificaciones | 溶液或乳膏：均为 1%。阴道栓：每个含药 50mg 或 100mg。栓剂：1%；洗剂：1%。<br>Emulsión o crema: 1%. Supositorio vaginal: cada uno contiene 50mg o 100mg de ciclopirox olamina. Supositorios: 1%; Loción; 1%. |
| **药品名称 Drug Names** | 联苯苄唑 Bifonazolo |
| 适应证<br>Indicaciones | 用于体癣、股癣、手足癣、花斑癣、红癣及皮肤念球菌病等表浅皮肤真菌感染及短小杆状菌引起的皮肤念球菌性外阴道炎。<br>Contra las tiñas corporal, inguinal, de manos y pies, versicolor, la eritrasma, la candidiasis cutánea y otras infecciones por hongos en la superficie de la piel, y contra la candidiasis vulvovaginal causada por bacilos cortos y pequeños. |
| 用法、用量<br>Administración y dosis | 涂患处，一日 1 次，2～4 周为一疗程。阴道给药，于睡前将阴道片放入阴道深处，一日 1 次，一次 1 片。<br>Aplique sobre la parte afectada, una vez al día. El periodo de tratamiento dura dos a cuatro semanas. Por vía vaginal, ponga la tableta vaginal en el fondo de la vagina a la hora de acostarse. Una vez al día, cada vez una tableta. |
| 剂型、规格<br>Formulaciones y especificaciones | 溶液：1%。乳膏：1%。凝胶：1%。阴道片：每片 100mg。<br>Loción; 1%; Crema: 1%. Gel: 1%. Tableta vaginal: 100mg/tableta. |
| **药品名称 Drug Names** | 酞丁安 Ftibamzona |
| 适应证<br>Indicaciones | 用于带状疱疹、单纯疱疹、尖锐湿疣、浅部真菌感染及各型沙眼等。<br>Se usa como auxiliar para el herpes zoster, herpes simplex, verrugas genitales, infecciones fúngicas superficiales, varios tipos del tracoma etc. |
| 用法、用量<br>Administración y dosis | 涂患处，一日 2～3 次，体癣、股癣连用 3 周，手足癣连用 4 周；滴眼，一次 1～2 滴，一日 3～4 次，连用 4 周。<br>Sólo para uso externo, 2 o 3 veces al día, uso constante de 3 semanas para la tiña corporal y la inguinal, 4 semanas para la tiña de manos y pies; gotas a los ojos, una vez 1 a 2 gotas, 3 a 4 veces al día, uso constante de 4 semanas. |
| 剂型、规格<br>Formulaciones y especificaciones | 软膏或乳膏：1%。搽剂：0.5%（5ml）。滴眼液：0.1%。<br>Ungüento o crema:1%.Linimento:0.5%(5ml).gotas para los ojos：0.1%. |
| **药品名称 Drug Names** | 克罗米通 Crotamitón |
| 适应证<br>Indicaciones | 用于治疗疥疮、皮肤瘙痒及继发性皮肤感染。<br>Se usa como auxiliar para la sarna, el prurito de la piel e infecciones secundarias de la piel. |

**续　表**

| 用法、用量<br>Administración y dosis | （1）疥疮：治疗前应洗澡并擦干，将本品从颈部以下涂搽全身皮肤，特别应涂搽在手足、指趾间、腋下和腹股沟；24小时后涂第2次，再隔48小时洗澡将药洗去，更换干净衣服和床单。必要时，1周后重复1次；也可一日涂搽1次，连续5～10日。<br>（2）瘙痒症：局部涂于患处，一日3次。<br>（3）脓性皮肤病：将患处用浸渍本品的敷料覆盖。<br><br>(1) Para la sarna: antes de aplicar el tratamiento, se bañe y seque completamente, aplique este medicamento desde el cuello hasta todo el cuerpo, con aplicación especial en las manos, pies, espacios entre los dedos y los dedos del pie, las axilas y la ingle; vuelva a aplicar después de 24 horas, tras 48 horas se bañe, cambie de ropa y sábana. En caso necesario, repite la aplicación una semana después; o aplique este medicamento una vez al día, uso continuo de 5 a 10 días.<br>(2) Para el prurito: que se aplica tópicamente a la zona afectada 3 veces al día.<br>(3) Para enfermedad purulenta de la piel: El área afectada se cubre con vendajes impregnados con este medicamento. |
|---|---|
| 剂型、规格<br>Formulaciones y especificaciones | 片剂：每片10mg；20mg。乳膏或软膏：0.025%；0.05%；0.1%。凝胶剂：0.05%。乙醇溶液：0.05～0.1%。<br><br>Tabletas: Cada tableta es de 10 mg; 20 mg. Crema o ungüento: 0.025%; 0.05%; 0.1%. Gel: 0.05%. Solución de etanol: 0.05 a 0.1%. |

| 药品名称 Drug Names | 维 A 酸 Tretinoína |
|---|---|
| 适应证<br>Indicaciones | 适用于寻常痤疮、扁平苔藓、白斑、毛发红糠疹和面部单纯糠疹。还用作银屑病的辅助治疗，亦用于治疗多发性寻常疣以及角化异常类的各种皮肤病如鱼鳞病、毛囊角化异常。<br><br>Se usa para el acné vulgar, liquen plano, la leucoplasia, la pitiriasis rubra pilaris y la pitiriasis facial simple. Se utiliza como tratamiento adyuvante de la psoriasis, también para el tratamiento de múltiples verrugas y varias dermatosis de queratosis anormal, tales como Ictiosis y queratosis folicular anormal. |
| 用法、用量<br>Administración y dosis | 口服：一日2～3次，一次10mg。外用0.025%乳膏或软膏治疗痤疮、单纯面部糠疹；0.1%乳膏或软膏治疗扁平苔藓、毛发红糠疹、白斑等皮肤病，一日涂药2次，或遵医嘱。<br><br>Oral: 2 a 3 veces al día, una vez 10mg. Tópico: 0.025% de crema o ungüento para el acné, la pitiriasis facial simple; 0,1% en crema o ungüento para el liquen plano, la pitiriasis rubra pilaris, la leucoplasia y otras dermatosis, frote 2 veces al día, o según las indicaciones. |
| 剂型、规格<br>Formulaciones y especificaciones | 片剂：每片10mg；20mg。软膏或乳膏：0.025%；0.05%；0.1%。凝胶：0.05%。乙醇溶液：0.05%～0.1%。<br><br>Tabletas: Cada tableta es de 10 mg; 20 mg. Ungüento o crema: 0.025%; 0.05%; 0.1%. Gel: 0.05%. solución de etanol: 0.05% a 0.1%. |

| 药品名称 Drug Names | 异维 A 酸 Isotretinoína |
|---|---|
| 适应证<br>Indicaciones | 用于其他药物治疗无效的严重痤疮，尤其是囊肿性痤疮及聚合性痤疮。<br><br>Se usa para el acné severo que los otros medicamentos utilizados se han resultado ineficaces, especialmente el acné quístico y acné conglobata. |
| 用法、用量<br>Administración y dosis | 口服：开始量为一日0.5mg/kg，4周后改用维持量，按每日0.1～1mg/kg计，视患者耐受性决定，但最高一日不超过1mg/kg。饭间或饭后服用，用量大时分次服用，一般16周为一疗程。如需要，停药8周后再进行下一疗程。局部外用：取适量涂于患处，每晚睡前涂一次。<br><br>Oral: volumen de inicio es 0.5mg/kg diario, 4 semanas después cambie a la dosis de mantenimiento, 0.1 ~ 1mg/kg al día, dependiendo de la tolerancia del paciente, pero no supera el máximo 1mg/kg diario. Tómelo con o después de la comida, en dosis divididas en cuanto necesita ingerir gran cantidad, por lo general 16 semanas consisten en un sólo tratamiento. Si es necesario, siga el siguiente curso 8 semanas después de detención de la medicación. Tópico: aplique en la zona afectada, frote una vez todas las noches antes de acostarse. |
| 剂型、规格<br>Formulaciones y especificaciones | 胶丸：每粒5mg；10mg。凝胶：0.05%。<br><br>Cápsulas: Cada una es de 5 mg; 10 mg. Gel: 0.05%. |

续 表

| 药品名称 Drug Names | 糠酸莫米松 Furoato de mometasona |
|---|---|
| 适应证<br>Indicaciones | 用于缓解对皮质激素有效的湿疹、接触性皮炎、特应性皮炎。神经性皮炎及皮肤瘙痒症等。<br>Se usa como auxiliar para el alivio del eczema, dermatitis por contacto, dermatitis atópica que son eficaces para los corticosteroides. Neurodermatitis y prurito en la piel. |
| 用法、用量<br>Administración y dosis | 涂患处，一日 1 次，不应封闭敷裹。<br>Aplique en la zona afectada, una vez al día, no se recomienda cubrirse cerrado. |
| 剂型、规格<br>Formulaciones y especificaciones | 乳膏或软膏：0.1%。<br>Crema o ungüento: 0.1%. |

19.4 眼科用药 Medicamentos oftálmicos

| 药品名称 Drug Names | 吡诺克辛 Pirenoxina |
|---|---|
| 适应证<br>Indicaciones | 用于老年性白内障、外伤性白内障、轻度糖尿病性白内障、并发性白内障和先天性白内障。<br>Se usa para catarata senil, catarata traumática, catarata diabética leve, catarata complicada y cataratas congénitas. |
| 用法、用量<br>Administración y dosis | 滴眼，用前摇匀，一日 3 ～ 5 次，一次 1 ～ 2 滴。<br>Gotas: agítelo bien antes de usar, 1 a 2 goteos una vez, 3 a 5 veces al día. |
| 剂型、规格<br>Formulaciones y especificaciones | 滴眼液：含药片 7.5mg，溶剂 15ml 溶解药片后，浓度为 0.005%。<br>Gotas: contienen comprimidos de 7.5 mg, cuando se disuelvan en disolvente de 15 ml, la concentración es de 0.005%. |

| 药品名称 Drug Names | 布林佐胺 Brinzolamida |
|---|---|
| 适应证<br>Indicaciones | 用于治疗原发性及继发性开角型青光眼和高眼压症。也可用于防止激光手术后的眼压升高。<br>Se usa para el glaucoma de ángulo abierto primario y secundario y la hipertensión ocular. También se puede utilizar para evitar que la presión intraocular se levante después de la cirugía láser. |
| 用法、用量<br>Administración y dosis | 用前摇匀，滴眼，一日 2 ～ 3 次，一次 1 滴，滴于结膜囊内，滴后用手指压迫眦泪囊部 3 ～ 5 分钟。<br>Agite bien antes de usar, gotas a los ojos, 1 goteo a la vez, 2 a 3 veces al día, gotee en el saco conjuntival, y luego presione con dedos en el saco lagrimal canthus 3 a 5 minutos. |
| 剂型、规格<br>Formulaciones y especificaciones | 滴眼液：每支 1%（5ml）。<br>Gotas: cada una es de 1% (5 ml). |

| 药品名称 Drug Names | 拉坦前列腺素 Latanoprost |
|---|---|
| 适应证<br>Indicaciones | 用于治疗青光眼、高眼压症和其他各种眼压升高。<br>Se usa como auxiliar para el glaucoma, hipertensión ocular y otros tipos de elevación de presión intraocular. |
| 用法、用量<br>Administración y dosis | 滴眼，一日一次，一次 1 滴，最好在睡前用。<br>Gotas: 1 goteo a la vez, una vez al día, será mejor utilizarlo antes de acostarse. |
| 剂型、规格<br>Formulaciones y especificaciones | 滴眼液：每支 125μg（2.5ml）。<br>Gotas: Cada uno es de 125μg (2.5 ml). |

| 药品名称 Drug Names | 托吡卡胺 Tropicamida |
|---|---|
| 适应证<br>Indicaciones | 用于散瞳检查眼底和散瞳验光。<br>Se usa para el examen del fondo de ojo dilatado y optometría dilatada. |

**续　表**

| | |
|---|---|
| 用法、用量<br>Administración y dosis | 滴眼，一次 1 滴，间隔 5 分钟滴第二次，即可满足散瞳检查之需。<br>Gotas: 1 goteo a la vez, cinco minutos después gotee otra vez, lo cual se puede satisfacer las necesidades de examen de ojos dilatados. |
| 剂型、规格<br>Formulaciones y especificaciones | 滴眼液：每支 0.25%（6ml）；0.5%（6ml）；1%（8ml）。<br>Gotas: cada uno es de 0.25% (6 ml); 0.5% (6 ml); 1% (8 ml). |
| **药品名称 Drug Names** | 玻璃酸钠 Hialuronato de sodio |
| 适应证<br>Indicaciones | 滴眼用于防治干眼症、眼疲劳、斯 - 约综合征等内因性疾病和术后药物性、外伤、光线对眼造成的刺激及戴软性接触镜引起的外因性疾病。眼科手术用其注射液。<br>Gotas: Se usa para la prevención y el tratamiento de las enfermedades internas tales como el ojo seco, la fatiga ocular, Síndrome de Stevens-Johnson, y las enfermedades exógenas que se causan por los medicamentos después de la cirugía, trauma, estimulación de la luz y el contacto con las lentillas. La inyección del medicamento se utiliza en la cirugía del ojo. |
| 用法、用量<br>Administración y dosis | 前房内注射，一次 0.5 ～ 0.75ml。滴眼，一日 4 ～ 6 次，一次 1 ～ 2 滴。<br>Inyección de la cámara anterior, 0.5 ~0.75 ml a la vez. Gotas, 1 a 2 gotas a la vez, 4 a 6 veces al día. |
| 剂型、规格<br>Formulaciones y especificaciones | 注射液：每支 5mg（0.5ml）。滴眼液：每支 0.1%（5ml）。<br>Inyección: Cada uno es de 5 mg (0.5 ml). Gotas: cada uno es de 0.1% (5 ml). |

19.5　耳鼻喉科和口腔科用药 Medicamentos para otorrinolaringologia y dental

| | |
|---|---|
| **药品名称 Drug Names** | 羟甲唑啉 Oximetazolina |
| 适应证<br>Indicaciones | 用于急性鼻炎、慢性单纯性鼻炎、慢性肥厚性鼻炎、变态反应性鼻炎（过敏性鼻炎）、鼻息肉、航空性鼻炎、航空性中耳炎、鼻出血、鼻阻塞性打喷嚏或其他鼻阻塞性疾病。<br>Se usa para rinitis aguda, rinitis crónica sencilla, rinitis hipertrófica crónica, rinitis alérgica, pólipos nasales, rinitis media aérea, otitis aérea, epistaxis, estornudo obstructivo nasal u otras enfermedades obstructivas nasales. |
| 用法、用量<br>Administración y dosis | 每揿定量为 0.065ml。将 1/4 喷头伸入鼻孔内，揿压喷鼻。成人和 6 岁以上儿童，一次一侧 1 ～ 3 喷，早晨和睡前各一次；或滴鼻，一日 2 ～ 3 次，一次 1 ～ 2 滴。若需长期用药，可采用连续用于 7 日停药一段时间在用药的间歇用药方式。<br>La cantidad de cada pulsación es de 0.065ml. Inserta una cuarta boquilla en la ventana de la nariz, deprima aerosol nasal. Adultos y niños mayores de 6 años, 1 a 3 echadas por cada lado por una vez, cada vez por la mañana y antes de acostarse; O gotas a la nariz, 1 a 2 gotas a la vez, 2 o 3 veces al día. En caso de la medicación a largo plazo, puede tomar el modo intermitente de la administración de medicamento, es decir, 7 días de medicación continua, a continuación, retención de medicamentos por un período, y luego vuelva a utilizarlo. |
| 剂型、规格<br>Formulaciones y especificaciones | 滴鼻剂：每支 1.5mg（3ml）；2.5mg（5ml）；5mg（10ml）。喷雾剂：每支 2.5mg（5ml）；5mg（10ml）。<br>Nasal: cada uno es de 1.5 mg (3 ml); 2.5 mg (5 ml); 5mg (10 ml). Atomozador: Cada uno es de 2.5 mg (5 ml), 5 mg (10 ml). |
| **药品名称 Drug Names** | 西地碘 Cidiodina |
| 适应证<br>Indicaciones | 用于治疗慢性咽喉炎、白念珠菌性口炎、口腔溃疡、慢性牙龈炎及糜烂扁平苔藓等。<br>Se usa para la laringitis crónica, estomatitis de candidiasis albicante, úlceras en la boca, la gingivitis crónica, liquen plano erosivo etc. |
| 用法、用量<br>Administración y dosis | 含化，一次 1.5mg，一日 3 ～ 5 次。<br>Fusión en la boca, 1.5 mg a la vez, 3 a 5 veces al día. |

**续 表**

| 剂型、规格<br>Formulaciones y especificaciones | 含片：每片 1.5mg。<br>Tabletas: Cada tableta es de 1.5 mg. |
|---|---|
| **药品名称 Drug Names** | **氯霉素滴耳液 Gotas para los oidos de cloranfenicol** |
| 适应证<br>Indicaciones | 用于外耳炎、中耳炎。<br>Se usa para la otitis externa, otitis media. |
| 用法、用量<br>Administración y dosis | 滴耳，一日 3 次。宜遮光保存。<br>Gotas a los oídos, 3 veces al día. Consérvese en lugar sombreado. |
| 剂型、规格<br>Formulaciones y especificaciones | 氯霉素 2g，乙醇 16ml，甘油加至 100ml。<br>2g de cloranfenicol, 16 ml de etanol, el glicerol se añade hasta 100 ml. |
| **药品名称 Drug Names** | **氧氟沙星滴耳液 Gotas para los oidos de ofloxacina** |
| 适应证<br>Indicaciones | 用于化脓性中耳炎。<br>Se usa para la otitis media supurativa. |
| 用法、用量<br>Administración y dosis | 耳浴，一日 1～2 次。<br>Baño de orejas, 1 a 2 veces al día. |
| 剂型、规格<br>Formulaciones y especificaciones | 氧氟沙星 0.3g，醋酸适量，甘油 20ml，乙醇（70%）加至 100ml。<br>0.3 g de ofloxacina, cantidad oportuna de ácido acético, 20 ml de glicerol, etanol (70%) se añade hasta 100 ml. |
| **药品名称 Drug Names** | **酚甘油滴耳剂 Gotas para los oidos de fenol-glicerol** |
| 适应证<br>Indicaciones | 有消炎杀菌及镇痛作用，用于急性及慢性中耳炎及外耳道炎。<br>Tiene los efectos anti-inflamatorio y analgésico, tanto para la otitis media aguda y crónica como para la otitis externa. |
| 用法、用量<br>Administración y dosis | 滴耳，一日 3 次。<br>Gotas a los oídos, 3 veces al día. |
| 剂型、规格<br>Formulaciones y especificaciones | 酚 2g，甘油加至 100ml。<br>2g de fenol, se añade glicerol hasta 100 ml. |
| **药品名称 Drug Names** | **硼酸滴耳液 Gotas para los oidos deácido bórico** |
| 适应证<br>Indicaciones | 用于慢性化脓性中耳炎。<br>Se usa para la otitis media supurativa crónica. |
| 用法、用量<br>Administración y dosis | 滴耳，一日 3 次。<br>Gotas a los oídos, 3 veces al día. |
| 剂型、规格<br>Formulaciones y especificaciones | 硼酸 2～3g，乙醇（70%）加至 100ml。<br>2～3g de ácido bórico, etanol (70%) se añade hasta 100 ml. |
| **药品名称 Drug Names** | **碳酸氢钠滴耳液 ( 耵聍液 )Gotas para los oídos de bicarbonato de sodio(líquidocerumen)** |
| 适应证<br>Indicaciones | 软化耵聍（耳垢）及冲洗耳道。<br>Se usa para ablandar el cerumen (la cerilla) y lavar el conducto auditivo. |

**续 表**

| 用法、用量<br>Administración y dosis | 滴耳，一日 3 次。每次用量要大，应将药液充满耳内。<br>Gotas a los oídos, 3 veces al día. Se recomienda una gran cantidad para cada vez, debe llenar toda la oreja con el líquido. |
|---|---|
| 剂型、规格<br>Formulaciones y especificaciones | 碳酸氢钠 5g，甘油 30ml，蒸馏水加至 100ml。<br>5 g de bicarbonato sódico, 30 ml de glicerol, se añade agua destilada hasta 100 ml. |

| 药品名称 Drug Names | 碘甘油 Iodoglicerina |
|---|---|
| 适应证<br>Indicaciones | 有防腐消毒作用，用于咽部慢性炎症及角化症，也可用于慢性萎缩性鼻炎。<br>Tiene los efectos anticorrosivo y desinfectante, se usa tanto para la inflamación crónica de la faringe como para rinitis atrófica crónica. |
| 用法、用量<br>Administración y dosis | 涂患处，一日 2 ～ 3 次。<br>Aplique sobre la zona afectada, 2 a 3 veces al día. |
| 剂型、规格<br>Formulaciones y especificaciones | 碘 2g，碘化钾 1g，甘油加至 100ml。<br>2 g del yodo, 1 g de yoduro de potasio, se añade glicerol hasta 100 ml. |

| 药品名称 Drug Names | 呋喃西林 / 盐酸麻黄碱滴鼻液 Gotas nasales de furacilina y clorhidrato deefedrina |
|---|---|
| 适应证<br>Indicaciones | 用于鼻炎或鼻黏膜肿胀。<br>Se usa para la rinitis y la hinchazón de la mucosa nasal. |
| 用法、用量<br>Administración y dosis | 滴鼻，一日 3 次，遮光保存。<br>Gotas a la nariz, 3 veces al día, consérvese en lugar sombreado. |
| 剂型、规格<br>Formulaciones y especificaciones | 盐酸麻黄碱 10g，羟苯乙酯 0.3g，0.01% 呋喃西林溶液加至 1000ml。<br>10g de clorhidrato de efedrina, 0.3g de etilparabeno, la solución de Nitrofurazone de concentración de 0.01% se añade hasta 1000ml. |

| 药品名称 Drug Names | 复方薄荷滴鼻液 Gotas nasales de compuesto de mentol |
|---|---|
| 适应证<br>Indicaciones | 用于干燥性鼻炎、萎缩性鼻炎、鼻出血，有除臭及滋养黏膜的作用。<br>Se usa para rinitis seca, rinitis atrófica y epistaxis, tiene los efectos desodorante y nutritivo para la mucosa. |
| 用法、用量<br>Administración y dosis | 滴鼻或涂鼻。<br>Gotas a la nariz o aplique a la nariz. |
| 剂型、规格<br>Formulaciones y especificaciones | 薄荷脑 1g，樟脑 1g，液状石蜡加至 100ml。<br>1g de mentol, 1 g de alcanfor, se añade parafina líquida hasta 100 ml. |

| 药品名称 Drug Names | 盐酸麻黄碱 滴鼻液 Gotas nasales de clorhidrato de efedrina |
|---|---|
| 适应证<br>Indicaciones | 有收缩血管作用，用于急性鼻炎、鼻窦炎、慢性肥大性鼻炎。<br>Se usa para rinitis aguda, sinusitis, y rinitis hipertrófica crónica como se auxilia a la vasoconstricción. |
| 用法、用量<br>Administración y dosis | 滴鼻，一日 3 次。<br>Gotas a la nariz, 3 veces al día. |
| 剂型、规格<br>Formulaciones y especificaciones | 盐酸麻黄碱 10g，氯化钠 0.6g，羟苯乙酯 0.03g，蒸馏水加至 1000ml。<br>10g de clorhidrato de efedrina, 0.6g de cloruro de sodio, 0.3g de etilparabeno, se añade agua destilada hasta 1000 ml. |

续　表

| 药品名称 Drug Names | 复方硼砂漱口片 Tabletas de Borax Compuesto(Gargarizar) |
|---|---|
| 适应证<br>Indicaciones | 用于口腔炎、咽喉炎及扁桃体炎等。<br>Se usa para estomatitis, faringitis y amigdalitis. |
| 用法、用量<br>Administración y<br>dosis | 一片加温开水一杯（60～90ml）溶后含漱，一日数次。<br>Haga gárgara de un vaso de agua templada (60~90ml) donde se haya derretido una tableta, varias veces al día. |
| 剂型、规格<br>Formulaciones y<br>especificaciones | 每片含：硼砂 0.324g，碳酸氢钠 0.162g，氯化钠 0.162g，麝香草酚 0.0032g。<br>Cada tableta contiene 0.324g de bórax, 0.162g de bicarbonato sódico, 0.162g de cloruro de sodio, y 0.0032g del timol. |

## 20. 其他类药物 Otros medicamentos

### 20.1　妇产科外用药 Medicamentos topica para ginecología y obstetricia

| 药品名称 Drug Names | 硝呋太尔制霉素阴道软胶囊 Nifuratel/Nistatina(Para uso vaginal) |
|---|---|
| 适应证<br>Indicaciones | 硝呋太尔制霉素在体外具有抗真菌、抗滴虫、抗细菌的广谱活性。用于细菌性阴道病、滴虫性阴道炎、念珠菌性外阴阴道炎、阴道混合感染。<br>Nifuratel nistatina in vitro tiene amplio espectro de actividad tales como anti-hongos, anti-tricomoniasis y anti-bacterial. Se usa para la vaginosis bacteriana, tricomoniasis vaginal, candidiasis vulvovaginal y las infecciones mixtas vaginales. |
| 用法、用量<br>Administración y<br>dosis | 阴道给药，每晚一粒，连用 6 日。亦可遵医嘱调整。<br>Aplique en la vagina, cada noche una tableta, uso continuo de 6 días. También se puede ajustar de acuerdo con el consejo del médico. |
| 剂型、规格<br>Formulaciones y<br>especificaciones | 每粒含硝呋太尔 0.5g，制霉素 20 万 U。<br>Cada tableta contiene 0.5g de nifuratel y20 mil unidades de nistatina. |

### 20.2　解毒药 Antídoto

| 药品名称 Drug Names | 谷胱甘肽 Glutatión |
|---|---|
| 适应证<br>Indicaciones | 临床上用于：①解毒：对丙烯腈、氟化物、一氧化碳、重金属及有机溶剂等的中毒均有解毒作用。对红细胞膜有保护作用，故防止溶血，从而减少高铁血红蛋白。②对某些损伤的保护作用：由于放射线治疗、放射性药物或由于使用肿瘤药物所引起白细胞减少症及由于放射线引起的骨髓组织炎症，本品均可改善其症状。③保护肝脏：能抑制脂肪肝的形成，也能改善中毒性肝炎和感染性肝炎的症状。④抗过敏：能纠正乙酰胆碱、胆碱酯酶的不平衡，从而消除由于 这种不平衡所引起的过敏症状。⑤改善某些疾病的症状：对缺氧血症的不适、恶心、呕吐、瘙痒等症状及由于肝脏疾病引起的其他症状，均有改善作用。⑥防止皮肤色素沉着：可防止新的黑色素形成并减少其氧化。⑦眼科疾病：可抑制晶体蛋白质巯基的不稳定，因而可以抑制进行性白内障及控制角膜及视网膜疾病的发展等。<br>Se usa para el tratamiento clínico de: ① desintoxicación: puede desintoxicar a los envenenamientos del acrilonitrilo, el fluoruro, el monóxido de carbón, los metales pesados y los disolventes orgánicos. Protegiendo a los eritrocitos, a través de evitar la hemólisis, reduce las metahemoglobinas. ② Protección a unos ciertos daños: puede mejorar los síntomas de la leucopenia causada por la terapia de radiación, los radiofármacos o uso de medicamentos para el cáncer, y los síntomas de la inflamación de tejido óseo causada por la radiación. ③ Protección al hígado: puede inhibir la formación de hígado graso, también puede mejorar los síntomas de la hepatitis tóxica y la hepatitis infecciosa. ④ contra alergia: Puede corregir el desequilibrio entre la acetilcolina y la colinesterasa, por lo tanto eliminar los síntomas de la alergia causados por este desequilibrio. ⑤ Mejoramiento de los síntomas de ciertas enfermedades: los síntomas de la anoxemia, tales como el malestar, náuseas, vómitos, pruritos, y otros síntomas causados por la enfermedad de hígado. ⑥ Prevención de la pigmentación de la piel: puede prevenir la formación de la melanina nueva y reducir su oxidación. ⑦ Enfermedades de los ojos: puede suprimir la inestabilidad de tiol de proteínas cristalinas, por lo tanto puede suprimir la catarata y controlar el desarrollo de enfermedades de la córnea y la retina. |

**续 表**

| | |
|---|---|
| 用法、用量<br>Administración y dosis | 肌内或静脉注射，用本品注射剂所附的 2ml 维生素 C 注射液溶解后使用。肝病患者一般 30 日为一个疗程，其他情况根据病情决定。滴眼，一次 1 ～ 2 滴，一日 4 ～ 8 次。<br><br>La inyección intramuscular o intravenosa, se usa después de la disolución de la adjunta inyección de la vitamina C de 2 ml. Para los pacientes hepáticos, generalmente 30 días consisten en un curso de tratamiento, en otros casos depende de la condición de la enfermedad. Gotas a los ojos, 1 a 2 gotas a la vez, 4 ～ 8 veces al día. |
| 剂型、规格<br>Formulaciones y especificaciones | 注射剂：每支 300mg；600mg。<br>Inyección: Cada una es de 300 mg; 600 mg. |
| 药品名称 Drug Names | 二巯丙醇 Dimercaprol |
| 适应证<br>Indicaciones | 对砷、汞及金的中毒有解救作用，但治疗慢性汞中毒效果差。对锑中毒的作用因锑化合物的不同而异，它能够减轻酒石酸锑钾的毒性而能增加锑波芬与新斯锑波散等的毒性。能减轻镉对肺的损害，故使用时要注意掌握。它还能减轻发泡性砷化合物战争毒气所引起的损害。<br><br>Puede desintoxicar a los envenenamientos del arsénico, el mercurio y el oro, pero resulta poco eficaz para la intoxicación crónica de mercurio. Y los efectos al envenenamiento de antimonio varían según los compuestos de antimonio. Puede reducir la toxicidad de tartrato potásico de antimonio mientras tanto aumentar la toxicidad del estibofeno y onda dispersada de Antimonio Neostigmina. Puede reducir el daño que el cadmio dé a los pulmones, por lo que tenga en cuenta la cantidad de uso. También puede aliviar el daño causado por el gas de guerra química tales como los compuestos de arsénico espumosos. |
| 用法、用量<br>Administración y dosis | 成人，肌内注射，按体重 2 ～ 3mg/kg，最初 2 日，每 4 小时注射 1 次。第三日，每 6 小时注射一次，以后每 12 小时注射 1 次，一个疗程为 10 日。小儿用量同成人。治疗小儿铅脑病，与依地酸钙钠同用。<br><br>Para los adultos, inyección intramuscular, 2 ~ 3mg/kg de acuerdo al peso corporal. En los primeros 2 días, haga 1 inyección por cada 4 horas, en el tercer día, 1 inyección por cada 6 horas, después 1 inyección cada 12 horas, completamente 10 días consisten en un curso de tratamiento. Para los niños la cantidad es la misma. También se usa como el tratamiento para niños con encefalopatía por plomo, junto con el uso de calcio edetato de sodio. |
| 剂型、规格<br>Formulaciones y especificaciones | 注射液：每支 0.1g/1ml，0.2g/ml。<br>Inyección: Cada una es de 0.1g/1ml, 0.2g/ml. |
| 药品名称 Drug Names | 二巯丁二钠 Dimercaptosuccinato sodio |
| 适应证<br>Indicaciones | 用于治疗锑、铅、汞、砷、铜的中毒（治疗汞中毒的效果不如二巯丙磺钠）及预防镉、钴、镍中毒，对肝豆状核变性病有驱铜及减轻症状的作用。<br><br>Se usa como el tratamiento de los envenenamientos del antimonio, plomo, mercurio, arsénico y cobre (para el envenenamiento de mercurio es menos eficaz que sodio dimercapto sulfonato) y la prevención de los envenenamientos del cadmio, cobalto, níquel, tiene los efectos de decopper y aliviar los síntomas para la enfermedad de Wilson o degeneración hepatolenticular. |
| 用法、用量<br>Administración y dosis | （1）成人解毒：1g，临用时配成 10% 溶液，立即缓慢静脉注射，10 ～ 15 分钟注射完毕。<br>（2）急性锑中毒引起的心律失常：本品首次剂量为 2g，用 5% 葡萄糖液 20ml 溶解后，静脉缓慢注射。以后每小时 1g，共 4 ～ 5 次。用于亚急性金属中毒：每次 1g，一日 2 ～ 3 次，共用 3 ～ 5 日。用于慢性中毒，一日 1g，共 5 ～ 7 日，或一日 1g，连续 3 日，停药 4 日为一疗程，按病情可用 2 ～ 4 疗程。<br>（3）小儿常用量：按体重 20mg/kg。<br><br>(1) Desintoxicación para los adultos: 1 g, justamente antes de usarlo se combine con una solución de la concentración de 10%, haga la inyección intravenosa lenta de inmediato, la cual dure 10 a 15 minutos.<br>(2) la arritmia provocada por la intoxicación aguda de antimonio: por la primera vez la dosis es de 2g, se combine con 20ml de la solución de glucosa con la concentración de 5%, haga la inyección intravenosa lenta. Después 1g por cada hora, totalmente son 4 o 5 veces. Se usa para la intoxicación subaguda de metal, 1g por cada vez, 2 o 3 veces al día, totalmente 3 a 5 días. Se usa para la intoxicación crónica, 1g al día, totalmente 5 a 7 días, o 1g al día, uso continuo de 3 días, retirada de 4 días, lo cual consiste en un curso de tratamiento, puede tomar 2 a 4 cursos de tratamiento de acuerdo con la condición de la enfermedad.<br>(3) la dosis normal para los niños: 20mg/kg de acuerdo con el peso corporal. |

**续　表**

| | |
|---|---|
| 剂型、规格<br>Formulaciones y especificaciones | 注射剂：每支：0.5g；1g。<br>Inyección: Cada una es de 0.5 g; 1g. |
| 药品名称 Drug Names | 去铁胺 Deferoxamina |
| 适应证<br>Indicaciones | 本品主要用于急性铁中毒和海洋性贫血、铁粒幼细胞贫血、溶血性贫血、再生障碍性贫血或其他慢性贫血，因反复输血引起的继发性含铁血黄素沉着症；亦用于特发性血色病有放血禁忌症者。对慢性肾衰竭伴有铝过量负荷引起的脑病、骨病和贫血，在进行透析过程中亦可应用。本品还可用作铁负荷试验。<br><br>Se usa principalmente para la intoxicación aguda por hierro, la talasemia, la anemia sideroblástica, la anemia hemolítica, la anemia aplásica y otras anemias crónicas, y la hemosiderosis secundaria provocada por las transfusiones de sangre repetidas. También se usa para hemocromatosis idiopática y las contraindicaciones de sangría. Para la encefalopatía, enfermedad ósea y anemia provocadas por la insuficiencia renal crónica asociada con la sobrecarga de aluminio, se puede aplicar durante el proceso de diálisis. También se utiliza en la prueba de carga de hierro. |
| 用法、用量<br>Administración y dosis | （1）成人：①急性铁中毒：肌内注射，首次 0.5～1g，隔 4 小时 0.5g，共 2 次，以后根据病情 4～12 小时 1 次，24 小时总量不超过 6g。静脉滴注，一次 0.5g，加入 5%～10% 葡萄糖注射液 50～500ml 中滴注，滴注速度，按体重 1 小时不超过 15mg/kg，24 小时总量不超过 90mg/kg。②慢性铁负荷过量，肌内注射，一日 0.5～1g。腹壁皮下注射，按体重 20～40mg/kg，8～24 小时，以微型泵作动力。<br>（2）小儿：①急性铁中毒：按体重一次 20mg/kg。②慢性铁负荷过量，按体重一日 10mg/kg，腹壁皮下注射，8～12 小时或 24 小时，用微型泵作动力。③慢性肾衰伴铁负荷过量：按体重 20mg/kg，1 周 1～2 次，在透析初 2 小时通过动脉导管滴注，1 周总量一般不超过 6g。铁负荷试验：成人肌肉注射本品 0.5g。注射前，排空膀胱内剩余尿，注射后留 6 小时尿。尿铁超过 1mg，提示有过量铁负荷；超过 1.5mg，对机体可引起病理性损害。<br><br>(1) para los adultos: ① la intoxicación aguda por hierro, haga la inyección intramuscular, 0.5g a 1g por la primera vez, 4 horas después 0.5g, completamente son 2 veces, en el futuro 4 a 12 horas por cada vez según la condición de la enfermedad, en 24 horas la dosis total no debe superar 6g. La infusión intravenosa, 0.5g por cada vez, se añade 50 a 500 ml de la inyección de glucosa, de acuerdo con el peso corporal la velocidad de infusión no supera 15mg/kg por hora, en 24 horas la dosis total no supera 90mg/kg. ② sobrecarga crónica de hierro, haga la inyección intramuscular, 0.5 a 1g al día. Hágalo en el subcutánea abdominal, de acuerdo con el peso corporal 20~40mg/kg, 8 a 24 horas, tome los microbombas como poder.<br>(2) para los niños: ① la intoxicación aguda por hierro, de acuerdo con el peso corporal cada vez 20mg/kg. ② sobrecarga crónica de hierro, de acuerdo con el peso corporal 10mg/kg al día, inyección subcutánea en la pared abdominal, 8 a 12 horas o 24 horas, inyección de microbombas. ③ Insuficiencia renal crónica con sobrecarga de hierro: administración según peso corporal 20mg/kg, 1 a 2 veces a la semana, haga la infusión por ductus arterioso en las primeras 2 horas después de la diálisis, normalmente la dosis total de una semana no supera 6g. En la prueba de carga de hierro, haga la inyección intramuscular 0.5g para los adultos. Después de la inyección, orina todo en la vejiga, permanezca la orina 6 horas después de la inyección. Si el hierro en la orina supera de 1 mg, lo que sugiere una sobrecarga de hierro; si excede de 1.5 mg, puede causar daños patológicos al cuerpo. |
| 剂型、规格<br>Formulaciones y especificaciones | 注射剂：0.5g。<br>Inyección: 0.5g. |
| 药品名称 Drug Names | 碘解磷定 Pralidoxima yoduro |
| 适应证<br>Indicaciones | 有机磷中毒。<br>Intoxicación por organofosforados. |
| 用法、用量<br>Administración y dosis | （1）治疗轻度中毒：成人 0.4～0.8g/ 次，以葡萄糖液或生理盐水稀释后静脉滴注或缓慢静脉注射，必要时 2～4 小时重复一次。小儿 1 次 15mg/kg。<br>（2）治疗中度中毒：成人首次 0.8～1.6g，缓慢静注，以后每 1 小时重复 0.4～0.8g，肌颤缓解和血液胆碱酯酶活性恢复至正常的 60% 以上后酌情减量或停药。或以静脉滴注给药维持，每小时给 0.4g，共 4～6 次。小儿 1 次 20～30mg/kg。 |

| | |
|---|---|
| **续 表** | |
| | （3）治疗重度中毒：成人首次用 1.6～2.4g，缓慢静脉注射，以后每小时重复 0.8～1.6g，肌颤缓解和血液胆碱酯酶活性恢复至正常以后的 60% 以上后酌情减量或停药。小儿 1 次 30mg/kg。 |
| | (1) Para la intoxicación leve: para los adultos 0.4 a 0.8g cada vez, haga la infusión intravenosa o la inyección intravenosa lenta con la combinación diluida por la solución de glucosa o suero fisiológico, en caso necesario repítalo 2 a 4 horas después. Para los niños 15 mg/kg una vez. |
| | (2) Para la intoxicación moderada: para los adultos por la primera vez, haga la inyección intravenosa lenta de 0.8 a 1.6g, después cada hora repita 0.4 a 0.8g, cuando el alivio de temblores musculares y la actividad de colinesterasa en la sangre regresen a 60% por encima de lo normal, puede reducir o retirar el medicamento según la situación. O haga la infusión intravenosa como la administración, 0.4g por hora, completamente 4 a 6 veces. Para los niños 20 a 30mg/kg cada vez. |
| | (3) Para la intoxicación grave: para los adultos por la primera vez aplique 1.6 a 2.4g, haga la inyección intravenosa lenta, después repita 0.8 a 1.6g por hora, cuando el alivio de temblores musculares y la actividad de colinesterasa en la sangre regresen a 60% por encima de lo normal, puede reducir o retirar el medicamento según la situación. Para los niños 30mg/kg cada vez. |
| 剂型、规格<br>Formulaciones y especificaciones | 注射剂：每支 0.4g；注射液 0.4g/10ml。<br><br>Inyección: cada una es de 0.4g; solución inyectable: cada una es de 0.4 g/10ml. |
| **药品名称 Drug Names** | 氯解磷定 Cloruro pralidoxima |
| 适应证<br>Indicaciones | 有机磷中毒。<br><br>Intoxicación por organofosforados. |
| 用法、用量<br>Administración y dosis | （1）成人：①轻度中毒：0.5～0.75g 肌内注射，必要时 1 小时后重复一次。②中度中毒：首次 0.75～1.5g，肌注或稀释后缓慢静注，以后每小时重复以后每小时重复 0.5～1.0g，肌颤消失或胆碱酯酶活性恢复至正常的 60% 以上后酌情减量或停药。③重度中毒：成人首次用 1.5～2.5g 分两处肌注或稀释后缓慢静脉注射，以后每 0.5～1 小时重复 1.0～1.5g，肌颤消失或血液胆碱酯酶活性恢复至正常以后的 60% 以上后酌情减量或停药。<br><br>（2）小儿：用法与成人同，①轻度中毒：按体重 15～20mg/kg；②中度中毒：按体重 20～30mg/kg；③重度中毒：按体重 30mg/kg。<br><br>(1) Para los adultos: ① intoxicación leve: haga la inyección intramuscular de 0.5 a 0.75g, si es necesario, repítalo después de una hora. ② intoxicación moderada: por la primera vez 0.75 a 1.5g, haga la inyección intramuscular o la intravenosa lenta después de dilución, después repita 0.5 a 1.0g por hora, cuando el alivio de temblores musculares y la actividad de colinesterasa en la sangre regresen a 60% por encima de lo normal, puede reducir o retirar el medicamento según la situación. ③ intoxicación grave: por la primera haga la inyección intramuscular en 2 diferentes lugares o la intravenosa lenta después de dilución, después cada media o 1 hora repita 1.0 a 1.5g, cuando el alivio de temblores musculares y la actividad de colinesterasa en la sangre regresen a 60% por encima de lo normal, puede reducir o retirar el medicamento según la situación.<br><br>(2) Para los niños: la aplicación es la mismo con la de los adultos, ① intoxicación leve: de acuerdo con el peso corporal 15 a 20 mg/kg; ② intoxicación moderada: de acuerdo con el peso corporal 20 a 30mg/kg. ③ intoxicación grave: de acuerdo con el peso corporal 30mg/kg. |
| 剂型、规格<br>Formulaciones y especificaciones | 注射液：0.5g/2ml。<br><br>solución inyectable: cada una es de 0.5 g/2ml. |
| **药品名称 Drug Names** | 阿托品 Atropina |
| 适应证<br>Indicaciones | 做解毒药使用时：①治疗有机磷类（包括有机磷农药及军用神经性毒剂）与氨基甲酸酯类农药中毒。应与胆碱酯酶复活剂合用，单独使用效果差（除西维因中毒外）。②治疗胃肠型毒蕈（如捕蝇蕈）中毒。③治疗中药乌头中毒。④治疗锑剂中毒引起的心律失常与钙通道阻滞剂引起的心动过缓。<br><br>Cuando se usa como antídoto: ① para el envenenamiento de fósforo orgánico (incluidos los Plaguicidas organofosforados y agentes nerviosos militares) y las intoxicaciones por pesticidas carbamatos. Debe utilizarse en combinación con el revivificador de la colinesterasa, tiene pobre efecto cuando se usa solamente (excepto envenenamiento del Carbaryl). ② para el envenemiento de seta venenosa gastrointestinal (por ejemplo Amanita muscaria). ③ para el envenenamiento de Aconitum ④ para la arritmia caucada por el envenenamiento del agente de antimonio y la bradicardia provocada por antagonistas del calcio. |

**续　表**

| | |
|---|---|
| 用法、用量<br>Administración y<br>dosis | 静脉注射或静脉点滴。<br>（1）成人：①治疗有机磷中毒：首次，轻度中毒，2.0～4.0mg；中度中毒，4.0～10mg；重度中毒，10～20mg。重复用药剂量为其半数，重复的次数依病情而异，达到阿托品化后减量或改用维持量。②治疗氨基甲酸酯类农药中毒，根据病情给药，首次应给足量，用量范围为0.5～3.0mg，经口严重中毒可用5mg；如毒蕈碱症状未消失，可重复给0.5～1mg，除经口严重中毒外，一般不需达到阿托品化。③治疗锑剂中毒引起的阿-斯综合征，立即静脉注射1.0～2.0mg，15～30分钟后在注射1mg。④治疗乌头中毒及钙拮抗剂过量，按消化系统用药的用量给药，一次0.5～1mg，肌内注射，1～4小时一次，至中毒症状缓解为止。<br>（2）小儿：用量可根据体重折算，用法与成人同。<br>Haga la inyección intravenosa o la infusión intravenosa.<br>(1) para los adultos: ① para la intoxicación por organofosforados: por la primera vez, intoxicación leve, 2.0 a 4.0mg; intoxicación moderada, 4.0 a 10mg; intoxicación grave, 10 a 20mg. La dosis de los medicamentos de repetición es la mitad de la primera vez, las veces repetidas dependen de la condición de la enfermedad, reduzca la dosis o mantenga la misma cuando aparezca los rendimientos de atropinalización. ② para la Intoxicación por plaguicidas carbamatos. Haga la administración según la enfermedad, por la primera vez debe aplicar la dosis suficiente, cuya categoría es de 0.5 a 3mg, puede utilizar 5g para la intoxicación grave por la boca; Si los síntomas de muscarina no desaparecen, repita 0,5～1mg, normalmente no hace falta llegar a la atropinalización excepto la intoxicación grave por la boca. ③ para el síndrome de Adams-Stokes provocado por el envenenamiento del agente de antimonio, haga la inyección intravenosa inmediatamente 1,0 a 2,0 mg, 15～30 minutos después haga otra de 1 mg. ④ para el envenenamiento de Aconitum y el exceso de los antagonistas del calcio, la cantidad de medicamento administrado se decide por el sistema digestivo, 0.5 a 1mg por cada vez, haga la inyección intramuscular, 1 a 4 horas por cada vez, hasta que los síntomas de intoxicación se alivien.<br>(2)para los niños: la cantidad puede ser calculada de acuerdo con el peso corporal, el uso se comparte con el para los adultos. |
| 剂型、规格<br>Formulaciones y<br>especificaciones | 注射液：每支0.5mg/1ml；1mg/2ml；5mg/1ml。<br>Inyección: Cada 0.5mg/1ml; 1mg/2ml; 5mg/1ml. |
| **药品名称Drug Names** | 东莨菪碱 Escopolamina |
| 适应证<br>Indicaciones | 有机磷农药类中毒的治疗。<br>Se usa como el tratamiento para las intoxicaciones por plaguicidas organofosforados |
| 用法、用量<br>Administración y<br>dosis | 成人首次为：轻度中毒：0.3～0.5mg；中度中毒：0.5～1.0mg；重度中毒：2.0～4.0mg。重复用药量0.3～0.6mg。<br>Para los adultos por la primera vez: envenenamiento leve: 0.3 a 0.5 mg; envenenamiento moederado: 0.3 a 0.5 mg; Envenenamiento grave: 2.0 a 4.0 mg. La dosis de la repetición es de 0.3 a 0.6g. |
| 剂型、规格<br>Formulaciones y<br>especificaciones | 注射液：1ml：0.3mg；1mg：0.5mg。<br>Solución inyectable: 1ml：0.3mg；1mg：0.5mg. |
| **药品名称Drug Names** | 亚甲蓝 Cloruro de metiltioninio |
| 适应证<br>Indicaciones | （1）治疗亚硝酸盐及苯胺类引起的中毒。<br>（2）治疗氰化物中毒。<br>(1) para la intoxicación del nitrito y la anilina.<br>(2) para la intoxicación por cianuro. |
| 用法、用量<br>Administración y<br>dosis | （1）治疗亚硝酸盐中毒：用1%溶液5～10ml（1～2mg/kg），稀释于25%葡萄糖溶液20～40ml中，缓慢静脉注射（10分钟注完）。若注射后30～60分钟发绀不消退，可重复注射首次剂量宜同前。3～4小时后，根据病情还可注射半量。若口服本品，可用150～250mg，每4小时1次。<br>（2）治疗氰化物中毒用1%溶液50～100ml（5～10mg/kg），以25%葡萄糖溶液稀释后缓慢注射，尔后，再注入25%硫代硫酸钠20～40ml。严重者二者交替使用。 |

**续 表**

| | |
|---|---|
| | (1) Se usa para la intoxicación por nitritos: se diluye la solución de 1% de 5 ~ 10ml (1 ~ 2mg/kg) en solución de glucosa de 25% de 20~40ml, haga la inyección intravenosa lenta (termínalo en 10 minutos). Si la cianosis no remite 30 a 60 minutos después de la inyección, puede repetir la dosis de la primera vez. 3 o 4 horas después, puede tomar media dosis de inyección según la enfermedad. Si toma la administración oral, puede utilizar 150 a 250mg por cada 4 horas.<br><br>(2) para la intoxicación por cianuro, después de la dilución de la solución de 1% de 50~100ml (5~10mg/kg) con la solución de glucosa de 25%, haga la inyección lenta, más tarde, se inyecta la solución del tiosulfato de sodio de 25% 20 ~ 40 ml. En los casos graves, los dos se utilizan indistintamente. |
| 剂型、规格<br>Formulaciones y especificaciones | 注射液：20mg/2ml。<br>Solución inyectable: 20mg/2ml. |
| 药品名称 Drug Names | 硫代硫酸钠 Tiosulfato de sodio |
| 适应证<br>Indicaciones | ①抢救氰化物中毒。②抗过敏。③治疗降压药硝普钠过量中毒。④治疗可溶性钡盐（如硝酸钡）中毒。⑤治疗砷、汞、铋、铅等金属中毒。<br><br>① el rescate del envenenamiento por cianuro. ② alergia.  ③ la intoxicación por el excesivo de nitroprusiato.  ④ el envenenamiento de sal de bario soluble, por ejemplo el nitrato de bario.  ⑤ los envenenamientos por metales, tales como el arsénico, mercurio, bismuto y plomo. |
| 用法、用量<br>Administración y dosis | （1）成人：①抢救氰化物中毒：由于本品解毒作用较慢，须先用作用迅速的亚硝酸钠、亚硝酸异戊酯或亚甲蓝，然后缓慢静脉注射 10 ~ 30g（25% ~ 50% 溶液 40 ~ 60ml），每分钟 5ml 以下。必要时，1 小时后再与高铁血红蛋白形成剂合用半量至全量。口服中毒者，还须用 5% 溶液洗胃，洗后留本品溶液适量于胃内。②硝普钠过量中毒：单独使用 25% 溶液 20 ~ 40ml，缓慢静脉注射。③可溶性钡盐中毒：缓慢静脉注射 25% 溶液 20 ~ 40ml。④治疗砷、汞铋。铅等金属中毒：静脉注射，0.5 ~ 1.0g/ 次。⑤抗过敏：0.5 ~ 1.0g（5%10 ~ 20ml）静脉注射，一日一次，10 ~ 14 日为一疗程。<br><br>（2）小儿：按体重计算，25% 溶液 1.0 ~ 1.5ml/kg（250 ~ 375mg/kg）。<br><br>(1) para los adultos:  ① para el rescate del envenenamiento por cianuro: como este medicamento tiene su efecto de desintoxicación muy lenta, es necesario utilizar primero el nitrito de sodio, el nitrito de amilo y el cloruro de metiltioninio, los cuales tienen una eficacia rápida. Y luego haga la inyección intravenosa lenta de 10 ~ 30g (solución al 25% ~ 50% de 40 ~ 60 ml), 5 ml por minuto o menos. En caso necesario, se combina con el agente formador de la metahemoglobina a la mitad de la dosis o la entera una hora después. En caso del envenenamiento oral, hace falta el lavado gástrico con la solución 5%, dejando una cierta cantidad de solución en el estómago. ② sobredosis de nitroprusiato de sodio: use sólo la solución de 25% de 20 ~ 40 ml, inyecte lentamente por la vena. ③ el envenenamiento por sal de bario soluble:haga la inyección intravenosa lenta de 25% de 20 ~ 40 ml. ④ para el envenenamiento por metales, tales como el arsénico, mercurio, bismuto y plomo:haga la inyección intravenosa, 0.5 ~ 1.0g cada vez. ⑤ contra la alergia: 0.5 ~ 1.0 g (5% 10 ~ 20 ml) de inyección intravenosa, una vez al día, 10 a 14 días consisten en un curso de tratamiento.<br><br>(2) para los niños: se calcule de acuerdo con el peso corporal, solución de 25% de 1.0 ~ 1.5ml/kg (250 ~ 375mg/kg). |
| 剂型、规格<br>Formulaciones y especificaciones | 注射用硫代硫酸钠：有无水物 0.32g（相当于含结晶水者 0.5g），无水物 0.64g（相当于含结晶水者 1.0g）；注射液：每支 0.5g/10ml，1.0g/20ml。<br><br>Tiosulfato de sodio para la inyección: contiene 0.32g de sustancia anhidra(equivalente a 0.5g de sustancia con agua de cristalización), contiene 0.64g de sustancia anhidra(equivalente a 1.0g de sustancia con agua de cristalización); solución inyectable: cada una es de 0.5g/10ml, 1.0g/20ml. |
| 药品名称 Drug Names | 亚硝酸钠 Nitrito de sodio |
| 适应证<br>Indicaciones | 治疗氰化物中毒及硫化氢中毒。<br>Se usa para la intoxicación por el cianuro y el sulfuro de hidrógeno. |
| 用法、用量<br>Administración y dosis | （1）成人，静脉注射：每次 3% 溶液 10 ~ 15ml（或 6 ~ 12mg/kg），注射速度宜慢（按 2ml/mim）。和用氯化钠注射液稀释至 100ml 后静脉注射（5 ~ 20 分钟），随后静脉注射 25% 硫代硫酸钠 40ml（硫化氢中毒不需要注射硫代硫酸钠）。必要时，0.5 ~ 1 小时后可重复给半量或全量。 |

**续　表**

（2）小儿：按体重 3% 溶液 0.15 ～ 0.3mg/kg。本品 3% 溶液，仅供静脉注射用，每次 10 ～ 20ml，每分钟注射 2 ～ 3ml；需要时在 1 小时后重复半量或全量。

(1) para los adultos, haga la inyección intravenosa: Cada vez use la solución de 3% de 10 ～ 15 ml (o 6 ～ 12mg/kg), con una velocidad lenta (2ml/min). Inyecte por la vena 5 a 20 minutos con la disolución de 1000ml de ésta con la solución de cloruro de sodio, más tarde inyecta por la vena tiosulfato de sodio de 25% de 40ml (no hace falta la inyección de tiosulfato de sodio para la intoxicación por el sulfuro de hidrógeno). En caso necesario, 0.5 a 1 hora, o se puede repetir la mitad de la cantidad o la total después de media o 1 hora.

(2) para los niños: multiplique el peso corporal con la disolución de 3% de 0.15~0.3mg/kg. La solución de 3% sólo se usa para la inyección intravenosa, 10 ～ 20 ml por cada vez, 2 ～ 3 ml por minuto. Se reitera la mitad o toda la cantidad o después de 1 hora cuando se necesite.

| | |
|---|---|
| 剂型、规格<br>Formulaciones y especificaciones | 注射液：0.3g/10ml。<br>Solución inyectable: 0.3g/10ml. |
| **药品名称 Drug Names** | 氟马西尼 Flumazenil |
| 适应证<br>Indicaciones | 苯二氮䓬类药物之中毒解救。也可用于乙醇中毒之解救。<br>Se usa para el rescate del envenenamiento de tanto benzodiacepina como el etanol. |
| 用法、用量<br>Administración y dosis | 成人常用量 0.5 ～ 2mg，静脉注射。小儿常用量：0.01mg/kg，静脉注射。最大剂量 1mg。①麻醉后：因苯二氮䓬类常用于术前的麻醉诱导和术中的麻醉维持。本药则于术后使用，以终止 BZD 类的镇静作用。开始用量是 15 秒内缓慢静脉注射 0.2mg，如 30 秒内尚未清醒，可再注射 0.1 ～ 0.3mg，必要时，60 秒重复一次，直至总量达 3mg 为止。通常使用 0.3 ～ 0.6mg 即可。②急救：对原因不明的神志丧失患者，可用本品来鉴别是否为苯二氮䓬类所致，如反复给药也不能使意识或呼吸功能改善，则可判定为非苯二氮䓬类所致。开始用量是 0.2mg，以氯化钠注射液或 5% 葡萄糖注射液稀释后静脉注射；重复给药每次增加 0.1mg，或每小时 0.1 ～ 0.4mg/h，滴速个体化，直至清醒为止。<br><br>Dosis habitual para adultos es de 0.5 ～ 2 mg, inyección intravenosa. Dosis usual para niños: 0.01mg/kg, inyección intravenosa, la dosis máxima de 1 mg. ① Después de la anestesia: como las benzodiacepinas se usan con frecuencia en la inducción de la anestesia preoperatoria y el mantenimiento de la anestesia en cirugía. Este medicamento se usa después de la cirugía, para terminar la sedación de BZD. La dosis del incio es inyección intravenosa lenta de 0.2mg en 15 segundos. Si aún no despierta en 30 segundos, puede volver a la inyección de 0.1 ～ 0.3 mg. Si es necesario, repítalo cada 60 segundos, hasta que llegue la cantidad total de 3 mg. Por lo general, se usa 0.3 ～ 0.6 mg. ② Primeros auxilios: Para los pacientes desmayados por causa inexplicable, puede utilizarse para identificar si es provocado por las benzodiacepinas. Si la administración repetida no puede mejorar la función respiratoria, se puede determinar la razón real no es las benzodiazepinas. La dosis en el principio es de 0.2mg, haga la inyección intravenosa con la solución disuída por la inyección del Cloruro de Sodio o 5% de inyección de dextrosa; la dosis repetida incrementa de 0.1 mg cada vez, o 0.1 a 0.4 mg por hora, la velocidad de gotear puede ser discrecional, hasta que se despierta completamente. |
| 剂型、规格<br>Formulaciones y especificaciones | 注射液：每支 0.5mg/5ml，1mg/10ml。<br>Solución inyectable: cada una es de 0.5mg/5ml，1mg/10ml. |
| **药品名称 Drug Names** | 纳洛酮 Naloxona |
| 适应证<br>Indicaciones | ①治疗阿片类药物及其他麻醉性镇痛药（如哌替啶、阿法罗定、美沙酮、芬太尼、二氢埃托啡、依托尼嗪等）中毒。②治疗镇静催眠药与急性酒精中毒。③阿片类及其他麻醉性镇痛药依赖性的诊断。<br><br>① los envenenamientos de fármacos opioides y otros analgésicos narcóticos, tales como la petidina, alfaprodina, metadona, fentanilo, dihidroetorfina, etonitazene. ② el envenenamiento de sedantes-hipnóticos e intoxicación alcohólica aguda. ③ el diagnóstico de la pendencia a los opioides y otros analgésicos narcóticos. |

| | |
|---|---|
| 用法、用量<br>Administración y dosis | 成人：静脉注射 0.4 ～ 0.8mg（小儿用量与成人同）。治疗阿片类。镇静催眠药类与急性酒精中毒，首剂 0.4 ～ 0.8mg，无效时可重复一次。因纳洛酮的作用只能持续 45 ～ 90 分钟，以后必须根据病情重复用药，以巩固疗效。<br><br>Para adultos: haga la inyección intravenosa de 0.4 ～ 0.8 mg (para niños se usa la misma cantidad). Se usa como tratamiento de opioide, el envenenamiento de sedantes-hipnóticos e intoxicación alcohólica aguda. La primera dosis es de 0.4 ～ 0.8 mg, si resulta inválido puede repetir una vez. Debido a que la eficacia de la naloxona sólo dura 45 a 90 minutos, después debe repetir la administración según el desarrollo de la enfermedad, a fin de consolidar el efecto curativo. |
| 剂型、规格<br>Formulaciones y especificaciones | 注射液：0.4mg/1ml。<br>Solución inyectable: 0.4mg/1ml. |
| 药品名称 Drug Names | 乙酰半胱氨酸 Acetilcisteína |
| 适应证<br>Indicaciones | 对乙酰氨基酚中毒。<br>Se usa para el envenenamiento por acetaminofeno. |
| 用法、用量<br>Administración y dosis | 5% 乙酰半胱氨酸水溶液加果汁内服，如服后 1 小时呕吐，可在补服一次，如连续呕吐可下胃管将药液直接导入十二指肠内。用量：140mg/kg 为起始量，70mg/kg 为后续量，每 4 小时一次，17 次可达解救的负荷量。静脉滴注：成人，第 1 阶段，140mg/kg 加入葡萄糖液 200ml 中，静滴 15 ～ 20 分钟。第二阶段，70mg/kg 加入 5% 葡萄糖液 500ml 中静滴。每 4 小时 1 次，共给 17 次。儿童，根据患儿的年龄和体重调整用量，解毒剂量同成人，但需按体重折算（将成人剂量按 50 ～ 69kg 折算成每千克的剂量）。<br><br>Se toma oralmente la disolución de zumo y acetilcisteína de 5%. Si vomita una hora después de la administración, puede tomarse otra vez. Si vuelve a vomitar puede usar la sonda nasogástrica al duodeno. La dosis: 140mg/kg es la dosis inicial, 70mg/kg es la cantidad de seguimiento, hágalo cada 4 horas, tras 17 veces puede alcanzar la carga para el rescate. La infusión intravenosa: para adultos, en la primera etapa, se diluye 200ml de solución de glucosa de 140mg/kg, haga la infusión intravenosa de 15 a 20 minutos. En la segunda etapa, haga la infusión intravenosa con la combinación de ésta y 500ml de solución de glucosa de 5%. Haga una infusión de cada cuatro horas, totalmente son 17 veces. Para niños, se ajuste la dosis según la edad y el peso corporal del niño, la dosis de desintoxicación es la misma para adultos pero se convierte al peso corporal. ( se convierte la dosis para adultos por 50 ～ 69kg a la dosis por kilogramo). |
| 剂型、规格<br>Formulaciones y especificaciones | 颗粒剂：100mg，泡腾片：600mg。<br>Gránulos: 100 mg, comprimidos efervescentes: 600mg. |
| 药品名称 Drug Names | 亚叶酸钙 Folinato cálcio |
| 适应证<br>Indicaciones | 用于抗叶酸代谢药过量中毒和甲醇中毒。<br>Por sobredosis de drogas de metabolismo Anti-folato y la intoxicación por metanol. |
| 用法、用量<br>Administración y dosis | （1）抗叶酸代谢药过量中毒：用量相当于抗叶酸代谢药的剂量（15 ～ 100mg），静脉注射。以后，如为甲氨蝶呤过量中毒，每 3 ～ 6 小时再注射或口服 15mg，共 8 次；如为甲氧苄啶过量中毒，口服 15mg，一日 1 次，共 5 ～ 7 日。<br>（2）甲醇中毒：亚叶酸钙 50mg，静脉注射，每 4 小时 1 次，共 2 日。<br><br>(1) para sobredosis de drogas del metabolismo anti-folato: la cantidad es equilavente a la de droga del metabolismo anti-folato, 15~100mg, haga la inyección intravenosa. Más tarde, si resulta que es la sobredosis de metotrexato, se inyecta o se toma por vía oral 15 mg cada 3 a 6 horas, totalmente son 8 veces; si resulta que es la sobredosis de trimetoprima, se toma la administración oral 15mg, una vez al día, totalmente son 5 a 7 veces.<br>(2) para la intoxicación por metanol, haga la inyección intravenosa con 50mg de la leucovorina, una vez cada 4 horas, totalmente 2 días. |
| 剂型、规格<br>Formulaciones y especificaciones | 片剂：5mg，15mg，25mg；注射液：50mg，100mg，300mg；胶囊：25mg。<br>Comprimidos: 5 mg, 15 mg, 25 mg; inyección: 50 mg, 100 mg, 300 mg; cápsula: 25 mg. |

**续 表**

### 20.3　诊断用药 Agentes de diagnosetico

| 药品名称 Drug Names | 碘海醇 Iohexol |
| --- | --- |
| 适应证<br>Indicaciones | 心血管造影、冠状动脉造影、尿路造影、CT 增强扫描及脊髓造影等。<br><br>Se usa para la angiografía, arteriografía coronaria, urografía, Mejoramiento del contraste CT y la mielografía. |
| 用法、用量<br>Administración y dosis | ①脊髓造影：腰椎穿刺注入造影剂 7 ～ 10ml。②泌尿系造影（300mgI/ml）：成人，静脉注射 40 ～ 80ml；儿童，＜ 7kg，3ml/kg；＞ 7kg，2ml/kg（最高 40ml）。③主动脉血管造影：注射 30 ～ 40ml/ 次。④ CT 增强扫描（300mgI/ml）：成人，100 ～ 180ml 静脉注射；儿童，按 1.5 ～ 2mg/kg 体重计。<br><br>① Mielografía: inyecte el contraste radiológico 7 ~ 10 ml con la punción lumbar. ② Urografía(300mgI/ml): para adultos, haga la inyección intravenosa de 40~80ml; para niños, ＜ 7kg, 3ml/kg；＞ 7kg,2ml/kg(no supera 40ml). ③ Angiografía aórtica: 30~40ml de inyección por cada vez. ④ Mejoramiento del contraste CT(300mgI/ml): para adultos, 100~180ml de inyección intravenosa; para niños, multiplique 1.5~2mg/kg con el peso corporal. |
| 剂型、规格<br>Formulaciones y especificaciones | 注射液：每支 20ml。<br><br>Solución inyectable: cada una es de 20ml. |
| 药品名称 Drug Names | 碘佛醇 Yoversol |
| 适应证<br>Indicaciones | 心血管造影、冠状动脉造影、尿路造影、CT 增强扫描及脊髓造影等。<br><br>Se usa para la angiografía, arteriografía coronaria, urografía, Mejoramiento del contraste CT y la mielografía. |
| 用法、用量<br>Administración y dosis | ①脊髓造影：腰椎穿刺注入造影剂 7 ～ 10ml。②泌尿系造影（300mgI/ml）：成人，静脉注射 40 ～ 80ml；儿童，＜ 7kg，3ml/kg；＞ 7kg，2ml/kg（最高 40ml）。③主动脉血管造影：注射 30 ～ 40ml/ 次。④ CT 增强扫描（300mgI/ml）：成人，100 ～ 180ml 静脉注射；儿童，按 1.5 ～ 2mg/kg 体重计。<br><br>① la mielografía: inyecte el contraste radiológico 7 ~ 10 ml con la punción lumbar. ② Urografía(300mgI/ml): para adultos, haga la inyección intravenosa de 40~80ml; para niños, ＜ 7kg, 3ml/kg；＞ 7kg, 2ml/kg(no supera 40ml). ③ Angiografía aórtica: 30~40ml de inyección por cada vez. ④ Mejoramiento del contraste CT(300mgI/ml): para adultos, 100~180ml de inyección intravenosa; para niños, multiplique 1.5~2mg/kg con el peso corporal. |
| 剂型、规格<br>Formulaciones y especificaciones | 注射液：20ml，50ml，100ml。<br><br>Solución inyectable: 20ml, 50ml, 100ml. |
| 药品名称 Drug Names | 碘帕醇 Iopamidol |
| 适应证<br>Indicaciones | 主要适用于腰、胸及颈段脊髓造影，脑血管造影，周围动、静脉造影，心血管造影，冠状动脉造影，尿路、关节造影及 CT 增强扫描等。<br><br>Principalmente se aplica a mielografía lumbar, torácica y cervical, la angiografía cerebral, arteriografía periférica, venografía periférica, angiografía cardiovascular, la arteriografía coronaria, urografia, artrografía y mejoramiento del contraste CT. |
| 用法、用量<br>Administración y dosis | 脊髓造影，成人用浓度为 200 ～ 300mgI/ml 溶液 5 ～ 15ml。大脑血管造影用 300mgI/ml 溶液 5 ～ 10ml（成人）。3 ～ 7ml（儿童）。周围动静脉造影用 300mgI/ml 溶液 20 ～ 50ml（成人）。冠状动脉造影用 370mgI/ml 溶液 4 ～ 8ml（成人）。主动脉造影（逆行）用 370mgI/ml 溶液 50 ～ 80ml（成人）。尿路造影用 300 ～ 370mgI/ml 溶液 20 ～ 50ml（成人），1 ～ 2.5ml（儿童）。CT 扫描用 300 ～ 370mgI/ml 溶液 50 ～ 100ml（成人）等。<br><br>La mielografía: para adultos se usa la solución de 200~300mgI/ml de 5 ～ 15ml. La angiografía cerebral: para adultos se usa la solución 300mgI/ml de 5~10ml, para niños 3~7ml. La arteriografía periférica y la venografía periférica: se usa la solución de 300mgI/ml de 20~50ml. La arteriografía coronaria: para adultos se usa la solución de 370mgI/ml de 4~8ml. La angiografía aórtica (retrógrado): para adultos se usa la solución 370mgI/ml de 50~80ml. La urografía: para adultos se usa solución de 300~370mgI/ml de 20~50ml, para niños 1~2.5ml. Mejoramiento del contraste CT: para adultos se usa la solución de 300~370mgI/ml de 50~100ml. |

**续　表**

| 剂型、规格<br>Formulaciones y especificaciones | 注射液：每支 20ml，50ml，100ml。<br>Solución inyectable: cada una es de 20ml, 50ml, 100ml. |
|---|---|

| 药品名称Drug Names | 碘克沙醇 Iiodixanol |
|---|---|
| 适应证<br>Indicaciones | 成人的心、脑血管造影（常规的与 i.a.DSA）、外周动脉造影（常规的与 i.a.DSA）腹部血管造影（i.a.DSA）尿路造影、静脉造影及 CT 增强检查。<br><br>Para adultos: la angiografía cardiovascular y cerebral (lo convencional y lo de i.a.DSA), arteriografía periférica(lo convencional y lo de i.a.DSA), angiografía abdominal (i.a.DSA), urografía, venografía y el mejoramiento del contraste CT. |
| 用法、用量<br>Administración y dosis | 用药剂量取决于检查类型、年龄、体重、心排血量和患者全身情况及所使用的技术。<br><br>La dosis depende del tipo de examen, la edad, el peso corporal, el gasto cardíaco, el estado general de los pacientes, y la tecnología utilizada. |
| 剂型、规格<br>Formulaciones y especificaciones | 注射液：150mg/ml（50ml；200ml）；270mg/ml（20ml；50ml；100ml）；320mg/ml（20ml；50ml；100ml）。<br><br>Solución inyectable: 150mg/ml(50ml；200ml)；270mg/ml(20ml；50ml；100ml)；320mg/ml(20ml；50ml；100ml). |

| 药品名称Drug Names | 硫酸钡 Sulfato de Bario |
|---|---|
| 适应证<br>Indicaciones | 适用于上、下消化道造影。<br>Se aplica a contraste gastrointestinal superior e inferior. |
| 用法、用量<br>Administración y dosis | （1）上消化道造影，根据检查部位和检查方法不同，加适量水调成不同浓度的混悬液，通常成人使用量食管：检查方法：经口，浓度为 100%～180%（W/V），用量为 50～150ml；胃、十二指肠：检查方法：经口，浓度为 100%～180%（W/V），用量为 50～150ml。<br>（2）下消化道造影：经肛门灌入肠内。灌前准备：按常规肠清洗（控制饮食、大量饮水、加用泻剂），肌内注射解痉灵（可根据医院临床经验及习惯选择）。使用前，加适量水调成 180%（W/V）浓度混悬液，按照自动灌肠机操作程序进行，250～300ml/次。<br><br>(1) contraste gastrointestinal superior: Dependiendo del método de examen y el posición de la inspección, se añade cierta cantidad de agua para tener suspensiones a diferentes concentraciones. Por lo general para adultos se usa esófago: métodos de inspección: por vía oral, a una concentración de 100%～180% (W / V), en una cantidad de 50～150 ml; estómago, duodeno: Método de inspección: por vía oral, a una concentración de 100%～180% (W / V), en una cantidad de 50～150 ml.<br>(2) contraste gastrointestinal inferior: Vierte en el intestino a través del ano. Preparación de Riego: limpieza intestinal convencional (dieta control, beber mucha agua, uso de laxantes), inyección muscular de la escopolamina Butilbromuro (puede seleccionar de acuerdo con la experiencia clínica y hábitos de hospital). Antes de el uso, agregue la cantidad apropiada de agua en una suspensión de concentración de 180% (W / V), de conformidad con los procedimientos de la máquina automática, 250～300 ml / veces. |
| 剂型、规格<br>Formulaciones y especificaciones | 混悬液：（W/V）100%，120%，130%，140%。<br>Suspensión: (W/V) 100%, 120%, 130%, 140%. |

| 药品名称Drug Names | 碘化油 Yodado de Aceite |
|---|---|
| 适应证<br>Indicaciones | 主要用于支气管及子宫、输卵管、瘘管、腔道等的造影检查，亦用于肝癌的栓塞治疗及地方性甲状腺肿。<br><br>Se utiliza principalmente para la angiografía bronquial y el útero, las trompas de Falopio, fístula, cavidad etc, también se utilizan para la embolización de cáncer de hígado y el bocio endémico. |
| 用法、用量<br>Administración y dosis | ①支气管造影：经气管导管直接注入气管或支气管腔内。成人单侧 15～20ml（40%），双侧 30～40ml；小儿酌减。注入应缓慢，采用体位使各叶支气管充盈。②子宫输卵管造影：经宫颈管直接注入子宫腔内，5～12ml（40%）。③各种腔室（如鼻旁窦、腮腺管、泪腺管等）和窦道、瘘管造影：依据病灶大小酌量直接注入。④肝癌栓塞治疗：先作选择性或超选择性肝动脉插管造影，将与抗癌药混合的碘化油 5～10ml 注入肿瘤供血动脉内。⑤预防地方甲状腺肿： |

**续　表**

多用肌内注射，亦可口服（应用其胶丸剂）。肌内注射：学龄前儿童 1 次剂量 0.5ml，学龄期儿童或成人 1 次量 1ml，每 2～3 年注射 1 次；口服，学龄前儿童每次服 0.2～0.3g，学龄期至成人服 0.4～0.6g，每 1～2 年服 1 次。

　　① broncografía: a través del tubo endotraqueal directamente vierte en la tráquea o los bronquios lumen. Para adultos 15～20 ml (40%) a lado unilateral, 30～40 ml a bilateral; para niños reduce la dosis discrecionalmente. La inyección debe ser lenta, utilizando posiciones para llenar cada lóbulo del bronquio.　② histerosalpingografía, HSG: a través del canal cervical se inyecta directamente en la cavidad uterina, 5～12 ml (40%). ③ angiografía de diferentes cámaras (por ejemplo senos paranasales, glándula parótida, conducto lagrimal) y angiografía sinusal y Fístula: inyección directa proporcionalmente en base al tamaño de la lesión.　④ el tratamiento de la embolización de cáncer de hígado: en primer lugar hacer una angiografía selectiva de la arteria hepática o super-selectiva, inyecte en las arterias tumorales suministradoras con 5～10 ml de la combinación del yodado de aceite y el medicamento para el cáncer.　⑤ Prevención del bocio endémico: se usa frecuentemente la inyección intramuscular, la administración oral también se usa (debe usar los agentes Cápsulas). la inyección intramuscular: para niños de edad preescolar la dosis es 0.5ml a la vez, para niños en edad escolar o adultos la dosis es 1 ml a la vez, haga 1 inyección cada 2 a 3 años; si se toma la administración oral, para niños de edad preescolar se toma 0.2~0.3g a la vez, para niños de edad escolar o adultos se toma 0.4~0.6g a la vez, se toma una vez cada 1 a 2 años.

| 剂型、规格<br>Formulaciones y especificaciones | 油注射液：每支 10ml（含碘 40%）；胶丸剂：每丸 0.1g，0.2g。<br>Inyección de aceite: Cada una contiene 10 ml (40% de yodo); cápsulas: Cada una es de 0.1 g, 0.2 g. |
|---|---|
| **药品名称 Drug Names** | 复方泛影葡胺 Compuesto meglumina diatrizoato |
| 适应证<br>Indicaciones | 常用于尿路造影，也可用于肾上腺肾盂、心、脑血管等的造影。<br>Se usa con frecuencia en urografía, también se puede usar en pielografía, angiografía cardiovascular y cerebral. |
| 用法、用量<br>Administración y dosis | ①逆行肾盂造影：20%，6～10ml。②尿路造影 50%，20～30ml。③脑血管造影：45% 以下溶液，10ml。④心脏大血管造影：50%，40ml。<br>① Pielografía retrógrada: 20%, 6~10ml.　② urografía: 50%, 20~30ml. ③ angiografía cerebral: solución por debajo de 45%, 10 ml. ④ Angiografía cardíaca: 50%, 40ml. |
| 剂型、规格<br>Formulaciones y especificaciones | 注射液：60%20ml；76%20ml。<br>Inyección: 60% 20 ml, el 76% 20ml. |
| **药品名称 Drug Names** | 钆喷酸葡胺 Gadopentetato dimetiglumina |
| 适应证<br>Indicaciones | 本品适用于中枢神经（脑脊髓）、腹、盆腔、四肢等人体脏器和组织的磁共振成像。还可替代 X 线含碘造影剂，用于不能使用者。<br>Se usa para las imágenes por resonancia magnética de los órganos y tejidos humanos, tales como el sistema nervioso central (cerebro y médula espinal), el abdomen, la pelvis y las extremidades. También puede reemplazar agentes de contraste de rayos X que contienen yodo, para los que no pueden usar tales agentes. |
| 用法、用量<br>Administración y dosis | （1）静脉注射：成人及 2 岁以上儿童，按体重一次 0.2ml/kg（或 0.1mmol/kg），最大用量为按体重一次 0.4ml/kg。颅脑及脊髓磁共振成像：为获得充分的强化，可按体重一次 0.4ml/kg 给药。最佳强化时间，一般在注射后数分钟之内（不超过 45 分钟）。<br>（2）将 1ml 钆喷酸葡胺（相当于 2mmol/L GD-DTPA）加 2449ml 氯化钠注射液或用 1mlGD-DTPA 加 49ml 氯化钠注射液稀释后，可直接用于体腔的造影，如关节造影或腹腔造影等。<br>（3）将 1ml 钆喷酸葡胺 +15g/L 甘露醇和 25mmol/L 缓冲剂枸橼酸钠配合，有较佳效果，胃肠涂布穿透力强，不易产生腔内浓缩的胃肠道阳性磁共振造影剂。尽管钆喷酸葡胺在大鼠脑池内注射的神经毒性，低于泛影葡胺及优维显等含碘造影剂，但目前仍不主张将它用于直接鞘内注射造影。<br>（4）利用钆喷酸葡胺中 Gd 元素原子序数高（157.3）有吸收 X 线的特点，可用于碘过敏病人的肾动脉 X 线造影或肾排泄性造影（即代替 X 线含碘造影剂）。 |

**续 表**

|  | (1) inyección intravenosa: para adultos y niños mayores que 2 años, multiplique 0.2mg/kg o 0.1mmol/kg con el peso corporal para una vez, la dosis máxima para una vez es la multiplicación 0.4ml/kg con el peso corporal. imágenes por resonancia magnética para el Cerebro y la médula espinal: para tener suficiente fortalecimiento, el resultado de la multiplicación de 0.4ml/kg con el peso corporal es la dosis para una vez. Normalmente la mejor hora de fortalecimiento está dentro de unos minutos después de la inyección (no más de 45 minutos).<br>(2) Diluye 1ml de Gd-DTPA (equivalente a 2mmol/L GD-DTPA) en 2449 ml de solución de cloruro de sodio, o diluye 1ml de Gd-DTPA en 49ml de solución de cloruro de sodio, la disolución puede usarse directamente en la angiografía de la cavidad corporal, tales como la artrografía o angiografía abdominal.<br>(3) Tiene mejor efectos si se combina 1ml de Gd-DTPA con el manitol de 15g/L y el tampón químico citrato de sodio de 25mmol/L, el revestimiento gastrointestinal se penetra mucho, es difícil producir agentes de contraste de MRI de Gastrointestinal positivo que se contensa en la cavida. Aunque Gd-DTPA tiene menos neurotoxicidad que los agentes de contraste que contienen yodo, tales como el diatrizoato y ultravist, cuando se inyecta a la cisterna cerebral de rata, por el momento no se recomienda la aplicación directa de la inyección intratecal de contraste.<br>(4) Aprovechándose de la característica de que el elemento Gd absorbe muy bien rayos X, lo cual existe en el Gd-DTPA, se puede usar en la arteriografía renal con rayos X y el contraste de la excreción renal para los pacientes alérgicos al yodo. (en vez de agentes de contraste de rayos X que contienen yodo). |
|---|---|
| 剂型、规格<br>Formulaciones y especificaciones | 注射液：每支 7.42g（20ml）；5.57g（15ml）；3.71g（10ml）。<br>Solución Inyectable: Cada una es de 7.42 g (20 ml); 5.57 g (15 ml); 3.71 g (10 ml). |

| 药品名称 Drug Names | 吲哚菁绿 Verde de indocianina |
|---|---|
| 适应证<br>Indicaciones | 本品用于诊断肝硬化、肝纤维化、韧性肝炎，对职业和药物中毒性肝病的诊断极有价值。也可用于循环系统功能（心排血量、平均循环时间或异常血流量）的检查测定。<br><br>Se usa para el diagnóstico de la cirrosis, fibrosis hepática, la tenacidad de la hepatitis, mientras tanto tiene mucho valor en el diagnóstico de la enfermedad hepática tóxica ocupacional y la inducida por fármacos. También se puede utilizar en la inspección y medición de las funciones del sistema circulatorio (gasto cardiaco, el tiempo de ciclo promedio o el flujo de sangre anormal). |
| 用法、用量<br>Administración y dosis | 静脉注射：①血浆消失率及血中停滞率的测定：0.5mg/kg，用蒸馏水稀释为 5mg/ml 浓度，在 30 秒从肘静脉慢慢注入。②肝血流量的测定：将本品 25mg 用少量蒸馏水溶解后，稀释成 2.5～5.90mg/ml 浓度，开始时，注射相当于 3mg 的此浓度溶液，以后再 50 分钟内慢慢静滴至采血完毕。③用于循环功能检查：通常从前臂静脉注入，成人 1 次量 5～10mg，小儿按体重酌减。<br><br>Inyección intravenosa: ① Determinación de la tasa de desaparición del plasma y de la tasa de estancamiento de sangre:se diluye 0.5mg/kg de este producto con agua destilada a una concentración de 5mg/ml, en 30 segundos se inyecta lentamente de la vena cubital. ② Determinación del flujo sanguíneo hepático: se disuelve este producto en agua destilada con una pequeña cantidad de 25 mg, a una concentración entre 2.5～5.90mg/ml. Inicialmente, inyecta la solución de esta concentración de 3ml, y después haga la inyección intravenosa lenta dentro de 50 minutos hasta la finalización de la recogida de sangre. ③ para las pruebas de función cíclicos: Por lo general, hag la inyección en la vena del antebrazo, la cantidad de adultos es de 5～10 mg a la vez, la dosis para niños se reduce de acuerdo con el peso corporal. |
| 剂型、规格<br>Formulaciones y especificaciones | 注射剂：每支 25mg（附注射用水 10ml）。<br>Inyección: Cada una es de 25 mg (adjunto el agua para inyección de 10ml). |

| 药品名称 Drug Names | 荧光素钠 Fluoresceína sódica |
|---|---|
| 适应证<br>Indicaciones | ①滴眼液用于眼科诊断，正常角膜不显色，异常角膜显色。②针剂用于测血液循环时间，静脉注射后，在紫外线灯下观察，以 10～15 秒唇部黏膜能见到黄绿色荧光为正常。<br><br>① Estas gotas para los ojos se usa en el diagnóstico, si no está cromogénico, resulta córnea normal, si está cromogénico, resulta córnea anormal. ② la inyección se usa para medir el tiempo de circulación de la sangre: Después de la inyección intravenosa, lo observe bajo la luz ultravioleta, si se ve la fluorescencia amarillo-verde en la mucosa del labio dentro 10 a 15 segundos, resulta normal. |

**续　表**

| | |
|---|---|
| 用法、用量<br>Administración y<br>dosis | ①滴眼后于角膜显微镜下观察颜色。②测血循环时间，于臂静脉注 2ml，每次用量 0.4 ～ 0.8g （2 ～ 4ml）。<br><br>① observe el color bajo un microscopio corneal después de las gotas a los ojos. ② mida el tiempo de circulación de la sangre, haga la inyección de 2 ml en la vena del brazo, cada dosis de 0,4 ～ 0,8 g (2 ～ 4 ml). |
| 剂型、规格<br>Formulaciones y<br>especificaciones | 滴眼液：2% 注射液：0.4g（2ml）。<br>Gotas a los ojos: solución inyectable es de 2%: 0.4 g (2 ml). |

20.4　生物制品 Productos biológicos

| 药品名称 Drug Names | 人用狂犬病疫苗 (vero 细胞 ) Vacunas antirrábicas para uso humano (vero cell) |
|---|---|
| 适应证<br>Indicaciones | 用于预防狂犬病。凡被狂犬或其他疯动物咬伤、抓伤时，不分年龄、性别均应立即处理局部伤口（用清水或肥皂水反复冲洗后，再用碘酊或酒精消毒数次），并及时按暴露后免疫程序注射本疫苗；凡有接触狂犬病病毒危险的人员（如兽医、动物饲养员、林业从业人员、屠宰厂工人、狂犬病实验人员等），按暴露前免疫程序预防接种。<br><br>Para la prevención de la rabia. Cuando se muerde o se arañe por perros rabiosos u otros animales rabiosos, sea lo que sea la edad y el género, la herida tópica debe ser tratada inmediatamente (Después de repetidos lavados con agua o agua jabonosa, y luego desinfecte varias veces con el yodo o alcohol), haga la vacunación oportuna según el programa de vacunación de post-exposición; para el personal que tenga muchas ocaciones de ponerse a la exposición de la virus de la rabia(tales como los veterinarios, ganaderos, profesionales forestales, trabajadores de mataderos, personal de laboratorio de la rabia), haga la vacunación oportuna según el programa de vacunación previa a la exposición. |
| 用法、用量<br>Administración y<br>dosis | （1）于上臂三角肌处肌内注射，幼儿可在大腿前外侧区肌内注射。<br>（2）暴露后免疫程序：一般咬伤者于 0 日（第 1 日，当日）、3 日（第 4 日，以下类推）7 日、14 日和 28 日各注射本疫苗 1 剂，全程免疫共注射 5 剂，儿童用量相同。对有下列情况之一的，建议首剂狂犬疫苗剂量加倍给予：①注射疫苗前一日或更早一些时间内，注射过狂犬病人免疫球蛋白或狂犬病血清的慢性患者。②先天性或获得性免疫缺陷患者。③接受免疫抑制剂（包括抗疟疾药物）治疗的患者。④老年人。⑤于暴露后 48 小时或更长时间后才注射狂犬病疫苗的人员。⑥暴露后免疫程序按下述伤及程度分级处理：Ⅰ级暴露：触摸动物，被动物舔及无破损皮肤，一般不需处理，不必注射狂犬疫苗。Ⅱ级暴露：未出血的皮肤咬伤、抓伤，应按暴露后免疫程序接种狂犬病疫苗。Ⅲ级暴露：一处或多处皮肤出血性咬伤或被抓伤出血，可疑或确诊的疯动物唾液污染黏膜，破损的皮肤被舔，应按暴露后程序立即接种狂犬病疫苗和抗狂犬病血清或抗狂犬病人免疫球蛋白按 20U/kg 给予。将尽可能多的抗狂犬病血清或抗狂犬病人免疫球蛋白做咬伤局部浸润注射，剩余部分做肌内注射，抗狂犬病血清或抗狂犬病人免疫球蛋白仅为单次应用。<br>（3）暴露前免疫程序：按 0 日、7 日、21 日或 28 日各注射 1 剂，全程免疫共注射 3 剂。<br>（4）对曾经接种过狂犬病疫苗的一般患者，再需接种疫苗的建议：①1 年内进行全程免疫，被可疑疯动物咬伤者，应于 0 日或 3 日各注射 1 剂疫苗。②1 年前进行过全程免疫，被可疑疯动物咬伤者，则应全程接种疫苗。③3 年内进行过全程免疫，并且进行过加强免疫，被可疑疯动物咬伤者，应于 0 日或 3 日各注射 1 剂疫苗。④3 年前进行过全程免疫，并且进行过加强免疫，被可疑疯动物咬伤者，应全程接种疫苗。<br><br>(1) Haga la inyección intramuscular en los deltoides del antebrazo, para niños en la zona anterolateral del muslo.<br>(2)Programa de vacunación de post-exposición: normalmente el mordido haga 1 inyección de la vacuna en el mismo día, el tercer día, el séptimo día, el decimocuarto día y el día 28, totalmente son 5 inyecciones, la dosis es la misma para niños. Para los pacientes quienes se conformen con una de estas situaciones, se recomienda que por la primera vez la dosis se doble: ① Un día o más tiempo antes de la vacunación, los pacientes se ha inyectado la inmunoglobulina antirrábica o serum rabia. ② Pacientes de inmunodeficiencia congénita o adquirida. ③ quienes reciban el tratamiento del inmunosupresor (incluidos los medicamentos antimaláricos). ④ los mayores. ⑤ quienes que no se inyecten hasta 48 horas o más tiempo despúes. ⑥ Programa de vacunación de post-exposición se clasifica de acuerdo con los siguientes grados de las lesiones: Ⅰ nivel de exposición: tocar animales, ser lamido por los animales sin daño en la piel, por lo general no hace falta el tratamiento, ni la vacuna contra la rabia. Ⅱ nivel de |

exposición: las picaduras o los rasguños de la piel sin sangría , debe recibir la vacuna antirrábica de acuerdo con el programa de vacunación post-exposición. Ⅲ nivel de exposición: una o más mordeduras o arañazos hemorrágico en la piel, sospechosa o confirmada contaminación de saliva mucosa de animales rabiosos, la piel dañada siendo lamiendo, debe recibir la vacuna antirrábica y el suero antirrábico inmediatamente, o dando la inmunoglobulina antirrábica de acuerdo con 20U/kg. Haga inyección de infiltración en la zona afectada con lo más suero antirrábico o inmunoglobulina antirrábica, haga la inyección intramuscular con el resto, el suero antirrábico o inmunoglobulina antirrábica se pueden usar por una sola vez.

(3) Programa de inmunización previa a la exposición: en el primer día, el séptimo día, el día 21 y el día 28, haga la vacunación en cada dicho día, completamente son 3 vacunaciones.

(4) para los pacientes quienes han sido vacunados contra la rabia, y si requieren vacunación las recomendaciones son: ① Llevar a cabo la inmunización completa en 1 año, si mordido por sopechosos animales rabiosos, debe ser sido vacunado en el mismo día y en el tercer día. ② hace un año que ha realizado la inmunización completa, si mordido por sopechosos animales rabiosos, debe llevar a cabo la inmunización completa. ③ dentro de 3 años ha realizado la inmunización completa y el fortalecimiento inmunológico, si mordido por sopechosos animales rabiosos, debe ser sido vacunado en el mismo día y en el tercer día. ④ hace 3 años que ha realizado la inmunización completa y el fortalecimiento inmunológico, si mordido por sopechosos animales rabiosos, debe llevar a cabo la inmunización completa.

| 剂型、规格<br>Formulaciones y especificaciones | 注射液：每瓶 1ml，每人 1 次用量为 1ml。狂犬病疫苗效价应不低于 2.5U。<br><br>Inyección: cada botella es de 1 ml, la dosis para una persona para una sola vez es de 1 ml. La potencia de la vacuna antirrábica debe ser no menos de 2.5U. |
| --- | --- |
| **药品名称 Drug Names** | **破伤风抗毒素 Tétanos antitoxina** |
| 适应证<br>Indicaciones | 本品用于预防和治疗破伤风。已出现破伤风或可疑症状时，应在进行外科处理及其他疗法的同时，及时使用抗毒素治疗。开放性外伤（特别是伤口深、污染严重者）有感染破伤风的危险时，应注射抗毒素进行紧急预防。凡已接受过破伤风的危险时，应在再受伤后，再注射 1 剂疫苗，以加强免疫，不必注射抗毒素；如受伤者未接受过破伤风疫苗免疫或免疫史不清者，须注射抗毒素预防，但也应同时开始疫苗预防注射，以获得持久免疫。<br><br>Se usa para la prevención y el tratamiento del tétanos. Cuando se haya producido el tétanos o síntomas sospechosos, debe llevar el tratamiento quirúrgico u otros tratamientos, al mismo tiempo se usa oportunamente un tratamiento anti-toxina. Cuando el trauma abierto (especialmente para las heridas profundas con una contaminación grave) pueda infectar el tétanos, debe inyectarse la antitoxina como la prevención de emergencias. Cuando se haya expuesto bajo el riesgo de tétanos , después de una nueva lesión, debe inyectarse con una vacuna más para mejorar la inmunidad, no tiene que inyectar la antitoxina; Si la persona lesionada no ha recibido la vacuna contra el tétanos o la historia de la inmunización no está claro, se requiere la inyección de antitoxina, pero también deben comenzar la inyección de la vacuna para obtener la inmunidad de larga duración. |
| 用法、用量<br>Administración y dosis | (1) 预防用：皮下或肌内注射，一次 1500～3000U，儿童与成人用量相同；伤势严重者可增加用量 1～2 倍。经 5～6 日，如破伤风感染危险还未消除，应重复注射。<br>(2) 治疗用：肌内注射或静脉注射，第 1 次肌内或静脉注射 50 000～200 000U，儿童与成人用量相同；以后视病情决定注射剂量和间隔时间，同时还可将适量的抗毒素注射于伤口周围的组织中。初生儿破伤风，24 小时内分次或 1 次肌内或静脉注射 20 000～100 000U。皮下注射应在上臂三角肌处，同时注射疫苗时，注射部位应分开。肌内注射应在上臂三角肌处或臀部。只有经过皮下或肌内注射未发生异常反应者，方可作静脉注射。静脉注射应缓慢，开始每分钟不超过 1ml，以后每分钟亦不宜超过 4ml。一次静脉注射总量不应超过 40ml。儿童每千克体重不宜超过 0.8ml。亦可将抗毒素加入葡萄糖注射液或氯化钠注射液等溶液中静脉点滴。静脉注射前应将安瓿置温水浴中加温至接近体温，注射中如发现异常反应，应立即停止。<br>(1) se usa para prevención: reciba la inyección subcutánea o intramuscular, 1500~3000U a la vez, la dosis es la misma para niños y adultos; los con lesiones graves pueden aumentar la cantidad de 1 a 2 veces. Después de 5 a 6 días, si el riesgo de infección por tétanos todavía no se ha eliminado, debe repetir las inyecciones. |

**续　表**

| | |
|---|---|
| | (2) se usa como el tratamiento: reciba la inyección intramuscular o inyección intravenosa, la de primera vez la cantidad es 50 000~200 000U, la dosis es la misma para niños y adultos; Después, la dosis inyectada y los intervalos se deciden de acuerdo con la condición, mientras que puede hacer la inyección de una cantidad apropiada de la antitoxina para el tejido que rodea la herida. El tétanos para los bebé recién nacidos, reciba la inyección intravenosa de 20 000~100 000U de una vez o se divide en varias veces durante 24 horas. La inyección subcutánea debe estar en deltoides del antebrazo, si recibe la vacunación en el mismo tiempo, debe separar el lugar de las 2 inyecciones. La inyección intramuscular debe estar en deltoides del antebrazo o en la nalga. Sólo los que no tenga reacción anomal a la inyección subcutánea y la inyección intramuscular, pueden tener la intravenosa. La inyección intravenosa debe ser muy lenta, en el incio no supera 1ml por minuto, después no supera 4ml por minuto. La cantidad total de una inyección no debe superar 40ml. Para niños no debe superar 0.8ml por kilo de peso corporal. También se puede recibir la inyección intravenosa con la disolución de la antitoxina y la solución de glucosa o la de cloruro de sodio. Antes de la inyección intravenosa deben poner ampollas en un baño de agua caliente para calentar a una temperatura establecida cerca de la temperatura corporal, durante la inyección si se ocurren reacciones anormales debe interrumpirse inmediatamente. |
| 剂型、规格<br>Formulaciones y especificaciones | 750μl ： 1.5mU，2.5ml ： 1wU。<br>750μl ： 1.5mU，2.5ml ： 1wU. |
| **药品名称 Drug Names** | 抗蛇毒血清 Antiveneno |
| 适应证<br>Indicaciones | 用于毒蛇咬伤中毒。<br>Se usa para la intoxicación de mordedura de serpiente. |
| 用法、用量<br>Administración y dosis | 稀释后静脉注射或静脉滴注，也可肌内或皮下注射。用量根据被咬伤者的受毒量及血清效价而定。以下为中和一条毒蛇的剂量：①抗蝮蛇毒血清：主要用于蝮蛇咬伤的治疗，对竹叶青和烙铁头毒蛇也有交叉中和作用。一次用 6000～16 000U，以氯化钠或25% 葡萄糖注射液稀释1倍，缓慢静脉注射。②抗五步蛇毒血清：主要用于五步蛇咬伤的治疗，对蝮蛇蛇毒也有交叉中和作用。每次用 8000U，以氯化钠注射液稀释1倍，缓慢静脉注射。③抗银环蛇毒血清：主要用于银环蛇咬伤的治疗，一次用 10 000U，缓慢静脉注射。④抗眼镜蛇毒血清：主要用于眼镜蛇咬伤的治疗，对其他科的毒蛇蛇毒也有交叉中和作用。一次用 2500 ～ 10 000U，缓慢静脉注射。<br><br>Haga la infusión intravenosa después de la dilución, también puede recibir la inyección intramuscular o subcutánea. La dosis depende de la cantidad de tóxico mordido y la potencia del suero. La siguiente es la dosis para neutralizar el tóxico de una serpiente: ① suero de anti-Venom: se usa principalmente como el tratamiento de la mordedura de la víbora, también tiene efecto de neutralización cruzada para el trimeresurus y el mucrosquamatus. Se diluye a media concentración 6000~16 000U de este producto con la solución de cloruro de sodio o la de glucosa de 25% por una vez, y luego haga la inyección intravenosa lenta. ② suero contra el tóxico de acutus: se usa principalmente como el tratamiento de la mordedura de acutus, también tiene efecto de neutralización cruzada para el tóxico de víbora. Se diluye a media concentración 8000U de este producto con la solución de cloruro de sodio, y luego haga la inyección intravenosa lenta. ③ suero contra el tóxico de Bungarus multicinctus: se usa principalmente como el tratamiento de la mordedura de Bungarus multicinctus, haga la inyección intravenosa lenta, 10 000U a la vez. ④ suero contra el tóxico de naja: se usa principalmente como el tratamiento de la mordedura de la naja, también tiene efecto de neutralización cruzada para los tóxicos de otras ramas de víboras. Haga la inyección intravenosa lenta, 2500~10 000U a la vez. |
| 剂型、规格<br>Formulaciones y especificaciones | 注射液：①抗蝮蛇蛇毒血清：每瓶含抗蝮蛇毒血清6000U。②抗五步蛇蛇毒血清：每瓶含抗眼镜蛇毒血清：2000U。③抗银环蛇毒血清：每瓶含抗银环蛇毒血清：10 000U。④抗眼镜蛇毒血清：每瓶含抗眼镜蛇毒血清：1000U。<br><br>Solución inyectable: ① suero de anti-Venom: cada botella contiene el suero de anti-Venom 6000U. ② suero contra el tóxico de acutus: cada botella contiene el suero contra el tóxico de acutus 2000U. ③ suero contra el tóxico de Bungarus multicinctus: cada botella contiene el suero contra el tóxico de Bungarus multicinctus 10 000U. ④ suero contra el tóxico de naja:cada botella contiene suero contra el tóxico de naja 1000U. |

**续　表**

| 药品名称 Drug Names | 人血白蛋白 Albúmina humana |
| --- | --- |
| 适应证<br>Indicaciones | 用于治疗因失血、创伤及烧伤等引起的休克，脑水肿及大脑损伤所致的脑压增高，防治低蛋白血症及肝硬化或肾病引起的水肿和腹水，有较好的疗效。<br><br>Se usa para el choque provocado por la pérdida de sangre, trauma y quemadura, el aumento de la presión intracraneal causado por el edema y el daño cerebrales, en prevención de tanto la hipoproteinemia como el edema y ascitis provocados por la cirrosis o enfermedades renales. |
| 用法、用量<br>Administración y<br>dosis | 静脉滴注，用量由医师酌定。一般因严重烧伤或失血等所致的休克可直接注射本品 5 ～ 10g，隔 4 ～ 6 小时重复注射一次。在治疗肾病及肝硬化等慢性白蛋白缺乏症时，可每日注射本品 5 ～ 10g，直至水肿消失、血清白蛋白恢复正常为止。<br><br>Haga la infusión intravenosa, la cantidad se decide por el médico. Por lo general para el choque provocados por quemaduras graves o la pérdida de sangre, puede inyectarse este producto 5~10g, repita la inyección cada 4 a 6 horas. En cuanto a tratar la deficiencia crónica de albúmina tales como enfermedades renales o la cirrosis, puede inyectarse este medicamento 5~10g, hasta que el edema se desparezca y la albúmina de suero se vuelva a nivel normal. |
| 剂型、规格<br>Formulaciones y<br>especificaciones | 注射液：1g（10ml）；2g（10ml）；2.5g（10ml）；5g（10ml）；10g（50ml）；12.5g（50ml）；25g（125ml）。冻干品：10g；20g。<br><br>Inyección: 1 g (10 ml); 2g (10 ml); 2,5 g (10 ml); 5 g (10 ml); 10g (50ml); 12,5 g (50 ml); 25 g (125 ml). Liofilizado: 10g; 20g. |
| 药品名称 Drug Names | 人免疫球蛋白 Inmunoglobulina humana |
| 适应证<br>Indicaciones | 主要用于预防麻疹和甲型肝炎等病毒性感染。<br>Se utiliza principalmente para la prevención del sarampión y la hepatitis A y otras infecciones virales. |
| 用法、用量<br>Administración y<br>dosis | （1）预防麻疹：0.05 ～ 0.15ml/kg 或 5 岁以内儿童注射 1.5 ～ 3ml，成人不得超过 6ml，预防效果为 1 个月。<br>（2）预防甲型肝炎：按每千克体重注射 0.05 ～ 0.1ml/kg 或儿童每次注射 1.5 ～ 3ml，成人每次注射 3ml。1 次注射，预防效果为 1 个月。<br><br>(1) prevención del sarampión: 0.05~0.15ml/kg o 1.5~3ml de inyección para niños menor que 5 años, para adultos no supera 6ml, se dura 1 mes;<br>(2) prevención de la hepatitis A: 0.05~0.1ml/kg o para niños 1.5~3ml de inyección a la vez, para adultos 3ml de inyección a la vez. Una inyección tiene su efecto preventivo para 1 mes. |
| 剂型、规格<br>Formulaciones y<br>especificaciones | 注射液：10%/1.5ml（150mg）；10%/3ml（300mg）。<br>Solución inyectable: 10%/1.5ml (150mg); 10%/3ml(300mg). |
| 药品名称 Drug Names | 乙型肝炎人免疫球蛋白 Inmunoglobulina humana de Hepatitis B |
| 适应证<br>Indicaciones | 用于乙型肝炎的预防。主要适用于：①乙型肝炎表面抗原阳性母亲的新生儿。②预防意外感染人群，如血友病患者、肾透析患者、医务人员或皮肤破损被乙型肝炎表面抗原阳性的血液或分泌物污染的人员等。③与乙型肝炎患者或携带者密切接触的易感人群。<br><br>Se usa para la prevención de la hepatitis B. Principalmente se aplica a: ① bebés cuyas madres tienen el antígeno positivo en la superficie de la hepatitis B; ② las personas que previene la infección accidental, tales como los hemofílicos, pacientes de diálisis renal, el personal médico etc; ③ las poblaciones susceptibles en estrecho contacto con los pacientes o portadores de la hepatitis B. |
| 用法、用量<br>Administración y<br>dosis | （1）母婴阻断：乙型肝炎表面抗原阳性母亲的婴儿出生 24 小时内，肌内注射 100 ～ 200U，同时联合乙型肝炎疫苗，按乙型肝炎疫苗注射程序全程注射（按照 0、1、6、个月或医生推荐的适宜方案）；亦可在婴儿出生 24 小时内肌内注射 100 ～ 200U，1 个月时在注射一次，同时按乙型肝炎疫苗注射程序全程注射。单独使用乙型肝炎免疫球蛋白很少获得满意结果，如果单独使用应多次注射，每 3 ～ 4 周 1 次，每次肌内注射 100 ～ 200U。<br>（2）乙型肝炎预防：用于预防意外暴露时，注射越早越好，一般应在 24 小时内进行肌内注射，最迟不超过 7 日。一次注射量，儿童为 100U，成人为 200U，必要时剂量可加倍，每 3 ～ 4 周再注射 1 次，必要时按注射程序全程注射乙型肝炎疫苗。 |

续　表

| | (1) Interdicción de la transmisión materno-neonatal (PTMI): para bebés cuyas madres tienen el antígeno positivo en la superficie de la hepatitis B, haga la inyección intramuscular de 100 ~ 200 UI dentro de las 24 horas siguientes al nacimiento, mientras haga la inyección de la vacuna contra la hepatitis B, según el procedimiento de vacunación de hepatitis B por toda la inyección (inyecciones regulares de conformidad con 0,1,6, meses o soluciones apropiadas recomiendas por médicos); o haga una inyección intramuscular de 100 ~ 200 U dentro de las 24 horas siguientes al nacimiento, y una otra cuando cumpla 1 mes, mientras haga la inyección de la vacuna contra la hepatitis B completa de acuerdo con el procedimiento de vacunación de hepatitis B. Es raro que el uso solo de la inmunoglobulina de hepatitis B pueda tener resultados satisfactorios, si se aplica el uso solo, debe repetirse muchas veces, haga la inyección intramuscular de 100 ~ 200 U cada tres o cuatro semanas.<br><br>(2) prevención de la Hepatitis B: se utiliza para prevenir la exposición accidental, haga la inyección lo antes posible, por lo general debe hacer la inyección intramuscular en 24 horas, no más de 7 días. La dosis de una sola vez para niños es 100U, para adultos es 200U, en caso necesario la dosis puede doblarse. Haga la inyección intramuscular cada tres o cuatro semanas, haga la vacunación completa contra la hepatitis B según el procedimiento de inyección cuando sea necesario. |
|---|---|
| 剂型、规格<br>Formulaciones y especificaciones | 注射液（冻干）：乙型肝炎免疫球蛋白　100U；200U；400U。<br>Inyección (liofilizada): inmunoglobulina antihepatitis B 100 U; 200 U; 400 U. |
| 药品名称 Drug Names | 破伤风人免疫球蛋白 Inmunoglobulina humana de tétanos |
| 适应证<br>Indicaciones | 用于预防和治疗破伤风，尤其适用于对破伤风抗毒素（TAT）有过敏反应的患者。<br>Se usa para la profilaxis y el tratamiento del tétanos, especialmente adecuado para pacientes con reacciones alérgicas a la antitoxina tetánica (TAT). |
| 用法、用量<br>Administración y dosis | 肌内注射。①预防用：儿童、成人一次用量均为250U。创面严重或创面严重和感染严重者可加倍注射。②治疗用：3000 ~ 6000U。可多点注射。<br>La inyección intramuscular.　① se usa para prevención: para niños y adultos, la cantidad es igualmente de 250 U a la vez. Para los que tenga herida grave y infecciones severas pueden duplicarse inyección. ② se usa como el tratamiento: 3000 ~ 6000U. Inyección en multipuntos. |
| 剂型、规格<br>Formulaciones y especificaciones | 注射液：100U；200U；250U。注射剂（冻干品）：100U；200U；250U。<br>Inyección: 100 U; 200 U; 250 U. Agente inyectable (producto liofilizado): 100 U; 200 U; 250 U. |
| 药品名称 Drug Names | 狂犬病人免疫球蛋白 Inmunoglobulina rabia humana |
| 适应证<br>Indicaciones | 本品主要配合狂犬病疫苗使用，当被狂犬或其他疯动物严重咬伤者，进行狂犬病疫苗预防注射的同时，配合使用本品，对狂犬病做紧急的被动免疫，以提高预防性治疗效果。<br>Se usa principalmente en combinación con la vacuna de la rabia, Cuando mordidos gravemente por perros o animales rabiosos, haga la inyección de la vacuna de la rabia en combinación con este medicamento como la inmunización pasiva contra la rabia de emergencia para mejorar el tratamiento preventivo. |
| 用法、用量<br>Administración y dosis | 肌内注射：动物咬伤部位及时清创后，于受伤部位用本品总剂量的1/2做皮下浸润注射，余下制剂进行肌内注射（头部咬伤者可于背部肌内注射），按体重每千克20U（或遵医嘱），一次注射，如所需总剂量大于10ml，可于1 ~ 2日分次注射。同时或随后即可进行狂犬病疫苗注射，但两种制品的注射部位和器具应严格分开。<br>La inyección intramuscular: después de desbridamiento oportuno en la zona mordida por los animales, en la zona lesionada se usa la mitad de esta dosis total para la inyección de la infiltración subcutánea, las preparaciones restantes se usa como inyección intramuscular (si la mordedura está en el cerebro, puede recibir la inyección intramuscular en la espalda), multiplique 20U con el peso corporal o según las recomiendas del médico. Si la dosis total de una inyección supera 10 ml, se puede dividir en varias veces de inyección en 1 a 2 días. La vacunación contra rabia puede llevarse a cabo de forma simultánea o un momento después, pero los puntos y los utensilios de inyección deben ser estrictamente separados. |
| 剂型、规格<br>Formulaciones y especificaciones | 注射液：100U；200U；500U。注射剂（冻干品）：100U；200U；500U。<br>Inyección: 100 U; 200 U; 500 U. Agente Inyectable (producto liofilizado): 100 U; 200 U; 500 U. |

| 药品名称Drug Names | 人纤维蛋白原 Fibrinógeno humana |
|---|---|
| 适应证<br>Indicaciones | （1）遗传性纤维蛋白原减少症，包括遗传性异常纤维蛋白原血症或遗传性纤维蛋白原缺乏症。<br>（2）获得性纤维蛋白原减少症，主要见于严重肝损害所致的纤维蛋白原合成不足及局部或弥散性血管内凝血导致纤维蛋白原消耗量增加。<br><br>(1) Trombocitopenia hereditaria de fibrinógeno, incluye la disfibrinogenemia hereditaria o la deficiencia hereditaria de fibrinógeno.<br>(2) Trombocitopenia adquirida de fibrinógeno, principalmente se ve en la falta de la síntesis de fibrinógeno provocada por lesiones hepáticas graves y el aumento del consumo del fibrinógeno causado por la coagulación intravascular localizada o diseminada. |
| 用法、用量<br>Administración y<br>dosis | 静脉注射：其用量视血浆纤维蛋白原水平及要达到止血所学的纤维蛋白原水平（1g/L）而定。由于纤维蛋白原的生物半衰期长达 96 ～ 144 小时，故开始每 1 ～ 2 日，以后每 3 ～ 4 日，滴注 1 次即可。能够按每 2g 纤维蛋白原可使血浆纤维蛋白原水平升至 0.5g/L 的原则推算所需剂量，一般首次用量 1 ～ 2g，必要时可加量。大出血时应立即给予 4 ～ 8g。<br><br>Inyección intravenosa: la dosis se decide por el nivel de fibrinógeno y el nivel necesario del fibrinógeno para hemostasia (1g/L). Como la vida media biológica de fibrinógeno es de 96 a 144 horas, de tal modo que en el inicio basta con una infusión cada 1 a 2 días, después una cada 3 a 4 días. Calcule la dosis requerida de acuerdo con el principio de que cada 2g de fibrinógeno pueda aumentar el nivel de fibrinógeno de plasma de 0.5g/L, normalmente la dosis de la primera vez es de 1~2g, cuando sea necesario puede aumentar el volumen. En caso de hemorragia masiva debe dar de inmediato 4 ~ 8 g. |
| 剂型、规格<br>Formulaciones y<br>especificaciones | 注射剂（冻干品）：每支 0.5g。<br><br>Agente inyectable (producto liofilizado): Cada uno es de 0.5 g. |
| 药品名称Drug Names | 重组人干扰素 α - 1b Interferón α -1b de recombinante humana |
| 适应证<br>Indicaciones | 用于病毒性疾病和某些恶性肿瘤。①已批准用于治疗慢性乙型肝炎、丙型肝炎和毛细胞血友病。②已有临床试验结果或文献报道，用于病毒性疾病，如带状疱疹、尖锐湿疣、流行性出血热和小儿呼吸道合胞病毒肺炎等。③用于治疗恶性肿瘤，如慢性粒细胞白血病、黑色素瘤、淋巴瘤等。④滴眼液，可用于眼部病毒性疾病。<br><br>Se usa para enfermedades de carácter viral y algunos tumores malignos. ① Ha sido aprobado usarse como el tratamiento de la hepatitis B crónica, la hepatitis C y la hemofilia de células pilosas.　② ha sido reportado en la literatura o los resultados de ensayos clínicos que se usa para enfermedades de carácter viral, tales como herpes zoster, verrugas genitals, fiebre hemorrágica epidémica, la neumonía por virus sincicial respiratorio en niños etc.　③ se usa para los tumores maglinos tales como la leucemia granulocítica crónica, melanoma, linfoma etc.　④ Gotas para los ojos: puede usarse para las enfermedades virales de los ojos. |
| 用法、用量<br>Administración y<br>dosis | （1）慢性乙型肝炎：一次 30 ～ 50µg，隔日一次，疗程 4 ～ 6 个月，可根据病情延长疗程至 1 年，也可进行诱导治疗，即在治疗开始时，每日用药 1 次，0.5 ～ 1 个月后改为每周 3 次，直到疗程结束。<br>（2）慢性丙型肝炎：一次 30 ～ 50µg，隔日一次疗，程 4 ～ 6 个月，无效者停用。有效者可继续治疗至 12 个月。根据病情需要，可延长至 18 个月。在治疗的第 1 个月，一日 1 次。疗程结束后随访 6 ～ 12 个月。急性丙型肝炎，应及早使用本品治疗，可减少慢性化。<br>（3）慢性粒细胞白血病：一次 30 ～ 50µg，一日 1 次，连续用药 6 个月以上。可根据病情适当调整，缓解后可改为隔日注射。<br>（4）肿瘤：视病情可延长疗程。如患者未出现病情恶化或严重不良反应，应当在适当剂量下继续用药。<br><br>(1) para la hepatitis B crónica: 30 ~ 50µg a la vez, se usa cada dos días, el curso de tratamiento dura 4 a 6 meses, puede extenderse a un año de acuerdo con la condición de la enfermedad. También puede tener la terapia de inducción, que en el inicio del tratamiento, una vez de medicación al día, medio mes o un mes después, 3 veces de medicación a la semana hasta el final del tratamiento.<br>(2) para la hepatitis C crónica: 30 ~ 50µg a la vez, se usa cada dos días, el curso de tratamiento dura 4 a 6 meses, si resulta ineficaz, deje de la medicación; si resulta eficaz, siga el curso de tratamiento hasta 12 meses. Según la condición de los pacientes, el curso de tratamiento se puede extender a 18 meses. En el primer mes de tratamiento, una vez al día. Después de tratamiento, continua el seguimiento de 6 a 12 meses. Para la hepatitis C aguda, debe usar este tratamiento lo antes posible para reducir la posibilidad de ser crónica. |

**续 表**

| | |
|---|---|
| | (3) para la leucemia granulocítica crónica: 30～50μg a la vez, se usa al día, medicación continua durante 6 meses o más tiempo. Puede ajustarse de acuerdo a la enfermedad, después del alivio se puede cambiar a una inyección de cada 2 días.<br><br>(4) para tumores: el curso de tratamiento se puede extender de acuerdo con la condición de enfermos. Si no se producen la progresión de la enfermedad o las reacciones adversas graves, el tratamiento debe continuar en las dosis adecuadas. |
| 剂型、规格<br>Formulaciones y especificaciones | 注射剂（冻干品）：10μg（10 万 U）；20μg（20 万 U）；30μg（30 万 U）；50μg（50 万 U）。<br>Agente inyectable (liofilizado): 10μg (100 mil U); 20 microgramos (200 mil U); 30μg (300 mil U); 50 microgramos (500 mil U). |
| 药品名称 Drug Names | 重组人白细胞介素 -2 Interleucina-2 recombinante humana |
| 适应证<br>Indicaciones | ①用于肾细胞癌、黑色素瘤，用于控制晚期腹水及其他晚期肿瘤。②用于先天或后天免疫缺陷症，如艾滋病等。③对某些病毒性、细菌性疾病、胞内寄生感染性疾病，如乙型肝炎、麻风病、肺结核、白念珠菌感染等，有一定作用。<br><br>① Se usa para el carcinoma de células renales, melanoma, controlar ascitis avanzada y otros tumores avanzados. ② se usa para síndrome de inmunodeficiencia congénita o adquirida, como el SIDA. ③ también tiene ciertos efectos para las enfermedades virales y bacterianas, enfermedades infecciosas parasitarias intracelulares tales como La hepatitis B, la lepra, la tuberculosis pulmonar, la infección de Candida albicans. |
| 用法、用量<br>Administración y dosis | 皮下注射：20 万～ 40 万 U/m² 加入灭菌注射用水 2ml，一日 1 次，每周注射 4 日，4 周为 1 疗程。肌内注射：慢性乙型肝炎，一次 20 万 U，隔日 1 次。静脉滴注：20 万～ 40 万 U/m²，加入注射用生理盐水 500ml，每日 1 次，每周连用 4 日，4 周为 1 疗程。腔内注射：先抽去腔内积液，再将本品 40 万～ 50 万 U/m² 加入注射用生理盐水 20ml 注入，一周 1 ～ 2 次，3 ～ 4 周为 1 疗程。瘤内、瘤周注射：10 万～ 30 万 U 加入注射用生理盐水 3 ～ 5ml，分多点注射到瘤内或瘤周，一周 2 次，连用 2 周为 1 个疗程。<br><br>Inyección subcutánea: haga una inyección al día con la disolución de 200 mil a 400 mil U/m² con 2ml de agua estéril para inyección, 4 veces a la semana, 4 semanas consisten en un curso de tratamiento. Inyección intramuscular: para hepatitis B crónica, haga la inyección de 200 mil U cada dos días. Infusión intravenosa: haga una inyección al día con la disolución de 200 mil a 400 mil U/m² con 500 ml de solución salina para inyección, uso continuo de 4 días a la semana, 4 semanas consisten en un curso de tratamiento. Inyección en la cavidad: en primer lugar elimine la efusión en la cavidad, y luego haga una inyección en multipuntos Intratumorales o peritumorales con la disolución de 400 mil a 500 mil U/m² con 3~5 ml de solución salina para inyección, 2 veces a la semana, uso continuo de 2 semanas constituye un curso de tratamiento. |
| 剂型、规格<br>Formulaciones y especificaciones | 注射剂（冻干品）：每支 50 万 U；100 万 U；200 万 U；1800 万 U。<br>Agente inyectable (liofilizado): Cada uno es de 500 mil U, 1 millón de U ; 2 millón de U; 18 millones de U. |
| 药品名称 Drug Names | 结核菌素纯蛋白衍生物 Derivado proteínico purificado de la tuberculina (TB-PPD) |
| 适应证<br>Indicaciones | 本品 5U 用于结核病的临床诊断，卡介苗接种对象的选择及卡介苗接种后机体免疫反应的监测。2U 制品用于临床诊断及流行病学监测。<br><br>5U de este medicamento se usa para el diagnóstico clínico de la tuberculosis, selección del objeto de la vacunación BCG y la vigilancia de la respuesta inmunitaria a la vacunación con BCG. 2U de este medicamento se usa para el diagnóstico clínico y la vigilancia epidemiológica. |
| 用法、用量<br>Administración y dosis | ①婴儿、儿童及成人均可用。②皮内注射，吸取本品 0.1ml（5U），皮内注射于前臂掌侧，于注射后 48 ～ 72 小时检查注射部位反应。测量应以硬结的横径及其垂直径的 mm 数记录之。5U 制品反应平均直径应不低于 5mm 为阳性反应。凡有水疱、坏死、淋巴管炎者均属阳性反应，应详细注明。<br><br>① Es medicamento adecuado para los bebés, niños y adultos. ② La inyección intradérmica: absorba 0,1 ml del medicamento (5U), haga la inyección intradérmica por vía intradérmica a lado palmar en el antebrazo, 48 a 72 horas después de la inyección, compruebe las reacciones en la zona de inyección. Se debe medir y registrar el diámetro y el diámetro vertical de induración en milímetros. Si el diámetro promedio de las reacciones de 5U es no menos que 5mm, resulta reacción positiva. Si se aparecen las ampollas, necrosis, linfangitis, resulta reacción positiva, debe especificarse en detalle. |

| | |
|---|---|
| 剂型、规格<br>Formulaciones y especificaciones | 注射剂：每瓶 1ml；2ml。①每一次人用剂量为 0.1ml 含 5UTB-PPD。②每一次人用剂量为 0.1ml 含 2U TB-PPD。<br><br>Agente inyectable: cada botella es de 1 ml; 2 ml. ① La dosis de una persona de una sola vez es de 0.1 ml, que contiene 5UTB-PPD. ② La dosis de una persona de una sola vez es de 0.1 ml, que contiene 2U TB-PPD. |
| 药品名称 Drug Names | 布氏菌纯蛋白衍生物 Derivado proteico purificado de brucelina (BR-PPD) |
| 适应证<br>Indicaciones | 可用于布氏疫苗接种对象的选择及布氏疫苗接种后机体免疫反应的监测和布氏菌的临床诊断与流行病学调查。<br><br>Se usa para la selección del objeto de la vacunación de brucellin, la vigilancia de la respuesta inmunitaria a la vacunación de Brucellin, el diagnóstico clínico de brucellin y la vigilancia epidemiológica. |
| 用法、用量<br>Administración y dosis | 用药途径：吸取本品 0.1ml（1U）皮内注射于前臂掌侧。于注射后 48～72 小时的检查注射部位反应，测量时应以硬节的横径及其垂直径的 mm 数记录之。反应平均直径应不低于 5mm 为阳性。凡有水疱、坏死、淋巴管炎者均属阳性反应，应详细注明。<br><br>Manera de administración: absorba 0.1 ml del medicamento (1U), haga la inyección intradérmica por vía intradérmica a lado palmar en el antebrazo, 48 a 72 horas después de la inyección, compruebe las reacciones en la zona de inyección. Se debe medir y registrar el diámetro y el diámetro vertical de induración en milímetros. Si el diámetro promedio de las reacciones es no menos que 5mm, resulta reacción positiva. Si se aparecen las ampollas, necrosis, linfangitis, resulta reacción positiva, debe especificarse en detalle. |
| 剂型、规格<br>Formulaciones y especificaciones | 注射液：每支 1ml；2ml。每人用量为 0.1ml 含 1U UBR-PPD。<br><br>Solución inyectable: Cada una es de 1 ml; 2 ml. La dosis por persona es de 0.1 ml, incluyendo 1U UBR-PPD. |

# 第 5 章

# 中、英、法、西班牙文对照麻醉药品和精神药品目录

## A List of Narcotic Drugs and Psychotropic Drugs in Chinese, English, French and Spanish

### 麻醉药品品种目录 (2013 年版 )
### Narcotic Drugs List(The 2013 Edition)

| 药品名称 | Drug Names | Dénomination du Médicament | Denominación del Medicamento |
|---|---|---|---|
| 1. 醋托啡 | Acetorphine | Acétorphine | Acetorfina |
| 2. 乙酰阿法甲基芬太尼 | Acetylalphamethylfentanyl | Acétylalphaméthylfentanyl | Acetialfametilfentanilo |
| 3. 醋美沙多 | Acetylmethadol | Acétylméthadol | Acetilmetadol |
| 4. 阿芬太尼 | Alfentanil | Alfentanil | Alfentanilo |
| 5. 烯丙罗定 | Allylprodine | Allylprodine | Alilprodina |
| 6. 阿醋美沙多 | Alphacetylmethadol | Alphacétylméthadol | Alfacetilmetadol |
| 7. 阿法美罗定 | Alphameprodine | Alphaméprodine | Alfameprodina |
| 8. 阿法美沙多 | Alphamethadol | Alphaméthadol | Alfametadol |
| 9. 阿法甲基芬太尼 | Alphamethylfentanyl | Alphaméthylfentanyl | Alfametilfentanilo |
| 10. 阿法甲基硫代芬太尼 | Alphamethylthiofentanyl | Alphaméthylthiofentanyl | Alfametiltiofentanilo |
| 11. 阿法罗定 | Alphaprodine | Alphaprodine | Alfaprodina |
| 12. 阿尼利定 | Anileridine | Aniléridine | Anileridina |
| 13. 苄替啶 | Benzethidine | Benzéthidine | Benzetidina |
| 14. 苄吗啡 | Benzylmorphine | Benzylmorphine | Benzilmorfina |
| 15. 倍醋美沙多 | Betacetylmethadol | Betacétylmethadol | Betacetilmetadol |
| 16. 倍他羟基芬太尼 | Betahydroxyfentanyl | Betahydroxyfentanyl | Betahidroxifentanilo |
| 17. 倍他羟基 -3- 甲基芬太尼 | Betahydroxy-3-methylfentanyl | Betahydroxy-3-méthylfentanyl | Betahidroxi-3-metilfentanilo |
| 18. 倍他美罗定 | Betameprodine | Betaméprodine | Betameprodina |
| 19. 倍他美沙多 | Betamethadol | Betaméthadol | Betametadol |
| 20. 倍他罗定 | Betaprodine | Betaprodine | Betaprodina |
| 21. 贝齐米特 | Bezitramide | Bezitramide | Bezitramida |
| 22. 大麻和大麻树脂与大麻浸膏和酊 | Cannabis and Cannabis Resin, and Extrats and Tinctures of Cannabis | Cannabis et Résine de Cannabis, et Extraits de Cannabis, Teinture de Cannabis | Cannabis y Resina de Cannabis, y Extracto de Cáñamo, y Tintura de Cáñamo |
| 23. 氯尼他秦 | Clonitazene | Clonitazene | Clonitazeno |
| 24. 古柯叶 | Coca Leaf | Feuilles de Coca | Hoja de Coca |
| 25. 可卡因 * | Cocaine | Cocaine | Cocaina |

**续 表**

| 药品名称 | Drug Names | Dénomination du Médicament | Denominación del Medicamento |
| --- | --- | --- | --- |
| 26. 可多克辛 | Codoxime | Codoxime | Codoxima |
| 27. 罂粟秆浓缩物 * | Concentrate of poppy Straw | Concentrés de Paille de Pavot | Concentrado de Paja de Amapola |
| 28. 地索吗啡 | Desomorphine | Desomorphine | Desomorfina |
| 29. 右吗拉胺 | Dextromoramide | Dextromoramide | Dextromoramida |
| 30. 地恩丙胺 | Diampromide | Diampromide | Diampromida |
| 31. 二乙噻丁 | Diethylthiambutene | Diéthylthiambutene | Dietiltiambutena |
| 32. 地芬诺辛 | Difenoxin | Difénoxine | Difenoxina |
| 33. 二氢埃托啡 * | Dihydroetorphine | Dihydroetorphine | Dihidroetorfina |
| 34. 双氢吗啡 | Dihydromorphine | Dihydromorphine | Dihidromorfina |
| 35. 地美沙多 | Dimenoxadol | Diménoxadol | Dimenoxadol |
| 36. 地美庚醇 | Dimepheptanol | Dimepheptanol | Dimefeptanol |
| 37. 二甲噻丁 | Dimethylthiambutene | Diméthylthiambutene | Dimetiltiambutena |
| 38. 吗苯丁酯 | Dioxaphetylbutyrate | Dioxaphetylbutyrate | Dioxafetilbutirato |
| 39. 地芬诺酯 * | Diphenoxylate | Diphénoxylate | Difenoxilato |
| 40. 地匹哌酮 | Dipipanone | Dipipanone | Dipipanona |
| 41. 羟蒂巴酚 | Drotebanol | Drotebanol | Drotebanol |
| 42. 芽子碱 | Ecgonine | Tilline | Tiofilina |
| 43. 乙甲噻丁 | Ethylmethylthiambutene | Ethylméthylthiambutene | Etilmetiltiambutena |
| 44. 依托尼秦 | Etonitazene | Etonitazene | Etonitazena |
| 45. 埃托啡 | Etorphine | Etorphine | Etorfina |
| 46. 依托利定 | Etoxeridine | Etoxeridine | Etoxeridina |
| 47. 芬太尼 * | Fentanyl | Fentanyl | Fentanilo |
| 48. 呋替啶 | Furethidine | Furethidine | Furetidina |
| 49. 海洛因 | Heroin | Héroïne | Heroína |
| 50. 氢可酮 * | Hydrocodone | Hydrocodone | Hidrocodona |
| 51. 氢吗啡醇 | Hydromorphinol | Hydromorphinol | Hidromorfinol |
| 52. 氢吗啡酮 | Hydromorphone | Hydromorphone | Hidromorfona |
| 53. 羟哌替啶 | Hydroxypethidine | Hydroxypethidine | Hidroxipetidina |
| 54. 异美沙酮 | Isomethadone | Isomethadone | Isometadona |
| 55. 凯托米酮 | Ketobemidone | Ketobemidone | Ketobemidona |
| 56. 左美沙芬 | Levomethorphan | Lévométorfène | Levometorfano |
| 57. 左吗拉胺 | Levomoramide | Levomoramide | Levomoramida |
| 58. 左芬啡烷 | Levophenacylmorphan | Levophenacylmorphane | Levofenacilmorfano |
| 59. 左啡诺 | Levorphanol | Levorphanol | Levorfanol |
| 60. 美他佐辛 | Metazocine | Metazocine | Metazocina |

**续　表**

| 药品名称 | Drug Names | Dénomination du Médicament | Denominación del Medicamento |
|---|---|---|---|
| 61. 美沙酮 * | Methadone | Methadone | Metadona |
| 62. 美沙酮中间体 | Methadone Intermediate | Méthadone Intermédiaire | Metadona Intermediaria |
| 63. 甲地索啡 | Methyldesorphine | Méthyldésorphine | Metildesorfina |
| 64. 甲二氢吗啡 | Methyldihydromorphine | Méthyldihydromorphine | Metildihidromorfina |
| 65. 3- 甲基芬太尼 | 3-methylfentanyl | 3-methylfentanyl | 3-metilfentanilo |
| 66. 3- 甲基硫代芬太尼 | 3-methylthiofentanyl | 3-methylthiofentanyl | 3-metiltiofentanilo |
| 67. 美托酮 | Metopon | Metopone | Metopona |
| 68. 吗拉胺中间体 | Moramide Intermediate | Moramide Intermédiaire | Moramida Intermediaria |
| 69. 吗哌利定 | Morpheridine | Morpheridine | Morferidina |
| 70. 吗啡 * | Morphine | Morphine | Morfina |
| 71. 吗啡甲溴化物及其它五价氮吗啡衍生物 | Morphine Methobromide and other pentavalent nitrogen morphine derivatives | Bromure de Méthyle de Morphine et Autres Dérivés de la Morphine de l'Azote Pentavalent | Bromuro Metílico de Morfina y Otros Derivados de la Morfina del Nitrógeno Pentavalente |
| 72. 吗啡 - N - 氧化物 | Morphine-N-oxide | Morphine-N-oxide | Morfina-N-oxida |
| 73. 1- 甲基 -4- 苯基 -4- 哌啶丙酸酯 | 1-Methyl-4-phenyl-4-piperidinol propionate(ester) (MPPP) | Propionate de 1-méthyl-4-phényl-4- pipéridinyle(esters) | Propionato de 1-metil-4-fenil-4- piperidilo(ester) |
| 74. 麦罗啡 | Myrophine | Myrophine | Mirofina |
| 75. 尼可吗啡 | Nicomorphine | Nicomorphine | Nicomorfina |
| 76. 诺美沙多 | Noracymethadol | Noracymethadol | Noracimetadol |
| 77. 去甲左啡诺 | Norlevorphanol | Norlevorphanol | Norlevorfanol |
| 78. 去甲美沙酮 | Normethadone | Normethadone | Normetadona |
| 79. 去甲吗啡 | Normorphine | Normorphine | Normorfina |
| 80. 诺匹哌酮 | Norpipanone | Norpipanone | Norpipanona |
| 81. 阿片 * | Opium | Opium | Opio |
| 82. 奥列巴文 | Oripavine | Oripavine | Oripavina |
| 83. 羟考酮 * | Oxycodone | Oxycodone | Oxicodona |
| 84. 羟吗啡酮 | Oxymorphone | Oxymorphone | Oximorfona |
| 85. 对氟芬太尼 | Para-fluorofentanyl | Para-fluorofentanyl | Para-fluorofentanilo |
| 86. 哌替啶 * | Pethidine | Pethidine | Petidina |
| 87. 哌替啶中间体 A | Pethidine intermediate A | Pethidine Intermédiaire A | Petidina Intermediaria A |
| 88. 哌替啶中间体 B | Pethidine intermediate B | Pethidine Intermédiaire B | Petidina Intermediaria B |
| 89. 哌替啶中间体 C | Pethidine intermediate C | Pethidine Intermédiaire C | Petidina Intermediaria C |
| 90. 苯吗庚酮 | Phenadoxone | Phenadoxone | Fenadoxona |
| 91. 非那丙胺 | Phenampromide | Phenampromide | Fenampromida |

续 表

| 药品名称 | Drug Names | Dénomination du Médicament | Denominación del Medicamento |
|---|---|---|---|
| 92. 非那佐辛 | Phenazocine | Phenazocine | Fenazocina |
| 93. 1-苯乙基-4-苯基-4-哌啶乙酸酯 | 1-phenethyl-4-phenyl-4--piperidinol acetate(ester) | Acétate de 1-phényléthyl-4-phényl- 4-pipéridinol(esters) | Acetato de 1-feniletil-4-fenil-4- piperidinol(ester) |
| 94. 非诺啡烷 | Phenomorphan | Phenomorphane | Fenomorfano |
| 95. 苯哌利定 | Phenoperidine | Phenoperidine | Fenoperidina |
| 96. 匹米诺定 | Piminodine | Piminodine | Piminodina |
| 97. 哌腈米特 | Piritramide | Piritramide | Piritramida |
| 98. 普罗庚嗪 | Proheptazine | Proheptazine | Proheptazina |
| 99. 丙哌利定 | Properidine | Properidine | Properidina |
| 100. 消旋甲啡烷 | Racemethorphan | Racemethorphane | Racemetorfano |
| 101. 消旋吗拉胺 | Racemoramide | Racemoramide | Racemoramida |
| 102. 消旋啡烷 | Racemorphan | Racemorphane | Racemorfano |
| 103 瑞芬太尼 * | Remifentanil | Remifentanyl | Remifentanilo |
| 104. 舒芬太尼 * | Sufentanil | Sufentanyl | Sufentanilo |
| 105. 醋氢可酮 | Thebacon | Thebacon | Tebacon |
| 106. 蒂巴因 * | Thebaine | Thebaine | Tebaina |
| 107. 硫代芬太尼 | Thiofentanyl | Thiofentanyl | Tiofentanilo |
| 108. 替利定 | Tilidine | Tilidine | Tilidina |
| 109. 三甲利定 | Trimeperidine | Trimeperidine | Trimeperidina |
| 110. 醋氢可待因 | Acetyldihydrocodeine | Acetyldihydrocodeine | Acetildihidrocodeina |
| 111. 可待因 * | Codeine | Codeine | Codeina |
| 112. 右丙氧芬 * | Dextropropoxyphene | Dextropropoxyphene | Dextropropoxifeno |
| 113. 双氢可待因 * | Dihydrocodeine | Dihydrocodeine | Dihidrocodeina |
| 114. 乙基吗啡 * | Ethylmorphine | Ethylmorphine | Etilmorfina |
| 115. 尼可待因 | Nicocodine | Nicocodine | Nicocodina |
| 116. 烟氢可待因 | Nicodicodine | Nicodicodine | Nicodicodina |
| 117. 去甲可待因 | Norcodeine | Norcodeine | Norcodeina |
| 118. 福尔可定 * | Pholcodine | Pholcodine | Folcodina |
| 119. 丙吡兰 | Propiram | Propiram | Propiram |
| 120. 布桂嗪 * | Bucinnazine | Bucinnazine | Bucinazina |
| 121. 罂粟壳 * | Poppy Shell | Coquilles de Pavot | Cáscara de Amapola |

注 (Note):
1. 上述品种包括其可能存在的盐和单方制剂 ( 除非另有规定 )。
The above drugs included their salt and prescribed preparation that probably exist.(Unless otherwise specified).
2. 上述品种包括其可能存在的化学异构体及酯、醚 ( 除非另有规定 )。
The above drugs included their chemical isomers, ester and ether that probably exist.(Unless otherwise specified).
3. 品种目录有 "*" 的麻醉药品为我国生产及使用的品种 .
The above drugs of * are produced and used in China.

# 精神药品品种目录 (2019 年版 )
# Psychotropic Drugs List(The 2019 Edition)

| 药品名称 | Drug Names | Dénomination du Médicament | Denominación del Medicamento |
|---|---|---|---|
| 第一类精神药品 | Class I Psychotropic Drugs | Médicaments Psychotropes de Catégorie I | Medicamentos Psicotrópicas de la Categoría I |
| 1. 布苯丙胺 | Brolamfetamine (DOB) | Brolamfetamine (DOB) | Brolamfetamina (DOB) |
| 2. 卡西酮 | Cathinone | Cathinone | Catinona |
| 3. 二乙基色胺 | 3-[2-(Diethylaminoethyl) indole (DET) | 3-[2-(Diethylaminoethyl)indole (DET) | 3-[2-(Dietilaminoetil)indol (DET) |
| 4. 二甲氧基安非他明 | 2,5-dimethoxy-α-methylphene-thylamine (DMA) | 2,5-dimethoxy-α-methylphene-thylamine (DMA) | 2,5-dimetoxi-α-metilfeno-tilamina (DMA) |
| 5.（1，2-二甲基庚基）羟基四氢甲基二苯吡喃 | Dimethylheptyl-tetrahydro-trimethyl—6H-dibenzopyran-ol (DMHP) | Dimethylheptyl-tetrahydro-trimethyl—6H-dibenzopyran-ol (DMHP) | Dimetilheptil-tetrahidro-trimetil—6H -dibenzopiran-ol (DMHP) |
| 6. 二甲基色胺 | Dimethylamino-ethyl-indole (DMT) | Dimethylamino-ethyl-indole (DMT) | Dimetilamino-etil-indol (DMT) |
| 7. 二甲氧基乙基安非他明 | Ethyl-dimethoxy-α-methylphene-thylamine (DOET) | Ethyl-dimethoxy-α-methylphene-thylamine (DOET) | Etil-dimetoxi-α-metilfeno-tilamina (DOET) |
| 8. 乙环利定 | Eticyclidine (PCE) | Eticyclidine (PCE) | Eticiclidina (PCE) |
| 9. 乙色胺 | Etryptamine | Etryptamine | Etriptamina |
| 10. 羟芬胺 | α-methyl-methylenedioxy-phenethyl - hydroxylamine, (N-hydroxyl MDA) | α-methyl-methylenedioxy-phenethyl-hydroxylamine,(N-hydroxyl MDA) | α-metil-metilenedioxi-fenetil-hidroxilamina, (N-hidroxil MDA) |
| 11. 麦角二乙胺 | (+)-Lysergide (LSD) | (+)-Lysergide (LSD) | (+)-Lisergida (LSD) |
| 12. 乙芬胺 | Ethyl-α- methyl -methylenedioxy-phenethylamine,(N-ethyl,MDA) | Ethyl-α- methyl -methylenedioxy-phenethylamine,(N-ethyl,MDA) | Etil-α- metil -metilenedioxi-fenetilamina,(N-etil,MDA) |
| 13. 二亚甲基双氧安非他明 | α-methyl—methylenedioxy-phene thylamine,( MDMA) | α-methyl—methylenedioxy-phene thylamine,( MDMA) | α-metil—metilenedioxi- fene tilamina,( MDMA) |
| 14. 麦司卡林 | Mescaline | Mescaline | Mescalina |
| 15. 甲卡西酮 | Methcathinone | Methcathinone | Metcatinona |
| 16. 甲米雷司 | 4-methylaminorex | 4-methylaminorex | 4-metilaminorex |
| 17. 甲羟芬胺 | Methoxy-α-methyl-methylened-ioxy - phenethylamine , (MMDA) | Methoxy-α- methyl- methylenedi-oxy - phenethylamine , (MMDA) | Metoxi-α- metil-metilenedioxi -fenetilamina , (MMDA) |
| 18. 4- 甲基硫基安非他明 | 4-methylthioamfetamine | 4-methylthioamfetamine | 4-metiltioamfetamina |
| 19. 六氢大麻酚 | Parahexyl | Parahexyl | Parahexilo |
| 20. 副甲氧基安非他明 | P-methoxyα-methylphenethyla-mine（PMA） | P-methoxyα-methylphenethyl-amine（PMA） | P-metoxilα-metilfenetilamina (PMA) |
| 21. 赛洛新 | Psilocine | Psilocine | Psilocina |
| 22. 赛洛西宾 | Psilocybine | Psilocybine | Psilocibina |
| 23. 咯环利定 | Rolicyclidine,(PHP) | Rolicyclidine,(PHP) | Roliciclidina,(PHP) |

**续　表**

| 药品名称 | Drug Names | Dénomination du Médicament | Denominación del Medicamento |
|---|---|---|---|
| 24. 二甲氧基甲苯异丙胺 | Dimethyoxy-α- dimethylphe-nethy lamine (STP ) | Dimethyoxy-α- dimethylphe-nethy lamine (STP ) | Dimetioxi-α- dimetilfenetila-mina (STP ) |
| 25. 替苯丙胺 | Tenamfetamine (MDA) | Tenamfetamine (MDA) | Tenamfetamina (MDA) |
| 26. 替诺环定 | Tenocyclidine(TCP) | Tenocyclidine(TCP) | Tenociclidina(TCP) |
| 27. 四氢大麻酚（包括其同分异构物及其立体化学变体） | Tetrahydrocannabinol | Tetrahydrocannabinol | Tetrahidrocannabinol |
| 28. 三甲氧基安非他明 | Trimethoxyl-α-methylphenethy lamine (TMA) | Trimethoxyl-α-methylphenethy lamine (TMA) | Trimetoxil-α-metilfenetilamina (TMA) |
| 29. 苯丙胺 | Amfetamine | Amfetamine | Amfetamina |
| 30. 氨奈普汀 | Amineptine | Amineptine | Amineptina |
| 31. 2,5- 二甲氧基 -4- 溴苯乙胺 | 4-bromo-2,5-dimethoxyphe-nethy-lamine(2-CB) | 4-bromo-2,5-dimethoxyphe-nethy-lamine(2-CB) | 4-bromo-2,5-dimetoxifenetila-mina (2-CB) |
| 32. 右苯丙胺 | Dexamfetamine | Dexamfetamine | Dexamfetamina |
| 33. 屈大麻酚 | Dronabinol | Dronabinol | Dronabinol |
| 34. 芬乙茶碱 | Fenetylline | Fenétylline | Fenetilina |
| 35. 左苯丙胺 | Levamfetamine | Levamfétamine | Levamfetamina |
| 36. 左甲苯丙胺 | Levomethamfetamine | Levomethamfétamine | Levometamfetamina |
| 37. 甲氯喹酮 | Mecloqualone | Mecloqualone | Mecloqualona |
| 38. 去氧麻黄碱 | Metamfetamine | Metamfétamine | Metamfetamina |
| 39. 去氧麻黄碱外消旋体 | Metamfetamine Racemate | Metamfétamine Racéate | Metamfetamina Racemato |
| 40. 甲喹酮 | Methaqualone | Methaqualone | Metaqualona |
| 41. 哌醋甲酯 * | Methylphenidate | Methylphénidate | Metilfenidato |
| 42. 苯环利定 | Phencyclidine (PCP) | Phencyclidine (PCP) | Fenciclidina (PCP) |
| 43. 芬美曲秦 | Phenmetrazine | Phenmétrazine | Fenmetrazina |
| 44. 司可巴比妥 * | Secobarbital | Secobarbital | Secobarbital |
| 45. 齐培丙醇 | Zipeprol | Zipeprol | Zipeprol |
| 46. 安非拉酮 | Amfepramone | Amfepramone | Amfepramona |
| 47. 苄基哌嗪 | Benzylpiperazine(BZP) | Benzylpipérazine(BZP) | Benzilpiperazina(BZP) |
| 48. 丁丙诺啡 * | Buprenorphine | Buprenorphine | Buprenorfina |
| 49. 丁基萘甲酰基吲哚 | Butyl-naphthoyl-indole (JWH-073) | Butyl-naphthoyl-indole (JWH-073) | Butil-naftoil-indol(JWH-073) |
| 50. 恰特草 | Catha edulis Forssk(Khat) | Catha edulis Forssk(Khat) | Cata edulis Forssk(Khat) |
| 51. 二甲氧基碘苯乙胺 | Dimethoxyiodophenethylamine(2C-I) | Dimethoxyiodophenethylamine(2C-I) | Dimetoxyiodofenetilamina (2C-I) |

**续　表**

| 药品名称 | Drug Names | Dénomination du Médicament | Denominación del Medicamento |
|---|---|---|---|
| 52. 二甲氧基苯乙胺 | Dimethoxyphenethylamine (2C-H) | Dimethoxyphenethylamine (2C-H) | Dimetoxifenetilamina(2C-H) |
| 53. 二甲基安非他明 | Dimethylamfetamine | Dimethylamfetamine | Dimetilamfetamina |
| 54. 依他喹酮 | Etaqualone | Etaqualone | Etaqualona |
| 55. 氟戊基 -1H- 吲哚碘苯基甲酮 | Fluoropentyl-1H-indole-iodobenzoyl-keton(AM-694) | Fluoropentyl-1H-indole-iodobenzoyl-keton(AM-694) | Fluoropentil-1H-indol-iodobenzoil-keton(AM-694) |
| 56. 氟戊基 - 萘甲酰基 -1H- 吲哚 | Fluoropentyl--naphthoyl-1H-indole(AM-2201) | Fluoropentyl-naphthoyl-1H-indole(AM-2201) | Fluoropentil--naftoil -1H-indol (AM-2201) |
| 57. γ - 羟丁酸 * | γ-hydroxybutyrate (GHB) | γ-hydroxybutyrate (GHB) | γ-hidroxibutirato (GHB) |
| 58. 氯胺酮 * | Ketamine | Ketamine | Ketamina |
| 59. 马吲哚 * | Mazindol | Mazindol | Mazindol |
| 60. 甲氧基苯基 - 戊基 -1H- 吲哚 - 基 - 乙酮 | Methoxyphenyl-pentyl-1H-indol-yl-ethanone(JWH-250) | Methoxyphenyl-pentyl-1H-indol-yl-ethanone(JWH-250) | Metoxifenil-pentil-1H-indol-il-etanona(JWH-250) |
| 61. 亚甲基二氧吡咯戊酮 | Methylenedioxypyrovalerone (MDPV) | Methylenedioxypyrovalerone (MDPV) | Metilenedioxipirovalerona (MDPV) |
| 62. 甲基乙卡西酮 | Methylethcathinone(4-MEC) | Methylethcathinone(4-MEC) | Metiletcatinona(4-MEC) |
| 63. 甲基甲卡西酮 | Methylmethcathinone(4-MMC) | Methylmethcathinone(4-MMC) | Metilmetcatinona(4-MMC) |
| 64. 亚甲二氧基甲卡西酮 | Methylenedioxy-methcathinone (Methylone) | Methylenedioxy-methcathinone (Methylone) | Metilenedioxi-metcatinona (Metilona) |
| 65. 莫达非尼 | Modafinil | Modafinile | Modafinilo |
| 66. 戊基 - 萘甲酰基 - 吲哚 | Pentyl- naphthoyl -indole (JWH-018) | Pentyl- naphthoyl -indole (JWH-018) | Pentil- naftoil -indol (JWH-018) |
| 67. 他喷他多 | Tapentadol | Tapentadol | Tapentadol |
| 68. 三唑仑 * | Triazolam | Triazolam | Triazolam |
| 69. 口服固体制剂每剂量单位含羟考酮碱大于 5mg，且不含其他麻醉药品、精神药品或药品类易制毒化学品的复方制剂 * | Oral solid preparation of oxycodone (>5mg/dose unit), and it didn't contain any other narcotic drugs, psychotropic drugs or a compound preparation(belonging to the category of drugs) of precursor chemicals (easily manufacturing drugs). | Préparations orales solides d'oxycodone (> 5mg/ unité de dose), et Il ne contient pas d'autres stupéfiants et substances psychotropes ou préparations composées (appartenant à la catégorie des médicaments) de précurseurs chimiques (Il est facile de fabriquer des drogues). | Preparación oral sólida de oxicodona(> 5mg/unidad de dosis), y no contiene otros estupefacientes, sustancias psicotrópicas o preparados compuestos (perteneciente a la categoría de los medicamentos) de precursores químicos (fácil fabricación de drogas). |
| 第二类精神药品 | Class Ⅱ Psychotropic Drugs | Médicaments Psychotropes de Catégorie Ⅱ | Medicamentos Psicotrópicas de la Categoría Ⅱ |
| 1. 异戊巴比妥 * | Amobarbital | Amobarbital | Amobarbital |
| 2. 布他比妥 | Butalbital | Butalbital | Butalbital |
| 3. 去甲伪麻黄碱 * | Cathine | Cathine | Catina |
| 4. 环己巴比妥 | Cyclobarbital | Cyclobarbital | Ciclobarbital |
| 5. 氟硝西泮 | Flunitrazepam | Flunitrazépam | Flunitrazepam |

**续 表**

| 药品名称 | Drug Names | Dénomination du Médicament | Denominación del Medicamento |
|---|---|---|---|
| 6. 格鲁米特 * | Glutethimide | Glutethimide | Glutetimida |
| 7. 喷他佐辛 * | Pentazocine | Pentazocine | Pentazocina |
| 8. 戊巴比妥 * | Pentobarbital | Pentobarbital | Pentobarbital |
| 9. 阿普唑仑 * | Alprazolam | Alprazolam | Alprazolam |
| 10. 阿米雷司 | Aminorex | Aminorex | Aminorex |
| 11. 巴比妥 * | Barbital | Barbital | Barbital |
| 12. 苄非他明 | Benzfetamine | Benzfetamine | Benzfetamina |
| 13. 溴西泮 | Bromazepam | Bromazépam | Bromazepam |
| 14. 溴替唑仑 | Brotizolam | Brotizolam | Brotizolam |
| 15. 丁巴比妥 | Butobarbital | Butobarbital | Butobarbital |
| 16. 卡马西泮 | Camazepam | Camazépam | Camazepam |
| 17. 氯氮䓬 * | Chlordiazepoxide | Chlordiazépoxide | Clordiazepoxida |
| 18. 氯巴占 | Clobazam | Clobazam | Clobazam |
| 19. 氯硝西泮 * | Clonazepam | Clonazépam | Clonazepam |
| 20. 氯拉䓬酸 | Clorazepate | Clorazépate | Clorazepato |
| 21. 氯噻西泮 | Clotiazepam | Clotiazépam | Clotiazepam |
| 22. 氯噁唑仑 | Cloxazolam | Cloxazolam | Cloxazolam |
| 23. 地洛西泮 | Delorazepam | Delorazépam | Delorazepam |
| 24. 地西泮 * | Diazepam | Diazépam | Diazepam |
| 25. 艾司唑仑 * | Estazolam | Estazolam | Estazolam |
| 26. 乙氯维诺 | Ethchlorvynol | Ethchlorvynol | Etclorvinol |
| 27. 炔己蚁胺 | Ethinamate | Ethinamate | Etinamato |
| 28. 氯氟䓬乙酯 * | Ethyl Loflazepate | Ethyl Loflazepate | Etil Loflazepato |
| 29. 乙非他明 | Etilamfetamine | Etilamfétamine | Etilamfetamina |
| 30. 芬坎法明 | Fencamfamin | Fencamfamine | Fencamfamina |
| 31. 芬普雷司 | Fenproporex | Fenproporex | Fenproporex |
| 32. 氟地西泮 | Fludiazepam | Fludiazépam | Fludiazepam |
| 33. 氟西泮 * | Flurazepam | Flurazépam | Flurazepam |
| 34. 哈拉西泮 | Halazepam | Halazépam | Halazepam |
| 35. 卤沙唑仑 | Haloxazolam | Haloxazolam | Haloxazolam |
| 36. 凯他唑仑 | Ketazolam | Ketazolam | Ketazolam |
| 37. 利非他明 | Lefetamine | Lefetamine | Lefetamina |

**续　表**

| 药品名称 | Drug Names | Dénomination du Médicament | Denominación del Medicamento |
|---|---|---|---|
| 38. 氯普唑仑 | Loprazolam | Loprazolam | Loprazolam |
| 39. 劳拉西泮 * | Lorazepam | Lorazépam | Lorazepam |
| 40. 氯甲西泮 | Lormetazepam | Lormetazépam | Lormetazepam |
| 41. 美达西泮 | Medazepam | Medazépam | Medazepam |
| 42. 美芬雷司 | Mefenorex | Méfénorex | Mefenorex |
| 43. 甲丙氨酯 * | Meprobamate | Meprobamate | Meprobamato |
| 44. 美索卡 | Mesocarb | Mesocarb | Mesocarb |
| 45. 甲苯巴比妥 | Methylphenobarbital | Methylphénobarbital | Metilfenobarbital |
| 46. 甲乙哌酮 | Methyprylon | Methyprylon | Metiprilon |
| 47. 咪达唑仑 * | Midazolam | Midazolam | Midazolam |
| 48. 尼美西泮 | Nimetazepam | Nimetazépam | Nimetazepam |
| 49. 硝西泮 * | Nitrazepam | Nitrazépam | Nitrazepam |
| 50. 去甲西泮 | Nordazepam | Nordazépam | Nordazepam |
| 51. 奥沙西泮 * | Oxazepam | Oxazépam | Oxazepam |
| 52. 奥沙唑仑 | Oxazolam | Oxazolam | Oxazolam |
| 53. 匹莫林 * | Pemoline | Pémoline | Pemolina |
| 54. 苯甲曲秦 | Phendimetrazine | Phéndimétrazine | Fendimetrazina |
| 55. 苯巴比妥 * | Phenobarbital | Phénobarbital | Fenobarbital |
| 56. 芬特明 | Phentermine | Phéntérmine | Fentermina |
| 57. 匹那西泮 | Pinazepam | Pinazépam | Pinazepam |
| 58. 哌苯甲醇 | Pipradrol | Pipradrol | Pipradrol |
| 59. 普拉西泮 | Prazepam | Prazepam | Prazepam |
| 60. 吡咯戊酮 | Pyrovalerone | Pyrovalerone | Pirovalerona |
| 61. 仲丁比妥 | Secbutabarbital | Secbutabarbital | Secbutabarbital |
| 62. 替马西泮 | Temazepam | Témazépam | Temazepam |
| 63. 四氢西泮 | Tetrazepam | Tétrazépam | Tetrazepam |
| 64. 乙烯比妥 | Vinylbital | Vinylbital | Vinilbital |
| 65. 唑吡坦 * | Zolpiden | Zolpiden | Zolpiden |
| 66. 阿洛巴比妥 | Allobarbital | Allobarbital | Alobarbital |
| 67. 丁丙诺啡透皮贴剂 * | Buprenorphine Transdermal Patch | Parements Transcutanés de Buprénorphine | Parches Transdérmicos de Buprenorfina |
| 68. 布托啡诺及其注射剂 * | Butorphanol and its Injection | Butorfanol et ses Injections | Butorfanol y sus Inyectables |

| 药品名称 | Drug Names | Dénomination du Médicament | Denominación del Medicamento |
|---|---|---|---|
| 69. 咖啡因 * | Caffeine | Cafeine | Cafeina |
| 70. 苯甲酸钠咖啡因 * | Caffeine Sodium Benzoate (CNB) | Benzoate de Sodium et de Caféine | Benzoato de Sodio y Cafeína |
| 71. 右旋芬氟拉明 | Dexfenfluramine | Dexfenfluramine | Dexfenfluramina |
| 72. 地佐辛及其注射剂 * | Dezocine and its Injection | Dezocine et ses Injections | Dezocine y sus Inyectables |
| 73. 麦角胺咖啡因片 * | Ergotamine and Caffeine Tablet | Ergotamine et Comprimés de Caféine | Ergotamina y Tabletas de Cafeína |
| 74. 芬氟拉明 | Fenfluramine | Fenfluramine | Fenfluramina |
| 75. 呋芬雷司 | Furfenorex | Furfenorex | Furfenorex |
| 76. 纳布啡及其注射剂 | Nalbuphine and its Injection | Nalbuphine et ses Injections | Nalbufina y sus Inyectables |
| 77. 氨酚氢可酮片 * | Paracetamol and Hydrocodone Bitartrate Tablet | Comprimés de Paracetamol et Hydrocodone Bitartrique | Tabletas de Paracetamol y Hidrocodona Bitartárico |
| 78. 丙己君 | Propylhexedrine | Propylhexedrine | Propilhexedrina |
| 79. 曲马多 * | Tramadol | Tramadol | Tramadol |
| 80. 扎来普隆 * | Zaleplone | Zaleplone | Zaleplona |
| 81. 佐匹克隆 * | Zopiclone | Zopiclone | Zopiclona |
| 82. 含可待因复方口服液体制剂（包括口服溶液剂、糖浆剂）* | Compound oral liquid preparation containing codeine (including oral solution and syrup). | Préparations orales liquides composées contenant de la codeine (y compris les solutions orales et les préparations sirop). | Preparados líquidos orales compuestos que contengan codeína (incluidos los preparados de solución oral y los preparados de jarabe). |
| 83. 口服固体制剂每剂量单位含羟考酮碱不超过 5mg，且不含其他麻醉药品、精神药品或药品类易制毒化学品的复方制剂 * | Oral solid preparation of oxycodone ( ≤ 5mg/dose unit), and it didn't contain any other narcotic drugs, psychotropic drugs or a compound preparation(belonging to the category of drugs) of precursor chemicals (easily manufacturing drugs). | Préparations orales solides d'oxycodone( ≤ 5mg/ unité de dose), et Il ne contient pas d'autres stupéfiants et substances psychotropes ou préparations composées (appartenant à la catégorie des médicaments) de précurseurs chimiques (Il est facile de fabriquer des drogues). | Preparación oral sólida de oxicodona( ≤ 5mg/unidad de dosis), y no contiene otros estupefacientes, sustancias psicotrópicas o preparados compuestos (perteneciente a la categoría de los medicamentos) de precursores químicos (fácil fabricación de drogas). |
| 84. 丁丙诺啡的复方口服固体制剂 * | A compound oral solid preparation of buprenorphine | Préparations orales solides composées de buprénorphine | Preparados sólidos orales compuestos de buprenorfina |
| 85. 纳洛酮的复方口服固体制剂 * | A compound oral solid preparation of naloxone | Préparations orales solides composées de naloxone | Preparado compuesto de naloxona para administración oral sólida |

注 (Note)：
1. 上述品种包括其可能存在的盐和单方制剂（除非另有规定）。
   The above drugs included their salt and prescribed preparation that probably exist.(Unless otherwise specified).
2. 上述品种包括其可能存在的化学异构体及酯、醚（除非另有规定）。
   The above drugs included their chemical isomers, ester and ether that probably exist.(Unless otherwise specified).
3. 品种目录有 "*" 的麻醉药品为我国生产及使用的品种.
   The above drugs of * are produced and used in China.

# 第 6 章
# 中、英、法、西班牙文对照妊娠危险等级药品目录

## A List of Drugs Dangerous to Pregnancy in Chinese, English, French and Spanish

| 药品名称 | Drug Name | Dénomination du médicament | Denominación del medicamento | 给药途径<br>Administration Route<br>Voie dàdministration<br>Vía de administración | 对妊娠危险性分级<br>Classification of pregnancy risk<br>Classification des risques liés à la grossesse Clasificación del riesgo de embarazo |
|---|---|---|---|---|---|
| 阿巴卡韦 | Abacavir | Abacavir | Abacavir | 口服给药，Oral | C |
| 阿苯达唑 | Albendazole | Albendazole | Albendazol | 口服给药，Oral | C |
| 阿达木单抗 | Adalimumab | Adalimumab | Adalimumab | 肠道外给药，Parentaral | B |
| 阿达帕林 | Adapalene | Adapalene | Adapalena | 局部 / 皮肤外用<br>Local/Skin( External Use) | C |
| 阿德福韦酯 | Adefovir Dipivoxil | Adefovir Dipivoxil | Adefovir Dipivoxil | 口服给药，Oral | C |
| 阿地白介素 | Aldesleukin | Aldesleukine | Aldesleukina | 肠道外给药，Parentaral | C |
| 阿伐斯汀 | Acrivastine | Acrivastine | Acrivastina | 口服给药，Oral | B |
| 阿芬太尼 | Alfentanil | Alfentanil | Alfentanilo | 肠道外给药，Parentaral | C；D- 如在临近分娩时长期大量使用<br>D-For example, long-term used in large doses near delivery. |
| 阿夫唑嗪 | Alfuzosin | Alfuzosine | Alfuzosina | 口服给药，Oral | B |
| 阿加曲班 | Argatroban | Argatroban | Argatroban | 肠道外给药，Parentaral | B |
| 阿卡波糖 | Acarbose | Acarbose | Acarbosa | 口服给药，Oral | B |
| 阿坎酸 | Acamprosate | Acamprosate | Acamprosato | 口服给药，Oral | C |
| 阿立哌唑 | Aripiprazole | Aripiprazole | Aripiprazol | 口服给药，Oral | C |
| 阿氯米松 | Alclometasone | Alclometasone | Alclometasona | 局部 / 皮肤外用<br>Local/Skin( External Use) | C |
| 阿仑膦酸 | Alendronate | Alendronate | Alendronato | 口服给药，Oral | C |
| 阿仑珠单抗 | Alemtuzumab | Alemtuzumab | Alemtuzumab | 肠道外给药，Parentaral | C |
| 阿米卡星 | Amikacin | Amikacine | Amikacina | 肠道外给药，Parentaral | D |
| 阿米洛利 | Amiloride | Amiloride | Amilorida | 口服给药，Oral | B；D- 如用于妊娠高血压患者<br>D-For example, for patients with gestational hypertension. |
| 阿米替林 | Amitriptyline | Amitriptyline | Amitriptilina | 口服给药，Oral | C |
| | | | | 肠道外给药，Parentaral | C |

**续　表**

| 药品名称 | Drug Name | Dénomination du médicament | Denominación del medicamento | 给药途径<br>Administration Route<br>Voie dàdministration<br>Vía de administración | 对妊娠危险性分级<br>Classification of pregnancy risk<br>Classification des risques liés<br>à la grossesse Clasificación<br>del riesgo de embarazo |
|---|---|---|---|---|---|
| 阿莫沙平 | Amoxapine | Amoxapine | Amoxapina | 口服给药，Oral | C |
| 阿莫西林 | Amoxicillin | Amoxicilline | Amoxicilina | 口服给药，Oral | B |
| 阿那格雷 | Anagrelide | Anagrelide | Anagrelida | 口服给药，Oral | C |
| 阿那曲唑 | Anastrozole | Anastrozole | Anastrozol | 口服给药，Oral | D |
| 阿普唑仑 | Alprazolam | Alprazolam | Alprazolam | 口服给药，Oral | D |
| 阿奇霉素 | Azithromycin | Azithromycine | Azitromicina | 口服给药，Oral | B |
| 阿曲库铵 | Atracurium | Atracurium | Atracurium | 肠道外给药，Parentaral | C |
| 阿瑞匹坦 | Aprepitant | Aprepitant | Aprepitant | 口服给药，Oral | B |
| 阿司咪唑 | Astemizole | Astemizole | Astemizol | 口服给药，Oral | C |
| 阿司帕坦 | Aspartame | Aspartame | Aspartam | 口服给药，Oral | B；C- 如用于苯丙酮尿症患者<br>C-For example, for patients with phenylketonuria. |
| 阿司匹林 | Aspirin | Aspirine | Aspirina | 口服给药，Oral | C；D- 如在妊娠晚期大量使用<br>D-For example, large dose used in late stage of pregnancy. |
| 阿糖胞苷 | Cytarabine | Cytarabine | Citarabina | 肠道外给药，Parentaral | D |
| 阿糖苷酶 | Alglucerase | Alglucerase | Alglucerasa | 肠道外给药，Parentaral | C |
| 阿糖腺苷 | Vidarabine | Vidarabine | Vidarabina | 眼部给药<br>Ophthalmic Drug Delivery | C |
| 阿替洛尔 | Atenolol | Atenolol | Atenolol | 口服给药，Oral | D |
| 阿替普酶 | Alteplase | Alteplase | Alteplasa | 肠道外给药，Parentaral | C |
| 阿托伐醌 | Atovaquone | Atovaquone | Atovaquona | 口服给药，Oral | C |
| 阿托伐他汀 | Atorvastatin | Atorvastatine | Atorvastatina | 口服给药，Oral | X |
| 阿托品 | Atropine | Atropine | Atropina | 眼部给药<br>Ophthalmic Drug Delivery | C |
|  |  |  |  | 口服给药，Oral | C |
|  |  |  |  | 肠道外给药，Parentaral | C |
| 阿维 A | Acitretin | Acitretine | Acitretina | 口服给药，Oral | X |
| 阿维 A 酯 | Eretinate | Eretinate | Eretinato | 口服给药，Oral | X |
| 阿昔单抗 | Abciximab | Abciximab | Abciximab | 肠道外给药，Parentaral | C |
| 阿昔洛韦 | Aciclovir | Aciclovir | Aciclovir | 口服给药，Oral | B |
|  |  |  |  | 肠道外给药，Parentaral | B |
|  |  |  |  | 局部 / 皮肤外用<br>Local/Skin( External Use) | B |
| 阿扎那韦 | Atazanavir | Atazanavir | Atazanavir | 口服给药，Oral | B |

**续 表**

| 药品名称 | Drug Name | Dénomination du médicament | Denominación del medicamento | 给药途径<br>Administration Route<br>Voie dàdministration<br>Vía de administración | 对妊娠危险性分级<br>Classification of pregnancy risk<br>Classification des risques liés à la grossesse Clasificación del riesgo de embarazo |
|---|---|---|---|---|---|
| 阿扎他定 | Azatadine | Azatadine | Azatadina | 口服给药，Oral | B |
| 艾司美拉唑 | Esomeprazole | Esomeprazole | Esomeprazol | 口服给药，Oral | B |
| 艾司洛尔 | Esmolol | Esmolol | Esmolol | 肠道外给药，Parentaral | C |
| 艾斯西酞普兰 | Escitalopram | Escitalopram | Escitalopram | 口服给药，Oral | C |
| 艾司唑仑 | Estazolam | Estazolam | Estazolam | 口服给药，Oral | X |
| 安非拉酮 | Amfepramone | Amfepramone | Amfepramona | 口服给药，Oral | B |
| 安非他酮 | Bupropion | Bupropione | Bupropion | 口服给药，Oral | C |
| 安普尼定 | Apraclonidine | Apraclonidine | Apraclonidina | 眼部给药<br>Ophthalmic Drug Delivery | C |
| 安他唑啉 | Antazoline | Antazoline | Antazolina | 眼部给药<br>Ophthalmic Drug Delivery | C |
| 安西奈德 | Amcinonide | Amcinonide | Amcinonida | 局部/皮肤外用<br>Local/Skin( External Use) | C |
| 氨苯蝶啶 | Triamterene | Triamterene | Triamterena | 口服给药，Oral | C；D- 如用于妊娠高血压患者<br>D-For example, for patient with gestational hypertension. |
| 氨苯砜 | Dapsone | Dapsone | Dapsona | 口服给药，Oral | C |
| 氨苯磺胺 | Sulfanilamide | Sulfanilamide | Sulfanilamida | 阴道给药<br>Vaginal Administration | C；D- 如在临近分娩时使用<br>D-For example, used for near delivery. |
| 氨苄西林 | Ampicillin | Ampicillin | Ampicilina | 口服给药，Oral | B |
| 氨茶碱 | Aminophylline | Aminophylline | Aminofilina | 口服给药，Oral | C |
|  |  |  |  | 肠道外给药，Parentaral | C |
|  |  |  |  | 直肠给药，<br>Rectal Administration | C |
| 氨基己酸 | Aminocaproic Acid | Acide Aminocaproique | Acido Aminocaproico | 口服给药，Oral | C |
|  |  |  |  | 肠道外给药，Parentaral | C |
| 氨甲环酸 | Tranexamic Acid | Acide Tranexamique | Acido Tranexamico | 口服给药，Oral | B |
|  |  |  |  | 肠道外给药，Parentaral | B |
| 氨力农 | Amrinone | Amrinone | Amrinona | 肠道外给药，Parentaral | C |
| 氨磷汀 | Amifostine | Amifostine | Amifostina | 肠道外给药，Parentaral | C |
| 氨鲁米特 | Aminoglute-thimide | Aminoglutethi-mide | Aminogluteti-mida | 口服给药，Oral | D |

**续 表**

| 药品名称 | Drug Name | Dénomination du médicament | Denominación del medicamento | 给药途径 Administration Route Voie dàdministration Vía de administración | 对妊娠危险性分级 Classification of pregnancy risk Classification des risques liés à la grossesse Clasificación del riesgo de embarazo |
|---|---|---|---|---|---|
| 氨氯地平 | Amlodipine | Amlodipine | Amlodipina | 口服给药，Oral | C |
| 氨普那韦 | Amprenavir | Amprenavir | Amprenavir | 口服给药，Oral | C |
| 氨曲南 | Aztreonam | Aztreonam | Aztreonam | 肠道外给药，Parentaral | B |
| 胺碘酮 | Amiodarone | Amiodarone | Amiodarona | 口服给药，Oral | D |
| | | | | 肠道外给药，Parentaral | D |
| 昂丹司琼 | Ondansetron | Ondansetron | Ondansetron | 口服给药，Oral | B |
| | | | | 肠道外给药，Parentaral | B |
| 奥布卡因 | Oxybuprocaine | Oxybuprocaine | Oxibuprocaina | 眼部给药 Ophthalmic Drug Delivery | C |
| 奥氮平 | Olanzapine | Olanzapine | Olanzapina | 口服给药，Oral | C |
| 奥芬君 | Orphenadrine | Orphenadrine | Orfenadrina | 口服给药，Oral | C |
| | | | | 肠道外给药，Parentaral | C |
| 奥卡西平 | Oxcarbazepine | Oxcarbazèpine | Oxcarbazepina | 口服给药，Oral | C |
| 奥利司他 | Oristat | Oristat | Oristat | 口服给药，Oral | B |
| 奥洛他定 | Olopatadine | Olopatadine | Olopatadina | 眼部给药 Ophthalmic Drug Delivery | C |
| 奥马珠单抗 | Omalizumab | Omalizumab | Omalizumab | 肠道外给药，Parentaral | B |
| 奥美拉唑 | Omeprazole | Omèprazole | Omeprazol | 口服给药，Oral | C |
| | | | | 肠道外给药，Parentaral | C |
| 奥美沙坦酯 | Olmesartan Medoxomil | Olmèsartan Mèdoxomil | Olmesartan Medoxomil | 口服给药，Oral | C；D- 如在妊娠中、晚期用药 D-For example, used in middle and late stage of pregnancy. |
| 奥匹哌醇 | Opipramol | Opipramol | Opipramol | 口服给药，Oral | C |
| 奥曲肽 | Octreotide | Octrèotide | Octreotida | 肠道外给药，Parentaral | B |
| 奥赛米韦 | Oseltamivir | Osèltamivir | Oseltamivir | 口服给药，Oral | C |
| 奥沙拉嗪 | Olsalazine | Olsalazine | Olsalazina | 口服给药，Oral | C |
| 奥沙利铂 | Oxaliplatin | Oxaliplatine | Oxaliplatina | 肠道外给药，Parentaral | D |
| 奥沙普秦 | Oxaprozin | Oxaprozine | Oxaprozina | 口服给药，Oral | C；D- 如在妊娠晚期或临近分娩时用药 D-For example, used in late stage of pregnancy or for near delivery. |
| 奥沙西泮 | Oxazepam | Oxazèpam | Oxazepam | 口服给药，Oral | D |
| 奥昔布宁 | Oxybutynin | Oxybutynine | Oxibutinina | 口服给药，Oral | B |
| 巴氨西林 | Bacampicillin | Bacampicilline | Bacampicilina | 口服给药，Oral | B |

**续 表**

| 药品名称 | Drug Name | Dénomination du médicament | Denominación del medicamento | 给药途径<br>Administration Route<br>Voie dàdministration<br>Vía de administración | 对妊娠危险性分级<br>Classification of pregnancy risk<br>Classification des risques liés à la grossesse Clasificación del riesgo de embarazo |
|---|---|---|---|---|---|
| 巴利昔单抗 | Basiliximab | Basiliximab | Basiliximab | 肠道外给药，Parentaral | B |
| 巴龙霉素 | Paromomycin | Paromomycine | Paromomicina | 口服给药，Oral | C |
| 巴氯芬 | Baclofen | Baclofène | Baclofeno | 口服给药，Oral | C |
|  |  |  |  | 肠道外给药，Parentaral | C |
| 白蛋白 | Albumin | Albumine | Albumina | 肠道外给药，Parentaral | C |
| 白陶土 | Kaolin | Kaolin | Kaolin | 口服给药，Oral | B |
| 白消安 | Busulfan | Busulfane | Busulfano | 口服给药，Oral | D |
| 保泰松 | Phenylbutazone | Phènylbutazone | Fenilbutazona | 口服给药，Oral | C；D- 如在妊娠晚期或临近分娩时用药<br>D-For example, used in late stage pregnancy or for near delivery. |
| 贝卡普勒明 | Becaplermin | Becaplèrmine | Becaplermina | 局部／皮肤外用<br>Local/Skin( External Use) | C |
| 贝那普利 | Benazepril | Benazèpril | Benazepril | 口服给药，Oral | C；D- 如在妊娠中、晚期用药<br>D-For example, used in middle and late stage of pregnancy. |
| 倍氯米松 | Beclometasone | Beclomètasone | Beclometasona | 吸入，Inhalation | C |
|  |  |  |  | 鼻腔给药，Nasal Delivery | C |
| 倍他洛尔 | Betaxolol | Bétaxolol | Betaxolol | 眼部给药<br>Ophthalmic Drug Delivery | C |
|  |  |  |  | 口服给药，Oral | C；D- 如在妊娠中、晚期用药<br>D-For example, used in middle and late pregnancy. |
| 倍他米松 | Betamethasone | Betamèthasone | Betametasona | 口服给药，Oral | C；D- 如在妊娠早期用药<br>D-For example, used in first trimester of pregnancy. |
|  |  |  |  | 肠道外给药，Parentaral | C；D- 如在妊娠早期用药<br>D-For example, used in first trimester of pregnancy. |
|  |  |  |  | 局部／皮肤外用<br>Local/Skin( External Use) | C；D- 如在妊娠早期用药<br>D-For example, used in first trimester of pregnancy. |
| 苯巴比妥 | Phenobarbital | Phènobarbital | Fenobarbital | 肠道外给药，Parentaral | D |
| 苯丙醇胺 | Phenylpropa-nolamine | Phènylpropa-nolamine | Fenilpropanola-mina | 口服给药，Oral | C |
| 苯丁胺氮芥 | Chlorambucil | Chlorambucil | Clorambucil | 口服给药，Oral | D |

**续 表**

| 药品名称 | Drug Name | Dénomination du médicament | Denominación del medicamento | 给药途径<br>Administration Route<br>Voie dàdministration<br>Vía de administración | 对妊娠危险性分级<br>Classification of pregnancy risk<br>Classification des risques liés à la grossesse Clasificación del riesgo de embarazo |
|---|---|---|---|---|---|
| 苯海拉明 | Diphenhydramine | Diphènhydramine | Difenhidramina | 口服给药，Oral | B |
| | | | | 肠道外给药，Parentaral | B |
| 苯海索 | Trihexyphenidyl | Trihèxyphénidyl | Trihexifenidil | 口服给药，Oral | C |
| 苯磺顺阿曲库铵 | Cisatracurium Besilate | Cisatracurium Bèsilate | Cisatracurio Besilato | 肠道外给药，Parentaral | B |
| 苯甲曲秦 | Phendimetrazine | Phéndimétrazine | Fendimetrazina | 口服给药，Oral | C |
| 苯托沙敏 | Phenyltoloxamine | Phényltoloxamine | Feniltoloxamina | 口服给药，Oral | C |
| 苯妥英 | Phenytoin | phénytoïne | Fenitoina | 口服给药，Oral | D |
| | | | | 肠道外给药，Parentaral | D |
| 苯乙肼 | Phenelzine | Phénélzine | Fenelzina | 口服给药，Oral | C |
| 苯佐卡因 | Benzocaine | Bénzocaine | Benzocaina | 口腔咽喉给药，Oral Cavity and Throat Administration | C |
| 苯唑西林 | Oxacillin | Oxacillin | Oxacilina | 口服给药，Oral | B |
| 比卡鲁胺 | Bicalutamide | Bicalutamide | Bicalutamida | 口服给药，Oral | X |
| 比马前列素 | Bimatoprost | Bimatoprost | Bimatoprost | 眼部给药<br>Ophthalmic Drug Delivery | C |
| 比哌立登 | Biperiden | Bipéridene | Biperidena | 口服给药，Oral | C |
| | | | | 肠道外给药，Parentaral | C |
| 比沙可啶 | Bisacodyl | Bisacodyl | Bisacodil | 口服给药，Oral | B |
| | | | | 直肠给药<br>Rectal Administration | B |
| 比索洛尔 | Bisoprolol | Bisoprolol | Bisoprolol | 口服给药，Oral | C；D- 如在妊娠中、晚期用药<br>D-For example, used in middle and late stage of pregnancy. |
| 吡多辛 | Pyridoxine | Pyridoxine | Piridoxina | 口服给药，Oral | A |
| | | | | 肠道外给药，Parentaral | A |
| 比格列酮 | Pioglitazone | Pioglitazone | Pioglitazona | 口服给药，Oral | C |
| 吡喹酮 | Praziquantel | Praziquantel | Praziquantel | 口服给药，Oral | B |
| 吡罗昔康 | Piroxicam | Piroxicam | Piroxicam | 口服给药，Oral | C；D- 如在妊娠晚期或临近分娩时用药<br>D-For example, used in late stage of pregnancy or for near delivery. |

| 药品名称 | Drug Name | Dénomination du médicament | Denominación del medicamento | 给药途径<br>Administration Route<br>Voie dàdministration<br>Vía de administración | 对妊娠危险性分级<br>Classification of pregnancy risk<br>Classification des risques liés à la grossesse Clasificación del riesgo de embarazo |
|---|---|---|---|---|---|
| 吡美莫司 | Pimecrolimus | Pimécrolimus | Pimecrolimus | 局部 / 皮肤外用<br>Local/Skin( External Use) | C |
| 吡嗪酰胺 | Pyrazinamide | Pyrazinamide | Pirazinamida | 口服给药，Oral | C |
| 苄氟噻嗪 | Bendroflumethi-azide | Bendroflumethi-azide | Bendroflumeti-azida | 口服给药，Oral | C；D- 如用于妊娠高血压患者<br>D-For example, for patient with gestational hypertension. |
| 苄青霉素 | Benzylpenici-llin | Benzylpenicilline | Benzilpenicilina | 肠道外给药，Parentaral | B |
| 苄星青霉素 | Benzathine Benzylpenici-llin | Benzathine Benzylpenicilline | Benzilpenicilina Benzatina | 肠道外给药，Parentaral | B |
| 表柔比星 | Epirubicin | Epirubicine | Epirubicina | 肠道外给药，Parentaral | B |
| 别嘌醇 | Allopurinol | Allopurinol | Alopurinol | 口服给药，Oral | D |
|  |  |  |  | 肠道外给药，Parentaral | C |
| 丙吡胺 | Disopyramide | Disopyramide | Disopiramida | 口服给药，Oral | C |
|  |  |  |  | 肠道外给药，Parentaral | C |
| 丙泊酚 | Propofol | Propofol | Propofol | 肠道外给药，Parentaral | C |
| 丙环定 | Procyclidine | Procyclidine | Prociclidina | 口服给药，Oral | B |
| 丙磺舒 | Probenecid | Probenecid | Probenecid | 口服给药，Oral | C |
| 丙卡巴肼 | Procarbazine | Procarbazine | Procarbazina | 口服给药，Oral | C |
| 丙硫氧嘧啶 | Propylthiour-acil | Propylthiouracil | Propiltiouracil | 口服给药，Oral | D |
| 丙氯拉嗪 | Prochlorper-azine | Prochlorperazine | Proclorperazina | 口服给药，Oral | D |
|  |  |  |  | 肠道外给药，Parentaral | C |
|  |  |  |  | 直肠给药<br>Rectal Administration | C |
| 丙美卡因 | Proxymetaca-ine | Proxymetacaine | Proximetacaina | 眼部给药<br>Ophthalmic Drug Delivery | C |
| 丙米嗪 | Imipramine | Imipramine | Imipramina | 口服给药，Oral | C |
|  |  |  |  | 肠道外给药，Parentaral | C |
| 丙嗪 | Promazine | Promazine | Promazina | 口服给药，Oral | C |
| 丙戊酸 | Valproic Acid | Acide Valproïque | Ácido Valproico | 口服给药，Oral | D |
|  |  |  |  | 肠道外给药，Parentaral | D |
| 波生坦 | Bosentan | Bosentan | Bosentan | 口服给药，Oral | X |

**续 表**

| 药品名称 | Drug Name | Dénomination du médicament | Denominación del medicamento | 给药途径 Administration Route Voie dàdministration Vía de administración | 对妊娠危险性分级 Classification of pregnancy risk Classification des risques liés à la grossesse Clasificación del riesgo de embarazo |
|---|---|---|---|---|---|
| 波希鼠李皮 | Cascara | Cascara | Cascara | 口服给药，Oral | C |
| 伯胺喹 | Primaquine | Primaquine | Primaquina | 口服给药，Oral | C |
| 泊利噻嗪 | Polythiazide | Polythiazide | Politiazida | 口服给药，Oral | C；D- 如用于妊娠高血压患者 D-For example, for patients with gestational hypertension. |
| 博来霉素 | Bleomycin | Bleomycine | Bleomicina | 肠道外给药，Parentaral | D |
| 布比卡因 | Bupivacaine | Bupivacaine | Bupivacaina | 肠道外给药，Parentaral | C |
| 布地奈德 | Budesonide | Budesonide | Budesonida | 吸入，Inhalation | B |
| | | | | 鼻腔给药，Nasal Delivery | B |
| | | | | 口服给药，Oral | C |
| | | | | 直肠给药 Rectal Administration | C |
| 布康唑 | Butoconazole | Butoconazole | Butoconazol | 阴道给药 Vaginal Administration | C |
| 布可利嗪 | Buclizine | Buclizine | Buclizina | 口服给药，Oral | C |
| 布林佐胺 | Brinzolamide | Brinzolamide | Brinzolamida | 眼部给药 Ophthalmic Drug Delivery | C |
| 布洛芬 | Ibuprofen | Ibuprofène | Ibuprofeno | 口服给药，Oral | B；D- 如在妊娠晚期或临近分娩时用药 D-For example, used in late stage of pregnancy or for near delivery. |
| 布美他尼 | Bumetanide | Bumétanide | Bumetanida | 口服给药，Oral | C |
| | | | | 肠道外给药，Parentaral | C |
| 布他比妥 | Butalbital | Butalbital | Butalbital | 口服给药，Oral | C；D- 如在临近分娩时长期大量使用 D-For example, long-term used in large doses near delivery. |
| 布替林 | Butriptyline | Butriptyline | Butriptilina | 口服给药，Oral | C |
| 布托啡诺 | Butorphanol | Butorphanol | Butorfanol | 鼻腔给药，Nasal Delivery | C；D- 如在临近分娩时长期大量使用 D-For example, long-term used in large doses near delivery. |
| | | | | 肠道外给药，Parentaral | C；D- 如在临近分娩时长期大量使用 D-For example, long-term used in large doses near delivery. |
| 茶苯海明 | Dramamine | Dramamine | Dramamina | 肠道外给药，Parentaral | B |

续　表

| 药品名称 | Drug Name | Dénomination du médicament | Denominación del medicamento | 给药途径<br>Administration Route<br>Voie dàdministration<br>Vía de administración | 对妊娠危险性分级<br>Classification of pregnancy risk<br>Classification des risques liés à la grossesse Clasificación del riesgo de embarazo |
|---|---|---|---|---|---|
| 茶碱 | Theophylline | Théophylline | Teofilina | 口服给药，Oral | C |
|  |  |  |  | 肠道外给药，Parentaral | C |
| 长春碱 | Vinblastine | Vinblastine | Vinblastina | 肠道外给药，Parentaral | D |
| 长春瑞滨 | Vinorelbine | Vinorélbine | Vinorelbina | 肠道外给药，Parentaral | D |
| 长春新碱 | Vincristine | Vincristine | Vincristina | 肠道外给药，Parentaral | D |
| 雌二醇 | Estradiol | Estradiol | Estradiol | 口腔咽喉给药，Oral Cavity and Throat Administration | X |
|  |  |  |  | 口服给药，Oral | X |
|  |  |  |  | 经皮给药，Transdermal Drug Delivery | X |
|  |  |  |  | 阴道给药 Vaginal Administration | X |
| 雌莫司汀 | Estramustine | Estramustine | Estramustina | 口服给药，Oral | X |
| 雌酮 | Estrone | Estrone | Estrona | 肠道外给药，Parentaral | X |
| 促红素 | Erythropoietin | Erythropoiétin | Eritropoyetina | 肠道外给药，Parentaral | C |
| 促卵泡素 α | Follitropin Alfa | Follitropine Alfa | Folitropina Alfa | 肠道外给药，Parentaral | X |
| 促卵泡素 β | Follitropin Beta | Follitropine Beta | Folitropina Beta | 肠道外给药，Parentaral | X |
| 促皮质素 | Corticotrophin | Corticotrophine | Corticotrofina | 肠道外给药，Parentaral | C |
| 醋丁洛尔 | Acebutolol | Acébutolol | Acebutolol | 口服给药，Oral | B；D-如在妊娠中、晚期使用药 D-For example, used in middle and late stage of pregnancy. |
| 醋磺己脲 | Acetohexamide | Acétohexamide | Acetohexamida | 口服给药，Oral | C |
| 醋甲唑胺 | Methazolamide | Méthazolamide | Metazolamida | 口服给药，Oral | C |
| 醋酸吡布特罗 | Pirbuterol Acetate | Acétate de Pirbutérol | Acetato de Pirbuterol | 吸入，Inhalation | C |
| 醋酸奋乃静 | Thiopropazate | Thiopropazate | Tiopropazato | 口服给药，Oral | C |
| 醋酸钙 | Calcium Acetate | Acétate de Calcium | Acetato de Calcio | 肠道外给药，Parentaral | C |
| 醋竹桃霉素 | Troleandomycin | Troléandomycine | Troleandomicina | 口服给药，Oral | C |
| α 达贝泊汀 | Darbepoetin Alfa | Darbépoétine Alfa | Darbepoetina Alfa | 肠道外给药，Parentaral | C |
| 达肝素钠 | Dalteparin Sodium | Daltéparine Sodique | Dalteparina Sódica | 肠道外给药，Parentaral | B |

**续 表**

| 药品名称 | Drug Name | Dénomination du médicament | Denominación del medicamento | 给药途径<br>Administration Route<br>Voie dàdministration<br>Vía de administración | 对妊娠危险性分级<br>Classification of pregnancy risk<br>Classification des risques liés à la grossesse Clasificación del riesgo de embarazo |
|---|---|---|---|---|---|
| 达卡巴嗪 | Dacarbazine | Dacarbazine | Dacarbazina | 肠道外给药，Parentaral | C |
| 达那肝素钠 | Danaparoid Sodium | Danaparoide Sodique | Danaparoida Sódica | 肠道外给药，Parentaral | B |
| 达那唑 | Danazol | Danazol | Danazol | 口服给药，Oral | X |
| 达托霉素 | Daptomycin | Daptomycine | Daptomicina | 肠道外给药，Parentaral | B |
| 大观霉素 | Spectinomycin | Spéctinomycine | Spectinomicina | 肠道外给药，Parentaral | B |
| 丹曲林 | Dantrolene | Dantroléne | Dantrolena | 口服给药，Oral | C |
| | | | | 肠道外给药，Parentaral | C |
| 单硝酸异山梨酯 | Isosorbide Mononitrate | Mononitrate d' Isosorbide | Mononitrato de Isosorbida | 口服给药，Oral | C |
| 胆骨化醇 | Colecalciferol | Colécalciférol | Colecalciferol | 口服给药，Oral | A；D- 如剂量超过美国的每日推荐摄入量<br>D-For example, the dosage exceeded the daily intake recommended by United States. |
| 胆碱水杨酸镁 | Choline Magnesium Trisalicylate | Choline Trisalicylate de Magnésium | Trisalicilato de colina y Magnesio | 口服给药，Oral | C；D- 如在妊娠晚期或临近分娩时用药<br>D-For example, used in late stage of pregnancy or for near delivery. |
| 氮卓斯汀 | Azelastine | Azélastine | Azelastina | 眼部给药<br>Ophthalmic Drug Delivery | C |
| 氮芥 | Chlormethine | Chlorméthine | Clormetina | 肠道外给药，Parentaral | D |
| 地尔硫卓 | Diltiazem | Diltiazém | Diltiazem | 口服给药，Oral | C |
| | | | | 肠道外给药，Parentaral | C |
| 地芬诺酯 | Diphenoxylate | Diphénoxylate | Difenoxilato | 口服给药，Oral | C |
| 地氟烷 | Desflurane | Désflurane | Desflurano | 吸入，Inhalation | B |
| 地高辛 | Digoxin | Digoxine | Digoxina | 口服给药，Oral | C |
| 地红霉素 | Dirithromycin | Dirithromycin | Diritromicina | 口服给药，Oral | C |
| 地拉韦啶 | Delavirdine | Délavirdine | Delavirdina | 口服给药，Oral | C |
| 地氯雷他定 | Desloratadine | Désloratadine | Desloratadina | 口服给药，Oral | C |
| 地美环素 | Demeclocycline | Déméclocycline | Demeclociclina | 口服给药，Oral | D |
| 地诺前列酮 | Dinoprostone | Dinoprostone | Dinoprostona | 阴道给药<br>Vaginal Administration | C |
| 地匹福林 | Dipivefrine | Dipivéfrine | Dipivefrina | 眼部给药<br>Ophthalmic Drug Delivery | B |

**续　表**

| 药品名称 | Drug Name | Dénomination du médicament | Denominación del medicamento | 给药途径<br>Administration Route<br>Voie dàdministration<br>Vía de administración | 对妊娠危险性分级<br>Classification of pregnancy risk<br>Classification des risques liés à la grossesse Clasificación del riesgo de embarazo |
|---|---|---|---|---|---|
| 地塞米松 | Dexamethasone | Déxaméthasone | Dexametasona | 眼部给药<br>Ophthalmic Drug Delivery | C |
| | | | | 口服给药，Oral | C；D- 如在妊娠早期用药<br>D-For example, used in the first trimester of pregnancy. |
| | | | | 肠道外给药，Parentaral | C；D- 如在妊娠早期用药<br>D-For example, used in the first trimester of pregnancy. |
| 地索奈德 | Desonide | Désonide | Desonida | 局部 / 皮肤外用<br>Local/Skin( External Use) | C |
| 地西卢定 | Desirudin | Désirudine | Desirudina | 肠道外给药，Parentaral | C |
| 地西泮 | Diazepam | Diazépam | Diazepam | 口服给药，Oral | D |
| | | | | 肠道外给药，Parentaral | D |
| | | | | 直肠给药<br>Rectal Administration | D |
| 地昔帕明 | Desipramine | Désipramine | Desipramina | 口服给药，Oral | C |
| 碘 | Iodine | l'iode | Yodo | 口服给药，Oral | D |
| 碘达胺 | Iodamide | Iodamide | Iodamida | 肠道外给药，Parentaral | D |
| 碘甘油 | Iodinated Glycerol | Iodoglycérol | Iodoglicerol | 口服给药，Oral | X |
| 碘苷 | Idoxuridine | Idoxuridine | Idoxuridina | 眼部给药<br>Ophthalmic Drug Delivery | C |
| 碘化钾 | Potassium Iodide | Iodure de Potassium | Yoduro de Potasio | 口服给药，Oral | D |
| 碘化钠 | Sodium Iodide | Iodure de Sodium | Yoduro Sódico | 口服给药，Oral | X；D- 如作为祛痰药使用<br>D-For example, when used as an expectorant. |
| 碘塞罗宁 | Liothyronine | Liothyronine | Liotironina | 口服给药，Oral | A |
| 丁苯那嗪 | Tetrabenazine | Tétrabénazine | Tetrabenazina | 口服给药，Oral | C |
| 丁丙诺啡 | Buprenorphine | Buprénorphine | Buprenorfina | 肠道外给药，Parentaral | C |
| 丁卡因 | Tetracaine | Tétracaine | Tetracaina | 眼部给药<br>Ophthalmic Drug Delivery | C |
| 丁螺环酮 | Buspirone | Buspirone | Buspirona | 口服给药，Oral | B |
| 东莨菪碱 | Scopolamine (Hyoscine) | Scopolamine | Scopolamina | 口服给药，Oral | C |
| | | | | 肠道外给药，Parentaral | C |
| | | | | 经皮给药，Transdermal Drug Delivery | C |

**续 表**

| 药品名称 | Drug Name | Dénomination du médicament | Denominación del medicamento | 给药途径<br>Administration Route<br>Voie dàdministration<br>Vía de administración | 对妊娠危险性分级<br>Classification of pregnancy risk<br>Classification des risques liés à la grossesse Clasificación del riesgo de embarazo |
|---|---|---|---|---|---|
| 毒扁豆碱 | Physostigmine | Physostigmine | Fisostigmina | 眼部给药<br>Ophthalmic Drug Delivery | C |
| | | | | 肠道外给药，Parentaral | C |
| 度他雄胺 | Dutasteride | Dutastéride | Dutasterida | 口服给药，Oral | X |
| 对乙酰氨基酚 | Paracetamol | Paracétamol | Paracetamol | 口服给药，Oral | B |
| 多巴胺 | Dopamine | Dopamine | Dopamina | 肠道外给药，Parentaral | C |
| 多巴酚丁胺 | Dobutamine | Dobutamine | Dobutamina | 肠道外给药，Parentaral | B |
| 多库酯钠 | Docusate Sodium | Docusate de Sodium | Docusato Sódico | 口服给药，Oral | C |
| 多拉司琼 | Dolasetron | Dolasétron | Dolasetron | 口服给药，Oral | B |
| | | | | 肠道外给药，Parentaral | B |
| 多奈哌齐 | Donepezil | Donépézil | Donepezil | 口服给药，Oral | C |
| 多黏菌素 B | Polymyxin B | Polymyxine B | Polimixina B | 局部 / 皮肤外用<br>Local/Skin( External Use) | B |
| 多柔比星 | Doxorubicin | Doxorubicine | Doxorubicina | 肠道外给药，Parentaral | D |
| 多塞平 | Doxepin | Doxépine | Doxepina | 口服给药，Oral | C |
| 多沙普伦 | Doxapram | Doxapram | Doxapram | 肠道外给药，Parentaral | B |
| 多沙唑嗪 | Doxazosin | Doxazosine | Doxazosina | 口服给药，Oral | C |
| 多西环素 | Doxycycline | Doxycycline | Doxiciclina | 口服给药，Oral | D |
| 多西拉敏 | Doxylamine | Doxylamine | Doxilamina | 口服给药，Oral | A |
| 多西他赛 | Docetaxel | Docétaxel | Docetaxel | 肠道外给药，Parentaral | D |
| 多佐胺 | Dorzolamide | Dorzolamide | Dorzolamida | 眼部给药<br>Ophthalmic Drug Delivery | C |
| 鹅去氧胆酸 | Chenodeoxycholic Acid | Acide Chénodéoxycholique | Acido Cenodeoxicolico | 口服给药，Oral | X |
| 厄贝沙坦 | Irbesartan | Irbésartan | Irbesartan | 口服给药，Oral | C；D- 如在妊娠中、晚期用药<br>D-For example, used in middle and late stage of pregnancy. |
| 厄洛替尼 | Erlotinib | Erlotinib | Erlotinib | 口服给药，Oral | D |
| 厄他培南 | Ertapenem | Ertapénem | Ertapenem | 肠道外给药，Parentaral | B |
| 恩夫韦地 | Enfuvirtide | Enfuvirtide | Enfuvirtida | 肠道外给药，Parentaral | B |
| 恩氟烷 | Enflurane | Enflurane | Enflurano | 吸入，Inhalation | B |
| 恩他卡朋 | Entacapone | Entacapone | Entacapona | 口服给药，Oral | C |

**续　表**

| 药品名称 | Drug Name | Dénomination du médicament | Denominación del medicamento | 给药途径<br>Administration Route<br>Voie dàdministration<br>Vía de administración | 对妊娠危险性分级<br>Classification of pregnancy risk<br>Classification des risques liés à la grossesse Clasificación del riesgo de embarazo |
|---|---|---|---|---|---|
| 二苯西平 | Dibenzepin | Dibénzépine | Dibenzepina | 口服给药，Oral | C |
| 二氮嗪 | Diazoxide | Diazoxide | Diazoxida | 口服给药，Oral | C |
|  |  |  |  | 肠道外给药，Parentaral | C |
| 二氟尼柳 | Diflunisal | Diflunisal | Diflunisal | 口服给药，Oral | C；D- 如在妊娠晚期或临近分娩时用药<br>D-For example, used in late stage of pregnancy or for near delivery. |
| 二甲双胍 | Metformin | Métformine | Metformina | 口服给药，Oral | B |
| 二甲茚定 | Dimethindene | Diméthindéne | Dimetindena | 口服给药，Oral | B |
| 二羟丙茶碱 | Diprophylline | Diprophylline | Diprofilina | 口服给药，Oral | C |
| 伐他那非 | Vardenafil | Vardénafil | Vardenafil | 口服给药，Oral | B |
| 伐地昔布 | Valdecoxib | Valdécoxib | Valdecoxib | 口服给药，Oral | C |
| 伐昔洛韦 | Valaciclovir | Valaciclovir | Valaciclovir | 口服给药，Oral | B |
| 法莫替丁 | Mamotidine | Mamotidine | Mamotidina | 口服给药，Oral | B |
| 番泻叶苷 A 和 B | Sensenoside A and B | Scinosine A et B | Escinosina A y B | 口服给药，Oral | C |
| 泛酸 | Pantothenic Acid | Acide Pantothenique | Acido Pantotenico | 口服给药，Oral | A；C- 如剂量超过美国的每日推荐摄入量<br>C-For example, the dosage exceeded the daily intake recommended by United States. |
| 泛昔洛韦 | Famciclovir | Famciclovir | Famciclovir | 口服给药，Oral | B |
| 放线菌素 | Actinomycin | Actinomycine | Actinomicina | 肠道外给药，Parentaral | C |
| 非格司亭 | Filgrastim | Filgrastim | Filgrastim | 肠道外给药，Parentaral | C |
| 非洛地平 | Felodipine | Félodipine | Felodipina | 口服给药，Oral | C |
| 非那吡啶 | Phenazopyridine | Phénazopyridine | Fenazopiridina | 口服给药，Oral | B |
| 非那西汀 | Phenacetin | Phénacétine | Fenacetina | 口服给药，Oral | B |
| 非那雄胺 | Finasteride | Finastéride | Finasterida | 口服给药，Oral | X |
| 非尼拉敏 | Pheniramine | Phéniramine | Feniramina | 口服给药，Oral | C |
| 非诺贝特 | Fenofibrate | Fénofibrate | Fenofibrato | 口服给药，Oral | C |
| 非诺洛芬 | Fenoprofen | Fénoprofène | Fenoprofeno | 口服给药，Oral | B；D- 如在妊娠晚期或临近分娩时用药<br>D-For example, used in late stage of pregnancy or for near delivery. |
| 非诺特罗 | Fenoterol | Fénotérol | Fenoterol | 肠道外给药，Parentaral | B |

**续　表**

| 药品名称 | Drug Name | Dénomination du médicament | Denominación del medicamento | 给药途径 Administration Route Voie dàdministration Vía de administración | 对妊娠危险性分级 Classification of pregnancy risk Classification des risques liés à la grossesse Clasificación del riesgo de embarazo |
|---|---|---|---|---|---|
| 非索非那定 | Fexofenadine | Féxofénadine | Fexofenadina | 口服给药，Oral | C |
| 芬氟拉明 | Fenfluramine | Fénfluramine | Fenfluramina | 口服给药，Oral | C |
| 芬太尼 | Fentanyl | Féntanyl | Fentanilo | 口含，Keep in the mouth | C；D- 如在临近分娩时长期大量使用 D-For example, long-term used in large doses near delivery. |
|  |  |  |  | 肠道外给药，Parentaral | C；D |
|  |  |  |  | 经皮给药，Transdermal Drug Delivery | C；D |
| 芬特明 | Phentermine | Phéntérmine | Fentermina | 口服给药，Oral | C |
| 酚苄明 | Phenoxybenzamine | Phénoxybénzamine | Fenoxibenzamina | 口服给药，Oral | C |
|  |  |  |  | 肠道外给药，Parentaral | C |
| 酚酞 | Phenolphthalein | Phénolphthaléine | Fenolftaleina | 口服给药，Oral | C |
| 酚妥拉明 | Phentolamine | Phéntolamine | Fentolamina | 肠道外给药，Parentaral | C |
| 奋乃静 | Perphenazine | Pérphénazine | Perfenazina | 口服给药，Oral | C |
| 呋喃妥因 | Nitrofurantoin | Nitrofurantoine | Nitrofurantoina | 口服给药，Oral | B |
| 呋喃唑酮 | Furazolidone | Furazolidone | Furazolidona | 口服给药，Oral | C |
| 呋塞米 | Furosemide | Furosémide | Furosemida | 口服给药，Oral | C；D- 如用于妊娠高血压患者 D-For example, for patients with gestational hypertension. |
|  |  |  |  | 肠道外给药，Parentaral | C；D- 如用于妊娠高血压患者 D-For example, for patients with gestational hypertension. |
| 伏立康唑 | Voriconazole | Voriconazole | Voriconazol | 口服给药，Oral | D |
|  |  |  |  | 肠道外给药，Parentaral | D |
| 氟胞嘧啶 | Flucytosine | Flucytosine | Flucitosina | 口服给药，Oral | C |
| 氟比洛芬 | Flurbiprofen | Flurbiproféne | Flurbiprofeno | 眼部给药 Ophthalmic Drug Delivery | C；D- 如在妊娠晚期或临近分娩时用药 D-For example, used in late stage of pregnancy or for near delivery. |
|  |  |  |  | 口服给药，Oral | B；D- 如在妊娠晚期或临近分娩时用药 D-For example, used in late stage of pregnancy or for near delivery. |
| 氟达拉滨 | Fludarabine | Fludarabine | Fludarabina | 肠道外给药，Parentaral | D |

**续　表**

| 药品名称 | Drug Name | Dénomination du médicament | Denominación del medicamento | 给药途径<br>Administration Route<br>Voie dàdministration<br>Vía de administración | 对妊娠危险性分级<br>Classification of pregnancy risk<br>Classification des risques liés à la grossesse Clasificación del riesgo de embarazo |
|---|---|---|---|---|---|
| 氟伐他汀 | Fluvastatin | Fluvastatine | Fluvastatina | 口服给药，Oral | X |
| 氟奋乃静 | Fluphenazine | Fluphénazine | Flufenazina | 口服给药，Oral | C |
|  |  |  |  | 肠道外给药，Parentaral | C |
| 氟伏沙明 | Fluvoxamine | Fluvoxamine | Fluvoxamina | 口服给药，Oral | C |
| 氟甲睾酮 | Fluoxymesterone | Fluoxymésterone | Fluoximesterona | 口服给药，Oral | X |
| 氟卡尼 | Flecainide | Flecainide | Flecainida | 口服给药，Oral | C |
|  |  |  |  | 肠道外给药，Parentaral | C |
| 氟康唑 | Fluconazole | Fluconazole | Fluconazol | 口服给药，Oral | C |
|  |  |  |  | 肠道外给药，Parentaral | C |
| 氟可龙 | Fluocortolone | Fluocortolone | Fluocortolona | 局部 / 皮肤外用<br>Local/Skin( External Use) | C |
| 氟马西尼 | Flumazenil | Flumazénil | Flumazenilo | 肠道外给药，Parentaral | C |
| 氟米龙 | Fluorometholone | Fluorométholone | Fluorometolona | 眼部给药<br>ophthalmic drug delivery | C |
| 氟尼缩松 | Flunisolide | Flunisolide | Flunisolida | 吸入，Inhalation | C |
| 氟尿苷 | Floxuridine | Floxuridine | Floxuridina | 肠道外给药，Parentaral | D |
| 氟尿嘧啶 | Fluorouracil | Fluorouracil | Fluorouracilo | 肠道外给药，Parentaral | D |
|  |  |  |  | 局部 / 皮肤外用<br>Local/Skin( External Use) | X |
| 氟哌啶醇 | Haloperidol | Halopéridol | Haloperidol | 口服给药，Oral | C |
|  |  |  |  | 肠道外给药，Parentaral | C |
| 氟哌利多 | Droperidol | Dropéridol | Droperidol | 肠道外给药，Parentaral | C |
| 氟哌噻吨 | Flupentixol | Flupéntixol | Flupentixol | 口服给药，Oral | C |
|  |  |  |  | 肠道外给药，Parentaral | C |
| 氟氢可的松 | Fludrocortisone | Fludrocortisone | Fludrocortisona | 口服给药，Oral | C |
| 氟轻松醋酸酯 | Fluocinolone Acetonide | Acétate Fluocinolone | Acetato Fluocinolona | 局部 / 皮肤外用<br>Local/Skin( External Use) | C |
| 氟他胺 | Flutamide | Flutamide | Flutamida | 口服给药，Oral | D |
| 氟替卡松 | Fluticasone | Fluticasone | Fluticasona | 吸入，Inhalation | C |
|  |  |  |  | 鼻腔给药，Nasal Delivery | C |
|  |  |  |  | 局部 / 皮肤外用<br>Local/Skin( External Use) | C |

**续　表**

| 药品名称<br>Drug Name | Dénomination<br>du médicament | Denominación<br>del<br>medicamento | 给药途径<br>Administration Route<br>Voie dàdministration<br>Vía de administración | 对妊娠危险性分级<br>Classification of pregnancy risk<br>Classification des risques liés<br>à la grossesse Clasificación<br>del riesgo de embarazo |
|---|---|---|---|---|---|
| 氟西泮 | Flurazepam | Flurazépam | Flurazepam | 口服给药，Oral | X |
| 氟西汀 | Fluoxetine | Fluoxétine | Fluoxetina | 口服给药，Oral | C |
| 福莫特罗 | Formoterol | Formotérol | Formoterol | 吸入，Inhalation | C |
| 福辛普利 | Fosinopril | Fosinopril | Fosinopril | 口服给药，Oral | C；D- 如在妊娠中、晚期用药<br>D-For example, used in middle<br>and late stage of pregnancy. |
| 钆喷酸 | Gadopentetic<br>Acid | Acide<br>Gadopéntétique | Acido<br>Gadopentetico | 肠道外给药，Parentaral | C |
| 甘精胰岛素 | Insulin Glargine | Insuline Glargine | Insulina<br>Glargina | 肠道外给药，Parentaral | C |
| 甘露醇 | Mannitol | Mannitol | Manitol | 肠道外给药，Parentaral | C |
| 杆菌肽 | Bacitracin | Bacitracine | Bacitracina | 眼部给药<br>Ophthalmic Drug Delivery | C |
|  |  |  |  | 肠道外给药，Parentaral | C |
|  |  |  |  | 局部 / 皮肤外用<br>Local/Skin( External Use) | C |
| α 干扰素 | Interferon Alfa | Interféron Alfa | Interferon Alfa | 肠道外给药，Parentaral | C |
| β 干扰素 | Interferon Beta | Interféron Beta | Interferon Beta | 肠道外给药，Parentaral | C |
| γ 干扰素 | Interferon<br>Gamma | Interféron Gamma | Interferon<br>Gamma | 肠道外给药，Parentaral | C |
| 肝素 | Heparin | Héparine | Heparina | 肠道外给药，Parentaral | C |
| 高血糖素 | Glucagon | Glucagon | Glucagon | 肠道外给药，Parentaral | B |
| 睾酮 | Testosterone | Téstostérone | Testosterona | 口服给药，Oral | X |
|  |  |  |  | 肠道外给药，Parentaral | X |
|  |  |  |  | 局部 / 皮肤外用<br>Local/Skin( External Use) | X |
|  |  |  |  | 经皮给药，Transdermal<br>Drug Delivery | X |
| 戈那瑞林 | Gonadorelin | Gonadoréline | Gonadorelina | 肠道外给药，Parentaral | B |
| 戈舍瑞林 | Goserelin | Goséréline | Goserelina | 肠道外给药，Parentaral | X |
| 格拉司琼 | Granisetron | Granisétron | Granisetron | 口服给药，Oral | B |
|  |  |  |  | 肠道外给药，Parentaral | B |
| 格列本脲 | Glibenclamide | Glibénclamide | Glibenclamida | 口服给药，Oral | C |
| 格列吡嗪 | Glipizide | Glipizide | Glipizida | 口服给药，Oral | C |
| 格列美脲 | Glimepiride | Glimépiride | Glimepirida | 口服给药，Oral | C |

**续 表**

| 药品名称 | Drug Name | Dénomination du médicament | Denominación del medicamento | 给药途径<br>Administration Route<br>Voie dàdministration<br>Vía de administración | 对妊娠危险性分级<br>Classification of pregnancy risk<br>Classification des risques liés à la grossesse Clasificación del riesgo de embarazo |
|---|---|---|---|---|---|
| 格帕沙星 | Grepafloxacin | Grépafloxacine | Grepafloxacina | 口服给药，Oral | C |
| 更昔洛韦 | Ganciclovir | Ganciclovir | Ganciclovir | 眼球内给药<br>Intraocular Administration | C |
|  |  |  |  | 口服给药，Oral | C |
|  |  |  |  | 肠道外给药，Parentaral | C |
| 骨化二醇 | Calcifediol | Calcifediol | Calcifediol | 口服给药，Oral | C；D- 如剂量超过美国的每日推荐摄入量<br>D-For example, the dosage exceeded the daily intake recommended by United States. |
| 骨化三醇 | Calcitriol | Calcitriol | Calcitriol | 口服给药，Oral | C；D- 如剂量超过美国的每日推荐摄入量<br>D-For example, the dosage exceeded the daily intake recommended by United States. |
|  |  |  |  | 肠道外给药，Parentaral | C；D- 如剂量超过美国的每日推荐摄入量<br>D-For example, the dosage exceeded the daily intake recommended by United States. |
| 胍法辛 | Guanfacine | Guanfacine | Guanfacina | 口服给药，Oral | B |
| 胍乙啶 | Guanethidine | Guanethidine | Guanetidina | 口服给药，Oral | C |
| 鬼臼毒素 | Podophyllotoxin | Podophyllotoxine | Podofilotoxina | 局部 / 皮肤外用<br>Local/Skin( External Use) | C |
| 鬼臼属 | Podophyllum | Podophyllum | Podofilum | 局部 / 皮肤外用<br>Local/Skin( External Use) | C |
| 桂利嗪 | Cinnarizine | Cinnarizine | Cinarizina | 口服给药，Oral | C |
| 过氧苯甲酰 | Benzoyl Peroxide | Peroxyde de Benzoyle | Peróxido de Benzoilo | 局部 / 皮肤外用<br>Local/Skin( External Use) | C |
| 核黄素 | Riboflavin | Riboflavine | Riboflavina | 口服给药，Oral | A；C- 如剂量超过美国的每日推荐摄入量<br>C-For example, the dosage exceeded the daily intake recommended by United States. |
| 红霉素 | Erythromycin | Erythromycine | Eritromicina | 口服给药，Oral | B |
|  |  |  |  | 肠道外给药，Parentaral | B |
|  |  |  |  | 局部 / 皮肤外用<br>Local/Skin( External Use) | B |

**续 表**

| 药品名称 | Drug Name | Dénomination du médicament | Denominación del medicamento | 给药途径<br>Administration Route<br>Voie dàdministration<br>Vía de administración | 对妊娠危险性分级<br>Classification of pregnancy risk<br>Classification des risques liés à la grossesse Clasificación del riesgo de embarazo |
|---|---|---|---|---|---|
| 红细胞生成素 | Erythropoietin | Erythropoietin | Eritropoyetina | 肠道外给药，Parentaral | C |
| 后马托品 | Homatropine | Homatropine | Homatropina | 眼部给药<br>Ophthalmic Drug Delivery | C |
| 琥珀雌三醇 | Estriol Succinate | Succinate de Estriol | Succinato de Estriol | 口服给药，Oral | X |
| 华法林 | Warfarin | Warfarine | Warfarina | 口服给药，Oral | X |
| 环孢素 | Ciclosporin | Ciclosporine | Ciclosporina | 口服给药，Oral | C |
| | | | | 肠道外给药，Parentaral | C |
| 环苯扎林 | Cyclobenzaprine | Cyclobénzaprine | Ciclobenzaprina | 口服给药，Oral | B |
| 环吡酮 | Ciclopirox | Ciclopirox | Ciclopirox | 局部/皮肤外用<br>Local/Skin( External Use) | B |
| 环丙沙星 | Ciprofloxacin | Ciprofloxacine | Ciprofloxacina | 眼部给药<br>Ophthalmic Drug Delivery | C |
| | | | | 口服给药，Oral | C |
| | | | | 耳部给药<br>Ear Drug Delivery | C |
| | | | | 肠道外给药，Parentaral | C |
| 环磷酰胺 | Cyclophospha-mide | Cyclophosphamide | Ciclofosfamida | 口服给药，Oral | D |
| | | | | 肠道外给药，Parentaral | D |
| 环喷脱脂 | Cyclopentolate | Cyclopéntolate | Ciclopentolato | 眼部给药<br>Ophthalmic Drug Delivery | C |
| 环丝氨酸 | Cycloserine | Cyclosérine | Cicloserina | 口服给药，Oral | C |
| 环戊噻嗪 | Cyclopenthia-zide | Cyclopénthiazide | Ciclopentiazida | 口服给药，Oral | C；D- 如用于妊娠高血压患者 D-For example, for patients with gestational hypertension. |
| 黄酮哌酯 | Flavoxate | Flavoxate | Flavoxato | 口服给药，Oral | B |
| 磺胺苯酰 | Sulfabenzamide | Sulfabénzamide | Sulfabenzamida | 阴道给药<br>Vaginal Administration | C；D- 如在临近分娩时使用 D-For example, used for near delivery. |
| 磺胺醋酯 | Sulfacetamide | Sulfacétamide | Sulfacetamida | 眼部给药<br>Ophthalmic Drug Delivery | C |
| | | | | 局部/皮肤外用<br>Local/Skin( External Use) | C |
| 磺胺甲噁唑 | Sulfamethoxazole | Sulfaméthoxazole | Sulfametoxazol | 口服给药，Oral | C；D- 如在临近分娩时使用 D-For example, used for near delivery. |

**续　表**

| 药品名称 | Drug Name | Dénomination du médicament | Denominación del medicamento | 给药途径 Administration Route Voie dàdministration Vía de administración | 对妊娠危险性分级 Classification of pregnancy risk Classification des risques liés à la grossesse Clasificación del riesgo de embarazo |
|---|---|---|---|---|---|
| 磺胺甲二唑 | Sulfamethizole | Sulfaméthizole | Sulfametizol | 口服给药，Oral | C；D- 如在临近分娩时使用 D-For example, used for near delivery. |
| 磺胺曲美 | Sulfametrole | Sulfamétrole | Sulfametrol | 口服给药，Oral | C；D- 如在临近分娩时使用 D-For example, used for near delivery. |
| 磺胺嘧啶 | Sulfadiazine | Sulfadiazine | Sulfadiazina | 口服给药，Oral | C；D- 如在临近分娩时使用 D-For example, used for near delivery. |
| 磺胺异噁唑 | Sulfafurazole | Sulfafurazole | Sulfafurazol | 口服给药，Oral | C；D- 如在临近分娩时使用 D-For example, used for near delivery. |
| 磺达肝癸钠 | Fondaparinux Sodium | Fondaparinux de Sodium | Fondaparinux Sódico | 肠道外给药，Parentaral | B |
| 灰黄霉素 | Griseofulvin | Griseofulvine | Griseofulvina | 口服给药，Oral | C |
| 吉非贝齐 | Gemfibrozil | Gemfibrozil | Gemfibrozil | 口服给药，Oral | C |
| 吉非替尼 | Gefitinib | Gefitinib | Gefitinib | 口服给药，Oral | D |
| 吉西他滨 | Gemcitabine | Gemcitabine | Gemcitabina | 肠道外给药，Parentaral | D |
| 己二烯雌酚 | Dienestrol | Dienestrol | Dienestrol | 局部 / 皮肤外用 Local/Skin( External Use) | X |
| 己酸羟孕酮 | Hydroxyproge-sterone Caproate | Caproate d'Hydroxyproge-stérone | Caproato de Hidroxiprogeste-rona | 肠道外给药，Parentaral | D |
| 己酮可可碱 | Pentoxifylline | Pentoxifylline | Pentoxifilina | 口服给药，Oral | C |
| 己烯雌酚 | Diethylstilbestrol | Diethylstilbestrol | Dietilstilbestrol | 口服给药，Oral | X |
| 加巴喷丁 | Gabapentin | Gabapentine | Gabapentina | 口服给药，Oral | C |
| 加兰他敏 | Galantamine | Galantamine | Galantamina | 口服给药，Oral | B |
| 加尼瑞克 | Ganirelix | Ganirelix | Ganirelix | 肠道外给药，Parentaral | X |
| 加替沙星 | Gatifloxacin | Gatifloxacine | Gatifloxacina | 眼部给药 Ophthalmic Drug Delivery | C |
| 甲氨蝶呤 | Methotrexate | Methotrexate | Metotrexato | 口服给药，Oral | X |
|  |  |  |  | 肠道外给药，Parentaral | X |
| 甲苯达唑 | Mebendazole | Mebendazole | Mebendazol | 口服给药，Oral | C |
| 甲苯磺丁脲 | Tolbutamide | Tolbutamide | Tolbutamida | 口服给药，Oral | C |
| 甲丙氨酯 | Meprobamate | Meprobamate | Meprobamato | 口服给药，Oral | D |
| 甲地嗪 | Methdilazine | Methdilazine | Metdilazina | 口服给药，Oral | C |

**续 表**

| 药品名称 | Drug Name | Dénomination du médicament | Denominación del medicamento | 给药途径<br>Administration Route<br>Voie dàdministration<br>Vía de administración | 对妊娠危险性分级<br>Classification of pregnancy risk<br>Classification des risques liés à la grossesse Clasificación del riesgo de embarazo |
|---|---|---|---|---|---|
| 甲地孕酮 | Megestrol | Mégéstrol | Megestrol | 口服给药，Oral | X |
| 甲芬那酸 | Mefenamic Acid | Acide Mefénamique | Acido Mefenamico | 口服给药，Oral | C；D- 如在妊娠晚期或临近分娩时用药<br>D-For example, used in late stage of pregnancy or for near delivery. |
| 甲氟喹 | Mefloquine | Méfloquine | Mefloquina | 口服给药，Oral | C |
| 甲睾酮 | Methyltestoste-rone | Méthyltéstosterone | Metiltestosterona | 口服给药，Oral | X |
| 甲磺酸本扎托品 | Benzatropine Mesilate | Mésilate de Bénzatropine | Mesilato Benzatropina | 口服给药，Oral | C |
| | | | | 肠道外给药，Parentaral | C |
| 甲磺酸钠黏菌素 | Colostomethate Sodium | Colostométhate de Sodium | Colostometato Sodico | 肠道外给药，Parentaral | C |
| 甲基多巴 | Methyldopa | Méthyldopa | Metildopa | 口服给药，Oral | B |
| | | | | 肠道外给药，Parentaral | B |
| 甲氯酚那酸 | Meclofenamic Acid | Acide Méclofénamique | Acido Meclofenamico | 口服给药，Oral | B；D- 如在妊娠晚期或临近分娩时用药<br>D-For example, used in late stage of pregnancy or for near delivery. |
| 甲氯噻嗪 | Methyclothiazide | Méthyclothiazide | Meticlotiazida | 口服给药，Oral | B；D- 如用于妊娠高血压患者<br>D-For example, for patients with gestational hypertension. |
| 甲哌卡因 | Mepivacaine | Mépivacaine | Mepivacaina | 肠道外给药，Parentaral | C |
| 甲泼尼龙 | Methylpredui-solone | Méthylpréduisolone | Metilpreduisolona | 口服给药，Oral | C |
| | | | | 肠道外给药，Parentaral | C |
| 甲羟孕酮 | Medroxyproge-sterone | Médroxyprogéste-rone | Medroxiprogeste-rona | 肠道外给药，Parentaral | X |
| 甲巯咪唑 | Thiamazole | Thiamazole | Tiamazol | 口服给药，Oral | D |
| 甲炔诺酮 | Norgestrel | Norgéstrel | Norgestrel | 口服给药，Oral | X |
| 甲硝唑 | Metronidazole | Métronidazole | Metronidazol | 口服给药，Oral | B |
| | | | | 肠道外给药，Parentaral | B |
| | | | | 局部 / 皮肤外用<br>Local/Skin( External Use) | B |
| 甲氧苄啶 | Trimethoprim | Trimèthoprime | Trimetoprim | 口服给药，Oral | C |
| 甲氧氯普胺 | Metoclopramide | Mètoclopramide | Metoclopramida | 口服给药，Oral | B |
| | | | | 肠道外给药，Parentaral | B |

**续　表**

| 药品名称 | Drug Name | Dénomination du médicament | Denominación del medicamento | 给药途径 Administration Route Voie dàdministration Vía de administración | 对妊娠危险性分级 Classification of pregnancy risk Classification des risques liés à la grossesse Clasificación del riesgo de embarazo |
|---|---|---|---|---|---|
| 甲氧沙林 | Methoxsalen | Mèthoxsalène | Metoxsalena | 口服给药，Oral | C |
| | | | | 局部 / 皮肤外用 Local/Skin( External Use) | C |
| 甲状腺素 | Thyroid | Thyroide | Tiroida | 口服给药，Oral | A |
| 间羟胺 | Metaraminol | Mètaraminol | Metaraminol | 肠道外给药，Parentaral | C |
| 降钙素 | Calcitonin | Calcitonine | Calcitonina | 鼻腔给药，Nasal Delivery | C |
| | | | | 肠道外给药，Parentaral | C |
| 金刚烷胺 | Amantadine | Amantadine | Amantadina | 口服给药，Oral | C |
| 金硫丁二钠 | Sodium Aurothiomalate | Aurothiomalate deSodium | Aurotiomalato deSodio | 口服给药，Oral | C |
| 金霉素 | Chlortetracycline | Chlortètracycline | Clortetraciclina | 眼部给药 Ophthalmic Drug Delivery | D |
| 金诺酚 | Auranofin | Auranofine | Auranofina | 口服给药，Oral | C |
| 肼苯哒嗪 | Hydralazine | Hydralazine | Hidralazina | 口服给药，Oral | C |
| | | | | 肠道外给药，Parentaral | C |
| 枸橼酸钾 | Potassium Citrate | Citrate de Potassium | Citrato de potasio | 口服给药，Oral | A |
| 聚苯乙烯磺酸钙 | Calcium Polystyrene Sulfonate | Polystyrène sulfonate de calcium | Sulfonato de poliestireno de calcio | 口服给药，Oral | C |
| | | | | 直肠给药 Rectal Administration | C |
| 聚苯乙烯磺酸钠 | Sodium Polystyrene Sulfonate | Polystyrène Sulfonate de sodium | Sulfonato de Poliestireno sódico | 口服给药，Oral | C |
| | | | | 直肠给药 Rectal Administration | C |
| 聚维酮碘 | Povidone-iodine | Polyvidone iode | Polividona yodada | 局部 / 皮肤外用 Local/Skin( External Use) | D |
| 卷曲霉素 | Capreomycin | Capreomycine | Capreomicina | 肠道外给药，Parentaral | C |
| 咖啡因 | Caffeine | Caffèine | Cafeína | 口服给药 ,Oral | B |
| 卡巴胆碱 | Carbachol | Carbachol | Carbachol | 眼部给药 Ophthalmic Drug Delivery | C |
| 卡巴沙明 | Carbinoxamine | Carbinoxamine | Carbinoxamina | 口服给药 ,Oral | C |
| 卡巴胂 | Carbarsone | Carbarsone | Carbarsona | 口服给药，Oral | D |

**续 表**

| 药品名称 | Drug Name | Dénomination du médicament | Denominación del medicamento | 给药途径<br>Administration Route<br>Voie dàdministration<br>Vía de administración | 对妊娠危险性分级<br>Classification of pregnancy risk<br>Classification des risques liés à la grossesse Clasificación del riesgo de embarazo |
|---|---|---|---|---|---|
| 卡比多巴 | Carbidopa | Carbidopa | Carbidopa | 口服给药 , Oral | C |
| 卡比马唑 | Carbimazole | Carbimazole | Carbimazol | 口服给药 , Oral | D |
| 卡泊芬净 | Caspofungin | Caspofungine | Caspofungina | 肠道外给药 , Parentaral | C |
| 卡泊三醇 | Calcipotriol | Calcipotriol | Calcipotriol | 局部 / 皮肤外用<br>Local/Skin( External Use) | C |
| 卡铂 | Carboplatin | Carboplatine | Carboplatina | 肠道外给药 , Parentaral | D |
| 卡立普多 | Carisoprodol | Carisoprodol | Carisoprodol | 口服给药 , Oral | C |
| 卡马西平 | Carbamazepine | Carbamazèpine | Carbamazepina | 口服给药 , Oral | D |
| 卡麦角林 | Cabergoline | Cabèrgoline | Cabergolina | 口服给药 , Oral | B |
| 卡那司汀 | Carmustine | Carmustine | Carmustina | 口服给药 , Oral | D |
| | | | | 肠道外给药 , Parentaral | D |
| 卡尼汀 | Carnitine | Carnitine | Carnitina | 口服给药 , Oral | B |
| | | | | 肠道外给药 , Parentaral | B |
| 卡培他滨 | Capecitabine | Capècitabine | Capecitabina | 口服给药 , Oral | D |
| 卡前列腺素 | Carboprost | Carboprost | Carboprost | 肠道外给药 , Parentaral | C |
| 卡替洛尔 | Carteolol | Cartèolol | Carteolol | 口服给药 , Oral | C；D- 如在妊娠中、晚期用药<br>D-For example, used in middle and late stage of pregnancy. |
| 卡托普利 | Captopril | Captopril | Captopril | 口服给药 , Oral | C；D- 如在妊娠中、晚期用药<br>D-For example, used in middle and late stage of pregnancy. |
| 卡维地洛 | Carvedilol | Carvèdilol | Carvedilol | 口服给药 , Oral | C；D- 如在妊娠中、晚期用药<br>D-For example, used in middle and late stage of pregnancy. |
| 坎地沙坦 | Candesartan | Candèsartan | Candesartan | 口服给药 , Oral | C；D- 如在妊娠中、晚期用药<br>D-For example, used in middle and late stage of pregnancy. |
| 抗坏血酸 | Ascorbic Acid | Acide Ascorbique | Ácido Ascórbico | 口服给药 , Oral | A；C- 如剂量超过美国的每日推荐摄入量<br>C-For example, the dosage exceeded the daily intake recommended by United States. |
| 抗凝血酶 III | Antithrombin III | Antithrombine III | Antitrombina III | 肠道外给药 , Parentaral | B |
| 抗凝血抑制复合物 | Anti-Coagulant Inhibitory Complex | Complèxe Anti- Coagulant d' Inhibiteur | Complejo anti- Coagulante Inhibidor | 肠道外给药 , Parentaral | C |

续　表

| 药品名称 | Drug Name | Dénomination du médicament | Denominación del medicamento | 给药途径<br>Administration Route<br>Voie dàdministration<br>Vía de administración | 对妊娠危险性分级<br>Classification of pregnancy risk<br>Classification des risques liés à la grossesse Clasificación del riesgo de embarazo |
|---|---|---|---|---|---|
| 考来替泊 | Colestipol | Colèstipol | Colestipol | 口服给药，Oral | B |
| 考来烯胺 | Colestyramine | Colèstyramine | Colestiramina | 口服给药，Oral | C |
| 可待因 | Codeine | Codèine | Codeina | 口服给药，Oral | C；D- 如在临近分娩时长期大量使用<br>D-For example, long-term used in large doses near delivery. |
| | | | | 肠道外给药，Parentaral | C；D- 如在临近分娩时长期大量使用<br>D-For example, long-term used in large doses near delivery. |
| 可的松 | Cortisone | Cortisone | Cortisona | 口服给药，Oral | C；D- 如在妊娠早期用药<br>D-For example, used in the first trimester of pregnancy. |
| | | | | 肠道外给药，Parentaral | C；D- 如在妊娠早期用药<br>D-For example, used in the first trimester of pregnancy. |
| 可乐定 | Clonidine | Clonidine | Clonidína | 硬膜外给药<br>Epidural Administration | C |
| | | | | 口服给药，Oral | C |
| | | | | 肠道外给药，Parentaral | C |
| | | | | 经皮给药，Transdermal Drug Delivery | C |
| 克拉霉素 | Clarithromycin | Clarithromycine | Claritromicina | 口服给药，Oral | C |
| | | | | 肠道外给药，Parentaral | C |
| 克拉屈滨 | Cladribine | Cladribine | Cladribina | 肠道外给药，Parentaral | D |
| 克拉维酸 | Clavulanic Acid | Acide Clavulanique | Acido Clavulanico | 口服给药，Oral | B |
| 克利库铵 | Clidinium Bromide | Bromure Clidinium | Clidinio Bromuro | 口服给药，Oral | C |
| 克林霉素 | Clindamycin | Clindamycine | Clindamicina | 口服给药，Oral | B |
| | | | | 肠道外给药，Parentaral | B |
| | | | | 局部 / 皮肤外用<br>Local/Skin( External Use) | B |
| | | | | 阴道给药<br>Vaginal Administration | B |
| 克罗米通 | Crotamiton | Crotamitone | Crotamiton | 局部 / 皮肤外用<br>Local/Skin( External Use) | C |

**续 表**

| 药品名称 | Drug Name | Dénomination du médicament | Denominación del medicamento | 给药途径<br>Administration Route<br>Voie dàdministration<br>Vía de administración | 对妊娠危险性分级<br>Classification of pregnancy risk<br>Classification des risques liés à la grossesse Clasificación del riesgo de embarazo |
|---|---|---|---|---|---|
| 克霉唑 | Clotrimazole | Clotrimazole | Clotrimazol | 局部 / 皮肤外用<br>Local/Skin( External Use) | B |
| | | | | 阴道给药<br>Vaginal Administration | B |
| 奎尼丁 | Quinidine | Quinidine | Quinidina | 口服给药，Oral | C |
| | | | | 肠道外给药，Parentaral | C |
| 奎宁 | Quinine | Quinine | Quinina | 口服给药，Oral | C |
| 喹硫平 | Quetiapine | Quetiapine | Quetiapina | 口服给药，Oral | C |
| 奎那普利 | Quinapril | Quinapril | Quinapril | 口服给药，Oral | C；D- 如在妊娠中、晚期用药<br>D-For example, used in middle and late stage of pregnancy. |
| 拉贝洛尔 | Labetalol | Labetalol | Labetalol | 口服给药，Oral | C；D- 如在妊娠中、晚期用药<br>D-For example, used in middle and late stage of pregnancy. |
| | | | | 肠道外给药，Parentaral | C；D- 如在妊娠中、晚期用药<br>D-For example, used in middle and late stage of pregnancy. |
| 拉布立酶 | Rasburicase | Rasburicase | Rasburicase | 肠道外给药，Parentaral | C |
| 拉米夫定 | Lamivudine | Lamivudine | Lamivudina | 口服给药，Oral | C |
| 拉莫三嗪 | Lamotrigine | Lamotrigine | Lamotrigina | 口服给药，Oral | C |
| 醋酸格拉太咪尔 | Glatiramer Acetate | Acétate de Glatiramer | Acetato de Glatiramer | 肠道外给药，Parentaral | B |
| 拉坦前列素 | Latanoprost | Latanoprost | Latanoprost | 眼部给药<br>Ophthalmic Drug Delivery | C |
| 来氟米特 | Leflunomide | Léflunomide | Leflunomida | 口服给药，Oral | X |
| 来匹卢定 | Lepirudin | Lépirudine | Lepirudina | 肠道外给药，Parentaral | B |
| 来曲唑 | Letrozole | Létrozole | Letrozol | 口服给药，Oral | D |
| 赖氨酸加压素 | Lypressin | Lypréssin | Lipresina | 鼻腔给药，Nasal Delivery | C |
| 赖普胰岛素 | Insulin Lispro | Insuline Lispro | Insulina Lispro | 肠道外给药，Parentaral | B |
| 赖诺普利 | Lisinopril | Lisinopril | Lisinopril | 口服给药，Oral | C；D- 如在妊娠中、晚期用药<br>D-For example, used in middle and late stage of pregnancy. |
| 兰索拉唑 | Lansoprazole | Lansoprazole | Lansoprazol | 口服给药，Oral | B |
| 莨菪碱 | Hyoscyamine | Hyoscyamine | Hiosciamina | 口服给药，Oral | C |
| 劳拉西泮 | Lorazepam | Lorazepam | Lorazepam | 口服给药，Oral | D |
| | | | | 肠道外给药，Parentaral | D |

续　表

| 药品名称 | Drug Name | Dénomination du médicament | Denominación del medicamento | 给药途径<br>Administration Route<br>Voie dàdministration<br>Vía de administración | 对妊娠危险性分级<br>Classification of pregnancy risk<br>Classification des risques liés à la grossesse Clasificación del riesgo de embarazo |
|---|---|---|---|---|---|
| 雷贝拉唑 | Rabeprazole | Rabéprazole | Rabeprazol | 口服给药，Oral | B |
| 雷洛昔芬 | Raloxifene | Raloxiféne | Raloxifeno | 口服给药，Oral | X |
| 雷米普利 | Ramipril | Ramipril | Ramipril | 口服给药，Oral | C；D- 如在妊娠中、晚期用药<br>D-For example, used in middle and late stage of pregnancy. |
| 雷尼替丁 | Ranitidine | Ranitidine | Ranitidina | 口服给药，Oral | B |
|  |  |  |  | 肠道外给药，Parentaral | B |
| 锂 | Lithium | Lithium | De litio | 口服给药，Oral | D |
| 利巴韦林 |  |  |  | 吸入，Inhalation | X |
|  | Ribavirin | Ribavirine | Ribavirina | 口服给药，Oral | X |
|  |  |  |  | 肠道外给药，Parentaral | X |
| 利多卡因 | Lidocaine | Lidocaine | Lidocaina | 肠道外给药，Parentaral | B；作为局麻药或抗心律失常药使用时<br>When used as a local anesthetic or antiarrhythmic. |
|  |  |  |  | 局部 / 皮肤外用<br>Local/Skin( External Use) | B |
| 利福布丁 | Rifabutin | Rifabutine | Rifabutina | 口服给药，Oral | B |
| 利福喷丁 | Rifapentine | Rifapéntine | Rifapentina | 口服给药，Oral | C |
| 利福平 | Rifampicin | Rifampicine | Rifampicina | 口服给药，Oral | C |
|  |  |  |  | 肠道外给药，Parentaral | C |
| 利鲁唑 | Riluzole | Riluzole | Riluzol | 口服给药，Oral | C |
| 利美索龙 | Rimexolone | Rimexolone | Rimexolona | 眼部给药<br>Ophthalmic Drug Delivery | C |
| 利奈孕酮 | Lynestrenol | Lynestrénol | Linestrenol | 口服给药，Oral | D |
| 利奈唑胺 | Linezolid | Linézolide | Linezolida | 口服给药，Oral | C |
|  |  |  |  | 肠道外给药，Parentaral | C |
| 利培酮 | Risperidone | Rispéridone | Risperidona | 口服给药，Oral | C |
| 利塞膦酸 | Risedronic Acid | Acide Risedronique | Acido Risedronico | 口服给药，Oral | C |
| 利斯的明 | Rivastigmine | Rivastigmine | Rivastigmina | 口服给药，Oral | B |
| 利托君 | Ritodrine | Ritodrine | Ritodrina | 口服给药，Oral | B |
|  |  |  |  | 肠道外给药，Parentaral | B |
| 利托那韦 | Ritonavir | Ritonavir | Ritonavir | 口服给药、Oral | B |
| 利妥昔单抗 | Rituximab | Rituximab | Rituximab | 肠道外给药，Parentaral | C |

**续 表**

| 药品名称 | Drug Name | Dénomination du médicament | Denominación del medicamento | 给药途径<br>Administration Route<br>Voie dàdministration<br>Vía de administración | 对妊娠危险性分级<br>Classification of pregnancy risk<br>Classification des risques liés à la grossesse Clasificación del riesgo de embarazo |
|---|---|---|---|---|---|
| 利血平 | Reserpine | Reserpine | Reserpina | 口服给药，Oral | C |
| 利扎曲坦 | Rizatriptan | Rizatriptan | Rizatriptan | 口服给药，Oral | C |
| 链激酶 | Streptokinase | Streptokinase | Streptokinase | 肠道外给药，Parentaral | C |
| 链霉素 | Streptomycin | Streptomycine | Streptomicina | 肠道外给药，Parentaral | D |
| α 链球菌 DNA 酶 | Domase Alfa | Domase Alfa | Domase Alfa | 肠道外给药，Parentaral | B |
| 两性霉素 B | Amphotericin B | Amphotericine B | Amfotericina B | 肠道外给药，Parentaral | B |
| | | | | 局部 / 皮肤外用<br>Local/Skin( External Use) | B |
| 亮丙瑞林 | Leuprorelin | Leuproreline | Leuprorelina | 肠道外给药，Parentaral | X |
| 林旦 | Lindane | Lindane | Lindano | 局部 / 皮肤外用<br>Local/Skin( External Use) | C |
| 林可霉素 | Lincomycin | Lincomycine | Lincomicina | 口服给药，Oral | B |
| | | | | 肠道外给药，Parentaral | B |
| 磷霉素 | Fosfomycin | Fosfomycine | Fosfomicina | 口服给药，Oral | B |
| 膦甲酸钠 | Foscarnet Sodium | Foscarnete de Sodium | Foscarneto Sódico | 肠道外给药，Parentaral | C |
| 硫胺 | Thiamine | Thiamine | Tiamina | 口服给药，Oral | A；C- 如剂量超过美国的每日推荐摄入量<br>C-For example, the dosage exceeded the daily intake recommended by United States. |
| 硫利达嗪 | Thioridazine | Thioridazine | Tioridazina | 口服给药，Oral | C |
| 硫鸟嘌呤 | Tioguanine | Tioguanine | Tioguanina | 口服给药，Oral | D |
| 硫喷妥钠 | Thiopental Sodium | Thiopental Sodique | Tiopental Sódico | 肠道外给药，Parentaral | C |
| | | | | 局部 / 皮肤外用<br>Local/Skin( External Use) | C |
| 硫普罗宁 | Tiopronin | Tiopronine | Tiopronina | 口服给药，Oral | C |
| 硫酸镁 | Magnesium Sulfate | Sulfate de Magnésium | Sulfato de Magnesio | 肠道外给药，Parentaral | B |
| 硫酸哌嗪雌酮 | Estropipate | Estropipate | Estropipato | 口服给药，Oral | X |
| | | | | 阴部给药<br>Vaginal Drug Delivery | X |
| 硫酸鱼精蛋白 | Protamine Sulfate | Sulfate de Protamine | Sulfato de Protamina | 肠道外给药，Parentaral | C |

**续 表**

| 药品名称 | Drug Name | Dénomination du médicament | Denominación del medicamento | 给药途径<br>Administration Route<br>Voie dàdministration<br>Vía de administración | 对妊娠危险性分级<br>Classification of pregnancy risk<br>Classification des risques liés à la grossesse Clasificación del riesgo de embarazo |
|---|---|---|---|---|---|
| 硫糖铝 | Sucralfate | Sucralfate | Sucralfato | 口服给药，Oral | B |
| 硫唑嘌呤 | Azathioprine | Azathioprine | Azatioprina | 口服给药，Oral | D |
| | | | | 肠道外给药，Parentaral | D |
| 柳氮磺吡啶 | Sulfasalazine | Sulfasalazine | Sulfasalazina | 口服给药，Oral | B；D- 如在临近分娩时使用 D-For example, used for near delivery. |
| | | | | 直肠给药 Rectal Administration | B；D- 如在临近分娩时使用 D-For example, used for near delivery. |
| 六甲蜜胺 | Altretamine | Altrétamine | Altretamina | 口服给药，Oral | D |
| 六氯酚 | Hexachlorophene | Héxachlorophéne | Hexaclorofeno | 局部 / 皮肤外用 Local/Skin( External Use) | C |
| 氯草酸钾 | Dipotassium Clorazepate | Clorazépate de Dipotassium | Clorazepato de Dipotasio | 口服给药，Oral | D |
| 氯胺酮 | Ketamine | Kétamine | Ketamina | 肠道外给药，Parentaral | B |
| 氯贝胆碱 | Bethanechol Chloride | Chlorure de Béthanechol | Cloruro de Betanecol | 口服给药，Oral | C |
| | | | | 肠道外给药，Parentaral | C |
| 氯贝丁酯 | Clofibrate | Clofibrate | Clofibrato | 口服给药，Oral | C |
| 氯倍他索 | Clobetasol | Clobétasol | Clobetasol | 局部 / 皮肤外用 Local/Skin( External Use) | C |
| 氯苯那敏 | Chlorphenamine | Chlorphénamine | Clorfenamina | 口服给药，Oral | B |
| 氯吡格雷 | Clopidogrel | Clopidogrél | Clopidogrel | 口服给药，Oral | B |
| 氯丙嗪 | Chlorpromazine | Chlorpromazine | Clorpromazina | 口服给药，Oral | C |
| | | | | 肠道外给药，Parentaral | C |
| 氯氮草 | Chlordiazepoxide | Chlordiazepoxide | Clordiazepoxida | 口服给药，Oral | D |
| | | | | 肠道外给药，Parentaral | D |
| 氯氮平 | Clozapine | Clozapine | Clozapina | 口服给药，Oral | B |
| 氯法齐明 | Clofazimine | Clofazimine | Clofazimina | 口服给药，Oral | C |
| 氯胍 | Proguanil | Proguanil | Proguanilo | 口服给药，Oral | B |
| 氯化铵 | Ammonium Chloride | Chlorure d'ammonium | Cloruro de Amonio | 口服给药，Oral | B |
| 氯化钙 | Calcium Chloride | Chlorure d'Calcium | Cloruro de Calcio | 肠道外给药，Parentaral | C |
| 氯化琥珀胆碱 | Suxamethonium Chloride | Chlorure d' Suxamethonium | Cloruro de Suxametonio | 肠道外给药，Parentaral | C |

**续　表**

| 药品名称 | Drug Name | Dénomination du médicament | Denominación del medicamento | 给药途径<br>Administration Route<br>Voie dàdministration<br>Vía de administración | 对妊娠危险性分级<br>Classification of pregnancy risk<br>Classification des risques liés à la grossesse Clasificación del riesgo de embarazo |
|---|---|---|---|---|---|
| 氯化钾 | Potassium Chloride | Chlorure d'Potassium | Cloruro Potásico | 口服给药，Oral | A |
| 氯化筒箭毒碱 | Tubocurarine Chloride | Chlorure d'Tubocurarine | Cloruro de Tubocurarina | 肠道外给药，Parentaral | C |
| 氯环力嗪 | Chloreyclizine | Chloreyclizine | Cloreiclizina | 口服给药，Oral | C |
| 氯磺丙脲 | Chlorpropamide | Chlorpropamide | Clorpropamida | 口服给药，Oral | C |
| 氯己定 | Chlorhexidine | Chlorhexidine | Clorhexidina | 口腔咽喉给药，Oral Cavity and Throat Administration | B |
| 氯喹 | Chloroquine | Chloroquine | Cloroquina | 口服给药，Oral | C |
|  |  |  |  | 肠道外给药，Parentaral | C |
| 氯雷他定 | Loratadine | Loratadine | Loratadina | 口服给药，Oral | B |
| 氯马斯汀 | Clemastine | Clémastine | Clemastina | 口服给药，Oral | B |
| 氯霉素 | Chloramphenicol | Chloramphénicol | Cloramfenicol | 眼部给药 Ophthalmic Drug Delivery | C |
|  |  |  |  | 耳部给药 Ear Drug Delivery | C |
|  |  |  |  | 肠道外给药，Parentaral | C |
| 氯米芬 | Clomifene | Clomiféne | Clomifeno | 口服给药，Oral | X |
| 氯米帕明 | Clomipramine | Clomipramine | Clomipramina | 口服给药，Oral | C |
| 氯普噻吨 | Chlorprothixene | Chlorprothixéne | Clorprotixeno | 口服给药，Oral | C |
| 氯噻嗪 | Chlorothiazide | Chlorothiazide | Clorotiazida | 口服给药，Oral | C;D- 如用于妊娠高血压患者 D-For example, for patients with gestational hypertension. |
| 氯噻酮 | Chlortalidone | Chlortalidone | Clortalidona | 口服给药，Oral | B;D- 如用于妊娠高血压患者 D-For example, for patients with gestational hypertension. |
| 氯沙坦 | Losartan | Losartan | Losartan | 口服给药，Oral | C;D- 如在妊娠中、晚期给药 |
| 氯替泼诺 | Loteprednol | Lotéprednol | Loteprednol | 眼部给药 Ophthalmic Drug Delivery | C |
| 氯烯雌醚 | Chlorotrianisene | Chlorotrianiséne | Clorotrianisena | 口服给药，Oral | X |
| 氯硝西泮 | Clonazepam | Clonazépam | Clonazepam | 口服给药，Oral | D |
|  |  |  |  | 肠道外给药，Parentaral | D |
| 氯乙酰胆碱 | Acetylcholine Chloride | Chlorure d'Acetylcholine | Cloruro de Acetylcholina | 眼部给药 Ophthalmic Drug Delivery | C |
| 氯唑沙宗 | Chlorzoxazone | Chlorzoxazone | Clorzoxazona | 口服给药，Oral | C |

**续　表**

| 药品名称 | Drug Name | Dénomination du médicament | Denominación del medicamento | 给药途径 Administration Route Voie dàdministration Vía de administración | 对妊娠危险性分级 Classification of pregnancy risk Classification des risques liés à la grossesse Clasificación del riesgo de embarazo |
|---|---|---|---|---|---|
| 氯唑西林 | Cloxacillin | Cloxacilline | Cloxacilina | 口服给药，Oral | B |
| 罗非昔布 | Rofecoxib | Rofécoxib | Rofecoxib | 口服给药，Oral | C;D- 如在妊娠晚期或临近分娩时用药 D-For example, used in late stage of pregnancy or for near delivery. |
| 罗格列酮 | Rosiglitazone | Rosiglitazone | Rosiglitazona | 口服给药，Oral | C |
| 罗库溴铵 | Rocuronium Bromide | Bromure de Rocuronium | Bromuro de Rocuronio | 肠道外给药，Parentaral | C |
| 罗匹尼罗 | Ropinirole | Ropinirole | Ropinirol | 口服给药，Oral | C |
| 螺内酯 | Spironolactone | Spironolactone | Spironolactona | 口服给药，Oral | C;D- 如用于妊娠高血压患者 D-For example, for patients with gestational hypertension. |
| 螺旋霉素 | Spiramycin | Spiramycine | Spiramicina | 口服给药，Oral | C |
|  |  |  |  | 肠道外给药，Parentaral | C |
|  |  |  |  | 直肠给药 Rectal Administration | C |
| 洛度沙胺 | Lodoxamide | Lodoxamide | Lodoxamida | 眼部给药 Ophthalmic Drug Delivery | B |
| 洛伐他汀 | Lovastatin | Lovastatine | Lovastatina | 口服给药，Oral | X |
| 洛拉卡比 | Loracarbef | Loracarbef | Loracarbef | 口服给药，Oral | B |
| 洛美沙星 | Lomefloxacin | Lomefloxacine | Lomefloxacina | 眼部给药 Ophthalmic Drug Delivery | C |
|  |  |  |  | 口服给药，Oral | C; 禁用于妊娠早期 Prohibited to use, especially in the first trimester of pregnancy. |
| 洛莫司汀 | Lomustine | Lomustine | Lomustina | 口服给药，Oral | D |
| 洛哌丁胺 | Loperamide | Loperamide | Loperamida | 口服给药，Oral | B |
| 洛匹那韦 | Lopinavir | Lopinavir | Lopinavir | 口服给药，Oral | C |
| 洛沙平 | Loxapine | Loxapine | Loxapina | 口服给药，Oral | C |
| 麻黄碱 | Ephedrine | Ephedrine | Efedrina | 口服给药，Oral | C |
| 马拉硫磷 | Malathion | Malathion | Malation | 局部 / 皮肤外用 Local/Skin( External Use) | B |
| 马普替林 | Maprotiline | Maprotiline | Maprotilina | 口服给药，Oral | B |
| 马吲哚 | Mazindol | Mazindol | Mazindol | 口服给药，Oral | C |

续 表

| 药品名称 | Drug Name | Dénomination du médicament | Denominación del medicamento | 给药途径<br>Administration Route<br>Voie dàdministration<br>Vía de administración | 对妊娠危险性分级<br>Classification of pregnancy risk<br>Classification des risques liés à la grossesse Clasificación del riesgo de embarazo |
|---|---|---|---|---|---|
| 吗啡 | Morphine | Morphine | Morfina | 口服给药，Oral | C;D- 如在临近分娩时长期大量使用<br>D-For example, long-term used in large doses near delivery. |
| | | | | 肠道外给药，Parentaral | C;D- 如在临近分娩时长期大量使用<br>D-For example, long-term used in large doses near delivery. |
| 吗茚酮 | Molindone | Molindone | Molindona | 口服给药，Oral | C |
| 麦角胺 | Ergotamine | Ergotamine | Ergotamina | 口含，Keep in the Mouth | X |
| | | | | 口服给药，Oral | X |
| | | | | 直肠给药<br>Rectal Administration | X |
| 麦角骨化醇 | Ergocalciferol | Ergocalciferol | Ergocalciferol | 口服给药，Oral | A;D- 如剂量超过美国的每日推荐摄入量<br>D-For example, the dosage exceeded the daily intake recommended by United States. |
| | | | | 肠道外给药，Parentaral | A;D- 如剂量超过美国的每日推荐摄入量<br>D-For example, the dosage exceeded the daily intake recommended by United States. |
| 麦角新碱 | Ergometrine | Ergometrine | Ergometrina | 肠道外给药，Parentaral | X |
| 麦考酚酸 | Mycophenolic Acid | Acide Mycophenolique | Ácido Micofenóico | 口服给药，Oral | D |
| | | | | 肠道外给药，Parentaral | D |
| 毛果芸香碱 | Pilocarpine | Pilocarpine | Pilocarpina | 眼部给药<br>Ophthalmic Drug Delivery | C |
| | | | | 口服给药，Oral | C |
| 毛花苷 C | Lanatoside C | Lanatoside C | Lanatoside C | 口服给药，Oral | C |
| 美雌醇 | Mestranol | Mestranol | Mestranol | 口服给药，Oral | X |
| 美法仑 | Melphalan | Melphalan | Melfalano | 口服给药，Oral | D |
| | | | | 肠道外给药，Parentaral | D |
| 美格司他 | Miglustat | Miglustat | Miglustat | 口服给药，Oral | X |
| 美金刚 | Memantine | Mémantine | Memantina | 口服给药，Oral | B |
| 美克洛嗪 | Meclozine | Méclozine | Meclozina | 口服给药，Oral | B |

续　表

| 药品名称 | Drug Name | Dénomination du médicament | Denominación del medicamento | 给药途径 Administration Route Voie dàdministration Vía de administración | 对妊娠危险性分级 Classification of pregnancy risk Classification des risques liés à la grossesse Clasificación del riesgo de embarazo |
|---|---|---|---|---|---|
| 美罗培南 | Meropenem | Méropénem | Meropenem | 肠道外给药，Parentaral | B |
| 美洛西林 | Mezlocillin | Mézlocilline | Mezlocilina | 肠道外给药，Parentaral | B |
| 美洛昔康 | Meloxicam | Méloxicam | Meloxicam | 口服给药，Oral | C;D- 如在妊娠晚期或临近分娩时用药 D-For example, used in late stage of pregnancy or for near delivery. |
| 美沙拉嗪 | Mesalazine | Mésalazine | Mesalazina | 口服给药，Oral | B |
|  |  |  |  | 直肠给药 Rectal Administration | B |
| 美沙酮 | Methadone | Méthadone | Metadona | 口服给药，Oral | C;D- 如在临近分娩时长期大量使用 D-For example, long-term used in large doses near delivery. |
|  |  |  |  | 肠道外给药，Parentaral | C;D- 如在临近分娩时长期大量使用 D-For example, long-term used in large doses near delivery. |
| 美司钠 | Mesna | Mésna | Mesna | 肠道外给药，Parentaral | B |
| 美索巴莫 | Methocarbamol | Méthocarbamol | Metocarbamol | 口服给药，Oral | C |
| 美索比妥 | Methohexital | Méthohexital | Metohexital | 肠道外给药，Parentaral | B |
|  |  |  |  | 直肠给药 Rectal Administration | B |
| 美索达嗪 | Mesoridazine | Mésoridazine | Mesoridazina | 口服给药，Oral | C |
| 美托拉宗 | Metolazone | Métolazone | Metolazona | 口服给药，Oral | B;D- 如用于妊娠高血压患者 D-For example, for patients with gestational hypertension. |
| 美托洛尔 | Metoprolol | Métoprolol | Metoprolol | 口服给药，Oral | C;D- 如在妊娠中、晚期给药 D-For example, used in middle and late stage of pregnancy. |
|  |  |  |  | 肠道外给药，Parentaral | C;D- 如在妊娠中、晚期给药 D-For example, used in middle and late stage of pregnancy. |
| 美西律 | Mexiletine | Méxiletine | Mexiletina | 口服给药，Oral | C |
| 门冬酰胺酶 | Asparaginase | Asparaginase | Asparaginase | 肠道外给药，Parentaral | C |
| 门冬胰岛素 | Insulin Aspart | Insuline Aspart | Insulina Aspart | 肠道外给药，Parentaral | B |
| 孟鲁司特 | Montelukast | Montelukast | Montelukast | 口服给药，Oral | B |

**续 表**

| 药品名称 | Drug Name | Dénomination du médicament | Denominación del medicamento | 给药途径<br>Administration Route<br>Voie dàdministration<br>Vía de administración | 对妊娠危险性分级<br>Classification of pregnancy risk<br>Classification des risques liés à la grossesse Clasificación del riesgo de embarazo |
|---|---|---|---|---|---|
| 咪达唑仑 | Midazolam | Midazolam | Midazolam | 口服给药，Oral | D |
| | | | | 肠道外给药，Parentaral | D |
| 咪康唑 | Miconazole | Miconazole | Miconazol | 局部 / 皮肤外用<br>Local/Skin( External Use) | C |
| | | | | 阴道给药<br>Vaginal Administration | C |
| 咪喹莫特 | Imiquimod | Imiquimod | Imiquimod | 局部 / 皮肤外用<br>Local/Skin( External Use) | B |
| 米氮平 | Mirtazapine | Mirtazapine | Mirtazapina | 口服给药，Oral | C |
| 米多君 | Midodrine | Midodrine | Midodrina | 口服给药，Oral | C |
| 米非司酮 | Mifepristone | Mifepristone | Mifepristona | 口服给药，Oral | X |
| 米力农 | Milrinone | Milrinone | Milrinona | 肠道外给药，Parentaral | C |
| 米诺地尔 | Minoxidil | Minoxidil | Minoxidil | 口服给药，Oral | C |
| 米诺环素 | Minocycline | Minocycline | Minociclina | 牙科给药<br>Dental Drug Delivery | D |
| | | | | 口服给药，Oral | D |
| | | | | 肠道外给药，Parentaral | D |
| 米索前列醇 | Misoprostol | Misoprostol | Misoprostol | 口服给药，Oral | X |
| 米托蒽醌 | Mitoxantrone | Mitoxantrone | Mitoxantrona | 肠道外给药，Parentaral | D |
| 免疫球蛋白 | Immunoglobulin | Immunoglobuline | Imunoglobulina | 肠道外给药，Parentaral | C |
| 莫达非尼 | Modafinil | Modafinil | Modafinil | 口服给药，Oral | C |
| 莫罗克隆 CD3 | Muromonab CD3 | Muromonab CD3 | Muromonab CD3 | 肠道外给药，Parentaral | C |
| 莫米松 | Mometasone | Mométasone | Mometasona | 鼻腔给药，Nasal Delivery | C |
| | | | | 局部 / 皮肤外用<br>Local/Skin( External Use) | C |
| 莫匹罗星 | Mupirocin | Mupirocine | Mupirocina | 鼻腔给药，Nasal Delivery | B |
| | | | | 眼部给药<br>Ophthalmic Drug Delivery | B |
| | | | | 局部 / 皮肤外用<br>Local/Skin( External Use) | B |
| 莫西沙星 | Moxifloxacin | Moxifloxacine | Moxifloxacina | 眼部给药<br>Ophthalmic Drug Delivery | C |
| | | | | 口服给药，Oral | C |
| | | | | 肠道外给药，Parentaral | C |

**续　表**

| 药品名称 | Drug Name | Dénomination du médicament | Denominación del medicamento | 给药途径<br>Administration Route<br>Voie dàdministration<br>Vía de administración | 对妊娠危险性分级<br>Classification of pregnancy risk<br>Classification des risques liés à la grossesse Clasificación del riesgo de embarazo |
|---|---|---|---|---|---|
| 莫昔普利 | Moexipril | Moéxipril | Moexipril | 眼部给药<br>Ophthalmic Drug Delivery | C;D- 如在妊娠中、晚期用药<br>D-For example, used in middle and late stage of pregnancy. |
| 那法瑞林 | Nafarelin | Nafaréline | Nafarelina | 鼻腔给药，Nasal Delivery | X |
| 那格列奈 | Nateglinide | Natéglinide | Nateglinida | 口服给药，Oral | C |
| 那拉曲坦 | Naratriptan | Naratriptan | Naratriptan | 口服给药，Oral | C |
| 那屈肝素钙 | Nadroparin Calcium | Nadroparine Calcique | Nadroparina Cálcica | 肠道外给药，Parentaral | B |
| 那他霉素 | Natamycin | Natamycine | Natamicina | 眼部给药<br>Ophthalmic Drug Delivery | C |
| 纳布啡 | Nalbuphine | Nalbuphine | Nalbufina | 肠道外给药，Parentaral | B;D- 如在临近分娩时长期大量使用<br>D-For example, long-term use in large doses near delivery. |
| 纳多洛尔 | Nadolol | Nadolol | Nadolol | 口服给药，Oral | C;D- 如在妊娠中、晚期用药<br>D-For example, used in middle and late stage of pregnancy. |
| 纳洛酮 | Naloxone | Naloxone | Naloxona | 肠道外给药，Parentaral | B |
| 纳曲酮 | Naltrexone | Naltréxone | Naltrexona | 口服给药，Oral | C |
| 奈多罗米 | Nedocromil | Nédocromil | Nedocromil | 吸入，Inhalation | B |
|  |  |  |  | 眼部给药<br>Ophthalmic Drug Delivery | B |
| 奈非那韦 | Nelfinavir | Néfenavir | Nelfinavir | 口服给药，Oral | B |
| 奈替米星 | Netilmicin | Nétilmicine | Netilmicina | 肠道外给药，Parentaral | D |
| 奈韦拉平 | Nevirapine | Névirapine | Nevirapina | 口服给药，Oral | B |
| 奈丁美酮 | Nabumetone | Nabumetone | Nabumetona | 口服给药，Oral | C;D- 如在妊娠晚期或临近分娩时用药<br>D-For example, used in late stage of pregnancy or for near delivery. |
| 萘啶酸 | Nalidixic Acid | Acide Nalidixique | Ácido Nalidixico | 口服给药，Oral | C |
| 萘夫西林 | Nafcillin | Nafcilline | Nafcilina | 肠道外给药，Parentaral | B |
| 萘普生 | Naproxen | Naproxène | Naproxeno | 口服给药，Oral | B;D- 如在妊娠晚期或临近分娩时用药<br>D-For example, used in late stage of pregnancy or for near delivery. |
| 尼古丁 | Nicotine | Nicotine | Nicotina | 口服给药，Oral | C |
|  |  |  |  | 经皮给药<br>Transdermal drug delivery | D |

**续　表**

| 药品名称 | Drug Name | Dénomination du médicament | Denominación del medicamento | 给药途径<br>Administration Route<br>Voie dàdministration<br>Vía de administración | 对妊娠危险性分级<br>Classification of pregnancy risk<br>Classification des risques liés à la grossesse Clasificación del riesgo de embarazo |
|---|---|---|---|---|---|
| 尼卡地平 | Nicardipine | Nicardipine | Nicardipina | 口服给药，Oral | C |
| 尼鲁米特 | Nilutamide | Nilutamide | Nilutamida | 口服给药，Oral | C |
| 尼莫地平 | Nimodipine | Nimodipine | Nimodipina | 口服给药，Oral | C |
| | | | | 肠道外给药，Parentaral | C |
| 尼扎替丁 | Nizatidine | Nizatidine | Nizatidina | 口服给药，Oral | B |
| 尿促卵泡素 | Urofollitropin | Urofollitropine | Urofolitropina | 肠道外给药，Parentaral | X |
| 尿促性素 | Menotrophin | Ménotrophine | Menotrofina | 肠道外给药，Parentaral | X |
| 尿激酶 | Urokinase | Urokinase | Urokinasa | 肠道外给药，Parentaral | B |
| 凝血因子 IX | Blood Coagulation Factor IX | Facteur de Coagulation IX | Factor de coagulación IX | 肠道外给药，Parentaral | C |
| 凝血因子VIII | Blood Coagulation Factor VIII | Facteur de Coagulation VIII | Factor de coagulación VIII | 肠道外给药，Parentaral | C |
| 凝血因子XIII | Blood Coagulation Factor XIII | Facteur de Coagulation XIII | Factor de coagulación XIII | 肠道外给药，Parentaral | C |
| 诺氟沙星 | Norfloxacin | Norfloxacine | Norfloxacina | 眼部给药 Ophthalmic Drug Delivery | C; 妊娠期妇女慎用，尤其是妊娠早期 Use with caution in pregnancy, especially in the first trimester. |
| | | | | 口服给药，Oral | C; 妊娠期妇女慎用，尤其是妊娠早期 Use with caution in pregnancy, especially in the first trimester |
| 诺龙 | Nandrolone | Nandrolone | Nandrolona | 肠道外给药，Parentaral | X |
| 帕利珠单抗 | Palivizumab | Palivizumab | Palivizumab | 肠道外给药，Parentaral | C |
| 帕罗西汀 | Paroxetine | Paroxétine | Paroxetina | 口服给药，Oral | D |
| 帕米膦酸 | Pamidronic Acid | Acide Pamidronique | Acido Pamidronico | 肠道外给药，Parentaral | D |
| 哌甲酯 | Methylphenidate | Méthylphénidate | Metilfenidato | 口服给药，Oral | C |
| 哌拉西林 | Piperacillin | Pipéracilline | Piperacilina | 肠道外给药，Parentaral | B |
| 哌立度酯 | Piperidolate | Pipéridolate | Piperidolato | 口服给药，Oral | C |
| 哌嗪 | Piperazine | Pipérazine | Piperazina | 口服给药，Oral | B |

**续 表**

| 药品名称 | Drug Name | Dénomination du médicament | Denominación del medicamento | 给药途径<br>Administration Route<br>Voie dàdministration<br>Vía de adminístración | 对妊娠危险性分级<br>Classification of pregnancy risk<br>Classification des risques liés à la grossesse Clasificación del riesgo de embarazo |
|---|---|---|---|---|---|
| 哌替啶 | Pethidine | Péthidine | Petidina | 口服给药，Oral | B;D- 如在临近分娩时长期大量使用<br>D-For example, long-term used in large doses near delivery. |
| | | | | 肠道外给药，Parentaral | B;D- 如在临近分娩时长期大量使用<br>D-For example, long-term used in large doses near delivery. |
| 哌唑嗪 | Prazosin | Prazosine | Prazosina | 口服给药，Oral | C |
| 泮库溴铵 | Pancuronium Bromide | Bromure de Pancuronium | Bromuro de Pancuronio | 肠道外给药，Parentaral | C |
| 泮托拉唑 | Pantoprazole | Pantoprazole | Pantoprazol | 口服给药，Oral | B |
| | | | | 肠道外给药，Parentaral | B |
| 培哚普利 | Perindopril | Périndopril | Perindopril | 口服给药，Oral | C;D- 如在妊娠中、晚期用药<br>D-For example, used in middle and late stage of pregnancy. |
| 聚乙二醇干扰素 α-2a | Peginterferon Alfa-2a | Péginterferon Alfa-2a | Peginterferón α-2a | 肠道外给药，Parentaral | C |
| 聚乙二醇干扰素 α-2b | Peginterferon Alfa-2b | Péginterferon Alfa-2b | Peginterferón α-2b | 肠道外给药，Parentaral | C |
| 培高利特 | Pergolide | Pérgolide | Pergolida | 口服给药，Oral | B |
| 培美曲塞 | Pemetrexed | Pemétréxede | Pemetrexeda | 肠道外给药，Parentaral | D |
| 喷布洛尔 | Penbutolol | Pénbutolol | Penbutolol | 口服给药，Oral | C;D- 如在妊娠中、晚期用药<br>D-For example, used in middle and late stage of pregnancy. |
| 喷他脒 | Pentamidine | Péntamidine | Pentamidina | 吸入，Inhalation | C |
| | | | | 肠道外给药，Parentaral | C |
| 喷他佐辛 | Pentazocine | Péntazocine | Pentazocina | 口服给药，Oral | C;D- 如在临近分娩时长期大量使用<br>D-For example, long-term used in large doses near delivery. |
| | | | | 肠道外给药，Parentaral | C;D- 如在临近分娩时长期大量使用<br>D-For example, long-term used in large doses near delivery. |
| | | | | 直肠给药<br>Rectal Administration | C;D- 如在临近分娩时长期大量使用<br>D-For example, long-term used in large doses near delivery. |

**续 表**

| 药品名称 | Drug Name | Dénomination du médicament | Denominación del medicamento | 给药途径<br>Administration Route<br>Voie dàdministration<br>Vía de administración | 对妊娠危险性分级<br>Classification of pregnancy risk<br>Classification des risques liés à la grossesse Clasificación del riesgo de embarazo |
|---|---|---|---|---|---|
| 喷昔洛韦 | Penciclovir | Pénciclovir | Penciclovir | 局部 / 皮肤外用<br>Local/Skin( External Use) | B |
| 硼替佐米 | Bortezomib | Bortézomib | Bortezomib | 肠道外给药，Parentaral | D |
| 匹莫林 | Pemoline | Pémoline | Pemolina | 口服给药，Oral | B |
| 匹莫齐特 | Pimozide | Pimozide | Pimozida | 口服给药，Oral | C |
| 泼尼松 | Prednisone | Prédnisone | Prednisona | 口服给药，Oral | C;D- 如在妊娠早期给药<br>D-For example, used in the first trimester of pregnancy. |
| 泼尼松龙 | Prednisolone | Prédnisolone | Prednisolona | 眼部给药<br>Ophthalmic Drug Delivery | C |
|  |  |  |  | 口服给药，Oral | C;D- 如在妊娠早期给药<br>D-For example, used in the first trimester of pregnancy. |
|  |  |  |  | 肠道外给药，Parentaral | C;D- 如在妊娠早期给药<br>D-For example, used in the first trimester of pregnancy. |
| 扑米酮 | Primidone | Primidone | Primidona | 口服给药，Oral | D |
| 扑灭司林 | Permethrin | Permethrine | Permetrina | 局部 / 皮肤外用<br>Local/Skin( External Use) | B |
| 葡萄糖酸钾 | Potassium Gluconate | Gluconate de Potassium | Gluconato de Potasio | 口服给药，Oral | A |
| 葡萄糖酸钙 | Calcium Gluconate | Gluconate de Calcium | Gluconato de Calcio | 肠道外给药，Parentaral | C |
| 普伐他汀 | Pravastatin | Pravastatine | Pravastatina | 口服给药，Oral | X |
| 普拉克索 | Pramipexole | Pramipexole | Pramipexol | 口服给药，Oral | C |
| 普鲁卡因胺 | Procainamide | Procainamide | Procainamida | 口服给药，Oral | C |
|  |  |  |  | 肠道外给药，Parentaral | C |
| 普鲁卡因青霉素 | Procaine Penicillin | Procaine Penicilline | Procaina Penicilina | 肠道外给药，Parentaral | B |
| 普罗布考 | Probucol | Probucol | Probucol | 口服给药，Oral | B |
| 普罗帕酮 | Propafenone | Propafenone | Propafenona | 口服给药，Oral | C |
| 普罗瑞林 | Protirelin | Protireline | Protirelina | 肠道外给药，Parentaral | C |
| 普萘洛尔 | Propranolol | Propranolol | Propranolol | 口服给药，Oral | C;D- 如在妊娠中、晚期用药<br>D-For example, used in middle and late stage of pregnancy. |
|  |  |  |  | 肠道外给药，Parentaral | C;D- 如在妊娠中、晚期用药<br>D-For example, used in middle and late stage of pregnancy. |

**续　表**

| 药品名称 | Drug Name | Dénomination du médicament | Denominación del medicamento | 给药途径<br>Administration Route<br>Voie dàdministration<br>Vía de administración | 对妊娠危险性分级<br>Classification of pregnancy risk<br>Classification des risques liés à la grossesse Clasificación del riesgo de embarazo |
|---|---|---|---|---|---|
| 齐多夫定 | Zidovudine | Zidovudine | Zidovudina | 口服给药，Oral | C |
| 齐拉西酮 | Ziprasidone | Ziprasidone | Ziprasidona | 口服给药，Oral | C |
| 前列地尔 | Alprostadil | Alprostadil | Alprostadil | 肠道外给药，Parentaral | X |
|  |  |  |  | 尿道给药<br>Urethral Drug Delivery | C |
| 羟保泰松 | Oxyphenbuta-zone | Oxyphenbutazone | Oxifenbutazona | 口服给药，Oral | C；D- 如在妊娠晚期或临近分娩时用药<br>D-For example, used in late stage of pregnancy or for near delivery. |
| 羟钴素 | Hydroxocoba-lamin | Hydroxocobala-mine | Hidroxocobala-mina | 肠道外给药，Parentaral | C；D- 如剂量超过美国的每日推荐摄入量<br>D-For example, the dosage exceeded the daily intake recommended by United States. |
| 羟基脲 | Hydroxycarba-mide | Hydroxycarbamide | Hidroxicarbamida | 口服给药，Oral | D |
| 羟甲烯龙 | Oxymetholone | Oxymetholone | Oximetolona | 口服给药，Oral | X |
| 羟甲唑啉 | Oxymetazoline | Oxymetazoline | Oximetazolina | 鼻腔给药，Nasal Delivery | C |
|  |  |  |  | 眼部给药<br>Ophthalmic Drug Delivery | C |
| 羟氯喹 | Hydroxychloro-quine | Hydroxychloro-quine | Hidroxicloroquina | 口服给药，Oral | C |
| 羟嗪 | Hydroxyzine | Hydroxyzine | Hidroxizina | 口服给药，Oral | C |
| 青霉胺 | Penicillamine | Penicillamine | Penicilamina | 口服给药，Oral | D |
| 青霉素 V | Phenoxymethylp-enici-llin | Phenoxymethylpe-nici-lline | Fenoximetilpeni-cilina | 口服给药，Oral | B |
| 氢氟噻嗪 | Hydroflumethia-zide | Hydroflumethia-zide | Hidroflumetiazida | 口服给药，Oral | C；D- 如用于妊娠高血压患者<br>D-For example, for patients with gestational hypertension. |
| 氢化可的松 | Hydrocortisone | Hydrocortisone | Hidrocortisona | 眼部给药<br>Ophthalmic Drug Delivery | C；D- 如在妊娠早期用药<br>D-For example, used in the first trimester of pregnancy. |
|  |  |  |  | 口服给药，Oral | C；D- 如在妊娠早期用药<br>D-For example, used in the first trimester of pregnancy. |
|  |  |  |  | 耳部用药<br>Ear Drug Delivery | C；D- 如在妊娠早期用药<br>D-For example, used in the first trimester of pregnancy. |

**续 表**

| 药品名称 | Drug Name | Dénomination du médicament | Denominación del medicamento | 给药途径<br>Administration Route<br>Voie dàdministration<br>Vía de administración | 对妊娠危险性分级<br>Classification of pregnancy risk<br>Classification des risques liés<br>à la grossesse Clasificación<br>del riesgo de embarazo |
|---|---|---|---|---|---|
| | | | | 肠道外给药，Parentaral | C；D- 如在妊娠早期用药<br>D-For example, used in the first trimester of pregnancy. |
| | | | | 局部／皮外用药<br>Local/Skin( External Use) | C；D- 如在妊娠早期用药<br>D-For example, used in the first trimester of pregnancy. |
| 氢可酮 | Hydrocodone | Hydrocodone | Hidrocodona | 口服给药，Oral | C；D- 如在临近分娩时长期大量使用<br>D-For example, long-term used in large doses near delivery. |
| 氢氯噻嗪 | Hydrochlorothi-azide | Hydrochlorothia-zide | Hidroclorotiazida | 口服给药，Oral | B；D- 如用于妊娠高血压患者<br>D-For example, for patients with gestational hypertension. |
| 氢吗啡酮 | Hydromorphone | Hydromorphone | Hidromorfona | 肠道外给药，Parentaral | C |
| 氢溴酸依来曲坦 | Eletriptan Hydrobromide | Hydrobromide d'Elétriptan | Hidrobromida de Eletriptan | 口服给药，Oral | C |
| 氰钴胺 | Cyanocobalamin | Cyanocobalamine | Cianocobalamina | 鼻腔给药，Nasal Delivery | C |
| 庆大霉素 | Gentamicin | Gentamicine | Gentamicina | 眼部给药<br>Ophthalmic Drug Delivery | C |
| | | | | 耳部给药<br>Ear Drug Delivery | C |
| | | | | 肠道外给药，Parentaral | C |
| | | | | 局部／皮外用药<br>Local/Skin( External Use) | C |
| γ - 球蛋白 | Gamma Globulin | Gamma Globuline | Gamma Globulina | 肠道外给药，Parentaral | C |
| 秋水仙碱 | Colchicine | Colchicine | Colcicina | 口服给药，Oral | D |
| | | | | 肠道外给药，Parentaral | D |
| 巯嘌呤 | Mercaptopurine | Mercaptopurine | Mercaptopurina | 口服给药，Oral | D |
| 曲安西龙 | Triamcinolone | Triamcinolone | Triamcinolona | 吸入，Inhalation | C |
| | | | | 鼻腔给药，Nasal Delivery | C |
| | | | | 口服给药，Oral | C；D- 如在妊娠早期用药<br>D-For example, used in the first trimester of pregnancy. |
| | | | | 肠道外给药，Parentaral | C；D- 如在妊娠早期用药<br>D-For example, used in the first trimester of pregnancy. |
| | | | | 局部／皮肤外用<br>Local/Skin( External Use) | C |

**续　表**

| 药品名称 | Drug Name | Dénomination du médicament | Denominación del medicamento | 给药途径 Administration Route Voie dàdministration Vía de administración | 对妊娠危险性分级 Classification of pregnancy risk Classification des risques liés à la grossesse Clasificación del riesgo de embarazo |
|---|---|---|---|---|---|
| 曲吡那敏 | Tripelennamine | Tripelennamine | Tripelenamina | 口服给药，Oral | B |
| 曲伐沙星 | Trovafloxacin | Trovafloxacine | Trovafloxacina | 口服给药，Oral | C |
| 曲伏前列素 | Travlprost | Travlprost | Travlprost | 眼部给药 Ophthalmic Drug Delivery | C |
| 曲氟尿苷 | Trifluridine | Trifluridine | Trifluridina | 眼部给药 Ophthalmic Drug Delivery | C |
| 曲马多 | Tramadol | Tramadol | Tramadol | 口服给药，Oral | C |
| | | | | 肠道外给药，Parentaral | C |
| 曲米帕明 | Trimipramine | Trimipramine | Trimipramina | 口服给药，Oral | C |
| 曲普利啶 | Triprolidine | Triprolidine | Triprolidina | 口服给药，Oral | C |
| 曲普瑞林 | Triptorelin | Triptoreline | Triptorelina | 肠道外给药，Parentaral | X |
| 曲妥珠单抗 | Trastuzumab | Trastuzumab | Trastuzumab | 肠道外给药，Parentaral | B |
| 去唑酮 | Trazodone | Trazodone | Trazodona | 口服给药，Oral | C |
| 去氨加压素 | Desmopressin | Desmopressine | Desmopresina | 鼻腔给药，Nasal Delivery | B |
| | | | | 口服给药，Oral | B |
| | | | | 肠道外给药，Parentaral | B |
| 去甲肾上腺素 | Norepinephrine | Norepinephrine | Norepinefrina | 肠道外给药，Parentaral | C |
| 去甲替林 | Nortriptyline | Nortriptyline | Nortriptilina | 口服给药，Oral | C |
| 去羟肌苷 | Didanosine | Didanosine | Didanosina | 口服给药，Oral | B |
| 去羟米松 | Desoximetasone | Desoximetasone | Desoximetasona | 局部 / 皮肤外用 Local/Skin( External Use) | C |
| 去铁胺 | Deferoxamine | Deferoxamine | Deferoxamina | 肠道外给药，Parentaral | C |
| 去氧肾上腺素 | Phenylephrine | Phenylephrine | Fenilefrina | 口服给药，Oral | C |
| 去乙酰毛花苷 | Deslanoside | Deslanoside | Deslanosida | 口服给药，Oral | C |
| 炔雌醇 | Ethinyl Estradiol | Ethinyl Estradiol | Etinil Estradiol | 口服给药，Oral | X |
| 炔诺酮 | Norethisterone | Norethisterone | Noretisterona | 口服给药，Oral | X |
| 炔孕酮 | Ethisterone | Ethisterone | Etisterona | 口服给药，Oral | D |
| 群多普利 | Trandolapril | Trandolapril | Trandolapril | 口服给药，Oral | C；D- 如在妊娠中、晚期用药 D-For example, used in middle and late stage of pregnancy. |
| 人免疫球蛋白 | Human Immunoglobulin | Human Immunoglobuline | Human Imunoglobulina | 肠道外给药，Parentaral | C |

**续 表**

| 药品名称 | Drug Name | Dénomination du médicament | Denominación del medicamento | 给药途径<br>Administration Route<br>Voie dàdministration<br>Vía de administración | 对妊娠危险性分级<br>Classification of pregnancy risk<br>Classification des risques liés à la grossesse Clasificación del riesgo de embarazo |
|---|---|---|---|---|---|
| 壬二酸 | Azelaic Acid | Acide Azelaique | Acido Azelaico | 局部 / 皮肤外用<br>Local/Skin( External Use) | B |
| 绒促性素 | Chorionic Gonadotrophin | Gonadotropine de Chorion | Gonadotropina Coriónica | 肠道外给药，Parentaral | X |
| 柔红霉素 | Daunorubicin | Daunorubicine | Daunorubicina | 肠道外给药，Parentaral | D |
| 鞣酸加压素 | Vasopressin Tannate | Tannin Vasopressin | Tanina Vasopresina | 肠道外给药，Parentaral | B |
| 乳果糖 | Lactulose | Lactulose | Lactulosa | 口服给药，Oral | B |
| 乳酸钙 | Calcium Lactate | Lactate de Calcium | Lactato de Calcio | 口服给药，Oral | C |
| 瑞肝素钠 | Reviparin Sodium | Réviparine Sodique | Reviparina Sódica | 肠道外给药，Parentaral | B |
| 瑞格列奈 | Repaglinide | Répaglinide | Repaglinida | 口服给药，Oral | C |
| 瑞舒伐他汀 | Rosuvastatin | Rosuvastatine | Rosuvastatina | 口服给药，Oral | X |
| 塞来昔布 | Celecoxib | Célecoxib | Celecoxib | 口服给药，Oral | C;D- 如在妊娠晚期或临近分娩时用药<br>D-For example, used in late stage of pregnancy or for near delivery. |
| 塞替派 | Thiotepa | Thiotepa | Tiotepa | 肠道外给药，Parentaral | D |
| 赛利洛尔 | Celiprolol | Céliprolol | Celiprolol | 口服给药，Oral | B;D- 如在妊娠中、晚期用药<br>D-For example, used in middle and late stage of pregnancy. |
| 噻康唑 | Tioconazole | Tioconazole | Tioconazol | 阴道给药<br>Vaginal Administration | C |
| 噻氯匹定 | Ticlopidine | Ticlopidine | Ticlopidina | 口服给药，Oral | B |
| 噻吗洛尔 | Timolol | Timolol | Timolol | 眼部给药<br>Ophthalmic Drug Delivery | C |
| | | | | 口服给药，Oral | C;D- 如在妊娠中、晚期用药<br>D-For example, used in middle and late stage of pregnancy. |
| 噻托溴铵 | Tiotropium Bromide | Bromure de Tiotropium | Bromuro de Tiotropio | 吸入，Inhalation | C |
| 赛庚啶 | Cyproheptadine | Cyprohéptadine | Ciproheptadina | 口服给药，Oral | B |
| 赛克利嗪 | Cyclizine | Cyclizine | Ciclizina | 口服给药，Oral | B |
| 三氟拉嗪 | Trifluoperazine | Trifluopérazine | Trifluoperazina | 口服给药，Oral | C |
| 三甲曲沙 | Trimetrexate | Trimétrexate | Trimetrexato | 肠道外给药，Parentaral | D |

**续　表**

| 药品名称 | Drug Name | Dénomination du médicament | Denominación del medicamento | 给药途径 Administration Route Voie dàdministration Vía de administración | 对妊娠危险性分级 Classification of pregnancy risk Classification des risques liés à la grossesse Clasificación del riesgo de embarazo |
|---|---|---|---|---|---|
| 三氯噻嗪 | Trichlormethiazide | Trichlorméthiazide | Triclormetiazida | 口服给药，Oral | C;D- 如用于妊娠高血压患者 D-For example, for patients with gestational hypertension. |
| 三唑仑 | Triazolam | Triazolam | Triazolam | 口服给药，Oral | X |
| 色甘酸 | Cromoglicic Acid | Acide Cromoglicique | Acido Cromoglicico | 吸入，Inhalation | B |
| 沙丁胺醇 | Salbutamol | Salbutamol | Salbutamol | 吸入，Inhalation | C |
| | | | | 口服给药，Oral | C |
| | | | | 肠道外给药，Parentaral | C |
| 沙格司亭 | Sargramostim | Sargramostim | Sargramostim | 肠道外给药，Parentaral | C |
| 沙奎那韦 | Saquinavir | Saquinavir | Saquinavir | 口服给药，Oral | B |
| 沙利度胺 | Thalidomide | Thalidomide | Talidomida | 口服给药，Oral | X |
| 沙美特罗 | Salmeterol | Salméterol | Salmeterol | 吸入，Inhalation | C |
| 舍曲林 | Sertraline | Sértraline | Sertralina | 口服给药，Oral | C |
| 肾上腺素 | Epinephrine | Epinéphrine | Epinefrina | 鼻腔给药，Nasal Delivery | C |
| | | | | 眼部给药 Ophthalmic Drug Delivery | C |
| | | | | 肠道外给药，Parentaral | C |
| 生长激素 | Somatropin | Somatropine | Somatropina | 肠道外给药，Parentaral | B |
| 生长抑素 | Somatostatin | Somatostatine | Somatostatina | 肠道外给药，Parentaral | B |
| 舒芬太尼 | Sufentanil | Sufentanil | Sufentanilo | 肠道外给药，Parentaral | C;D- 如在临近分娩时长期大量使用 D-For example, long-term used in large doses near delivery. |
| 舒林酸 | Sulindac | Sulindaque | Sulindaco | 口服给药，Oral | C;D- 如在妊娠晚期或临近分娩时用药 D-For example, used in late stage of pregnancy or for near delivery. |
| 舒马普坦 | Sumatriptan | Sumatriptan | Sumatriptan | 鼻腔给药，Nasal Delivery | C |
| | | | | 口服给药，Oral | C |
| | | | | 肠道外给药，Parentaral | C |
| 鼠李蒽酚 | Casanthranol | Casanthranol | Casantranol | 口服给药，Oral | C |
| 双硫仑 | Disulfiram | Disulfiram | Disulfiram | 口服给药，Oral | C |
| 双氯非那胺 | Dichlorphenamide | Dichlorphenamide | Diclorfenamida | 口服给药，Oral | C |

| 药品名称 | Drug Name | Dénomination du médicament | Denominación del medicamento | 给药途径<br>Administration Route<br>Voie dàdministration<br>Vía de administración | 对妊娠危险性分级<br>Classification of pregnancy risk<br>Classification des risques liés à la grossesse Clasificación del riesgo de embarazo |
|---|---|---|---|---|---|
| 双氯芬酸 | Diclofenac | Diclofenac | Diclofenaco | 眼部给药<br>Ophthalmic Drug Delivery | C;D- 如在妊娠晚期或临近分娩时用药<br>D-For example, used in late stage of pregnancy or for near delivery. |
| | | | | 口服给药，Oral | B;D- 如在妊娠晚期或临近分娩时用药<br>D-For example, used in late stage of pregnancy aor for near delivery. |
| | | | | 肠道外给药，Parentaral | B;D- 如在妊娠晚期或临近分娩时用药<br>D-For example, used in late stage of pregnancy or for near delivery. |
| | | | | 局部 / 皮肤外用<br>Local/Skin( External Use) | C |
| 双氯西林 | Dicloxacillin | Dicloxacilline | Dicloxacilina | 口服给药，Oral | B |
| 双嘧达莫 | Dipyridamole | Dipyridamole | Dipiridamol | 口服给药，Oral | B |
| 双氢麦角胺 | Dihydroergota-mine | Dihydroergotamine | Dihidroergota-mina | 口服给药，Oral | X |
| 双氢速甾醇 | Dihydrotachyst-erol | Dihydrotachysterol | Dihidrotacosterol | 口服给药，Oral | A;D- 如剂量超过美国的每日推荐摄入量<br>D-For example, the dosage exceeded the daily intake recommended by United States. |
| 双水杨酯 | Salsalate | Salsalate | Salsalato | 口服给药，Oral | C;D- 如用于妊娠晚期<br>D-For example, used in late stage of pregnancy. |
| 水合氯醛 | Chloral Hydrate | Hydrate de Chloral | Hidrato de Cloral | 口服给药，Oral | C |
| | | | | 直肠给药<br>Rectal Administration | C |
| 水杨酸铋 | Bismuth Salicylate | Salicylate de Bismuth | Salicilato de Bismuto | 口服给药，Oral | C |
| 顺铂 | Cisplatin | Cisplatine | Cisplatina | 肠道外给药，Parentaral | D |
| 司来吉兰 | Selegiline | Selegiline | Selegilina | 口服给药，Oral | C |
| 司帕沙星 | Sparfloxacin | Sparfloxacine | Sparfloxacina | 口服给药，Oral | C; 禁用于妊娠早期<br>Prohibited to use, especially in the first trimester of pregnancy. |
| 司他夫定 | Stavudine | Stavudine | Stavudina | 口服给药，Oral | C |

**续 表**

| 药品名称 | Drug Name | Dénomination du médicament | Denominación del medicamento | 给药途径<br>Administration Route<br>Voie dàdministration<br>Vía de administración | 对妊娠危险性分级<br>Classification of pregnancy risk<br>Classification des risques liés à la grossesse Clasificación del riesgo de embarazo |
|---|---|---|---|---|---|
| 司坦唑醇 | Stanozolol | Stanozolol | Stanozolol | 口服给药，Oral | X |
| 司维拉姆 | Sevelamer | Sevelamer | Sevelamer | 口服给药，Oral | C |
| 四环素 | Tetracycline | Tétracycline | Tetraciclina | 眼部给药<br>Ophthalmic Drug Delivery | D |
| | | | | 口服给药，Oral | D |
| | | | | 局部／皮肤外用<br>Local/Skin( External Use) | B |
| 羧苄西林 | Carbenicillin | Carbénicilline | Carbenicilina | 口服给药，Oral | B |
| 缩宫素 | Oxytocin | Oxytocine | Oxitocina | 肠道外给药，Parentaral | X |
| 索他洛尔 | Sotalol | Sotalol | Sotalol | 口服给药，Oral | B;D- 如在妊娠中、晚期用药<br>D-For example, used in middle and late stage of pregnancy. |
| | | | | 肠道外给药，Parentaral | B;D- 如在妊娠中、晚期用药<br>D-For example, used in middle and late stage of pregnancy. |
| 他达拉非 | Tadalafil | Tadalafil | Tadalafil | 口服给药，Oral | B |
| 他克林 | Tacrine | Tacrine | Tacrina | 口服给药，Oral | C |
| 他克莫司 | Tacrolimus | Tacrolimus | Tacrolimus | 口服给药，Oral | C |
| | | | | 肠道外给药，Parentaral | C |
| | | | | 局部／皮肤外用<br>Local/Skin( External Use) | C |
| 他莫昔芬 | Tamoxifen | Tamoxiféne | Tamoxifeno | 口服给药，Oral | D |
| 他扎罗汀 | Tazarotene | Tazaroténe | Tazarotena | 局部／皮肤外用<br>Local/Skin( External Use) | X |
| 泰利霉素 | Telithromycin | Télithromycine | Telitromicina | 口服给药，Oral | C |
| 坦洛新 | Tamsulosin | Tamsulosine | Tamsulosina | 口服给药，Oral | B |
| 碳酸钙 | Calcium Carbonate | Carbonate de Calcium | Carbonato de Calcio | 口服给药，Oral | C |
| 碳酸氢钠 | Sodium Bicarbonate | Bicarbonate de Sodium | Bicarbonato Sodica | 口服给药，Oral | C |
| 特比萘芬 | Terbinafine | Terbinafine | Terbinafina | 口服给药，Oral | B |
| | | | | 局部／皮肤外用<br>Local/Skin( External Use) | B |
| 特布他林 | Terbutaline | Terbutaline | Terbutalina | 吸入，Inhalation | B |
| | | | | 口服给药，Oral | B |
| | | | | 肠道外给药，Parentaral | B |

**续　表**

| 药品名称 | Drug Name | Dénomination du médicament | Denominación del medicamento | 给药途径<br>Administration Route<br>Voie dàdministration<br>Vía de administración | 对妊娠危险性分级<br>Classification of pregnancy risk<br>Classification des risques liés à la grossesse Clasificación del riesgo de embarazo |
|---|---|---|---|---|---|
| 特非那定 | Terfenadine | Terfenadine | Terfenadina | 口服给药，Oral | C |
| 特康唑 | Terconazole | Terconazole | Terconazol | 阴道给药<br>Vaginal Administration | C |
| 特拉唑嗪 | Terazosin | Terazosine | Terazosina | 口服给药，Oral | C |
| 特立帕肽 | Teriparatide | Teriparatide | Teriparatida | 肠道外给药，Parentaral | C |
| 替奥噻吨 | Tiotixene | Tiotixene | Tiotixena | 口服给药，Oral | C |
| 替加色罗 | Tegaserod | Tegaserode | Tegaseroda | 口服给药，Oral | B |
| 替卡西林 | Ticarcillin | Ticarcilline | Ticarcilina | 肠道外给药，Parentaral | B |
| 替鲁膦酸 | Tiludronic Acid | Acide Tiludronique | Acido Tiludronico | 口股给药，Oral | C |
| 替马西泮 | Temazepam | Temazepam | Temazepam | 口服给药，Oral | X |
| 替米沙坦 | Telmisartan | Telmisartan | Telmisartan | 口股给药，Oral | C;D- 如在妊娠中、晚期用药<br>D-For example, used in middle and late stage of pregnancy. |
| 替莫唑胺 | Temozolomide | Temozolomide | Temozolomida | 口服给药，Oral | D |
| 替尼泊苷 | Teniposide | Teniposide | Teniposida | 肠道外给药，Parentaral | D |
| 替特普酶 | Tenecteplase | Tenecteplase | Tenecteplasa | 肠道外给药，Parentaral | C |
| 萜品醇 | Terpin Hydrate | Hydrate de Terpine | Hydrato de Terpina | 口股给药，Oral | D |
| 亭扎肝素钠 | Tinzaparin Sodium | Tinzaparine Sodique | Tinzaparina Sódica | 肠道外给药，Parentaral | B |
| 酮康唑 | Ketoconazole | Ketoconazole | Ketoconazol | 口服给药，Oral | C |
|  |  |  |  | 局部 / 皮肤外用<br>Local/Skin( External Use) | C |
| 酮咯酸 | Ketorolac | Kétorolaque | Ketorolaco | 眼部给药<br>Ophthalmic Drug Delivery | C |
|  |  |  |  | 口服给药，Oral | C;D- 如在妊娠晚期或临近分娩时用药<br>D-For example, used in late stage of pregnancy or for near delivery. |
|  |  |  |  | 肠道外给药，Parentaral | C;D- 如在妊娠晚期或临近分娩时用药<br>D-For example, used in late stage of pregnancy or for near delivery. |
| 酮洛芬 | Ketoprofen | Kétoproféne | Ketoprofeno | 口服给药，Oral | B;D- 如在妊娠晚期或临近分娩时用药<br>D-For example, used in late stage of pregnancy or for near delivery. |

**续　表**

| 药品名称 | Drug Name | Dénomination du médicament | Denominación del medicamento | 给药途径<br>Administration Route<br>Voie dàdministration<br>Vía de administración | 对妊娠危险性分级<br>Classification of pregnancy risk<br>Classification des risques liés à la grossesse Clasificación del riesgo de embarazo |
|---|---|---|---|---|---|
| 酮替芬 | Ketotifen | Kétotiféne | Ketotifeno | 眼部给药<br>Ophthalmic Drug Delivery | C |
| 头孢氨苄 | Cefalexin | Céfalexine | Cefalexina | 口股给药，Oral | B |
| 头孢吡肟 | Cefepime | Céfepime | Cefepima | 肠道外给药，Parentaral | B |
| 头孢丙烯 | Cefprozil | Céfprozil | Cefprozil | 口服给药，Oral | B |
| 头孢泊肟 | Cefpodoxime | Céfpodoxime | Cefpodoxima | 口股给药，Oral | B |
| 头孢布烯 | Ceftibuten | Céftibutene | Ceftibuteno | 口服给药，Oral | B |
| 头孢地尼 | Cefdinir | Céfdinir | Cefdinir | 口服给药，Oral | B |
| 头孢呋辛 | Cefuroxime | Céfuroxime | Cefuroxima | 口服给药，Oral | B |
| | | | | 肠道外给药，Parentaral | B |
| 头孢克洛 | Cefaclor | Céfaclor | Cefaclor | 口服给药，Oral | B |
| 头孢克肟 | Cefixime | Céfixime | Cefixima | 口服给药，Oral | B |
| 头孢拉定 | Cefradine | Céfradine | Cefradina | 口服给药，Oral | B |
| | | | | 肠道外给药，Parentaral | B |
| 头孢雷特 | Ceforanide | Céforanide | Ceforanida | 肠道外给药，Parentaral | B |
| 头孢美唑 | Cefmetazole | Céfmetazole | Cefmetazol | 肠道外给药，Parentaral | B |
| 头孢孟多 | Cefamandole | Céfamandole | Cefamandol | 肠道外给药，Parentaral | B |
| 头孢尼西 | Cefonicid | Céfonicid | Cefonicid | 肠道外给药，Parentaral | B |
| 头孢哌酮 | Cefoperazone | Céfoperazone | Cefoperazona | 肠道外给药，Parentaral | B |
| 头孢匹林 | Cefapirin | Céfapirine | Cefapirina | 肠道外给药，Parentaral | B |
| 头孢羟氨苄 | Cefadroxil | Céfadroxil | Cefadroxil | 口服给药，Oral | B |
| 头孢曲秦 | Cefatrizine | Céfatrizine | Cefatrizina | 口服给药，Oral | B |
| 头孢曲松 | Ceftriaxone | Céftriaxone | Ceftriaxona | 肠道外给药，Parentaral | B |
| 头孢噻吩 | Cefalotin | Céfalotine | Cefalotina | 肠道外给药，Parentaral | B |
| 头孢噻肟 | Cefotaxime | Céfotaxime | Cefotaxima | 肠道外给药，Parentaral | B |
| 头孢他啶 | Ceftazidime | Céftazidime | Ceftazidima | 肠道外给药，Parentaral | B |
| 头孢替坦 | Cefotetan | Céfotetan | Cefotetan | 肠道外给药，Parentaral | B |
| 头孢托仑 | Cefditoren | Céfditorene | Cefditorena | 口服给药，Oral | B |
| 头孢西丁 | Cefoxitin | Céfoxitine | Cefoxitina | 肠道外给药，Parentaral | B |
| 头孢唑林 | Cefazolin | Céfazoline | Cefazolina | 肠道外给药，Parentaral | B |
| 头孢唑肟 | Ceftizoxime | Céftizoxime | Ceftizoxima | 肠道外给药，Parentaral | B |
| 土霉素 | Oxytetracycline | Oxytétracycline | Oxitetraciclina | 口服给药，Oral | D |

续 表

| 药品名称 | Drug Name | Dénomination du médicament | Denominación del medicamento | 给药途径<br>Administration Route<br>Voie dàdministration<br>Vía de administración | 对妊娠危险性分级<br>Classification of pregnancy risk<br>Classification des risques liés à la grossesse Clasificación del riesgo de embarazo |
|---|---|---|---|---|---|
| 吐根 | Ipecacuanha | Ipécacuanha | Ipecacuanha | 口服给药，Oral | C |
| 托吡卡胺 | Tropicamide | Tropicamide | Tropicamida | 眼部给药<br>Ophthalmic Drug Delivery | C |
| 托吡酯 | Topiramate | Topiramate | Topiramato | 口服给药，Oral | C |
| 托卡朋 | Tolcapone | Tolcapone | Tolcapona | 口服给药，Oral | C |
| 托拉塞米 | Torasemide | Torasémide | Torasemida | 口服给药，Oral | B |
| | | | | 肠道外给药，Parentaral | B |
| 托美汀 | Tolmetin | Tolmetine | Tolmetina | 口服给药，Oral | C;D- 如在妊娠晚期或临近分娩时用药<br>D-For example, used in late stage of pregnancy or for near delivery. |
| 托莫西汀 | Atomoxetine | Atomoxetine | Atomoxetina | 口服给药，Oral | C |
| 托瑞米芬 | Toremifene | Toremifene | Toremifeno | 口服给药，Oral | D |
| 托特罗定 | Tolterodine | Tolterodine | Tolterodina | 口服给药，Oral | C |
| 托西溴苄铵 | Bretylium Tosilate | Tosilate de Bretylium | Tosilato de Bretylio | 肠道外给药，Parentaral | C |
| 妥布霉素 | Tobramycin | Tobramycine | Tobramicina | 吸入，Inhalation | D |
| | | | | 眼部给药<br>Ophthalmic Drug Delivery | B |
| | | | | 肠道外给药，Parentaral | D |
| 妥卡胺 | Tocainide | Tocainide | Tocainida | 口服给药，Oral | C |
| 妥拉磺脲 | Tolazamide | Tolazamide | Tolazamida | 口服给药，Oral | C |
| 妥拉唑林 | Tolazoline | Tolazoline | Tolazolina | 肠道外给药，Parentaral | C |
| 拓泊替康 | Topotecan | Topotecan | Topotecan | 肠道外给药，Parentaral | D |
| 万古霉素 | Vancomycin | Vancomycine | Vancomicina | 口服给药，Oral | B |
| | | | | 肠道外给药，Parentaral | C |
| 维甲酸 | Tretinoin | Tretinoine | Tretinoina | 口服给药，Oral | D；禁用于妊娠早期<br>Prohibited to use, especially in the first trimester of pregnancy. |
| | | | | 局部 / 皮肤外用<br>Local/Skin( External Use) | C |
| 维库溴铵 | Vecuronium Bromide | Bromure de Vecuronium | Bromuro de Vecuronio | 肠道外给药，Parentaral | C |
| 维拉帕米 | Verapamil | Verapamil | Verapamilo | 口服给药，Oral | C |
| | | | | 肠道外给药，Parentaral | C |

续　表

| 药品名称 | Drug Name | Dénomination du médicament | Denominación del medicamento | 给药途径<br>Administration Route<br>Voie dàdministration<br>Vía de administración | 对妊娠危险性分级<br>Classification of pregnancy risk<br>Classification des risques liés à la grossesse Clasificación del riesgo de embarazo |
|---|---|---|---|---|---|
| 维生素 D | Vitamin D | Vitamine D | Vitamina D | 口服给药，Oral | A;D- 如剂量超过美国的每日推荐摄入量<br>D-For example, the dosage exceeded the daily intake recommended by United States. |
| 维生素 E | Vitamin E | Vitamine E | Vitamina E | 口服给药，Oral | A;C- 如剂量超过美国的每日推荐摄入量<br>C-For example, the dosage exceeded the daily intake recommended by United States. |
| 维替泊芬 | Verteporfin | Verteporfine | Verteporfina | 肠道外给药，Parentaral | C |
| 伪麻黄碱 | Pseudoephedrine | Pseudoephedrine | Pseudoefedrina | 口服给药，Oral | C |
| 文拉法辛 | Venlafaxine | Venlafaxine | Venlafaxina | 口服给药，Oral | C |
| 乌洛托品 | Methenamine | Methenamine | Metenamina | 口服给药，Oral | C |
| 乌诺前列酮 | Unoprostone | Unoprostone | Unoprostona | 眼部给药<br>Ophthalmic Drug Delivery | C |
| 戊巴比妥 | Pentobarbital | Pentobarbital | Pentobarbital | 肠道外给药，Parentaral | D |
| 戊四硝酯 | Pentaerithrityl Tetranitrate | Tétranitrate de Pentaérythritol | Tetranitrato de Pentaeritritol | 口服给药，Oral | C |
| 西地那非 | Sildenafil | Sildenafil | Sildenafil | 口服给药，Oral | B |
| 西多福韦 | Cidofovir | Cidofovir | Cidofovir | 肠道外给药，Parentaral | C |
| 西甲硅油 | Simeticone | Simeticone | Simeticona | 口服给药，Oral | C |
| 西拉普利 | Cilazapril | Cilazapril | Cilazapril | 口服给药，Oral | C;D- 如在妊娠中、晚期用药<br>D-For example, used in middle and late stage of pregnancy. |
| 西立伐他汀钠 | Cerivastatin Sodium | Cerivastatine Sodique | Cerivastatina Sódica | 口服给药，Oral | X |
| 西罗莫司 | Sirolimus | Sirolimus | Sirolimus | 肠道外给药，Parentaral | C |
| 西洛他唑 | Cilostazol | Cilostazole | Cilostazol | 口服给药，Oral | C |
| 西咪替丁 | Cimetidine | Cimetidine | Cimetidina | 口服给药，Oral | B |
|  |  |  |  | 肠道外给药，Parentaral | B |
| 西诺沙星 | Cinoxacin | Cinoxacine | Cinoxacina | 口服给药，Oral | C |
| 西曲瑞克 | Cetrorelix | Cetrorelix | Cetrorelix | 肠道外给药，Parentaral | X |
| 西沙必利 | Cisapride | Cisapride | Cisaprida | 口服给药，Oral | C |
| 西司他丁 | Cilastatin | Cilastatine | Cilastatina | 肠道外给药，Parentaral | C |
| 西酞普兰 | Citalopram | Citalopram | Citalopram | 口服给药，Oral | C |

**续　表**

| 药品名称 | Drug Name | Dénomination du médicament | Denominación del medicamento | 给药途径<br>Administration Route<br>Voie dàdministration<br>Vía de administración | 对妊娠危险性分级<br>Classification of pregnancy risk<br>Classification des risques liés<br>à la grossesse Clasificación<br>del riesgo de embarazo |
|---|---|---|---|---|---|
| 西替利嗪 | Cetirizine | Cetirizine | Cetirizina | 口服给药，Oral | B |
| 西妥昔单抗 | Cetuximab | Cetuximab | Cetuximab | 肠道外给药，Parentaral | C |
| 烯丙吗啡 | Nalorphine | Nalorphine | Nalorfina | 肠道外给药，Parentaral | D |
| 腺苷 | Adenosine | Adenosine | Adenosina | 肠道外给药，Parentaral | C |
| 香豆素 | Coumarin | Coumarine | Coumarina | 口服给药，Oral | X |
| 硝苯地平 | Nifedipine | Nifedipine | Nifedipina | 口服给药，Oral | C |
| 硝普钠 | Sodium Nitroprusside | Nitroprusside de Sodium | Nitroprusida Sódico | 肠道外给药，Parentaral | C |
| 硝酸甘油 | Glyceryl Trinitrate | Trinitrate de Glycérides | Trinitrato de Glicerol | 舌下给药<br>Sublingual Administration | C |
| | | | | 经皮给药，Transdermal Drug Delivery | C |
| 硝酸异山梨酯 | Isosorbide Dinitrate | Dinitrate d'Isosorbide | Dinitrato de Isosorbida | 口含，Keep in the Mouth | C |
| | | | | 口服给药，Oral | C |
| | | | | 肠道外给药，Parentaral | C |
| | | | | 经皮给药，Transdermal Drug Delivery | C |
| 缬更昔洛韦 | Valganciclovir | Valganciclovir | Valganciclovir | 口服给药，Oral | C |
| 缬沙坦 | Valsartan | Valsartan | Valsartan | 口服给药，Oral | C;D- 如在妊娠中、晚期用药<br>D-For example, used in middle and late stage of pregnancy. |
| 辛伐他汀 | Simvastatin | Simvastatine | Simvastatina | 口服给药，Oral | X |
| 新霉素 | Neomycin | Neomycine | Neomicina | 口服给药，Oral | C |
| 新斯的明 | Neostigmine | Neostigmine | Neostigmina | 口服给药，Oral | C |
| | | | | 肠道外给药，Parentaral | C |
| A 型肉毒毒素 | Botulinum Toxin A | Toxine Botulique A | Toxina Botulínica A | 肠道外给药，Parentaral | C |
| 胸腺法新 | Thymalfasin | Thymalfasine | Timalfasina | 肠道外给药，Parentaral | C |
| 熊去氧胆酸 | Ursodesoxycholic Acid | Acide Ursodesoxycholique | Acido Ursodesoxicolico | 口服给药，Oral | B |
| 溴苯那敏 | Brompheniramine | Brompheniramine | Bromfeniramina | 口服给药，Oral | C |
| 溴吡斯的明 | Pyridostigmine Bromide | Bromure de Pyridostigmine | Bromuro de Piridostigmina | 口服给药，Oral | C |
| | | | | 肠道外给药，Parentaral | C |

**续　表**

| 药品名称 | Drug Name | Dénomination du médicament | Denominación del medicamento | 给药途径<br>Administration Route<br>Voie dàdministration<br>Vía de administración | 对妊娠危险性分级<br>Classification of pregnancy risk<br>Classification des risques liés à la grossesse Clasificación del riesgo de embarazo |
|---|---|---|---|---|---|
| 溴丙胺太林 | Propantheline Bromide | Bromure de Propantheline | Bromuro de Propantelina | 口服给药，Oral | C |
| 溴美喷酯 | Mepenzolate Bromide | Bromure de Mepenzolate | Bromuro de Mepenzolato | 口服给药，Oral | C |
| 溴莫尼定 | Brimonidine | Brimonidine | Brimonidina | 眼部给药<br>Ophthalmic Drug Delivery | B |
| 溴隐亭 | Bromocriptine | Bromocriptine | Bromocriptina | 口服给药，Oral | B |
| 血管加压素 | Vasopressin | Vasopressin | Vasopresina | 肠道外给药，Parentaral | B |
| 亚胺培南 | Imipenem | Imipenem | Imipenem | 肠道外给药，Parentaral | C |
| 亚叶酸钙 | Caleium Folinate | Folinate de Calcium | Folinato de Calcio | 口服给药，Oral | C |
|  |  |  |  | 肠道外给药，Parentaral | C |
| 烟醇 | Nicotinyl Alcohol | Alcool Nicotinique | Alcohol Nicotílico | 口服给药，Oral | C |
| 烟酰胺 | Nicotinamide | Nicotinamide | Nicotinamida | 口服给药，Oral | A；C- 如剂量超过美国的每日推荐摄入量<br>C-For example, the dosage exceeded the daily intake recommended by United States. |
| 盐酸阿洛司琼 | Alosetron Hydrochloride | Chlorhydrate de Alosetron | Clorhidrato de Alosetron | 口服给药，Oral | B |
| 盐酸吡布特罗 | Pirbuterol Hydrochloride | Chlorhydrate de Pirbuterol | Clorhidrato de Pirbuterol | 吸入，Inhalation | C |
| 盐酸奈法唑酮 | Nefazodone Hydrochloride | Chlorhydrate de Nefazodone | Clorhidrato de Nefazodona | 口服给药，Oral | C |
| 盐酸曲恩汀 | Trientine Hydrochloride | Chlorhydrate de Trientine | Clorhidrato de Trientina | 口服给药，Oral | C |
| 盐酸瑞芬太尼 | Remifentanil Hydrochloride | Chlorhydrate de Remifentanil | Clorhidrato de Remifentanil | 肠道外给药，Parentaral | C |
| 盐酸罂粟碱 | Papaverine Hydrochloride | Chlorhydrate de Papaverine | Clorhidrato de Papaverina | 口服给药，Oral | C |
| 洋地黄毒苷 | Digitoxin | Digitoxine | Digitoxina | 口服给药，Oral | C |
| 氧氟沙星 | Ofloxacin | Ofloxacine | Ofloxacina | 眼部给药<br>Ophthalmic Drug Delivery | C；妊娠期妇女慎用，尤其是妊娠早期<br>Use with caution in pregnancy, especially in the first trimester. |
|  |  |  |  | 口服给药，Oral | C；妊娠期妇女慎用，尤其是妊娠早期<br>Use with caution in pregnancy, especially in the first trimester. |

续 表

| 药品名称 | Drug Name | Dénomination du médicament | Denominación del medicamento | 给药途径<br>Administration Route<br>Voie dàdministration<br>Vía de administración | 对妊娠危险性分级<br>Classification of pregnancy risk<br>Classification des risques liés à la grossesse Clasificación del riesgo de embarazo |
|---|---|---|---|---|---|
|  |  |  |  | 耳部给药<br>Ear Drug Delivery | C；妊娠期妇女慎用，尤其是妊娠早期<br>Use with caution in pregnancy, especially in the first trimester. |
|  |  |  |  | 肠道外给药，Parentaral | C；妊娠期妇女慎用，尤其是妊娠早期<br>Use with caution in pregnancy, especially in the first trimester. |
| 氧烯洛尔 | Oxprenolol | Oxprenolol | Oxprenolol | 口服给药，Oral | C；D- 如在妊娠中、晚期用药<br>D-For example, used in middle and late stage of pregnancy. |
| 氧雄龙 | Oxandrolone | Oxandrolone | Oxandrolona | 口服给药，Oral | X |
| 叶酸 | Folic Acid | Acide Folique | Ácido Fólico | 口服给药，Oral | A；C- 如剂量超过美国的每日推荐摄入量<br>C-For example, the dosage exceeded the daily intake recommended by United States. |
| 伊班膦酸 | Ibandronaic Acid | Acide Ibandronaique | Acido Ibandronaico | 口服给药，Oral | C |
| 伊达比星 | Idarubicin | Idarubicine | Idarubicina | 肠道外给药，Parentaral | D |
| 伊拉地平 | Isradipine | Isradipine | Isradipina | 口服给药，Oral | C |
| 伊立替康 | Irinotecan | Irinotecan | Irinotecan | 肠道外给药，Parentaral | D |
| 伊洛前列素 | Iloprost | Iloprost | Iloprost | 吸入，Inhalation | C |
| 伊马替尼 | Imatinib | Imatinib | Imatinib | 口服给药，Oral | D |
| 伊米苷酶 | Imiglucerase | Imiglucerase | Imiglucerasa | 肠道外给药，Parentaral | C |
| 伊曲康唑 | Itraconazole | Itraconazole | Itraconazol | 口服给药，Oral | C |
|  |  |  |  | 肠道外给药，Parentaral |  |
| 伊维菌素 | Ivermectin | Ivermectine | Ivermectina | 口服给药，Oral | C |
| 依发韦仑 | Efavirenz | Efavirenz | Efavirenz | 口服给药，Oral | D |
| 依法珠单抗 | Efalizumab | Efalizumab | Efalizumab | 肠道外给药，Parentaral | C |
| 依酚氯铵 | Edrophonium Chloride | Chlorures de Edrophonium | Cloruro de Edrofonio | 肠道外给药，Parentaral | C |
| 依美斯汀 | Emedastine | Emedastine | Emedastina | 口服给药，Oral | B |
| 依那普利 | Enalapril | Enalapril | Enalapril | 口服给药，Oral | C；D- 如在妊娠中、晚期用药<br>D-For example, used in middle and late stage of pregnancy. |
| 依诺肝素 | Enoxaparin | Enoxaparine | Enoxaparina | 肠道外给药，Parentaral | B |

**续　表**

| 药品名称 | Drug Name | Dénomination du médicament | Denominación del medicamento | 给药途径<br>Administration Route<br>Voie dàdministration<br>Vía de administración | 对妊娠危险性分级<br>Classification of pregnancy risk<br>Classification des risques liés à la grossesse Clasificación del riesgo de embarazo |
|---|---|---|---|---|---|
| 依诺沙星 | Enoxacin | Enoxacine | Enoxacina | 口服给药，Oral | C |
| 依匹斯汀 | Epinastine | Epinastine | Epinastina | 眼部给药<br>Ophthalmic Drug Delivery | C |
| 依前列醇 | Epoproslenol | Epoproslenol | Epoproslenol | 肠道外给药，Parentaral | B |
| 伊索庚嗪 | Ethoheptazine | Ethoheptazine | Etoheptazina | 口服给药，Oral | C |
| 依他尼酸 | Etacrynic Acid | Acide de Etacrynique | Acido de Etacrinico | 口服给药，Oral | B；D- 如用于妊娠高血压患者<br>D-For example, for patients with gestational hypertension. |
| | | | | 肠道外给药，Parentaral | B；D- 如用于妊娠高血压患者<br>D-For example, for patients with gestational hypertension. |
| 依他凝血素α | Eptacog Alfa(activated) | Eptacog Alfa(activé) | Eptacog Alfa(activado) | 肠道外给药，Parentaral | C |
| 依他西普 | Etanercept | Etanercept | Etanercept | 肠道外给药，Parentaral | B |
| 依替巴肽 | Eptifibatide | Eptifibatide | Eptifibatida | 肠道外给药，Parentaral | B |
| 依替膦酸 | Etidronic Acid | Acide de Etidronique | Acido de Etidronico | 口服给药，Oral | B |
| | | | | 肠道外给药，Parentaral | C |
| 依托泊苷 | Etoposide | Etoposide | Etoposida | 肠道外给药，Parentaral | D |
| 依托度酸 | Etodolic Acid | Acide Etodolique | Acido Etodolico | 口服给药，Oral | C；D- 如在妊娠晚期或临近分娩时用药<br>D-For example, used in late stage of pregnancy or for near delivery. |
| 依托咪酯 | Etomidate | Etomidate | Etomidato | 肠道外给药，Parentaral | C |
| 依西美坦 | Exemestane | Exemestane | Exemestano | 口服给药，Oral | D |
| 依折麦布 | Ezetimibe | Ezetimibe | Ezetimibe | 口服给药，Oral | C |
| 胰岛素 | Insulin | Insuline | Insulina | 肠道外给药，Parentaral | B |
| 胰脂肪酶 | Pancrelipase | Pancrelipase | Pancrelipasa | 口服给药，Oral | C |
| 乙胺丁醇 | Ethambutol | Ethambutol | Etambutol | 口服给药，Oral | B |
| 乙胺嘧啶 | Pyrimethamine | Pyrimethamine | Pirimetamina | 口服给药，Oral | C |
| 乙琥氨 | Ethosuximide | Ethosuximide | Etosuximida | 口服给药，Oral | C |
| 乙硫异烟胺 | Ethionamide | Ethionamide | Etionamida | 口服给药，Oral | C |
| 乙酰半胱氨酸 | Acetylcysteine | Acetylcysteine | Acetilcisteina | 吸入，Inhalation | B |
| | | | | 口服给药，Oral | B |
| | | | | 肠道外给药，Parentaral | B |

续 表

| 药品名称 | Drug Name | Dénomination du médicament | Denominación del medicamento | 给药途径<br>Administration Route<br>Voie dàdministration<br>Vía de administración | 对妊娠危险性分级<br>Classification of pregnancy risk<br>Classification des risques liés à la grossesse Clasificación del riesgo de embarazo |
|---|---|---|---|---|---|
| 乙酰唑胺 | Acetazolamide | Acetazolamide | Acetazolamida | 口服给药，Oral | C |
| | | | | 肠道外给药，Parentaral | C |
| 异丙碘铵 | Isopropamide Iodide | Iodure de Isopropamide | Yoduro de Isopropamida | 口服给药，Oral | C |
| 异丙嗪 | Promethazine | Promethazine | Prometazina | 口服给药，Oral | C |
| | | | | 肠道外给药，Parentaral | C |
| 异丙肾上腺素 | Isoprenaline | Isoprenaline | Isoprenalina | 肠道外给药，Parentaral | C |
| 异丙托溴铵 | Ipratropium Bromide | Bromure d'Ipratropium | Bromuro de Ipratropio | 吸入，Inhalation | B |
| 异环磷酰胺 | Ifosfamide | Ifosfamide | Ifosfamida | 肠道外给药，Parentaral | D |
| 异克舒令 | Isoxsuprine | Isoxsuprine | Isoxsuprina | 口服给药，Oral | C |
| 异美汀 | Isometheptene | Isometheptene | Isometeptena | 口服给药，Oral | C |
| 异炔诺酮 | Noretynodrel | Noretynodrel | Noretinodrel | 口服给药，Oral | X |
| 异A维酸 | Isotretinoin | Isotretinoine | Isotretinoina | 口服给药，Oral | X |
| 异戊巴比妥 | Amobarbital | Amobarbital | Amobarbital | 口服给药，Oral | D |
| 异烟肼 | Isoniazid | Isoniazide | Isoniazida | 口服给药，Oral | C |
| | | | | 肠道外给药，Parentaral | C |
| 抑肽酶 | Aprotinin | Aprotinine | Aprotinina | 肠道外给药，Parentaral | B |
| 益康唑 | Econazole | Econazole | Econazol | 局部/皮肤外用<br>Local/Skin( External Use) | C；不宜使用，尤其是妊娠早期 Unfavorable use, especially in the first trimester of pregnancy. |
| | | | | 肠道给药，<br>The Intestinal Drug Delivery. | C；不宜使用，尤其是妊娠早期 Unfavorable use, especially in the first trimester of pregnancy. |
| 吲哚洛尔 | Pindolol | Pindolol | Pindolol | 口服给药，Oral | B；D- 如在妊娠中、晚期用药 D-For example, used in middle and late stage of pregnancy. |
| 吲哒帕胺 | Indapamide | Indapamide | Indapamida | 口服给药，Oral | B；D- 如用于妊娠高血压患者 D-For example, for patients with gestational hypertension. |
| 吲哚美辛 | Indometacin | Indometacine | Indometacina | 眼部给药<br>Ophthalmic Drug Delivery | B；D- 如持续使用超过48小时，或在妊娠34周以后用药 D-For example, when the drug was administered continuously for more than 48 hours or after 34 weeks of gestation. |

**续　表**

| 药品名称 | Drug Name | Dénomination du médicament | Denominación del medicamento | 给药途径<br>Administration Route<br>Voie dàdministration<br>Vía de administración | 对妊娠危险性分级<br>Classification of pregnancy risk<br>Classification des risques liés à la grossesse Clasificación del riesgo de embarazo |
|---|---|---|---|---|---|
|  |  |  |  | 口服给药，Oral | B; D-如持续使用超过 48 小时，或在妊娠 34 周以后用药<br>D-For example, when the drug was administered continuously for more than 48 hours or after 34 weeks of gestation. |
|  |  |  |  | 肠道外给药，Parentaral | B; D-如持续使用超过 48 小时，或在妊娠 34 周以后用药<br>D-For example, when the drug was administered continuously for more than 48 hours or after 34 weeks of gestation. |
|  |  |  |  | 直肠给药<br>Rectal Administration | B; D-如持续使用超过 48 小时，或在妊娠 34 周以后用药<br>D-For example, when the drug was administered continuously for more than 48 hours or after 34 weeks of gestation. |
| 茚地那韦 | Indinavir | Indinavir | Indinavir | 口服给药，Oral | C |
| 英利昔单抗 | Infliximab | Infliximab | Infliximab | 肠道外给药，Parentaral | B |
| 荧光素 | Fluorescein | Fluoresceine | Fluoresceina | 眼部给药<br>Ophthalmic Drug Delivery | C |
|  |  |  |  | 肠道外给药，Parentaral | C |
| 左芬氟拉明 | Dexfenflura-mine | Dexfenfluramine | Dexfenfluramina | 口服给药，Oral | C |
| 右氯苯那敏 | Dexchlorpheni-ramine | Dexchlorphenir-amine | Dexclorfenira-mina | 口服给药，Oral | B |
| 右美沙芬 | Dextrometho-rphan | Dextrométorfène | Dextrometor-fano | 口服给药，Oral | C |
| 右美托咪定 | Dexmedetomi-dine | Dexmedetomidine | Dexmedetomi-dina | 肠道外给药，Parentaral | C |
| 右溴苯那敏 | Dexbrompheni-ramine | Dexbromphénira-mine | Dexbromfenira-mina | 口服给药，Oral | C |
| 右旋糖酐 | Dextran | Dextrane | Dextrano | 肠道外给药，Parentaral | C |
| 右旋糖酐铁 | Iron Dextran | Dextranate de Fer | Dextrano de Hierro | 肠道外给药，Parentaral | C |
| 愈创甘油醚 | Guaifenesin | Guaifenesine | Guaifenesina | 口服给药，Oral | C |
| 孕酮 | Progesterone | Progesterone | Progesterona | 口服给药，Oral | B |

续　表

| 药品名称 | Drug Name | Dénomination du médicament | Denominación del medicamento | 给药途径 Administration Route Voie dàdministration Vía de administración | 对妊娠危险性分级 Classification of pregnancy risk Classification des risques liés à la grossesse Clasificación del riesgo de embarazo |
|---|---|---|---|---|---|
| 扎鲁司特 | Zafirlukast | Zafirlukast | Zafirlukast | 口服给药，Oral | B |
| 扎那米韦 | Zanamivir | Zanamivir | Zanamivir | 吸入，Inhalation | C |
| 扎西他滨 | Zalcitabine | Zalcitabine | Zalcitabina | 口服给药，Oral | C |
| 樟脑 | Camphor | Camphre | Alcanfor | 局部/皮肤外用 Local/Skin( External Use) | C |
| 植物甲萘醌 | Phytomenadione | Phytomenadione | Fitomenadiona | 口服给药，Oral | C |
| | | | | 肠道外给药，Parentaral | C |
| 制霉菌素 | Nystatin | Nystatine | Nistatina | 口腔咽喉给药，Oral Cavity and Throat Administration | C |
| | | | | 口服给药，Oral | C |
| | | | | 局部/皮肤外用 Local/Skin( External Use) | C |
| | | | | 阴道给药 Vaginal Administration | A |
| 珠氯噻醇 | Zuclopenthixol | Zuclopenthixol | Zuclopentixol | 口服给药，Oral | C |
| | | | | 肠道外给药，Parentaral | C |
| 紫杉醇 | Paclitaxel | Paclitaxel | Paclitaxel | 肠道外给药，Parentaral | D |
| 左布比卡因 | Levobupivacaine | Levobupivacaine | Levobupivacaina | 肠道外给药，Parentaral | B |
| 左布诺洛尔 | Levobunolol | Levobunolol | Levobunolol | 眼部给药 Ophthalmic Drug Delivery | C |
| 左甲状腺素钠 | Levothyroxine Sodium | Lévothyroxine Sodique | Levotiroxina Sódica | 口服给药，Oral | A |
| 左卡巴斯汀 | Levocabastine | Lévocabastine | Levocabastina | 眼部给药 Ophthalmic Drug Delivery | C |
| 左炔诺孕酮 | Levonorgestrel | Lévonorgéstrel | Levonorgestrel | 口服给药，Oral | X |
| | | | | 皮下给药，Subcutaneous | X |
| 左西替利嗪 | Levocetirizine | Lévocétirizine | Levocetirizina | 口服给药，Oral | B |
| 左旋多巴 | Levodopa | Lévodopa | Levodopa | 口服给药，Oral | C |
| 左旋咪唑 | Levamisole | Lévamisole | Levamisol | 口服给药，Oral | C |
| 左氧氟沙星 | Levofloxacin | Lévofloxacine | Levofloxacina | 眼部给药 Ophthalmic Drug Delivery | C；禁用，尤其是妊娠早期 Prohibited to use, especially in the first trimester of pregnancy. |

续　表

| 药品名称 | Drug Name | Dénomination du médicament | Denominación del medicamento | 给药途径 Administration Route Voie dàdministration Vía de administración | 对妊娠危险性分级 Classification of pregnancy risk Classification des risques liés à la grossesse Clasificación del riesgo de embarazo |
|---|---|---|---|---|---|
|  |  |  |  | 口服给药，Oral | C；禁用，尤其是妊娠早期 Prohibited to use, especially in the first trimester of pregnancy. |
|  |  |  |  | 肠道外给药，Parentaral | C；禁用，尤其是妊娠早期 Prohibited to use, especially in the first trimester of pregnancy. |
| 左乙拉西坦 | Levetiracetam | Lévoétiracetam | Levetiracetam | 口服给药，Oral | C |
| 佐米曲普坦 | Zolmitriptan | Zolmitriptane | Zolmitriptan | 口服给药，Oral | C |
| 唑吡坦 | Zolpidem | Zolpidem | Zolpidem | 口服给药，Oral | B |
| 唑来膦酸 | Zoledronic Acid | Acide Zolédronique | Acido Zoledronico | 肠道外给药，Parentaral | D |

# 第 7 章

# 中、英、法、西班牙文对照运动员禁忌药品目录 *

A List of Contraindicated Drugs for Athlets in Chinese, English, French and Spanish

| 药品分类 | 药品名称 | Drug Name | Dénomination du médicament | Denominación del medicamento |
|---|---|---|---|---|
| 1. 蛋白同化激素制剂；<br>Hydroxystenozole;<br>Préparations hormonales d'assimilation des protéines;<br>Agents hormonales de asimilación de proteínas. | 克仑特罗 | Clenbuterol | Clenbutérol | Clenbuterol |
| | 达那唑 | Danazol | Danazole | Danazol |
| | 乙雌烯醇 | Ethylestrenol | Ethylestrénol | Etilestrenol |
| | 氟甲睾酮 | Fluoxymesterone | Fluoxymestérone | Fluoximesterona |
| | 孕三烯酮 | Gestrinone | Géstrinone | Gestrinona |
| | 美雄诺龙 | Mestanolone | Méstanolone | Mestanolona |
| | 美睾酮 | Mesterolone | Mestérolone | Mesterolona |
| | 美雄酮 | Methandienone | Méthandienone | metandienona |
| | 美替诺龙 | Metenolone | Métenolone | Metenolona |
| | 美雄醇 | Methandriol | Méthandriol | Metandriol |
| | 甲诺睾酮 | Methylnortestosterone | Methylnortéstostérone | Metilnortestosterona |
| | 甲睾酮 | Methyltestosterone | Methyltéstostérone | Metiltestosterona |
| | 羟甲睾酮 | Oxymesterone | Oxyméstérone | Oximesterona |
| | 羟甲烯龙 | Oxymetholone | Oxymétholone | Oximetolona |
| | 普拉睾酮 | Prasterone | Prastérone | Prasterona |
| | 司坦唑醇 | Stanozolol | Stanozolole | Stanozolol |
| | 睾酮 | Testosterone | Testostérone | Testosterona |
| | 替勃龙 | Tibolone | Tibolone | Tibolona |
| 2. 肽类激素制剂；<br>Peptide hormone preparation;<br>Préparations hormonales à base de peptides;<br>Preparados hormonales de los péptidos. | 艾瑞莫瑞林 | Alexamorelin | Alexamoreline | Alexamorelina |
| | 布舍瑞林 | Buserelin | Busereline | Buserelina |
| | 促皮质素类 | Corticotrophins | Corticotrophines | Clase de Corticotropina |
| | 可的瑞林 | Corticorelin | Corticoreline | Corticorelina |
| | 达贝泊汀 | Darbepoetin(Depo) | Darbepoetine(Depo) | Darbepoetina(Depo) |
| | 地洛瑞林 | Deslorelin | Desloreline | Deslorelina |
| | 促红素 (EPO) 类 | Erythropoietins(EPO) | Erythropoietines(EPO) | Clase de Eritropoietina (EPO) |
| | 促红素受体激动剂类 | Erythropoietin-Receptor Agonists | Classe des Agonistes du Récepteur d'Erythropoietin | Clase de Agonistas del Receptor de Eritropoyetina |

**续　表**

| 药品分类 | 药品名称 | Drug Name | Dénomination du médicament | Denominación del medicamento |
|---|---|---|---|---|
| | 成纤维细胞生长因子类 | Fibroblast Growth Factors(Fgfs) | Sous-Catégorie des Facteurs de Croissance des Fibroblastes | Categoría del Factor de Crecimiento de los Fibroblastos |
| | GATA 抑制剂类 | GATA Inhibitors | Inhibiteurs de GATA | Clase de Inhibidores de GATA |
| | 生长激素释放肽类 (GHRPs) | GH-Releasing Peptides(Ghrps) | Les Peptides Libérateurs d'Hormones de Croissance | Los Peptidos Liberadores de la Hormona del Crecimiento |
| | 戈那瑞林 | Gonadorelin | Gonadoreline | Gonadorelina |
| | 戈舍瑞林 | Goserelin | Gosereline | Goserelina |
| | 生长因子类 | Growth Factors | Facteurs de Croissance | Factores de Crecimiento |
| | 生长因子调节剂类 | Modulators Growth | Modulateurs du facteur de croissance | Moduladores del Factor de Crecimiento |
| | 生长激素 (GH) | Growth Hormone(GH) | Hormones de Croissance | Hormona del crecimiento |
| | 生长激素释放因子类 | Growth Hormone Releasing Factors | Facteurs de Libération de Hormones de Croissance | Factor Liberador de la Hormona del Crecimiento |
| | 生长激素释放激素 (GHRH) 及其类似物 | Growth Hormone Releasing Hormone (GH-RH) and Its Analogues | Hormones Libérantes d'Hormones de Croissance et Leurs Analogues | Hormonas Liberadoras de la Hormona del Crecimiento y Sus Análogos |
| | 肝细胞生长因子 (HGF) | Hepatocyte Growth Factor(HGF) | Facteur de Croissance Hépatique | Factor de recimiento de células del Hígado |
| | 胰岛素类 | Insulins | Insuline | Insulina |
| | 亮丙瑞林 | Leuprorelin | Leuproreline | Leuprorelina |
| | 罗特西普 | Luspatercept | Luspatercept | Luspatercept |
| | 甲氧基聚乙二烯乙二醇红细胞生成素 β（培促红素 β） | Methoxy Polyethylene Glycol-Erythropoietin Beta(Micera) | Méthoxy Polyéthylène Glycol Erythropoietin β | Metoxi Polietileno Glicol Eritropoyetina β |
| | 那法瑞林 | Nafarelin | Nafareline | Nafarelina |
| | 肽类激素和激素调节剂类 | Peptide Hormones and Hormone Modulators | Hormones de Peptides et des Modulateurs d'Hormones | Hormonas Péptidas y Moduladores de Hormonas de la Clase |
| | 血小板衍生生长因子 (PDGF) | Platelet-Derived Growth Factor(PDGF) | Facteurs de Croissance Dérivés des Plaquettes | Factores de Crecimiento Derivados de las Plaquetas |
| | 舍莫瑞林 | Sermorelin | Sermoreline | Sermorelina |
| | 替莫瑞林 | Tesamorelin | Tesamoreline | Tesamorelina |
| | 曲普瑞林 | Triptorelin | Triptoreline | Triptorelina |
| | 血管内皮生长因子 (VEGF) | Vascular-Endothelial Growth Factor(VEGF) | Facteur de Croissance Endotheliale Vasculaire | Factor de Crecimiento Endotelial Vascular |

**续 表**

| 药品分类 | 药品名称 | Drug Name | Dénomination du médicament | Denominación del medicamento |
|---|---|---|---|---|
| 3. 麻醉药品；<br>Narcotic drugs;<br>Narcóticos. | 大麻制品 | Cannabis | Cannabis | Cannabis |
| | 可卡因 | Cocaine | Cocaïne | Cocaína |
| | 芬太尼及其衍生物 | Fentanyl and Its Derivatives | Fentanyl et ses Dérivés | Fentanilo y sus Derivados |
| | 氢吗啡酮 | Hydromorphone | Hydromorphone | Hidromorfona |
| | 大麻 | Marijuana | Marijuana | Marihuana |
| | 美沙酮 | Methadone | Methadone | Metadona |
| | 吗啡 | Morphine | Morphine | Morfina |
| | 尼可吗啡 | Nicomorphine | Nicomorphine | Nicomorfina |
| | 羟考酮 | Oxycodone | Oxycodone | Oxicodona |
| | 羟吗啡酮 | Oxymorphone | Oxymorphone | Oximorfona |
| | 哌替啶 | Pethidine | Pethidine | Petidina |
| 4. 刺激剂（含精神药品）；<br>Stimulants (including psychotropic drugs);<br>Agents irritants (y compris les substances psychotropes);<br>Irritantes (incluidas las sustancias psicotrópicas) | 安非拉酮 | Amfepramone | Amfepramone | Amfepramona |
| | 苯丙胺 | Amfetamine | Amfetamine | Amfetamina |
| | 安非他尼 | Amfetaminil | Amfetaminil | Amfetaminil |
| | 阿米苯唑 | Amiphenazole | Amiphenazole | Amifenazol |
| | 丁丙诺啡 | Buprenorphine | Buprenorphine | Buprenorfina |
| | 去甲伪麻黄碱 | Cathine | Cathine | Catina |
| | 卡西酮 | Cathinone | Cathinone | Catinona |
| | 肾上腺素（肾上腺素与局麻药合用或局部使用如鼻、眼等不禁用） | Epinephrine (Adrenaline) | Adrénaline | Adrenalina |
| | 芬布酯 | Fenbutrazate | Fenbutrazate | Fenbutrazato |
| | 芬氟拉明 | Fenfluramine | Fenfluramine | Fenfluramina |
| | 左甲苯丙胺 | Levmetamfetamine | Levmetamfetamine | Levmetamfetamina |
| | 美索卡 | Mesocarb | Mesocarb | Mesocarb |
| | 甲基苯丙胺（右旋） | Metamfetamine(D-) | Metamfetamine(D-) | Metamfetamina(D-) |
| | 哌甲酯 | Methylphenidate | Methylphenidate | Metilfenidato |
| | 莫达非尼 | Modafinil | Modafinil | Modafinil |
| | 尼可刹米 | Nikethamide | Nikethamide | Niketamida |
| | 匹莫林 | Pemoline | Pemoline | Pemolina |
| | 喷他佐辛 | Pentazocine | Pentazocine | Pentazocina |
| | 戊四氮 | Pentetrazol | Pentetrazole | Pentetrazol |
| | 司来吉兰 | Selegiline | Selegiline | Selegilina |
| | 西布曲明 | Sibutramine | Sibutramine | Sibutramina |

**续　表**

| 药品分类 | 药品名称 | Drug Name | Dénomination du médicament | Denominación del medicamento |
|---|---|---|---|---|
| 5. 易制备毒品的药物；<br>A drugs that readily produces narcotic drugs;<br>Médicaments pour lesquels les drogues sont faciles à préparer;<br>Medicamentos que facilitan la preparación de drogas. | 麻黄碱 | Ephedrine | Ephedrine | Efedrina |
| | 甲基麻黄碱 | Methylephedrine | Methylephedrine | Metilefedrina |
| | 伪麻黄碱 | Pseudoephedrine | Pseudoephedrine | Pseudoefedrina |
| 6. 医用毒性药品；<br>Toxic medical drug;<br>Médicaments toxiques à usage médical;<br>Medicamentos tóxicos para uso médico. | 士的宁 | Strychnine | Strychnine | Strychnina |
| 7. 其他药品；<br>Other drugs;<br>Autres produits pharmaceutiques;<br>Otros productos farmacéuticos. | 醋丁洛尔 | Acebutolol | Acebutolol | Acebutolol |
| | 乙酰唑胺 | Acetazolamide | Acetazolamide | Acetazolamida |
| | 阿普洛尔 | Alprenolol | Alprenolol | Alprenolol |
| | 阿米洛利 | Amiloride | Amiloride | Amilorida |
| | 氨鲁米特 | Aminoglutethimide | Aminoglutethimide | Aminoglutetimida |
| | 阿那瑞林 | Anamorelin | Anamoreline | Anamorelina |
| | 阿替洛尔 | Atenolol | Atenolol | Atenolol |
| | 倍他米松 | Betamethasone | Betamethasone | Betametasona |
| | 倍他洛尔 | Betaxolol | Betaxolol | Betaxolol |
| | 比索洛尔 | Bisoprolol | Bisoprolol | Bisoprolol |
| | 布地奈德 | Budesonide | Budesonide | Budesonida |
| | 布美他尼 | Bumetanide | Bumetanide | Bumetanida |
| | 坎利酮 | Canrenone | Canrenone | Canrenona |
| | 卡替洛尔 | Carteolol | Carteolol | Carteolol |
| | 卡维地洛 | Carvedilol | Carvedilol | Carvedilol |
| | 塞利洛尔 | Celiprolol | Celiprolol | Celiprolol |
| | 氯噻嗪 | Chlorothiazide | Chlorothiazide | Clorotiazida |
| | 氯噻酮 | Chlortalidone | Chlortalidone | Clortalidona |
| | 氯米芬 | Clomifene | Clomifene | Clomifena |
| | 可的松 | Cortisone | Cortisone | Cortisona |
| | 地夫可特 | Deflazacort | Deflazacort | Deflazacort |
| | 去氨加压素 | Desmopressin | Desmopressine | Desmopresina |
| | 地塞米松 | Dexamethasone | Dexamethasone | Dexametasona |

**续 表**

| 药品分类 | 药品名称 | Drug Name | Dénomination du médicament | Denominación del medicamento |
|---|---|---|---|---|
| | 艾司洛尔 | Esmolol | Esmolol | Esmolol |
| | 依他尼酸 | Etacrynic Acid | Acide Ethanique | Ácido Etanínico |
| | 依西美坦 | Exemestane | Exemestane | Exemestana |
| | 非诺特罗 | Fenoterol | Fenoterol | Fenoterol |
| | 氟替卡松 | Fluticasone | Fluticasone | Fluticasona |
| | 福莫特罗（吸入，24 小时内最大摄入剂量不超过 54ug） | Formoterol (inhaled, maximum human dose within 24 hours not exceeding 54ug) | Formoterol (par inhalation, la dose maximale absorbée par l'homme ne dépasse pas 54ug sur une période de 24 heures) | Formoterol (por inhalación, la dosis máxima en el ser humano no excede de 54ug en 24 horas) |
| | 呋塞米 | Furosemide | Furosemide | Furosemida |
| | 去甲乌药碱 | Higenamine | Higenamine | Higenamina |
| | 氟维司群 | Fulvestrant | Fulvestrant | Fulvestrant |
| | 氢氯噻嗪 | Hydrochlorothiazide | Hydrochlorothiazide | Hidroclorotiazida |
| | 氢化可的松 | Hydrocortisone | Hydrocortisone | Hidrocortisona |
| | 茚达特罗 | Indacaterol | Indacaterol | Indacaterol |
| | 吲达帕胺 | Indapamide | Indapamide | Indapamida |
| | 拉贝洛尔 | Labetalol | Labetalol | Labetalol |
| | 兰度戈珠单抗 | Landogrozumab | Landogrozumab | Landogrozumab |
| | 来曲唑 | Letrozole | Letrozole | Letrozol |
| | 左布诺洛尔 | Levobunolol | Levobunolol | Levobunolol |
| | 甲泼尼龙 | Methylprednisolone | Methylprednisolone | Metilprednisolona |
| | 美替洛尔 | Metipranolol | Metipranolol | Metipranolol |
| | 美托拉宗 | Metolazone | Metolazone | Metolazona |
| | 美托洛尔 | Metoprolol | Metoprolol | Metoprolol |
| | 肌抑素抑制剂类 | Myostatin Inhibitors | Inhibiteurs de la Myostatine | Inhibidores de la Myostatina |
| | 肌抑素结合蛋白类 | Myostatin-Binding Proteins | Protéines liées à la Myostatine | Proteínas unidas a la Myostatina |
| | 肌抑素中和抗体类 | Myostatin- Neutralizing Antibodies | Anticorps Neutralisants de la Myostatine | Anticuerpos Neutralizantes de la Myostatina |
| | 纳多洛尔 | Nadolol | Nadolol | Nadolol |
| | 奥达特罗 | Olodaterol | Olodaterol | Olodaterol |
| | 吲哚洛尔 | Pindolol | Pindolol | Pindolol |
| | 泼尼松龙 | Prednisolone | Prednisolone | Prednisolona |
| | 泼尼松 | Prednisone | Prednisone | Prednisona |

续　表

| 药品分类 | 药品名称 | Drug Name | Dénomination du médicament | Denominación del medicamento |
|---|---|---|---|---|
| | 丙磺舒 | Probenecid | Probenecide | Probenecida |
| | 丙卡特罗 | Procaterol | Procaterol | Procaterol |
| | 普萘洛尔 | Propranolol | Propranolol | Propranolol |
| | 雷洛昔芬 | Raloxifene | Raloxifene | Raloxifena |
| | 瑞普特罗 | Reproterol | Epirubicina | Reproterol |
| | 罗沙司他 ( 缺氧诱导因子——脯氨酸羟化酶抑制剂 ) | Roxadustat(FG-4592) (Hypoxia inducing factor--proline hydroxylase inhibitors) | Roxadustat (Facteurs induisant l'hypoxia--Inhibiteur de la proline hydroxylase) | Roxadustat Factores de inducción de la hipoxia--Inhibidor de la prolina hidroxilasa) |
| | 沙丁胺醇 ( 吸入，24 小时内最多不超过 1600μg，任意 12 小时不超过 800μg) | Salbutamol (Inhale, no more than 1600μg for 24 hours, no more than 800μg in any 12 hours) | Salbutamol (Par inhalation, jusqu'à 1600μg sur une période de 24 heures, Pas plus de 800μg par période de 12 heures) | Salbutamol (Por inhalación, hasta UN máximo de 1600μg en UN período de 24 horas,no más de 800μg en cualquier período de 12 horas) |
| | 沙美特罗 ( 吸入，24 小时内最多不超过 200μg) | Salmeterol (Inhale, no more than 200μg for 24 hours) | Salmeterol (Par inhalation, jusqu'à 200μg sur 24 heures) | Salmeterol (Por inhalación, no más de 200μg en 24 horas) |
| | 索他洛尔 | Sotalol | Sotalol | Sotalol |
| | 螺内酯 | Spironolactone | Spironolactone | Spironolactona |
| | 他莫瑞林 | Tabimorelin | Tabimoreline | Tabimorelina |
| | 他莫昔芬 | Tamoxifen | Tamoxifene | Tamoxifena |
| | 特布他林 | Terbutaline | Terbutaline | Terbutalina |
| | 噻吗洛尔 | Timolol | Timolol | Timolol |
| | 托伐普坦 | Tolvaptan | Tolvaptan | Tolvaptan |
| | 托瑞米芬 | Toremifene | Toremifene | Toremifena |
| | 曲安西龙 | Triamcinolone | Triamcinolone | Triamcinolona |
| | 氨苯蝶啶 | Triamterene | Triamterene | Triamterena |
| | 曲美他嗪 | Trimetazidine | Trimetazidine | Trimetazidina |
| | 妥洛特罗 | Tulobuterol | Tulobuterol | Tulobuterol |
| | 维兰特罗 | Vilanterol | Vilanterol | Vilanterol |

* 1. 本表中药品名称源自中国国家体育总局等部门联合发布的《2019 年兴奋剂目录》。

　　The drug names in this table are from 《The 2019 analeptic list》 jointly issued by The General Administration of Sport and other Departments of China.

2. 本表中药品仅选取了该目录中部分临床常用药品。

　　Only some drugs commonly used in clinical practice were selected from the Catalogue.

3. 用于运动员治疗及有特殊说明的药品，请仔细查阅相关文件。

　　For some drugs used to treat athlete and had special instructions, please consult the relevant documents carefully.

# 第8章
# 常用中成药临床使用说明（中文）

Medication Instructions of Clinical Commonly Used Chinese Patent Medicine（Chinese）

（按拼音排序）

A

| 编号 | 药品名称 | 用法用量 | 功能主治 | 制剂及规格 |
|---|---|---|---|---|
| 1 | 安宫牛黄丸 | 口服。一次1丸.一日1次；小儿三岁以内一次1/4丸，四岁至六岁一次1/2丸，一日1次.或遵医嘱。 | 清热解毒，镇惊开窍。用于热病，邪入心包，高热惊厥，神昏谵语；中风昏迷及脑炎、脑膜炎、中毒性脑病、脑出血、败血症见上述证候者。 | 丸剂 3g/丸 |
| 2 | 安脑丸 | 口服。一次1～2丸，一日2次，或遵医嘱，小儿酌减。 | 清热解毒，醒脑安神，豁痰开窍，镇惊息风。用于高热神昏，烦躁谵语，抽搐惊厥，中风窍闭，头痛眩晕。亦用于高血压及一切急性炎症伴有的高热不退，神志昏迷等。 | 丸剂 3g/丸 |
| 3 | 安神补脑液 | 口服，一次1支，一日2次。 | 生精补髓，益气养血，强脑安神。用于肾精不足、气血两亏所致的头晕、乏力、健忘、失眠；神经衰弱症见上述证候者。 | 口服溶液 10ml |
| 4 | 安坤颗粒 | 开水冲服。一次10g，一日2次。 | 滋阴清热，健脾养血。用于放环后引起的出血，月经提前、量多或月经紊乱，腰骶酸痛，下腹坠痛，心烦易怒，手足心热。 | 颗粒 10g |

B

| 编号 | 药品名称 | 用法用量 | 功能主治 | 制剂及规格 |
|---|---|---|---|---|
| 5 | 柏子养心丸 | 口服。一次60粒（6g），一日2次。 | 补气，养血，安神。用于心气虚寒，心悸易惊，失眠多梦，健忘。 | 丸剂 60g |
| 6 | 补中益气丸 | 口服，一次6g，一日2～3次。 | 补中益气，升阳举陷。用于脾胃虚弱、中气下陷所致的泻泄，症见体倦乏力、食少腹胀、便溏久泻、肛门下坠。 | 丸剂 6g |
| 7 | 百乐眠胶囊 | 口服，一次4粒，一日2次，14天为一个疗程。 | 滋阴清热，养心安神。用于阴虚火旺型失眠症，症见入睡困难、多梦易醒、醒后不眠、头晕乏力、烦躁易怒、心悸不安等。 | 胶囊剂 0.27g |
| 8 | 板蓝根颗粒* | 口服，一次1～2袋，一日3～4次。 | 清热解毒，凉血利咽。用于肺胃热盛所致的咽喉肿痛、口咽干燥；急性扁桃体炎见上述证候者。 | 颗粒剂 5g（有糖） 3g（无糖） |
| 9 | 保济丸* | 口服，一次1.85～3.7g，一日3次。 | 解表，祛湿，和中。用于暑湿感冒，症见发热头痛，腹痛腹泻，恶心呕吐，肠胃不适；亦可用于晕车晕船。 | 丸剂 3.7g |
| 10 | 鼻渊通窍颗粒 | 开水冲服，一次15g（1袋），一日3次。 | 疏风清热，宣肺通窍。用于急鼻渊（急性鼻窦炎）属外邪犯肺证，证见：前额或颧骨部压痛，鼻塞时作，流涕黏白或黏黄，或头痛，或发热，苔薄黄或白，脉浮。 | 颗粒 15g |

**续　表**

| 编号 | 药品名称 | 用法用量 | 功能主治 | 制剂及规格 |
|---|---|---|---|---|
| 11 | 鼻炎康片 * | 口服。一次 4 片，一日 3 次。 | 清热解毒，宣肺通窍，消肿止痛。用于风邪蕴肺所致的急、慢性鼻炎，过敏性鼻炎。 | 片剂 每 片 重 0.37g（含马来酸氯苯那敏 1mg） |
| 12 | 冰黄肤乐软膏 | 外用，涂搽患处，每日 3 次。 | 清热燥湿，活血祛风，止痒消炎。用于湿热蕴结或血热风燥引起的皮肤瘙痒；神经性皮炎、湿疹、足癣及银屑病等瘙痒性皮肤病见上述证候者。 | 软膏 20g |
| 13 | 八正片 | 口服。一次 4 片，一日 3 次。 | 清热，利尿，通淋。用于湿热下注，小便短赤，淋沥涩痛，口燥咽干。 | 片剂 0.39g |

C

| 编号 | 药品名称 | 用法用量 | 功能主治 | 制剂及规格 |
|---|---|---|---|---|
| 14 | 柴桂解表颗粒 | 开水冲服。每次 1～2 袋，一日 2 次；高热者每次 2 袋，一日 4 次。 | 清热解毒，表里双解。用于各种感冒。 | 颗粒剂 10g（有糖）5g（无糖） |
| 15 | 柴银口服液 | 口服，一次 1 瓶，一日 3 次，连服 3 日。 | 清热解毒，利咽止咳。用于上呼吸道感染外感风热症，症见：发烧恶风，头痛，咽痛，汗出，鼻塞流涕，咳嗽，舌边尖红，苔薄黄等症。 | 口服液 20ml |
| 16 | 苁蓉益肾颗粒 | 口服。一次 1 袋，一日 2 次。 | 补肾填精。用于肾气不足，腰膝痠软，记忆减退，头晕耳鸣，四肢无力。 | 颗粒 2g |
| 17 | 肠泰合剂 | 口服，一次 10～20ml，一日 3 次。 | 益气健脾，消食和胃。用于脾胃气虚所致的神疲懒言，体倦无力，食少腹胀，大便稀溏。 | 合剂 10ml |
| 18 | 创可贴 | 清洁创面，使药带贴于创面，松紧适当即可。 | 止血，镇痛，消炎，愈创。用于小面积开放性创伤。 | 贴剂 1cm×8cm |

D

| 编号 | 药品名称 | 用法用量 | 功能主治 | 制剂及规格 |
|---|---|---|---|---|
| 19 | 防风通圣丸 * | 口服，一次 1 袋，一日 2 次。 | 解表通里，清热解毒。用于外寒内热，表里俱实，恶寒壮热，头痛咽干，小便短赤，大便秘结，风疹湿疮。 | 丸剂 6g |
| 20 | 冬凌草片 | 口服，一次 2～5 片，一日 3 次。 | 清热解毒，消肿散结，利咽止痛。用于热毒壅盛所致咽喉肿痛、声音嘶哑；扁桃体炎、咽炎、口腔炎见上述证候者及癌症的辅助治疗。 | 片剂 255mg |
| 21 | 大活络丸 | 口服，1 丸／次，1～2 次／日。 | 祛风止痛，除湿豁痰，舒筋活络。用于中风痰厥引起的瘫痪，足萎痹痛，筋脉拘急，腰腿疼痛及跌打损伤，行走不便，胸痹等症。 | 丸剂 3.6g |
| 22 | 大黄䗪虫胶囊 | 口服，一次 4 粒，一日 2 次；或遵医嘱。 | 活血化瘀，通经消癥。用于瘀血内停，腹部肿块，肌肤甲错，目眶黯黑，潮热羸瘦，经闭不行。 | 胶囊剂 0.4g |
| 23 | 地榆升白片 | 口服，一次 2～4 粒，一日 3 次。 | 升高白细胞。用于白细胞减少症。 | 片剂 0.1g |
| 24 | 丹七片 | 口服，一次 3～5 片，一日 3 次。 | 活血化瘀，通脉止痛。用于瘀血闭阻所致的胸痹心痛，眩晕头痛，经期腹痛。 | 片剂 0.3g |
| 25 | 代温灸膏 | 外用。根据病证，按穴位贴一张。 | 温通经脉，散寒镇痛。用于风寒阻络所致的痹病，症见腰背、四肢关节冷痛；寒伤脾胃所致的脘腹冷痛、虚寒泄泻；慢性风湿性关节炎、慢性胃肠炎见上述证候者。 | 贴膏 5cm×7cm |

E

| 编号 | 药品名称 | 用法用量 | 功能主治 | 制剂及规格 |
|---|---|---|---|---|
| 26 | 二妙丸 | 口服。一次6～9g(约1／2瓶盖)，一日2次。 | 燥湿清热。用于湿热下注，足膝红肿热痛，下肢丹毒，白带，阴囊湿痒。 | 丸剂 120g |

F

| 编号 | 药品名称 | 用法用量 | 功能主治 | 制剂及规格 |
|---|---|---|---|---|
| 27 | 枫蓼肠胃康分散片 | 口服。一次2粒，一日3次。浅表性胃炎15天为一个疗程。 | 理气健胃，除湿化滞。用于中运不健、气滞湿困而致的急性胃肠炎及其所引起的腹胀、腹痛和腹泻等消化不良症。 | 分散片 0.6g |
| 28 | 复方丹参滴丸* | 口服或舌下含服，一次10丸，一日3次，4周为一个疗程；或遵医嘱。 | 活血化瘀，理气止痛。用于气滞血瘀所致的胸痹，症见胸闷、心前区刺痛；冠心病心绞痛见上述证候者。 | 滴丸 25mg |
| 29 | 复方益肝灵片 | 口服。一次4片，一日3次，饭后服用。 | 益肝滋肾，解毒祛湿。用于肝肾阴虚，湿毒未清引起胁痛，纳差，腹胀，腰酸乏力，尿黄等症；或慢性肝炎转氨酶增高者。 | 片剂，每片含水飞蓟素以水飞蓟宾计为21mg |
| 30 | 复方红豆杉胶囊 | 口服。一次2粒，一日3次，21日为一疗程。 | 祛邪散结。用于气虚痰瘀所致的中晚期肺癌化疗的辅助治疗。 | 胶囊 300mg |
| 31 | 复方草珊瑚含片 | 含服。一次1片（大片），每隔2小时1次，一日6次。 | 疏风清热，消肿止痛，清利咽喉。用于外感风热所致的喉痹，症见咽喉肿痛、声哑失音；急性咽喉炎见上述证候者。 | 片剂 1g |
| 32 | 复方皂矾丸 | 口服。一次7～9丸，一日3次，饭后即服。 | 温肾健髓，益气养阴，生血止血。用于再生障碍性贫血，白细胞减少症，血小板减少症，骨髓增生异常综合征及放疗和化疗引起的骨髓损伤、白细胞减少属肾阳不足、气血两虚证者。 | 丸剂 200mg |
| 33 | 复方金钱草颗粒 | 一次1～2袋、一日3次。 | 清热利湿，通淋排石。用于湿热下注所致的热淋、石淋，症见尿频、尿急、尿痛、腰痛；泌尿系结石、尿路感染见上述证候者。 | 颗粒剂（无糖）3g |
| 34 | 复方鳖甲软肝片 | 口服。一次4片，一日3次，6个月为一疗程，或遵医嘱。 | 软坚散结，化瘀解毒，益气养血。用于慢性乙型肝炎肝纤维化，以及早期肝硬化属淤血阻络、气血亏虚兼热毒未尽证。症见：胁肋隐痛或肋下痞块，面色晦黯，脘腹胀满，纳差便溏，神疲乏力，口干口苦，赤缕红丝等。 | 片剂 500mg |
| 35 | 复方夏天无片 | 口服。一次2片，一日3次，小儿酌减。 | 祛风逐湿，舒筋活络，行血止痛。用于风湿淤血阻滞，经络不通引起的关节肿痛、肢体麻木、屈伸不利、步履艰难；风湿性关节炎、坐骨神经痛、脑血栓形成后遗症及小儿麻痹后遗症见上述证候者。 | 片剂 320mg |
| 36 | 复方苁蓉益智胶囊 | 口服。一次4粒，一日3次。 | 益智养肝，活血化浊，健脑增智。用于轻、中度血管性痴呆肝肾亏虚兼痰瘀阻络证。症见智力减退、思维迟钝、神情呆滞、健忘，或喜怒不定、腰膝酸软、头晕耳鸣、失眠多梦等。 | 胶囊 300mg |

**续　表**

| 编号 | 药品名称 | 用法用量 | 功能主治 | 制剂及规格 |
|---|---|---|---|---|
| 37 | 复方青黛胶囊 | 胶囊：口服。一次 4 粒，一日 3 次。丸：口服。一次 10 丸，一日 3 次。 | 清热解毒，化瘀消斑，祛风止痒。用于血热挟瘀、热毒炽盛证；进行期银屑病、玫瑰糠疹、药疹见上述证候者。 | 胶囊、500mg丸剂200mg |
| 38 | 复方斑蝥胶囊 | 口服，一次 3 粒，一日 2 次。 | 破血消瘀，攻毒蚀疮。用于原发性肝癌，肺癌，直肠癌，恶性淋巴瘤，妇科恶性肿瘤等。 | 胶囊250mg |
| 39 | 复方枣仁胶囊 | 口服，一次 1 粒，睡前服。 | 养心安神。用于心神不安，失眠，多梦，惊悸。 | 胶囊400mg |
| 40 | 复方地龙胶囊 | 口服。一次 2 粒，一日 3 次，饭后服用。 | 化瘀通络，益气活血。用于缺血性中风中经络恢复期气虚血瘀证，症见半身不遂，口舌歪斜，言语塞涩或不语，偏身麻木，乏力，心悸气短，流涎，自汗等。 | 胶囊280mg |
| 41 | 复方鲜竹沥液 | 口服。一次 20ml，一日 2～3 次。 | 清热化痰，止咳。用于痰热咳嗽，痰黄黏稠。 | 口服液20ml |
| 42 | 复方小活络丸 | 温黄酒或温开水送服，一次 1～2 丸，一日 2 次。 | 舒筋活络、散风止痛。用于风寒湿邪引起的风寒湿痹，肢节疼痛，麻木拘挛，半身不遂、行走艰难。 | 丸剂3g |
| 43 | 附子理中丸 * | 口服，一次 1 丸，一日 2～3 次。 | 温中健脾。用于脘腹冷痛，肢冷便溏。 | 丸剂9g |
| 44 | 复方阿胶浆 | 口服，一次 20ml，一日 3 次。 | 补气养血。用于气血两虚，头晕目眩，心悸失眠，食欲不振及白细胞减少症和贫血。 | 胶浆20ml |
| 45 | 风油精 | 外用，涂擦于患处。口服，一次 4～6 滴。 | 清凉，止痛，驱风，止痒。用于蚊虫叮咬及伤风感冒引起的头痛，头晕，晕车不适。 | 擦剂3ml |
| 46 | 肺力咳胶囊 | 合剂：口服。七岁以内一次 10ml，七岁至十四岁一次 15ml，成人一次 20ml，一日 3 次；或遵医嘱。胶囊：口服，一次 3～4 粒，一日 3 次；或遵医嘱。 | 止咳平喘，清热解毒，顺气祛痰。用于咳喘痰多，呼吸不畅，以及急、慢性支气管炎，肺气肿见上述证候者。 | 胶囊300mg |

G

| 编号 | 药品名称 | 用法用量 | 功能主治 | 制剂及规格 |
|---|---|---|---|---|
| 47 | 固本益肠片 * | 口服，一次 8 片，一日 3 次。30 日为一疗程，连服 2～3 个疗程。 | 健脾温肾，涩肠止泻。用于脾肾阳虚所致的泄泻，症见腹痛绵绵，大便清稀或有黏液及黏液血便，食少腹胀，腰酸乏力，形寒肢冷，舌淡苔白，脉虚；慢性肠炎见上述证候者。 | 片剂0.6g |
| 48 | 更年安片 * | 口服，一次 6 片，一日 2～3 次。 | 滋阴清热，除烦安神。用于肾阴虚所致的绝经前后诸证，症见烦热出汗、眩晕耳鸣、手足心热、烦躁不安；更年期综合征见上述证候者。 | 片剂0.3g |
| 49 | 根痛平片 | 口服，一次 5 片，一日 3 次；饭后服用。颗粒：开水冲服。一次 1 袋，一日 2 次。饭后服用。或遵医嘱。 | 活血、通络、止痛。用于风寒阻络所致颈椎病，症见肩颈疼痛，活动受限，上肢麻木。 | 片剂300mg颗粒（无糖型）8g |

**续表**

| 编号 | 药品名称 | 用法用量 | 功能主治 | 制剂及规格 |
|---|---|---|---|---|
| 50 | 感冒清热颗粒* | 开水冲服。一次1袋，一日2次。 | 疏风散寒，解表清热。用于风寒感冒，头痛发热，恶寒身痛，鼻流清涕，咳嗽咽干。 | 颗粒剂<br>12g（有糖）<br>6克（无糖） |
| 51 | 桂林西瓜霜含片 | 含服，一次2片，一日5次，5～7日为一个疗程。 | 清热解毒，消肿止痛。用于咽喉肿痛，口舌生疮，牙龈肿痛或出血，口疮；急、慢性咽炎，扁桃体炎，口腔溃疡见上述证候者。 | 片剂<br>0.6g |
| 52 | 桂枝茯苓胶囊 | 口服。一次3粒，一日3次。饭后服。前列腺增生疗程8周，其余适应症疗程12周，或遵医嘱。 | 活血，化瘀，消癥。用于妇人瘀血阻络所致癥块、经闭、痛经、产后恶露不尽，子宫肌瘤，慢性盆腔炎包块，痛经，子宫内膜异位症，卵巢囊肿见上述证候者；也可用于女性乳腺囊性增生病属瘀血阻络证，症见乳房疼痛、乳房肿块、胸胁胀闷；或用于前列腺增生属瘀阻膀胱证，症见小便不爽、尿细如线、或点滴而下、小腹胀痛者。 | 胶囊<br>310mg |
| 53 | 骨疏康胶囊 | 口服，一次4粒，一日2次。疗程6个月。 | 补肾益气，活血壮骨。用于肾虚兼气血不足所致的原发性骨质疏松症，症见腰背疼痛、腰膝酸软、下肢痿弱、步履艰难、神疲、目眩、舌质偏红或淡，脉平或濡细。 | 胶囊<br>320mg |
| 54 | 狗皮膏 | 外用。用生姜擦净患处皮肤，将膏药加温软化，贴于患处或穴位。 | 祛风散寒，活血止痛。用于风寒湿邪、气血瘀滞所致的痹病，症见四肢麻木、腰腿疼痛、筋脉拘挛，或跌打损伤、闪腰岔气、局部肿痛；或寒湿瘀滞所致的脘腹冷痛、行经腹痛、寒湿带下、积聚痞块。 | 贴膏<br>8/4.5cm*4 |
| 55 | 骨通贴膏 | 外用，整片撕去盖衬，贴于患处，弹力布弹力方向与关节活动方向一致，每次1贴/患处，7天为一疗程。 | 祛风散寒，活血通络，消肿止痛。用于寒湿阻络兼血瘀证之局部关节疼痛、肿胀、麻木重着、屈伸不利或活动受限。 | 贴剂<br>7cm*10cm |

H

| 编号 | 药品名称 | 用法用量 | 功能主治 | 制剂及规格 |
|---|---|---|---|---|
| 56 | 藿胆丸* | 口服。一次3～6g，一日2次。 | 芳香化浊，清热通窍。用于湿浊内蕴、胆经郁火所致的鼻塞、流清涕或浊涕、前额头痛。 | 滴丸<br>6g |
| 57 | 黄氏响声丸* | 口服。炭衣丸：一次6丸（每丸重0.133g），一日3次，饭后服用；儿童减半。 | 疏风清热，化痰散结，利咽开音。用于风热外束、痰热内盛所致的急、慢性喉瘖，症见声音嘶哑、咽喉肿痛、咽干灼热、咽中有痰，或寒热头痛、或便秘尿赤；急慢性喉炎及声带小结、声带息肉初起见上述证候者。 | 丸剂<br>0.133g |
| 58 | 黄葵胶囊 | 口服。一次5粒，一日3次；8周为一疗程。 | 清利湿热，解毒消肿。用于慢性肾炎之湿热证，症见：浮肿、腰痛、蛋白尿、血尿、舌苔黄腻等。 | 胶囊<br>500mg |
| 59 | 藿香正气 | 软胶囊：口服，一次2～4粒，一日2次。<br>口服液：口服，一次5～10ml，一日2次，用时摇匀。 | 解表化湿，理气和中。用于外感风寒、内伤湿滞或夏伤暑湿所致的感冒，症见头痛昏重、胸膈痞闷、脘腹胀痛、呕吐泄泻；胃肠型感冒见上述证候者。 | 胶囊<br>0.45g<br>口服液<br>10ml |
| 60 | 回生第一丹胶囊* | 用温黄酒或温开水送服，一次1g，一日2～3次。 | 活血散瘀，消肿止痛。用于跌打损伤，闪腰岔气，伤筋动骨，皮肤青肿，血瘀疼痛。 | 胶囊剂<br>0.2g |

**续　表**

| 编号 | 药品名称 | 用法用量 | 功能主治 | 制剂及规格 |
|---|---|---|---|---|
| 61 | 红药片 | 贴膏：外用，洗净患处，贴敷，1～2日天更换一次。<br>片：黄酒或温开水送服，一次5～6片，一日3次。<br>气雾剂：外用。喷于患处，每日4～6次。 | 贴膏：祛瘀生新，活血止痛。用于跌打损伤，筋骨瘀痛。<br>红药片：活血止痛，去瘀生新，用于跌打损伤，瘀血肿痛，风湿麻木。<br>气雾剂：活血逐瘀、消肿止痛。用于跌打损伤，局部瘀血肿胀，筋骨疼痛。 | 贴膏<br>7×10cm²<br>片剂<br>0.26g<br>气雾剂<br>每瓶装<br>60g |
| 62 | 黄芪片 | 口服。一次4片，一日2次。 | 补气固表，利尿，托毒排脓，生肌。用于气短心悸，虚脱，自汗，体虚浮肿，慢性肾炎，久泻，脱肛，子宫脱垂，痈疽难溃，疮口久不愈合。 | 片剂<br>0.41g |
| 63 | 虎力散胶囊 | 口服。一次1粒，一日1～2次，开水或温酒送服。外用。将内容物撒于伤口处。 | 驱风除湿，舒筋活络，行瘀，消肿定痛。用于风湿麻木，筋骨疼痛，跌打损伤，创伤流血。 | 胶囊<br>300mg |
| 64 | 化痔栓 | 患者取侧卧位，置入肛门2～2.5厘米深处，一次1粒，一日1～2次。 | 清热燥湿，收涩止血，用于大肠湿热所致的内外痔，混合痔疮 | 栓剂<br>1.4g |
| 65 | 华蟾素 | 胶囊：口服。一次3～4粒，一日3～4次。<br>注射液：肌内注射，一次2～4ml（2/5～4/5支），一日2次；静脉滴注，一日1次，一次10～20ml（2～4支），用5%的葡萄糖注射液500ml稀释后缓缓滴注，用药7日，休息1～2日，四周为1个疗程，或遵医嘱。 | 解毒，消肿，止痛。用于中、晚期肿瘤，慢性乙型肝炎等症。 | 胶囊<br>300mg<br>250mg<br>注射液<br>5ml |
| 66 | 活血止痛膏 | 外用，贴患处。 | 活血止痛，舒筋通络。用于筋骨疼痛，肌肉麻痹，痰核流注，关节酸痛。 | 贴膏<br>6.5cm×5cm |

J

| 编号 | 药品名称 | 用法用量 | 功能主治 | 制剂及规格 |
|---|---|---|---|---|
| 67 | 京制咳嗽痰喘丸 | 口服。一次30粒，一日2次，8岁以内小儿酌减。 | 散风清热，宣肺止咳，祛痰定喘。用于外感风邪，痰热阻肺，咳嗽痰盛，气促哮喘，不能躺卧，喉中作痒，胸膈满闷，老年痰喘。 | 丸剂<br>每瓶装180粒 |
| 68 | 京万红软膏 | 用生理盐水清理创面. 涂敷本品或将本品涂于消毒纱布上，敷盖创面，消毒纱布包扎，每日换药一次。 | 活血解毒，消肿止痛，去腐生肌。用于轻度水、火烫伤，疮疡肿痛，创面溃烂。 | 软膏<br>20g |
| 69 | 加味逍遥丸* | 口服，一次6g，一日2次。 | 舒肝清热，健脾养血。用于肝郁血虚，肝脾不和，两胁胀痛，头晕目眩，倦怠食少，月经不调，脐腹胀痛。 | 水丸<br>6g |
| 70 | 健胃消食片 | 口服。一次3片，一日3次。 | 健胃消食。用于脾胃虚弱所致的食积，症见不思饮食、嗳腐酸臭、脘腹胀满、消化不良见上述证候者。 | 片剂<br>800mg |

续　表

| 编号 | 药品名称 | 用法用量 | 功能主治 | 制剂及规格 |
|---|---|---|---|---|
| 71 | 急支糖浆 | 口服，一次 20～30ml，一日 3～4 次，小儿酌减。 | 清热化痰，宣肺止咳。用于外感风热所致的咳嗽，症见发热、恶寒、胸膈满闷、咳嗽咽痛；急性支气管炎、慢性支气管炎急性发作见上述证候者。 | 糖浆剂 200ml |
| 72 | 金匮肾气丸 * | 口服，一次 4～5g，一日 2 次。 | 温补肾阳，化气行水。用于肾虚水肿，腰膝酸软，小便不利，畏寒肢冷。 | 丸剂 6g |
| 73 | 金莲花 | 颗粒：开水冲服，一次 3g，一日 2～3 次，小儿酌减。分散片：加水分散后口服或直接嚼碎服。一次 3 片，一日 24 次 | 清热解毒。用于上呼吸道感染，咽炎，扁桃体炎。 | 颗粒 3g（无糖型）分散片 0.7g |
| 74 | 金莲清热颗粒 | 口服。成人一次 5g，一日 4 次，高热时每四小时服 1 次；小儿 1 岁以下每次 2.5g，一日 3 次，高热时每日 4 次；1～15 岁每次 2.5～5g，一日 4 次，高热时每 4 小时 1 次，或遵医嘱。 | 清热解毒，生津利咽，止咳祛痰。用于感冒热毒壅盛证，症见高热、口渴、咽干、咽痛、咳嗽、痰稠；流行性感冒、上呼吸道感染见有上述证候者。 | 颗粒 5g |
| 75 | 解痉镇痛酊 | 涂擦患处，一日 2 次。 | 活血通经、止痛。用于治疗软组织损伤而引起的颈、肩、腰、腿痛。对冻疮也有一定疗效。 | 酊剂 30ml |

K

| 编号 | 药品名称 | 用法用量 | 功能主治 | 制剂及规格 |
|---|---|---|---|---|
| 76 | 克咳胶囊 | 口服，一次 3 粒，一日 2 次。 | 止嗽，定喘，祛痰。用于咳嗽，喘急气短。 | 胶囊 0.3g |
| 77 | 康复新液 | 口服，一次 10ml，一日 3 次，或遵医嘱。外用，用医用纱布浸透药液后敷于患处，感染创面先清创后再用本品冲洗，并用浸透本品的纱布填塞或敷用。 | 通利血脉，养阴生肌。内服：用于瘀血阻滞，胃痛出血，胃、十二指肠溃疡；以及阴虚肺痨，肺结核的辅助治疗。外用：用于金疮、外伤、溃疡、瘘管、烧伤、烫伤、压疮之创面。 | 溶液 100ml 50ml |
| 78 | 康力欣胶囊 | 口服，一次 2～3 粒，一日 3 次；或遵医嘱。 | 扶正去邪，软坚散结。用于消化道恶性肿瘤，乳腺恶性肿瘤，肺恶性肿瘤见于气血瘀阻证者。 | 胶囊 500mg |
| 79 | 坤宝丸 | 口服。一次 50 粒，一日 2 次。 | 滋补肝肾，镇静安神，养血通络。用于妇女绝经前后，肝肾阴虚引起的月经紊乱，潮热多汗，失眠健忘，心烦易怒，头晕耳鸣，咽干口渴，四肢酸楚，关节疼痛。 | 水蜜丸 每袋装 50 粒（5g） |

L

| 编号 | 药品名称 | 用法用量 | 功能主治 | 制剂及规格 |
|---|---|---|---|---|
| 80 | 六味地黄丸 | 口服，一次 2 粒，一日 2 次。 | 滋阴补肾，用于肾阴亏虚所致的头晕耳鸣，腰膝酸软，骨蒸潮热，盗汗。 | 丸剂 360 丸 |
| 81 | 雷公藤多苷 | 口服：每日每千克体重 1～1.5mg，分 3 次饭后服。 | 祛风解毒，除湿消肿，舒筋通络，有抗炎及抑制细胞免疫和体液免疫等作用。用于风湿热瘀，毒邪阻滞所致的类风湿关节炎，肾病综合症，白塞氏三联症，麻风反应，自身免疫性肝炎等。 | 片剂 10mg |

**续　表**

| 编号 | 药品名称 | 用法用量 | 功能主治 | 制剂及规格 |
|---|---|---|---|---|
| 82 | 六君子丸 * | 口服，1 次 9g，一日 2 次。 | 补脾益气，燥湿化痰。用于脾胃虚弱，食量不多，气虚痰多，腹胀便溏。 | 水丸<br>9g |
| 83 | 连花清瘟 | 颗粒：口服，一次 1 袋，一日 3 次。<br>胶囊：口服，一次 4 粒，一日 3 次。 | 清瘟解毒，宣肺泄热。用于治疗流行性感冒属热毒袭肺证，症见：发热或高热，恶寒，肌肉酸痛，鼻塞流涕，咳嗽，头痛，咽干咽痛，舌偏红，苔黄或黄腻等。 | 颗粒<br>6g<br>胶囊<br>每粒装 0.35g |
| 84 | 龙血竭 | 散：用酒或温开水送服，一次 1.2g，一日 4 ~ 5 次；水煎服，1 次 4.8 ~ 6.0g，一日 1 次；外用适量，敷患处或用酒调敷患处。<br>片：口服。1 次 4 ~ 6 片，一日 3 次；或遵医嘱。 | 活血散瘀，定痛止血，敛疮生肌。用于跌打损伤，瘀血作痛，妇女气血凝滞，外伤出血，脓疮久不收口。 | 散剂<br>1.2g<br>片剂<br>400mg |

### M

| 编号 | 药品名称 | 用法用量 | 功能主治 | 制剂及规格 |
|---|---|---|---|---|
| 85 | 麻仁胶囊 | 口服，一次 2 ~ 4 粒，早晚各一次或睡前服用。 | 润肠通便。用于肠燥便秘。 | 胶囊剂<br>0.35g |
| 86 | 麻仁润肠丸 | 口服，一次 1 ~ 2 丸，一日 2 次。 | 润肠通便。用于肠胃积热，胸腹胀满，大便秘结。 | 丸剂<br>每丸重 6g |
| 87 | 蜜炼川贝枇杷膏 * | 口服，一次 22g，一日 3 次。 | 清热润肺，止咳平喘，理气化痰。适用于肺燥之咳嗽，痰多，胸闷，咽喉痛痒，声音沙哑。 | 膏剂<br>每瓶装 138g |
| 88 | 摩罗丹 | 口服。一次 8 丸，一日 3 次。 | 和胃降逆，健脾消胀，通络定痛。用于慢性萎缩性胃炎症见胃痛，胀满，痞闷，纳呆，嗳气等症。 | 浓缩丸<br>每 8 丸重 1.84g |
| 89 | 脉血康胶囊 | 口服。一次 2 ~ 4 粒，一日 3 次。 | 破血逐瘀，通脉止痛。用于中风，半身不遂，癥瘕痞块，血瘀经闭，跌扑损伤。 | 胶囊<br>0.25g |
| 90 | 木丹颗粒 | 饭后半小时服用，用温开水冲服。一次 1 袋，一日 3 次。4 周为 1 个疗程，可连续服用 2 个疗程。 | 益气活血，通络止痛。用于治疗糖尿病性周围神经病变属气虚络阻证，临床表现为四肢末梢及躯干部麻木、疼痛及感觉异常，或见肌肤甲错、面色晦暗、倦怠乏力、神疲懒言、自汗等。 | 颗粒<br>每袋装 7g |
| 91 | 迈之灵片 | 饭后口服。成人每日 2 次，早、晚各 1 次，每次 1 ~ 2 片。病情较重或治疗初期，每日 2 次，每次 2 片，或遵医嘱服用。20 日为一疗程。可长期服用。 | 1. 用于慢性静脉功能不全、静脉曲张、深静脉血栓形成及血栓性静脉炎后综合症引起的下肢肿胀、痉挛、瘙痒、灼热、麻木、疼痛、疲劳沉重感、皮肤色素沉着、郁血性炎、溃疡、精索静脉曲张引起的肿痛等。<br>2. 用于手术后、外伤、创伤、烧烫伤、所致的软组织肿胀、静脉性水肿。<br>3. 痔静脉曲张引起的内、外痔急性发作症状。如肛门潮湿、瘙痒、便血、疼痛等。 | 片剂<br>每片含马栗提取物 150mg |
| 92 | 明目地黄丸 | 口服。一次 1 丸，一日 2 次。 | 滋肾，养肝，明目。用于肝肾阴虚，目涩畏光，视物模糊，迎风流泪。 | 丸剂<br>9g |

N

| 编号 | 药品名称 | 用法用量 | 功能主治 | 制剂及规格 |
|------|----------|----------|----------|------------|
| 93 | 诺迪康胶囊 | 口服。一次1~2粒，一日3次。 | 益气活血，通脉止痛。用于气虚血瘀所致胸痹，症见胸闷，刺痛或隐痛，心悸气短，神疲乏力，少气懒言，头晕目眩；冠心病、心绞痛见上述证候者。 | 胶囊剂 280mg |
| 94 | 尿毒清颗粒（无糖型） | 温开水冲服。每日4次，6、12、18时各服一袋，22时服2袋，每日最大服用量8袋，也可另定服药时间，但2次服药间隔勿超过8小时。 | 通腹降浊、健脾利湿、活血化瘀。用于慢性肾功能衰竭，氮质血症期和尿毒症早期、中医辨证属脾虚湿浊症和脾虚血瘀症者。可降低肌酐、尿素氮，稳定肾功能，延缓透析时间。对改善肾性贫血，提高血钙、降低血磷也有一定的作用。 | 颗粒5g |
| 95 | 宁泌泰胶囊 | 口服，一次3~4粒，一日3次；7日为一个疗程，或遵医嘱。 | 中医：清热解毒，利湿通淋。用于湿热蕴结所致淋证，证见：小便不利，淋漓涩痛，尿血，以及下尿路感染、慢性前列腺炎见上述证候者。 | 胶囊 380mg |
| 96 | 牛黄降压丸 | 大蜜丸：口服，一次1~2丸。 | 清心化痰，平肝安神。用于心肝火旺、痰热壅盛所致的头晕目眩、头痛失眠、烦躁不安；高血压病见上述证候者。 | 丸剂 1.6g |
| 97 | 牛黄解毒丸 | 口服。一次1丸，一日2~3次。 | 清热解毒。由于火热内盛，咽喉肿痛，牙龈肿痛，口舌生疮，目赤肿痛。 | 丸剂 3g |
| 98 | 牛黄上清丸 | 口服，一次1丸，一日2次。 | 清热泻火，散风止痛。用于热毒内盛、风火上攻所致的头痛眩晕、目赤耳鸣、咽喉肿痛、口舌生疮、牙龈肿痛、大便燥结。 | 丸剂 6g |
| 99 | 牛黄清心丸 | 口服。一次1丸，一日1次。 | 清心化痰，镇惊祛风。用于风痰阻窍所致的头晕目眩、痰涎壅盛、神志混乱、言语不清及惊风抽搐、癫痫。 | 丸剂 3g |
| 100 | 牛黄清火丸 | 口服。一次2丸，一日2次。 | 清热，散风，解毒。用于肝胃肺蕴热引起的头晕目眩、口鼻生疮、风火牙疼、咽喉肿痛、疖腮红肿、耳鸣肿痛。 | 丸剂 3g |
| 101 | 脑得生丸 | 口服。一次2g，一日3次。 | 活血化瘀，通经活络。用于瘀血阻络所致的眩晕、中风，症见肢体不用；语言不利及头晕目眩；脑动脉硬化，缺血性脑中风及脑出血后遗症见上述证候者。 | 丸剂 2g |
| 102 | 脑安胶囊 | 口服，一次2粒，一日2次，疗程4周，或遵医嘱。 | 活血化瘀，益气通络。用于脑血栓形成急性期，恢复期属气虚血瘀症候者，症见急性起病，半身不遂，口舌歪斜，舌强语謇，偏身麻木，气短乏力，口角流涎，手足肿胀，舌暗或有瘀斑，苔薄白等。 | 胶囊 0.4g |
| 103 | 脑心通胶囊 | 口服，一次2~4粒，一日3次，或遵医嘱。 | 益气活血、化瘀通络。用于气虚血滞、脉络瘀阻所致中风中经络，半身不遂、肢体麻木、口眼歪斜、舌强语謇及胸痹心痛、胸闷、心悸、气短；脑梗死、冠心病心绞痛属上述症候者。 | 胶囊 400mg |

续　表

| 编号 | 药品名称 | 用法用量 | 功能主治 | 制剂及规格 |
|---|---|---|---|---|
| 104 | 牛黄清胃丸 | 口服。一次 2 丸，一日 2 次。 | 清胃泻火. 润燥通便。用于心胃火盛，头晕目眩，口舌生疮，牙龈肿痛，乳蛾咽痛，便秘尿赤。 | 丸剂<br>6g |
| 105 | 暖宫七味丸 | 口服，一次 11～15 丸，一日 1～2 次。 | 调经养血，温暖子宫，驱寒止痛。用于心、肾"赫依"病，气滞腰痛，小腹冷痛，月经不调，白带过多。 | 丸剂<br>2g |

P

| 编号 | 药品名称 | 用法用量 | 功能主治 | 制剂及规格 |
|---|---|---|---|---|
| 106 | 普济痔疮栓 | 直肠给药。一次 1 粒。一日 2 次、或遵医嘱。 | 清热解毒，凉血止血，用于热证便血。对各期内痔、便血及混合痔肿胀等有较好的疗效。 | 栓剂<br>1.3g |
| 107 | 盘龙七片 | 口服。一次 3～4 片，一日 3 次。 | 活血化瘀，祛风除湿，消肿止痛。用于风湿性关节炎，腰肌劳损，骨折及软组织损伤。 | 片剂<br>0.3g |
| 108 | 皮肤康洗液 | 皮肤湿疹：取适量药液直接涂抹于患处，有糜烂面者可稀释 5 倍量后湿敷，一日 2 次。<br>妇科病：先用清水冲洗阴道，取适量药液用温开水稀释 5～10 倍，用阴道冲洗器将药液注入阴道内保留几分钟。或坐浴，每日 2 次。或遵医嘱。 | 清热解毒，凉血除湿，杀虫止痒。主治湿热阻于皮肤所致湿疹，见有瘙痒、红斑、丘疹、水疱、渗出、糜烂等和湿热下注所致阴痒，白带过多。皮肤湿疹及各类阴道炎见有上述证候者。 | 洗剂<br>50ml |
| 109 | 普乐安片* | 口服，一次 3～4 片，一日 3 次。 | 补肾固本。用于肾气不固所致的腰膝酸软、排尿不畅、尿后余沥或失禁；慢性前列腺炎及前列腺增生症见上述证候者。 | 片剂<br>0.57g |

Q

| 编号 | 药品名称 | 用法用量 | 功能主治 | 制剂及规格 |
|---|---|---|---|---|
| 110 | 杞菊地黄丸 | 口服，一次 8 丸，一日 3 次。 | 滋肾养肝。用于肝肾阴亏，眩晕耳鸣，羞明畏光，迎风流泪，视物昏花。 | 丸剂<br>每 8 丸相当于原药材 3 克 |
| 111 | 千柏鼻炎片 | 口服，一次 3～4 片，一日 3 次。 | 清热解毒，活血祛风，宣肺通窍。用于风热犯肺，内郁化火，凝滞气血所致的鼻塞、鼻痒气热、流涕黄稠，或持续鼻塞、嗅觉迟钝；急慢性鼻窦炎，见上述证候者。 | 片剂<br>0.3g |
| 112 | 千山活血膏 | 外用，将膏药加温软化，贴于患处或相关穴位上（请参阅背面穴位图）；或遵医嘱。 | 活血化瘀、舒筋活络、消肿止痛。用于肌肤、关节肿胀、疼痛、活动不利，以及跌打损伤，腰、膝部骨性关节炎见上述症状者。 | 贴膏<br>5g |
| 113 | 全天麻胶囊 | 口服，一次 2～6 粒，一日 3 次。 | 平肝，息风。用于肝风上扰所致的眩晕、头痛、肢体麻木。 | 胶囊<br>0.5g |
| 114 | 芪苈强心胶囊 | 口服，一次 4 粒，一日 3 次。 | 益气温阳，活血通络，利水消肿。用于冠心病、高血压病所致轻、中度充血性心力衰竭证属阳气虚乏，络瘀水停者，症见心慌气短，动则加剧，夜间不能平卧，下肢浮肿，倦怠乏力，小便短少，口唇青紫，畏寒肢冷，咳吐稀稀白痰等。 | 胶囊<br>300mg |

**续　表**

| 编号 | 药品名称 | 用法用量 | 功能主治 | 制剂及规格 |
|---|---|---|---|---|
| 115 | 祛风止痛丸 | 口服。一次 2.2g，一日 2 次。 | 祛风寒，补肝肾，壮筋骨。用于风寒湿邪闭阻、肝肾亏虚所致的痹病，症见关节肿胀、腰膝疼痛、四肢麻木。 | 丸剂<br>2.2g |
| 116 | 强力定眩胶囊 | 口服。一次 4～6 粒，一日 3 次。 | 降压、降脂、定眩。用于高血压，动脉硬化，高血脂症以及上述诸病引起的头痛，头晕，目眩，耳鸣，失眠等症。 | 胶囊<br>400mg |
| 117 | 强骨胶囊 | 饭后用温开水送服。一次 1 粒.一日 3 次。3 个月为一疗程。 | 补肾，强骨、止痛。用于肾阳虚所致的骨痿。症见骨脆易折、腰背或四肢关节疼痛、畏寒肢冷或抽筋、下肢无力、夜尿频多；原发性骨质疏松症、骨量减少见上述证候者。 | 胶囊<br>250mg |
| 118 | 前列舒通胶囊 | 口服，一次 3 粒，一日 3 次。 | 清热利湿，化瘀散结。用于慢性前列腺炎、前列腺增生属湿热瘀阻证，证见：尿频、尿急、尿淋沥、会阴、下腹或腰骶部坠胀或疼痛，阴囊潮湿等。 | 胶囊<br>0.4g |
| 119 | 清热解毒口服液 | 口服，一次 10～20ml，一日 3 次。 | 清热解毒。用于热毒壅盛所致发热面赤，烦躁口渴，咽喉肿痛；流感、上呼吸道感染见上述证候者。 | 口服液<br>每支装 10ml |
| 120 | 清凉油 | 外用，需要时涂于太阳穴或患处。 | 清凉散热，醒脑提神，止痒止痛。用于伤暑引起的头痛，晕车，蚊虫叮咬。 | 软膏<br>3g |
| 121 | 青鹏软膏 | 外用。取本品适量涂于患处，一日 2 次。 | 藏医：活血化瘀，消炎止痛。用于痛风、风湿、类风湿关节炎，热性"冈巴""黄水"病变引起的关节肿痛、扭挫伤肿痛、皮肤瘙痒、湿疹。中医：活血化瘀，消肿止痛。用于风湿性关节炎、类风湿关节炎、骨关节炎、痛风、急慢性扭挫伤、肩周炎引起的关节、肌肉肿胀疼痛及皮肤瘙痒、湿疹。 | 软膏<br>20g |
| 122 | 清肝降压胶囊 | 口服。一次 3 粒，一日 3 次，或遵医嘱。 | 清热平肝，补益肝肾。用于高血压病，肝火亢盛、肝肾阴虚证，症见眩晕、头痛、面红目赤、急躁易怒、口干口苦、腰膝酸软、心悸不寐、耳鸣健忘、便秘溲黄。 | 胶囊<br>500mg |
| 123 | 清脑复神液 | 口服，轻症一次 10ml，重症一次 20ml，一日 2 次。 | 清心安神，化痰醒脑，活血通络。用于神经衰弱，失眠，顽固性头痛，脑震荡后遗症所致头痛、眩晕、健忘、失眠等症。 | 口服溶液<br>10ml |

## R

| 编号 | 药品名称 | 用法用量 | 功能主治 | 制剂及规格 |
|---|---|---|---|---|
| 124 | 乳癖消 | 口服，一次 3 片，一日 3 次。 | 软坚散结，活血消痛，清热解毒。用于痰热互结所致的乳癖、乳痈，症见乳房结节、数目不等、大小形态不一、质地柔软，或产后乳房结块、红热疼痛；乳腺增生、乳腺炎早期见上述证候者。 | 片剂<br>0.67g |
| 125 | 乳癖散结胶囊 | 口服。一次 4 粒，一日 3 次，45 日为 1 个疗程，或遵医嘱。 | 行气活血，软坚散结。用于气滞血瘀所致的乳腺增生病，症见乳房疼痛、乳房肿块、烦躁易怒、胸胁胀满等。 | 胶囊<br>530mg |

**续　表**

| 编号 | 药品名称 | 用法用量 | 功能主治 | 制剂及规格 |
|---|---|---|---|---|
| 126 | 人参归脾丸 | 口服，一次 1 丸，一日 2 次。 | 益气补血，健脾养心。用于气血不足，心悸，失眠，食少乏力，面色萎黄，月经量少，色淡。 | 丸剂<br>9g |
| 127 | 仁丹 | 含化或用温开水送服。一次 10 ~ 20 粒。 | 清暑开窍。用于伤暑引起的恶心胸闷，头昏，晕车晕船。 | 丸剂<br>0.3g |
| 128 | 人参健脾丸 | 口服。一次 2 丸，一日 2 次。 | 健脾益气，和胃止泻。用于脾胃虚弱所致的饮食不化、脘闷嘈杂、恶心呕吐、腹痛便溏、不思饮食、体弱倦怠。 | 丸剂<br>6g |
| 129 | 如意珍宝丸 | 口服。一次 8 ~ 10 丸，一日 2 次。 | 清热，醒脑开窍，舒筋通络，干黄水。用于瘟热、陈旧热症、白脉病、四肢麻木、瘫痪、口眼歪斜、神志不清、痹症、痛风、肢体强直、关节不利。对白脉病有良效。 | 丸剂<br>0.25g |
| 130 | 仁青芒觉 | 研碎开水送服。一次 1 丸，一日 1 次。 | 清热解毒，益肝养胃，明目醒神，愈疮，滋补强身。用于自然毒、食物毒、配制毒等各种中毒症；"培根木布"，消化道溃疡，急慢性胃肠炎，萎缩性胃炎，腹水，麻风病等。 | 丸剂<br>1g |

S

| 编号 | 药品名称 | 用法用量 | 功能主治 | 制剂及规格 |
|---|---|---|---|---|
| 131 | 麝香保心丸* | 口服，一次 1 ~ 2 丸，一日 3 次；或症状发作时服用。 | 芳香温通，益气强心。用于气滞血瘀所致的胸痹，症见心前区疼痛、固定不移；心肌缺血所致的心绞痛、心肌梗死见上述证候者。 | 丸剂 22.5mg |
| 132 | 麝香海马追风膏 | 贴患处。 | 驱风散寒，活血止痛。用于风寒麻木，腰腿疼痛，四肢不仁。 | 贴膏剂<br>5cm×6.5cm |
| 133 | 麝珠明目滴眼液 | 滴眼。取本品 1 支（0.3g）倒入装有 5ml 生理盐水的滴眼瓶中，摇匀，即可滴眼，每次 3 滴（每滴 1 滴闭眼 15 分钟），1 日 2 次。 | 消翳明目，用于老年性初、中期白内障。 | 滴眼剂<br>0.3g |
| 134 | 麝香壮骨膏 | 外用。贴患处。将患处皮肤表面洗净，擦干，撕去覆盖在膏布上的隔离层，将膏面贴于患处的皮肤上。天冷时，可辅以按摩与热敷。 | 镇痛，消炎。用于风湿痛，关节痛，腰痛，神经痛，肌肉酸痛，扭伤，挫伤。 | 橡胶膏剂<br>6cm×10cm |
| 135 | 松龄血脉康胶囊* | 口服。一次 3 粒，一日 3 次。 | 平肝潜阳，镇心安神。用于肝阳上亢所致的头痛、眩晕、急躁易怒、心悸、失眠；高血压病及原发性高脂血症见上述证候者。 | 胶囊剂<br>0.5g |
| 136 | 舒肝和胃丸* | 口服，大蜜丸一次 2 丸，一日 2 次。 | 舒肝解郁，和胃止痛。用于肝胃不和，两胁胀满，胃脘疼痛，食欲不振，呃逆呕吐，大便失调。 | 丸剂<br>6g |
| 137 | 舒肝颗粒 | 颗粒：口服。一次 1 袋，一日 2 次，用温开水或姜汤送服。 | 舒肝理气，散郁调经。用于肝气不舒的两胁疼痛，胸腹胀闷，月经不调，头痛目眩，心烦意乱，口苦咽干，以及肝郁气滞所致的面部黧黑斑（黄褐斑）。 | 颗粒<br>3g |
| 138 | 速效救心丸* | 含服。4 ~ 6 粒 / 次，3 次 / 日。急性发作时 10 ~ 15 粒 / 次。 | 行气活血，祛瘀止痛，增加冠脉血流量，缓解心绞痛。用于气滞血瘀型冠心病，心绞痛。 | 丸剂<br>40mg |

续　表

| 编号 | 药品名称 | 用法用量 | 功能主治 | 制剂及规格 |
|---|---|---|---|---|
| 139 | 四磨汤口服液 | 口服。成人一次 20ml，一日 3 次，疗程一周；新生儿一次 3～5ml，一日 3 次，疗程 2 日；幼儿一次 10ml，一日 3 次，疗程 3～5 日。 | 顺气降逆，消积止痛。用于婴幼儿乳食内滞证，症见腹胀、腹痛、啼哭不安、厌食纳差、腹泻或便秘；中老年气滞、食积证，症见脘腹胀满、腹痛、便秘。以及腹部手术后促进肠胃功能的恢复。 | 口服液 10ml |
| 140 | 参芍片 | 口服，一次 4 片，一日 2 次。 | 活血化瘀，益气止痛。用于气虚血瘀所致的胸闷，胸痛，心悸，气短。 | 片剂 每片重 0.3g |
| 141 | 参苓白术丸 | 丸剂：口服。一次 6g，一日 3 次。 | 健脾、益气。用于体倦乏力，食少便溏。 | 丸剂 6g |
| 142 | 参松养心胶囊 | 口服。一次 2～4 粒，一日 3 次。 | 益气养阴，活血通络，清心安神。用于治疗冠心病室性早搏属气阴两虚，心络瘀阻证，症见心悸不安，气短乏力，动则加剧，胸部闷痛，失眠多梦，盗汗，神倦懒言。 | 胶囊剂 0.4g |
| 143 | 舒眠胶囊 | 口服。一次 3 粒，一日 2 次；晚饭后、临睡前各服用 1 次。疗程为 4 周。 | 疏肝解郁、宁心安神。用于肝郁伤神所致的失眠症，症见：失眠多梦，精神抑郁或急躁易怒，胸胁苦满或胸膈不畅，口苦目眩，舌边尖略红，苔白或微黄，脉弦。 | 胶囊剂 0.4g |
| 144 | 生脉饮（党参方、人参方）* | 口服，一次 10ml，一日 3 次。 | 益气，养阴生津，用于气阴两亏，心悸气短，自汗。 | 口服液 10ml |
| 145 | 双黄连 | 颗粒：口服或开水冲服。一次 10g，一日 3 次；6 个月以下，一次 2～3g；6 个月至一岁，一次 3～4g；一岁至三岁，一次 4～5g；三岁以上儿童酌量或遵医嘱。口服液：口服。一次 10ml（1 支），一日 3 次；小儿酌减或遵医嘱。 | 疏风解表，清热解毒。用于外感风热所致的感冒，症见发热、咳嗽、咽痛。 | 颗粒剂 5g 口服液 10ml |
| 146 | 参芪降糖颗粒 | 颗粒：口服。一次 1g，一日 3 次，一个月为一个疗程。效果不显著或治疗前症状较重者，每次用量可达 3g，一日 3 次。 | 益气养阴，滋脾补肾。主治消渴症，用于Ⅱ型糖尿病。 | 颗粒剂 3g |
| 147 | 生血宝合剂 | 合剂：口服。一次 15ml，一日 3 次。用时摇匀。 | 滋补肝肾，益气生血。用于肝肾不足、气血两虚所致的神疲乏力、腰膝酸软、头晕耳鸣、心悸气短、失眠、咽干、纳差食少；放、化疗所致的白细胞减少，缺铁性贫血见上述证候者。 | 合剂 100ml |
| 148 | 生血丸 | 口服。一次 5g，一日 3 次；小儿酌减。 | 补肾健脾，填精养血。用于脾肾虚弱所致的面黄肌瘦、体倦乏力、眩晕、食少、便溏；放、化疗后全血细胞减少及再生障碍性贫血见上述证候者。 | 丸剂 5g |
| 149 | 苏黄止咳胶囊 | 口服。一次 3 粒，一日 3 次。疗程 7～14 日。 | 疏风宣肺，止咳利咽。用于风邪犯肺，肺气失宣所致的咳嗽，咽痒，痒时咳嗽，或呛咳阵作，气急，遇冷空气、异味等因素突发或加重，或夜卧晨起咳剧，多呈反复发作，干咳无痰或少痰，舌苔薄白等。感冒后咳嗽及咳嗽变异型哮喘见上述症候者。 | 胶囊剂 0.45g |

**续　表**

| 编号 | 药品名称 | 用法用量 | 功能主治 | 制剂及规格 |
|---|---|---|---|---|
| 150 | 伤科灵喷雾剂 | 外用。将喷头对准患处距 15～20cm，连续按压喷头顶部，使药液均匀喷至创面。对软组织损伤所致皮肤瘀血、肿胀、疼痛等症，可直接喷于患处或将药液喷于药棉上，用药棉贴于患处，每日喷 2～6 次。对新鲜烧烫伤创面，连续喷药 3～4 次即可止痛，如有水泡，将其刺破，泡皮不须剥落。止痛后，每日用药 2～6 次（视其轻重，每日也可多喷数次）至痂皮脱落痊愈。 | 苗医：抬赊抬凯：轮官、轮洗，劳冲，凯豆。中医：清热凉血、活血化瘀、消肿止痛。用于软组织损伤、骨伤，Ⅱ度烧烫伤，湿疹、疱疹。 | 喷雾剂 100ml |

T

| 编号 | 药品名称 | 用法用量 | 功能主治 | 制剂及规格 |
|---|---|---|---|---|
| 151 | 天王补心丸 * | 口服。小蜜丸一次 9g，一日 2 次。 | 滋阴养血，补心安神。用于心阴不足之心悸健忘、失眠多梦、大便干燥。 | 丸剂 9g |
| 152 | 天芪降糖胶囊 | 口服。一次 5 粒，一日 3 次，8 周为一疗程，或遵医嘱。 | 益气养阴、清热生津。用于 2 型糖尿病气阴两虚证，症见：倦怠乏力，口渴喜饮，五心烦热，自汗，盗汗，气短懒言，心悸失眠。 | 胶囊剂 0.32g |
| 153 | 天丹通络胶囊 | 口服。一次 5 粒，一日 3 次。 | 活血通络，息风化痰。用于中风中经络，风痰瘀血痹阻脉络证，症见半身不遂、偏身麻木、口眼歪斜、语言謇涩。脑梗死急性期、恢复早期见上述证候者。 | 胶囊剂 0.4g |
| 154 | 头痛宁胶囊 | 口服。一次 3 粒，一日 3 次。 | 息风涤痰，逐瘀止痛。用于偏头痛，紧张性头痛属痰瘀阻络证，证见：痛势甚剧，或攻冲作痛，或痛如锥刺，或连及目齿，伴目眩畏光，胸闷脘胀，恶心呕吐，急躁易怒，反复发作。 | 胶囊剂 0.4g |
| 155 | 通心络胶囊 * | 口服。一次 2～4 粒，一日 3 次。 | 益气活血，通络止痛。用于冠心病心绞痛属心气虚乏、血瘀络阻证，症见胸部憋闷，刺痛、绞痛，固定不移，心悸自汗，气短乏力，舌质紫暗或有瘀斑，脉细涩或结代。亦用于气虚血瘀络阻型中风病，症见半身不遂或偏身麻木，口舌歪斜，言语不利。 | 胶囊剂 0.26g |
| 156 | 通便灵胶囊 | 口服。一次 5～6 粒，一日 1 次。 | 泻热导滞，润肠通便。用于热结便秘，长期卧床便秘，一时性腹胀便秘，老年习惯性便秘。 | 胶囊剂 0.25g |
| 157 | 通滞苏润江片 | 口服。一次 3～4 片，一日 2 次。 | 开通阻滞，消肿止痛。用于关节骨痛，风湿病，类风湿关节炎，坐骨神经痛。 | 片剂 0.52g |
| 158 | 通天口服液 | 口服。用于瘀血阻滞、风邪上扰所致的偏头痛，第一日：即刻、服药 1 小时后、2 小时后、4 小时后各服 10ml，以后每 6 小时服 10ml。第二日、三日：一次 10ml，一日 3 次，三日为一疗程，或遵医嘱；用于轻度中风病（轻度脑梗死）恢复期瘀血阻络挟风证，一次 20ml，一日 3 次，疗程为 4 周。 | 活血化瘀，祛风止痛。用于瘀血阻滞、风邪上扰所致的偏头痛，症见头部胀痛或刺痛、痛有定处，反复发作、头晕目眩、或恶心呕吐、恶风，用于轻度中风病（轻度脑梗死）恢复期瘀血阻络挟风证，症见半身不遂、口舌歪斜、言语不利、肢体麻木等。 | 口服液 10ml |

**续　表**

| 编号 | 药品名称 | 用法用量 | 功能主治 | 制剂及规格 |
|---|---|---|---|---|
| 159 | 痛风定胶囊 | 口服。一次 4 粒，一日 3 次。 | 清热祛湿，活血通络定痛。用于湿热瘀阻所致的痹痛，症见关节红肿热痛，伴有发热、汗出不解、口渴心烦、小便黄、舌红苔黄腻、脉滑数；痛风见上述症候者。 | 胶囊剂 0.4g |
| 160 | 通宣理肺丸 | 口服。一次 2 丸，一日 2～3 次。 | 解表散寒，宣肺止嗽。用于风寒束表、肺气不宣所致的感冒咳嗽，症见发热、恶寒、咳嗽、鼻塞流涕、头痛、无汗、肢体酸痛。 | 丸剂 6g |

W

| 编号 | 药品名称 | 用法用量 | 功能主治 | 制剂及规格 |
|---|---|---|---|---|
| 161 | 温胃舒胶囊 | 口服。一次 3 粒，一日 2 次。 | 温中养胃，行气止痛。用于中焦虚寒所致的胃痛，症见胃脘冷痛、腹胀嗳气、纳差食少、畏寒无力；浅表性胃炎见上述证候者 | 胶囊剂 0.4g |
| 162 | 胃苏颗粒 *（无糖型） | 用适量开水冲服，搅拌至全溶。若放置时间长有少量沉淀，摇匀即可。一次 1 袋，一日 3 次。15 日为一个疗程。 | 理气消胀，和胃止痛。主治气滞型胃脘痛，症见胃脘胀痛，窜及两胁，得嗳气或矢气则舒，情绪郁怒则加重，胸闷食少，排便不畅及慢性胃炎见上述证候者。 | 颗粒剂 5g |
| 163 | 乌鸡白凤丸 | 口服。大蜜丸一次 6g，一日 2 次。 | 补气养血，调经止带。用于气血两虚，身体瘦弱，腰膝酸软，月经不调，带下。 | 丸剂 6g |
| 164 | 维 C 银翘片 | 口服。一次 2 片，一日 3 次。 | 疏风解表，清热解毒。用于外感风热所致的流行性感冒，症见发热、头痛、咳嗽、口干、咽喉疼痛。 | 片剂 / |
| 165 | 翁沥通胶囊 | 饭后服。一次 3 粒，一日 2 次。 | 清热利湿，散结祛瘀。用于证属湿热蕴结，痰瘀交阻之前列腺增生症，证见尿频、尿急，或尿细，排尿困难等。 | 胶囊剂 0.4g |
| 166 | 胃复春片 | 口服。一次 4 片，一日 3 次。 | 健脾益气、活血解毒。用于治疗胃癌癌前期病变、胃癌手术后辅助治疗。慢性浅表性胃炎属脾胃虚弱证者。 | 片剂 0.36g |
| 167 | 稳心颗粒 | 开水冲服。一次 1 袋，一日 3 次。或遵医嘱。 | 益气养阴，活血化瘀。用于气阴两虚，心脉瘀阻所致的心悸不宁、气短乏力、胸闷胸痛；室性早搏、房性早搏见上述症候者。 | 颗粒剂 5g |
| 168 | 五加生化胶囊 | 口服。一次 6 粒，一日 2 次。温开水送服，疗程 3 日或遵医嘱。 | 益气养血、活血祛瘀。适用于经期及人流术后、产后气虚血瘀所致阴道流血，血色紫暗或有血块，小腹疼痛按之不减、腰背酸痛、自汗、心悸气短、舌淡、兼见瘀点，脉沉弱等。 | 胶囊剂 0.4g |
| 169 | 乌灵胶囊 | 口服。一次 3 粒，一日 3 次。 | 补肾健脑，养心安神。用于心肾不交所致的失眠、健忘、心悸心烦、神疲乏力、腰膝酸软、头晕耳鸣、少气懒言、脉细或沉无力；神经衰弱见上述证候者。 | 胶囊剂 0.33g |

X

| 编号 | 药品名称 | 用法用量 | 功能主治 | 制剂及规格 |
|------|---------|---------|---------|-----------|
| 170 | 西黄丸 | 口服，一次 3g，一日 2 次。 | 清热解毒，消肿散结。用于热毒壅结所致的痈疽疔毒、瘰疬、流注，癌肿。 | 丸剂 3g |
| 171 | 小儿豉翘清热颗粒 | 开水冲服。6 个月～1 岁：一次 1～2g（半袋～1 袋）；1～3 岁：一次 2～3g（1 袋～1 袋半）；4～6 岁：一次 3～4g（1 袋半～2 袋）；7～9 岁：一次 4～5g（2 袋～2 袋半）；10 岁以上：一次 6g（3 袋）；一日 3 次。 | 疏风解表，清热导滞。用于小儿风热感冒挟滞证，证见：发热咳嗽，鼻塞流涕，咽红肿痛，纳呆口渴，脘腹胀满，便秘或大便酸臭，溲黄等。 | 颗粒剂 2g |
| 172 | 小儿消积止咳口服液 * | 口服，1 岁以内，每次 5ml；1～2 岁，每次 10ml；3～4 岁，每次 15ml；5 岁以上，每次 20ml；一日 3 次，疗程 5 日。 | 清热肃肺，消积止咳。用于小儿饮食积滞、痰热蕴肺所致的咳嗽、夜间加重、喉间痰鸣、腹胀、口臭。 | 口服液 10ml |
| 173 | 心宝丸 | 口服。慢性心功能不全按心功能 1、2、3 级一次分别服用 120、240、360mg，3 次/日，一疗程为 2 个月，在心功能正常后改为日维持量 60～120mg。病窦综合征病情严重者 300～600mg/次，3 次/日，疗程为 3～6 个月。其他心律失常（期外收缩）及房颤、心肌缺血或心绞痛 120～240mg/次，3 次/日，一疗程为 1～2 个月。 | 温补心肾，益气助阳，活血通脉。用于治疗心肾阳虚、心脉瘀阻引起的慢性心功能不全，窦房结功能不全引起的心动过缓，病窦综合征以及缺血性心脏病引起的心绞痛及心电图缺血性改变。 | 丸剂 60mg |
| 174 | 仙灵骨葆胶囊 | 口服。一次 3 粒，一日 2 次；4～6 周为一疗程；或遵医嘱。 | 滋补肝肾，接骨续筋，强身健骨。用于骨质疏松和骨质疏松症，骨折，骨关节炎，骨无菌性坏死等。 | 胶囊剂 0.5g |
| 175 | 消渴丸 * | 口服，一次 5～10 丸，一日 2～3 次。饭前用温开水送服。或遵医嘱。 | 滋肾养阴，益气生津。用于气阴两虚所致的消渴病，症见多饮、多尿、多食、消瘦、体倦乏力、眠差、腰痛；2 型糖尿病见上述证候者。 | 丸剂 0.25g |
| 176 | 消炎利胆片 | 口服。一次 6 片，一日 3 次。 | 清热，祛湿，利胆。用于肝胆湿热引起的口苦，胁痛和急性胆囊炎，胆管炎。 | 片剂 |
| 177 | 消风止痒颗粒 | 口服。1 岁以内一日 1 袋；1～4 岁一日 2 袋；5～9 岁一日 3 袋；10～14 岁一日 4 袋；15 岁以上一日 6 袋。分 2～3 次服用；或遵医嘱。 | 消风清热，除湿止痒。主治丘疹样荨麻疹，也用于湿疹、皮肤瘙痒症。 | 颗粒剂 15g |
| 178 | 心脑欣片 | 口服。一次 2 片，一日 2 次；饭后服。 | 益气养阴，活血化瘀。用于气阴不足，瘀血阻滞所引起头晕，头痛，心悸，气喘，乏力，缺氧引起的红细胞增多症见上述证候者。 | 片剂 0.5g |
| 179 | 消痛贴膏 | 外用。将小袋内润湿剂均匀涂在药垫表面，润湿后直接敷于患处或穴位。每贴敷 24 小时。 | 活血化瘀，消肿止痛。用于急慢性扭挫伤、跌打瘀痛、骨质增生、风湿及类风湿疼痛，亦用于落枕、肩周炎、腰肌劳损和陈旧性伤痛等。 | 贴膏剂 9cm×12cm |
| 180 | 血脂康胶囊 * | 口服。一次 2 粒，一日 2 次，早晚饭后服用；轻、中度患者一日 2 粒，晚饭后服用。或遵医嘱。 | 化浊降脂，活血化瘀，健脾消食。用于痰阻血瘀所致的高脂血症，症见气短、乏力、头晕、头痛、胸闷、腹胀、食少纳呆；也可用于高脂血症及动脉粥样硬化所致的其他的心脑血管疾病的辅助治疗。 | 胶囊剂 0.3g |

**续 表**

| 编号 | 药品名称 | 用法用量 | 功能主治 | 制剂及规格 |
|---|---|---|---|---|
| 181 | 血塞通 | 颗粒：开水冲服。一次1～2袋，一日3次。<br>胶囊：口服，一次100mg（1粒），一日3次。 | 活血祛瘀，通脉活络，抑制血小板聚集和增加脑血流量。用于脑络瘀阻，中风偏瘫，心脉瘀阻，胸痹心痛；脑血管后遗症、冠心病心绞痛属上述证候者。 | 颗粒剂<br>1.5g<br>胶囊<br>0.1g |
| 182 | 血府逐瘀软胶囊 | 口服。一次4粒，一日2次。 | 活血祛瘀，行气止痛。用于瘀血内阻证，证见头痛或胸痛，内热瞀闷，失眠多梦，心悸怔忡，急躁善怒。 | 软胶囊<br>0.5g |
| 183 | 香砂和胃丸* | 口服。一次6g，一日2次。 | 健脾开胃，行气化滞。用于脾胃虚弱，消化不良引起的食欲不振，脘腹胀痛，吞酸嘈杂，大便不调。 | 丸剂<br>每100粒重6g |
| 184 | 眩晕宁片 | 口服。一次2～3片，一日3～4次。 | 健脾利湿，益肝补肾。用于痰湿中阻、肝肾不足引起的头昏头晕。 | 片剂<br>每片重0.38g（相当于原药材6g） |
| 185 | 消癌平滴丸 | 口服。一次8～10丸，一日3次。 | 抗癌，消炎，平喘。用于食管癌、胃癌、肺癌，对大肠癌、宫颈癌、白血病等多种恶性肿瘤，亦有一定疗效，亦可配合放疗、化疗及手术后治疗。并用于治疗慢性气管炎和支气管哮喘。 | 滴丸<br>0.35g |
| 186 | 新清宁片 | 口服。一次3～5片，一日3次；必要时可适当增量；学龄前儿童酌减或遵医嘱；用于便秘，临睡前服5片。 | 清热解毒，泻火通便。用于内结实热所致的喉肿、牙痛、目赤、便秘、发热。 | 片剂<br>0.31g |
| 187 | 辛芩颗粒 | 开水冲服。一次1袋，一日3次，20日为1个疗程。 | 益气固表，祛风通窍。用于肺气不足、风邪外袭所致的鼻痒、喷嚏、流清涕、易感冒；过敏性鼻炎见上述证候者。 | 颗粒剂<br>5g |

Y

| 编号 | 药品名称 | 用法用量 | 功能主治 | 制剂及规格 |
|---|---|---|---|---|
| 188 | 愈风宁心片 | 口服。一次5片，一日3次。 | 解痉止痛，增强脑及冠脉血流量。用于高血压头晕，头痛，颈项头痛，冠心病，心绞痛，神经性头痛，早期突发性耳聋。 | 片剂<br>0.28g |
| 189 | 咽炎颗粒 | 口服：每次1～2袋，一日2次。冲服。 | 清热滋阴，利咽消肿。用于急慢咽炎。 | 颗粒剂<br>10g（有糖）<br>5g（无糖） |
| 190 | 元胡止痛滴丸* | 口服，一次20～30丸，一日3次。 | 理气，活血，止痛。用于行经腹痛，胃痛，胁痛，头痛。 | 滴丸<br>每10丸重0.5g。 |
| 191 | 养心氏片 | 口服。一次2～3片，一日3次。 | 益气活血，化瘀止痛。用于气虚血瘀所致的胸痹，症见心悸气短、胸闷、心前区刺痛；冠心病心绞痛见于上述证候者。 | 片剂<br>0.6g |

续　表

| 编号 | 药品名称 | 用法用量 | 功能主治 | 制剂及规格 |
|---|---|---|---|---|
| 192 | 养正消积胶囊 | 口服。一次 4 粒，一日 3 次。 | 健脾益肾、化瘀解毒。适用于不宜手术的脾肾两虚、瘀毒内阻型原发性肝癌辅助治疗，与肝内动脉介入灌注加栓塞化疗合用，有助于提高介入化疗疗效，减轻对白细胞、肝功能、血红蛋白的毒性作用，改善患者生存质量、改善脘腹胀满、纳呆食少、神疲乏力、腰膝酸软、溲赤便溏、疼痛。 | 胶囊 0.39g |
| 193 | 养血安神丸 | 口服。一次 50 粒（6g），一日 3 次。 | 养血安神。用于失眠多梦，心悸头晕。 | 丸剂 每 100 粒重 12g |
| 194 | 银杏叶片 | 口服。一次 1 片，一日 3 次；或遵医嘱。 | 活血化瘀通络。用于瘀血阻络引起的胸痹心痛、中风、半身不遂、舌强语謇；冠心病稳定型心绞痛、脑梗死见上述证候者。 | 片剂 每片含总黄酮醇苷 9.6mg、萜类内酯 2.4mg |
| 195 | 云南白药 | 胶囊：1. 口服。2. 外用涂于患处：取药粉用酒调匀敷患处。 气雾剂：外用。喷于伤患处。使用云南白药气雾剂，一日 3 ～ 5 次。凡遇较重闭合性跌打损伤者，先喷云南白药气雾剂保险液，若剧烈疼痛仍不缓解，间隔 1 ～ 2 分钟重复给药，一日使用不得超过 3 次。喷云南白药气雾剂保险液间隔 3 分钟后，再喷云南白药气雾剂。 | 胶囊：止血化瘀、活血止痛。解毒消肿。用于跌打损伤、瘀血肿痛、吐血、咳血、便血、痔疮、崩漏下血、疮疡肿毒、软组织挫伤、闭合性骨折、支气管扩张及肺结核咳血，溃疡病出血，以及皮肤感染性疾病。 气雾剂：活血散瘀，消肿止痛。用于跌打损伤，瘀血肿痛，肌肉酸痛及风湿性关节疼痛等症。 | 胶囊剂 0.25g 气雾剂 85g/30g |
| 196 | 越鞠保和丸 | 口服。一次 6g，一日 1 ～ 2 次。 | 舒肝解郁，开胃消食。用于气食郁滞所致的胃痛，症见脘腹胀痛、倒饱嘈杂、纳呆食少、大便不调；消化不良见上述证候者。 | 丸剂 6g |
| 197 | 益母草颗粒 | 开水冲服，一次 15g，一日 2 次。 | 活血调经。用于血瘀所致的月经不调，症见经水量少。 | 颗粒剂 15g |
| 198 | 益心舒胶囊 | 口服。一次 3 粒，一日 3 次。 | 益气复脉，活血化瘀，养阴生津。用于气阴两虚，瘀血阻脉所致的胸痹，症见胸痛胸闷、心悸气短、脉结代，冠心病心绞痛见上述证候者。 | 胶囊 0.4g |
| 199 | 野菊花栓 | 肛门给药，每次 1 粒，一日 1 ～ 2 次；或遵医嘱。 | 抗菌消炎。用于前列腺炎及慢性盆腔炎等疾病。 | 栓剂 2.4g |
| 200 | 鱼石脂软膏 | 外用，一日 2 次，涂患处。 | 用于疖肿。 | 软膏剂 10g（10%） |
| 201 | 茵栀黄颗粒（口服液） | 颗粒：开水冲服。一次 2 袋，一日 3 次。 口服液：口服。一次 10ml（一支），一日 3 次。 | 清热解毒，利湿退黄。用于肝胆湿热所致的黄疸，症见面目悉黄、胸胁胀痛、恶心呕吐、小便黄赤；急、慢性肝炎见上述症候者。 | 颗粒 3g 口服液 10ml |

Z

| 编号 | 药品名称 | 用法用量 | 功能主治 | 制剂及规格 |
|------|---------|---------|---------|-----------|
| 202 | 至灵胶囊 | 口服，一次 2～3 粒，一日 2～3 次，或遵医嘱。 | 补肺益气。用于肺肾两虚所致咳喘、浮肿等症，亦可用于各类肾病、慢性支气管哮喘、慢性肝炎及肿瘤的辅助治疗。 | 胶囊剂 0.25g |
| 203 | 致康胶囊 | 口服，一次 2～4 粒，一日 3 次；或遵医嘱。 | 清热凉血止血，化瘀生肌定痛。用于创伤性出血，崩漏、呕血及便血等。 | 胶囊剂 0.3g |
| 204 | 贞芪扶正胶囊 | 口服。一次 6 粒，一日 2 次。 | 补气养阴，用于久病虚损，气阴不足。配合手术、放疗治疗、化学治疗，促进正常功能恢复。 | 胶囊剂 每 6 粒相当于原生药 12.5g |
| 205 | 祖师麻膏药 | 温热软化后贴于患处。 | 祛风除除湿，活血止痛。用于风寒湿痹、瘀血痹阻经脉。症见：肢体关节肿痛、畏寒肢冷、局部肿胀有硬结或瘀斑。 | 贴膏剂 每张净重 10g |
| 206 | 正心泰颗粒 | 开水冲服。一次 1 袋，一日 3 次。 | 补气活血，通脉益肾。用于冠心病、心绞痛表现为气虚血瘀或兼肾虚证候者，证见胸闷、心悸、乏力眩晕，腰膝酸软等。 | 颗粒 5g |
| 207 | 知柏地黄丸 | 口服，一次 6 克，一日 2 次。 | 滋阴降火。用于阴虚火旺，潮热盗汗，口干咽痛，耳鸣遗精，小便短赤。 | 丸剂 每 30 粒重 6g |
| 208 | 泽桂癃爽胶囊 | 口服。每次 2 粒，一日 3 次；30 日为 1 个疗程。 | 行瘀散结，化气利水。用于膀胱瘀阻型良性前列腺增生及慢性前列腺炎，症见夜尿频多、排尿困难、小腹胀满，或小便频急，排尿不尽，少腹、会阴或腰骶疼痛或不适、睾丸坠胀不适、尿后滴白等。 | 胶囊 0.44g |
| 209 | 正红花油 | 外用。擦于患处，一日 4～6 次。 | 祛风止痛。用于风湿性骨关节痛，跌打损伤，感冒头痛，蚊虫叮咬。 | 搽剂 20ml |
| 210 | 扎冲十三味丸 | 口服，一次 5～9 粒，一日 1 次，晚间临睡前服，或遵医嘱。 | 祛风通窍，舒筋活血，镇静安神，除湿。用于半身不遂，口眼斜、四肢麻木、腰腿不利、语言不清、筋骨疼痛、神经麻痹、风湿，关节疼痛等症。 | 丸剂 每 10 粒重 2g |

说明：＊为国家基本药品目录收载品种

# 附录 A  临床用药常用英制与公制单位换算表

| | |
|---|---|
| 温度 | 50 华氏（F）=10 摄氏（℃）<br>F=（℃ ×9/5）+32<br>℃ =5/9×（F-32） |
| 长度 | 1 英寸 =2.54 厘米<br>1 厘米 =1/2.54 英寸<br>（1 英尺 =12 英寸） |
| 重量 | 1 磅 =0.454545 千克<br>1 千克 =2.2 磅<br>1 盎司 =0.02835 千克<br>1 千克 =35.2734 盎司 |
| 面积 | 1 平方英寸 =6.4516 平方厘米<br>1 平方厘米 =0.1550 平方英寸 |
| 体积 | 1 英国加仑 =4.5461 升<br>1 升 =0.2200 英国加仑 |

# 附录 B  临床用药常用计算公式

每次用药量（mg）= 体表面积

体表面积（m²）=（4× 体重 +7）/（体重 +90）=5.99× [体重（g）× 身长（cm）]<sup>1/2</sup>

小儿体表面积（m²）=0.0061× 身高（cm）+0.0128× 体重（kg）－ 0.1529

1～30kg 小儿体表面积：

1～5kg：m²=0.05× 体重（kg）+0.05

6～10kg：m²=0.04× 体重（kg）+0.1

11～20kg：m²=0.03× 体重（kg）+0.2

21～30kg：m²=0.02× 体重（kg）+0.4

> 30kg 小儿体表面积计算：体重每增加 5kg，体表面积增加 0.1

不便直接获得的小儿体重

1—6 个月：体重（kg）=3（kg）+ 月龄 ×0.6

7—12 个月：体重（kg）=3（kg）+ 月龄 ×0.5

1 岁以上：体重（kg）=8（kg）+ 月龄 ×2

儿童用药量计算

• 按体表面积计算

小儿用药剂量 = 成人剂量 /1.73（m²）× 小儿体表面积（m²）

• 按体重计算

小儿用药剂量 = 成人剂量 × 小儿体重（kg）/60

• 按年龄计算法

| 初生—1 个月 | 成人剂量的 1/18～1/14 |
| --- | --- |
| 1—6 个月 | 成人剂量的 1/14～1/7 |
| 6 个月—1 岁 | 成人剂量的 1/7～1/5 |
| 1—2 岁 | 成人剂量的 1/5～1/4 |
| 2—4 岁 | 成人剂量的 1/4～1/3 |
| 4—6 岁 | 成人剂量的 1/3～2/5 |
| 6—9 岁 | 成人剂量的 2/5～1/2 |
| 9—14 岁 | 成人剂量的 1/2～2/3 |
| 14—18 岁 | 成人剂量的 2/3～全量 |

肾功能不全者用药时肾小球滤过率

（GFR）计算

• 肾小球滤过率（Cockcroft-Gault）计算法

Ccr=（140－年龄）× 体重（kg）/[72×Scr（mg•dl）] 或 Ccr=[（140－年龄）× 体重（kg）]/[0.818×Scr（umol/L）]

Ccr 为内生肌酐清除率，Scr 为血清肌酐（mg/dl），女性按计算结果 ×0.85。

· 肾功能损害程度评定

正常值：GFR ≥ 90ml/（min•1.73m$^2$）

轻度损害：GFR 为 60 ～ 89ml/（min•1.73m$^2$）

中度损害：GFR 为 30 ～ 59ml/（min•1.73m$^2$）

重度损害：GFR ＜ 30ml/（min•1.73m$^2$）

# 附录 C　处方常用缩略语

## Abbreviations commonly used in prescriptions
## Abréviations couramment utilisées dans les prescriptions
## Abreviaturas comúnmente utilizadas en la prescripción

| 中文 | Abbreviations/Abréviations/abreviaturas |
|---|---|
| 【给药次数和时间】 | 【Drug administration time】 |
| 每日 1 次 | q.d. |
| 每日 2 次 | b.i.d. |
| 每日 3 次 | t.i.d. |
| 每日 4 次 | q.i.d. |
| 隔日 1 次 | q.o.d. |
| 每晚 1 次 | q.n. |
| 每小时 | q.h. |
| 每 3 小时 | q.3h. |
| 【给药途径】 | 【Drug delivery route】 |
| 口服 | p.o |
| 灌肠 | p.r |
| 静脉注射 | i.v |
| 肌内注射 | i.m |
| 皮下注射 | i.h/s.c |
| 皮内注射 | i.c |
| 腹腔注射 | i.p |
| 皮试 | c.t |
| 外用 | Ad us.ext./pro us.ext. |
| 静脉滴注 | i.v.gtt/i.v.drip |
| 【剂型】 | 【Preparation】 |
| 复方 | Co. / Comp. |
| 片剂 | Tab. |
| 胶囊剂 | Caps. |
| 注射剂 | Inj. |
| 丸剂 | Pil. |

续　表

| 中文 | Abbreviations/Abréviations/abreviaturas |
|---|---|
| 颗粒剂 | Gran. |
| 栓剂 | Supp. |
| 滴剂 | Gtt. |
| 洗剂 | Lot. |
| 喷雾剂 | Neb. |
| 合剂 | Mist. |
| 溶液剂 | Liq. / Sol. |
| 乳剂 | Em. / Emuls. |
| 软膏剂 | Ung. |
| 硬膏剂 | Emp. |
| 糖浆剂 | Syr. |
| 搽剂 | Lin. |
| 【其他】 | 【Others】 |
| 请取 | Rp. |
| 紧急 | Cit. |
| 注明用法；标记 | S.i.g. |
| 应服用 | Cap. |
| 立即 | Stat. / st. |
| 必要时 | p.r.n. |
| 需要时 | s.o.s. |
| 遵医嘱 | Ut Dict |
| 发热时 | Feb. urg |
| 足够量 | q.s. |

# 附录 D 缩略语对照表

| 缩略语 | 全称 | 缩略语 | 全称 |
|---|---|---|---|
| 17-OHCS | 17- 羟皮质醇 | ALG | 抗淋巴细胞球蛋白 |
| 2，5-OAS | 2，5- 寡腺苷酸合成酶（抗病毒活性指标） | ALP（AKP） | 碱性磷酸酶 |
| | | ALS | 抗淋巴细胞血清 |
| 3-OMD | 3-O- 甲基多巴 | ALT | 丙氨酸氨基转移酶 |
| 4-ABA | 4- 氨基苯甲酰 - β - 丙氨酸 | AMI | 急性心肌梗死 |
| 5'-DFUR | 5'- 脱氧 -5- 氟尿苷 | AML | 急性髓细胞白血病 |
| 5-ASA | 5- 氨基水杨酸 | ANA | 抗核抗体 |
| 5-dFCR | 5'- 脱氧 -5- 氟胞苷 | ANC | 中性粒细胞绝对计数 |
| 5-FU | 氟脲嘧啶 | Ang Ⅱ | 血管紧张素 Ⅱ（Angiotensin Ⅱ） |
| 5-HIAA | 5- 羟基吲哚醋酸 | ANH | 急性等容血液稀释 |
| 5-HT | 5- 羟色胺 | AOP | 阿霉素、长春新碱和泼尼松联合化疗方案 |
| 5-HT1a | 5- 羟色胺 -1A | | |
| 5-HT3 | 5- 羟色胺 3 | APC | 活化蛋白 C |
| 6-MNA | 6- 甲氧基 -2- 萘乙酸 | APD | 动作电位时间 |
| 6-MP | 巯嘌呤 | APH | 腺垂体激素 |
| **A** | | APL | 急性早幼粒细胞白血病 |
| AA | 花生四烯酸 | Apo A | 载脂蛋白 A |
| ABVD | 阿霉素、博来霉素、长春碱和达卡巴嗪联合化疗方案 | Apo B | 载脂蛋白 B |
| | | APP | 淀粉样蛋白 β - 淀粉样前体蛋白 |
| ABW | 实际体重（actual body weight） | APSCA | 链激酶复合物缩略语全称 |
| ACE | 血管紧张素转换酶 | APTT | 激活的部分凝血活酶时间 |
| ACEI | 血管紧张素转换酶抑制药 | ARA | 血管紧张素 Ⅱ 受体拮抗药 |
| Ach | 乙酰胆碱 | Ara-C | 阿糖胞嘧啶 |
| AchE | 乙酰胆碱酯酶 | ARDS | 急性呼吸窘迫综合征 |
| ACP | 阿霉素、环磷酰胺和顺铂联合化疗方案 | ARF | 急性肾衰竭 |
| | | ARN | 急性视网膜坏死综合征 |
| ACT | 活化全血凝固时间 | ART | 辅助生育技术（助孕技术） |
| ACTH | 促肾上腺皮质激素 | AST | 天门冬氨酸氨基转移酶 |
| ACV | 阿昔洛韦 | AT-3 | 抗凝血酶Ⅲ |
| AC | 阿霉素和阿糖胞苷联合化疗方案 | AT1 | 血管紧张素 Ⅱ -1 型受体 |
| AD | 肾上腺素 | AT2 | 血管紧张素 Ⅱ -2 型受体 |
| ADCC | 抗体依赖的细胞介导的细胞毒反应 | ATG | 抗胸腺细胞球蛋白 |
| ADH | 血管升压素（抗利尿激素） | ATP | 三磷酸腺苷 |
| ADMC | 抗体依赖性巨噬细胞的细胞毒作用 | AUC | 曲线下面积 |
| ADP | 二磷酸腺苷 | AVP | 精氨酸加压素 |
| ADW | 矫正体重 | AZT | 叠氮脱氧胸苷 |
| AFP | 甲胎蛋白 | **B** | |
| AIDS | 获得性免疫缺陷综合征（艾滋病） | BAL | 二巯基丙醇 |
| ALAAD | 芳香族氨基酸脱羧酶 | BCR | 断裂点成簇区 |

| 缩略语 | 全称 | 缩略语 | 全称 |
|---|---|---|---|
| BDZ | 苯二氮䓬类 | CMV | 巨细胞病毒 |
| bFGF | 碱性成纤维细胞生长因子 | CNS | 中枢神经系统 |
| BFU-E | 红系爆式集落形成单位 | COC | 复方口服避孕药 |
| bid. | 一日2次（每日2次） | CODP 方案 | 环磷酰胺、长春新碱、柔红霉素和泼尼松联合化疗方案 |
| BMD | 骨矿物质密度 | | |
| BMI | 体重指数 | COMP 方案 | 环磷酰胺、长春新碱、甲氨蝶呤和泼尼松联合化疗方案 |
| Bolus | 弹丸注射 | | |
| BOOP | 闭塞性毛细支气管炎 | COMT | 儿茶酚 - 氧位 - 甲基转移酶 |
| BPH | 前列腺增生 | Coomb's 方案 | 直接抗球蛋白试验 |
| BSP | 磺溴酞钠 | COPD | 慢性阻塞性肺疾病 |
| BT | 出血时间 | COPP 方案 | 氮芥或环磷酰胺、长春新碱、泼尼松及丙卡巴肼联合化疗方案 |
| BU | Batroxobin Unit（为酶活性单位） | | |
| BUN | 血尿素氮 | COX | 环氧化酶 |
| BZ | 苯二氮类药物 | COX-1 | 环氧化酶 -1 |
| BZR | 苯二氮受体 | COX-2 | 环氧化酶 -2 |
| | | CPK | 肌酸磷酸激酶 |
| **C** | | CPR | 心脏停搏 |
| C1 | 纤溶酶激活补体 | Cr | 肌酐 |
| CABG | 冠状动脉旁路移植术 | CRF | 慢性肾衰竭 |
| CAF 方案 | 环磷酰胺、阿霉素和氟脲嘧啶联合化疗方案 | CRH | 下丘脑促皮质素释放激素 |
| | | Crohn 病 | 克罗恩病 |
| cAMP | 环磷酸腺苷 | CSF | 集落刺激因子 |
| CAPD | 持续性非卧床腹膜透析 | CSII | 持续皮下胰岛素输注 |
| CAST | 心律失常抑制试验 | CT | 凝血时间 |
| CBFV | 脑血流速度 | CTP | 三磷酸胞苷 |
| Ccr | 内生肌酐清除率 | CTX | 环磷酰胺 |
| CDC | 美国疾病控制和预防中心 | CTZ | 中枢催吐化学感受区 |
| CDCA | 鹅去氧胆酸 | CVP | 中心静脉压 |
| CDK | 细胞周期依赖性激酶 | CY-VA-DIC 方案 | 环磷酰胺、长春新碱、阿霉素和达卡巴嗪联合化疗方案 |
| CER | 雌激素受体 | | |
| CFU-E | 红系集落形成单位 | CYP | 细胞色素 P450 |
| cGMP | 环一磷酸鸟苷 | CYP 2C9 | 细胞色素 P4502C9 |
| CHF | 充血性心力衰竭 | CYP 3A4 | 细胞色素 P4503A4 |
| CHO | 胆固醇 | CysLT1 | 半胱氨酰白三烯 |
| CHOP 方案 | 环磷酰胺、阿霉素、长春新碱和泼尼松联合化疗方案 | **D** | |
| CI | 心脏指数 | DA | 多巴胺 |
| CK | 肌酸激酶 | DAMP 方案 | 柔红霉素、阿糖胞苷、巯嘌呤或硫鸟嘌呤和泼尼松联合化疗方案 |
| CL | 清除率 | | |
| Cmax | 血药浓度峰值（峰值血药浓度） | DDA | 双脱氧腺苷 |
| CMC 方案 | 洛莫司汀、甲氨蝶呤和环磷酰胺联合化疗方案 | DDI | 双去氧肌苷 |
| | | DDW | 用药体重 |
| CME | 黄斑囊样水肿 | dGTP | 2'- 脱氧鸟苷三磷酸 |
| CMF 方案 | 环磷酰胺、甲氨蝶呤和氟尿嘧啶联合化疗方案 | DHA | 二十六碳六烯酸 |
| | | DHODH | 二氢乳清酸脱氢酶 |
| CmL | 慢性髓细胞白血病 | DHT | 双氢睾酮 |
| CMML | 慢性粒 - 单细胞白血病 | DIC | 弥散性血管内凝血 |

| 缩略语 | 全称 |
| --- | --- |
| DM | 弥散型美多巴 |
| DOAP 方案 | 柔红霉素、长春新碱、阿糖胞苷和泼尼松联合化疗方案 |
| DOPAC | 二羟苯乙酸 |
| DTP | 白喉、破伤风类毒素和百日咳菌苗三联疫苗 |
| DU | 十二指肠溃疡 |
| DUB | 功能失调性子宫出血 |
| DVT | 深静脉血栓 |

## E

| 缩略语 | 全称 |
| --- | --- |
| E1 | 雌酮 |
| E2 | 雌二醇 |
| EAA | 必需氨基酸 |
| EB 病毒 | 非淋巴细胞瘤病毒 |
| ECG | 心电图 |
| ECHO | 超声波心动描记法 |
| ECL | 胃黏膜轻度肠嗜铬样 |
| ECP | 嗜酸粒细胞阳离子蛋白 |
| ED | 勃起功能障碍 |
| EEG | 脑电图 |
| EFAD | 必需脂肪酸缺乏症 |
| EGFR | 表皮生长因子受体 |
| Eh | 电位 |
| EHC | 肠肝循环 |
| Ekbom 综合征 | 不宁腿综合征 |
| ELT | 优球蛋白溶解时间 |
| EPA | 二十五碳五烯酸 |
| EPL | 必需磷脂 |
| EPO | 促红细胞生成素 |
| EPS | 锥体外系综合征 |
| ER | 孕激素 |
| ERCP | 内镜逆行胰胆管造影 |
| ERG | 视网膜电流图 |
| ERP | 有效不应期 |
| ERPF | 有效肾血浆流量 |
| ERSD | 晚期肾病 |
| ESR | 红细胞沉降率 |
| ESRD | 终末期肾病 |
| ET-1 | 内皮素 -1 |
| ETEC | 产肠毒素大肠杆菌 |
| EURP | 胰蛋白酶灭活单位 |

## F

| 缩略语 | 全称 |
| --- | --- |
| FAM 方案 | 氟脲嘧啶、阿霉素、丝裂霉素联合化疗方案 |
| FD | 功能性消化不良 |
| FDA | 美国食品药品监督管理局 |

| 缩略语 | 全称 |
| --- | --- |
| FDP | 纤维蛋白原降解产物 |
| FdUMP | 活性型氟苷单磷酸盐 |
| FEV1 | 第一秒用力呼气量 |
| FMN | 黄素单核苷酸 |
| FSH | 促卵泡素（卵泡刺激素） |
| FT3 | 血清游离三碘甲状腺素原氨酸 |
| FT4 | 血清游离甲状腺素 |
| FVC | 用力肺活量 |
| F Ⅷ | 凝血因子Ⅷ |
| F Ⅷ a | 活化的凝血因子Ⅷ |
| F Ⅸ a | 凝血因子Ⅸ a |

## G

| 缩略语 | 全称 |
| --- | --- |
| G-6PD | 葡萄糖 -6- 磷酸脱氢酶 |
| GABA | γ - 氨基丁酸 |
| GCS | 谷氨酰半胱氨酸合成酶 |
| GERD | 胃食管反流性疾病 |
| GF | 生长因子 |
| GFR | 肾小球滤过率 |
| GH | 生长激素 |
| GIST | 胃肠道间质细胞瘤 |
| GM-CSF | 粒细胞 - 单核巨噬细胞集落刺激因子 |
| GMP | 鸟苷酸 |
| GnRH | 促性腺激素释放激素 |
| GnRH-a | 促性腺激素释放激素激动剂 |
| GP | 糖蛋白 |
| GS | 葡萄糖注射液 |
| GSH | 谷胱甘肽 |
| GSSG | 氧化型谷胱甘肽 |
| GTP | 三磷酸鸟苷 |
| GU | 胃溃疡 |
| GVHD | 输血相关的移植物抗宿主病 |
| GVHR | 移植物抗宿主反应 |
| GX | 甘氨酰二甲苯胺 |

## H

| 缩略语 | 全称 |
| --- | --- |
| Hb | 血红蛋白 |
| HbAlc | 糖化血红蛋白 |
| HBeAg | 乙型肝炎 e 抗原 |
| HBG | 性激素结合球蛋白 |
| HBIG | 乙型肝炎免疫球蛋白 |
| HBsAg | 乙型肝炎表面抗原 |
| HBV | 乙型肝炎病毒 |
| HCG | 绒毛膜促性腺激素 |
| HCT | 血细胞比容 |
| HCV | 丙型肝炎病毒 |
| HDCV | 人类二倍体细胞狂犬病疫苗 |
| HDL | 高密度脂蛋白 |

| 缩略语 | 全称 | 缩略语 | 全称 |
|--------|------|--------|------|
| HDL-C | 高密度脂蛋白胆固醇 | IGT | 糖耐量减低 |
| HER-2 | 人表皮生长因子受体 -2 | IL-1 | 白细胞介素 -1 |
| hGH | 人生长激素 | IL-2 | 白细胞介素 -2 |
| HGPRT | 黄嘌呤 - 鸟嘌呤磷酸核糖基转移酶 | IL-6 | 白细胞介素 -6 |
| HIV | 人类免疫缺陷病毒（艾滋病病毒） | INR | 国际标准化比值 |
| HL | 肝脂酶 | IR | 即释剂 |
| HLA | 人类白细胞组织相容性抗原 | IRDS | 婴儿呼吸窘迫综合征 |
| HLA- Ⅱ | 人类白细胞组织相容性抗原 Ⅱ | ITP | 特发性血小板减少性紫癜 |
| HMD | 透明膜肺 | | **K** |
| HMG | 尿促性素 | Ki | 抑制常数 |
| HMG-CoA | 羟甲基戊二酸单酰辅酶 A | KIU | 激肽释放酶灭活单位 |
| HoFH | 纯合子型家族性高胆固醇血症 | | **L** |
| HP | 幽门螺杆菌 | LAK | 淋巴细胞激活的杀伤细胞 |
| HPA | 下丘脑 - 腺垂体 - 肾上腺皮质轴 | LCA | 石胆酸 |
| HPLC | 高效液相色谱法 | LCT | 长链三酰甘油 |
| HPV | 人乳头瘤病毒 | LDH | 乳酸脱氢酶 |
| HR | 心率 | LDL | 低密度脂蛋白 |
| HSC | 肝星状细胞 | LDL-C | 低密度脂蛋白胆固醇 |
| HSD | 羟甾脱氢酶 | LDW | 瘦体重（lean bodyweight） |
| HSP70 | 热休克蛋白 70 | LES | 食管下括约肌 |
| HSV | 单纯疱疹病毒 | LESP | 食管下端括约压 |
| HSV- Ⅰ | 单纯疱疹病毒 Ⅰ | LH | 黄体生成素 |
| HSV- Ⅱ | 单纯疱疹病毒 Ⅱ | LMV 方案 | 洛铂、甲氨蝶呤和长春碱联合化疗方案 |
| HVA | 高香草酸 | | |
| HZV | 带状疱疹病毒 | LMWH | 低分子量肝素 |
| | **I** | LNG | 左炔诺孕酮 |
| i.d. | 皮内注射 | Lp（a） | 脂蛋白（a） |
| i.h. | 皮下注射 | LPL | 脂蛋白脂酶 |
| i.m. | 肌内注射 | LPS | 脂多糖 |
| i.v. | 静脉注射 | LTs | 白三烯 |
| i.v.gtt. | 静脉滴注 | LV | 亚叶酸钙 |
| IBW | 理想体重 | LVEDP | 左心室舒张末压 |
| ICAM | 细胞间黏附分子 | LVEDV | 左室舒张末容积 |
| ICE 方案 | 异环磷酰胺、足叶乙苷、卡铂联合化疗方案 | LVEF | 左心室射血分数 |
| | | Lyell 综合征 | 中毒性表皮坏死溶解症 |
| ICU | 重症监护 | | **M** |
| ID50 | 50% 抑制量 | MAC | 最低肺泡有效浓度 |
| IDU | 碘苷 | MACC 方案 | 甲氨蝶呤、阿霉素、环磷酰胺和洛莫司汀联合化疗方案 |
| IDV | 茚地那韦 | | |
| IFO | 异环磷酰胺 | MAO | 单胺氧化酶 |
| IgA | 免疫球蛋白 A | MAOI | 单胺氧化酶抑制剂 |
| IgD | 免疫球蛋白 D | MAP | 平均动脉压 |
| IgE | 免疫球蛋白 E | MBC | 最低杀菌浓度 |
| IGF-1 | 胰岛素样生长因子 -1 | MCT | 中链三酰甘油 |
| IgG | 免疫球蛋白 G | MDF | 心肌抑制因子 |
| IgM | 免疫球蛋白 M | MDS | 骨髓增生异常综合征 |

| 缩略语 | 全称 | 缩略语 | 全称 |
|---|---|---|---|
| MEGX | 单乙基甘氨酰二甲苯胺 | PAI | 纤维蛋白溶解酶原激活剂抑制因子 |
| MFO | 多功能氧化酶 | PAI-1 | 纤溶酶原激活剂抑制因子 1 |
| MIC | 最小抑菌浓度 | PAN | 聚丙烯腈 |
| MMP-1 | 间质胶原酶 | PaO2 | 动脉血氧分压 |
| MPA | 霉酚酸 | PBI | 血清蛋白结合碘 |
| MPAG | 酚化葡萄糖苷酸 | PBP1 | 青霉素结合蛋白 1 |
| MPAP | 平均肺动脉压 | PBP3 | 青霉素结合蛋白 3 |
| mRNA | 信使核糖核酸 | PBPs | 青霉素结合蛋白 |
| MRS | 耐甲氧西林葡萄球菌 | PC | 抗凝蛋白 C |
| MRSA | 耐甲氧西林金黄色葡萄球菌 | PCI | 经皮冠状动脉介入治疗 |
| MSSA | 对甲氧西林敏感的金黄色葡萄球菌 | PCOS | 多囊卵巢综合征 |
| MTD | 日均最高耐受剂量 | PCR | 聚合酶链反应 |
| MTX | 甲氨蝶呤 | PCWP | 肺小动脉楔压 |
| MUGA | 多通道放射性核素血管造影 | PDE5 | 磷酸二酯酶 5 型 |
| **N** | | PDGF | 血小板衍化生长因子 |
| NAD | 烟酰胺腺核苷酸 | PE | 肺栓塞 |
| NADH | 还原型烟酰胺腺嘌呤二核苷酸 | PEMA | 苯乙基丙二酰胺 |
| NADP+（辅酶Ⅱ） | 烟酰胺腺嘌呤二核苷酸磷酸 | PEP | 射血前期 |
| NADPH | 还原型烟酰胺腺嘌呤二核苷酸磷酸 | PER | 呼气峰流速 |
| NE（NA） | 去甲肾上腺素 | PF3 | 血小板第 3 因子 |
| NEAA | 非必需氨基酸 | PF4 | 血小板第 4 因子 |
| NHL | 非霍奇金淋巴瘤 | PG | 前列腺素 |
| NK | 自然杀伤细胞 | PGE | 前列腺素 E |
| NMDA | N- 甲基 -D- 天冬氨酸 | PGE1 | 前列腺素 E1 |
| NMS | 恶性综合征 | PGE2 | 前列腺素 E2 |
| NO | 一氧化氮 | PGI2 | 前列环素 |
| NOS | 一氧化氮合成酶 | PIC | α2 纤溶酶抑制物 - 纤溶酶复合物 |
| NPH | 中性低精蛋白锌胰岛素 | PIE 综合征 | 嗜酸粒细胞增多性肺浸润 |
| NPN | 非蛋白氮 | PIVKA | 无活性前体蛋白 |
| NRTI | 核苷类逆转录酶抑制药 | PL | 磷脂 |
| NS | 0.9% 氯化钠注射液（生理盐水） | PLA2 | 磷脂酶 A2 |
| NSAID | 非甾体抗炎药 | PMN | 多形核白细胞 |
| NYHA | 纽约心脏病学会心功能分级 | PN | 哌拉西林 |
| **O** | | PNMT | 苯乙胺 -N- 甲基转移酶 |
| OH | 游离羟基 | PPAR | 过氧化物增殖体激活受体 |
| OHA | 口服降糖药 | PPARγ | 过氧化物酶体增殖激活受体 γ |
| OHSS | 卵巢过度刺激综合征 | PPD | 结核菌素试验 |
| ORS | 口服补液盐 | PPX | 哌可二甲代苯胺 |
| **P** | | PR | 孕激素受体 |
| p.o. | 口服给药 | PRPP | 磷酸核糖焦磷酸 |
| PABA | 对氨基苯甲酸 | PSA | 前列腺特异性抗原 |
| PaCO2 | 动脉血二氧化碳分压 | PSP | 酚磺酞排泄试验 |
| PADAM | 雄激素缺乏综合征 | PSVT | 阵发性室上性心动过速 |
| PAE | 抗生素后效应 | PT | 凝血酶原时间 |
| PAF | 抑制血小板活化因子 | PTCA | 经皮穿刺腔内冠状动脉成形术 |
| Paget's 病 | 变形性骨炎 | PTH | 甲状旁腺素 |

| 缩略语 | 全称 | 缩略语 | 全称 |
|---|---|---|---|
| PTN | 哌拉西林 - 他唑巴坦 | **T** | |
| PTT | 凝血激酶时间 | t-PA | 组织型纤维蛋白溶酶原激活剂 |
| **Q** | | t-RNA | 转移核糖核酸 |
| q.n1 ～ n2h | 每 n1 ～ n2 小时 1 次 | T3 | 三碘甲状腺原氨酸 |
| q.nh | 每 n 小时 1 次 | T4 | 四碘甲状腺原氨酸 |
| qd. | 一日 1 次（每日 1 次） | T1/2 | 半衰期 |
| qid. | 一日 4 次（每日 4 次） | T1/2 α | 半衰期 α 相（分布半衰期） |
| qod. | 隔日 1 次 | T1/2 β | 半衰期 β 相（清除半衰期） |
| QT | 复极 | TAT | 凝血酶 - 抗凝血酶复合物 |
| **R** | | TBG | 甲状腺激素结合球蛋白 |
| RA-APL 综合征 | 维 A 酸 - 急性早幼粒细胞白血病综合征 | TC | 总胆固醇 |
| RAAS | 肾素 - 血管紧张素 - 醛固酮系统 | TCAs | 三环类抗抑郁药 |
| RAR | 视黄醛酸受体 | TD | 迟发性运动障碍 |
| RBC | 红细胞 | TBW | 总体重（total body weight） |
| RDS | 呼吸窘迫综合征 | TeBG | 睾酮雌激素结合球蛋白 |
| RE | 视黄醇当量 | TEM | 烷化剂三乙烯三聚氰胺（癌宁） |
| REMS | 快眼动相睡眠 | TEN | 暴发型中毒性表皮融解坏死 |
| rhGH | 重组人生长激素 | TENS | 经皮电神经刺激 |
| RK 手术 | 非穿透性放射状角膜切开术 | TG | 三酰甘油 |
| RSV | 呼吸道合胞病毒 | TGF-β | 转化生长因子 - β |
| rt-PA | 组织型纤溶酶 | TH | 甲状腺激素 |
| rT3 | 反 T3 | Th 细胞 | 辅助性 T 细胞 |
| RVA | 狂犬病疫苗 | TIA | 短暂性脑缺血发作 |
| RXR | 视黄醛 X 受体 | tid. | 一日 3 次 |
| **S** | | Tmax | 血药浓度达峰时间（药物浓度达峰时间） |
| SCF | 干细胞因子（Stemcell factor） | TMP | 甲氧苄啶 |
| SCID | 免疫缺陷病 | TNF-a | 肿瘤坏死因子 a |
| SGOT | 谷草氨基转移酶 | TNF-α | 肿瘤坏死因子 α（α - 肿瘤坏死因子） |
| SGPT | 谷丙氨基转移酶 | Tourette 综合征 | 抽动 - 秽语综合征 |
| SH | 肝素钠 | TP | 5'- 三磷酸酯 |
| SHBG | 性激素结合球蛋白（血浆性激素蛋白） | TPMT | 硫嘌呤甲基转移酶 |
| SIADH | 血管升压素（抗利尿激素）分泌异常综合征 | TPN | 完全胃肠外营养 |
| Sjogren 综合征 | 干燥综合征 | TRH | 促甲状腺素释放激素 |
| SLE | 系统性红斑狼疮 | TS | 胸苷酸合成酶 |
| SMON | 亚急性脊髓神经症 | TSB | 血清胆红素 |
| SP | 磺胺吡啶 | TSH | 促甲状腺素 |
| SPAG | 微粒气雾发生器 | TT | 凝血酶时间 |
| SR | 缓释剂 | TTP | 血栓性血小板减少性紫癜 |
| SSRI | 选择性 5- 羟色胺重吸收抑制药 | TTT | 麝香草酚浊度 |
| STZ | 链脲霉素 | TXA2 | 血栓烷 A2 |
| SU | 磺酰脲类 | TXB2 | 血栓烷 B2 |
| SV | 每搏量 | **U** | |
| | | UBT | 尿素呼吸试验 |
| | | UDCA | 熊去氧胆酸 |
| | | ULN | 最高上限 |

| 缩略语 | 全称 | 缩略语 | 全称 |
|---|---|---|---|
| UVA | 长波紫外线 | 房扑 | 心房扑动 |
| UVB | 中波紫外线 | 房室阻滞 | 房室传导阻滞 |
| **V** | | 房速 | 房性心动过速 |
| VCAM | 血管细胞黏附分子 | 放疗 | 放射治疗 |
| VCR | 长春新碱 | 肺气肿 | 阻塞性肺气肿 |
| Vd | 表观分布容积 | 肺心病 | 肺源性心脏病 |
| VLDL | 极低密度脂蛋白 | 风心病 | 风湿性心脏病 |
| VLDL-C | 极低密度脂蛋白胆固醇 | 呼衰 | 呼吸衰竭 |
| VMA | 香草基杏仁酸 | 急非淋白血病 | 急性非淋巴细胞白血病 |
| vWD | 血管性血友病 | 急淋白血病 | 急性淋巴细胞白血病 |
| **W** | | 甲减 | 甲状腺功能减退症 |
| WBC | 白细胞 | 甲亢 | 甲状腺功能亢进症 |
| West's 综合征 | 婴儿痉挛症 | 金葡菌 | 金黄色葡萄球菌 |
| WFN | 世界神经病学联盟 | 利伯病 | 家族遗传性球后视神经炎 |
| WHO | 世界卫生组织 | 慢粒白血病 | 慢性粒细胞白血病 |
| Wilson 病 | 肝豆状核变性 | 慢淋白血病 | 慢性淋巴细胞白血病 |
| WPW 综合征 | 预激综合征 | 慢支炎 | 慢性支气管炎 |
| | | 室内阻滞 | 室内传导阻滞 |
| β-TG | 血浆 β-血栓球蛋白 | 室速 | 室性心动过速 |
| γ-GT | γ-谷氨酸转肽酶 | 哮喘 | 支气管哮喘 |
| 病窦综合征 | 病态窦房结综合征 | 再障 | 再生障碍性贫血 |
| 房颤 | 心房颤动 | 窦房阻滞 | 窦房传导阻滞 |

# 中文药品名称索引

（以药名首字汉语拼音为序）

# 英文药品名称索引

# 法文药品名称索引

## E

## Q

## R

# 西班牙文药品名称索引

## D

## H

## I